15

FIFTEENTH EDITION

# Handbook of Nonprescription Drugs

## *An Interactive Approach to Self-Care*

15

FIFTEENTH EDITION

# Handbook of Nonprescription Drugs

## *An Interactive Approach to Self-Care*

ROSEMARY R. BERARDI
LISA A. KROON
JUNE H. McDERMOTT
GAIL D. NEWTON
MICHAEL A. OSZKO
NICHOLAS G. POPOVICH
TAMI L. REMINGTON
CAROL J. ROLLINS
LESLIE A. SHIMP
KAREN J. TIETZE

APhA
American Pharmacists Association™
Improving medication use. Advancing patient care.

Development Editor/Managing Editor
**Linda L. Young**

Editorial Services
**Dorothy Hoffman, Eileen Kreitman**

Composition Services
**Roy A. Barnhill**

Cover Design
**Jody Billert, Kristen Fernekes, Design Literate, Inc.**

Anatomic Drawings
**Marie A. Dauenheimer, Aaron Hilmers, Walter Hilmers, Jr., Judith M. Guenther, Alexa L. Chun**

Printing
**Banta Book Group**

Library of Congress Cataloging-in-Publication Data:
Main entry under the title: Handbook of Nonprescription Drugs

ISSN 0889-7816
ISBN 1-58212-074-9
ISBN-13 978-1-58212-074-4


APhA was founded in 1852 as the American Pharmaceutical Association

Published by the American Pharmacists Association
2215 Constitution Avenue, NW
Washington, DC 20037
www.aphanet.org

To comment on this book by e-mail, send your message to the publisher at aphabooks@aphanet.org.


**How To Order This Book**
By phone: 800-878-0729 (domestic)
Online: www.pharmacist.com
VISA®, MasterCard®, and American Express® cards accepted.

# Contents

## SECTION V

**Gastrointestinal Disorders**
*Editor:* Rosemary R. Berardi



## SECTION VI

**Nutrition and Nutritional Supplementation**
*Editor:* Carol J. Rollins



## SECTION VII

**Ophthalmic, Otic, and Oral Disorders**
*Editor:* Michael A. Oszko

## SECTION VIII
**Dermatologic Disorders**
*Editor:* Gail D. Newton



## SECTION IX
**Other Medical Disorders**
*Editor:* Lisa A. Kroon



## SECTION X
**Home Medical Equipment**
*Editor:* Leslie A. Shimp

## SECTION XI

**Complementary and Alternative Medicine**
*Editor:* June H. McDermott



## Appendix I



## Appendix II

# Foreword

Self-care is defined as "the action individuals take for themselves and their families to stay healthy and manage minor and chronic conditions based on their knowledge and the information available." (Further information is available at http://www.pagb.co.uk/pagb/primarysections/selfcare/selfcare.htm. Accessed October 19, 2005). These activities can be initiated by individuals on their own behalf or recommended by health care professionals. The concept of individuals taking responsibility for their own health requires the expertise and support of all health care professionals as it relates to both nonpharmacologic (e.g., diet, lifestyle) and pharmacologic (e.g., nonprescription medications) treatment. (The pharmacist's role in self-medication is discussed at http://www.pjonline.com/Editorial/19980912/forum/fip.html. Accessed October 19, 2005.)

Self-care should be viewed as a continuum of self-initiated behaviors that enhance the health and independent functioning of individuals, rather than as a failure of the individual to use professional medical services. Self-care behaviors can be classified as (1) healthful lifestyle behaviors intended to promote health and prevent disease, (2) medical self-care behaviors that relate to symptoms and treatment, and (3) behaviors that relate to improving quality of life and daily living in individuals with disabling limitations associated with physical or cognitive function, or chronic disease. The use of nonprescription medications, complementary and alternative therapies, nonpharmacologic measures, diagnostic tests, and medical devices are integral parts of self-care.

Today, many individuals take an active role in their own health care. Numerous factors have contributed to the growing self-care movement in the United States, including an increase in direct-to-consumer advertising of prescription and nonprescription medications. Information obtained from television commercials, newspaper and magazine advertisements, the Internet, and health-related articles serves to empower consumers to make decisions about their own health care. However, individuals embracing self-care may not have adequate information to determine if their medical condition is amenable to self-treatment and if the self-selected treatments are appropriate for the condition.

Individuals who wish to self-treat minor health disorders are faced with a staggering number of single-entity and combination nonprescription products. The Consumer Healthcare Products Association indicates that "retail sales of nonprescription medications in the United States in 2004 exceeded $15.1 billion (excluding sales at WalMart), reflecting an increase from $2.9 billion in 1971. (Further information is available at http://www.chpa-info.org/web/press_room/statistics/otc_retail_sales.aspx. Accessed October 19, 2005.) Other similar surveys confirm the increased use of nonprescription medications. Sales may be boosted further by the Internal Revenue Service Revenue Ruling 2003-102, which went into effect October 1, 2003. This ruling allows employers to reimburse properly substantiated nonprescription medication expenses, but not dietary supplements, from flexible health care spending accounts. (Full text of ruling is available at http://www.irs.gov/pub/irs-drop/rr-03-102.pdf. Accessed October 19, 2005.)

The anticipated increase in the number of prescription medications that will be reclassified as nonprescription will further confound the patient's dilemma in selecting appropriate self-treatment. All health care practitioners should be able to assist individuals in the management of their own self-care. However, pharmacists, because of their accessibility and expertise with respect to nonprescription and prescription medications, are in a unique position to fulfill the self-care needs of most individuals with minor health ailments.

Complementary medicines (e.g., botanical and nonbotanical natural medicines) and alternative therapies (e.g., homeopathic remedies) are also experiencing exponential growth in the United States and reflect societal changes in attitude toward natural and preventive medicine. Patients use these therapies as (1) adjuncts to conventional prescription medications, (2) treatment for minor health conditions, and (3) preventive measures to foster good health. In the past, complementary and alternative medicines have been primarily distributed through health food stores and by mail order. However, these therapies are sold in mainstream mass-market outlets today, including grocery stores and pharmacies. Unlike nonprescription medications, however, no federal regulatory agency evaluates the safety and effectiveness of complementary and alternative therapies.

Homeopathic therapies, another alternative to traditional medicine, have been used for years in this country. In the past, most homeopathic products were distributed through health food stores and by mail order. Today, homeopathic therapies are regulated by the federal government, homeopathic manufacturers are subject to inspection—as are the conventional pharmaceutical companies—and there is an official homeopathic national formulary.

The increased use of complementary and alternative medicines—as well as the paucity of clinical evidence as to their safety and effectiveness, and the potential for serious adverse events when these products are combined with each other or with nonprescription and prescription medications—demands that health care practitioners be knowledgeable about alternatives to traditional medications and be able to provide therapeutic information and guidance to the consumer.

John A. Gans, PharmD
Executive Vice President & CEO
American Pharmacists Association

# Preface

This new (fifteenth) edition of the *Handbook of Nonprescription Drugs: An Interactive Approach to Self-Care* is a comprehensive and authoritative textbook on self-care and nonprescription medications. The goal for this edition has been to provide an up-to-date reference that is not only helpful to all health care professionals and students—but also is user-friendly. This edition remains true to the spirit of previous editions—namely to assist students and practitioners in developing problem-solving skills needed to

- Assess a patient's health status; medical problems; current use of nonprescription and prescription medications, herbs, and dietary supplements; and other demographics such as pregnancy.
- Determine whether self-care is appropriate.
- If applicable, recommend appropriate self-care measures.

Written and reviewed by experts, this edition of the *Handbook* continues to serve as an authoritative source for students and practitioners who guide and care for individuals undertaking self-treatment.

## Highlights of New Features and Revisions

Considerable time and effort have been invested by the editors in improving the fifteenth edition. We are hopeful that the following changes continue to improve the quality and usability of the book, and to provide increased clarity and convenience for students and practitioners.

- New chapter
  - Meal Replacement and Functional Foods
- Chapters that have undergone major revisions
  - Asthma
  - Diabetes Mellitus
  - Heartburn and Dyspepsia
  - Headache
  - Musculoskeletal Injuries and Disorders
  - Sports Nutrition and Performance-enhancing Nutrients
  - Prevention of Pregnancy and Sexually Transmitted Infections
- Redundancy has been reduced by deleting repetition of basic drug information in chapters discussing drugs that treat multiple disorders. The following chapters have been designated as the primary chapter for discussing basic drug information for a given drug class. Other chapters that discuss the use of these drugs focus on drug information relevant to a specific disorder and cross reference the primary chapter for basic drug information.

| Agent/Class | Primary Chapter |
|---|---|
| Systemic analgesics | Headache |
| Antihistamines | Disorders Related to Cold and Allergy |
| Antacids, histamine$_2$-receptor antagonists, proton pump inhibitors | Heartburn and Dyspepsia |
| Topical hydrocortisone | Contact Dermatitis |
| Laxatives, stool softeners | Constipation |
| Fiber | Essential and Conditionally Essential Nutrients |
| Oral rehydration solutions | Diarrhea |

- Case assessment model was revised to include the following:
  - Increased emphasis on assessment and triage
  - New tables added to help differentiate diseases with similar symptoms
  - New headings: Information Gathering, Assessment and Triage, Plan, and Patient Education
  - New cases added and many others revised
- Disease-related chapters were revised to include the following:
  - Key points replace the conclusions at the end of chapters and highlight important concepts
  - Streamlined headings in Pharmacologic Therapy section by placing adverse effects, interactions, contraindications, and precautions under the new heading Safety Considerations
  - Information and references updated throughout
  - Improved cross-referencing among chapters
  - New and improved figures

## Chapter Content

All disease-oriented chapters in this edition include the following features and information:

- Nonprescription medications, herbs, and dietary supplements
- Treatment algorithms that provide a visual representation of triage and treatment
- Patient education boxes that highlight the major points in self-treating a specific disorder
- Self-care exclusion criteria

- Case-assessment format that facilitates and guides student development and learning
- Prescription to nonprescription conversions
- Self-care therapeutic issues and controversies
- Self-care treatment or prevention guidelines
- Nonprescription drug withdrawals from the market
- Product tables with examples of specific nonprescription products

## Chapter Features

Chapter features from the fourteenth edition remain unchanged. Most of these features support the interactive therapeutic approach to self-care. Students and practitioners can use these features to develop or improve problem-solving and critical-thinking skills.

- Disease-oriented chapters are grouped primarily according to body systems. These chapters begin with a discussion of the epidemiologic, etiologic, and pathophysiologic characteristics and clinical manifestations of the disorder, followed by a comprehensive discussion of the self-care options. The inclusion of selected herbs, dietary supplements, homeopathic products, and nonpharmacologic and preventive measures completes the discussion of self-care options.
- Elements such as the cases, treatment algorithms, discussions of therapeutic comparisons of self-treatments, patient education boxes, and product selection guidelines foster an interactive therapeutic approach to learning.
- Evaluation of patient outcomes sections reinforce follow-up of self-treating patients. This section defines the parameters for confirming successful self-treatment and those that indicate medical referral.
- The list of FDA pregnancy risk categories and information on lactation for selected nonprescription medications and nutritional supplements in Appendix I provide critical information for pregnant women and nursing mothers. The table format allows quick access to the categories of the most common nonprescription products. Appendix II lists botanical medicines to avoid in pregnancy and lactation.
- Chapters include tables that list interactions (drug–drug, drug–herb, drug–nutrient), and dosage and administration guidelines.
- Authors provide therapeutic comparisons of agents based on available clinical studies of safety and effectiveness, as well as product selection guidelines based on patient factors and preferences.
- Authors discuss the place of nonprescription therapies within a context of the whole spectrum of therapy for a specific disorder and describe other options in the event that nonprescription therapy fails or is not indicated.
- The book's organization and content allow students and practitioners to quickly find all the information needed to make a treatment recommendation and to counsel patients.

## Acknowledgments

We would like to acknowledge the many individuals who contributed to the new edition of this textbook. We are grateful to the 77 authors and co-authors and 121 reviewers who contributed to this comprehensive and authoritative textbook. These individuals were selected from many practice settings and health professions throughout the country. Their scholarship and clinical experience reflect a broad perspective and interdisciplinary approach to patient care. The dedication of the authors and reviewers in ensuring that chapters were up-to-date, accurate, thorough, clear, balanced, and relevant and of the highest quality is deeply appreciated. We thank Debbie Wagner for reviewing/updating the FDA pregnancy risk categories for selected nonprescription medications and nutritional supplements, and for compiling lactation risk categories for these products.

We would like to convey a special thanks to Linda Young, our managing/development editor. Linda provided invaluable guidance and support to the editors and authors in all aspects related to the publication of this edition of the textbook. She substantively edited the chapters and managed the design, editorial, and composition stages of the book. Without her experience and attention to detail, the improvements in this edition would not have been possible.

We are confident that the combined efforts of these individuals will enable the *Handbook of Nonprescription Drugs: An Interactive Approach to Self-Care* to continue to serve as the worldwide standard and teaching resource on self-care and nonprescription products.

Rosemary R. Berardi
Lisa A. Kroon
June H. McDermott
Gail D. Newton
Michael A. Oszko
Nicholas G. Popovich
Tami L. Remington
Carol J. Rollins
Leslie A. Shimp
Karen J. Tietze

January, 2006

# Editors

## Editor in Chief and Section Editor

**Rosemary R. Berardi, PharmD, FCCP, FASHP**
Professor of Pharmacy, Department of Clinical Sciences, The University of Michigan College of Pharmacy, Ann Arbor

## Section Editors

**Lisa A. Kroon, PharmD, CDE**
Associate Professor of Clinical Pharmacy, Department of Clinical Pharmacy, University of California-San Francisco School of Pharmacy

**June H. McDermott, MS Pharmacy, MBA, FASHP**
Adjunct Clincial Assistant Professor, Program on Integrative Medicine, Department of Physical Medicine and Rehabilatation, University of North Carolina School of Medicine, Chapel Hill

**Gail D. Newton, PhD, RPh**
Associate Professor, Department of Pharmacy Practice, Purdue University School of Pharmacy and Pharmacal Sciences, West Lafayette, Indiana

**Michael A. Oszko, PharmD, BCPS**
Associate Professor, Department of Pharmacy Practice, University of Kansas School of Pharmacy, Kansas City

**Nicholas G. Popovich, PhD**
Professor and Head, Department of Pharmacy Administration, University of Illinois at Chicago College of Pharmacy

**Tami L. Remington, PharmD**
Clinical Pharmacist, Department of Pharmacy, The University of Michigan Hospitals and Health System; Clinical Associate Professor, Department of Clinical Sciences, The University of Michigan College of Pharmacy, Ann Arbor

**Carol J. Rollins, MS, RD, PharmD, BCNSP**
Associate Clincal Professor, Department of Pharmacy Practice and Science, University of Arizona College of Pharmacy, Tucson; Coordinator, Nutrition Support Pharmacy, University Medical Center, Tucson, Arizona

**Leslie A. Shimp, PharmD, MS**
Professor of Pharmacy, Department of Clinical Sciences, The University of Michigan College of Pharmacy, Ann Arbor

**Karen J. Tietze, PharmD**
Professor of Clinical Pharmacy, Department of Pharmacy Practice, Philadelphia College of Pharmacy, University of the Sciences in Philadelphia, Philadelphia, Pennsylvania

# Contributors

## Authors

*Note:* Numbers in parentheses denote the chapters authored or co-authored.


**Robert J. Anderson, PharmD (49)**
Professor (Emeritus), Department of Clinical and Administrative Sciences, Mercer University Southern School of Pharmacy, Atlanta, Georgia

**Mitra Assemi, PharmD (47)**
Director, UCSF Fresno Pharmacy Education Program (PEP), Fresno, California; Associate Professor of Clinical Pharmacy, Department of Clinical Pharmacy, University of California-San Francisco School of Pharmacy

**Cathy L. Bartels, PharmD, FAAIM (27)**
Associate Professor, Department of Pharmacy Practice, Creighton University School of Pharmacy and Health Professions, Omaha, Nebraska

**Rosemary R. Berardi, PharmD, FCCP, FASHP (18)**
Professor of Pharmacy, Department of Clinical Sciences, The University of Michigan College of Pharmacy, Ann Arbor

**Daphne B. Bernard, PharmD, CACP (42)**
Associate Professor, Department of Pharmacy Practice, Howard University College of Pharmacy, Nursing, and Allied Health Sciences, Washington, DC

**Ilisa B. G. Bernstein, PharmD, JD (4)**
Senior Advisor for Regulatory Policy, Office of Policy, Food and Drug Administration, Rockville, Maryland

**Suzanne G. Bollmeier, PharmD, AE-C (13)**
Assistant Professor of Pharmacy Practice, St. Louis College of Pharmacy, St. Louis, Missouri

**John D. Bowman, MS, BCPS (41)**
Associate Professor, Department of Pharmacy Practice, Samford University McWhorter School of Pharmacy, Birmingham, Alabama

**Geneva Clark Briggs, PharmD, BCPS (51)**
Clinical Associate, MedOutcomes, Inc., Richmond, Virginia

**Lawrence M. Brown, PharmD, PhD (2)**
Assistant Professor, Department of Pharmaceutical Sciences, College of Pharmacy; Assistant Professor, Department of Preventive Medicine, College of Medicine, University of Tennessee Health Sciences Center, Memphis

**Wayne Buff, PharmD (37)**
Clinical Associate Professor and Associate Dean, Department of Pharmacy Practice and Outcomes Sciences, University of South Carolina College of Pharmacy, Columbia

**Demetris M. Butler, PharmD (16)**
Director of Clinical Pharmacy Programs, Clinical Pharmacy Associates, Inc., Laurel, Maryland

**Dana G. Carroll, PharmD, BCPS (39, 40)**
Assistant Professor, University of Oklahoma College of Pharmacy, Oklahoma City

**Juliana Chan, PharmD (18)**
Clinical Assistant Professor, Department of Pharmacy Practice, College of Pharmacy, and Department of Medicine, Sections of Digestive and Liver Diseases, University of Illinois at Chicago College of Pharmacy

**Katherine H. Chessman, PharmD, FCCP, BCNSP, BCPS (26)**
Associate Professor, Department of Pharmacy Practice and Clinical Sciences; Clinical Pharmacy Specialist, Pediatrics/Pediatric Surgery; Residency Program Director, Pediatric Pharmacy Practice, Medical University of South Carolina College of Pharmacy, Charleston

**Cynthia W. Coffey, PharmD (38, 45)**
Clinical Assistant Professor, Department of Clinical and Administrative Sciences, Mercer University Southern School of Pharmacy, Atlanta, Georgia

**Michael Colvard, DDS, MTS, MS, MO M RCS(Ed) (31)**
Assistant Professor, Department of Oral Medicine and Diagnostic Sciences; Director, Disaster Emergency Medicine Readiness Training (DEMRT) Center, Department of Oral Medicine and Diagnostic Sciences, University of Illinois at Chicago College of Dentistry

**Robin L. Corelli, PharmD (50)**
Associate Professor of Clinical Pharmacy, Department of Clinical Pharmacy, University of California-San Francisco School of Pharmacy

**Kimberly M. Crosby, PharmD (39, 40)**
Clinical Assistant Professor, Department of Clinical and Administrative Pharmacy, The University of Oklahoma College of Pharmacy, Oklahoma City; Staff Pharmacist, Mays Drugs Stores Inc., Tulsa, Oklahoma

**Barbara Insley Crouch, PharmD, MSPH (21)**
Director, Utah Poison Control Center; Professor (Clinical), Department of Pharmacy Practice; University of Utah, Salt Lake City

**Clarence E. Curry, Jr., PharmD (16)**
Associate Professor of Pharmacy Practice, Department of Clinical and Administrative Pharmacy Sciences, Howard University College of Pharmacy, Nursing, and Allied Health Sciences, Washington, DC

**Janet P. Engle, PharmD, RPh, FAPhA (29)**
Associate Dean for Academic Affairs and Clinical Professor of Pharmacy Practice, University of Illinois at Chicago College of Pharmacy

**Joli D. Fermo, PharmD, BCPS, BC-ADM, CDE (20)**
Associate Professor, Department of Pharmacy and Clinical Sciences; Clinical Coordinator and Specialist, Department of Pharmacy Services; Ambulatory Care Residency Program Director, Medical University of South Carolina College of Pharmacy, Charleston

**Richard G. Fiscella, RPh, MPH (28)**
Clinical Professor, Department of Pharmacy Practice; Adjunctive Assistant Professor, Department of Ophthalmology; University of Illinois at Chicago College of Pharmacy

**Karla T. Foster, PharmD (38, 45)**
Clinical Assistant Professor, Department of Clinical and Administrative Sciences, Mercer University Southern School of Pharmacy, Atlanta, Georgia

**Cliff Fuhrman, PhD (37)**
Assistant Dean and Clinical Associate Professor, University of South Carolina College of Pharmacy, Columbia

**Jeffrey A. Goad, PharmD, BCPS (19)**
Assistant Professor of Clinical Pharmacy; Co-Coordinator, Community Pharmacy Program; Director, Community Care Pharmacy Practice Residence, University of Southern California School of Pharmacy, Los Angeles; Travel Health Consultant, University Park Health Center, Los Angeles, California

**Charles S. Greene, BS, DDS (32)**
Clinical Professor, Department of Oral Medicine and Diagnostic Sciences; Director of Orofacial Pain Studies, University of Illinois at Chicago College of Dentistry

**Jennifer L. Hardman, PharmD (10)**
Pharmacotherapist and Clinical Assistant Professor, Department of Pharmacy Practice, University of Illinois at Chicago College of Pharmacy

**Michael D. Hogue, PharmD (46)**
Assistant Professor, Department of Pharmacy Practice, Samford University McWhorter School of Pharmacy, Birmingham, Alabama

**Yvonne Huckleberry, RD, PharmD (23)**
Clinical Staff Pharamcist, Department of Pharmacy, University Medical Center, Tucson, Arizona; Clinical Assistant Professor, College of Pharmacy, University of Arizona, Tucson

**Karen Suchanek Hudmon, DrPH, MS, RPh (50)**
Assistant Professor of Epidemiology, Department of Epidemiology and Public Health, Yale University School of Medicine, New Haven, Connecticut

**Anne Lamont Hume, PharmD, FCCP, BCPS (53)**
Professor of Pharmacy, Department of Pharmacy Practice, University of Rhode Island College of Pharmacy, Kingston

**Brian J. Isetts, PhD, BCPS, FAPhA (2)**
Associate Professor, Peters Institute of Pharmaceutical Care, Department of Pharmaceutical Care and Health Systems, University of Minnesota College of Pharmacy, Minneapolis

**Michael Kirk Jensen, RPh, MS (28)**
Clinical Pharmacist, Level IV Ambulatory Care, Moran Eye Center, Department of Pharmacy Services, University of Utah Hospital, Salt Lake City

**Kenneth R. Keefner, RPh, PhD (35)**
Associate Professor and Vice Chair, Department of Pharmacy Sciences, Creighton University School of Pharmacy and Health Professions, Omaha, Nebraska

**Cynthia K. Kirkwood, PharmD, BCPP (48)**
Associate Professor of Pharmacy, Vice Chair for Education, Virginia Commonwealth University, Richmond

**Gary D. Klasser, DMD (31, 32)**
Visiting Adjunct Clinical Assistant Professor, Department of Oral Medicine and Diagnostic Sciences, University of Illinois at Chicago College of Dentistry

**Wendy Klein-Schwartz, PharmD, MPH (21)**
Coordinator of Research and Education, Maryland Poison Center; Associate Professor, Department of Pharmacy Practice and Science, University of Maryland School of Pharmacy, Baltimore

**Lisa A. Kroon, PharmD, CDE (50)**
Associate Professor of Clinical Pharmacy, Department of Clinical Pharmacy, University of California-San Francisco School of Pharmacy

**Linda Krypel, PharmD (30)**
Associate Professor of Pharmacy Practice, Department of Pharmacy Practice, Drake University College of Pharmacy and Health Sciences, Des Moines, Iowa

**Begabati Lennihan, RN, CCH (55)**
Director, Teleosis School of Homeopathy, Teleosis School of Homeopathy and East-West Health Services, Cambridge, Massachusetts

**Robert W. Martin III, MD (33, 34)**
Department of Dermatology, Arnett Clinic, West Lafayette, Indiana

**Cydney E. McQueen, PharmD (54)**
Assistant Director, Natural Product Information, UMKC Drug Information Center; Clinical Assistant Professor, Department of Pharmacy Practice, University of Missouri-Kansas City School of Pharmacy

**Patrick D. Meek, PharmD, MS (15)**
Assistant Professor, Albany College of Pharmacy, Albany, New York

**Sarah T. Melton, PharmD, BCPS, BCPP (48)**
Consultant Pharmacist, Melton Healthcare Consulting, LLC, Lebanon, Virginia

**Sarah J. Miller, PharmD (27)**
Professor of Clinical Pharmacy, Department of Pharmacy Practice, The University of Montana School of Pharmacy, Missoula

**Candis M. Morello, PharmD, CDE (47)**
Assistant Professor of Clinical Pharmacy, University of California San Diego School of Pharmacy and Pharmaceutical Sciences, La Jolla, California

**Lawrence Neinstein, MD (19)**
Professor of Pediatrics and Medicine, University of Southern California Keck School of Medicine, Los Angeles; Director, University Park Health System; Associate Dean of Student Affairs, University of Southern California, Los Angeles

**Mark A. Newnham, PharmD, BCPS, BCNSP (25)**
Clinical Affiliate Assistant Professor, NOVA Southeastern University College of Pharmacy, Fort Lauderdale, Florida; Clinical Coordinator, Lawnwood Regional Medical Center, Fort Pierce, Florida

**Gail D. Newton, PhD, RPh (43, 44)**
Associate Professor, Department of Pharmacy Practice, Purdue University School of Pharmacy and Pharmacal Sciences, West Lafayette, Indiana

**Gloria J. Nichols-English, BSP, MEd, PhD (3)**
Research Fellow, Georgia Institute for the Prevention of Human Disease and Accidents, Department of Pediatrics, Georgia Prevention Institute Medical College of Pharmacy, Augusta, Georgia

**Diane Nykamp, PharmD (49)**
Professor of Pharmacy, Department of Clinical and Administrative Sciences, Mercer University Southern School of Pharmacy, Atlanta, Georgia

**Christine K. O'Neil, PharmD, BCPS, FCCP, CGP (52)**
Associate Professor of Clinical Pharmacy, Department of Pharmacy Practice, Duquesne University Mylan School of Pharmacy, Pittsburgh, Pennsylvania

**Victor A. Padrón, RPh, PhD (36)**
Associate Professor of Pharmacy Sciences, Creighton University School of Pharmacy and Health Professions, Omaha, Nebraska

**Somnath Pal, BS (Pharm), MBA, PhD (1)**
Professor, Department of Pharmacy and Administrative Sciences, St. John's University College of Pharmacy and Allied Health Professions, Jamaica, New York

**Louise Parent-Stevens, PharmD, BCPS (10)**
Clinical Assistant Professor, Department of Pharmacy Practice; Pharmacotherapist, Family Medicine Center, University of Illinois at Chicago College of Pharmacy

**Nicholas G. Popovich, PhD (43, 44)**
Professor and Head, Department of Pharmacy Administration, University of Illinois at Chicago College of Pharmacy

**Theresa R. Prosser, PharmD, FCCP, BCPS, AE-C (13)**
Professor of Pharmacy Practice, St. Louis College of Pharmacy, St. Louis, Missouri

**Tami L. Remington, PharmD (5)**
Clinical Pharmacist, Department of Pharmacy, The University of Michigan Hospitals and Health System; Clinical Associate Professor, Department of Clinical Sciences, The University of Michigan College of Pharmacy, Ann Arbor

**Lee A. Reussner, MD (30)**
Director, Kansas Voice Center, Lawrence; Assistant Professor, University of Kansas School of Medicine, Lawrence

**Edward D. Rickert, JD, RPh (4)**
Partner, Smith, Rickert, and Smith, Downers Grove, Illinois; Instructor, Adjunct Professor, Pharmacy Law, Department of Pharmacy Administration, University of Illinois at Chicago College of Pharmacy

**June E. Riedlinger, RPh, PharmD (55)**
Adjunct Associate Professor, Southwest College of Naturopathic Medicine and Health Sciences, Tempe, Arizona; Adjunct Associate Professor, Massachusetts College of Pharmacy and Health Sciences, Boston

**Magaly Rodriguez de Bittner, PharmD, BCPS, CDE (3)**
Associate Professor, Department of Pharmacy Practice and Science, University of Maryland School of Pharmacy, Baltimore

**Carol J. Rollins, MS, RD, PharmD, BCNSP (23, 24)**
Associate Clinical Professor, Department of Pharmacy Practice and Science, University of Arizona College of Pharmacy, Tucson; Coordinator, Nutrition Support Pharmacy, University Medical Center, Tucson, Arizona

**Wendy Munroe Rosenthal, PharmD (51)**
President, MedOutcomes, Inc., Richmond, Virginia

**Kelly L. Scolaro, PharmD (11)**
Clinical Assistant Professor, Department of Pharmacy Practice, University of Florida College of Pharmacy, Gainesville; Assistant Campus Director-St. Petersburg Campus, Distance Continuing and Executive Education, University of Florida-St. Petersburg College of Pharmacy, Seminole

**Steven A. Scott, PharmD (33, 34)**
Associate Professor of Clinical Pharmacy and Associate Head, Department of Pharmacy Practice, Purdue University School of Pharmacy and Pharmacal Sciences, West Lafayette, Indiana

**Joan Lerner Selekof, RN, BSN, CWOCN (22)**
Certified Wound Ostomy Continence Nurse, University of Maryland Medical Center, Baltimore

**Laura Shane-McWhorter, PharmD, BCPS, FASCP, CDE, BC-ADM (20)**
Professor (Clinical), Department of Pharmacy Practice, University of Utah College of Pharmacy, Salt Lake City

**Leslie A. Shimp, PharmD, MS (8, 9)**
Professor of Pharmacy, The University of Michigan College of Pharmacy, Ann Arbor

**Nicole M. Stack, PharmD (8)**
Assistant Professor of Pharmacy Practice-Primary Care, Albany College of Pharmacy, Albany, New York; Clinical Pharmacy Specialist, Family Medical Group, Rensselaer, New York

**Kathryn Michele Strong, PharmD, RPh (53)**
Medical Liaison-Neuroscience Division, Medical Sciences Department, Solvay Pharmaceuticals, Inc., Washington, DC

**Liza Takiya, PharmD, CDE, BCPS (6)**
Assistant Professor of Clinical Pharmacy, Department of Pharmacy Practice and Pharmacy Administration, Philadelphia College of Pharmacy, University of the Sciences in Philadelphia, Pennsylvania

**Karen J. Tietze, PharmD (12)**
Professor of Clinical Pharmacy, Department of Pharmacy Practice and Pharmacy Administration, Philadelphia College of Pharmacy, University of the Sciences in Philadelphia, Pennsylvania

**Paul C. Walker, PharmD (17)**
Clinical Associate Professor, Department of Clinical Sciences, The University of Michigan College of Pharmacy; Manager of Clinical Services, Department of Pharmacy, The University of Michigan Health System, Ann Arbor

**Sharon Wilson, PharmD (22)**
Clinical Specialist-Surgery/Transplantation, University of Maryland Medical Center, Baltimore; Clinical Assistant Professor, Department of Pharmacy Services, University of Maryland School of Pharmacy, Baltimore

**Eric A. Wright, PharmD, BCPS (7)**
Assistant Professor, Department of Pharmacy Practice, Wilkes University Nesbitt School of Pharmacy, Wilkes-Barre, Pennsylvania

**Ann Zweber, RPh (14)**
Instructor, Department of Pharmacy Practice, Oregon State University College of Pharmacy, Corvallis

## Reviewers

*Note:* Chapters in parentheses denote the chapters reviewed.

**Ami Abel, OD (29)**
Director, Contact Lens Services, Contact Lens Clinic; Assistant Professor, University of Alabama at Birmingham School of Optometry, Birmingham, Alabama

**Renee Ahrens, PharmD, MBA (18)**
Associate Professor, Department of Pharmacy Practice, Shenandoah University Bernard J. Dunn School of Pharmacy, Winchester, Virginia

**Robert J. Anderson, PharmD (2)**
Professor (Emeritus), Department of Clinical and Administrative Sciences, Mercer University Southern School of Pharmacy, Atlanta, Georgia

**Kenneth A. Bachmann, PhD, FCP (49)**
Distinguished University Professor, Department of Pharmacology, The University of Toledo College of Pharmacy, Toledo, Ohio

**Rebecca K. Baer, BS, PharmD (40)**
Assistant Professor, South Dakota State University College of Pharmacy, Brookings

**Danial E. Baker, PharmD, FASHP, FASCP (2)**
Associate Dean for Clincial Programs, Professor of Pharmacotherapy, Department of Pharmacotherapy, Washington State University-Spokane College of Pharmacy

**Jeffrey L. Barnett, MD (18)**
Private Practitioner, Huron Gastroenterology Associates, Ypsilanti, Michigan

**Jimmy D. Bartlett, OD (28)**
Interim Chair, Department of Optometry, Professor of Optometry, School of Optometry; Professor of Pharmacology, School of Medicine, University of Alabama at Birmingham

**Robert W. Bennett, MS (38)**
Associate Professor of Clinical Pharmacy, Director of Continuing Professional Education, Purdue University School of Pharmacy and Pharmacal Sciences, West Lafayette, Indiana

**Hildegarde J. Berdine, BS, PharmD, BCPS (7)**
Clinical Assistant Professor, Department of Clinical, Social, and Administrative Sciences, Duquesne University Mylan School of Pharmacy, Pittsburgh, Pennsylvania

**Christine A. Berger, PharmD (5)**
Clinical Assistant Professor, Department of Pharmacy Practice, University of Kansas School of Pharmacy, Lawrence

**Tricia M. Berry, PharmD, BCPS (43, 46)**
Associate Professor, Division of Pharmacy Practice, St. Louis College of Pharmacy, St. Louis, Missouri

**Karen Beth Bohan, PharmD, BCPS (45)**
Assistant Professor, Wilkes University Nesbitt School of Pharmacy, Wilkes-Barre, Pennsylvania

**Heather Boon, BScPhm, PhD (55)**
Assistant Professor, University of Toronto Faculty of Pharmacy, Toronto, Ontario

**John A. Borneman, BS, RPh (55)**
President, Homoeopathic Pharmacopoeia of the United States, Wayne, Pennsylvania

**Donald J. Brideau, MD, MMM (50)**
Family Physician, Springfield Family Medicine, Alexandria, Virginia; Assistant Clinical Professor, Georgetown University and George Washington University Schools of Medicine, Washington, DC

**Tina Penick Brock, RPh, MS, EdD (50)**
Department of Practice and Policy, University of London School of Pharmacy, London, United Kingdom; Clinical Associate Professor, University of North Carolina at Chapel Hill School of Pharmacy

**Ashley Butler, PharmD (10)**
Assistant Professor of Pharmacy Practice, St. Louis College of Pharmacy, St. Louis, Missouri

**Stephen M. Caiola, MS (15, 51)**
Associate Professor, Director, Postgraduate/Continuing Education Program and Community Pharmacy Residency Program, University of North Carolina at Chapel Hill School of Pharmacy

**Marla J. Campbell, PharmD (53)**
Assistant Clinical Professor, The University of Connecticut School of Pharmacy, Storrs; Clinical Faculty, Ambulatory Care, Bristol Hospital, Bristol, Connecticut

**Bruce C. Carlstedt, PhD (11)**
Professor, Department of Pharmacy Practice, Purdue University School of Pharmacy and Pharmacal Sciences, West Lafayette, Indiana

**R. Frank Chandler, Bsc Pharm, MSc, PhD (53)**
Professor and Director (Retired), Dalhousie University; President, Chandler Herbal Consulting, Halifax, Nova Scotia

**Hae Mi Choe, PharmD, CDE (12)**
Clinical Assistant Professor, Department of Pharmacy Practice, The University of Michigan College of Pharmacy, Ann Arbor

**Peter A. Chyka, PharmD (21)**
Professor of Pharmacy, University of Tennessee Health Sciences Center College of Pharmacy, Memphis

**Kevin Clauson, PharmD (54)**
Assistant Professor, Department of Pharmacy Practice, Drug Information Specialist, Nova Southeastern University-West Palm Beach College of Pharmacy, Palm Beach Gardens, Florida

**Elizabeth Clements, PharmD (5)**
Clinical Specialist-Emergency Medicine, Pharmacy Department, Spectrum Health System, Grand Rapids, Michigan

**Martha D. Cobb, MS, MEd, CWOCN (22)**
Clinical Associate Professor (Emeritus), University of Arizona College of Nursing, Tucson

**Susan Cornell, PharmD, CDE, CDM (47)**
Clinical Pharmacist and Educator, Dominick's Pharmacy, Oakbrook, Illinois; Assistant Professor, Midwestern University-Chicago College of Pharmacy, Downers Grove, Illinois

**Catherine M. Crill, PharmD, BCPS, BCNSP (26)**
Assistant Professor, Department of Pharmacy, The University of Tennessee Health Science Center College of Pharmacy, Memphis

**Lourdes M. Cuellar, MS, RPh, FASHP (3)**
Executive Director, Medical Support and Pharmacy Services, TIRR, Houston, Texas

**Lawrence W. Davidow, PhD (1)**
Clinical Assistant Professor; Director, Integrated Laboratory, Department of Pharmacy Practice, Kansas University School of Pharmacy, Lawrence

**Jeffrey C. Delafuente, MS, FCCP, FASCP (11)**
Professor, Director of Geriatric Programs; Interim Director, Community Pharmacy Programs, Virginia Commonwealth University School of Pharmacy, Richmond

**Joseph T. DiPiro, PharmD (17)**
Professor and Head, Department of Clinical and Administrative Pharmacy, The University of Georgia College of Pharmacy; Clinical Professor of Surgery, The Medical College of Georgia, Augusta

**Michael B. Doherty, PharmD (47)**
Assistant Professor of Clinical Pharmacy Practice, University of Cincinnati College of Pharmacy; Clinical Service Coordinator, Cincinnati Health Department, Cincinnati, Ohio

**Jeremiah Duby, PharmD (25)**
Critical Care Pharmacist
Kaiser Permanente
Vallejo, California

**B. DeeAnn Dugan, PharmD (6)**
Assistant Professor of Community Pharmacy Practice and Interim Director of Experiential Programs, Department of Pharmacy Practice and Administration, Palm Beach Atlantic University School of Pharmacy, West Palm Beach, Florida

**Herbert L. DuPont, MD (17)**
Chief, Internal Medicine Service, St. Luke's Episcopal Hospital; Director, Center for Infectious Diseases, University of Texas School of Public Health; Clinical Professor and Vice-Chairman of the Department of Medicine, Baylor College of Medicine, Houston, Texas

**Marilyn Edwards, PhD, RD (25)**
Associate Professor, Department of Internal Medicine, Division of Gastroenterology, Hepatology, and Nutrition, The University of Texas Medical School, Houston

**Robert Emerson, RPh (30)**
Clinical Assistant Professor, Coordinator, Integrated Laboratories, Department of Pharmacy Practice, The University of Kansas School of Pharmacy, Lawrence

**Elizabeth Ewing, (23, 27)**
Department of Oral Medicine and Diagnostic Sciences, Methodist LeBonheur Healthcare-Germantown Hospital, Germantown, Tennessee

**Stefanie P. Ferreri, PharmD, CDE (16)**
Clinical Assistant Professor, Department of Pharmacotherapy, University of North Carolina at Chapel Hill School of Pharmacy

**Richard Finkel, PharmD (48)**
Assistant Professor, Department of Pharmaceutical Sciences, Nova Southeastern University College of Pharmacy, Fort Lauderdale, Florida

**Karla T. Foster, PharmD (20, 33)**
Clinical Assistant Professor, Department of Clinical and Administrative Sciences, Mercer University Southern School of Pharmacy, Atlanta, Georgia

**Andrea R. Franks, PharmD, BCPS (18)**
Assistant Professor, Departments of Pharmacy and Family Medicine, University of Tennessee Health Science Center, Colleges of Pharmacy and Medicine, Memphis

**Conchetta W. Fulton, PharmD (7)**
Clinical Assistant Professor, Department of Pharmacy Practice, Xavier University of Louisiana College of Pharmacy, New Orleans

**Diane B. Ginsburg, MS, RPh, FASHP (3)**
Clinical Associate Professor, Regional Director, Internship Program, Division of Pharmacy Practice, The University of Texas at Austin College of Pharmacy

**Jeffrey A. Goad, PharmD, BCPS (17)**
Assistant Professor of Clinical Pharmacy; Co-Coordinator, Community Pharmacy Program; Director, Community Care Pharmacy Practice Residence, University of Southern California School of Pharmacy, Los Angeles; Travel Health Consultant, University Park Health Center, Los Angeles, California

**William C. Gong, PharmD, FASHP, FCSHP (2)**
Associate Professor of Clinical Pharmacy; Director, Residency and Fellowship Training, University of Southern California School of Pharmacy, Los Angeles

**Nicholas E. Hagemeier, PharmD (39, 41)**
Community Practitioner, West Lafayette, Indiana

**Lea Ann Hansen, PharmD, BCOP (22)**
Associate Professor of Pharmacy, Virginia Commonwealth University School of Pharmacy, Richmond

**Jan K. Hastings, PharmD (3)**
Associate Professor, Department of Pharmacy Practice, University of Arkansas for Medical Sciences College of Pharmacy, Little Rock

**Metta Lou Henderson, RPh, PhD (1)**
Professor Emerita of Pharmacy, Raabe College of Pharmacy, Ohio Northern University, Ada

**Thomas J. Holmes, PhD (44)**
Associate Dean and Professor, Medicinal/Pharmaceutical Chemistry/Pharmacognosy, Campbell University School of Pharmacy, Buies Creek, North Carolina

**James Hoover, DPM (44)**
Private Practitioner, Lafayette, Indiana

**David Hughes, PharmD, BCPS, CDE (51)**
Clinical Assistant Professor, University of Wisconsin-Madison School of Pharmacy

**Daniel A. Hussar, BS Pharmacy, MS, PhD (2)**
Remington Professor of Pharmacy, Philadelphia College of Pharmacy, University of the Sciences in Philadelphia, Pennsylvania

**Pramodini B. Kale-Pradhan, PharmD (12, 20)**
Associate Clinical Professor, Department of Pharmacy Practice, Eugene Applebaum College of Pharmacy and Health Sciences, Wayne State University, Detroit, Michigan; Department of Pharmacy Services, St. John Hospital and Medical Center, Detroit, Michigan

**William D. King, RPh, MPH, DrPH (20, 21)**
Division Director and Professor of Pediatrics, Department of Pediatrics, The University of Alabama at Birmingham

**Teresa Bailey Klepser, PharmD (35)**
Associate Professor, Kalamazoo Center for Medical Studies-Michigan State University; Director of Managed Care Pharmacy Practice Residency, Ferris State University College of Pharmacy, Kalamazoo, Michigan

**Jeffrey Kreitman, PharmD (6)**
Disease Management Pharmacist, McKesson Specialty Pharmacy, New Orleans, Louisiana

**David J. Kroll, PhD (53, 54)**
Senior Research Pharmacologist, Natural Products Laboratory, Research Triangle Institute (RTI), Research Triangle Park, North Carolina

**Thomas E. Lackner, PharmD (52)**
Professor, Experimental and Clinical Pharmacology and Institute for the Study of Geriatric Pharmacotherapy, University of Minnesota College of Pharmacy, Minneapolis

**Lisa A. Lawson, PharmD (7)**
Associate Professor of Clinical Pharmacy, Philadelphia College of Pharmacy, University of the Sciences in Philadelphia, Pennsylvania

**Michele A. Leady, PharmD (21)**
Clinical Pharmacist, Ephraim McDowell Regional Medical Center, Danville, Kentucky

**Anne Y. Lin, PharmD (45)**
Dean and Professor, Midwestern University College of Pharmacy-Glendale, Arizona

**Howard Maibach, MD (33, 34, 37)**
Dermatology Department, University of California Hospital, San Francisco

**Patricia Marshik, PharmD (13)**
Associate Professor of Pharmacy; Director, Pediatric Asthma Outreach Clinics, University of New Mexico Health Sciences Center School of Pharmacy, Albuquerque

**Beth A. Martin, MS, RPh (50)**
Clinical Assistant Professor, University of Wisconsin-Madison School of Pharmacy

**Robert W. Martin III, MD (37)**
Department of Dermatology, Arnett Clinic, West Lafayette, Indiana

**Marsha McFalls-Stringert, RPh, PharmD (41)**
Instructor of Pharmacy Practice; Director, Center for Pharmacy Practice, Department of Clinical, Social, and Administrative Sciences, Duquesne University Mylan School of Pharmacy, Pittsburgh, Pennsylvania

**Stephen Messer, NMD (55)**
Southwest College of Naturopathic Medicine and Health Sciences, Tempe, Arizona

**Emily K. Meuleman, RN, C, MS (8, 9)**
Nurse Practitioner, Department of Family Medicine, The University of Michigan, Chelsea Family Practice, Chelsea

**Susan M. Meyer, BS Pharmacy, MS, PhD (51)**
Senior Vice President, American Association of Colleges of Pharmacy, Alexandria, Virginia

**Jane R. Mort, PharmD (16)**
Professor of Clinical Pharmacy, Department of Clinical Pharmacy, South Dakota State University College of Pharmacy, Brookings

**Stephanie Olson, RD (23)**
Clinical Dietitian, Nutrition Services, University Medical Center, Tucson, Arizona

**Patricia L. Orlando, PharmD (6, 42, 43)**
Associate Professor (Clinical), Department of Pharmacy Practice, University of Utah College of Pharmacy, Salt Lake City

**Nicole Paolini, PharmD (31, 32)**
Clinical Assistant Professor, Department of Pharmacy Practice; UB-Rite Aid Program Director, Ambulatory Care Practice Initiative; UB-Lifetime Health Program Director, Pharmacotherapy Education and Research Program, The State University of New York at Buffalo

**Karen Steinmetz Pater, PharmD, BCPS, CDE (5)**
Clinical Assistant Professor, University of Illinois at Chicago College of Pharmacy

**Charles D. Ponte, PharmD, CDE, BCPS, BC-ADM, FASHP, FCCP, FAPhA (10, 38)**
Professor of Clinical Pharmacy and Family Medicine, Departments of Clinical Pharmacy and Family Medicine, West Virginia University Robert C. Byrd Health Sciences Center Schools of Pharmacy and Medicine, Morgantown

**David R. Potts, MD (42)**
Private Practitioner
Lafayette, Indiana

**Pamela Dee Reiter, PharmD, BCPS (26)**
Pediatric Critical Care Pharmacy Specialist, Department of Pharmacy, The Children's Hospital, Denver, Colorado; Adjoint Assistant Professor, University of Colorado Health Sciences Center School of Pharmacy, Denver

**Ronald J. Ruggiero, PharmD (9, 10)**
Clinical Professor (Emeritus), Departments of Clinical Pharmacy and Obstetrics, Gynecology, and Reproductive Sciences, Schools of Pharmacy and Medicine, The UCSF National Center of Excellence in Women's Health, The Medical Center at University of California-San Francisco

**Carolyn Sampselle, PhD, MSN (52)**
Professor of Nursing and Associate Dean for Research and The Carolyn K. Davis Collegiate Professor of Nursing, Professor of Women's Studies, Professor of Obstetrics and Gynecology, University of Michigan School of Nursing, Ann Arbor

**Philip Schneider, PharmD (16, 20)**
Director of Pharmacy, Olathe Medical Center, Olathe, Kansas; Adjunct Clinical Assistant Professor, Department of Pharmacy Practice, University of Kansas School of Pharmacy, Lawrence

**Kelly L. Scolaro, PharmD (51)**
Clinical Assistant Professor, Department of Pharmacy Practice, University of Florida College of Pharmacy, Gainesville; Assistant Campus Director-St. Petersburg Campus, Distance Continuing and Executive Education, University of Florida-St. Petersburg College of Pharmacy, Seminole

**Debra Sibbald, BSc Phm, MA, PhD [candidate] (36)**
Coordinator, Pharmaceutical Care I, University of Toronto Faculty of Pharmacy, Mississauga, Ontario

**John K. Siepler, PharmD, BCNSP, FCCP (14)**
Research Specialist, Nutrishare, Inc., Elk Grove, California; Clinical Professor, University of California at San Francisco School of Pharmacy

**Heather Skillman, MS, RD, CSP, CNSD (26)**
Pediatric Critical Care Dietitian, The Children's Hospital, Denver, Colorado

**Carl F. Skrabacz, RPh, FASCP (52)**
Chief Executive Officer, Omnicare of Northern Illinois, Des Plaines

**Mindy Smith, MD, MS (8, 10)**
Professor of Family Medicine, Michigan State University College of Human Medicine, Lansing

**Susan Claire Smolinske, PharmD (21)**
Poison Control Center, Children's Hospital of Michigan, Detroit

**Jenelle L. Sobotka, PharmD (1)**
Manager, Professional Relations, The Procter and Gamble Company, Cincinnati, Ohio

**E. John Staba, PhD (53)**
Professor Emeritus, Pharmacognosy, Department of Medicinal Chemistry, University of Minnesota College of Pharmacy and Medicinal Chemistry, Minneapolis

**Vanessa A. Stanford, MS, RD, CSCS (25)**
Research Specialist, Sr., Department of Nutritional Sciences, University of Arizona College of Agriculture and Life Sciences, Tucson

**Mark Stiling, PharmD (13)**
Clinical Science Liaison, Yamaguchi Pharma America, Rock Hill, South Carolina

**Donald L. Sullivan, PhD (51)**
Associate Professor of Pharmacy Practice, Department of Pharmacy Practice, Ohio Northern University College of Pharmacy, Ada

**Larry N. Swanson, PharmD, FASHP (27, 34)**
Professor and Chairman, Department of Pharmacy Practice, Campbell University School of Pharmacy, Buies Creek, North Carolina

**Keith A. Swanson, PharmD (48)**
Associate Professor, Director, Pharmacy Student Services, Department of Pharmacy Practice, University of Oklahoma College of Pharmacy, Oklahoma City

**Jane Takagi, PharmD, BCNSP (27)**
Adjunct Associate Professor of Pharmacy Practice, University of Southern California School of Pharmacy, Los Angeles; Assistant Clinical Professor, Department of Clinical Pharmacy, University of California at San Francisco School of Pharmacy; Kaiser Permanente Drug Information Services, Downey, California

**Andrea D. Tassone, PharmD, CDM, RPh (47)**
Associate Category Manager-Diagnostics, Walgreen Company, Deerfield, Illinois; Clinical Assistant Professor, Department of Pharmacy Practice, University of Illinois at Chicago College of Pharmacy

**Jeff G. Taylor, PhD (11)**
Associate Professor of Pharmacy, University of Saskatchewan College of Pharmacy and Nutrition, Saskatoon, Saskatchewan

**Michael S. Torre, MS, RPh, CDE (47)**
Clinical Professor of Pharmacy, Department of Clinical Pharmacy Practice, St. John's University College of Pharmacy and Allied Health Professions, Jamaica, New York

**Renee M. Trewyn, PharmD (12)**
Clinical Pharmacy Coordinator
Mercy Health System–Kansas
Fort Scott and Independence, Kansas

**Dominic P. Trombetta, PharmD (46)**
Assistant Professor of Pharmacy Practice, Wilkes University Nesbitt School of Pharmacy, Wilkes-Barre, Pennsylvania; Allied Services Rehabilitation Hospital & Outpatient Centers, Scranton, Pennsylvania

**Candy Tsourounis, PharmD (48)**
Associate Professor of Clinical Pharmacy, Department of Clinical Pharmacy, University of California at San Francisco School of Pharmacy

**Jesse C. Vivian, BS Pharm, JD (4)**
Professor, Department of Pharmacy Practice, Wayne State University Eugene Applebaum College of Pharmacy and Health Sciences, Detroit, Michigan

**Paul C. Walker, PharmD (19, 36)**
Clinical Associate Professor, Department of Clinical Sciences, The University of Michigan College of Pharmacy; Manager of Clinical Services, Department of Pharmacy, The University of Michigan Health System, Ann Arbor

**Geoffrey C. Wall, RPh, PharmD, BCPS (14)**
Assistant Professor of Pharmacy Practice, College of Pharmacy and Health Sciences, Drake University; Internal Medicine Clinical Pharmacist and Director, Pharmacy Practice Residency Program, Iowa Methodist Medical Center; Clinical Assistant Professor of Pharmacology/Physiology, Des Moines University of Osteopathic Medicine, Des Moines, Iowa

**C. Wayne Weart, PharmD (14)**
Professor, Department of Pharmacy and Clinical Sciences, Associate Professor of Family Medicine, Medical University of South Carolina College of Pharmacy, Charleston

**Tara R. Whetsel, PharmD (14)**
Clinical Assistant Professor, Robert C. Byrd Health Sciences Center West Virginia University School of Pharmacy, Morgantown

**Amy L. Whitaker, PharmD (28, 29, 40)**
Assistant Professor, Department of Pharmacy, Virginia Commonwealth University School of Pharmacy, Richmond

**David Williams, DDS (31, 32)**
Private Practitioner, Shawnee, Kansas

**G. Thomas Wilson, RPh, JD (4)**
Assistant Professor, Department of Pharmacy Practice, Purdue University School of Pharmacy and Pharmacal Sciences, West Lafayette, Indiana

**Michael Z. Wincor, PharmD, BCPP (49)**
Associate Professor of Clinical Pharmacy, Psychiatry, and the Behavioral Sciences; Associate Dean, External Programs, University of Southern California Schools of Pharmacy and Medicine, Los Angeles

**Eric T. Wittbrodt, PharmD, BCPS, FCCM (13)**
Associate Professor of Clinical Pharmacy, Department of Pharmacy Practice and Pharmacy Administration, Philadelphia College of Pharmacy, University of the Sciences in Philadelphia, Pennsylvania

**Robert Wolk, PharmD (23)**
Manager, Clinical and Education, Department of Pharmacy, Tucson Medical Center, Tucson, Arizona

**Supakit Wongwiwatthananukit, PharmD, PhD (50)**
Assistant Professor, Department of Clinical Pharmacy, Chulalongkorn University Faculty of Pharmaceutical Sciences, Bangkok, Thailand

**David P. Wrzesniewski, RPh (50)**
Pharmacy Specialist, East Region, Giant Food Stores LLC, Carlisle, Pennsylvania

**John R. Yuen, PharmD (28, 29)**
Pharmacist Specialist, Los Angeles Medical Center Kaiser Permanente, Los Angeles, California

**Ann Zweber, RPh (15)**
Instructor, Department of Pharmacy Practice, Oregon State University College of Pharmacy, Corvallis

# How to Use the Case Problem-solving Model

## Rationale for Case Format

Use of a problem-solving model is one mechanism for developing problem-solving skills. Repeated exposure to a model in a variety of contexts aids students in learning the model and applying it in various circumstances. Use of the model in each disease-related chapter of this text provides repeated exposure and reinforces learning.

## Case Format Description

The new case format is based on the guided-design instructional format that models the steps of decision making. This format facilitates student development of a framework for the organization and application of acquired information to the solution of novel problems. The basic steps used in the guided-design decision-making format are as follows.

- Gather information pertinent to the problem and its solution.
- Identify the problem.
- Identify exclusions for self-treatment.
- Patient assessment and triage.
- Identify alternative solutions.
- Select an optimal solution.
- Prepare and implement a plan to solve the problem.
- Provide patient education.
- Evaluate patient outcome.
- When outcome does not meet the self-treatment goal, start the process again from the beginning.

### *Steps 1 and 2: Gather Information*

When an individual presents to a practitioner and is in need of self-care advice, the practitioner must collect information about the patient that may be pertinent to solving the patient's problem. This information falls into two general categories: (1) information about the symptoms that prompted the patient to seek assistance and (2) information about the patient's history. The first two steps in the new case format direct the student to elicit this type of information.

It may be argued that it is unnecessary to collect all the patient's background characteristics to solve every patient problem. However, it should be remembered that novice problem solvers do not yet have the expertise to selectively elicit the most pertinent information to a specific situation. Thus, the model prompts them to ask about all of the listed characteristics to avoid overlooking information that is critical to the solution of the problem.

### *Step 3: Identify the Problem*

The third step involves the evaluation of information gathered in the previous steps to identify the patient's problem, its severity, and its most probable cause. Clear articulation of the symptoms is critical to (1) assist with differentiation among conditions with similar symptoms and (2) determine the goals of self-treatment. A comparison of the patient's symptoms to the usual or typical presentation of symptoms for a particular disease will help to differentiate and determine the most likely primary problem. For example, it is inadequate to conclude that a patient's problem is a common cold. In this instance, the therapeutic goal—to relieve the cold—is too vague to be useful because there are dozens of symptoms that may or may not be associated with the common cold and there are even more alternatives for symptomatic relief. On the other hand, if the patient's problem is nasal congestion, the goal would be to relieve the congestion: This goal is a much more useful criterion against which to evaluate a more limited set of potential therapeutic options.

### *Step 4: Identify Exclusions for Self-Treatment*

There are several reasons why it may be inappropriate for an individual to self-treat the symptoms or problems they are experiencing, which include (1) symptoms should not be self-treated as medical referral is necessary (e.g., eye pain); (2) patient is not an appropriate candidate for self-care (e.g., woman with diabetes who develops a vaginal candidal infection); (3) symptoms are too severe or long-lasting for self-treatment; or (4) effective nonprescription therapy is not available, or nonprescription dosages or duration of treatment are inadequate to treat the disorder.

Assessing the severity and determining the most likely primary problem a patient is experiencing is essential in making appropriate recommendations for treatment or referral. For example, a patient who complains of a cough associated with a cold is often a candidate for self-care. However, if the cough is significantly hampering the patient's ability to sleep or carry out routine activities or if the cough produces pain in the chest area, referral to a primary care provider may be appropriate. In another instance, a patient who complains of a mild cough may not be a candidate for self-care if other information about the condition (e.g., history of tobacco use and emphysema) suggests an etiology that is not amenable to self-management.

### Step 5: Identify Alternative Solutions

The fifth step involves formulation of a list of possible approaches to the patient's problem. At this point, no alternative should be prejudged or omitted. There are four general options available to practitioners who are advising patients about self-care: (1) recommend self-care with drug, nondrug, and/or complementary therapies, (2) refer patient to an appropriate primary care provider for treatment, (3) recommend self-care until an appropriate primary care provider can be consulted and (4) take no action. In the context of self-treatment, all potentially plausible product categories, dosage forms, and nondrug products and measures should be included in the list. Similarly, all potentially useful sources of care (e.g., urgent care clinic, dentist, emergency department) should be considered.

Critics of this approach have sometimes indicated that including no action at all as an option is unconscionable or not in the best interest of patients. In fact, there are situations in which this option may be preferred. For example, consider a situation involving a patient on a limited income who suffers from an asymptomatic, common wart that is in a location where it is neither noticeable nor likely to be spread easily to others. Given that most common warts resolve spontaneously without treatment and that the patient has limited income to pay for a nonprescription product, no action at all may indeed be an optimal solution in this instance. Further, the crucial point often overlooked by critics is that at this point in the decision-making process all ideas are listed and none are prejudged. Thus, it is entirely appropriate to consider no action, even if it turns out to be an inappropriate alternative.

### Step 6: Select an Optimal Solution

During the sixth step, each of the plausible solutions is evaluated to determine whether and to what extent each achieves the intended goal and is concordant with the patient's preferences in terms of goals of therapy, cost of therapy, and overall approach (e.g., personal philosophy, health beliefs) to self-care. Next, one of the alternatives that may adequately achieve the goal is selected on the basis of a variety of patient-specific and therapy-specific variables. Therapy-specific variables include dosage forms, ingredients, side effects, adverse reactions, relative effectiveness, and price. Patient-specific variables may include age, sex, medication history, concurrent medical conditions, patient preferences, and economic status.

### Steps 7 and 8: Prepare and Implement a Plan

These steps involve the communication of a therapeutic plan to the patient. The plan should include a summary of the condition and the reasons for treatment. The patient should be made aware of the available treatment options and their relative merits. When the recommended solution involves drug therapy, the plan should include monitoring parameters.

### Steps 9-11: Educate Patient

Patient education is designed to provide a clear and concise description of administration of the treatment, side effects and precautions, expected outcomes, and guidelines for appropriate use. When appropriate, the plan should include nondrug measures, including dietary and lifestyle modifications, and additional information resources.

The practitioner should ensure that the patient understands the plan by having the patient repeat it and by correcting any misunderstandings. Finally, after answering any remaining questions from the patient, the practitioner should encourage the patient to call or return if the symptoms fail to resolve. If symptoms are not resolved, the entire decision-making procedure begins anew.

SECTION I

# The Practitioner's Role in Self-Care

CHAPTER 1

# Self-Care and Nonprescription Pharmacotherapy

*Somnath Pal*

Self-care is defined as the diagnosis, treatment, and prevention of one's own illness without having professional expertise. It is a form of drug experimentation practiced by young and old alike, and often occurs when a person is suffering from illness. In the last five decades, a self-care movement has become solidly established in this country and many consumers practice self-care without consulting a health care professional. Given the increase in the aging population, restricted access to prescribers through health management organizations, and the increasing costs of health care, self-care will continue to escalate in the future.

Nonprescription drugs remain integral to the self-care industry. The emerging concept of nonprescription drugs in disease management, particularly chronic conditions, such as osteoporosis, gives more reason and opportunity for the pharmacist to continue to incorporate nonprescription drug therapy into his or her practice. People have always used the services of others in treating and preventing illness. Village elders, medicine men or women, priests, barbers, midwives, apothecaries, and physicians have been available in the community to provide services and preparations intended to restore health throughout time. People always have attempted to diagnose and treat themselves. Today, self-diagnosis and treatment are more common than ever before because of the availability of nonprescription drugs and a high proportion of underinsured or uninsured people in the U.S. population.

In the 21st century, nonprescription products will continue to be essential, cost-effective components of the U.S. health care system. Nonprescription drugs are appropriate for the prevention, treatment, symptomatic relief, or cure of diseases, injuries, and other conditions that consumers can self-diagnose and treat with or without the assistance of pharmacists and other health care practitioners. Nonprescription drugs are effective for their intended uses, and the recommended doses provide a good margin of safety as a safeguard against the consequences of inappropriate use by consumers. For example, ranitidine 300 mg is a prescription drug, whereas its nonprescription version is 75 mg. However, the possibility of patient misadventure always exists.

Usually, an individual from each American household takes a leading role in adopting a course of action to address a health crisis situation in a family. Such a course of action could include decision-making as to when to consult a physician; which physician to consult; when to self-medicate; what conditions to self-medicate; and whether the self-therapy should involve use of home remedies, nonprescription drugs, dietary supplements, and/or homeopathic medications. In 1990, 32% of the households had only two persons, a fourfold increase over two centuries.[1] With the growth of the U.S. geriatric population, and the decreasing number of persons per household, the number of individuals (each representing a household) selecting the most appropriate self-therapy options is increasing. Therefore, it is important for pharmacists to be conversant with the various options beyond nonprescription products, including homeopathics, herbals, and dietary supplements.

## Self-Medication

Many consumers are taking active roles in addressing their own health care needs. Hundreds of health-related self-help books, newspaper feature articles, television and radio programs, instructional audio and videotapes, and Internet sites and portals are evidence of the proliferation of interest in self-medication. Although a consumer may find this information overwhelming and confusing, the practicing pharmacist has the expertise to filter/screen the information and apply it to individual health care needs. Consumers need to know which self-care practices to use and how and why to do so. Health care practitioners should incorporate this concept into their daily practice.

According to the 2003 National Opinion Survey many people take various kinds of medicines and remedies. Fifty-nine percent of Americans have taken a nonprescription drug in the past 6 months as opposed to 54% who have taken prescription drugs during the same period. Even with the aging population, consumers took an average of 2.2 nonprescription medications compared with 3 prescription medications per month.[2] This number will change as the Food and Drug Administration (FDA) permits more prescription drug products to be switched to the nonprescription drug category.

A survey conducted for the National Council on Patient Information and Education (NCPIE)[2] found a majority of Americans take nonprescription drugs routinely for a variety of common ailments, including the following:

- Pain (78%)
- Cough/cold/flu/sore throat (52%)

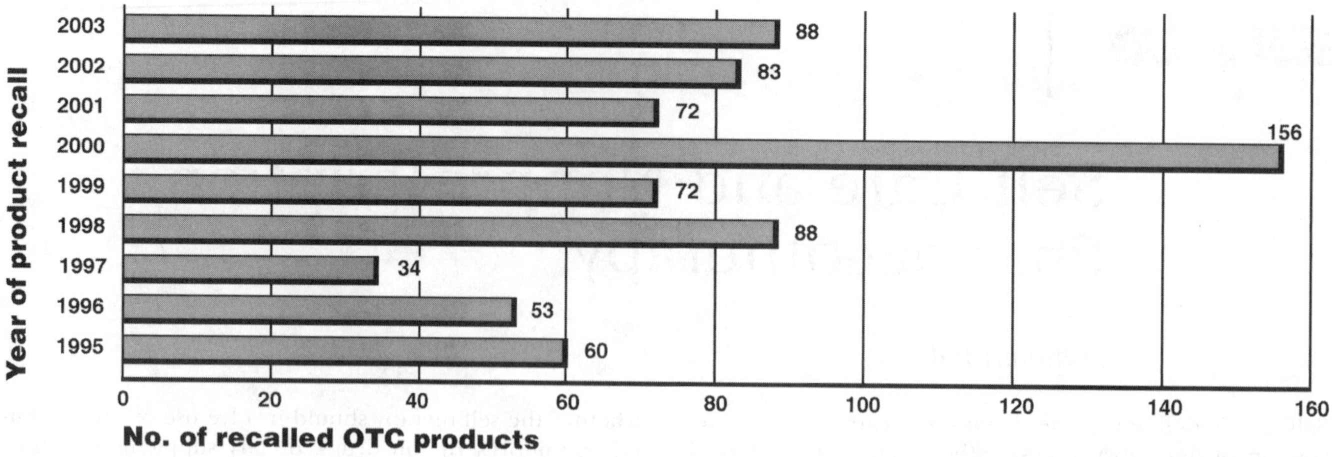


**FIGURE 1-1** Pharmaceutical nonprescription products recalled, 1995-2004. (*Source:* Compiled from several News Alert Bulletins issued by FDA. Available at: http://www.fda.gov.)

- Allergy/sinus problems (45%)
- Heartburn, indigestion (37%)
- Constipation/diarrhea/gas (21%)
- Minor infections (12%)
- Skin problems (10%)

Because nonprescription drug products are under the aegis of the FDA, consumers assume those on the market are pure, safe, and effective for the intended use. However, over the past 10 years product recalls have increased (Figure 1-1). Patients should therefore be made aware that all drugs, whether prescription or nonprescription, have equal probability of not being pure, safe, or effective. Patients must be reminded to refrain from taking or administering any drug product that seem to be of questionable purity, safety, or effectiveness and encouraged to notify their pharmacist as soon as suspicion arises. Some of the "out of ordinary" product features that should arouse suspicion are abnormal smells, color change, texture differences, and abnormal shape of the solid dosage forms of nonprescription drugs. Before any product is used, the consumer should read the label and check the expiration date that appears on the product label. In summary, as self-care with nonprescription medication continues to increase, the pharmacist should promote the concept that nonprescription drugs, like prescription drugs, must be taken with care and diligence.

### *Options for Self-Medication*

Nonprescription drugs provide self-care options to treat more than mere aches and pains (see Chapters 5 and 7); some products can prevent diseases, such as tooth decay (see Chapter 32), cure infections such as athlete's foot (see Chapter 43), and, with medical supervision, help manage recurrent conditions such as vulvovaginal candidiasis (see Chapter 8) and control the minor pain of arthritis (see Chapter 7). Nonprescription drugs are also used to treat reproductive (see Section III), respiratory (see Section IV), gastrointestinal (see Section V), otic (see Section VII), and dermatologic (see Section VIII) disorders. Nonprescription drugs promote healthy lifestyles and general wellness, in addition to preventing skin cancer (see Chapter 39) and helping smokers "kick the habit" (see Chapter 50). Generally, nonprescription drugs, herbals, and/or dietary/nutritional supplements (see Section VI) are used safely and effectively by millions of Americans every day and are found in nearly every household medicine cabinet. Complementary and alternative medicine (e.g., homeopathic medicines; see Chapter 55) is an important, though sometimes controversial, area of self-care. This area of self-care has had worldwide sales of $150 billion,[3] and helped build up a $19.8 billion dietary supplement industry in the United States by 2003.[4] With new opportunities in self-medication come new responsibilities and an increased need for knowledge. As people live longer, work longer, and take a more active role in their own health care, they need to become better informed about self-care options.

Consumption of nonprescription drugs has increased for all the major therapeutic categories. However, the nonprescription drugs available in pharmacies and retail outlets are not for every situation or every patient. Thus, pharmacists must embrace an important advisory role in the use of the nonprescription drugs and dietary supplements or be able to triage patients to consult their physician before undertaking self-therapy.

Since 1994, sales of dietary supplements have been increasing steadily at an average annual rate of 8.5%, but annual sales of nonprescription drugs increased at a significantly slower rate of 3.1%. So the annual sales (in dollars) of dietary supplements have been more than those of nonprescription drugs since 2000.[5] In 2003, dietary supplements netted sales of $19.8 billion while nonprescription drugs sales were $17.5 billion. According to the *Chain Drug Review*, 42%, 32%, and 26% of total nonprescription drug sales were made through discount stores, drugstores, and supermarkets, respectively, in 2003.[6] Sales of the top 10 therapeutic categories of nonprescription drugs for the years 2002 through 2004 are available on the Consumer Healthcare Products Association's Web site (see reference 7). Cough/cold medications netted the highest dollar sales for all 3 years, followed by nonprescription drugs used for treatment/mitigation of all types of pains. Migraine was the most prevalent form of headaches encountered by women, more so than men. Lip remedies made it to the top 10 list with sales of $326 million.[7] From 2004 to 2003, dollar sales dropped in excess of 5% in each of the four therapeutic categories (i.e., cough/cold products, analgesics, first aids, and laxatives). However, nonprescription drug product sales in the heartburn therapeutic category rose by 13.3% in 2004.

### *Influences on Self-Medication*

The Internal Revenue Service ruling 2003-102-§105 allows reimbursement of medically substantiated nonprescription drugs with pretax dollars through health care flexible spending accounts.[8] Reimbursable expenses include "nonprescription drugs" defined in the 1938 Food Drug & Cosmetics Act (FDC Act) as "alleviating or treating" personal injuries/illness, but only those that make therapeutic claims on their labels. Also qualified for pretax health care dollar reimbursement are dietary supplements if the patient's physician has suggested their use for the treatment/mitigation of an illness, such as iron for iron-deficiency anemia. Dietary supplements such as vitamins, minerals, herbals, and botanicals, which are "merely beneficial to the general health," are not eligible as pretax expenses.

The implication of the deductibility of nonprescription drug costs from income tax is far reaching, especially considering that several insurance providers do not cover prescription drugs when nonprescription versions (generally of a lower strength) are available for safe and effective treatment. The medical expense "pretax" deduction is becoming increasingly popular as Americans pay more for "out-of-pocket" health care costs. In 2004, 5.02% of taxpayers claimed medical expense deductions, up from 4.3% in 1997.[9] Therefore, employees have an economic incentive to use low-cost nonprescription drugs (rather than expensive prescription drugs with insurance copayment plans), giving pharmacists greater opportunity to play a role in therapeutic counseling.

Americans are aging, and patients of advanced age consume a disproportionately larger share of nonprescription drugs. New projections illustrate the magnitude of the still-to-come elderly boom. The percentage of older Americans has been increasing gradually since the 1950s, but in 2001 it started to increase sharply as the baby boom generation approached the 65 and older age group.[10] Individuals reaching age 65 are expected to live an additional 17.9 years based on the average life expectancy. By 2030, 20% (i.e., 70 million) of the U.S. population will be over 65 years, up from 12.4% (i.e., 35 million) in 2000.[11] The growth of this age group provides opportunities for health care practitioners, especially pharmacists. Self-medication has also become one of the most common forms of medical care among persons of advanced age. Patients over the age of 65 purchase 30% of all prescription drugs and 40% of all nonprescription drugs.[12]

Increased use of nonprescription drugs by older Americans can be attributed to the following:

1. Conditions for which nonprescription drugs are used, such as arthritis pain, insomnia, and constipation, become more prevalent with advancing age.
2. Nonprescription drugs provide low-cost alternatives to more expensive primary care visits and prescription drugs.
3. Accessibility to pharmacists in the community setting makes nonprescription drugs an acceptable alternative to scheduling visits to primary care providers.

The fastest-growing segment of the elderly are those older than 85 years.[10] In 2000, 2% of the population was older than 85, and in the coming years people 85 and older will make up nearly 25% of the older population.[13] They are projected to total six million as early as 2010—twice their 1990 level. Because these patients tend to be in poorer health and require more services than those between 65 and 85 years, they will have a bigger impact on the future of the U.S. health care system. Currently, people of advanced age account for at least 25% of nonprescription drug use, even though they make up only 13% (34.2 million) of the population.[14]

Following are some of the findings of a consumer survey on self-medication among older Americans:[15]

- Within a given 3-month period, 37% of those over 65 years of age have been ill.
- Self-diagnosing and self-treating were preferred by 48% of those 65 or older.
- Before going to a primary care provider, 66% of those over 65 had a good idea of the diagnosis.
- Forty-two percent of those over 65 were receptive of the idea of treating certain serious conditions with nonprescription drugs if they were made available with proper labeling.

Increased access to nonprescription medicine is especially important for the aging population. Figure 1-2 demonstrates the prevalence of the most common health problems in persons 65 years and older. Some of these chronic conditions are treated by nonprescription drugs alone, or by nonprescription drugs serving as an adjunct to prescription drug therapy. As the number of people over 65 doubles by 2030, the consumption of nonprescription drugs will also rise.[11]

As is true worldwide, there are more women than men of advanced age in the United States. The percentage of the female population increases with age and more women than men suffer from minor illnesses that are self-treatable with nonprescription drugs. Figure 1-3 shows that, across the board, more women than men (in the range of 31% to 65%) self-treat for each of the six ailments. For example, self-treatment of skin conditions was performed by 65% more women than men, and constipation/diarrhea was self-treated by 62% more women than their male counterparts. But the magnitude of difference between women and men was smallest (31% more women than men) for self-treatment of muscle aches and/or joint or back pain. It can be inferred that older women will probably be utilizing more nonprescription drug products than older men.

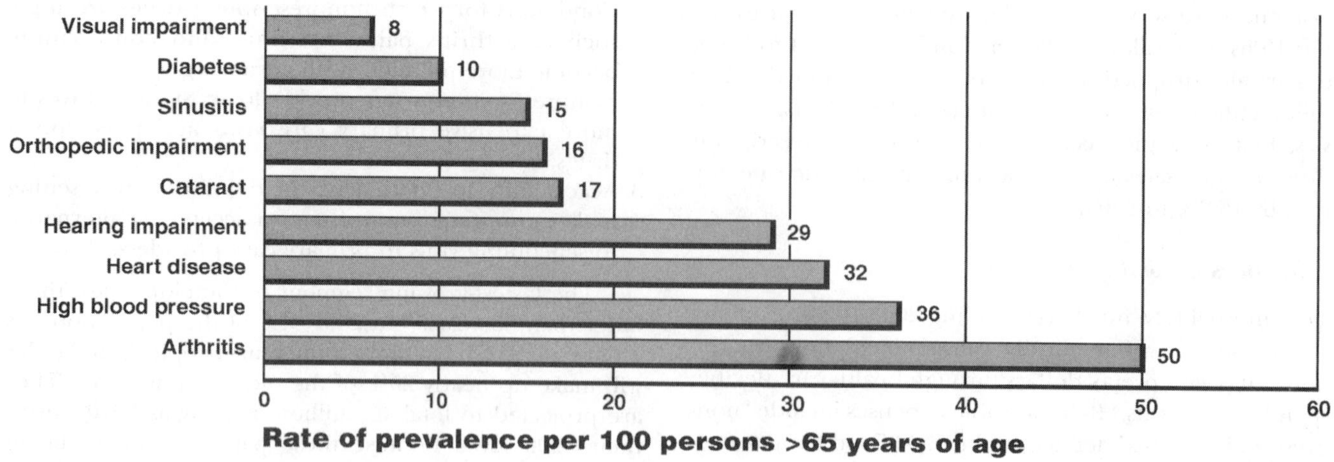


FIGURE 1-2 Common health problems for persons age 65 and older (*Source:* Aging and health: the role of self-medication. Available at: http://www.chpa-info.org/publications/aging_and_health.asp. Accessed February 23, 2005.)

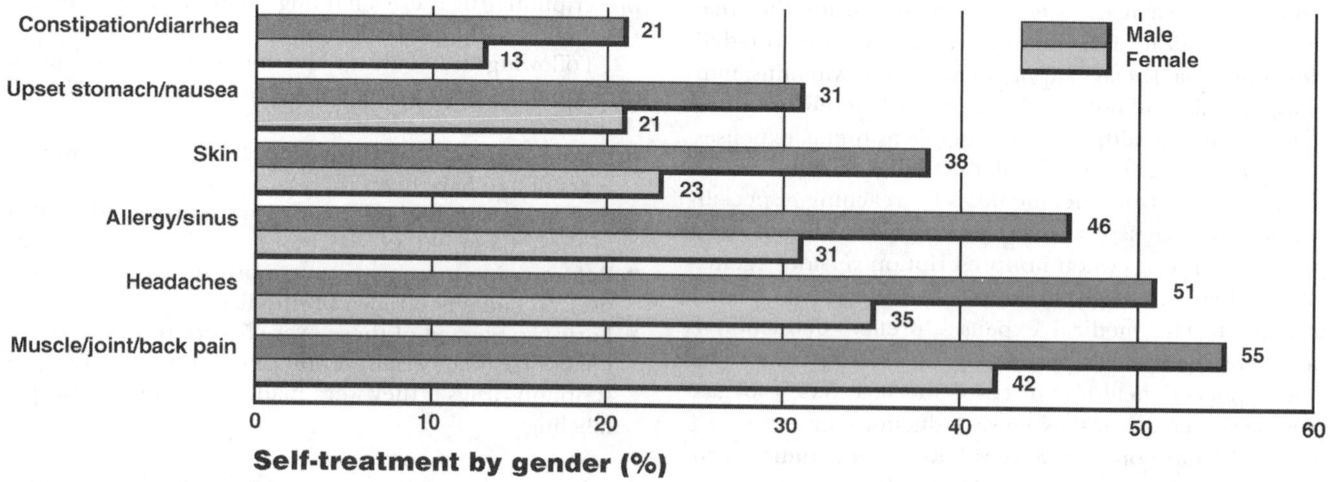


FIGURE 1-3 Selected ailments self-treated by men and women. (*Source: Consumer Healthcare Products Association Roper Starch Worldwide Study.* Available at: http://www.chpa-info.org/web/press_room/statistics/pdfs/women_final.pdf, Accessed February 25, 2005.)

However, before taking any prescription drugs, men and women should inform their primary care providers, including the pharmacist, of any nonprescription drugs they use, such as laxatives, aspirin, diet aids, calcium supplements, treatments for vaginal infections, and sleep aids. The following survey results reveal interesting information about self-treatment among older men and women:[16]

- In the past 3-month period, 44% of men and 52% of women were ill.
- In the past 1-year period, 47% of men and 31% of women did not seek the help of a primary care provider for their health problems.
- In the past 6-month period, 82% of women and 71% of men used a nonprescription drug to treat one ailment.
- In the past 6-month period, 46% of men and 60% of women used a dietary supplement.
- Pharmacists were regarded as the primary resource for minor health problems by 44% of women and 46% of men.

### *Accessibility to Nonprescription Drug Products for Self-Medication*

Health care–related information is readily accessible on the Internet. These resources can be accessed globally, and information updated in the privacy and comfort of a patient's home. The major drawback is lack of quality control, which in many instances compromises patients' welfare.[17] Because no one individual or group owns the Internet, no single organization is accountable for the quality and accuracy of the information available on Web sites.[18] Because many sites contain inadequate or incomplete information, it is not safe to simply "surf" and self-medicate.[19] In response to public safety concerns, the National Association of Boards of Pharmacy (NABP) has started to evaluate the credentials of online pharmacies (also known as e-pharmacies) through the Verified Internet Pharmacy Practice Sites (VIPPS) program.[20]

The VIPPS program is voluntary, and an e-pharmacy must agree to strict conditions to be certified by NABP under its auspices. The program also includes a provision for NABP inspections. Each e-pharmacy that meets the NABP standards is entitled to use the VIPPS logo on its Web page. The logo gives credibility to the information posted on the site. The influence of the Internet on self-care and acquisition of health care information creates a new challenge for health care professionals. Pharmacists have great potential to reach more than 100 million Americans on the Internet.[21] According to a study by MedStat, 52% of U.S. households surfed the Internet for information on a specific health problem and 7% surfed the Internet for specific drug information.[22]

There are 12 VIPPS-approved Web site addresses in the entire United States. Though all of them dispense prescription drugs, some dispense nonprescription drugs, homeopaths/vitamins/nutraceuticals, and medical devices. All of these sites provide "next day delivery" and have "on site" medical/pharmaceutical information available for patients. However, only a few have links to medical/pharmaceutical information, and even fewer provide "same day delivery."[2] The NABP lists the names of the Verified Internet Pharmacy Sites for each state, and which ones dispense nonprescription drugs and vitamins/nutrients. The number of e-pharmacies "dispensing nonprescription drugs" ranged from a high of 21 in the state of Alabama to as few as 10 in Michigan. As for e-pharmacies providing "Web links for access to medical/pharmaceutical information," South Carolina topped the list with 18, while Michigan had only seven. South Carolina had the highest number of e-pharmacies "dispensing vitamins/nutrients," while five states—Florida, Georgia, Massachusetts, New Jersey, and Wisconsin—tied for listing the lowest number of e-pharmacies (i.e., four).[23]

FDA has the final authority to categorize a drug as prescription or nonprescription based on the provisions of the 1951 Durham-Humphrey amendment to the Food, Drug, and Cosmetics Act of 1938. Prescription drugs are safe and effective when used according to the prescriber's instructions. On the other hand, nonprescription drugs are judged by FDA as safe and effective even if used without a prescriber's directive and oversight. FDA has the final word in reclassifying a drug from prescription to nonprescription status if three questions can be answered in the affirmative:

1. Can the patient adequately self-diagnose the clinical abnormality?
2. Can the clinically abnormal condition be successfully self-treated?
3. Is the self-treatment product safe and effective for consumer use, under conditions of actual use?

The Center for Drug Evaluation and Research (CDER), a division of FDA, oversees the formulation, production, and distribution of nonprescription drugs to ensure that they are labeled properly and the benefits associated with their use outweigh the risks. Easy access to nonprescription drugs plays a vital role in America's health care system.

Currently, the use of nonprescription pseudoephedrine products to illicitly manufacture methamphetamine is a public health concern that must be aggressively addressed by law enforcement. However, recent legislative and regulatory proposals advocate allowing pseudoephedrine to be sold only in pharmacies, in some cases by regulating pseudoephedrine as a Schedule V controlled substance (see Chapter 4). These actions will place unnecessary burdens on pharmacies while giving pharmacists authority to monitor the clinical need for a third class of nonprescription drugs.

More than 700 nonprescription products on the market at present use ingredients or dosages that were available only by prescription 25 years ago.[24] Table 1-1 shows the product categories of pharmaceuticals switched from prescription to nonprescription category between 2000 and 2004. In the year 2002, four drugs were switched, two having one ingredient in common. In the year 2003, only one switch was approved and none in 2004. Ideally, the pharmacist is situated and accessible to advise patients on appropriate choices of nonprescription drugs, especially the newer drugs that have been "switched" from prescription status.

- A female patient can save as much as $80 by using switched nonprescription vaginal antifungal products for recurring yeast infections, according to the American Pharmacists Association. While a nonprescription drug can be obtained for less than $20, a physician's visit and prescription-only vaginal antifungal drug can cost almost $100. Savings can be even higher when indirect (e.g., travel, lost time from work) costs are considered.[24]
- A survey found that consumers benefit by up to $750 million a year as a result of nonprescription cough-cold drugs once available only by prescription. The same study demonstrated that physician visits for the common cold dropped by 110,000 a year between 1976 and 1989.[24] This further demonstrates the success of FDA's policy of switching cold medicines to nonprescription status.

## Pharmacists' Role in Nonprescription Drug Therapy

With numerous clinical and economic factors fostering the growth of nonprescription drug therapy, the pharmacy profession needs to continue expanding its professional and business roles. The following are some of the justifications for such expansion:

- The public is becoming increasingly health conscious and desires a better understanding of disease and disease management.
- While prescription drugs are available at approximately 55,000 pharmacies nationwide, nonprescription drugs are conveniently available for patients at over 750,000 retail outlets in the United States.[15]
- Of approximately 3.5 billion health problems treated annually, some 2 billion (i.e., 57%) are treated with nonprescription drugs, according to the American Pharmacists Association.[25]
- The pharmacist is educated formally in drug pharmacotherapy, and thus can play a very important role in helping the patient with proper nonprescription drug selection.

**TABLE 1-1 Prescription-to-Nonprescription Switches, 2000-2004**

| Year of Approval | Ingredient | Adult Dosage | Product Category | Product Examples |
|---|---|---|---|---|
| 2000 | Ibuprofen | 200 mg | Migraine | Motrin Migraine Pain; Advil Migraine Liqui-gel |
| | Docosanol | 10% cream | Cold sore/fever blister | Abreva Cream |
| | Famotidine | 10 mg | Heartburn | Pepcid Complete |
| | Calcium carbonate, magnesium hydroxide | Calcium carbonate 800 mg; magnesium hydroxide 165 mg | Acid indigestion | |
| 2001 | Butenafine hydrochloride | 1% cream | Athlete's foot; jock itch; ringworm | Lotrimin Ultra |
| 2002 | Ibuprofen–pseudoephedrine HCl (suspension) | Ibuprofen 100 mg and pseudoephedrine HCl 15 mg per 5 mL; 4 times daily | Analgesic/decongestant | Children's Advil Cold |
| | Nicotine polacrilex troche/lozenge | 2 and 4 mg | Smoking cessation | Commit |
| | Loratadine | 10 mg | Antihistamine | Claritin |
| | Loratadine, ephedrine sulfate | 240 mg | Antihistamine/decongestant | Claritin-D |
| 2003 | Omeprazole magnesium | 20 mg | Acid reducer | Prilosec OTC |
| 2004 | None | | | |

Key: OTC, over-the-counter.

- It is estimated that patients save $20 billion in health care costs each year using nonprescription drugs in treatment of 12 common health conditions. Savings accrue from avoiding prescription costs, primary care provider visits, loss of wages, and lost productivity, among other factors.[26] The rising cost of prescription drugs is making it difficult to provide an affordable broad-based prescription benefit. Its relative safety and effectiveness at lower cost increase the value of nonprescription drug therapy.

As accessibility of nonprescription drugs increases, so does the potential for drug interactions. Many nonprescription drugs have active ingredients that interact with the human body in different ways in a few individuals. In addition, diet and lifestyle can have a significant impact on a drug's ability to work in the body. Certain foods, beverages (e.g., grapefruit juice), alcohol, caffeine, and even cigarette smoking can interact with drugs. These interactions may make the drugs less effective or may cause dangerous side effects or other therapeutic problems. Patients should therefore consult pharmacists in selecting herbals, dietary supplements, or nonprescription drugs. Table 1-2 lists a few of the commonly used nonprescription drugs and their interactions with food, alcohol, other nonprescription drugs, and certain disease conditions.[27-31]

Self-care with nonprescription drugs is often the most sought-after first level of care. The self-medication revolution focuses on the development of knowledge and skill in promoting wellness, as well as in treating medical conditions with nonprescription drugs. Informed, appropriate, and responsible use of nonprescription drugs is a large part of self-medication. Data suggest that most patients respect these drugs, recognize their limitations, and read labeling information carefully.[32] Yet, many patients do not understand the circumstances under which nonprescription drugs should be discontinued. For example, for self-treatment of itching skin, if the condition worsens or symptoms persist for more than 7 days or clear up and recur within a few days, patients should stop using hydrocortisone (1%) cream and seek medical attention. Casual and inappropriate use of nonprescription drugs can lead to serious adverse direct effects (e.g., liver toxicity with prolonged intake of high doses of acetaminophen), drug-drug interactions, and indirect effects (e.g., from delay in seeking appropriate medical attention). The FDA, pharmaceutical manufacturers, pharmacy organizations, and pharmacists should discourage casual and inappropriate use of nonprescription drugs through the following measures:

1. Adequate package labeling
2. More emphasis on "indications for use," rather than promotion of nonprescription drugs in direct-to-consumer advertising
3. Patient education and counseling by pharmacists about the consequences of casual and inappropriate use of nonprescription drugs

Pharmacists are uniquely qualified to serve the public interest in nonprescription pharmacotherapy because they receive university-level education and skill development, with in-depth instruction in the basic pharmaceutical sciences. Furthermore, they are accessible in the community to provide drugs and information on how to maximize

**TABLE 1-2 Potential Interactions With Selected Nonprescription Drugs**

**Drug–Drug Interactions[27]**

| OTC Drug | OTC Drug | Potential Adverse Effect |
|---|---|---|
| Aluminum-containing antacids | Ascorbic acid | ↓ Aluminum absorption |
| Antidiabetic agents (metformin) | Psyllium | ↓ Metformin absorption |
| Aspirin | Products containing aluminum, calcium, or magnesium | ↓ Aspirin blood concentration by increasing aspirin elimination |
| Cimetidine | Antacids | ↓ Cimetidine absorption |
| Iron | Products containing aluminum, calcium, or magnesium | ↓ Iron absorption |
| Mineral oil | Docusate | ↑ Mineral oil absorption |

**Drug–Food/Beverage Interactions**

| OTC Drug | Food/Beverage | Potential Adverse Effect |
|---|---|---|
| Acetaminophen | Garlic | Delays acetaminophen absorption[28] |
| Aspirin | Garlic | ↑ Risk of bleeding[29] |
| Calcium | Oxalic acid foods (spinach, rhubarb); phytic acid foods (bran/whole cereal) | Alters calcium absorption[30] |
| Zinc | Caffeine; dairy products (milk) | ↓ Zinc absorption[31] |

**Drug–Disease Interactions[27]**

| OTC Drug | Condition | Mechanism |
|---|---|---|
| Aspirin | Hyperuricemia | ↓ Renal excretion of uric acid |
| Naproxen; ketoprofen | Peptic ulcer disease | Changes gastric mucosal barrier |
| Doxylamine succinate; phenylephrine HCl | Glaucoma | Obstructs aqueous outflow |
| Pheniramine maleate; naphazoline HCl; nicotine | Hypertension | ↑ Vascular resistance |

**Drug–Alcohol Interactions[27]**

| OTC Drug | Potential Adverse Effect | Mechanism |
|---|---|---|
| Aspirin | ↑ GI blood loss | Bleeding time prolongation |
| Diphenhydramine HCl | ↑ Sedation | Central nervous system depression |
| Insulin | ↑ Hypoglycemia | ↓ Hepatic gluconeogenesis |
| Ketoconazole (topical) | Vomiting, tachycardia | Disulfiramlike reaction |
| Yohimbine | ↑ Blood pressure | ↑ Norepinephrine level |

Key: GI, gastrointestinal; OTC, over-the-counter.

their value while minimizing any potential adverse consequences.

In the initial encounter with a patient seeking assistance with nonprescription drugs, the pharmacist should

- assess, by interview and observation, the patient's physical complaint/symptoms and medical condition (see Chapter 2)
- differentiate self-treatable conditions from those requiring a primary care provider's intervention
- advise and counsel the patient on the proper course of action (i.e., no drug treatment, self-treatment with nonprescription drugs, referral to a primary care provider or other health care professional)
- advise the patient on the outcome of the selected course of action
- assure the patient that the desired therapeutic outcome can be achieved if nonprescription drugs are taken as directed on the label and/or recommended by the physician/pharmacist

- reinforce the concept that the pharmacist and physician are qualified to perform follow-up assessment of the treatment

If self-treatment with nonprescription drugs is in the best interest of the patient, then the pharmacist can be consulted for the following services:

- Assisting in product selection
- Assessing patient risk factors (e.g., contraindications, warnings, precautions, comorbidities, age, organ function)
- Counseling the patient about proper drug use (e.g., dosage, administration technique, monitoring parameters, duration of self-therapy)
- Maintaining an accurate patient drug profile that includes nonprescription and prescription drugs
- Assessing the potential of nonprescription drugs to mask symptoms of a more serious condition
- Preventing delays in seeking appropriate medical attention

The public's ability to discern critical information about the condition being treated and the clinical risk and benefit of the product is highly variable. The array of product choices, line extensions, and overstated, vague, or misleading marketing messages create consumer confusion. Generally, package labeling is limited in the breadth and depth of the message it communicates; it can never address the informational needs of patients in all clinical circumstances. Moreover, comorbidity and polypharmacy create an infinite number of special considerations in ensuring safe, appropriate, and effective use of nonprescription drugs. Thus, the pharmacist-patient interaction is vital to optimal nonprescription drug therapy. Although the pharmacist's active involvement in self-care usually costs the patient nothing directly, and no universal reimbursement scheme exists, this is still an important area of consumer-oriented pharmaceutical care that can be viewed as other disease management services. The need to develop reimbursement strategies for pharmacists' expertise and knowledge is high. In the meantime, the underlying goal of pharmacists' service is to ensure that the patient gets correct, practical information and understands it in the context of the ailment being treated. Validation of the patient's understanding is critically important. The pharmacist should always encourage the patients to ask questions and learn more.

## Nonprescription Drug Therapy

A host of professional, economic, and public interest issues and opportunities are converging to increase the prominence of nonprescription drug therapy within health care delivery and financing. Americans benefit economically from the wide range of therapeutic products available without a prescription. Table 1-3 lists some medical disorders that can be self-treated with nonprescription drugs. However, these products must be used properly to ensure they are safe and effective. For example, FDA's advisory panel concluded that the side effects (e.g., drowsiness) of nonprescription antihistamines should be listed on the label as a specific warning for consumers. This requirement was imposed even though 850 million packages of antihistamine have been sold over the last 10 years and no significant correlation has been found between their use and serious accidents.[33] But with safety as an FDA priority, it is highly probable that patients will see more product warnings on labels (commonly called the black box) in the near future. They have a right to know the health risks their drug products pose. Clinically proven benefits-versus-risks must ultimately be weighed in selecting any herbal/dietary supplement/drug products.

Pharmacists should also reinforce the importance of not exceeding the recommended dosage regimen (on nonprescription drug labels) during patient counseling. Patients should be instructed to seek medical attention if symptoms persist after use of the nonprescription drugs. Prolonged use of any nonprescription drug, unless otherwise advised by the physician or pharmacist, should be discouraged even with symptomatic relief. On the other hand, some nonprescription drugs are intended for continued use (e.g. daily aspirin for stroke prevention, daily psyllium for cholesterol lowering effects).

Inactive ingredients in nonprescription drugs, such as binders, disintegrants, fillers, and preservatives, are not threatening to most consumers. However, these can cause allergic reactions in a few individuals. For the safety of the very few who may encounter an allergic reaction, the FDA requires inactive ingredients be listed on the label so patients will know what they are ingesting. Table 1-4 lists some of the inactive ingredients with known adverse effects found in drug formulations.

### *Importance of Nonprescription Drug Labeling*

To assist consumers in distinguishing between similar and therapeutically different self-care drug products, FDA has mandated use of a standard label format for each of the product categories, namely, herbals, dietary supplements, and nonprescription drugs.[39] The standard product label, titled "Drug Facts," has specific sections for active ingredients, uses, warnings, when to use the product, directions, and inactive ingredients (see Chapter 4). In addition, the wording in the Drug Interactions area has been changed to "Ask your physician or pharmacist." Chances are, if a patient had an upset stomach, a runny nose, or muscle aches over the last year, he or she has already seen the "Drug Facts" label on most nonprescription drugs since May 15, 2002, and all nonprescription drugs since May 15, 2005. The advantage of "Drug Facts" is that it easier to read. All relevant information the patient needs when taking the drug appears on all package labels in the same sequence, enabling patients to find information in a familiar spot on the label. The label informs the reader exactly what medicine he or she is taking, how much to take, when to take it, when not to take it, when to consult a health care professional, what side effects may occur, how to store the medicine, and much more. Now, whether buying a bottle of pain relievers or a box of cough medicine, the patient will be able to find the information needed to make

**TABLE 1-3 Selected Medical Disorders Amenable to Nonprescription Drug Therapy***

| | | | |
|---|---|---|---|
| Abrasions | Colds (viral upper respiratory infection) | Gastritis | Ostomy care |
| Aches and pains (general, mild to moderate) | Congestion (chest, nasal) | Gingivitis | Ovulation prediction |
| Acidity | Constipation | Hair loss | Periodontal disease |
| Acne | Contact lens care | Halitosis | Pharyngitis |
| Albumin testing | Contraception | Hangover morning relief | Pinworm infestation |
| Allergic reactions | Corns | Head lice | Premenstrual syndrome |
| Allergic rhinitis | Cough | Headache | Pregnancy (diagnostic) |
| Anemia | Cuts (superficial) | Heartburn | Prickly heat |
| Arthralgia | Dandruff | Hemorrhoids | Psoriasis |
| Asthma | Deficiency disorders | Herpes | Ringworm |
| Athlete's foot | Dental care | Impetigo | Seborrhea |
| Bacterial infection | Dermatitis (contact) | Indigestion | Sinusitis |
| Blisters | Diabetes mellitus (insulin, monitoring equipment, supplies) | Ingrown toenails | Smoking cessation |
| Blood pressure monitoring | Diaper rash | Insect bites and stings | Sprains |
| Boils | Diarrhea | Insomnia | Strains |
| Bowel preparation (diagnostic) | Dry skin | Jet lag | Stye (hordeolum) |
| Burns (minor, thermal) | Dysmenorrhea | Jock itch | Sunburn |
| Calluses | Dyspepsia | Migraine | Teething |
| Candidal vaginitis | Dyslipidemia | Motion sickness | Thrush |
| Canker sores | Feminine hygiene | Myalgia | Toothache |
| Carbuncles | Fever | Nausea | Vomiting |
| Chapped skin | Flatulence | Nutrition (infant) | Warts (common and plantar) |
| Cold sores | | Obesity | Xerostomia |
| | | Occult blood in feces (detection) | Wound care |

* The pertinent nonprescription drug(s) for a particular disorder may serve as primary or major adjunctive therapy.

**TABLE 1-4 Adverse Effects of Some Inactive Ingredients Used in Drug Preparations**

| Inactive Ingredient | Use | Found in | Adverse Events |
|---|---|---|---|
| Aspartame | Sweetener | Liquid sucrose-free preparations | Headaches, hallucinations, panic attacks[34] |
| Benzalkonium chloride | Preservative | Antiasthmatic drugs, nasal decongestants | Airway constriction[27] |
| Benzyl alcohol | Preservative | Liquid preparations | Neonatal deaths, severe respiratory and metabolic complications[27] |
| Lactose | Filler | Capsules and tablets | Diarrhea, dehydration, cramping[27] |
| Propylene glycol | Solubilizes drugs | Liquid preparations | Respiratory problems, irregular heartbeat, low blood pressure; seizure, skin rashes[35] |
| Saccharin | Sweetener | Liquid preparations | Cross-sensitivity with sulfonamides, dermatologic reactions, pruritis[36] |
| Sulfites | Antioxidant | Antiasthmatic drugs; anti-inflammatories | Wheezing, breathing difficulties[37] |
| Yellow tartrazine | Coloring agent | Solid/liquid preparations | Allergic reaction similar to that of aspirin[38] |

an informed choice at the store and to use the product safely to its maximum benefit. The difficulty is getting patients to read this important information, according to the NCPIE Survey.[2]

The best way to become informed is to read and understand the information on nonprescription drug labels. In the ambulatory care setting, noncompliance to the therapeutic regimen, inappropriate choice of drug, and poor health outcomes with nonprescription drugs are particularly pronounced when patients lack information, have limited reading skills, and have language barriers. The National Adult Literacy Survey found that nearly 44 million Americans cannot read and write,[40] and 90 million adults have difficulty understanding information related to health care. Health illiteracy's impact is particularly profound on Medicaid recipients, 90% of whom have reading skills at the fifth-grade level. Such a low level of literacy adversely affects the health care outcome of patients using nonprescription drugs. Medicaid recipients also encounter difficulty in understanding the information provided by health care professionals.

The Omnibus Budget Reconciliation Act of 1990 mandates pharmacists to "offer to counsel" on prescription drugs they dispense. Nonprescription drugs, however, are exempted from this provision. Understanding what is on the label is critical for self-care that includes self-diagnosis and self-treatment, and pharmacists are well positioned to answer patients' questions after they have read the label. To increase patient safety, FDA is requiring every container of medicines (including nonprescription drugs) to be labeled with a bar code, to ensure (for hospital patients) that nurses and health care professionals dispense the right drug(s) in the right amount and at the right time.

While the FDA's requirement has the greatest impact on prescription drugs, nonprescription drugs intended to be used in institutional settings are also affected. Twenty percent of all prescription and nonprescription drugs are dispensed in error, 7% leading to potentially serious problems. The Institute of Medicine estimated that 7300 people died in 1993 because of medication errors, a number that could be rising. In these cases, accidental poisoning by drugs, medications, and biologicals was the result of acknowledged errors by patients or medical personnel.[41] Another study reported that the total cost of preventable drug errors is between $17 billion and $29 billion per year.[42] To reduce medication errors, several devices have been marketed to assist ambulatory patients in complying with their therapeutic regimens. These devices include beeping pillboxes, tablet dispensers, alphanumeric electronic pagers, automated medication dispensers, handheld medication reminder devices, talking wristwatches, and a device that is attached to the bottom of a tablet container for the patient to listen to the caregiver's message.

### Handling and Storage of Nonprescription Drugs

For the consumer to benefit optimally from nonprescription drug therapy, the drug has to have the potency stated on the label when it is used (assuming this occurs before the drug's expiration date). To retain its potency, a drug has to be stored properly. Prescription and nonprescription drugs are mistakenly stored in bathroom cabinets, often above the sink. Humidity and heat from the shower and sink are easily trapped in the cabinet, accelerating the degradation of the drugs even if they are in a prescription vial or bottle. Consumers need to be aware that all drugs should be stored in a cool, dark, dry place to ensure they retain their potency and effectiveness. Further, all drugs should preferably be stored on a closet or cabinet shelf that is high enough to be out of children's reach. Table 1-5 lists some nonprescription drugs and health care products generally kept on hand to treat minor ailments or injuries with storage recommendations. It is good practice to encourage patients to purge medicine cabinets at least once every 6 months. Drugs should be checked for expiration dates and a pharmacist/health care provider should be consulted before they are discarded.

**TABLE 1-5 Recommended Storage Places of Selected Nonprescription Health Care Products**

| Closet/Kitchen Cabinet or Shelf | Bathroom Medicine Cabinet |
|---|---|
| Analgesics (relieve pain) | Adhesive bandages |
| Antacids (relieve upset stomach) | Adhesive tape |
| Antibiotic ointments (reduce risk of infection) | Alcohol wipes |
| Antihistamines (relieve allergy symptoms) | Calibrated measuring spoon |
| Antipyretics (adult and child) | Dental floss |
| Antiseptics (help stop infection) | Disinfectant |
| Decongestants (relieve stuffy nose and cold) | Gauze pads |
| Hydrocortisone (relieve itching and inflammation) | Thermometer |

*Source:* Adapted from Lewis C. Your medicine cabinet needs an annual checkup, too. *FDA Consumer.* 2000;34(2):25-8.

## Complementary and Alternative Therapies

The Dietary Supplement Health and Education Act of 1994 (DSHEA) defines *dietary supplement* as a product taken by mouth that contains a dietary ingredient intended to supplement the diet. The term *dietary ingredient* includes vitamins, minerals, herbs, amino acids, and/or enzymes. While much remains unknown about many dietary supplements (e.g., their health benefits and potential risks), patients can count on one thing: the availability of a wide range of such products. According to the *Nutrition Business Journal*'s 2004 *Healthcare Distribution Management Association Industry Profile & Healthcare Factbook* (available at www.nutritionbusiness.com; accessed February 23, 2005), the revenue generated from the sales of nonprescription drugs used to treat/mitigate gastrointestinal disorders and symptoms of cold/flu exceed the sales of dietary supplements. But when it comes to sports/energy/weight loss products, the dietary supplements generate significantly more revenue than nonprescription drugs. But the differential in sales is relatively small for products sold for the treatment/mitigation of ailments related to the heart and joints. As for insomnia, the sales of nonprescription drugs were marginally greater than those of dietary supplements.

Patients taking advantage of the availability of dietary supplements should do so with care, making sure they have the necessary information and consult with their primary care provider and/or their pharmacist as needed. The Medstat Pulse Survey (available at www.nutritionbusiness.com; accessed February 23, 2005) has compiled data on the percentage of people who use alternative medicines for the treatment of some common ailments. Topping the list are back pain (35.8%) and migraines (28.9%), for which no traditional medications (prescription and nonprescription drugs) have yet provided a "magic bullet" rather than symptomatic relief. Following these are alternative medicines for foot problems (28.1%), stomach problems (27%), allergies (26.5), and asthma (25.5). These percentages are not mutually exclusive, as patients may suffer for multiple ailments. Some dietary supplement manufacturers are responsible and careful, but, as with all products on the market, patients need to be discriminating. Caution should be exercised in the use of dietary supplements as more evidence documents their interactions with prescription and nonprescription drugs.

Dietary supplements are recognized as a subset of foods under the federal law and are therefore regulated by FDA and the Federal Trade Commission. DSHEA, which regulates dietary supplements, requires that manufacturers substantiate all claims made on product labeling (see Chapter 4 for further discussion). The dietary supplement industry and health care professionals play important roles in providing safe products, but patients must also take responsibility for learning all they can about dietary supplements. The Introduction to Botanical and Nonbotanical Natural Medicines discusses quality verification programs for dietary supplements, whose purpose is to ensure that dietary supplements contain the ingredients and quantities stated on the labels, and are free of contaminants.

## Key Points for Self-Care and Nonprescription Pharmacotherapy

- Nonprescription drugs are used by millions of Americans each year because they offer safe and effective relief for a variety of common health care ailments.
- Health care professionals and the FDA agree that nonprescription drugs, though safe and effective, bear some risks associated with not reading and closely following the label instructions when taking the medications.
- It is critical for the patients to keep on mind that improper use or intentional abuse of nonprescription drugs, for example, taking more than is recommended or for a longer period of time than recommended, may result in serious health consequences.
- Self-care will play an increasingly important role in health care, and nonprescription pharmacotherapy represents a significant element in the self-care process.
- Patients, manufacturers, governmental agencies, and professional groups, particularly pharmacists, should become even more intent on recognizing that each group fulfills essential functions in ensuring the safe, appropriate, effective, and economical use of nonprescription drugs.

## References

1. US Department of Commerce, Bureau of the Census. Statistical Abstracts of the United States. Historical statistics of US colonial times to 1990. Washington, DC: US Government Printing Office; 1995.
2. Attitudes and beliefs about the use of over-the-counter medicines: A dose of reality: A national survey of consumers and health professionals. Harris Interactive, Inc; Bethesda, Md: National Council on Patient Information and Education; 2002. Available at: www.bemedwise.org/survey/final_survey.pdg. Accessed August 12, 2005.
3. Nutrition Business Journal Welcome; Available at: http://www.nutritionbusiness.com/index.cfm. Accessed February 23, 2005.
4. Nutrition Business Journal's Supplement Business Report 2004. Available at: http://store.yahoo.com/nbj/nbsupbusrep2.html. Accessed February 23, 2005.
5. Consumer Healthcare Products Association. OTC retail sales (1964-2004). Available at: http://www.chpa-info.org/web/press_room/statistics/otc_retail_sales.aspx. Accessed February 25, 2005.
6. Healthcare Distribution Management Association: 2004 industry profile & healthcare factbook. *Chain Drug Review*.Jan 5, 2004: Table 229; 99.
7. Consumer HealthCare Products Association: OTC sales by category: 2001-2004. Available at: http://www.chpa-info.org/web/press_room/statistics/otc_sales.aspx. Accessed August 10, 2005.
8. Internal Revenue Service, Department of Treasury; Over-the-counter drugs to be covered by health care flexible spending accounts. Available at: http://www.irs.gov/newsroom/article/0,,id=112623,00.html. Accessed February 23, 2005.
9. Consumer HealthCare Products Association: FAQs about the OTC Medicine Tax Fairness Act and making OTCs tax deductible. Available at: http://www.chpa-info.org/web/press_room/faqs/tax_fairness_act.aspx. Accessed February 23, 2005.
10. US Census Bureau. *Statistical Abstract of the United States:2004-2005: Decennial Census and Projections.* Available at: http://www.census.gov/prod/2004pubs/04statab/pop.pdf. Accessed on February 23, 2005.
11. As elderly population explodes, study published in JAMA calls for increase in geriatric training programs in US medical schools. *Ascribe Newswire: Health.* December 12, 2002: 4; 3.
12. WebMd Health: Medications and older adults. Available at: http://my.webmd.com/content/article/6/1680_51638.htm. Accessed on February 23, 2005.
13. US Department of Commerce, US Census Bureau. *The 65 Years and Over Population: 2000. Census 2000 Brief.* Available at: http://www.census.gov/prod/2001pubs/c2kbr01-10.pdf. Accessed February 23, 2005.
14. Federal Interagency Forum on Aging-Related Statistics. Older Americans 2004: key indicators of well-being. Available at: http://www.agingstats.gov/chartbook2004/population.html. Accessed February 25,2005.
15. Roper Starch report: Self-care trends among older Americans. Available at: http://www.chpa-info.org/web/press_room/statistics/pdfs/older_americans_final.pdf. Accessed February 25, 2005.
16. Self-care trends among women and men [fact sheet]. Available at: http://www.chpa-info.org/web/press_room/statistics/pdfs/women_final.pdf. Accessed February 25, 2005.
17. Henkel J. Buying drugs online: it's convenient and private, but beware of "rogue sites." *FDA Consumer.* 2000;34(1):5-9.
18. Anderson C. A call for Internet pharmacies to comply with quality standards. *Qual Safety Health Care.* 2003;12:86.
19. Bessell TL, Anderson JN, Silagy CA, et al. Surfing, self-medicating and safety: buying non-prescription and complementary medicines via the Internet. *Qual Safety Health Care.* 2002;11:88-92.
20. Verified Internet Pharmacy Practice Sites™ (VIPPS®) Program and PayPal® information. Available at: http://www.nabp.net/vipps/intro.asp. Accessed February 23, 2005.
21. Felkey B, Hotchkiss B. Incorporating the Internet into everyday practice. *J Am Pharm Assoc (Wash).* 1999;39:575-6.

22. Healthcare Facts & Figures: Reason for Using Health Information Services. Available at: http://www.medstat.com/healthcare/medfact17.asp. Accessed February 21, 2005.
23. Compiled from VIPPS® Database Search. Available at: http://www.nabp.net/vipps/consumer/search.asp. Accessed February 23, 2005.
24. The Switch Process. Available at: http://www.chpa-info.org/web/advocacy/general_issues/switch/switch_process.aspx. Accessed February 25, 2005.
25. OTC medicines are convenient and increasingly popular with Americans. Available at: http://www.chpa-info.org/web/advocacy/general_issues/advancing_quality_healthcare.aspx. Accessed February 25, 2005.
26. Consumer Healthcare Products Association. OTC facts and figures. Available at: http://www.chpa-info.org/web/press_room/statistics/otc_facts_figures.aspx. Accessed February 25,2005.
27. Novak KN, Kastrup EK, Wickersham RM, eds. *Drug Facts and Comparisons* [monthly loose-leaf updates]. St. Louis: Wolters Kluwer Health, Inc; 2005.
28. Divoll M, Greenblatt DJ, Ameer B, et al. Effect of food on acetaminophen absorption in young and elderly subjects. *J Clin Pharmacol.* 1982;22:571-6.
29. Kiesewetter H, Jung F, Jung EM, et al. Effect of garlic on platelet aggregation in patients with increased risk of juvenile ischemia attack. *Eur J Clin Pharmacol.* 1993;45:333-6.
30. Orwoll ES. The milk-alkali syndrome: current concepts. *Ann Intern Med.* 1982;97:242-8.
31. Pecoud A, Donzel P, Schelling JL. Effect of foodstuffs on the absorption of zinc sulfate. *Clin Pharmacol Ther.* 1975;17:469-74.
32. Drug facts label. Available at: http://www.chpa-info.org/Consumers/Drug_Label/index.aspx. Accessed February 25, 2005.
33. Russell C, Edenhart D. CHPA details safety, effectiveness of antihistamines at NTSB/FDA meeting: consumers, government agencies reminded of the importance of reading medicine labels. CHPA News release November 14, 2001. Available at: http://www.chpa-info.org/web/press_room/news_releases/2001/8_01_ntsb_nov_2001_final.pdf. Accessed February 23, 2005.
34. Schiffman SS, Buckley CE, Sampson A. Aspartame and susceptibility to headache. *N Engl J Med.* 1987;317:1181-5.
35. MacDonald MG, Getson PR, Mathison DA. Propylene glycol: increased incidence of seizures in low birth weight infants. *Pediatrics.* 1987;79:622-5.
36. Cohen SM. Saccharin: past, present and future. *J Am Diet Assoc.* 1986;86:929-31.
37. Freedman BJ. Asthma induced by sulfur dioxide, benzoate and tartrazine contained in orange drinks. *Clin Allergy.* 1997;7:407-15.
38. Stevenson DD, Simon RA, Lumry WR, et al. Adverse reactions to tartrazine. *J Allergy Clin Immunol.* 1986;78:182-91.
39. Drug facts label. Available at: http://www.chpa-info.org/Consumers/Drug_Label/index.aspx. Accessed February 25, 2005.
40. Kirsch I, Jungeblut A, Jenkins L, et al. *Adult Literacy in America: A First Look at the Findings of the National Adult Literacy Survey.* Washington, DC: National Center for Education Statistics, US Department of Education; 1993.
41. Philips DP, Christenfeld N, Glynn LM. Increase in US medication error deaths between 1983 and 1993. *Lancet.* 1998;351:643-4.
42. Johnson WG, Brennan TA, Newhouse JP, et al. The economic consequences of medical injuries. *JAMA.* 1992;267:2487-92.

CHAPTER 2

# Patient Assessment and Consultation

*Brian J. Isetts and Lawrence M. Brown*

The development of viable pharmaceutical care business models are helping pharmacists more effectively respond to the drug-related needs of patients. One important development relates to the use of a clearly defined patient care process to fulfill a patient's self-care needs. In addition, decisions made by pharmacists functioning to identify, resolve, and prevent drug therapy problems are valid, or clinically credible, as judged by panels of physicians and pharmaceutical care practitioners. This chapter describes the consistent and systematic process used to meet the drug-related needs of patients with self-care concerns.

The patient care process pertaining to medication therapy management includes assessment, care planning, and evaluation. Assessment represents the first set of clinical judgments made by a practitioner when caring for a patient. The purpose of assessment is to determine, describe, and define the patient's drug-related needs, including the goals of therapy and identification of drug therapy problems the patient may be experiencing. Assessment provides the practitioner with a basis for consulting with a patient to decide which of the patient's drug therapy problems the practitioner will help resolve. A care plan is a detailed schedule of responsibilities for achieving treatment goals and resolving and preventing drug therapy problems, whereas follow-up evaluation represents an accounting of actual patient outcomes.

Patients expect pharmacists to assist them with many health care concerns and to help them interpret treatment options within the health care delivery system. This chapter is divided into six sections: (1) a brief review of the demands for self-care; (2) an introduction to the consistent and systematic patient care process practitioners use when assuming responsibility for a patient's drug-related needs; (3) a description of the rational and ordered process for conducting an assessment, developing a care plan, and completing a follow-up evaluation of a patient's drug-related needs; (4) a discussion of the skills necessary to care for patients with self-care needs; (5) a summary of special considerations when caring for selected high-risk and special patient populations (infants and children, persons of advanced age, and pregnant and breast-feeding women); and (6) key points for integrating these principles into pharmacy practice. Because the federal government has equated the terms "pharmaceutical care" and "medication therapy management" (MTM), these terms will be used synonymously in this chapter. The term MTM first appeared in federal legislation introduced, but not passed, in the late 1990s, proposing to compensate pharmacists for pharmaceutical care services. In addition, a case-based format is used to demonstrate how a pharmacist can apply the information contained in this chapter to the care of patients with self-care needs.

## Demand for Self-Care

The U.S. health care system is very dynamic and marked by rapid change. Access, cost, and quality of health care are extensively debated at a public policy level. Our complicated, diverse, and fractionated health care system can leave consumers frustrated when confronted with personal health care concerns. Fortunately, patients have come to trust and depend on their pharmacist when faced with their own personal health care needs.

Pharmacists, who are often on the front line of the health care delivery system, are called on to help patients evaluate therapeutic options. In most cases, the pharmacist can help patients by (1) recommending no treatment at all, (2) recommending self-care therapy, or (3) referring patients to other health care professionals. Several chapters in this book contain information and tables on exclusions for self-care treatment that pharmacists may find helpful in deciding when to refer patients to other health care professionals. In addition, issues relating to special populations such as infants and young children, persons of advanced age, and pregnant or breast-feeding women are also addressed in this text.

Self-care, self-diagnosis, and self-medication are important components of the health care system in the United States. Instead of seeking the advice of a medical care provider, many people self-diagnose and treat their symptoms with a vast array of self-care options ranging from nonprescription drugs, herbal products, and home remedies to yoga, meditation, and spiritual healing, among others. Survey data show that 73% of Americans prefer self-care treatment options to seeing a primary care provider when ill.[1] Nonprescription drugs allow individuals to manage their many medical problems rapidly, economically, and conveniently, and may prevent unnecessary visits to a primary care provider or specialist. Patients often believe products that move from prescription to nonprescription status are more effective than other nonprescription drugs, and 87% of Americans believe that nonprescription drugs are safe when used as directed.[2] The demand for and shift toward self-medication are further described and documented in Chapter 1.

The appropriate use of a nonprescription product, like the use of any other drug, requires attention to the intended use, effectiveness, safety, and convenience of administration. Although warnings are required on the labels of such products, labeling alone may be inadequate, and the patient may need assistance in selecting and properly using nonprescription drugs. Inappropriate use and misuse of nonprescription drugs can increase the risk of drug misadventures,[3] resulting in increased health care costs and more serious illness. Thus, the pharmacist's role is crucial in assessing a patient's need for nonprescription medications.

The magnitude of drug misadventures, or drug therapy problems, has been described in terms of drug-induced morbidity and mortality.[4,5] In addition, one category of drug therapy problems, referred to as medication safety, has received extensive national attention in reports such as those issued through the Institute of Medicine and the work of organizations such as the Institute for Safe Medication Practices. From 1995 to 2000, the cost of drug therapy problems more than doubled.[5] Drug therapy problems are defined as any aspect of a patient's drug therapy that is interfering with a desired, positive therapeutic outcome.[6] A patient who requires a nonprescription medication pursuant to a self-care consultation with a pharmacist is experiencing a drug therapy problem because he or she has an untreated medical condition and requires the intervention of a pharmacist. A pharmacist's interpretation that use of a nonprescription product can help the patient achieve a desired therapeutic outcome is an intervention intended to resolve the patient's drug therapy problem (i.e., patient needs additional drug therapy). In addition, it is noted that 23% of all drug therapy problems involve one or more nonprescription drug products, either as the cause of the drug therapy problem or in its resolution.[6]

Many patients do not appreciate, or are not aware of, the need for professional assistance in selecting nonprescription drugs. The presence of a pharmacist differentiates the nonprescription drug department in a pharmacy from a similar department in a nonpharmacy outlet. To serve patients better, pharmacists need to maximize the personal service they offer. Patient inquiries should be referred to pharmacists, who must actively promote the value of their guidance in selecting and monitoring treatment with a nonprescription drug. It is essential to increase a patient's awareness of the importance of consulting a pharmacist, not only when considering a drug for the first time but also when making subsequent purchases.

A patient's primary patronage motive, or choice of pharmacy, is convenience, followed by price and service.[7] A random-sample telephone interview survey of 1505 adults found that 84% of Americans agree that pharmacists are a good source of information for minor health problems. Nevertheless, only 7% of those interviewed seek information from a pharmacist when treating minor health care problems; they are more likely to consult family and friends (27%), physicians (20%), and medical books (10%).[1]

The principles of pharmaceutical care are available to help practitioners more effectively address patients' self-care needs. A consistent and systematic patient care process helps practitioners to be complete and concise when assuming responsibility for a patient's self-care needs. In addition, use of the systematic patient care process is important in obtaining compensation for the pharmacist's care.

## Introduction to Pharmaceutical Care

Until recently, the issue of classifying pharmacists as health care practitioners or health care providers has been contentious. One of the reasons used to restrict payment to pharmacists for pharmaceutical care was the fact that they were not explicitly listed as practitioners in the Medicare program and most Medicaid programs. The two federal laws significantly affecting pharmacist practitioner classification are the Health Insurance Portability and Accountability Act[8] and the Medicare Modernization Act.[9] These two laws helped the profession of pharmacy work with the American Medical Association (AMA) and the Centers for Medicare and Medicaid Services (CMS) to establish pharmacists' professional service billing codes described in *Current Procedural Terminology* (i.e., CPT codes), and include pharmacies as a "Place of Service" in the 15th edition of the *CPT Manual*.[10] The significance of these new developments to the future of pharmacy is highlighted throughout this chapter.

Pharmaceutical care has fulfilled an unmet need in the health care delivery system by providing a systematic approach for consistently achieving intended drug therapy treatment goals while avoiding adverse, unintended, and ineffective medication consequences. In addition, pharmaceutical care has clarified the responsibilities of pharmacists as health care practitioners, and defined the relationship between the profession and society. In 1990, a landmark article titled "Opportunities and Responsibilities in Pharmaceutical Care" described the theoretical constructs necessary for pharmacists to take responsibility for a patient's drug therapy outcomes.[11] Now that pharmacists are officially classified as health care practitioners eligible for patient care compensation, the principles of pharmaceutical care will be important to the growing number of pharmacists building and expanding patient care practices.

The established characteristics of a pharmaceutical care practice were based on the rules governing the conduct of other professional practices. A practice may be viewed as the application of knowledge, guided by a commonly held social purpose, to the resolution of specific problems in a standard manner accepted and recognized by society. The definition of a pharmaceutical care practice, developed through analysis of other professional practices, is "a practice in which the practitioner takes responsibility for all of a patient's drug-related needs and is held accountable for this commitment."[6] The reader is referred to *Pharmaceutical Care Practice: The Clinician's Guide,* by Cipolle, Strand, and Morley, for a thorough discussion of these practice components.[6] A reference is also available for pharmacists seeking information on constructing a pharmaceutical care practice management system, including an example of a detailed practice management plan.[12]

The goal when assuming responsibility for a patient's drug-related needs is to help the patient achieve the intended therapeutic goals and ensure a positive outcome. A standard problem-solving process, originally termed the Pharmacist's Workup of Drug Therapy and now referred to as the Pharmacotherapy Workup, was developed to help pharmacists systematically address all of a patient's drug-related needs.[13] This standard problem-solving process is designed to move the pharmacist through an ordered sequence of decisions related to the intended use, effectiveness, safety, and convenience of use of the patient's drug therapies. The purpose of defining a common patient care process is to accomplish positive patient care objectives, not to constrain the freedoms or decisions of individual practitioners. In fact, pharmacists who have established patient care businesses have been found to execute the standard patient care process slightly differently.[14]

Pharmacists must use a systematic, comprehensive, and efficient process to take responsibility for a patient's drug-related needs. To meet this objective, the patient care process involves the following three major steps:[6]

1. Assess, or systematically review, the patient's drug-related needs, including identifying any and all drug therapy problems.
2. Create a care plan or detailed schedule outlining both the practitioner's and the patient's activities and responsibilities designed to resolve any drug therapy problems, achieve treatment goals, and prevent any potential drug therapy problems.
3. At planned follow-up intervals, evaluate the patient's outcome and current status.

The care plan and evaluation provide the accountability and results that are often lacking in the health care delivery system. The following section focuses on conducting an assessment of a patient's drug-related needs, with an emphasis on assessing the drug-related needs of patients presenting with self-care concerns.

## Assessment of a Patient's Drug-related Needs

Identifying drug therapy problems is a primary clinical decision made by the practitioner. From a historical perspective, this new health care responsibility for pharmacists represents a shift in societal expectations that has occurred within a relatively short period of time. Until 1963, pharmacists were precluded by the American Pharmacists Association's (previously known as the American Pharmaceutical Association) Code of Ethics from informing the patient of the name of the medication being dispensed, much less the intended actions and adverse reactions. The consumer movement of the 1970s and 1980s then prompted pharmacists to begin providing the name, action, and adverse drug events of the medications being dispensed to patients.

From a consumer perspective, pharmaceutical care is a new and emerging concept. Patients are now seeking the personal attention of a trusted professional to help them achieve drug therapy treatment goals, while avoiding or minimizing the adverse consequences of taking medications. The rational and ordered process for conducting an assessment helps the pharmacist, functioning as a health care practitioner, maintain a disciplined approach when confronted with this changing societal demand.

Before presenting specific examples of how to use the information presented in this chapter, it is important to discuss the realities of providing self-care consultations during the course of a typical day for a pharmacist working in the dispensing business of a pharmacy, compared with consulting a patient in a professional services reimbursement group through the patient care business of a pharmacy. Obviously, pharmacists asked to conduct a self-care consultation when fulfilling prescription dispensing responsibilities will have less time to devote to working with the patient than pharmacists working in the patient care business. For those pharmacists who have not yet worked in the patient care business of a pharmacy, it is important to point out that there are a number of proven strategies and approaches for starting a patient care business in juxtaposition to a pharmacy's traditional prescription dispensing business. Payment for pharmaceutical care is a reality, and pharmacists who desire a future focused on working in a pharmacy's patient care business can now seek out these types of employment opportunities. In fact, a recent independent analysis of resource needs conducted by the Lewin Group, Inc. compiled, and suggested, a $2.00 to $3.00 per minute compensation level is necessary to sustain the delivery of medication therapy management services within a pharmaceutical care practice.[15]

## Skills Necessary to Care for Patients with Self-Care Needs

Advising patients on self-treatment is an important part of a pharmacist's professional responsibilities. When pharmacists use a standard care process to address a patient's self-care needs, they serve in the role of a primary care practitioner. Often the pharmacist is a patient's first contact with the health care system, and the pharmacist can evaluate the situation and recommend a course of action. This role may include recommending a nonprescription drug, dissuading patients from buying a medication when drug therapy is not indicated, recommending a nondrug treatment, or referring patients to another health care practitioner. If the pharmacist deters healthy people from using more costly health care services or products and refers more seriously ill patients to other primary care providers, health care delivery in the United States can be improved and health care resources can be conserved.

The following case study, presented in five parts, illustrates a few important pharmacotherapy assessment skills necessary to care for patients with self-care needs.

### PATIENT-PHARMACIST CONSULTATION

**General Patient Presentation**

Mrs. E.J. is a 66 year-old female patient in good medical condition taking three prescription medications (lisinopril, atenolol, and lovastatin) to manage two chronic medical conditions (hypertension and dyslipidemia). Mrs. E.J.'s primary concern relates to the fact that she has been finding it a little more difficult to initiate a bowel movement.

Regardless of whether a pharmacist is working in a busy dispensing pharmacy or caring for patients during scheduled appointments, working with patients to identify their drug-related needs is at the center of the pharmacist's communication process during interaction with the patient. Drug-related needs are defined as those health care needs of a patient that have some relationship to drug therapy and for which the practitioner is able to offer professional assistance.[6] Patients will tell their story or present a picture (e.g., "When I urinate, I feel as though I am going to pass out") in a random fashion. It is the pharmacist's job to interpret a patient's explicit and implicit drug-related needs. This skill is somewhat analogous to throwing a deck of cards into the air and reassembling the deck by suits.

In the case of Mrs. E.J., the pharmacist will listen to the patient's concerns to ascertain the nature and extent of her problem. The pharmacist will also want to know the patient's current medications to determine whether or not the condition may be caused by a medication, and to select a product appropriate for the patient. A pharmacist working in a pharmaceutical care practice will then move forward to assess all of the patient's current medications, supplements, and remedies for indication, effectiveness, safety, and convenience of use. Proceeding systematically in this order is critical to avoid missing an important piece of information or jumping to an erroneous conclusion. Patients express their drug-related needs as understanding (or sometimes as a lack of understanding), expectations, concerns, and behavior (noncompliance). The pharmacist translates a patient's expression of drug-related needs into an assessment of drug therapy problems.

A final determination of drug therapy problems is conducted in consultation and agreement with the patient. Pharmacists cannot force their will on patients. For instance, a 54-year-old female who smokes two cigarettes in the gazebo while her husband conducts business out of town 1 day per month might not believe she has a drug therapy problem. Pushing a smoking cessation intervention onto the patient may be detrimental to the therapeutic relationship. A therapeutic relationship is a partnership between the practitioner and the patient formed for the purpose of identifying the patient's drug-related needs.[6] When pharmacists care for patients using this systematic process, physicians and pharmaceutical care practitioners have been found to agree with 94.2% of all their clinical decisions made to identify, resolve, and prevent drug therapy problems, and to achieve intended drug therapy treatment goals.[16]

## Communication

Interactions by pharmacists through consultation and effective assessment strategies can enhance patient outcomes. Patients' expression of their drug-related needs is one of the most important sources of information pharmacists need to provide pharmaceutical care related to nonprescription drugs. Each step of the patient care process involves communicating with the patient, gathering information from the patient, and transmitting information back to the patient. This process is particularly important during the assessment step, because these data form the basis for the care plan and subsequent follow-up evaluation. Good communication between a pharmacist and patient are essential in the practice of pharmacy.

**PATIENT-PHARMACIST CONSULTATION**

**Translation of Patient Concerns Into an Assessment of Drug Therapy Problems**

Mrs. E.J.'s primary concern relates to the fact that she has been finding it a little more difficult to initiate a bowel movement. She informs you that she doesn't want anything too strong because a friend of hers became dependent on laxatives. The pharmacist also finds out that the patient has not started any new medications within the last 6 months and has not had any changes in her diet. A decision is made to start Mrs. E.J. on the stool softener docusate 100 mg once daily for 1 week. This patient's primary concern has been translated into a need for additional drug therapy.

Interaction between the pharmacist and the patient establishes a therapeutic relationship, or an alliance, needed to identify the patient's drug-related needs. It is characterized by trust, empathy, respect, authenticity, and responsiveness. This relationship allows the pharmacist to gather detailed, sometimes intimate, information from patients. In return, patients rely on the pharmacist to use knowledge, skills, and experience to ensure safe and effective drug therapy. Scheduled patient follow-up and reassessment are vital components of this therapeutic relationship and are used to determine actual patient outcomes and progress toward meeting therapeutic objectives. These components allow a pharmacist to reassess whether a patient is experiencing drug therapy problems. In the case of Mrs. E.J., the goal of therapy is a return to the patient's normal bowel movement pattern within 1 week. In a dispensing pharmacy, the patient is responsible for taking action if goals of therapy are not achieved, while in a pharmaceutical care practice the pharmacist assumes responsibility for following up with the patient in 1 week to determine progress toward achieving goals of therapy.

The patient-pharmacist relationship is dynamically affected by numerous variables. A positive interaction one day could be followed by a negative interaction a few days later for reasons unrelated to the practitioner's care. The pharmacist must become adept at interpreting nonverbal cues (e.g., facial expression or body position), as well as at responding to voice tones, inflection, and mood.[17] If a patient has a drug-related need, but does not have the time or inclination to discuss it during a particular encounter, the pharmacist should schedule an alternative time to gather additional information to assess the patient's drug-related needs and determine an appropriate intervention. The potential severity of a drug therapy problem will dictate the timetable for these actions.

### General Principles of Communication

To establish an effective therapeutic relationship with the patient, the pharmacist must be capable of demonstrating empathy to objectively identify with the patient's affective state.[18] Because the pharmacist's underlying attitude toward the patient will influence the quality of communication, the pharmacist must eliminate barriers by avoiding biases toward a patient's level of education, socioeconomic or cultural background, interests, or attitudes. In addition, the pharmacist must assure patients that any information they discuss will be kept in strict confidence.

A first step in a patient encounter is to assess what the patient already knows and determine where gaps in knowledge exist. This step is important because patients may resent being told what they already know and may be confused if the pharmacist wrongly assumes that they understand more than they do. When interacting with patients, the pharmacist should use words that a layperson can understand.

Effective communication occurs when the receiver of a message hears and understands exactly what the sender wants to communicate. One way to ensure understanding is through active listening, a process in which the receiver repeats the information back to the sender. As information is exchanged, the participants change roles as receivers and senders of information. The message received is influenced by its content and context, as well as by how it is sent. Communications can be improved by paying attention to the interaction between sender and receiver.

## Effective Questioning

Skillful questioning is a mark of a good communicator. Patients should feel that the pharmacist's questions convey a genuine interest in them and a desire to help. Because a patient may be uncooperative if the questions suggest only superficial curiosity, the pharmacist should explain the reason for asking personal questions (e.g., "I want to obtain additional information so I can determine if a nonprescription medication will help treat your specific problem."). It is important to avoid interrupting, or cutting off the patient in the middle of a response, which can occur when thinking ahead to the next question without adequately processing the current response.

When the pharmacist is unfamiliar with the patient, he or she should start the patient encounter by stating, "My name is ____, and I'm the pharmacist." The pharmacist should begin the exchange with an open-ended query such as, "How can I help you?" or "Would you please tell me more about the symptoms/problems you have?" Such valuable open-ended queries allow for increased flexibility and provide greater information than will questions that can be answered with only a yes or no response. Such open-ended queries enable a good practitioner to collect information efficiently and to establish better communications. If a patient's response wanders, however, the pharmacist must keep the interaction focused. To be sure that a patient understands dosage instructions, the pharmacist could ask, "So I know that I haven't forgotten to tell you anything, would you please tell me how you plan to take this medicine?"

Summarizing the important points or redirecting the interaction with closed-ended question is useful. A question such as, "How long have you had this pain?" may help the pharmacist gather specific information or clarify information obtained through earlier open-ended questions. It is important to ask one question at a time; asking two questions in rapid succession or multiple-choice questions will cause confusion and restrict communication. It is also important to avoid leading questions or judgmental questions such as, "You don't smoke, do you?"

## Effective Listening

Effective listening is a vital component of communication. When the pharmacist really listens, patients are free to state their problem completely and are assured of receiving the pharmacist's undivided attention. The pharmacist must focus on the patient and exclude distractions such as a telephone or a computer screen. The pharmacist may need to clarify the details of a patient's problem and should be receptive to a patient's response to questions. The pharmacist should respond with empathy, perhaps by paraphrasing a patient's words or by reflecting on what was said in terms of the patient's own experience. For instance, after listening to a complaint of pain, the pharmacist could say, "You have a sharp, stabbing pain in your wrist; is that right?" and end with a statement such as, "That must be very uncomfortable." Interrupting or demonstrating lack of interest or disapproval may inhibit a patient's discussion of problems and concerns. Encouraging a patient to talk, exploring a patient's comments, and expressing understanding all facilitate communication. The pharmacist should reinforce wise decisions a patient has made while reserving judgment about any potentially unhealthy behaviors.

## Nonverbal Communication

Nonverbal communication skills are important when conducting an assessment. A pharmacist's body language, such as posture and facial expression, communicates strong, direct messages.[17] Pharmacists should be aware of their own nonverbal behavior as well as that of the patient. An open body posture—facing the patient with arms and legs uncrossed—indicates openness, honesty, and a willingness to communicate and listen. Maintaining an appropriate distance from a patient will facilitate confidential communication without making patients uncomfortable. If a patient backs away or moves closer, the pharmacist should maintain the new distance the patient has established. Pharmacists should maintain eye contact with a patient and control their facial expressions to avoid showing negative emotions such as disapproval or shock.

The patient's nonverbal communication is equally important. If a patient has a closed body posture—arms crossed, legs crossed, body turned away—the pharmacist may need to find out why the patient is uncomfortable and then try to allay any concerns. The pharmacist should watch a patient's facial expressions for signs of anxiety, nervousness, and physical symptoms such as pain.

## Physical Barriers to Communication

High counters, glass separators, and elevated platforms inhibit communication and provide physical barriers. Pharmacists should try to be at eye level with the patient. A tall pharmacist may need to sit on a stool or lower his or her body position to avoid "hovering over" the patient. Discussions between patient and pharmacist should be as private and uninterrupted as possible. If the pharmacist expects or perceives that a patient is uncomfortable discussing the problem, a quiet semiprivate or private consultation area should be sought and used. Ideally, a specific, private area should be designated for patient consultations.

### Communication Techniques for Special Populations

Special communication techniques may be required with some patients.[19] Writing or printing out the information to provide a quality copy may be necessary if the patient is deaf or hearing impaired. If a patient who is hearing impaired reads lips, the pharmacist should be physically close to, and directly in front of, the patient and maintain eye contact while speaking. The pharmacist should speak slowly and distinctly in a low-pitched, moderate tone because yelling further distorts the sound and might embarrass the patient. A quiet, well-lit environment is essential because background noise and dimness can markedly diminish a hearing-impaired individual's ability to communicate. The pharmacist may use visual reinforcement, such as pointing to the part of the body that hurts or to the directions on a container. Using written or printed information alone can create misunderstandings with language that confuses the patient and requires further explanation. However, using printed information in conjunction with patient discussions has been found to be more effective than using written information alone.[19]

When interacting with a patient who is blind or visually impaired, the pharmacist should first state, "I am the pharmacist." Because a blind patient cannot perceive most nonverbal communication, the pharmacist should depend on tone of voice and verbal feedback to convey empathy and interest in the patient's problem. If the pharmacist needs to touch the patient to obtain additional information about the patient's condition, such as might be the case with a sprained ankle, or to obtain a fingerstick blood glucose measurement, permission should first be obtained.

An estimated 13% to 40% of Americans are illiterate, and another 20% are considered marginally literate.[19] For these patients, written information or directions on a label are barriers, and the pharmacist cannot rely on them to reinforce information provided orally. Patients with reading impairments may be less inclined to ask questions or express their concerns. Although some common characteristics of illiteracy are related to age, education, and employment status, [19] an understanding of the patient's literacy status may take time to determine through the development of a therapeutic relationship.

The pharmacist must build a caring relationship to provide effective communication and consultation. The pharmacist can facilitate communication by using simple language and pictorial labels. Language and cultural barriers to communication may occur when interacting with patients of unfamiliar ethnic backgrounds.[20] For patients who are unable to communicate well in English, pharmacists may need to take extra time to demonstrate proper use of medication (e.g., eyedrops, inhalers) and develop visual aids (e.g., pictorial labels, illustrations) or pamphlets in the patient's language. Interpreters are also available as a resource in some communities and medical care facilities, and pharmacists may ask questions related to cultural beliefs to assess how these beliefs influence the patient's use of medications (see Chapter 3). Similarly, cultural behaviors may result in failure to make eye contact and should not be interpreted as a lack of interest or understanding.

## Patient Consultation

Interacting with a patient regarding self-treatment is a primary care activity that carries a great professional responsibility. Patients with self-care needs present differently from those who have already gotten a treatment decision from a medical care provider. To obtain assurances that a particular drug product is appropriate for a patient, the pharmacist needs to perform an assessment by eliciting information from the patient, integrating these data to determine if any drug therapy problems exist, and then develop a patient care plan. As mentioned previously, pharmacists functioning in the dispensing business of a pharmacy, as well as pharmacists being reimbursed for providing pharmaceutical care, both start from the same point in interacting with a patient with self-care concerns (i.e., nature and extent of the patient's problem, current medications, and other medical conditions).

The self-care encounter in a pharmacy can be initiated by either the patient or the pharmacist (Figure 2-1). Although patients often initiate the consultation, an increasing number of pharmacists greet patients who are entering the self-care section of the premises and initiate an assessment of the patient's self-care concerns and drug-related needs. The patient may approach the pharmacist with a symptom, often in the form of a question such as, "What do you recommend for ... ?" Or the patient may ask a product-related question, such as "Which of these two products do you recommend?"

### *Information-gathering Process*

Before formulating a plan for self-treatment or medical referral, the pharmacist must obtain enough information to identify and assess the patient's medical condition and drug therapy problem(s). Important data include the patient's perceived needs and concerns, demographics (i.e., patient-related variables), diseases, and medications. With experience, the pharmacist will be able to gather the necessary information to assess a particular condition within a relatively short period of time.

In a pharmaceutical care practice, the pharmacist will also conduct a general review of systems. A verbal review of the patient's physiologic systems, from head to toe, can help account for all of a patient's drug-related needs. The Pharmacotherapy Workup provides pharmacists with a complete listing of the 15 body organ systems needed to conduct this review of systems: neurologic, psychological, eye-ear-nose-throat, endocrine, vital signs, cardiovascular, hematology, pulmonary, musculoskeletal, gastrointestinal (GI), fluid/electrolyte status, renal, hepatic, genitourinary/reproductive, and skin.

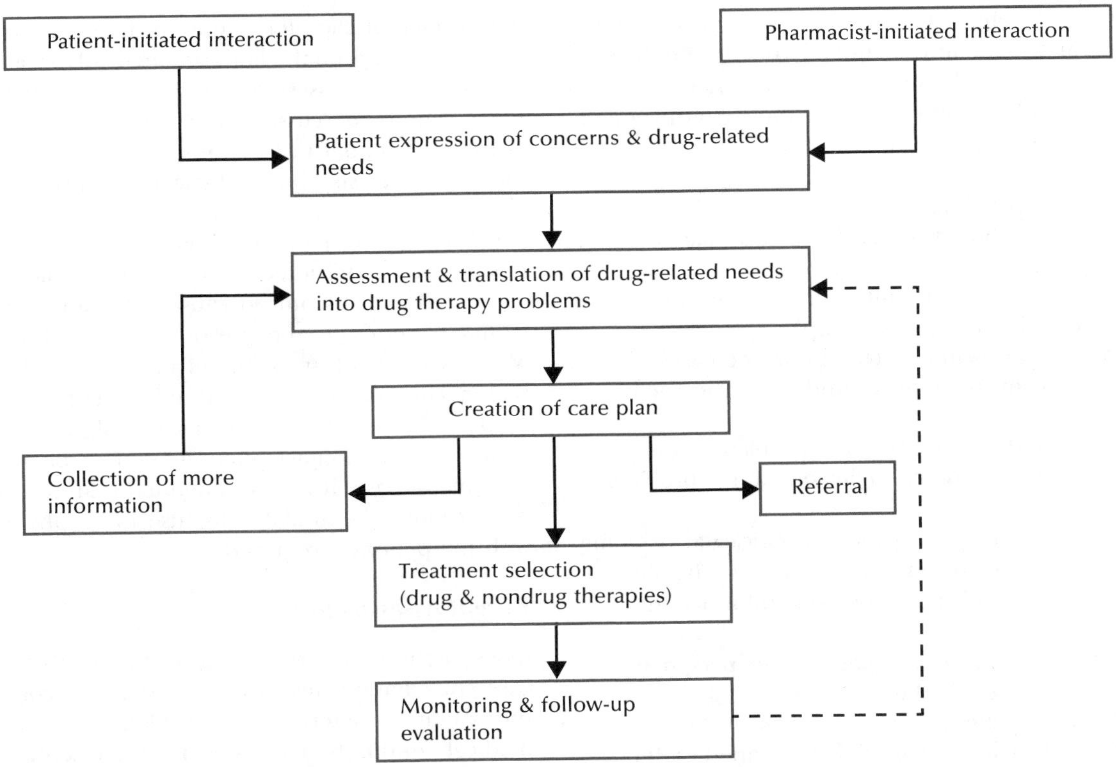


**FIGURE 2-1** Patient–pharmacist consultation process.

Other important information is an accurate accounting of each medication a patient is using to treat all medical conditions. This list includes prescription, nonprescription, and herbal products, vitamins, and dietary supplements. Thorough questioning is important because patients tend to underreport use of nonprescription medications and dietary supplements.[21] If possible, the pharmacist may find it helpful to have the patient's medication history available at the start of the patient consultation.

The pharmacist can explain the need to review all medications by saying, "I would like to review each of the medications you are currently taking so that the drug product we might select for you fits with your current therapy. Here is a list of medications you have received at our pharmacy. Let's take a minute to see which ones you are currently taking, as well as what other medications you may be using." It may also be helpful for the pharmacist to have patients describe their daily activities and medication schedule in case they have difficulty recalling the names of all the medications they are taking.

When an accurate picture of the patient's active medication list has been obtained, the pharmacist in a pharmaceutical care practice will tie all active medications to each of the patient's medical conditions. A patient's drug allergies and relative medical history may be taken at this point. The assessment process is dictated by the patient's knowledge level, as well as by the amount of time available to continue the interaction. Thus, to obtain the needed information quickly and efficiently, the pharmacist should approach the problem logically and keep the questioning direct and to the point.

Fortunately, within the context of providing pharmaceutical care, the pharmacist need not try to obtain all relevant information in one encounter. The planned follow-up evaluation extends the initial assessment process and allows the pharmacist to obtain additional information. The weight of a 13-year-old child, the smoking history of a patient with emphysema, the allergy history of a patient with a sinus infection, and the calcium intake of a postmenopausal woman are examples of information that may be important during the patient encounter but may also be obtained during the follow-up evaluation. With continual practice, the pharmacist will learn to use every patient encounter to gather important additional information. The pharmacist will develop a sense, based on the patient's expression of needs, for when to bring the initial assessment to a close and, in a pharmaceutical care practice, how to establish appropriate follow-up.

### *Patient History*

After the pharmacist has accounted for the patient's other medications and drug-related needs, it is time to return to the patient's initial presentation of his or her self-care concerns. If the patient is not using any medications, supplements, or remedies, the pharmacist commences the self-care encounter with a broad overview of the patient's health to determine the nature and extent of the problem. This overview of the patient's health enables the pharmacist to understand the patient's condition and make the most appropriate recommendation, regardless of whether a drug is included. Pharmacists should start by determining a patient's needs with an open-ended question such as, "How may I help you?" Patients may initially present incomplete and vague information. To determine the specific symptoms and whether they are amenable to self-treatment, the pharmacist can pose the following open-ended queries or requests:

- Describe your problem.
- Describe to me how your problem has changed over time.
- How does the problem limit your daily activities (e.g., sleeping, eating, working, walking)?
- How has this problem affected you in the past?
- Tell me about any foods, drugs, and/or physical activities that make the problem worse.
- What have you done to relieve this problem in the past?
- What have you been doing so far to treat the problem?

The next step is to gather patient-specific data, including demographic information and medical history. The pharmacist should selectively elicit the following information:

- Who is the patient? Is the patient the person in the pharmacy or someone else?
- How old is the patient?
- Is the patient male or female? If the patient is female, is she pregnant or breast-feeding?
- Does the patient have any other medical problems that may alter the expected effects of a nonprescription drug or be aggravated by the drug's effects? Is the complaint related to a chronic illness?
- Does the patient have any allergies?
- Is the patient on a special diet? Does the patient have special nutritional requirements?
- Is the patient using any prescription, nonprescription, or social drugs (e.g., vitamins or food supplements, caffeine, nicotine, alcohol, or marijuana)? How long has the patient been taking the drugs?
- Has the patient experienced adverse drug reactions in the past?
- Who is responsible for administering medication (the patient or a caregiver)?

Throughout the encounter, the pharmacist is formulating a clinical decision-making hypothesis based on identifying actual or potential drug therapy problems. The pharmacist should determine whether the patient has misinterpreted the condition, done any harm by waiting to seek advice, or worsened the condition by previous attempts at self-treatment.

### Observed Physical Data

Besides the historical data, physical data are helpful in determining the patient's self-care needs. Physical data include pulse rate, heart sounds, respiration rate, age, and weight. Depending on training and skills, the pharmacist can collect physical data by all or some of the following techniques: observation or inspection, palpation or manipulation, percussion, and auscultation. The importance of each technique in the process of data collection depends on the body system involved. For example, the skin is easily assessed by inspection and palpation, the lungs require percussion and auscultation, and all four skills are essential in examining the abdomen. However, most pharmacists obtain physical data primarily through observation.

Many clues to a patient's general health and the seriousness of a condition can come from simple observation. The degree of discomfort caused by pain may be judged from a patient's facial expressions or lack of use of a limb. Manifestations of an infection may include lethargy and pallor. The practitioner needs to inspect the patient's skin before offering advice about a skin rash, which may result from a simple contact phenomenon or be suggestive of systemic disease. It is recommended that nonlatex examination gloves be available for use when physical contact with the patient is required.

### Patient Assessment

Assessment of a patient's drug-related needs during a self-care consultation involves evaluating data collected from the patient to determine the etiology and severity of the medical condition. This assessment is essential for reaching appropriate conclusions about treatment or the need for referral. Methods of assessing severity will vary, depending on the problem. Pharmacists and students learning how to conduct an assessment have found it useful to view the initial patient interaction as having a flow consisting of three broad, general phases: (1) establishing a therapeutic relationship, including determining the patient's primary concerns about his or her health care in general and use of medications specifically; (2) reviewing all of the patient's active medications/remedies to assess indication, effectiveness, safety, and convenience of use; and (3) conducting a verbal review of systems to ensure that no drug-related needs have been overlooked.[22]

Assessing the severity of the patient's condition is an important component of deciding on treatment or referral. Many times, however, the etiology and severity of a condition cannot be conclusively determined because data are not accessible. Referral may be required when available information suggests that a certain etiology is responsible or a condition may be particularly severe. For example, an acutely inflamed joint that is swollen, warm to the touch, tender, and painful may be caused by trauma, bacterial infection, gout, or rheumatoid arthritis. Because a final assessment may require examination of the joint fluid, such a patient should be referred to a medical care provider. In general, the more severe the problem, the greater is the potential for referral.

Patients of advanced age, infants, children, patients with chronic diseases such as diabetes or renal or heart disease, patients with multiple medical conditions, those taking multiple medications, recently hospitalized patients, and patients who are receiving treatment from several medical care providers are at greater risk for complications and require more careful evaluation.

### *Care Plan Development*

After collecting all available information, evaluating the patient's condition, and assessing the patient's drug-related needs, the pharmacist formulates a care plan. Regardless of practice setting, a care plan is simply an understanding of the intended goals of therapy with accompanying time frame for achieving these goals. The patient and pharmacist work together to establish realistic and observable goals. In a pharmaceutical care practice, a care plan is a detailed schedule outlining the activities and responsibilities of practitioner and patient.[6]

A care plan is constructed for the following three purposes:

1. Resolve drug therapy problems identified during the assessment.
2. Meet the goals for each of the patient's medical conditions.
3. Prevent future drug therapy problems from developing.

A pharmacist may create a care plan without having all desired information. Areas of uncertainty may exist, but a well-designed plan can help the patient properly manage his or her medical conditions. For a more detailed description of documentation systems and principles pertinent to recording a patient's care plan, the reader is referred to texts that review these subjects in detail.[6,12] The importance of documenting care delivered to a patient cannot be overstated. Developing a sound care plan for a patient with self-care needs will most likely include the following five steps:

1. Collect additional information.
2. Refer the patient to a primary care provider, if warranted.
3. Select self-treatment, if appropriate.
4. Advise the patient about self-treatment.
5. Evaluate progress toward achieving treatment goals.

#### Collect Additional Information

The practitioner may need more information to assess the patient's condition, which may require specific action such as either talking to a parent/caregiver or calling a medical care provider. Communication between the pharmacist and medical care provider is often desirable to avoid conflict in managing the patient and to overcome problems of overlapping responsibilities. When such communication becomes necessary, the pharmacist should do the following:

- Obtain data on preexisting medical conditions to determine whether self-treatment is appropriate.
- Determine whether the medical care provider wants to address the patient's problem over the telephone.
- Determine whether the medical care provider wants to see the patient or whether the patient should be referred to an urgent care center or a hospital emergency department.
- Provide information on the reason for referral.

#### Refer Patient

When enough information is available to evaluate the condition, the pharmacist must decide whether to refer the patient to a medical care provider or to advise on self-treatment. If the plan involves a medical referral, the pharmacist must consider both the type of treatment center to which the patient will be referred (physician's office or emergency care facility) and the urgency for treatment. Some conditions do not require the immediate attention or extensive evaluation by emergency care personnel.

When advising a patient to see a medical care provider, the pharmacist should discuss with the patient why the referral is being made. The pharmacist must use tact and firmness so the patient is not unnecessarily frightened but is convinced of the need for concern. Medical referral is indicated in the following situations:

- The symptoms are too severe to be endured by the patient without definitive diagnosis and treatment.
- The symptoms are minor but persistent and do not appear to be the result of some easily identifiable cause.
- The symptoms have repeatedly returned with no readily recognizable cause.
- The pharmacist is in doubt about the patient's medical condition.

**PATIENT-PHARMACIST CONSULTATION**

**Collecting Additional Information and Referring Patient**

Mrs. E.J. returns to your pharmacy 1 month after accepting your decision to start a stool softener inquiring about which iron product is best to "help give her more red blood cells." During the course of the assessment, the patient reveals that she has felt a little rundown because she has been losing a little blood in her stools. As you collect additional information, the patient reports that this condition started about a week ago and she has had three instances in which she noted blood in the stool. Without alarming the patient, you recommend that she consult her physician and offer to help her set an appointment with her primary care provider.

In the case of Ms. E.J., the pharmacist collected additional information from the patient to address her concerns about fecal blood loss. However, her condition is persistent (lasting 1 week), there is no readily recognizable cause, and the pharmacist is in doubt about the patient's condition without a definitive medical diagnosis. Therefore, a referral for medical evaluation is warranted.

#### Select Self-Treatment

Selecting self-treatment in collaboration with a patient requires the pharmacist to consider several factors. First, the pharmacist must identify a measurable and achievable therapeutic objective, based on the patient's condition and clinical status. A therapeutic modality—either drug or nondrug—may then be recommended. For example, a patient who has a productive cough, but is having difficulty expectorating his/her sputum may need to use an expectorant, such as guaifenesin, as a complement to drinking plenty of water. However, for a patient with a dry, nonproductive, and bothersome nighttime cough (that is not an adverse reaction to a drug such as an angiotensin converting enzyme inhibitor), the therapeutic objective may be to quiet the cough for a few nights, in which case a cough suppressant may be selected. Choosing a specific treatment requires reviewing drug variables (e.g., dosage forms, ingredients, adverse reactions, relative effectiveness, and price) and matching them with patient variables (e.g., age, gender, drug history, other physiologic problems, and ability to pay).

If self-treatment without the use of a medication is indicated, selection of the nondrug modality would similarly be modified using patient variables. For example, the pharmacist may suggest that a patient with vomiting and diarrhea consider only drinking fluids for a brief period of time to provide bowel rest. However, if the patient has insulin-dependent diabetes, the pharmacist must modify this possible course of action because patients with diabetes have specific caloric requirements. Communicating with the patient, and possibly another medical care provider, about modifying the dose of insulin to compensate for changes in caloric intake would be prudent in this situation.

To measure the success of treatment, the pharmacist should set goals and measurement parameters based on the therapeutic objective, the toxic or adverse effects of treatment, the nature and severity of the condition, the patient's ability to understand the condition and its treatment, and the anticipated time to symptom resolution. The objective in treating sinusitis with decongestants, for example, is to facilitate drainage and relieve symptoms such as headache. Ways to facilitate drainage can be determined by observing or asking about the nature of nasal discharge (e.g., quantity, color, and viscosity), whereas relief of symptoms such as headache can be achieved by simply asking about the headache. Toxicity includes those symptoms associated with an excessive dose or an untoward reaction. The pharmacist should identify toxicities that suggest the problem may be worsening and require special attention. Finally, queries relating to the patient's understanding of the condition and its treatment can include determining the appropriateness of the patient's questions to the pharmacist as well as the patient's response to those questions.

### Advise Patient on Self-Treatment

The fourth step in the care plan is to advise the patient about self-treatment. The primary purposes are to develop a plan of action with the patient and obtain the consent necessary to enact the plan. Specifically, the pharmacist should provide advice in the following areas:

- Reasons for self-treatment
- Description of the drug and/or treatment
- Administration of the drug and/or treatment
- Adverse reactions and precautions
- General treatment guidelines

In advising the patient about a suggested treatment plan, the pharmacist should summarize the patient's condition, explain the significance of the symptoms, and outline the reasons for treatment. The pharmacist should clearly explain the therapeutic objectives and provide a realistic time frame for achieving the objectives. If the patient desires information on alternative treatments, the pharmacist should be prepared to present such information about their relative merits and drawbacks without biasing the information and jeopardizing the patient-medical care provider relationship. The pharmacist should then discuss the nonprescription drugs selected, describing in lay terms both the therapeutic action of the ingredients (e.g., decongestants, antihistamines, laxatives) and the effect the products will have on the patient's symptoms and condition. The pharmacist should inform the patient about various dosage forms and the availability of any generic product.

The pharmacist should explain administration guidelines clearly and concisely. Because many patients may remember only part of the information, some thought should be given to deciding what is most important for the patient to remember. Covering a few of the most important points is better than overwhelming a patient with a lot of information. In addition, patients will remember dosage instructions better if administration is linked to specific times of the day, rather than just "three times daily." Having a patient review normal daily activities will help establish the best times to take the medication. It is also important to include information about the duration of treatment.

The patient should be told the most common adverse reactions associated with a drug and be instructed on how to manage them. The pharmacist should describe activities, other drugs, foods, or beverages that should be avoided, as well as discuss which of the patient's medical conditions may be complicated by use of the drug. Information should be written down if it is extensive or complex.

The pharmacist should offer the patient some general treatment guidelines that may be helpful in managing the condition. These guidelines might include lifestyle changes, additional products or services, informational sources, and a list of signs and symptoms that indicate whether the drug is working, whether it is causing adverse effects, and when a medical care provider's advice is needed. The patient should be informed about the expected response time to the treatment, the time required for the condition to resolve, and what to do if response is delayed.

**PATIENT-PHARMACIST CONSULTATION**

**Advising Patient on Treatment and Care Plan Development**

Mrs. E.J. visits her primary care provider for assessment of blood loss and returns to your pharmacy 1 week later with a copy of her laboratory results. She presents a note from the physician asking you to help the patient select an iron product for the patient to take twice a day that is easy on the stomach. On questioning, the patient indicates that her physician did a full medical workup related to blood in her stools and she is happy to report that she does not have any type of serious anemia and her doctor gave her "a clean bill of health." In collaboration with the patient, you determine that the patient will begin taking ferrous gluconate 325 mg twice daily. Mrs. E.J. then reports that she is scheduled for follow-up blood work in the clinic in 3 weeks.

### Evaluate Progress Toward Achieving Treatment Goals

The final area in the patient care process is follow-up evaluation. Evaluation is defined as the practitioner's determination—at planned intervals of follow-up—of the patient's outcome and current status.[6] The purpose of the evaluation is to determine whether previous drug therapy problems have been resolved, to evaluate the patient's progress toward achieving therapeutic goals, and to assess whether new problems have developed from the drug therapy.

> **PATIENT-PHARMACIST CONSULTATION**
>
> **Evaluation of Patient Outcomes**
>
> You determined that the use of ferrous gluconate, rather than ferrous sulfate, may cause Mrs. E.J. less gastric irritation. In a busy dispensing pharmacy, the pharmacist would advise the patient on the proper use of ferrous gluconate and possibly look at the patient's laboratory results and encourage the patient to return to the clinic in 3 weeks to see how the medication is working. In a pharmaceutical care practice, the pharmacist would review the patient's copy of her laboratory results to set goals of therapy and the anticipated time frame for achieving those goals. A follow-up appointment would then be made with Mrs. E.J. after her clinic appointment to account for progress toward achieving goals of therapy and reassess her for additional drug-related needs.

Documentation systems used by pharmacists in a pharmaceutical care practice typically have a way of tracking the safety and effectiveness of drug therapies that may include an evaluation of outcomes for each of the patient's medical conditions and a resolution status of drug therapy problems. Pharmacists may also include a brief progress note in a patient's pharmaceutical care chart after each patient encounter. Evaluation notes help pharmacists convey important aspects of the patient's care in a clear and concise manner to fellow practitioners.

Aspects of patient care that pharmaceutical care practitioners convey, in written format, may include the patient's expression of drug-related needs, goals of therapy, monitoring parameters, assessment of drug therapy problems, and a plan for resolving and preventing drug therapy problems and achieving treatment goals. An evaluation note can take on an appearance similar to the SOAP (subjective, objective, assessment, plan) format used in medicine for the problem-oriented medical record system. Within a pharmaceutical care practice, the pharmacist assumes responsibility for all the patient's drug-related needs within each of the patient's medical conditions, and the evaluation note may reflect this holistic approach to care.

Follow-up allows the pharmacist to determine whether self-treatment has resulted in an appropriate therapeutic response and whether the patient has used medications appropriately or experienced any drug therapy problems, including drug-related toxicity. On follow-up, the pharmacist may determine the need to reassess the patient's drug therapy and either modify or develop a new patient care plan. The patient may decide to take responsibility for initiating the follow-up encounter after an appropriate time interval, or the patient and the pharmacist may decide to schedule a follow-up appointment, either in person or over the telephone.

Follow-up provides feedback that allows pharmacists to determine whether their communication skills require modification and whether useful information has been provided. At the same time, the patient will sense that the pharmacist cares. The pharmacist's concern for the correct use of nonprescription drugs will also reinforce the notion that these products are drugs and must be used carefully.

## Pharmaceutical Care for High-risk and Special Groups

Pharmaceutical care should be an important part of health care for all of our patients, but it is especially important for vulnerable populations. Certain groups of patients—infants and children, persons of advanced age, pregnant and breast-feeding women—may experience a higher incidence of drug therapy problems than other patients. Because such problems can have dire consequences, these high-risk patients require special attention. Awareness of the physiologic state, possible pathologic conditions, and social context of these patients is necessary to properly assess their medical conditions and recommend appropriate treatment.

In many respects, persons of advanced age, infants, and children require surprisingly similar considerations. They all have a need for drug dosages that are different from those for other age groups because of the following:

- They have altered pharmacokinetic parameters.
- Their ability to cope with illness or adverse drug events is decreased because of physiologic changes associated with either normal aging or child development.
- Their patterns of judgment are impaired because of either altered sensory function or immaturity.
- They have drug effects and potential adverse reactions that are unique to their age groups.
- They have a need for special consideration in administering medications.

Yet, because each of these groups of patients is heterogeneous, it is important to consider these features for each individual patient.

### *Special Considerations in Infants and Children*

A study of the prevalence of nonprescription drug use in 3-year-old children found that 53.7% had been given a nonprescription drug within the past 3 months. The most commonly used medications were acetaminophen and cough or cold products.[23] An analysis of vitamin supplement use found that 54.4% of 3-year-olds in the United States were given vitamin and mineral supplements within the past 3 months. Providing pharmaceutical care to pediatric patients is challenging because of differences in physiology and pharmacokinetics, lack of clinical data, insufficient drug labeling, and problems associated with drug dosing and administration.[24] In considering nonprescription drugs for infants and children, the pharmacist should note that the pediatric population may vary substantially among age groups. It is appropriate to differentiate among relatively distinctive pediatric ages as follows:[25,26]

- *Premature*: gestational age of less than 36 weeks
- *Neonate*: first postnatal month of life
- *Infant* (*baby*): ages 1 to 12 months
- *Toddler*: ages 1 to 3 years
- *Preschool or early childhood*: ages 3 to 6 years
- *Middle childhood*: ages 6 to 12 years
- *Adolescence*: ages 13 to 18 years

For most products, the Food and Drug Administration (FDA) recommends against self-medication in children younger than 2 years of age. Pharmacists can provide recommendations regarding drugs with which they are familiar and for which dosage guidelines are readily available (e.g., pediatric acetaminophen products), but should recommend primary care provider evaluation for medical conditions or drugs for which they do not have pediatric experience. Case 2-1 illustrates the assessment of a patient in this age group. Some package labeling provides dosage guidelines by age group rather than by weight.

## CASE 2-1

| Relevant Evaluation Criteria | Scenario/Model Outcome |
|---|---|
| **Information Gathering** | |
| 1. Gather essential information about the patient's symptoms, including: | |
| a. description of symptom(s) (i.e., nature, onset, duration, severity, associated symptoms) | Patient has suffered from a fever for the past 12 hours. The patient's mother says that the child was hot to the touch during the night, and that he does not seem to be as active as he normally is. The mother wants to know how much of the acetaminophen drops she should give him. |
| b. description of any factors that seem to precipitate, exacerbate, and/or relieve the patient's symptom(s) | None |
| c. description of the patient's efforts to relieve the symptoms | The mother says that rubbing his body with a cool wet cloth helped. She has also been giving him lots of water. |
| 2. Gather essential patient history information: | |
| a. patient's identity | Chauncey Jordan |
| b. age, sex, height, and weight | 10 months old, M, 29", 26 lb |
| c. patient's occupation | N/A |
| d. patient's dietary habits | Baby food, rice, and formula |
| e. patient's sleep habits | Averages 8-9 hours per night |
| f. concurrent medical conditions, prescription and nonprescription medications, and dietary supplements | None |
| g. allergies | NKA |
| h. history of other adverse reactions to medications | None |
| i. other (describe)_______ | This is the first time Chauncey has had a fever, and this is the mother's first child. |
| **Assessment and Triage** | |
| 3. Differentiate the patient's signs/symptoms and correctly identify the patient's primary problem(s). | Fever of unknown etiology. Patient's forehead, neck, arms, and legs still very hot to the touch. |
| 4. Identify exclusions for self-treatment. | Fever of unknown etiology in child less than 2 years of age |
| 5. Formulate a comprehensive list of therapeutic alternatives for the primary problem to determine if triage to a medical practitioner is required, and share this information with the patient. | Options include:<br>(1) Refer Chauncey to pediatrician for care.<br>(2) Recommend an OTC antipyretic product.<br>(3) Take no action. |

## CASE 2-1 (continued)

| Relevant Evaluation Criteria | Scenario/Model Outcome |
|---|---|
| **Plan** | |
| 6. Select an optimal therapeutic alternative to address the patient's problem, taking into account patient preferences. | Refer patient to pediatrician for care. |
| 7. Describe the recommended therapeutic approach to the patient. | N/A |
| 8. Explain to the patient the rationale for selecting the recommended therapeutic approach from the considered therapeutic alternatives. | Seeing his pediatrician is necessary because of the unknown cause of his fever and because there are no OTC antipyretic products that are FDA approved for use in children less than 2 years of age without consulting a physician. |
| **Patient Education** | |
| 9. When recommending self-care with nonprescription medications and/or nondrug therapy, convey accurate information to the patient, including: | Criterion does not apply in this case. |
| 10. Solicit follow-up questions from patient. | Can I give him ibuprofen drops instead? |
| 11. Answer patient's questions. | No. Not without first going to see his pediatrician. However, it is recommended that you keep a thermometer at home, because that is a more accurate way to tell whether a fever is present or not. |

Key: N/A, not applicable; NKA, no known allergies; OTC, over-the-counter.

### Physiologic and Pharmacokinetic Differences

Pediatric patients are at risk for drug therapy problems because their body and organ functions are in a continuous state of development. Not only are the pharmacokinetic properties of drugs different in children compared with adults, but these properties can undergo rapid change as children grow and mature.[26] Furthermore, illness in children is potentially more serious than in adults because their physiologic state is less tolerant of changes. Fever, vomiting, and diarrhea represent greater potential risks to children because they are more susceptible to the effects of fluid loss. Therefore, the pharmacist should consider primary care provider referral for a condition in a child sooner than for an adult with the same condition.

### Other Potential Drug Therapy Problems

The pharmacist should be sensitive to the potential for drug therapy problems among children. In some illnesses such as diarrhea, nondrug therapy is often more appropriate than therapy with nonprescription antidiarrheal drugs. In some situations, specific drugs are contraindicated; for example, aspirin should not be administered to young children with certain viral illnesses (especially influenza and varicella) because of its association with Reye's syndrome (see Chapter 6). After warnings against using aspirin in children with viral illnesses were issued, the number of cases of Reye's syndrome dropped dramatically.[27] Pharmacists should counsel parents of children and adolescents with febrile viral illnesses against using aspirin. For younger children, solid dosage forms are inappropriate, and the pharmacist will need to guide parents to liquid medications or chewable tablets.

*Inaccurate Dosing* Labeling on nonprescription drugs generally uses age-based guidelines for determining dosages; however, many products do not provide dosage information for children younger than 6 years. Following the nonprescription drug's label, instructions for dosing a child older than 6 years can result in too high a dose and potential toxicity for the younger child. Inaccurate dosing by parents can result from determining an incorrect dose from the label instructions, by measuring out an incorrect amount, or both. A study of 200 children, 10 years of age and younger, who had been given a dose of acetaminophen or ibuprofen in the past 24 hours, found that 51% of them had been given an incorrect dose by their caregiver.[28] Pharmacists must better educate parents about dosing and administering nonprescription drugs by helping parents interpret labels and demonstrating the appropriate use of measuring devices.

*Improper Administration/Dosage Forms* Selecting the proper drug and dosage is not beneficial unless a medication is actually administered. Proper administration of medications to pediatric patients requires an appreciation of dosage forms, delivery methodology, routes of administration, palatability, and other factors. The discussion that follows focuses on oral medications.

Liquids are relatively easy to administer, and the dose can be titrated to the patient's weight; therefore, liquid medications are often used in pediatric populations. Because elixirs and syrups can have high alcohol and sugar content, respectively, these liquid forms may be less desirable than suspensions and solutions. A suspension may also mask the disagreeable taste of a drug.

Problems with drug administration can result in the child receiving the wrong dose. In a mock dosing scenario in which caregivers had the choice of using teaspoons, tablespoons, syringes, droppers, measuring cups, and measuring tubes, only 67% of the caregivers accurately measured the dose they intended to administer.[28] The volume delivered by household teaspoons ranges from 2.5 to 7.8 mL and may also vary greatly when the same spoon is used by different individuals. The American Academy of Pediatrics Committee on Drugs highly recommends the use of appropriate devices for liquid administration, such as a medication cup, cylindrical dosing spoon, oral dropper, or oral syringe. Ease of administration and accuracy should be considered when choosing a dosing device. Plastic medication cups are fairly accurate for volumes of exact multiples of 5 mL (i.e., 5 mL, 10 mL, 15 mL). An oral syringe is preferable to the other oral dosing devices for higher viscosity liquids because the syringe completely expels the total measured dose. Potent liquid medications should be administered with an oral syringe to ensure that the correct dose is given; the pharmacist should briefly explain to caregivers how to use and read an oral syringe. However, drawing up the dose in the syringe requires dexterity.

The use of precision devices for oral dosing helps ensure adequate therapeutic response by reducing the incidence of underdoses and eliminating adverse drug effects from potential overdoses. These devices may also enhance acceptance of medication by infants and children. Parents or caregivers may need instructions on using these devices to measure doses accurately, as well as advice on giving medications to reluctant or struggling children. The pharmacist may need to demonstrate to parents and older children how to take the medication.

A child older than 4 years of age can usually swallow tablets or capsules. Tablets that are not sustained-release or enteric-coated formulations may be crushed. Most capsules may be opened and the contents sprinkled on small amounts of food (applesauce, jelly, or pudding) to ensure that all the drug is taken. If the child does not eat the full portion, underdosing can occur. If multiple drugs are prescribed, the child may be more cooperative if allowed to choose what flavored drink to use and which medication to take first. Table 2-1 presents selected guidelines for administering oral medications to pediatric patients.

**TABLE 2-1 Selected Medication Administration Guidelines for Oral Medications**

**Infants**

- Use a calibrated dropper or oral syringe.
- Support the infant's head while holding the infant in the lap.
- Give small amounts of medication to prevent choking.
- If desired, crush nonenteric-coated or nonsustained-release tablets into a powder and sprinkle them on small amounts of food.
- Provide physical comforting while administering medications to help calm the infant.

**Toddlers**

- Allow the toddler to choose a position in which to take the medication.
- If necessary, disguise the taste of the medication with a small volume of flavored drink or small amounts of food. A rinse with a flavored drink or water will help remove an unpleasant aftertaste.
- Use simple commands in the toddler's jargon to obtain cooperation.
- Allow the toddler to choose which of the medications (if multiple) to take first.
- Provide verbal and tactile responses to promote cooperative taking of medication.
- Allow the toddler to become familiar with the oral dosing device.

**Preschool Children**

- If possible, place a tablet or capsule near the back of the tongue; then provide water or a flavored liquid to aid the swallowing of the medication.
- If the child's teeth are loose, do not use chewable tablets.
- Use a straw to administer medications that could stain teeth.
- Use a follow-up rinse with a flavored drink to help minimize any unpleasant medication aftertaste.
- Allow the child to help make decisions about dosage formulation, place of administration, medication to take first, and type of flavored drink to use.

*Adverse Drug Effects* Adverse reactions are another potential drug therapy problem in children. Adverse drug events in children may be different from those in adults. For example, as in the older population, antihistamines and central nervous system (CNS) depressants may cause excitation in children. Except for Claritin (loratadine) syrup, FDA recommends not administering antihistamines to children younger than 6 years of age.[29] In contrast, sympathomimetics such as pseudoephedrine may cause drowsiness in children. In the United States, drug-induced acute liver failure is most commonly caused by acetaminophen, and about 18 percent of those cases were a result of accidental overdose. Additionally, administration of acetaminophen at doses above the recommended daily dose over a period of 2 to 4 days can result in hepatotoxicity in children.[30]

*Noncompliance* Noncompliance may occur when children refuse to take medication or when caregivers give up before the child receives the entire dose. Adherence may be improved by recommending a sweetly flavored product because children may be more willing to take a medication

**TABLE 2-2 Six Steps for Improving Medication Use in Children[33]**

Pharmacists should use a patient-centered style that focuses on the following steps:

1. Educating both the child and parents about the medication.
2. Investigating any concerns or fears that the child or parents may have about the medication.
3. Asking the child and parents about priorities for improved quality of life.
4. Following up with the child and parents to learn if they consider the child's treatment effective.
5. Offering to follow up with the pediatrician to improve the child's therapy (if needed).
6. Encouraging the child or parents to ask questions about the medication.

if they like the flavor, consistency, or texture.[31] Noncompliance can also occur when caregivers do not understand instructions or do not pass them on to day care providers, teachers, or school nurses. A 2003 survey study of 82 child day care centers found that 52% of centers reported missing a dose during the past year, and 49% reported that the child's medication was not available.[32]

*Assessment and Consultation* Assessment and consultation for pediatric patients usually involve the parents or caregivers. A 2003 article by Sleath and coworker, lists six overall steps for communicating with children and improving their medication use process[33] (Table 2-2). One should remember that it is important to include the child and parent during the patient counseling process and that the child's and parents' concerns or fears about the medication should be taken into consideration.

### *Special Considerations in Persons of Advanced Age*

Social, economic, physiologic, and age-related health factors place persons of advanced age at high risk for medical problems and prompt them to be large consumers of nonprescription drugs. Indeed, this population as a group consumes more drugs than any other age segment of our society. While individuals 65 years of age and older take on average 1.8 nonprescription drugs daily, geographic area, race/ethnicity, and gender affect this number.[34] Nonprescription drug use in this population is highest in the midwestern United States, in Caucasians, and in women. Analgesics, laxatives, and nutritional supplements are the most common nonprescription drugs used by persons of advanced age. A study in 86 women who were 65 and older reported an average use of 3.8 nonprescription drugs per person.[35] In the 45% of women who used herbal products, the average number of herbal products was 2.5. The response to drug therapy by older patients is more scattered and unpredictable than that of other populations. Pharmacokinetic, pharmacodynamic, and various nonpharmacologic factors predispose these patients to potential problems with nonprescription drugs. Preexisting medical conditions in older persons may affect the use of some non-prescription drugs. For example, antihistamines should be avoided in patients with emphysema, bronchitis, glaucoma, and urinary retention from prostatic hypertrophy. Although nasal and oral decongestants can be used without adverse effect in many older persons, caution may be necessary in some patients with heart disease, hypertension, thyroid disease, and diabetes because of potential adverse effects of sympathomimetics on blood pressure, heart rate, and blood glucose.

#### Physiologic and Pharmacokinetic Differences

Persons of advanced age often suffer from impaired vision (e.g., difficulty reading and differentiating colors) and hearing loss. The pharmacist should be aware of patient behaviors that indicate visual or hearing loss and should take these impairments into consideration when communicating with older patients. Additional instructions for nonprescription drugs may need to be provided in larger, high-contrast, dark print. Asking the patient to repeat counseling instructions can ensure that the directions were heard correctly and understood.

Subtle changes in mental status, such as confusion, may be anticipated in older patients who are anxious about their state of health. Older patients with cognitive impairments may have difficulty comprehending directions. Patients may not remember the names of all their medications or may not be able to remember instructions. Because of memory lapses, some older patients may require special drug delivery systems (e.g., transdermal patches or sustained-release preparations) to help them adhere to their dosage regimen. Older patients with cognitive impairments are less likely to read and interpret labels correctly,[36] which further emphasizes their need for special dosage-form considerations.

Older patients are believed to confuse at least one third of their problems with age-associated problems and, therefore, misreport their symptoms. Accurate perception and reporting of symptoms is vital to the successful use of any drug. In addition, older patients are often reluctant to share health information with others.

The aging process, as well as many chronic diseases, can alter a patient's nutritional status. Older patients who are most at risk for undernourishment or malnutrition are homebound patients and nursing home residents. Poverty, multiple chronic diseases, multiple drug therapy, or a combination of these factors may cause malnutrition in these patients. The patient's nutritional status and weight are important because they can alter the pharmacokinetics and pharmacodynamics of drugs.

Aging alters the absorption, distribution, metabolism, and elimination of certain drugs, increasing the susceptibility of older patients to drug therapy problems. Pharmacokinetic changes, which have been well described in literature, are caused not only by advancing age but also by the effects of disease states and often by multiple drug use.

Older persons appear to have more sensitivity to some drugs, particularly to anticholinergic drugs, which may relate in part to alterations in cholinergic transmission.[37] Nonprescription drugs with anticholinergic effects, such as antihistamines, may worsen preexisting medical conditions such as angina, congestive heart failure, constipation, diabetes mellitus, glaucoma, urinary dysfunction, sleep disturbance, and dementia.[37] The risk of accidents such as falls may also increase as a result of pupillary dilatation induced by anticholinergic drugs and the inability to accommodate the effect.

Both subjective and objective evidence indicates that older patients have an enhanced CNS sensitivity to drugs, especially CNS depressants such as sedatives and antidepressants. Increased brain sensitivity and other changes (e.g., decreased coordination, prolongation of reaction time, impairment of short-term memory) manifest as increased frequency of confusion, urinary incontinence, and number of falls, especially among older women. Drug therapy may exaggerate all these changes, particularly if drugs are used in the "usual" dose or if multiple drugs are used.

Control of bowel and bladder function lessens with advancing age. A further decrease in efficiency is likely with laxative use. Anticholinergic drugs and CNS drugs may reduce neurologic control. Antihistamines have sedative properties that may reduce bladder control in older persons.[37] Adverse effects of nonprescription drugs often increase when such drugs are added to an existing medication regimen.

Nonsteroidal anti-inflammatory drugs (NSAIDs) are widely used, especially by patients with osteoarthritis and rheumatoid arthritis. The absolute number of events of NSAID-related toxicity is greater for older patients because of their frequent use of NSAIDs and the increased prevalence of comorbid conditions coupled with concomitant drug therapies.[38] These patients may be especially susceptible to NSAID-associated peptic ulcer disease as well as congestive heart failure in susceptible individuals.[39] There is also some evidence that the chronic use of NSAIDs may elevate blood pressure in women ages 31 to 50.[40] Many patients were switched from NSAIDs to a cyclooxygenase-2 (COX-2) inhibitor, which were thought to be safer because they caused fewer GI-related adverse events. However, recent evidence suggests that the risk of cardiac events from taking Rofecoxib, such as thrombotic stroke and myocardial infarction, far outweigh the beneficial GI profile. Rofecoxib has already been withdrawn from the market because of the increased risk of cardiac events.[41]

### Other Potential Drug Therapy Problems

*Duplicate Therapy* Patients of advanced age can receive unnecessary drug therapy when drugs are added to their therapeutic regimen without a reevaluation of the entire regimen to determine whether certain drugs should be deleted. Duplicate therapy may occur if these patients are seeing multiple health care providers for their various medical problems, or using multiple pharmacies. Use of a single pharmacy can significantly lower the risk of inappropriate drug combinations. Nonprescription drugs commonly involved in drug interactions in older persons include aspirin, other NSAIDs, antacids, cimetidine, and antihistamines.[42] Many older patients have serious and multiple diseases such as coronary artery disease, chronic renal failure, or congestive heart failure, which can be aggravated by concurrent therapy for other acute problems. Concomitant illnesses or certain drugs may contraindicate the use of other drugs. It is important to consider whether an older patient is requesting a nonprescription drug to treat an adverse reaction from another medication.

*Inaccurate Dosing/Dosage Forms* Normal drug doses of analgesics and sedating antihistamines may be too high for patients of advanced age because of their impaired hepatic and renal function. These situations would necessitate either lowering the dose or increasing the dosing interval. Furthermore, older patients may experience difficulty with some dosage forms (e.g., swallowing large calcium or vitamin tablets, using inhalers) because of physical impairments. Older patients may have difficulty opening and closing containers because of arthritis or tremors. Child-resistant containers may be especially difficult for older patients to open if they have deficits in physical dexterity. A pharmacist should direct older patients to products without child-resistant containers, but should warn them of the potential poisoning hazard for visiting grandchildren or other young visitors.

*Noncompliance* The prevalence of noncompliance with medications is high in the advanced-age population and is often the result of inadequate understanding of their medication regimen. Poor adherence may result from difficulty swallowing or administering the drug. It may also result from an inability to afford the drug because of a limited or fixed income. Older patients may lack a social support network to supply the aid required by an illness. Pharmacists may need to involve caregivers in medication administration.

## Special Considerations in Pregnant Patients

Drug therapy during pregnancy may be necessary to treat medical conditions or to manage common complaints of pregnancy such as vomiting or constipation. However, because most drugs cross the placenta to some extent, a mother who takes a drug might expose her fetus to it. Thus, the desire to ease the mother's discomfort must be balanced with concern for the developing fetus.

A 2001 study found that 13% of pregnant women, from an academic setting birthing center, used dietary supplements.[43] Of these women, 25% reported using supplements to relieve nausea and vomiting, and 25% reported stopping the use of these products because of concern for their fetus. The authors concluded that although the use of dietary supplements was low among these women, the lack of safety data for these products is of concern. In another study, women attending an antenatal clinic reported using an average of 2.3 to 2.6 nonprescription drugs in the three pregnancy trimesters, which was slightly higher than nonprescription drug use in the 3 months prior to pregnancy.[45] The most frequently taken medications were analgesics, vitamin and mineral supplements, and GI medications. Approximately 10% of pregnant women used herbal products.

### Potential Drug Therapy Problems

Pregnant women should never presume that a nonprescription medication is safe to use during pregnancy. They should first consult with a pharmacist or primary care provider to determine whether a medication is teratogenic (i.e., causes abnormal embryo development). Nausea and vomiting can cause another medication-related problem: difficulty in taking oral dosage forms of medications.

*Teratogenic Effects* Several factors are important in determining whether a drug taken by a pregnant woman will adversely affect the fetus. Two such factors are the stage of pregnancy and the ability of the drug to pass from maternal to fetal circulation through the placenta. The first trimester, when organogenesis occurs, is the period of greatest risk for inducing major anatomic malformations. However, exposure at other periods of gestation may be no less important because the exact critical period depends on the specific drug in question.

Drug therapy problems are also important considerations for the pregnant patient. Although dosage guidelines for some prescription drugs (e.g., phenytoin) differ for the pregnant patient, no information on dosage adjustments exists for nonprescription drugs. Unnecessary drug therapy should be avoided. Nondrug therapy is often more appropriate than drug therapy for pregnant women. Use of cigarettes and ingestion of alcohol should be avoided or limited because they have been associated with increased risk to the fetus.[45] Consumption of moderate doses of caffeine appears to be safe.[46]

In the pregnant patient, the primary concern is related to drug safety. All pharmacists should be familiar with the A-B-C-D-X system for evaluating the safety of drugs in pregnancy.[46] Often the issue is not whether a more effective drug is available but whether a safer drug is available. For example, evidence exists that aspirin is associated with congenital defects, incidence of stillbirths, neonatal deaths, and reduced birth weight.[43,46] Use of aspirin late in pregnancy has been associated with increases in length of gestation and duration of labor. These effects are related to aspirin's inhibition of prostaglandin synthesis. In addition, because aspirin affects platelet function, perinatal aspirin ingestion has been found to increase the incidence of hemorrhage in both the pregnant woman and the newborn during and following delivery. Therefore, a woman should avoid using aspirin during pregnancy, especially during the last trimester. Instead, because acetaminophen is generally considered safe for use during pregnancy, it is the nonprescription drug of choice for antipyresis and analgesia when taken in standard therapeutic doses.[43] NSAIDs such as ibuprofen and naproxen can be taken early in pregnancy.[46] However, they should not be used late in pregnancy because they are potent prostaglandin synthetase inhibitors. Not only can they cause problems in the newborn, but they can also affect the duration of gestation and labor. Chronic use of large doses of antitussive products that contain codeine may cause withdrawal in the newborn after delivery.[46] Severe CNS depression and hypoventilation at birth have been reported following maternal use of diphenhydramine, which was taken for several weeks prior to delivery for severe itching.[47]

*Noncompliance* Nausea and vomiting associated with pregnancy may make it difficult for the pregnant woman to adhere to instructions for taking oral medications. Pharmacists can recommend eating small meals, frequent snacks, and crackers to alleviate or minimize nausea and vomiting. The patient should avoid foods, smells, or situations that cause vomiting. If necessary, an effervescent glucose or buffered carbohydrate solution, or the use of ginger may be effective. Only if those measures are ineffective should an antihistamine or antiemetic be considered. Consultation with a primary care provider may be indicated at this point.

*Management of the Pregnant Patient* The pharmacist can aid the self-treating pregnant woman in deciding which drug or nondrug treatments she should consider and when self-treatment may be harmful to her or her unborn child. The decision to suggest a drug must be based on both an up-to-date knowledge of the literature and a critical risk-benefit evaluation of the mother and the fetus. Pharmacists should consult a reference such as the Drugs in Pregnancy and Lactation by Briggs and others to check for the safety of medications in this population.[46]

When the pharmacist has a choice between two drugs, the preferred drug will be the one that has been in use for a longer time. Ascertaining the trimester of pregnancy is important because it is a factor in determining whether some nonprescription drugs can be used safely. The pharmacist should discourage pregnant women from self-medicating with nonprescription drugs without receiving counseling from a primary care provider or pharmacist. The assessment and management of the pregnant patient require observation of the following principles.

First, the pharmacist must be alert to the possibility of pregnancy in any woman of childbearing age who has certain key symptoms of early pregnancy, such as nausea, vomiting, and frequent urination. Any woman who fits this description should be warned not to take a drug that might be of questionable safety if she is pregnant.

Second, the pharmacist should advise the pregnant patient to avoid using drugs, in general, at any stage of pregnancy unless the patient's primary care provider deems such use essential. Also, because the safety and effectiveness of homeopathic and herbal remedies in pregnancy have not been established, their use should be discouraged.

Third, the pharmacist should advise the pregnant patient to increase her reliance on nondrug modalities as treatment alternatives (see Noncompliance).

Fourth, the pharmacist should refer the patient to a primary care provider for certain problems that carry increased risk of poor outcomes in pregnancy (e.g., high blood pressure, vaginal bleeding, urinary tract infections, rapid weight gain, and edema).

### Special Considerations in the Nursing Mother

A mother's drug use while breast-feeding can have an adverse effect on the infant. The concentration of a drug in the mother's milk depends on a number of factors, including the drug's concentration in the mother's blood, the drug's molecular weight, lipid solubility, degree of ionization, degree of binding to plasma and milk protein, and the drug's active secretion into the milk. Other important considerations include the relationship between the time of taking a drug and the time of breast-feeding, as well as the drug's potential for causing toxicity in infants. Also, some drugs (e.g., decongestants) may decrease milk supply.

When advising a nursing mother on self-care, the pharmacist should decide whether a drug is really necessary, recommend the safest drug (e.g., acetaminophen instead of aspirin) if one is necessary, and advise the mother to take the medication just after breast-feeding or just before the infant's lengthy sleep periods.[48,49] It is preferable to select a drug that has been in use for a long time that has shown no apparent harm to nursing infants. If appropriate, topical or local therapy may be preferred to oral systemic therapy. In general, advise against medications that are extra strength, maximum strength, or long acting, or products that contain a variety of active ingredients.[49]

When taken in therapeutic dosages, most drugs are not present in breast milk in sufficient amounts to cause significant harm to the infant. However, several drugs are contraindicated for use while breast-feeding, and others should be used with caution by nursing mothers. The amount of caffeine in caffeine-containing beverages is not harmful, but higher doses (i.e., more than 1 g daily) have been reported to cause irritability and poor sleep patterns in infants.[49] Many nonprescription drugs exist for which there are no data on their transfer into breast milk and their possible clinical effects.

Nonprescription drugs that are usually considered compatible with breast-feeding include the following:[46,50]

- *Analgesics:* acetaminophen, ibuprofen, naproxen, and ketoprofen
- *Antacids*
- *Antidiarrheals:* kaolin-pectin, attapulgite, and loperamide
- *Antihistamines:* brompheniramine, chlorpheniramine, diphenhydramine, and triprolidine
- *Antisecretory agents*: cimetidine, famotidine, ranitidine, and nizatidine
- *Cough preparations*: dextromethorphan
- *Cromolyn sodium*
- *Decongestants*: phenylephrine and pseudoephedrine
- *Fluoride*
- *Laxatives*: bran type, bulk-forming type, docusate, glycerin suppositories, magnesium hydroxide, and senna
- *Vitamins*

## Key Points for Patient Assessment and Consultation

The use of nonprescription drugs represents an important component of the health care system. Under ideal conditions, consumers can diagnose their own symptoms, select a nonprescription drug product, and monitor their own therapeutic response. If properly used, nonprescription drugs can relieve patients' minor physical complaints and permit primary care providers to concentrate on more serious illnesses. If used improperly, however, nonprescription products can create a multitude of drug therapy problems. The key points discussed in this chapter include the following:

- Twenty-three percent of all drug therapy problems experienced by patients have a cause or resolution associated with the use of nonprescription drugs.
- Interacting with patients to address self-care needs requires attention to the principles of communication discussed in this chapter.
- A systematic patient care process has been established to effectively address a patient's self-care needs.
- The consistent and systematic patient care process helps practitioners be complete and concise when assuming responsibility for a patient's self-care needs.
- A pharmacist working in a busy dispensing pharmacy can establish a relationship with the patient, determine the patient's self-care needs, and ascertain a list of the patient's current medications and medical conditions before recommending an appropriate course of action.
- The extent to which pharmaceutical care is implemented and documented, regarding patients with self-care needs, ultimately depends on compensation for services.
- Compensation for the provision of medication therapy management services provided within pharmaceutical care practices is a reality.
- In a pharmaceutical care practice, the pharmacist devotes attention to assessing patients' drug-related needs in which the identification of drug therapy problems and establishment of treatment goals take place.
- Addressing the special drug-related needs of selected high-risk groups such as infants and children, people of advanced age, and pregnant and breast-feeding women have been highlighted in this chapter.

To be of greatest service to patients, pharmacists must continually expand their therapeutic knowledge and must improve their interpersonal communication skills. As pharmacists strive to fulfill their responsibilities as health care practitioners and continue to expand their patient care services, people will learn of those services and seek their pharmacist's assistance whenever they are in doubt about self-treatment. The result will be better informed patients who will not only use the professional services of pharmacists but also recognize pharmacists' contributions to health care.

## References

1. Roper Starch Worldwide Inc. Self-care in the new millennium: American attitudes toward maintaining personal health and treatment. Report prepared for the Consumer Healthcare Products Association. Available at:http://www.chpa-info.org/pdfs/CHPA%20Final%20Report%20revised%20(03-20).pdf. Accessed February 10, 2005.

2. OTC Facts and Figures. Consumer Healthcare Products Association. Available at: http://www.chpa-info.org/web/press_room/statistics/otc_facts_figures.aspx. Accessed March 1, 2005.
3. Manasse HR Jr. Medication use in an imperfect world: drug misadventuring as an issue of public policy: parts 1 and 2. *Am J Hosp Pharm.* 1989;46:929-44, 1141-52.
4. Johnson JA, Bootman JL. Drug-related morbidity and mortality: a cost of illness model. *Arch Intern Med.* 1995;155:949-56.
5. Ernst FR, Grizzle AJ. Drug-related morbidity and mortality: updating the cost-of-illness model. *J Am Pharm Assoc.* 2001;41:192-9.
6. Cipolle RJ, Strand LM, Morley PC. *Pharmaceutical Care Practice: A Clinician's Guide.* 2nd ed. New York: McGraw Hill Inc; 2004.
7. Stergachis A, Maine LL, Brown LM. The 2001 national pharmacy consumer survey. *J Am Pharm Assoc.* 2002;42:568-76.
8. Public Law No. 108-173: Medicare Prescription Drug, Improvement, and Modernization Act of 2003.
9. Federal *Register.* Thursday, August 17, 2000, Part III, 45 CFR Parts 160 and 162: Health Insurance Reform: Standards for Electronic Transactions; Announcement of Designated Standard Maintenance Organizations; Final Rule and Notice, p. 50331.
10. Pharmacist Services Technical Advisory Coalition. Medication Therapy Management Services CPT Billing Codes [press release]. Available at: http://www.pstac.org/aboutus/profsvc.html. Accessed August 20, 2005.
11. Hepler CD, Strand LM. Opportunities and responsibilities in pharmaceutical care. *Am J Hosp Pharm.* 1990;47:533-43.
12. Isetts BJ. Pharmaceutical care. In: Mueller B, ed. *Pharmacotherapy Self-Assessment* Program—*The Science and Practice of Pharmacotherapy I.* 4th ed. Book 5. Kansas City, Mo: American College of Clinical Pharmacy; 2002: 147-2.
13. Cipolle RJ, Strand LM, Morley PC. *Pharmaceutical Care Practice.* 2nd ed. New York: McGraw Hill Inc; 2004.
14. Willink DP, Isetts B.J. Becoming 'indespensible:' developing innovative community pharmacy practices. *J Am Pharm Assoc.* 2005:45;376-89.
15. Dobson A, DaVanzo J, Koenig L, Book R. *Medication Therapy Management Services: A Critical Review.* Washington, DC: Final Report of The Lewin Group, Inc.; May 17, 2005.
16. Isetts BJ, Brown LM, Schondelmeyer SW, et al. Quality assessment of a collaborative approach for decreasing drug-related morbidity and achieving therapeutic goals. *Arch Intern Med.* 2003;163:1813-20.
17. Purtillo RB, Haddad A. *Health Professional and Patient Interaction.* Philadelphia: WB Saunders; 1996.
18. Berger BA. Communication Skills for Pharmacists: Building Relationships Improving Patient Care. Washington, DC: American Pharmacists Association; 2002.
19. Rantucci MJ. Pharmacists Talking with Patients: A Guide to Patient Counseling. Baltimore: Williams & Wilkins; 1997.
20. Siganga WW, Huynh TC. Barriers to the use of pharmacy services: the case of ethnic populations. *J Am Pharm Assoc.* 1997;37:335-40.
21. Hensrud DD, Engle DD, Scheitel SM. Underreporting the use of dietary supplements and nonprescription medications among patients undergoing periodic health examination. *Mayo Clin Proc.* 1999;74:443-7.
22. Isetts BJ, Sorensen TD. Use of a student-driven, university-based pharmaceutical care clinic to define the highest standards of patient care. *Am J Pharm Educ.* 1999;63:443-9.
23. Kogan MD, Pappas G, Yu SM, et al. Over-the-counter medication use among U.S. preschool-age children. *JAMA.* 1994;272:1025-30.
24. Zenk KE. Challenges in providing pharmaceutical care to pediatric patients. *Am J Hosp Pharm.* 1994;51:688-94.
25. Wong DL. Developmental influences on child health promotion. In: Wong DL, ed. *Essentials of Pediatric Nursing.* 5th ed. St. Louis: Mosby; 1997:83-103.
26. Skaer TL. Dosing considerations in the pediatric patient. *Clin Ther.* 1991;13:526-44.
27. Belay ED, Bresee JS, Holman RC, et al. Reye's syndrome in the United States from 1981 through 1997. *N Engl J Med.* 1999;340:1377-82.
28. Li SF, Lacher B, Crain EF. Acetaminophen and ibuprofen dosing by parents *Pediatr Emerg Care.* 2000;16:394-7.
29. Pray WS. The pharmacist as self-care advisor. *J Am Pharm Assoc.* 1996;36:329-41.
30. Larsen OM, Ostapowicz G, Fontana RJ, et al. Outcome of acetaminophen-induced liver failure in the USA in suicidal vs accidental overdose: preliminary results of a prospective multicenter trial. *Hepatology.* 2000;32:396A.
31. Compounding for the pediatric patient. *Pharma Compounding.* 1997;1:84-6.
32. Sinkovits HS, Kelly MW, Ernst ME. Medication administration in day care centers for children. *J Am Pharm Assoc.* 2003;43:379-82.
33. Sleath B, Bush PJ, Pradel FG. Communicating with children about medicines: a pharmacist's perspective. *Am J Health-Syst Pharm.* 2003;60:604-7.
34. Hanlon JT, Fillenbaum GG, Ruby CM, et al. Epidemiology of over-the-counter drug use in community dwelling elderly: United States perspective. *Drugs Aging.* 2001;18:123-31.
35. Yoon SJ, Horne CH. Herbal products and conventional medicine used by community-residing older women. *J Adv Nurs.* 2001;33:51-9.
36. Meyer ME, Schuna HH. Assessment of geriatric patients' functional ability to take medication. *Drug Intell Clin Pharm.* 1989;23:171-4.
37. Mintzer J, Burns A. Anticholinergic side-effects of drugs in elderly patients. *J R Soc Med.* 2000;93:457-62.
38. Solomon DH, Gurwitz JH. Toxicity of nonsteroidal anti-inflammatory drugs in the elderly: is advanced age a risk factor? *Am J Med.* 1997;1:208-15.
39. Page J, Henry D. Consumption of NSAIDs and the development of congestive heart failure in elderly patients: an underrecognized public health problem. *Arch Intern Med.* 2000;160(6):777-84.
40. Curhan GC, Willett WC, Rosner B, et al. Frequency of analgesic use and risk of hypertension in younger women. *Arch Intern Med.* 2002;162:2204-8.
41. FitzGerald GA. Coxibs and cardiovascular disease. *N Engl J Med.* 2004;351:1709-11.
42. Seymour RM, Routledge PA. Important drug-drug interactions in the elderly. *Drugs Aging.* 1998;12:485-94.
43. Tsui B, Dennehy CE, Tsourounis C. A survey of dietary supplement use during pregnancy at an academic medical center. *Am J Obstet Gynecol.* 2001;185:433-37.
44. Henry A, Crowther C. Patterns of medication use during and prior to pregnancy: the M A P study. *Aust N Z J Obstet Gynaecol.* 2000;40:165-72.
45. Wagner CL, Katikaneni LD, Cox TH, et al. The impact of prenatal drug exposure on the neonate. *Obstet Gynecol Clin North Am.* 1998;25:169-94.
46. Briggs GG, Freeman RK, Yaffe SJ. *Drugs in Pregnancy and Lactation: A Reference Guide to Fetal and Neonatal Risk.* 5th ed. Baltimore: Williams & Wilkins; 1998:73a-81a, 125c-31c, 254c-5c, 524i-6i, 757n-8n.
47. Miller AA. Diphenhydramine toxicity in a newborn: a case report. *J Perinatol.* 2000;20:390-1.
48. American Academy of Pediatrics Committee on Drugs. Transfer of drugs and other chemicals into human milk. *Pediatrics.* 2001;108:776-89.
49. Dillon AE, Wagner CL, Wiest D, et al. Drug therapy in the nursing mother. *Obstet Gynecol Clin North Am.* 1997;24:675-96.
50. Nice FJ, Snyder JL, Kotansky BC. Breastfeeding and over-the-counter medications. *J Hum Lact.* 2000;16:319-31.

CHAPTER 3

# Multicultural Aspects of Self-Care

*Magaly Rodriguez de Bittner and Gloria J. Nichols-English*

Culture influences beliefs about the health care system and may impact patients' decisions regarding self-care. This chapter addresses important aspects of patients' health beliefs and use of nonprescription products to help guide pharmacists in the delivery of pharmaceutical care and the counseling of patients from diverse backgrounds and cultures.

The ability of pharmacists to gather information, assess patient complaints, guide a patient's product selection, and/or advise patients to seek care from another health care provider is an important component of pharmaceutical care. Through data collection and proper assessment of the patient's symptoms, important health issues can be identified and solved. However, if cultural issues are not taken into account during the patient interview, it may be difficult for a health care provider to assess or counsel a patient effectively. Practitioners can choose a more appropriate self-care plan for the health issue presented if they understand the patient's cultural framework and incorporate the patient's health care beliefs into the formulation of the care plan.

This chapter highlights common issues and challenges faced by individuals of diverse backgrounds in self-care management of health conditions involving the use of nonprescription products and the decision to use complementary and alternative medicines (CAMs). Barriers to participating in medical decision making are also discussed, and approaches to promoting the exchange of ideas about alternative care strategies and recommendations for optimizing patient outcomes and quality of care are delineated. In addition, practical approaches to providing care and counseling of patients of diverse cultural backgrounds are presented.

Major shifts in the composition of the U.S. population are reviewed to illustrate the relevance of cultural issues in health and the overall delivery of health care. Emphasis is placed on defining and listing important cultural terms and theoretical frameworks for cross-cultural pharmaceutical care so that pharmacists are able to better understand the cultural framework of patients. Characteristics of the four major ethnic/minority groups in the United States are discussed, as well as differences in cultural approaches to seeking care, particularly self-care. Emphasis is placed on cultural assessment techniques and communication strategies to assist pharmacists in communicating effectively with patients of diverse cultures and developing a culturally competent self-care plan.

In this chapter the terms *Western, American,* or *conventional* medicine are used synonymously to mean evidence-based therapy, including prescription and nonprescription products. The terms *complementary, alternative,* or *traditional* medicine encompass a large array of health practices from all over the world, consisting of essentially natural therapies and products ranging from relatively new modalities to ancient skills and traditions such as magnetotherapy, acupuncture, herbs, mind/body techniques, homeopathy, and massage therapy.

## Demographic Changes in the U.S. Population

In the past decade, the rapid growth of the racial and ethnic minorities in the United States has resulted in a significant shift of the composition of the U.S. population. According to projections of the U.S. Census Bureau, racial and ethnic minorities constituted 30.7% of the total population in 2005 and will grow to 47.2% by 2050.[1] Some predictions state that minority populations in the United States will constitute the majority population by the next century, surpassing the white, non-Hispanic population. By 2050, it is estimated that Hispanics will number 102.6 million and constitute 25% of the U.S. population, surpassing all other minority groups.[1] In 2004, it was reported that 34.2 million people in the United States were foreign-born. This figure represents 12% of the total U.S. population.[2]

For statistical purposes, the U.S. Census classifies ethnic minorities as Hispanics or Latino, black or African American, Asian, Native Hawaiian and other Pacific Islanders, and American Indian and Alaska Natives.[1] Because ethnic groups can be racially diverse, further classifications were made during the 2000 census to more accurately estimate the composition of the U.S. population. For the first time in the history of the United States, population estimates were published by race and Hispanic origin categories. Race and Hispanic origin are considered two separate categories; Hispanics may be of any race or races. People can also be classified racially as non-Hispanic white, Hispanic white, non-Hispanic black, Hispanic black, American Indian and Alaska Natives, Asian, and Native Hawaiian and Pacific Islander. In addition, people were allowed to define themselves as belonging to more than one racial group in the 2000 census.

It is important to keep in mind the heterogeneity of these classifications. The groups included in the classification of Asian American and Pacific Islanders have great variability within them. The same holds true for the Hispanic American classification, which includes four diverse groups: Mexican Americans, Puerto Ricans, Cubans, and others (e.g., Central Americans, South Americans, Spaniards). Many people in the United States may belong to two or more ethnic groups, making the issue of race and ethnic background very complex.

In addition to racial/ethnic characteristics, the U.S. population is diverse based on gender, age, physical disabilities, religious preference, and sexual orientation. These demographic changes have penetrated most areas in the United States that have been considered to be homogeneous in culture, making the importance of cultural competence a national issue. Therefore, pharmacists in every practice setting are likely to interact with patients from diverse cultures and backgrounds.

One important aspect of these changes in demographics is that the current racial/ethnic composition of health professionals in the United States does not reflect the changes observed in the general population. Statistics on the health professions estimate that in the United States in 1990 there were approximately 186,269 pharmacists of all races.[3] Of these, 86% were white, 4.2% were African American, 3.1 % were Hispanic, 0.2% were American Indian or Alaska Native, and 6.6% were Asian and Pacific Islanders. Asian Americans are the only minority group overrepresented in the pharmacy profession compared with the racial/ethnic composition of the U.S. population: Asian Americans account for 3.6% of the U.S. population, but constitute 6.6% of all U.S. pharmacists. This fact is also true in the student population at pharmacy schools, where it is estimated that 18.6% of professional pharmacy degrees conferred between 1998 and 1999 were awarded to Asian-American students.[3]

These statistics indicate that white health care providers are caring for the majority of the patients from minority groups. This highlights the need for pharmacists of all races to understand the influences of culture in health care and for schools of pharmacy to institute curricular content that incorporates cultural competency. Many health care providers, including pharmacists, have no formal training in cultural competence and usually undergo only "on-the-job" training. This training may not contain the didactic content, teaching techniques, or skills the pharmacist needs to deliver effective, culturally competent care. The lack of formal training may jeopardize the practitioner's relationship with patients and lead to unintentional misunderstandings and negative health outcomes.

## Definition of Culture

First, it is important to define what is considered culture in the context of this chapter. Cultural identity is developed based on characteristics such as ethnicity, gender, age, race, country of origin, language, sexual orientation, and religious and spiritual beliefs. For the purpose of this chapter, *culture* is defined as the sum total of socially inherited characteristics of a human group, and comprises socially transmitted assumptions about the nature of the physical, social, and supernatural world, as well as the goals of life and the permissible means that one can take to achieve them.[2] Culture is a learned set of values, beliefs, and meanings that guide decisions, attitudes, and action. It is important to remember that unique individuals with slightly different characteristics or beliefs may belong to the same cultural group. Individual differences must be considered when dealing with patients from specific ethnic or cultural groups. There is a great risk in making generalizations or assumptions that a person within a group will always behave in the same manner. This is known as stereotyping.

Variations in behaviors among members of a group become more important when people belonging to a specific cultural group migrate and live in places that have a different, but dominant culture. In this case, the effect of acculturation or assimilation can be observed. *Acculturation,* also referred to as *assimilation,* is an involuntary process by which members of a specific cultural group begin to incorporate behaviors and beliefs of the dominant culture.[2] Subsequently, people influenced by the dominant culture may behave differently from the culture group's norm. The underlying assumption is that persons lose or modify their cultural identity to acquire a new identity that differs from their original cultural group. In many instances, these behaviors and adaptations may cause internal conflicts among members of the cultural group. For example, conflicts can arise when younger members of a cultural group do not follow the traditions. One may often observe differences in behavior and beliefs between members of the group who are first- or second-generation immigrants compared with their parents. The later generations are more adapted to the U.S. culture and may behave in a manner more consistent with the dominant culture. In many instances, the second-generation children of immigrants do not even speak their parents' native language.

Culture can influence an individual's beliefs and attitudes toward health, illness, and treatment, which will influence the person's decisions regarding health issues. The inability of a pharmacist to understand an individual's culture may impede the effective delivery of pharmaceutical care and the achievement of optimal health outcomes. Incongruent beliefs and expectations between the practitioner and the patient may lead to misunderstandings, confusion, and, ultimately, undesirable therapeutic outcomes.

## Effects of Culture on Health Practices in Self-Care

Different cultural groups seek health care in significantly different ways. Definitions of health, perceptions of illness, and health habits differ among individuals of various cultural groups. These differences stem from group differences in verbal and nonverbal communication, differences in experiences with the health care system, and lack of indoctrination into the use of the Western health care system. Providing effective care to culturally diverse populations requires that providers understand how culture influences the way patients use and respond to mainstream American medical care. Some patients accept the American health care system and others may blend it with their cultural medical practices to create their own unique system. In many instances, patients are afraid to share with the practitioner these health care practices for fear of ridicule or misunderstanding.

### *Sociocultural Framework for Self-Care Practices*

Practitioners who give little or no consideration to the beliefs and expectations of their patients will likely encounter resistance to their professional advice. Expecting patients to respond to the practitioner's advice based solely on biomedical principles is naïve and could evoke considerable frustration for the patient and the practitioner. Each patient may have different social support needs and concerns related to making decisions about self-care behaviors and their medication use. The group's cultural beliefs provide the criteria by which the group judges whether or not a person is really sick, if the patient should seek care from the health system, or if it is more appropriate to use the folk system.[4] The folk system of many cultural groups involves the use of home remedies, herbs, or other alternative treatments that are passed down from generation to generation.[4]

There is a significant contrast between the ethnomedical model of health and illness beliefs and the biomedical model. The biomedical model relies on scientific research and technology to diagnose and treat patients.[5] Rarely does the biomedical model take into account a person's beliefs, attitudes, or social influences when considering causes and remedies for an illness. In the ethnomedical model, cultural interpretations are taken into account when searching for clues to the origin of the disease and presenting options for treatment.[5] Lay definitions that are based on perceptions, feelings, and norms and expected behaviors are taken into consideration and referenced by cultural meanings. By using familiar words and phrases and understanding the patient's cultural background, a practitioner can make a patient feel comfortable discussing health care issues and treatment options. If a practitioner does not understand cultural issues or folk medicine or employ certain cultural terms, a patient might feel disappointed and misunderstood and not wish to participate in the interview or follow the recommended treatment plan. Therefore, the therapeutic outcomes will not be met.

Communication within the framework of the patient's culture helps break down barriers and facilitate a trust and understanding between the patient and practitioner. Through this knowledge, the pharmacist is able to lead a patient successfully away from harmful practices and provide safe culturally sensitive alternatives. Subsequently, the practitioner can develop interventions (even biomedical ones) within the context of the patient's belief system. If the folk practices are not harmful or even found to be beneficial to the patient, the practitioner is encouraged to accept them as aspects of the treatment plan so the effects can be monitored and taken into consideration when evaluating patient outcomes. For example, a patient who is being monitored and treated through Western or conventional medicine might also use a folk healer. Some common healing methods include prayers, massage, and aromatherapy. Because these practices may be harmless and potentially additive to Western medicine, the practitioner may want to accept and even encourage their use. It may be helpful if the pharmacist maintains consistent communications with the patient, folk healer, and other health care practitioners throughout the treatment.

Interpretations of illnesses are usually influenced by religious beliefs, family and social contacts, cultural expectations, educational training, and personal experiences. According to Kleinman, the patient's understanding of a disease is based on a consensus of beliefs, information, and expectations pertaining to the illness that is shared with a social network.[6] This consensus constitutes the criteria for interpreting conditions for sickness and healing. These normative beliefs are generated by social interaction and personal experiences and may be completely different from a biomedical understanding. For example, the group may view "hypertension" as caused by "bad nerves" or "high excitement," but may not understand that the disease is the chronic elevation of arterial blood pressure. The group may not perceive the risk factors of obesity, family history, or dietary sodium intake as precursors to the development of coronary artery disease and stroke.[6]

Patients are responsible for taking care of the day-to-day management of their illness. Consequently, better methods need to be developed to determine the patient's health-seeking behaviors, informational needs, preferences, and expectations about treatment management approaches. The pharmacist can use the ethnomedical model of care to understand how patients interpret discrete episodes of illness in reference to disease causation, onset of symptoms, the anatomic nature of the disease, and the course of sickness and treatment.[6] Through these methods, the adverse impact of miscommunication, misinformed decisions, and harmful health behaviors can be reduced or eliminated.

### *The Practice of Folk Medicine*

*Home remedies, folk medicine,* and *herbal remedies* or *therapies* have a variety of definitions. Home remedies are defined as any substance not usually sold for a medical purpose that is used in the cure, treatment, mitigation, or prevention of disease or adverse health-related symptoms, or any drug product purchased without a prescription and used for medical purposes in a manner not indicated on the product label.[7] Herbal remedies are considered to be those remedies derived from natural products such as certain wild herbs and berries used in the treatment of health conditions (e.g., licorice root used to treat cough, sore throats, and colds).[2] The National Institutes of Health (NIH) and U.S. federal agencies use the term *complementary and alternative medicine,* defined as "a group of diverse medical and health care systems, practices, and products that are not presently considered to be part of conventional medicine."[8] Differences between complementary and alternative medicine are further defined: "*Complementary* medicine is used *together with* conventional medicine. An example of a complementary therapy is using aromatherapy to help lessen a patient's discomfort following surgery"; "*alternative* medicine is used *in place of* conventional medicine." An example of an alternative therapy is treating cancer with a special diet instead of undergoing surgery, radiation, or chemotherapy recommended by a conventional doctor.[8]

Use of home remedies or the practice of folk medicine has a variety of important clinical implications. First, many

**TABLE 3-1 Examples of Cultural Behaviors Observed Among Selected Ethnic Groups**

| Group | General Characteristics |
|---|---|
| Hispanic Americans | ■ Family is very important (family members are deeply involved in the care of the patient)<br>■ Use curanderos (healers)<br>■ Use home remedies (mostly tea or herbal remedies) that contain one ingredient<br>■ Use religious medals for good luck<br>■ Believe that health is a matter of "luck"<br>■ Have pessimistic attitude toward recovery ("fatalism")<br>■ Believe illnesses are classified as hot and cold (treatment is chosen depending on the classification of the disease) |
| Asian Americans | ■ Family is important<br>■ Balance between forces defines health ("ying" and "yang")<br>■ Believe illnesses are caused by an imbalance of cold and hot forces<br>■ Use alternative medicine<br>■ Use Chinese herbal products (mostly a blend of a variety of herbs)<br>■ May have a distrust of Western medicine |
| African Americans | ■ Use home remedies and folk medicine<br>■ Distrust the health care system based on previous experiences with the health care system<br>■ Religion is important in achieving cure<br>■ Family is also very important |
| American Indians | ■ Use sweat lodges as a method of cure<br>■ Use herbal medicine/natural roots<br>■ Use prayer for cure of illnesses<br>■ Believe that health is a harmony with "Mother Earth"<br>■ Use healers (medicine man) |

home remedies contain herbs with active ingredients that have pharmacologic properties. These ingredients can interact with a prescribed medication and, for example, may potentiate or inhibit its effect. Second, use of home remedies may discourage the patient from taking a prescribed medication because of added costs, side effects, or scheduling issues. In addition, home remedies may contain alcohol or sugar to improve flavor. These ingredients can cause additive effects when taken with prescribed medications or affect the control of chronic conditions such as diabetes or hypertension. Use of folk or home remedies should always be considered in the medication use interview.

### *General Description of Beliefs by Different Population Groups*

Table 3-1 lists some of the characteristics shared by people in the major ethnic/minority groups in the United States (i.e., Hispanic Americans, Asian Americans, American Indians, African Americans).[2] These differences in beliefs and attitudes may alter perceptions of drug therapy response and actual responses to therapy.[4,9] It is imperative to clarify that these are generalizations. It is not safe to assume that every member of an ethnic or cultural group will conform to these attitudes and beliefs. This chapter uses examples of these beliefs and attitudes in an attempt to help sensitize practitioners to aspects of health behavior they may encounter with some patients. These beliefs and behaviors are documented in the literature.[2,4,6] Awareness of these differences in beliefs and expectations allows the pharmacist to provide pharmaceutical care in a more effective and culturally competent manner.

Religious beliefs are also important in patients' acceptance of the diagnosis and treatment. The set of beliefs, attitudes, and expectations of illness and treatment based on religion may cause friction with the health care system and the health care team. A typical example of how religion affects the acceptance of a treatment modality is the case of the Jehovah's Witnesses. Members of this religious group oppose the use of blood transfusions as a means of medical treatment. In some instances, attending physicians and/or health care institutions have initiated legal action to force a patient or his/her parents to allow the administration of a life-saving blood transfusion. This example illustrates the complexity of the issue and incongruity between Western medicine and some religious beliefs.

Individuals from different cultures may choose to treat illnesses using different rituals and religious items that are outside the realm of Western medicine. For example, Hispanic patients may use home remedies or other artifacts recommended by the *curandera(o)*. The *curandera(o)* are spiritual healers and members of the community. On many occasions, these healers may use a combination of herbal remedies and religious rituals. Practitioners can better tailor therapy to the patient's needs if they understand these rituals and the belief systems. When practitioners appear nonjudgmental about different approaches, they can better understand how and when the patient plans to use drug therapy or another alternative treatment method. Knowing this information can help the pharmacist determine what prior treatments the patient used or is going to use, or if there are major interactions between the nonprescription product to be recommended and the patient's alternative treatment.

Recent research findings showed trends of increasing use of alternative or folk and herbal remedies on a regular basis in the United States patient population.[10] Factors associated with herbal use among urban multiethnic patients were identified in a group of primary care clinics in Houston, Texas.[11] The results of this study indicated that racial/ethnic differences existed in the use of herbal remedies. A total of 36% of the surveyed patients indicated use of herbs, with 50% of Hispanics, 50% of Asians, 41% of whites, and 22% of African Americans admitting herbal use. About 40% of the respondents indicated they believed taking prescription medications and herbal medicines together would increase the effectiveness of each product.[11] Whites were more likely to disclose herbal medicine use to other health care providers (67%) than African Americans (45%), Hispanics (31%), or Asians (31%).[11] In this survey, 41% of the Hispanic patients reported that herbal medications were superior to prescription medications, compared to 12% of the white patients. While the use of these agents varies among ethnic groups, alternative remedies represent an important approach to health care for many individuals in these groups. The increasing use of alternative medicine influences treatment decisions and has also been associated with severe adverse reactions and significant drug interactions.[12] When securing a drug history, pharmacists should elicit the patient's current use of complementary/alternative approaches and herbal therapies during all clinical encounters.

### *Use of Nonprescription Medications by Culturally Diverse Patients*

Limited data in the literature assess the use of nonprescription products among patients of diverse cultural groups or patients with diverse sexual, gender, or religious preferences. It is known that for many cultural groups, especially those without drug coverage, nonprescription products represent the most frequently used treatments prior to consulting a primary care provider.[10] Because of monetary constraints, fear of the health care system, and cultural beliefs, some immigrants will use the pharmacist as the first source of care. In many countries, the pharmacist plays a very important and significant role in assessing patient symptoms and triaging the patient to appropriate medical care.

Because of the limited access to health care facilities in many countries, pharmacists have served as primary care providers. It is important that pharmacists understand a large number of patients from other countries may be seeking their involvement in their care with this understanding of the pharmacist's primary care role. Patients' expectations may include the belief that the pharmacist will provide them with prescription medications such as antibiotics without a prescription. Failure to do so may negatively influence the patients' expectations of the pharmacist. Understanding these expectations will allow the pharmacist to be prepared for the encounter and effectively communicate to the patient the rationale for his or her therapeutic recommendations.

### *Suboptimal Responses to Nonprescription Drug Therapy*

The improper use of nonprescription products places vulnerable populations at an increased risk for adverse drug reactions, drug–drug interactions, and toxicities from long-term exposure.[13] Therefore, the misuse and abuse of drugs that are available for self-treatment may outweigh the benefit–risk ratio in some high-risk patients.[14] Increased use of nonprescription products by minority groups may create another challenge in self-care management. The need for quick relief may prompt more frequent use of nonprescription medicines and, thus, raises the risk of overmedication and a tendency for people to self-medicate for nonpathologic conditions. Lowered tolerance for discomfort can also lead people to rely on medications instead of seeking longer-term, behaviorally oriented strategies. An example of this behavior is the use of vitamins, laxatives, and antacids to counteract poor eating habits. What is more important to realize is that these self-management strategies can mask symptoms and complicate the diagnosis of serious diseases.

Several other factors contribute to the increased vulnerability of low-income minority patients to the harmful effects of overuse of nonprescription products.[15] First, patients with poor health status, low education, and low income are most likely to reduce consumption of prescription drugs when their costs increase. Second, many uninsured patients seek nonprescription products as alternatives to prescription drugs. Third, these same patients may seek medical care only for the most recognizable and urgent symptoms, delaying regular, routine visits to their primary care provider's office. Practitioners who counsel patients on the use of nonprescription products can help prevent delays in seeking needed medical care. In addition, many medical conditions are considered "silent," such as hypertension and hyperlipidemia. Nonprescription products may be used by patients to treat minor symptoms associated with these conditions such as headache, nosebleeds, or chest discomfort. The more serious conditions may not be diagnosed until the patient experiences a negative consequence or complication.

### *Pharmacogenetics and Drug Response*

Culturally diverse populations have been underrepresented in clinical research trials. This problem has been addressed in part by the NIH Revitalization Act of 1993, which requires that ethnic minorities and women be included in clinical research studies funded by NIH.[16] More research is needed on the pharmacokinetics and pharmacodynamic differences in drug metabolism among different ethnic/racial groups. There are also very little data available concerning differences in response to nonprescription drugs among patients of diverse cultural groups.

To date, researchers are discovering that variability in drug responses can be determined by racial or ethnic background, but the data are limited in scope.[17,18] The field of pharmacogenetics or pharmacogenomics uses genome-wide approaches to study the inherited basis of differences between persons in the response to drugs.[19] The genetic makeup of a race or ethnic group may be such that many people within that group are simply unable to produce certain enzymes needed to adequately metabolize a drug. It is estimated that genetics account for 20% to 95% of variability of drug disposition and effects.[19] This inherited variability in drug response has been associated with variants in the genes encoding drug-metabolizing enzymes, drug transporters, or drug targets. These differences in drug response do not change over time; they remain stable throughout the patient's life. Drug safety and efficacy are compromised when genetic variability in drug response is coupled with other nongenetic factors such as age, organ function, gender, concomitant therapy, drug interactions, and environmental factors.[17-19]

Armed with specific education and skill development, pharmacists can assist in the detection and reporting of unexpected adverse drug reactions and atypical drug responses from nonprescription drug interactions and adverse affects in ethnic minorities. Therefore, it is important for pharmacy educators and pharmacy institutions to provide this education and skill development in the pharmacy curricula and in continuing education programs. In addition, practitioners can inform their ethnic minority patients of the need for their participation in pharmacodynamic and pharmacokinetic studies to gather more data in this area.

## Providing Care to Culturally Diverse Groups

Barriers to care presented by differences in language and culture are challenges that health care providers confront every day in their practice. Providing services in cross-cultural situations can be extremely challenging and rewarding. In some cases, small differences in the interpretation of language, gesture, or eye contact may lead to misunderstandings between people of different cultures and their health care providers. In many cases, the health care provider's lack of cultural competency may impede the delivery of appropriate care and triage.

In addition, major health disparities among members of minority groups have been identified.[20] It is well known that people of some minority groups do not equally experience long life spans, good health, and access to health services. Current data from the U.S. Census and the Department of Health and Human Services indicate that index measures of the health status of the U.S. population show marked disparities in the health of different racial and ethnic groups.[20-23] In many cases, these health disparities cannot be explained solely on the basis of current information about the biologic and genetic characteristics of African Americans, Hispanic Americans, American Indians, Alaska Natives, Asians, Native Hawaiians, and Pacific Islanders. They may be the result of the complex interactions among genetic variations, environmental factors, socioeconomic factors, and specific health beliefs and behaviors.[24]

African Americans comprised 12% of the U.S. population in 2000. It is estimated that African Americans' life expectancy is 6 years shorter than that of whites at birth and 2 years shorter at the age of 65.[23] For example, compared with the white non-Hispanic majority, African Americans suffer higher rates of hypertension, diabetes, tuberculosis, and infant mortality, and experience higher rates of death resulting from heart disease, lung cancer, breast cancer, and stroke.[21,24,25] Heart disease death rates are more than 40% higher for African Americans than for whites. The death rate for all cancers is 30% higher for African Americans than for whites; for prostate cancer, it is more than double that for whites.[25] African-American women have a higher death rate from breast cancer despite having a mammography screening rate that is nearly the same as that for white women.[23] The death rate from HIV/AIDS for African Americans is more than seven times higher than that for whites.[23]

In 2000, Hispanics accounted for 12.5% of the U.S. population, and estimates indicate that this population will be the second largest racial/ethnic group (after non-Hispanic whites) in 2010.[26] Currently, Hispanics living in the United States are almost twice as likely to die from diabetes as are non-Hispanic whites. It is interesting that although constituting only 11% of the total population in 1996, Hispanics accounted for 20% of the new cases of tuberculosis. Hispanics also have higher rates of high blood pressure and obesity than non-Hispanic whites.[25] The Commonwealth Fund survey in 2001 found that, regardless of their language skills, Hispanics had great difficulty understanding and/or communicating with their physicians.[27] It is important to highlight that within the Hispanic population there are differences in the rate and prevalence of some diseases depending on the group (i.e., Puerto Rican, Mexican, Central America, Cuban). Even though this population is grouped together, there are important differences between the groups.

American Indians and Alaska Natives constituted 0.9% of the total population in 2000.[1] An infant death rate almost double that of whites has been reported. The rate of diabetes for this population group is more than twice that of non-Hispanic whites.[25] The Pima of Arizona have one of the highest rates of diabetes in the world.[28] American Indians and Alaska Natives also have disproportionately high death rates from unintentional injuries and suicide. Access to care among this population is lacking in many areas. Preventive care is an issue among many of the members of the American Indian communities.

Asians and Pacific Islanders made up 3.6% of the total U.S. population in 2000.[28] On average, Asians and Pacific Islanders are one of the healthiest population groups in the United States. However, there is great diversity within this population, and health disparities for some specific segments are quite marked. Women of Vietnamese origin, for example, suffer from cervical cancer at a rate nearly five times higher than that of white women.[28] New cases of hepatitis and tuberculosis also are higher in Asians and Pacific Islanders living in the United States than in non-Hispanic whites.

The federal government has implemented a public policy to address the health needs of minority groups and reduce racial and ethnic health disparities. These efforts are well summarized in the publication *Healthy People 2010*, which established goals aimed at decreasing disparities in health care and outcomes of therapy for all Americans,

**TABLE 3-2 Broad Goals for *Healthy People 2010***

1. Improve access to comprehensive, high-quality health care services.
2. Eliminate health disparities among segments of the population, including differences that occur by gender, race, ethnicity, education, income, disability, geographic location, or sexual orientation.

with a special focus on decreasing health disparities among minority groups.[25] Table 3-2 summarizes the major goals to decrease health disparities among minority groups. In addition, a Center for Minority Health and Health Disparities (www.ncmhd.nih.gov) is a part of the NIH. These national initiatives have created an interest among the health care system, health care providers, and government agencies in identifying those factors that contribute to health disparities and develop strategies to decrease the gap that currently exists.

One of the factors identified by many government agencies and health care groups as a cause of health disparities is the lack of awareness of cultural issues and health disparities among health care providers. This may be attributed to lack of formalized training on cultural issues in health care at many higher education institutions. Cultural issues are not an integral part of the curricula or textbooks used in many curricula. In addition, there are few opportunities for practitioners to receive skill development as part of continuing professional education because of the limited number of courses devoted to this topic. A recent report from the Institute of Medicine highlighted the need to train culturally competent health care providers to decrease the racial and ethnic health disparities observed among different minority groups.[29] In addition, in 1997, the Office of Minority Health developed the National Standards for Culturally and Linguistically Appropriate Services in Health Care.[30] These standards are based on an in-depth review of the literature, regulations, laws, and standards currently used in the federal and state agencies. One of the goals of the standards is to provide criteria for accreditation and credentialing agencies to assess and compare the level of culturally competent care that providers and institutions have provided. Some of these agencies include the Joint Commission on Accreditation of Healthcare Organizations and the National Committee on Quality Assurance.

To ensure effective delivery of culturally and linguistically appropriate care in cross-cultural settings, practitioners need to understand cultural issues related to health and illness, health disparities among different groups, and communication strategies to deal with culturally diverse patients.

## Communication With Culturally Diverse Groups

### *Data Gathering*

When preparing to interact with patients from different cultures, practitioners must use specific communication skills aimed at elucidating the patient's cultural beliefs. Some of the required communication skills include (1) an openness to alternative viewpoints and approaches, (2) a clear understanding of one's own prejudices and biases (self-awareness), (3) engagement to identify the patient's beliefs, expectations, and barriers to treatment, (4) understanding of the influences of the patient's beliefs and attitudes in the treatment plan, and (5) an ability to negotiate treatment that is acceptable to the patient and the practitioner. Preestablished trust and effective communication are essential for this process to succeed. Trust is essential to gaining awareness of the issues involved in the interaction, and appropriate language is crucial to effective communication.

Many techniques have been suggested to improve care in cross-cultural settings. Berlin proposed and described a model for individual and institutional cultural development.[31] This technique, described with the acronym "LEARN," may be used in all clinical encounters to assist the health care provider. The acronym of LEARN refers to the following:

- *L*isten with sympathy and understanding to the patient's perception of the problem.
- *E*xplain your perceptions of the problem.
- *A*cknowledge and discuss the differences and similarities.
- *R*ecommend treatment.
- *N*egotiate agreement.

Tables 3-3 and 3-4 provide guidelines to help the practitioner communicate better with culturally diverse patients. In many instances, the communication barrier may include the patient's inability to speak English. Table 3-5 lists some approaches that the practitioner can use with patients who speak another language. On many occasions practitioners may need to work with an interpreter. An interpreter provides a means of dealing with a language barrier, but this approach has limitations. On many occasions, problems may arise when family members are used as interpreters. The patient and family members may be put in an uncomfortable position. This becomes more critical when a younger family member, sometimes a child, is asked to interpret for his or her parents or grandparents in a clinical encounter. This is an unacceptable position of responsibility that leads to family conflicts by altering the hierarchy within the family. It also places an undue burden on the child. The use of family members or untrained personnel to interpret may lead to receiving or transmitting inaccurate information because of the lack of training or failure to translate in a proper manner. The health care provider may fail to detect relevant, critical information or the information provided by the clinician may be mistranslated between clinician, interpreter and patient. These problems may be avoided when the health care provider uses trained translators who are prepared in medical language and in interpretation and familiar with the provider and his or her practice.

Many health professionals are aware that patients may use alternative health care and self-prescribed medicinal products as well as prescribed or recommended medications.

| TABLE 3-3 | Recommended Actions to Develop Effective Cross-cultural Communication |
|---|---|

- Acknowledge that diversity exists.
- Understand that culture is part of what makes individuals unique.
- Respect people or cultures that may be unfamiliar or different from one's own.
- Conduct a self-assessment to identify one's own cultural beliefs and biases.
- Recognize that there are differences in the way people define and value health and illness.
- Be patient, flexible, and willing to modify health care delivery to meet the cultural needs of the patient.
- Allow for differences among members of the same cultural group (do not expect all individuals from a cultural group to behave identically at all times).
- Appreciate the richness of culture.
- Embrace diversity.
- Understand that cultural beliefs and values are difficult to change and in many instances are learned from birth.

*Source:* Adapted with permission from Schrefer S. *Quick Reference to Cultural Assessment.* St. Louis: Mosby; 1994:IV.

| TABLE 3-4 | Guidelines for Communicating With Culturally Diverse Patients |
|---|---|

- Assess your personal beliefs surrounding persons from different cultures.
- Assess your own biases and prejudices.
- Assess communication variables from a cultural perspective (language barriers, nonverbal communication, use of interpreters, beliefs, and feelings).
- Plan care based on communicated needs and cultural background. Adapt care to meet the cultural needs of the patient.
- Modify communication approaches to meet cultural needs (use more than one method to communicate the stated plan).

*Source:* Adapted with permission from Schrefer S. *Quick Reference to Cultural Assessment.* St. Louis: Mosby; 1994:33.

| TABLE 3-5 | Communication Strategies for Non–English-speaking Patients |
|---|---|

- Use a caring tone of voice and facial expression (demonstrate your interest in the patient).
- Speak slowly and clearly, not loudly. Do not yell.
- Use gestures, pictures, and other role-playing techniques to help the patient understand.
- Repeat the message in many ways, using different communication approaches.
- Avoid using medical terms, slang terms or jargon, and/or abbreviations.
- Keep the message simple, and repeat it in several ways.

*Source:* Adapted with permission from Schrefer S. *Quick Reference to Cultural Assessment.* St. Louis: Mosby; 1994:34.

Some are supportive and respectful of their patient's choice. However, misinformation or omission of the patient's self-medication decisions in the counseling encounter and confusion on the patient's part as to how much and when to inform the physicians about alternative care practices can lead to negative outcomes. Health providers must initiate a dialogue about alternative therapies, or use systematic methods to capture this information from their patients and document it appropriately in the pharmaceutical care database.

## Assessment of Cultural Issues on Patient Adherence

Practitioners can assess the role that culture may play in a patient's acceptance of the diagnosis and treatment of an illness by following the recommendations listed in Table 3-6. These recommendations will help the health care provider conduct a better assessment of the impact that cultural health beliefs and perceptions may have on the patient's acceptance of a diagnosis or treatment. For example, many Hispanic patients may have the perception that injectable dosage forms are more effective than oral tablets. This belief is probably a result of the fact that in many Hispanic countries, particularly Central America, primary care providers employ injectable drugs with repository drug delivery forms to provide more sustained drug delivery. This technique is used to deal with the geographical distances many patients have to travel to receive care and helps achieve a more predictable duration of treatment. Further, this form of drug delivery ensures adherence with treatment. Because a cure is most likely achieved, the patient associates effectiveness with this method of drug administration.

In the United States, however, injectable dosage forms are not commonly and routinely employed. Therefore, Hispanic patients may leave a health facility with a prescription for a tablet or capsule believing that the treatment is not going to be effective. This lack of trust in the therapy may affect adherence with the regimen and impair achievement of a cure. If health care providers are aware of this particular cultural belief and take the time to assess the patient's preferences or beliefs to a variety of treatments, they can modify the treatment plan or educate the patient about the benefit of the oral dosage form. Even though this approach seems simplistic, it is a very complex process that requires time and individual assessment of the patient's beliefs and preferences.

## Development of a Self-Care Plan

The information gathered in the interview process and the physical assessment needs to be incorporated into the development of a self-care plan. The self-care plan must take into consideration the cultural differences and beliefs identified by the patient. These beliefs, as well as the role of the family in the patient's care, will help dictate the most appropriate treatment recommendation for the patient. The pharmacist will be able to design strategies that maximize the patient's goals and expectations of therapy. These strategies can achieve better adherence to the drug therapy and treatment recommendations.

**TABLE 3-6 Cultural Assessment of Diagnosis and Treatment of Illness**

| Diagnosis | Treatment |
|---|---|
| What is the patient's understanding of the diagnosis?<br>What does this diagnosis mean to the patient? | What motivates the patient to recover?<br>Why does the patient want to recover?<br>For whom does the patient want to recover? |
| How does the patient interpret the illness?<br>Does the patient believe that the diagnosis is terminal? | What are the patient's feelings and beliefs about the treatment?<br>How will the treatment affect the patient's relationship with his/her family?<br>What are the expectations of the family regarding the treatment? |
| How is the patient accepting the diagnosis?<br>Is the patient in denial? | What is the role of the family in the treatment?<br>Is the family involved in administration of the medications or treatment? |
| How does the patient think others view/feel about the illness?<br>How will the diagnosis affect the patient's social status or social acceptance within their culture? | What effect does the treatment have in the patient's religious and/or cultural beliefs?<br>Is there a concordance between the patient's beliefs and the treatment plan? |

*Source:* Adapted with permission from Schrefer S. *Quick Reference to Cultural Assessment*. St. Louis: Mosby; 1994:35-36.

The assessment of the problem must take into consideration the patient's beliefs, values, and expectations of treatment. The practitioner must then use this information to delineate and develop his or her self-care recommendations and patient education strategies. In addition, there should be communication with other health care providers, particularly with the physician, about the cultural beliefs and preferences of the patient. A collaborative approach ensures that all health care providers involved in the care of this particular patient are aware of his or her cultural preferences. For example, when developing a plan of care for the treatment of a self-limiting illness that requires nonprescription drug therapy, the practitioner must

1. Take into account the patient's beliefs and perceptions of the problem.
2. Find out if the patient has treated the problem with any nonprescription or herbal products/alternative treatments.
3. Identify any communication issues that cast doubt on whether the patient understood the questions being asked and/or whether the data gathered are accurate.
4. Identify any cultural/religious beliefs that may influence the patient's acceptance or willingness to use a specific product.
5. Identify the patient's perceptions/acceptance of the recommended treatment.
6. Identify other methods/resources to help the patient better understand the appropriate use of the product. For example, is a family member present who can understand the instructions and explain them to the patient? Is an interpreter available? Are materials written in the patient's language available? Can diagrams be used to communicate the information?
7. Make sure that the patient knows what to do if the product/treatment does not solve the problem.
8. Make sure that the patient knows when to contact the practitioner again or seek the care of a primary care provider.

## Decision Making and Nonprescription Products

The market for nonprescription drugs is expanding and patient autonomy concerning health care extends to taking part in the decision making for the need for treatment, monitoring treatment progress, and using nonprescription medications, home monitoring devices, and diagnostic kits at intervals during the treatment process. Because there are higher rates of chronic conditions and diseases within minority populations, drugs (even nonprescription drugs) to treat these conditions and symptoms will be more widely used.[10]

To facilitate decision making for self-care, health care providers must examine the reasons their patients are attracted to the use of CAM in conjunction with or in opposition to, conventional therapies for self-care treatment. Parallel to conventional medicine, most folk systems provide explanations, remedies, diagnostic aids, and curative measures.[32] Scientific evidence from rigorous research is not the driving force behind the CAM movement as an aspect of self-care. CAM use stems from an appeal to emotional factors, for example, personal healing.[33] Rejection of science and technology, distrust of established systems for health care delivery, and the spiritual dimension (i.e., the emphasis of holism) may be what is appealing to many minority group populations as these factors validate their views of health, illness, and healing. These alternative methods in many cases are more congruent with the patient's beliefs and expectations of treatment. Therefore, patients are more attracted to these alternative therapies.

Practitioners may also observe differences in the types of CAM therapy used among different ethnic groups. For example, Asian Americans use mostly Chinese herbal medicines, which tend to be combinations of herbals. These combinations contain a variety of active ingredients that make it difficult for pharmacists to decide which ingredients may interact with the prescription medications the patient is taking. In addition, this combination of active ingredients may increase the likelihood of adverse events with these products. In contrast, the herbal products used in the Hispanic community tend to contain a single ingredient, and these are mostly teas of seeds or herbs. This makes it easier to identify the active ingredient(s) in the product. It is also important to point out that in many instances Hispanic patients may use the home remedy in addition to their prescription medications and not as a substitute.

On many occasions, the use of home remedies does not need to be discouraged. They can serve as palliative therapy for symptoms commonly observed in self-limiting illnesses such as the common cold or the flu. One example is the use of chamomile tea, which can provide hydration and comfort. Many Hispanic patients use this tea to treat colds, the flu, and nervous conditions, or to "calm the nerves."

Pharmacists can help the patient in the decision to use nonprescription products by conducting thorough assessments to determine whether or not the patient has the proper skills and motivation to follow through on a recommended self-care plan. Pharmacists should plan to interact with the patient at regular, usually brief, intervals during prescription refills to reinforce nonprescription product selection decisions, make adjustments to the self-care plan, and detect possible adverse effects. Pharmacists may be the health care providers best suited to orient patients toward appropriate referral and self-care behavior.

### Provider–Patient Relationships

The early self-care movement gave rise to a shift in provider–patient relationships whereby the patient became the center of the health encounter.[34] Patients are encouraged to assume responsibility of being an active participant in their own care. The continued success of this trend will depend on how well the consumer exercises judgment about how and when to self-treat, and how effectively health care professionals can assist consumers in the management of their self-care needs.

Competencies needed by health care providers to participate effectively in informed decision making for self-care include awareness of the ideas and information that the patient may have or need before seeking health care, or where the patient is on the pathway to deciding to self-medicate. Some self-medication transactions (steps) include the following:[35]

1. The patient detects a health problem.
2. The patient determines what he or she thinks is wrong using a series of diagnostic indicators (e.g., feeling of pain or discomfort, fever, presence of inflammation).
3. The patient experiences the progressive nature of the illness.
4. The patient uses certain criteria to decide if the problem is mild, serious, or an emergency situation.
5. The patient makes decisions about a course of action to follow (which includes "doing nothing," "taking something," or "applying a therapeutic substance using a device").
6. The patient decides to consult with family members and/or his or her social network.
7. The patient decides whether to ask for medical advice from a health care professional or from a folk or traditional healer.

## *Concordance in the Consultation Process*

A British work group dealing with medication-taking issues recommends that *concordance* should replace the term *compliance*.[36] This change in terminology denotes the role of the patient as a decision maker and partner in the consultation process. Concordance implies that the patient and provider can reach an agreement about what health action is to be taken and review these decisions regularly.[36] To ensure an adequate interchange of information for concordance in treatment decisions, practitioners must be aware of a patient's beliefs about the cause, threat, and severity of illness, as well as the patient's beliefs about the diagnosis and prognosis, including the course and timing of symptoms. Culture significantly influences these factors. If the patient disagrees with the practitioner's suggested treatments, the patient's decision must be respected and incorporated into the plan.

As a result of professional training and different backgrounds and experiences, practitioners, as well as patients, bring certain beliefs and expectations to the provider–patient encounter.[37] For example, if a person believes that taking a medication is a good thing and expects it to work, then he or she will have a favorable attitude toward taking the medication. Alternatively, if a health provider believes a patient is difficult to understand, just does not listen, or ignores directions, he or she may not take the time to counsel more effectively about the correct use of the medication or give advice for alternative options.

There are several barriers to concordance in the provider–patient relationship. First, concordance between patients and health professionals on when and how to share information on concurrent use of nonprescription products or CAM is low. Second, most providers have no formal methods of capturing patients' preferences for how they best receive health information. Third, little time is taken to assess the impact of patient's characteristics, values, lifestyle, and cultural preferences and beliefs on prescription adherence and choices for alternative therapies. Strategies to address these barriers and improve the provider's consulting style can effectively bring about better provider–patient concordance and increase patient satisfaction with the care.[38]

Improving cultural competence among health care providers may enhance the quality of health care for minority populations. However, it is important to mention that racial concordance (patient and provider are from the same racial, ethnic, or cultural background) contributes significantly to greater patient satisfaction and more effective use of the health care system.[39] This reinforces the need to increase the number of minority health providers. They play an important role in helping reduce the disparities in health outcomes of minority patients by their presence and the unique type of care they provide to underserved communities.

## Barriers to Self-Care Management

### Financial Concerns

Economic factors such as lack of health insurance are widely recognized as playing an important role in health-seeking behaviors and the decisions related to drug use.[40] When examining financial concerns, one should consider the political and historical context, poverty status, refugee status, past discrimination, and lack of access to care of the cultural group to which the patient belongs. Providers should also keep in mind that, although a patient may currently be enjoying a stable socioeconomic status, research shows that a disadvantaged history has continuing negative repercussions on a person's health.[41]

The young, particularly those with poor health status, low education, and low income, are most likely to decrease consumption of prescription drugs when copayments or out-of-pocket expenses increase.[15] These economic factors could increase the use of nonprescription products as substitutes for prescription drugs to treat health problems, resulting in negative health consequences. For example, because of financial circumstances, some people must decide between meeting basic needs and seeking medical care. In some households in which more than one person is ill, a conscious decision is often made to purchase medications and health care for the one who is most seriously ill. Other problems may evolve as some patients self-regulate their medicine to stretch their supplies to the end of the month. Many of these patients may seek nonprescription products (because of their lower cost) as alternative treatments for their chronic diseases.[40,41]

When patients encounter financial burden, it is appropriate for the pharmacist to serve as a source of advice and help the patient seek alternatives to acquire medications. One of these alternatives may be to educate the patient about the differences between brand names and generics and the impact of these differences on the cost of the medications or the amount of the copayment. Generic alternatives to brand-name drugs may be a solution for patients with no health insurance or with financial constraints. In addition, the pharmacist could work with drug companies to help patients take advantage of discount cards or indigent patient programs within the company.

### Fear and Mistrust of Health Care Providers

Mistrust of providers creates a barrier to self-care management because patients tend to avoid following the practitioner's advice or prescribed therapeutic plan. Patients may feel that practitioners did not consider their concerns and, therefore, their expectations were not met.

### Language Barriers and Unfamiliarity With Medical Terms

Inability to speak or read English makes it difficult for many patients to communicate with their health care providers or to read instructions on an nonprescription product label. This creates a significant barrier to seeking self-care or the advice of a health care provider such as the pharmacist. Because of language barriers, many patients rely on television advertisements (on channels in their language of origin) or on the recommendations of family members or relatives. Problems in interpreting professional jargon are important factors that may impede effective self-care management.

In many cultures, patients may express their symptoms in a different manner than what is typically encountered in a Western medical system. It is not uncommon to observe patients of different cultural groups express pain or symptoms of mental illnesses differently from the typical white patient. One example of this situation occurs when a practitioner asks Hispanic patients if they are depressed. The patient most likely will answer "no" and may get upset with the inference that she or he may be depressed. On further questioning, the patient may say, "I have little or no energy" or other statements that may lead to the practitioner to realize that the patient is depressed. If the practitioner asks if the patient is "feeling down or blue," the patient may not understand this expression. In such cases, the use of validated questionnaires to determine diagnosis may not be useful in capturing the patient's feelings because of cultural differences in the meaning of the words. In this example, the term "feeling blue" has no cultural meaning to the Hispanic patient and will be interpreted as a very confusing and silly question. The practitioner should seek out and use questionnaires that have been validated for use in the languages of the populations being served.

Another example is the interpretation and expressions of pain by patients of Asian descent. Many Asian-American patients do not request pain relief medications even when they are in extreme pain. It has been reported that Asian Americans exhibit a higher tolerance of pain. This may lead to undertreatment of pain in many of these patients.

### Health Illiteracy

The lack of health literacy is an important barrier to self-management and decision making about nonprescription products. The prerequisite requirements of the Food and Drug Administration (FDA) Durham-Humphrey (1951) and Kefauver-Harris (1962) amendments, used in evaluating new drug applications for proposed nonprescription drugs, demonstrate the need for improved health literacy. The required criteria for nonprescription approval include demonstrated evidence that (1) patients can recognize and diagnose themselves for the condition specified in the proposed indication, (2) patients can read the product label and extract the key information necessary to use the drug properly, (3) the drug is effective when used as recommended, and (4) the drug is safe when used as instructed. The consumer must be able to read and understand the information on the label to know the proper dose, recognize warnings and contraindications, and determine whether or not contraindications apply. New FDA labeling requirements beginning in 2002 are intended to make it easier for patients to read and understand nonprescription drug labels. Manufacturers are required to use large print, simple language, and an easy-to-read format on the nonprescription drug labels to help patients with product selection and dosage instruction. In addition to these requirements, pharmacists and other health care providers should be on the alert to meet the educational needs of all patients, particularly those with poor reading skills.

Illiteracy is a pervasive, but often unrecognized, problem that affects all population groups and threatens the health of millions of Americans. Health illiteracy is more prevalent in minority groups because of high poverty and school dropout rates. People with low literacy skills are less likely to adhere to medication regimens and appointments or to present for care in the course of treatment of a disease. In a study of hospitalized patients, 49% of patients with hypertension and 44% of those with diabetes were found to have inadequate health literacy for managing their self-care treatment plans.[42]

Studies have documented a relationship between poor reading skills and poor health.[43] Twenty-five percent of U.S. adults (approximately 90 million) read with only marginal literacy skills. It is estimated that 40 million are functionally illiterate, making it difficult or impossible for them to understand routine written information such as dosage instruction on medication bottles, poison warnings, appointment slip reminders, or consent forms.[43]

Low literacy has been called "a quiet disability" because many patients do not acknowledge the problem.[44] People who cannot read often hide their illiteracy because of shame, embarrassment, low self-esteem, and fear. As a result of this behavior, many pharmacists and other health care providers often overlook this potential source of nonadherence to prescription drugs and misinformation concerning nonprescription products.

To detect literacy problems, the practitioner should be sensitive to cues that indicate patient difficulty with reading. For example, patients may say they "forgot their glasses" when asked to read something, or ask you "to fill out a form for me." Poor readers do not like to be exposed and may never join a group education or support group session. Instead, such patients may prefer one-on-one consultations with their health care providers.

Practitioners are encouraged to assess health literacy when developing a self-care plan by using the Test of Functional Health Literacy in Adults (TOFHLA), which is available in English and Spanish,[45] or the Rapid Estimate of Adult Literacy in Medicine (REALM).[46] The TOFHLA tests include items that assess the patient's ability to understand labeled prescription vials, blood glucose test results, clinic appointment slips, and financial information forms. REALM tests a person's ability to read through a list of medical words, moving from short and easy words to difficult and multiple-syllable words. It correlates well with reading tests and offers a good marker for literacy levels. The National Work Group on Literacy recommends that educational materials be developed at a fifth-grade level, and that a variety of media be used to get the message across.[47]

**TABLE 3-7 Concepts of Cultural Competence**

- Demonstrate understanding of and respect for the values, beliefs, and expectations of patients.
- Modify communication approaches, allowing for incorporation of a variety of communication techniques to meet the cultural needs of patients.
- Apply new knowledge and skills to each patient encounter to improve outcomes.
- Apply new knowledge of cultural preferences and drug response variability among patients of different cultures/races to the selection of the best therapy for the patient.
- Adapt and modify the treatment plan based on negotiated agreements.

## Ensuring Cultural Competence in Health Care

### *Elements of Cultural Competency*

Cultural competence has been defined as a set of congruent behaviors and attitudes among professionals that enables them to work effectively in cross-cultural situations.[48] Cultural competence is a continuous process undertaken to ensure that care is delivered in an appropriate manner among diverse populations of patients and practitioners while avoiding cultural generalizations.[49] Development of cultural competency in pharmaceutical care has the potential to increase effectiveness and favorably affect health outcomes, and it helps the practitioner understand the treatment of choice and the monitoring parameters to follow. This is very important in the area of self-care, when the patient has the opportunity to select his or her therapy of choice. By having knowledge in the area of cultural competence and possessing the skills to assess patient's cultural beliefs, the practitioner can help the patient choose treatment options that are congruent with the patient's cultural beliefs. It is believed that this action will lead to better adherence with the treatment and optimal outcomes. Some important elements related to cultural competence are listed in Table 3-7.

At Georgetown University, researchers have described a series of stages that define the continuum of cross-cultural process toward achieving cultural proficiency.[50] The six stages are as follows:

1. *Cultural destructiveness:* This is the beginning of the continuum and represents the most negative stage, in which there is bigotry, racism, discrimination, and exploitation that can harm other cultures and the patients within them. Cultural destructiveness could be an intentional or unintentional behavior. Many health care systems are in this stage but simply do not realize they are. They have policies that can harm patients from different cultures.
2. *Cultural incapacity:* In this stage, an organization or health care practitioner does not have any programs or services available to respond to the needs of patients from other cultures. There is a sense of ethnocentrism in which the dominant culture assumes a paternalistic stance toward other cultures.

3. *Cultural blindness:* In this stage, organizations or individuals try to remain unbiased. They believe that culture or race makes no difference and they treat everyone the same. This is probably the stage that prevails in many health care organizations. In this stage the organization does not have any programs or policies addressing cultural needs of different groups.
4. *Cultural precompetence:* This stage is the first on the positive end of the continuum. Organizations or individuals start to reach out to other cultures by hiring a diverse workforce, hiring translators, or translating materials into different languages. Organizations at this stage of the continuum limit their efforts to one or two initiatives and, at times, they become frustrated with the lack of progress.
5. *Cultural competence:* In this stage, there is an ongoing acceptance and respect for the differences among cultural groups. Practitioners and organizations are continually increasing their knowledge and skills in the area of cultural competence. Models to deliver culturally appropriate care are implemented and there is true commitment to cultural competence and to improving the outcomes of patients from diverse cultures.
6. *Cultural proficiency:* This is the highest level in the continuum. The organizations and practitioners in this stage have a true commitment to culturally competent practices by engaging in research, evaluating new therapies and approaches to care, publishing their findings, conducting training, and disseminating their findings. They have a true commitment to achieving cultural proficiency and value the positive impact that culture has in health care.

To achieve cultural competence, health professionals and the health care systems in which they work will increasingly be expected to undertake major initiatives aimed at achieving changes in awareness, attitude, skills, and behaviors that will enable them to provide effective culturally competent care. This can be achieved only by having a true commitment to change, a real conviction of the significance of the task, and an in-depth assessment of the beliefs and attitudes of the personnel and the institution. The first step in this effort is to conduct a self-assessment of the level of cultural competence in the institution and the care being provided by practitioners. The literature describes many self-assessment instruments. One of these instruments, created by the Georgetown Center on Cultural Competence, is a survey containing a series of questions and statements aimed at having the institution and the practitioner assess current activities in the area of cultural competence. This survey can be found at http://www.aafp.org/fpm/20001000/58cult.html.

Important elements of a culturally competent practice include dissemination of cultural knowledge and skills as well as advocacy. The dissemination of cultural knowledge and skills should be targeted at decreasing racism or other forms of bias and increasing awareness among practitioners of the influence of culture in health. Advocacy efforts should involve recognition of racism in the health care provider and actions taken by the health care provider to reverse racism. Only by incorporating these two final elements can a practitioner deliver culturally competent care.

To develop a service or program that is culturally competent, the practitioner may want to follow the recommendations included in the publication *Getting Started...and Moving On,* which outlines the steps in developing a comprehensive community mental health service for children and family. Even though the recommendations are for a mental health service, the steps can be incorporated into any community outreach program. A copy can be found at http://www.georgetown.edu/research/gucdc/nccc/documents/Getting_Started_SAMHSA.pdf. A practical guide to the development of culturally competent health promotion materials can be found at http://www.georgetown.edu/research/gucdc/nccc/documents/Materials_Guide.pdf.

Unfortunately, cultural competence often requires on-the-job training because of a lack of formalized training in this area in many health care professional schools. An increased level of cultural competence training in the health professions schools and continuing education programming is needed.

The case scenarios on the following pages illustrate important aspects of cultural competence care in the area of self-care. These cases are examples of issues that are commonly observed in community practice.

## Key Points for Multicultural Aspects of Self-Care

- Major shifts in the demographics of the U.S. population are affecting the delivery of care to patients.
- Currently, minority populations are experiencing a broad range of health disparities compared with their white counterparts. A disproportionately high number of minority patients are experiencing increased rates of complications with chronic diseases compared with other populations.
- Cultural issues affect patients' attitudes and behaviors toward health and illness, as well as their acceptance and adherence to treatment plans.
- The inability of health care providers, including pharmacists, to deliver effective culturally competent care can affect the health outcome of diverse patient populations.
- To become culturally competent, health care providers need to evaluate their biases and prejudices, and acquire the knowledge and skills to become culturally competent. Cultural competence implies that the health care provider has the knowledge and skills to deal effectively with diverse patient populations and is able to apply these to the care of patients.
- Delivering culturally competent pharmaceutical care should be a goal of every health care provider, particularly in the area of self-care. Self-care lends itself very well to the practice of culturally competent pharmaceutical care. Many minority groups seek nonprescription products and herbal and alternative therapies as their main source of care.

### CASE 3-1
### CULTURAL COMPETENCE IN SELF-CARE

**Patient Complaint/History**

Mr. Truong is a 63-year-old Korean man, who comes to the pharmacy on a Friday afternoon complaining of stomach pains. The patient enters the pharmacy and is waiting to have the opportunity to ask the pharmacist for an nonprescription product recommendation. He speaks limited English and is afraid to interrupt the pharmacist to ask the question. After approximately 25 minutes of waiting, a clerk realizes that the patient is waiting and asks if he needs help. The patient proceeds to tell the clerk that he would like to talk to the pharmacist. The pharmacist comes from behind the counter and proceeds to ask the patient about his condition. The patient looks down and answers with "yes" and "no" responses. The pharmacist elicits the following information: the patient has lost a lot of weight (15 pounds in 2 months) because of his inability to eat, he has had epigastric pain for the last 3 months, and he denies using alcohol or smoking. He moved to this country 8 months ago. Currently, he is in a lot of pain, but states he "is OK." The patient wants to know "Which pain medicine is better to treat my pain?"

*What would be an appropriate action at this time?*
*What do you think is going on with Mr. Truong?*

**Clinical/Cultural Considerations**

Mr. Truong may have different beliefs and perceptions concerning his pain. It is important to assess what his beliefs are and what other treatment (alternative treatments or herbals) he has tried already. This patient is of Asian descent, which puts him at a high risk for stomach cancer. It is important to assess the patient's symptoms and understand that in many Asian countries patients are taught to tolerate pain quietly. Pain perception is also influenced to a very large extent by our cultural definition of pain. How pain and discomfort are presented varies among cultures. The fact that Mr. Truong is seeking medications implies that the symptoms are very severe and he has probably tried other alternative treatments that have failed. All of these factors indicate that this patient needs to be referred for further evaluation. Analgesics are not an appropriate alternative at this time. The options concerning his treatment must be explained to the patient.

### CASE 3-2
### CULTURAL COMPETENCE IN SELF-CARE

**Patient Complaint/History**

Mrs. Gonzalez is a 48-year-old Hispanic woman who comes to the pharmacy asking to speak to the pharmacist. The patient asks the pharmacist for antibiotics to treat her cold. The pharmacist indicates that she needs a prescription for antibiotics. The patient is insistent and becomes angry when the pharmacist refuses to give her an antibiotic.

*What would be an appropriate action at this time?*
*What do you think is going on with Mrs. Gonzalez?*

**Clinical/Cultural Considerations**

Mrs. Gonzalez obviously has different beliefs and perceptions concerning the treatment of the common cold. In her country of origin (Mexico), it is a common practice for a patient to go to the pharmacy seeking treatment for a variety of symptoms. In many provinces in Mexico, the dispensing of antibiotics does not require a prescription. This patient is not familiar with the laws in the United States and the differences in the health care system. It is important for the pharmacist not to criticize the health care system in her country of origin (this will create a negative environment and jeopardize the pharmacist–patient relationship) and to educate the patient about the differences in the laws of both countries. The pharmacist must welcome the patient's trust in the pharmacist and congratulate the patient for seeking advice. The patient must be informed that there are other nonprescription products designed to alleviate the symptoms of the common cold and the pharmacist would be pleased to recommend one of these products. The patient needs to be assured that the symptoms should subside in approximately 48 to 72 hours and she can come back to see the pharmacist if she does not get relief. The patient must feel there is *respeto* (respect) and *confianza* (trust) in her relationship with the pharmacist. Hispanic patients value these two components of their relationships with health care providers.

## References


1. US Census Bureau, US Department of Commerce. *United States Census 2000.* Available at: http://census.gov/popest/estimates.php. Accessed August 8, 2005.
2. Spector RE. *Cultural Diversity in Health and Illness.* 6th ed. Upper Saddle River, NJ: Pearson Prentice Hall; 2004.
3. Report of the Ad Hoc Committee on Affirmative Action and Diversity. *Am J Pharm Educ.* 2000;64(suppl): 53-7S.
4. Pachter DO. Culture and clinical care: folk illness beliefs and behaviors and their implications for health care delivery. *JAMA.* 1994;271:690-4.
5. Kleinman A, Eisenberg L, Good B. Culture, illness, and care: clinical lessons from anthropologic and cross cultural research. *Ann Intern Med.* 1978:88:251-8.
6. Kleinman, A. *Patients and Healers in the Context of Culture.* Berkeley: University of California Press; 1980.
7. Boyd EL, Shimp LA, Hackney MJ. *Home* Remedies *and the Black Elderly: A Reference Manual for Health Care Providers.* Ann Arbor: Institute of Gerontology and the University of Michigan College of Pharmacy; 1984.
8. National Center for Complementary and Alternative Medicine. What Is Complementary and Alternative Medicine (CAM)? Available at: http://nccam.nih.gov/health/whatiscam/. Accessed February 25, 2005.
9. Seidl HM, Ball JW, Dains JE, et al. Cultural awareness. In: *Mosby's Guide to Physical Examination.* 4th ed. St. Louis: Mosby; 1999.
10. Eisenberg DM, Davis RB, Ettner SL, et al. Trends in alternative medicine use in the United States. 1990-1997: results of a follow up national survey. *JAMA.* 1998;280:1569-75.
11. Kuo GM, Hawley ST, Weiss LT, et al. Factors associated with herbal use among urban multiethnic primary care patients: a cross-sectional study. *BMC Complementary Alternative Med.* 2004,4:18.
12. Bates DW, Cullen DJ, Laird N, et al. Incidence of adverse events and potential adverse drug events. *JAMA.* 1995;274:29-34.
13. Brass EP. Drug therapy: changing the status of drugs from prescription to over-the-counter availability. *N Engl J Med.* 2001;345:810-6.
14. Oborne CA. Luzac ML. Over-the-counter medicine use prior to and during hospitalization. *Ann Pharmacother.* 2005;39:268-73.

## CASE 3-3
## CULTURAL COMPETENCE IN SELF-CARE

### Patient Complaint/History

Ms. Jones is a 35-year-old African American with a history of hypertension and diabetes. She comes to the pharmacy asking the pharmacist for a product called "Noni Juice." Her cousin recommended that she get this product because she saw on television that it cures diabetes. The patient's mother has diabetes and is currently undergoing kidney dialysis, and her father has hypertension and diabetes. The patient is concerned about her diseases and wants a cure. She has tried other alternative treatments, including home remedies, with little success.

*What would be an appropriate action at this time?*
*What do you think is going on with Ms. Jones?*

### Clinical/Cultural Considerations

Ms. Jones may have different beliefs and perceptions concerning the etiology and pathophysiology of her disease. She has a strong family history for diabetes and hypertension. In many African-American families, it is common for family members to share medications and use home remedies. Family is very important and the advice of a family member is taken seriously. Obviously, this patient is having issues coping with her diseases and has a fear of complications. Therefore, it is important to assess what her issues are with her current treatment and emphasize the need for adherence with therapy to prevent complications associated with her medical conditions. How is this done? The pharmacist must explain the limited amount of scientific data on the effectiveness and safety available for many herbal products. The patient needs to be assured that her relative had her well-being in mind, but there are no data supporting the use of "Noni Juice" in the treatment of diabetes. Many herbal products contain active ingredients that can make the patient's condition worse or interact with the medications the patient is taking. The pharmacist must offer the patient assistance in managing her conditions.


15. Lundberg L, Johannesson M, Isacson D. The effects of user charges on the use of prescription medicines in different socioeconomic groups. *Health Policy.* 1998;44:123-34.
16. National Institutes of Health, US Department of Health and Human Services. *NIH Guidelines on the Inclusion of Women and Minorities as Subjects* Available at: http://grants.nih.gov/grants/funding/women_min/women_min.htm. Accessed August 10, 2005.
17. US Food and Drug Administration, Center for Drug Evaluation and Research. *Guidance for Industry: Population Pharmacokinetics.* February 1999. Available at: http://www.fda.gov/cder/guidance/index.htm. Accessed August 10, 2005.
18. Evans WE, McLeod HL. Pharmacogenomics: drug disposition, drug targets, and side effects. *N Engl J Med.* 2003;348:538-49.
19. Kalow W, Tang BK, Endrenyi I. Hypothesis: comparisons of inter- and intra-individual variations can substitute for twin studies in drug research. *Pharmacogenetics.* 1998;8:283-9.
20. US Department of Health and Human Services. Eliminating racial and health disparities in health. *Public Health Rep.* 1998;113:372.
21. Keppel KG, Pearcy JN, Wagener DK. Trends in racial and ethnic-specific rates for health status indicators: United States, 1990-98. In: *Healthy People Statistical Notes No. 23.* Hyattsville, Md: National Center for Health Statistics; January 2002.
22. US Department of Health and Human Services. The President's Initiative on Race, Healthcare Rx: Access for All. Barriers to Healthcare for Racial and Ethnic Minorities: Access, Workforce Diversity and Cultural Competence. Washington, DC: US Department of Health and Human Services; 1998.
23. US Census Bureau, Census 2000. *Summary File 1.* Available at: http://www.factfinder.census.gov. Accessed August 10, 2005.
24. Pappas G, Queen S, Hadden W, et al. The increasing disparity in mortality between socioeconomic groups in the United States, 1960-1986. *N Engl J Med.* 1993;329:103-9.
25. *Healthy People 2010.* Available at: http://www.healthypeople.gov. Accessed August 10, 2005.
26. US Census Bureau. Population projections of the United States by age, sex, race, and Hispanic 12origin: 1995 to 2050. In: *Current Populations Reports, 1996.* Available at: http://www.census.gov/prod/1/pop/p25-1130. Accessed August 10, 2005.
27. Collins KS, Hughes DL, Doty MM, et al. Diverse Communities, Common Concerns: Assessing Health Care Quality for Minority Americans. Findings from the Commonwealth Fund 2001 Health Care Quality Survey. New York: The Commonwealth Fund; 2002. Pub No. 523.
28. Eberhardt MS, Ingram DD, Makuc DM, et al. *Health, United States, 2001, with Urban and Rural Health Chartbook.* Hyattsville, Md: National Center for Health Statistics; 2001.
29. Smedley BD, Stith AY, Nelson AR, eds. Committee on Understanding and Eliminating Racial and Ethnic Disparities in Health Care, Board on Health Sciences Policy. Unequal Treatment: Confronting Racial and Ethnic Disparities in Health Care. Washington, DC: National Academy Press; 2002.
30. US Department of Health and Human Services, Office of Minority Health. *National Standards for Culturally and Linguistically Appropriate Services in Health Care: Final Report.* Washington, DC: US Department of Health and Human Services;March 2001. P3-20. Available at: http://www.omhrc.gov/omh/programs/2pgprograms/finalreport.pdf. Accessed February 25, 2005.
31. Berlin EA, Fowkes WC Jr. A teaching framework for cross-cultural care: application in family practice in cross cultural medicine. *West J Med.* 1983;12:93-8.
32. Bensoussan A. Complementary medicine—where lies its appeal [editorial]. *Med J Aust.* 1999;170:247-8.
33. Kaptchuk TJ, Eisenberg D. The persuasive appeal of alternative medicine. *Ann Intern Med.* 1998;129:1061-5.
34. Shoor S, Lorig KR. Self-care and the doctor-patient relationship. *Med Care.* 2002;40(4 suppl):II40-4.
35. Rogers A, Entwistle V, Pencheon D. A patient led NHS: managing demand at the interface between lay and primary care. *BMJ.* 1998;316:1816-9.
36. *From Compliance to Concordance: Achieving* Shared *Goals in Medicine Taking.* London: Royal Pharmaceutical Society of Great Britain, and Merck Sharp and Dohme; 1997.
37. Stewart M, Brown JB, Boon H, et al. Evidence on patient-doctor communication. *Cancer Prev Control.* 1999;3:25-30.
38. Nichols-English G, Poirier S. Optimizing adherence to pharmaceutical care plans. *J APhA.* 2000;40:475-85.
39. Somnath S, Komaromy M, Koepsell TD, et al. Patient-physician racial concordance and the perceived quality and use of health care. *Arch Intern Med.* 1999;159:997-1004.
40. Stuart B, Grana J. Ability to pay and the decision to medicate. *Med Care.*1998:36:202-11.
41. McRae K. Socioeconomic deprivation and health and the ecological fallacy. *BMJ.* 1994;309:1478-9.
42. Williams MV, Baker DW, Parker RM, et al. Relationship of functional health literacy to patient's knowledge of their chronic disease: a study of patients with hypertension and diabetes. *Arch Intern Med.* 1998;158:166-72.

43. Baker DS, Parker RM, Williams MV, et al. The relationship of patient reading ability to self-reported health and use of health services. *Am J Public Health.* 1997;87:1027-30.
44. Parikh NS, Parker RM, Nurss JR, et al. Shame and health literacy: the unspoken connection. *Patient Educ Couns.* 1996;27:33-9.
45. Parker RM, Baker DW, Williams MV, et al. The test of functional health literacy in adults: a new instrument for measuring patients' literacy skills. *J Gen Intern Med.* 1995;10:537-41.
46. Davis TC, Crouch MA, Long SW, et al. Rapid assessment of literacy levels of adult primary care patients. *J Fam Med.* 1991;23: 433-5.
47. Weiss BD. Communicating with patients who have limited literacy skills: report of the National Work Group on Literacy and Health. *J Fam Pract.* 1998;46:168-76.
48. Cohen E, Goode TD. *Policy Brief 1:Rationale for* Cultural *Competence in Primary Health Care.* Washington, DC: National Center for Cultural Competence; 1999.
49. Kim-Godwin YS, Clarke PN, Burton L. A model for the delivery of culturally competent community care. *J Adv Nurs.* 2001;35: 918-25.
50. Cross TL, Bazron BJ, Dennis KW, et al. Towards a Culturally Competent System of Care: A Monograph on Effective Services for Minority Children Who Are Severely Emotionally Disturbed. Washington, DC: Child and Adolescent Service System Program, Technical Assistance Center, Center for Child Health and Mental Health Policy, Georgetown University Child Development Center; 1989.

CHAPTER 4

# Legal and Regulatory Issues in Self-Care Pharmacy Practice

*Ilisa B. G. Bernstein and Edward D. Rickert*

This chapter analyzes the federal laws and regulations that govern the manufacturing, distribution, labeling, and marketing of the products patients commonly use for self-care. There are differences in the way nonprescription drugs are regulated compared with prescription-only drugs and other consumer health care products, such as dietary supplements and homeopathic medicines. It is important that health care providers have a basic understanding of these regulations so they can respond to their patients' questions and concerns about the self-care products they use.

## Regulation of Nonprescription Drugs

The first major federal legislation enacted in the United States to regulate drugs was the Pure Food and Drug Act of 1906. "Unsafe" and "nonefficacious" drug products were not actually prohibited by the statute; drugs were required to meet only the standards of strength, quality, and purity claimed by the manufacturers. Laws did not mandate drug safety until passage of the 1938 Federal Food, Drug, and Cosmetic Act (FD&C Act). In 1951, an amendment to the FD&C Act in essence established two classes of drugs: prescription-only and nonprescription (also referred to as over-the-counter, or OTC). Before that time, manufacturers were free to determine to which category their drug product belonged. Drugs that could be used safely without medical supervision and had labeling that included adequate directions for use could be marketed without a prescription. In 1962, a major amendment to the FD&C Act was enacted, requiring that all new drugs be shown to be effective, as well as safe, for their intended uses. As a result of this amendment, the Food and Drug Administration (FDA) undertook a review of the effectiveness of 4500 new drug products, including 512 nonprescription drugs that had been approved only for safety since 1938.

In 1972, FDA initiated a massive scientific review of the 700 active ingredients in 300,000 nonprescription drug formulations to ensure that they were safe and effective, and bore fully informative labeling. This review process, which is still underway, is often referred to as the "OTC Drug Review."

FDA is also responsible for the labeling of nonprescription drugs and reclassifying (i.e., switching) drugs from prescription to nonprescription status. Consequently, nonprescription drugs that are on the market today fall into one of the three following categories (from a legal and regulatory perspective):

1. Approved via the drug approval process and either (a) reclassified (i.e., switched) from prescription to nonprescription or (b) approved directly as a nonprescription drug
2. Approved via the monograph process (described in OTC Monograph Process later in this chapter)
3. On the market pending a determination under the OTC Drug Review monograph process of the drug's disposition

### Drug Approval Process

The FD&C Act of 1938, as amended in 1962, requires that all new drugs introduced for marketing be cleared in advance through a new drug application (NDA), which requires that the drugs be proven safe and effective for human use before being marketed. Products marketed before 1938 were exempted from the NDA requirement under a grandfather clause. Some currently marketed nonprescription drugs, such as aspirin, still fall under this clause. However, FDA's Office of Nonprescription Products has evaluated, or is in the process of evaluating, all nonprescription drugs for safety, effectiveness, and labeling, regardless of the date of marketing entry.[1]

A new chemical entity never before marketed in the United States would be classified as a new drug and, in most cases, initially be approved for prescription use only. An NDA for a nonprescription drug product can also be approved directly (without reclassification), which is what occurred with ibuprofen 200 mg (a dose that was never available by prescription). When a new drug is used for many years by many patients (referred to in the FD&C Act as "used for a material time and material extent"), it may be considered generally recognized as "safe and effective" and qualifies for marketing as a nonprescription drug. Additionally, under new regulations, certain data regarding the safety, efficacy, and use of the product in a foreign country can be used to determine if a drug can be marketed as a nonprescription product in the United States.[2]

Some drugs are available by prescription-only and nonprescription in the same strength, but marketed for different uses. For example, nonprescription meclizine is available for motion sickness, which is easy to diagnose,

**Editor's Note:** Views presented in this chapter do not necessarily reflect those of the Food and Drug Administration.

and by prescription for vertigo, which is a complex condition that is not easy to diagnose and treat.

### New Drug Application

An NDA is necessary for a drug the FD&C Act defines as not recognized as safe and effective until it has been reviewed and approved by FDA.[3] The approved NDA is manufacturer specific and allows only the sponsor (applicant) to market the product. Any other manufacturer interested in marketing a similar product would first need to seek FDA approval through its own NDA. In some cases, a full NDA is not necessary for the second manufacturer; an abbreviated NDA (ANDA) may be submitted instead, eliminating the need for duplicative testing. All NDAs must contain complete labeling information, with final printed labeling being the usual last step before approval (see Drug Facts Labeling for Nonprescription Drugs).

### OTC Monograph Process

An OTC monograph is developed for therapeutic classes of ingredients that are generally recognized as safe and effective (also referred to as "GRAS/E"). A manufacturer desiring to market a product containing an ingredient covered under an OTC monograph need not seek FDA's prior approval. In this case, marketing is not exclusive; any manufacturer may market a similar product without specific approval. Under the monograph approach, all data and information supporting safety and efficacy of the product and its nonprescription status are publicly available. The FDA Office of Nonprescription Products has established the monographs through a complex administrative process called rulemaking, which allows for comments from the general public, manufacturers, and other interested parties. Each individual rulemaking has resulted in an administrative record that is extensive. Figure 4-1 illustrates the process by which the OTC drug monographs are reviewed.

Under a final OTC monograph, the manufacturer has considerable flexibility in labeling. All the required monograph labeling must be included; for example, antacids must include terms such as heartburn, acid indigestion, and sour stomach. In addition, certain language not included in the monograph may be used in specific places on the label without prior approval. For example, *hospital-tested* or *pleasant-tasting antacid* are terms considered outside the scope of the monograph, but permissible in antacid labeling. However, even though these permissible terms are not precleared, they are subject to the general labeling provision of the FD&C Act and may not be false or misleading.

Monographs primarily address active ingredient(s) in the product and, in most cases, final formulations are not subject to monograph specifications. Manufacturers are free to include any inactive ingredients that serve a pharmaceutical purpose, provided those ingredients are safe and do not interfere with either product effectiveness or any required final product testing. In a few instances, even though the product contains generally recognized safe and effective ingredients, it may need to meet a monograph-testing procedure; for example, antacids must pass an acid-neutralizing test.

Because the drugs in the OTC monograph system are GRAS/E, there is no legal or regulatory requirement to report adverse events associated with these products. Historically, any changes in ingredient status and labeling have occurred as a result of adverse drug findings reported in the literature or through similar public mechanisms. FDA's MedWatch program is a safety information and adverse event reporting system for medical products, including nonprescription drugs. Health care professionals and consumers are encouraged by FDA to report serious adverse events that they suspect are associated with the drugs they dispense, prescribe, or use. Reporting can be done online or by telephone, fax, or mail. The Web site is www.fda.gov/medwatch.[4] FDA uses this information to examine adverse trends and, if necessary, take appropriate action (see Adverse Event Reporting).

## Labeling and Packaging Issues

### "Drug Facts" Labeling for Nonprescription Drugs

It is essential that the labeling of nonprescription drug products clearly communicate to the patient the important information on how to use the product safely and effectively. In recent years, FDA and consumers have been concerned about the adequacy of labeling for nonprescription drugs. This concern is heightened because an increasing number of prescription drugs are being switched from prescription to nonprescription status. Many of these "switch" drugs require the patient to perform more sophisticated self-diagnostic and self-monitoring evaluations. Therefore, to provide adequate directions and safety information, a greater number of sophisticated messages must be communicated through the nonprescription label.

Recognizing these concerns, FDA has changed nonprescription drug labeling requirements. FDA regulations now require a standardized content and format for the labels on the estimated 100,000 nonprescription drugs on the market.[5] Nonprescription drug labels have an area on the package designated as the "Drug Facts" box, which contains the information required by FDA to be on the label.[6] A nonprescription product that lacks this new area may be considered misbranded and subject to the same enforcement approach that FDA can take with other misbranded drugs, including issuance of a warning letter, product seizures, and injunctions.

The nonprescription labeling regulations make it easier for consumers to read and understand information about the product's benefits and risks and how it should be taken. It also helps consumers select the right product to meet their needs. The format enables consumers to determine readily and easily whether a product contains ingredients they need, do not need, or should not take. It also makes it easy for consumers to compare similar products to determine which has the appropriate ingredients for their symptoms or personal health situation.

The Drug Facts labeling format, with standardized headings and subheadings, also uses terms that are familiar to consumers, for example, *uses* instead of *indications*. Lay

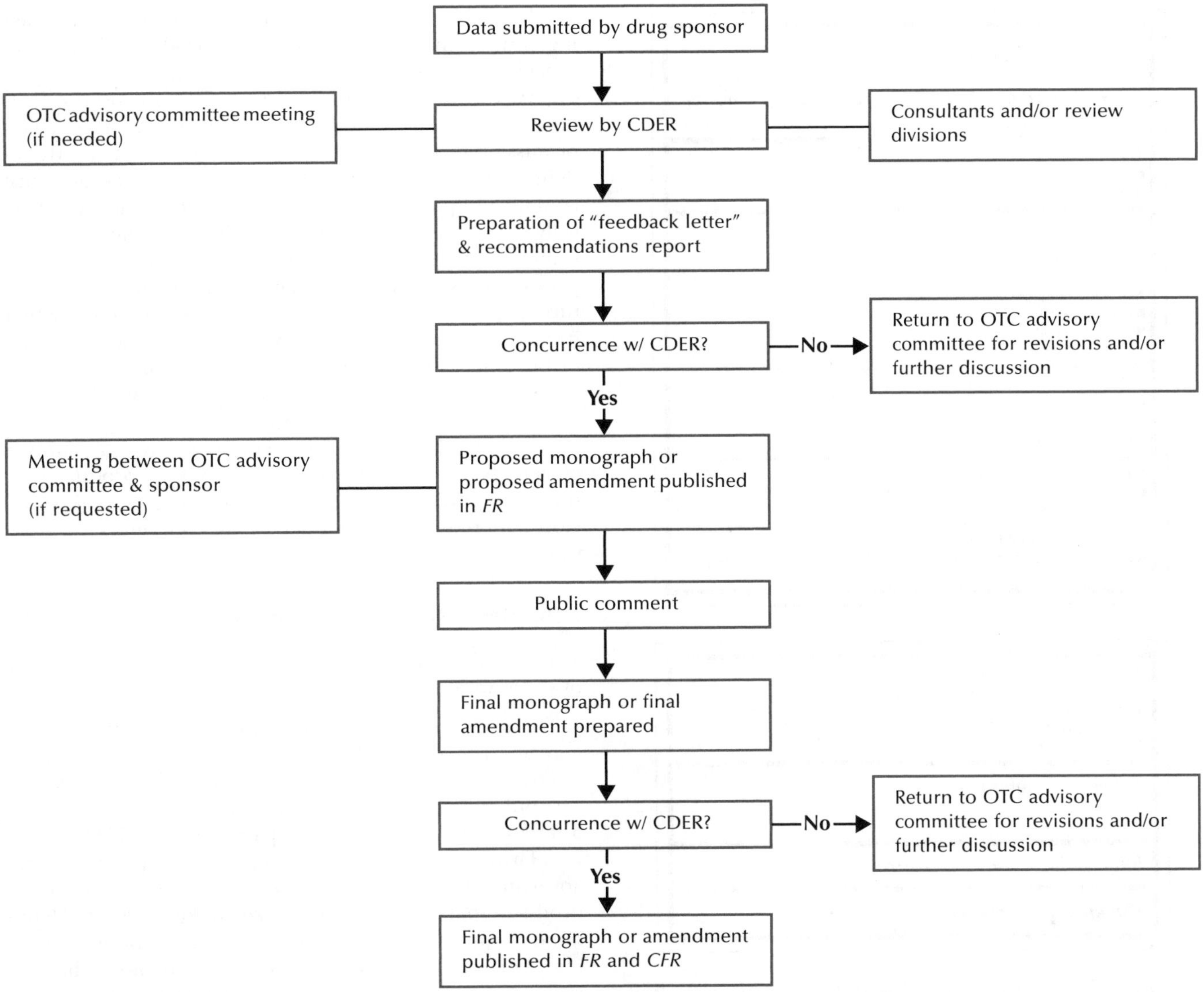


**FIGURE 4-1** OTC drug monograph review process, showing how CDER determines the safety and effectiveness of OTC drug products. Key: CDER, Center for Drug Evaluation and Research; *CFR, Code of Federal Regulations; FR, Federal Register*; OTC, over-the-counter. (*Source:* http://www.fda.gov/cder/handbook/otc.htm. Accessed October 7, 2003.)

terms are also used instead of medical jargon (e.g., *lung* instead of *pulmonary*).

The population of persons 65 years of age or older is increasing. Older people are significant users of nonprescription products, and they may have greater difficulty reading product labels because of decreasing visual functioning. The labeling requirements set a minimal type size that labels must use, and labels cannot use any type smaller than the minimal standard. An easy-to-read font style is also required, as are other graphical features that enhance the ability to read the information on the label clearly.

Pharmacists should be familiar with the Drug Facts format. It is an essential counseling tool for nonprescription drugs. The Drug Facts format allows pharmacists to readily find information on the label and point it out to the patient. Figure 4-2 illustrates the basic Drug Facts format and the standardized headings and order of information. Figures 4-3 and 4-4 show examples of the Drug Facts format.

Dietary supplements are not regulated as "drugs" under the FD&C Act. Consequently, they do not follow the Drug Facts format. Dietary supplements must be labeled in accordance with the regulations discussed in Dietary Supplements.

### *Expiration Date Labeling*

Most nonprescription drug products are required to include an expiration date on the labeling.[7] This is the date beyond which the product should not be used because the stability, potency, strength, or quality may have been affected over time. FDA regulations govern how this date is determined and tested. Most nonprescription drug product labels must also include any special storage conditions or requirements for the product. nonprescription drug products that do not have a dosage limit and are stable for at least 3 years are exempt from the requirement to include the expiration date on the label. Such products

**Drug Facts**

| **Active ingredient (in each dosage unit)** | **Purpose** |
|---|---|
| xxxxxxxxxxxxxxx mg | xxxxxxxxxx |

**Uses**
- xxxxxxxxxxxxxx
- xxxxxxxxxxxxxx

**Warnings**

**Do not use** xxxxxxxxxxxxxxxxxxxxxxxxxxxxxxxxxxxxxxx

**Ask a doctor before use if you have**
- xxxxxxxxxxxxxx
- xxxxxxxxxxxxxx

**Ask a doctor or pharmacist before use if you are** xxxxxxxxxxxxxx

**When using this product**
- xxxxxxxxxxxxxx
- xxxxxxxxxxxxxx

**Stop use and ask a doctor if**
- xxxxxxxxxxxxxx
- xxxxxxxxxxxxxx

**If pregnant or breast-feeding,** ask a health professional before use.
**Keep out of reach of children.** In case of overdose, get medical help or contact a Poison Control Center right away.

**Drug Facts** (continued)

**Directions**
- xxxxxxxxxxxxxx
- xxxxxxxxxxxxxx

**Other information**
- xxxxxxxxxxxxxx
- xxxxxxxxxxxxxx

**Inactive ingredients** xxxxxxxxxxxxxx

**Questions?** 123-555-1234

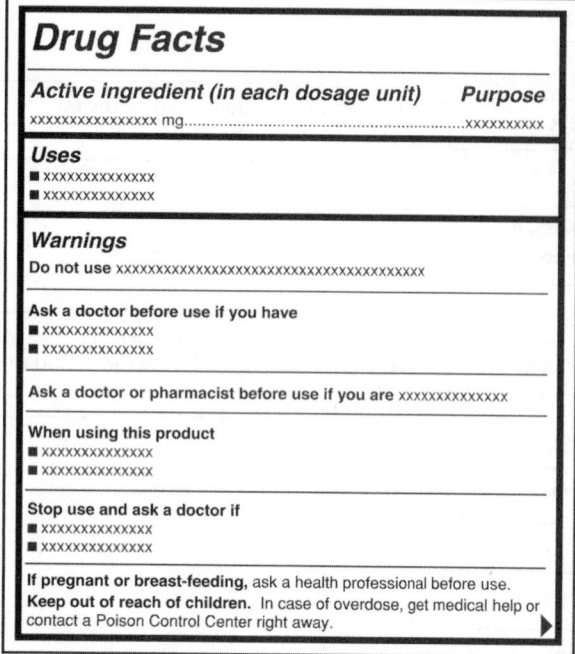

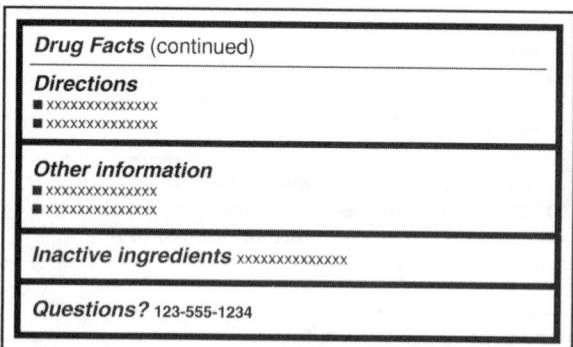

FIGURE 4-2 Drug facts labeling outline. (*Source:* 21 CFR 201.66.)

include certain topical drugs, skin protectants, lotions, and astringents.

Health care providers should remind patients to check their nonprescription product labels periodically to ensure that the expiration date has not passed. Patients often ask whether a nonprescription drug product they have at home is still good if the expiration date has passed. Although safety issues rarely arise from using a drug that is modestly past its expiration date, the patient should be advised that the product has probably lost some of its ability to work as effectively as possible for the particular symptom or medical problem and it should be discarded.

### Tamper-evident Packaging

In the wake of several high-profile tampering incidents involving nonprescription drug products, FDA instituted several packaging, labeling, and manufacturing requirements to protect consumers. Historically, the term *tamper-resistant* was used to describe methods used to prevent tampering. The focus has shifted to "tamper-evident," to heighten consumer awareness of any evidence of tampering, rather than attempt to make products difficult to breach or tamper-proof.

With few exceptions, nonprescription drug products must have one or more barriers to entry that, if breached or missing from the package, provide consumers with evidence that tampering may have occurred.[8] Packages must contain unique designs or other characteristics that typically cannot be duplicated. Additionally, to alert the consumer to the specific tamper-evident features, the retail package must contain a statement that identifies the feature, is prominently placed on the package, in a way that it will be unaffected if the tamper-evident feature is missing or breached. For example, the statement on a bottle with a shrink band might say, "For your protection, this bottle has an imprinted seal around the neck."

Patients should be educated to check for the tamper-evident features on every nonprescription product they purchase and, if the features are missing or look suspicious, to return the product to the pharmacy or store where it was purchased as soon as possible.

## Drug Reclassification: Prescription-to-OTC Switch

Traditionally, a prescription-to-OTC switch occurs in one of three ways:

1. The drug is switched through the nonprescription drug review process.
2. The manufacturer requests the switch by submitting a supplemental application to its approved NDA.
3. The manufacturer or other party petitions FDA.

Through the OTC drug review process, panels of nongovernment experts are reviewing the prescription drug products that were on the market before 1962 to determine if some are appropriate for nonprescription marketing. This ongoing process has produced more than 40 reclassifications from prescription-only to nonprescription status since the 1970s.

Another common way that a prescription drug is switched to nonprescription status is for the manufacturer to submit data to FDA, in the form of a supplemental NDA, demonstrating that the drug is appropriate for self-administration. Typically, these applications include studies showing that the product's labeling can be read, understood, and followed by a consumer without the guidance of a health care provider.[10] FDA reviews this information, along with any information known about the drug from its prescription use history. All of this information is usually presented to FDA's Nonprescription Drug Advisory Committee, which is composed of nongovernment experts. This committee serves as a forum for the exchange of ideas and recommends to FDA whether the drug in question should be switched to nonprescription status. The FDA is not bound by the committee's recommendation, but usually it follows the committee's advice.

Overall, more than 700 nonprescription drug products are on the market today that use ingredients or dosages once available only by prescription.[9] The categories of drug products that have seen the most activity in this area are analgesics, $H_1$ and $H_2$ histamine receptor antagonists,

**Drug Facts**

| **Active ingredient (in each tablet)** | **Purpose** |
|---|---|
| Chlorpheniramine maleate 2 mg | Antihistamine |

**Uses** temporarily relieves these symptoms due to hay fever or other upper respiratory allergies: ■ sneezing ■ runny nose ■ itchy, watery eyes ■ itchy throat

**Warnings**

**Ask a doctor before use if you have**
■ glaucoma ■ a breathing problem such as emphysema or chronic bronchitis
■ trouble urinating due to an enlarged prostate gland

**Ask a doctor or pharmacist before use if you are** taking tranquilizers or sedatives

**When using this product**
■ you may get drowsy ■ avoid alcoholic drinks
■ alcohol, sedatives, and tranquilizers may increase drowsiness
■ be careful when driving a motor vehicle or operating machinery
■ excitability may occur, especially in children

**If pregnant or breast-feeding,** ask a health professional before use.
**Keep out of reach of children.** In case of overdose, get medical help or contact a Poison Control Center right away.

**Directions**

| | |
|---|---|
| adults and children 12 years and over | take 2 tablets every 4 to 6 hours; not more than 12 tablets in 24 hours |
| children 6 years to under 12 years | take 1 tablet every 4 to 6 hours; not more than 6 tablets in 24 hours |
| children under 6 years | ask a doctor |

**Drug Facts** (continued)

**Other information** ■ store at 20-25°C (68-77°F) ■ protect from excessive moisture

**Inactive ingredients** D&C yellow no. 10, lactose, magnesium stearate, microcrystalline cellulose, pregelatinized starch

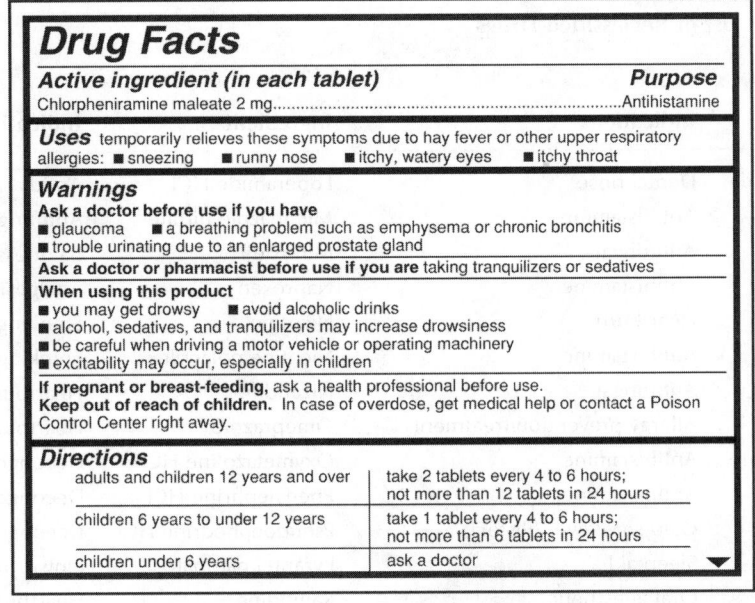

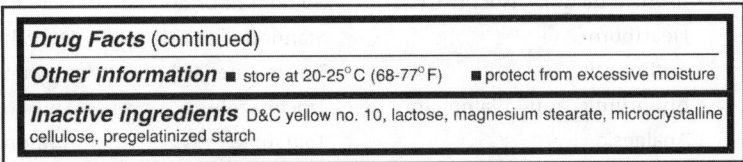

FIGURE 4-3 Drug facts labeling example. (*Source*: 21 CFR 201.66.)

antifungal medications, smoking deterrents, and topical medications used to treat minor skin conditions. Drug products in these categories are good candidates for prescription to nonprescription switching because they are used to treat self-limiting conditions that are easily identified by laypersons, with or without the assistance of a health care provider.

A company, usually the manufacturer, can also petition FDA to switch a drug or class of drugs to nonprescription status. In recent years, however, FDA has received petitions originating not from the drug's manufacturer, but from third-party payers.[11] Citing FDA's statutory authority under Section 503(b) of the FD&C Act to remove the prescription requirement for a drug when doing so will not create a threat to public health, third-party payers have petitioned FDA, seeking to have certain drugs switched from prescription to nonprescription status. Three recent examples include the nonsedating antihistamines loratadine, fexofenadine, and cetirizine. In 2002, loratadine was switched to nonprescription status after the manufacturer dropped its original opposition to the switch. However, fexofenadine and cetirizine have retained their prescription-only status.

It is easy to understand why third-party payers, employers, and state and federal health care programs have taken a strong interest in increasing the number of prescription-to-OTC switches. The availability of nonprescription products for self-treatment may save consumers millions of dollars in health care costs by reducing the number of physician visits, preventing unnecessary sick days from work, and decreasing costs associated with the advancement of

**Drug Facts**

| **Active ingredient** | **Purpose** |
|---|---|
| Selenium sulfide 1% | Antidandruff |

**Use** controls scalp itching and flaking due to dandruff

**Warnings**
**For external use only**

**Ask a doctor before use if you have**
■ seborrheic dermatitis that covers a large area of the body

**When using this product**
■ do not get into eyes. If contact occurs, rinse eyes thoroughly with water.

**Stop use and ask a doctor if**
■ condition worsens or does not improve after regular use

**Keep out of reach of children.** If swallowed, get medical help or contact a Poison Control Center right away.

**Directions**
■ shake well ■ for best results, use at least 2 times a week

**Inactive ingredients** water, ammonium laureth sulfate, ammonium lauryl sulfate, cocamide MEA, glycol disterate, ammonium xylenesulfonate, dimethicone, tricetylmonium chloride, cetyl alcohol, DMDM hydantoin, sodium chloride, stearyl alcohol, hydroxypropyl methylcellulose, FD&C red no. 4

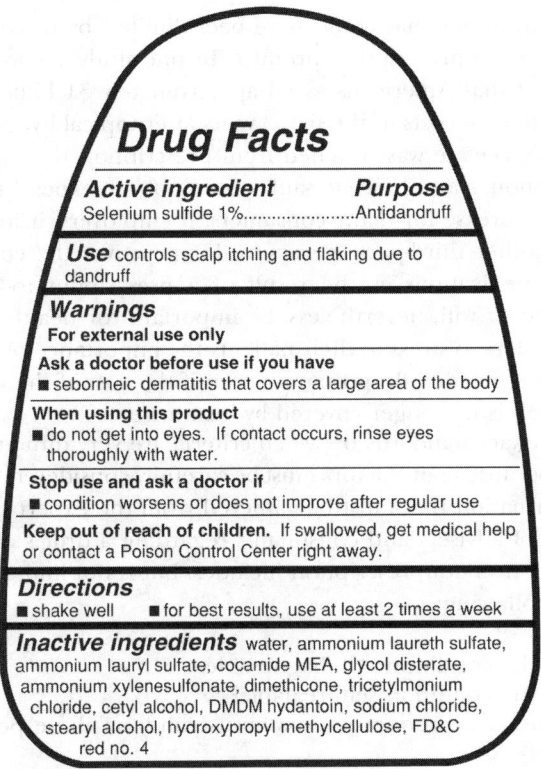

FIGURE 4-4 Drugs facts labeling example. (*Source: Federal Register.* 1999;64:13301).

**TABLE 4-1 Selected List of Reclassified Drugs**

| Ingredient | Indications | Ingredient | Indications |
|---|---|---|---|
| Acidulated phosphate fluoride | Dental rinse | Loperamide HCl | Antidiarrheal |
| Brompheniramine maleate | Antihistamine | Miconazole nitrate | Antifungal |
| Butoconazole nitrate | Antifungal | Minoxidil | Baldness |
| Chlorpheniramine maleate | Antihistamine | Naproxen | Analgesic |
| Cimetidine | Heartburn | Nicotine | Smoking cessation |
| Clemastine fumarate | Antihistamine | Nicotine polacrilex | Smoking cessation |
| Clotrimazole | Antifungal | Nizatidine | Heartburn |
| Cromolyn sodium | Allergy prevention/treatment | Omeprazole | Heartburn (proton pump inhibitor) |
| Dexbrompheniramine maleate | Antihistamine | Oxymetazoline HCl | Decongestant |
| Diphenhydramine HCl | Antihistamine | Phenylephrine HCl | Decongestant |
| Docosanol | Cold sore/fever blister | Pseudoephedrine HCl | Decongestant |
| Doxylamine succinate | Sleep aid | Pyrantel pamoate | Pinworm treatment |
| Dyclonine HCl | Oral anesthetic | Ranitidine | Heartburn |
| Ephedrine sulfate | Bronchodilator, vasoconstrictor | Sodium fluoride | Dental rinse |
| Famotidine | Heartburn | Stannous fluoride | Dental rinse or gel |
| Haloprogin* | Antifungal | Terbinafine HCl | Antifungal |
| Hydrocortisone | Antipruritic, anti-inflammatory | Tioconazole | Antifungal |
| Ibuprofen | Analgesic | Tolnaftate | Antifungal |
| Ketoconazole | Antifungal (shampoo only) | Triclosan | Antigingivitis |
| Ketoprofen | Analgesic | Triprolidine HCl | Antihistamine |
| Loratadine | Nonsedating antihistamine | Xylometazoline HCl | Decongestant |

disease states that could have been limited by treatment with a nonprescription product. In one study, it was estimated that Americans saved approximately $1 billion in health care costs in the first 3 years after topical hydrocortisone acetate was switched from prescription to nonprescription status.[12] That said, out-of-pocket expenditures may increase for many consumers, if employers, insurers, and other third-party payers no longer cover the cost of the medications as the result of a prescription-to-OTC switch. It will, nevertheless, be important for health care providers to stress to their patients the importance of continuing needed drug therapy, even if the cost of the medication is no longer covered by insurance.

Exact standards or switch criteria are very difficult to set because many factors must be carefully considered. The information that must be gathered from the expert opinions of advisers and consultants regarding a drug's classification as nonprescription includes, but is not limited to, the following:

- Is the condition self-diagnosable?
- Is the condition self-treatable?
- Does the product possess misuse and/or abuse potential?
- Is the product habit forming?
- Do methods of use preclude nonprescription availability?
- Do the benefits of availability outweigh the risks?
- Can adequate directions for use be written?

Further scientific scrutiny typically addresses the following questions as well:

- Does the reclassification candidate have an adequate margin of safety?
- Has the reclassification candidate been used for a sufficiently long time (e.g., 3-5 years) on the prescription market to yield a full characterization of its safety profile?
- Has a vigorous risk analysis been performed? If so, what are the results?
- Has the efficacy literature been reviewed in a way that supports the expected use and labeling of the reclassification candidate?
- Have potential drug interactions for the reclassification candidate been characterized?

Table 4-1 lists some of the prescription drugs reclassified as nonprescription since 1975. The most recent addition to this list is omeprazole, a proton pump inhibitor. FDA had initially rejected omeprazole for nonprescription status on the basis of concerns about the ability of the average consumer to comprehend the proposed labeling and concerns about the efficacy of the nonprescription dosage proposed by the petitioner, which was 10 mg, or half of the prescription dose.[13] FDA's concerns were addressed by the petitioner, and the drug is now available without prescription in the same 20 mg dosage as was previously available only by prescription.[14]

Other drugs that have been considered for a switch to nonprescription status include two of the "statins," lovastatin and pravastatin. The issue of whether a cholesterol-lowering drug should be granted nonprescription status has raised concerns, including the ability of the public to understand cholesterol in general and the need for routine blood testing in particular. Also, if approved for nonprescription status, the statins would be the first nonprescription drugs indicated for long-term use to manage and control a potentially life-threatening condition, as opposed to short-term use to control symptoms, such as a runny nose or heartburn. The manufacturers for these recently rejected drugs have renewed their petitions seeking nonprescription status for their products.

In January, 2005, a joint FDA advisory committee, made up of both the Nonprescription Drugs and the Endocrinologic and Metabolic advisory committees, soundly rejected Merck's application seeking nonprescription approval for a 20 mg, once daily strength of lovastatin. While the joint committee had no concerns about the safety and efficacy of lovastatin, it felt that the current U.S. nonprescription system is inadequate for patients to appropriately assess whether they would require a cholesterol-lowering drug for use on a chronic basis.

Interestingly, many committee members stated that they would have voted for nonprescription status had there been a behind-the-counter class of drugs, as there is in the United Kingdom.[15] Although a third class of drugs that are available without a prescription, but only from a pharmacist, would address the concerns raised with drugs such as the statins, FDA has taken the view that "at this time there is no public health concern that would justify the creation of a third class of drugs."[16] A de facto third class of drugs has been created and currently exists, however. For example, the sale of certain Schedule V controlled substances is permitted without a prescription, but only from a pharmacist. Also, many states have passed laws permitting pharmacists to prescribe in certain circumstances, often through a collaborative practice arrangement with a physician. Evidence that consumers have benefitted and pharmacists have successfully managed risks in these areas could be used as support for a broader, federally sanctioned third class of drugs.

Activity in the area of prescription-to-OTC switches seems certain to increase in the coming years. Health care providers can reasonably expect that more prescription drugs will be subjected to review, as payers, the pharmaceutical industry, and FDA continue to grapple with the difficult task of balancing economic pressures with safety concerns. As more drugs are switched to nonprescription status, health care providers will be called on to play a greater role in assessing the need for treatment and monitoring the use of these drugs.

## Regulation of Methamphetamine Precursors

Over the past several years, state and federal regulators have taken steps for increasingly stringent regulation of sale of nonprescription products containing pseudoephedrine. Federal law requires sellers of these products to monitor and report sales above a certain threshold amount, and to prohibit sales in quantities that exceed certain thresholds. State lawmakers have enacted laws restricting the sale of cough and cold products containing pseudoephedrine, in some cases requiring that such products be purchased only from the pharmacy. These laws were enacted to combat the growing problem of illicit methamphetamine labs, operated by "garage chemists" who use pseudoephedrine as the precursor in the manufacturing process.

Under federal law, the Comprehensive Methamphetamine Control Act of 1996 (MCA) regulates the sale of pseudoephedrine-containing products by limiting the quantities that can be purchased in a single transaction and by imposing certain recordkeeping and reporting requirements on sellers, including pharmacies.[17] Pseudoephedrine, along with other substances that can be used in manufacturing illegal drugs, are regulated as List I chemicals, and sellers of these substances are required to register with the Drug Enforcement Administration (DEA). Pharmacies that possess a valid DEA registration for dispensing controlled substances are not required to obtain a separate List I registration, but are required to comply with the recordkeeping and other requirements under the act. Threshold quantities have been set for sales of listed chemicals contained in drug products. If the pharmacy engages in any above-threshold retail transactions of pseudoephedrine (9 g), phenylpropanolamine (PPA) (9 g), combination ephedrine (24 g) and single-entity ephedrine drug products, it must maintain a record of these transactions for 2 years. Pharmacies must also obtain proof of identity from customers and report suspicious above-threshold retail transactions to DEA. The regulations exempt single transactions of regulated products packaged in blister packs from being treated as "regulated transactions,"[18] but caution that such sales of pseudoephedrine and PPA products, regardless of packaging, should be below the 9 g threshold. However, occasional above-threshold sale of blister packs are not subject to the MCA recordkeeping requirement. The DEA Drug Diversion Web site, www.deadiversion.usdoj.gov, has additional information regarding the MCA, including a chart showing what quantity of pseudoephedrine-, ephedrine-, and PPA-containing products would exceed the threshold.

In addition to federal law, many states have enacted their own laws to regulate the sale of methamphetamine precursors. For example, in March 2005, the state of Iowa enacted a law that requires customers to show identification and sign their names on a sales log, including their name and address, with every purchase of any medicine containing pseudoephedrine. In addition, the law limits the purchase of pseudoephedrine-containing products by an individual to one package in a 24-hour period and 7500 mg of pseudoephedrine every 30 days. The law also requires that pseudoephedrine-containing products be kept behind the pharmacy counter, or in a locked cabinet if on the sales floor.[19]

As of August 2005, at least 25 states have passed similar laws restricting he sale of pseudoephedrine, ephedrine, and PPA.[20] Many other states have similar laws pending, and in 2005, the U.S. Senate and House of Representatives were considering federal legislation that would severely limit access to methamphetamine precursors.[21] Practitioners will need to monitor legislative activities in their states, to ensure compliance with applicable laws. Even in the absence of a law, however, it is incumbent on all health care practitioners to try to ensure, as best as possible, that medications, whether prescription or nonprescription, are sold for legitimate medical purposes.

## Marketing Issues

### *Product Line Extensions*

Increasingly, product line extensions are becoming more commonplace in the nonprescription market. Product line extensions include new strengths, formulations, combinations of ingredients, and even a totally different therapeutic entity (e.g., a device) of a brand name product that was originally marketed as a single-ingredient product at a specific dose to treat a specific symptom. In developing product line extensions, manufacturers hope to capitalize on the loyalty created by consumer recognition and trust of a brand name.

Product line extensions can create consumer confusion and inappropriate drug selection and use. Pharmacists must be familiar with the range of products within a brand name to recommend safely and correctly and to counsel patients on these products. Particular care must be taken with respect to the active ingredients because these often differ within a product line. Some product line extensions that carry the original brand name as the prefix retain the active ingredient of the original product, but strengths may vary. Some manufacturers with many product line extensions continue to use the original brand name as the prefix, but use none of the active ingredients of the original products and attach a suffix for differentiation (e.g., PM, EX, DM, AF, Cold and Flu, Non-Drowsy, Extra, Allergy-Sinus-Headache, Advanced Formula, PH, Day/Night, and Plus).

### *Nonprescription Drug Advertising*

The Federal Trade Commission (FTC) is responsible for matters involving claims made in advertisements for nonprescription drug products. FDA handles most matters involving the labeling, as opposed to the advertisement, of nonprescription drugs. In the 1970s, the FTC Act was amended to prohibit advertisers from using language to describe the therapeutic benefits of a nonprescription drug product that differs from language approved by FDA for use in the product labeling.

The FTC Act requires that advertising be truthful and nondeceptive. Depending on the claim, advertisers may be required to back up their representations with competent and reliable scientific evidence, including tests, studies, or other objective data.

In 1973, the National Association of Broadcasters and the Consumer Healthcare Products Association developed a code of guidelines for manufacturers to follow in creating television advertisements for nonprescription drugs.[22] The guidelines, which are updated periodically, set standards for truthfulness and honesty, and suggest that an advertisement should, among other things, do the following:

- Comply with all relevant applicable laws and regulation.
- Urge the consumer to read and follow label directions.
- Contain no claims of product effectiveness that are unsupported by clinical or other scientific evidence, responsible medical opinion, or experience through use.
- Present no information in a manner that suggests the product prevents or cures a serious condition that must be treated by a licensed practitioner.
- Emphasize the uses, results, and advantages of the particular product.
- Reference no doctors, hospitals, or nurses, unless such representations can be supported by independent evidence.
- Present no negative or unfair reflections about competing nonprescription drug products, unless those reflections can be supported scientifically and presented in a manner that consumers can perceive differences in the uses.

Consumers should be analytical when listening to or reading marketing messages, particularly because some can be subjective, superficial, vague, or potentially misleading. Health care professionals, particularly the pharmacist and the primary care provider, are well positioned to assist patients in separating fact from ambiguity with regard to nonprescription drug use and serve the public interest as an objective, informed source of nonprescription drug information.

## Vitamins, Minerals, Botanical Medicines, and Other Dietary Supplements

During the past decade, one of the fastest growing areas of consumer self-care has been the use of vitamins, minerals, botanical medicines, and other dietary supplements (collectively referred to as "dietary supplements"). It is important for consumers, as well as health care providers, to understand that dietary supplements are *not* drugs. Unlike drugs, dietary supplements are not intended to diagnose, cure, or treat a medical disease or condition. Nor are dietary supplements regulated by FDA, or any other state or federal governmental agency, as stringently as are prescription and nonprescription drugs.

Dietary supplements are regulated under the federal Dietary Supplement Health and Education Act of 1994 (DSHEA). DSHEA became law in recognition that many consumers believe dietary supplements have health benefits. The law represented a balance between consumer access to dietary supplements and the authority of the FDA to withdraw dangerous products and address false and misleading claims. FDA's authority to regulate dietary supplements is significantly less than that for prescription and nonprescription products.

DSHEA established a formal definition of *dietary supplement* using several criteria. According to DSHEA, a dietary supplement is a product (other than tobacco) that is[23]

- intended to supplement the diet that bears or contains one or more of the following dietary ingredients: a vitamin, a mineral, an herb or other botanical, an amino acid, a dietary substance for use in supplementing the diet by increasing the total daily intake, or a concentrate, metabolite, constituent, extract, or combinations of these ingredients
- intended for ingestion in pill, capsule, tablet, or liquid form
- not represented for use as a conventional food or as the sole item of a meal or diet
- labeled as a "dietary supplement"

### Regulatory Oversight of Dietary Supplements

FDA regulates dietary supplements differently from the way it regulates prescription and nonprescription drugs. Before DSHEA, dietary supplements were generally subjected to the same regulatory requirements that applied to food products. DSHEA amended the FD&C Act, prohibiting Congress or FDA from regulating supplements as food additives or drugs.[24]

The regulations applicable to dietary supplements under DSHEA are far less stringent than those that apply to drugs. First, unlike prescription and nonprescription drugs, which must be proven to be safe and effective by the manufacturer before the product can be marketed and sold in the United States, dietary supplement manufacturers are responsible for determining only the safety of their products. There is no efficacy requirement. Moreover, the dietary supplement regulations do not require the manufacturer to submit safety data to FDA for review and approval prior to marketing their products, as is required for drug manufacturers. If FDA has concerns about the safety of a dietary supplement and wants the product removed from the market, DSHEA places the burden on FDA to prove that the supplement is unsafe.[25]

Next, unlike drug manufacturers, dietary supplement manufacturers generally do not need to register with FDA. As a result, FDA does not maintain a list of manufacturers, distributors, or the dietary supplement products sold in the market, as it does with prescription and nonprescription drugs.

This is not to say, however, that FDA has no role in regulating dietary supplements. Under DSHEA, FDA has the authority to stop the sale of dietary supplements proven to be unsafe after they reach the market. FDA monitors safety through postmarketing surveillance, including voluntary dietary supplement adverse event reporting and product information, such as labeling, claims, package inserts, and accompanying literature.

FDA also has the authority to prescribe, through regulation, good manufacturing practices, including regulations addressing potency and stability of products and the cleanliness of manufacturing facilities. In 2003, FDA exercised its authority under DSHEA and took the first formal step toward establishing current good manufacturing practices aimed at reducing the risks associated with adulterated and misbranded dietary supplement products.[26] FDA published a proposed regulation that would require the use of industrywide standards in the manufacturing, packing, and holding of dietary supplements and ensure that the identity, purity, quality, strength, and composition of dietary supplements are accurately reflected on the product label.[27] FDA received diverse comments on this proposed regulation, particularly from the dietary supplement industry and at the time of publication has not issued final regulations.

### Labeling of Dietary Supplements

Under DSHEA, supplement manufacturers are permitted to make certain claims on their labels, as long as the claims are accurate and truthful. DSHEA prohibits "disease claims" that explicitly or implicitly indicate the product can be used to prevent, treat, cure, mitigate, or diagnose a disease. Disease claims are reserved for drug products, and,if a dietary supplement label makes a disease claim, FDA can step in and regulate the dietary supplement as a drug. "Structure/function" claims, on the other hand, are permitted under DSHEA. A structure/function claim describes the role that the supplement plays in affecting the normal structure or function of the human body.[28] Thus, for example, it may be permissible for a manufacturer to claim that its product helps improve mood, but not that it can be used to treat depression. Dietary supplements can also make statements related to a classical nutrient deficiency disease and state the prevalence of the disease in the United States.

In addition, when a manufacturer makes a permissible claim, it must also include the following disclaimer: "This statement has not been evaluated by FDA. This product is not intended to diagnose, treat, cure, or prevent any disease." Manufacturers making structure/function claims must also notify FDA of its use of the specific claim no later than 30 days after marketing the product, and must have support that any labeling claims it makes are truthful and not misleading. However, there is no requirement that FDA approve labeling before a supplement is marketed.

For herbal products, the label must also state the part of the plant used in the product (e.g., root, stem, or leaf). Figure 4-5 illustrates the standard label format. A standardized format provides the patient with certain minimum information about the product prior to consumption.

### Advertising and Promotion of Dietary Supplements

FTC regulates advertising of dietary supplements and other products marketed to consumers in any media. Its reach includes traditional magazine advertising, television and radio, "infomercials," catalogs and similar direct marketing materials, and advertising and promotion over the Internet. The role of FTC, which enforces federal laws prohibiting "unfair or deceptive acts or practices," is to ensure that consumers get accurate information about dietary supplements so they can make informed decisions about these products.[29]

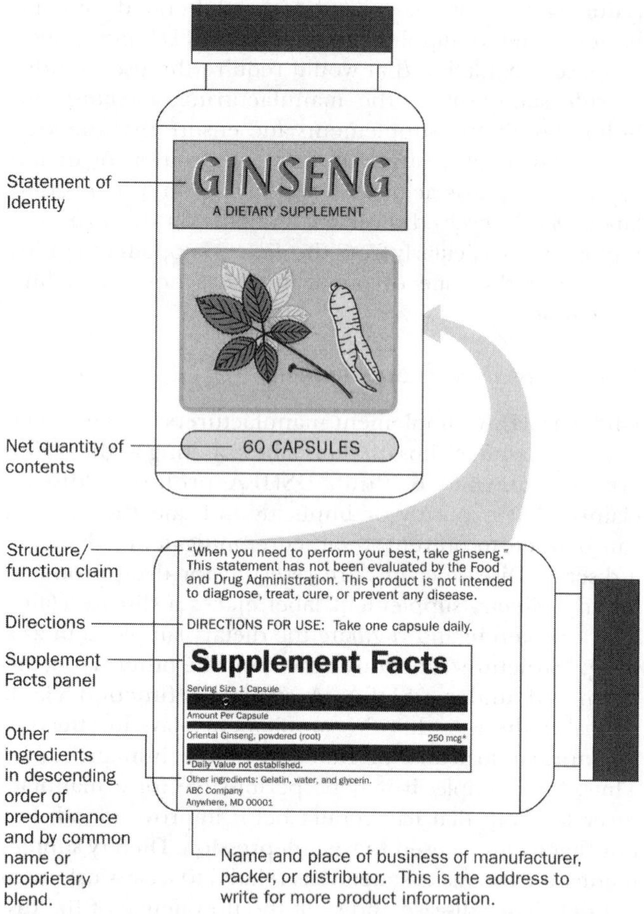
Statement of Identity
GINSENG
A DIETARY SUPPLEMENT
Net quantity of contents
60 CAPSULES
Structure/function claim
"When you need to perform your best, take ginseng." This statement has not been evaluated by the Food and Drug Administration. This product is not intended to diagnose, treat, cure, or prevent any disease.
Directions
DIRECTIONS FOR USE: Take one capsule daily.
Supplement Facts panel
Supplement Facts
Serving Size 1 Capsule
Amount Per Capsule
Oriental Ginseng, powdered (root)
250 mcg*
*Daily Value not established.
Other ingredients in descending order of predominance and by common name or proprietary blend.
Other ingredients: Gelatin, water, and glycerin.
ABC Company
Anywhere, MD 00001
Name and place of business of manufacturer, packer, or distributor. This is the address to write for more product information.

**FIGURE 4-5** Statutory labeling format for certain dietary supplements. (*Source:* US Food and Drug Administration. *Anatomy of the New Requirements for Dietary Supplement Labels.* Available at: http://www.cfsan.fda.gov/~acrobat/fdsuppla.pdf. Accessed August 24, 2005.)

FTC works with FDA under a longstanding liaison agreement governing the division of responsibilities between the two agencies. As applied to dietary supplements, FDA, through its Center for Food Safety and Applied Nutrition, has primary responsibility for claims on product labeling, including packaging, inserts, and other promotional materials distributed at the point of sale, whereas FTC has primary responsibility for claims in advertising.

## Homeopathy

Homeopathic medicines include substances that have evoked positive images (e.g., chamomile, marigold, daisy, onion) as well as those that are considered the cruelest of creations (e.g., poison ivy, mercury, arsenic, pit viper venom, hemlock). Based on a medical theory that potency increases with dilution, homeopathy has been practiced for more than 200 years.[30] Homeopathic medicines are made from a variety of sources (e.g., plants, minerals, animals). Their use is based on a person's genetic history, personal health history, body type, and present status inclusive of all physical, emotional, and mental symptoms.

Some homeopathic remedies are so dilute that the molecules of the healing substance are difficult and sometimes impossible to identify, even using some of the most sophisticated technologies of the 21st century. Homeopaths, however, believe that the substance leaves its imprint or a "spiritlike" essence that stimulates the body to heal itself. (See Chapter 55 for a discussion of homeopathic concepts and techniques.)

### *FDA Regulation of Homeopathic Products*

It is widely believed that Senator Royal Copeland of New York, a homeopathic primary care provider and the chief sponsor of the FD&C Act, was responsible for writing into the act the recognition of any product listed in the *Homeopathic Pharmacopoeia of the United States* (*HPUS*).[31] Homeopathic drugs are recognized as drugs under the FD&C Act, which defines the term *drug* as "articles recognized in the official United States Pharmacopoeia, official Homeopathic Pharmacopoeia of the United States, or official National Formulary, (i) or any supplement to any of them…."[32] Further, the act provides that whenever a drug is recognized in both the *United States Pharmacopoeia* and the *HPUS*, it is subject to the requirements of the *United States Pharmacopoeia* unless it is labeled and offered for sale as a homeopathic drug, in which case it is subject to the provisions of the *HPUS*.

FDA regulates homeopathic remedies under provisions of the FD&C Act, but in significantly different ways from other drugs. Manufacturers of homeopathic drugs are not required to submit an NDA to FDA before marketing their products. Furthermore, these products are exempt from good manufacturing practice requirements related to expiration dating and from finished product testing for identity and strength. This disparity exists because homeopathic products contain little or no active ingredient, and so there is a diminished concern for safety or toxicity. Another disparity is in the concentration of alcohol in the preparation. Conventional drugs for adults can contain no more than 10% alcohol and the amount is even less in medications intended for pediatric use.[33] Homeopathic products, however, are exempt from these limits and can contain much higher amounts of alcohol.

Homeopathic products are not, however, exempt from all FDA regulations. If a homeopathic drug claims to treat a serious disease (e.g., cancer), it can be sold only by prescription. Only products sold for the so-called self-limiting conditions—colds, headaches, and other minor health problems that eventually resolve on their own—can be sold as nonprescription items.

### *Labeling of Homeopathic Products*

Homeopathic products are subject to the same labeling provisions of the FD&C Act as are other drug products. However, if these products are labeled in accordance with the existing Compliance Policy Guide for homeopathic products, they will not be subject to regulatory action.[34] Labeling requirements include an ingredients list, instructions for safe use, at least one major indication, and dilution (for example 2X for one part per hundred, 3X for one part per thousand).

The FDA is focusing on educating the homeopathic industry about FDA regulations. FDA is aware of a few reports of illness associated with the use of homeopathic products. Investigation of such reports revealed that the homeopathic product was not the cause of the adverse reaction. In one instance, arsenic, which is a recognized homeopathic ingredient, was implicated, but, as would be expected, the FDA analysis revealed the concentration of arsenic was so minute that no cause-effect relationship could be established. Even with the lack of clinical research, homeopathy's popularity in the United States is growing.

### Drug–Cosmetic Products

Some nonprescription drug products are also considered cosmetic products.[35] The claim(s) that are made for the product determine whether it is a drug, a cosmetic, or a drug-cosmetic. Labeling and marketing requirements differ depending on how a product is classified. Often this distinction is not apparent to the consumer, but a consumer may wonder why a product they considered to be a cosmetic contains Drug Facts labeling. If a product has a "drug"-intended use and a "cosmetic"-intended use, it is considered a drug-cosmetic. For example, a shampoo is a cosmetic because its intended use is to clean the hair, which is a cosmetic claim. An antidandruff shampoo is a drug because its intended use is to treat dandruff, which is considered a drug claim. Therefore, an antidandruff shampoo that claims to clean the hair and treat dandruff would be a drug-cosmetic and have OTC Drug Facts labeling. Other drug-cosmetic products include toothpastes that contain fluoride, deodorants that are also antiperspirants, and moisturizers and some makeup that are marketed with sun-protection claims.

## Identifying and Removing Potentially Dangerous Products from the Market

### *Adverse Event Reporting*

The pharmacist stands out as the one health care provider who has the most frequent and ready access to consumers of prescription and nonprescription drugs. Through counseling of patients in the pharmacy or assisting a customer in selecting the appropriate nonprescription treatment for some health-related condition, pharmacists often obtain information that suggests a drug or other FDA-related product, including dietary supplements, may be causing unintended and unexpected adverse health consequences. Pharmacists play a critical role in helping FDA and industry manage the risks associated with regulated products. To fulfill this responsibility, it is important for the pharmacist to understand FDA's adverse event reporting system.

The FDA MedWatch program is a voluntary adverse event reporting system that allows health care providers and consumers to report serious adverse drug reactions directly to the agency. FDA analyzes trends and correlations between drug use and adverse reports from information submitted to MedWatch. There is no cost to either the health care professional or the consumer for filing a report. Though the program is voluntary, it is ineffective unless properly utilized. Health care providers should take their role in patient safety seriously and, as part of that responsibility, make sure that serious adverse drug reactions suspected to be associated with drugs are reported to FDA. Official reporting forms are available from FDA by calling 1-800-FDA-1088. Reports can also be submitted online by accessing the MedWatch Web site at http://www.fda.gov/medwatch/index.html. FDA safety alerts and product recall information are also accessible at this site.

It is important to understand that submitting a report to FDA does not constitute a legal claim, nor does it in any way constitute an acknowledgment that there has even been an adverse drug reaction associated with use of the product. The identities of the practitioners and the patients are confidential. Health care providers are encouraged to report all suspected adverse reactions and to ensure effective review of the reports. FDA asks that practitioners describe the reaction, the exposure to the regulated product, the time between exposure and reaction, and the underlying disease.

### *Product Recalls*

When a product regulated by FDA is identified as a potential risk to the public, it may be necessary to have that product removed from the market. Products may pose a risk for a variety of reasons, including adulteration or misbranding or because an unacceptable risk of adverse effects is discovered through postmarket surveillance.

FDA has two methods available to force the removal of a product from the market. First, if the drug is misbranded or adulterated, the FD&C Act allows FDA to seize the product and order that it be held pending a review by the court concerning its safety.[36] Next, FDA can also seek a court injunction, preventing further distribution or sale of the product. Both of these remedies are potentially expensive and time-consuming and, more important, do not address the issue of retrieving drugs that have already been purchased.

A third avenue FDA may pursue is to request the manufacturer to recall their product from the market. FDA has no statutory authority to order a recall, but when potentially serious health risks are associated with the use of a drug product, typically, manufacturers are more than willing to institute a recall. If a recall is instituted, FDA does have the authority to prescribe the procedures to which the recall must conform. This cooperation between FDA and its regulated industries has proven over the years to be the quickest and most reliable method for removing potentially dangerous products from the market. This method has been successful because it is in the interest of both FDA and the industry to get unsafe and defective products out of consumer hands as soon as possible. FDA guidelines governing product recalls make clear that FDA expects manufacturers to take full responsibility for product recalls, including follow-up checks to ensure that recalls are successful. Under the guidelines, companies are expected to notify FDA when recalls are started, to make reports to FDA on their progress, and to undertake recalls when asked to do so.[37]

The guidelines categorize all recalls into one of three classes according to the level of hazard associated with the product at issue:

- *Class I* recalls are for dangerous or defective products that predictably could cause serious health problems or death.
- Class *II* recalls are for products that might cause a temporary health problem, or pose only a slight threat of a serious nature.
- *Class III* recalls are for products that are unlikely to cause any adverse health reaction, but that violate FDA labeling or manufacturing regulations.

The manufacturer is responsible for notifying sellers of the recall. The sellers, including pharmacists, are responsible for contacting customers, if necessary. A pharmacist is also responsible for knowing what drugs or other regulated products have been recalled. Failing to remove a recalled product from the shelf—and subsequently providing the product to a consumer—may violate the FD&C Act and also exposes the pharmacist to civil liability in the event that someone is injured by use of the product.

FDA issues general information about new recalls it is monitoring through FDA Enforcement Reports, a weekly publication available on FDA's Internet page at http://www.fda.gov.

## OTC Products and Civil Liability

OTC drug products are, by nature, deemed to be safe and effective for use by the general public for self-care, without the oversight of a health care practitioner. However, no drug, whether prescription or nonprescription, is completely safe. As with any product, injuries can result from the use of a nonprescription product. For example, a patient can have an allergic reaction to an ingredient in a nonprescription product, can become injured as a result of an interaction between a nonprescription product and another drug, or suffer injury resulting from a side effect associated with the use of the drug. The fact that these types of injuries can and do occur, however, does not mean that the drugs causing the problem are inherently dangerous or unsafe, or that they should not be available without a prescription.

Whether a health care practitioner can be held liable for money damages for recommending or selling a nonprescription drug that causes an injury is an issue that is decided under state law, and legislation varies from state to state. A complete analysis of the nuances of the various theories of liability is beyond the scope of this chapter. There are, however, some general principles that practitioners may find useful to understand and guard against potential civil liability.

Initially, it is important to note that regardless of what a court may decide in any given case, the primary obligation of a health care provider is to provide health care. This obligation may include recommending or selling appropriate nonprescription products for patient self-care. A health care provider who refuses to recommend or sell a product for fear of incurring civil liability is not providing health care, and is doing a disservice to himself or herself, the profession, and the patient.

### *Theories of Civil Liability*

The body of law concerning civil liability is guided by the general principle that in a civilized society, people are responsible for their actions. If one's actions cause an injury to another person, the law may require that the injured person be compensated, or made whole. In the U.S. justice system, an injured person who seeks compensation for the injuries he or she has sustained as a result of another's actions has the right to bring a civil lawsuit against the person who caused the injury. Typically, the injured party (the "plaintiff") will ask the court to award money damages to be paid by the party causing the injury (the "defendant"). For example, a plaintiff who sustains an injury after taking a nonprescription medication recommended by a pharmacist can file a lawsuit against the pharmacist, seeking monetary compensation for the injuries. The plaintiff may seek compensation for the past, present, and future medical bills he or she has incurred or will incur as a result of the injury, for income lost from missing work, for the pain and suffering endured, and for any permanent injury or damage.

The mere fact that an injury occurred does not, however, entitle the plaintiff to damages. The plaintiff has the burden of proving that he or she has satisfied each of the elements required to be proved under the theory of liability alleged in the complaint. The theories of liability that can be alleged against a health care provider in connection with an injury caused by a nonprescription drug include negligence, breach of warranty, and strict product liability.

#### Negligence

The mere fact that an injury has occurred does not mean that a party can found liable for negligence. Similarly, even if a health care provider makes a mistake, that action alone does not necessarily entitle the injured party to compensation. To prevail in a case alleging negligence of a health care provider, the plaintiff must prove four elements: (1) that the defendant owed the plaintiff a duty of care, (2) that the defendant by his or her conduct breached that duty, (3) that the breach caused the injury complained of, and (4) that, in fact, the plaintiff sustained some cognizable injury or damage. If the plaintiff cannot prove all of these elements, there can be no liability.

The first element, duty, is decided by the court. The relevant inquiry is whether the health care provider failed to exercise the degree of care a reasonable and prudent person would have used under similar circumstances. Courts will examine the relationship between the parties, the foreseeability that the defendant's actions, or failure to act, could cause an injury, and the gravity of harm that resulted from the act or failure to act. After the court defines the duty, the jury will decide whether the duty has been breached by the health care provider.

In one very old case addressing liability for injuries resulting from a pharmacist's recommendation of a nonprescription product, the court defined the duty as requiring the pharmacist to exercise a high degree of care in advising the purchaser of the injurious effects of the recommended nonprescription product.[38] In that case, the patient presented the pharmacist with a prescription for a product to treat poison ivy. The pharmacist advised the patient to use a nonprescription product instead of the product prescribed by the doctor. A reaction between the nonprescription ointment and a residue present on the patient's skin caused the skin to turn black. The court stated

> In the discharge of their functions, druggists, apothecaries, and other persons dealing in drugs, poisons, and medicines, are required, not only to be skillful, but also exceedingly cautious and prudent, in view of the terrific consequences which may attend the least inattention on their part. The highest degree of care known among practical men must be used by them to prevent injury from the use of their compounds, and they are held to a special degree of responsibility corresponding with their superior knowledge and are generally held liable for the slightest negligence.

The court sustained a jury verdict awarding money damages to the plaintiff, finding that the recommendation of the nonprescription product and the recommendation that the plaintiff continue to use the product even after she began to notice that her skin was turning black constituted a breach of the standard of care owed to the patient.

Although each state's law differs, and the ruling in any case is dependent on the facts presented, it is likely that courts will hold pharmacists and other health care providers to a high standard of care in connection with the recommendation of nonprescription products. A reasonable pharmacist would likely not, for example, recommend that a patient discontinue all antidepressant medications and take St. John's wort to treat clinical depression. Nor would a reasonable health care provider recommend that a patient take aspirin, if it is known that the patient is also on warfarin therapy. The health care provider must act reasonably, and make recommendations that are in the patient's best interest. If, despite the exercise of due care, an injury results, a provider likely would not be held liable for negligence.

Of course, even if a duty and breach are found, the provider would not be liable for injuries that were not caused by the negligent conduct. If, for example, the evidence in the poison ivy case described above showed that the patient's skin turned black not because of any reaction between the product recommended by the pharmacist, but because of some inherent condition the patient suffered from, which coincidentally manifested itself at the same time as the patient began using the nonprescription ointment, the pharmacist would not be held liable. Again, the plaintiff must prove all four elements—duty, breach, causation, and injury—to prevail.

### Breach of Warranty

Liability for breach of warranty is based on the theory that the defendant violated either an express or implied agreement concerning the quality of the product in connection with its sale. Express warranties arise out of specific statements made by the seller, whereas implied warranties are created by and imposed by law. Keep in mind that warranty liability can arise only if the health care provider sold the product that fails to perform. Thus, a recommendation by a health care provider that the patient buy a certain cough and cold preparation that causes injury will not result in warranty liability if the provider merely recommended, but did not sell the product.

The Uniform Commercial Code (UCC), which has been adopted by nearly every state, defines an express warranty as "an affirmation of fact or promise made to the buyer, that relates to the goods and becomes a basis of the bargain."[39] In one of the few published cases addressing the breach of an express warranty made by a pharmacist in connection with the sale of a drug product, the court found the representation that the product sold "was the same as what the plaintiff's prescription called for" created an express warranty, and when the product sold was in fact different, and caused an injury, the pharmacist was held liable.[40] Using the poison ivy case again as an example, the pharmacist advised the plaintiff that the blackened skin that resulted after the first use of the nonprescription product would clear up with continued use of the ointment. Instead, it got worse. On those facts, the plaintiff likely could have stated a claim for breach of express warranty.

Express warranties should not be confused with "sales talk," or puffery, which are statements made to induce a sale that do not specifically relate to the ability of the product. For example, a statement such as "this is the best ointment you will ever buy" would likely be viewed as sales talk, and not an express warranty.

Implied warranties are created by law. Two implied warranties included in the UCC should most concern health care providers who sell goods—the implied warranty of fitness for a particular purpose and the implied warranty of merchantability. When a seller recommends a particular product to meet the buyer's specific needs, it is implied that the product recommended is fit for that purpose. Thus, for example, if a health care provider recommends and sells a product to treat a specific condition, and it turns out that the product should not have been used to treat that condition, the plaintiff could claim the provider breached the warranty of fitness for a particular purpose.

The implied warranty of merchantability states that the product sold is fit for all general purposes for which the product typically is sold. Included within this warranty is the understanding that the products sold and their containers meet certain minimum quality standards. If a pharmacist sells a product that is outdated, contaminated, or subpotent, he has breached the implied warranty of merchantability.

Warranty claims often are brought against not just the immediate seller of the product, but also against the product's manufacturer. However, if the condition that has rendered the product unfit for ordinary purposes was caused by the manufacturer, and not the seller, that would not necessarily relieve the seller of responsibility. State laws vary in this area, with some states having laws that limit the liability of the seller in those circumstances. In general, to avoid warranty liability, the provider must be mindful of the source and origin of the products it sells.

### Strict Product Liability

The last type of liability that will be discussed is strict product liability. Unlike a negligence or warranty theory, strict liability is imposed when a product causes an injury to the user, even if the seller was not negligent and made no express or implied representations regarding the product. Although this type of case is typically brought against the manufacturer, it remains a viable theory of recover against retail sellers of products in many states. The theory is based on the idea that a seller of a product that has profited from the sale should also be required to compensate victims who are injured by the product, even if the seller was not in any way negligent in causing the injury. The mere sale of a product that is found to be defective, even if the defect is unknown or even unknowable to the seller, can form the basis for imposing strict liability.

When the product involved is a prescription product, courts have almost universally held that pharmacists cannot be held strictly liable for injuries caused by products they dispense. However, when a pharmacist acts as a retailer and sells goods that cause injuries, the theory may remain viable. Again, many states have laws that will automatically pass liability up the chain, past the retailer to the manufacturer.

Again, the most important rule that a pharmacist or any health care provider can follow to avoid civil liability is to simply practice health care as it should be practiced. Caring for the patient and acting in the patient's best interest to improve the patient's health and well being should be the primary concern of all health care providers and, more often than not, adherence to that general principal will provide a defense in the event that a patient claims that the provider's conduct in connection with the recommendation or sale of a product caused an injury.

## Key Points for Legal and Regulatory Issues in Self-Care Pharmacy Practice

- Although nonprescription drug products are readily available, they are subject to regulatory and legal requirements to ensure their safety and efficacy.
- The Drug Facts labeling panel is a useful consumer counseling tool for pharmacists.
- Dietary supplements and homeopathic products are not regulated the same way as prescription and nonprescription drugs.
- Pharmacists play a critical role in helping FDA and industry manage risks associated with nonprescription drugs and should voluntarily report adverse events to FDA's MedWatch program or the manufacturer.
- With increasing frequency, FDA is approving product switches from prescription to nonprescription status. Health care providers play a crucial role in educating their patients as to the safe and proper use of recently switched products.
- Although liability risks may be associated with the sale of a nonprescription product, health care providers must remember that their primary role is to provide health care, and that the best way to protect themselves is to act reasonably and in the best interest of their patient when recommending a nonprescription product.

## References


1. US Food and Drug Administration, Center for Drug Evaluation and Research. Rulemaking History for OTC Drug Products: Drug Category List. Available at: http://www.fda.gov/cder/otcmonographs/rulemaking_index.htm. Accessed October 3, 2003.
2. 67 *Federal Register* 3060 (2002) (codified at 21 CFR §330.14).
3. US Food and Drug Administration, Center for Drug Evaluation and Research. Drug Applications. Available at: http://www.fda.gov/cder/regulatory/applications/nda.htm. Accessed October 3, 2003.
4. US Food and Drug Administration. Reporting Adverse Reactions and Medical Product Problems to the FDA. Available at: http://www.fda.gov/medwatch/how. Accessed October 3, 2003.
5. *Federal Register.* 1999;64:13254. Available at: http://www.fda.gov/cder/consumerinfo/OTClabel.htm. Accessed October 7, 2003.
6. 21 CFR §201.66.
7. 21 CFR §211.137.
8. 21 CFR §211.132. (Exceptions include dermatologicals, dentifrice, insulin, and lozenge products.)
9. US Food and Drug Administration. Over-the-counter medicines: What's right for you? Available at: http://www.fda.gov/cder/consumerinfo/WhatsRightForYou.pdf. Accessed August 1, 2005.
10. Norberg, T. Now available without a prescription. *FDA Consumer.* November 1996.
11. Newton GD, Benninghoff AJ, Popovich NG. New OTC drugs and devices: a selective review. *J Am Pharm Assoc.* 2002;42:267-77.
12. Shih YT, Prasad M, Luce BR. The effect on social welfare of a switch of second-generation antihistamines from prescription to over-the-counter status: a microeconomic analysis. *Clin Ther.* 2002;24:701-16.
13. Erickson A. RX-to-OTC switches offer golden opportunity. *Pharmacy Today.* 2002;8:1, 5, 35.
14. FDA approves Prilosec OTC to treat frequent heartburn [press release]. Available at: http://www.fda.gov/bbs/topics/news/2003/NEW00916.html. Accessed September 24, 2003.
15. Mevacor Daily OTC Switch Rejected Based on Patient Inability to Self Select. *FDA Advisory Committee.com.* Available at: http://www.fdaadvisorycommittee.com/FDC/AdvisoryCommittee/Committees/Endocrinologic+and+Metabolic+Drugs/011305_Mevacor1/011405_MevacorR2.htm. Accessed March 11, 2005.
16. US Food and Drug Administration. Rx to OTC: the switch is on. Available at: http://www.fda.gov/bbs/topics/CONSUMER/CN00012c. html. Accessed August 1, 2005.
17. *DEA Pharmacist's Manual.* (An excellent summary of the provisions of the Methamphetamine Control Act as it relates to pharmacists and pharmacies engaged in the sale of these products.) Available at: http://www.deadiversion.usdoj.gov/pubs/manuals/. Accessed March 15, 2005.
18. 21 CFR 1300.02(b)(28).
19. Iowa Senate File 169, 81st General Assembly, Sect. 124.212, subsect. 4, Code 2005.

20. *National Association of Boards of Pharmacy Newsletter.* August 2005; 34(7).
21. Senate Bill 103, the Combat Meth Act of 2005. Available at: http://thomas.loc.gov. Accessed August 5, 2005.
22. Consumer Healthcare Products Association. Voluntary codes and guidelines of the self-care industry, Code of advertising practices for nonprescription medicines. Available at: http://www.chpa-info.org/web/about_chpa/voluntary_codes_guidelines.aspx #Advertising%20Practices. Accessed August 1, 2005
23. 21 USC §321(ff).
24. Fink J, Vivian J, Bernstein, I. *Pharmacy Law Digest.* 40th ed. St. Louis: Facts and Comparisons; 2006:89-90.
25. 21 USC §350b(a)(2).
26. *Federal Register.* 2003;68:12157-263.
27. FDA proposes manufacturing and labeling standards for all dietary supplements [press release]. Available at: http://www.fda.gov/bbs/topics/NEWS/dietarysupp/background.html. Accessed April 24, 2003.
28. *Federal Register.* 2000;65:1000.
29. Federal Trade Commission. Dietary supplements: an advertising guide for industry. Available at: http://www3.ftc.gov/bcp/conline/pubs/buspubs/dietsupp.htm#Introduction. Accessed September 25, 2003.
30. Stehlin, I. Homeopathy: Real medicine or empty promises? *FDA Consumer.* November 1996. Available at: http://www.fda.gov/fdac/features/096_home.html. Accessed August 15, 2005).
31. Junod SW. An alternative perspective: homeopathic drugs, Royal Copeland and federal drug regulation. *Food Drug Law J.* 2000; 55:161-83.
32. 21 USC §321(g)(1).
33. 21 CFR §328.
34. *Federal Register.* 53:21728; Conditions under which homeopathic drugs may be marketed. *FDA Compliance Policy Guide.* Sect. 7132.15. Rockville, Md: US Food and Drug Administration.
35. US Food and Drug Administration. Is it a cosmetic, a drug, or both? July 8, 2002. Available at: http://www.cfsan.fda.gov/~dms/cos-218.html. Accessed October 3, 2003.
36. 21 USC §304.
37. 21 CFR §7.40.
38. *Fuhs v. Barber,* 36 P2d 962 (Kan 1934).
39. Uniform Commercial Code, Article 2, §2313; *See also,* Fink J, Vivian J, Bernstein I. *Pharmacy Law Digest.* 40th ed. St. Louis: Facts and Comparisons; 2006:287-8.
40. *Jacobs Pharmacy Co. v. Gibson,* 159 SE2d 171 (Ga 1967).

SECTION II

# Pain and Fever Disorders

CHAPTER 5

# Headache

*Tami L. Remington*

Headache is a very common pain complaint, with more than 90% of people experiencing headache at some time during their lives.[1] In an international survey of people seeking primary care, 22% reported experiencing pain for at least 6 months during the preceding year, with 45% reporting headache.[2] There are many types of headaches, and it is not uncommon for patients to experience more than one type over time. Many headache sufferers do not seek medical attention and self-treat with nonprescription remedies. Nearly half of patients using nonprescription pain relievers do not read the labeling on the container, and 43% of people surveyed were unaware of the risks associated with taking these agents with prescription medications.[3] Clearly, an opportunity to improve medication use exists among patients self-treating for various pain syndromes.

Headaches are generally classified as primary or secondary.[4] Primary headaches (approximately 90% of headaches) are not associated with an underlying illness. Examples include episodic and chronic tension-type headaches, migraine headache with and without aura, cluster headaches, and medication overuse headaches. Secondary headaches are symptoms of an underlying condition such as head trauma, vascular defects (e.g., infarction, intracerebral hemorrhage, aneurysm), substance abuse or withdrawal, bacterial and viral diseases, and disorders of craniofacial structures.

This chapter focuses on the most common headaches that are amenable to self-treatment: tension-type headache, diagnosed migraine (vascular) headache, and sinus headache. Nonprescription analgesics are useful in treating headache, either as monotherapy or as adjuncts to nonpharmacologic or prescription therapy. Throughout this chapter, the abbreviation NSAID will be used to denote the class of nonsalicylate nonsteroidal anti-inflammatory agents (ibuprofen, naproxen, ketoprofen).

## Epidemiology of Headache

Tension-type headaches, also called muscle contraction headaches and stress headaches, can be episodic or chronic. More than 75% of the U.S. population will experience tension-type headaches at some time, with the 1-year prevalence being 38%.[1,5]

Migraine headaches are experienced by 20% to 25% of the U.S. population although only about half of them have been diagnosed with migraine headache.[1,5] Migraine without aura occurs almost twice as frequently as migraine with aura, and many individuals may have both types of headaches. Women have a three times higher incidence of migraine headaches than do men.[1] Among children, boys and girls are affected equally, but attacks usually disappear in boys after puberty.[5] Up to 70% of patients with migraine have family histories of migraine, suggesting that this disease is influenced by heredity. Onset usually begins in the first three decades of life, with greatest prevalence during the fifth decade.

Sinus headache is a frequently reported symptom in patients with acute or chronic sinusitis. These patients will also experience other sinus symptoms such as toothache in the upper teeth, nasal stuffiness, and nasal discharge. It is now recognized that many patients who believe they are suffering sinus headache may actually be experiencing migraine headache.

## Anatomy and Physiology of Headache

Pain is an unpleasant sensory and emotional experience associated with actual or potential tissue damage or described in terms of such damage. The definition recognizes that pain can have physical, affective, and learned components and is not necessarily a result of physical injury.

The sensory component of pain derives from a process during which messages are transmitted from the site of injury to the brain, where they are detected as pain (Figure 5-1). Initially, damaged tissues release chemical substances such as prostaglandins, bradykinin, serotonin, substance P, and histamine, which stimulate or sensitize nociceptive neurons.

In a matter of milliseconds, nociceptors deliver electrical impulses from the site of injury to the spinal cord. This process involves neuronal depolarization, which depends on transport of sodium, potassium, and other ions across cell membranes. The afferent nerve impulses are transmitted to ascending spinal cord neurons, which deliver nociceptive impulses to various centers of the brain. Here, the impulses are consciously recognized as pain.

In response to pain, neurons in the brainstem release inhibitory transmitters, including endogenous opioids (endorphins and enkephalins), norepinephrine, serotonin, gamma-aminobutyric acid, and neurotensin. These substances block pain transmissions from the periphery, thereby modulating the sensation of pain.[6]

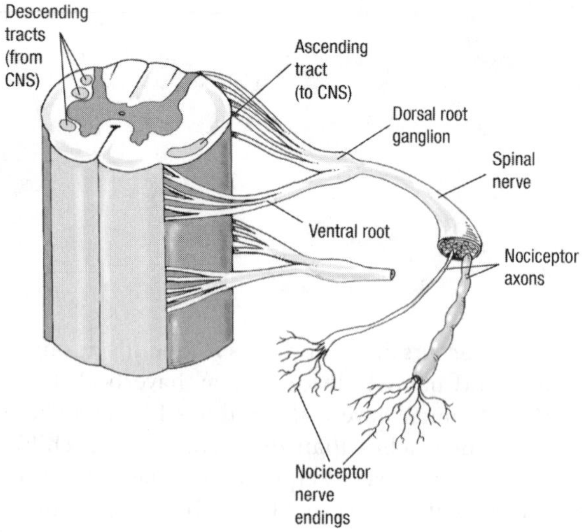


**FIGURE 5-1** Peripheral and central pain pathways.

## Etiology of Headache

*Tension-type headaches* are a type of myofascial pain (originates in muscles or the overlying fascial tissue) that manifests in response to stress, anxiety, depression, emotional conflicts, fatigue, and repressed hostility. Tight muscles in the upper back, head, and neck area can cause headaches. Referred pain from remote trigger points can also initiate or exacerbate headaches.

*Migraine headaches* have up to four phases and probably arise from a complex interaction of neuronal and vascular factors. Stress, fatigue, oversleeping, fasting or missing a meal, vasoactive substances in food, caffeine, alcohol, menses, and changes in barometric pressure and altitude may trigger migraine. Medications (reserpine, nitrates, indomethacin, oral contraceptives, and postmenopausal hormones) can also trigger migraine. Although still debated, personality features of migraine sufferers include perfectionism, rigidity, and compulsiveness. Menstrual migraines appear at the menstrual stage of the ovarian cycle and occur in fewer than 10% of women.[7] Most affected women suffer attacks in the premenstrual period and, for some women, migraine headaches recur at specific times before, after, or during the menstrual cycle.

Migraine and tension-type headaches may coexist. Patients with this disorder have daily tension headaches and occasional migraines. Most headache specialists view headaches across a spectrum, with tension-type on one end and migraine headaches on the other end. The current opinion is that either type of headache can precipitate the other.

Sinus headache occurs when infection or blockage of the paranasal sinuses causes inflammation or distention of the sensitive sinus walls (see Chapter 11).

Although a number of medications can cause headache as a side effect, issues discussed here relate to overuse (rebound) and withdrawal of agents used for analgesia. Medication-overuse headaches are a challenging area for clinicians. Agents associated with them are acetaminophen, aspirin, caffeine, triptans, opioids, butalbital, and ergotamine formulations.[8] Medication-overuse headaches are usually associated with use for 3 months or longer and occur within hours of stopping the agent; readministration provides relief. Symptomatology shifts from the baseline headache type to a nearly continuous headache, particularly noticeable on awakening. This continuous headache may be punctuated by periodic headaches of the baseline type; some patients note an increased frequency of their baseline headache type. When medication-overuse headache is suspected, use of offending agent(s) should be tapered and subsequently eliminated. Most often, this should be done with medical supervision because use of prescription therapies may be needed to combat the increased headaches that temporarily ensue during the days to weeks of the withdrawal period.[8,9]

## Pathophysiology of Headache

The pathophysiology of tension-type and migraine headaches is not well elucidated. Historically, it was thought that these two headache types had distinct pathologies, but this may not be the case. Many now believe that migraine and tension-type headaches are different manifestations of a single pathophysiology. This would help account for the observation that most people suffering migraine headaches also experience episodic tension-type headaches.[10,11]

Most investigation into the pathophysiology of headache has centered on migraine headache. The best evidence suggests that migraine occurs through a neuronal dysfunction of the trigeminovascular system rather than a vascular disturbance as once believed. Neuronal hyperexcitability has been proposed as the trigger for aura. Stimulation (by an axon reflex) of trigeminal sensory fibers in the large cerebral and dural vessels causes neuropeptide release with concomitant neurogenic inflammation, vasodilatation, and platelet and mast cell activation. A reduction of blood flow has been reported only in patients who experience migraine with aura. This reduction occurs initially in the cortical region identified as responsible for aura symptoms then spreads anteriorly.[12] Magnesium deficiency may contribute to this state and predispose the brain to spontaneous initiation of spreading depression, an event that occurs early in migraine.[13,14] Previously, it was felt that tension-type headaches originated from an abnormality in neck and pericranial muscles; however, recent investigations have failed to establish a link.[11]

## Signs and Symptoms of Headache

Headaches can be differentiated by their signs and symptoms (Table 5-1). Tension-type headaches commonly present as bilateral, diffuse pain of the head that may radiate to other areas, such as the neck and shoulders. Patients often describe the pain as "tight" or "pressing," as if a band is constricting the head. The pain is usually more gradual in onset than the pain of vascular headaches. Shivering or cold temperatures may increase the pain. Chronic tension-type headaches occur at least 15 days per month for at least 6 months; these headaches are often a manifestation of psychologic conflict, depression, or anxiety, and may be associated with sleep disturbances, shortness

TABLE 5-1 Characteristics of Tension-type, Migraine, and Sinus Headaches[4]

| | Tension-type Headache | Migraine Headache | Sinus Headache |
|---|---|---|---|
| Location | Bilateral<br>Over the top of the head, extending to the base of the skull | Usually unilateral | Face, forehead or periorbital area |
| Nature | Diffuse aching<br>Tight, pressing, constricting pain | Throbbing<br>May be preceded by an aura | Pressure behind eyes or face |
| Onset | More gradual | Sudden | Simultaneous with sinus symptoms, including purulent nasal discharge |
| Duration | Minutes to days | Hours to 2 days | Resolves with sinus symptoms |

of breath, constipation, weight loss, fatigue, decreased sexual drive, palpitations, and menstrual changes. The severity of pain associated with tension-type headaches is variable; some headaches are so mild as to not require treatment, while others are severe enough to be disabling.[1]

Migraine headaches are recurrent and are classified as migraine either with or without aura. The aura associated with migraine manifests as a series of neurologic symptoms: shimmering or flashing areas or blind spots in the visual field, difficulty speaking, visual and auditory hallucinations, and (usually) one-sided muscle weakness. These symptoms may last for up to 30 minutes, and the throbbing headache pain that follows may last from several hours to 2 days. Migraines without aura begin immediately with the throbbing headache pain. Both forms of migraine are often associated with nausea, vomiting, photophobia, phonophobia, tinnitus, light-headedness, vertigo, and irritability and are aggravated by routine physical activity. A migraine attack may have a prodrome of a burst of energy or fatigue, extreme hunger, and nervousness. Migraine pain tends to be much more severe than that associated with tension-type headaches, with 80% of migraineurs reporting their pain as severe.[1] Migraine headache is a significant cause of absenteeism and lost productivity in the workplace and affects relationships with family and friends.[5]

Sinus headache is usually localized to facial areas over the sinuses. Pain tends to occur on awakening and may subside gradually after the patient has been upright for a while. Stooping or blowing the nose often intensifies the pain. Persistent sinus pain and/or discharge suggests possible infection and requires referral for further medical evaluation.

## Treatment of Headache

### *Treatment Goals*

The goals of treating headache are to (1) alleviate acute pain; (2) restore normal functioning; (3) prevent relapse; and (4) minimize side effects. For chronic headache, an additional goal is to reduce the frequency of headaches.

### *General Treatment Approach*

Most patients with episodic headaches respond adequately to self-treatment with nonpharmacologic interventions and/or nonprescription medications. Some patients with episodic headaches and most with chronic headaches are candidates for prescription treatments. However, these patients will often use nonprescription therapies adjunctively.

Episodic tension-type headaches often respond well to nonprescription analgesics, especially when an appropriate analgesic is taken as soon as the headache starts. If nonprescription analgesics are used to treat chronic headache, use should be episodic to prevent medication-overuse headache. Chronic tension-type headaches usually benefit from physical therapy and relaxation exercises in addition to nonprescription or prescription medication. The algorithm in Figure 5-2 outlines the self-treatment of headaches and lists exclusions for self-treatment.

Many patients use the term migraine to denote any bad headache. Therefore, a clinician's diagnosis is required to ensure that the headache is truly a migraine before treatment is suggested. Taking an analgesic at the onset of symptoms can abort a mild or moderate migraine headache. Once a migraine has evolved, analgesics sometimes will relieve the pain. Migraine sufferers who can predict the occurrence of the headache (e.g., during menstruation) should take an analgesic (usually an NSAID) before the event known to trigger the headache as well as throughout the duration of the event.

For patients with coexisting tension and migraine headaches, treatment of the initiating headache type can abort the mixed headache problem. It is not always necessary to treat both types.

For patients with sinus headache, decongestants (e.g., pseudoephedrine) are often useful in facilitating drainage of the sinuses (see Chapter 11). Concomitant use of decongestants and nonprescription analgesics can relieve the pain of sinus headache.

### *Nonpharmacologic Therapy*

Chronic tension-type headaches often respond to relaxation exercises and physical therapy emphasizing stretching and strengthening of the affected muscles. General treatment measures for migraine include (1) maintaining a regular schedule for sleeping and eating meals to avoid fatigue, oversleeping, or hunger and (2) practicing methods for coping with stress. Some migraine patients benefit from use of ice (ice bags or cold packs) combined with pressure applied to the forehead or temple areas to reduce pain associated with acute migraine attacks.

Nutritional strategies are intended to prevent migraine and are based on (1) dietary restriction of foods that contain triggers, (2) avoidance of hunger and low blood glucose (a trigger of migraine), and (3) magnesium supplementation. Advocates of nutritional therapy recommend avoidance of foods with vasoactive substances such as nitrites, tyramine (found in red wine and aged cheese), phenylalanine (found in the artificial sweetener aspartame), monosodium glutamate (often found in Asian food), caffeine (in coffee, tea, cola beverages, and chocolate), and theobromines (in chocolate). Any food allergen can also be a trigger.[15]

### *Pharmacologic Therapy*

Available nonprescription analgesics for management of headache include acetylated salicylate (aspirin), nonacetylated salicylates (magnesium salicylate, choline salicylate, and sodium salicylate), acetaminophen, and NSAIDs (ibuprofen, ketoprofen, and naproxen). Although these agents are available without a prescription, they are not benign; selection of an analgesic should be based on a careful review of a patient's medical and medication histories.

#### Acetylated and Nonacetylated Salicylates

*Mechanism of Action* Salicylates inhibit prostaglandin synthesis from arachidonic acid by inhibiting both isoforms of the enzyme cyclooxygenase (COX-1 and COX-2). The resulting decrease in prostaglandins reduces the sensitivity of pain receptors to the initiation of pain impulses at sites of inflammation and trauma. Although some evidence suggests that aspirin also produces analgesia through a central mechanism, its site of action is primarily peripheral.

*Pharmacokinetics* Salicylates are absorbed by passive diffusion of the nonionized drug in the stomach and small intestine. Factors affecting absorption include dosage

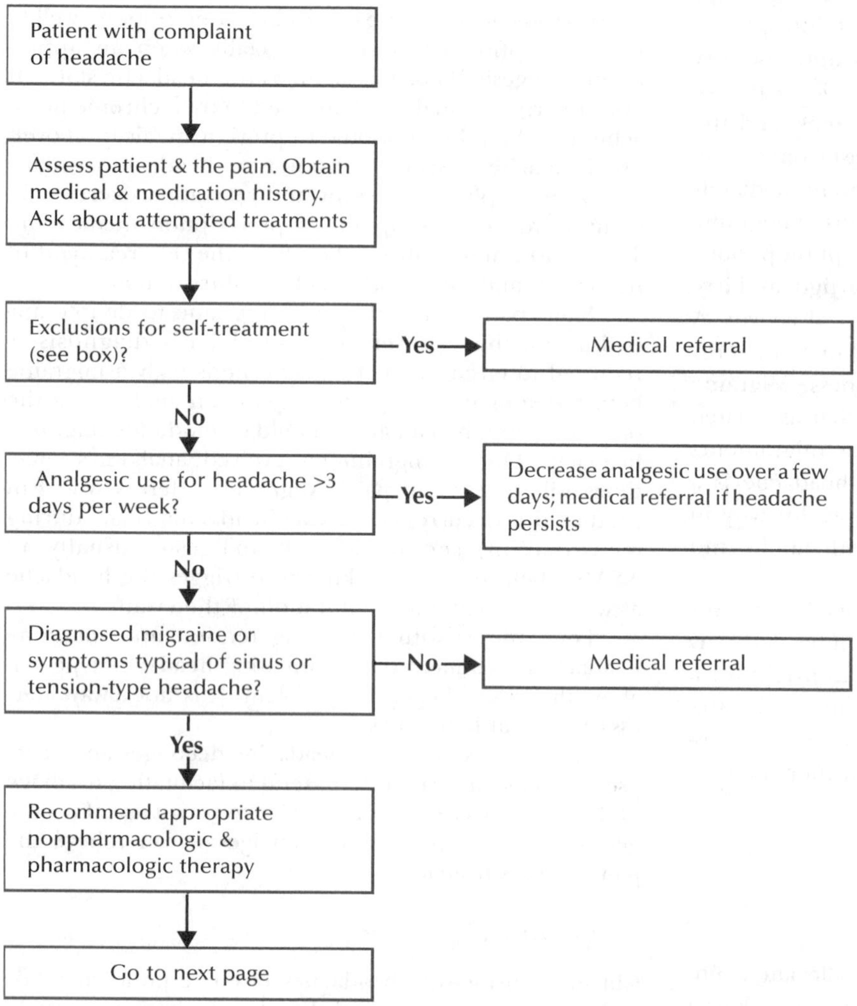


**Exclusions for Self-Treatment**

- Severe head pain
- Headaches that persist for 10 days with or without treatment
- Last trimester of pregnancy
- ≤7 years of age
- High fever or signs of serious infection
- History of liver disease or consumption of ≥3 alcoholic drinks per day
- Headache associated with underlying pathology (secondary headache)
- Symptoms consistent with migraine, but no formal diagnosis of migraine headache

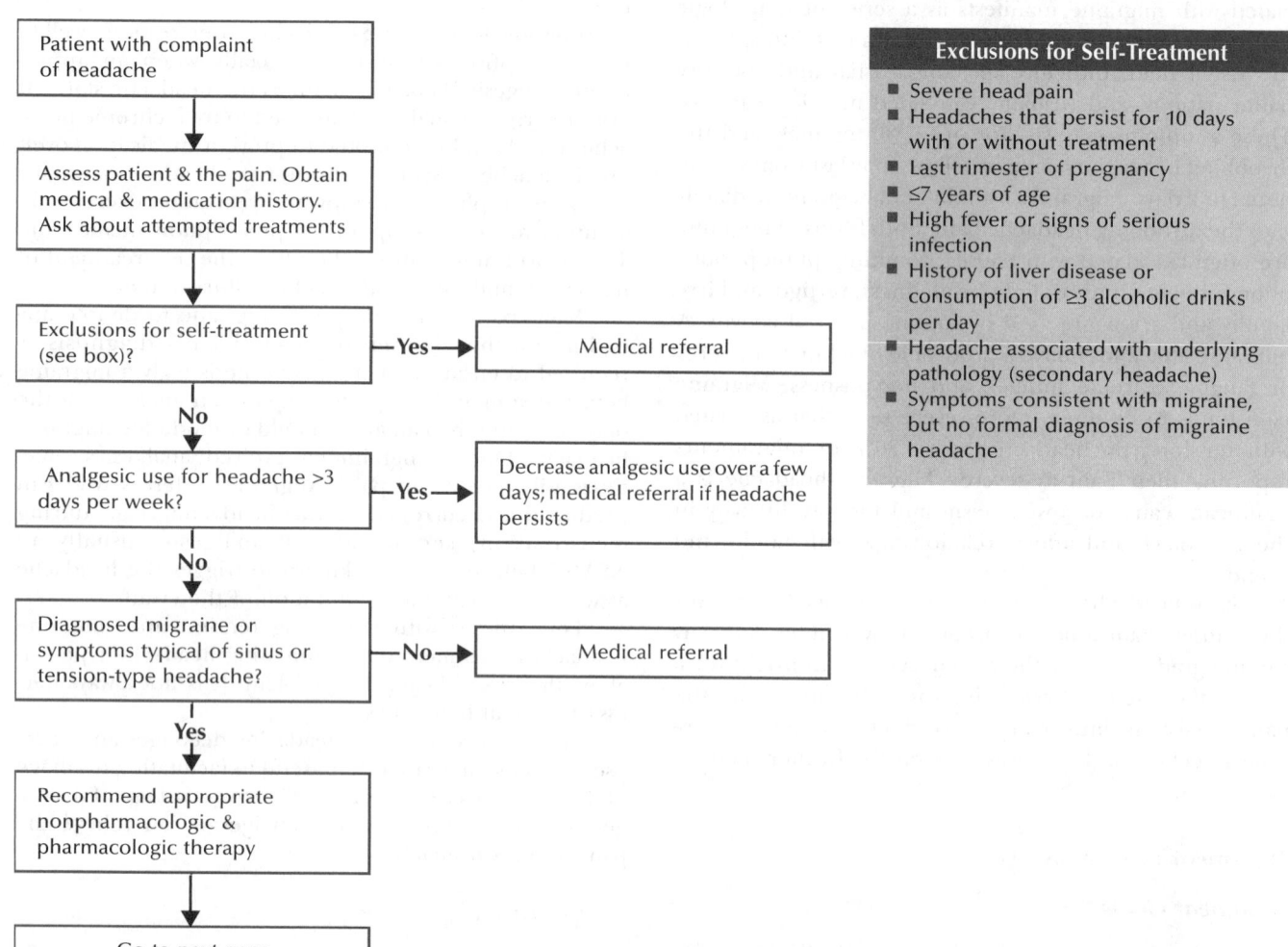

**FIGURE 5-2** Self-care of headache. Key: CHF, congestive heart failure; GI, gastrointestinal; HBP, high blood pressure; NSAID, nonsteroidal anti-inflammatory drug; OTC, over-the-counter.

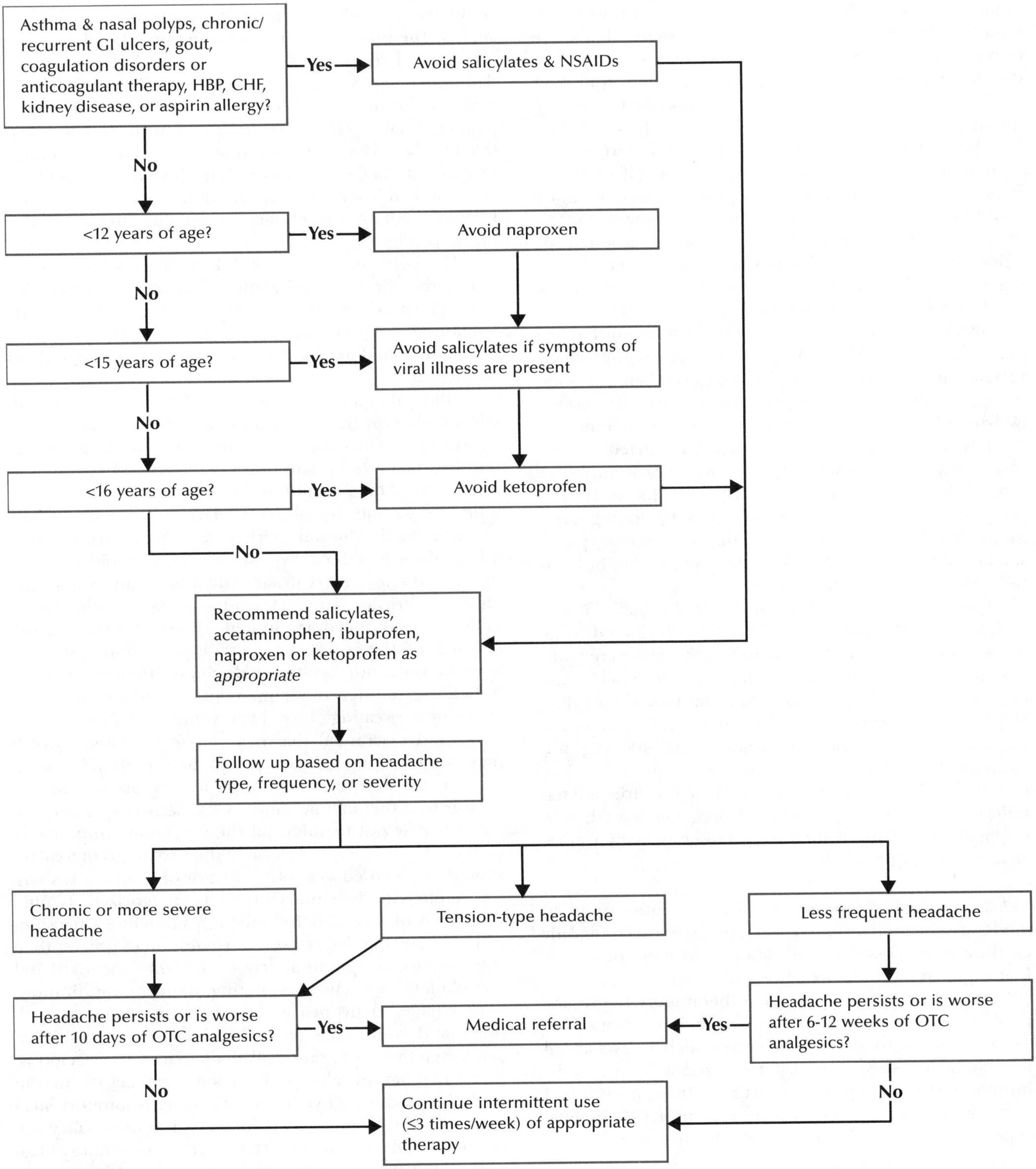


**FIGURE 5-2 (continued)**

form, gastric pH, gastric emptying time, dissolution rate, and the presence of antacids or food. Absorption from immediate-release aspirin products is complete. Choline salicylate is more water soluble than aspirin and offers the advantage of being stable in an oral solution. It is absorbed from the stomach more rapidly than aspirin tablets, but this difference may not be clinically important. Rectal absorption of salicylate is slow and unreliable, and proportional to rectal retention time.

Dosage form alterations include enteric coating, buffering, and sustained release. Such formulations were developed to change the rate of absorption and/or reduce the potential for gastrointestinal (GI) toxicity. Enteric-coated aspirin is absorbed only from the small intestine; its absorption is markedly slowed by food, attributed to prolonged gastric emptying time. For patients requiring rapid pain relief, enteric-coated aspirin is inappropriate because of the delay in absorption and the time to analgesic effect.

Buffered aspirin products are absorbed more rapidly than nonbuffered products, but onset of effect is not improved appreciably. Buffered aspirin products are available in both tablet and solution forms. Common buffers include aluminum hydroxide, magnesium carbonate or oxide, calcium carbonate, and sodium bicarbonate. Different combinations of buffers are used in various products.

Effervescent aspirin solutions (e.g., Alka-Seltzer) are rapidly absorbed because disintegration does not have to occur. However, there is no evidence that such products produce more rapid or effective analgesia than oral solid dosage forms of salicylates. Moreover, some effervescent aspirin solutions contain large amounts of sodium and must be avoided by patients requiring restricted sodium intake (e.g., patients with hypertension, heart failure, or renal failure). Sustained-release aspirin is formulated to prolong the product's duration of action by slowing dissolution and absorption. Because of this delayed absorption, such products are not useful for rapid pain relief but may be useful as bedtime medication.

Once absorbed, aspirin is hydrolyzed to salicylic acid in 1 to 2 hours. Salicylic acid is widely distributed to all tissues and fluids in the body including the central nervous system (CNS), breast milk, and fetal tissue. Protein binding is concentration dependent. At concentrations lower than 100 mg/mL, approximately 90% is bound to albumin, whereas at concentrations greater than 400 mg/mL approximately 75% is bound. Salicylic acid is largely eliminated through the kidney. The pH of the urine determines the amount of unchanged drug eliminated, with urinary concentrations increasing substantially in a more alkaline urine (pH ~8).

*Indications* Salicylates are effective in treating mild to moderate pain and fever. These agents are most commonly used for musculoskeletal indications, but they are usually ineffective in pain of visceral origin.

In addition, aspirin possesses other important uses for indications unrelated to pain syndromes. It is indicated for prevention of thromboembolic events, such as myocardial infarction and stroke, in high-risk patients owing to its inhibitory effects on platelet function.[16] It has been noted that risk for recurrent colon cancer is reduced in colorectal cancer survivors who regularly use aspirin.[17]

*Dosage and Administration Guidelines* Tables 5-2 and 5-3 list pediatric and adult dosages of selected trade-name nonprescription salicylates. Table 5-4 provides selected salicylate products. Aspirin dosages in the range of 4 to 6 g/day are often needed to produce anti-inflammatory effects. Because the maximum analgesic dosage for self-medication with aspirin is 4 g/day, anti-inflammatory activity often will not occur unless the drug is used at the high end of the acceptable dosage range. Therefore, NSAIDs may be preferred for self-treatment of inflammatory disorders such as rheumatoid arthritis or acute muscle injury.

A 5 mL dose of choline salicylate (174 mg/mL, or 870 mg) is equivalent to 650 mg of aspirin in salicylate content. For patients who find the fishy odor of the liquid product unacceptable, the oral solution of choline salicylate may be mixed with fruit juice, a carbonated beverage, or water just before administration. However, it should not be mixed with any alkaline solution, including antacids, because liberation of choline exaggerates the fishy odor of the product.

The salicylate content of 377 mg of magnesium salicylate tetrahydrate is equivalent to 325 mg of sodium salicylate. The maximum 24-hour dose of magnesium salicylate contains 264 mg (11 mEq) of magnesium. The product is sodium-free and may be used in patients requiring sodium restriction.

Mild salicylate intoxication (salicylism) occurs with chronic therapy that produces toxic salicylate plasma concentrations. Chronic intoxication in adults generally requires taking salicylate doses of 90 to 100 mg/kg/day for at least 2 days. Conditions that predispose patients to salicylate toxicity include (1) marked renal or hepatic impairment (i.e., uremia, cirrhosis, or hepatitis), (2) metabolic disorders (i.e., hypoxia or hypothyroidism), (3) unstable disease (i.e., cardiac arrhythmias, intractable epilepsy, or brittle diabetes), and (4) status asthmaticus. Patients of advanced age in general are at increased risk because of the incidence of multiple-system disorders. Symptoms include headache, dizziness, tinnitus, difficulty in hearing, dimness of vision, mental confusion, lassitude, drowsiness, sweating, thirst, hyperventilation, nausea, vomiting, and occasional diarrhea. These symptoms, which may mimic signs and symptoms of the disease being treated, are all reversible on lowering the plasma concentration to a therapeutic range. Clinicians remember that patients may not manifest all the signs and symptoms of toxicity. Tinnitus, typically one of the early signs of toxicity, should not be used as a sole indicator of salicylate toxicity.

Acute salicylate intoxication is categorized as mild (ingestion of less than 150 mg/kg), moderate (ingestion of 150 to 300 mg/kg), or severe (ingestion of greater than 300 mg/kg). Symptoms are concentration dependent and include lethargy, nausea, vomiting, dehydration, tinnitus, hemorrhage, tachypnea and pulmonary edema, convulsions, and coma. Acid-base disturbances are prominent and range from respiratory alkalosis to metabolic acidosis. Initially, salicylate affects the respiratory center in the medulla, producing hyperventilation and respiratory alkalosis. In severely intoxicated adults and in most salicylate-poisoned children younger than 5 years, respiratory alkalosis rapidly progresses to metabolic acidosis. Children are more prone than adults to develop high fever in salicylate poisoning. Hypoglycemia resulting from increased glucose utilization may be especially serious in children. Bleeding may occur from the GI tract or mucosal surfaces, and petechiae are a prominent feature at autopsy.

Emergency management of acute salicylate intoxication is directed toward preventing absorption of salicylate from the GI tract and supportive care. Activated charcoal should be used at home only if recommended by

**TABLE 5-2 Recommended Pediatric Dosages for Nonprescription Analgesics[18,19]**

| Agent | Dose by Body Weight (mg/kg) | Weight or Age | Single Dose (mg) |
|---|---|---|---|
| Acetaminophen* | 10-15 | 6-11 lb | 40 |
| | | 12-17 lb | 80 |
| | | 18-23 lb | 120 |
| | | 24-35 lb | 160 |
| | | 36-47 lb | 240 |
| | | 48-59 lb | 320 |
| | | 60-71 lb | 400 |
| | | 72-95 lb | 480 |
| | | ≥96 lb | 650 |
| Aspirin* | 10-15 | <24 lb | As directed by primary care provider |
| | | 24-35 lb | 162 |
| | | 36-47 lb | 243 |
| | | 48-59 lb | 324 |
| | | 60-71 lb | 405 |
| | | 72-95 lb | 486 |
| | | ≥96 lb | 648 |
| Ibuprofen† | 7.5 | 12-17 lb | 50 |
| | | 18-23 lb | 75 |
| | | 24-35 lb | 100 |
| | | 35-47 lb | 150 |
| | | 48-59 lb | 200 |
| | | 60-71 lb | 250 |
| | | 72-95 lb | 300 |
| | | >95 lb | 200-400 mg (maximum 1200 mg/day) |
| Naproxen sodium | | <12 years | Not recommended |
| | | >12 years | 220 mg q8-12h (maximum 660 mg/day) |
| Ketoprofen | | <16 years | Not recommended |
| | | >16 years | 12.5 mg q4-6h (dose may be repeated after 1 hour if needed; maximum 75 mg/day) |

* Individual doses may be repeated q4-6h as needed, not to exceed five doses in 24 hours.

† Individual doses may be repeated q6-8h as needed, not to exceed four doses in 24 hours.

**TABLE 5-3 Recommended Adult Dosages of Nonprescription Analgesics[18]**

| Agent | Dosage Forms | Usual Adult Dosage (Maximum Daily Dosage) |
|---|---|---|
| Aspirin | Immediate-release, buffered, enteric-coated, film-coated, effervescent, and chewable tablets; caplets; suppositories; chewing gum | 650-1000 mg q4-6h (4000 mg) |
| Choline salicylate | Oral solution | 870 mg q3-4h (5220 mg) |
| Magnesium salicylate | Caplets, tablets | 650 mg q4h or 1000 mg q6h (4000 mg) |
| Acetaminophen | Immediate-release, extended-release, effervescent, dissolving and chewable tablets; caplets; gel caps and gel tabs; liquid drops; elixir; suspension; solution; suppositories | 325-1000 mg q4-6h (4000 mg) |
| Ibuprofen | Immediate-release and chewable tablets; capsules; gelcaps; suspension; liquid drops | 200-400 mg q4-6h (1200 mg) |
| Naproxen sodium | Tablets | 220 mg q8-12h (660 mg) |
| Ketoprofen | Tablets | 12.5-25 mg q4-6h (75 mg) |

**TABLE 5-4 Selected Single-entity Salicylate Products**

| Trade Name | Primary Ingredients |
|---|---|
| **Pediatric Formulations** | |
| Bayer Low-Dose Children's Chewable Aspirin Tablets | Aspirin 81 mg |
| **Adult Formulations of Aspirin Products** | |
| Alka-Seltzer Original Effervescent Tablets | Aspirin 325 mg |
| Bayer Aspirin Extra Strength Caplets/Tablets | Aspirin 500 mg |
| Bayer Full-Dose Aspirin Tablets | Aspirin 325 mg |
| Bufferin Tablets | Aspirin 325 mg |
| Ecotrin Adult Low Strength Tablets | Aspirin 81 mg |
| Ecotrin Maximum Strength Enteric-Coated Tablets | Aspirin 500 mg |
| Ecotrin Regular Strength Enteric-Coated Tablets | Aspirin 325 mg |
| **Adult Formulations of Salicylate Products** | |
| Arthropan Liquid | Choline salicylate 870 mg/5 mL |
| Doan's Extra Strength Caplets | Magnesium salicylate 500 mg |
| Momentum Backache Relief Coated Tablets | Magnesium salicylate tetrahydrate 580 mg |

poison control or emergency department personnel. When the patient is seen in an emergency department, gastric lavage or activated charcoal may be used, depending on the clinician's preference and the clinical situation. Enhancing renal elimination can be accomplished through alkalinization of the urine. Further guidelines and dosing recommendations on the use of activated charcoal in preventing absorption of salicylate are included in Chapter 21.

*Safety Considerations* Aspirin produces GI mucosal damage by penetrating the protective mucous and bicarbonate layers of the gastric mucosa and permitting back diffusion of acid, thus causing cellular and vascular erosion. Two distinct mechanisms cause this problem: (1) a local irritant effect resulting from the drug contacting the gastric mucosa and (2) a systemic effect from prostaglandin inhibition.

Gastritis is a local effect that can occur without risk of ulceration. Conversely, ulceration is caused by systemic activity and can be asymptomatic until it is advanced. Acute injury occurs within 1 to 2 hours after ingestion of 600 mg of aspirin, causing gastric petechiae and erosions.[20] Endoscopic studies using lower doses of 300 mg/day for 14 days also show gastric and duodenal petechiae, erosions, and endoscopic ulcers. Gastric mucosal bleeding has been demonstrated in patients taking 75 mg/day. Other data have shown that 10% of patients taking daily doses of 10 to 300 mg for 12 weeks have documented gastric ulcers (one patient was receiving the 10 mg dose).[21]

GI blood loss with aspirin is dose dependent. Normal subjects with no aspirin exposure lose approximately 0.5 mL of blood per day in the stool. Moderate aspirin intake increases this amount to 2 to 6 mL per day, and up to 15% of patients will lose in excess of 10 mL per day. Chronic GI bleeding of this magnitude can deplete total body iron and produce iron deficiency anemia.

Patients of advanced age and those with alcoholic liver disease or a history of gastric ulceration or bleeding are at increased risk for acute hemorrhagic gastritis with aspirin use and, therefore, should avoid self-treatment with aspirin. In addition, patients should be advised that ingesting aspirin with alcohol appears to increase the incidence of GI bleeding. Risk factors identified for the development of salicylate-related ulcers include age (≥60 years), history of ulcer, higher dose, short duration of therapy (<2 weeks), and serious systemic illness. Concomitant use of corticosteroids and anticoagulants should be evaluated. Smoking, alcohol use, and the presence of *Helicobacter pylori* infections are less clear in their role as risk factors.

Various aspirin formulations may have different rates of GI side effects. Enteric coating may reduce occurrence of mucosal lesions identified by endoscopy as well as decrease local gastric irritation.[22] For major upper GI bleeding that results in hematemesis or melena, no difference in risk among plain, enteric-coated, and buffered products has been identified.[20,21] Endoscopic evaluation comparing gastric damage produced by buffered and nonbuffered aspirin products suggests similar rates of gastric damage.[21] However, enteric coating eliminates the local gastric irritation produced by aspirin, making it a preferred dosage form for patients requiring chronic therapy with medium to high doses.[20,22]

Clinically important aspirin intolerance is uncommon, and consists of two types: urticaria-angioedema type and bronchospastic type. Manifestations of aspirin intolerance include urticaria, angioedema, difficulty in breathing, bronchospasm, profuse rhinorrhea, and shock. These adverse effects usually occur within 3 hours of aspirin ingestion. The mechanism is not immunologically mediated and does not preclude use of nonacetylated salicylates.

Risk factors for aspirin intolerance include chronic urticaria for urticaria-angioedema type and asthma with nasal polyps for bronchospastic type. In patients with one of these conditions, the incidence of aspirin intolerance has been reported to range from 10% to 30%. Severity of the intolerance is variable, ranging from minor to severe.

Patients intolerant to aspirin may also cross-react to other chemicals or drugs. Up to 15% of patients who are intolerant to aspirin may cross-react when exposed to tartrazine (Food Drug and Cosmetic yellow dye No. 5), which can be found in many drugs and foods. Cross-reaction rates for acetaminophen, ibuprofen and naproxen in documented aspirin-intolerant patients are 7%, 98%, and 100%, respectively.[23] High cross-reaction rates in aspirin-intolerant patients are also reported with some prescription NSAIDs. The proposed mechanism of cross-sensitivity between aspirin and NSAID involves shunting arachidonic metabolism down the lipoxygenase pathway (because of inhibition of the cyclooxygenase pathway), resulting in accumulation of leukotrienes that can cause bronchospasm and anaphylaxis. Thus, patients with a history of aspirin intolerance should be advised to avoid all aspirin- and NSAID-containing products and to use acetaminophen preferentially for analgesic self-medication.

The cross-reaction rate for acetaminophen is low, but aspirin-intolerant patients may exhibit urticarial or bronchospastic symptoms with this drug. Usually a mild reaction, it occurs more often with higher doses (1000 mg).[24] Other nonprescription analgesics that have a low risk of cross-reactivity include sodium salicylate and choline salicylate.[25]

Nonprescription salicylates interact with several other important drugs and drug classes. Table 5-5 lists clinically important drug interactions reported for salicylates.[18] A large number of additional drug–drug interactions have been documented, many of which are not as clinically significant as those listed. Clinicians should review current drug interaction references for newly identified interactions when monitoring the therapy of patients taking high-dose salicylates.

Additive effects can occur with other agents or diseases with similar adverse effects, such as bleeding complications or GI irritation. Aspirin in doses greater than 3 g/day can have a hypoprothrombinemic effect that can be additive to that produced by oral anticoagulants such as warfarin. In addition, GI erosion and inhibition of platelet aggregation produced by as little as 500 mg/day of aspirin may further increase the bleeding risk when used concurrently with an oral anticoagulant such as warfarin. Thus, patients receiving oral anticoagulants should be cautioned to avoid self-treatment of pain with all nonprescription analgesic products containing aspirin or other salicylates and to consider acetaminophen as an appropriate nonprescription analgesic alternative.[25]

Concomitant use of ethanol with salicylates increases risk of gastropathy and fecal blood loss. This effect results from the GI erosive effects of alcohol and aspirin and an extended bleeding time prolonged by alcohol's potentiation of aspirin's antiplatelet effect. In one study, ingestion of alcohol plus 1000 mg of aspirin 1 hour after a standard breakfast significantly elevated blood alcohol concentrations, compared with those of subjects who did not receive aspirin. In such patients, alcohol bioavailability is increased because gastric alcohol dehydrogenase is inhibited, thus allowing greater GI absorption of alcohol.[26] Clinicians should advise patients not to consume alcohol and aspirin together because of the potential for enhanced GI irritation or bleeding and exaggerated neurologic impairment from increased alcohol absorption.

The hypoglycemic effect of sulfonylurea oral antidiabetic agents may be enhanced by concurrent administration of more than 2 g/day of any salicylate that increases insulin secretion. Decreased protein binding of the sulfonylurea may also play a role. Patients taking sulfonylureas to control diabetes should avoid self-treatment with all salicylate-containing products and consider acetaminophen as an appropriate alternative.

The uricosuric effect of probenecid and sulfinpyrazone may be antagonized by salicylates, resulting in worsening hyperuricemia and possible exacerbation of gout. The magnitude of this effect is salicylate dose dependent. Aspirin doses of greater than 3 g/day are uricosuric. Although intermittent use of salicylate is unlikely to cause serious problems in patients taking uricosuric drugs, self-treatment with all salicylates should be avoided to minimize risk. Acetaminophen is the best nonprescription alternative.

Salicylates are known to displace some drugs from their protein-binding sites. Analgesic doses of aspirin may increase the free fraction of valproic acid in plasma, causing enhanced neurologic symptoms such as drowsiness and behavioral disturbances. The mechanism appears to be a combination of protein-binding displacement and decreased clearance of valproic acid. Patients taking valproic acid should avoid self-treatment with salicylates; naproxen and acetaminophen are safe nonprescription analgesic alternatives.

Salicylates may increase the toxicity of methotrexate by displacing the drug from protein-binding sites and decreasing its renal excretion. Serious sequelae, including pancytopenia, have been reported with this drug combination. Patients taking methotrexate must be warned against self-medication with any salicylate-containing product. Acetaminophen has been safely used concurrently with methotrexate.

Aspirin ingestion may produce positive results on fecal occult blood testing; therefore, its use should be discontinued for at least 3 days before testing.

Aspirin can potentiate bleeding from capillary sites such as those found in the GI tract (with ulcers), tonsillar beds (after tonsillectomy), and tooth sockets (after dental extractions). A single 650 mg dose of aspirin can double bleeding time, and low doses also increase bleeding time. Aspirin should be discontinued at least 48 hours before surgery and should not be used to relieve the pain after tonsillectomy, dental extraction, or other surgical procedures, except under the close supervision of a primary care provider or dentist.

Because of the effect on hemostasis, aspirin is contraindicated in patients with hypoprothrombinemia, vitamin

**TABLE 5-5 Clinically Important Drug Interactions with Nonprescription Analgesic Agents[18]**

| Analgesic/Antipyretic | Drug | Potential Interaction | Management/Preventive Measures |
|---|---|---|---|
| Acetaminophen | Alcohol | ↑ Risk of hepatotoxicity | Avoid concurrent use if possible; minimize alcohol intake when using acetaminophen |
| Aspirin | Valproic acid | Displacement from protein-binding sites and inhibition of oxidation of valproic acid; up to 30% reduction in clearance | Avoid concurrent use. Use naproxen instead of aspirin (no interaction) |
| Aspirin | NSAIDs, including COX-2 inhibitors | ↑ Risk of gastroduodenal ulcers | Avoid concurrent use if possible; consider use of gastroprotective agents (e.g., PPIs) |
| NSAIDs (some) | Phenytoin | Phenytoin displaced from serum protein–binding sites if phenytoin metabolism is saturated or folate levels are low | Monitor unbound phenytoin levels; adjust dose, if indicated; ensure patient has sufficient folate |
| NSAIDs (several) | Digoxin | Inhibited renal clearance of digoxin | Monitor digoxin levels; adjust doses as indicated |
| Salicylates and NSAIDs (several) | Antihypertensive agents, β-blockers, ACE inhibitors, vasodilators, diuretics | Antihypertensive effect antagonized; hyperkalemia possible with potassium-sparing diuretics and ACEIs | Monitor blood pressure, cardiac function, and potassium levels |
| Salicylates and NSAIDs | Anticoagulants | ↑ Risk of bleeding, especially GI | Avoid concurrent use, if possible; lowest risk with salsalate and choline magnesium trisalicylate |
| Salicylates and NSAIDs | Alcohol | ↑ Risk of GI bleeding | Avoid concurrent use, if possible; minimize alcohol intake when using salicylates and NSAIDs |
| Salicylates and NSAIDs (several) | Methotrexate | ↓ Methotrexate clearance | Avoid salicylates and NSAIDs with high-dose methotrexate therapy; monitor levels with concurrent treatment |
| NSAIDs (several) | Bisphosphonates | ↑ Risk of GI or esophageal ulceration | Use caution with concomitant use |
| Salicylates (moderate to high doses) | Sulfonylureas | ↑ Hypoglycemic activity | Avoid concurrent use, if possible; Monitor blood glucose levels when changing salicylate dose |
| Salicylates | Corticosteroids | Salicylate clearance possibly increased with long-term, high-dose corticosteroid therapy | Monitor salicylate levels when changing steroid dose; adjust salicylate dose, if indicated |

Key: ACE, angiotensin-converting enzyme; COX, cyclooxygenase; GI, gastrointestinal; NSAID, nonsteroidal anti-inflammatory drug; PPI, proton pump inhibitor.

K deficiency, hemophilia, history of any bleeding disorder, or history of peptic ulcer disease. When peripheral anti-inflammatory activity is not needed and aspirin's effect on hemostasis is a concern, acetaminophen is an appropriate analgesic for self-medication. Prescription salicylate compounds salsalate and choline magnesium trisalicylate do not have appreciable effects on platelet aggregation and are reasonable alternatives when a peripheral anti-inflammatory agent is indicated. Sodium salicylate does not affect platelets, but it does increase prothrombin time.

The maximum 4 g dose of sodium salicylate contains 560 mg (25 mEq) of sodium. Consequently, patients on strict sodium restriction should avoid using sodium salicylate. Patients with compromised renal function have the potential for decreased renal excretion of magnesium, allowing accumulation of toxic levels.

All salicylates should be avoided in patients with a history of gout or hyperuricemia because of their effects on renal uric acid handling. The resulting effect on plasma uric acid is dose related. Doses of 1 to 2 g/day inhibit tubular uric acid secretion without affecting reabsorption and may increase plasma uric acid levels, which can precipitate or worsen an attack of gout. Moderate doses of 2 to 3 g/day have little effect on uric acid secretion. High doses of more than 5 g/day may decrease plasma uric acid by increasing its renal excretion, but because these are toxic salicylate doses, they should not be used in the clinical management of gout or hyperuricemia.

Reye's syndrome is an acute, potentially fatal illness occurring almost exclusively in children younger than 15 years. Although the cause of Reye's syndrome is unknown, viral and toxic agents, especially salicylates, have been associated with it. It is characterized by vomiting, progressive CNS damage, hepatic injury (fatty liver with encephalopathy), and hypoglycemia. The onset usually follows a viral infection with influenza (type A or B) or varicella zoster (e.g., chickenpox). Within 1 to 7 days, persistent vomiting generally occurs along with stupor, possibly progressing to generalized convulsions and coma. Other neurologic symptoms include listlessness, lethargy, disorientation, hostility, combativeness, inability to recognize family members, incessant moaning or screaming, twitching, and jerking. The mortality rate may be as high as 50%.

The American Academy of Pediatrics, the Food and Drug Administration (FDA), the Centers for Disease Control and Prevention, and the Surgeon General issued warnings that aspirin and other salicylates should be avoided in children and young adults who have influenza or chickenpox. The following contraindication is listed on labels of nonprescription aspirin and aspirin-containing products:

> Aspirin should not be used in children and teenagers for viral infections, with or without fever, because of the risk of Reye's syndrome with concomitant use of aspirin in certain viral illnesses.

In addition, FDA has extended this contraindication to include all nonprescription oral and rectal products containing bismuth subsalicylate or nonaspirin salicylates; new warnings on the packaging of most of these products were implemented in 2004.[27] Therefore, it is imperative that clinicians warn against giving any salicylate product to children and teenagers with viral illness. In such cases, acetaminophen is the preferred nonprescription analgesic/antipyretic. Although a simple viral upper respiratory infection (e.g., a common cold) is not a contraindication to aspirin use, it can be difficult to differentiate symptoms of this type of infection from influenza and chickenpox. Many clinicians therefore recommend a conservative approach of avoiding aspirin whenever symptoms resembling influenza are present. The use of aspirin as a pediatric antipyretic has all but ceased in the United States, as have reports of Reye's syndrome.

Since 1999, FDA has required a warning label regarding alcohol use on all nonprescription analgesic/antipyretic products for adult use. Concurrent use of aspirin with alcohol increases the risk of adverse GI events, including stomach bleeding. Patients who consume three or more alcoholic drinks daily should be counseled about the risks and referred to their primary care provider before they use these products.

Patients with preexisting coagulopathies should be cautious because salicylate use can impair hemostasis. Patients with asthma or nasal polyps may experience bronchospasm when using salicylates. Patients with renal or hepatic dysfunction should use salicylates with caution, as should patients taking anticoagulants.

### Acetaminophen

*Mechanism of Action* Acetaminophen is an effective analgesic and antipyretic, but does not possess anti-inflammatory activity. Unlike salicylates, acetaminophen produces analgesia through a central rather than a peripheral inhibition of prostaglandin synthesis.

*Pharmacokinetics* Acetaminophen is rapidly absorbed from the GI tract and extensively metabolized in the liver to inactive glucuronic and sulfuric acid conjugates. In addition, acetaminophen is metabolized to a hepatotoxic intermediate metabolite by the cytochrome P-450 enzyme system. This intermediate metabolite is detoxified by glutathione. Rectal bioavailability of acetaminophen is approximately 50% to 60% of that achieved with oral administration.

*Indications* Acetaminophen is effective in relieving mild to moderate pain of nonvisceral origin. Randomized, double-blind, placebo-controlled studies have documented superiority of acetaminophen 1000 mg over placebo in patients with migraine and tension-type headache.[28,29]

*Dosage and Administration Guidelines* Recommended pediatric and adult dosages of acetaminophen are provided in Tables 5-2 and 5-3. Table 5-6 lists selected tradename products.

Acetaminophen is available for administration in various oral liquid and solid dosage forms and as rectal suppositories. Acetaminophen oral capsules contain tasteless

**TABLE 5-6 Selected Single-entity Acetaminophen Products**

| Trade Name | Acetaminophen Content |
|---|---|
| **Pediatric Formulations** | |
| Children's Tylenol Meltaway tablets | 80 mg |
| FeverAll Infants' Suppositories | 80 mg |
| FeverAll Children's Suppositories | 160 mg |
| FeverAll Junior Strength Suppositories | 325 mg |
| Jr Tylenol Meltaway tablets | 160 mg |
| Tylenol Children's Suspension Liquid | 160 mg/5 mL |
| Tylenol Infants' Concentrated Drops | 80 mg/0.8 mL |
| **Adult Formulations** | |
| BromoSeltzer Effervescent Tablets | 650 mg |
| FeverAll Suppositories | 650 mg |
| Tylenol Arthritis Pain Extended Relief Caplets | 650 mg |
| Tylenol Extra Strength Adult Liquid | 1000 mg/30 mL |
| Tylenol Extra Strength Tablets/Caplets/Gelcaps/Geltabs | 500 mg |
| Tylenol Regular Strength Tablets | 325 mg |

granules that can be emptied onto a spoon containing a small amount of drink or soft food. Patients and parents should not add contents of the capsules to a glass of liquid because large numbers of granules may adhere to the side of the glass. Mixing with a hot beverage can result in a bitter taste.

Acetaminophen poisoning is a major reason for contacting poison control centers and the leading cause of acute liver failure in the United States.[30,31] The actual incidence of acetaminophen-induced hepatotoxicity cannot be determined because the drug is widely available and the number of acetaminophen users cannot be quantified. It is extremely uncommon for hepatotoxicity to occur at recommended doses of acetaminophen,[32] but it is probably dose related. In a prospective study, 83% of patients presenting with acetaminophen hepatotoxicity had taken more than 4 g/day.[31] Unintended chronic overdose may be associated with worse clinical outcomes, perhaps relating to later presentation for medical care, compared with intentional overdoses. It has been proposed that malnutrition and alcohol intake are risk factors for acetaminophen-induced hepatic injury, but this is refuted owing to the paucity of clinical evidence supporting the relationships.[33,34] In an attempt to reduce the occurrence of accidental overdose, FDA recommended labeling changes for prescription products containing acetaminophen and is considering labeling changes for nonprescription products as well.[35] In the United Kingdom, limiting package size to 16 tablets has reduced deaths attributable to acetaminophen overdose.[36]

Early symptoms of acetaminophen intoxication can include nausea, vomiting, drowsiness, confusion, and abdominal pain, but these symptoms may be absent, belying the potential gravity of the exposure. Serious clinical manifestations of hepatotoxicity begin 2 to 4 days after acute ingestion of acetaminophen and include increased plasma aspartate and alanine aminotransferase, increased plasma bilirubin with jaundice, prolonged prothrombin time, and obtundation. In the majority of cases, hepatic damage is reversible over a period of weeks or months,[31] but fatal hepatic necrosis can occur.

Because of the potential seriousness of acetaminophen overdose, all cases should be referred to a poison control center or medical personnel experienced in managing such cases. In addition to supportive care, activated charcoal (or other method of gut decontamination) is used to reduce the absorption of acetaminophen in cases presenting within a short time of an acute overdose. When acetaminophen serum levels exceed those known to cause hepatic injury, administration of acetylcysteine is warranted.[37] Prompt administration is important because its effectiveness is reduced when administration is delayed beyond 8 hours after an acute ingestion. For patients with chronic ingestions of greater than 4 g/day, administration of acetylcysteine is indicated until liver toxicity is ruled out by assessing liver enzymes and function tests.

*Safety Considerations* Side effects of acetaminophen are uncommon. Rarely, nephropathy, blood dyscrasias, and anemia have occurred. Compared with salicylates and NSAIDs, acetaminophen has no effect on urinary excretion of uric acid, prothrombin synthesis, or platelet aggregation and bleeding time. In addition, it produces less GI irritation, erosion, and bleeding than aspirin or other salicylates.Acetaminophen has a very low incidence of cross-reactivity in aspirin-intolerant patients. Thus, for patients who cannot take aspirin or another salicylate because of allergy, intolerance, or interactions, acetaminophen is an appropriate nonprescription analgesic alternative.

Clinically important drug interactions of acetaminophen are listed in Table 5-5. Although acetaminophen is considered the analgesic of choice in patients taking warfarin, doses in excess of 2275 mg/week have been associated with increases in international normalized ratio. Periodic increases in acetaminophen usage should be discouraged in patients on anticoagulant regimens. Patients who may require higher scheduled doses (e.g., those with osteoarthritis) should have their international normalized ratio monitored and warfarin adjusted as acetaminophen doses are titrated.

Use of acetaminophen is contraindicated in patients who are hypersensitive to it.

Acetaminophen is potentially hepatotoxic in doses exceeding 4 g/day, especially with chronic use. Patients should be cautioned against exceeding this dose limit. More conservative dosing (i.e., <2 g/day) or avoidance may be warranted in patients at increased risk for acetaminophen-induced hepatotoxicity, including those with preexisting liver disease, concurrent use of other potentially hepatotoxic drugs, poor nutritional intake, or ingestion of three or more alcoholic drinks per day.[38] Patients with glucose-6-phosphate dehydrogenase deficiency should also use caution when medicating with acetaminophen.

## Nonsteroidal Anti-inflammatory Drugs

*Mechanism of Action* NSAIDs relieve pain through peripheral inhibition of COX and subsequent inhibition of prostaglandin synthesis.

*Pharmacokinetics* All nonprescription NSAIDs are rapidly absorbed from the GI tract with consistently high bioavailability. They are extensively metabolized to inactive compounds in the liver, mainly by glucuronidation. Elimination occurs primarily through the kidneys. Naproxen sodium has an onset of activity similar to other nonprescription NSAIDs, but its duration of action may be somewhat longer.

*Indications* The labeled indications for nonprescription nonsteroidal anti-inflammatory analgesics include relieving minor pain associated with headache, the common cold, toothache, muscle ache, backache, arthritis, and menstrual cramps. They are all approved as antipyretics. NSAIDs have analgesic, antipyretic, and anti-inflammatory activity, and are useful in managing mild to moderate pain of nonvisceral origin. Three agents (all propionic acid–derivative NSAIDs) are approved for nonprescription use: ibuprofen (1984), naproxen sodium (1994), and ketoprofen (1995).

TABLE 5-7 Selected Single-entity Nonsteroidal Anti-inflammatory Drugs

| Trade Name | Primary Ingredients |
|---|---|
| **Pediatric Formulations of Ibuprofen Products** | |
| Advil Children's Suspension | Ibuprofen 100 mg/5 mL |
| Advil Children's Chewable Tablets | Ibuprofen 50 mg |
| Advil Junior Strength Chewable Tablets | Ibuprofen 100 mg |
| Advil Junior Strength Coated Tablets | Ibuprofen 100 mg |
| Motrin Children's Chewable Tablets | Ibuprofen 50 mg |
| Motrin Children's Suspension | Ibuprofen 100 mg/5 mL |
| Motrin Infants' Drops | Ibuprofen 50 mg/1.25 mL |
| Motrin Junior Strength Caplets | Ibuprofen 100 mg |
| Motrin Junior Strength Chewable Caplets | Ibuprofen 100 mg |
| **Adult Formulations of Ibuprofen Products** | |
| Advil Migraine Liquid Filled Capsules | Ibuprofen 200 mg |
| Advil Tablets/Caplets/Gelcaps/LiquiGels | Ibuprofen 200 mg |
| Motrin IB Tablets/Caplets/Gelcaps and Migraine Pain | Ibuprofen 200 mg |
| **Ketoprofen Products** | |
| Orudis KT Tablets | Ketoprofen 12.5 mg |
| **Naproxen Products** | |
| Aleve Tablets/Capsules/Gelcaps | Naproxen sodium 220 mg |
| Pamprin Maximum Strength All Day Relief | Naproxen sodium 220 mg |

*Dosage and Administration Guidelines* Tables 5-2, 5-3, and 5-7 list pediatric and adult doses and selected trade-name products of nonprescription NSAIDs. A dose–effect relationship has been demonstrated for ibuprofen analgesia in the range of 100 to 400 mg. On a milligram-to-milligram basis, ibuprofen is approximately 3.5 times more potent than aspirin as an analgesic, and the analgesic effect may last up to 6 hours.

Naproxen sodium can be used for patients 12 years and older; doses should be taken 8 to 12 hours apart. Patients older than 65 years should not take more than one tablet every 12 hours unless directed to do so by a primary care provider. Children younger than 12 years of age should use the drug only under the supervision of a primary care provider.

Ketoprofen 12.5 mg appears to be equivalent to ibuprofen 200 mg. The drug is recommended for patients 16 years and older. No pediatric dosing recommendations are available.

If a patient misses a dose and it is almost time for the next regular dose, the patient should skip the missed dose and resume taking medication at the next scheduled time. These medications may be taken with food, milk, or antacids if they upset the stomach. Tablets should be taken with a full glass of water, suspensions should be shaken thoroughly, and enteric-coated or sustained-release preparations should be neither crushed nor chewed.

Overdoses of NSAIDs usually produce minimal symptoms of toxicity and are rarely fatal. In a prospective study of 329 cases of ibuprofen overdose, it was found that GI and CNS symptoms (in 42% and 30% of patients, respectively) were most common and included nausea, vomiting, abdominal pain, lethargy, stupor, coma, nystagmus, dizziness, and light-headedness. Hypotension, bradycardia, tachycardia, dyspnea, and painful breathing were also reported. In this study, 43% of ibuprofen-overdose patients were asymptomatic.[39]

*Safety Considerations* The most frequent adverse effects of NSAIDs involve the GI tract and include dyspepsia, heartburn, nausea, anorexia, and epigastric pain, even among children using pediatric formulations. These agents produce less GI upset and bleeding than aspirin. A meta-analysis ranked relative risk of GI toxicity among salicylates and NSAIDs. Ibuprofen was lowest, aspirin and naproxen were intermediate, and ketoprofen was higher although these rankings may not correlate directly with nonprescription use (<10 days and adherence to nonprescription dosage).[24] Other adverse effects include dizziness, fatigue, headache, or nervousness. Rashes or itching may occur in some patients, and some cases of photosensitivity have been reported. Fluid retention can occur and, in some cases, edema develops. At normal nonprescription doses, these effects are usually rare.

There may be an association between NSAIDs and risk for cardiovascular and cerebrovascular events. Naproxen was associated with a 50% increase in cardiovascular events, compared with placebo in an ongoing study investigating the ability of the drug to prevent Alzheimer disease. The study was halted prematurely and highlights the possibility that NSAIDs (at least when used for longer periods of time) may increase risk for cardiovascular and cerebrovascular events. Further study of this association is needed before a definitive link can be established.[40] However, FDA has issued a public health advisory emphasizing the need for medical supervision if a nonprescription NSAID is taken for more than 10 days.[40] Furthermore, the agency mandated labeling changes for all NSAIDs to include warnings about possible increased risk for heart attack or stroke with long-term continuous use.[41]

Clinically important drug–drug interactions of NSAIDs are listed in Table 5-5. A brief discussion of drug–drug interactions with ibuprofen, naproxen, and ketoprofen follows.

Digoxin Ibuprofen has been reported to increase plasma digoxin concentrations in patients receiving digoxin. The clinical significance of this interaction is uncertain. Worsening heart failure with fluid overload and blunting of furosemide responsiveness may occur with administration of ibuprofen to patients with congestive heart failure. Because of the uncertainty of a possible ibuprofen–digoxin interaction and the potential for ibuprofen-induced furosemide refractoriness with symptomatic deterioration, clinicians should advise patients with a history of congestive heart failure to avoid self-medicating with any ibuprofen-containing products.

Antihypertensive Drugs NSAIDs antagonize the blood pressure–lowering effects of certain antihypertensive drugs, including diuretics, angiotensin-converting enzyme inhibitors, β-blockers, and centrally acting antihypertensives. Usually an effect on blood pressure is not observed with treatment for less than a week.[24] Thus, clinicians should advise hypertensive patients who are selecting a nonprescription analgesic that NSAIDs may antagonize their blood pressure medication if used more than several days and that acetaminophen is a good alternative.

Methotrexate A potentially serious interaction exists between methotrexate and NSAIDs. Pancytopenia and acute renal failure have been reported. All nonprescription NSAIDs have been reported to affect methotrexate levels, sometimes with fatal consequences. The exact mechanism is not fully known but may relate to competition of the NSAID with methotrexate for renal proximal tubular secretion, causing decreased renal clearance of methotrexate and resulting in nephrotoxicity. Displacement from protein binding may also be involved if a salicylate is combined with methotrexate. Patients receiving methotrexate must be warned not to use nonprescription analgesics containing NSAIDs or aspirin without medical supervision. For such patients, acetaminophen is the only nonprescription analgesic considered safe.

NSAIDs are contraindicated in patients with a history of intolerance to aspirin or to any other NSAID. Cross-reactivity with ibuprofen and naproxen are reported to be 98% and 100%, respectively, in patients with documented aspirin intolerance. Patients with a history of aspirin intolerance and asthma may experience a worsening of their bronchospastic symptoms with NSAIDs. According to FDA class-labeling requirements, all NSAIDs carry the same warning about cross-reactivity. Nonacetylated salicylates are better tolerated than NSAIDs in patients with a documented aspirin intolerance.

Patients should be cautioned that ibuprofen increases bleeding time by inhibiting platelet aggregation. However, ibuprofen's effect on platelet aggregation, unlike that of aspirin, is reversible within 24 hours after medication is discontinued.[24] In doses of 1200 to 2400 mg/day, ibuprofen does not appear to affect the hypoprothrombinemia produced by warfarin. However, ibuprofen should not be recommended for self-medication to patients who are concurrently taking anticoagulants because it can displace plasma protein-bound warfarin and its antiplatelet activity could increase GI bleeding.

As with other nonprescription analgesics, patients who have three or more alcoholic drinks per day should be cautioned about increased risk of adverse GI events, including stomach bleeding, and be referred to their primary care provider regarding use.

Patients with preexisting renal impairment or congestive heart failure should also use NSAIDs cautiously. These agents may decrease renal blood flow and glomerular filtration rate as a result of inhibition of renal prostaglandin synthesis. Consequently, increased blood urea nitrogen and serum creatinine values, often with concomitant sodium and water retention, can occur. Advanced age, hypertension, diabetes, atherosclerotic cardiovascular disease, and use of diuretics appear to increase risk of renal toxicity with ibuprofen use. As a result, patients with a history of impaired renal function, congestive heart failure, or diseases that compromise renal hemodynamics should not self-medicate with NSAIDs.

## Combination Products

Many nonprescription analgesics are available as combination products containing aspirin, ibuprofen, or acetaminophen as primary ingredients plus caffeine or an antihistamine. Combination products containing two nonprescription analgesics are also available (Table 5-8).

The adjuvant ingredients are claimed to enhance analgesic efficacy of the product. Some evidence supports the enhanced efficacy of such combination products. Other studies have failed to demonstrate a benefit from the adjuvants. An analgesic effect for caffeine alone has been supported by some studies but not others. When combined with other nonprescription analgesics (aspirin, acetaminophen, or ibuprofen), a synergistic analgesic effect is demonstrated.

Studies have shown that Excedrin Migraine is superior to placebo in alleviating pain associated with migraine headaches.[42] Because this product contains caffeine, patients should be counseled about the possibility of

TABLE 5-8 Selected Combination Analgesic Products

| Trade Name | Primary Ingredients |
|---|---|
| Advil Cold & Sinus Tablets | Ibuprofen 200 mg; pseudoephedrine 30 mg |
| Aleve Sinus and Headache | Naproxen sodium 220 mg; pseudoephedrine 120 mg |
| Alka-Seltzer Morning Relief | Aspirin 500 mg; caffeine 65 mg |
| Anacin Caplets/Coated Tablets | Aspirin 400 mg; caffeine 32 mg |
| Excedrin Aspirin Free Caplets/Geltabs/Quick Tabs | Acetaminophen 500 mg; caffeine 65 mg |
| Excedrin Extra Strength Caplets/Tablets/Geltabs and Excedrin Migraine | Acetaminophen 250 mg; aspirin 250 mg; caffeine 65 mg |
| Goody's Extra Strength Headache Powder | Acetaminophen 260 mg; aspirin 520 mg; caffeine 32.5 mg |
| Pamprin Maximum Strength Menstrual Pain Relief Caplets | Acetaminophen 250 mg; magnesium salicylate 250 mg |
| Saleto Tablets | Acetaminophen 115 mg; aspirin 210 mg; caffeine 16 mg; salicylamide 65 mg |
| Tylenol Sinus Daytime Caplets, Geltabs, Gelcaps | Acetaminophen 500 mg; pseudoephedrine 30 mg |
| Vanquish Caplets | Acetaminophen 194 mg; aspirin 227 mg; caffeine 33 mg |

medication-overuse headaches. Patients who use this combination for more than three episodes weekly should be referred to a headache specialist for further evaluation. Efficacy of caffeine/analgesic combinations has also been demonstrated for a variety of conditions including dental pain, postpartum pain, cancer pain, sore throat, and headache, both tension-type and migraine.

In addition, enhanced analgesia has been reported for various antihistamine–analgesic combinations, including orphenadrine–acetaminophen and phenyltoloxamine–acetaminophen. Although these combinations have demonstrated superior efficacy in acute pain, compared with acetaminophen alone, their use is limited by the sedating effects of the antihistamines.

Combination dosage forms containing a decongestant and either acetaminophen or an NSAID are also available. Such combinations appear logical for use in sinus headaches or other indications in which both analgesia and decongestion are needed.

## Pharmacotherapeutic Comparison

*Aspirin Versus Nonacetylated Salicylates* Although definitive clinical data are lacking, aspirin and nonacetylated salicylates are believed to be equal in anti-inflammatory potency, but aspirin is thought to be a superior analgesic and antipyretic.[43]

*Aspirin Versus Acetaminophen* Numerous controlled studies have demonstrated the equivalent analgesic efficacy of aspirin and acetaminophen on a milligram-for-milligram basis in various pain models, including postoperative pain, cancer pain, episiotomy pain, and oral surgery pain. In a placebo-controlled trial involving 542 patients, single doses of acetaminophen 500 mg and 1000 mg and aspirin 500 mg and 1000 mg were compared for the treatment of tension-type headache. Two hours after taking the study medication, both aspirin groups and acetaminophen 1000 mg produced superior pain relief, compared with placebo. Although the study was not powered to detect differences between active treatment arms, the percentage of patients reporting adequate or total relief were similar among these three groups.[29]

*Aspirin Versus Ibuprofen* Ibuprofen has been shown to be at least as effective as aspirin in treating various types of pain, including dental extraction pain, dysmenorrhea, and episiotomy pain.

*NSAID Versus Acetaminophen* For episodic tension-type headache, acetaminophen 1000 mg appears to provide relief that is equivalent to ketoprofen 25 mg or naproxen 375 mg.[44,45] For moderate to severe (dental or sore throat) pain in children, single doses of acetaminophen 7 to 15 mg/kg produced similar pain relief, compared with ibuprofen 5 to 10 mg/kg. Both drugs were well-tolerated.[46]

*Naproxen Versus Ibuprofen* Naproxen sodium 220 mg appears to be similar in efficacy to ibuprofen 200 mg. The onset of activity is similar between the two NSAIDs. Naproxen sodium's duration of action is somewhat longer than that of ibuprofen, but the clinical significance of that difference is not clear. Nonetheless, some patients report better response to one NSAID than to another for reasons that are unclear. It is possible that such differences will be apparent at nonprescription doses of NSAIDs.

## Product Selection Guidelines

*Special Population Considerations* Salicylates should be avoided during viral illness in children because of the risk of Reye's syndrome (see Safety Considerations in Acetylated and Nonacetylated Salicylates).

Aspirin consumption during pregnancy may produce adverse maternal effects, including anemia, antepartum or postpartum hemorrhage, and prolonged gestation and labor. Aspirin ingestion on a regular basis during pregnancy may increase risk for complicated deliveries, including cesarean sections, as well as breech and forceps deliveries. However, definitive data supporting this concern are lacking.

In 1990, FDA required oral and rectal nonprescription drug products that contain aspirin to carry labels that warn against using the drugs during the last 3 months of pregnancy unless the patient is directed to do so by a medical provider.

Aspirin readily crosses the placenta and can be found in higher concentrations in the neonate than in the mother. Salicylate elimination is slow in the neonate because of the liver's immaturity and underdeveloped capacity to form glycine and glucuronic acid conjugates and because of reduced urinary excretion resulting from low glomerular filtration rates.

Fetal effects of in utero aspirin exposure include intrauterine growth retardation, congenital salicylate intoxication, decreased albumin-binding capacity, and increased perinatal mortality. In utero mortality results, in part, from antepartum hemorrhage or premature closure of the ductus arteriosus. In utero aspirin exposure within 1 week of delivery can produce hemorrhagic episodes and/or pruritic rash in the neonate. Reported neonatal bleeding complications include petechiae, hematuria, cephalhematoma, subconjunctival hemorrhage, and bleeding after circumcision. An increased incidence of intracranial hemorrhage in premature or low-birth-weight infants has also been reported after maternal aspirin use near birth.[47] The relationship between maternal aspirin ingestion and congenital malformation is unresolved. An association between maternal aspirin ingestion, oral clefts, and congenital heart disease has been reported. However, other studies have failed to confirm increased risk for fetal malformation resulting from maternal aspirin exposure.

Aspirin and other salicylates are excreted into breast milk in low concentrations. After single-dose oral salicylate ingestion, peak milk levels occur at about 3 hours, producing a milk-to-maternal plasma ratio of 3:8. Although no adverse effects on platelet function in the nursing infant exposed to aspirin through the mother's milk have been reported, they still must be considered a potential risk.[47] Women should be advised to avoid aspirin during pregnancy, especially during the last trimester, and when breast-feeding. During pregnancy, acetaminophen is the preferred analgesic for self-medication. Acetaminophen is also the preferred agent for nursing mothers; however, ibuprofen can be used.

Use of acetaminophen in the pediatric population is complicated by the various available strengths and formulations. Unintended over- or underdosing can occur when parents switch between infant drops (80 mg/0.8 mL) and elixir (160 mg/5 mL), incorrectly assuming they are the same concentration. In addition, rapidly growing infants quickly outgrow previous dose requirements. Therefore, recalculation of the pediatric dose according to present age and body weight is appropriate at the time of each treatment course.

Acetaminophen crosses the placenta, but is considered safe for use during pregnancy.[47] It appears in breast milk, producing a milk-to-maternal plasma ratio of 0.5:1.0. On the basis of a 1 g maternal dose, the estimated maximum infant dose is 1.85% of the maternal dose. The only adverse effect reported in nursing infants exposed to acetaminophen through breast milk is a rarely occurring maculopapular rash, which subsides when drug exposure is discontinued. Acetaminophen use is considered to be compatible with breast-feeding.[47]

No evidence exists that NSAIDs are teratogenic in either humans or animals. However, use of these agents is contraindicated during the third trimester of pregnancy because all potent prostaglandin synthesis inhibitors can cause delayed parturition, prolonged labor, and increased postpartum bleeding. These agents can also have adverse fetal cardiovascular effects (e.g., delayed closure of the ductus arteriosus). Lactating women taking up to 2.4 g of ibuprofen per day showed no measurable excretion of ibuprofen into breast milk, and ibuprofen is considered compatible with breast-feeding.[47]

Naproxen is also considered compatible with breast-feeding.[47] No evidence of teratogenicity or toxicity to embryos has been uncovered in studies of pregnant animals given high doses of ketoprofen. No evidence exists of adverse effects on fertility. The product labeling, however, recommends that nursing mothers not use this drug.

*Patient Factors* Age is an important consideration when selecting an appropriate nonprescription medication. Parents of patients younger than 2 years should seek the advice of their pediatrician on what treatment option to pursue. Children older than 2 years may use acetaminophen or ibuprofen. Naproxen sodium has been approved for use in patients at least 12 years of age, and ketoprofen is approved for individuals 16 years of age or older. Parents should not use aspirin or aspirin-containing products in children younger than 15 years, unless directed to do so by a primary care provider, because of the risk for Reye's syndrome.

Salicylates and NSAIDs should be avoided in the last trimester of pregnancy. Acetaminophen is a safe and effective alternative during this time. Acetaminophen, ibuprofen, and naproxen are compatible with breast-feeding, whereas current labeling advises against aspirin and ketoprofen use in nursing mothers.[47]

Persons of advanced age are at increased risk for many adverse effects of salicylates and NSAIDs. Preexisting comorbidities, impaired renal function, and use of other medications may contribute to the increased risk. In particular, older adults are more vulnerable to serious GI toxicity,[48] as well as to the hypertensive and renal effects of these agents. For this reason, acetaminophen is generally recognized as the treatment of choice for management of mild to moderate pain in older adults.[49]

Patients with renal impairment should exercise caution when using NSAIDs or salicylates. Clinically important alterations in renal blood flow resulting in acute reduction in renal function can result from use of even short courses of NSAIDs or salicylates. These patients should be referred for medical evaluation for assistance in selecting an analgesic.

*Patient Preferences* Nonprescription analgesics are available in a number of dosage forms. During the patient assessment, clinicians should determine which dosage form will provide the patient with an optimum outcome. In the majority of cases, patients will have a preference for route of administration and dosage form (e.g., oral or rectal, capsule or tablet).

TABLE 5-9 Selected Complementary/Alternative Medicines Used to Treat Headache

| Agent | Risks | Uses/Effectiveness |
|---|---|---|
| **Botanical Medicines (Scientific Name)** | | |
| Butterbur (*Petasites hybridus*) | Belching; avoid during pregnancy and lactation; avoid products with UPA constituents; UPA-free products seem safe for use ≤16 weeks | Prevention of migraine headache; PC RT demonstrated ≥50 mg/day may reduce frequency by ~50% |
| Feverfew (*Tanacetum parthenium*) | Possible rebound headache with chronic use; mouth ulceration with direct contact with leaves; possible anticoagulant effect | Treatment and prevention of migraine headache; mixed results from clinical trials, possibly because of differences in formulations |
| Peppermint oil (*Mentha piperita*) | Skin irritation at application site; avoid during pregnancy and lactation | Topical treatment of tension headache; preliminary evidence suggests peppermint oil applied to forehead and temples may relieve tension headaches |
| **Nonbotanical Natural Medicines** | | |
| Coenzyme Q10 | Avoid during pregnancy and lactation; minor GI disturbances most common side effects | Prevention of migraine headache; small, open label trial demonstrated 150 mg/day reduced frequency by ~33% |
| **Nutritional Supplements** | | |
| Magnesium | Diarrhea; GI upset | Treatment and prevention of migraine headache; PC, blinded RTs of 20-24 mmol/day yielded mixed results for prevention; patients with hypomagnesemia may respond to IV magnesium administered during acute attack |
| Riboflavin | Diarrhea; polyuria | Prevention of migraine headache; small RT of 400 mg/day showed reduced frequency of migraine headaches |

Key: GI, gastrointestinal; IV, intravenous; PC, placebo-controlled; RT, randomized trial; UPA, unsaturated pyrrolizidine alkaloid.

One area in which the clinician can be instrumental in affecting outcomes is in determining which dosing frequency will be needed for an individual patient. Naproxen sodium can be taken two to three times daily and may improve patient compliance. Ketoprofen may be effective given three to four times daily. Conversely, acetaminophen, ibuprofen, and salicylates may require dosing as frequently as every 4 hours.

### *Complementary Therapies*

Patients may seek other therapies for headache because they want to avoid drugs or have had unsuccessful treatment (Table 5-9). Feverfew is the herbal that has received the most study in preventing migraine headache. Several randomized, placebo-controlled, double-blind trials have shown feverfew is more effective than placebo although one of the better designed trials found no significant difference. No significant problems with its use are reported, but it may cause medication-overuse headaches on discontinuation. The usual dose for migraine prophylaxis is 100 to 250 mg/day standardized to contain 0.2% parthenolide.

Acupuncture has been used to treat headache including migraine, tension-type, and mixed forms. A review of 27 criteria-selected trials showed benefit was achieved in 23, leading the authors to conclude that acupuncture seems promising in spite of methodologic difficulties in evaluation.[50]

## Assessment of Headache: A Case-based Approach

Before a nonprescription medication can be recommended, the clinician must assess the patient's headache—the type, severity, location, frequency, intensity over time, and age at onset—and obtain a medical and psychosocial history. All current medications should be inventoried, and all past and present headache treatments should be reviewed, with emphasis on determining which treatments, if any, were successful or preferred.

As noted previously, secondary headaches other than minor sinus headache are excluded from self-treatment. A brief description of the signs and symptoms of some secondary headaches is presented here to aid in differentiating between primary and secondary headaches. Headache associated with seizures, confusion, drowsiness, or intellectual impairment may be a sign of brain tumor, subdural hematoma, or subarachnoid hemorrhage. Headache accompanied by nausea, vomiting, fever, and stiff neck may indicate brain abscess (arising from bacterial, fungal, or parasitic infection) or meningitis. The presence of headache with night sweats, aching joints, fever, weight loss, and visual symptoms (such as blurring) in patients with a history similar to rheumatoid arthritis may indicate cranial arteritis. Headache associated with localized facial pain, muscle tenderness, and limited motion of the jaw may indicate temporomandibular joint disorder. Case 5-1 illustrates assessment of a patient with headache.

## CASE 5-1

| Relevant Evaluation Criteria | Scenario/Model Outcome |
|---|---|
| **Information Gathering** | |
| 1. Gather essential information about the patient's symptoms, including: | |
| a. description of symptom(s) (i.e., nature, onset, duration, severity, associated symptoms) | Patient has headaches that have been increasing in frequency and severity over the last 2 months; currently, he is experiencing two to three headaches per week. The headaches worsen gradually over the course of an afternoon, beginning over and behind the eyes, and spreading to include the top and back of the head by evening. Pain is constant and vicelike and sometimes accompanied by sensitivity to light. Patient reports it is difficult for him to continue working when the headaches occur. |
| b. description of any factors that seem to precipitate, exacerbate, and/or relieve the patient's symptom(s) | Symptoms began about the same time the patient was reassigned to desk work. Lying down and resting his eyes lessen the pain. |
| c. description of the patient's efforts to relieve the symptoms | Self-treatment with a nonprescription pain reliever (Excedrin QuickTabs) was partially effective for two headache episodes. |
| 2. Gather essential patient history information: | |
| a. patient's identity | Richard Perkins |
| b. age, sex, height, and weight | 62 y/o M, 5'10", 210 lb |
| c. patient's occupation | Public safety officer, recently reassigned to desk duty |
| d. patient's dietary habits | Mixture of healthful and processed foods; about 2 cups of coffee daily during the work week; drinks two to three alcoholic drinks two or three times per month |
| e. patient's sleep habits | Sleeps about 6-7 hours nightly during the week; stays up late and sleeps in on weekends |
| f. concurrent medical conditions, prescription and nonprescription medications, and dietary supplements | For hypertension, he is taking atenolol and felodipine. |
| g. allergies | NKA |
| h. history of other adverse reactions to medications | Cough from enalapril |
| i. other (describe)______ | |
| **Assessment and Triage** | |
| 3. Differentiate the patient's signs/symptoms and correctly identify the patient's primary problem(s) (see Table 5-1). | Mr. Perkins appears to be experiencing episodic tension headaches related to eye or muscle strain from his new job responsibilities. |
| 4. Identify exclusions for self-treatment (see Figure 5-2). | Mr. Perkins has no conditions excluding him from self-treatment. |
| 5. Formulate a comprehensive list of therapeutic alternatives for the primary problem to determine if triage to a medical practitioner is required and share this information with the patient. | Options include:<br>(1) Refer Mr. Perkins for medical evaluation.<br>(2) Recommend a nonprescription single-entity analgesic such as acetaminophen, a salicylate, or an NSAID.<br>(3) Suggest nondrug measures, alone or in combination with drug therapy.<br>(4) Take no action. |
| **Plan** | |
| 6. Select an optimal therapeutic alternative to address the patient's problem, taking into account patient preferences. | Improving the lighting or ergonomics of his work area may help alleviate muscle and eye strain. Self-treatment can be used; acetaminophen may be preferred because of its safety in patients with concomitant hypertension. |

CASE 5-1 (continued)

| Relevant Evaluation Criteria | Scenario/Model Outcome |
|---|---|
| 7. Describe the recommended therapeutic approach to the patient. | Your headaches may be caused by muscle or eye strain from desk work. Try adjusting your work environment to improve the lighting and your posture to help reduce eye and muscle strain. If drug treatment is needed, take acetaminophen early in the course of a headache. |
| 8. Explain to the patient the rationale for selecting the recommended therapeutic approach from the considered therapeutic alternatives. | Most episodic tension-type headaches are amenable to self-treatment. Your headache does not warrant medical attention at this time. Although any OTC analgesic would be expected to be helpful, acetaminophen is likely to be the safest for you. Other nonprescription pain medications could raise your blood pressure, cause swelling of your legs and feet, or irritate your stomach lining. Avoid using Excedrin QuickTabs because they have caffeine that you might not need. |
| **Patient Education** | |
| 9. When recommending self-care with nonprescription medications and/or nondrug therapy, convey accurate information to the patient, including: | |
| a. appropriate dose and frequency of administration | Acetaminophen 325-1000 mg every 4-6 hours as needed for headache, up to a maximum of 4 g/day |
| b. maximum number of days the therapy should be employed | Use acetaminophen up to 3 days per week. |
| c. product administration procedures | Take it as soon as possible after the start of a headache. Do not drink alcohol while using acetaminophen. |
| d. expected time to onset of relief | Pain relief can be expected to begin within 15-60 minutes. |
| e. degree of relief that can be reasonably expected | Complete resolution of the headaches is a reasonable expectation for this treatment. |
| f. most common side effects | Because you did not have side effects with Excedrin QuickTabs, you will probably be able to take acetaminophen without problems. |
| g. side effects that warrant medical intervention should they occur | Discontinue use of acetaminophen and seek medical attention if you experience nausea, vomiting, drowsiness, confusion, or abdominal pain. |
| h. patient options in the event that condition worsens or persists | If acetaminophen is not effective for the headaches, or you need medication more than 3 days per week, then you should see your primary care provider. Don't try other nonprescription pain relievers unless you are monitoring your blood pressure with your primary care provider. |
| i. product storage requirements | Keep acetaminophen in a tightly closed container and away from children. |
| j. specific nondrug measures | See comments in step 6 regarding altering work environment. |
| 10. Solicit follow-up questions from patient. | (1) Can I double the dose of acetaminophen to get better more quickly?<br>(2) Why can't I take medications more than 3 days per week? |
| 11. Answer patient's questions. | You should not take more than 1000 mg of acetaminophen in a single dose. Taking more will only increase your risk of suffering unwanted side effects.<br>Using headache medicines more than 3 days per week can cause rebound headaches. Also, frequent headaches may be better treated with preventive medications that are available by prescription only. |

Key: NKA, no known allergies; NSAID, nonsteroidal anti-inflammatory drug.

## Patient Counseling for Headache

To optimize outcomes from therapy, the practitioner should instruct patients to take an appropriate dose of analgesic early in the course of the headache. The use of nonprescription analgesics to preempt or abort migraine headaches should also be explained to migraine sufferers whose headaches are predictable. Patients who have headaches with some frequency should be encouraged to keep a log of their headaches to document triggers; frequency, intensity, and duration of episodes; and response to treatment. This may also be helpful in identifying factors that can improve headache prevention and treatment. Patients

## PATIENT EDUCATION FOR HEADACHE

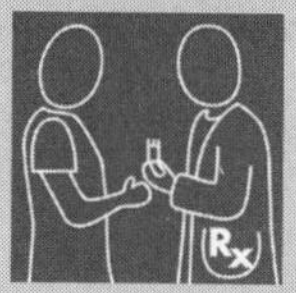

The objectives of self-treatment are to (1) relieve the pain of self-treatable headaches once they have set in, (2) prevent or abort migraine headaches when possible, and (3) prevent medication-overuse headaches by avoiding chronic use of nonprescription analgesics. For most patients, carefully following product instructions and the self-care measures listed here will help ensure optimal therapeutic outcomes.

### Tension-type Headaches

- Nonprescription pain relievers (analgesics) are usually effective for episodic tension-type headaches. However, consult a primary care provider before using them for chronic tension-type headache.
- If nonprescription pain relievers are used for chronic headaches, keep records of how often they are used, and share this information with your primary care provider.
- Do not use products containing caffeine because of the risk of caffeine-withdrawal headaches.

### Migraine Headache

- Avoid substances (food, caffeine, alcohol, medications) or situations (stress, fatigue, oversleeping, fasting, or missing meals) that you know can trigger a migraine.
- Use the following nutritional strategies to prevent migraine:
  - Avoid foods or food additives known to trigger migraines, including red wine, aged cheese, aspartame, monosodium glutamate, coffee, tea, cola beverages, and chocolate.
  - Avoid foods to which you are allergic.
  - Eat regularly to avoid hunger and low blood glucose.
  - Consider taking magnesium supplements.
- If onset of migraines is predictable (e.g., headache occurs during menstruation), take a salicylate (such as aspirin) or NSAID (ibuprofen, ketoprofen, or naproxen) to prevent the headache. Start taking the analgesic 2 days before menstruation and continue scheduled use during menses.
- Try to abort a migraine by taking acetaminophen, aspirin, or an NSAID at the onset of headache pain.
- If desired, use an ice bag or cold pack applied with pressure to the forehead or temples to reduce the pain associated with acute migraine attacks.

### Other Headaches

- If you have coexisting migraine and tension-type headaches, avoid caffeine-containing analgesics and other medications such as opioids that cause dependency. These substances can cause medication-overuse headache.
- Consider using a combination of a decongestant and nonprescription analgesics to relieve the pain of sinus headache.

### Precautions for Nonprescription Analgesics

- If you are pregnant or breast-feeding, consult a primary care provider before taking any nonprescription drugs.
- Obtain medical advice before taking any of these medications if you have a medical condition or are taking prescription medications. Nonprescription analgesics are known to interact with several medications.
- Do not take these medications for longer than 10 days unless a primary care provider has recommended prolonged use.
- Do not take these medications if you consume three or more alcoholic beverages daily.
- Do not exceed recommended dosages.
- Products containing aspartame and/or phenylalanine (usually chewable tablets) should not be given to individuals with phenylketonuria.

### *Salicylates and NSAIDs*

- Do not take aspirin during the last 3 months of pregnancy unless a primary care provider is supervising such use. Unsupervised use of this medication could harm the unborn child or cause complications during delivery.
- Do not give aspirin or other salicylates to children 15 years or younger who are recovering from chickenpox or the symptoms of influenza. To avoid the risk of Reye's syndrome, a rare but potentially fatal condition, use acetaminophen for pain relief.
- Do not take aspirin or NSAIDs if you are allergic to aspirin or have asthma and nasal polyps. Take acetaminophen instead.
- Do not take aspirin or NSAIDs if you have stomach problems or ulcers, liver disease, kidney disease, or heart failure.
- Do not take aspirin if you are taking medication for bleeding problems (anticoagulants), gout, diabetes mellitus, or arthritis, unless such use is supervised by a primary care provider.
- Do not take salicylates or NSAIDs if you are taking anticoagulants.
- Do not take magnesium salicylate if you have kidney disease.
- Do not take sodium salicylate if you are on a sodium-restricted diet.
- Do not give ketoprofen to a child younger than 16 years.
- Do not give naproxen to a child younger than 12 years.
- Stop taking aspirin or NSAIDs and seek medical attention if any of the following symptoms occur:
  - Headache, dizziness, ringing in the ears, difficulty in hearing, dimness of vision, mental confusion, lassitude, drowsiness, sweating, thirst, hyperventilation, nausea, vomiting, or occasional diarrhea. These symptoms indicate mild salicylate toxicity.
  - Dizziness, nausea and mild stomach pain, constipation, ringing in the ears, or swelling in the feet or legs. These symptoms are common side effects of salicylates and NSAIDs.
  - Rash or hives, or red, peeling skin; swelling in the face or around the eyes; wheezing or trouble breathing; bloody or black tarry stools; severe stomach pain or bloody vomit; bloody or cloudy urine; or unexplained bruising and bleeding. These symptoms require immediate medical attention.

### *Acetaminophen*

- To avoid possible damage to the liver, do not take more than 4 g of acetaminophen a day.
- Do not drink alcohol while taking this medication.
- If you have had an adverse reaction to acetaminophen or have a history of liver disease, do not take acetaminophen. These factors increase the risk of toxicity from acetaminophen.
- Follow dosage instructions for acetaminophen carefully if you have glucose-6-phosphate dehydrogenase deficiency.

Stop taking acetaminophen and seek medical attention in the following situations:

- Nausea, vomiting, drowsiness, confusion, and abdominal pain occur.
- New symptoms develop.
- A headache gets worse or lasts more than 10 days.

should be advised that continuing or escalating pain can be a sign of a more serious problem and that prompt medical attention is warranted. The box Patient Education for Headache lists specific information to provide patients. The clinician should explain appropriate drug and non-drug measures for treating headaches. Frequent use of nonprescription analgesics is not appropriate because of the risk for medication-overuse headache. It should be conveyed that nonprescription analgesics are potent medications with accompanying potential adverse effects, interactions, and precautions/warnings.

## Evaluation of Patient Outcomes for Headache

Appropriate follow-up will depend on headache type, frequency, and severity and patient factors. For patients with less frequent headaches, a trial of 6 to 12 weeks may be needed to assess efficacy of treatment. For frequent or more severe headaches, clinicians should communicate with patients within 10 days of initiation of self-treatment to assess efficacy and tolerability. If headaches persist or become worse despite self-treatment, the patient should seek medical attention.

It is notable that more than half of patients suffering from migraine headache use only nonprescription medications, despite the severity of pain.[5] Patients with migraine headaches that are not adequately self-treated should be referred for a medical evaluation because effective prescription therapies are available that can substantially limit pain and disability.

## Key Points for Headache

- Most tension-type, migraine, and sinus headaches are amenable to treatment with nonprescription drugs.
- Patients with symptoms suggestive of secondary or undiagnosed migraine headaches should be referred for medical attention.
- Many patients with frequent headaches may improve by identifying and modifying environmental, behavioral, nutritional, or other triggers for their headaches.
- The choice of nonprescription analgesic for an individual patient depends on patient preferences, presence of precautionary or contraindicating conditions, concomitant medications, cost, and other factors.
- Pharmacists have been identified as key sources of information for nonprescription analgesics users to reduce risk for acetaminophen-induced hepatotoxicity and NSAID-induced GI bleeding and nephrotoxicity.
- Use of nonprescription analgesics for headache should be limited to 3 days per week to prevent medication-overuse headache.

## References


1. Smith TR. Epidemiology and impact of headache: an overview. *Prim Care Clin Office Pract.* 2004;31:237-41.
2. Gureje O, Von Korff M, Simon GE, et al. Persistent pain and well-being: a World Health Organization study in primary care. *JAMA.* 1998;280:147-51.
3. Consumers uninformed about nonprescription pain relievers. *Am J Health-Syst Pharm.* 1998;55:2597.
4. Headache Classification Subcommittee of the International Headache Society. The international classification of headache disorders, 2nd edition. *Cephalalgia.* 2004;24 (suppl 1):1-160.
5. Mannix LK. Headache: epidemiology and impact of primary headache disorders. *Med Clin N Am.* 2001;85:887-95.
6. Pasero C, Paice JA, McCaffery M. Basic mechanisms underlying the causes and effects of pain. In: McCaffery M, Pasero C, eds. *Pain: Clinical Manual.* 2nd ed. St. Louis: Mosby, Inc; 1999:18-23.
7. Schoenen J, de Noordhout AM. Headache. In: Wall PD, Melzack R, eds. *Textbook of Pain.* 4th ed. Edinburgh, Scotland: Churchill Livingstone; 1999.
8. Diener H-C, Limmroth V. Medication-overuse headache: a worldwide problem. *Lancet* Neurol. 2004;3:475-83.
9. Ward TN. Medication overuse headache. *Prim Care Clin Office Pract.* 2004;31:369-80.
10. Krusz JC. Tension-type headaches: what they are and how to treat them. *Prim Care Clin Office Pract.* 2004;31:293-311.
11. Schreiber CP. The pathophysiology of primary headache. *Prim Care Clin Office Pract.* 2004;31:261-76.
12. Goadsby PJ. Current concepts of the pathophysiology of migraine. *Neurol Clinics.* 1997;15:27-42.
13. Welch KMA. Current opinions in headache pathogenesis: introduction and synthesis. *Curr Opin Neurol.* 1998;11:193-7.
14. Mauskop A, Altura BM. Role of magnesium in the pathogenesis and treatment of migraines. *Clin Neurosci.* 1998;5:24-7.
15. Loder E. Migraine diagnosis and treatment. *Prim Care Clin Office Pract.* 2004;31:277-92.
16. U.S. Food and Drug Administration. Internal analgesic, antipyretic, and antirheumatic drug products for over-the-counter human use. *Code of Federal Regulations.* Title 21, vol. 5 (21CFR343. 80). Revised April 1, 2003.
17. Sandler RS, Halabi S, Baron JA, et al. A randomized trial of aspirin to prevent colorectal adenomas in patients with previous colorectal cancer. *N Engl J Med.* 2003;348:883-90.
18. Drug *Facts and Comparisons.* St. Louis: Facts and Comparisons; 2005.
19. Lexi-Comp [database online]. Hudson, Ohio: Lexi-Comp; 2005.
20. Kelly JP, Kaufman DW, Jurgelon JM, et al. Risk of aspirin-associated major upper-gastrointestinal bleeding with enteric-coated or buffered product. *Lancet.* 1996;348:1413-6.
21. Lanas AI. Current approaches to reducing gastrointestinal toxicity of low-dose aspirin. *Am J Med.* 2001;110 (1A):70-3S.
22. Dammann HG, Burkhardt F, Wolf N. Enteric coating of aspirin significantly decreases gastroduodenal mucosal lesions. *Aliment Pharmacol Ther.* 1999;13:1109-14.
23. Jenkins C, Costello J, Hodge L. Systematic review of prevalence of aspirin induced asthma and its implications for clinical practice. *BMJ.* 2004;328:434-40.
24. Hersh EV, Moore PA, Ross GI. Over-the-counter analgesics and antipyretics: a critical assessment. *Clin Ther.* 2000;22:500-48.
25. American Society of Health-System Pharmacists. ASHP therapeutic position statement on the safe use of oral nonprescription analgesics. *Am J Health-Syst Pharm.* 1999;56:1126-31.
26. Roine R, Gentry RT, Hernandez-Munoz R, et al. Aspirin increases blood alcohol concentrations in humans after ingestion of ethanol. *JAMA.* 1990;264:2406-8.
27. Department of Health and Human Services, Food and Drug Administration. Labeling for oral and rectal over-the-counter products containing aspirin and nonaspirin salicylates; Reye's Syndrome warning. *Federal Register.* 2003;68:18861-9.
28. Lipton RB, Baggish JS, Stewart WF, et al. Efficacy and safety of acetaminophen in the treatment of migraine. *Arch Intern Med.* 2000;160:3486-92.

29. Steiner TJ, Lange R, Voelker M. Aspirin in episodic tension-type headache: placebo-controlled dose-ranging comparison with paracetamol. *Cephalalgia.* 2003;23:59-66.
30. Watson WA, Litovitz TL, Klein-Schwartz W, et al. 2003 Annual report of the American Association of Poison Control Centers toxic exposure surveillance system. *Am J Emerg Med.* 2004;22:335-404.
31. Ostapowicz G, Fontana RJ, Schiodt RV, et al. for the U.S. Acute Liver Failure Study Group. Results of a prospective study of acute liver failure at 17 tertiary care centers in the United States. *Ann Intern Med.* 2002;137:947-54.
32. Bolesta S, Haber SL. Hepatotoxicity associated with chronic acetaminophen administration in patients without risk factors. *Ann Pharmacother.* 2002;36:331-3.
33. Rumack BH. Acetaminophen misconceptions. *Hepatology.* 2004; 40:10-15.
34. Prescott LF. Paracetamol, alcohol and the liver. *Br J Clin Pharmacol.* 2000;49:291-301.
35. US Food and Drug Administration. Letter to state boards of pharmacy: acetaminophen hepatotoxicity and nonsteroidal anti-inflammatory drug (NSAID)-related gastrointestinal and renal toxicity. Center for Drug Evaluation and Research; January 22, 2004.
36. Hawton K, Simkin S, Deeks J, et al. UK legislation on analgesic packs: before and after study of long term effect on poisonings. *BMJ.* 2004;329:1076-80.
37. Zed PJ, Krenzelok EP. Treatment of acetaminophen overdose. *Am J Health-Syst Pharm.* 1999;56:1081-93.
38. Farrell GC. Liver disease caused by drugs, anesthetics, and toxins. In: Feldman M, Friedman LS, Sleisenger MH, eds. *Sleisenger & Fordtran's Gastrointestinal and Liver Disease.* 7th ed. Philadephia, Pa: Saunders; 2002:1403-47.
39. McElwee N, Veltri JC, Bradford DC, et al. A prospective, population-based study of acute ibuprofen overdose: complications are rare and routine serum levels not warranted. *Ann Emerg Med.* 1990;19:657-62.
40. US Food and Drug Administration. Public health advisory: nonsteroidal anti-inflammatory drug products (NSAIDs). Rockville, Md: Center for Drug Evaluation and Research; December 23, 2004.
41. US Food and Drug Administration. Request to sponsors of nonprescription NSAIDs: revised supplemental request letter and labeling template. Rockville, Md: Center for Drug Evaluation and Research; July 18, 2005.
42. Lipton R, Steward W, Saper J, et al. Efficacy and safety of acetaminophen, aspirin, and caffeine in alleviating migraine headache pain: three double-blind, randomized, placebo-controlled trials. *Arch Neurol.* 1998;55:210-7.
43. Altman RD. Salicylates in the treatment of arthritic disease: how safe and effective? *Postgrad Med.* 1988;84:206-10.
44. Prior MJ, Cooper KM, May LG, Bowen DL. Efficacy and safety of acetaminophen and naproxen in the treatment of tension-type headache: a randomized, double-blind, placebo-controlled trial. *Cephalalgia.* 2002;22:740-8.
45. Steiner TJ, Lange R. Ketoprofen (25 mg) in the symptomatic treatment of episodic tension-type headache: double-blind placebo-controlled comparison with acetaminophen (1000 mg). *Cephalalgia.* 1998;18:38-43.
46. Perrott DA, Piira T, Goodenough B, Champion D. Efficacy and safety of acetaminophen vs ibuprofen for treating children's pain or fever. *Arch Pediatr Adolesc Med.* 2004;158:521-6.
47. Briggs G, Freeman R, Yaffe S, eds. *Drugs in Pregnancy and Lactation.* 6th ed. Baltimore: Williams & Wilkins; 2002.
48. Wolfe MM, Lichtenstein Dr, Singh G. Gastrointestinal toxicity of nonsteroidal anti-inflammatory drugs. *N Engl J Med.* 1999;340: 1888-99.
49. AGS Panel on Persistent Pain in Older Persons. The management of persistent pain in older persons. *J Am Geriatr Soc.* 2002;6:S205-24.
50. Manias P, Tagaris G, Karageorgiou K. Acupuncture in headache: a critical review. *Clin J Pain.* 2000;16:334-9.

## Additional Information Resources

www.ahrq.gov/ (Agency for Healthcare Research and Quality)
www.ampainsoc.org (American Pain Society)
www.fda.gov/cder/consumerinfo/otc_all_resources.htm (U.S. Food and Drug Administration consumer education on nonprescription medicine)

CHAPTER 6

# Fever

*Liza Takiya*

Fever is defined as a body temperature higher than the normal core temperature of 100°F (37.8°C). It is important to distinguish "fever" from "hyperthermia" and "hyperpyrexia." Fever is a regulated rise in body temperature maintained by the hypothalamus in response to a pyrogen; it is a sign of an increase in the body's thermoregulatory set point. In contrast, hyperthermia represents a malfunctioning of the normal thermoregulatory process at the hypothalamus level.[1] Because of their different mechanisms, treatment of fever versus hyperthermia also varies. Hyperpyrexia is a body temperature greater than 106°F (41.1°C) that typically results in mental and physical consequences.

Most fevers are self-limited and nonthreatening; however, fever can cause a great deal of discomfort and, in some cases, may indicate serious underlying pathology (e.g., acute infectious process) for which prompt medical evaluation is indicated. The principal reason for treating fever is to alleviate discomfort; however, the underlying cause should be identified before treatment. Serious complications of fever are uncommon; overly aggressive fever management may be more dangerous than the fever itself. Because the symptomatology of fever and hyperthermia are very similar, this chapter will focus on fever and will also discuss hyperthermia briefly.

## Epidemiology of Fever

Fever is the 16th most common reason patients seek medical care.[2] In 2002, patients primarily complaining of fever made approximately 12,250,000 medical office visits, with men making a slightly greater number of visits.[2] Fever is also one of the most common reasons that parents seek medical care for their children. One of every five emergency room visits for children is related to fever, and 19% to 30% of children presenting to their pediatrician's office have fever as a complaint.[3] Overall, 69.6% of all fevers in children younger than 5 years of age are referred to a health care provider for medical evaluation; however, only 57.2% of patients with fever in the total population seek medical care.[2] Children suffer from fevers more often than adults. The rate of reported fevers in children younger than 5 years of age is 10 in 100 persons versus the rate of 0.5 in 100 adults. Nonetheless, the rate of fever does not seem to differ significantly when distinguishing among gender, race, or geographic area of residence in the United States.[2] Of all the therapeutic classifications of drugs on the market, antipyretics are the 14th most commonly mentioned drugs at medical office visits, and acetaminophen is the most commonly discussed generic agent.[2]

## Physiology of Body Thermoregulation

Core temperature refers to the temperature of the blood that surrounds the hypothalamus, which may differ from the surrounding body or skin temperature. Core temperature is regulated by a feedback system that involves information transmitted between the thermoregulatory center located in the anterior hypothalamus and the thermosensitive neurons located in the skin and central nervous system (CNS). Physiologic and behavioral mechanisms regulate body temperature within the normal range. Behavioral adaptations to temperature changes include wearing additional clothing, rubbing the hands together, adjusting air conditioning, and seeking shade for relief from the hot sun. Compensatory physiologic mechanisms such as heat dissipation (e.g., sweating, vasodilation, hyperventilation) in response to heat, as well as heat production or conservation (e.g., shivering, goose bumps, vasoconstriction) in response to cold, are mediated by alterations in the secretion of various hormones, such as thyroxine, aldosterone, serotonin, and catecholamines.[4] Therefore, although skin temperature may fluctuate greatly in response to environmental conditions, the core temperature is regulated within a very narrow range.

Normal thermoregulation prevents wide fluctuations in body temperature; the average temperature is usually maintained between 97.5°F and 98.9°F (36.4°C and 37.2°C). Temperature maintained in this range is considered to be the "set point," or the point at which the physiologic or behavioral mechanisms are not activated. Normal body temperature varies throughout the day, peaking daily between 5 PM and 7 PM and reaching its lowest point between 3 AM and 5 AM.[5] This consistent rhythm occurs at ages older than 2 years and is more pronounced in children than in adults. Body temperature can vary by as much as 1.8°F (1°C) in adults and as much as 2.58°F (1.48°C) in children each day, depending on normal circadian rhythm and activity level. Children and adults may have elevated temperatures after vigorous activity or exercise. Because circadian variation continues during febrile illness, patients may be described incorrectly as afebrile when they have a relatively normal temperature in the early morning, and a moderately high evening temperature may be misinterpreted as fever. The average rectal temperature for an 18-month-old baby is 100°F (37.8°C); therefore, 50% of infants have normal rectal temperatures above 100°F (37.8°C). Rectal temperatures of healthy children may approach 101°F (38.3°C) in the late afternoon or after physical activity.[6] A patient's ability to perceive fever varies

TABLE 6-1 Selected Medications That Induce Hyperthermia[1,9,10]

| Anti-infectives | Antineoplastics | Cardiovascular | CNS Agents | Other Agents |
|---|---|---|---|---|
| Aminoglycosides | Bleomycin | Epinephrine | Amphetamines | Allopurinol |
| Amphotericin B | Chlorambucil | Hydralazine | Barbiturates | Atropine |
| Cephalosporins | Cytarabine | Methyldopa | Benztropine | Azathioprine |
| Clindamycin | Daunorubicin | Nifedipine | Carbamazepine | Cimetidine |
| Chloramphenicol | Hydroxyurea | Procainamide | Haloperidol | Corticosteroids |
| Imipenem | l-Asparaginase | Quinidine | Lithium | Folate |
| Isoniazid | 6-Mercaptopurine | Streptokinase | MAOIs | Inhaled anesthetics |
| Macrolides | Procarbazine | | Nomifensine | Interferon |
| Mebendazole | Streptozocin | | Phenytoin | Iodides |
| Nitrofurantoin | | | Phenothiazines | Levamisole |
| Para-aminosalicylic acid | | | SSRIs | Metoclopramide |
| Penicillins | | | Trifluoperazine | Propylthiouracil |
| Rifampin | | | Thioridazine | Prostaglandin $E_2$ |
| Streptomycin | | | TCAs | Ritodrine |
| Sulfonamides | | | | Salicylates |
| Tetracyclines | | | | Tolmetin |
| Vancomycin | | | | |

Key: MAOIs, monoamine oxidase inhibitors; SSRIs, selective serotonin reuptake inhibitors; TCAs, tricyclic antidepressants.

because of the many variables. Some individuals quite accurately perceive elevations in their body temperature, whereas others (e.g., those who are immunosuppressed) may not be as sensitive to temperature changes.

## Etiology of Fever

An increase in body temperature may be idiopathic or can be caused by a variety of mechanisms, including an infectious process, a response to certain drugs, physiologic processes, or vigorous activity.

### *Microbe-induced Fever*

Most febrile episodes are caused by microbial infections (i.e., viruses, bacteria, fungi, yeasts, or protozoa). Elevated temperatures associated with bacterial infections generally are higher than those associated with viral infections, but there is no absolute temperature at which these infections can be differentiated. Also, there is no basis for differentiating viral from bacterial infections according to the magnitude of temperature reduction from antipyretic drug therapy. Fever is often less intense in patients of advanced age than in younger individuals. Consequently, infection may not be recognized easily in older patients if fever is the primary assessment criterion.[7] Microbe-induced fever is common in neutropenic patients, and the underlying cause should be treated aggressively once identified.

### *Pathology-induced Fever*

Noninfectious pathologic causes of increases in temperature include malignancies, tissue damage (e.g., myocardial infarction or surgery), antigen–antibody reactions, dehydration, heat stroke, CNS inflammation, and metabolic disorders such as hyperthyroidism or gout. Many of these processes actually may cause hyperthermia rather than fever because they interfere with the hypothalamic regulation of temperature. Tissue damage, antigen–antibody reactions, and CNS inflammation allow release of endogenous pyrogens, resulting in fever; however, hyperthyroidism, dehydration, and heat stroke cause hyperthermia by interfering with either metabolic rate or heat dissipation.

### *Drug-induced Fever*

Drug-induced fever, more appropriately termed *drug-induced hyperthermia*, occurs via a variety of mechanisms. Its incidence is unknown, but this type of fever may account for more than 3% of all adverse drug reactions and occurs in up to 10% of all hospitalized patients (Table 6-1).[8] Failure to discontinue the offending drug can result in substantial morbidity and even mortality. However, drug-induced hyperthermia often goes unrecognized because of inconsistent signs and symptoms.[9]

Drug-induced hyperthermia is independent of atopy, gender, age, or existing medical conditions. It has been attributed to one of the following mechanisms: (1) altered thermoregulation, (2) pharmacologic action, (3) drug administration, (4) hypersensitivity, or (5) an idiosyncrasy; all of which lead to the body's inability to maintain core temperature.[10] The most common mechanism is hypersensitivity; however, many drugs are known to interfere with peripheral heat dissipation or to increase basal metabolic rate. Other drugs cause fever by invoking a cellular immune response, mimicking the structure of endogenous pyrogens, or inflicting direct tissue damage.

Some drugs elevate body temperature by altering normal thermoregulatory mechanisms, causing hyperthermia. Large doses of phenothiazines, tricyclic antidepressants, or drugs with anticholinergic properties decrease sweating and thus reduce heat dissipation. Sympathomimetics such as amphetamines and epinephrine also decrease heat dissipation by inducing vasoconstriction. Thyroid hormones may increase the metabolic rate and thus increase heat generation. Other drugs may modify the behavioral response to the climatic temperature. For example, obtundation (dulling of body sensations) from sedatives may impair the normal behavioral withdrawal response from high environmental temperature.

Fever may be a direct result of the pharmacologic effect of a drug. The release of endotoxin from bacteria after the initiation of antibiotic therapy (e.g., penicillin for syphilis) can result in high fever, chills, hypotension, myalgia, and leukocytosis. This phenomenon (Jarisch–Herxheimer reaction) may occur within hours after parenteral antibiotic therapy is begun. Fever may also result from the release of endogenous pyrogens associated with cellular injury or death after cancer chemotherapy. Similarly, the administration of drugs that possess oxidizing activity, such as aspirin or sulfamethoxazole, to individuals who have a glucose-6-phosphate dehydrogenase deficiency may cause fever as a result of the release of endogenous pyrogens from damaged erythrocytes.

Another possibility related to drug-induced hyperthermia may be the administration or the vehicle of the drug. In the past, some products, such as vancomycin, contained impurities that could be toxins themselves, or the impurities could trigger the release of endogenous pyrogens. Also, cephalothin, a first-generation cephalosporin, may cause venous irritation, resulting in the release of endogenous pyrogens.

Drug-induced hyperthermia is also attributed to the formation of antibody–antigenic complexes. Some drugs or their metabolites, as well as some biological preparations such as infliximab, streptokinase, or vaccine products, have antigenic properties that produce a hypersensitivity reaction from the release of antibody–antigen complexes. Drug fever usually develops after 7 to 10 days of treatment. Fever and other symptoms may occur shortly after initiation of therapy if previous exposure to the drug occurred.[10] Drug-induced hyperthermia caused by antineoplastic agents often occurs within 7 days of initiation of therapy. However, vaccine-associated drug fever usually occurs within 48 hours of administration.

Drug-induced hyperthermia can be differentiated from other causes by establishing a temporal relationship between the fever and the administration of a drug, observing a temperature elevation despite improvement of the underlying disorders, and identifying possible "allergic" symptoms. Symptoms associated with drug fever vary. One study of drug-induced fever identified skin rash in only 18% of patients, with fewer than half experiencing urticaria (hives); mild eosinophilia was present in only 22% of the patients.[10] The presence of high temperature and shaking chills may make differentiation of drug fever from infection difficult. Drug-induced hyperthermia may also be associated with a shift to the left in the white blood cell differential count.[10] Diurnal temperature variation in drug fever is often minimal.

Increased temperature secondary to idiosyncratic reactions such as malignant hyperthermia and neuroleptic malignant syndrome (NMS) are rare, but potentially life threatening.[11,12] Malignant hyperthermia is characterized by temperature greater than 104°F (40°C), muscle rigidity, and metabolic acidosis, typically in the presence of general anesthetics such as succinylcholine or inhaled anesthetics.[9] NMS typically presents with high temperature, muscle rigidity, abnormal body movements, sweating, tachycardia, high or low blood pressure, incontinence, and altered consciousness including delirium, stupor, or coma.[9] NMS occurs most commonly in young males or dehydrated patients taking neuroleptic medications (e.g., phenothiazines, butyrophenones, thioxanthenes).

The management of drug-induced hyperthermia involves discontinuing the suspected drug whenever possible. If feasible, all medications should be temporarily discontinued. If the hyperthermia is drug-induced, the patient's temperature will generally decrease within 24 to 72 hours after the offending drug is withdrawn. After patient safety and the identification of the offending drug have been considered, each medication may be restarted, one at a time, while monitoring for fever recurrence. If an implicated drug cannot be discontinued, supportive care including oxygen, external cooling, and systemic corticosteroids may be given to decrease the temperature and to minimize other allergic symptoms. Dosage reduction of phenothiazines, anticholinergic agents, and thyroid hormone may decrease temperature and should be considered if these drugs are suspected of causing fever, particularly in older patients. Patients exhibiting symptoms of malignant hyperthermia or NMS should be referred immediately for medical evaluation and should discontinue the offending medication immediately.

## Pathophysiology of Fever

Pyrogens are fever-producing substances that activate the body's host defenses, resulting in an increase in the hypothalamic heat regulatory set point. Pyrogens can be exogenous, originating outside the body, such as microbes or toxins; or they can be endogenous, originating within the body, such as immune cytokines. Most exogenous pyrogens are proteins or breakdown products of proteins released from microbes. The most common microbial toxins are the lipopolysaccharide endotoxins produced by gram-negative bacteria and the toxic shock syndrome enterotoxin produced by *Staphylococcus*.[13,14] Exogenous pyrogens do not independently increase the hypothalamic temperature set point. They stimulate the release of endogenous pyrogens and thereby increase the core temperature.[4,13,14] Endogenous pyrogens are products released in response to or from damaged tissue such as interleukins, interferons, and tumor necrosis factor.

Prostaglandins of the $E_2$ series ($PGE_2$) are produced in response to circulating pyrogens and elevate the thermoregulatory set point in the hypothalamus.[4] Within hours, body temperature reaches this new set point and fever occurs. During the period of upward temperature readjustment, the patient experiences chills caused by peripheral vasoconstriction and muscle rigidity to maintain homeostasis. Because the new set point is regulated by negative feedback, body temperature rarely exceeds 106°F (41.1°C).[4] The antipyretic activity of nonsteroidal anti-inflammatory drugs (NSAIDs) and acetaminophen is mediated by inhibiting the synthesis of $PGE_2$ in the CNS in response to endogenous pyrogens.

## Signs and Symptoms of Fever

Fever is a symptom of a larger underlying process, whether it is an infection, abnormal metabolism, or drug-induced. Therefore, once the symptom of fever is established, investigation into the underlying cause is important. Signs and symptoms that typically accompany fever and cause a great deal of discomfort include headache, diaphoresis, generalized malaise, chills, tachycardia, arthralgia, myalgia, irritability, and anorexia. Symptoms such as sweating, tachycardia, and chills are directly related to the adjustment in temperature set point during fever, while symptoms such as myalgias and arthralgias are related more to the release of endogenous pyrogens. High body temperature dulls intellectual function and causes disorientation and delirium, especially in individuals with preexisting dementia, cerebral arteriosclerosis, or alcoholism. Patients who are unable to describe their symptoms (e.g., children, patients with dementia) and those who have temperatures greater than 104°F (40°C) should be referred to a clinician for further evaluation. Because the symptoms of fever are nonspecific and do not occur in all patients, the etiology of the fever is difficult to determine from the symptomatology. The most important sign of fever is an elevated temperature; thus, accurate temperature measurement is paramount.

**TABLE 6-2 Body Temperature Range Depending on Site of Measurement[15]**

| Site of Measurement | Normal | Fever |
|---|---|---|
| Rectal | 97.9°F-100.4°F (36.6°C-38°C) | >101.8°F (38.8°C) |
| Oral | 95.9°F-99.5°F (35.5°C-37.5°C) | >100°F (37.8°C) |
| Axillary | 94.5°F-99.0°F (34.7°C-37.2°C) | >99.0°F (37.2°C) |
| Tympanic | 96.4°F-100.4°F (35.8°C-38°C) | >100.4°F (38.0°C) |

**TABLE 6-3 Selected Temperatures in °Celsius and Equivalent °Fahrenheit**

| Celsius | Fahrenheit |
|---|---|
| 36° | 96.8° |
| 37° | 98.6° |
| 38° | 100.4° |
| 39° | 102.2° |
| 40° | 104.0° |
| 41° | 105.8° |
| 42° | 107.6° |

Conversion formulas:
Celsius = 5/9 (°F – 32); Fahrenheit = (9/5 × °C) + 32.

## Detection of Fever

Subjective assessment of fever typically involves feeling a part of the body, such as the forehead, for warmth. Although this method may identify an increase in skin temperature, it does not accurately detect a rise in core temperature. The most accurate method of detecting fever is measuring body temperature with a thermometer using proper techniques. The patient's age and level of physical and emotional stress, environmental temperature, time of day, and anatomic site at which the temperature is measured are important considerations because these factors can affect the results of temperature measurement.

Core body temperature cannot be measured directly in the outpatient setting because it involves identifying the temperature near the hypothalamus. Therefore, core temperature is estimated with various types of thermometers used at the rectal, axillary, oral, temporal, or ear canal sites. Body temperature should be measured with the same thermometer at the same site over the course of an illness because the readings from different thermometers or sites may vary (Table 6-2). The rectal method is considered the "gold standard" measurement because it most consistently estimates core body temperature. However, most patients prefer other methods of temperature measurement because of comfort and ease of use. A rectal temperature above 101.8°F (38.8°C), an oral temperature above 100°F (37.8°C), or an axillary temperature above 99°F (37.2°C) are considered elevated.[15] Rectal temperatures are 0.8° to 1.8°F (0.4°C to 0.9°C) higher than oral readings, and oral temperature readings may be up to 1.6°F (0.8°C) higher than tympanic readings.[16] Axillary temperatures range from 0.7°F to 3.6°F (0.4°C to 2°C) lower than rectal temperatures. The discrepancy between the various sites of temperature measurement is normal and should not be ascribed to improper measurement technique. As noted previously, normal body temperature may range 1.8°F to 2.5°F (1°C to 1.5°C) from these norms, and diurnal rhythm causes variances in body temperature during the day.

The conversion between the Celsius and Fahrenheit scales often causes confusion about the presence of a fever (Table 6-3). The normal variations in temperature among rectal, oral, and axillary sites of measurement can also confuse patients or caregivers. These differences should be emphasized when instructing individuals on the proper use of fever thermometers.

### *Types of Thermometers*

Over the past several years, there have been many advances in the types of thermometers available for use. Although most people are familiar with the mercury-in-glass thermometers, more recent innovations include electronic, infrared, and color-change thermometers. Many of these innovations may have stemmed from the Environmental Protection Agency's (EPA) position on reducing the number of mercury-based products in the United States.[17] Many states have banned the sale of mercury-in-glass thermometers, and many retail pharmacies have voluntarily phased out the sale of these thermometers. Along with the EPA, the American Academy of Pediatrics also supports the elimination of mercury-in-glass thermometers.[18] To properly dispose of mercury-in-glass thermometers, patients should contact their local municipality. Mercury-in-glass, electronic, and infrared thermometers are all accurate and reliable, if used appropriately.

#### Mercury-in-glass Thermometers

Mercury-in-glass thermometers detect body temperature by using the thermal expansion of mercury as a measure. Oral mercury-in-glass thermometers have a long, thin bulb designed to reach well under the tongue. In contrast, the bulb of the rectal thermometer is short and thick, permitting insertion in the rectum with little risk of breakage. Although a rectal thermometer can be used for oral temperature measurement, an oral thermometer should never be inserted into the rectum because the more fragile oral thermometers may break and injure rectal tissue. The same thermometer should never be used both rectally and orally because effective disinfection is difficult.

The advantages of mercury-in-glass thermometers include patient familiarity, low cost, light weight, and compact size. However, they can break, are difficult to read, and take up to 5 minutes for an accurate reading. Although elemental mercury is nonabsorbable from the gastrointestinal tract and nontoxic, it may vaporize at room temperature and may be toxic when inhaled. Glass fragments can be dangerous, and chipped thermometers should be discarded. If mercury leaks onto a hard surface, it should be removed with an eyedropper and placed in a hard, airtight container for disposal. In addition, these thermometers register slowly and must be disinfected before each use. They should be stored in a cool location and out of direct sunlight because they may be damaged by excessive heat. These thermometers are being phased out of distribution and may be difficult to obtain.

#### Electronic Thermometers

Electronic probe thermometers are available for oral, rectal, and axillary temperature measurements. The probes have an electronic transducer that provides a temperature reading in about 30 to 60 seconds. The oral electronic probes are available in both pen and pacifier shape. The pacifier-shaped electronic thermometer is for oral use only and takes about 4 minutes to provide a reading, but it is useful in infants who are unable to hold probes under their tongue. The pen-shaped probe may be used in the oral, rectal, or axillary area. Advantages of the electronic thermometers include quick readings and the elimination of glass breakage, mercury toxicity, and risk of cuts. The use of disposable covers with these thermometers also eliminates the need for disinfection after their use. In addition, the electronic digital temperature display makes these thermometers easier to read than the traditional glass thermometers. Most electronic thermometers require batteries and need to be calibrated periodically.

#### Infrared Thermometers

Infrared thermometers are available for tympanic and temporal temperature measurements. These thermometers use infrared technology to detect heat from the arterial blood supply. Therefore, they must be placed directly in sight of a blood supply, whether near the temporal artery or the tympanic membrane. Infrared thermometers measure body temperature in less than 5 seconds and are considered very accurate, if used appropriately. The major problem with these thermometers is that they are not always placed appropriately and thus give inaccurate readings. The tympanic and temporal thermometers are relatively expensive and require batteries and routine calibration, but many families with young children prefer them because of their convenience and noninvasive nature.

#### Color-change Thermometers

Color-change thermometers are easy to use; however, they are not sufficiently accurate or reliable. The thermometer is an adhesive strip containing heat-sensitive material that changes color in response to different temperature gradients. The strip may be placed anywhere on the skin, but the forehead is used most often because skin has less variation in temperature than other parts of the body. Although this method may detect changes in skin temperature, it does not reliably detect changes in core temperature. Skin temperature is influenced by many factors, including environment temperature and skin perfusion. Color-change thermometers may be useful in noting temperature trends but not absolute temperature.

### *Routes of Temperature Measurement*

Different types of thermometers may be used through different routes to detect temperature. Each thermometer should be used correctly to obtain an accurate reading. Patient-related factors may preclude use of a particular type of thermometer through a given route. Although there are a variety of routes of temperature measurement, rectal temperature measurement still remains the gold standard because of its reliability and accuracy. Oral, tympanic, and temporal routes are all appropriate for temperature measurements as long as the proper procedure is followed.

#### Oral

Table 6-4 describes the proper methods of taking oral measurements with glass and electronic thermometers.[15] Oral temperature should not be taken when an individual

**TABLE 6-4 Guidelines for Oral Temperature Measurements**

**Glass Thermometers**

1. Inspect the thermometer for cracks or imperfections before taking a temperature.
2. Disinfect the thermometer by drawing it through a swab moistened with an antiseptic such as alcohol or povidone–iodine solution.
3. Rinse the thermometer with cool water. Never use hot water, which may break the thermometer. Rotate the thermometer at or slightly below eye level to confirm that the displayed temperature is below 96°F (35.6°C). If the reading is higher, shake the thermometer over a bed, carpet, or other soft surface, using a rapid, downward, snapping motion until the mercury column falls below the 96°F (35.6°C) level.
4. Place the thermometer under the tongue, and position it slightly to one side of the mouth.
5. Keep the lips closed around the thermometer to hold it in place and prevent air from flowing over the thermometer.
6. Leave the thermometer in place for a minimum of 3-4 minutes.
7. Remove saliva from the thermometer by wiping it with tissue from the stem to the bulb.
8. After the temperature is recorded, shake the mercury down to less than the 96°F (35.6°C) level.
9. Disinfect the thermometer as described in step 2.

**Electronic Thermometers**

1. Remove the probe from the thermometer base in which it is stored.
2. Verify that the temperature set point is as specified by the manufacturer.
3. Insert the thermometer probe into a disposable cover.
4. Insert the probe into the mouth as described in steps 4 and 5 for oral glass thermometer.
5. After the thermometer indicates the temperature has been measured (usually after 10-60 seconds), remove it from the mouth.
6. Discard the disposable cover.
7. Record the displayed temperature.
8. Reset the thermometer by returning the probe to the base.

**TABLE 6-5 Guidelines for Rectal Temperature Measurements**

**Glass Thermometers**

1. Use a mercury-in-glass thermometer designed for rectal, *not* oral, use. Inspect the thermometer for cracks or imperfections before taking a temperature.
2. Follow steps 2 and 3 for glass thermometers listed in Table 6-4.
3. Apply a water-soluble lubricant to the bulb of the thermometer to allow for easy passage through the anal sphincter and to reduce the risk of trauma.
4. For infants or young children, place child face down over your lap, separate the buttocks with the thumb and forefinger of one hand, and insert the thermometer gently in the direction of the child's umbilicus with the other hand. For infants, insert the thermometer to the length of the bulb. For young children, insert it about 1 in. into the rectum.
5. For adults, have the patient lie on one side with the legs flexed to about a 45° angle from the abdomen. Insert the bulb 0.5-2 in. into the rectum by holding the thermometer 0.5-2 in. away from the bulb and inserting it until the finger touches the anus. Have the patient take a deep breath during this process to facilitate proper positioning of the thermometer.
6. Hold the thermometer in place for a minimum of 5 minutes.
7. Remove the thermometer. Clean by wiping away from the stem toward the bulb.
8. After the temperature is recorded, shake the mercury down to less than the 96°F (35.6°C) level.
9. Disinfect the thermometer as before.
10. Wipe away any remaining lubricant from the anus.

**Electronic Thermometers**

1. Follow steps 1-3 for electronic thermometers listed in Table 6-4.
2. Follow steps 3-5 for rectal glass thermometers listed above.
3. After the thermometer indicates the temperature has been measured, gently remove the probe.
4. Discard the disposable cover.
5. Record the displayed temperature.
6. Wipe away any remaining lubricant from the anus.
7. Reset the thermometer by returning the probe to the base.

is mouth breathing or hyperventilating; has recently had oral surgery; is not fully alert; or is uncooperative, lethargic, or confused. Mercury-in-glass oral thermometers are not appropriate for use in most children younger than 3 years because they find it difficult to maintain a tight seal around the thermometer and keep the thermometer under the tongue for long periods of time, in which case pacifier thermometers may be recommended. Pacifier thermometers provide reliable temperature readings with a sensitivity of approximately 72% and specificity of 98%, compared with rectal measurements; however, in children younger than 3 months, pacifier thermometers are less accurate.[19,20] Electronic oral thermometers can be used for children as young as 3 years because these instruments are not breakable if bitten, pose no risk of accidental cuts, and are more efficient than mercury-in-glass thermometers, but young children may still have a difficult time keeping the probe in place. To ensure reliable measurement, the patient should neither engage in vigorous physical activity nor heat nor cool the oral cavity artificially by smoking or drinking hot or cold beverages for a minimum of 5 minutes before temperature is measured.

## Rectal

Table 6-5 describes the proper methods of taking rectal temperatures in children and adults with mercury-in-glass and electronic thermometers. Rectal temperature measurement is the gold standard because of its predictable rise and high sensitivity and specificity, compared with the body's core temperature. Although the rectal route is the closest estimate of the core temperature, its intrusive nature can be very frightening to young children. In children

| TABLE 6-6 | Guidelines for Tympanic Temperature Measurements |
|---|---|

1. Place a clean disposable lens cover over the ear probe.
2. Turn on the thermometer and wait until it is ready for use.
3. For children younger than 1 year, pull the ear backward to straighten the ear canal. Place the ear probe into the canal, and aim the tip of the probe toward the patient's eye.
4. For anyone older than 1 year, pull the ear backward and up to straighten the ear canal. Place the ear probe into the canal, and aim the tip of the probe toward the patient's eye.
5. Press the button for temperature measurement (usually for only 1-5 seconds).
6. Read and record the temperature.
7. Discard the lens cover.

| TABLE 6-7 | Guidelines for Temporal Temperature Measurements[28] |
|---|---|

1. Disinfect the thermometer by drawing it through a swab moistened with an antiseptic such as alcohol or povidone–iodine solution.
2. Place the probe on one side of the forehead (near the temporal area).
3. Turn on the thermometer and wait until it is ready for use.
4. Sweep the thermometer across the hairline to the other side of the forehead. Make sure the probe remains in contact with the skin at all times.
5. Lift the thermometer from the forehead, and read and record the temperature.
6. Turn off the thermometer.

less than 6 months of age, however, rectal temperature is the preferred method of estimating fever. Risks associated with taking a rectal temperature include retention of the thermometer, rectal or intestinal perforation, and peritonitis. The patient should never be left unattended while the rectal thermometer remains in place because a positional change may cause the thermometer to be expelled or broken. Rectal temperature measurement is relatively contraindicated in patients who are neutropenic, have had recent rectal surgery or injury, or have rectal pathology (e.g., obstructive hemorrhoids, diarrhea). Rectal temperature measurement is slow to measure changes in body temperature because of the large muscle mass and poor blood flow to the area; therefore, the thermometer must be left in place for a minimum of 5 minutes.[15,21,22] The most common sources of error in rectal temperature measurement include stool impaction and poor technique in taking or reading the temperature.[23]

### Tympanic/Aural

Table 6-6 describes the proper method of using tympanic thermometers, which varies slightly, depending on the age of the patient. Tympanic thermometers have digital readouts, and many can be set to provide either a rectal or an oral temperature equivalent. The tip of the tympanic thermometer, which is placed in the ear canal, measures body temperature by sensing infrared heat from the blood vessels in the eardrum. The tympanic membrane is close to the hypothalamus, and the blood supply to these two anatomic areas is at the same temperature, providing an accurate reading of the body core temperature. The thermometer must be positioned in the ear canal properly to ensure that the measured infrared radiation is from the tympanic membrane and not from the ear canal or adjacent areas. In clinical trials, accuracy of tympanic thermometers has varied, compared with the rectal and oral routes.[24-26] Variations in temperature assessment have been attributed to cerumen impaction, inflammation in the ear canal (otitis media), age of patient (size of ear canal), and inappropriate technique.[16] Comparisons of tympanic and rectal measurements showed tympanic measurement to be 94.8% to 100% specific but only 58% to 68.3% sensitive for fever detection.[24,27] Tympanic thermometers are not recommended in infants younger than 6 months because the ear canal is not developed fully, leading to inappropriate technique and inaccurate readings. However, if used correctly, tympanic thermometry is found to be more reliable in measuring core temperature in adults than axillary or oral thermometry.[21]

### Temporal

Temporal thermometers are placed on the side of the forehead directly over the temporal artery and moved across the forehead (Table 6-7). The temporal artery is one of the few arteries close enough to the skin surface to detect heat changes. The thermometer is capable of providing a temperature reading in a few seconds. Its rapid, noninvasive nature makes it a preferable route of temperature measurement, and the temporal thermometer is significantly more sensitive than the tympanic thermometer for detecting fever.[28] However, compared with rectal temperature measurement, temporal measurement is close to 100% sensitive but has variable specificity (40%-86%), thereby still indicating that rectal temperature measurement is the most accurate. Temporal temperature measurement may differ from rectal temperature measurement by ± 1.3°C.[20,29] The presence of hair near the temporal area may confound the temperature reading, so hair must be pushed away before a reading is taken.

### Axillary

Axillary temperature measurement performed with mercury-in-glass and electronic thermometers (Table 6-8) is not recommended routinely because it is not as reliable in detecting fever, compared with the oral and rectal routes. In clinical studies, axillary temperature measurement was found to be only 63.5% to 75% sensitive and 64% to 92.6% specific in detecting fever, compared with rectal measurement.[24,27] Large variations in temperatures have been reported with axillary measurements attributable to inappropriate placement of the thermometer, movement of arms during measurement leading to a poor seal around the thermometer, and measurements taken for a shorter period of time.[23] Axillary temperature should not be taken directly after vigorous activity or bathing since both can affect body temperature.

**TABLE 6-8 Guidelines for Axillary Temperature Measurements**

**Glass Thermometer**

1. Use an oral mercury-in-glass thermometer to take axillary temperatures. Inspect the thermometer for cracks or imperfections before taking a temperature.
2. Disinfect the thermometer by drawing it through a swab moistened with an antiseptic such as alcohol or povidone–iodine solution. If disinfectants are not available, rinse the thermometer with *tepid* water.
3. Rotate the thermometer at or slightly below eye level to confirm that the displayed temperature is below 96°F (35.6°C). If the reading is higher, shake the thermometer over a bed, carpet, or other soft surface, using a rapid, downward, snapping motion until the mercury column falls below the 96°F (35.6°C) level.
4. Place the tip of the thermometer in the armpit. Make sure the armpit is clean and dry.
5. Gently press the arm against the body for at least 5-10 minutes.
6. Read and record the temperature.

**Electronic Thermometer**

1. Remove the probe from the thermometer base in which it is stored.
2. Verify the temperature set point is as specified by the manufacturer.
3. Insert the thermometer probe into a disposable cover.
4. Place the tip of the thermometer in the armpit. Make sure the armpit is clean and dry.
5. Gently press the arm against the body for 10-60 seconds.
6. Read and record the temperature.
7. Discard the disposable cover.

## Complications of Fever

The presence of fever is a cause of great concern although in most cases fever may be self-limiting and serious complications are rare. In one study, 56% of caregivers were "very worried" about the potential complications of fever, and 34% were "somewhat worried." There is less concern about complications of fever now than 20 years ago; however, 67% of interviewed caregivers still list seizures, brain damage, and death as the main complications of fever.[30] Overall, the major risks of fever are rare but include acute complications such as seizures, dehydration, and change in mental status.

Febrile seizures are defined as a seizure accompanied by fever in the absence of another cause such as an acute metabolic disorder or CNS inflammation. These seizures occur in 2% to 5% of all children from the ages of 6 months to 5 years.[31] The most common seizures associated with fever are simple febrile seizures, which are characterized by nonfocal movements generally lasting less than 15 minutes. Significant neurologic sequelae (e.g., impaired intellectual development, epilepsy) are unlikely after a single pediatric febrile seizure. High, rapidly increasing temperatures have been associated with febrile seizures. Although both the magnitude and rate of temperature increase appear to be critical determinants in precipitating febrile seizures, the temperature at which a particular child will seize is unpredictable. Most initial febrile seizures occur in children younger than 3 years. Seizures occurring after that age are usually unrelated to fever. The risk of recurrence is increased in children who have experienced a previous febrile seizure (especially if it occurred before 1 year of age or was a complex febrile seizure), who have documented seizure or other CNS disorder, or whose family history includes febrile seizures.[31,32] Prophylaxis against simple febrile seizures with antiepileptic or antipyretic drugs is not recommended by the American Academy of Pediatrics.[32]

Serious detrimental effects (e.g., dehydration, delirium, seizures, coma, irreversible neurologic or muscle damage) occur more often in patients with hyperpyrexia [temperatures greater than 106°F (41.1°C)], which is usually associated with hyperthermia and not fever. It is rare that a febrile person will have temperatures exceeding 106°F (41.1°C) owing to the homeostatic mechanisms of the hypothalamus. However, even lower body temperature elevations may be life threatening in patients with heart disease and pulmonary dysfunction. Increased risk of complications exists in infants and patients with brain tumors or hemorrhage, CNS infections, preexisting neurologic damage, and decreased ability to dissipate heat attributed to lower tolerance of elevated body temperature. Patients of advanced age are at a higher risk for fever-related complications because of their decreased thirst perception and perspiration ability.[6,33]

## Treatment of Fever

Fever is a sign of an underlying process. Treatment of fever should focus on the underlying cause instead of the temperature reading. No correlation exists between the magnitude and pattern of temperature elevation (i.e., persistent, intermittent, recurrent, or prolonged) and the underlying etiology or severity of the disease. Therefore, it is difficult to determine the cause of the fever on the sole basis of the temperature reading. Patient discomfort associated with fever is the main indication for antipyretic therapy, but arguments against such treatment include the generally benign and self-limited course of fever, the possible elimination of a diagnostic or prognostic sign, the attenuation of enhanced host defenses (i.e., possible therapeutic effect of fever), and the untoward effects of antipyretic drugs.

The decision to treat fever is based on a patient-specific risk–benefit ratio. Fever increases oxygen consumption, production of carbon dioxide, and cardiac output. However, fever is not associated with many harmful effects unless the temperature exceeds 106°F (41.1°C), and there is evidence that fever is an adaptive response and that elevated body temperature may be beneficial. Certain microbes are thermolabile; therefore, their growth is impaired by higher than normal temperatures. Clinical reports suggest that treating chicken pox with acetaminophen and rhinovirus with aspirin may increase the duration of the symptoms, compared with no treatment.[34] Thus, overtreatment of fever may also be detrimental. Furthermore, low-grade fever may have beneficial effects on host defense mechanisms (e.g., antigen recognition, T-helper lymphocyte function, leukocyte motility), but these effects have not been shown to favorably alter the course of infectious diseases.[4] Because there is not an overwhelming amount of data to support either the beneficial or harmful effects of fever, it is important to take other patient-specific factors into consideration when recommending treatment.

### Treatment Goals

The major goal of self-treatment is to alleviate the discomfort of fever by reducing the body temperature to a normal level.

### General Treatment Approach

General management of fever consists of antipyretic medication taken round the clock and continued for at least 24 hours, along with nonpharmacologic measures (Figure 6-1). Self-care measures are appropriate for most patients; however, an initial medical evaluation may be appropriate for patients with comorbid conditions and other exclusions for self-treatment. Patients with conditions that cause impaired oxygen utilization, those with impaired immune function, and those with CNS damage should be referred to their practitioner before self-care therapy is recommended. These patients are at a higher risk of developing fever-related complications than those without comorbid conditions. Referral for further evaluation should be considered immediately in children predisposed to seizures, infants younger than 6 months with a rectal temperature of 101°F (38.3°C) or greater, any patient exhibiting symptoms of an infection or a rectal temperature greater than 104°F (40°C), or patients with comorbid conditions and a rectal temperature greater than 102°F (38.8°C).

Fever exceeding 101°F (38.3°C) orally should be treated with antipyretic agents (see Chapter 5, Tables 5-2 and 5-3) as well as nonpharmacologic measures. Treatment with antipyretics may be indicated at lower temperatures if the patient experiences discomfort or is of advanced age. Studies suggest that for each decade increase in age, average temperature is decreased by 0.14°F (0.8°C); temperatures less than 101°F (38.3°C) may indicate fever in older populations.[33] The discomfort associated with a fever of less than 101°F (38.3°C) may be the primary indication for any of the nonprescription antipyretic medications since all of these agents are also analgesics.

### Nonpharmacologic Therapy

Nonpharmacologic therapy mainly consists of adequate fluid intake to prevent dehydration. Sponging or baths have limited utility in the management of fever. Body sponging with tepid water may facilitate heat dissipation because only a small temperature gradient between the body and the sponging medium is necessary to achieve an effective antipyretic response. However, sponging is not routinely recommended for those with a temperature below 104°F (40°C) because usually it is uncomfortable and often induces shivering, which could further raise the temperature. Ice-water baths or sponging with hydroalcoholic solutions (e.g., isopropyl or ethyl alcohol) is uncomfortable, unnecessary, and not recommended. Alcohol poisoning can result from cutaneous absorption or inhalation of topically applied alcohol solutions. Unlike acetaminophen and NSAIDs, sponging does not reduce the hypothalamic set point, thus sponging should follow oral antipyretic therapy by 1 hour to permit the appropriate reduction of the hypothalamic set point and a more sustained temperature-lowering response.[35]

Other nonpharmacologic interventions, regardless of the temperature, include wearing light clothing, removing blankets, maintaining room temperature at 78°F (25.6°C), and drinking sufficient fluid to replenish insensible losses. Fluid intake in febrile children should be increased by at least 30 to 50 mL (1 oz) of fluids per hour (e.g., sports drinks, fruit juice, water, other fluids) and by at least 50 to 100 mL (2-3 oz) per hour in adults, unless fluids are contraindicated.

### Pharmacologic Therapy

Antipyretics inhibit $PGE_2$ synthesis, which decreases the feedback between the thermoregulatory neurons and the hypothalamus, reducing the hypothalamic set point during fever. All antipyretics decrease the production of $PGE_2$ by inhibiting the cyclooxygenase (COX) enzyme. NSAIDs and aspirin inhibit the COX enzyme in the periphery and CNS, whereas acetaminophen mainly inhibits the COX enzyme in the CNS.[36] Chapter 5 provides an in-depth discussion of the pharmacokinetics, dosing, adverse effect profile, interactions, contraindications, and precautions of the antipyretic agents.

Although NSAIDs and acetaminophen are very safe and effective when used at low doses for a short duration of time, as in the treatment of fever, recent reports of medication errors and increased adverse events involving these agents has led the Food and Drug Administration (FDA) to encourage health care providers to take preventive actions. FDA recommendations include a patient education campaign to decrease medication errors as well as increase awareness of side effects and contraindications (Table 6-9). Common medication errors include overdosing

**TABLE 6-9 FDA Recommendations for Improving Safety of Antipyretic Agents[40]**

Health care providers should educate patients actively on antipyretic agents, including the following measures:

- A wide variety of different strengths, formulations, and combinations of acetaminophen- and NSAID-containing products are available over the counter or by prescription.
- Any nonprescription analgesic is a drug, and should be taken and stored appropriately. Specific precautions include:
  - The correct dosing frequency for each of the acetaminophen or the NSAID formulations
  - The correct weight-based dose for each child.
  - Use of the correct measuring device for the liquid formulations.
  - Risks of taking nonprescription analgesics with prescription or other nonprescription medications.
  - Signs and symptoms of self-recognizable side effects.
  - Potential problems associated with simultaneous use of more than one pain reliever product.

Key: NSAID, nonsteroidal anti-inflammatory drug.

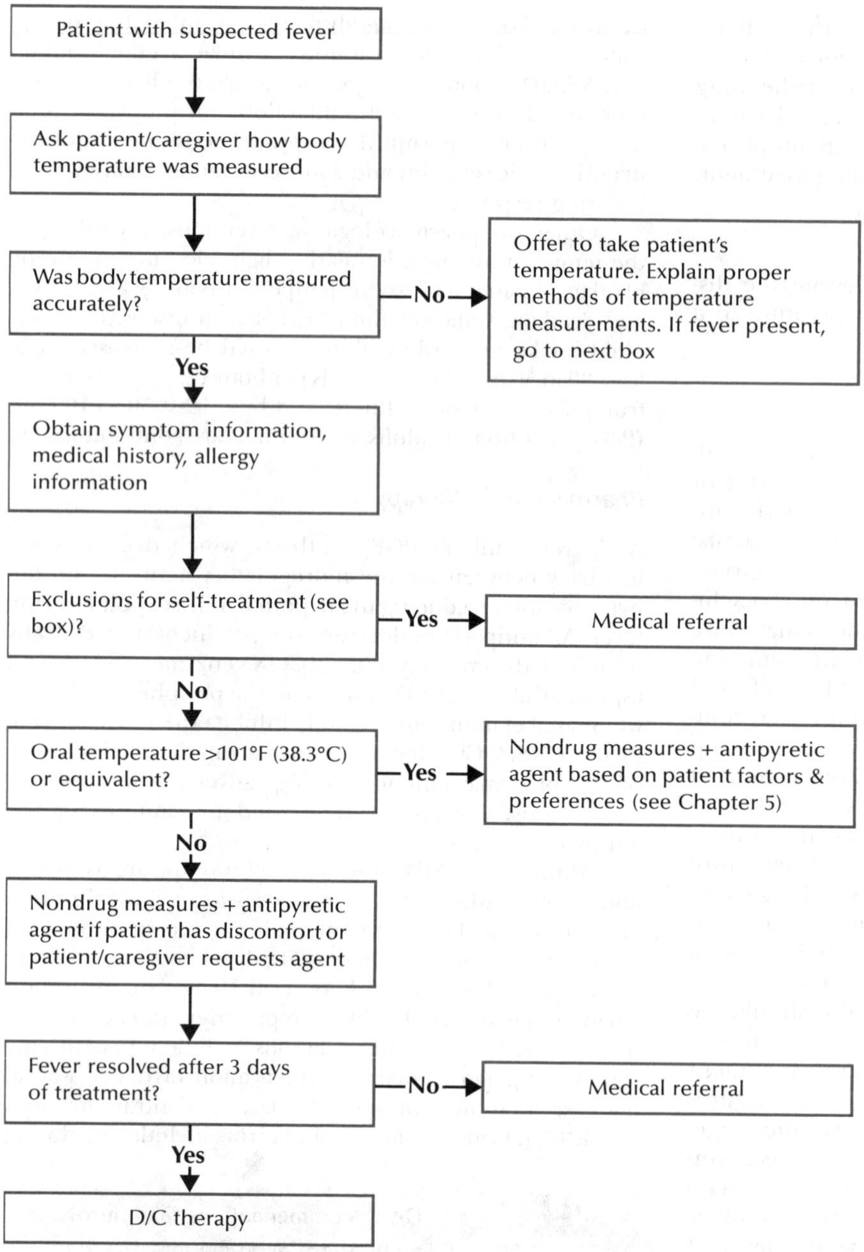


**Exclusions for Self-Treatment**

- Patients >6 months of age with rectal temperature ≥104°F (40°C) or equivalent
- Children <6 months of age with rectal temperature ≥101°F (38.3°C)
- Symptoms of infection
- Risk for hyperthermia
- Impaired oxygen utilization (e.g., severe COPD, respiratory distress, heart failure)
- Impaired immune function (e.g., cancer, HIV)
- CNS damage (e.g., head trauma, stroke)
- Children with history of febrile seizures or seizures

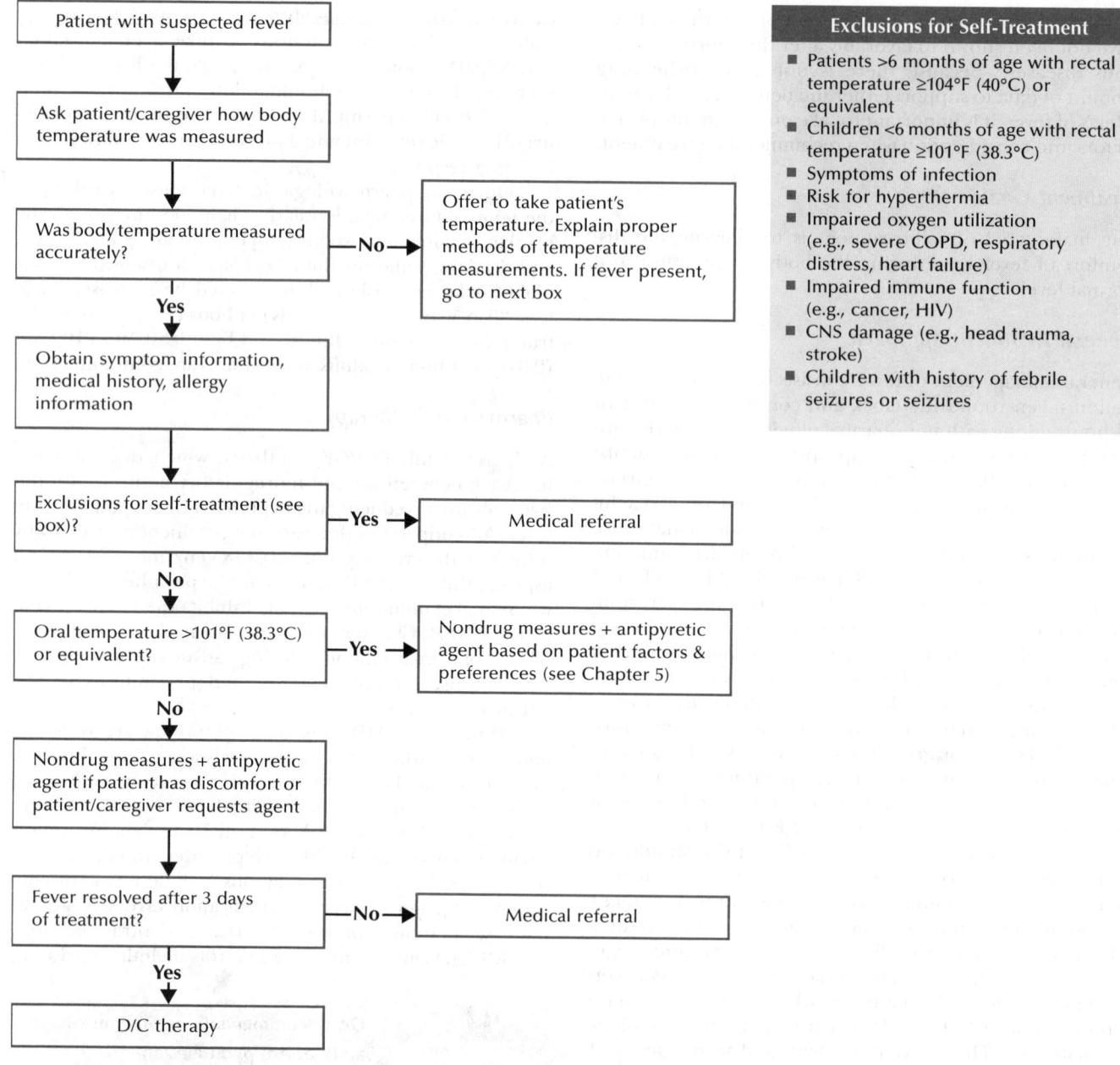

**FIGURE 6-1** Self-care of fever. Key: CNS, central nervous system; COPD, chronic obstructive pulmonary disease; D/C, discontinue; HIV, human immunodeficiency virus.

or duplicating therapy when using multiple products with similar ingredients and inappropriate dosing for pediatric patients attributed to mathematical errors in calculating a weight-based dose. Many of the antipyretic agents are present in combination products for multisymptom relief. For the relief of fever alone, combination products are not necessary and their use may lead to overdosing of medications. Alternating acetaminophen and NSAID therapy (i.e., ibuprofen) to lower fever is also practiced, but not recommended by the American Academy of Pediatrics because of the risk of overdose, medications errors, and increased side effects.[37] Significant side effects are gastrointestinal bleeding from NSAID- and aspirin-containing products and hepatotoxicity with acetaminophen, especially when used at high-doses and for long periods in patients who drink more than 3 alcoholic beverages per day.[38] In general, low-dose antipyretics control fever and should not be used more than 3 days to treat fever without referring for further evaluation to determine the underlying cause.

## Pharmacotherapeutic Comparison

In clinical studies, ibuprofen has demonstrated comparable efficacy and safety profiles, compared with acetaminophen, and has a longer duration of action at normal doses.[39] However, any of the nonprescription analgesic/antipyretic medications (i.e., acetaminophen, aspirin, ibuprofen, naproxen sodium, ketoprofen) are appropriate and indicated for treating fever.[40,41]

**TABLE 6-10 Selected Complementary/Alternative Medicines Used to Treat Fever[42,43]**

| Agent | Risks | Effectiveness |
|---|---|---|
| **Botanical Medicines (Scientific Name)** | | |
| Angelica (*Angelica archangelica*) | Photosensitivity | Approved by Commission E monographs for fever and colds |
| Arnica (*Arnica montana*) | Skin rashes; cardiac toxicity if used internally | Approved by Commission E monographs for fever and colds |
| Echinacea (*Echinacea* sp.) | Nausea, vomiting, hypotension | Approved by Commission E monographs for fever and colds |
| English plantain (*Plantago lanceolata*) | None known | Approved by Commission E monographs for fever and colds |
| European elder (*Sambucus nigra*) | None known | Approved by Commission E monographs for fever and colds; increases bronchial secretions and causes diaphoresis |
| German chamomile (*Matricaria recutita*) | Contact dermatitis, conjunctivitis, vomiting | Approved by Commission E monographs for fever and colds |
| Japanese mint (*Mentha arvensis*) | Gallbladder inflammation and liver dysfunction | Approved by Commission E monographs for fever and colds |
| Larch (*Larix decidua*) | Possible kidney, liver, and CNS damage | Approved by Commission E monographs for fever and colds |
| Meadowsweet (*Filipendula ulmaria*) | GI upset, nausea, salicylate toxicity | Approved by Commission E monographs for fever and colds |
| Scotch pine (*Pinus* sp.) | Bronchial spasms, kidney damage, cardiac insufficiency | Approved by Commission E monographs for fever and colds |
| Spruce (*Picea* sp.) | Bronchial spasms, cardiac insufficiency | Approved by Commission E monographs for fever and colds |
| **Nonbotanical Natural Medicines** | | |
| Vitamin C | | Not studied specifically for fever |
| Zinc | Metallic taste, constipation | Not studied specifically for fever |
| **Homeopathic Medicines** | | |
| Aconite | Arrhythmias, acidosis, confusion. | Not recommended |
| Belladonna | Anticholinergic effects: blurred vision, urinary retention, constipation, changes in mental status | Not recommended |
| Nux vomica | Liver dysfunction, fatigue, restlessness, convulsions, acidosis, rhabdomylosis | Not recommended |
| Pulsatilla | Dermatitis, GI irritation | Helpful to treat, but not prevent influenza and related fever |
| Oscillococcinum (Anas barbariae hepatis) | Nausea, vomiting, diarrhea | Helpful to treat, but not prevent influenza and related fever |

Key: CNS, central nervous system; GI, gastrointestinal.

### *Complementary Therapies*

A multitude of complementary remedies are marketed for the treatment of fever including herbal agents, homeopathic agents, and home remedies. Although limited efficacy or safety data exist to support use of these agents, some patients may prefer these remedies to traditional therapies.

#### Botanical Medicines

Table 6-10 lists the risks and effectiveness of selected herbal remedies for fever. The German Commission E has approved the following agents for the treatment of fever and cold: angelica, arnica, *Echinacea*, English plantain, European elder, German chamomile, Japanese mint, larch, meadowsweet, Scotch pine, and spruce. (See Chapter 53 for further discussion of these products.) Other agents such as divi-divi and wormwood have been used in a variety of countries for years, but are not supported with clinical data. Common agents marketed for the treatment of fever in the United States are boneset (*Eupatorium perfoliatum*) and German chamomile.[42] Agents such as *Echinacea* and wild indigo stimulate the immune response but are not known to specifically reduce fever. Angelica, boneset, German chamomile, and Jacob's ladder are used primarily for their fever-reducing properties. Dogwood, peppermint, and European five-finger grass are used for the treatment of fever attributed to their cooling properties. Many commercial products contain multiple ingredients. It is important to be aware of these products; they may increase the potential for overdosing or duplicating therapy.

### Nonbotanical Natural Medicines

Vitamin C and zinc are commonly used home remedies to treat fever. Vitamin C and zinc enhance the immune system and therefore may assist in reducing fever if the underlying cause is infectious; however, they are not direct antipyretic agents.

### Homeopathy

Aconite, Belladonna, Nux vomica, and Pulsatilla are common homeopathic agents used to treat fever (see Chapter 54).[43] Aconite and Belladonna typically are used in febrile patients who feel warm, whereas Nux vomica is used mainly when the patient notices chills, and Pulsatilla is used in patients who feel irritable during their fever episode. These agents should be used cautiously because all have substantial side effects if used at supratherapeutic doses. Belladonna and Nux vomica have anticholinergic properties and therefore may inhibit diaphoresis when used in excess. However, homeopathic doses are typically low and thus may not interfere with natural cooling processes. Oscillococcinum is a natural product that has been marketed for the treatment of influenza. In clinical studies, oscillococcinum has reduced fever by 32.7°F (0.38°C) in patients with existing influenza.[44]

## Assessment of Fever: A Case-based Approach

The first step in assessing a patient with a complaint of fever is to obtain an objective temperature measurement to determine if fever actually is present. Subjective or inaccurate temperature measurement must be ruled out. If fever is present, assessment of its severity, the seriousness of the underlying cause, and other associated symptoms is indicated. Children who are capable of providing and understanding information should be included in any dialogue concerning their care. Cases 6-1 and 6-2 give examples of the assessment of patients with fever.

### CASE 6-1

| Relevant Evaluation Criteria | Scenario/Model Outcome |
|---|---|
| **Information Gathering** | |
| 1. Gather essential information about the patient's symptoms, including: | |
| a. description of symptom(s) (i.e., nature, onset, duration, severity, associated symptoms) | Day care staff reported to a mother that her son has an oral temperature of 101 °F (38.3°C) and that he complains that "his body hurts." The mother noticed that he seemed extra tired this morning, but she did not notice any other symptoms. |
| b. description of any factors that seem to precipitate, exacerbate, and/or relieve the patient's symptom(s) | The mother has not tried anything yet to relieve the temperature or discomfort. The child is unable to describe what worsens his symptoms. |
| c. description of the patent's efforts to relieve the symptoms | Day care staff noticed that the child continually asked for water because he was "thirsty" and wanted to "sleep all day." |
| 2. Gather essential patient history information: | |
| a. patient's identity | Michael Bates |
| b. age, sex, height, and weight | 5 y/o M, 3'8", 44 lb |
| c. patient's occupation | Student |
| d. patient's dietary habits | Normal healthy diet with occasional junk food. However, he has not eaten much all day today and continually asks for water to drink. |
| e. patient's sleep habits | Sleeps approximately 10 hours per day, including one 1-hour nap. However, today he seemed very tired at day care and had a longer nap (2 hours). |
| f. concurrent medications and medical conditions | Flinstone's Vitamins |
| g. allergies | NKA |
| h. history of other adverse reactions to medications | None |

## CASE 6-1 (continued)

| Relevant Evaluation Criteria | Scenario/Model Outcome |
|---|---|
| i. other (describe) _______ | Michael seems very cranky and tired while in your pharmacy. He did not participate in many activities at day care today. His mother and he deny nasal congestion, vomiting, diarrhea, or productive cough. In the pharmacy, his oral temperature is 100.°F (37.7°C). |
| **Assessment and Triage** | |
| 3. Differentiate patient's signs/symptoms and correctly identify the patient's primary problem(s). | Patient has a low-grade fever with some discomfort, possibly related to a virus transmitted in day care. He does not exhibit any symptoms of bacterial infection. |
| 4. Identify exclusions for self-care (see Figure 6-1). | None |
| 5. Formulate a comprehensive list of therapeutic alternatives to address the primary problem to determine if triage to a medical practitioner is required and share this information with the caregiver. | Options include:<br>(1) Refer Michael to a clinician.<br>(2) Monitor his symptoms and rely on nonpharmacologic interventions.<br>(3) Recommend self-care with an appropriate OTC product combined with nonpharmacologic interventions.<br>(4) Take no action. |
| **Plan** | |
| 6. Select an optimal therapeutic alternative to address the patient's problem, taking into account patient preferences. | Michael has no symptoms of infection or other exclusions for self-treatment (see Figure 6-1); therefore, self-care with an NSAID or acetaminophen combined with nonpharmacologic interventions is appropriate for this patient. His age contraindicates the use of aspirin-containing products. |
| 7. Describe the recommended therapeutic approach to the caregiver. | See Table 5-2 in Chapter 5 for recommended product dosages. If fever or discomfort persists after 3 days of treatment, take your son to his clinician (see box Patient Education for Fever). |
| 8. Explain to the caregiver the rationale for selecting the recommended therapeutic alternatives that were considered. | Seeing a clinician is not necessary at this time because Michael is otherwise fairly healthy and has a low-grade fever without other symptoms of infection. Using nondrug interventions alone is also not recommended because Michael is in discomfort. |
| **Patient Education** | |
| 9. When recommending self-care with over-the-counter medications, convey accurate information to the caregiver, including: | |
| a. appropriate dose and frequency of administration | Acetaminophen syrup 240 mg (7.5 mL of liquid formulation) orally every 4-6 hours (see Chapter 5, Tables 5-2 and 5-6). |
| b. maximum number of days the therapy should be employed | If symptoms do not resolve in 3 days with therapy, take Michael to his clinician for further evaluation. |
| c. product administration procedures | Use dosing spoon or syringe to administer appropriate amount of syrup. |
| d. expected time to onset of relief | With proper dosing and usage of medication, noticeable improvement may be observed within 1-2 hours of therapy. |
| e. degree of relief that can be reasonably expected | Complete resolution of symptoms may take anywhere from 2 days to 3 weeks, depending on the underlying cause of the fever. |
| f. most common side effects | Rare; possible rash |
| g. side effects that warrant medical intervention should they occur | If gastrointestinal upset occurs, give medication with food. If a skin rash appears, stop giving medication. |
| h. patient options in the event that condition worsens or persists | A clinician should be consulted if symptoms worsen or if symptoms persist after 3 days of drug therapy. |
| i. product storage requirements | Keep medication in a tightly closed container away from dampness or extreme heat and child. |

## CASE 6-1 (continued)

| Relevant Evaluation Criteria | Scenario/Model Outcome |
|---|---|
| j. specific nondrug measures | Drinking sufficient fluids (50 mL every hour) and wearing lightweight clothing are important in conjunction with drug therapy (see box Patient Education for Fever). |
| 10. Solicit follow-up questions from caregiver. | May I give Michael both acetaminophen and ibuprofen so he will get better more quickly? |
| 11. Answer caregiver's questions. | No. There is no evidence that using alternating doses of acetaminophen and ibuprofen provides a better response than using either alone. Using the products together may become confusing and may increase the risk of suffering unwanted side effects.[37] |

Key: NKA, no known allergies; NSAID, nonsteroidal anti-inflammatory drug; OTC, over-the-counter.

## CASE 6-2

| Relevant Evaluation Criteria | Scenario/Model Outcome |
|---|---|
| **Information Gathering** | |
| 1. Gather essential information about the patient's symptoms, including: | |
| a. description of symptom(s) (i.e., nature, onset, duration, severity, associated symptoms) | Your neighbor tells you that she hasn't been feeling well for the past 2 days. She complains of feeling tired and warm all over. She denies chest pain and runny nose, vomiting, and diarrhea, but complains of shortness of breath from coughing and muscle aches. |
| b. description of any factors that seem to precipitate, exacerbate, and/or relieve the patient's symptom(s) | She cannot pinpoint any particular factor that makes her pain or fatigue worse, but says that she has been sleeping more over the past 2 days because of the fatigue. |
| c. description of the patent's efforts to relieve the symptoms | She has tried a muscle rub for the muscle pain without much relief. She was thinking about trying some aspirin for her pain, but wanted to consult with you first. |
| 2. Gather essential patient history information: | |
| a. patient's identity | Emily Shaw |
| b. age, sex, height, and weight | 76 y/o F, 5'8", 162 lb |
| c. patient's occupation | Retired sales clerk |
| d. patient's dietary habits | Normal healthy diet. However, she has not eaten much (only soups and sandwiches) over the past 2 days because she is too tired to cook. |
| e. patient's sleep habits | Sleeps approximately 6 hours per night, but over the past 2 days she has taken naps throughout the day |
| f. concurrent medications and medical conditions | Hypertension and heart failure<br>Medications: digoxin 0.125 mg by mouth once daily, lisinopril 40 mg by mouth once daily, furosemide 40 mg by mouth once daily, atenolol 50 mg by mouth once daily, aspirin 81 mg by mouth once daily, Centrum silver 1 tablet once daily |
| g. allergies | NKA |
| h. history of other adverse reactions to medications | None |
| i. other (describe)_______ | She seems quite tired and short of breath while speaking with you. You take her oral temperature, which is 101.1°F (38.4°C). |

**CASE 6-2 (continued)**

| Relevant Evaluation Criteria | Scenario/Model Outcome |
|---|---|
| **Assessment and Triage** | |
| 3. Differentiate patients's signs/symptoms and correctly identify the patient's primary problem(s). | Emily has a fever with some discomfort. Since older adult patients typically have lower temperatures than younger patients, a temperature of 101.1°F (38.8°C) may be of concern. Fever may be related to an infection (from viral or bacterial sources). Shortness of breath may be from her heart failure condition or a symptom of respiratory infection. |
| 4. Identify exclusions for self-treatment (see Figure 6-1). | Patient has history of heart failure which is an exclusion for self-care. |
| 5. Formulate a comprehensive list of therapeutic alternatives to address the primary problem to determine if triage to a medical practitioner is required and share this information with the patient. | Options include:<br>(1) Refer Emily for medical evaluation.<br>(2) Monitor her symptoms and rely on nonpharmacologic interventions.<br>(3) Recommend a proper OTC product combined with nonpharmacologic interventions.<br>(4) Take no action. |
| **Plan** | |
| 6. Select an optimal therapeutic alternative to address the patient's problem, taking into account the patient's preferences. | Refer patient for further medical evaluation. Patient has an exclusion for self-care (see Figure 6-1). |
| 7. Describe the recommended therapeutic approach to the patient. | N/A |
| 8. Explain to the patient the rationale for selecting the recommended therapeutic approach from the considered therapeutic alternatives. | Your age and your heart condition (heart failure) may predispose you to complications of fever (dehydration and delirium). Your shortness of breath may indicate signs of respiratory infection and needs further medical evaluation. |
| **Patient Education** | |
| 9. When recommending self-care with over-the-counter medications, convey accurate information to the patient. | N/A |
| 10. Solicit follow-up questions from patient. | If I am unable to see my clinician today or tomorrow, is there anything I can do to feel better? |
| 11. Answer patient's questions. | Continue to drink fluids and wear light clothing because fever can cause dehydration. If the discomfort persists, you can use acetaminophen temporarily until you see your clinician. Do not use aspirin-containing products or NSAIDs such as ibuprofen because they may worsen your heart failure or high blood pressure. If you are begin to feel worse, you should seek care at an urgent care facility. |

Key: NKA, no known allergies; N/A, not applicable; NSAID, nonsteroidal anti-inflammatory drug; OTC, over-the-counter.

## Patient Counseling for Fever

Although fever is a common symptom, it often is misunderstood and poorly treated. Studies suggest that fever is considered a disease associated with detrimental consequences rather than a symptom; frequently is treated inappropriately; and is evaluated improperly.[45,46] Many parents and caregivers have "fever phobia" that results in heightened anxiety and inappropriate treatment of fever.[30,47] Clinicians can improve patient outcomes by educating patients and caregivers about fever, and by teaching patients self-assessment skills and the proper methods for measuring body temperature. Such instruction should include demonstration of temperature measurement techniques. Practitioners should also explain the appropriate nonpharmacologic

## PATIENT EDUCATION FOR FEVER

The primary objectives of treating fever are to (1) relieve the discomfort of fever by returning the body temperature to the normal level and (2) prevent complications associated with fever. For most patients, carefully following product instructions and the self-care measures listed here will help to ensure optimal therapeutic outcomes.

### Temperature Measurement

- Do not rely on feeling the body for fever. Take a temperature reading with an appropriate thermometer.
- For children up to 6 months of age, the rectal method of temperature measurement is preferred (see Table 6-5). Use of a tympanic thermometer is not recommended because of the size and shape of the infant's ear canal.
- For children ages 6 months to 5 years, the rectal method is still preferred; however, the tympanic, temporal, or oral pacifier method may be used if proper technique is followed (see Tables 6-6 and 6-7).
- For individuals older than 5 years, the oral, temporal, or tympanic method is appropriate (see Tables 6-4, 6-6, and 6-7).

### Nondrug Measures

- Do not use isopropyl or ethyl alcohol in body sponging. Alcohol poisoning can result from skin absorption or inhalation of topically applied alcohol solutions.
- For all degrees of fever, wear light clothing, remove blankets, and maintain room temperature at 78°F (25.6°C).
- Unless advised otherwise, drink or provide sufficient fluids to replenish body fluid losses. For children, increase fluids by at least 1 oz per hour. Sports drinks, fruit juice, or water are acceptable.

### Nonprescription Medications

- Nonprescription analgesics/antipyretics (see Chapter 5, Tables 5-2 and 5-3) help in alleviating discomfort associated with fever and reducing the temperature.
- Nonprescription analgesics/antipyretics may take up to 6 hours to decrease temperature and possibly longer to decrease discomfort.
- Monitor level of discomfort and body temperature using the same thermometer at the same body site two to three times per day during a febrile illness.
- Use single-entity nonprescription analgesics/antipyretics at low doses for up to 3 days for treatment of fever (see Chapter 5, Tables 5-2 and 5-3 for dosages), unless you have an exclusion to self-care (see Figure 6-1).
- If you are pregnant or have uncontrolled high blood pressure, congestive heart failure, renal failure, or an allergy to aspirin avoid use of nonsteroidal anti-inflammatory drugs (ibuprofen, ketoprofen, naproxen sodium) or aspirin-containing products.
- Avoid using aspirin and aspirin-containing products for fever in children younger than 12 years because of the possible risk of Reye's syndrome.
- Do not use more than one product to treat the fever to prevent overdosing.

Seek medical attention if fever or discomfort persists or worsens after 3 days of drug treatment.

and pharmacologic treatments for fever and when to seek further medical care. Discussions of pharmacologic treatments should highlight methods for safe use of antipyretics (Table 6-9).

## Evaluation of Patient Outcomes for Fever

The main monitoring parameters of febrile patients include temperature and discomfort. In one study, 52% of caregivers said that they would check a patient's temperature at least every hour in a febrile patient.[30] Overaggressive monitoring may result from "fever phobia." Pharmacologic therapy for fever may take up to 1 day to result in a temperature drop; therefore, body temperature should be monitored only two to three times a day. Associated symptoms including headache, diaphoresis, generalized malaise, chills, tachycardia, arthralgia, myalgia, irritability, and anorexia should also be monitored daily. If symptoms are not improving or are worsening over the course of 3 days with self-treatment regardless of a drop in temperature, a practitioner should be consulted either by phone or appointment for further evaluation. Timeliness of patient follow-up with medical care is important in determining the presence of a non–self-limiting underlying cause.

## Key Points for Fever

- Fever is self-limiting and rarely poses severe consequences unless the oral temperature is greater than 104°F (40°C).
- The main treatment goal of fever is to eliminate the underlying cause as well as to alleviate the associated discomfort.
- Fever should be confirmed only by using a thermometer and appropriate measurement techniques.
- Rectal temperature measurement is the most accurate method; however, oral, tympanic, and temporal measurements are also accurate if taken appropriately.
- Patients should be referred for further evaluation if their temperature is greater than 102°F (38.9°C), they have a history of febrile seizures, they have comorbid conditions compromising their health, or they are younger than 6 months.
- Sponge baths and the use of topical isopropyl alcohol to reduce fever should be discouraged.
- Referral for further medical evaluation is appropriate to detect an underlying cause if 3 days of self-treatment is not successful.

- Clinicians should counsel patients on the proper use of nonprescription antipyretic agents to limit medication errors and side effects.

## References


1. Halloran LL, Bernard DW. Management of drug-induced hyperthermia. *Current Opinion Pediatr.* 2004;16:211-5.
2. National Ambulatory Medical Care Survey; 2002 Summary. Advance Data: From Vital and Health Statistics. Washington, DC: US Department of Health and Human Services. Series No. 346. Available at: URL: http://www.cdc.gov/nchs/data/ad/ad346.pdf. Accessed December 19, 2004.
3. Rehm KP. Fever in infants and children. *Curr Opin Pediatr.* 2001; 13:83-8.
4. Mackowiak PA. Concepts of fever. *Arch Intern Med.* 1998;158:1870-81.
5. Porat R, Dinarello CA. Pathophysiology and treatment of fever. In: UpToDate. Version 9.1. Wellesley, Mass: UpToDate, Inc; 2001.
6. Guyton AC, Hall JE. Textbook of Medical Physiology. 10th ed. Philadelphia: WB Saunders; 2000:830-2.
7. Norman DC. Fever in the elderly. *Clin Infect Dis.* 2000;31: 148-51.
8. DiPiro JT, Ownby DR, Schlesselman LS. Allergic and pseudoallergic drug reactions. In: DiPiro JT, Talbert RL, Yee GC, et al., eds. *Pharmacotherapy: A Pathophysiologic Approach.* 5th ed. New York: McGraw-Hill, Inc; 2002:1588.
9. McDonald M, Sexton DJ. Drug fever. In: UpToDate. Version 9.1. Wellesley, Mass: UpToDate, Inc; 2001.
10. Johnson DH, Cunha BA. Drug fever. *Infect Dis Clin North Am.* 1996;10:85-91.
11. Chan T, Evans S, Clark R. Drug-induced hyperthermia. *Crit Care Clin.* 1997;13:785-809.
12. Velammor V. Neuroleptic malignant syndrome: recognition, prevention, and management. Drug Saf. 1998;19:73-82.
13. Dinarello CA, Bunn PA. Fever. *Semin Oncol.* 1997;24: 288-98.
14. Netea MG, Kullberg BJ, Van der Meer JW. Circulating cytokines as mediators of fever. *Clin Infect Dis.* 2000;31: S178-84.
15. How to take a child's temperature. Available at: http://www.ps.ca/english/carekids/childhoodillnesses/temperature.htm. Accessed July 21, 2001.
16. Rabinowitz RP, Cookson ST, Wasserman SS, et al. Effects of anatomic site, oral stimulation, and body position on estimates of body temperature. *Arch Intern Med.* 1996; 156:777-80.
17. US Environmental Protection Agency. Product stewardship: mercury in products. Available at: http://www.epa. gov/epaoswer/non-hw/reduce/epr/products/mfed.html. 2002. Accessed March 12, 2003.
18. American Academy of Pediatrics. AAP supports elimination of mercury-containing thermometers. Available at: http://www.aap.org/advocacy/archives/julymerc.htm. 2001. Accessed March 12, 2003.
19. Press S. Quinn BJ. The pacifier thermometer: comparison of supralingual with rectal temperatures in infants and young children. *Arch Pediatr Adolesc Med.* 1997;151:551-4.
20. Callanan D. Detecting ferver in young infants: reliability of perceived, pacifier, and temporal artery temperatures in infants younger than 3 months of age. *Pediatr Emerg Care.* 2003;19:240-3.
21. Robinson JL, Seal RF, Spady DW, et al. Comparison of esophageal, rectal, axillary, bladder, tympanic, and pulmonary artery temperatures in children. *J Pediatr.* 1998; 133:553-6.
22. Greenes DS. Fleisher GR. When body temperature changes, does rectal temperature lag? *J Pediatr.* 2004;144:824-6.
23. Bernardo LM, Henker R, O'Connor J. Temperature measurement in pediatric trauma patients: a comparison of thermometry and measurement routes. *J Emerg Nurs.* 1999;25:327-9.
24. Wilshaw R, Beckstrand R, Waid D, et al. A comparison of the use of tympanic, axillary, and rectal thermometers in infants. *J Ped Nurs.* 1999;14:88-93.
25. Craig JV, Lancaster GA, Taylor S, et al. Infrared ear thermometry compared with rectal thermometry in children: a systematic review. *Lancet.* 2002;360:603-9.
26. Varney SM, Manthey DE, Culpepper VE, et al. A comparison of oral, tympanic, and rectal temperature measurement in the elderly. *J Emerg Med.* 2002:22:153-7.
27. Jean-Mary MB, Dicanzio J, Shaw J, et al. Limited accuracy and reliability of infrared axillary and aural thermometers in a pediatric outpatient population. *J Pediatr.* 2002;141:671-6.
28. Greenes DS, Fleisher GR. Accuracy of a noninvasive temporal artery thermometer for use in infants. *Arch Pediatr Adolesc Med.* 2001;155:376-81.
29. Siberry GK, Diener-West M, Schappell E, et al. Comparison of temple temperatures with rectal temperatures in children under two years of age. *Clin Pediatr.* 2002;41:405-14.
30. Crocetti M, Moghbeli N, Serwint J. Fever phobia revisited: have parental misconceptions about fever changed in 20 years? *Pediatrics.* 2001;107:1241-6.
31. Baumann RJ, D'Angelo SL. The neurodiagnostic evaluation of the child with a first simple febrile seizure. *Pediatrics.* 1996;97: 773-5.
32. Practice parameter: long-term treatment of the child with simple febrile seizures. *Pediatrics.* 1999;103:1307-9.
33. Roghmann MC, Warner J, Mackowiak PA. The relationship between age and fever magnitude. *Am J Med Sci.* 2001; 322:68-70.
34. Plaisance KI, Mackowiak PA. Antipyretic therapy: physiologic rationale, diagnostic implications, and clinical consequences. *Arch Intern Med.* 1996;160:449-56.
35. Axelrod P. External cooling in the management of fever. *Clin Infect Dis.* 2000;31(suppl 5):S224-9.
36. Aronoff DM, Neilson EG. Antipyretics: mechanisms of action and clinical use in fever suppression. *Am J Med.* 2001;111:304-15.
37. Mayoral CE., Marino RV, Rosenfeld W, Greensher J. Alternating antipyretics: is this an alternative? *Pediatrics.* 2000;105:1009-12.
38. Safety concerns associated with over-the-counter drug products containing analgesic/antipyretic active ingredients for internal use. 2004. Food and Drug Administration Science Background. Available at: URL: http://www.fda.gov/cder/drug/analgesics/SciencePaper.pdf. Accessed February 20, 2005.
39. Perrott DA, Piira R, Goodenough B, Champion GD. Efficacy and safety of acetaminophen versus ibuprofen for treating children's pain or fever: a meta-analysis. *Arch Pediatr Adolesc Med.* 2004; 158(6):521-6.
40. Wong A, Sibbald A, Ferrero F, et al. Antipyretic effects of dipyrone versus ibuprofen versus acetaminophen in children: results of a multinational, randomized, modified double-blind study. *Clin Pediatr.* 2001;40:313-24.
41. McIntyre J, Hull D. Comparing efficacy and tolerability of ibuprofen and paracetamol in fever. *Arch Dis Child.*1996;74:164-7.
42. PDR for Herbal Medicines. 2nd ed. Montvale, NJ: Medical Economics Co; 2000.
43. Cummings S, Ullman D. *Everybody's Guide to Homeopathic Medicines.* 3rd ed. New York: Penguin Putnam;1997:48-61.
44. Vickers AJ, Smith C. Homeopathic oscillococcinum for preventing and treating influenza and influenza-like syndromes. Cochrane Database of Systematic Reviews. 2005. Updated June 11, 2004.
45. Ey JL. Fever commentary. *Clin Pediatr.* 2002;41:14-6.
46. Lagerlov P, Helseth S. Holager T. Childhood illnesses and the use of paracetamol: a qualitative study of parent' management of common childhood illnesses. *Fam Practice.* 2003;20:717-23.
47. Parkinson GW, Gordon KE, Camfield CS, Fitzpatrick EA. Anxiety in parents of young febrile children in a pediatric emergency department: why is it elevated? *Clin Pediatr.* 1999;38:219-26.

CHAPTER 7

# Musculoskeletal Injuries and Disorders

*Eric Wright*

Pain is one of the most common symptoms that prompt a visit to a health care professional.[1] Because pain is a common symptom of disease, patients often seek medical attention although many seek to relieve the pain without notifying their health care provider. Much of the pain for which people attempt self-treatment arises from the musculoskeletal system. Musculoskeletal pain may be felt in the affected tissue itself, or it may be referred from another anatomic source (e.g., hip pain referred from its primary source in the lower back).[2]

Musculoskeletal pain arises from the muscles (myalgia), bones, joints (arthralgia), or connective tissue. Similar to other types of pain phenomena, musculoskeletal pain can be idiopathic, iatrogenic, or related to injury. Musculoskeletal pain includes pain from stable degenerative joint disease (osteoarthritis), as well as acute sports or strain injuries (e.g., tendonitis, strains, and sprains). Unfortunately, this term is also used to describe regional discomfort arising from any soft tissue source (including the skin), which leads to confusion among clinicians and in the medical literature. Table 7-1 describes other types of musculoskeletal complaints/disorders.

Use of nonprescription analgesics and external counterirritants remain high, with over $2 billion spent per year in the United States on these nonprescription remedies.[3] In addition, nearly 80% of adults admit to taking a pain reliever at least once a week.

This high medication use presents a significant challenge for providers. Under the best circumstances, a patient experiencing pain will ask a clinician to assist in selecting a nonprescription or prescription product. Clinicians need to understand the types of pain for which patients are seeking treatment and communicate effectively with patients to better understand the nature of a specific individual's pain complaint. They must also be ready to provide reasonable recommendations for either treatment or further evaluation.

## Epidemiology of Musculoskeletal Injuries and Disorders

Despite the ubiquitous nature of pain, surprisingly little research has addressed its prevalence. Studies of generalized pain in the community show occurrences ranging from 7% to 64%, with many experiencing recurrent, persistent, or severe pain.[4] Acute musculoskeletal injury and pain are less often observed by clinicians and generally self-treated. Hence, the incidence and prevalence of reported skeletal muscle injuries may be underestimated.

Chronic musculoskeletal complaints are associated with rheumatoid arthritis, osteoarthritis, and less common diseases such as fibromyalgia and other muscle, bone, or connective tissue diseases. Malignant pain conditions (e.g., cancer) and nonmalignant neuropathic pain are reported less often than chronic pain of the muscles, connective tissue, or joints.[5]

Musculoskeletal and connective tissue disorders are the third and fifth leading cause of lost work days in men and women, respectively.[6] Only workplace injury and respiratory system disease consistently cause a greater number of lost workdays. Musculoskeletal complaints also result in a significant amount of work limitations and loss of employment, and are believed to be the greatest contributors to the economic burden of chronic pain estimated to cost the U.S. economy more than $60 billion annually.[7] Backache and osteoarthritis are highly prevalent pain complaints with approximately one half of the U.S. population over the age of 70 having osteoarthritis.[8] Approximately one tenth of the working population is being treated for arthritis with prescription medications, while many choose to self-treat and go unreported.[9] Hence, the incidence and prevalence of reported skeletal muscle injuries may be underestimated.

## Anatomy and Physiology of the Musculoskeletal System

The musculoskeletal system includes the muscles, tendons, ligaments, cartilage, and bones. Muscles are attached to bones by tendons, and ligaments connect bone to bone. Under normal conditions, tendons and ligaments have limited ability to stretch and twist. Because of their tensile strength, tendons and ligaments rarely rupture unless subjected to intense forces, but may become damaged when hyperextended or overused.

Cartilage functions as protective pads between bones in many joints and in the vertebral column. Skeletal, or striated muscle, is composed of cells (myocytes) in which two constituents (actin and myosin) are primarily responsible for contraction. Muscle contraction also involves several electrolytes within the muscle tissue, including calcium and potassium. Pain receptors are located in skeletal muscle and the overlying fascia, and can be stimulated as

**TABLE 7-1 Common Musculoskeletal Complaints and Disorders**

*Myofascial pain* or *musculoskeletal pain* refers to pain that can be elicited from specific points in the muscle or fascia.

*Myalgia* is a term used to describe muscle pain.

*Fibromyalgia* is a condition characterized by diffuse muscle and joint pain.

*Fibrositis* implies that a trigger point, or a specific point from which pain can be evoked, lies within a palpable band of fibrous tissue.

*Strain* is an injury to a muscle or tendon caused by overuse or improper use.

*Sprain* is an injury to a ligament caused by joint overextension.

*Muscle spasm* is an involuntary contraction of muscle.

*Muscle cramp* is a prolonged muscle spasm that produces painful sensations.

*Muscle stiffness* is a common term used to describe muscle discomfort that results in a decreased range of motion.

a result of overuse or injury to the muscle or surrounding structures. Chapter 5 reviews neurological pain transmission.

Pain relating to the musculoskeletal system is described in this chapter and its presentation and treatment will be discussed according to the tissue affected.

## Etiology of Musculoskeletal Injuries and Disorders

### *Myalgia*

Muscle injuries can be categorized as strains, contusions caused by blunt trauma, and delayed-onset muscle soreness. Ischemic muscle pain is caused by intramuscular pressure during activity that reduces blood supply to the muscle. Normally, this effect disappears within seconds of muscle relaxation. Ischemic muscle pain lasting for longer periods is probably the effect of histamine, acetylcholine, serotonin, and bradykinin. Potassium and adenosine may also contribute.

Overexertion or repeated unaccustomed eccentric muscle contraction is associated with delayed-onset (8 hours or more) muscle soreness, which can last for days, usually peaking at 24 to 48 hours. This pain reflects muscle damage that was presumably initiated by force generated in the muscle fibers. The mechanism by which delayed-onset muscle pain is generated is unknown. Prolonged tonic contraction produced by exercise, tension, or poor posture and by body mechanics can also produce muscle pain.

Myalgia can also result from systemic infections (e.g., influenza, Coxsackievirus, measles, other illnesses), chronic disorders (e.g., fibromyalgia and polymyalgia rheumatica), and medications (e.g., by some cholesterol-lowering agents such as statins).[10] Abuse of alcohol may precipitate acute alcoholic myopathy. Bone and muscle pain (from osteomalacia) may also occur as a result of dietary deficiency of vitamin D.

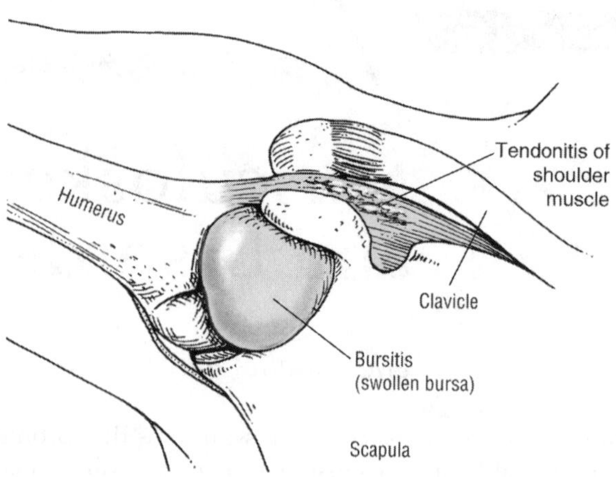


**FIGURE 7-1** Bursitis and tendonitis. These two painful injuries, which often result from overuse of a joint or tendon, can cause inflammation, swelling, and tenderness in the injured area. (Reprinted with permission from *US Pharm.* January 1995;20:1.)

### *Tendonitis and Bursitis*

Tendonitis is the inflammation of a tendon, which results from acute injuries or chronic overuse of a body part (Figure 7-1). An example of the latter is carpal tunnel syndrome, a condition characterized by tingling or numbness of the first digits of the hand caused by repetitive use of hands and wrists. Tendon sheaths become inflamed and constrict the median nerve as it passes through a narrow channel between wrist bones. In industry, factors such as poorly designed equipment, awkward working positions, lack of job variation, long work hours, and inadequate rest breaks contribute to its development. In athletics, contributing factors for tendonitis can include increased age, poor technique, improper conditioning, exercise of prolonged intensity or duration, and poorly designed equipment for specific activities (e.g., poor cushioning of athletic shoes).

Bursitis is a common cause of localized pain, tenderness, and swelling, which is worsened by any movement of the structure adjacent to the bursa (Figure 7-1). Pain caused by either macro- or microtrauma may be acute. When pain is accompanied by presence of a puncture site (may be from intra-articular injection), an adjacent source of infection, or severe inflammation, an infectious cause should be suspected and ruled out before self-treatment.

### *Sprains, Strains, and Cramps*

The most common problem with ligaments is a sprain, which is characterized by degree. First-degree sprains result from excessive stretching, second-degree sprains are a partial tear, and third-degree sprains involve a complete tear of the tissue. The tear or rupture of a ligament is more common than that of a tendon. Examples of ligament sprains include inversion of the ankle (turning inward at an extreme angle) and tearing of the anterior cruciate ligament of the knee during rotation or twisting motions. Anterior cruciate ligament tears are relatively common injuries in sports such as basketball, volleyball, football, tennis, and skiing, in which knees are involved in both propelling and pivoting the body.

Tendons can become strained when their stretch capacity is exceeded, such as in a hyperextension injury of an arm or leg. Eccentric contraction of the muscle while the muscle is lengthening causes the injury. To explain the etiology of the muscle damage and repair, researchers have hypothesized a number of mechanisms that involve disturbances of calcium homeostasis, inflammatory response, and synthesis of stress (heat shock) proteins.[11] No single hypothesis is favored or proven.

Similarly, at least five causes have been hypothesized to explain exercise-induced muscle cramps, including inherited abnormal substrate metabolism, abnormal fluid balance, abnormal serum electrolyte concentrations, extremes of heat or cold, and abnormal spinal reflex activity.[12]

### Lower Back Pain

Unlike the overuse injuries described previously, this regional musculoskeletal disorder is caused primarily by a sedentary lifestyle (particularly one disrupted by bursts of activity), as well as poor posture, improper shoes, excess body weight, poor mattresses and sleeping posture, and improper technique in lifting heavy objects. Thus, back pain is primarily a disease of living. Although most patients recover within a few days to a few weeks with conservative treatment, lower back pain is likely to recur if the initial episode of pain is severe, and if the patient had multiple prior episodes.[13]

In 30% to 90% of patients, low back pain is postural because of supporting muscle and/or ligament injury. Other causes include (1) congenital anomalies, (2) osteoarthritis, (3) vertebral fractures and compressions, (4) spinal tuberculosis, and (5) referred pain from diseased kidneys, pancreas, liver, or prostate.

### Joint Pain

Pain from arthritis has been attributed to a number of sources, including joint instability, increased pressure in the spaces between bones, inflammatory synovitis, periarticular involvement (e.g., bursitis), muscle atrophy, periosteal elevation, fibromyalgia, pain amplification, or central pain mechanisms. Even in the same individual, the pain may arise from different sources at any given time. For instance, rheumatoid arthritis is often associated with "flares," in which pain and inflammation increases, followed by a period of remission.

Osteoarthritis is characterized by a gradual softening and destruction of the cartilage between bones. Cartilage and bone are destroyed in the joint spaces and regenerated, causing a rearrangement of the synovial architecture. Often referred to as a disease of "old age" or "degenerative joint disease," it is caused by genetic, metabolic, and environmental factors. Heavy physical activity, repetitive movement, and lifting heavy weights may aggravate this condition, whereas light to moderate activity does not and is generally helpful.[14]

## Pathophysiology of Musculoskeletal Injuries and Disorders

Somatic pain occurs when pain impulses are transmitted from peripheral nociceptors to the CNS by nociceptive nerve fibers. Common sites of origin of somatic pain are muscles, fascia, bones, and nerves. Somatic pain is most commonly myofascial or musculoskeletal as in arthritis. Trigger points, which can occur following injury or immobility of the affected tissues, cause a reproducible, referred pain pattern when pressed. (See Chapter 5 for a discussion of transduction, transmission, perception, and modulation of pain.)

Mechanoreceptors and chemoreceptors mediate muscle pain. These nerve endings are heterogeneous in that only a single chemical can stimulate some, whereas a variety of chemical, mechanical, and thermal triggers can stimulate others. Bradykinin, serotonin, and histamine, as well as potassium and hydrogen ions, are the primary chemical stimuli.

Erythema or redness, edema, and tenderness or hyperalgesia at the affected site characterize the inflammatory response, which develops through participation of multiple mediators, including histamine, bradykinin, serotonin, leukotrienes, and prostaglandins of the E series. Opioid receptors in peripheral tissues may play a role in the inflammatory response and may exert antihyperanalgesic activity.[15] Because pain and inflammation increase prostaglandin production, drugs that inhibit peripheral production of prostaglandins (e.g., nonsteroidal anti-inflammatory drugs, or NSAIDs) reduce the transmission of pain impulses from the periphery to the CNS.

## Signs and Symptoms of Musculoskeletal Injuries and Disorders

Table 7-2 lists many of the presenting signs and symptoms of musculoskeletal disorders and also differentiates among other factors. Pain is a common symptom in all the musculoskeletal disorders. In addition to the pain induced by a sprain, a greater range of motion when manipulated is also common. If visibly deformed, a joint is probably ruptured or fractured, and requires emergency assistance. Sprains and strains (unlike ruptures and fractures) are likely to allow limited use of the affected limbs.

Patients with carpal tunnel syndrome often experience a sense of heat or cold, a sense their hands are swollen when they are not, weakness, and a tendency to drop things. Symptoms persist during sleep and even when the hand is not being used, a characteristic that can distinguish this disorder from others.

The pain of osteoarthritis does not directly correlate to the degree of joint damage. Pain is often referred, and proximal muscles could be involved if a person with osteoarthritis guards the affected joint by changing the gait to reduce discomfort. The pain caused by chronic osteoarthritis often limits the patient's activities of daily living (ADLs; e.g., unable to grip containers or walk more than a short distance). It is unclear which joint structures are responsible for the pain and discomfort, but the pain has variably been ascribed to derangements of bone, cartilage,

**TABLE 7-2 Differentiation of Musculoskeletal Disorders**

| Criterion | Osteoarthritis | Rheumatoid Arthritis | Myalgia |
|---|---|---|---|
| Location | Weight-bearing joints, knees, hip, spine, hands | Symmetric presentation typically in small joints of fingers, wrists, feet | Body muscles |
| Signs | Noninflammatory joints; joint space narrowing; restructuring of bone and cartilage (resulting in joint deformities); possible joint swelling | Joint swelling and deformities (e.g. swan-neck, boutonniere), (+) rheumatoid factor, increased ESR, rheumatoid nodules, anemia, low-grade fever | Possible swelling (rare) and increase in CPK |
| Symptoms | Dull joint pain relieved by rest; joint stiffness <20-30 minutes; symptoms localized to joint | Pain worse in morning (usually lasting >30 minutes); joints possibly swollen, tender, warm, limited in motion; pain aggravated by movement; systemic symptoms of fatigue, weakness, loss of appetite | Dull, constant ache; sharp pain relatively rare; weakness and fatigue of muscles also common |
| Onset | Insidious development over years | Insidious development over weeks to months, 20% of patients develop disease abruptly | Depends on cause: trauma = acute; drug-induced = insidious |
| Etiology | Degeneration of joint space related to genetic, metabolic, and environmental factors | Unknown initiating event; systemic inflammatory response | Trauma; overuse; infection; drug- or alcohol-induced |
| Exacerbating factors | Obesity; lack of activity; heavy physical activity; repetitive movement; trauma | Movement of affected joints | Contraction of muscle |
| Modifying factors | Continuous exercise (light to moderate activity); weight loss; systemic or topical analgesics | Joint rest; physical therapy; treatment with NSAIDs, steroids, and DMARDs | Eliminating cause; rest; topical or systemic analgesics |

Key: ESR, erythrocyte sedimentation rate; CPK, creatinine phosphokinase; DMARD, disease-modifying antirheumatic drug; NSAID, nonsteroidal anti-inflammatory drug; RICE, rest, ice, compression, elevation.

muscle, connective tissue, and nerves supplying the affected joint or joints. Pain and tightness in the lower back also often results from posture, muscle support, and degenerative changes and often limits a patient's ability to bend, move, sit, or walk. Low back pain can be neuropathic and involve the sciatic nerve, causing sharp deferred pain into one or both of the patient's legs.

Signs and symptoms that preclude self-treatment are listed in Figure 7-2.

## Complications of Musculoskeletal Injuries and Disorders

Complications of untreated pain-inducing injuries include further tissue damage and, in advanced arthritis, bone and cartilage remodeling. The worst complication of poorly managed pain is disability and loss of function. Pain is associated with significant limitations including a reduction of ADLs, loss of work time, and physical impairments such as insomnia. Complications may also arise if the etiology of the pain is misdiagnosed or misjudged. It is important to look for warning signs (Figure 7-2) indicating the pain cannot be managed with nonprescription analgesics.

## Treatment of Musculoskeletal Injuries and Disorders

Acute pain is the body's alarm system; it signals injury by trauma, disease, muscle spasms, or inflammation. Chronic pain conversely may or may not be indicative of injury and requires a primary care provider's assessment before treatment should be initiated.

### *Treatment Goals*

Treatment of the patient with musculoskeletal complaints encompasses many goals, including: (1) decrease the subjective intensity (severity) and duration of the pain; (2) minimize suffering, functional limitation, and disability (i.e., improve ADLs); and (3) prevent acute pain from becoming chronic persistent pain.

### *General Treatment Approach*

Patients with musculoskeletal injuries or disorders present with similar symptoms, especially pain and swelling of the affected area. These conditions have similar self-treatment approaches. The algorithm in Figure 7-2 presents a stepwise approach to self-management of pain associated with these complaints for patients who do not meet the criteria for exclusion for self-care.

| Tendonitis/Bursitis | Sprain/Strain | Cramp |
|---|---|---|
| Joints | Sprain: joint; strain: muscle | Muscles (calf and abdominal muscles are most susceptible) |
| Warmth, edema, erythema, and possible crepitus | Swelling; bruising | Cramped muscle is generally firm to palpation and may be visibly distorted |
| Tenderness; pain similar to arthritis; constant pain in bursitis; exercise improves tendonitis; pressure over joint capsule induces bursitis pain | Pain; loss of some function and gradual stiffening over time; impairment of function, allodynia, paresthesia, numbness, and hyperesthesia may occur | Pain of mild to severe intensity lasting seconds to minutes, which often recurs in affected muscle |
| Acute with injury; can often be recurrent with precipitant use of joint | Acute with injury | See etiology below; leg cramps frequently occur at night during sleep |
| Trauma and excessive wear/use; septic bursitis (most frequently preceded by trauma and caused by *Staphylococcus aureus*) presents with fever and acute painful swelling | Sprain, hyperextension of joint; Strain: excessive stretch of muscle | Overexertion; electrolyte imbalance; water imbalance; symptom of alcoholism, anemia, or arthritis |
| Movement of affected joints | Improper protection (i.e., elastic wrap); lack of proper care after injury | Exercise in "hot" environments; exercise soon after eating; immersion into cold water; food poisoning; diuretic-induced hypokalemia |
| Joint rest; immobilization; topical or systemic analgesics | RICE; protective wraps (e.g., ankle tape, knee brace, cane); topical counterirritants; systemic analgesics | Proper hydration and electrolyte balance; waiting to exercise or swim after eating; limiting overexertion |

## Myalgia

Nonprescription analgesics are often appropriate for managing acute muscle pain, if it is not too severe and if the complaints are not suggestive of a serious underlying disorder.

Acute muscle pain usually responds well to nonprescription analgesics, especially when used in conjunction with heat and/or massage. Nonprescription analgesics should be initiated soon after the injury, taken on a regular schedule while the noxious stimulus is present, and administered in sufficient doses. Benefit from salicylates and NSAIDs occurs during early treatment particularly for pain control (first 1 to 3 days); however, longer-term treatment may have little benefit and in some instances may even delay the repair process.

Chronic muscle pain is often inappropriately treated with pharmacotherapeutic agents. Analgesic medications, as well as other central nervous system (CNS) depressant drugs, are not effective as primary treatment modalities. These agents can produce adverse effects and may actually worsen pain. Patients with severe (chronic nonmalignant) pain often take excessive doses of nonprescription analgesics, which can lead to toxicities. The management of chronic nonmalignant pain often requires an interdisciplinary approach. Nonprescription analgesics may be useful adjuncts for some chronic nonmalignant pain, but these drugs are of limited value in most such syndromes. Physical therapy and behavioral therapies are the main treatment modalities for this type of pain.

## Tendonitis and Bursitis

Injury from playing sports or exercising is preventable by warming up and stretching muscles before exertion. Warming and stretching muscles are particularly important steps for preventing reinjury. Health care providers recommend preventing repetitive strain by exercising the muscles vulnerable to injury. The other major preventive measure is to use ergonomic controls that reduce risk of predisposing factors, such as a chair that is specially designed to improve posture. In addition, Achilles tendonitis can be treated with heel lifts and better-fitting shoes.

Rest, ice, compression, and elevation (RICE) therapy applied to the affected area and nonprescription systemic and topical analgesics are the recommended self-treatment of tendonitis and bursitis (Table 7-3). RICE is also the mainstay of conservative treatment of repetitive strain injury, with emphasis placed on resting the affected area. RICE treatment includes the use of splints or braces (if appropriate). NSAIDs and topical analgesics may help

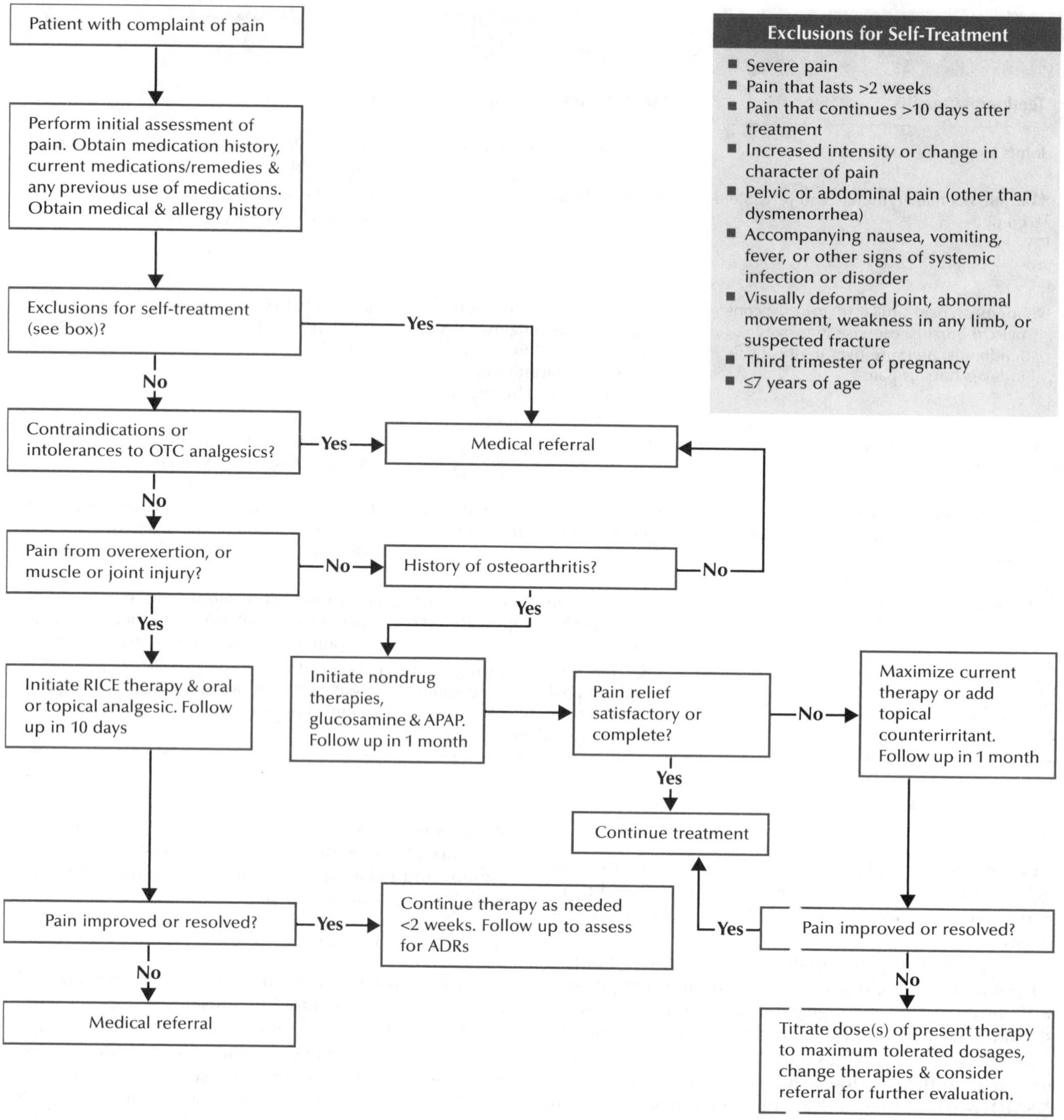


**FIGURE 7-2** Self-care of musculoskeletal injuries and disorders. Key: APAP, acetaminophen; ADR, adverse drug reaction; OTC, over-the-counter; RICE, rest, ice, compression, elevation. (Adapted from Self-care of self-limited pain. In: Albrant DH, ed. *The American Pharmaceutical Association Drug Treatment Protocols*. 2nd ed. Washington, DC: American Pharmaceutical Association; 2001:424-5.)

reduce pain and swelling. An exercise program administered by a physical therapist following acute RICE therapy can be helpful. If pain persists, a primary care provider may inject an anesthetic or corticosteroid (to shrink swollen tissues). A discussion of other alternative treatments is beyond the scope of this chapter, but invasive options are available.

Because of documentation on fluoroquinolone antibiotics causing tendonitis and tendon rupture, any patient showing signs of tendon pain or inflammation (particularly of the Achilles tendon) should immediately discontinue use of the drug and refrain from exercise until the diagnosis of tendonitis is excluded.[16] Those patients particularly at risk include older adults (>60 years) and those concurrently taking corticosteroids.

### Strains, Sprains, and Cramps

RICE therapy, systemic analgesics, and topical analgesics are appropriate self-treatments for Grade I sprains and strains. Grade II sprains involve abnormal joint movement and should be treated by a primary care provider. A visibly deformed joint (Grade III sprain) indicates a possible ruptured or fractured joint and requires emergency treatment.

The healing process for a tendon or ligament strain is slow, and may take weeks or months, depending on the area affected and the extent of the injury. Ice applied immediately after such an injury may reduce inflammation, and anti-inflammatory medications can also be used within the first 6 hours of an injury. After that period, anti-inflammatory drugs may suppress chronic inflammatory processes but will not exert a clinically important effect on the acute process.

For muscle cramps, stretching and massaging the affected area immediately followed by rest or at least reduced activity will loosen the muscle. Stretching must be done cautiously to avoid muscle strain. For persistent cramps, heat should be applied to the area in the form of a warm wet compress, heating pad, or hot-water bottle. Warming up and stretching muscles prior to physical activity, drinking sufficient fluids, and not exercising to the point of exhaustion may prevent cramps. For electrolyte depletion, appropriate oral supplementation of wasted electrolytes can be employed with the selection of fluids containing potassium, sodium, or magnesium.

### Lower Back Pain

Self-treatment of back pain is limited to acute lower back pain. Chronic pain (i.e., lasting more than 6 to 7 weeks) requires medical evaluation and treatment. Management of acute back pain includes rest and ice, nonprescription oral analgesics, and nonprescription topical analgesics. Approaches to chronic low back pain also include therapeutic interventions such as heat therapy, massage with traction (contraindicated for pregnant women and people with osteoporosis, tumor, or spine infection), and most important, mobilization (a program of techniques and exercises to restore back mechanics and movement) and exercise. Chiropractic manipulation and acupuncture (often with electrical stimulation) are also commonly employed for the treatment of back pain, with some positive results.[17]

### Osteoarthritis

Rheumatoid arthritis, gouty arthritis, Lyme arthritis, and osteoarthritis all cause arthritic pain, but only the pain of osteoarthritis is approved for self-treatment after an initial medical diagnosis. General treatment approach includes appropriate lifestyle changes (including physical therapy and weight loss) and systemic therapy with standard doses of acetaminophen or lower-dose NSAIDs with or without topical therapy.[18] Acetaminophen is the drug of first choice for osteoarthritis when inflammation is not a major consideration because of its reduced side effect profile, compared with NSAIDs (i.e., less gastrointestinal toxicity). Acetaminophen may not be as effective as NSAIDs, cyclooxygenase-2 (COX-2) inhibitors (e.g., prescription celecoxib), or other anti-inflammatory drugs, such as glucocorticoids, for patients with moderate to severe pain from osteoarthritis or an inflamed joint. Topical counterirritants are used as adjunctive therapy for osteoarthritic pain. Glucosamine sulfate has demonstrated benefit in reducing not only the pain, but also the progression of the disease, making it an attractive therapeutic choice early in the treatment of osteoarthritis.[19]

## *Nonpharmacologic Therapy*

RICE therapy promotes healing and helps reduce swelling and inflammation of muscle and joint injuries (Table 7-3). Ice should not be applied for more than 10 minutes as excessive icing (e.g., more than 10 to 15 minutes) can cause significant vasoconstriction and reduce vascular clearance of inflammatory mediators from the damaged area. Ice therapy should be applied as close to the injury time as possible and three to four times a day until the swelling decreases, generally 12 to 24 hours, but may continue for 48 to 72 hours for more severe injuries

**TABLE 7-3 Guidelines for RICE Therapy**

- Rest the injured area, using slings or splints if necessary.
- Apply ice as soon as possible to the injured area in 10-minute increments, 3-4 times/day. Continue the ice-pack therapy for 12-24 hours (48-72 hours for more severe injuries).
- Apply compression to the injured area with an elastic support or an elasticized bandage as follows:
  - Choose the appropriate size bandage for the injured body part. If preferred, purchase a product specifically designed for the appropriate body part.
  - Unwind about 12-18 in. of bandage at a time and allow the bandage to relax.
  - If ice is also being applied to the injured area, soak the bandage in water to aid the transfer of cold.
  - Wrap the injured area by overlapping the previous layer of bandage by about one third to one half its width.
  - Tightly wrap the point most distal from the injury. For example, if the ankle is injured, begin wrapping just above the toes.
  - Decrease the tightness of the bandage as you continue to wrap. If the bandage feels tight or uncomfortable or circulation is impaired, remove the compression bandage and rewrap it. Cold toes or swollen fingers would indicate a bandage is too tight.
  - After using the bandage, wash it in lukewarm, soapy water; do not scrub it. Rinse the bandage thoroughly and allow to air dry on a flat surface.
  - Roll up the bandage to prevent wrinkles and store it in a cool, dry place. Do not iron the bandage to remove wrinkles.
- Elevate the injured area at or above the level of the heart to decrease swelling and relieve pain.

(e.g., ankle sprains). In addition, postexercise icing is often appropriate to reduce the likelihood of inflammation and reduce pain. Ice, as well as heat, at temperatures outside the skin's threshold for tolerance can be damaging and result in blistering or burning, and therefore should not be applied directly to the skin. Compression and elevation also assist in reducing the swelling and pain.

Heat therapy is an alternative for patients who develop pain of a noninflammatory nature. Although its mechanism of action is not fully understood, heat may help reduce pain by increasing blood flow to the affected area. Heat is applied for 15 to 20 minutes three to four times a day. Ease of use may be simplified by newer heat-generating adhesive products (e.g., Thermacare). Heat should not be applied to areas recently injured (less than 48 hours) or inflamed, as it will intensify vasodilation and exacerbate vascular leakage and tissue damage. Also, heat should not be used with other topical agents, or over broken skin. A heating device should not be used on an area of skin with decreased sensation; this practice can lead to a skin burn.

Physical and rehabilitative therapies have been used to treat acute pain from sports injuries as well as chronic pain. Physical therapy can assist in building up supporting muscle structures, such as the abdominal muscles that support the lower back. Physical therapy is often supplemented with deep tissue heating and ultrasound, which have demonstrated some positive results.[17]

Chronic muscle pain often requires structured physical therapy to isolate and stretch affected muscles. Although it may be appropriate to rest an injured muscle for a few days, failure to mobilize the area once the acute injury begins to heal will often result in the muscle becoming tight, weak, and overly contracted (guarded). Once guarding happens, patients can develop a tight band of muscle tissue. The tight bands, referred to as trigger points, can arise in any muscle but are most commonly seen in large muscle groups. If muscle pain becomes chronic, the painful area may require application of ice or vapocoolant sprays, or injections, typically using local anesthetics (trigger point injections [TPIs]) to facilitate remobilization. Analgesics and TPIs facilitate physical therapy for chronic muscle pain syndromes; however, the drugs are not curative. Clinicians should keep in mind that physical therapy should occur within 2 hours of a TPI and patients should be counseled appropriately.

### *Pharmacologic Therapy*

#### Systemic Analgesics

NSAIDs and acetaminophen are commonly used nonprescription analgesics, and are often employed in the initial treatment of musculoskeletal injuries. Scheduled doses of typical strengths are instituted early in the course of an injury, followed by quick tapering of dose and interval as the injury improves (generally in 1 to 3 days). Analgesic therapy should be limited to 10 days of self-care use, and patients should seek appropriate medical care if the condition continues past this time or worsens during the course of treatment. (See Chapter 5 for dosages and properties of nonprescription analgesics.)

*Pharmacotherapeutic Comparison* Current guidelines for the treatment of osteoarthritis recommend acetaminophen as first-line therapy versus other NSAIDs.[18] Acetaminophen and NSAIDs have limited placebo-controlled trial information, and much of the data are limited to pain reduction and functional improvements over a few weeks to months. Comparatively, NSAIDs improve pain slightly over acetaminophen in patients with osteoarthritis of the hip and knee.[20,21] It should be noted, however, that responses to analgesics do vary from patient to patient, and initial treatment recommendations may be better made on drug safety than efficacy, while adjusting drug therapy based on patient response.[22] Acetaminophen has a proven safety record if given in recommended dosage (see Chapter 5). Chapter 5 also described the safety of NSAIDs. Concerns over kidney damage, gastrointestinal (GI) bleeds, and most recently of cardiac events, limit NSAIDs from first-line therapy for OA.[23]

#### Topical Products

Topical analgesics may have local analgesic, anesthetic, antipruritic, or counterirritant effects. (See Chapters 37 and 41 for discussion of topical analgesics, anesthetics, and antipruritics.) Counterirritants are specifically approved for the topical treatment of minor aches and pains of muscles and joints (simple backache, arthritis pain, strains, bruises, and sprains).[24]

Topical counterirritants are included with the topical analgesics because they are topically applied to relieve pain. The difference between counterirritants and other external analgesics (anesthetics, analgesics, antipruritics) is that the pain relief is caused by more nerve stimulation rather than depression.[24] Counterirritation is the paradoxical pain-relieving effect achieved by producing a less severe pain to counter a more intense one. Based on topical effects, four types of counterirritants exist (Table 7-4). Table 7-5 lists selected trade-name products.

Because percutaneous absorption of counterirritant drugs is generally undesirable, the finished product should consist of ingredients and vehicles that keep skin penetration to a minimum. The ideal topical drug vehicle should be (1) easy to apply and remove; (2) nontoxic, nonirritating, and nonallergenic; (3) cosmetically acceptable, nongreasy, and nondehydrating; (4) homogeneous; (5) bacteriostatic; (6) chemically stable; and (7) pharmacologically inert.

The Food and Drug Administration (FDA) has published no final ruling on counterirritants to date. All regulations and labeling are therefore based on the detailed previous proposed rule-making documents published in the *Federal Register* in 1979 and 1983.[24,25] FDA has recognized the ingredients in Table 7-4 as safe and effective (Category I) counterirritants for use in adults and children ages 2 years or older.[25] Although allyl isothiocyanate, ammonia water, turpentine oil, and histamine dihydrochloride are classified by FDA as Category I counterirritants, few commercially available preparations contain these ingredients. Tables 7-4 and 7-5 describe the commonly used counterirritants currently available in the United States.

**TABLE 7-4 Classification and Dosage Guidelines* for Nonprescription Counterirritant External Analgesics**

| Group | Mechanism of Action | Ingredients | Concentration (%) | Frequency/Duration of Use |
|---|---|---|---|---|
| A | Rubefacients | Allyl isothiocyanate<br>Ammonia water<br>Methyl salicylate<br>Turpentine oil | 0.5-5.0<br>1.0-2.5<br>10-60<br>6-50 | For all counterirritants: apply no more often than 3-4 times/day for up to 7 days |
| B | Produce cooling sensation | Camphor<br>Menthol | 3-11<br>1.25-16.0 | As above in group A |
| C | Cause vasodilation | Histamine dihydrochloride<br>Methyl nicotinate | 0.025-0.1<br>0.25-1.0 | As above in group A |
| D | Incite irritation without rubefaction; are equal in potency to Group A ingredients | Capsicum<br>Capsicum oleoresin<br>Capsaicin | 0.025-0.25<br>0.025-0.25<br>0.025-0.25 | Acute pain: as above in group A<br>Chronic pain: apply 3-4 times/day for duration of pain (often long-term) |

* Dosages approved for adults and children ages ≥2 years.

*Source:* Reference 24.

*Methyl Salicylate* Methyl salicylate occurs naturally as wintergreen oil or sweet birch oil; gaultheria oil and teaberry oil are other names for the natural compound. In some areas of the United States, it is still referred to as "mountain tea." Synthetic methyl salicylate is prepared by the esterification of salicylic acid with methyl alcohol. In either form, methyl salicylate is the most widely used counterirritant.

Mechanism of Action/Pharmacokinetics When applied to the skin at pain sites, methyl salicylate and other counterirritants produce a mild, local, inflammatory reaction, which provides relief at another site that is usually adjacent to, or underlying, the skin surface being treated. These induced sensations distract from the deep-seated pain in muscles, joints, and tendons. Pain is only as intense as it is perceived to be, and the perception of other sensations caused by the counterirritant or its application (e.g., massage, warmth, or redness) causes the sufferer to disregard the sensation of pain. The result is that the patient's attention is diverted from the muscular or visceral structure by the application of the counterirritant drug.

Methyl salicylate is also a rubefacient, which results in vasodilation of cutaneous vasculature producing reactive hyperemia; it is hypothesized that this increase in blood pooling and/or flow is accompanied by an increase in localized skin temperature, which then may exert a counterirritant effect. Table 7-4 groups counterirritants according to their specific mechanism of action.

Undoubtedly, the action of counterirritants in relieving pain has a psychologic component. These agents may exert a placebo effect through pleasant odors or the sensation of warmth or coolness they produce on the skin. Other factors, which influence the intensity of response to the counterirritation, include the irritant used, its concentration, the solvent in which it is dissolved, and the duration of its contact with the skin.

The exact mechanism by which methyl salicylate produces its analgesic effect is not known, but in addition to the preceding mechanisms, it is generally accepted that both central and peripheral inhibition of prostaglandin synthesis occur. Studies on the rate and extent of percutaneous absorption of various commercially available methyl salicylate preparations show direct tissue penetration rather than redistribution by the systemic blood supply, indicating a localized effect of the topical product.[26] However, systemic bioavailability increases with use of occlusive dressings, multiple applications, and the timing of the agents' application to different areas of the body in this order: plantar, heel, instep, forearm, and abdomen.[27]

Indications Labels for methyl salicylate and other counterirritants indicate the drug's use for "the temporary relief of minor aches and sprains of muscles and joints." In addition, labeling recommended by most members of the FDA review panel includes claims indications for "simple backache, arthritis pain, strains, bruises, and sprains."[24] Product labels may contain descriptors such as "external analgesic," "topical," or "pain-relieving" cream, lotion, or ointment. However, these terms are not necessarily similar to the manufacturer's advertising claims.[25]

It is acceptable to use terms describing certain physical or chemical qualities of the counterirritant preparations as long as the terms do not imply any therapeutic effects occur. Terms such as nongreasy, soothing, cooling action, penetrating relief, warming relief, and cool comforting relief are considered acceptable in labeling.

As with all nonprescription drug products, counterirritants are intended to achieve a beneficial effect within a reasonable period of time. However, claims related to product performance are unacceptable unless they can be substantiated by scientific data. Claims such as fast, quick, prompt, swift, immediate, and remarkable are misleading

TABLE 7-5 Selected External Analgesic Products

| Trade Name | Primary Ingredients |
|---|---|
| **Menthol-containing Products** | |
| Absorbine Jr. Extra Strength Liquid | Menthol 4% |
| Absorbine Jr. Original Liniment | Menthol 1.27% |
| BenGay S.P.A. Cream | Menthol 10% |
| Icy Hot Patch | Menthol 5% |
| Therapeutic Mineral Ice Gel | Menthol 2% |
| **Camphor-containing Products** | |
| JointFlex Cream | Camphor 3.1% |
| **Capsaicin-containing Products** | |
| Capzasin-HP Lotion/Cream | Capsaicin 0.075% |
| Capzasin-P Lotion/Cream | Capsaicin 0.025% |
| Icy Hot Arthritis Therapy Gel | Capsaicin 0.025% |
| Zostrix Cream | Capsaicin 0.025% |
| Zostrix Sports/Zostrix-HP Cream | Capsaicin 0.075% |
| **Trolamine Salicylate–containing Products** | |
| Aspercreme Cream/Lotion | Trolamine salicylate 10% |
| Aspergel | Trolamine salicylate 10% |
| Myoflex Cream | Trolamine salicylate 10% |
| Sportscreme Cream/Lotion | Trolamine salicylate 10% |
| **Combination Products** | |
| Absorbine Arthritis Strength Liquid | Menthol 4%; capsaicin 0.025% (from capsicum oleoresin) |
| ArthriCare Pain Relieving Rub Cream | Menthol 1.25%; methyl nicotinate 0.25%; capsicum oleoresin 0.025% |
| ArthriCare for Women Multi-Action Cream | Menthol 1.25%; capsicum oleoresin (capsaicin 0.025%), methyl nicotinate 0.25% |
| Arthritis Hot Cream | Methyl salicylate 15%; menthol 10% |
| BenGay Original Formula Pain Relieving Ointment | Methyl salicylate 18.3%; menthol 16% |
| BenGay Ultra Strength Pain Relieving Cream | Methyl salicylate 30%; menthol 10%; camphor 4% |
| Dura-patch | Menthol 4%; capsaicin 0.075% |
| Flexall Ultra Plus Gel | Menthol 16%; methyl salicylate 10%; camphor 3.1% |
| Icy Hot Chill Stick | Methyl salicylate 30%; menthol 10% |
| Menthacin Cream/Menthacin EZ Lotion | Menthol 4%; capsaicin 0.025% |
| Mentholatum Deep Heating Arthritis Formula Cream | Methyl salicylate 30%; menthol 8% |
| Mentholatum Deep Heating Lotion | Methyl salicylate 20%; menthol 6% |
| Mentholatum Ointment | Camphor 9%; natural menthol 1.3% |
| Sloan's Liniment | Turpentine oil 47%; capsaicin 0.025% (from capsicum oleoresin) |

and do not signal any property that is important to the safe and effective use of these products.[25]

Dosage and Administration Guidelines Table 7-4 contains dosing information. The longer methyl salicylate or any counterirritant remains in contact with the skin, the longer its duration of action. Little agreement exists on how long the counterirritants should remain in contact with the skin for optimal results; however, a practical guideline is that preparations should be applied no more than four times a day.

At very low concentrations (0.04%), methyl salicylate is used in oral preparations for its pleasant flavor and aroma. Although an FDA survey found that oral ingestion of methyl salicylate formulated as ointments caused no deaths and few cases manifested severe symptoms,[24] regulations require the use of child-resistant containers for liquid preparations containing concentrations greater than 5%.[28]

Safety Considerations Localized (i.e., skin irritation, rash) and systemic reactions (i.e., salicylate toxicity) may occur with the use of methyl salicylate.

Concomitant use of salicylate-containing external analgesics and maintenance warfarin therapy has been implicated in prolonging prothrombin time.[29] Both methyl salicylate and trolamine salicylate were implicated. A later study showed that 11 patients had an abnormally elevated international normalized ratio after significant usage of topical methyl salicylate ointment.[30] Chapter 5 describes other potential drug interactions for salicylates.

Strong irritation may cause local reactions such as erythema, blistering, neurotoxicity, or thermal hyperalgesia. No evidence exists that the risk of adverse reactions to counterirritants increases when the application site is lightly bandaged; however, tight bandaging or occlusive dressing does increase the risk of irritation, redness, or blistering.[25,31] Heating pads used in conjunction with counterirritants containing methyl salicylate have produced the elevated temperature, vasodilation, and occlusion necessary to greatly enhance percutaneous absorption of menthol and methyl salicylate, causing full-thickness skin and muscle necrosis as well as persistent interstitial nephritis.[32] In addition, heat exposure and exercise after applying methyl salicylate have shown a threefold increase in systematic availability of salicylate. This resultant increase in absorption could lead to adverse systemic reactions.[33] Therefore, patients should be cautioned against using heating pads or other heating devices in conjunction with any external analgesics.

Because percutaneous absorption can occur, methyl salicylate should be avoided in children and used with caution in individuals who are sensitive to aspirin or suffer from severe asthma or nasal polyps.

*Camphor* Although camphor occurs naturally and is obtained from the camphor tree, approximately three fourths of the camphor used is prepared synthetically. The natural product is dextrorotatory; the synthetic product is optically active.

Mechanism of Action In concentrations of 0.1% to 3.0%, camphor depresses cutaneous receptors and is used as a topical analgesic, anesthetic, and antipruritic. In concentrations exceeding 3%, particularly when combined with other counterirritant ingredients, camphor stimulates the nerve endings in the skin and induces relief of pain and discomfort by masking moderate to severe deeper visceral pain with a milder pain arising from the skin at the level of innervation. When applied vigorously, it produces a rubefacient reaction.

Indications See Indications under Methyl Salicylate.

Dosages and Administration Guidelines Table 7-4 contains dosing information. Higher concentrations than those recommended are not more effective and can cause more serious adverse reactions if accidentally ingested.[25] The risk of toxicity relates to both the concentration of camphor in the ingested product and the rate of absorption of camphor into the body. Accordingly, preparations with camphor concentrations exceeding 11%, such as camphorated oil (camphor liniment), which is a solution of 20% camphor in cottonseed oil, are not considered safe for nonprescription use and have been removed from the market.

In children, 5 mL of a 20% camphor liniment is a potentially lethal dose, and death resulting from respiratory depression or complications of status epilepticus can occur.[34]

Safety Considerations High doses of camphor can cause nausea, vomiting, colic, headache, dizziness, delirium, convulsion, and coma.

Placing camphor into the nostrils of an infant may cause immediate respiratory collapse. In 1994, the American Academy of Pediatrics Committee on Drugs noted that, although nonprescription camphor-containing preparations cannot exceed concentrations of 11%, camphor toxicity continues. The academy advised parents to be aware of this potential danger and recommended use of modalities that do not contain camphor.[35]

*Menthol* Menthol is either extracted from peppermint oil (which contains a 30% to 50% concentration of menthol) or prepared synthetically. Menthol may be used safely in small quantities as a flavoring agent and has found wide acceptance in candy, chewing gum, cigarettes, cough drops, toothpaste, nasal sprays, and liqueurs. Menthol is usually combined with other ingredients with antipruritic or analgesic properties, such as camphor.

Mechanism of Action/Pharmacokinetics At concentrations below 1%, menthol depresses cutaneous receptor response (i.e., acts as an anesthetic), whereas it stimulates response in concentrations above 1.25% (i.e., acts as a counterirritant). Applied to the skin, menthol stimulates the nerves that perceive cold while depressing the nerves that perceive pain. The initial feeling of coolness is soon followed by a sensation of warmth. An experimental study demonstrated that exposure to 2% menthol solution caused the threshold for warmth to rise significantly, whereas the threshold for pain caused by heat remained unchanged.[36] Theories of menthol's action on the perception of pain involve calcium movement in thermoreceptors and activation of κ-opioid receptors.[37,38]

Indications See Indications under Methyl Salicylate.

Dosage and Administration Guidelines Table 7-4 contains dosing information. The fatal dose of menthol in humans is approximately 2 g.[39] In acute studies however, menthol appears to be a substance of very low toxicity.[40]

Safety Considerations A review of reactions to menthol has been published.[41] Although occurrence is rare, sensitization to menthol in certain individuals causes symptoms such as urticaria, erythema, and other cutaneous lesions.[42]

Peppermint-flavored toothpaste has even been implicated in exacerbating wheezing and dyspnea in a young woman with a history of asthma.[43] Although menthol is commonly used for upper respiratory congestion and rhinitis (in cough drops and vapo-rubs), additional evidence suggests menthol may provide symptomatic relief of dyspnea.[44]

Menthol is contraindicated in patients with hypersensitivity to the agent. Treatment should be discontinued if the patient develops irritation, rash, burning, stinging, swelling, or infection.

*Methyl Nicotinate* Methyl nicotinate is a safe and effective counterirritant if used according to FDA's guidelines.

Mechanism of Action/Pharmacokinetics Although nicotinic acid is inactive topically, methyl nicotinate readily penetrates the cutaneous barrier. Vasodilation and elevation of skin temperature result from very low concentrations, with higher penetration rates seen with hydrophilic mediums (i.e., gels). Studies have shown that indomethacin, ibuprofen, and aspirin significantly depress the skin's vascular response to methyl nicotinate. Because these three drugs suppress prostaglandin biosynthesis, it was concluded that the vasodilator response to methyl nicotinate is mediated, at least in part, by prostaglandin biosynthesis.[45]

Indications See Indications under Methyl Salicylate.

Dosage and Administration Guidelines See Table 7-4 for dosing information.

Safety Considerations Generalized vascular dilation can occur when methyl nicotinate passes through the skin into the circulation system.

Susceptible patients who apply methyl nicotinate over large areas may experience a drop in blood pressure and pulse rate and syncope caused by generalized vascular dilation.

*Capsicum Preparations* Capsicum preparations (capsaicin, capsicum, and capsicum oleoresin) are derived from the fruit of various species of plants of the nightshade family. Capsicum contains about 1.5% of an irritating oleoresin, the major component of which is capsaicin (0.02%). Capsaicin is the major pungent ingredient of hot (chile) pepper.

Mechanism of Action/Pharmacokinetics When applied to normal skin, capsaicin elicits a transient feeling of warmth. More concentrated solutions produce a sensation of burning pain. However, as a result of tachyphylaxis, this local effect diminishes with repeated applications. Capsicum preparations do not cause blistering or reddening of the skin, even in high concentrations, because they do not act on capillaries or other blood vessels.

The mechanism of action is thought to be directly related to its effects on substance P. Substance P is found in slow-conducting, unmyelinated type C neurons that innervate the dermis and epidermis. It is released in the skin in response to endogenous (stress) and exogenous (trauma or injury) factors. It appears that pruritic stimuli along with pain impulses are conveyed to central processing centers by type C fibers in the skin, for which capsaicin has selective activity. Local application of capsaicin to the peripheral axon appears to affect substance P primarily by depleting it from sensory neurons that have been implicated in mediating cutaneous pain. The depletion occurs both peripherally and centrally, presumably as the result of impulse initiation. When substance P is released, burning pain and redness occur initially but abate with repeated applications. The net effect may be analogous to cutting a nerve or ligating it, which also depletes the substance P content of the neuron.[46] No evidence exists to date, however, that topical application of low concentrations of capsaicin causes any permanent neurologic injury.

Indications See Indications under Methyl Salicylate.

Dosage and Administration Guidelines Table 7-4 lists dosing information for capsaicin. The optimal dose of this agent, however, may vary among patients. It appears that efficacy decreases and local discomfort increases when capsaicin is applied less often, because the drug's duration of action is 4 to 6 hours. Pain relief is usually noted within 14 days after therapy has begun but will occasionally be delayed by as much as 4 to 6 weeks. Notably, because capsicum lots vary, the concentration range for capsaicin cannot be expressed as a percentage and must be calculated for each lot.

Once capsaicin has begun to relieve pain, its use must continue regularly three or four times a day to keep the pain from returning. If capsaicin treatment is stopped and pain returns, treatment can be resumed.

Overdose with use of capsaicin is not noted, but use of topical preparations greater than 1% have been associated with neurotoxicity and hyperalgesia.

Efficacy Capsaicin is used to reduce the pain, but not the inflammation, of rheumatoid arthritis and osteoarthritis, and is used in a wide variety of other pain disorders (e.g., postherpetic neuralgia, psoriasis, and diabetic neuropathy). The efficacy of capsaicin is difficult to assess, compared with placebo, because the burning and stinging sensations make it difficult to carry out a blinded clinical trial. For the treatment of musculoskeletal pain, capsaicin 0.025% used for 4 weeks would improve pain by at least 50% in one out of every eight patients treated. Improved efficacy is seen with 0.075% used in the treatment of neuropathic pain, suggesting dose-related effects.[47]

Capsaicin also enhances the penetration of naproxen through human skin, which would suggest improved efficacy with combined therapy versus that produced by either agent alone.[48] However, this combined efficacy is only speculative, since it has not been clinically studied and topical NSAIDs are not yet approved for use in the United States.

Safety Considerations Burning and stinging occur with the application of capsaicin in 40% to 70% of patients. However, this effect generally diminishes in intensity with continued use. If capsaicin gets into eyes or on other sensitive areas of the body, it will cause a burning sensation.

Concentrations over 0.025% have also been associated with a cough.[47]

Use in patients with hypersensitivity to capsaicin is contraindicated. The agent should be discontinued temporarily if skin breaks down (weeping, red, small ulcers) and should not be applied to wounds or damaged skin.

*Nonmonograph Agents* Eucalyptus oil, trolamine salicylate, and topical NSAIDs are currently classified as Category III ingredients (insufficient data are available to establish safety and efficacy). Several commercial products containing trolamine salicylate as the primary ingredient are available (Table 7-5).

Eucalyptus Oil Eucalyptus oil may produce some minor counterirritant effects, but it is not recommended for use as a counterirritant because of inconclusive efficacy data. Eucalyptus is often noted as an inactive ingredient in some products because of its characteristic odor.

Trolamine Salicylate Trolamine salicylate, although a salicylate salt, is not a counterirritant analgesic. Trolamine salicylate is absorbed through the skin and results in synovial fluid salicylate concentrations slightly below that of oral aspirin. The recommended topical dosage of trolamine salicylate for adults and children 2 years and older is a 10% to 15% concentration applied to the affected area not more than three or four times a day.

Trolamine salicylate has the same drug interactions as other salicylates (see Chapter 5). Use is contraindicated in patients with renal insufficiency or hypersensitivity to trolamine or salicylates. Patients with liver disease, hypoprothrombinemia (a deficiency of thrombin in the blood), or vitamin K deficiency, who are scheduled for surgery, or who are chronic alcohol users should not use this agent. The agent should not contact the eyes or mucous membranes.

Several studies led FDA to conclude that topical trolamine salicylate does not show any significant benefit over placebo in the treatment of musculoskeletal pain. Reports published after the review have shown limited effectiveness in alleviating neuralgia caused by unaccustomed strenuous exercise[49] and muscle soreness induced by a reproducible program of weight training.[50] Trolamine salicylate has also demonstrated improved playing time in musicians with localized pain in the arms, wrists, hands, and fingers, and improved pain and stiffness in patients with osteoarthritis of the hands.[51,52]

Trolamine salicylate is still available over the counter, and may be most useful to those patients who do not favor the localized irritation, or the scent of other Category I counterirritants.

### Combination Products

General guidelines for nonprescription drug combination products state that Category I active ingredients from the same therapeutic category ordinarily should not be combined unless the combination is deemed safer or more effective and has enhanced patient acceptance or quality of formulation.[25] Four separate chemical and/or pharmacologic groups of counterirritants provide four qualitatively different types of irritation. Many marketed preparations aim for at least two such effects when greater potency is desired. Table 7-4 lists the individual ingredients and classifies them according to their relative potency and acceptable concentration ranges. Manufacturers may combine active ingredients from one group of counterirritants with one, two, or three other active ingredients, provided that each active ingredient is from a different group.

It is irrational to combine counterirritants with local anesthetics, topical antipruritics, or topical analgesics. Because these agents depress sensory cutaneous receptors, their effects oppose the counterirritant stimulation of cutaneous sensory receptors. It is also irrational to combine counterirritants with skin protectants because the protectants oppose and may nullify counterirritant effects.

Preparation labels must list the active ingredients, including their concentrations, and must identify them by their officially recognized, established names. Also, manufacturers have voluntarily listed inactive ingredients on the label. It is noteworthy that many manufacturers of combination products list only some of the active ingredients under the "active" heading, and many of the other pharmacologically viable products in the inactive ingredient section (e.g., TheraPatch lists methyl salicylate; Bengay Vanishing Scent lists camphor under inactive ingredients). Although the concentrations of inactive ingredients are not listed, they are generally below therapeutically determined amounts, and are added for reasons other than pain-relieving effects. The manner of usage and the frequency of applications should also be indicated.[24]

### Product Selection Guidelines

*Special Population Considerations* No significant variability in response has been noted among patients of different ages or racial background.

*Patient Factors* The choice of treatment for acute pain syndromes and chronic conditions such as osteoarthritis is patient dependent. In addition to nonpharmacologic treatment, oral therapy is often employed. One should take into consideration the patient's history, taking note of exclusions for self-treatment, other medications the patient is taking, and any known allergies to medications. Topical therapy is used as an adjunct or substitute to oral therapy. If a counterirritant is selected, one with Category I ingredients should be recommended. Patients with precautions to the use of individual counterirritants should be cautioned about the use of certain products, particularly combination products. Product concentrations are variable and, in general, the lowest effective dose should be recommended for the shortest duration needed.

*Patient Preferences* Factors that impact product selection include dosage form, ease of use, cost, and even odor of the preparation. Dosage forms available include solutions, liniments, gels, lotions, ointments, creams, and patches. Oleaginous preparations (ointments and oil-based liniments) may have greater potency than solutions, gels, lotions, and creams, but are greasy and generally less acceptable to patients. The use of patches is becoming more popular because of their simple application and duration of action, but their use eliminates any benefit of a therapeutic rubbing action.[3] With the exception of patches and solutions, topical products should be rubbed into the skin. Alcoholic liniments and gels may produce a more intense response than equal quantities in other preparations, and excessive rubbing should be avoided to reduce the risk of unpleasant burning sensations with these preparations. Additional information about formulation characteristics are described elsewhere.[53,54]

### Emerging Treatments

Topical NSAIDs are not currently available over the counter in the United States, but have been marketed for a number of years in Europe. Topical NSAIDs are not counterirritants and presumably act locally in a manner analogous to their systemic mechanism of action. Their application on acute soft tissue strains and sprains, where the target tissue is situated closer to the skin surface, are reported to provide the benefits of oral NSAIDs with minimal systemic side effects.

Systematic reviews have concluded that topical NSAIDs may be more effective than placebo in the treatment of musculoskeletal pain for short-term use but lose effectiveness beyond 2 weeks.[55,56] A well-designed trial of 1.5% topical diclofenac solution applied four times a day demonstrated symptomatic improvement in osteoarthritis of the knee following 12 weeks of treatment.[57] Dimethyl sulfoxide (DMSO) was used to help improve diclofenac penetration, and also was present in the placebo. No significant gastrointestinal side effects were noted in the trial, but localized dryness and rash were more prevalent in the treatment group. Evidence to date suggests that the use of topical NSAIDs may provide symptomatic relief of musculoskeletal pain with little systemic side effects.

### *Complementary Therapies*

A variety of complementary therapies containing many different compounds and ingredients are marketed for the management of pain. It is difficult to find controlled clinical trials of these agents in humans although some of the substances have undergone animal trials to identify their active components and the pharmacology of these components.[58] Table 7-6 lists some of the many complementary therapies available without prescription for the management of pain and discomfort.

Glucosamine is a glycoprotein either derived from marine exoskeletons or produced synthetically. It is found endogenously and is required for the synthesis of the structural components of joint connective tissue. Glucosamine has been used for the treatment of osteoarthritis for some time, but evidence supporting its use had been inconclusive. Two well-designed studies have supported the effectiveness of glucosamine sulfate for the treatment of osteoarthritis.[20,59] Both trials were double-blinded, randomized, placebo-controlled trials designed to establish the efficacy of oral glucosamine sulfate on subjective pain improvement as well as the primary objective to measure joint structural changes. Results showed that 1500 mg once daily of a crystallized powder formulation improved pain scores and reduced joint space narrowing of the knee after a 3-year follow-up. These results confirm that glucosamine sulfate is a beneficial agent in the treatment of osteoarthritis, and unlike other FDA-approved medications (i.e., acetaminophen or NSAIDs), glucosamine sulfate curtails the disease process. Glucosamine's tolerability is favorable and despite reports of increased plasma glucose levels in rats given high-dose parenteral glucosamine, clinical trials in humans show insignificant effect on glucose in diabetic patients.[60] Although the support for clinically significant pain improvement in osteoarthritis patients is not without contrary evidence[61] and the latest 2000 osteoarthritis guidelines by the American College of Rheumatology do not recommend therapy with glucosamine,[19] the result of recent well-controlled studies showing reductions in pain and disease progression as well as the tolerability of the product, provide justification for the use of glucosamine as a first-line agent for the treatment of osteoarthritis of the knee.[62]

Chondroitin sulfate also is a popular complementary agent used in the treatment of osteoarthritis and often is combined with glucosamine in commercially available products. No evidence to date proves the combination is superior to glucosamine alone, but a large, randomized, controlled trial currently in progress is comparing the combination with each agent alone and with placebo.[63] Pain improvement and a reduced progression of disease has been noted in clinical trials.[64] A recent meta-analysis highlights the data to date of glucosamine and chondroitin in the treatment of osteoarthritis of the knee.[65]

The efficacy of avocado/soybean unsaponifiables, peppermint, methyl-sulfonyl-methane (MSM), and S-adenosyl-L-methionine (SAMe) also are summarized in Table 7-6. Additional information on these and other complementary agents have been described elsewhere and are discussed in greater detail in Chapters 53 and 54.[66-68]

## Assessment of Musculoskeletal Injuries and Disorders: A Case-based Approach

Routinely, the clinician should inventory all past and present medications, including pain medications, and should note the patient's satisfaction with or preference for past treatments. The clinician should also inquire into the patient's medical history that bears directly on either the origin or treatment of pain.

Before an attempt is made to treat a pain complaint, the clinician should qualify and quantify the pain. Inquiry about the cause, duration, location, and severity of pain, as well as factors that relieve and exacerbate it will help the clinician assess the pain. An alphabetical mnemonic can assist in remembering the components required when evaluating pain. "P" represents the *precipitating factors* associated with pain, such as stress or physical exertion. "Q" denotes *quality* of the pain, that is, whether the pain is sharp, dull, constant, aching, shooting, and so forth. "R" represents *region* and is used to describe the location of the pain. "S" is the subjective description by the patient of the pain's *severity*, and whether activities are being altered

TABLE 7-6 Selected Complementary Medications Used for the Treatment of Musculoskeletal Pain

| Agent | Risks | Effectiveness |
|---|---|---|
| **Botanical Medicines (Scientific Name)** | | |
| Avocado/soybean unsaponifiables (oral) | Mild GI complaints | Improved pain in stable hip OA and reduced NSAID use[66] |
| Peppermint (*Mentha piperita*) | Allergic reactions; respiratory collapse | Topical efficacy similar to menthol (contains menthol) |
| **Nonbotanical Natural Medicines** | | |
| Chondroitin sulfate | Mild GI pain and nausea | Improvement in pain similar to glucosamine and improved pain relief when added to NSAID;[65,67] reduction in disease progression likely[64] |
| Glucosamine sulfate | Mild GI complaints | Probable improvement in pain;[61,65,67] reduced disease progression[20,59] |
| Methyl-sulfonyl-methane (MSM) | Nausea, diarrhea, headache, pruritus, and allergy symptoms | Efficacy for acute and chronic pain (arthritis, bursitis, tendonitis) not established |
| S-adenosyl-L-methionine (SAMe) | Multiple dose–dependent GI complaints | Improves functional limitation of osteoarthritis similar to NSAIDs, but with delayed response and less pain improvement[65,66] |

Key: GI, gastrointestinal; NSAID, nonsteroidal anti-inflammatory drug; OA, osteoarthritis.

as a result of the pain. For example, does the pain make the patient wake up at night? Has the patient suffered loss of appetite? Finally, “T” represents the *time-related* nature of the pain. It is useful to ask the patient whether the pain is related to any particular daily activity or to any weekly or monthly cycles.

Pain scales help in objectively measuring a patient’s pain. With the numerical pain scale, the clinician asks patients to rank the present pain on a scale of 0 to 10, with 0 being no pain and 10 being pain as bad as the patient can imagine. Scores greater than 3 indicate the need for an intervention, as do any scores that increase 2 or more points on the 10-point scale. Initially, pain scores establish a baseline for pain before treatment. In addition, a high pain score can be used to screen for patients who would be better served by seeking an appropriate medical evaluation. Pain scores also serve as a measuring stick for therapeutic outcomes. In general, nonprescription medications are appropriate for numerical rating scale scores of 1 to 3. These medications may also be appropriate for scores of 4 or 5. Scores of 6 or higher indicate pain that requires medical referral. Other scales are available for pain rating in children (Faces Pain Scale), adolescents, non-English speakers, and other special populations.

A chronic painful condition presents a different set of challenges. An observant clinician should intervene with a patient who frequently or regularly purchases aspirin, other NSAID products, or acetaminophen to evaluate the nature of the pain complaint. If additional interviewing indicates an inadequately treated pain problem, a referral to a primary care provider should be made. This will prevent unwanted long-term adverse consequences of drug therapy (e.g., renal impairment) as well as assist the patient in receiving the appropriate care for the pain problem. Education should be offered regarding the risks of inadequate treatment as well as overuse of medications.

On the basis of information collected, the clinician can appropriately determine whether the patient may self-treat or be referred for further evaluation (Figure 7-2). Cases 7-1 and 7-2 illustrate assessment of patients with musculoskeletal injuries and disorders.

## Patient Counseling for Musculoskeletal Injuries and Disorders

Consultation with the patient should include the expected benefit of any recommended medication, the appropriate dose and drug administration schedule, potential adverse reactions, potential drug-drug or drug-disease interactions, and self-monitoring techniques for assessing response to therapy. The consequences of nonadherence should be emphasized. Printed materials reinforce verbal information. Many such pamphlets or single-page handouts are available from national professional societies (e.g., www.arthritis.org), including those that educate persons on various chronic pain syndromes such as osteoarthritis. These materials offer advice on exercise, diet, and sleep habits, and the advantages as well as disadvantages of pharmacologic therapy. Generally, these materials can be obtained for free or for a nominal delivery fee. Clinicians may wish to design their own supplementary materials.

Patients taking NSAIDs should be warned about possible drug-drug interactions, including with antihypertensive medications, warfarin, aspirin, and phenytoin. Patients should be cautioned not to take more than the recommended nonprescription dose or duration of the medication. Duplication of acetaminophen and NSAIDs is probably more common than recognized, as patients often

## CASE 7-1

| Relevant Evaluation Criteria | Scenario/Model Outcome |
|---|---|
| **Information Gathering** | |
| 1. Gather essential information about the patient's symptoms, including: | |
| a. description of symptom(s) (i.e., nature, onset, duration, severity, associated symptoms) | Patient complains of muscle soreness and pain over his hand and wrist. He continues to have full range of motion of his wrist, but admits to some tenderness and pain on a scale of 3/10. He denies any other problems. Patient's wrist is not visibly deformed, but does have some clean surface abrasions over the joint. |
| b. description of any factors that seem to precipitate, exacerbate, and/or relieve the patient's symptom(s) | Patient arrives about 2 hours after a mountain biking accident when he fell over his handlebars. |
| c. description of the patient's efforts to relieve the symptoms | Patient has not self-treated the pain yet, but is inquiring about the use of a topical product. |
| 2. Gather essential patient history information: | |
| a. patient's identity | Randy Travels |
| b. age, sex, height, and weight | 24 y/o M, 6'3", 210 lb |
| c. patient's occupation | Radon inspector |
| d. patient's dietary habits | Patient eats 3 meals plus pizza or another snack at midnight each night and occasionally uses alcohol. |
| e. patient's sleep habits | Without complaints |
| f. concurrent medical conditions, prescription and nonprescription medications, and dietary supplements | Albuterol 90 μg, 2 puffs 4 times/day as needed for asthma after exercise |
| g. allergies | Aspirin (wheezing) |
| h. history of other adverse reactions to medications | N/A |
| i. other (describe)______ | Patient is right-handed. |
| **Assessment and Triage** | |
| 3. Differentiate the patient's signs/symptoms and correctly identify the patient's primary problem(s) (see Table 7-2). | Patient with an acute muscle injury caused by traumatic event. Primary problem is the patient's pain and soreness of the wrist. |
| 4. Identify exclusions for self-treatment (see Figure 7-2). | None |
| 5. Formulate a comprehensive list of therapeutic alternatives for the primary problem to determine if triage to a medical practitioner is required, and share this information with the patient. | Options include:<br>(1) Refer patient to PCP for further assessment.<br>(2) Recommend nonpharmacologic treatment (e.g., clean abrasion, RICE therapy).<br>(4) Recommend oral nonprescription analgesic (e.g., acetaminophen).<br>(5) Recommend topical counterirritant.<br>(6) Take no action. |
| **Plan** | |
| 6. Select an optimal therapeutic alternative to address the patient's problem, taking into account patient preferences. | Proper cleansing of the abrasion over the wrist (see Chapter 42). Applying ice at 10-minute increments 3-4 times/day for another 24 hours to help reduce swelling and pain. The patient should also rest the hand as much as possible over the next couple days. This may be difficult considering he is right-handed, but reasonable rest of the affected hand should be attempted. Use acetaminophen at 650-1000 mg every 6 hours as needed for the pain. |

**CASE 7-1 (continued)**

| Relevant Evaluation Criteria | Scenario/Model Outcome |
|---|---|
| 7. Describe the recommended therapeutic approach to the patient. | Take acetaminophen 650 mg 4 times/day as needed for pain for 10 days maximum. |
| 8. Explain to the patient the rationale for selecting the recommended therapeutic approach from the considered therapeutic alternatives. | Acetaminophen should help with the pain you are experiencing. Because of your history of asthma and reaction to aspirin in the past with wheezing, I would not recommend any other pain product besides acetaminophen to avoid the risk of this reaction happening with other anti-inflammatory drugs. Because of the abrasions you have on your wrist after the fall, you should avoid placing any medicated pain formula on the site until the abrasions are healed. Proper wound care also should be instituted (see Chapter 42). |
| **Patient Education** | |
| 9. When recommending self-care with nonprescription medications and/or nondrug therapy, convey accurate information to the patient, including: | |
| a. appropriate dose and frequency of administration | Acetaminophen 650-1000 mg 4 times/day as need for pain (maximum of 4 g/day) |
| b. maximum number of days the therapy should be employed | 10 days |
| c. product administration procedures | Take 2 tablets every 6 hours as needed for your pain. Do not take more than a total of 4 g/day. |
| d. expected time to onset of relief | Improvement in pain should be noticeable 30-60 minutes following ingestion. |
| e. degree of relief that can be reasonably expected | Improvement in pain should occur following therapy, but complete resolution of pain may not occur until the patient's underlying injury is healed. |
| f. most common side effects | Not significant in doses less than 4 g/day |
| g. side effects that warrant medical intervention should they occur | At recommended doses, acetaminophen is not expected to cause any side effects that warrant medical attention. |
| h. patient options in the event that condition worsens or persists | If pain worsens or persists past 10 days, see your primary care provider. |
| i. product storage requirements | Keep product in a tightly closed container out of a child's reach. |
| j. specific nondrug measures | N/A |
| 10. Solicit follow-up questions from patient. | I have heard that acetaminophen can hurt my liver. Can it? |
| 11. Answer patient's questions. | Acetaminophen is a very safe product when taken as prescribed and at doses no more than 4 g/day. Please note that other pain products also often have acetaminophen in them, so always check the label. Never take two acetaminophen products at the same time; wait until the next dose time (i.e., 6 hours) to take the next dose. If you take higher doses, or if you are severely malnourished or drink consistent amounts of alcohol, you will be at a greater risk of liver damage. Therefore, I would recommend you continue your normal diet and refrain from alcohol use. |

Key: N/A, not applicable; PCP, primary care provider; RICE, rest, ice, compression, elevation.

do not realize that nonprescription products contain the same or similar drug as their prescription drug. Failure to recognize this duplication can significantly increase the risk of serious adverse events, and patients should be warned of the risk. In acute pain management, early administration of nonprescription analgesics should be employed to prevent escalating pain, with downward tapering of the analgesic doses as pain severity allows. This can usually take place 1 to 2 days after the precipitating event.

Patients should be instructed to notify their primary care provider whenever the pain changes in character or severity, or if new acute pain develops. Other sudden uncharacteristic pains may be harbingers of new tissue damage. Patients should be advised to obtain their prescriptions from as few prescribers as possible and to get their prescriptions drugs, nonprescription drugs, and complementary remedies at the same pharmacy to minimize the potential for drug interactions.

## CASE 7-2

| Relevant Evaluation Criteria | Scenario/Model Outcome |
|---|---|
| **Information Gathering** | |
| 1. Gather essential information about the patient's symptoms, including: | |
| a. description of symptom(s) (i.e., nature, onset, duration, severity, associated symptoms) | Patient admits to pain in her knees, and difficulty using her hands to open bottles. Patient has had the pain for over a year and notes the pain occurs mostly on walking and is reduced on rest. She rates the pain today as a 4 on a 10-point scale, but it ranges anywhere from 2-5. |
| b. description of any factors that seem to precipitate, exacerbate, and/or relieve the patient's symptom(s) | Patient notices improvement in joint movement after she walks short distances. Walking long distances or standing for long periods of time tends to worsen her symptoms. Her hands are not as much of a concern. They are stiffest in the morning, but improve within about 15 minutes after she wakes. |
| c. description of the patient's efforts to relieve the symptoms | Patient has used acetaminophen 650 mg 4 times/day with limited relief. She used ibuprofen, naproxen, and celecoxib in the past, but stopped them because of all the reports she has heard about them being "bad." |
| 2. Gather essential patient history information: | |
| a. patient's identity | Victoria Bird |
| b. age, sex, height, and weight | 68 y/o F, 5'3", 183 lb |
| c. patient's occupation | Retired housewife |
| d. patient's dietary habits | Eats three meals a day and snacks throughout the day on chips, cookies, and fruit |
| e. patient's sleep habits | Occasional restless nights because of the discomfort in her joints |
| f. concurrent medical conditions, prescription and nonprescription medications, and dietary supplements | Atenolol 50 mg every morning for postoperative MI; lisinopril 10 mg every morning for blood pressure, glyburide 10 mg every morning for type 2 DM; acetaminophen 650 mg 4 times/day for osteoarthritis diagnosed about 1 year ago |
| g. allergies | NKDA |
| h. history of other adverse reactions to medications | N/A |
| i. other (describe)_______ | N/A |
| **Assessment and Triage** | |
| 3. Differentiate the patient's signs/symptoms and correctly identify the patient's primary problem(s) (see Table 7-2). | Patient with joint problems of hands and knees indicating osteoarthritis. Rheumatoid arthritis is not likely because of the presentation of a patient advancing in age, arthritis in her knees, and the lack of inflammatory or systemic symptoms. |
| 4. Identify exclusions for self-treatment (see Figure 7-2). | Patient has had pain for a long period of time and has experienced unsatisfactory relief from scheduled acetaminophen. Since patient's condition is stable, additional self-treatment could be recommended. If, however, this patient's pain worsens or does not improve with recommended treatment, the patient should discuss her care with her PCP. |
| 5. Formulate a comprehensive list of therapeutic alternatives for the primary problem to determine if triage to a medical practitioner is required, and share this information with the patient. | Options include:<br>(1) Recommend nondrug measures (e.g., exercise, weight loss, use of cane).<br>(2) Recommend use of a topical counterirritant.<br>(3) Recommend oral OTC analgesic.<br>(4) Recommend glucosamine sulfate 1500 mg by mouth daily with or without chondroitin sulfate 1200 mg by mouth daily.<br>(5) Refer patient to PCP for further assessment and treatment.<br>(6) Take no action. |
| **Plan** | |
| 6. Select an optimal therapeutic alternative to address the patient's problem, taking into account patient preferences. | Exercise 3-5 times/week by walking, biking, and/or stretching. Take 1500 mg of glucosamine sulfate at the same time each day. Apply topical counterirritant with menthol, methyl salicylate, capsaicin, or camphor in a cream or gel formulation 3-4 times a day (see Table 7-4). Continue acetaminophen. |

## CASE 7-2 (continued)

| Relevant Evaluation Criteria | Scenario/Model Outcome |
|---|---|
| 7. Describe the recommended therapeutic approach to the patient. | Take glucosamine/chondroitin 1500 mg/1200 mg daily by mouth and apply Capsaicin Cr 0.025% topically. Apply a small layer of cream to the knee 3-4 times a day. You may continue taking acetaminophen 650 mg 4 times/day. I recommend products with easy-to-open lids. |
| 8. Explain to the patient the rationale for selecting the recommended therapeutic approach from the considered therapeutic alternatives. | To receive full benefits from this therapy, you must begin lifestyle changes (such as exercise) and take your medications as prescribed. Exercise will help circulate more blood to the damaged areas of your joints and also help strengthen the muscles around the joint to give you more support. In addition, exercise may lead to some weight loss with appropriate diet, which may reduce the stress to your joints and help with your diabetes. Glucosamine sulfate and chondroitin sulfate are complementary medicines that, in addition to exercise and weight loss, may help your pain and reduce the damage to your joints. The capsaicin helps in a different way. You likely will feel a slight burning sensation when you first apply it, but the burning should be minimal and will make your knee pain less bothersome. The burning should decrease each time you use the product. Continuous application of the product 3-4 times a day is needed for best results. You may continue to use acetaminophen if the previous use provided pain relief. |
| **Patient Education** | |
| 9. When recommending self-care with nonprescription medications and/or nondrug therapy, convey accurate information to the patient, including: | |
| a. appropriate dose and frequency of administration | See dosing in #7 above. |
| b. maximum number of days the therapy should be employed | You should always follow appropriate lifestyle changes (i.e., exercise and weight reduction) and should remain on glucosamine treatment long-term (years) to prevent further joint damage and improve pain. Treatment with topical products will depend on response. If no response is noted after an adequate trial of 1 month, another agent may be tried, or a dose increase may be attempted. A common reason for treatment failure with topical counterirritants is not following the regimen of applying the medication 3-4 times a day. Adherence to therapy should be considered before determining treatment failure. |
| c. product administration procedures | Take oral glucosamine/chondroitin at the same time of the day.<br>Apply a small amount of topical capsaicin cream and rub the joint during applications. Be sure to wash your hands before and after application, and do not use heat in conjunction with the topical medication.<br>See the box Patient Education for Musculoskeletal Injuries and Disorders. |
| d. expected time to onset of relief | With consistent use of topical and glucosamine/chondroitin therapy, relief may take up to and sometimes more than 1 month. |
| e. degree of relief that can be reasonably expected | Improvements in pain symptoms will be gradual over the first month of treatment. A reduction in disease worsening is expected with continued treatment and lifestyle changes. The goal is to improve your ability to do normal activities, reduce your pain to an acceptable level, and prevent further destruction of your joints. |
| f. most common side effects | Minor gastrointestinal effects such as nausea, dyspepsia, diarrhea, or heartburn. Some localized burning or stinging can be expected with the topical capsaicin, but diminish with continued use. |
| g. side effects that warrant medical intervention should they occur | Therapy typically is well tolerated, but, rarely, rash, itchiness, increased heart rate, and edema have been reported with glucosamine.<br>Localized rash and red or small ulcers with topical capsaicin are rare, but warrant discontinuation of therapy and consultation with your PCP, that is, primary care provider.<br>See the box Patient Education for Musculoskeletal Disorders and Injuries. |

**CASE 7-2 (continued)**

| Relevant Evaluation Criteria | Scenario/Model Outcome |
|---|---|
| h. patient options in the event that condition worsens or persists | See your PCP if symptoms worsen or do not improve after 1 month of therapy. At that time you may consider other prescription or OTC treatments for your arthritis. |
| i. product storage requirements | Place the medications in an easy-to-open container if they are not already, and be sure to keep products out of a child's reach. |
| j. specific nondrug measures | N/A |
| 10. Solicit follow-up questions from patient. | Will this glucosamine increase my glucose? |
| 11. Answer patient's questions. | Although the word glucosamine sounds like it has glucose in it or will affect your glucose, diabetic patients who are given glucosamine generally do not have any major increases in their blood glucose. However, you should monitor your blood glucose and report it to your PCP. More important, to ensure the best control of your diabetes, you should eat a proper diet (i.e., no snacking), exercise, and lose weight, which also will help your osteoarthritis. |

Key: DM, diabetes mellitus; MI, myocardial infarction; N/A, not applicable; NKDA, no known drug allergy; OTC, over-the-counter; PCP, primary care provider.

The box Patient Education for Musculoskeletal Injuries and Disorders lists specific information to provide patients about topical analgesics and preventive and nondrug measures.

## Evaluation of Patient Outcomes for Musculoskeletal Injuries and Disorders

The primary indicator of treatment effectiveness is the patient's perception of pain relief. If a patient reports the pain is still present or has worsened after 7 to 10 days of using nonprescription analgesics, the clinician should refer the patient for further evaluation. In many instances, the lack of a return visit indicates a successful treatment regimen. Patients with minor sprains or strains will not require a second visit as the tissues heal and return to normal function. If the clinician has a good relationship with the patient, he or she may call the patient in a few days to determine whether the complaint has resolved. However, a patient who does return with signs of continued swelling, pain, or inflammation should be directed to a primary care provider. The continued pain may indicate an ongoing process that could lead to long-term disability or decreased mobility.

## Key Points for Musculoskeletal Injuries and Disorders

- Self-treatment of patients presenting with pain secondary to injury or disorder of the musculoskeletal system should be limited to those with mild to moderate pain and no exclusions to self-treatment such as a visibly deformed joint or systemic symptoms (Figure 7-2).
- Self-treatment of acute musculoskeletal injuries should include nondrug therapy, such as rest, ice, compression, and elevation. Heat therapy may also provide benefit after swelling abates.
- Patients self-treating chronic pain of osteoarthritis should be advised to employ nondrug therapy such as weight loss, exercise and stretching, and use of assisting devices (i.e., cane).
- Clinicians should advise patients on the proper selection of a product for their musculoskeletal injury or disorder taking into account the patient's preferences.
- Systemic analgesics are valid first-line treatments for the majority of musculoskeletal injuries and disorders. Acetaminophen is preferred in noninflammatory diseases, where NSAIDs are preferred if inflammation is present. Side effects and drug interactions should be considered before therapy is chosen (see Chapter 5).
- Topical counterirritants are useful for treatment of acute musculoskeletal injuries and as an adjunct in the treatment of chronic musculoskeletal disorders. They are to be used only topically and on skin that is intact. Patients should be advised not to use heating devices with topical counterirritants or cover the counterirritant with a tight bandage.
- Alternative therapy with glucosamine may provide benefit in patients with mild to moderate osteoarthritis.
- Clinicians should monitor the outcome of self-treatments and advise patients who self-treat their acute musculoskeletal injury to contact their primary care provider if their symptoms do not improve after 10 days
- Clinicians can assist patients through direct support and education by counseling in a nonjudgmental way and providing other resources to help manage their pain.

## References

1. Loeser JD, Melzack R. Pain: an overview [review]. *Lancet.* 1999; 353:1607-9.
2. Mense S, Simons DG, Russell IJ. *Muscle Pain: Understanding Its Nature, Diagnosis and Treatment.* Baltimore: Lippincott William & Wilkins; 2001:1-20.

## PATIENT EDUCATION FOR MUSCULOSKELETAL INJURIES AND DISORDERS

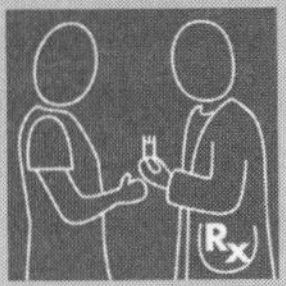

The objectives of self-treatment are to (1) reduce the severity and duration of pain, (2) restore function of the affected area, (3) prevent reinjury and disability, and (4) prevent acute pain from becoming chronic persistent pain. Certain nondrug measures and nonprescription counterirritants can relieve the symptoms of pain from a sudden and recent muscle, tendon, or ligament injury; an overuse injury (tendonitis, bursitis, or repetitive stress injury); lower back pain; or arthritis. For most patients, carefully following product instructions and the self-care measures listed here will help ensure optimal therapeutic outcomes.

### Nondrug Measures

- For pain related to a muscle or joint injuries, begin treatment with RICE therapy (see Table 7-3).
- For periodic muscle cramps, stretch and massage the affected area immediately; then rest or reduce activity of the muscle to allow it to loosen.
- For persistent cramps, apply heat to the affected area in the form of a warm wet compress, a heating pad, or a hot-water bottle.
- For osteoarthritis, try a combination of nondrug measures, including applying heat or cold to the affected area, supporting the area with splints, and doing range-of-motion and strength maintenance exercises.

### Preventive Measures

- To prevent muscle or joint strains and sprains, do warm-up and stretching exercises before playing sports or exercising, and wrap injured muscle or joint with protective bandage or tape.
- To prevent repetitive strain, exercise the muscles vulnerable to injury and use ergonomic controls to adjust posture, stresses, motions, and other damaging physical factors.
- To prevent cramps, warm up and stretch muscles before physical activity, drink sufficient fluids, and do not exercise to the point of exhaustion. To help prevent nocturnal leg cramps, raise the foot of the bed. If you suffer from Achilles tendonitis, try wearing better-fitting shoes and heel lifts to reduce the symptoms.
- To prevent or reduce the occurrence of lower back pain, do exercises to strengthen the muscles of the lower back and use assistive devices (i.e., cane or walker) if needed.
- To prevent or reduce the occurrence of osteoarthritis, avoid a sedentary lifestyle, keep the joints active, lose weight if overweight, and use assistive devices if needed.

### Nonprescription Medications

- For mild to moderate muscle pain, take a nonprescription analgesic for no longer than 10 days (see Chapter 5 for listing of nonprescription analgesics) and/or a topical counterirritant (see Table 7-4 for recommended dosages of counterirritants).
- Do not use counterirritants if your skin is abraded, sunburned, or otherwise damaged.
- When using counterirritants, wash your hands before touching your eyes or mucous membranes or before handling contact lenses.
- Gently rub a thin layer of counterirritant product into affected muscles or joints until you cannot see the product. Thick application of the product does not make the product work better.
- Do not put a tight bandage or dressing over an area treated with a counterirritant. Do not use warming devices with counterirritants.
- Do not treat a child younger than 2 years of age with counterirritants unless a primary care provider supervises the use.
- If you suffer from arthritis, consult your primary care provider before attempting to treat your pain with counterirritants or with topical or internal analgesics.
- If you have asthma, and symptoms of wheezing and shortness of breath worsen while you are using a mentholated formulation, stop using it.
- Do not use any product containing salicylates (including aspirin, methyl salicylate, and trolamine salicylate) if you are receiving anticoagulation therapy (especially warfarin).
- If a counterirritant causes excessive redness and blistering or hives and vomiting, stop using it.

⚠ If you experience nausea, vomiting, colic, and other unusual symptoms while using a product containing camphor, seek medical care immediately.

⚠ If the pain was present for more than 2 weeks before you sought treatment, consult a primary care provider.

⚠ If the symptoms persist after more than 10 days of treatment or if the pain is constant and felt in any position, consult a primary care provider.


3. Hamacher Research Group. Analgesics: the relentless search for relief. *Drug Topics* [serial online]. December 13, 2004. Available at: http://www.drugtopics.com/drugtopics/article/articleDetail.jsp?id=138083. Accessed November 2, 2005.
4. Crombie IK. Epidemiology of persistent pain. In: Jensen TS, Turner JA, Wiesenfeld-Hallin Z, eds. *Proceedings of the 8th World Congress on Pain, Progress in Pain Research and Management.* Seattle, Wash: IASP Press; 1997:53-5.
5. Loeser JD. Economic implications of pain management [review]. *Acta Anaesthesiol Scand.* 1999;43:957-9.
6. Benson V, Marano MA. Current estimates from the national health interview survey. *Vital Health Statistics.* Series 10, No. 199. Washington, DC: US Department of Health and Human Services. 1-428. 10-1-1998. DHSS Pub No. PHS 98-1527.
7. Stewart WF, Ricci JA, Chee E, et al. Lost productive time and cost due to common pain conditions in the US workforce [see comment]. *JAMA.* 2003;290:2443-54.
8. Pendleton A, Arden N, Dougados M, et al. EULAR recommendations for the management of knee osteoarthritis: report of a task force of the Standing Committee for International Clinical Studies Including Therapeutic Trials (ESCISIT) [see comment]. *Ann Rheum Dis.* 2000;59:936-44.
9. Burt VL, Harris T. The third National Health and Nutrition Examination Survey: contributing data on aging and health. *Gerontologist.* 1994;34:486-90.
10. *Meyler's Side Effects of Drugs.* 14th ed. Oxford: Elsevier Science; 2000.
11. Clarkson PM, Sayers SP. Etiology of exercise-induced muscle damage [review]. *Can J Applied Physiol.* 1999;24:234-48.

12. Schwellnus MP, Derman EW, Noakes TD. Aetiology of skeletal muscle 'cramps' during exercise: a novel hypothesis [review]. *J Sports Sci.* 1997;15:277-85.
13. Carey TS, Garrett JM, Jackman A, et al. Recurrence and care seeking after acute back pain: results of a long-term follow-up study. North Carolina Back Pain Project. *Med Care.* 1999;37:157-64.
14. McAlindon TE, Wilson PW, Aliabadi P, et al. Level of physical activity and the risk of radiographic and symptomatic knee osteoarthritis in the elderly: the Framingham study. *Am J Med.* 1999;106:151-7.
15. Yaksh TL. Pharmacology and mechanisms of opioid analgesic activity [review]. *Acta Anaesthesiol Scand.* 1997;41(1 pt 2):94-111.
16. van der Linden PD, Sturkenboom MC, Herings RM, et al. Fluoroquinolones and risk of Achilles tendon disorders: case-control study. *BMJ.* 2002;324:1306-7.
17. Wright A, Sluka KA. Nonpharmacological treatments for musculoskeletal pain [see comment] [review]. *Clin J Pain.* 2001;17:33-46.
18. Recommendations for the medical management of osteoarthritis of the hip and knee: 2000 update. American College of Rheumatology Subcommittee on Osteoarthritis Guidelines [see comment]. *Arthritis Rheum.* 2000;43:1905-15.
19. Reginster JY, Deroisy R, Rovati LC, et al. Long-term effects of glucosamine sulphate on osteoarthritis progression: a randomised, placebo-controlled clinical trial [see comment]. *Lancet.* 2001;357:251-6.
20. Wegman A, van der WD, van TM, et al. Nonsteroidal antiinflammatory drugs or acetaminophen for osteoarthritis of the hip or knee? A systematic review of evidence and guidelines [see comment] [review]. *J Rheumatol.* 2004;31:344-54.
21. Lee C, Straus WL, Balshaw R, et al. A comparison of the efficacy and safety of nonsteroidal antiinflammatory agents versus acetaminophen in the treatment of osteoarthritis: a meta-analysis. *Arthritis Rheum.* 2004;51:746-54.
22. Nikles CJ, Yelland M, Del MC, et al. The role of paracetamol in chronic pain: an evidence-based approach [review]. *Am J Ther.* 2005;12:80-91.
23. Hippisley-Cox J, Coupland C. Risk of myocardial infarction in patients taking cyclo-oxygenase-2 inhibitors or conventional non-steroidal anti-inflammatory drugs: population based nested case-control analysis. *BMJ.* 2005;330:1366.
24. Department of Health and Human Services. External analgesic products for over-the-counter human use; establishment of a monograph and notice of proposed rulemaking. *Federal Register.* 1979;44:69768-874.
25. Department of Health and Human Services. External analgesic drug products for over-the-counter human use: tentative final monograph. *Federal Register.* 1983;48:5852-69.
26. Cross SE, Anderson C, Roberts MS. Topical penetration of commercial salicylate esters and salts using human isolated skin and clinical microdialysis studies. *Br J Clin Pharmacol.* 1998;46:29-35.
27. Roberts MS, Favretto WA, Meyer A, et al. Topical bioavailability of methyl salicylate. *Aust New Zealand J Med.* 1982;12:303-5.
28. Methyl salicylate. In: Reynolds JEF, ed. *Martindale The Extra Pharmacopoeia.* 33 ed. London: The Royal Pharmaceutical Society; 2002:1090-1.
29. Littleton F Jr. Warfarin and topical salicylates. *JAMA.* 1990;263: 2888.
30. Yip AS, Chow WH, Tai YT, et al. Adverse effect of topical methylsalicylate ointment on warfarin anticoagulation: an unrecognized potential hazard. *Postgrad Med J.* 1990;66:367-9.
31. Bell AJ, Duggin G. Acute methyl salicylate toxicity complicating herbal skin treatment for psoriasis. *Emerg Med* (Fremantle, Wash). 2002;14:188-90.
32. Heng MC. Local necrosis and interstitial nephritis due to topical methyl salicylate and menthol. *Cutis.* 1987;39:442-4.
33. Danon A, Ben-Shimon S, Ben-Zvi Z. Effect of exercise and heat exposure on percutaneous absorption of methyl salicylate. *Eur J Clin Pharmacol.* 1986;31:49-52.
34. Siegel E, Wason S. Camphor toxicity [review]. *Pediatr Clin North Am.* 1986;33:375-9.
35. Camphor revisited: focus on toxicity. Committee on Drugs. American Academy of Pediatrics. *Pediatrics.* 1994;94:127-8.
36. Green BG. Menthol inhibits the perception of warmth. *Physiol Behav.* 1986;38:833-8.
37. Schafer K, Braun HA, Rempe L. Discharge pattern analysis suggests existence of a low-threshold calcium channel in cold receptors. *Experientia.* 1991;47:47-50.
38. Galeotti N, Di Cesare ML, Mazzanti G, et al. Menthol: a natural analgesic compound. *Neurosci Lett.* 2002;322:145-8.
39. Menthol. In: Reynolds JEF, ed. *Martindale The Extra Pharmacopoeia.* 33 ed. London: The Royal Pharmaceutical Society; 2002: 1043-4.
40. Eccles R. Menthol and related cooling compounds [review]. *J Pharm Pharmacol.* 1994;46:618-30.
41. Fisher AA. Reactions to menthol. *Cutis.* 1986;38:17-8.
42. Blondeel A, Oleffe J, Achten G. Contact allergy in 330 dermatological patients. *Contact Dermatitis.* 1978;4:270-6.
43. Spurlock BW, Dailey TM. Shortness of (fresh) breath toothpaste-induced bronchospasm [see comment]. *N Engl J Med.* 1990;323: 1845-6.
44. Eccles R. Menthol: effects on nasal sensation of airflow and the drive to breathe [review]. *Curr Allerg Asthma Rep.* 2003;3:210-4.
45. Wilkin JK, Fortner G, Reinhardt LA, et al. Prostaglandins and nicotinate-provoked increase in cutaneous blood flow. *Clin Pharmacol Ther.* 1985;38:273-7.
46. Fitzgerald M. Capsaicin and sensory neurones a review [review]. *Pain.* 1983;15:109-30.
47. Mason L, Moore RA, Derry S, et al. Systematic review of topical capsaicin for the treatment of chronic pain[see comment] [review]. *BMJ.* 2004;328:991.
48. Degim IT, Uslu A, Hadgraft J, et al. The effects of Azone and capsaicin on the permeation of naproxen through human skin. *Int J Pharm.* 1999;179:21-5.
49. Politino V, Smith SL, Waggoner WC. A clinical study of topical 10% trolamine salicylate for relief of delayed-onset exercise-induced arthralgia/myalgia. *Curr Ther Res.* 1985;38:321-7.
50. Hill DW, Richardson JD. Effectiveness of 10% trolamine salicylate cream on muscular soreness induced by a reproducible program of weight training. *J Orthop Sports Phys Ther.* 1989;11:19-23.
51. Hochberg FH, Lavin P, Portney R, et al. Topical therapy of localized inflammation in musicians: a clinical evaluation of aspercreme versus placebo. *Med Prob Performing Arts.* 1988;3:9-14.
52. Rothacker DQ, Lee I, Littlejohn TW. Effectiveness of a single topical application of 10% trolamine salicylate cream in the symptomatic treatment of osteoarthritis. *J Clin Rheumatol.* 1998; 4:12.
53. Block LH. Medicated topicals. In: Hoover JE, ed. *Remington: The Science and Practice of Pharmacy.* 20 ed. Easton, Pa: Mack Publishing; 2000:836-57.
54. Nairn JG. Solutions, emulsions, suspensions, and extracts. In: Hoover JE, ed. *Remington: The Science and Practice of Pharmacy.* 20 ed. Easton, Pa: Mack Publishing; 2000:721-52.
55. Moore RA, Tramer MR, Carroll D, et al. Quantitative systematic review of topically applied non-steroidal anti-inflammatory drugs [see comment; erratum appears in *BMJ* 1998;316:1059]. *BMJ* 1998;316:333-8.
56. Lin J, Zhang W, Jones A, et al. Efficacy of topical non-steroidal anti-inflammatory drugs in the treatment of osteoarthritis: meta-analysis of randomised controlled trials [see comment]. *BMJ.* 2004;329:324.

57. Roth SH, Shainhouse JZ. Efficacy and safety of a topical diclofenac solution (pennsaid) in the treatment of primary osteoarthritis of the knee: a randomized, double-blind, vehicle-controlled clinical trial. *Arch Intern Med.* 2004;164:2017-23.
58. *PDR for Herbal Medicines.* Montvale, NJ: Medical Economics; 1998.
59.Pavelka K, Gatterova J, Olejarova M, et al. Glucosamine sulfate use and delay of progression of knee osteoarthritis: a 3-year, randomized, placebo-controlled, double-blind study. *Arch Intern Med.* 2002;162:2113-23.
60. Scroggie DA, Albright A, Harris MD. The effect of glucosamine-chondroitin supplementation on glycosylated hemoglobin levels in patients with type 2 diabetes mellitus: a placebo-controlled, double-blinded, randomized clinical trial [see comment]. *Arch Intern Med.* 2003;163:1587-90.
61. Towheed TE, Anastassiades TP. Glucosamine and chondroitin for treating symptoms of osteoarthritis: evidence is widely touted but incomplete [see comment]. *JAMA.* 2000;283:1483-4
62. Hochberg MC. What a difference a year makes: reflections on the ACR recommendations for the medical management of osteoarthritis [review]. *Curr Rheumatol Rep.* 2001;3:473-8.
63. Towheed TE, Anastassiades TP. Glucosamine and chondroitin for treating symptoms of osteoarthritis: evidence is widely touted but incomplete. [see comment]. *JAMA.* 2000;28:1483-4.
64. Michel BA, Stucki G, Frey D et al. Chondroitins 4 and 6 sulfate in osteoarthritis of the knee: a randomized, controlled trial. *Arthritis & Rheumatism.* 2005;52:779-86.
65. Richy F, Bruyere O, Ethgen O, et al. Structural and symptomatic efficacy of glucosamine and chondroitin in knee osteoarthritis: a comprehensive meta-analysis [see comment]. *Arch Intern Med.* 2003;163:1514-22.
66. Little CV, Parsons T. Herbal therapy for treating osteoarthritis [review] [50 refs]. *Cochrane Database of Systematic Reviews.* 2001; CD002947:(1).
67. Soeken KL. Selected CAM therapies for arthritis-related pain: the evidence from systematic reviews [review] [24 refs]. *Clinical Journal of Pain.* 2004;13-8.
68. Usha PR, Naidu MU. Randomised, double-blind, parallel, placebo-controlled study of oral glucosamine, methylsulfonylmethane and their combination in osteoarthritis. *Clinical Drug Investigation.* 2004;24:353-63.

SECTION III

# Reproductive and Genital Disorders

CHAPTER 8

# Vaginal and Vulvovaginal Disorders

*Nicole M. Stack and Leslie A. Shimp*

Vaginal symptoms are among the most common health concerns of women of reproductive age and older. Vaginal symptoms may be experienced by women from all walks of life: married or single, sexually active or sexually abstinent, homosexual or heterosexual, and premenopausal or postmenopausal.[1] Vaginal discharge is among the top 25 reasons that women seek medical care and accounts for more than 10 million office visits annually.[2] It is estimated that about 65% of women who experience vaginal symptoms have a vaginal infection caused by one of the three most common vaginal infections: bacterial vaginosis (BV), vulvovaginal candidiasis (VVC), and trichomoniasis.[1] Infections may also be mixed, with more than one causative organism.

Vaginal infections are generally perceived as minor health problems. However, bacterial vaginosis and trichomoniasis have been linked to significant health problems.[3,4] In view of the large number of women seeking diagnosis and treatment for vaginal infections and the approval of nonprescription vaginal antifungal compounds for the treatment of VVC, it is imperative that practitioners understand the therapeutic management of these three vaginal infections and the appropriate patient education for VVC.

Women may also self-treat noninfectious vaginal symptoms such as vaginal dryness, atrophic vaginitis, and allergic or chemical dermatologic reactions.[1,3] Many women use douches for routine vaginal hygiene. Unfortunately, women are not always knowledgeable about normal vaginal health and the consequences of improper douching methods. Therefore, consumers and health care providers need to understand vaginal health to make informed and appropriate decisions about self-care for vaginal symptoms and vaginal hygiene.

## ANATOMY AND PHYSIOLOGY OF THE VAGINA

The vagina is an elastic fibromuscular tube that extends 8 to 10 cm from the vulva to the uterus. The upper end of the vagina is closed except for the cervical os, the opening to the cervix. Anatomically, the vagina lies between the urinary bladder and the rectum. At the lower (vulvar) end of the vagina are the Bartholin's glands, which produce secretions in response to sexual stimulation. At puberty, under the influence of estrogen, the vagina is lined by stratified squamous epithelium, which contains glycogen. This glycogen is acted on by *Lactobacillus* bacteria to form lactic acid, which creates an acidic pH of about 4 to 4.5. This acidic pH and the production of hydrogen peroxide by these bacteria help protect the vagina from infection with other bacteria. After menopause, thinning of the vaginal lining occurs, the lactobacilli decline, and the pH rises.[5]

The mature vagina is colonized by a variety of organisms. *Lactobacillus* species predominate, accounting for 90% to 95% of the vaginal flora. Another five to 10 species of bacteria (e.g., *Corynebacteria*, Streptococcus, *Staphylococcus epidermidis, Gardnerella vaginalis, Peptostreptococcus,* and *Bacteroides*) are present in small quantities, with anaerobes being more common than aerobes.[3,6] *Candida albicans* and *Escherichia coli* may also be isolated in the absence of active infection in about 20% of women.[6,7]

Various factors influence the vaginal ecosystem (i.e., the number and type of endogenous organisms, vaginal pH, and glycogen concentration), including hormonal fluctuations of the menstrual cycle, aging, certain diseases (e.g., diabetes mellitus), use of various medications (e.g., contraceptive preparations, hormones, antibiotics), douching, and number of sex partners (increasing exposure to additional organisms).

The healthy vagina is cleansed daily by secretions that lubricate the vaginal tract. Normal vaginal discharge (leukorrhea) consists of about 1.5 g of vaginal fluid daily, which is odorless, clear or white, and viscous or sticky.[7] This physiologic discharge consists of endocervical mucus, serum transudate from vaginal capillary beds, endogenous vaginal flora, and epithelial cells.[6,7] An increase in vaginal secretions is normal during ovulation, during pregnancy, following menses, and with sexual excitement or emotional flares. An alteration in vaginal secretions may also occur in response to vaginal irritants (e.g., feminine hygiene deodorant products, vaginal douches, and other cleansing products), contraceptive products and devices, or use of tampons.

## DIFFERENTIATION OF COMMON VAGINAL INFECTIONS

The signs and symptoms for various vaginal infections may be similar and the characteristic symptoms that often help distinguish infections may be absent. Both patients and clinicians may have difficulty accurately determining the type of infection on the sole basis of symptoms.[8,9]

Accurately distinguishing VVC from BV and trichomoniasis is especially important because of the availability of nonprescription antifungal therapy. In addition, BV and trichomoniasis are associated with potential complications such as pelvic inflammatory disease (PID), urinary tract infections, cervicitis, endometriosis, and tubal infertility in addition to the facilitation of transmission of human immunodeficiency virus (HIV).[4,10,11]

Given the availability of nonprescription topical vaginal antifungal preparations and the cost and inconvenience of an office evaluation, many patients prefer to self-treat empirically for presumed VVC. In a study by Foxman et al.,[12] women with at least one physician-diagnosed episode and a reported presumed episode of VVC within the preceding 2 months were as likely to self-diagnose VVC as to contact a prescriber by phone or via an office visit. Women who reported having four or more episodes of VVC were the most likely to self-diagnose.

Sales of nonprescription vaginal antifungals are greater than the predicted number of VVC cases, illustrating the difficulty with accurate self-diagnosis.[13] Recent studies indicate that many women have trouble identifying VVC based on their symptoms.[8,14] One study found that when women who had previously been diagnosed with VVC read a description of the classic symptoms of the infection, only 35% could accurately recognize it.[15] Similarly among a group of women who purchased a nonprescription vaginal antifungal to self-treat for vaginal symptoms only about half had a candidal infection when they were evaluated by a primary care provider.[14] Ferris and coworkers[14] found that women with a greater number of lifetime vaginal candidal infections were more likely to make an error in self-diagnosis.

The symptom most apt to differentiate a candidal vaginal infection from that of bacterial vaginosis and trichomoniasis is the absence of an offensive odor of the vaginal discharge.[16]

Noninfectious conditions that may be confused with vaginal infections are vulvovaginal irritation or pruritus caused by allergic or hypersensitivity reactions. These reactions may be a result of allergy to latex, spermicides, vaginal lubricants containing potential irritants (e.g., propylene glycol), or anesthetics (used by males to delay ejaculation) or of irritation secondary to douches, feminine hygiene products, soaps/detergents, or frequent use of panty liners or sanitary napkins.[3] In addition, urethral irritation and dysuria resulting from vulvovaginitis may be mistaken for a urinary tract infection.

Inappropriate use of vaginal antifungal products does have some risks, including (1) unnecessary use of the antifungal agent and (2) delay in effective treatment and possible delay in treatment of a serious condition. The risks of exposure to the vaginal antifungals in the absence of VVC are minor—primarily local irritation and the cost of therapy.[13] Labeling instructions advise patients to seek help for persistent symptoms and, if these guidelines are followed, the delay in treatment from misdiagnosis will likely present few serious consequences for most women. However, repeated use of nonprescription agents for persistent or recurring symptoms can delay appropriate therapy with potentially significant health implications and may allow transmission of infections. Use of nonprescription vaginal pH self-testing devices by patients has been examined as an option to reduce this inappropriate use of antifungals.[17] This study evaluated the use of pH devices in symptomatic women. Nearly 57% of women who believed they had a yeast infection did not, which was confirmed by self-testing with the pH device and an exam by a health care provider. The use of pH self-testing devices may be beneficial in reducing inappropriate self-treatment with antifungals. These devices are inexpensive (e.g., pHEM-ALERT, Fem Exam) and available at many pharmacies or can be purchased online.

Table 8-1 describes the classic symptoms of the three common vaginal infections as well as the symptoms that women typically experience.[1,2,4,10,11,18-20]

## VULVOVAGINAL CANDIDIASIS

### Epidemiology of VVC

Vulvovaginal candidiasis (also referred to as "yeast infection" and "moniliasis") is the second most common vaginal infection, accounting for approximately 20% to 25% of cases of vaginitis. VVC is uncommon prior to menarche, but by age 25 about 50% of women will have had one or more episodes of VVC.[6] A study of 2000 women found that 6.5% of women 18 years of age and older reported experiencing an episode of VVC within the previous 2 months.[12] Black women reported three times the number of VVC episodes (17.4% of women) as did white women (5.8%) or women of other races or ethnic groups (4.8%).[12] Recurrent infections (defined as four or more infections within a 1-year period) occur in fewer than 5% of women.[4] About 20% of women may be colonized with *Candida albicans* without experiencing vaginal symptoms.[8]

### Etiology of VVC

*Candida* fungi are the causative organisms of this vaginal infection, with about 80% to 92% of cases caused by *C. albicans*.[4] The incidence of non–*C. albicans* infections has increased in the past two decades; *C. glabrata, C. tropicalis,* and *Saccharomyces cerevisiae* now account for a significant minority of candidal vaginal infections.[4,7] This increase may be a result of the widespread use of nonprescription antifungals, short courses of azole therapy, and long-term suppressive therapy with azole antifungals.[4]

No precipitating factor is identified for most episodes of VVC. However, a number of physiologic and behavioral factors have been studied as possible risk factors for VVC. The risk factors discussed below are not consistently associated with symptomatic candidal vaginitis, and their presence does not clearly establish an increased likelihood of VVC in a patient with vaginal symptoms. Most women with sporadic and infrequent candidal vaginitis do not have a readily apparent "cause" for the infection.[4] Modification of factors linked to VVC is not warranted for most patients.[1]

Pregnancy, high-dose estrogen oral contraceptives, and estrogen replacement therapy (ERT) may increase vaginal susceptibility to candidal infections by increasing the glycogen content of the vagina. However, studies do not support an increased risk for candidal infections with low-dose estrogen oral contraceptives, and studies on risk during pregnancy or use of postmenopausal ERT are inconsistent.[21,22] Vaginal pH increases during menstruation; this may predispose menstruating women to cyclic fungal vaginal infections. At menopause, the decline in glycogen leads to a decrease in lactic acid and an increase in vaginal pH, which can alter vaginal ecology and may also predispose to vaginal infections. Women with diabetes mellitus are known to be at greater risk for skin and vaginal candidal infections, particularly if glycemic control is poor.

A number of patients (25% to 70% in several studies) report developing candidal vaginal infections during or just after treatment with broad-spectrum antibiotics such as tetracycline, ampicillin/amoxicillin, and cephalosporins.[23,24] The proposed mechanism is a decrease in normal vaginal flora, especially lactobacilli, allowing an overgrowth of *Candida* organisms. However, neither an increase in vaginal *Candida* organisms nor a decrease in lactobacilli occurs in all women who have taken antibiotics.

Patients who are taking systemic corticosteroid, antineoplastic, or immunosuppressant drugs may be at increased risk for developing candidal infections. This risk is well known for certain patient populations such as recipients of an organ transplant and patients with HIV infection.

An increased frequency of VVC is associated with the onset of regular sexual activity. However, neither the number of sexual partners nor the frequency of sexual intercourse is related to the occurrence of VVC episodes.[4] There is some evidence suggesting an increase in risk associated with receptive oral sex.[1] In addition, use of an intrauterine device (IUD) or vaginal sponge contraceptive has been shown to increase the risk for VVC.[4]

Studies do not demonstrate a consistent association between tight-fitting, nonabsorbent clothing or pantyhose and vaginal candidal infections. However, clothing of this type may increase risk by creating a warm and moist environment. Some studies have suggested that foods that may increase urinary sugar (e.g., dietary sugars, refined carbohydrates, milk, artificial sweeteners) may increase risk for candidal vaginal infections.[1,2] It has been suggested that consumption of yogurt may have a potential prophylactic benefit against VVC.[25] More studies are needed to determine the influence of diet as a preventive or risk factor for candidal vaginal infections.

The treatment of candidal vaginal infections does not typically include treatment of the male partner. No controlled studies have shown that treatment of male partners prevents recurrence of candidal vaginal infections in women. However, in cases of recurrent infections, male partners may be treated with a topical imidazole.

## Signs and Symptoms of VVC

The characteristic symptoms of VVC are described in Table 8-1.

## Treatment of VVC

The treatment of VVC is determined by the severity of symptoms and the frequency of episodes. VVC can be categorized as uncomplicated or complicated; recurrent VVC is a type of complicated infection.[16] Complicated infections occur in only about 5% of women. These more severe infections may occur because of host factors—an inability of normal factors to prevent candidal colonization—or the presence of fungal organisms more resistant to azole antifungal therapy.

### Treatment Goals

The goals of therapy for vaginal fungal infections are (1) relief of symptoms and eradication of the infection and (2) reestablishment of normal vaginal flora.

A single course of drug therapy is effective in achieving these goals for virtually all patients. However, a small percentage of patients will experience persistent or recurrent infections and require prolonged therapy or higher doses of medication.

### General Treatment Approach

Self-treatment of VVC with nonprescription antifungal therapy can be appropriate for patients with uncomplicated disease (infrequent episodes, mild to moderate symptoms), whereas women with complicated (more severe symptoms, concurrent predisposing illness or medications) or recurrent infections should be referred for assessment and treatment by a primary care provider. (See Figure 8-1 for a list of exclusions for self-care.)

By definition, recurrent VVC occurs when a woman experiences at least four (documented) infections within a 12-month period.[4] Patients with such symptoms should be evaluated for the possibility of a mixed infection or a strain of candidal infection other than *C. albicans*, which may be resistant to standard therapy. Recurrent candidal infections often require long-term suppressive prophylactic therapy. About two thirds of surveyed physicians report seeing patients who had delayed treatment because of inappropriate use of nonprescription products.[24] In addition, frequent or recurrent episodes of VVC may be an early sign of HIV infection or diabetes. The Food and Drug Administration (FDA) now requires labels of nonprescription products to include a warning similar to the following:

> If your symptoms return within 2 months or if you have infections that do not clear up easily with proper treatment, consult your doctor. You could be pregnant, or there could be a serious underlying medical cause for your infections, such as diabetes or a damaged immune system (including damage from infection with HIV, the virus that causes AIDS).

Preventive measures are not a standard part of therapy for vaginal fungal infections. However, women with infections that are more frequent or are not responsive to antifungal therapy may try dietary changes, nondrug measures (e.g., avoidance of nonabsorbent clothing), or alteration in other drug therapy known to be a risk factor for VVC. A 3-to-4-month trial of these approaches will reveal whether they are useful for individual patients.[1] Figure 8-1 outlines the appropriate approach to treating the patient with vaginal symptoms.

**TABLE 8-1 Differentiation of Common Vaginal Infections**

| Classic Symptoms[1] | Differentiating Signs and Symptoms | Etiology and Epidemiology[1] |
|---|---|---|
| **Bacterial Vaginosis** | | |
| Thin (watery), off-white or discolored (green, gray, tan), sometimes foamy discharge; unpleasant "fishy" odor that increases after sexual intercourse or with elevated vaginal pH (e.g., menses) | Vaginal irritation, dysuria, and itching less frequent with BV than with VVC or trichomoniasis[19]<br>Malodor strongly associated with BV; absence of malodor virtually rules out BV<br>Increased vaginal discharge ("wetness") more common with BV than with VVC or trichomoniasis | Polymicrobial infection resulting from imbalance in normal vaginal flora with increase in *G. vaginalis* and anaerobes (*Peptostreptocccus, Mobiluncus, Prevotella,* and *Mycoplasma hominis*) and decrease in *Lactobacilli*<br>Risk factors: new sexual partner, African American race, use of IUD, douching, receptive oral sex, tobacco use (smoking alters vaginal flora), and prior pregnancy<br>Possible protective factors: use of female hormones, including OC, and condoms<br>Responsible for 33% of vaginal symptoms<br>Predominately affects young sexually active women but can arise spontaneously regardless of sexual activity; found in 12% of virginal adolescents; lower prevalence in postmenopausal women, even with use of postmenopausal hormones |
| **Trichomoniasis** | | |
| Copious, malodorous, yellow-green (or discolored) discharge<br>pruritus; vaginal irritation; dysuria<br>No symptoms initially in ~50% of affected women<br>Most men are asymptomatic and serve as reservoirs of the disease | Erythema and vulvar edema can occur with this infection[18]<br>Yellow discharge: increased likelihood of trichomoniasis | STI caused by *Trichomonas vaginalis*, a protozoan<br>Risk factors: multiple sex partners, new sexual partner, nonuse of barrier contraceptives, and presence of other STIs<br>Responsible for 15%-20% of vaginal infections |
| **Vulvovaginal Candidiasis** | | |
| Thick, white ("cottage cheese") discharge with no odor; normal pH (see text for detailed information; also referred to as "yeast infection" or "moniliasis") | Presence of erythema, itching, and/or vulvar edema, and absence of malodor: increased likelihood of VVC; thick, "cheesy" discharge: strongly predictive of VVC[18,20] | Organisms: *C. albicans, C. glabrata, C. tropicalis,* and *Saccharomyces*<br>Some medications: antibiotics, immunosuppressants<br>No identifiable cause for most infections<br>Responsible for 20%-25% of vaginal infections |

Key: BV, bacterial vaginosis; HIV, human immunodeficiency virus; IUD, intrauterine device; OC, oral contraceptives; PID, pelvic inflammatory disease; STI, sexually transmitted infection; UTI, urinary tract infection; VVC, vulvovaginal candidiasis.

### *Nonpharmacologic Therapy*

Decreased consumption of sucrose and refined carbohydrates, as well as consumption of yogurt containing live cultures (see Complementary Therapies) have been suggested as measures to decrease VVC, particularly for women who experience recurrent infections.[1,2,25]

Discontinuing a drug known to increase susceptibility to vaginal fungal infections might be effective in decreasing the incidence of this disorder. Low-dose oral contraceptives are unlikely to contribute to the occurrence of VVC, but they might be discontinued to see whether the frequency of infection is altered. Patients taking broad-spectrum antibiotics or immunosuppressants should consult their primary care provider before discontinuing these medications.

### *Pharmacologic Therapy (Vaginal Antifungals)*

Currently, a nonprescription imidazole (butoconazole, clotrimazole, miconazole, or tioconazole) product is the recommended initial therapy for uncomplicated VVC. These products are available as vaginal creams, suppositories, and tablets (Table 8-2).

Studies have shown the imidazoles to be equally effective, with effectiveness rates of approximately 80% to 90%.[4,6] Different treatment durations have been studied. Miconazole single-dose and 7-day treatments were

| Complications[2,4,10,11] | Treatment |
|---|---|
| PID, UTI, cervicitis, endometriosis, and infections after gynecologic surgical procedures<br>Risks for pregnant patients: preterm labor and low-birth-weight infants<br>May facilitate transmission of HIV | Topical 2% clindamycin inserted vaginally for 7 days or metronidazole 0.75% gel 5 g inserted vaginally twice daily for 5 days<br>Oral metronidazole single 2 g dose<br>7-day oral course of metronidazole 500 mg twice daily or clindamycin 300 mg twice daily<br>Povidine–iodine 5 g vaginal suppositories inserted twice daily for 14-28 days<br>Oral/vaginal<br>*L. acidophilus* or yogurt<br>Routine treatment of sexual partners not warranted |
| Increased risk for low-birth-weight infants and tubal infertility<br>May facilitate transmission of HIV | Metronidazole 2 g as single dose or 500 mg twice daily for 7 days<br>Tinidazole 2 g as single dose (new option for metronidazole-resistant infections)<br>Successful treatment requires concurrent treatment of sexual partner(s) and avoidance of sexual intercourse until patient and partner(s) have completed therapy and are asymptomatic |
| Increased risk of other infections | Typically does not include male partners (see Table 8-2) |

compared, resulting in similar overall cure rates with significantly faster rates of symptom relief by day 3 in the ovule group compared with the 7-day treatment groups.[26] Butoconazole nitrate 2% single dose cream has also been compared with miconazole 7-day treatment, resulting in nonsignificant differences in cure rates.[27] Seven-day regimens of clotrimazole and miconazole, 3-day regimens of butoconazole, clotrimazole, and miconazole, and 1-day regimens of clotrimazole, miconazole, and tioconazole are available without a prescription. Monistat 1 has also been approved for insertion in the morning or at bedtime. This change in timing of administration has resulted in similar cure rates of infection between the daytime and bedtime treatments.[28] Table 8-2 lists the recommended nonprescription dosage regimens for products containing these ingredients. Information on currently available prescription and nonprescription products and regimens for acute infections, recurrent infections, and prophylactic therapy is presented in several reviews.[1,2,4,16]

Several nonspecific, nonprescription vaginal preparations, including Vagisil and Yeast-Gard (benzocaine and resorcinol), and Vaginex (tripelennamine), are also available. However, use of these agents for VVC is rarely, if ever, appropriate given the obvious advantages of the azole antifungals, including superior efficacy, improved patient compliance associated with ease of use, less frequent local reactions, and shorter treatment durations. The nonspecific products and medicated douches are more appropriate for vaginal and vulvar irritation and itching. They should be used for a limited time or on the advice of a

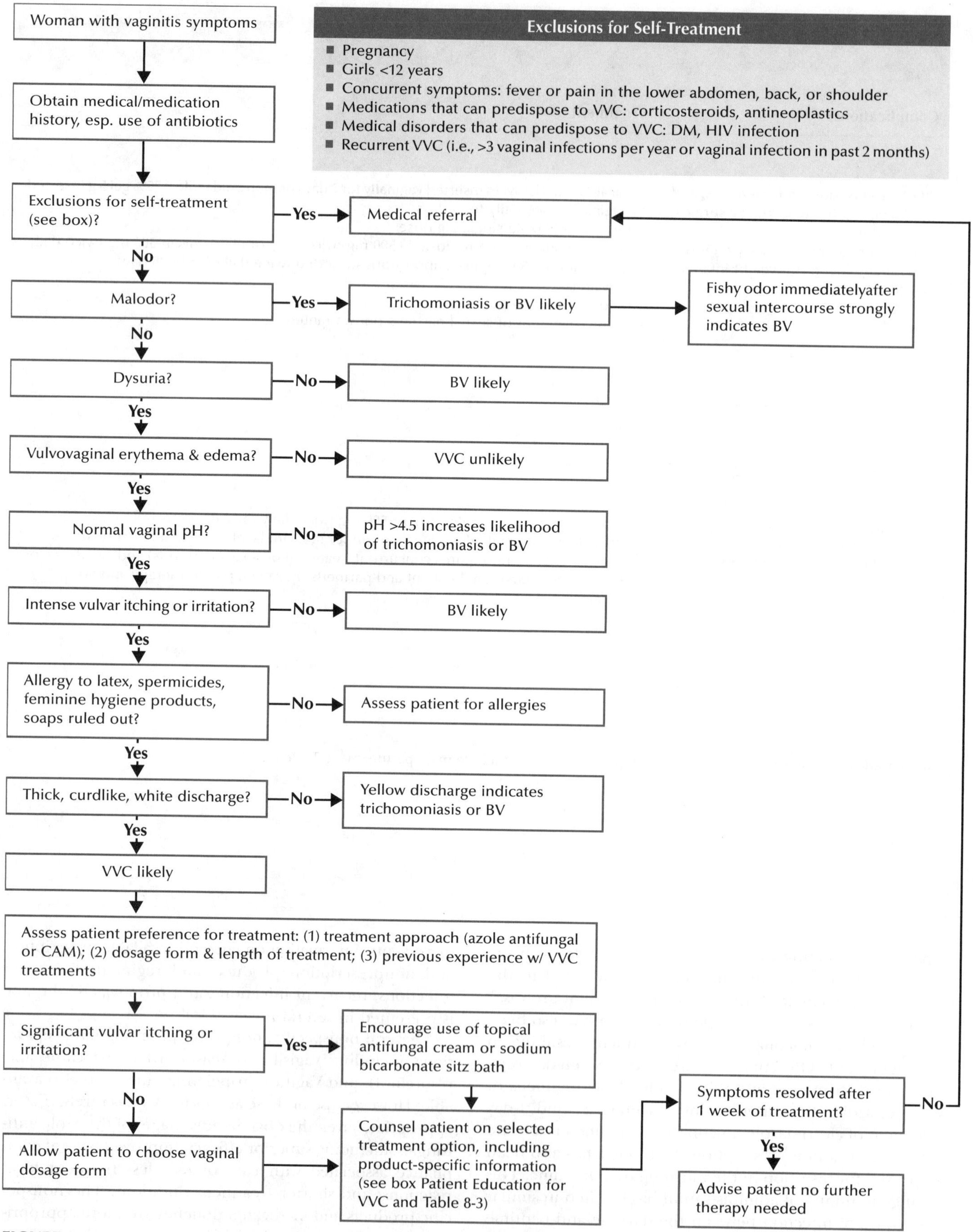


**FIGURE 8-1** Self-care of vulvovaginal candidiasis.[18-20] Key: CAM, complementary and alternative medicine; DM, diabetes mellitus; HIV, human immunodeficiency virus; VVC, vulvovaginal candidiasis.

TABLE 8-2 Selected Vaginal Antifungal Products and Their Dosages

| Trade Name | Primary Ingredient | Dosage |
|---|---|---|
| **Butoconazole Nitrate Products** | | |
| Mycelex-3 Cream | Butoconazole nitrate 2% | Insert cream into vagina daily for 3 days; apply to vulva twice daily as needed for itching. |
| **Clotrimazole Products** | | |
| Gyne-Lotrimin 7 Cream<br>Mycelex-7 Cream | Clotrimazole 1% | Insert cream into vagina daily for 7 days; apply to vulva twice daily as needed for itching. |
| Mycelex-7 Combination Pack | Tablet: clotrimazole 100 mg<br>Cream: clotrimazole 1% | Insert tablet into vagina daily for 7 days; apply cream to vulva twice daily for itching. |
| Gyne-Lotrimin 3 Cream | Clotrimazole 2% | Insert cream into vagina daily for 3 days; apply to vulva twice daily for itching. |
| **Miconazole Nitrate Products** | | |
| Monistat 1 Combination Pack<br>Monistat 1 Daytime Ovule | Cream: miconazole nitrate 2%<br>Suppository: miconazole nitrate 1200 mg | Apply cream to vulva twice daily as needed for itching; insert suppository into vagina daily (morning or at bedtime) for 1 day. |
| Monistat 3 Cream* | Miconazole nitrate 4% | Insert cream into vagina daily for 3 days; apply to vulva twice daily as needed for itching. |
| Monistat 3 Combination Pack*<br>M-zole 3 Combination Pack | Cream: miconazole nitrate 2%<br>Suppository: miconazole nitrate 200 mg | Apply cream to vulva twice daily as needed for itching; insert suppository into vagina daily for 3 days. |
| Monistat 7 Suppository | Miconazole nitrate 100 mg | Insert suppository into vagina daily for 7 days. |
| Monistat 7 Cream<br>Femizole-M Cream | Miconazole nitrate 2% | Insert cream into vagina daily for 7 days; apply to vulva twice daily as needed for itching. |
| Monistat 7 Combination Pack<br>M-zole 7 Combination Pack | Cream: miconazole nitrate 2%<br>Suppository: miconazole nitrate 100 mg | Apply cream to vulva twice daily as needed for itching; insert suppository into vagina daily for 7 days. |
| **Tioconazole Products** | | |
| Vagistat-1 Ointment<br>1-Day Ointment | Tioconazole 6.5% | Insert ointment into vagina daily for 1 day. |

* Prefilled applicators are available for this product.

primary care provider. (See Table 8-3 for additional examples of these products.)

### Mechanism of Action

The major antifungal effect of the imidazole compounds is accomplished by altering the membrane permeability of the fungi. These agents inhibit cytochrome P-450 enzymes in the fungal cell membrane, thereby decreasing synthesis of the essential fungal sterol ergosterol. The reduced membrane ergosterol content is accompanied by a corresponding increase in lanosterol-like methylated sterols. These lanosterol-like sterols cause structural damage to fungal membranes, resulting in the loss of normal membrane function.

### Pharmacokinetics

The topical vaginal imidazole preparations are not appreciably absorbed. Studies of butoconazole, clotrimazole, and tioconazole found that about 5%, between 3% and 10%, and negligible amounts of a vaginal dose were systemically absorbed, respectively. Fungicidal clotrimazole concentrations are detectable in the vaginal fluid for up to 3 days after a single 500 mg intravaginal dose.

### Indications

Nonprescription imidazoles are FDA approved for local treatment of VVC and relief of external vulvar itching and irritation associated with the infection.

### Dosage and Administration Guidelines

Table 8-4 describes proper administration of vaginal antifungals.

### Safety Considerations

Side effects from topical imidazoles are minimal and include vulvovaginal burning, itching, and irritation in 3% to 7% of patients.[22] These side effects are more likely to occur with the initial application of the vaginal preparation and are similar to symptoms of the vaginal infection.

**TABLE 8-3 Selected Products for Vaginal Itching and Irritation**

| Trade Name | Primary Ingredients |
|---|---|
| **Benzocaine Products*** | |
| Lanacane Crème | Benzocaine 6%; benzethonium chloride 0.1% |
| Vagi-Gard Advanced Sensitive Cream<br>Vagisil Anti-itch Original Formula | Benzocaine 5%; resorcinol 2% |
| Vagisil Maximum Strength<br>Vagi-Gard Maximum Strength Cream | Benzocaine 20%; resorcinol 3% |
| Vagi-Gard Cream | Benzocaine 5%; benzalkonium chloride 0.13% |
| **Hydrocortisone Products†** | |
| Cortef Feminine Itch Cream<br>Massengill Medicated Towelette | Hydrocortisone 0.5% |
| Gyne-cort Female Cream | Hydrocortisone 1% |
| **Povidone–Iodine Products** | |
| Betadine Medicated Suppository‡ | Povidone–iodine 10% |
| Betadine Premixed Medicated Disposable Douche<br>Massengill Medicated Disposable Douche<br>Summer's Eve Special Care Medicated Douche | Povidone–iodine 0.3% (in disposable bottles) |
| **Homeopathic Products** | |
| Yeast-Gard Suppository§ | Pulsatilla (28X); Candida albicans (28X) Candida parapsilosis (28X) |
| Yeast-X Suppository‖ | Pulsatilla (28X) |
| **Other Products** | |
| Summer's Eve Feminine Powder¶ | Cornstarch; aloe; mineral oil |
| Vaginex# | Tripelennamine |
| Vagisil Feminine Powder¶ | Cornstarch; aloe; mineral oil |

* Apply benzocaine products externally.
† Apply hydrocortisone products externally; avoid prolonged use; may use concomitantly with antifungal products.
‡ Use 1 povidone–iodine suppository nightly for 7 days.
§ Use 1 Yeast-Gard suppository daily for 7 days.
‖ Use 1 Yeast-X suppository daily as needed.
¶ Apply feminine powders externally to absorb moisture.
\# Apply Vaginex externally 3 or 4 times/day.

Abdominal cramps (3%), penile irritation, and allergic reactions (3%-7%) are uncommon, and headache may occur in up to 9% of women.[1]

Because of the limited absorption of topical antifungals, drug interactions are unlikely. However, a case report documented an interaction between miconazole vaginal suppositories (100-200 mg) and warfarin.[29] In this patient, international normalized ratio (INR) levels were significantly increased on two occasions when vaginal miconazole was used. Miconazole and warfarin are both metabolized by cytochrome P-450 2C9, and concurrent use may decrease the clearance of warfarin and increase unbound drug. Reducing the dose of warfarin during concurrent therapy may avoid an increase in INR. Nonprescription vaginal antifungal product information warns women using warfarin in combination with these products that bleeding or bruising might occur. Aside from an allergy to the imidazoles, there are no contraindications to use of the vaginal imidazoles.

## Product Selection Guidelines

Self-treatment of VVC is not appropriate for girls younger than 12 years. This condition is rare in premenarchal girls, and any vaginal symptoms in this age group warrant evaluation by a primary care provider.

The topical imidazole antifungals are generally safe for use during pregnancy. However, self-treatment during pregnancy is not appropriate. Prescriber assessment is important to evaluate for complications (e.g., elevated blood sugar) and to assess for other vaginal organisms because

**TABLE 8-4 Guidelines for Applying Vaginal Antifungal Products**

1. Start treatment at night before going to bed. Lying down will reduce leakage of the product from the vagina.
2. Wash the entire vaginal area with mild soap and water, and dry completely before applying the product.
3. *Vaginal cream*: (If prefilled applicators are being used, skip to step 4.) Unscrew the cap; place the cap upside down on the end of the tube. Push down firmly until the seal is broken. Attach the applicator to the tube by turning the applicator clockwise. Squeeze the tube from the bottom to force the cream into the applicator. Squeeze until the inside piece of the applicator is pushed out as far as possible and the applicator is completely filled with cream. Remove the applicator from the tube.
   *Vaginal tablets/suppositories*: Remove the wrapper and place the product into the end of the applicator barrel.
4. While standing with your feet slightly apart and your knees bent, as shown in drawing A, or while lying on your back with your knees bent, as shown in drawing B, gently insert the applicator into the vagina as far as it will go comfortably.

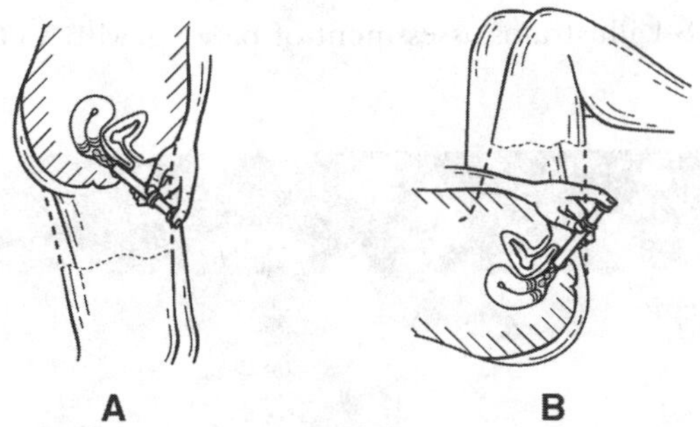


5. Push the inside piece of the applicator in and place the cream as far back in the vagina as possible. To deposit vaginal tablets/suppositories, insert the applicator into the vagina and press the plunger until it stops.
6. Remove the applicator from the vagina.
7. After use, recap the tube (if using cream). Then clean the applicator by pulling the two pieces apart and washing them with soap and warm water.
8. If desired, wear a sanitary pad to absorb leakage of the vaginal antifungal. Do not use a tampon to absorb leakage.
9. Continue using the product for the length of time specified in the product instructions. Use the product every day without skipping any days, even during menstrual flow.

bacterial vaginosis and trichomoniasis have the potential for adverse pregnancy outcomes. Breast-feeding women can use any of the nonprescription vaginal antifungals.[22]

*Patient Preferences* Selection of cream, tablet, or suppository formulations can be left to patient preference; some patients may prefer the convenience of prefilled applicators. Studies have found that women who have previously experienced VVC prefer shorter courses of therapy than do women who have not had a prior infection; physicians tend to prefer longer courses of therapy.[1] If vulvar symptoms are significant, a cream preparation or the combination of a cream with vaginal suppositories or tablets is preferred.

### *Alternative Therapies for Vaginitis*

An alternative approach to treating VVC is the use of *Lactobacillus acidophilus* preparations. The rationale for use of these preparations is to reestablish normal vaginal flora and inhibit overgrowth of *Candida* organisms. Data on the effectiveness of this approach are limited; one recent study examining the usefulness of *Lactobacillus* administered orally, vaginally, and via both routes found that none of these regimens protected against the development of post-antibiotic VVC.[30] However, eating yogurt with live cultures (8 oz daily) may be of some benefit in preventing recurrent VVC.[25,31,32]

Home remedies such as vaginal douches of yogurt or vinegar have also been used to treat this condition but are generally not effective. However, use of a sodium bicarbonate sitz bath (1 teaspoon in 1 pint of water; 2-4 tablespoons in 2 inches of bath water; sit in the sitz bath or bathtub for 15 minutes as needed for symptom control) may provide prompt relief of vulvar irritation associated with a candidal vaginal infection before antifungal agents can provide benefit.[21,33]

Some women may prefer herbal products to manage VVC. Herbal products reported for the treatment of VVC include garlic (orally and vaginally) and tea tree oil (vaginal preparations).[34,35] Garlic has both antibacterial and antifungal properties. The active ingredient is allicin, which is released when a clove of garlic is crushed. Garlic is typically administered as one crushed clove wrapped in unbleached gauze inserted vaginally at bedtime for 6 nights. Garlic may cause a burning sensation if significant irritation of the vaginal tissues is present because of the vaginitis; in this case using a whole uncut clove of garlic may be preferable. No serious side effects have been reported, although some women may experience an allergic reaction or chemical burns with prolonged intravaginal use.[34] Tea tree oil also has antibacterial and antifungal properties and *Lactobacillus* organisms are more resistant to tea tree oil than organisms associated with BV. The typical dose is 1 to 2 drops of tea tree oil in a capsule filled with calendula oil, vegetable oil, or water. It is administered as 2 capsules inserted vaginally at bedtime for 6 nights. A 200 mg vaginal suppository containing tea tree oil is also available commercially. It is used nightly for 6 nights. The possibility of allergic dermatitis exists.

### *Other Therapies*

Gentian violet (a dye) is an old treatment for VVC that is generally used today as therapy for resistant candidal infections. However, it is available on the nonprescription market and can be used as topical therapy; a tampon can be soaked in the dye and inserted into the vagina. The tampon is left in the vagina for several hours or overnight. Often a single application is adequate, but treated tampons can be used once or twice a day for up to 5 consecutive days. The major disadvantage of using gentian violet is that it can stain fabrics and skin.[22]

Another option for the treatment of VVC is boric acid. The regimen is boric acid 600 mg in a size 0 gelatin capsule inserted vaginally once or twice daily for 14 days. Boric acid 5% in lanolin can be applied topically for vulvar irritation.[2,4,36] Boric acid therapy is particularly useful for non–*C. albicans* infections, which are more likely to be resistant to the azole antifungals. High short-term cure rates have been reported (85%-95%) when boric acid is used following treatment failure with another antifungal.[36,37] For resistant cases, the therapy is used twice weekly for longer durations. Boric acid can be toxic and teratogenic; human fatalities have been reported from oral ingestion.[36] Counseling should be provided to explain that the capsule should not be ingested and pregnant women should not use boric acid.

## Assessment of VVC: A Case-based Approach

Many episodes of VVC are uncomplicated and can be effectively treated by topical antifungal agents.[4,21] In particular, women who experience episodes that are sporadic and uncomplicated (i.e., healthy women who are not immunocompromised and have no predisposing drug therapy) and women who predictably experience VVC following a course of antibiotic therapy are the best candidates for self-treatment.[21,23]

Determining the appropriateness of self-care and the likelihood of the presence of a candidal infection are important initial steps in advising a patient about the management of vaginal symptoms with nonprescription therapy.

Practitioners can advise patients when it is appropriate to self-treat for vaginal symptoms consistent with VVC, and when medical evaluation, including pelvic examination and laboratory examination of vaginal secretions, is indicated. Self-treatment is most appropriate when the woman meets the following three criteria:

1. Vaginal symptoms are infrequent (i.e., no more than three vaginal infections per year and no vaginal infection within the past 2 months).
2. At least one previous episode of VVC was medically diagnosed.
3. Current symptoms are mild to moderate, and consistent with the characteristic signs and symptoms of VVC—in particular, a nonmalodorous discharge.

Case 8-1 illustrates assessment of patients with VVC.

### CASE 8-1

| Relevant Evaluation Criteria | Scenario/Model Outcome |
|---|---|
| **Information Gathering** | |
| 1. Gather essential information about the patient's symptoms, including: | |
| a. description of symptom(s) (i.e., nature, onset, duration, severity, associated symptoms) | Patient is experiencing intense vulvar itching with mild pain and stinging when she urinates. |
| b. description of any factors that seem to precipitate, exacerbate, and/or relieve the patient's symptom(s) | Patient experienced sudden onset of symptoms late yesterday evening. |
| c. description of the patient's efforts to relieve the symptoms | She washed the perineal area, which relieved the itching for a short time. |
| 2. Gather essential patient history information: | |
| a. patient's identity | Elizabeth Reedy |
| b. patient's age, sex, height, and weight | 19 y/o F, 5'4", 124 lb |
| c. patient's occupation | College student |
| d. patient's dietary habits | Typically eats on the run on the way to class, usually high-carbohydrate foods |
| e. patient's sleep habits | Usually gets 5-6 hours of sleep per night |
| f. concurrent medical conditions, prescription and nonprescription medications, and dietary supplements | Alesse 1 daily; multivitamin 1 daily; ibuprofen 2 tablets (200 mg) every 4-6 hours as needed; Afrin 2 sprays in each nostril every 10-12 hours as needed. Also, finishing a course of amoxicillin 500 mg twice daily for a recent urinary tract infection |
| g. allergies | NKDA |
| h. history of other adverse reactions to medications | None |
| i. other (describe)______ | Elizabeth was diagnosed with a VVC infection 4 years ago and was also diagnosed with BV 1 1/2 years ago, and her current symptoms seem similar to her BV infection but there is a lack of odor. |

## CASE 8-1 (continued)

| Relevant Evaluation Criteria | Scenario/Model Outcome |
|---|---|
| **Assessment and Triage** | |
| 3. Differentiate the patient's signs/symptoms and correctly identify the patient's primary problem(s) (see Table 8-1). | Elizabeth has intense vulvar itching, discomfort with urination, and a lack of malodor consistent with a vaginal candidal infection. |
| 4. Identify exclusions for self-treatment (see Figure 8-1). | In a monogamous relationship and not at risk for STIs |
| 5. Formulate a comprehensive list of therapeutic alternatives for the primary problem to determine if triage to a medical practitioner is required, and share this information with the patient. | Options include:<br>(1) Refer Elizabeth for medical evaluation.<br>(2) Recommend self-treatment with an OTC vaginal antifungal product.<br>(3) Suggest Elizabeth consider the use of an OTC vaginal preparation for relief of her itching and irritation until she can see her PCP.<br>(4) Take no action. |
| **Plan** | |
| 6. Select an optimal therapeutic alternative to address the patient's problem, taking into account patient preferences. | Elizabeth has classic mild symptoms associated with VVC. She is completing a course of amoxicillin, which may predispose her to VVC. Her diet is high in carbohydrates, which may increase her risk of a VVC infection. She has no chronic medical problems and is a good candidate for self-treatment. |
| 7. Describe the recommended therapeutic approach to the patient. | You have several choices of OTC vaginal antifungal products. Since you have vulvar itching, a cream preparation or a combination pack will probably provide the best relief of your symptoms. See the box Patient Education for Vulvovaginal Candidiasis for instructions on proper use. |
| 8. Explain to the patient the rationale for selecting the recommended therapeutic approach from the considered therapeutic alternatives. | This treatment is appropriate because you have the characteristic symptoms of VVC, or vulvovaginal candidiasis, a fungal infection. Also, the antibiotic and your diet are likely predisposing factors (antibiotic and diet), your symptoms are mild to moderate, you have no contraindications to self-treatment, and you have infrequent vaginal infections. See your primary care provider if your symptoms do not improve within 3 days or are not gone within a week, if the vaginal discharge changes (particularly if it becomes malodorous), or if symptoms return within the next 2 months. |
| **Patient Education** | |
| 9. When recommending self-care with nonprescription medications and/or nondrug therapy, convey accurate information to the patient. | |
| a. appropriate dose and frequency of administration | Miconazole cream: insert vaginally once daily for 3 days; apply externally to the vulva as needed for itching. |
| b. maximum number of days the therapy should be employed | 3 days |
| c. product administration procedures | See Table 8-4. |
| d. expected time to onset of relief | Relief should occur in 24-48 hours; often some relief occurs within hours of the first application. |
| e. degree of relief that can be reasonably expected | All symptoms should be resolved within a week after beginning treatment. |
| f. most common side effects | Vulvovaginal burning and itching |
| g. side effects that warrant medical intervention should they occur | Significant stinging, burning, or itching that persists beyond the first 48 hours of treatment |
| h. patient options in the event that condition worsens or persists | See your primary care provider if symptoms do not improve in 3 days or worsen. |

**CASE 8-1 (continued)**

| Relevant Evaluation Criteria | Scenario/Model Outcome |
|---|---|
| i. product storage requirements | Product should be stored in a cool area; storage in the bathroom or bedside is appropriate for ease of use. |
| j. specific nondrug measures | None |
| 10. Solicit follow-up questions from patient. | (1) Are any of the nonprescription vaginal antifungal products better than any others? Are some regimens more effective than others?<br>(2) Will I develop VVC every time I use an oral antibiotic? |
| 11. Answer patient's questions. | (1) No. All of the products and regimens are equally effective.<br>(2) Not necessarily; however, you may be someone for whom oral antibiotic use will increase the likelihood of VVC. Daily intake of yogurt while taking an antibiotic can help reduce this risk of a VVC infection. |

Key: BC, bacterial vaginosis; NKDA, no known drug allergies; OTC, over-the-counter; STI, sexually transmitted infection; VVC, vulvovaginal candidiasis.

## Patient Counseling for VVC

Providers counseling patients considering self-treatment with the vaginal antifungals should emphasize the importance of (1) limiting self-treatment to appropriate circumstances such as the presence of mild to moderate classic symptoms, infrequent vaginal symptoms, and predictable antibiotic-associated VVC, and (2) seeking medical evaluation if symptoms persist beyond a week after treatment, if symptoms recur within 2 months, or if vaginal symptoms occur more than three times in a 12-month interval.

Patients should be informed that a short course of a nonprescription vaginal antifungal product will kill the "yeast" organisms that caused the infection. Label instructions should also be reviewed with the patient, stressing that the antifungal is to be used only once a day for the length of time specified on the label. The provider should advise the patient that symptomatic relief will likely begin within a day or so but that it may take a week for complete resolution of symptoms. The patient should also be advised of signs and symptoms that indicate medical attention is needed. The box Patient Education for Vulvovaginal Candidiasis lists specific information to provide patients.

## Evaluation of Patient Outcomes for VVC

Symptoms of VVC should improve within 2 to 3 days of initiation of therapy and resolve within 1 week. The length of treatment (particularly for 1-to-3-day treatments) does not directly correspond to the time of resolution of symptoms.

Follow-up with a phone call allows the provider to discuss treatment effectiveness (continued or altered symptoms) and the importance of adherence to the course of treatment. Persistent symptoms or new-onset symptoms that are incompatible with VVC are reasons for advising the patient to see her primary care provider.

# ATROPHIC VAGINITIS

Atrophic vaginitis is inflammation of the vagina related to atrophy of the vaginal mucosa secondary to decreased estrogen levels.

## Epidemiology of Atrophic Vaginitis

An estimated 10% to 40% of postmenopausal women have symptomatic atrophic vaginitis, but only 20% to 25% of symptomatic women seek treatment.[38] Dyspareunia, a symptom sometimes related to inadequate vaginal lubrication or atrophic vaginitis, is common. In one primary care study, 46% of sexually active women of all ages reported dyspareunia; this compares with other studies that reported a prevalence of 17% to 34% (a result of varying definitions of dyspareunia).[39]

## Etiology of Atrophic Vaginitis

During menopause, the postpartum period, and breastfeeding, the vaginal epithelium becomes thin and vaginal lubrication declines secondary to a decrease in estrogen levels. Women may experience atrophic vaginitis and associated dyspareunia during these intervals.[22,38] The most common cause of dyspareunia is a lack of adequate vaginal lubrication. Atrophic vaginitis may also occur among women with a decrease in ovarian estrogen production (e.g., radiation therapy, chemotherapy) or in women who are taking antiestrogenic medications such as clomiphene, medroxyprogesterone, tamoxifen, raloxifene, danazol, leuprolide, and nafarelin.[22,38] Rarely, a low-estrogen oral contraceptive may cause atrophic vaginitis secondary to an unphysiologic/undesirable estrogen–progestin balance.[9]

## Signs and Symptoms of Atrophic Vaginitis

Generally, a long-term decrease in estrogen levels is required for atrophic vaginitis to occur. An early symptom of atrophic vaginitis is a decrease in vaginal lubrication;[38] other symptoms include vaginal irritation, dryness, burning, itching, leukorrhea, and dyspareunia. A thin, watery (occasionally bloody), or yellow malodorous vaginal discharge or "spotting" may also be present.[4,7,38] Sexual activity may result in vaginal bleeding or spotting. Any postmenopausal vaginal bleeding needs to be evaluated, as it is presumed to be endometrial cancer until proven otherwise. Dyspareunia may result in emotional distress.

## PATIENT EDUCATION FOR VULVOVAGINAL CANDIDIASIS

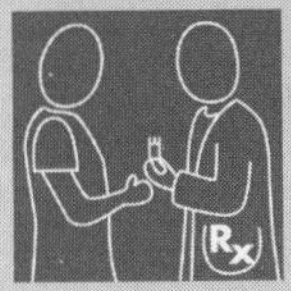

The goals of self-treatment are to (1) cure the vaginal fungal infection and (2) reestablish normal vaginal flora. Carefully following the product instructions and the self-care measures listed here will help ensure optimal therapeutic outcomes.

### Nondrug Measures

- If significant irritation of the vulva is present, use a sodium bicarbonate sitz bath to provide relief and give the antifungal medication time to become effective.
- If you have recurrent infections, try eating yogurt (1 cup per day of live culture yogurt) and decreasing sugar and refined carbohydrates in your diet.

### Nonprescription Medications

- Insert the antifungal product into the vagina once a day, preferably at bedtime to minimize leakage from the vagina. Use a sanitary pad or panty liner to avoid staining of underwear.
- See Table 8-4 for instructions on administering vaginal antifungals. You should have significant relief of symptoms within 24 to 48 hours. Some relief is often apparent within hours after the first dose. However, the length of treatment (particularly for 1- to 3-day treatments) does not directly correspond to the time of resolution of symptoms.
- Continue the therapy for the recommended length of time, even if your symptoms are gone. Stopping treatment early is one of the most common reasons for recurrence of vaginal symptoms and, possibly, occurrence of difficult to treat organisms.
- Note that vaginal antifungals can be used during a menstrual period. If desired, wait and treat the infection after menses end. Do not, however, interrupt a course of therapy because your period begins.
- Do not use tampons or douche while using a vaginal antifungal product and for 3 days after use.
- Although side effects are uncommon, the first dose of the antifungal may cause some vaginal burning and irritation and a few women (about 1 in 10) experience a headache.
- Refrain from sexual intercourse during treatment with the vaginal antifungal. Vaginal lubricants and vaginal spermicides should not be used at the same time as the vaginal antifungal. Vaginal antifungals can damage latex condoms and diaphragms, and may result in unreliable contraceptive effects. Do not use these contraceptives during therapy or for 3 days after therapy because the antifungal medication remains in the vagina for several days.
- Do not use vaginal antifungals if
  - You are less than 12 years old.
  - You are pregnant.
  - You have diabetes mellitus, are HIV positive or have AIDS, or have impaired immune function, including use of medications that may impair function of the immune system.
- If you are breast-feeding, consult a primary care provider before using a vaginal antifungal.

⚠ Seek medical attention if symptoms do not improve within 3 days or if symptoms persist beyond 7 days.

⚠ Seek medical attention if vaginal symptoms worsen or change, especially if the vaginal secretions become bad-smelling, frothy, or discolored, or if other symptoms (e.g., abdominal tenderness) occur. These events may indicate that the *Candida* ("yeast") organisms are resistant to the nonprescription therapy or that another type of vaginal infection is present.

## Treatment of Atrophic Vaginitis

Self-treatment of atrophic vaginitis is limited to alleviating the primary symptom, vaginal dryness, with lubricant products. Preventing vaginal dryness requires prescription ERT, a measure often recommended for women at menopause. Women who are breast-feeding or have recently given birth often have temporary declines in estrogen levels. Vaginal lubricants may be needed only until estrogen levels return to normal.

### *Treatment Goals*

The goal of therapy is to (1) reduce or eliminate the symptoms of vaginal dryness, burning, and itching and (2) eliminate dyspareunia, if vaginal dryness causes discomfort during or interferes with sexual intercourse.

### *General Treatment Approach*

Vaginal dryness can often be treated with nonprescription topical lubricants such as those listed in Table 8-5. One study found that about half of women with vaginal dryness tried "something," including substances such as butter, baby oil, and petroleum jelly (Vaseline), before seeking medical attention.[40] Among women with dyspareunia in one primary care study,[39] 10% had tried a nonprescription analgesic and 62% had done nothing; there was little use of personal lubricant products. Many women are likely to be inadequately treating dyspareunia given the apparent lack of knowledge about personal lubricant products.[39] Sexual arousal and intercourse can improve atrophic vaginitis, and women who are sexually active have fewer symptoms of atrophic vaginitis.[38]

Self-treatment is appropriate when the symptoms are mild to moderate, are confined to the vaginal area, and no bleeding is present. Self-treatment is most appropriate for women who have previously been able to maintain adequate vaginal lubrication. Severe vaginal dryness, dyspareunia, or bleeding warrants medical evaluation (Figure 8-2). In addition, products that may aggravate vaginal symptoms (e.g., irritants and allergens such as powders, perfumes, spermicides, and panty liners) should be avoided.[38]

Figure 8-2 outlines the treatment of vaginal dryness associated with atrophic vaginitis.

### *Pharmacologic Therapy (Vaginal Lubricants)*

A number of water-soluble products for vaginal lubrication (e.g., Astroglide, K-Y Jelly, Replens) are available on the nonprescription market. Personal lubricant products act to temporarily moisten vaginal tissues. These products provide

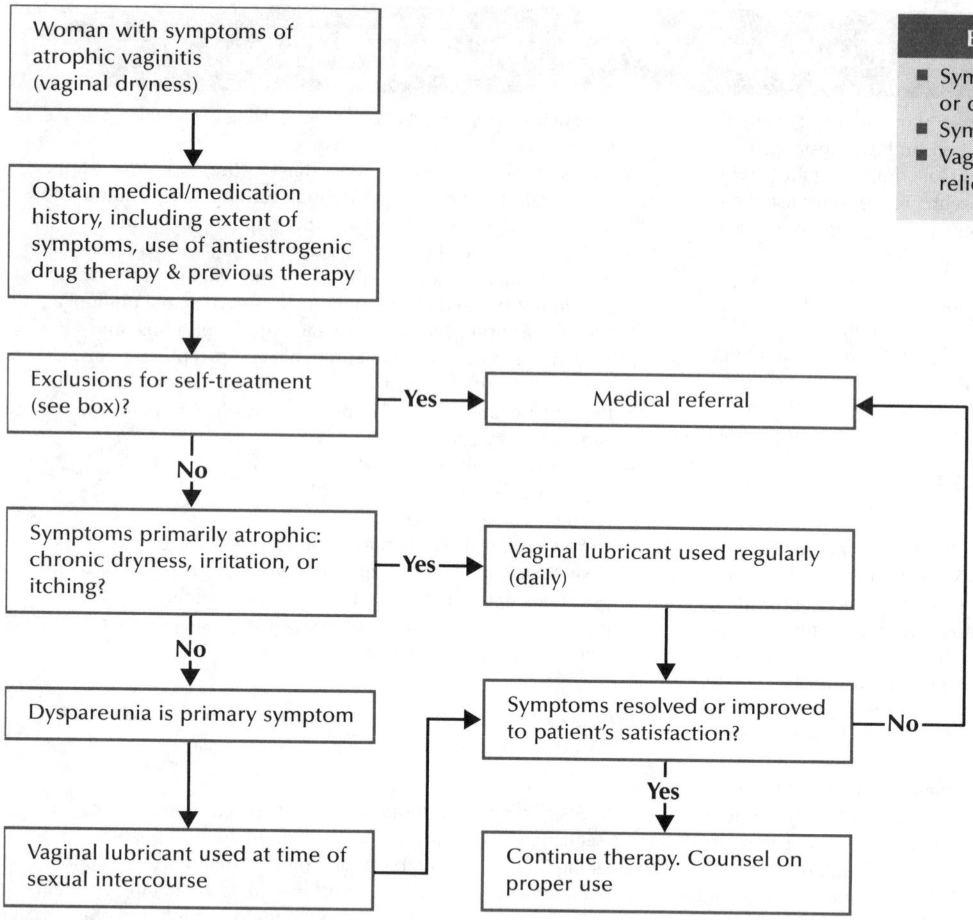

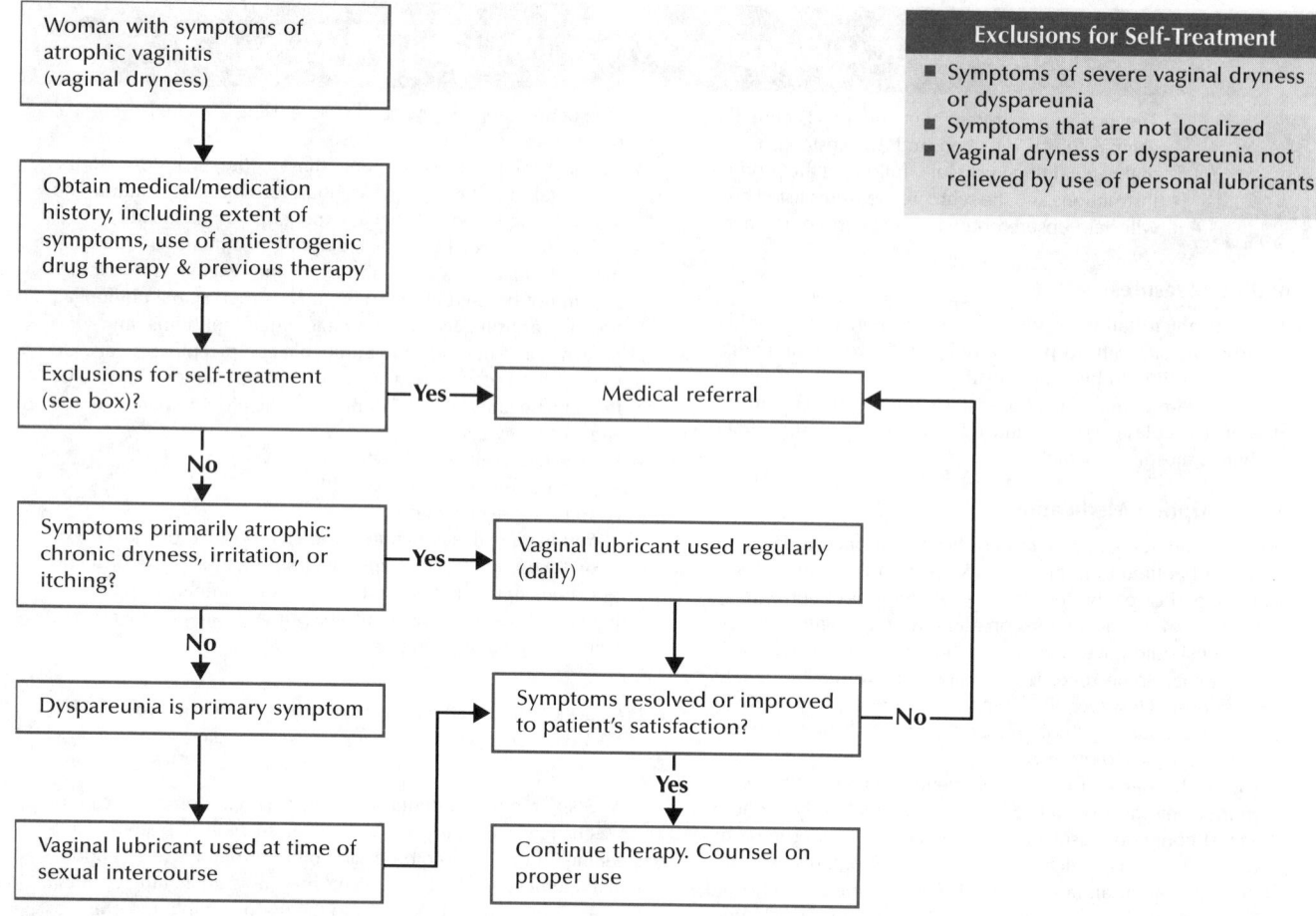

**FIGURE 8-2** Self-care of atrophic vaginitis.

**Exclusions for Self-Treatment**

- Symptoms of severe vaginal dryness or dyspareunia
- Symptoms that are not localized
- Vaginal dryness or dyspareunia not relieved by use of personal lubricants

**TABLE 8-5 Selected Vaginal Lubricants**

| Trade Name | Primary Ingredients |
|---|---|
| Astroglide | Glycerin; propylene glycol |
| H-R Lubricating Jelly | Hydroxypropyl methylcellulose |
| K-Y Jelly | Glycerin; hydroxyethylcellulose |
| K-Y Personal Lubricant Liquid | Glycerin; propylene glycol |
| K-Y Silk-E Vaginal Moisturizer | Vitamin E; propylene glycol gel |
| K-Y Warming Liquid Personal Lubricant | Propylene glycol; glycerin; acacia honey type O |
| Liquid Silk | Propylene glycol |
| Lubrin Suppositories | Caprylic/capric triglyceride; glycerin |
| Maxilube Jelly | Silicone oil; glycerin |
| Moist Again Vaginal Moisturizing Gel | Aloe vera; glycerin |
| Replens Gel | Glycerin; mineral oil |
| Surgel | Propylene glycol; glycerin |
| Vagisil Intimate Moisturizer Lotion* | Glycerin; propylene glycol |
| Women's Health Formula Lubricating Gel | Chlorhexidine gluconate; glycerin |

* Fragrance-free.

short-term improvement in atrophic vaginal symptoms, such as relief from burning and itching. Personal lubricants can also provide adequate vaginal lubrication to facilitate sexual intercourse.

Vaseline should not be used because it is difficult to remove from the vagina. If the patient is using a latex condom or diaphragm, only water-soluble lubricants should be used because other products (e.g., Vaseline) may damage the latex and impair the efficacy of these contraceptive methods. Water-soluble lubricant gels can be applied both externally and internally. Initially, the patient should be instructed to use a liberal quantity of lubricant (up to 2 tablespoons) and then to tailor the quantity and frequency of use to her specific needs. Most lubricant products provide an improvement in symptoms for less than 24 hours.[38] If the patient is treating dyspareunia, the lubricant should be applied to both the vaginal opening and the penis. If the use of nonprescription lubricants does not produce adequate benefit or is esthetically unappealing to the patient, she should be referred for medical evaluation.

## Assessment of Atrophic Vaginitis: A Case-based Approach

When discussing symptoms of vaginal dryness, patient assessment should include obtaining a description of symptoms (including the association with sexual intercourse) and their severity, as well as information about whether the woman has recently given birth, is lactating, or is perimenopausal or postmenopausal. The practitioner should question patients about the use of any vaginal or feminine hygiene products because such products may cause or worsen vaginal irritation and dyspareunia. Case 8-2 gives an example of assessment of patients with atrophic vaginitis.

### CASE 8-2

| Relevant Evaluation Criteria | Scenario/Model Outcome |
|---|---|
| **Information Gathering** | |
| 1. Gather essential information about the patient's symptoms, including: | |
| a. description of symptom(s) (i.e., nature, onset, duration, severity, associated symptoms) | Patient is experiencing vaginal dryness, irritation, and no vaginal bleeding. |
| b. description of any factors that seem to precipitate, exacerbate, and/or relieve the patient's symptom(s) | She is postmenopausal; she was taking oral estrogen but stopped because of concern about possible side effects. |
| c. description of the patient's efforts to relieve the symptoms | Previous use of oral estrogen |
| 2. Gather essential patient history information: | |
| a. patient's identity | Annette Warwick |
| b. patient's age, sex, height, and weight | 59 y/o F; 5'7", 160 lb |
| c. patient's occupation | Psychologist, counselor |
| d. patient's dietary habits | Healthy diet—limits red meat, dietary cholesterol, and fats; eats plenty of fruits and vegetables |
| e. patient's sleep habits | She reports that she is not getting enough sleep—too many hours at work; plans to cut back on her hours at work. |
| f. concurrent medical conditions, prescription and nonprescription medications, and dietary supplements | HCTZ 50 mg daily for hypertension; Zetia 10 mg daily for hypercholesterolemia; Quercetin-C 400 mg 3 times/day for allergies; SAMe 200 mg 3 times/day for arthritis |
| g. allergies | NKDA |
| h. history of other adverse reactions to medications | Statins—muscle aches, irritability |
| i. other (describe)______ | Discontinuation of Premarin 0.625 mg about 6 months ago |
| **Assessment and Triage** | |
| 3. Differentiate the patient's signs/symptoms and correctly identify the patient's primary problem(s). | AW is postmenopausal. She has vaginal dryness with no symptoms indicative of other vaginal infections. She had this symptom previously; it was treated with oral estrogen, which she recently discontinued. The symptom and her history are consistent with atrophic vaginitis. |

## CASE 8-2 (continued)

| Relevant Evaluation Criteria | Scenario/Model Outcome |
|---|---|
| 4. Identify exclusions for self-treatment (see Figure 8-2). | None |
| 5. Formulate a comprehensive list of therapeutic alternatives for the primary problem to determine if triage to a medical practitioner is required, and share this information with the patient. | Options include:<br>(1) Recommend self-treatment with a vaginal lubricant.<br>(2) Refer AW to her PCP for possible vaginal estrogen therapy.<br>(3) Suggest AW consider use of a vaginal lubricant for symptom improvement until she can see her PCP.<br>(4) Take no action. |
| **Plan** | |
| 6. Select an optimal therapeutic alternative to address the patient's problem, taking into account patient preferences. | Since AW has decided not to use oral estrogens, she should try a vaginal lubricant product. A lubricant product may provide adequate relief for generalized vaginal dryness. If it does not provide adequate relief, then she will have to discuss prescription (vaginal) estrogen with her PCP. |
| 7. Describe the recommended therapeutic approach to the patient. | See the box Patient Education for Atrophic Vaginitis. |
| 8. Explain to the patient the rationale for selecting the recommended therapeutic approach from the considered therapeutic alternatives. | A vaginal lubricant may relieve your symptoms. If it does not, you will likely have to consider use of a topical (vaginal) estrogen product (e.g., Estring). There are vaginal estrogen products with limited or no systemic estrogenic effects. |
| **Patient Education** | |
| 9. When recommending self-care with nonprescription medications and/or nondrug therapy, convey accurate information to the patient. | |
| a. appropriate dose and frequency of administration | See the box Patient Education for Atrophic Vaginitis. |
| b. maximum number of days the therapy should be employed | No limitations on length or dosing (quantity used) of lubricant therapy |
| c. product administration procedures | See the box Patient Education for Atrophic Vaginitis. |
| d. expected time to onset of relief | For generalized vaginal dryness, some relief should be apparent initially, but optimal effect will likely be noted only after the product has been used regularly for several weeks. |
| e. degree of relief that can be reasonably expected | Vaginal lubricants may decrease symptoms. However, these products are often unable to provide adequate relief of generalized vaginal dryness. |
| f. most common side effects | Leakage of product from vagina |
| g. side effects that warrant medical intervention should they occur | None |
| h. patient options in the event that condition worsens or persists | Referral for medical evaluation |
| i. product storage requirements | Product should be stored in a cool dry place. |
| j. specific nondrug measures | None |
| 10. Solicit follow-up questions from patient. | (1) How often can I apply the lubricant?<br>(2) If this doesn't work for me, will I have to take oral estrogen? |
| 11. Answer patient's questions. | (1) Vaginal lubricants can be applied as often as required in the quantity needed to keep you comfortable.<br>(2) Oral estrogen therapy is usually not necessary for the treatment of atrophic vaginitis; vaginal estrogen products (creams, tablets, or Estring) are options. Vaginal products are often effective when used only intermittently (e.g., twice a week). |

Key: HCTZ, hydrochlorothiazide; NKDA, no known drug allergies; OTC, over-the-counter; PCP, primary care provider.

## PATIENT EDUCATION FOR ATROPHIC VAGINITIS

The objective of self-treatment with vaginal lubricants is to relieve vaginal dryness or pain during sexual intercourse related to atrophic vaginitis. Carefully following product instructions and the self-care measures listed here will help ensure optimal therapeutic outcomes.

- Apply the vaginal lubricant as frequently as needed for relief of atrophic symptoms (vaginal dryness, irritation, burning, or itching) or inadequate vaginal lubrication.
- Begin treatment of atrophic symptoms with a liberal quantity of lubricant (2 tbsp); tailor subsequent doses to the quantity and frequency of use needed to provide relief.
- If using lubricants at the time of sexual intercourse, apply the lubricant to the vagina, particularly at the vaginal opening, and to the penis.
- Some leakage of product will occur. If desired, use a sanitary napkin or panty liner to avoid staining of underwear.

Relief of symptoms may be apparent within hours after the first dose. Regular application of a lubricant can reverse atrophic symptoms to some extent. If no improvement is noticeable within a week or if symptoms worsen or there is any vaginal bleeding, see a primary care provider.

### Patient Counseling for Atrophic Vaginitis

The practitioner should stress the short-term nature of atrophic vaginitis to women who are breast-feeding or who recently gave birth. Women who are perimenopausal or postmenopausal should know that long-term treatment with vaginal lubricants may be necessary. In either case, the practitioner should explain the proper use of the lubricants for treatment of vaginal dryness or dyspareunia. The box Patient Education for Atrophic Vaginitis lists specific information to provide to patients.

### Evaluation of Patient Outcomes for Atrophic Vaginitis

Symptoms of atrophic vaginitis should improve within a week. The practitioner should advise the patient to call to discuss treatment effectiveness if she has any questions or concerns and to call after 1 week of treatment to report progress in resolution of the symptoms. Symptoms that persist or the presence of bleeding requires medical evaluation.

## VAGINAL DOUCHING

### Prevalence of Douching

The 1995 National Survey of Family Growth reported that 27% of U.S. women douche on a regular basis. Douching rates were influenced by race, geographic region, socioeconomic status, and education. Race and education are important predictors of douching practices: among black women, 70% of those who had not completed high school douched compared with 40% of those with a college degree, whereas among white women, 53% of those who had not completed high school douched compared with only 9% of women with a college degree.[41] Geographic region was another strong predictor of douching. A telephone survey of southern U.S. women 18 to 88 years of age found that almost 80% had douched at some point during their lives and 60% had begun the practice before or at age 20.[42] Most women who report douching state that they began the practice as adolescents. A recent study of 250 black adolescents found that the mean age at which douching was initiated was 16 years.[43] Similar to the data for older women, adolescents residing in the South are more likely to douche. A study of Texas adolescents (mean age 18 years) found that 70% had douched and 51% douched at least once a week.[42] In 2002, gross sales of douche products were $58.1 million.[44]

The most frequently stated reason for douching is to achieve good vaginal hygiene. Because vaginal douches mechanically irrigate the vagina, clearing away mucus and other accumulated debris, they may be used as cosmetic cleansing agents. Among the women in a focus group study,[41] most considered it part of normal feminine hygiene, and most reported douching after menstruation and sexual intercourse. These women also stated that douching was done to ensure vaginal cleanliness and eliminate odors. Another reported reason for douching is to enhance the sexual experience. Over half of adolescents in one survey had heard that douching could dry and tighten the vagina for sexual purposes.[45]

### Potential Adverse Effects of Douching

Studies have not shown douching to be either safe or desirable. Conversely, although many studies have found an association between douching and adverse health outcomes, it is unclear if this is a causal relationship.[46] Frequent douching has been associated with an increased risk for PID, reduced fertility, ectopic pregnancy, vaginal infections (e.g., bacterial vaginosis), sexually transmitted infections, low birth weight, and cervical cancer.[41,43] Additional possible problems include irritation or sensitization from douche ingredients and disruption of normal vaginal flora and pH. Local irritation, sensitization, and contact dermatitis are also possible with many antimicrobial agents found in douches.

The effect of douches on vaginal flora varies depending on the douche ingredients and frequency. The most commonly used douche is a commercially prepared water–vinegar solution.[42,47] Studies have found that water–vinegar douches had little to no effect on lactobacilli, but inhibited some vaginal pathogens, whereas douches containing antiseptics inhibited all vaginal flora.[47,48] Povidone–iodine (e.g., Betadine) has a greater potential than acetic acid douches to reduce total bacteria, but may allow pathogenic species to proliferate, increasing the risk for vaginal infection.[49] Although few allergic reactions have been reported with intravaginal povidone–iodine, it may be systemically absorbed and should not be used by individuals allergic to iodine-containing products. Absorption poses a particular hazard to pregnant women; repeated vaginal applications may result in iodine-induced goiter and hypothyroidism in the fetus. Table 8-3 lists examples of douche products that contain povidone–iodine. Numerous nonmedicated douches are also available. Less frequent douching (less than once a week) was not associated with an increased risk of BV in a recent study.[47]

## Proper Use of Douche Equipment

Two types of syringes are available for douching purposes: douche bags and bulb douche syringes. The douche bag (fountain syringe or folding feminine syringe) holds 1 to 2 qt of fluid and comes with tubing and a shutoff valve. Two types of tips are supplied: one for enema use (the shorter rectal nozzle) and one for douching. The two tips are not interchangeable; vaginal infections may occur if a single tip is used for both douching and enemas.

Bulb douche syringes are available as both disposable and nondisposable products. The nondisposable units hold 8 to 16 oz of fluid, whereas the disposable units contain 3 to 9 oz. The flow rate is regulated by the amount of hand pressure exerted when the bulb is squeezed. Gentle pressure is recommended because excess pressure may force fluid through the cervix, causing uterine inflammation. Instructions for the proper use of these devices are found in Table 8-6.

## Patient Counseling for Douching

Practitioners should discuss a woman's reasons for douching. Women should be informed that douching is not necessary for cleansing of the vagina and that douching has potential adverse consequences. Douching for routine hygienic purposes should be discouraged, and douching is contraindicated during pregnancy. Douching should be delayed at least 6 to 8 hours after sexual intercourse if a vaginal spermicide was used as a contraceptive agent.

An alternative cleansing method for vaginal and perineal areas should be suggested, such as gently washing the vagina and the vulvar, perineal, and anal regions with the fingers using lukewarm water and mild soap. If a woman is douching to prevent or treat symptoms of a vaginal infection (e.g., an abnormal vaginal discharge), she should be counseled about more effective therapy or referred for medical evaluation, as appropriate.

Patients for whom douches have been prescribed or those who insist on douching for other reasons should be instructed on how to use these products safely, appropriately, and effectively. The box Patient Education for Douching lists specific information to provide these patients.

**TABLE 8-6 Administration Guidelines for Douches**

**Bulb Douche Syringe Method**

- Choose a douching position that is comfortable for you. Two positions are recommended: (a) sitting on the toilet or (b) standing in the shower. Whichever you choose, remember that douching is easier when you are relaxed.
- Gently insert the nozzle about 3 in. into your vagina. Avoid closing the lips of the vagina.
- Squeeze bottle gently, letting the solution cleanse the vagina and then flow freely from the body.
- After douching, throw away bottle and nozzle, if disposable.

**Douche Bag Method**

- Fill the douche bag with the prescribed solution or with a warm water and vinegar solution.
- Lie back in the tub with knees bent. Place the douche bag about 1 ft above the height of your hips. Do not place it or hang it any higher because such height will cause the pressure of fluid entering the vagina to be too high.
- Insert the nozzle several inches into the vagina. Aim the nozzle up and back toward the small of the back. While holding the labia closed around the nozzle, release the clamp slowly to allow fluid to enter the vagina. Rotate the tip and allow fluid to enter the vagina until the vagina feels full. Stop the flow of fluid; then hold the fluid in the vagina for about 30-60 seconds. Release and allow the fluid to flow out; repeat until the douche bag is empty.
- Wash the nozzle with mild soap and water.

## Key Points for Vaginal and Vulvovaginal Disorders

- Vaginal symptoms are often nonspecific, and it may be difficult to distinguish the three common vaginal infections. The symptom most likely to differentiate a candidal infection from BV and trichomoniasis is the absence of an offensive odor to the vaginal secretions. Measurement of vaginal pH (pH > 4.5 indicates a noncandidal infection) may also help to distinguish *Candida* and reduce inappropriate use of nonprescription antifungals.
- Vaginal candidal infections are typically caused by *Candida albicans*, but recently non–*C. albicans* infections have increased. These species of *Candida* may be more resistant to azole antifungals.
- Self-treatment for a vaginal candidal infection is most appropriate when the woman's symptoms are mild to moderate, there are no predisposing illnesses or medications, and symptoms are not recurrent. Recurrent infections are defined as four or more within a 12-month period and symptoms occurring within 2 months of previous vaginal symptoms.
- All of the azole antifungals are equally effective. Selection of length of regimen or time of day of administration can be determined by patient preference.
- Patients should be informed that symptoms typically improve shortly after application of the vaginal antifungals; symptoms should improve within 2 to 3 days after initiation of therapy and be resolved within a week. The

## PATIENT EDUCATION FOR DOUCHING

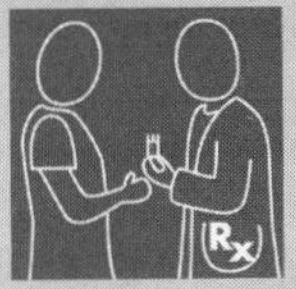

Improper methods of douching or too frequent douching can cause vaginal irritation. Douching can also increase the risk for pelvic inflammatory disease, ectopic pregnancy, and sterility. Strictly following the product instructions and the self-care measures listed here will help avoid these problems.

- Keep all douche equipment clean.
- Use lukewarm water to dilute products.
- Follow the appropriate instructions in Table 8-6 for the method of douching being used.
- Never instill a douche with forceful pressure.
- Do not use these products for birth control.
- Do not douche until at least 8 hours after intercourse during which a diaphragm, cervical cap, or contraceptive jelly, cream, or foam was used.
- Do not douche for at least 3 days after the last dose of vaginal antifungal medication.
- Do not douche for 48 hours before any gynecologic examination.
- Do not douche during pregnancy unless under the advice and supervision of a primary care provider.
- Use douches only as directed for routine cleansing.
- Do not douche more often than twice a week, except on the advice of a primary care provider.
- If vaginal dryness or irritation occurs, discontinue use of the douche.

length of the treatment regimen does not directly correspond to resolution of symptoms.

- Use of a sodium bicarbonate sitz bath can provide relief of itching and irritation prior to onset of benefit from the antifungal.
- Eating yogurt with live cultures (8 oz daily) may be of some benefit to patients in preventing recurrent VVC infections.
- Atrophic vaginitis, inflammation of the vagina secondary to decreased estrogen levels, can occur after menopause, postpartum, during breast-feeding, or as a result of antiestrogenic medications. Vaginal dryness and dyspareunia can be relieved by use of topical personal lubricant products. If symptoms do not improve within a week, medical evaluation is needed.
- Atrophic vaginitis may cause vaginal bleeding, however, any postmenopausal bleeding needs to be evaluated to rule out endometrial cancer.
- Douching is not necessary for vaginal cleansing, and adverse consequences of douching can occur. Douching is contraindicated during pregnancy and should be postponed until at least 8 hours after sexual intercourse if a vaginal spermicide was used for contraception.

## References


1. Reed BD. Vaginitis. In: Sloane PD, Slatt LM, Ebell MH, et al, eds. *Essentials of Family Medicine.* 4th ed. Philadelphia: Lippincott Williams & Wilkins; 2002.
2. Haefner HK. Current evaluation and management of vulvovaginitis. *Clin Obstet Gynecol.* 1999;42:184-95.
3. Cullins VA, Dominguez L, Guberski T, et al. Treating vaginitis. *Nurse Practitioner.* 1999;24:46-58.
4. Sobel JD. Vaginitis. *N Engl J Med.* 1997;337:1896-903.
5. Benjamin F. Anatomy, physiology, growth, and development. In: Seltzer VL, Pearse WH, eds. *Women's Primary Health Care.* New York: McGraw-Hill, Inc; 1995.
6. Cleveland A. Vaginitis: finding the cause prevents treatment failure. *Cleve Clin J Med.* 2000;67:634-46.
7. Quan M. Vaginitis: meeting the clinical challenge. *Clin Cornerstone.* 2000;3:36-47.
8. Nyirjesy P. Vaginitis in the adolescent patient. *Pediatr Clin North Am.* 1999;46:733-45.
9. Lipsky MS, Taylor C. The use of over-the-counter antifungal vaginitis preparations by college students. *Fam Med.* 1996;28:493-5.
10. Holzman C, Leventhal JM, Qui H, et al. Factors linked to bacterial vaginosis in nonpregnant women. *Am J Pub Health.* 2001;91:1661-70.
11. Soper D. Trichomoniasis: under control or undercontrolled? *Am J Obstet Gynecol.* 2004;190:281-90.
12. Foxman B, Barlow R, D'Arcy H, et al. Candida vaginitis: self-reported incidence and associated costs. *Sex Transm Dis.* 2000;27:230-5.
13. Thai L, Hart LL. Boric acid vaginal suppositories. *Ann Pharmacother.* 1993;27:1355-7.
14. Ferris DG, Dekle C, Litaker MS. Women's use of over-the-counter antifungal medications for gynecologic symptoms. *J Fam Pract.* 1996;42:595-600.
15. Moraes PSA, Taketomi EA. Allergic vulvovaginitis. *Ann Allergy Asthma Immunol.* 2000;85:253-67.
16. Coco A, Vandenbosche M. Infectious vaginitis: an accurate diagnosis is essential and attainable. *Postgrad Med.* 2000;107:63-74.
17. Roy S, Caillouette JC, Faden, JS, et al. Improving use of antifungal medications: the role of an over-the-counter vaginal pH self-test device. *Infect Dis Obstet Gynecol.* 2003;11(4):209-16.
18. Anderson MR, Caillouette JC, Faden, JS, et al. Evaluation of vaginal complaints. *JAMA.* 2004;291:1368-79.
19. Klebanoff M, Schwebke J, Zhang J, et al. Vulvovaginal symptoms in women with bacterial vaginosis. *Obstet Gynecol.* 2004;104:267-72.
20. Owen MK, Clenney TL. Management of Vaginitis. *Am Fam Physician.* 2004;70:2125-32, 2139-40.
21. Sobel JD, Faro S, Force RW, et al. VVC: epidemiologic, diagnostic, and therapeutic considerations. *Am J Obstet Gynecol.* 1998;178:203-11.
22. Suess JA, Holzman C. Vulvar and vaginal disease. In: Smith MA, Shimp LA, eds. *20 Common Problems in Women's Health Care.* New York: McGraw-Hill; 2000.
23. Sobel JD. *Candida* vulvovaginitis. *Semin Dermatol.* 1996;15:17-28.
24. ACOG Technical Bulletin (No. 226). Vaginitis. *Int J Gynaecol Obstet.* 1996;54:293-302.
25. Hilton E, Isenberg HD, Alperstein P, et al. Ingestion of yogurt containing *Lactobacillus acidophilus* as prophylaxis for candidal vaginitis. *Ann Intern Med.* 1992;116:353-7.
26. Upmalis DH, Cone FL, Lamia CA, et al. Single-dose miconazole nitrate vaginal ovule in the treatment of vulvovaginal candidiasis: two single-blind, controlled studies versus miconazole nitrate 100mg cream for 7 days. *J Women's Health Gender-based Med.* November 4 2000;9:421-9.

27. Brown D, Henzl MR, Kaufman RH, Gynazole Study Group. Butoconazole nitrate 2% for vulvovaginal candidiasis: new, single-dosed vaginal cream formulation vs. seven-day treatment with miconazole nitrate. *J Reprod Med.* November 1999;44(11):933-8.
28. Barnhart K. Safety and efficacy of bedtime versus daytime administration of the miconazole nitrate 1200mg vaginal ovule insert to treat vulvovaginal candidiasis. *Curr Med Res Opinions.* 2005;21: 127-34.
29. Elmer GW, Surawicz CM, McFarland LV. Biotherapeutic agents: a neglected modality for the treatment and prevention of selected intestinal and vaginal infections. *JAMA.* 1996;275:870-6.
30. Pirotta M, Gunn J, Chondros P, et al. Effect of lactobacillus in preventing post-antibiotic vulvovaginal candidiasis: a randomized controlled trial. *BMJ.* 2004;329(7465):548-51.
31. Shalev E, Battino S, Weiner E, et al. Ingestion of yogurt containing *Lactobacillus acidophilus* compared with pasteurized yogurt as prophylaxis for recurrent candidal vaginitis and bacterial vaginosis. *Arch Fam Med.* 1996;5:593-6.
32. Nyirjesy P, Seeney SM, Grody MH, et al. Chronic fungal infections: the value of cultures. *Am J Obstet Gynecol.* 1995;173(3 pt 1): 820-3.
33. Korenek P, Britt R, Hawkins C. Differentiation of the vaginosis-bacterial vaginosis, lactobacillosis, and cytolytic vaginosis. *Internet J Adv Nurs Pract.* 2003;6(1).
34. Van Kessel K, Assefi N, Marrazzo J, et al. Common complementary and alternative therapies for yeast vaginitis and bacterial vaginosis: a systematic review. *Obstet Gynecol Survey.* 2003;58(5): 351-8.
35. Reid G, Bocking A. The potential for probiotics to prevent bacterial vaginosis and preterm labor. *Am J Obstet Gynecol.* 2003;189: 1202-8.
36. Allen-Davis JT, Beck A, Parker R et al. Assessment of vulvovaginal complaints: accuracy of telephone triage and in-office diagnosis. *Obstet Gynecol.* 2002;99:18-22.
37. Ferris DG, Nyirjesy P, Sobel JD, et al. Over-the-counter antifungal drug misuse associated with patient-diagnosed vulvovaginal candidiasis. *Obstet Gynecol.* 2002;99:419-25.
38. Bachmann GA, Nevadunsky NS. Diagnosis and treatment of atrophic vaginitis. *Am Fam Physician.* 2000;61:3090-6.
39. Jamieson DJ, Steege JF. The prevalence of dysmenorrhea, dyspareunia, pelvic pain, and irritable bowel syndrome in primary care practices. *Obstet Gynecol.* 1996;87:55-8.
40. Sarazin SK, Seymour SF. Causes and treatment options for women with dyspareunia. *Nurse Pract.* 1991;16:30-41.
41. Lichtenstein B, Nansel TR. Women's douching practices and related attitudes: findings from four focus groups. *Women Health.* 2000;31:117-31.
42. Oh MK, Merchant JS, Brown P. Douching behavior in high-risk adolescents: what do they use, when and why do they douche? *J Pediatr Adolesc Gynecol.* 2002;15:83-8.
43. Schwebke JR, Desmond RA, Oh MK. Predictors of bacterial vaginosis in adolescent women who douche. *Sex Transm Dis.* 2004; 31:433-6.
44. ECRM-Online.com. Just the Facts Stats: Feminine Hygiene/Protection Overview. Available at: http://www. ecrm-epps.com/ Expose/V6_11/44.pdf. Accessed October 13, 2003.
45. Simpson T, Merchant J, Grimley Dm, et al. Vaginal douching among adolescents and young women: more challenges than progress. *J Pediatr Adolesc Gynecol.* 2004;17:249-55.
46. Monif GRG. The great douching debate: to douche, or not to douche. *Obstet Gynecol.* 1999;94:630-1.
47. Zhang J, Hatch M, Zhang D, et al. Frequency of douching and risk of bacterial vaginosis in African American women. *Obstet Gynecol.* 2004;104:756-60.
48. Pagvlova SI, Tao L. In vitro inhibition of commercial douche products against vaginal microflora. *Infect Dis Obstet Gynecol.* 2000; 8:99-104.
49. Onderdonk AB, Delaney ML, Hinkson PL, et al. Quantitative and qualitative effects of douche preparations on vaginal microflora. *Obstet Gynecol.* 1992;80:333-8.

CHAPTER 9

# Disorders Related to Menstruation

*Leslie A. Shimp*

The menstrual cycle is a regular physiologic event for women beginning during adolescence and usually continuing through late middle age. Women are able to self-treat for two common menstrual disorders: primary dysmenorrhea and premenstrual syndrome. Many women use nonprescription products and seek advice from practitioners on how best to manage symptoms of these disorders, including abdominal pain and cramping, irritability, and fluid retention. An understanding of the menstrual cycle will help both patients and practitioners make informed and appropriate decisions about self-care. Practitioners should also be familiar with common menstrual symptoms and disorders, as well as with the risks associated with menstrual products (e.g., toxic shock syndrome [TSS]).

## Physiology of the Menstrual Cycle

Menstruation results from the monthly cycling of female reproductive hormones. A single menstrual cycle is the time between the onset of one menstrual flow (menstruation or menses) and the beginning of the next.

The average age at which menarche (the initial menstrual cycle) occurs in U.S. women is 12 years; however, normal menarche may occur as early as age 10 or as late as age 16.[1] The onset of menstruation is influenced by a number of factors such as race, genetics, nutritional status, and body mass.

The menstrual cycle, on average, lasts 28 days; however, only 15% of women have a 28 day cycle.[2] Menstrual cycle length varies between 21 and 40 days.[2] Menses last, on average, 4 days (plus or minus 2 days).[3] Most of the blood loss occurs during days 1 and 2. The major components of menstrual fluid are endometrial cellular debris and blood. Average blood loss per cycle is 30 to 80 mL.[2] A loss of more than 80 mL per cycle or bleeding lasting longer than 7 days is considered abnormal and is associated with anemia.[2]

Two principal reproductive events, each hormonally controlled, occur during each menstrual cycle. The first event is the maturation and release of an ovum (egg) from the ovaries; the second is the preparation of the endometrial lining of the uterus for the implantation of a fertilized ovum. The events of the menstrual cycle (Figure 9-1) can be described in phases that reflect changes in either the ovary (follicular/ovulatory and luteal phases) or the uterine endometrium (menstrual/proliferative and secretory phases).[3] The follicular/ovulatory phase correlates with the menstrual/proliferative phase, and the luteal phase correlates with the secretory phase.

The menstrual cycle results from the hormonal activity of the hypothalamus, pituitary gland, and ovaries (hypothalamic-pituitary-ovarian axis). The hypothalamus plays the key role in regulating the menstrual cycle by producing gonadotropin-releasing hormone (GnRH). Low levels of estradiol and progesterone, present at the end of the previous menstrual cycle, stimulate the hypothalamus to release GnRH. GnRH stimulates pituitary gonadotroph cells to synthesize and secrete luteinizing hormone (LH) and follicle-stimulating hormone (FSH).

The first day of the menstrual flow is called day 1 of the cycle and is the beginning of the follicular phase in the ovary and of the menstrual/proliferative phase in the uterus. The follicular phase can range in length from several days to several weeks, but lasts an average of 14 days. During the follicular phase, FSH stimulates the maturation of a group of ovarian follicles. These maturing follicles secrete the estrogen estradiol, which promotes the growth of the uterine endometrium.

By about cycle day 8, a single ovarian follicle becomes dominant. The usual development of a single dominant follicle results in the ovulation of only one egg. The ovulatory phase of the cycle is approximately 3 days in length. During this phase, the LH surge (a 48-hour period when the pituitary secretes high levels of LH) occurs. The LH surge catalyzes the final steps in the maturation of the ovum, as well as stimulates production of prostaglandins and proteolytic enzymes necessary for ovulation (release of a mature ovum). Estradiol levels also decrease during the LH surge, sometimes with midcycle endometrial bleeding. Ovulation typically occurs within 24 to 36 hours after the LH surge begins.[4] Ovulation releases 5 to 10 mL of follicular fluid, which contains the oocyte mass; this event may cause abdominal pain (mittelschmerz) for some women.

The luteal phase is the time between ovulation and the beginning of menstrual blood flow. After the follicle ruptures, it is referred to as the corpus luteum. The luteal phase length is more constant, about 14 days (plus or minus 2 days), consistent with the functional period (about 10 to 12 days) of the corpus luteum.[3] The corpus luteum secretes progesterone, estradiol, and androgens. The increased levels of estrogen and progesterone alter the uterine endometrial lining; glands mature, proliferate, and become secretory (secretory phase) as the uterus prepares for the implantation of a fertilized egg. Progesterone and estrogen levels reach their peaks in the middle of the luteal phase, whereas levels of LH and FSH decline in response to the increased hormone levels. If pregnancy occurs,

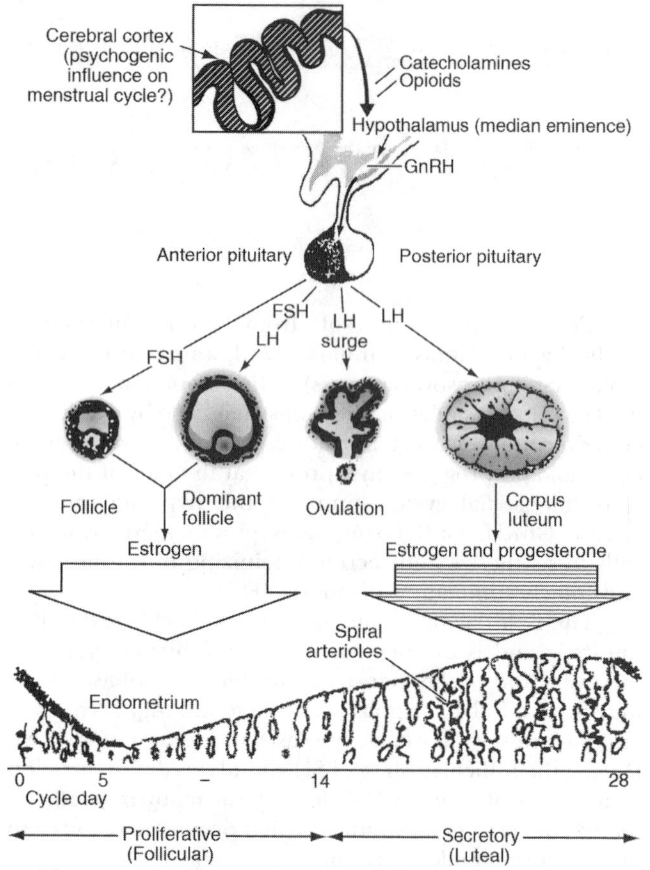


**FIGURE 9-1** Hormonal and anatomic relationships during menstrual cycle. There is also feedback from ovarian hormones estradiol and progesterone to the pituitary and the hypothalamus. (Reprinted with permission from Mattox JH. Normal and abnormal uterine bleeding. In: Mattox JH, ed. *Core Textbook of Obstetrics and Gynecology.* St. Louis: Mosby-Yearbook; 1998:397.)

human chorionic gonadotropin released by the developing embryo supports the function of the corpus luteum until the placenta develops enough to begin secreting estrogen and progesterone. If pregnancy does not occur, the corpus luteum ceases to function. Estrogen and progesterone levels then decline, causing the endometrial lining of the uterus to become edematous and necrotic. The decrease in progesterone also allows prostaglandin synthesis. Following prostaglandin-initiated vasoconstriction and uterine contractions, sloughing of the outer two endometrial layers occurs. The decline in estrogen and progesterone results in an increase in GnRH and in the renewed production of LH and FSH, which begins a new menstrual cycle.[3]

## DYSMENORRHEA

Dysmenorrhea (difficult or painful menstruation) is one of the most common gynecologic problems in the United States. Dysmenorrhea is divided into primary and secondary disease. Primary dysmenorrhea is idiopathic and associated with cramplike abdominal pain at the time of menstruation in the absence of pelvic disease. Secondary dysmenorrhea is usually associated with pelvic pathology.

### Epidemiology of Primary Dysmenorrhea

The prevalence of dysmenorrhea is highest in adolescence with up to 90% of young women being affected.[5] Primary dysmenorrhea usually develops within 6 to 12 months of menarche, generally affecting women during their teens and early 20s. Primary dysmenorrhea occurs only during ovulatory cycles; therefore, its prevalence increases between early and older adolescence as the regularity of ovulation increases.[6,7] Its prevalence decreases after the age of 25 years.

Approximately 15% of young women report that the pain associated with dysmenorrhea is severe.[6,7] Dysmenorrhea has been described as the single greatest cause of school absenteeism and lost working hours among adolescent girls and young women. Two large studies of adolescents found that 10% to 15% of girls reported missing school because of dysmenorrhea,[8] whereas a study of about 700 Hispanic girls found that 38% had missed school days because of dysmenorrhea.[9] Those reporting moderate or severe pain were two or four times as likely to miss school as those with mild pain. A study of freshman college women found that 25% of this group reported missing school, and 42% reported that at some time they had missed an activity because of dysmenorrhea.[8] In addition to school absence, girls with dysmenorrhea reported that it limited classroom concentration (59%), sports participation (51%), and going out with friends (46%).[9] Similarly, an estimated 600 million work hours are lost annually because of dysmenorrhea.[7]

The decrease in prevalence and severity in women in their late 20s and older may be partially explained by oral contraceptive use and pregnancy. Oral contraceptive use is more common after adolescence and is known to be an effective therapy for dysmenorrhea. During the last trimester of pregnancy, uterine adrenergic nerves virtually disappear and only a portion regenerate after childbirth.[7] This is believed to explain the disappearance of dysmenorrhea following childbirth for many women.

### Etiology of Primary Dysmenorrhea

The cause of primary dysmenorrhea is not fully understood, but it is known to be related to prostaglandin levels.[7,8] Both the endometrium and the myometrium of the uterus have the capacity to synthesize prostaglandins. Prostaglandin serum and endometrial levels are three to four times greater in women with dysmenorrhea than in women without dysmenorrhea and are highest during the first 2 days of menses, when dysmenorrhea commonly occurs.[8] Leukotrienes, inflammatory mediators known to cause vasoconstriction and uterine contractions, have also been found to be elevated in women with dysmenorrhea. It has been suggested that leukotrienes may contribute significantly to dysmenorrhea in women who do not respond to therapy with prostaglandin inhibitors (i.e., nonsteroidal anti-inflammatory drugs [NSAIDs]).[7] Similarly, vasopressin (a substance that can produce dysrhythmic uterine contractions) may play a role in the etiology of primary dysmenorrhea; circulating levels of vasopressin are fourfold higher in women with dysmenorrhea than in asymptomatic women.[7]

## Pathophysiology of Primary Dysmenorrhea

At the end of the luteal phase of the menstrual cycle, progesterone levels decrease, resulting in an increase in arachidonic acid, which is the precursor to both prostaglandins (notably $PGF_{2a}$) and leukotrienes. Prostaglandins stimulate uterine contractions and release vasopressin. Normal contractions and vasoconstriction help expel menstrual fluids and control bleeding as the endometrium sloughs.[6] However, the increased levels of prostaglandins, leukotrienes, and vasopressin present with dysmenorrhea can lead to strong uterine contractions and significant vasoconstriction, resulting in uterine ischemia and pain. During menses in women without dysmenorrhea, uterine contraction pressure is about 100 mm Hg. In women with dysmenorrhea, contractions occur often and pressures can reach 200 mm Hg.[10] Both intrauterine pressure and the frequency of uterine contractions contribute to ischemia and tissue hypoxia and, thus, to pain.

## Signs and Symptoms of Primary Dysmenorrhea

Primary dysmenorrhea pain is cyclic pain directly related to the onset of menstruation. It is typically experienced as a continuous dull aching pain with spasmodic cramping in the lower midabdominal or suprapubic region, which may radiate to the lower back and upper thighs. Uterine contractions can force prostaglandins into the systemic circulation, causing additional symptoms such as nausea, vomiting, fatigue, dizziness, irritability, diarrhea, and headache in about 50% of women.[6] The onset of pain is several hours prior to or coincident with the onset of menses and usually lasts less than 48 hours, but may persist up to 72 hours.[7] Primary dysmenorrhea usually initially occurs within the first 6 to 12 months after menarche, when ovulatory cycles are established.[5,7] This clinical presentation can be adequate for the diagnosis of primary dysmenorrhea if the pain is mild to moderate and the patient responds to NSAID therapy.

Secondary dysmenorrhea is suggested if dysmenorrhea initially begins years after menarche (at age 25 years or older); if pelvic pain occurs at times other than during menses and is not related to the first day of menses; or if the patient experiences irregular menstrual cycles, has menorrhagia (excessively prolonged or profuse menses), or a history of pelvic inflammatory disease (PID), dyspareunia, or infertility.[5,7] Causes of secondary dysmenorrhea include endometriosis, PID, ovarian cysts, uterine tumors, uterine fibroids, cervical os stenosis, inflammatory bowel disease, and congenital abnormalities.[7,11] Secondary dysmenorrhea may also be caused by the presence of an intrauterine device (IUD).

## Treatment of Primary Dysmenorrhea

Many women believe they are able to self-treat dysmenorrhea with nonprescription products. In one study,[12] 66% of women with dysmenorrhea did not see a clinician despite having moderate to severe symptoms, and 92% were satisfied with self-treatment.

### *Treatment Goals*

The goals of treating primary dysmenorrhea are to (1) provide relief or a significant improvement in symptoms and (2) minimize the disruption of usual activities.

### *General Treatment Approach*

An important initial step in managing dysmenorrhea is distinguishing between primary and secondary disease. Self-care is appropriate for an otherwise healthy young woman with a history consistent with primary dysmenorrhea who is not sexually active or a woman who has been diagnosed with primary dysmenorrhea.[5,6] Adolescents with pelvic pain who are sexually active (at risk for PID) and women with characteristics indicating secondary dysmenorrhea should be referred for medical evaluation. Table 9-1 compares primary and secondary dysmenorrhea.

Essentially all patients with primary dysmenorrhea can obtain adequate relief of symptoms with nondrug, nonprescription, or prescription drug therapy. Approximately 80% to 90% of women with primary dysmenorrhea can be successfully treated with NSAIDs, oral contraceptives, or both. Other treatment options include nonpharmacologic measures, such as use of topical heat, regular exercise, and discontinuation of tobacco smoking. These measures often serve as adjuncts to drug therapy although topical heat may be adequate as sole therapy for some women.

Figure 9-2 presents an algorithm for managing primary dysmenorrhea.

The patient with more severe dysmenorrhea, a change in the pattern or intensity of pain, intolerance to NSAIDs, or dysmenorrhea that does not respond to nonprescription therapy should be referred to her primary care provider. (Figure 9-2 lists exclusions for self-care.) A trial with other prescription NSAIDs or therapy with an oral contraceptive may be prescribed.

### *Nonpharmacologic Therapy*

Some adolescents do not use medication to manage dysmenorrhea and menstrual discomfort. One study of 289 adolescents found that common nondrug measures were rest (90% of respondents), heat (74%), wearing loose clothing (67%), exercise (57%), and rubbing or massaging where it hurt (54%). Respondents reported that heat, exercise, and rubbing/massage were about 50% effective in relieving their discomfort.[13] The use of heat is a commonly recommended nondrug therapy. An abdominal heat patch has been developed and tested for the treatment of dysmenorrhea.[14] The heat patch was significantly better (14% greater pain relief) than placebo and acetaminophen in relieving pain and cramping. Its analgesic effect had a faster onset than drug therapy, and it added to the relief provided by ibuprofen. Nondrug therapy may be especially useful for the estimated 15% of women who cannot tolerate or do not respond to nonprescription medications.[13]

**TABLE 9-1 Differentiation of Primary and Secondary Dysmenorrhea[5,6,11]**

| | Primary Dysmenorrhea | Secondary Dysmenorrhea |
|---|---|---|
| Age at onset of dysmenorrhea symptoms | Typically 6-12 months after menarche—age 12-13 years for most girls | Mid- to late 20s or older; usually 30s and 40s for women with secondary dysmenorrhea |
| Menses | More likely to be regular with normal blood loss | More likely to be irregular; menorrhagia more common |
| Pattern and duration of dysmenorrhea pain | Onset just prior to or coincident with onset of menses; pain with each or most menses, lasting only 2-3 days | Pattern and duration varies with cause; change in pain pattern or intensity also may indicate secondary disease |
| Pain at other times of menstrual cycle | No | Yes, may occur before, during, or after menses |
| Response to NSAIDs and/or oral contraceptives | Yes | No |
| Other symptoms | Nausea, vomiting, fatigue, dizziness, irritability, diarrhea, and headache may occur at same time as dysmenorrhea pain | Vary according to cause of the secondary dysmenorrhea; may include dyspareunia, pelvic tenderness |

Lifestyle alterations may alleviate symptoms to varying degrees. Smoking and exposure to secondhand smoke has been associated with more severe dysmenorrhea.[5] The severity reportedly increases with the number of cigarettes smoked per day. The basis for this effect is unknown, but it has been hypothesized that nicotine-induced vasoconstriction is involved. Evidence regarding the benefit of exercise is conflicting. Participation in regular exercise may lessen the symptoms of primary dysmenorrhea for some women.[5]

### *Pharmacologic Therapy*

The three nonprescription analgesic medications most commonly used by women to treat dysmenorrhea are acetaminophen, aspirin, and ibuprofen. A study[15] of adolescents (average age of 16 years) found that many more adolescents used acetaminophen than ibuprofen. Ninety-five percent reported using acetaminophen, 55% aspirin, and 42% ibuprofen; some used more than one agent. However, acetaminophen and aspirin are less effective than nonsalicylate NSAIDs for treating dysmenorrhea. In addition, aspirin is not recommended for use by adolescents because of its association with Reye's syndrome. In one study of girls who took acetaminophen or aspirin, only about one half found the administered analgesic to be effective.[16]

Furthermore, an evaluation of the doses and regimens used by adolescents showed that most tended not to use the maximum dosage recommended on nonprescription labels; only 31% took the recommended single dose (one to two pills) at the maximum suggested frequency of use (three to four times daily). A significant difference was found in the duration of discomfort between users who took recommended doses compared with those who took less, suggesting that adolescents may be experiencing discomfort from dysmenorrhea that could be relieved by more appropriate selection and dosage of nonprescription medications.[15] Delaying initiation of drug therapy may result in inadequate treatment or treatment failure.

Unfortunately, as these studies illustrate, many women with dysmenorrhea remain untreated or are inadequately treated. They continue to experience the pain and limitations on activity this condition imposes. The following sections outline the uses and properties of aspirin, acetaminophen, and the nonsalicylate NSAIDs as agents in the treatment of dysmenorrhea; Table 9-2 lists dosages for dysmenorrhea. Chapter 5 provides further discussion of their adverse effects, contraindications, and drug interactions, as well as a table describing all nonprescription internal analgesic products.

#### Aspirin

Aspirin may be adequate for treating mild symptoms of dysmenorrhea. However, in low doses, aspirin has only a limited effect on prostaglandin synthesis and is, therefore, only moderately effective in treating women with more than minimal symptoms of dysmenorrhea.[11] Aspirin may increase menstrual flow. In addition, adolescent girls should not use aspirin because of the potential for Reye's syndrome.

#### Acetaminophen

Like aspirin, acetaminophen may be adequate for treating only mild symptoms of dysmenorrhea. Acetaminophen, which has a minimal effect on prostaglandins, is known to be less effective than a nonsalicylate NSAID for the treatment of dysmenorrhea.[5,11]

#### Nonsalicylate NSAIDs

Three nonsalicylate NSAIDs are available as nonprescription products: ibuprofen 200 mg, naproxen sodium 220 mg, and ketoprofen 12.5 mg. In clinical trials, these NSAIDs were found to be effective in 66% to 90% of patients. However, clinical trial doses and currently recommended

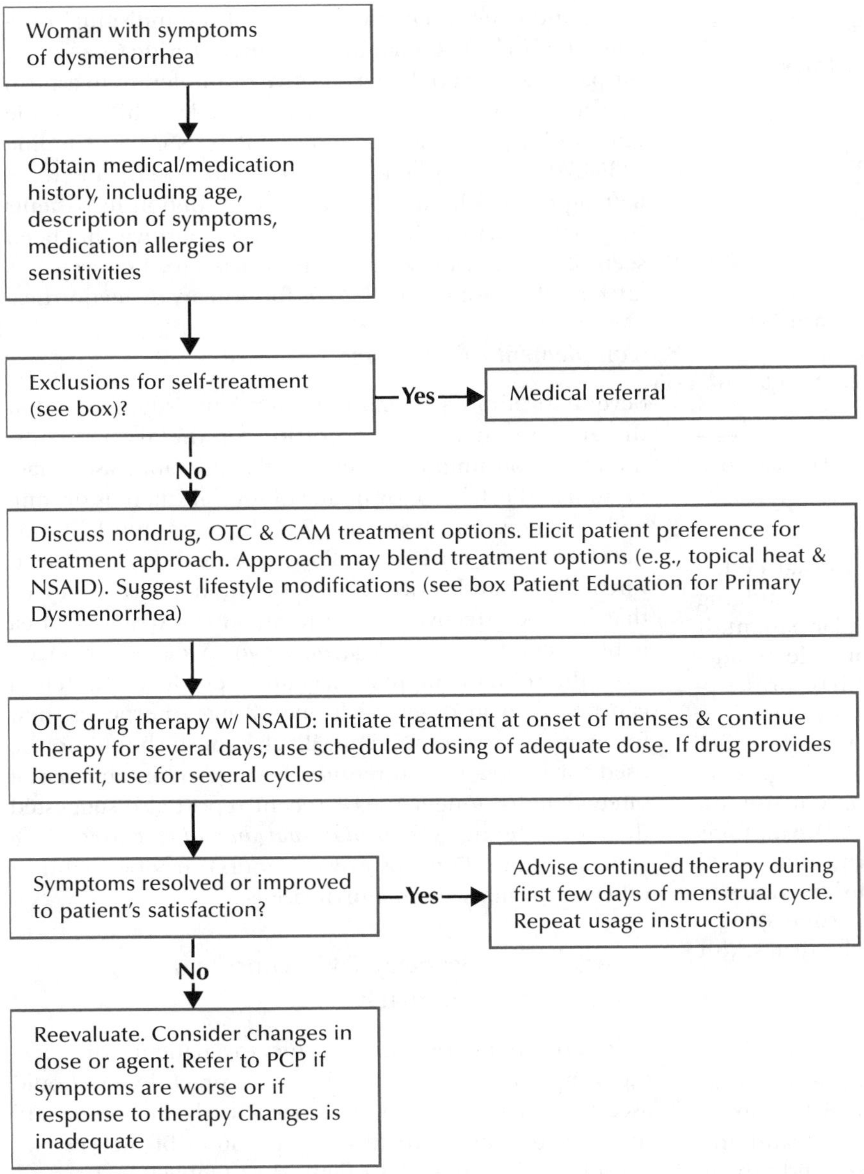

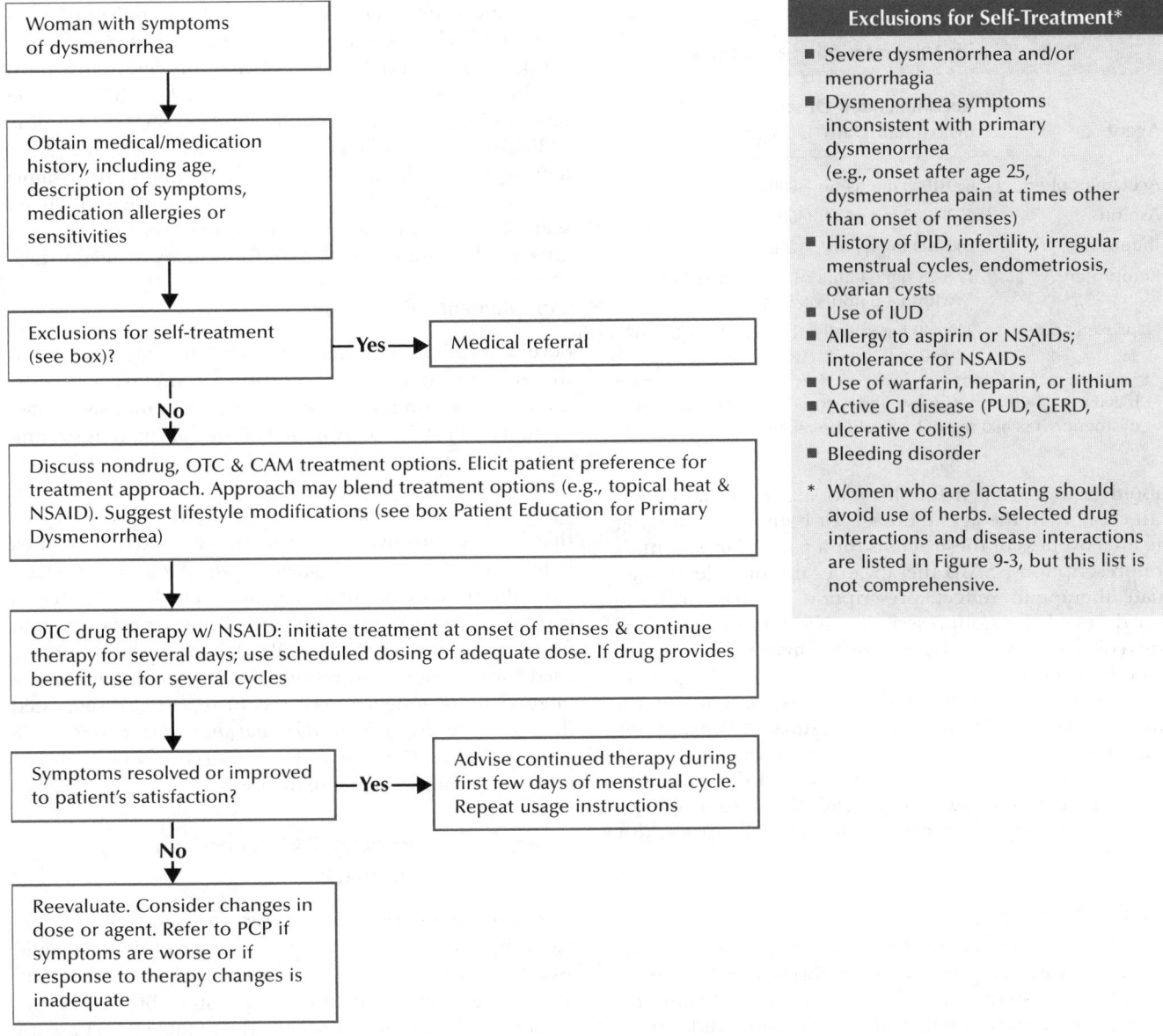

**Exclusions for Self-Treatment***

- Severe dysmenorrhea and/or menorrhagia
- Dysmenorrhea symptoms inconsistent with primary dysmenorrhea (e.g., onset after age 25, dysmenorrhea pain at times other than onset of menses)
- History of PID, infertility, irregular menstrual cycles, endometriosis, ovarian cysts
- Use of IUD
- Allergy to aspirin or NSAIDs; intolerance for NSAIDs
- Use of warfarin, heparin, or lithium
- Active GI disease (PUD, GERD, ulcerative colitis)
- Bleeding disorder

* Women who are lactating should avoid use of herbs. Selected drug interactions and disease interactions are listed in Figure 9-3, but this list is not comprehensive.

FIGURE 9-2 Self-care of primary dysmenorrhea. Key: CAM, complementary and alternative medicine; GERD, gastroesophageal reflux disease; GI, gastrointestinal; IUD, intrauterine device; NSAID, nonsteroidal anti-inflammatory drug; OTC, over-the-counter; PID, pelvic inflammatory disease; PCP, primary care provider; PUD, peptic ulcer disease.

prescription doses for the treatment of dysmenorrhea are often higher than the labeled nonprescription doses. Therefore, prescription therapy may be required if the maximum nonprescription dose does not provide adequate symptom relief.

Nonsalicylate NSAIDs are the principal nonprescription agents for treating primary dysmenorrhea. These agents inhibit the production and action of prostaglandins.

Therapy with nonsalicylate NSAIDs should begin at the onset of menses or pain; if inadequate pain relief occurs, treatment beginning 1 to 2 days before expected menses may improve symptom relief.[2] If the possibility of pregnancy exists, then therapy should be initiated only after menses begin. Patients should be instructed that the NSAID is used as much to prevent cramps as to relieve pain. Optimal pain relief is achieved when these agents are taken on a scheduled rather than an as-needed basis. Therefore, ibuprofen should be taken every 4 to 6 hours, ketoprofen every 4 to 8 hours, and naproxen sodium every 8 to 12 hours for the first 48 to 72 hours of menstrual flow because that time frame correlates with maximum prostaglandin release (Table 9-2). The therapeutic effect of these drugs is usually apparent within 30 to 60 minutes, and benefit will be optimal with continued regular dosing.

A patient with dysmenorrhea may respond better to one nonsalicylate NSAID than to another. If an adequate dose (or the maximum nonprescription dose) of one agent does not provide adequate benefit, then switching to another agent is recommended. The analgesic effect for most of these NSAIDs plateaus, so further dose increases may increase the risk of adverse drug effects rather than provide more benefit. Therapy with nonsalicylate NSAIDs

**TABLE 9-2 Treatment of Dysmenorrhea with Nonprescription Medications**

| Agent | Recommended Dosage (Maximum Daily Dosage) |
|---|---|
| Acetaminophen | 650-1000 mg q4-6h (4000 mg) |
| Aspirin | 650-1000 mg q4-6h (4000 mg) |
| Ibuprofen | 200-400 mg q4-6h* (1200 mg) |
| Ketoprofen | 12.5-25 mg q4-8h; not more than 25 mg within 4-6 hours (75 mg) |
| Naproxen sodium | 220-440 mg initially; then 220 mg q8-12h (660 mg) |

* If 200 mg q4-6h is ineffective, the recommended dosage for dysmenorrhea 400 mg q6h should be taken.

should be undertaken for three to six menstrual cycles, with changes in the agent, dosage, or both before judging the effectiveness of these agents for a particular patient. If nonprescription NSAID therapy does not provide an adequate therapeutic effect, prescription NSAIDs, prescription doses of the nonprescription NSAIDs, or use of an oral contraceptive or Depo-Provera may provide relief from dysmenorrhea.

Side effects from a few days of intermittent use are limited and usually include gastrointestinal (GI) symptoms (e.g., upset stomach, vomiting, heartburn, abdominal pain, diarrhea, constipation, anorexia) and side effects of the central nervous system (e.g., headache, dizziness). The GI side effects may be decreased by taking the drugs with food.

## Product Selection Guidelines

Nonsalicylate NSAIDs are the preferred nonprescription agents for treating primary dysmenorrhea. Selection of one of these agents should be based on cost and the patient's preference for the number of doses and tablets to take. Product selection should also be based on the side effect and drug interaction profile of the individual nonsalicylate NSAID. Acetaminophen may provide some relief for patients who are hypersensitive or intolerant to aspirin or who are intolerant to the GI and platelet-inhibition side effects of aspirin and the nonsalicylate NSAIDs. Choline (435-870 mg every 4 hours) or sodium salicylate (325-650 mg every 4 hours) may also be an option in patients hypersensitive to aspirin, since no cross-sensitivity has been seen. These nonprescription products are, however, less effective than aspirin or NSAIDs for primary dysmenorrhea.

### *Complementary Therapies*

Several preliminary small studies have suggested that dietary modifications—ingestion of dietary fish oils, increased consumption of eggs and fruit[17] (increased magnesium and calcium), or intake of several vitamins or minerals (magnesium,[18] vitamins $B_1$,[19] $B_{12}$,[20] vitamin E[21]) may decrease dysmenorrhea. All these potential therapies need further study and verification. A traditional herbal remedy that may be effective for the treatment of dysmenorrhea is black cohosh (*Cimicifuga racemosa*). A decoction made from the root, or the pharmaceutical product Remifemin can be taken in doses of 20 mg (2 mg triterpenes; new formulation) two times daily. Black cohosh should not be used for longer than 6 months because of an absence of safety data for longer use. A recent report also suggested that sweet fennel (*Foeniculum vulgare dulce*) extract (2% concentration; 25 drops every 4 hours) may be useful in relieving primary dysmenorrhea.[22]

## Assessment of Primary Dysmenorrhea: A Case-based Approach

Before recommending any product to a patient experiencing symptoms of dysmenorrhea, the practitioner should ascertain that the symptoms, particularly the onset and duration of pain in relation to the onset of menses, are consistent with primary dysmenorrhea (Table 9-1). Case 9-1 illustrates the assessment of patients with dysmenorrhea.

**CASE 9-1**

| Relevant Evaluation Criteria | Scenario/Model Outcome |
|---|---|
| **Information Gathering** | |
| 1. Gather essential information about the patient's symptoms, including: | |
| a. description of symptom(s) (i.e., nature, onset, duration, severity, associated symptoms) | Patient is experiencing significant menstrual cramps; she had to leave class at school today because of the pain. Her "period" started yesterday. This is the third month in the last four that her cramps were this severe. |
| b. description of any factors that seem to precipitate, exacerbate, and/or relieve the patient's symptom(s) | Her cramps are the worst at the beginning of her "period." Sometimes lying down for a while seems to help. The cramps occur only during the first 1-2 days of her period. |
| c. description of the patient's efforts to relieve the symptoms | She took some Tylenol. It did not help much and the school nurse suggested to her and her mother that she get something stronger at the pharmacy. |

## CASE 9-1 (continued)

| Relevant Evaluation Criteria | Scenario/Model Outcome |
|---|---|
| 2. Gather essential patient history information: | |
| a. patient's identity | Amanda Peterson |
| b. patient's age, sex, height, and weight | 14 y/o F; 5'4", 110 lb |
| c. patient's occupation | Student |
| d. patient's dietary habits | Healthy diet with some "junk food" |
| e. patient's sleep habits | She routinely gets enough sleep—sometimes she gets less sleep if she is up late doing school work. |
| f. concurrent medical conditions, prescription and nonprescription medications, and dietary supplements | Menarche about 6 months ago; multivitamin once daily |
| g. allergies | NKDA |
| h. history of other adverse reactions to medications | None |
| i. other (describe)_______ | N/A |
| **Assessment and Triage** | |
| 3. Differentiate the patient's signs/symptoms and correctly identify the patient's primary problem(s) (see Table 9-1). | Amanda appears to have primary dysmenorrhea—her pain fits the typical presentation of this condition—suprapubic cramping at the onset of her menses and it only occurs for the first 1-2 days of her menses. Her age is also consistent with the typical presentation of primary dysmenorrhea. |
| 4. Identify exclusions for self-treatment (see Figure 9-2). | None |
| 5. Formulate a comprehensive list of therapeutic alternatives for the primary problem to determine if triage to a medical practitioner is required, and share this information with the patient. | Options include:<br>(1) Recommend self-treatment with an NSAID, acetaminophen, or nonpharmacologic therapy.<br>(2) Refer AP to her PCP for evaluation.<br>(3) Suggest AP consider use of an NSAID for symptom improvement until she can see her PCP.<br>(4) Recommend a complementary therapy.<br>(5) Take no action. |
| **Plan** | |
| 6. Select an optimal therapeutic alternative to address the patient's problem, taking into account patient preferences. | Amanda's symptoms fit the typical presentation of primary dysmenorrhea and there are no exclusions for self-care. She might consider use of either topical heat via a heating pad or an abdominal heat patch or an NSAID. Acetaminophen would be a less optimal choice as she tried this agent and had inadequate symptom management. She has no contraindications to use of an NSAID. The efficacy of applicable complementary therapies is not well established. Therefore, self-treatment with either an NSAID or topical heat would be appropriate. |
| 7. Describe the recommended therapeutic approach to the patient. | See the box Patient Education for Primary Dysmenorrhea. |
| 8. Explain to the patient the rationale for selecting the recommended therapeutic approach from the considered therapeutic alternatives. | NSAIDs are the most effective nonprescription medications for management of primary dysmenorrhea. They are also well tolerated and can be taken for just 1-2 days per month. Onset of benefit is rapid. No other nonprescription agents are as well studied or of similar proven efficacy. She might also try a topical heat patch in place of or in combination with the NSAID, depending on how well each manages her symptoms when used as a single agent, and her preference with regard to therapeutic approach. If her symptoms are not adequately controlled, then she should see her PCP for evaluation. Prescription drug therapy may be necessary. |

**CASE 9-1 (continued)**

| Relevant Evaluation Criteria | Scenario/Model Outcome |
|---|---|
| **Patient Education** | |
| 9. When recommending self-care with nonprescription medications and/or nondrug therapy, convey accurate information to the patient, including: | |
| a. appropriate dose and frequency of administration | See the box Patient Education for Primary Dysmenorrhea. |
| b. maximum number of days the therapy should be employed | NSAID therapy should need to be taken only during the first several days of menses—but may be taken for as many days as her cramps usually last. NSAIDs should be taken on a schedule, not just when pain occurs. If there is no risk of pregnancy and her periods are predictable, she can begin the NSAID the day before her period. |
| c. product administration procedures | See the box Patient Education for Primary Dysmenorrhea. |
| d. expected time to onset of relief | You should feel some relief within an hour of the first dose of an NSAID if you take it early enough; optimal benefit will occur with regular dosing. |
| e. degree of relief that can be reasonably expected | Significant improvement or amelioration of pain and cramping |
| f. most common side effects | Gastrointestinal upset (e.g., nausea, vomiting, diarrhea, constipation), headache, and dizziness may occur. |
| g. side effects that warrant medical intervention should they occur | Severe gastrointestinal distress, significant bruising or fluid retention, rash, or wheezing/difficulty breathing |
| h. patient options in the event that condition worsens or persists | Referral for medical evaluation |
| i. product storage requirements | Product should be stored in a cool dry place. You can keep some with you for scheduled dosing. |
| j. specific nondrug measures | Local application of heat via heating pad or topical heat wrap product may also help improve symptoms. If you smoke tobacco, you should stop. |
| 10. Solicit patient's follow-up questions. | Why do I have to take the NSAID regularly; can't I just use it when my cramps are bad? |
| 11. Answer patient's questions. | The goal of NSAID therapy is to prevent cramping and pain. As-needed use will not relieve the pain and prevent cramping as well as regular on-time use. |

Key: N/A, not applicable; NKDA, no known drug allergies; NSAID, nonsteroidal anti-inflammatory drug; PCP, primary care provider.

## Patient Counseling for Primary Dysmenorrhea

Adolescents and young women who experience primary dysmenorrhea symptoms should be educated about this condition so that they (1) realize primary dysmenorrhea is normal, (2) recognize typical symptoms and symptoms that are inconsistent with primary dysmenorrhea and when to seek medical evaluation, and (3) understand that NSAIDs are preferred therapy because of their proven greater efficacy and how to use these agents for greatest benefit. Patients should also be advised that any of the nonprescription nonsalicylate NSAIDs can be appropriate for initial therapy, but not all women will respond to these agents. If response to the first agent is not adequate, the other nonsalicylate NSAIDs, as well as nondrug interventions, can be tried before a primary care provider is consulted. The practitioner should explain the proper use of these agents and their potential adverse effects. The box Patient Education for Primary Dysmenorrhea lists specific information to provide patients.

## Evaluation of Patient Outcomes for Primary Dysmenorrhea

Patient monitoring is accomplished by having the patient report whether the symptoms are resolved. Symptoms should improve within an hour or so of taking an NSAID if it is taken in time. The optimal effect of drug therapy may not be seen, however, until the woman has used the medication on a scheduled basis. The practitioner should follow up with a phone call to discuss treatment effectiveness (i.e., continued or altered symptoms) and the importance of scheduled dosing. The practitioner can also inquire about the dose of medication being taken and discuss an adequate dose. The patient with persistent symptoms should be advised to try another nonprescription nonsalicylate NSAID or to see a primary care provider for evaluation.

## PATIENT EDUCATION FOR PRIMARY DYSMENORRHEA

The objective of self-treatment is to relieve or significantly improve symptoms of dysmenorrhea so as to limit discomfort and the disruption of usual activities. For most patients, carefully following product instructions and the self-care measures listed here will help ensure optimal therapeutic outcomes.

### Nondrug Measures

- If effective, apply heat to the abdomen, lower back, or other painful area, using a heating pad or an abdominal heat patch.
- Stop smoking cigarettes.
- Participate in regular exercise if it lessens the symptoms.

### Nonprescription Medications

- Nonsalicylate NSAID nonprescription medications (ibuprofen, ketoprofen, and naproxen sodium) are the best type of nonprescription medication to treat primary dysmenorrhea. These medications stop or prevent the strong contractions (cramping) of the uterus.
- Start taking the medication when the menstrual period begins or when menstrual pain or other symptoms begin. Then take the medication at regular intervals following the product instructions instead of just when the symptoms are present.
- See Table 9-2 for recommended dosages of nonprescription nonsalicylate NSAIDs.
- Take a nonsalicylate NSAID with food to limit the most common side effects: upset stomach, heartburn, diarrhea, or constipation.
- Do not take nonsalicylate NSAIDs if you are allergic to aspirin or any nonsalicylate NSAID, or if you have peptic ulcer disease, gastroesophageal reflux disease, colitis, or any bleeding disorder.
- If you have hypertension, asthma, or congestive heart failure, watch for early symptoms that the nonsalicylate NSAID is causing fluid retention.
- Do not take a nonsalicylate NSAID if you are also taking anticoagulants or lithium.

⚠ If abdominal pain occurs at times other than just before or during the first few days of a menstrual period, seek medical attention.

⚠ Seek medical attention if the pain intensity increases or if new symptoms occur.

## PREMENSTRUAL SYNDROME

PMS is defined as a cyclic disorder composed of a combination of physical and emotional (mood) symptoms that occur during the luteal phase of the menstrual cycle, improve significantly or disappear within the first several days of menstrual flow, and are absent during the first week following menses. The diagnosis of PMS can be made based on physical or mood symptoms that occur cyclically.[23] Premenstrual dysphoric disorder (PMDD) is a severe form of PMS; the diagnosis of this condition requires that a specific constellation of symptoms occur on a cyclic basis and the symptoms are severe enough to cause functional impairment (interfere with social and/or occupational functioning).[23]

### Epidemiology of PMS

Almost all women experience some physical or mood changes before the onset of menses.[24] A normal sign of ovulatory cycles, these symptoms are referred to medically as molimina.[23,25] Symptoms vary among women but are typically constant for an individual woman. They may include physical symptoms, food cravings, and emotional lability or lowered mood. In addition, some women report positive changes, such as increased energy, creativity, work productivity, and sexual desire.[24] The majority of women with premenstrual symptoms experience only mild, primarily physical symptoms that do not interfere with their lives.

The number and severity of symptoms and the extent to which they interfere with functioning distinguish typical premenstrual symptoms, PMS, and PMDD. An estimated 40% of women with premenstrual symptoms describe them as bothersome, 10% to 15% report their symptoms as severe, and 3% to 5% report symptoms that cause significant impairment in daily life that interferes with relationships, lifestyle, or work[24] (Table 9-3[24,26,27]).

PMS can occur any time after menarche; symptoms usually originate when women are in their early 20s, but typically women wait to seek care until they are over age 30.[24,26,28] PMS symptoms occur only during ovulatory cycles. Symptoms disappear during events that interrupt ovulation, such as pregnancy and breast-feeding, and PMS symptoms disappear at menopause.

Among women, Caucasians and African Americans have a similar symptom experience. Asian women report a lower severity of PMS symptoms while Hispanic women report more severe PMS symptoms.[29] Factors that predict severe PMS or PMDD are a past history of depression, working outside the home, less education, and use of tobacco.[30] Current smokers are four times more likely to have a diagnosis of PMDD than nonsmokers.[30] Similarly, symptoms may also be more severe for current smokers.[29] This parallels the correlation between tobacco smoking and depression.[30]

Women with PMDD tend to be high utilizers of health care; use of both mental health practitioners and primary care providers is greater in women with PMDD than in the general population. Women with PMDD also have a significant rate of suicide attempts (15% report at least one attempt).[31]

### Etiology of PMS

The etiology of PMS is unknown. The current consensus is that normal ovarian function (and the consequent fluctuation of estrogen and progesterone levels) is the cyclic trigger for PMS/PMDD symptoms. There is no known

**TABLE 9-3 Differentiation of PMS and PMDD from Other Conditions with Luteal Phase Symptoms[24,26,27]**

| | |
|---|---|
| Typical premenstrual symptoms (molimina) | Mild physical (breast tenderness, bloating, lower backache, food cravings) or mood (emotional lability, lowered mood, increased energy or creativity) changes before the onset of menses that do not interfere with normal life functions |
| Premenstrual syndrome | At least one mood (e.g., depression, irritability, anger, anxiety) or physical (e.g., breast tenderness, abdominal bloating) symptom during the 5 days prior to menses. Symptoms are virtually absent during cycle days 5-10. The symptom or symptoms have a negative effect on social functioning or lifestyle, but the severity is mild to moderate. |
| Premenstrual dysphoric disorder | Five or more symptoms (mood or physical) present the last week of the luteal phase of the menstrual cycle with at least one symptom being significant depression, anxiety, affective lability or anger. The intensity of the symptoms interfere with work, school, social activities, and social relationships. Symptoms should be absent the week after menses and must not be an exacerbation of the symptoms of another disorder such as depression, panic disorder, or personality disorder. |
| Premenstrual exacerbation | A worsening of the symptoms of other, typically psychiatric, disorders such as depression and anxiety or panic disorders. Conditions such as endometriosis, hypothyroidism, attention deficit disorder, diabetes mellitus, migraine headaches, and perimenopause can also worsen premenstrually. However, symptoms do not occur only during the luteal phase of the menstrual cycle; there is no symptom-free interval. |

hormonal imbalance in women with PMS. It appears that some women are biologically vulnerable or predisposed to experience PMS because of a neurotransmitter sensitivity to physiologic changes in levels of hormones.[28] Women with PMS/PMDD may be predisposed to mood and anxiety symptoms caused by a difference in the sensitivity of the serotonin system. The neurotransmitter serotonin is affected by estrogen and progesterone levels and is involved in the pathogenesis of premenstrual irritability and dysphoria. Other neurotransmitters and systems that may be of potential importance are GABA, opiates (endorphins) and the β-adrenergic receptors.[23,28] Thys-Jacobs suggests that a difference in the cyclicity of calcium and of substances influencing calcium levels in the body (i.e., vitamin D, parathyroid hormone) may explain why some women experience PMS symptoms.[32] PMS symptoms are quite similar to symptoms of hypocalcemia. There is evidence of a genetic predisposition, and sociocultural factors may also influence PMS symptoms.[23] A recent study of twins found evidence for a genetic predisposition, but environmental influences (external stressors) correlated more strongly with symptoms.[33]

PMS does not appear to be simply a variant of depression: it is cyclic, it does not spontaneously remit, symptoms are not relieved by all types of antidepressants, and its primary symptoms are irritability and anxiety, not depression.[34] Early studies found an association between PMDD and mood disorders such as major depression; in one study, 58% of women with PMDD had a history of depression.[30] However, this association has been disputed except for evidence of an increased likelihood of postpartum depression among women with PMDD.[34]

Exogenous hormones may influence premenstrual symptoms. Women taking either oral contraceptives or postmenopausal hormone replacement therapy may experience adverse effects similar to PMS symptoms as a result of the altered hormone levels.[23] Conversely, oral contraceptive use may also protect against emotional symptoms. PMS scores for women using oral contraceptives were lower than for women not using them.[29,33]

## Pathophysiology of PMS

Fluctuations in ovarian hormones (estrogen and progesterone) give rise to biochemical changes in neurotransmitters. Serotonin levels are decreased in women with PMS.[23] A decrease in serotonin levels is associated with irritability, dysphoria, and food cravings; these symptoms are also associated with PMS/PMDD.

Central nervous system metabolism of steroids may also be different in women with PMS/PMDD. Levels of allopregnanolone, a progesterone metabolite that interacts with the GABA system, have been found to be lower during the luteal phase in women with PMS than in women without these symptoms. A decrease in allopregnanolone could increase anxiety. Also, selective serotonin reuptake inhibitors (SSRIs), which are known to relieve PMS/PMDD, have been found to affect the synthesis of allopregnanolone.[23]

Therefore, for symptoms severe enough to warrant prescription drug therapy, treatment is based on medications that affect the levels of serotonin or suppress ovulation and interrupt hormonal cycling.

## Signs and Symptoms of PMS

None of the symptoms of PMS or PMDD are unique to these conditions; however, the occurrence of specific symptoms and their fluctuation with the phases of the menstrual cycle are diagnostic. Premenstrual symptoms typically begin or intensify about a week prior to the onset of menses, peak the day before or on the first day of menses, and resolve within several days after the beginning of menses.[24] A woman with PMS or PMDD should experience essentially a symptom-free interval during days 4 to 12 of her menstrual cycle. Symptoms may also be experienced for 1 day at the time of ovulation.[25,26] Symptoms of PMS/PMDD appear to be worse early in reproductive life and tend to improve toward menopause, when ovulation may be intermittent and hormonal fluctuation perhaps lessens.[29]

**TABLE 9-4 Occurrence Rate of Common PMS Symptoms**

| Symptom | Occurrence in Women with PMS (%) |
|---|---|
| **Behavioral** | |
| Fatigue | 92 |
| Irritability | 91 |
| Labile mood with alternating sadness and anger | 81 |
| Depression | 80 |
| Oversensitivity | 69 |
| Crying spells | 65 |
| Social withdrawal | 65 |
| Forgetfulness | 56 |
| Difficulty concentrating | 47 |
| **Physical** | |
| Abdominal bloating | 90 |
| Breast tenderness | 85 |
| Acne | 71 |
| Appetite changes and food cravings | 70 |
| Swelling of the extremities | 67 |
| Headache | 60 |
| Gastrointestinal upset | 48 |

*Source:* Reprinted with permission from reference 15.

Common symptoms of PMS are listed in Table 9-4. In a recent study, the two most common premenstrual symptoms were bloating/weight gain and breast swelling/tenderness. Aside from these physical symptoms, affective symptoms (e.g., fatigue, anxiety, irritability) were more common than other physical symptoms.[33] For an individual woman, symptoms remain consistent across cycles.[25,26] Among women experiencing at least one PMS symptom frequently over the past 12 months, 55% reported that the symptom was present in almost all cycles.[31] The majority of women rate their symptoms as mild or moderate, and do not feel they interfere in their life or are limiting. Mood symptoms tend to cause more impairment than physical symptoms.[26]

Symptoms of PMDD are similar to those of PMS, but women with PMDD experience more symptoms, more severe symptoms, and symptoms that impair personal relationships and the ability to function well at work to a greater extent than women with PMS. Among women with PMDD the most common symptoms are affective: depressed mood/hopelessness/self-depreciation (90.5%), affective lability (89.7%), irritability/anger (81.5%), fatigability (78.6%), physical complaints (78.1%), anxiety/tension (67%), and decreased interest (63.3%).[31] Other symptoms of PMDD include difficulty concentrating, lethargy, hypersomnia or insomnia, and physical symptoms (e.g., breast tenderness, bloating). The severity of symptoms results in an average of 2.6 days of impairment or disability per month.[31] A daily rating of symptoms for several cycles establishes a diagnosis of PMDD, and these types of symptoms should have occurred during most menstrual cycles over the past year. PMDD symptoms during the late luteal phase (last 7 days of the cycle) should be at least 30% worse than those experienced during the mid-follicular phase (days 3 to 9 of the menstrual cycle).

It is important to distinguish PMS/PMDD from typical premenstrual symptoms (molimina) and also from premenstrual exacerbations of other disorders (PME), particularly mood disorders. A number of medical conditions can be aggravated during the premenstrual phase, including major depression, panic attacks, migraine headaches, asthma, and seizure disorders.[34] In addition, mood disorders not occurring solely during the luteal phase must be distinguished from cyclic mood symptoms (Table 9-3).

Lack of a symptom-free interval suggests that the patient has a psychiatric disorder (e.g., anxiety or panic disorder) or another health condition (e.g., perimenopause) rather than PMS.

## Treatment of PMS

PMS is a multisymptom disorder, involving behavioral and physical symptoms. A single therapeutic agent is unlikely to address all symptoms; thus, agents should be selected to address the patient's most bothersome symptoms. A symptom log/calendar is a very useful tool to document the most bothersome symptom(s) and the cyclic nature of this disorder. This information will also be useful in evaluating the efficacy of treatment. Patients with severe symptoms are less likely to have symptoms alleviated solely by use of nonprescription therapies. Additionally, PMS symptoms are chronic and in most cases will continue until menopause. Therefore, the cost of therapy, the fact that a woman may become pregnant, and the likelihood of adverse effects from therapy are important considerations in selecting therapy.[24,25]

### *Treatment Goals*

Two outcomes are desirable for women with PMS or PMDD: (1) to understand PMS and (2) to improve or resolve symptoms to reduce the impact on activities and interpersonal relationships. Typically, therapy is thought effective if symptoms are reduced by 50% or more.

### *General Treatment Approach*

The initial treatment of PMS symptoms is generally conservative, consisting of education and nondrug measures such as dietary modifications, physical exercise, and stress management. Women with symptoms of PMS should be educated about the syndrome and encouraged to identify techniques for coping with PMS symptoms and stress. Many women are engaged in multiple social roles, which can increase stress. Knowledge of this disorder can allow a woman to exert some control over her symptoms by anticipating and planning. For example, she might schedule more challenging tasks during the first half of the cycle, thus limiting the influence of this condition on her social and occupational functioning.

For symptoms that are not responsive to nondrug therapy, several nonprescription or complementary agents that are relatively nontoxic might be suggested. These agents include calcium, magnesium, vitamin E, pyridoxine, and chasteberry (*Vitex agnus*).

Prescription drug therapy should be considered if the treatments outlined in Figure 9-3 fail or the patient suffers from severe PMS or PMDD. Prescription therapy includes psychotropic medications (e.g., alprazolam, SSRIs) and menstrual cycle modifiers (e.g., oral contraceptives, danazol, GnRH agonists).

### Nonpharmacologic Therapy

Several nonpharmacologic therapies may provide some amelioration of PMS symptoms. These include aerobic exercise, dietary modifications, and cognitive-behavioral therapy.[27] Women who exercise may have fewer and less severe PMS symptoms compared with nonexercisers.[27,35] Although the benefit of nutritional therapy for PMS is largely unproven, many clinicians recommend a balanced diet combined with avoiding salty foods and simple sugars (which may cause fluid retention) as well as caffeine and alcohol (which can increase irritability). Consumption of caffeine-containing beverages has been associated with increased PMS symptoms.[35] Cravings for foods high in carbohydrates, which contain the serotonin precursor tryptophan, are common in women with PMS. A study of a carbohydrate-rich beverage, which increased tryptophan levels, demonstrated an improvement in mood scores (depression, tension, anger, confusion) for women with PMDD.[36] Consuming foods that are rich in complex carbohydrates (e.g., whole-grain foods) during the premenstrual interval may reduce symptoms. A strict low-fat diet may decrease breast pain.[34]

Stress is reported to increase PMS symptoms. Cognitive-behavioral therapy, which emphasizes relaxation techniques and coping skills, can help reduce PMS symptoms. These approaches may be helpful used singly or as adjuncts to other therapies.

### Pharmacologic Therapy

Surveys of women have found that 20% to 50% use some nonprescription medication for premenstrual symptoms, primarily analgesics and vitamins.[37] One study[38] of more than 1000 women ages 21 to 64 years found that 42% of those who had PMS-type symptoms (feeling more emotional, bloating, food cravings, pain) took medication for their symptoms; 80% were taking a nonprescription product. Among women taking a nonprescription product, the medications most commonly cited were Midol (24% of women), acetaminophen (19%), ibuprofen (16%), and Pamprin (14%). Other nonprescription therapies that may be effective are vitamins, minerals, and NSAIDs.

#### Pyridoxine

Vitamin $B_6$ has been suggested as a therapy for PMS. Many trials have found this agent to be ineffective. However, a meta-analysis found that $B_6$ was more effective than placebo in relieving overall PMS symptoms (mastalgia, irritability, fatigue, bloating, tension) and depression associated with PMS,[39] although no dose-response correlation was shown. It is recommended that the dose of pyridoxine be limited to 100 mg daily because of the potential for neuropathy. Risk of neuropathy is usually associated with high doses (2-6 g daily) but can occur with daily doses greater than 200 mg, although with lower doses the neuropathy is usually reversible.[39] Symptoms of this toxicity include paresthesia (a sensation of pricking, tingling, or creeping on the skin), bone pain, muscle weakness, and hyperesthesia (stinging, burning, itching sensations).

#### Vitamin E

Vitamin E (400 IU daily) is sometimes recommended for the symptom of breast tenderness. However, data on its effectiveness are unconvincing.

#### Calcium

A well-designed trial studied the effect of calcium (600 mg twice daily) in 466 women with moderate to severe PMS.[40] Symptoms were significantly reduced by the second month of therapy; by the third month, calcium had reduced overall symptoms by 48%. Emotional (e.g., mood swings, depression, anger), behavioral (e.g., food cravings), and physical symptoms (e.g., fluid retention, breast tenderness, backaches, abdominal cramping) were all reduced. More than 50% of the women taking calcium had a greater than 50% improvement in symptoms; 29% had a greater than 75% improvement in symptoms. Few women experienced adverse effects from calcium; five withdrew from the study because of nausea, and one woman in each group (calcium and placebo) developed kidney stones. The dose of calcium used in the trial is consistent with the recommended daily calcium intake for women of reproductive age. Similarly, a study comparing two doses of dietary calcium (587 or 1336 mg) found that women experienced less negative mood symptoms and fluid retention on the higher calcium diet.[41] Importantly, all health care providers should be reinforcing adequate calcium and vitamin D intake in women to help prevent osteoporosis.

#### Magnesium

One small trial has shown that magnesium (360 mg daily administered during the luteal phase) can relieve affective symptoms of PMS.[42] It has been hypothesized that magnesium deficiency may lead to PMS-type symptoms (e.g., irritability), and low magnesium levels in red blood cells have been found in women with PMS.[42] The dose of magnesium used in the trial was similar to the recommended dietary allowance (RDA) of magnesium for women (280 to 300 mg). About one half of women regularly consume less than that amount, and obtaining adequate magnesium from food may be difficult. Side effects from magnesium are uncommon; diarrhea is the most common side effect.

Woman with PMS symptoms

↓

Obtain medical/medication history, including type, severity & timing of symptoms. Ask about use of hormones & any association between onset of hormone use & onset or worsening of symptoms

↓

Discuss previous treatments, current use of calcium/other minerals, vitamins $B_6$ & E, diuretics & other OTC menstrual products

↓

Exclusions for self-treatment (see box)? — Yes → Medical referral

No ↓

Discuss nondrug, OTC & CAM treatment options. Elicit patient preference for treatment approach. An approach may blend treatment options (e.g., dietary modification & calcium). Suggest potentially helpful lifestyle modifications (see box Patient Education for Premenstrual Syndrome)

↓

OTC or herbal therapy: Advise use for several cycles before assessment of benefit; onset & maximum benefit of vitamins/minerals & herbal products occurs after several months of therapy

↓

Symptoms resolved to patient's satisfaction? — Yes → Continue therapy. Reinforce patient education about PMS

No ↓

Reevaluate. Consider trial w/ alternative OTC or herbal products or a combination of agents

↓

Symptoms resolved to patient's satisfaction? — Yes → Continue therapy. Reinforce patient education about PMS

No ↓

Medical referral

### Exclusions for Self-Treatment*

- Severe PMS or PMDD
- Uncertain pattern of symptoms (timing in relationship to menses), particularly for emotional/psychologic symptoms
- Onset of symptoms coincident with use of OCs or HRT
- Contraindications to specific agents:

| | |
|---|---|
| Caffeine/pamabron | Disease: PUD, anxiety/insomnia<br>Drugs: MAOI, xanthine medications |
| Ammonium chloride | Disease: renal or liver impairment |
| Chasteberry | Disease: hormone-sensitive cancers, in vitro fertilization procedures; may increase fertility<br>Drugs: OCs, HRT, dopamine agonists and antagonists |
| Black cohosh | Disease: hormone-sensitive cancers<br>Drugs: some chemotherapy agents (doxorubicin, docetaxol) |
| St. John's wort | Disease: Alzheimer's disease, depression, bipolar disorder, schizophrenia, infertility<br>Drugs: antidepressants (SSRI, TCA, or MAOI), narcotic analgesics, digoxin, dextromethorphan, OCs, warfarin, AIDS drugs |
| Ginkgo | Drugs: anticoagulants and antiplatelet agents, insulin, seizure threshold-lowering drugs, thiazide diuretics |

* Lactating women should not use herbs. Selected drug interactions and disease interactions are listed above; however, the list is not comprehensive.

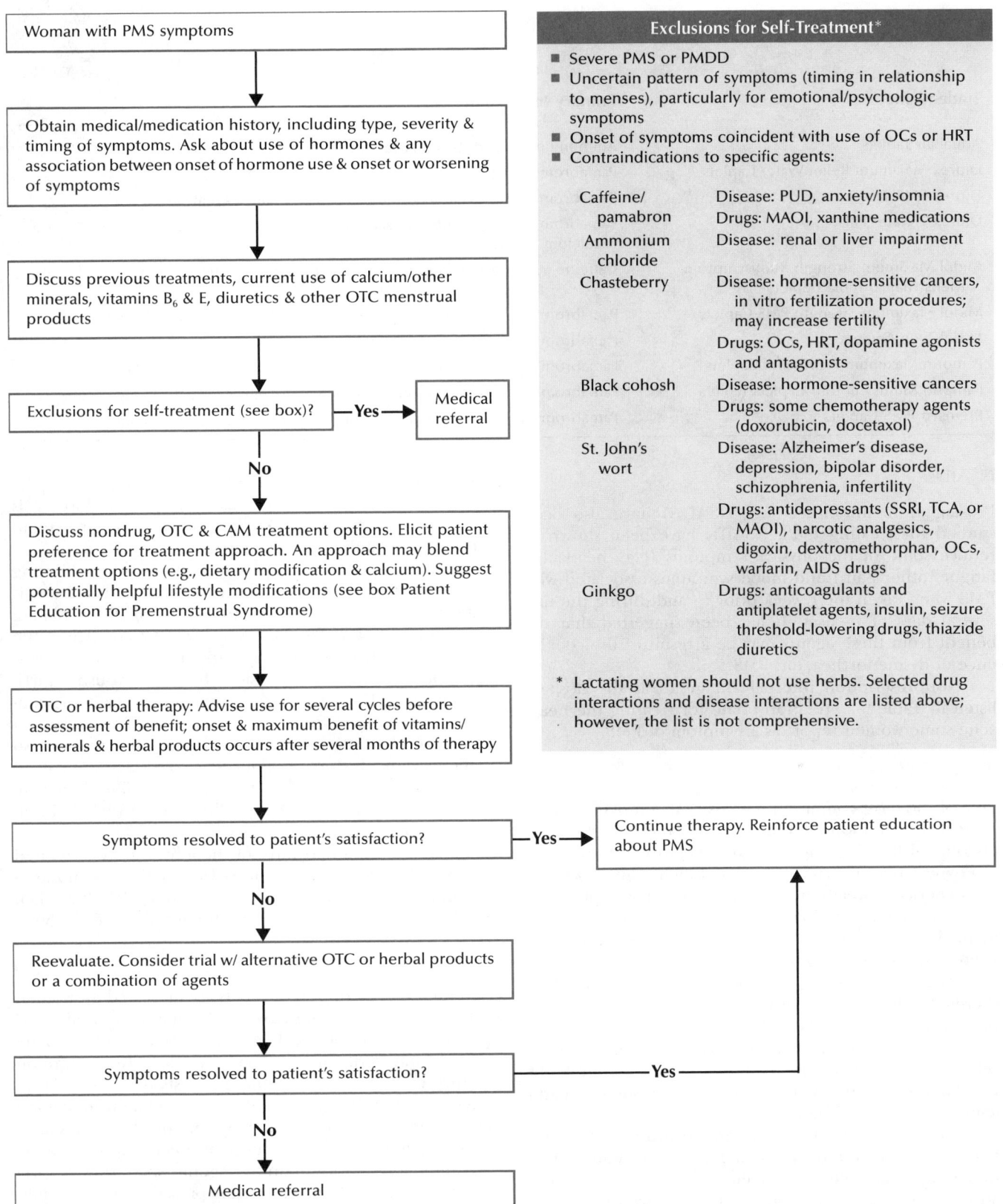

FIGURE 9-3 Self-care of premenstrual syndrome. Key: AIDS, acquired immunodeficiency syndrome; CAM, complementary and alternative medicine; HRT, hormone replacement therapy; MAOI, monoamine oxidase inhibitor; OC, oral contraceptive; OTC, over-the-counter; PMDD, premenstrual dysphoric disorder; PMS, premenstrual syndrome; PUD, peptic ulcer disease; SSRI, selective serotonin reuptake inhibitor; TCA, tricyclic antidepressant.

**TABLE 9-5 Selected Menstrual Products**

| Trade Name | Primary Ingredients |
|---|---|
| AquaBan Tablets | Ammonium chloride 325 mg; caffeine 100 mg |
| Diurex Maximum Relief Water Caplets | Pamabrom 50 mg |
| Diurex PMS Tablet | Pamabrom 25 mg; acetaminophen 500 mg; pyrilamine maleate 15 mg |
| Diurex-2 Water Pills | Pamabrom 25 mg; magnesium salicylate tetrahydrate 202 mg; calcium carbonate; calcium sulfate |
| Midol Maximum Strength Multisymptom Menstrual Formula Caplets | Caffeine 60 mg; acetaminophen 500 mg; pyrilamine maleate 15 mg |
| Midol Maximum Strength PMS Caplets | Pamabrom 25 mg; acetaminophen 500 mg; pyrilamine maleate 15 mg |
| Midol Teen Caplets | Pamabrom 25 mg; acetaminophen 400 mg |
| Pamprin Maximum Pain Relief Caplets | Pamabrom 25 mg; magnesium salicylate 250 mg; acetaminophen 250 mg |
| Pamprin Multisymptom Caplets/Tablets | Pamabrom 25 mg; acetaminophen 500 mg; pyrilamine maleate 15 mg |
| Premsyn PMS Caplets | Pamabrom 25 mg; acetaminophen 500 mg; pyrilamine maleate 15 mg |

### NSAIDs

Prostaglandin inhibitors (e.g., NSAIDs) have also been studied for treating PMS. NSAIDs have been shown to reduce some of the physical symptoms (e.g., headache, fatigue, other pain) and mood symptoms associated with PMS when taken for 1 week prior to and during the first several days of menses. It has been suggested that the benefit from these agents may be a result of the coexistence of dysmenorrhea and PMS.

Nonprescription internal analgesics at the dosages listed in Table 9-2 are appropriate for treating the headache some women report as a symptom of PMS.

### Diuretics

One of the most common premenstrual complaints is the subjective sensation of fluid accumulation, particularly abdominal bloating. However, the majority of women do not experience any true water or sodium retention and do not experience weight gain.[43] Two factors may explain the sense of abdominal bloating. First, a distinction must be made between fluid redistribution and fluid retention (detected by weight gain). The bloating and swelling observed with PMS are primarily caused by a fluid shift; therefore, diuretics—indicated for relieving fluid retention—are unlikely to be helpful for most PMS patients. Second, abdominal distension may occur secondary to relaxation of the gut muscle caused by progesterone.[43] For women who have true water retention and resultant weight gain, a diuretic may be useful.

The Food and Drug Administration (FDA) has approved three diuretics as useful for relieving water retention, weight gain, bloating, swelling, and feeling of fullness and safe for nonprescription use. These diuretics—ammonium chloride, caffeine, and pamabrom—are contained in commercially available menstrual products (Table 9-5).

Ammonium chloride is an acid-forming salt with a short duration of effect; it is taken in oral doses of up to 3 g/day (divided into three doses) for no more than 6 consecutive days. Larger doses of ammonium chloride (4-12 g/day) can produce significant adverse effects of the GI and central nervous systems. Ammonium chloride is contraindicated in patients with renal or liver impairment because metabolic acidosis may result.

Caffeine, a xanthine, promotes diuresis by inhibiting the renal tubular reabsorption of sodium and water. It is safe and effective as a diuretic in dosages of 100 to 200 mg every 3 to 4 hours. Patients may develop tolerance to the diuretic effect. Caffeine may also cause anxiety, restlessness, or insomnia. Additive side effects (nervousness, irritability, or tachycardia) might occur if other caffeine-containing beverages, foods, or medications are consumed concurrently. Caffeine may also cause GI irritation, so patients with a history of peptic ulcer disease should avoid it. Patients taking monoamine oxidase inhibitors or xanthine medications (e.g., theophylline) should avoid diuretics that contain caffeine.

Pamabrom, a derivative of theophylline, is contained in combination products (along with analgesics and antihistamines) marketed for the treatment of PMS. It is taken in doses of up to 200 mg/day (50 mg four times daily).

### Combination Products

Several nonprescription products are marketed for women with PMS-type symptoms. Two of the most commonly used products are Midol and Pamprin (acetaminophen, pamabrom, and pyrilamine). Pain is a relatively uncommon feature of PMS, and no evidence exists that the sedative effect of an antihistamine will provide benefit to women experiencing the emotional symptoms of PMS. Therefore, these types of nonprescription products should not be recommended. More definitive agents, such as those previously discussed, and referral for prescription drug therapy are more appropriate therapeutic recommendations.

### Product Selection Guidelines

Calcium, because it has overall health benefits and is generally well tolerated, can be suggested for the initial treatment of PMS symptoms. If this agent provides inadequate

**TABLE 9-6 Vitamins, Minerals, Herbs, and Dietary Supplements for the Treatment of PMS**

| Agent | Effectiveness | Comments |
|---|---|---|
| Vitamin $B_6$ | Likely effective | Limit dose to avoid neuropathy; insufficient evidence on effectiveness from high-quality studies; not first-line therapy |
| Vitamin E | Possibly effective for mastalgia | Minimal evidence of benefit; nontoxic in usual dose (400 IU/day) |
| Calcium | Effective | Good evidence on effectiveness from large randomized trials; improvement in both mood and physical symptoms; onset of benefit across several cycles; usual dose 1200-1500 mg/day |
| Magnesium | Likely effective | Limited data on effectiveness but biologic rationale exists; usual dose 200-400 IU/day |
| Manganese | Insufficient evidence | One small trial (10 women); used along with calcium |
| Potassium | Insufficient evidence | Uncontrolled case reports; dose: 600 mg of potassium gluconate |
| Evening primrose oil* | Not effective | Controlled trials did not show a benefit; use unwarranted |
| St. John's wort* | Possibly effective | Only one small study to date using 300 mg (0.3% standardized hypericin) daily; showed improvement in mood scores; herb may be beneficial because MOA is similar to SSRI antidepressants |
| Vitex (chasteberry)* | Likely effective | Several trials (some using 20-40 mg Ze440 extract) have shown herb reduces PMS symptoms, onset of benefit occurs over several cycles, and is well tolerated; GI symptoms and headache possible side effects; dosing depends on product |
| Black cohosh* | Possibly effective | Often beneficial for menopausal symptoms, may relieve PMS symptoms because of similarity of symptoms; dosing depends on product; Remifemin, enzymatic therapy, and phytopharmica products are standardized to 1 mg triterpene per 20 mg tablet; 40-80 mg twice daily used in many studies |
| Ginkgo* | Likely effective | Ginkgo shown in randomized trial to improve PMS symptoms, particularly breast tenderness and fluid retention; ginkgo's antiplatelet effects may increase risk for bleeding; interacts with a number of drugs including anticoagulants, antiplatelet agents, anticonvulsants, fluoxetine, omeprazole, trazodone, buspirone, and St. John's wort; usual dose is 80 mg twice daily beginning cycle day 16 until day 5 of the next cycle |

Key: GI, gastrointestinal; MOA, mechanism of action; PMS, premenstrual syndrome; SSRI, selective serotonin reuptake inhibitor.

* See Chapter 53 for more information.

relief, another agent or a combination of two or more agents may be tried. Women who experience bloating with documented weight gain might try pamabrom or caffeine. Caffeine may not be an appropriate choice for a woman who experiences irritability as a PMS symptom. Both xanthines (caffeine and pamabrom) are contraindicated in patients who have a history of peptic ulcer disease or are taking monoamine oxidase inhibitors or other xanthine medications (e.g., theophylline). NSAIDs should be reserved for women who experience both PMS and dysmenorrhea or headache symptoms. Use of combination products containing antihistamines should be discouraged; drowsiness may impair schoolwork and driving.

### *Complementary Therapies*

Trials have been conducted on several alternative therapies. Herbs studied for the treatment of PMS include evening primrose oil, St. John's wort (*Hypericum perforatum*), chaste tree or chasteberry (*Vitex agnus-castus*), black cohosh (*Cimicifuga racemosa*), and ginkgo (*Ginkgo biloba*) (Table 9-6).[44]

*Vitex* (chasteberry) has been used traditionally for managing menstrual cycle symptoms; the German Commission E monograph lists PMS, mastodynia, and menstrual rhythm abnormalities as indications for *Vitex*. Two trials using a standardized fruit extract ZE 440 of *Vitex* found a significant reduction in the symptoms of mood, irritability/anger, pain/headache, breast tenderness, and fluid retention.[45,46] Symptoms were progressively reduced over several cycles, and some benefit persisted for a few months after discontinuation; therapy was well tolerated with few side effects. Another uncontrolled trial of the *Vitex* preparation Femicur in 1634 patients found much or very much reduced symptoms for 80% of women; 42% of all women studied reported that the *Vitex* eliminated their symptoms, whereas 51% reported improvement, and only 6% reported no improvement.[47] In a trial in women diagnosed with PMDD, *Vitex* was compared with fluoxetine, an SSRI antidepressant known to be effective for the treatment of severe PMS and PMDD. A similar percentage of patients improved on both agents. *Vitex* was shown to decrease the following symptoms by over 50%— irritability, breast tenderness, swelling, food cravings, and cramps. In contrast, fluoxetine improved more mood symptoms; symptoms with a 50% reduction included depression, irritability, insomnia, nervous tension, feeling out of control, breast tenderness, and aches. *Vitex* was well tolerated; nausea and headache were the most common side effects of therapy. *Vitex* may offer more benefit for patients with less severe symptoms—mild to moderate PMS.[48] Vitex may have estrogenic or progestogenic activity; use should be avoided by women who may be pregnant or who are not using reliable contraception.

A placebo-controlled randomized trial of ginkgo (165 women) found it improved all PMS-related symptoms. Benefit was greatest for breast pain and fluid retention symptoms.[35,44]

Light therapy has also been studied. Bright light therapy has been shown to be effective in some mood disorders—most notably seasonal affective disorder. PMS/PMDD may show seasonal variation with worsening in the winter. A small study of 14 women rated subjects as very improved in 89% of bright white light cycles compared with dim light cycles.[49] Improvement was noted for both mood and physical symptoms.

## Assessment of PMS: A Case-based Approach

The practitioner should obtain a complete description of the patient's symptoms and their timing to determine whether the patient has PMS/PMDD or another disorder with PMS-type symptoms. The severity of PMS symptoms is another factor in self-treatment. As with any disorder, the practitioner should explore the use of medications that might be causing the symptoms or that might potentially interact with nonprescription agents used to treat PMS. Previous treatments of the symptoms should also be explored. Case 9-2 illustrates the assessment of patients with PMS.

### CASE 9-2

| Relevant Evaluation Criteria | Scenario/Model Outcome |
|---|---|
| **Information Gathering** | |
| 1. Gather essential information about the patient's symptoms, including: | |
| a. description of symptom(s) (i.e., nature, onset, duration, severity, associated symptoms) | For the past year she has been experiencing irritability, sadness, and breast tenderness each month for about a week prior to her menstrual periods. She feels "normal" the rest of the month. |
| b. description of any factors that seem to precipitate, exacerbate, and/or relieve the patient's symptom(s) | If she is stressed by things at work or in dealing with her two adolescent children, then her symptoms are worse. |
| c. description of the patient's efforts to relieve the symptoms | She has been exercising regularly and trying to get enough sleep. |
| 2. Gather essential patient history information: | |
| a. patient's identity | Marina Decker |
| b. patient's age, sex, height, and weight | 41 y/o F, 5'6", 132 lb |
| c. patient's occupation | Gardener, landscaper |
| d. patient's dietary habits | Her diet includes fruits and vegetables daily, she eats fish and poultry, includes nuts and legumes in her diet several times a week. Yogurt and cheese are also consumed regularly. For treats she eats dark chocolate and popcorn. She drinks six or more cups a day of black or green tea. |
| e. patient's sleep habits | She generally gets about 7 hours per night. |
| f. concurrent medical conditions, prescription and nonprescription medications, and dietary supplements | No chronic medical conditions; occasional colds and headaches, allergies in the fall; chlorpheniramine 4-6 mg once daily during allergy season; multivitamin |
| g. allergies | NKDA |
| h. history of other adverse reactions to medications | None |
| i. other (describe)______ | She tried Premsyn (pamabrom, acetaminophen, and pyrilamine) but it made her too sleepy during the day. |

## CASE 9-2 (continued)

| Relevant Evaluation Criteria | Scenario/Model Outcome |
|---|---|
| **Assessment and Triage** | |
| 3. Differentiate the patient's signs/symptoms and correctly identify the patient's primary problem(s) (see Table 9-3). | MD has typical symptoms of PMS. The symptoms occur cyclically and are mild to moderate. She has symptoms only during the luteal phase of the cycle. |
| 4. Identify exclusions for self-treatment (see Figure 9-3). | None |
| 5. Formulate a comprehensive list of therapeutic alternatives for the primary problem to determine if triage to a medical practitioner is required, and share this information with the patient. | Options include:<br>(1) Recommend self-treatment with a product such as a mineral or herb.<br>(2) Refer MD to her PCP for medical evaluation and prescription therapy.<br>(3) Suggest MD consider use of a nonprescription product for symptom improvement until she can see her PCP.<br>(4) Take no action. |
| **Plan** | |
| 6. Select an optimal therapeutic alternative to address the patient's problem, taking into account patient preferences. | MD is healthy and her symptoms are mild to moderate. It is appropriate for her to try nonprescription therapy. In addition. Learning more about PMS may help her cope with the symptoms. |
| 7. Describe the recommended therapeutic approach to the patient. | See the box Patient Education for Premenstrual Syndrome. |
| 8. Explain to the patient the rationale for selecting the recommended therapeutic approach from the considered therapeutic alternatives. | Several OTC therapies can help reduce the symptoms of PMS. These therapies have few side effects and some, like calcium, are good for overall health. |
| **Patient Education** | |
| 9. When recommending self-care with nonprescription medications and/or nondrug therapy, convey accurate information to the patient, including: | |
| a. appropriate dose and frequency of administration | See the box Patient Education for Premenstrual Syndrome. |
| b. maximum number of days the therapy should be employed | No limitations |
| c. product administration procedures | See the box Patient Education Premenstrual Syndrome. |
| d. expected time to onset of relief | The time to see a benefit will vary, but an optimal effect likely will be noted only after the product has been used regularly for several months. |
| e. degree of relief that can be reasonably expected | Degree of relief also will vary, but symptoms often are reduced by 30%-50%. |
| f. most common side effects | Most of the products have few side effects. |
| g. side effects that warrant medical intervention should they occur | None |
| h. patient options in the event that condition worsens or persists | See your primary care provider. |
| i. product storage requirements | Product should be stored in a cool dry place. |
| j. specific nondrug measures | Learn about PMS and ways to reduce stress. Continue exercising. Eating carbohydrates such as whole grain products during the week before menses may help. If tea causes irritability, decrease the amount you consume. |

## CASE 9-2 (continued)

| Relevant Evaluation Criteria | Scenario/Model Outcome |
| --- | --- |
| 10. Solicit patient's follow-up questions. | What do you recommend I try first, and how will I know if it helps? |
| 11. Answer patient's questions. | Calcium is a good therapy to try; it has been proven effective and is well tolerated. It also has other health benefits (bone health). List 3-5 of your PMS symptoms and rate them during your next menstrual cycle; then, in 2-3 months, rate them again. This process will allow you to see if the calcium has helped. |

Key: NKDA, no known drug allergies; NSAID, nonsteroidal anti-inflammatory drug; OTC, over-the-counter; PCP, primary care provider; PMS, premenstrual syndrome.

## PATIENT EDUCATION FOR PREMENSTRUAL SYNDROME

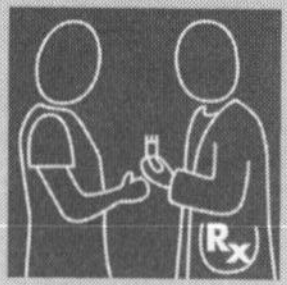

The objective of self-treatment is to achieve relief from or significant improvement in symptoms to limit discomfort, distress, and the disruption of personal relationships or usual activities. For most patients, carefully following product instructions and the self-care measures listed here will help ensure optimal therapeutic outcomes.

### Nondrug Measures

- Try to avoid stress, develop effective coping mechanisms for managing stress, and learn relaxation techniques.
- If possible, participate in regular aerobic exercise.
- During the 7 to 14 days before your menstrual period, reduce or eliminate intake of salt, caffeine, chocolate, and alcoholic beverages. Eating foods rich in carbohydrates and low in protein during the premenstrual interval may also reduce symptoms.

### Nonprescription Medications

- Nonprescription medications and lifestyle modifications may not improve symptoms for all women, and it may take several months to determine whether these therapies are working.
- Therapy with one nonprescription medication may improve only some of the symptoms; several medications may be needed for optimal symptom control. However, it is best to add one agent at a time so that it is possible to determine which agent causes benefit or side effects.
- Follow the guidelines here for the agents that best control your symptoms:
  - Take 1200 mg of calcium daily in divided doses. Take no more than 500 mg at one time. Calcium may cause stomach upset or constipation; if this occurs take with food.
  - Take 360 mg of magnesium daily during the premenstrual interval only. Magnesium may cause diarrhea.
  - Take 400 IU of vitamin E daily.
  - Take 100 mg of pyridoxine (vitamin B6) daily. Do not exceed this daily dosage or neurologic symptoms caused by vitamin B6 toxicity may occur.

⚠ If you are taking vitamin B6 and develop neurologic symptoms, such as a sensation of pricking, tingling, or creeping on the skin; bone pain; muscle weakness; and stinging, burning, or itching sensations, stop taking the vitamin and seek medical attention.

⚠ If the symptoms do not improve or if they worsen, seek medical attention.

## Patient Counseling for PMS

Educating women with PMS about the timing of symptoms (symptom log/calendar) and what might control them may increase compliance with recommended therapies. Practitioners should be prepared to discuss treatment of behavioral as well as physical symptoms of mild to moderate PMS. If the patient wants to use nonprescription medications or vitamins, the proper use and potential adverse effects of these agents should be explained. The patient should also be advised that treatment measures must be implemented during every menstrual cycle because it may take several cycles for symptomatic relief to occur. The box Patient Education for Premenstrual Syndrome lists specific information to provide patients.

## Evaluation of Patient Outcomes for PMS

Patient monitoring is accomplished by having the patient report whether the symptoms are resolved. It may take several menstrual cycles to ascertain if lifestyle changes or nonprescription therapies are reducing the symptoms of PMS. Comparing the symptom log/calendar for pre and post months can help determine the usefulness of a therapy. Follow-up with a phone call allows the practitioner to discuss treatment effectiveness (continued or altered symptoms) and to clarify information or answer any patient questions. Reasons for advising the patient to see a primary care provider are either persistent symptoms or symptoms that the patient reports as disruptive to personal relationships or the patient's ability to engage in usual activities or function productively at work.

## TOXIC SHOCK SYNDROME

Toxic shock syndrome was a term originally coined in 1978 to describe a severe multisystem illness characterized by high fever, profound hypotension, severe diarrhea, mental confusion, renal failure, erythroderma, and skin desquamation. In 1980, these symptoms were recognized as affecting a relatively large number of young, previously healthy, menstruating women, and the term *toxic shock syndrome* was applied to their illness. TSS is commonly divided into menstrual and nonmenstrual cases.

### Epidemiology of Menstrual TSS

Menstrual TSS has been found to affect primarily young women between 15 and 19 years of age; about 40% of cases of menstrual TSS still occur in women 13 to 19 years of age.[50] Menstrual TSS is associated with menstruation and tampon use (98% of cases), and is strongly linked to the use of high-absorbency tampons.[50]

During the TSS epidemic of 1979 to 1980, menstrual TSS accounted for 91% of TSS cases. More recently (1987-1996), menstrual TSS accounted for only 59% of all TSS cases.[50,51] Incidence rates have also declined from 10 per 100,000 for women ages 15 to 44 years old in 1980 to 2 to 4 per 100,000 currently.[50,51] The decrease in cases of menstrual TSS has been attributed to several factors: removal of superabsorbent tampons from the market, a change in the composition of tampons, an increased awareness of the recommendations for the frequency of tampon changing and the need to alternate tampon and pad use, and FDA-required standardized labeling of tampons.[50]

### Etiology of Menstrual TSS

TSS is a severe, life-threatening multisystem disease caused by the toxin-producing strains of *Staphylococcus aureus* or *Streptococcus pyogenes*. TSS is an inflammatory immune response to the enterotoxins produced by these bacteria. *S. aureus* is the cause of almost all cases of menstrual TSS.[52] Toxin-producing strains of *S. aureus* produce the superantigen (SAG) toxin TSST-1. Most adults have a protective level of antibodies against the TSST-1 toxin. Younger people who lack this antibody protection and who become infected with a toxin-producing strain of *S. aureus* may develop TSS.[52]

Risk factors for menstrual TSS have been identified. The strongest predictor of risk is the use of tampons. Since the early 1980s, when the association between tampon usage and TSS was first noted, the absorbency and composition of tampons have changed dramatically. Certain compositions were associated with a higher risk, and tampons with cross-linked carboxymethylcellulose and polyester foam were removed from the market. In addition, FDA changed the requirement for the labeling of tampons so that terms used to indicate the absorbency of tampons have a uniform meaning and indicate a specific range of fluid absorbed per tampon. Nonetheless, women who currently use tampons still have a 33-fold greater risk for TSS than nonusers. The greatest risk is associated with the use of higher absorbency tampons; for every 1-g increase in absorbency, the risk for TSS increases 34% to 37%. Continuous use of tampons for at least 1 day of menses has also been shown to correlate with an increased risk for menstrual TSS. Besides tampons, TSS has been associated with the use of barrier contraceptives, including diaphragms, cervical caps, and cervical sponges, and with IUDs.[52]

### Pathophysiology of Menstrual TSS

TSS develops in three phases: proliferation of toxin-producing bacteria, production of toxin, and engagement of the immune system. Menstrual blood can serve as a medium for bacterial growth, and the retention of blood in the vagina by the tampon can increase bacterial proliferation. Also, some tampons contain fibers that inhibit lactobacilli, thereby diminishing their ability to limit the proliferation of *S. aureus*. Four conditions promote toxin production: (1) elevated protein levels, (2) neutral pH, (3) elevated carbon dioxide levels, and (4) elevated oxygen levels.[50] During menses, menstrual blood provides an increase in protein and also increases vaginal pH to 7, neutral. Tampon use may create the environment for TSS by introducing oxygen into the vagina.[50] Hours after the introduction of a tampon the vagina returns to its anaerobic state with elevated carbon dioxide levels. In addition, tampons, IUDs, and contraceptive sponges have been shown to create microtrauma, and may increase exposure of the toxins to the circulation and immune system. Exposure of immune cells to TSST-1 initiates the inflammatory cascade involving interleukin-1 and tumor necrosis factor. This inflammatory response results in the signs and symptoms of TSS.[52]

### Signs and Symptoms of Menstrual TSS

By definition, menstrual TSS occurs within 2 days of the onset of menses, during menses or within 2 days after menses.[51] Prodromal symptoms (malaise, myalgias, and chills) occur for 2 to 3 days prior to TSS.[52] GI symptoms (vomiting, diarrhea, and abdominal pain) typically occur early in the illness and affect almost all patients. After that period of time, TSS characteristically evolves quite rapidly. Full-blown TSS includes high fever, myalgias, vomiting and diarrhea, erythroderma, decreased urine output, severe hypotension, and shock. Neurologic manifestations (headache, confusion, agitation, lethargy, and seizures) also occur in almost all cases. Acute renal failure, cardiac involvement, and adult respiratory distress syndrome are also common.

Dermatologic manifestations are characteristic of TSS; both early rash and subsequent skin desquamation are required for a definite diagnosis (Table 9-7). The early rash is often described as a sunburnlike, diffuse, macular erythroderma that is not pruritic. About 5 to 12 days after the onset of TSS, desquamation of the skin on the patient's face, trunk, and extremities, including the soles of the feet and the palms of the hands, occurs.

## PATIENT EDUCATION FOR TOXIC SHOCK SYNDROME

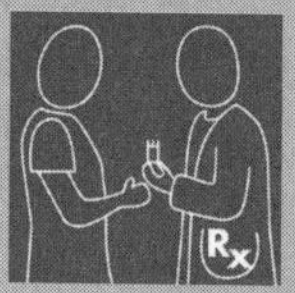

The objective of self-treatment is to reduce the risk of developing toxic shock syndrome (TSS) associated with the use of tampons or contraceptive devices. For most patients, carefully following product instructions and the self-care measures listed here will help ensure optimal therapeutic outcomes.

- To reduce the risk to almost zero, use sanitary pads instead of tampons during your period.
- To lower the risk while using tampons, use the lowest-absorbency tampons compatible with your needs. Also, alternate the use of menstrual pads with the use of tampons (e.g., use pads at night).
- Change tampons four to six times a day and at least every 6 hours; overnight use should be no longer than 8 hours.
- Wash your hands with soap before inserting anything into the vagina (e.g., tampon, diaphragm, contraceptive sponge, or vaginal medication). The bacteria causing TSS is usually found on the skin.
- Do not leave a contraceptive sponge, diaphragm, or cervical cap in place in the vagina longer than recommended; do not use any of them during menstruation.
- Do not use tampons, contraceptive sponges, or a cervical cap during the first 12 weeks after childbirth. It may also be best to avoid using a diaphragm.
- Read the insert on TSS enclosed in the tampon package and familiarize yourself with the early symptoms of this disorder.

⚠ If you develop symptoms of TSS (a high fever, muscle aches, a sunburnlike rash appearing after a day or two, weakness, fatigue, nausea, vomiting, and diarrhea), remove the tampon or contraceptive device immediately and seek emergency medical treatment. If left untreated, TSS can cause shock and even death.

**TABLE 9-7 Centers for Disease Control and Prevention Case Definition of TSS**

- Fever: oral temperature ≥102°F (38.9°C)
- Rash: diffuse macular erythroderma
- Desquamation: 1-2 weeks after onset of illness, particularly on palms and soles
- Hypotension: systolic blood pressure ≤90 mm Hg, orthostatic drop in diastolic ≥15 mm Hg; orthostatic syncope or dizziness
- Involvement of three or more of the following organ systems:
  - Gastrointestinal: vomiting or diarrhea at onset of illness
  - Muscular: severe myalgia or twice-normal creatine phosphokinase
  - Mucous membranes: vaginal, oropharyngeal, or conjunctival hyperemia
  - Renal: twice-normal blood urea nitrogen or creatinine or pyuria (more than five white blood cells in a high-power field)
  - Hepatic: twice-normal bilirubin or transaminases
  - Hematologic: platelets <1,000,000/mm$^3$
- Central nervous system: disorientation or alterations in consciousness without focal neurologic signs when fever and hypotension are absent
- Negative results on the following tests, if obtained:
  - Blood, throat, or cerebrospinal fluid cultures (blood culture may be positive for *S. aureus*)
  - Serologic tests for Rocky Mountain spotted fever, leptospirosis, or measles

## Prevention of Menstrual TSS

Women can reduce the risk of menstrual TSS to nearly zero by using sanitary pads instead of tampons during their menstrual cycle. Women who use tampons can reduce the risk by following the guidelines in the box Patient Education for Toxic Shock Syndrome.

Women who have had TSS are at risk for recurrence; TSS recurs in about 28% to 64% of women with menstrual TSS.[52] Recurrence rates are lower for women who are treated with antibiotics during TSS. Prevention of TSS for these patients includes avoiding tampons, IUDs, diaphragms, and contraceptive sponges.

## Assessment of Menstrual TSS: A Case-based Approach

Obtaining prompt medical attention is a very important aspect of care for patients with symptoms consistent with TSS. A practitioner can be alert to symptoms of TSS when patients seek nonprescription therapy for a severe "flu" (e.g., fever, vomiting, diarrhea, dizziness) or an unusual skin rash that occurs in conjunction with the previously described symptoms. If TSS is suspected, the patient should be advised to seek medical care immediately and avoid use of NSAIDs for fever and myalgias, as these agents may increase the progression of TSS by increasing the production of tumor necrosis factor.

## Patient Counseling for Menstrual TSS

Tampons are used by most (81%) women of all ages during the reproductive years.[53] Practitioners should counsel patients about the prevention of TSS as outlined in the box Patient Education for Toxic Shock Syndrome. In particular, the importance of washing the hands (organisms causing TSS are found on the skin) before inserting a tampon should be emphasized as only about half of women report doing so.[53] Similarly, about 18% to 36% of women report that they do not always change a tampon at least every 6 hours. The practitioner should emphasize, however, that the risk for this condition is quite small. If a patient presents with early symptoms of TSS, she should be advised to remove the tampon or any barrier contraceptive device and to seek emergency medical treatment.

## KEY POINTS FOR DISORDERS RELATED TO MENSTRUATION

- Self-care is appropriate for an otherwise healthy young woman with a history consistent with primary dysmenorrhea who is not sexually active or for a woman diagnosed with primary dysmenorrhea. Adolescents with pelvic pain who are sexually active (at risk for PID) and women with characteristics indicating secondary dysmenorrhea should be referred for medical evaluation
- NSAIDs are the drugs of choice for the management of primary dysmenorrhea. These medications should be taken at the onset, or just prior to menses and used in scheduled doses for several days for optimum reduction in pain and cramping.
- The use of local topical heat can also provide relief from dysmenorrhea. Its analgesic effect had a faster onset than drug therapy, and it can add to the relief provided by an NSAID. Nondrug therapy may be especially useful for women who cannot tolerate or who do not respond to nonprescription NSAIDs.
- It is important to distinguish PMS/PMDD from typical premenstrual symptoms and also from premenstrual exacerbations of other disorders (PME), particularly mood disorders.
- PMS/PMDD symptoms typically begin or intensify about a week prior to the onset of menses, peak the day before or on the first day of menses, and resolve within several days after the beginning of menses. A woman with PMS or PMDD experiences a symptom-free interval during days 4 to 12 of her menstrual cycle.
- PMS symptoms are chronic and in most cases will continue until menopause. Therefore, the cost of therapy, the fact that a woman may become pregnant, and the likelihood of adverse effects from therapy are important considerations in selecting therapy.
- Several nonprescription or complementary agents (calcium, magnesium, vitamin E, pyridoxine, and chasteberry [*Vitex agnus*]) might be suggested to reduce the symptoms of PMS. PMDD symptoms warrant prescription drug therapy.
- TSS has been linked to tampon use. To lower the risk for TSS while using tampons, women should use the lowest-absorbency tampons compatible with their needs and alternate the use of sanitary pads with the use of tampons (e.g., at night).

## References


1. Yussman SM, Klein JD. Adolescent health care. In Leppert PC, Peipert JF, eds. *Primary Care for Women.* 2nd ed. Philadelphia: Lippincott Williams & Wilkins; 2004.
2. Griswold D. Menstruation and related problems and concerns. In Youngkin EQ, Davis MS, eds. *Women's Health: A Primary Care Clinical Guide.* 3rd ed. Upper Saddle River, NJ: Prentice Hall 2004.
3. Letterie GS. Disorders of menstruation: from amenorrhea to menorrhagia. In Lemcke DP, Pattison J, Marshall LA, et al., eds. *Current Care of Women Diagnosis and Treatment.* New York: Lange Medical Books McGraw-Hill; 2004.
4. Leppert PC. The reproductive-age woman. In: Leppert PC, Peipert JF, eds. *Primary Care for Women.* 2nd ed. Philadelphia: Lippincott Williams & Wilkins; 2004.
5. Durain D. Primary dysmenorrhea: assessment and management update. *J Midwifery Women's Health.* 2004;49:520-8.
6. Slap GB. Menstrual disorders in adolescents. *Best Pract Res Clin Obstet Gynaecol.* 2003;17:75-92.
7. Howard FM. Dysmenorrhea. In Leppert PC, Peipert JF, eds. *Primary Care for Women.* 2nd ed. Philadelphia: Lippincott Williams & Wilkins; 2004.
8. Davis AR, Westhoff CL. Primary dysmenorrhea in adolescent girls and treatment with oral contraceptives. *J Pediatr Gynecol.* 2001; 14:3-8.
9. Banikarim C, Chacko MR, Kelder SH. Prevalence and impact of dysmenorrhea on Hispanic female adolescents. *Arch Pediatr Adolesc Med.* 2000;154:1226-9.
10. Marsden JS, Strickland CD, Clements TL. Guaifenesin as a treatment for primary dysmenorrhea. *J Am Board Fam Pract.* 2004;17: 240-6.
11. Mazza D. *Women's Health in General Practice.* Edinburgh: Butterworth Heinemann; 2004.
12. Hewison A, van den Akker OB. Dysmenorrhea, menstrual attitude, and GP consultation. *Br J Nurs.* 1996;5:480-4.
13. Campbell MA, McGrath PJ. Non-pharmacologic strategies used by adolescents for the management of menstrual discomfort. *Clin J Pain.* 1999;15:313-20.
14. Akin M, Price W, Rodriguez G Jr, et al. Continuous, low-level, topical heat wrap therapy as compared to acetaminophen for primary dysmenorrhea. *J Reprod Med.* 2004;49:739-45.
15. Campbell MA, McGrath PJ. Use of medication by adolescents for the management of menstrual discomfort. *Arch Pediatr Adolesc Med.* 1997;151:905-13.
16. Hillen TJ, Grbavac SL, Johnston PJ, et al. Primary dysmenorrhea in young western Australian women: prevalence, impact, and knowledge of treatment. *J Adolesc Health.* 1999;25:40-5.
17. Balbi C, Musone R, Menditto A, et al. Influence of menstrual factors and dietary habits on menstrual pain in adolescence age. *Eur J Obstet Gynecol Reprod Biol.* 2000;91:143-8.
18. Benassi L, Barletta FP, Baroncini L, et al. Effectiveness of magnesium pidolate in the prophylactic treatment of primary dysmenorrhea. *Clin Exp Obstet Gynecol.* 1992;19:176-9.
19. Wilson ML, Murphy PA. Herbal and dietary therapies for primary and secondary dysmenorrhea. *Cochrane Database Syst Rev.* 2001; CD002124.
20. Deutch B, Jorgensen EB, Hansen JC. Menstrual discomfort in Danish women reduced by dietary supplements of omega-3 PUFA and B-12 (fish oil or seal oil capsules). *Nutr Res.* 2000;20: 621-31.
21. Ziaei S, Faghihzadeh F, Sohrabvand M, et al. A randomized placebo-controlled trial to determine the effect of vitamin E in treatment of primary dysmenorrhea. *Br J Obstet Gynaecol.* 2001; 108:1181-3.
22. Jahromi BN, Tartifizadeh A, Khabnadideh S. Comparison of fennel and mefenamic acidfor the treatment of primary dysmenorrhea. *Int J Gynaecol Obstet.* 2003;80:153-7.
23. Kessel B. Premenstrual syndrome: advances in diagnosis and treatment. *Obstet Gynecol Clin North Am.* 2000;27:625-39.
24. Johnson SR. Premenstrual syndrome, premenstrual dysphoric disorder, and beyond: a clinical primer for practitioners. *Obstet Gynecol.* 2004;104845-59.
25. Ryden JR. Premenstrual syndrome. In: Ryden JR, Blumenthal PD, eds. *Practical Gynecology: A Guide for the Primary Care Physician.* Philadelphia: American College of Physicians; 2002.
26. Dell DL. Premenstrual syndrome, premenstrual dysphoric disorder, and premenstrual exacerbation of another disorder. *Clin Obstet Gynecol.* 2004;47:568-75.

27. Dickerson LM, Mazyck PJ, Hunter MH. Premenstrual syndrome. *Am Fam Physician.* 2003;67:1743-52.
28. Grady-Weliky TA, Lewis V. Premenstrual syndrome. In: Leppert PC, Peipert JF, eds. *Primary Care for Women.* 2nd ed. Philadelphia: Lippincott Williams & Wilkins; 2004.
29. Sternfeld B, Swindle R, Chawla A, et al. Severity of premenstrual symptoms in a health maintenance organization population. *Obstet Gynecol.* 2002;99:1014-24.
30. Cohen LS, Soares CN, Otto MW, et al. Prevalence and predictors of premenstrual dysphoric disorder (PMDD) in older premenopausal women: the Harvard study of moods and cycles. *J Affect Disord.* 2002;70:125-32.
31. Wittchen HU, Becker E, Lieb R, Krause P. Prevalence, incidence and stability of premenstrual dysphoric disorder in the community. *Psychol Med.* 2002;32:119-32.
32. Thys-Jacobs S. Micronutrients and the premenstrual syndrome: the case for calcium. *J Am Coll Nutr.* 2000;19: 220-7.
33. Treloar SA, Heath AC, Martin NG. Genetic and environmental influences in premenstrual symptoms in an Australian twin sample. *Psychol Med.* 2002;32:25-38.
34. Ulman KH, Carlson KJ. Premenstrual syndrome. In: Carlson KJ, Eisenstat SA, eds. *Primary Care of Women.* 2nd ed. St Louis: Mosby; 2002.
35. Dog TL. Integrative treatments for premenstrual syndrome. *Altern Ther Health Med.* 2001;7:32-9.
36. Sayegh R, Wurtman J, Spiers P, et al. The effect of a carbohydrate-rich beverage on mood, appetite, and cognitive function in women with premenstrual syndrome. *Obstet Gynecol.* 1995;86:520-8.
37. Steiner M, Pearlstein T. Premenstrual dysphoria and the serotonin system: pathophysiology and treatment. *J Clin Psychiatry.* 2000;61(suppl 12):17-21.
38. Singh B, Berman BM, Simpson RL, et al. Incidence of premenstrual syndrome and remedy usage: a national probability sample study. *Altern Ther Health Med.* 1998;4:75-9.
39. Wyatt KM, Dimmock PW, Jones PW, et al. Efficacy of vitamin $B_6$ in the treatment of premenstrual syndrome: systematic review. *BMJ.* 1999;318:1375-81.
40. Thys-Jacobs S, Starkey P, Bernstein D, et al. Calcium carbonate and the premenstrual syndrome: effect on premenstrual and menstrual symptoms. *Am J Obstet Gynecol.* 1998;179:444-52.
41. Penland JG, Johnson PE. Dietary calcium and manganese effects on menstrual cycle symptoms. *Am J Obstet Gynecol.* 1993;168:1417-23.
42. Facchinetti F, Borella P, Sances G, et al. Oral magnesium successfully relieves premenstrual mood changes. *Obstet Gynecol.* 1991;78:177-81.
43. O'Brien PMS, Ismail KMK, Dimmock P. Premenstrual syndrome. In: Shaw RW, Soutter WP, Stanton SL, eds. *Gynecology.* 3rd ed. Edinburgh: Churchill Livingstone; 2003.
44. Girman A, Lee R, Kligler B. An integrative medicine approach to premenstrual syndrome. *Am J Obstet Gynecol.* 2003;188:S56-65.
45. Schellenberg R. Treatment for the premenstrual syndrome with agnus castus fruit extract: prospective, randomized, placebo-controlled study. *BMJ.* 2001;322:134-7.
46. Berger D, Schaffner W, Schrader E, et al. Efficacy of *Vitex agnus* L. extract Ze 440 in patients with premenstrual syndrome (PMS). *Arch Gynecol Obstet.* 2000;264:150-3.
47. Loch EG, Selle H, Boblitz N. Treatment of premenstrual syndrome with a phytopharmaceutical formulation containing Vitex agnus castus. *J Women's Health Gend Based Med.* 2000;9:315-20.
48. Atmaca M, Kumru S, Tezcan E. Fluoxetine versus Vitex agnus castus extract in the treatment of premenstrual dysphoric disorder. *Hum Psychopharmacol Clin Exp.* 2003;18:191-5.
49. Lam RW, Carter D, Misri S, et al. A controlled study of light therapy in women with late luteal phase dysphoric disorder. *Psychiatry Res.* 1999;86:185-92.
50. McCormick JK, Yarwood JM, Schlievert PM. Toxic shock syndrome and bacterial superantigens: an update. *Annu Rev Microbiol.* 2001;55:77-104.
51. Schlievert PM, Tripp TJ, Perterson ML. Reemergence of Staphylococcal toxic shock syndrome in Minneapolis-St. Paul, Minnesota, during the 2000-2003 surveillance period. *J Clin Microbiol.* 2004;42:2875-6.
52. Reiss MA. Toxic shock syndrome. *Prim Care Update Obstet/Gynecol.* 2000;7:85-90.
53. Czerwinski BS. Variation in feminine hygiene practices as a function of age. *J Obstet Gynecol Neonatal Nurs.* 2000; 29:625-33.

CHAPTER 10

# Prevention of Pregnancy and Sexually Transmitted Infections

*Louise Parent-Stevens and Jennifer L. Hardman*

Unprotected sexual activity can result in unintended pregnancy and sexually transmitted infections (STIs), either of which can exact a high physical, psychological, and financial toll on those affected. This chapter discusses how nonprescription contraceptive products or methods, when properly used, can guard against the risks of these adverse outcomes.

According to the 2002 National Survey of Family Growth (NSFG), approximately 90% of sexually active 15- to 44-year-old U.S. women at risk for unintended pregnancy use some form of birth control.[1] Table 10-1 lists the percentage of women using each of the various contraceptive methods available. Some women use more than one method simultaneously. Approximately half of women using condoms do so in conjunction with another method such as hormonal or chemical agents.[1]

In the United States and worldwide, reliance on nonprescription methods of contraception for pregnancy and STI prevention is widespread. The fact that such products are readily accessible and relatively inexpensive makes them very important for those who do not have access to family-planning services, choose not to use primary care providers or clinics, or are unable or unwilling to use prescription contraceptives. Even if a prescription product is chosen as the primary contraceptive method, low-cost and low-risk nonprescription methods may be appropriate at different times during a person's sexually active life.

## Epidemiology of Pregnancy and STIs

Close to 50% of pregnancies in the United States are unintended.[3] Women with childbearing potential who engage in unprotected intercourse experience an annual pregnancy rate of approximately 85%. However, a survey of women with unintended pregnancies found that more than half had been using a method of contraception during the month in which they conceived.[3] This high rate of unintended pregnancy despite the use of contraception may be a result of either inherent method failure or incorrect or inconsistent use of the contraceptive method.

In the United States alone, an estimated 15 million persons are infected annually with one or more STIs and 65 million persons are living with STIs.[4,5] Most STIs involve individuals younger than 25 years.[5]

Of particular concern is the high risk of pregnancy and STIs in the adolescent population. The NSFG and the National Longitudinal Study of Adolescent Health found that approximately one half of high school students had experienced sexual intercourse.[6] Although the teenage pregnancy rate in the United States (9.7% of 15- to 19-year-olds in 1996) has declined in recent years, it remains the highest among developed countries.[7]

Adolescents, more than any other group, are particularly vulnerable to STIs. Reasons include having multiple sexual partners, unprotected intercourse, an inherent biologic susceptibility to infection, and barriers to health care utilization.[8] The economic, social, and personal costs of STIs are staggering. The direct and indirect costs associated with STIs, excluding the impact of human immunodeficiency virus (HIV) and acquired immunodeficiency syndrome (AIDS), are estimated to exceed $10 billion yearly.[4] AIDS, chlamydia, gonorrhea, and syphilis are the only STIs that are reportable in every state.[4] Protecting the public health requires the timely and accurate diagnosis of STIs and their appropriate treatment.

## Etiology of Pregnancy and STIs

Pregnancy can result only when a viable egg is available for fertilization by a sperm. (See Chapter 9 for a discussion of the reproductive process.) It is estimated that conception can occur during a 6-day window beginning 5 days before ovulation through the day of ovulation. The estimated risk of pregnancy from an unprotected coital act during this 6-day period in the middle of the menstrual cycle ranges from 5% to 45%, with peak risk occurring with intercourse the day before ovulation.[9] Pregnancy can occur even with the use of contraceptive products if the product is used incorrectly or it fails (e.g., condom breakage).

STIs are acquired through contact with infected genital tissues, mucous membranes, and/or body fluids. Causative agents typically include bacteria, viruses, and protozoa. Table 10-2 summarizes the major infections. Whereas STIs affect both genders, women are more likely to develop reproductive consequences including pelvic inflammatory disease, chronic pelvic pain, ectopic pregnancy, malignancies, and infertility. Intrauterine and perinatal morbidity and mortality also increase as a consequence of STIs during pregnancy.[5] These gender-biased

**Editor's Note:** This chapter is based, in part, on the 14th edition chapters "Prevention of Unintended Pregnancy," written by Louise Parent-Stevens and Jennifer L. Hardman, and "Prevention of Sexually Transmitted Infections," written by Charles D. Ponte.

**TABLE 10-1 Failure and Use Rates of Various Contraceptive Methods[1,2]**

| Method | Sexually Active Women at Risk for Unintended Pregnancy Using Method (%)* | Accidental Pregnancy in the First Year of Use (%) | |
|---|---|---|---|
| | | Typical Use† | Perfect Use‡ |
| No method | 10.2 | 85 | |
| Withdrawal | 3.4 | 27 | 4 |
| Natural family planning (periodic abstinence) | 12.4 | 25 | |
| Calendar (rhythm) method | | | 9 |
| Cervical mucus (ovulation) method | | | 3 |
| Symptothermal method | | | 2 |
| Basal body temperature (postovulation) method | | | 1 |
| Lactational amenorrhea method (first 6 months postpartum) | | | 2 |
| Spermicides (foam, gel, vaginal suppositories, vaginal film) | <0.8 | 29 | 18 |
| Cervical cap (with spermicide) | <0.8 | 32 (parous women)<br>16 (nulliparous women) | 26 (parous women)<br>9 (nulliparous women) |
| Diaphragm (with spermicide) | 0.3 | 16 | 6 |
| Contraceptive sponge | <0.8 | 32 (parous women)<br>16 (nulliparous women) | 20 (parous women)<br>9 (nulliparous women) |
| Male condom (without spermicide) | 15.3 | 15 | 2 |
| Female condom (without spermicide) | <0.8 | 21 | 5 |
| Prescription methods | 33.6 | 0.05-8 | ≤0.6 |
| Sterilization (male/female) | 35.2 | ≤0.5 | ≤0.5 |

* Percentage of sexually active 15- to 44-year-old women who are not pregnant, postpartum, nor attempting to become pregnant.

† Among typical couples who initiate use of a method (not necessarily for the first time), the percentage who experience an accidental pregnancy during the first year if they do not stop use for any other reason.

‡ Among typical couples who initiate use of a method (not necessarily for the first time) and who use it consistently and correctly, the percentage who experience an accidental pregnancy during the first year if they do not stop use for any other reason.

**TABLE 10-2 Sexually Transmitted Infections**

| Disease/Scientific Name (Type) | Incubation Period | Symptoms | Diagnosis/Treatment | Complications | Congenital Transmission/ Neonatal Complications |
|---|---|---|---|---|---|
| **Curable STIs** | | | | | |
| Genital chlamydia *Chlamydia trachomatis* (bacterium) | | M: range from asx to urethritis, proctitis, urogenital discharge, itching, dysuria<br>F: range from asx to vaginal discharge, postcoital bleeding, cervicitis | Culture of affected tissue/antibiotics | PID, ectopic pregnancy, infertility | Yes/ ophthalmia neonatorum, pneumonia |

**TABLE 10-2 Sexually Transmitted Infections (continued)**

| Disease/Scientific Name (Type) | Incubation Period | Symptoms | Diagnosis/Treatment | Complications | Congenital Transmission/ Neonatal Complications |
|---|---|---|---|---|---|
| Gonorrhea *Neisseria gonorrhea* (bacterium) | Up to 10 days | Urethritis, cervicitis, proctitis, pharyngitis M: mucopurulent urethral discharge F: often asx | Culture/antibiotics | Septic arthritis, perihepatitis, endocarditis, meningitis, PID, infertility, ectopic pregnancy | Yes/sepsis, meningitis, arthritis, ocular infections |
| Nongonococcal urethritis (males) Various, including *C. trachomatis, Ureaplasma urealyticum, Mycoplasma* sp. (bacteria) | 1-2 weeks | M: nonspecific urethritis, discharge, dysuria, pruritus | Nucleic acid amplification test/ antibiotics | Epididymitis, proctitis, proctocolitis, Reiter syndrome | — |
| Syphilis *Treponema pallidum* (spirochete) | 3 weeks | Primary syphilis: chancre | Darkfield microscopy or direct fluorescent antibody exam of tissue/antibiotics | Secondary syphilis: rash, lymphedema, hepatospleno-megaly, alopecia Tertiary syphilis: syphilitic tumors of vasculature, CNS, skin and skeleton | Yes/stillbirth, preterm labor, intrauterine growth restriction, hepatosplenomeg aly, failure to thrive, progression to neurosyphilis as adult |
| Trichomoniasis *Trichomonas vaginalis* (flagellated anaerobic protozoan) | | M: commonly asx F: ~50% asx, malodorous, frothy green vaginal discharge, itching, dyspareunia, postcoital bleeding | Microscopic exam of vaginal fluids Antibiotics | Pregnancy: preterm labor, low-birthweight, premature rupture of membranes | No |
| **Noncurable STIs** | | | | | |
| AIDS HIV (virus) | Up to 10 years | After initial flulike illness, asx until OI occur | Serologic antibody testing/antivirals, prophylaxis for OI | OI, malignancies, death | Yes, also transmitted via breast milk |
| Genital warts Human papilloma virus* (DNA virus) | 2-4 months (average) | Asx infections common, warts on external genitalia, rectum, anus, perineum, mouth, larynx, vagina, urethra, cervix | Colposcopy, serology, DNA/RNA probe/ cytoablation (chemical or physical), antivirals, antimetabolites, immunomodulators | Cervical dysplasia/ neoplasia | Yes |
| Genital herpes HSV (virus) | 6 days (average) | Vesicular/ulcerative lesions on mucus membranes | Culture/antivirals | Disseminated infection, pneumonitis, hepatitis, meningitis/ encephalitis | Yes |
| Hepatitis B virus (virus) | 6 weeks-6 months | Acute: self-limited, mild | Serology/antivirals | Cirrhosis, hepato-cellular cancer | Yes |
| Hepatitis C virus (virus) | 8-9 weeks | Asx or mild clinical illness | Serology/antivirals | Cirrhosis, hepato-cellular cancer | Yes |

Key: asx, asymptomatic; F, female; HIV, human immunodeficiency virus; HPV, human papilloma virus; HSV, herpes simplex virus; M, male; OI, opportunistic infections; PID, pelvic inflammatory disease.

* Self-clearance of HPM virus may occur.

complications may result from difficulties in diagnosis, lack of patient recognition of symptoms, and high probability of asymptomatic infection.[5] Women are also more likely than men to acquire an STI after a single unprotected coital act: Approximately 50% of women will become infected with gonorrhea after a single exposure with an infected man, whereas only 25% of men contract gonorrhea from a single exposure with an infected woman.[5]

According to the 2002 NSFG, approximately 20% of sexually active female teenagers engage in unprotected intercourse or use contraceptives only sporadically.[1] The reasons for low levels of contraceptive use in this population include lack of knowledge, denial, lack of planning, and infrequent or unpredictable intercourse. Approximately 20% of 15- to 19-year-olds did not use any contraception during their first sexual encounter. Among these, half became pregnant within a year after their first intercourse.[1,10] Of teenage pregnancies, 78% are unintended.[3] Often, a young woman does not use contraceptives until after she becomes pregnant. Repeat pregnancies are common, occurring in 17% to 35% of adolescent mothers, and are often associated with inadequate contraceptive use after the first pregnancy.[11] Women who are approaching menopause also experience a large number of unintended pregnancies. Failure to use contraceptive products also increases the risk of STIs in these populations.

## Prevention of Pregnancy and STIs

The goal of contraceptive use is to prevent unintended pregnancy and STIs in persons at risk with a minimum of adverse effects. No method of birth control is perfect. Contraceptive choices may change during a person's sexually active life. Major points to consider in selecting a contraceptive method should include safety, effectiveness, accessibility, and acceptability of the method to each sexual partner.

The primary safety factor to consider in choosing a method of contraception is the risk of side effects, including the potential for adverse effects on future fertility and on the fetus, if unintended conception occurs.

The effectiveness of a contraceptive method in preventing pregnancy is reported in two ways: the accidental pregnancy rate in the first year of *perfect* use (method-related failure rate) and in the first year of *typical* use (use-related failure rate) (Table 10-1). The lowest expected rate—that of perfect use—is very difficult to measure and indicates the method's theoretical effectiveness. It assumes accurate and consistent use of the method every time intercourse occurs. The more realistic rate of typical use includes pregnancies that may have occurred because of inconsistent or improper use of the method. Reported use-related failure rates vary, depending on the population studied. The 1995 NSFG found that women in low-income groups had higher levels of contraceptive failure than comparable women in higher-income groups; this finding may be related to lack of consistent access to contraception.[12] Effectiveness increases the longer a particular method is used. Decreased coital frequency and declining fertility in a population of older users may contribute to increased effectiveness rates.[2]

**TABLE 10-3 Prevention Strategies[5,8]**

- Abstain from sexual activity.
- Avoid intercourse with a known infected partner.
- Avoid intercourse with an individual having multiple sex partners.
- Use a new condom with each episode of anal, oral, or vaginal intercourse.
- Seek a mutually monogamous relationship with an uninfected partner.
- Discuss your partner's past sexual experiences.
- Examine your partner for genital lesions.
- Practice genital self-examination.
- Avoid sexual activity involving direct contact with blood, semen, or other body fluids.
- Choose safe and effective methods (e.g., mechanical or chemical barriers) to reduce the risk of STIs (consider adding more effective methods of pregnancy prevention when necessary).
- Avoid sexual activity if signs/symptoms of an STI are present.
- Consider vaccination if you are at high risk for a vaccine-preventable STI (e.g., HAV and HBV).

Key: HAV, hepatitis A virus; HBV, hepatitis B virus; STI, sexually transmitted infection.

The best way for an individual to avoid contracting an STI is either to abstain from risky sexual activity or to be involved in a long-term mutually monogamous sexual relationship with an uninfected partner.[8] For individuals who view abstinence or monogamy as unrealistic or unreasonable, preventive strategies in conjunction with use of selected contraceptives may provide the best alternative method for reducing risk of infection (Table 10-3, Table 10-4, and Figure 10-1).

### *Selection of a Contraceptive Method*

Acceptability of any given contraceptive method is vital for correct and consistent use of the method. Important acceptability factors include the user's religious beliefs and future reproductive plans, the partner's supportiveness, complexity of the method, degree of interruption of spontaneity, "messiness," and cost. To help their patients make informed decisions, practitioners should be aware of the safety, effectiveness, accessibility, acceptability, and relative cost of different contraceptive methods. The algorithm in Figure 10-1 can assist the practitioner in making appropriate contraceptive recommendations.

#### Nonprescription Contraceptive Products

Nonprescription contraceptive products, which include male condoms, female condoms, vaginal spermicides, and the contraceptive sponge, vary in effectiveness as protection against unintended pregnancy.

*Male Condoms* Condoms—also known as rubbers, sheaths, prophylactics, safes, skins, or pros—are the most important barrier contraceptive device in an era of STIs. Condom sales increased significantly after the Surgeon General's report on their benefit in preventing STIs.[13]

**TABLE 10-4 Contraceptive Methods and STI Risk**

| Method | Bacterial STI | Viral STI |
|---|---|---|
| Latex male condoms | Protective* | Protective* |
| Polyurethane male condoms | Probably protective* | Probably protective* |
| Natural membrane condoms | Protective* | Not protective* |
| Female condoms | Protective* | Protective* |
| Spermicides | Possibly increased risk | Possibly increased risk |
| Diaphragms (with spermicide) | Possibly protective against cervical infection* | Possibly protective against cervical dysplasia/cancer |
| Contraceptive sponge | Possibly protective* | Not protective |
| Intrauterine devices | Not protective. Risk of pelvic inflammatory disease during first month following insertion | Not protective |
| Hormonal methods | Not protective. Increase in cervical *Chlamydia* | Not protective |
| Fertility awareness-based methods (e.g., calendar, basal body temperature, etc.) | Not protective | Not protective |

* Improper or inconsistent use will significantly decrease the protection these contraceptive products provide against transmission of STIs.

According to the 2002 NSFG, condom use among women at first intercourse rose from 38.1% in the 1980s to 67.3% in 1999-2002.[1] Apart from its role as a contraceptive, the importance of condoms in disease prevention is second only to that of abstinence.

Composition/Features Condoms are available in latex, polyurethane, and lamb cecum (natural membrane or skin; Table 10-5).

Latex condoms come in various sizes, colors, styles, shapes, and thicknesses (ranging from 0.03 mm to approximately 0.11 mm). Other features include reservoir tips, ribs, studs, and lubrication. Spermicide-treated condoms are also available, but the amount of spermicide they contain is much less than that of a vaginal spermicide; evidence is lacking on the increased contraceptive efficacy of spermicide-treated condoms.[14] Latex condoms range in price from $0.25 to $3.00 each.

Two brands of polyurethane condoms are currently available, and others not yet on the market have been approved by the Food and Drug Administration (FDA). Polyurethane condoms conduct heat well, come prelubricated, and are not subject to degradation by oil-based products.[15] However, they are less stretchy and, at $1.50 to $2.00 each, are more expensive than latex condoms.

Condoms made from lamb cecum are labeled only for pregnancy prevention because the presence of pores in the membrane may allow passage of viral organisms, including HIV and hepatitis B virus.[16] They conduct heat well and are very strong. With a price of about $3.00 each, they are also more expensive than latex condoms. Only a few brands of natural membrane condoms are on the market.

Effectiveness Since 1976, condom quality has been under the purview of FDA. The Center for Devices and Radiological Health is responsible for monitoring the quality of domestically produced and imported condoms. The testing program was expanded in 1987 because of concerns about protection from AIDS. The United States uses a water-leak test as the standard for latex condoms. The failure rate per batch cannot exceed 0.25%.[16] The condoms are also air-burst tested.[17] There is currently no standard test for polyurethane condoms.

The true incidence of condom breakage is unknown, and breakage rates from studies vary widely, ranging from 0.41% to 7.9%.[18] In some studies, however, a limited group of study patients reported multiple incidences of breakage, indicating that breakage may be related as much to the individual user as it is to manufacturing defects. Behaviors that have been associated with an increased risk of condom breakage are (1) incorrect placement of the condom; (2) use of an oil-based lubricant with latex condoms; (3) reuse of condoms; (4) increased duration, intensity, or frequency of coitus; and (5) prior history of condom breakage.[13,18,19] One study found a decreased incidence of breakage with continued use, indicating that correct use may improve with experience. The benefit of using additional lubrication with lubricated condoms is unclear. One study found that additional lubricant use increased the risk of condom slippage. However, another study found that use of an additional water-based lubricant was associated with decreased breakage rates, but no increase in condom slippage rates. Factors that may affect the impact of additional lubrication include the type of lubricant, the site of application (vaginal or rectal), and the type of intercourse (vaginal or anal).[19] A review of comparative studies found that the polyurethane condom had a significantly higher breakage and slippage rate than the latex condom.[15,20] One study also reported a significantly higher pregnancy rate with the polyurethane condom than with latex condoms.[21] Because of these reports, polyurethane condom use should be reserved for individuals with intolerance to latex condoms.

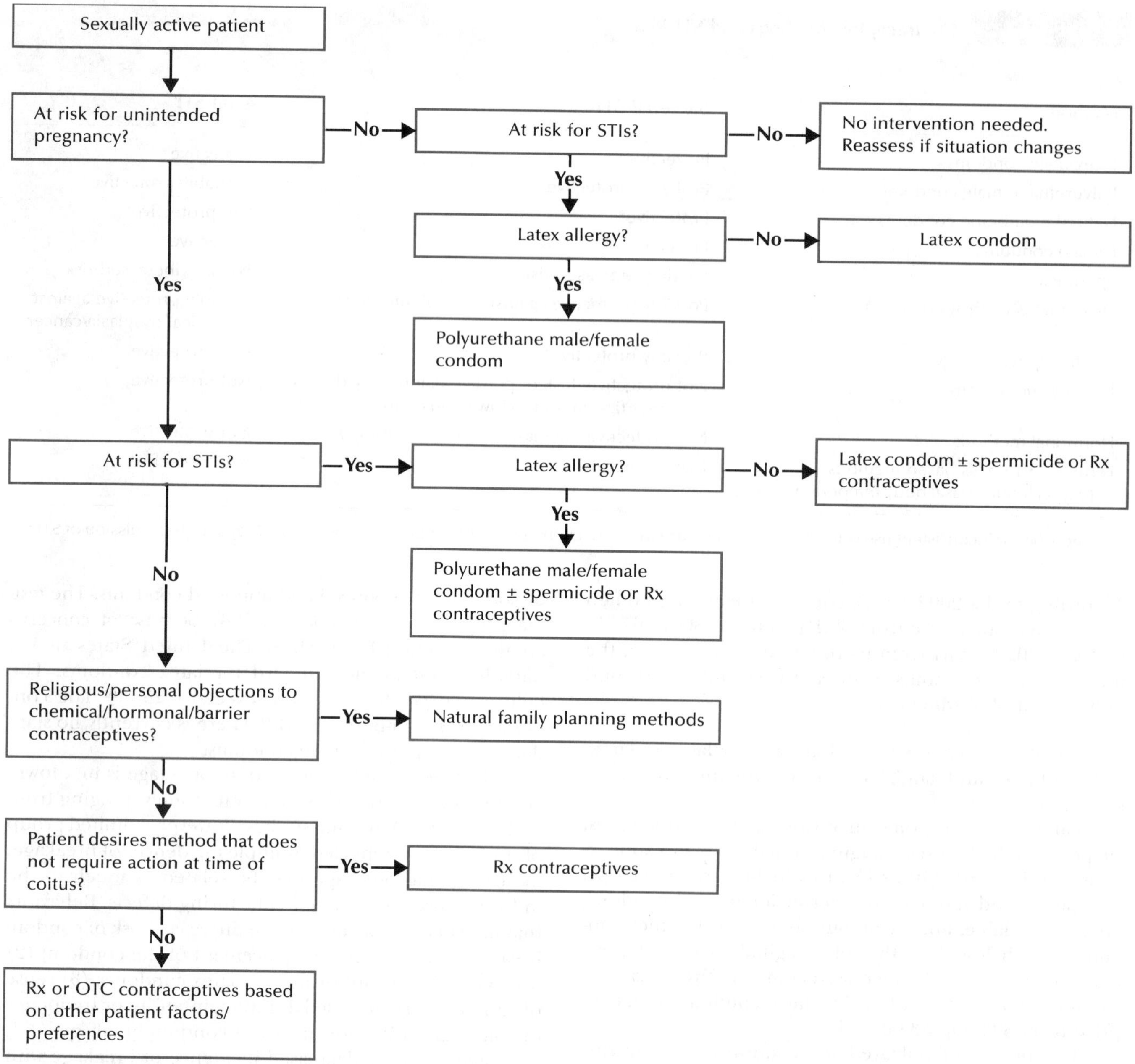


**FIGURE 10-1** Prevention of unintended pregnancy and sexually transmitted infections. Key: OTC, over-the-counter; Rx, prescription; STI, sexually transmitted infection.

The use-related failure rate for condoms is approximately 15 pregnancies per 100 women during the first year of use (Table 10-1). Efficacy of condoms regarding pregnancy prevention does appear to improve, however, with increasing duration of use.

In 2001, the National Institutes of Health Condom Effectiveness Conference concluded that male condoms reduced the risk of HIV infection in men and women by about 85% and gonorrhea in men by approximately 25% to 75%. HPV infection was not affected by condom use although HPV-related morbidity including condylomata in men and cervical neoplasia in women may be reduced.[17] Importantly, the evidence was inconclusive whether condoms affected the transmission of other STIs, including syphilis, chlamydia, trichomoniasis, genital herpes, gonorrhea in women, and chancroid. Studies suggest that nonoxynol-9–coated male condoms are no more effective than untreated condoms at preventing STIs, and their use as such has been discouraged because of possible increased risk of irritation and infection.[22] On the basis of this information, some manufacturers have discontinued production of spermicide-treated condoms.[14]

The most common cause of use-related failure with condoms, as with all other contraceptive methods, is lack of consistent, proper use.

Usage/Storage Guidelines Proper use of condoms is essential to their preventing pregnancy and STIs (Table

**TABLE 10-5 Selected Male Condoms**

| Trade Name | Product Features |
|---|---|
| **Polyurethane Condoms** | |
| Avanti | Lubricated; reservoir tip |
| Avanti Super Thin | Lubricated; reservoir tip |
| **Natural Membrane Condoms** | |
| Kling Tite Naturalamb | With or without spermicidal lubricant |
| Trojan Supra | With spermicidal lubricant |
| **Latex Condoms** | |
| Beyond Seven | Lubricated; with or without spermicide |
| Class Act Ribbed and Sensitive | Reservoir end; with or without spermicidal lubricant; ribbed surface |
| Durex Extra Sensitive | Reservoir end; lubricated; with or without spermicide |
| Kimono Microthin | Lubricated; with or without spermicide |
| LifeStyles: Assorted Colors, Form Fitting, or Studded | Colored; contour shaped; ribbed or rubber studded, large size |
| Night Light | Glow-in-the-dark |
| Trojan | Nonreservoir tip, nonlubricated |
| Trojan-Enz Large | Reservoir end; with or without spermicidal lubricant; large size |
| Trojan Magnum | Reservoir end; lubricated; large size |
| Trojan Pleasure Mesh | Surface texture; reservoir end; with or without spermicidal lubricant |
| Trojan Ribbed | Reservoir end; with or without spermicidal lubricant; ribbed/textured surface |
| Trojan Shared Pleasure | Reservoir tip, lubricated |
| Trojan Shared Sensation | Flared end with reservoir tip; lubricated; textured surface with bumps and ribs |
| Trojan Pleasure Mesh | Surface texture; reservoir end; with or without spermicidal lubricant |
| Vivid | Studded; extra thin; large size |

10-6). Patients using the polyurethane condom should be advised that it is not as elastic as the latex condom and will not fit as snugly. A space must be left at the tip when using condoms without a reservoir.

Prelubricated condoms are a good choice when lubrication is desired. Additional lubrication for use with any latex condom should be selected from products that do not harm or weaken the strength and integrity of the condom (Table 10-7).

Packaged condoms should be kept in their sealed packages until time of use and protected from light and excessive heat. Excessive heat or overexposure to ozone at levels found in some metropolitan areas will rapidly decrease the integrity of the latex. The shelf life of condoms under optimal conditions, as packaged by the manufacturers, is 3 to 5 years. FDA requires that latex condoms be labeled with an expiration date.[17] The user should always check for discoloration, brittleness, or stickiness, and should discard condoms displaying any of these characteristics, even if they are within the expiration date.

Safety Considerations The most frequent complaint about condoms is decreased sensitivity of the glans penis, resulting in decreased sexual pleasure for the male. Contact dermatitis caused by latex allergy is becoming a more common problem with condoms. An estimated 1% to 2% of the population and a higher percentage of health care workers may be sensitized to latex.[23] This condition, which can occur in the male or female partner, may be characterized by immediate localized itching and swelling (urticarial reaction) or by a delayed eczematous reaction. In patients with severe sensitivity, the reaction may spread beyond the area of physical contact with the latex.[24] The spermicide in spermicide-treated condoms may enhance latex allergy or cause sensitivity reactions itself.[13,14]

Product Selection Guidelines For most people, condoms are an effective, acceptable, inexpensive, safe, and nontoxic method of birth control. Given the wide variety of condoms available, patients should be encouraged to try a different style or brand if they are dissatisfied with the condom they have used previously. Before recommending a latex condom, health care providers should ask patients if they can wear rubber (latex) gloves or blow up a balloon without itching occurring. The sensitizers in latex condoms are usually antioxidants or accelerators used in processing the rubber. Because different manufacturers use different processes, changing brands may alleviate the

**TABLE 10-6 Usage Guidelines for Male Condoms**

- Use only condoms that are fresh (not previously opened), that are within their expiration date, and that have been stored in a dry, cool place (not a wallet or car glove compartment).
- Do not attempt to test the condom for leaks before using; this test only increases the risk of tearing.
- Condoms occasionally break. Have a vaginal spermicidal product (foam or jelly) available, and insert it as soon as possible if a condom break or spill occurs.
- Be aware that long fingernails or jewelry may easily tear condoms.
- As shown in drawing A, unroll the condom onto the erect penis before the penis comes into any contact with the vagina. If you start to put the condom on backward, discard that condom and use a fresh one. (Preejaculate secretions may contain sperm.)
- If you are not using a reservoir-tipped condom, leave 1/2 in. of space between the end of the condom and the tip of the penis by pinching the top of the condom as you unroll it (drawing B). This method leaves space for the ejaculate (drawing C) and decreases the risk of breakage.
- If your partner has vaginal dryness, use additional lubrication, if desired. This step will help decrease the risk of tears and breakage. Use only water-based lubricants; oil-based lubricants weaken latex condoms and increase the chance of breakage. Spermicidal agents may be used as lubricants with condoms and may also increase the effectiveness of the condom (see Table 10-9).
- After ejaculation, withdraw the penis immediately. To prevent the condom from slipping off, especially if you have used additional lubrication, hold on to the rim of the condom as you withdraw.
- Check the condom for tears and then discard.
- If a tear has occurred, immediately insert spermicidal foam or jelly containing a high concentration of spermicide into the vagina. Do not use suppositories or a vaginal film in these cases, because the delay time for dissolution may decrease the product's efficacy.

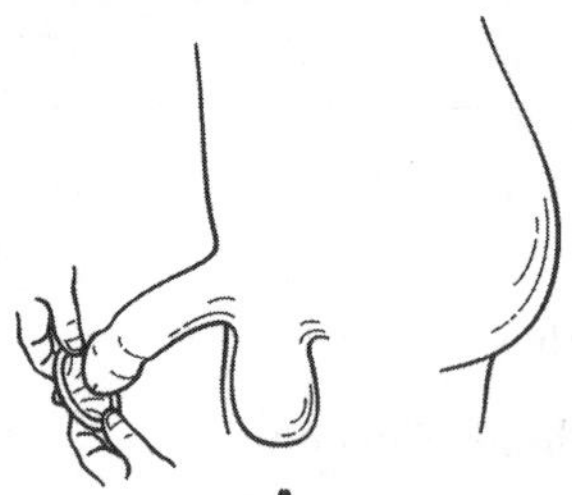
A

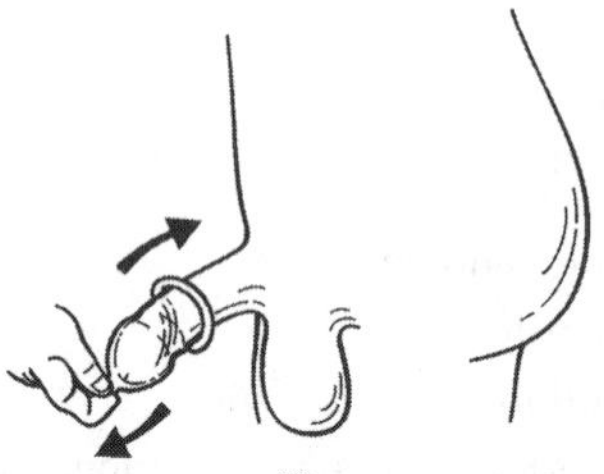
B

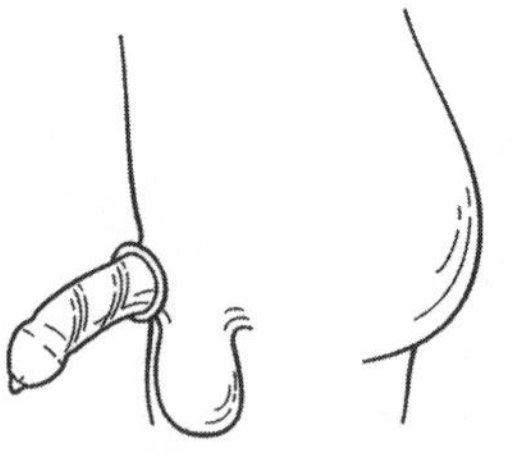
C

problem of allergic contact dermatitis. If switching brands does not eliminate the irritation, the patient may use polyurethane condoms. Natural skin condoms may also be used if the patient recognizes their limitations in preventing STIs. Also, some patients may be sensitized to components of the lubricant or spermicide. Changing brands or using a condom without spermicide may resolve the problem.[13]

The use of very thin condoms, ridged condoms, polyurethane condoms, or natural membrane condoms—in a monogamous relationship with an HIV-negative individual—may alleviate complaints of decreased sensitivity.

*Female Condoms* Although FDA approved the female condom in 1993, only one product—the F.C. Female Condom—is currently available.

Composition/Features The F.C. Female Condom is made of polyurethane rather than latex. It is prelubricated, comes with additional lubricant, and resists degradation by oil-based lubricants. The female condom consists of an outer ring, a sheath or pouch that fits over the vaginal mucosa, and an inner ring that secures the sheath by fitting like a diaphragm over the cervix. The female condom is designed for one-time use only. At a cost of $2.50 to $3.00 each, the female condom is significantly more expensive than the latex male condom, which has stimulated interest in its potential reuse. One study has shown that the female condom retains its integrity after multiple cycles of disinfection and washing.[25] However, reuse of female condoms is not recommended. Latex female condoms are in development.

Effectiveness The breakage rate of the female condom has been shown to be lower than that of latex male condoms, but slippage rates may be higher, especially with its initial uses.[18] The 6-month pregnancy failure rate among all users of the female condom is 12.4%, similar to that for users of diaphragms and cervical caps; among perfect users, however, 6-month pregnancy failure rates of 0.8 to 2.5% have been documented. The extrapolated annual pregnancy failure rate for the female condom is 25% for all users and 5% for perfect users (Table 10-1).[21]

The polyurethane composition of the female condom has been shown to be an effective barrier to sexually transmitted bacteria and viruses. Several studies have shown that female condoms are similar in efficacy to latex male condoms in decreasing the risk of STIs.[25]

Usage/Storage Guidelines Table 10-8 provides step-by-step instructions for proper use of the female condom. A high proportion of women report difficulty inserting the female condom during initial use; this resolves with practice and continued use.[25] The condom may be inserted up

**TABLE 10-7 Lubricants/Products That Are Safe or Unsafe to Use With Latex Condoms**

| Safe | Unsafe |
|---|---|
| Aloe-9 | Baby oils |
| Aqua-Lube | Bag Balm |
| Astroglide | Burn ointments |
| Contraceptive foams (e.g., Delfen, VCF Foam) | Coconut oil/butter |
| Contraceptive gels (e.g., Conceptrol) | Cold cream |
| DeLube | Corn Huskers |
| Duragel | Edible oils (e.g. olive, peanut, corn, canola, safflower) |
| Durex Play (More, Longer, Tingling) | Elbow Grease Cream |
| Egg white | Hemorrhoidal ointments |
| Elbow Grease Gel | Insect repellents |
| Eros Bodyglide | Margarine/dairy butter |
| ForPlay Lubricant | Massage oil |
| Glycerin (USP) | Mens Cream |
| ID Glide | Mineral oil |
| ID Millennium | Palm oil |
| Joe Lube | Petroleum jelly (e.g., Vaseline) |
| Juicy Lube | Rubbing alcohol |
| KY Jelly/Liquid | Shortening (e.g. Crisco) |
| Liquid Silk | Suntan oil/lotion |
| Lubrin Insert | Vaginal creams (e.g., Monistat, Estrace, Femstat, Vagisil, Premarin) |
| Probe | Wet Aromatherapy |
| Prepair Lubricant | Wet Oil-based lubricant |
| Purj | Zestra |
| Replens Inserts | |
| Saliva | |
| Vagi-gard | |
| Water | |
| Wet | |

to 8 hours before intercourse, but it is effective immediately on insertion.

Fresh condoms can be stored at room temperature in their unopened package. Before inserting the female condom, the woman should ensure that the product is within its expiration date.

Safety Considerations The most common complaints about the female condom are vaginal irritation and increased noise ("squeaking"). Additional lubrication may resolve these problems. Some women may complain of decreased sensation or discomfort caused by the outer ring during intercourse.

Product Selection Guidelines The female condom provides a method for women to protect themselves against pregnancy. It is thinner than many latex condoms and has a lower breakage rate than the male condom.[18] Compared with vaginal spermicides, the female condom can be inserted much earlier before intercourse and is less messy to use. However, some women find the female condom cumbersome and unattractive. Use of the female condom in conjunction with a male condom is not recommended because adherence between the two products might result in displacement of either condom.[26]

*Vaginal Spermicides* Vaginal spermicides use surface-active agents to immobilize (kill) sperm. For gels and foams, the spermicide vehicle also acts as a physical barrier against sperm. The effective spermicides include nonoxynol-9, octoxynol-9, and menfegol. In the United States, all currently available products contain nonoxynol-9 (Table 10-9). The cost of vaginal spermicides ranges from $1.00 to $3.00 per dose. Research on microbicidal agents that have the potential to inactivate sperm as well as prevent STI transmission is ongoing.[27]

Dosage Forms The vehicles for vaginal spermicides include gels, foams, suppositories, and film. Although onset and duration of action vary among dosage forms, the woman should delay douching for at least 6 hours after intercourse no matter which dosage form she uses. The following sections discuss the advantages and disadvantages of each dosage form.

Some vaginal gels (jellies) are labeled for use only in conjunction with a diaphragm or cervical cap. When selecting a vaginal jelly to use without a diaphragm or cervical cap, the person should be careful to choose a product with a higher concentration of spermicide, not one that has a lower concentration and is designed to use with barrier methods. Products with a higher concentration of spermicide may be used alone or with a diaphragm or cervical cap (Table 10-10).

For convenience, applicators may be prefilled before use. Prefilled unit-dose applicators are also available.

Vaginal foams, available in canisters or in prefilled applicators, distribute more evenly and adhere better to the cervical area and vaginal walls, but provide less lubrication than jellies. A new canister should always be available as it is difficult to know when the canister is nearly empty.

Vaginal suppositories are solid or semisolid dosage forms that are activated by moisture in the vaginal tract. Some occasions may exist when the suppository will not completely dissolve, resulting in an unpleasant, gritty sensation. Vaginal suppositories do not require refrigeration although in warmer climates, refrigeration may be desirable to prevent softening.[28]

Vaginal contraceptive film contains nonoxynol-9, 28%, as its active ingredient and is available in packets of 3, 6, or 12 paper-thin, 2-inch-square sheets. One film is used for each act of intercourse. The film is activated by vaginal secretions. The practice of inserting the film by placing it over the penis should be avoided because this method does not ensure proper placement and does not allow adequate time for dissolution. In one comparison of spermicide dosage formulations, the film was preferred widely. Although it was rated the most difficult to use, this difficulty decreased with continued use.[28] A similarly designed vaginal cleansing film does not contain spermicide and should not be used for contraception. Patients should be advised to verify that they are using the correct vaginal film product if they desire contraception.

Effectiveness Spermicides used alone have a relatively high typical usage failure rate among first-year users (Table 10-1). A comparative trial of five vaginal spermicidal dosage

**TABLE 10-8 Usage Guidelines for Female Condoms**

- Remove the condom from the package. One end of the condom is closed to form a pouch (drawing A).
- Gently rub the sides together to evenly distribute the lubricant. If needed, use additional lubrication at this point.
- Add a drop of lubricant on the outside of the pouch to improve the ease of insertion. Oil- or water-based lubricants can be used with this condom.
- To place the pouch properly, grasp the inner ring between the thumb and middle finger of one hand. Place the index finger on the sheath between the other two fingers (drawing B).
- Be careful that sharp fingernails or jewelry do not tear the condom.
- Squeeze the inner ring. Then insert the condom into the vagina as far as possible (drawing C).
- Be sure that the inner ring is placed beyond the pubic (pelvic) bone, that the pouch is not twisted, and that the outer ring is outside the vagina (drawing D).
- During intercourse, make sure that the penis enters the vagina inside the pouch and that the outer ring remains outside the vagina.
- If desired, add more lubricant during intercourse, without removing the condom.
- Remove the pouch before standing by twisting the outer ring and pulling gently (drawing E).
- Discard the used condom in a trash can, not a toilet.
- Insert a new condom for each act of intercourse.
- Do not use a male condom with the female condom. The increased friction could cause displacement of the female condom.

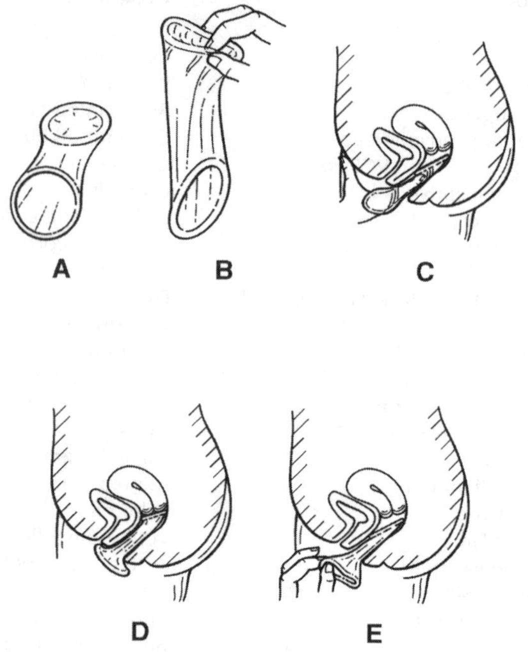


forms found a similar pregnancy rate between two gels, a suppository, and film, each containing 100 to 150 mg nonoxynol-9 per dose. However, a gel containing 52.5 mg nonoxynol-9 per dose was significantly less effective at preventing pregnancy than the higher-dose formulations.[29] (The 52.5 mg product is not currently available in the United States.)

Efficacy improves greatly if spermicides are used in conjunction with barrier methods such as diaphragms, cervical caps, or condoms.

Results concerning the ability of nonoxynol-9 (N-9) to prevent STIs are conflicting. In a recent randomized controlled trial, the compound was found to offer no protection against male to female transmission of gonococcal or chlamydial infection.[30] Importantly, various genital and rectal lesions have been observed after nonoxynol-9 use, which may increase risk for HIV infection.[8] Diaphragms with spermicide offer no protection against HIV infection, but may guard against cervical gonorrhea and chlamydia.[8,26] On the basis of current knowledge, if a risk of STIs exists, use of spermicides alone should not be recommended.

Administration Guidelines Table 10-10 provides guidelines for the proper administration of vaginal spermicides.

Safety Considerations Although allergic reactions are rare, either partner may experience such reactions to spermicides. Couples having oral–genital sex may find the taste of some products unpleasant. Frequent use or use of high-concentration products may irritate or damage vaginal and cervical epithelium,[27] which may be associated with an increased risk for STIs. Some people are concerned about a possible association between spermicide use and birth defects or miscarriage. However, currently available data do not support an increased risk of birth defects attributable to spermicides.[31]

Product Selection Guidelines The relatively low effectiveness of spermicides when used alone is their major disadvantage. However, studies suggest that simultaneous use of condoms and spermicides have efficacy rates similar to those of oral contraceptives and intrauterine devices (IUDs).[2] Their availability and ease of use make spermicides a good choice for women who need a backup method. Spermicides are not recommended for women with anatomic abnormalities that would preclude proper placement of the spermicide near the cervical opening.

Product selection depends on the individual. One study of spermicide formulations found that gel use was associated with excessive lubrication and women compensated by using less than a full dose, which may decrease product effectiveness.[28] If a patient complains of excessive lubrication, an alternative vehicle, such as foam or film, should be recommended.

*Contraceptive Sponge* The Today Vaginal Contraceptive Sponge, the first commercially available vaginal contraceptive sponge, was withdrawn from the market in 1995. In early 2005, the FDA approved its reintroduction to the U.S. market. Currently, three brands of contraceptive sponges are available in the United States through Internet sites (Table 10-11).

**TABLE 10-9 Selected Vaginal Spermicides**

| Trade Name | Spermicide (mg/dose) |
|---|---|
| **Spermicidal Foams** | |
| Delfen Foam | Nonoxynol-9, 12.5% (85 mg) |
| VCF Vaginal Contraceptive Foam | Nonoxynol-9, 12.5% (85 mg) |
| **Spermicidal Gels/Jellies** | |
| Advantage-S Bioadhesive Contraceptive Gel | Nonoxynol-9, 3.5% (70 mg) |
| Encare Contraceptive Gel | Nonoxynol-9, 4% (100 mg) |
| Ortho Options Conceptrol Gel | Nonoxynol-9, 4% (100 mg) |
| Ortho Options Gynol II Vaginal Contraceptive Jelly* | Nonoxynol-9, 2% (100 mg) |
| Ortho Options Gynol II Extra Strength Vaginal Contraceptive Jelly | Nonoxynol-9, 3% (150 mg) |
| **Spermicidal Suppositories** | |
| Encare Vaginal Contraceptive Inserts | Nonoxynol-9, 100 mg |
| **Spermicidal Film** | |
| VCF Vaginal Contraceptive Film | Nonoxynol-9, 28% film (72 mg) |
| Ortho Options Vaginal Contraceptive Film | Nonoxynol-9, 100 mg |

* Product formulated for use with a diaphragm or cervical cap; it should not be used alone.

Composition/Features The contraceptive sponge is a small, circular, disposable sponge made of polyurethane permeated with spermicide (Table 10-11). The sponge is believed to act as a contraceptive by (1) serving as a mechanical barrier, (2) providing a spermicide, and (3) absorbing semen. The contraceptive sponge ranges in price from $3 to $6 per sponge.

Effectiveness In two large trials, the failure rate for the contraceptive sponge ranged from 17.4 to 24.5 pregnancies per 100 women in the first year of use.[32] Women who had given birth previously (parous women) had a significantly higher pregnancy rate while using the sponge, compared with women who had never given birth (nulliparous women),[30] which may be related to poor fit in women who have delivered vaginally.

Use of a contraceptive sponge has been associated with a decreased risk of cervical infections with chlamydia and gonorrhea. However, protection against HIV infection has not been shown with use of the contraceptive sponge, and one study found an increased risk of HIV infection in women with frequent sponge use, possibly because of an increased incidence of vaginal ulceration from the spermicide.[33]

Usage/Storage Guidelines A woman must be able to locate her cervix and must be comfortable in doing so to correctly place the sponge. Table 10-11 provides instructions for properly using these products. However, the sponge may become dislodged during intercourse.

Some of the sponges have a loop attached to the convex side or slits to facilitate removal. Some women have difficulty removing the sponge, and it has been known to fragment on removal. The sponge should be stored in its unopened package in a cool place and used before its expiration date.

Safety Considerations Vaginal dryness is reported among sponge users. Although the incidence is rare, the contraceptive sponge has been associated with an increased risk of toxic shock syndrome (TSS).[26] Women should take special care to wash their hands before inserting the sponge, should not use the sponge during menstruation or for 6 weeks postpartum, and should not exceed the maximum recommended retention time. Women should also be advised to make sure the entire sponge is removed because fragments left in the vagina may serve as a focus for infection.

Product Selection Guidelines The contraceptive sponge is convenient, safe, and portable. Contraindications for use include spermicide sensitivity, anatomic abnormalities of the vagina, and a history of TSS. At this time, it may be prudent not to routinely recommend the contraceptive sponge to parous women because of possible problems with adequate cervical coverage.

### Natural Contraceptive Methods

Contraceptive methods that do not use a chemical or barrier to prevent conception include natural family planning (NFP), lactational amenorrhea, home ovulation prediction tests, and withdrawal. Many couples like the fact that these methods are nonchemical and nonhormonal, eliminating health risks to the couple (or to the fetus, should pregnancy occur). Others use these methods for financial or religious reasons. Most natural contraceptive methods cost little to no money, so they can be significantly less expensive than prescription methods. In some cases, natural contraceptive methods are used because of a lack of access to or knowledge of other methods of contraception. Disadvantages of natural methods include lack of STI protection and a need for periodic abstinence.

*Natural Family Planning* NFP methods, also called periodic abstinence, the rhythm method, or fertility awareness, use various techniques to determine a woman's period of fertility. The information provided by these techniques helps identify the fertile phase of the menstrual cycle. NFP methods have the positive effect of encouraging communication within a relationship and may be the only truly shared contraceptive method. NFP is widely used around the world and is the only method of contraception approved by the Roman Catholic Church.

NFP can be divided into five methods: calendar, basal body temperature (BBT), cervical mucus, standard days, and

**TABLE 10-10 Administration Guidelines for Vaginal Spermicides**

| Dosage Form* | Application Method | Onset/Duration of Action | Application Time Before Intercourse | Reapplication Requirements |
|---|---|---|---|---|
| Vaginal gel alone | Insert full dose near cervix | Immediate/1 hour | Up to 30-60 minutes | For each coital act |
| Vaginal gel used with diaphragm/ cervical cap | Fill barrier device one third full with gel and place it near cervix. Leave barrier in place for at least 6 hours after intercourse | Immediate/ diaphragm: 6 hours; cervical cap: 48 hours | Up to 1 hour | Diaphragm: for each coital act that occurs within 6 hours of initial insertion of device, reapply spermicide without removing device; for coitus after 6 hours of initial insertion, remove and wash device, fill with new spermicide, and reinsert device<br>Cervical cap: remove and wash device and reapply spermicide for each coital act that occurs 48 hours after initial insertion of device |
| Vaginal foam | Insert full dose near cervix | Immediate/1 hour | Up to 1 hour | For each coital act |
| Vaginal suppository | Insert suppository near cervix | 10-15 minutes/1 hour | 10-15 minutes | For each coital act |
| Vaginal contraceptive film | Drape film over fingertip; place film near cervix | 15 minutes/1-3 hours (brand-dependent) | 15 minutes | For each coital act |

* Delay douching for at least 6 hours after last coital act.

**TABLE 10-11 Contraceptive Sponges**

| Product | Spermicide | Instructions for Use | Onset/Duration | Removal |
|---|---|---|---|---|
| Today | Nonoxynol-9 100 mg | Moisten with tap water, insert convex side against cervix; can be inserted up to 24 hours before intercourse | Immediate onset/24 hours | Leave in for >6 hours after intercourse, no longer than 30 hours total; polyester loop to facilitate removal |
| Protectaid | F-5 gel* (nonoxynol-9 6.25 mg, benzalkonium chloride 6.25 mg, sodium cholate 25 mg | Does not need to be moistened before insertion; can be inserted up to 6 hours before intercourse | 15 minutes/ 12 hours | Leave in for >6 hours after intercourse; has finger slots to facilitate removal |
| Pharmatex | Benzalkonium chloride 60 mg* | Does not need to be moistened before insertion; can be inserted up to 22 hours before intercourse | Immediate onset/24 hours | Leave in for >2 hours after intercourse, no longer than 24 hours total |

* Not an FDA-approved spermicide.

symptothermal.[34] Each method requires the woman to keep detailed records of her menstrual cycles and other symptoms associated with cyclical hormonal levels on detailed monthly charts. After proper instruction, a woman can usually predict her most fertile time using the chart information. A couple can choose to abstain from sexual intercourse during that period if they want to avoid pregnancy.

Calendar Method The calendar method is based on records of monthly menstrual cycle lengths. A woman's fertile period is calculated from estimates of the viable life of ova (1 day) and sperm (3 to 5 days).[9,34] Because a woman's menstrual cycles may vary, menstrual cycle lengths should be recorded for 6 to 12 months to predict the likely range of fertile days. The first fertile day in a

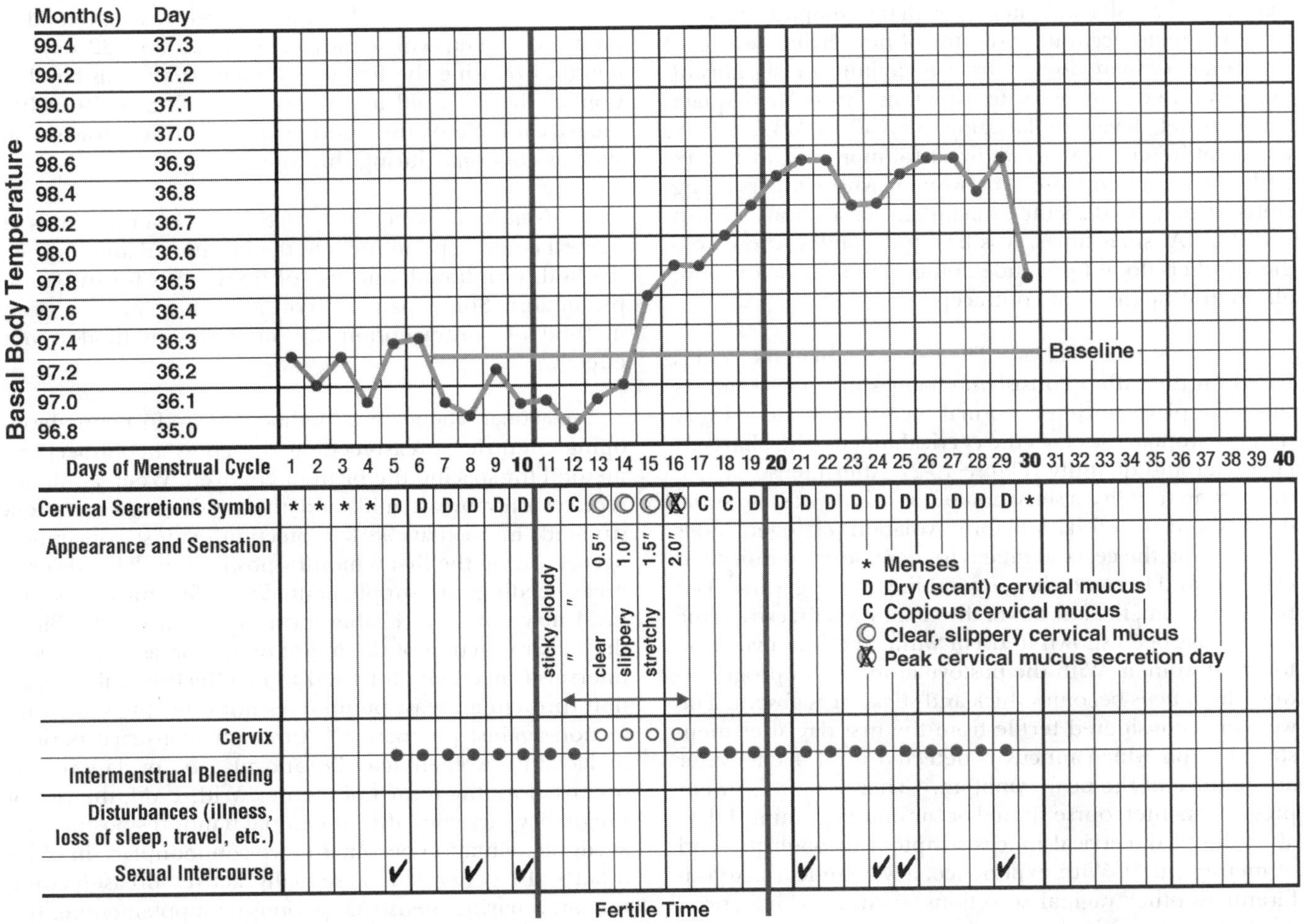


FIGURE 10-2 Symptothermal variations during a model menstrual cycle. (Reprinted with permission from Jennings VH, Arevalo M, Kowal D. Fertility awareness-based methods. In: Hatcher RA, Trussell J, Stewart F, et al., eds. *Contraceptive Technology*. 18th rev ed. New York: Ardent Media; 2004:327.)

woman's menstrual cycle is calculated by subtracting 18 from the number of days in her shortest cycle. The last fertile day is calculated by subtracting 11 from the number of days in her longest cycle.

Basal Body Temperature Method The BBT method is effective only at calculating the end of the fertile phase and therefore should be used only with another fertility awareness method (see Symptothermal Method below). In the BBT method, the woman measures and charts her body temperature every morning.[9,34] She takes her temperature, preferably with a digital thermometer calibrated in increments of 0.1°F (0.05°C). This thermometer allows her to detect small changes in body temperature. She must obtain her temperature before beginning any physical activity (i.e., she must check her temperature before getting out of bed) and at the same time every day. Oral or rectal temperature may be used, but one method should be selected and used consistently.

Electronic digital thermometers are more accurate than mercury thermometers and have a shorter recording time (45 to 90 seconds). Because the activity of shaking down a thermometer may cause the woman's body temperature to change, mercury thermometers must be shaken down each night rather than immediately before use in the morning. Also, because of safety concerns, mercury thermometers are no longer available for purchase. Patients who still have mercury thermometers at home should be encouraged to properly dispose of them and purchase a digital thermometer.

Daily temperatures should be recorded on a chart (Figure 10-2). In some women, onset of ovulation may be detected since the BBT may drop 12 to 24 hours before ovulation. At the time of ovulation, BBT rises by at least 0.4°F (0.2°C) above the lowest point (the nadir.)[34] This sharp rise, called the thermal shift, is caused by high progesterone levels. The safe (infertile) period begins once there have been 3 consecutive days of rising temperature and lasts until the end of menses.

For patients who believe they may have difficulty interpreting shifts in their BBT, a computerized monitor (e.g., Bioself SymptoTherm, OvuTherm) registers and stores the BBTs (see Chapter 51).[9] The monitors use the collected data to predict periods of infertility and fertility. However, these products are only as good as the information they record. A woman must still take her temperature at the same time every morning before any physical activity. Anything that affects her BBT will interfere with the computer's ability to generate an accurate indicator of her fertility levels.

Some women do not have a definite or significant temperature dip or rise with ovulation. Stress, inadequate sleep, travel, fever, or lactation may affect BBT.[34] Also, temperature changes are difficult to interpret just before and during menopause. For women who work rotating shifts, it may be difficult to maintain an accurate record of BBT.[34] At such times, it is best for couples whose religious beliefs do not preclude doing so to use one or more alternative methods of contraception.

Cervical Mucus Method The cervical mucus method is based on the rather consistent changes in cervical mucus that take place during a normal menstrual cycle.[34] Every day, the woman observes the cervical mucus; she charts its character and quantity (Figure 10-2). After menstruation, most women notice a sensation of vaginal dryness on some days. About 5 to 6 days before ovulation, estrogen levels rise, causing the cervical mucus to increase in quantity and elasticity and become clear, resembling raw egg white. The peak symptom, the last day of the clear, stretchy, estrogenic mucus, has been shown to occur within a day of ovulation for most women. With the postovulatory rise in progesterone, the mucus becomes thick and sticky or is absent. The woman is considered fertile from the first day after menstruation on which mucus is detected until 4 days after appearance of the peak symptom.[34] Therefore, to prevent pregnancy, intercourse should occur only beginning 4 days after the peak cervical mucus symptom through the end of menstruation. With experience, a woman learns to differentiate other vaginal secretions, such as an infectious discharge or seminal fluid, from normal mucus. Most women can learn this method after three cycles. This method of natural family planning is preferred over the BBT method for postpartum lactating women and women nearing menopause. Women who use this method are also apt to detect abnormalities in their normal mucus patterns that may be caused by infections, enabling them to seek early treatment. Women should be informed that vaginal foams, gels, creams, and douches will interfere with cervical mucus.

Another method of monitoring cervical secretions is called the TwoDay method.[35,36] On a day a woman is considering intercourse, she should think about whether she noticed any secretions that day or the day before. If she did not, she is probably not fertile. If she did notice secretions on either day, then she is likely to be fertile. The TwoDay method is a simple method that does not require keeping records or logs. Unfortunately, the exact effectiveness of this method is unknown and it should be used with caution.

Symptothermal Method The symptothermal method combines methods of fertility awareness to determine the fertile period. Usually BBT charting is combined with notations of changes in cervical mucus.[9,34] Most studies of this method's effectiveness use the thermal shift (the temperature rise after the nadir) of the BBT method to determine the postovulatory safe period, as well as the cervical mucus or calendar method to determine the end of the preovulatory or postmenstrual infertile period (Figure 10-2).

Standard Days Method This method is recommended only for women with cycles between 26 and 32 days in length. Counting the first day of menstruation as day 1, a woman should avoid intercourse on days 8 to 19 of her menstrual cycle or use another method of contraception such as condoms during this time.[34]

*Other Natural Contraceptive Methods* Other methods of natural contraception include the lactational amenorrhea method, withdrawal, and use of home tests for ovulation prediction. Some patients consider douching to be a method of contraception although this method is not effective.

Lactational Amenorrhea Method (LAM) In many developing countries, breast-feeding is used as a contraceptive method for spacing the birth of children. When an infant receives only breast milk and the mother has not menstruated, more than 98% protection against conception occurs during the first 6 months postpartum.[37] However, if breast-feedings are supplemented with feedings by bottle, LAM may not be a reliable form of contraception. Since the suckling action of the infant on the breast at frequent intervals is necessary for LAM to be effective, milk extraction through a breast pump does not offer the same protection against pregnancy.[38] Although menstrual periods in lactating women may be anovulatory, ovulation may occur before the return of menses. With LAM, the risk of pregnancy increases after the initial 6 months postpartum as supplementation becomes more commonplace in older infants. In general, if a sexually active, breast-feeding woman is having menstrual periods or supplementing her infant's diet, or is more than 6 months postpartum, she should use an additional method of contraception.[37,38]

Home Tests for Ovulation Prediction Ovulation prediction tests are designed to aid couples in conceiving by detecting the surge in luteinizing hormone that occurs shortly before ovulation (see Chapter 51).[34] These kits detect an increase in urinary excretion of the hormone, which usually occurs 8 to 40 hours before actual ovulation. Because the life expectancy of sperm may be longer than 72 hours, these ovulation predictors do not give warning of impending ovulation with enough accuracy to be effective contraceptive agents when used alone.

Withdrawal Coitus interruptus (withdrawal) involves coital activity until ejaculation is imminent, followed by withdrawal of the stimulated penis and ejaculation away from the vagina or vulva. Method failures (pregnancy even when the method is used correctly and consistently) occur in part because involuntary preejaculation secretions may contain millions of sperm. Disadvantages of this method include requirement of considerable self-control by the man, and potential for diminished pleasure for the couple because of interrupted lovemaking.

Douching Vaginal douches should never be considered a method of contraception. Under favorable conditions in the female reproductive tract, active sperm have been found in the cervical crypts and oviducts within minutes after ejaculation. Postcoital douching has no effect in removing sperm from the upper reproductive tract and could, in fact, force or propel sperm higher up in the tract.

*Effectiveness of Natural Contraceptive Methods* Overall, the pregnancy rate for typical use of natural family planning methods is approximately 25%.[2] The calendar method is considered the least effective of these methods, primarily because of natural variations in the length of a woman's normal menstrual cycle. Although it is still widely used as a sole contraceptive method, such reliance results in many unintended pregnancies, as shown in Table 10-1. Consequently, family planners do not recommend using the calendar method alone, but suggest instead using the calendar method in conjunction with other methods of NFP. Methods that specifically identify preovulatory and postovulatory changes, such as the symptothermal method, have much better outcomes. Table 10-1 shows that combinations of these methods have good predicted effectiveness; with perfect use, the annual failure rate is 2%.

For a woman who is breast-feeding an infant almost exclusively, studies have reported pregnancy rates of 0.5% to 2% for the 6-month period after delivery. However, once supplemental feedings begin, the efficacy rate falls significantly.[38] Efficacy rates on using home ovulation predictors are not available; however, assuming correct use, an efficacy rate similar to that seen with BBT monitoring could be expected. For couples who rely on withdrawal, accidental pregnancy rates range from 4 to 27 pregnancies per 100 couples in the first year of use.[2]

NFP methods do not provide any protection against STIs and should be recommended solely for non-STI–infected couples in mutually monogamous relationships.

### Emergency Contraception

Emergency contraception (EC) involves the use of pills or an IUD to prevent pregnancy after intercourse. Only the use of pills is discussed in this section. The dedicated emergency contraceptive product, Plan B, or oral contraceptive pills containing levonorgestrel or D,L-norgestrel may be used. Plan B costs about $25 to $30. The cost for emergency contraception using oral contraceptive pills ranges from about $25 to $40, depending on the pill selected and whether or not the patient requests brand or generic.

Currently, emergency contraceptive pills (ECPs) are available only by prescription. However, pharmacies in some states have collaborative practice agreements with physicians, and in California, state law allows pharmacists to provide EC to women directly without visiting their provider first. In addition, the makers of Plan B had filed an application to reclassify the product as nonprescription. On August 26, 2005, FDA announced its intent to publish an advance notice of proposed rulemaking to resolve the unique policy and regulatory questions posed by the application: (1) using age as a criterion to determine the availability status of a drug and (2) having an agent available as nonprescription and prescription for the same indication.[39] At press time, the application was still pending. Many organizations, including the American Medical Association and the American College of Obstetrics and Gynecology, believe this change will decrease the incidence of unplanned pregnancies.[40]

ECPs should be recommended for patients who had unprotected intercourse or experienced method failure (e.g., condom breakage).[41] The pills reduce the expected number of pregnancies by 74% to 89%. Providers should consider giving patients a prescription for ECPs for future use in case the patient has a problem with her regular method of contraception. The exact mechanism of action of ECPs is unknown, but is believed to result primarily from the suppression of ovulation.[42] Other possible mechanisms of action include interfering with fertilization, inhibiting transport of the fertilized egg to the uterus, or inhibiting implantation of the fertilized egg in the endometrium.

Emergency contraception using oral contraceptive pills is given in two doses.[41] For optimal efficacy, the first dose should be given as soon as possible after unprotected intercourse, and the second dose 12 hours later. Plan B may be given as one pill every 12 hours for two doses, but is often given as a single dose of two pills with equal effectiveness.[43,44] Although the initial recommendations were that the first dose of ECPs be given within 72 hours of unprotected intercourse, several studies have shown that ECPs are still effective if given within 5 days.[44,45] Therefore, women presenting within 120 hours of unprotected sex should be offered ECPs. Patients presenting between 5 to 7 days after unprotected intercourse should be referred to a physician for possible IUD insertion. Table 10-12 lists the available products used for emergency contraception. The

**TABLE 10-12 Oral Contraceptive Pills That May Be Used for Emergency Contraception**

| Trade Name | No. of Pills per Dose | Color of Pills to Take |
|---|---|---|
| Alesse | 5 | Pink |
| Aviane | 5 | Orange |
| Cryselle | 4 | White |
| Enpresse | 4 | Orange |
| Lessina | 5 | Pink |
| Levlen | 4 | Light orange |
| Levlite | 5 | Pink |
| Levora | 4 | White |
| Lo-Ovral | 4 | White |
| Low-Ogestrel | 4 | White |
| Lutera | 5 | White |
| Nordette | 4 | Light orange |
| Ogestrel | 2 | White |
| Ovral | 2 | White |
| Ovrette | 20 | Yellow |
| Portia | 4 | Pink |
| Seasonale | 4 | Pink |
| Tri-Levlen | 4 | Yellow |
| Triphasil | 4 | Yellow |
| Trivora | 4 | Pink |

| TABLE 10-13 | Counseling Points for Emergency Contraception |
|---|---|

- Make certain that the patient does not want to get pregnant.
- Explain how to take emergency contraception correctly. Patients may want to time the first dose to allow for a more convenient dosing time for the second dose. (Both doses of Plan B may be given at the same time.) It is best if the first dose is taken as soon as possible after unprotected intercourse; however, the method is effective when taken up to 120 hours after unprotected intercourse. Patients presenting between 5 and 7 days after unprotected intercourse should be referred to a physician for possible IUD insertion.
- Describe potential adverse effects and how to manage them. If the patient will be taking an antiemetic, she should take one dose 30 to 60 minutes before each dose of ECPs.
- Emphasize that emergency contraception is not to be used as a regular contraceptive method.
- Recommend that a sexually active woman use another form of contraception after taking ECPs. Emergency contraception may delay ovulation, so the risk of pregnancy may be high soon after treatment.
- Explain that emergency contraception does not protect against STIs.
- Tell the patient that her next period may be a few days early or late.
- Explain that emergency contraception can fail. If the patient's period does not come within 21 days after treatment, she should perform a home pregnancy test or contact her primary care provider.
- Provide written instructions.
- Encourage the patient to call if she has any questions.
- Make referrals to Child Protective Services, Planned Parenthood, domestic violence or rape relief resources, or other primary care providers as needed for ongoing contraception, IUD insertion, or STI evaluation and treatment.

*Source:* Adapted from reference 46, p. 11.

most common adverse effects reported are nausea and vomiting.[41] Nausea occurs in about 50% of women using combination EC and 25% of women using progesterone-only EC. Vomiting occurs in about 25% and 5% of combination and progesterone-only EC users, respectively. Headaches, breast tenderness, and dizziness have also been reported. Plan B has been found to be more effective and better tolerated than combination pills. Patients may choose to take an antiemetic before each dose of ECPs to minimize nausea and vomiting. Table 10-13 provides patient counseling information on ECPs.[46]

## Assessment of the Prevention of Pregnancy and STIs: A Case-based Approach

Before advising a patient on contraception and STI prevention, the practitioner must identify first the patient's level of knowledge about contraceptive methods. Before they can select a product or method that is appropriate, patients must understand their risk for pregnancy and STIs. Patients who prefer NFP methods must understand the reproductive cycle before they can use these methods effectively. Patients who prefer nonprescription contraceptive products must know how to use them properly and be prepared to use them with every act of intercourse. The practitioner should identify the patient's preferences for products or methods on the basis of the timing of use or on religious or cultural practices. Cases 10-1 and 10-2 illustrate the assessment of patients who are seeking advice on contraception.

## Patient Counseling for Prevention of Pregnancy and STIs

As the most accessible health care provider, pharmacists are in a distinctive position to impact the incidence and consequences of unintended pregnancy and STIs in their communities. The pharmacist should seek opportunities

### CASE 10-1

| Relevant Evaluation Criteria | Scenario/Model Outcome |
|---|---|
| **Information Gathering** | |
| 1. Gather essential information about the patient's symptoms, including: | |
| a. description of symptom(s) (i.e., nature, onset, duration, severity, associated symptoms) | Patient has been having recurrent vaginal itching without vaginal discharge after sexual intercourse. |
| b. description of any factors that seem to precipitate, exacerbate, and/or relieve the patient's symptoms. | Patient uses latex condoms with or without spermicide for prevention of pregnancy and STIs. Symptoms resolve in 2 to 3 days with or without intervention. |
| c. description of the patient's efforts to relieve the symptoms | She has tried several brands of condoms and has not noted much difference in the reaction between the different products. She also used an OTC antifungal product for yeast vaginitis but it did not clear her symptoms more rapidly than no intervention. |

## CASE 10-1 (continued)

| Relevant Evaluation Criteria | Scenario/Model Outcome |
|---|---|
| 2. Gather essential patient history information: | |
| a. patient's identity | Jo Harding |
| b. age, sex, height, and weight | 31 y/o F, 5'5", 160 lb |
| c. patient's occupation | Clerk in law office |
| d. patient's dietary habits | Generally healthy diet |
| e. patient's sleep habits | N/A |
| f. concurrent medical conditions, prescription and nonprescription medications, and dietary supplements | None |
| g. allergies | NKA |
| h. history of other adverse reactions to medications | None |
| i. other (describe)_______ | H/O chlamydia and trichomonas last year with previous partner; current partner with h/o genital Herpes; no prior h/o latex allergy |
| **Assessment and Triage** | |
| 3. Differentiate the patient's signs/symptoms and correctly identify the patient's primary problem(s) (see Table 10-2). | Risk for undesired pregnancy and STI; possible latex or spermicide allergy |
| 4. Identify exclusions for self-treatment. | None, however, patient should be referred to her PCP if she develops symptoms consistent with an STI, such as vaginal discharge or blisters. |
| 5. Formulate a comprehensive list of therapeutic alternatives for the primary problem to determine if triage to a medical practitioner is required, and share this information with the patient. | Options include:<br>(1) Recommend a different type of condom (nonspermicide-treated latex, polyurethane, or natural membrane)<br>(2) Recommend a female condom<br>(3) Recommend use of a spermicide alone (with or without barrier such as diaphragm or cervical cap), or a contraceptive sponge.<br>(4) Recommend a natural family planning method.<br>(5) Refer Jo to her PCP for prescription methods of contraception.<br>(6) Take no action. |
| **Plan** | |
| 6. Select an optimal therapeutic alternative to address the patient's problem, taking into account patient preferences. | Recommend polyurethane female condom because patient prefers female-controlled method. |
| 7. Describe the recommended therapeutic approach to the patient. | Use a polyurethane female condom with each act of sexual intercourse. |
| 8. Explain to the patient the rationale for selecting the recommended therapeutic approach from the considered therapeutic alternatives. | Your symptoms may be a result of spermicide or latex allergy. Since you have not obtained relief by trying different brands/types of latex condoms, nonlatex (polyurethane) condoms (either male or female) should avoid the adverse reactions seen with the latex condoms while still providing comparable STI prevention and contraceptive benefit. Natural membrane condoms should not be used as they are not as effective as latex and polyurethane condoms at preventing STIs. |
| **Patient Education** | |
| 9. When recommending self-care with nonprescription medications and/or nondrug therapy, convey accurate information to the patient, including: | |

## CASE 10-1 (continued)

| Relevant Evaluation Criteria | Scenario/Model Outcome |
|---|---|
| a. appropriate dose and frequency of administration | Use fresh condom with each act of sexual intercourse. See Table 10-8. |
| b. maximum number of days the therapy should be employed | N/A |
| c. product administration procedures | See Table 10-8. |
| d. expected time to onset of relief | Female condoms are effective immediately once correctly inserted and can be inserted up to 8 hours before intercourse. |
| e. degree of relief that can be reasonably expected | See Table 10-1 for efficacy rates of female condoms. |
| f. most common side effects | Vaginal irritation, increased noise (squeaking) |
| g. side effects that warrant medical intervention should they occur | Continued vaginal irritation |
| h. patient options in the event that condition worsens or persists | A PCP, that is, primary care provider, should be consulted if irritation is intolerable or persists after changing to polyurethane condom. |
| i. product storage requirements | See Table 10-8. |
| j. specific nondrug measures | None |
| 10. Solicit follow-up questions from patient. | Can I use lubricants or vaginal spermicides with the female condom? |
| 11. Answer patient's questions. | A PCP should be consulted if irritation is intolerable or persists after changing to polyurethane condom. |

Key: h/o, history of; N/A, not applicable; NKA, no known allergies; OTC, over-the-counter; PCP, primary care provider; STI, sexually transmitted infection.

## CASE 10-2

| Relevant Evaluation Criteria | Scenario/Model Outcome |
|---|---|
| **Information Gathering** | |
| 1. Gather essential information about the patient's symptoms, including: | |
| a. description of symptom(s) (i.e., nature, onset, duration, severity, associated symptoms) | Patient states that the condom broke last night during intercourse. She is not using any other contraceptive method. She does not desire to become pregnant. |
| b. description of any factors that seem to precipitate, exacerbate, and/or relieve the patient's symptoms. | N/A |
| c. description of the patient's efforts to relieve the symptoms | N/A |
| 2. Gather essential patient history information: | |
| a. patient's identity | Bethany Lewis |
| b. age, sex, height, and weight | 23 y/o F, 5'3", 125 lb |
| c. patient's occupation | Student |
| d. patient's dietary habits | Normal healthy diet |
| e. patient's sleep habits | Ibuprofen 400 mg by mouth 4 times/day as needed for menstrual cramps |
| f. concurrent medical conditions, prescription and nonprescription medications, and dietary supplements | NKA |

## CASE 10-2 (continued)

| Relevant Evaluation Criteria | Scenario/Model Outcome |
|---|---|
| g. allergies | None |
| h. history of other adverse reactions to medications | None |
| i. other (describe)_______ | |
| **Assessment and Triage** | |
| 3. Differentiate the patient's signs/symptoms and correctly identify the patient's primary problem(s) (see Table 10-2). | Patient is in need of emergency contraception for pregnancy prevention. |
| 4. Identify exclusions for self-treatment. | Emergency contraception is not available without a prescription. In some states, emergency contraception can be given out by pharmacies through collaborative agreements with a prescriber or a state itself (e.g., California). |
| 5. Formulate a comprehensive list of therapeutic alternatives for the primary problem to determine if triage to a medical practitioner is required, and share this information with the patient. | Patient may take Plan B or any other levonorgestrel or norgestrel containing oral contraceptive pill (see Table 10-12). |
| **Plan** | |
| 6. Select an optimal therapeutic alternative to address the patient's problem, taking into account patient preferences. | Patient should see her provider for emergency contraception. Patient may also obtain emergency contraception from a pharmacy in some states or online. |
| 7. Describe the recommended therapeutic approach to the patient. | Plan B, take 2 pills orally now. |
| 8. Explain to the patient the rationale for selecting the recommended therapeutic approach from the considered therapeutic alternatives. | This is the preferred method since it is easier to take and is better tolerated that using oral contraceptive pills. |
| **Patient Education** | |
| 9. When recommending self-care with nonprescription medications and/or nondrug therapy, convey accurate information to the patient, including: | |
| a. appropriate dose and frequency of administration | Patient will need to take only one dose of Plan B. Repeat doses are necessary only if unprotected intercourse occurs again. |
| b. maximum number of days the therapy should be employed | N/A |
| c. product administration procedures | N/A |
| d. expected time to onset of relief | N/A |
| e. degree of relief that can be reasonably expected | N/A |
| f. most common side effects | Nausea and vomiting |
| g. side effects that warrant medical intervention should they occur | Severe headache, abdominal pain, leg pain, or chest pain |
| h. patient options in the event that condition worsens or persists | N/A |
| i. product storage requirements | N/A |

**CASE 10-2 (continued)**

| Relevant Evaluation Criteria | Scenario/Model Outcome |
|---|---|
| j. specific nondrug measures | Patient should be sure to use condoms with intercourse. She should check a pregnancy test at home or come in for one if her menses does not occur within 3 weeks of taking emergency contraception. |
| 10. Solicit follow-up questions from patient. | Is emergency contraception 100% effective at preventing pregnancy? |
| 11. Answer patient's questions. | No. However, emergency contraception will reduce the likelihood of pregnancy by 75% to 89%. |

Key: N/A, not applicable; NKA, no known allergies.

to discuss specific diseases or prevention strategies with individuals who may be identified at high risk for unintended pregnancy and STIs.

Practitioners should thoroughly familiarize themselves with the proper use of currently available nonprescription contraceptive products and provide opportunities for consultation with patients by removing barriers that may prevent dialogue. In pharmacies, contraceptive products and information as well as STI-related consumer information should be available in an area where the patient can browse and the pharmacist can easily interact with the patient, such as next to or directly in front of the prescription counter.

In addition to the educational role, the practitioner may be able to assist an individual in gaining access to other needed medical and social supportive services. In cases of suspected domestic violence or sexual abuse, pharmacists should act on their role as mandatory reporters. A private area for education and counseling is important if adequate discussion is to take place.

Special efforts should be made to offer contraceptive information and services to adolescents. Clinicians who are uncomfortable discussing reproductive health with young people should refer adolescents to a clinic that specializes in services to young people, if one is available. Adolescents need clear, accurate information on all aspects of reproductive health. The practitioner should keep in mind that misconceptions about STI and pregnancy risk and proper contraceptive use are common, especially among adolescents; therefore, adequate education is very important. Particularly useful nonprescription methods for the sometimes impulsive adolescent might include condoms and contraceptive foam in prefilled applicators.

NFP may be best recommended for a couple in a stable relationship. NFP methods, especially the BBT and cervical mucus methods, require extensive training and support from health care professionals who have experience and training with these methods. The provider should be supportive and available to answer questions regarding such techniques. Besides stocking spermicidal products, BBT thermometers, and monitoring charts, the pharmacist may serve as a referral center for patients who want to use these methods of family planning. A pharmacist with the proper training might consider counseling patients on NFP as a unique practice possibility.

## Evaluation of Patient Outcomes Prevention of Pregnancy and STIs

Many sexually active patients are at risk for unintended pregnancy or STIs. Efficacy rates of contraceptives vary, but the most important factor affecting their ability to prevent pregnancy and STIs is correct and consistent use with each sexual encounter. Although any of the methods can be used for pregnancy prevention, the latex male condom and the female condom are the preferred methods for prevention of STIs. Individuals who experience an adverse reaction after use of a nonprescription contraceptive should switch to an alternate brand or agent. If the symptoms do not resolve or recur with the use of other agents, the patient should seek medical attention. A sexually active woman who misses a menstrual period should be encouraged to perform a home pregnancy test or seek medical attention. Symptoms of an STI in a sexually active individual also require medical referral (Table 10-2).

## Key Points for Prevention of Pregnancy and STIs

- No method of contraception is completely effective at preventing unintended pregnancy and STIs.
- Selection of a contraceptive product or method must be based on patient risk for undesired outcomes (pregnancy, STI) and efficacy, safety, and patient acceptability.
- Efficacy of nonprescription contraceptives is significantly increased by correct and consistent use of the product/method with each sexual encounter (Tables 10-6, 10-8, 10-10, and 10-11).
- Latex male condoms and female condoms are the preferred contraceptive products for patients at risk for STIs. The polyurethane condom may be used in persons with latex hypersensitivity.
- Currently available spermicides decrease risk of unintended pregnancy but may increase risk of STIs.
- Vaginal spermicides are available in a variety of dosage forms to improve patient acceptability.
- Natural family planning methods are an inexpensive, modestly effective method of contraception that can be used by non–STI-infected couples in a mutually monogamous relationship.

- Emergency contraception is an effective method of postcoital contraception that can decrease risk of unintended pregnancy, but it does not decrease risk of STIs.

## References


1. Mosher WD, Martinez GM, Chandra A, et al. Use of contraception and use of family planning services in the United States: 1982-2002. *Advance Data Vital Health Stat.* 2004;350:1-36.
2. Trussell J. The essentials of contraception: efficacy, safety, and personal considerations. In: Hatcher RA, Trussell J, Stewart F, et al., eds. *Contraceptive Technology.* 18th rev ed. New York: Ardent Media; 2004:221-52.
3. Henshaw SK. Unintended pregnancy in the United States. *Fam Plan Perspect.* 1998;30:24-9,46.
4. Cason C, Orrock N, Schmitt K at al. The impact of laws on HIV and STD prevention. *J Law Med Ethics.* 2002;30(3 suppl):139-45.
5. Cates W. Reproductive tract infections. In: Hatcher RA, Trussell J, Stewart F, et al., eds. *Contraceptive Technology.* 18th ed. New York: Ardent Media; 2004:191-220.
6. Biddlecom AE. Trends in sexual behaviours and infections among young people in the United States. *Sex Transm Infect.* 2004; 80(suppl):ii74-9.
7. Miller FC. Impact of adolescent pregnancy as we approach the new millennium. *J Pediatr Adolesc Gynecol.* 2000;13:5-8.
8. Centers for Disease Control and Prevention. Sexually transmitted diseases treatment guidelines 2002. *MMWR Morb Mortal Wkly Rep.* 2002;51(RR-6):1-78.
9. Sanford JB, White GL Jr, Hatasaka H. Timing intercourse to achieve pregnancy: current evidence. *Obstet Gynecol.* 2002;100: 1333-41.
10. Glei DA. Measuring contraceptive use patterns among teenage and adult women. *Fam Plan Perspect.* 1999;31:73-80.
11. Paukku M, Quan J, Barney P, et al. Adolescent's contraceptive use and pregnancy history: is there a pattern? *Obstet Gynecol.* 2003; 101:534-8.
12. Fu H, Darroch JE, Haas T, et al. Contraceptive failure rates: new estimates from the 1995 National Survey of Family Growth. *Fam Plan Perspect.* 1999;31:56-63.
13. Warner DL, Hatcher RA, Steiner MJ. Male condoms. In: Hatcher RA, Trussell J, Stewart F, et al., eds. *Contraceptive Technology.* 18th rev ed. New York: Ardent Media; 2004:331-53.
14. Condoms: Extra protection. *Consumer Rep.* 2005;70:34-5.
15. Nonlatex vs latex condoms: an update. *Contraception Report.* 2003; 14:10-3.
16. Carey RF, Lytle CD, Cyr WH. Implications of laboratory tests of condom integrity. *Sex Transm Dis.* 1999;26:216-20.
17. Workshop summary: scientific evidence on condom effectiveness for sexually transmitted disease (STD) prevention. July 20, 2001. Washington, DC: National Institute of Allergy and Infectious Diseases, National Institutes of Health, Department of Health and Human Services. Available at: http://www.niaid.nih.gov/dmid/stds/condomreport.pdf. Accessed March 9, 2005.
18. Valappil T, Kelaghan J, Macaluso M, et al. Female condom and male condom failure among women at high risk of sexually transmitted diseases. Sex *Transm Dis.* 2005;32:35-43.
19. Golombok S, Harding R, Sheldon J. An evaluation of a thicker versus a standard condom with gay men. *AIDS.* 2001;15:245-50.
20. Potter WD, de Villemeur M. Clinical breakage, slippage and acceptability of a new commercial polyurethane condom: a randomized, controlled study. *Contraception.* 2003;68:39-45.
21. Steiner MJ, Dominik R, Rountree W, et al. Contraceptive effectiveness of a polyurethane condom and a latex condom. *Obstet Gynecol.* 2003;101:539-47.
22. Roddy RE, Cordero M, Ryan KA, et al. A randomized controlled trial comparing nonoxynol-9 lubricated condoms with silicone lubricated condoms for prophylaxis. *Sex Transm Inf.* 1998;74:116-9.
23. Liss GM, Sussman GL. Latex sensitization: occupational versus general population prevalence rates. *Am J Ind Med.* 1999;35:196-200.
24. Levy DA, Khouaders S, Leynadier F. Allergy to latex condoms. *Allergy.* 1998;53:1107-8.
25. Hoffman S, Mantell J, Exner T, et al. The future of the female condom. *Perspect Sex Reprod Health.* 2004;3:120-6.
26. Cates Jr W, Stewart F. Vaginal barriers: the female condom, diaphragm, contraceptive sponge, cervical cap, Lea's shield and femcap. In: Hatcher, RA, Trussell J, Stewart F, et al., eds. *Contraceptive Technology.* 18th rev ed. New York: Ardent Media; 2004: 365-89.
27. Van Damme L. Clinical microbicide research: an overview. *Trop Med Int Health.* 2004;9:1290-6.
28. Coggins C, Elias CJ, Atisook R, et al. Women's preferences regarding the formulation of over-the-counter vaginal spermicides. *AIDS.* 1998;12:1389-91.
29. Raymond E, Chen PL, Luoto J. Contraceptive effectiveness and safety of five nonoxynol-9 spermicides: a randomized trial. *Obstet Gynecol.* 2004;103:430-9.
30. Roddy RE, Zekeng L, Ryan KA, et al. Effect of nonoxynol-9 gel on urogenital gonorrhea and chlamydial infection. *JAMA.* 2002; 287:1117-22.
31. Briggs G, Freeman RK, Yaffe SJ. *Drugs in Pregnancy* and *Lactation.* 6th ed. Philadelphia: Lippincott Williams & Wilkins; 2002:1010-3.
32. Kuyoh MA, Toroitich-Ruto C, Grimes DA, et al. Sponge versus diaphragm for contraception: a Cochrane review. *Contraception.* 2003;67:15-8.
33. Cook RL, Rosenberg MJ. Do spermicides containing nonoxynol-9 prevent sexually transmitted infections?: a meta-analysis. *Sex Tranms Dis.* 1998;25:144-50.
34. Jennings VH, Arevalo M, Kowal D. Fertility awareness-based methods. In: Hatcher RA, Trussell J, Stewart F, et al., eds. *Contraceptive Technology.* 18th rev ed. New York: Ardent Media; 2004:317-29.
35. Jennings V, Sinai I. Further analysis of the theoretical effectiveness of the TwoDay method of family planning. *Contraception.* 2001;64:149-53.
36. Arévalo M, Jennings V, Nikula M, et al. Efficacy of the new TwoDay Method of family planning. *Fertil Steril.* 2004;82:885-92.
37. Kennedy KI, Kotelchuck M. Policy considerations for the introduction and promotion of the lactational amenorrhea method: advantages and disadvantages of LAM. *J Hum Lact.* 1998;14:191-203.
38. Kennedy KI, Trussell J. Postpartum contraception and lactation. In: Hatcher RA, Trussell J, Stewart F, et al., eds. *Contraceptive Technology.* 18th rev ed. New York: Ardent Media; 2004:575-600.
39. FDA Takes Action on Plan B. Statement by FDA Commissioner Lester M. Crawford [press release]. Available at: http://www.fda.gov/bbs/topics/news/2005/NEW01223.html. Accessed December 19, 2005.
40. Johnson J. Obstructing Access to Emergency Contraception in Hospital Emergency Rooms. March 2005. Available at: http://www.plannedparenthood.org/pp2/portal/files/portal/medicalinfo/ec/fact-032102-obstructing.sml. Accessed October 18, 2005.
41. Stewart F, Trussell J, Van Look PFA. Emergency contraception. In: Hatcher RA, Trussell J, Stewart F, et al., eds. *Contraceptive Technology.* 18th rev ed. New York: Ardent Media; 2004:279-303.
42. Croxatto HB, Brache V, Pavez M, et al. Pituitary-ovarian function following the standard levonorgestrel emergency contraceptive dose or a single 0.75-mg dose given on the days preceding ovulation. *Contraception.* 2004;70:442-50.
43. von Hertzen H, Piaggio G, Ding J. Low dose mifepristone and two regimens of levonorgestrel for emergency contraception: a WHO multicentre randomized trial. *Lancet.* 2002;360:1803-10.
44. Ellertson C, Webb A, Blanchard K, et al. Modifying the Yuzpe regimen of emergency contraception: a multicenter, randomized controlled trial. *Obstet Gynecol.* 2003;101:1160-7.
45. Rodrigues I, Grou F, Joly J. Effectiveness of emergency contraceptive pills between 72 and 120 hours after unprotected sexual intercourse. *Am J Obstet Gynecol.* 2001;184:531-7.
46. American Pharmaceutical Association. *Emergency* Contraception*: The Pharmacist's Role.* Washington, DC: American Pharmaceutical Association; 2000.

SECTION IV

# Respiratory Disorders

CHAPTER 11

# Disorders Related to Colds and Allergy

*Kelly L. Scolaro*

Colds and allergic rhinitis are two of the most common conditions for which patients access the health care system. The chapter reviews the role of the plethora of nonprescription products patients may use to self-treat symptoms associated with these two disorders.

## Anatomy and Physiology of the Respiratory System

The respiratory system is divided into the upper respiratory system, which filters, warms, and humidifies inspired air, and the lower respiratory system, which directs the airflow and participates in gas exchange. Each breath enters the nose and passes through the respiratory structures in the following order: pharynx, larynx, trachea, bronchioles, alveolar ducts, and alveoli. Gas exchange takes place at the cellular level in the alveoli.

The nose contains the olfactory apparatus, many arteriovenous anastomoses, and the cavernous sinusoids. Vibrissae (coarse hairs) line the nostrils and remove large particles from inspired air. Each nostril ends in a cavity that is divided horizontally into three turbinates. Inspired air is warmed to approximately 91°F (33°C) and humidified by the well-perfused nasal mucosa.

Sensory, cholinergic, and sympathetic nerves innervate the nose. Sensory fibers respond to mechanical and thermal stimuli and to mediators such as histamine and bradykinin. Cholinergic stimulation dilates and sympathetic stimulation constricts arterial blood flow. Sympathetic nerves also innervate veins and venules. Cholinergic and sympathetic nerves innervate glands as well as the arteries that supply the glands. The cavernous sinusoids contain erectile tissue that engorges when the sympathetic tone is reduced or when the cholinergic system is stimulated. The sensory, cholinergic, and sympathetic nerves also respond to a variety of neuropeptide neurotransmitters.

The pharynx, divided into the nasopharynx, oropharynx, and hypopharynx, connects the nasal cavities to the larynx and esophagus. Four pairs of sinus cavities (paranasal sinuses) drain posteriorly into the pharynx. The nasopharynx is connected to the middle ears by the eustachian tubes. The vocal cords and epiglottis are located in the larynx.

The respiratory mucosa, a specialized membrane, lines the surfaces of the upper and lower respiratory tracts, including the sinuses. The respiratory mucosa contains ciliated epithelial cells, goblet cells, and mucus-secreting glands. The glands secrete a variety of enzymes, immunoglobulins, and other immunomodulatory factors. A double fluid layer covers the respiratory mucosa. Outermost is a thick, sticky layer that traps dust, bacteria, viruses, and other foreign materials. Innermost is a thinner, more aqueous layer in which ciliated epithelial cells beat in a synchronized, wavelike pattern, thus sweeping the thicker outer layer toward the larynx where the mucus is swallowed. The interstitial tissue contains lymphocytes, fibroblasts, and mast cells. Mast cells are located close to nerves and blood vessels, and are clustered in the epithelium just beneath the basement membrane. When stimulated, mast cells release histamine and other mediators that trigger inflammation and increased mucus production, causing some symptoms associated with colds and allergic rhinitis.

## COLDS

A cold, also known as the common cold, is a viral infection of the upper respiratory tract and is one of the top five illnesses diagnosed in the United States.[1] Studies show proper hand hygiene reduces the transmission of cold viruses, and the Centers for Disease Control (CDC) encourages frequent handwashing with soap or soap substitutes to help prevent colds.[2] Studies conducted in the 1980s found use of antiviral disinfectants such as Lysol (kills >99% of rhinoviruses after 1 minute) and antiviral tissues such as Kleenex Anti-Viral (10% fewer respiratory infections than a placebo group) may also help prevent colds.[3] However, to date no effective prophylactic treatment or cure for colds exists. Antibiotics, often prescribed for patients with colds, are ineffective against viral infections. Colds usually are self-limiting illnesses, but to treat symptoms, patients frequently self-medicate with nonprescription drugs, herbals, or other alternative remedies. Colds are the leading cause of work and school absenteeism. Patients spend approximately $299 million on nonprescription cold products.[4]

**Editor's Note:** This chapter is based, in part, on the 14th edition chapter with the same title, which was written by Karen J. Tietze.

## Epidemiology of Colds

According to some estimates, 1 billion cases of colds occur annually in the United States.[2] Children usually have six to 10 colds per year but may have as many as 12 colds annually, especially if they attend day care.[2] Adults (<60 years of age) typically have two to four colds per year.[2] Women, especially ages 20 to 30 years old, tend to have more colds than men and this may be because of more frequent contact with preschool or school-age children.[2] Colds may occur at any time, but in the United States cold season is from late August through early April.[2]

## Etiology of Colds

More than 200 viruses cause colds. The majority of colds in children and adults are caused by rhinoviruses.[2] Other pathogens shown to cause colds include coronaviruses, influenza viruses, parainfluenza viruses, adenoviruses, echoviruses, respiratory syncytial virus, and coxsackieviruses. Double viral infection and bacterial coinfection (usually with group A β-hemolytic streptococci) occur but are rare.

The most efficient mode of transmission is self-inoculation of the nasal mucosa or conjunctiva following contact with viral-laden secretions on animate (hands) or inanimate (doorknobs and telephones) objects. Aerosol transmission is also important. Smoking, allergic disorders affecting the nose or pharynx, increased population density, a sedentary lifestyle, less diverse social networks, and chronic (e.g., ≥1 month) psychologic stress increase susceptibility to colds.[5] Contrary to common belief, cold environments, sudden chilling, exposure to central heating, walking outside barefoot, teething, or enlarged tonsils or adenoids do not increase susceptibility to viral upper respiratory infections.[6,7]

## Pathophysiology of Colds

Rhinoviruses bind to intercellular adhesion molecule-1 receptors on respiratory epithelial cells in the nose and nasopharynx. Once inside the epithelial cells, the virus replicates and infection spreads to other cells.[8] Peak viral concentrations occur 2 to 4 days after initial infection, and viruses are present in the nasopharynx for 16 to 18 days. Infected cells release chemokine "distress signals" and cytokines activate inflammatory mediators and neurogenic reflexes, resulting in recruitment of additional inflammatory mediators, vasodilatation, transudation of plasma, glandular secretion, and stimulation of pain nerve fibers and sneeze and cough reflexes. Inflammatory mediators and parasympathetic nervous system reflex mechanisms cause hypersecretion of watery nasal fluid. Viral infection ends once enough neutralizing antibody (secretory immunoglobulin A or serum immunoglobulin G) leaks into the mucosa to end viral replication.

## Signs and Symptoms of Colds

A predictable sequence of symptoms appears 1 to 3 days after infection.[9] Sore throat is the first symptom to appear, followed by nasal symptoms, which dominate by day 2 or 3, and cough, although an infrequent symptom (<20%), appears by day 4 or 5. Physical assessment of a patient with a cold may yield the following findings: slightly red pharynx with evidence of postnasal drainage, nasal obstruction, and mildly to moderately tender sinuses on palpation. During the first 2 days of a cold, patients may report clear, thin nasal secretions. As the infection progresses, the secretions become thicker, and the color may change to yellow or green. When the cold begins to resolve, the secretions become clear and watery. Patients may have low-grade fever, but colds are rarely associated with a fever above 100°F (37.8°C). Rhinovirus cold symptoms persist for about 7 days.[9] Signs and symptoms of a cold may be confused with influenza and other respiratory illness (Table 11-1).

**TABLE 11-1 Differentiation of Colds and Other Respiratory Disorders**

| Illness | Signs and Symptoms |
|---|---|
| Allergic rhinitis | Watery eyes; itchy nose, eyes, or throat; repetitive sneezing; nasal congestion; watery rhinorrhea; red, irritated eyes with conjunctival injection |
| Asthma | Cough, dyspnea, wheezing |
| Bacterial throat infection | Sore throat, fever, exudate, tender anterior cervical adenopathy |
| Colds | Sore throat, nasal congestion, rhinorrhea, sneezing common; low-grade fever, chills, headache, malaise, myalgia, and cough possible |
| Croup | Fever, rhinitis, and pharyngitis initially, progressing to cough (may be "barking" cough), stridor, and dyspnea |
| Influenza | Myalgia, arthralgia, fever, sore throat, nonproductive cough, moderate-severe fatigue |
| Otitis media | Ear popping, ear fullness, otalgia, otorrhea, hearing loss, dizziness |
| Pneumonia or bronchitis | Chest tightness, wheezing, dyspnea, productive cough, changes in sputum color, persistent fever |
| Sinusitis | Tenderness over the sinuses, facial pain aggravated by Valsalva's maneuver or postural changes, fever >101.5°F (38.6°C), tooth pain, halitosis, upper respiratory tract symptoms for >7 days with poor response to decongestants |
| West Nile virus infection | Fever, headache, fatigue, rash, swollen lymph glands, and eye pain initially, possibly progressing to GI distress, CNS changes, seizures, or paralysis |
| Whooping cough | Initial catarrhal phase (rhinorrhea, sneezing, mild cough, sneezing) of 1-2 weeks, followed by 1-6 weeks of paroxysmal coughing |

CNS, central nervous system; GI, gastrointestinal.

## Complications of Colds

Most people do not have complications from colds. However, complications of colds may be severe and, rarely, life threatening. Complications include sinusitis, middle ear infections, bronchitis, bacterial pneumonia, and exacerbations of asthma or chronic obstructive pulmonary disease.

## Treatment of Colds

### *Treatment Goals*

Since there is no known cure or proven prophylactic treatment for colds, the goal of therapy is to reduce bothersome symptoms.

### *General Treatment Approach*

The mainstays of therapy include rest and adequate fluid intake. If a patient desires to self-treat, symptom-specific therapy with single-entity products is recommended (Figure 11-1).[10] Most cold symptoms are present sometime during the course of the cold; however, symptoms appear, peak, and resolve at different times. Combination products are convenient, but the convenience must be weighed against the risks from taking unnecessary drugs. Patient education regarding the administration of intranasal (Table 11-2) and ocular (see Chapter 28) drugs is important.

Not all patients should self-treat colds (refer to the exclusions for self-treatment listed in Figure 11-1). Patients with hypertension, ischemic heart disease, coronary artery disease, hyperthyroidism, diabetes mellitus, increased intraocular pressure, or prostatic hypertrophy should use decongestants only after consulting a primary care provider.

### *Nonpharmacologic Therapy*

Nondrug therapy includes increased fluid intake, adequate rest, a nutritious diet as tolerated, increased humidification with cool mist vaporizers or steamy showers, saline gargle, and nasal irrigation. Saline nasal sprays or drops soothe irritated mucosal membranes and loosen encrusted mucus. Simple, inexpensive foods such as tea with lemon and honey, chicken soup, and hot broths are soothing and increase fluid intake. Limited evidence suggests that chicken soup could have anti-inflammatory activity.[11] Milk products should not be withheld as there is no evidence that milk increases cough or congestion. Medical devices, such as Vicks Breathe Right nasal strips, are marketed for temporary relief from nasal congestion and stuffiness resulting from colds and allergies. These devices lift the nares open, enlarging the anterior nasal passages; mentholated strips produce a soothing odor, which may ease nasal irritation.

Nondrug therapy for infants includes upright positioning to enhance nasal drainage, maintaining an adequate fluid intake, increasing the humidity of inspired air, and irrigating the nose with saline drops. Also, since children typically cannot blow their own noses until about 4 years of age, carefully clearing the nasal passageways with a bulb syringe may be necessary if accumulation of mucus interferes with sleeping or eating.

**TABLE 11-2 Administration Guidelines for Nasal Drugs**

**Nasal Sprays**

- Gently insert the bottle tip into one nostril as shown in drawing A.
- Keep head upright. Sniff deeply while squeezing the bottle. Repeat with other nostril.

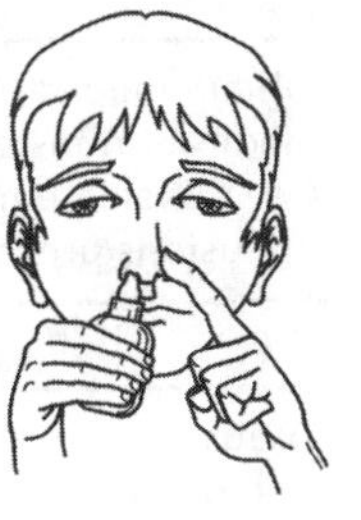

A

**Pump Nasal Sprays**

- Prime the pump before using the first time. Hold the bottle with the nozzle between the first two fingers and thumb on the bottom of the bottle.
- Tilt the head forward.
- Gently insert the nozzle tip into one nostril as shown in drawing B. Sniff deeply while depressing the pump once.
- Repeat with other nostril.

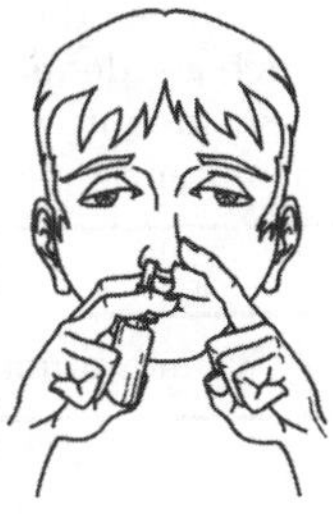

B

**Nasal Inhalers**

- Warm the inhaler in hand just before use.
- Gently insert the inhaler tip into one nostril as shown in drawing C. Sniff deeply while inhaling.
- Repeat with other nostril.
- Wipe the inhaler after each use. Make sure the cap is tightly in place between uses. Discard after 2-3 months even if the inhaler still smells medicinal.

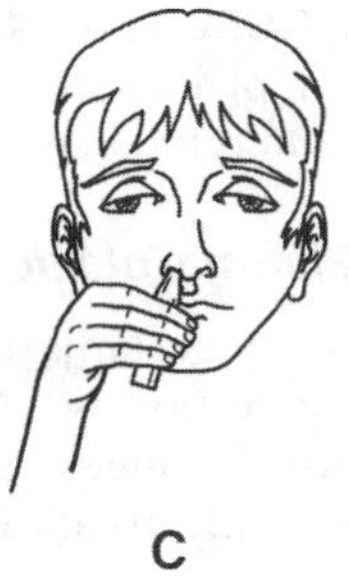

C

**Nasal Drops**

- Squeeze the bulb to withdraw medication from the bottle.
- Lie on bed with head tilted back over the side of the bed as shown in drawing D.
- Place the recommended number of drops into one nostril. Gently tilt head from side to side.
- Repeat with other nostril. Lie on bed for a couple of minutes after placing drops in the nose.
- Do not rinse the dropper.

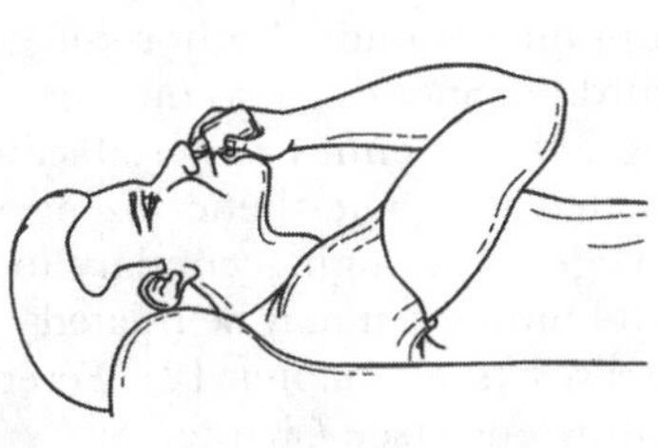

D

*Note:* Do not share the drug with anyone. Discard solutions if discolored or if contamination is suspected. Remove caps before use and replace after use. Do not use expired products. Clear nasal passages before administering the dose. Gently depress the other side of the nose with finger to close off the nostril not receiving the medication. Wait a few minutes after using the drug before blowing the nose.

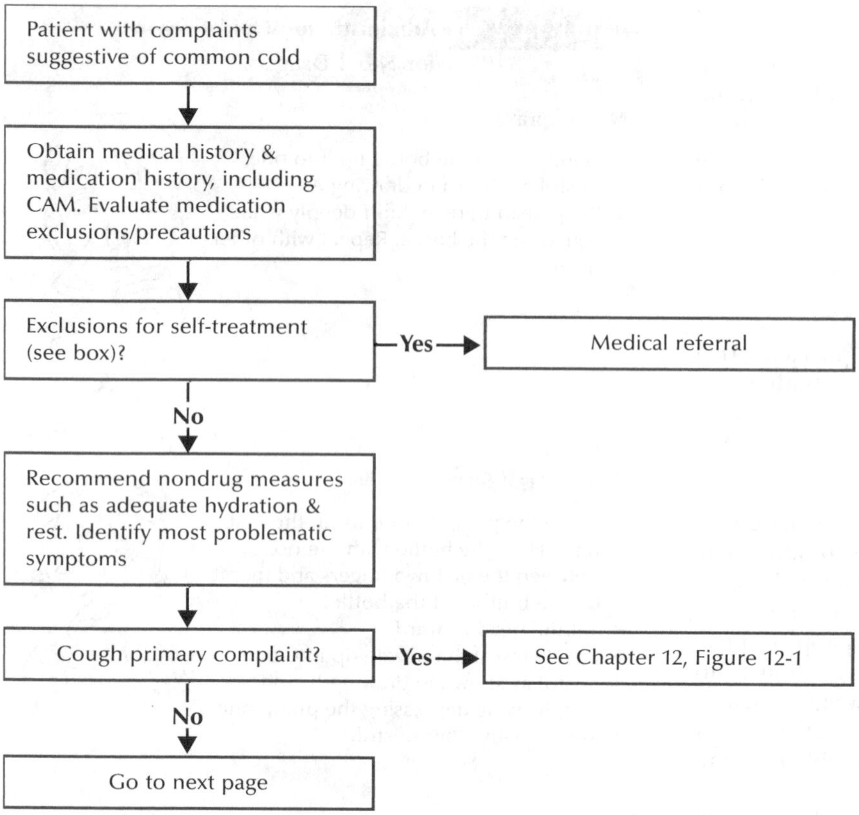


**Exclusions for Self-Treatment**

- Fever >101.5°F (38.6°C)
- Chest pain
- Shortness of breath
- Worsening of symptoms or development of additional symptoms during self-treatment
- Concurrent underlying chronic cardiopulmonary diseases (e.g., asthma, COPD, CHF)
- AIDS or chronic immunosuppressant therapy
- Frail patients of advanced age
- Infants <9 months of age
- Hypersensitivity to recommended OTC medications

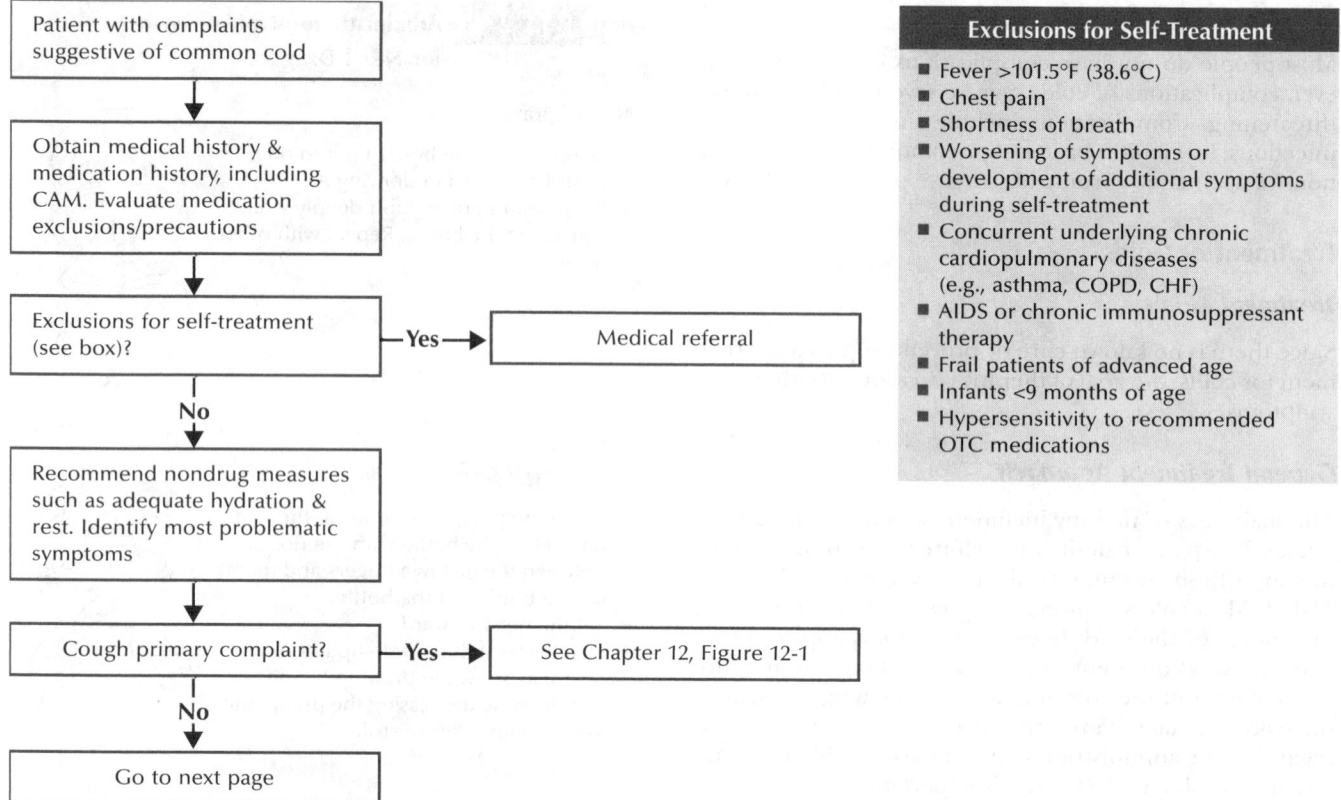

**FIGURE 11-1** Self-care of the common cold. Key: AH, antihistamine; AIDS, acquired immunodeficiency syndrome; CAM, complementary and alternative medicine; CHF, congestive heart failure; COPD, chronic obstructive pulmonary disease. (Adapted from reference 10.)

### *Pharmacologic Therapy*

Decongestants are the mainstay of therapy for colds. Nasal congestion is treated with topical or oral adrenergic agonist decongestants. Rhinorrhea is multifactorial and only partially treatable with available medications. Antihistamines with anticholinergic properties (sedating antihistamines) and the prescription anticholinergic drug ipratropium bromide both reduce rhinorrhea by about a third.[12,13] Sneezing is a common but minor symptom; sedating antihistamines may reduce sneezing.[13] Pharyngitis is treated with anesthetic lozenges or sprays and systemic analgesics. Cough secondary to postnasal drip is usually self-limiting but may be treated with decongestants or antitussives (see Chapter 12). Fever is treated with systemic antipyretics (see Chapter 6).

#### Decongestants

Decongestants (Table 11-3) specifically treat sinus and nasal congestion. Topical decongestants are convenient dosage forms but use should be limited to no more than 3 to 5 days to avoid rhinitis medicamentosa (rebound congestion).

*Mechanism of Action* Decongestants are adrenergic agonists (sympathomimetics). Stimulation of α-adrenergic receptors constricts blood vessels, thereby decreasing sinusoid vessel engorgement and mucosal edema. There are three types of decongestants. Direct-acting decongestants (phenylephrine, oxymetazoline, tetrahydrozoline) bind directly to adrenergic receptors. Indirect-acting decongestants displace norepinephrine from storage vesicles in prejunctional nerve terminals. Indirect-acting sympathomimetics have the slowest onset and longest duration of action; however, tachyphylaxis develops as stored neurotransmitter is depleted. Mixed decongestants (e.g., pseudoephedrine) have both direct and indirect activity.

*Pharmacokinetics* Systemic decongestants are rapidly metabolized by monoamine oxidase (MAO) and catechol-O-methyltransferase in the gastrointestinal (GI) mucosa, liver, and other tissues. Pseudoephedrine is well absorbed after oral administration; phenylephrine has a low oral bioavailability (approximately 38%). Both pseudoephedrine and phenylephrine have large volumes of distribution (2.6-5 L/kg) and short half-lives (6 hours for pseudoephedrine and 2.5 hours for phenylephrine); peak concentrations for both drugs occur at 0.5 to 2 hours following oral administration.

*Indications* Decongestants are indicated for temporary relief of nasal and eustachian tube congestion and cough associated with postnasal drip. As of April 11, 2007, nonprescription decongestants will no longer have an approved indication to be used to self-treat nasal congestion associated with sinusitis. FDA will require manufacturers of decongestants to remove the terms *sinusitis* and *associated with sinusitis* from all labeling.

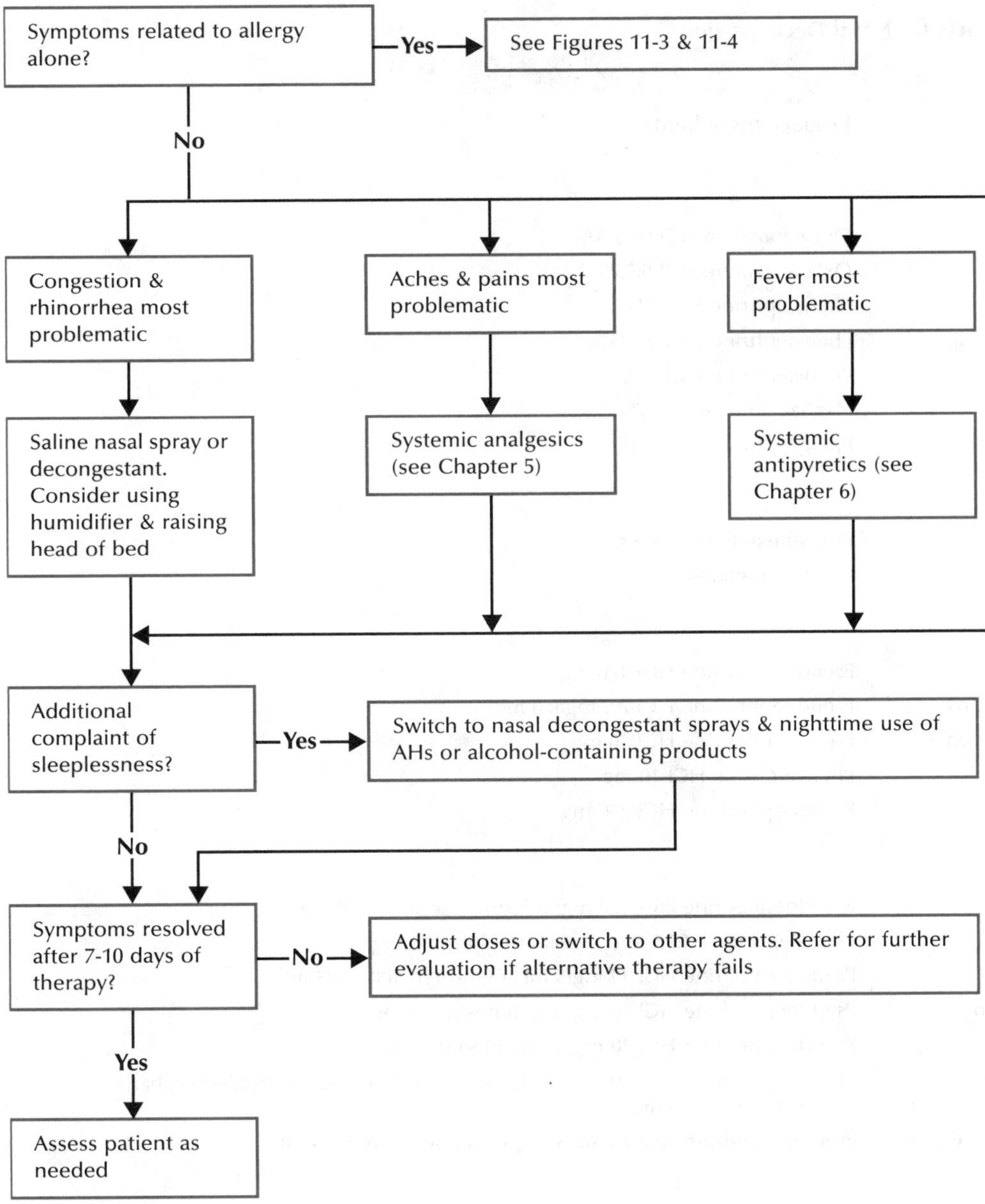

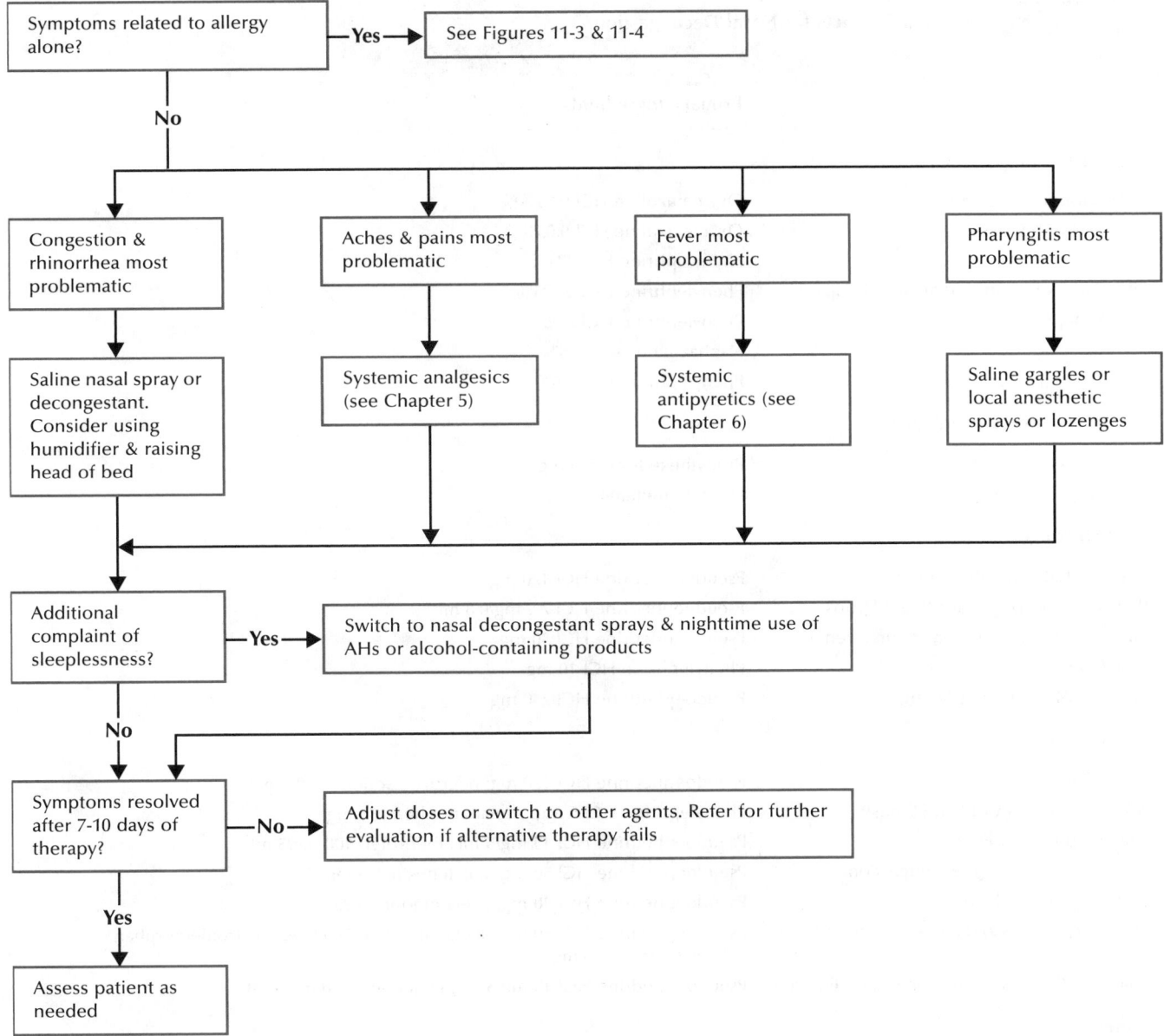

**FIGURE 11–1 (continued)**

*Dosage and Dosage Formulations* Food and Drug Administration (FDA)-approved dosages for decongestants are listed in Tables 11-4 and 11-5.[15] Nonprescription decongestants are marketed as systemic and topical (intranasal and ophthalmic) dosage formulations; many combination products are available. Topical drugs work locally but have little effect on systemic symptoms. The systemic nonprescription decongestants include pseudoephedrine and phenylephrine. The ophthalmic nonprescription decongestants include naphazoline, oxymetazoline, phenylephrine, and tetrahydrozoline (see Chapter 28). The intranasal nonprescription decongestants include the short-acting decongestants ephedrine, epinephrine, naphazoline, phenylephrine, and tetrahydrozoline; the intermediate-acting decongestant xylometazoline; and the long-acting decongestant oxymetazoline. Desoxyephedrine and propylhexedrine are available as nonprescription nasal inhalers.

Each nasal drug delivery dosage form has distinct advantages and disadvantages. Nasal sprays are simple to use, cover a large surface area, are relatively inexpensive, and have a fast onset of action. The disadvantages include imprecise dosage, a tendency for the tip to become clogged with repeated use, and a high risk of contamination from aspiration of nasal mucus into the bottle. Metered pump sprays deliver a more precise dose. Nasal drops are preferred for small children, but are awkward to use, cover a limited surface area, and pass easily into the larynx. There is also a high risk of contamination because of the tendency to touch the dropper to the nose during administration. Nasal inhalers are small and unobtrusive, but require an unobstructed airway and sufficient airflow to distribute the drug to the nasal mucosa. Nasal

**TABLE 11-3 Selected Products for Nasal Decongestion**

| Trade Name | Primary Ingredients |
|---|---|
| **Topical Decongestants** | |
| Afrin Original Nasal Spray | Oxymetazoline HCl 0.05% |
| Dristan 12-hr Nasal | Oxymetazoline HCl 0.05% |
| 4-Way Fast Acting | Phenylephrine HCl 1% |
| Little Noses Decongestant Nose Drops | Phenylephrine HCl 0.125% |
| Neo-Synephrine | Phenylephrine HCl 0.25% |
| Privine | Naphazoline HCl 0.05% |
| Vicks Sinex Ultra Fine Mist | Phenylephrine HCl 0.5% |
| **Nasal Decongestant Inhalers** | |
| Benzedrex Inhaler | Propylhexedrine 250 mg |
| Vicks Vapor Inhaler | Levmetamfetamine 50 mg |
| **Oral Decongestants** | |
| Drixoral 12-Hour Non-Drowsy* | Pseudoephedrine HCl 120 mg |
| PediaCare Decongestant Infant Drops† | Pseudoephedrine HCl 7.5 mg/0.8 mL |
| Sudafed Non-Drowsy Maximum Strength† | Pseudoephedrine HCl 30 mg |
| Sudafed PE | Phenylephrine HCl 10 mg |
| Sudafed 24 hour Long Acting | Pseudoephedrine HCl 240 mg |
| **Combination Products** | |
| Aleve Cold & Sinus | Pseudoephedrine HCl 120 mg; naproxen sodium 220 mg |
| Alka-Seltzer Plus Cold and Sinus‡§ | Phenylephrine HCl 5 mg; acetaminophen 250 mg |
| Dimetapp Cold & Fever | Pseudoephedrine HCl 15 mg/5 mL; ibuprofen 100 mg/5 mL |
| Robitussin Cold Severe Congestion | Pseudoephedrine HCl 30 mg; guaifenesin 200 mg |
| Sudafed Cold and Sinus | Pseudoephedrine HCl 30 mg; acetaminophen 325 mg |
| TheraFlu Severe Cold and Congestion‡§ | Pseudoephedrine HCl 60 mg; acetaminophen 1000 mg; dextromethorphan hydrobromide 30 mg |
| Triaminic Chest & Nasal Congestion liquid†‡‖ | Pseudoephedrine HCl 15 mg/5 mL; guaifenesin 50 mg/5 mL |
| **Other** | |
| Ocean Premium Saline Nasal Spray | Sodium chloride 0.65% |

*Dye-free; †contains sucrose; ‡contains sodium; §contains aspartame; ‖certified kosher by the Orthodox Union.

**TABLE 11-4 Dosage Guidelines for Nonprescription Systemic Nasal Decongestants[15]**

| | Dosage (Maximum Daily Dosage) | | |
|---|---|---|---|
| Drug | Adults/Children ≥12 Years | Children 6-12 Years | Children 2-6 Years |
| Phenylephrine | 10 mg q4h (60 mg) | 5 mg q4h (30 mg) | 2.5 mg q4h (15 mg) |
| Pseudoephedrine | 60 mg q4-6h (240 mg) | 30 mg q4-6h (120 mg) | 15 mg q4-6h (60 mg) |

**TABLE 11-5 Dosage Guidelines for Topical Nasal Decongestants[15]**

| Drug | Concentration (%) | Adults/Children ≥12 Years | Children 6-12 Years | Children 2-6 Years* |
|---|---|---|---|---|
| **Sprays/Drops** | | | | |
| Ephedrine | 0.5 | 2-3 drops/sprays not more often than q4h | 1-2 drops/sprays not more often than q4h | Not recommended for children <6 years except under advice of PCP |
| Naphazoline | 0.05 | 1-2 drops/sprays not more often than q6h | Not recommended for children <12 years except under advice of PCP | Not recommended for children <6 years except under advice of PCP |
| | 0.025 | — | 1-2 drops/sprays not more often than q6h | Not recommended for children <6 years except under advice of PCP |
| Oxymetazoline | 0.05 | 2-3 drops/sprays not more often than q10-12h (max 2 doses/24 hours) | 2-3 drops/sprays not more often than q10-12h (max 2 doses/24 hours) | Not recommended for children <6 years except under advice of PCP |
| | 0.025 | — | — | 2-3 drops/sprays not more often than q10-12h (max 2 doses/24 hours) |
| Phenylephrine | 1.0 | 2-3 drops/sprays not more often than q4h | Not recommended for children <12 years except under advice of PCP | Not recommended for children <6 years except under advice of PCP |
| | 0.5 | 2-3 drops/sprays not more often than q4h | Not recommended for children <12 years except under advice of PCP | Not recommended for children <6 years except under advice of PCP |
| | 0.25 | 2-3 drops/sprays not more often than q4h | 2-3 drops/sprays not more often than q4h | Not recommended for children <6 years except under advice of PCP |
| | 0.125 | — | — | 2-3 drops not more often than q4h |
| Xylometazoline | 0.1 | 2-3 drops/sprays not more often than q8-10h | Not recommended for children <12 years except under advice of PCP | Not recommended for children <6 years except under advice of PCP |
| | 0.05 | — | 2-3 drops/sprays not more often than q8-10h | 2-3 drops/sprays not more often than q8-10h |

Key: N/A, not applicable; PCP, primary care provider.

* No recommended dosages exist for children under 2 years of age, except under the advice and supervision of a PCP.

inhalers lose efficacy after 2 to 3 months even when tightly capped because of dissipation of the active ingredient. Nasal polyps, enlarged turbinates, and abnormalities such as septal deviation may reduce the efficacy of topical dosage forms.

*Overdosage* Systemic decongestant overdoses cause excessive central nervous system (CNS) stimulation, paradoxical CNS depression, cardiovascular collapse, shock, and coma. Treatment is supportive.

*Safety Considerations* Because topical decongestants are minimally absorbed, systemic side effects are generally infrequent and mild. However, adverse effects include cardiovascular stimulation (elevated blood pressure, tachycardia, palpitation, or arrhythmias) and CNS stimulation (restlessness, insomnia, anxiety, tremors, fear, or hallucinations). Children and older adults are more likely to experience adverse effects than other age groups.

More common problems include propellant- or vehicle-associated side effects (burning, stinging, sneezing, local dryness) and trauma from the dosage administration device. Rhinitis medicamentosa occurs when topical decongestants are administered longer than 3 to 5 days and is more common with the short-acting decongestants.

**TABLE 11-6 Decongestant and Antihistamine Drug Interactions**

| Drug | Effect |
|---|---|
| **Decongestants** | |
| MAOIs (phenelzine, tranylcypromine, isocarboxazid, furazolidone, procarbazine) | ↑ Blood pressure |
| Methyldopa | ↑ Blood pressure |
| TCAs (amitriptyline, nortriptyline, imipramine) | ↑ Blood pressure (direct-acting decongestant)<br>↓ Decongestant activity (indirect-acting decongestants) |
| Urinary acidifiers (ammonium chloride, potassium phosphate, sodium acid phosphate) | ↑ Elimination (pseudoephedrine) |
| Urinary alkalinizers (potassium acetate, sodium acetate, sodium bicarbonate, sodium citrate, sodium lactate, tromethamine, potassium citrate, citric acid) | ↓ Elimination (pseudoephedrine) |
| **Antihistamines** | |
| CNS depressants (alcohol, sedatives) | ↑ Sedation (sedating antihistamines) |
| MAOIs (phenelzine, tranylcypromine, isocarboxazid, furazolidone, procarbazine) | Prolonged and intensified anticholinergic and CNS depressive effects (sedating antihistamine)<br>↓ Blood pressure (dexchlorpheniramine) |
| Phenytoin | ↓ Phenytoin elimination (chlorpheniramine) |
| Ketoconazole, erythromycin, cimetidine | ↑ Loratadine plasma concentration |

Key: CNS, central nervous system; MAOI, monoamine oxidase inhibitor; TCA, tricyclic antidepressant.

Benzalkonium chloride, a common preservative in these products, may contribute to the problem.[16] Treatment consists of slowly withdrawing the topical decongestant (one nostril at a time); replacing the decongestant with topical normal saline, which soothes the irritated nasal mucosa; and, if needed, using topical corticosteroids and systemic decongestants. The mucous membrane returns to normal within 1 to 2 weeks.

Decongestants interact with numerous drugs, as summarized in Table 11-6.

Decongestants are contraindicated in patients who have a history of hypersensitivity or idiosyncratic reaction to a decongestant and in patients receiving concomitant MAO inhibitors (MAOIs). Some decongestants are contraindicated in children of varying ages (Tables 11-4 and 11-5). Product labels and inserts also carry this information.

Decongestants may exacerbate diseases sensitive to adrenergic stimulation, such as hypertension, hyperthyroidism, diabetes mellitus, coronary heart disease, ischemic heart disease, elevated intraocular pressure, and prostatic hypertrophy. Patients with hypertension should use decongestants only with medical advice. No clear evidence exists that any one agent is safer in patients with hypertension. Clinicians should educate patients who participate in organized sports that oral decongestants are considered “doping” products and should be used with caution. Clinicians also should be aware of patients wishing to purchase large quantities of pseudoephedrine, which is illegally used to produce methamphetamine. Ten states have enacted legislation to restrict sales of pseudoephedrine and in April 2004 Oklahoma changed its tablet form to a Schedule V drug.[17] The Consumer Healthcare Products Association and the National Association of Chain Drug Stores have created Meth Watch, www.methwatch.com/index.aspx, to provide assistance to clinicians.

### Antihistamines

Nonprescription sedating antihistamines decrease the rhinorrhea associated with colds by about one third and may reduce sneezing. Apart from questions of efficacy, an important issue is whether potential benefits of sedating antihistamines outweigh known risks associated with these drugs. Loratadine, a nonsedating antihistamine, has no anticholinergic activity and therefore no activity against rhinorrhea or sneezing. (See discussion of antihistamines in the allergic rhinitis section of this chapter).

### Local Anesthetics

Lozenges, troches, mouthwashes, and sprays containing local anesthetics (e.g., benzocaine, dyclonine hydrochloride) are available for the temporary relief of sore throats (Table 11-7). Local anesthetic products may be used every 3 to 4 hours. Some products contain local antiseptics (cetylpyridinium chloride, hexylresorcinol) and/or menthol or camphor. Local antiseptics are not effective for viral infections. The clinical efficacy of menthol or camphor is not well documented. Clinicians should counsel patients with a history of allergic reactions to anesthetics to avoid products with benzocaine.

**TABLE 11-7 Selected Products for Sore Throat**

| Trade Name | Primary Ingredients |
|---|---|
| **Lozenges** | |
| Cepacol Sore Throat Sugar Free* | Benzocaine 10 mg; menthol 4.5 mg |
| Chloroseptic Sore Throat | Benzocaine 6 mg; menthol 10 mg |
| Halls Fruit Breezers | Pectin 7 mg |
| Sucret's Maximum Strength | Dyclonine HCl 3 mg |
| **Throat Sprays** | |
| Cepacol Spray*† | Dyclonine 0.1% |
| Chloroseptic Sore Throat*† | Phenol 1.4% |
| Triaminic Sore Throat*† | Phenol 0.5% |
| **Oral Disintegrating Strips** | |
| Chloroseptic Sore Throat Relief Strips | Benzocaine 3 mg; menthol 3 mg |

*Sucrose free; †alcohol free.

### Systemic Analgesics

Systemic analgesics are effective for aches or fever sometimes associated with colds. When patients are feverish, a nonprescription antipyretic (e.g., aspirin, acetaminophen, ibuprofen, naproxen, or ketoprofen) is effective treatment. However, some research has shown that use of aspirin and acetaminophen may increase viral shedding and prolong illness.[18] Aspirin-containing products should not be used in children with viral illnesses because of the risk of Reye's syndrome (see Chapters 5 and 6).

### Antitussives

Cough, when present, is usually nonproductive and may be suppressed with antitussives (see Chapter 12). However, neither codeine[19] nor dextromethorphan[20] has been proven effective in natural colds. Guaifenesin, an expectorant, has not been proven effective in natural colds.[21]

### Combination Products

Decongestants and antihistamines are marketed in many combinations, including decongestant/antihistamine combinations and various combinations with analgesics, expectorants, and antitussives.

### Product Selection Guidelines

Product selection is based on the patient's symptoms, classification as a high-risk patient, concomitant illnesses, lifestyle, and preferences.

*Special Populations* Drug use during pregnancy and lactation is a balance between risk and benefit. Since most colds are self-limiting, with bothersome rather than life-threatening symptoms, many clinicians recommend non-drug therapy. When drugs are considered, those with a long record of safety in animals and humans are preferred. To minimize possible adverse effects on the fetus or newborn, pregnant or nursing mothers should be advised to avoid products labeled extra or maximum strength, long-acting, and combination products. Most of the active ingredients in FDA-approved cold medications are Pregnancy Category B or C. There is no clear association between birth defects and the use of systemic or intranasal decongestants during pregnancy.[22] However, systemic decongestants theoretically decrease fetal blood flow and should be avoided. Pseudoephedrine has also been linked to abdominal wall defects (gastroschisis) in newborns.[22] Oxymetazoline is poorly absorbed following intranasal administration and is the preferred topical decongestant during pregnancy. The American Academy of Pediatrics has found pseudoephedrine to be compatible with breast-feeding and to be the preferred decongestant.[23] Intranasal phenylephrine usually is safe in nursing mothers. Nasal preparations containing xylometazoline and naphazoline should be avoided in lactating mothers.[23] Since decongestants may decrease milk production, mothers should monitor their milk production and drink extra fluids as needed. Analgesics do not increase the risk for birth defects when taken in the first trimester, but analgesics with prostaglandin-inhibiting properties (aspirin, nonsteroidal anti-inflammatory drugs or NSAIDs) are associated with an increased risk for intracranial hemorrhage and premature closure of the patent ductus arteriosus and should be avoided during the third trimester. Aspirin should be avoided during lactation. Dextromethorphan, guaifenesin, benzocaine, dyclonine, camphor, and menthol have low risks for birth defects and have been found to be compatible with breast-feeding.[22,23]

Children younger than 1 year should not be given nonprescription cold medications except under the direction of a primary care provider.

## Complementary Therapies

Numerous complementary therapies are marketed for the treatment of colds (Table 11-8; see also Section XI).[24,25] Although there has been a great deal of interest in echinacea, high-dose vitamin C, and zinc lozenges, recent Cochrane Database Systematic Reviews of published studies cast doubt on the efficacy of these agents in the treatment of colds.[26-28] In addition to the more traditional complementary therapies for colds, new products that claim to help strengthen the immune system are gaining popularity.

According to the CDC, echinacea is one of the most commonly (40.3% of 31,044 adults) used herbs in the United States.[29] Three of the nine species of echinacea are reported to have immunostimulant properties such as increasing the number of circulating white blood cells, activation of phagocytosis, and elevation of body temperature. Formulations include single-entity and combination hydroalcoholic extracts, capsules, teas, and soups. Echinacea has not been shown to be effective in preventing colds,

**TABLE 11-8 Selected Complementary/Alternative Medicines Used to Treat Colds and Allergies[24,25]**

| Agent | Risks* | Effectiveness |
|---|---|---|
| **Botanical Medicines (Scientific Name)** | | |
| Coltsfoot (*Tussilago farfava*) | Hepatotoxicity | Demulcent effect for sore throat unproven |
| Devil's claw (*Harpagophytum procumbens*) | GI toxicity/ulcers (stimulates gastric secretions) | Anti-inflammatory effect in allergic rhinitis unproven |
| Echinacea (*Echinacea angustifolia, E. pallida, E. purpurea*) | Hepatotoxicity; metabolic Disturbances; immunosuppression (with prolonged use); aggravation of autoimmune disorders (e.g., multiple sclerosis, rheumatoid arthritis, lupus) | Immunostimulant effects in prevention or treatment of colds and flu unproven |
| Ephedra [ma-huang] (Ephedra sinica) | Tachycardia, hypertension, heart attack, stroke, seizure | Effective decongestant† |
| Feverfew (*Tanacetum parthenium*) | GI toxicity, mouth ulcers | Anti-inflammatory effect of active ingredient parthenolide in allergic rhinitis unproven |
| Goldenseal (*Hydrastis canadensis*) | Potentially toxic, especially in patients with glucose-6-dehydrogenase deficiency | Antibacterial and anti-inflammatory effects of active ingredient berberine for sore throat and colds unproven |
| Horehound (*Marrubium vulgare*) | None reported | Expectorant effect unproven |
| Licorice (*Glycyrrhiza glabia*) | Risk of pseudoaldosteronism | Expectorant and demulcent effects for cough and sore throat unproven |
| Marshmallow (*Althaea officinalis*) | Hypoglycemia; possible delayed absorption of concomitantly administered drugs | Demulcent effect for sore throat and cough unproven |
| Wild cherry (*Prunus serotina*) | Toxicity similar to cyanide poisoning caused by prunasin contained in all plant parts except fruit | Astringent and anti-inflammatory effects for cough and colds unproven |
| Yerba santa (*Eriodictyon californicum*) | None reported | Expectorant effect in colds unproven |
| **Homeopathic Medicines** | | |
| Zicam Cold Remedy liquid nasal gel (Zincum Gluconicum 2X) | Nasal irritation (e.g., burning, stinging); increased sneezing or nasal discharge | Anti-viral and immunostimulant effects in colds unproven |
| Zicam Cold Remedy Chewables‡ (Zincum Gluconicum 1X and Zincum Aceticum 2X) | GI upset | Anti-viral and immunostimulant effects in colds unproven |
| Zicam Allergy Relief Nasal Solution (Luffa Operculata 4x, 12x, 30x, Galphimia Glauca 12x, 30x, Histaminum Hydrochloricum 12x, 30x, 200x, Sulphur 12x, 30x, 200x | Anaphylaxis, increased nasal irritation, nose bleeds | Decongestant and antiallergy symptom effects unproven |

Key: GI, gastrointestinal.

* Herbal products should not be taken by children or by pregnant or lactating women.

† FDA banned sales of ephedra in 2004 (see Chapter 4).

‡ Contains sucrose.

and evidence of the herb's ability to significantly reduce the severity and duration of colds is conflicting.[30,31] Evidence does suggest that patients should not take echinacea for more than 8 weeks at a time.[24] It also should not be taken by breast-feeding or pregnant women or given to children younger than 2 years. Two recent randomized double-blind placebo-controlled trials found no difference in symptom severity or duration between groups treated with echinacea and with placebo.[30,31]

High local concentrations of zinc ions purportedly block the adhesion of human rhinovirus to the nasal epithelium and are also thought to inhibit viral replication by disrupting viral capsid formation. However, in vitro studies have shown only a modest antiviral effect. Formulations include tablets, capsules, chewing gums, lozenges, and various nasal gels, sprays, and swabs. The effectiveness of zinc has been highly debated. Clinical trials that concluded zinc decreased severity and/or duration of symptoms in adults used zinc gluconate lozenges containing at least 13.3 mg of elemental zinc with a rigorous administration schedule started within 24 to 48 hours of symptom onset (i.e., one lozenge every 2 hours for the duration of the cold). GI side effects (e.g., nausea, upset stomach, bitter taste) are common with the oral lozenges. A recent meta-analysis of eight trials showed zinc lozenges were not effective in reducing cold symptoms or duration.[32] Two recent randomized placebo-controlled trials using intranasal zinc have added to the conflicting evidence.[33,34] A 2002 study of one spray of zinc nasal gel (total daily zinc dose ~2.1 mg) in each nostril four times daily started within 24 hours of onset of symptoms showed duration was 2 days shorter and symptoms were significantly reduced by day 2 of treatment.[33] A 2001 study of one spray of Zicam (zinc gluconate 33 mM) in each nostril five times daily started 3 days prior to rhinovirus challenge showed no benefit.[34] Adverse effects related to intranasal zinc include headache, nasal tenderness, dry mouth, and nasal stinging or burning. Recently, case reports of anosmia (loss of smell) after use of zinc gluconate nasal gel and nasal spray have been published.[35]

Vitamin C supplementation does not reduce the number of cold episodes in the general population.[36] However, large doses (e.g., ≥1 g/day) of vitamin C started early in the course of a cold may decrease the duration of illness slightly (by less than 1 day) and decrease the severity of illness by about 20%.[36] The clinical significance and risk–benefit ratio of these effects are debatable. Doses of 4 g/day or greater are associated with diarrhea and other GI symptoms and should not be recommended.

Several new products that claim to strengthen the immune system are available. Larch arabinogalactan, traditionally used as a food additive, is now marketed as Natrol ImmunEnhancer. This product is thought to have probiotic properties and increase the activity of natural killer cells. Airborne effervescent tablets are a combination of 17 active ingredients including high doses of vitamins A and C, herbs (echinacea, ginger, and Chinese vitex), and amino acids (glutamine and lysine). The marketing for Airborne is unique. Patients are urged to take the product before entering crowded environments such as airplanes, offices, and classrooms. Despite the popularity of these new products, their safety and efficacy has not been proven.

## Assessment of Colds: A Case-based Approach

The practitioner should ask the patient what symptoms are most troublesome. If questions about the patient's medical history or medication use do not reveal exclusions for self-treatment, the practitioner should recommend medications that target the specific symptoms. The patient should also be asked about self-treatment of current and previous colds and about the effectiveness of the treatments. Case 11-1 illustrates assessment of patients with a cold.

### CASE 11-1

| Relevant Evaluation Criteria | Scenario/Model Outcome |
|---|---|
| **Information Gathering** | |
| 1. Gather essential information about the patient's symptoms, including: | |
| a. description of symptom(s) (i.e., nature, onset, duration, severity, associated symptoms) | Patient complains of sore throat that started yesterday and woke up with nasal congestion and rhinorrhea today. Patient feels slightly warm. |
| b. description of any factors that seem to precipitate, exacerbate, and/or relieve the patient's symptom(s) | The patient was exposed to several young children with similar symptoms 4 days ago. Patient cannot identify any exacerbating factors. No symptom relief noted. |
| c. description of the patient's efforts to relieve the symptoms | Patient has tried acetaminophen 500 mg in two doses and saline gargles with no relief of sore throat. |
| 2. Gather essential patient history information: | |
| a. patient's identity | Nancy Lewis |
| b. age, sex, height, and weight | 28 y/o F, 5'7", 170 lb |
| c. patient's occupation | Teacher |
| d. patient's dietary habits | Normal healthy diet with occasional fast food |
| e. patient's sleep habits | Sleeps 7-8 hours per night |
| f. concurrent medical conditions, prescription and nonprescription medications, and dietary supplements | Ortho-Tri-Cyclen Lo (patient just stopped last week and is trying to get pregnant) |

## CASE 11-1 (continued)

| Relevant Evaluation Criteria | Scenario/Model Outcome |
|---|---|
| g. allergies | Penicillin |
| h. history of other adverse reactions to medications | Rash with penicillin when patient was 12 y/o |
| i. other (describe)_______ | Patient checked her temperature this morning and it was 99.9°F (37.7°C). |
| **Assessment and Triage** | |
| 3. Differentiate the patient's signs/symptoms and correctly identify the patient's primary problem(s) (see Table 11-1). | The patient has signs/symptoms (nasal congestion preceded by sore throat and mild fever) of an uncomplicated cold. |
| 4. Identify exclusions for self-treatment (see Figure 11-1). | None |
| 5. Formulate a comprehensive list of therapeutic alternatives for the primary problem to determine if triage to a medical practitioner is required, and share this information with the patient. | Options include:<br>(1) Recommend a separate OTC product for each symptom; local anesthetic for sore throat; nasal saline or a nasal or systemic decongestant for nasal congestion; sedating antihistamine for sneezing and rhinorrhea. Recommending a combination product containing two or more active ingredients may be appropriate, depending on symptoms.<br>(2) Refer Nancy to her primary care provider for further evaluation and treatment.<br>(3) Recommend self-care until Nancy can consult her PCP.<br>(4) Take no action. |
| **Plan** | |
| 6. Select an optimal therapeutic alternative to address the patient's problem, taking into account patient preferences. | Symptomatic OTC treatment is appropriate for Nancy's cold symptoms. She has no exclusions for self-care (see Figure 11-1), so referral to a PCP is not necessary. |
| 7. Describe the recommended therapeutic approach to the patient. | For your sore throat, you should select a local anesthetic lozenge/spray that contains either benzocaine or dyclonine such as Chloroseptic Sore Throat lozenges (benzocaine 6 mg; menthol 10 mg). You may also continue the acetaminophen to help with the sore throat and mild fever. For your congestion, you may use a nasal decongestant such as Afrin Original nasal spray (oxymetazoline HCl 0.05%). |
| 8. Explain to the patient the rationale for selecting the recommended therapeutic approach from the considered therapeutic alternatives. | In case you are already pregnant, avoid products containing phenol and try to minimize use of systemic drugs. Since you don't have a cough, anticough medications are not necessary. |
| **Patient Education** | |
| 9. When recommending self-care with nonprescription medications and/or nondrug therapy, convey accurate information to the patient, including: | |
| a. appropriate dose and frequency of administration | Use the Chloroseptic Sore Throat lozenges every 2 hours as needed. Use two to three sprays in each nostril of Afrin not more often than every 10 to 12 hours. Do not exceed two doses (12 sprays) in 24 hours. |
| b. maximum number of days the therapy should be employed | The lozenges can be used for a maximum of 2 days unless otherwise directed by a primary care provider The Afrin should not be used more than 5 days. |
| c. product administration procedures | Allow the lozenge to dissolve slowly in your mouth (see box Patient Education for Colds). Clear the nasal passages before administering two or three sprays of Afrin in each nostril (see Table 11-2). |

CASE 11-1 (continued)

| Relevant Evaluation Criteria | Scenario/Model Outcome |
|---|---|
| d. expected time to onset of relief | Sore throat symptoms will diminish on contact with the lozenge. Nasal symptoms should significantly diminish in 10 minutes, and relief will last up to 10-12 hours after using Afrin. |
| e. degree of relief that can be reasonably expected | Sore throat symptoms will be temporarily relieved with each lozenge. Nasal congestion will persist for about a week. |
| f. most common side effects | The most common side effects of the lozenge include numbness of the mouth and tongue. Afrin may cause nasal stinging or burning. |
| g. side effects that warrant medical intervention should they occur | Lozenges: there is a risk of aspirating food or liquids if you eat while the throat and mouth are numb. Seek medical care if aspiration occurs and you have problems breathing or develop a persistent choking sensation. Afrin rarely increases heart rate or blood pressure. Seek medical care if you feel your heart racing or your blood pressure significantly increases. If you use Afrin for more than 5 days you may experience increased or worsened congestion. Seek medical attention if this occurs. |
| h. patient options in the event that condition worsens or persists | If your sore throat worsens or lasts more than 2 days and if your congestion significantly worsens or is not improved in 7-10 days, see your primary care provider. |
| i. product storage requirements | Store at room temperature. |
| j. specific nondrug measures | Dress normally, increase noncaffeinated fluids, maintain usual diet, and rest as much as possible. |
| 10. Solicit follow-up questions from patient. | Would zinc lozenges be better than Chloroseptic? |
| 11. Answer patient's questions. | Probably not. The zinc lozenges do not have an anesthetic in them and would not provide relief from pain as the Chloroseptic lozenges do. Zinc is thought to help prevent or shorten the duration of a cold, not treat sore throats. |

Key: OTC, over-the-counter; PCP, primary care provider.

## Patient Counseling for Colds

Nondrug measures may be effective in relieving the discomfort of cold symptoms. The practitioner should explain the appropriate nondrug measures for the patient's particular symptoms. For patients who prefer to self-medicate, the purpose of each medication should be described, and the patient should be counseled to take the appropriate medication as symptoms appear. Patients need an explanation of possible side effects, drug interactions, and precautions or warnings. Finally, the signs and symptoms that indicate the disorder is worsening and that medical care should be sought should be provided. (See the box Patient Education for Colds.)

## Evaluation of Patient Outcomes for Colds

Since most colds are self-limiting, symptoms will usually resolve on their own in 7 to 10 days. For the majority of patients, targeted nonprescription therapy will relieve their cold symptoms. Patients should be monitored for worsening symptoms and progression of complications by measuring temperature, assessing nasal secretions, assessing respirations for wheezing or shortness of breath, identifying productive cough, and asking about facial or neck pain. If complications are suspected, medical referral is necessary. Referral to primary care provider (PCP) is also required for patients who meet the exclusions for self-treatment in Figure 11-1 or the warnings section in the box Patient Education for Colds. Follow-up usually is not necessary for patients with uncomplicated colds, but a clinician may deem telephone follow-up in 7 to 10 days appropriate.

# ALLERGIC RHINITIS

Allergic rhinitis, a systemic disease with prominent nasal symptoms, is a worldwide problem that affects adults and children. An estimated 20% of adults and 40% of children in the United States have this disease, and the number of newly diagnosed cases in the country has been steadily increasing over the past three decades.[37] Approximately 9% of adults and 10% of children in the United States were newly diagnosed with allergic rhinitis in 2002.[38] Annual direct costs (e.g., medications, office visits) and indirect costs (e.g., lost school and work days) are estimated to be $2 to $5 billion.[39] Impaired quality of life creates additional significant, but yet to be quantified, intangible costs. An estimated 58% of U.S. nonprescription purchases are allergy/sinus medications.[4]

## PATIENT EDUCATION FOR COLDS

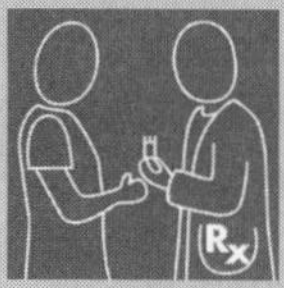

The objectives of self-treatment are to (1) reduce symptoms, (2) improve functioning and the sense of well-being, and (3) prevent the spread of the disease. For most patients, carefully following product instructions and the self-care measures listed here will help ensure optimal therapeutic outcomes.

### Nondrug Measures

- To prevent spreading a cold to others follow these steps: frequently wash your hands with soap for at least 15 seconds; use facial tissues to cover your mouth and nose when coughing or sneezing and then promptly throw the tissues away; and use antiviral products, such as Lysol, to clean surfaces you may have touched such as doorknobs and telephones.
- The following measures may provide relief for or speed up recovery from a cold:
  - Getting adequate rest may help you recover more quickly.
  - Drinking more fluids and using a humidifier may loosen mucus and promote sinus drainage.
  - Sucking on hard candy, gargling with salt water, or drinking fruit juices or hot tea with lemon may soothe a sore throat.

### Nonprescription Medications

- Ask a clinician to help you select medications that target the most bothersome symptoms.

### Sore Throat and Cough

- Sore throat may be treated with anesthetic lozenges or sprays and/or systemic analgesics:
  - Allow lozenges, or troches, to dissolve slowly in the mouth; do not chew or bite the lozenge/troche.
  - Benzocaine and dyclonine may numb the mouth and tongue. If these effects occur, do not eat or drink until they go away.
- Note that cough related to a runny nose (postnasal drip) should be treated with decongestants.

### Rhinorrhea (Runny Nose) and Sneezing

- See the box Patient Education for Allergic Rhinitis for treatment of rhinorrhea (runny nose) and sneezing.

### Nasal Congestion

- Nasal congestion may be treated with topical or systemic decongestants:
  - Do not touch the tips of spray or dropper bottles with the hands. Do not rinse droppers.
  - Do not use topical nasal decongestants longer than 3 to 5 days.
- Decongestants have the following side effects:
  - The most common side effects caused by systemic decongestants are cardiovascular stimulation (i.e., elevated blood pressure, rapid heart rate, palpitations, arrhythmias) and central nervous system stimulation (i.e., restlessness, insomnia, anxiety, tremors, fear, hallucinations). Central nervous system depression (i.e., lethargy, excessive fatigue, confusion) may also occur.
  - Topical decongestants may cause any of the side effects listed for systemic decongestants; however, less of the topical medication gets into the body so side effects are less common.
  - Topical decongestants may irritate the nose, or the bottle tip can injure the nose if used forcefully.
- Note the following precautions for use of decongestants in persons with other medical conditions:
  - Persons with hypertension should use decongestants only with medical advice.
  - Persons with hyperthyroidism, coronary heart disease, ischemic heart disease, elevated intraocular pressure, or an enlarged prostate may experience worsening symptoms of their underlying disease if they take decongestants.
  - Persons with diabetes may need to adjust their dose of insulin if they take decongestants.
  - Blood sugar concentrations need to be monitored closely.
- Note the following drug interactions for decongestants:
  - Persons taking MAOIs (e.g., tranylcypromine or phenelzine), the antibacterial furazolidone, and the anticancer drug procarbazine, should not take indirect-acting or mixed decongestants.
  - Persons taking rauwolfia alkaloids, methyldopa, and tricyclic antidepressants should use direct- and indirect-acting decongestants with caution. These medications interact with decongestants to increase blood pressure, sometimes to the point of causing strokes. Tricyclic antidepressants may increase or decrease blood pressure, depending on the specific decongestant.
  - Medications that decrease the pH of urine increase the elimination of pseudoephedrine.
  - Medications that increase the pH of urine decrease the elimination of pseudoephedrine.

Seek medical attention for the following situations:

- Sore throat persists more than several days, is severe, or is associated with persistent fever, headache, or nausea or vomiting.
- Cough does not improve within 7 to 10 days.
- Symptoms worsen while nonprescription medications are being taken.
- Signs and symptoms of bacterial infections develop (e.g., thick nasal or respiratory secretions that are not clear; temperature higher than 101.5°F [38.6°C]; shortness of breath; chest congestion; wheezing, rash, or significant ear pain).

## Epidemiology of Allergic Rhinitis

Symptoms of allergic rhinitis generally begin after the second year of life, and the disease is prevalent in adults ages 45 to 64 years.[40] After age 65, the number of cases decreases. The prevalence of allergic rhinitis is higher in the southern United States.[40] Allergic rhinitis is classified as seasonal or perennial, depending on the timing and duration of symptoms. The World Health Organization (WHO) has suggested that the terms seasonal allergic rhinitis and perennial allergic rhinitis be replaced with the terms intermittent allergic rhinitis and persistent allergic rhinitis, but these terms are not yet in widespread usage in the United States. Repetitive and predictable seasonal

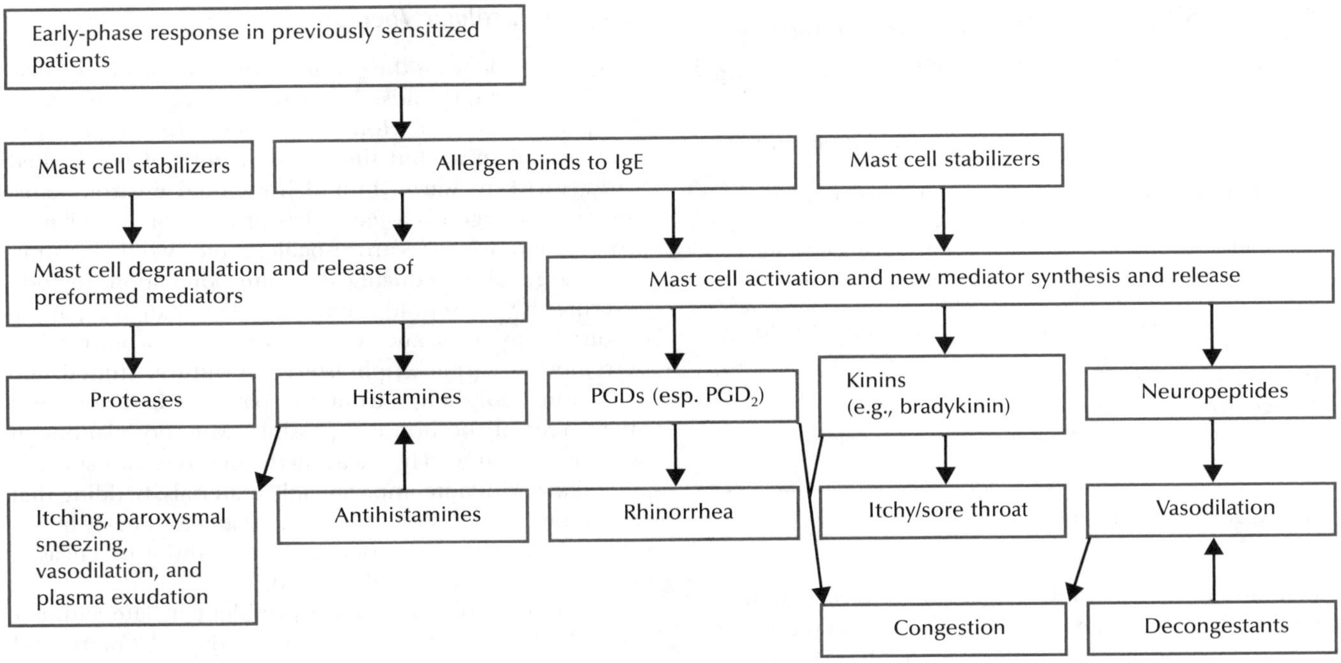


**FIGURE 11-2** Mediator-specific symptoms and targeted drug therapy.[40] Key: Ig, immunoglobulin; PGD, prostaglandin.

symptoms characterize seasonal allergic rhinitis (SAR), whereas symptoms that persist throughout the year without any obvious seasonal pattern characterize perennial allergic rhinitis (PAR). Symptoms of PAR overlap those of many nonallergic rhinitis disorders (e.g., vasomotor rhinitis, nonallergic rhinitis with eosinophilia syndrome); successful therapy requires careful diagnostic evaluation. Patients may experience relatively severe seasonal symptoms superimposed on more moderate perennial symptoms.

## Etiology of Allergic Rhinitis

Allergic rhinitis is triggered by aeroallergens (airborne environmental allergens). Common outdoor aeroallergens include pollen and mold spores; some nonaeroallergen pollens have been implicated. Pollutants (e.g., ozone, diesel exhaust particles) are considered environmental triggers and are becoming more of a concern in highly populated areas. Common indoor aeroallergens include house-dust mites, cockroaches, mold spores, cigarette smoke, and pet danders. Occupational aeroallergens include the following: wool dust, latex, resins, biological enzymes, organic dusts (e.g., flour), and various chemicals (e.g., isocyanate, glutaraldehyde).

## Pathophysiology of Allergic Rhinitis

The pathogenesis of allergic rhinitis is complex, involving numerous cells and mediators and consists of four phases.[41] First is the sensitization phase, which occurs on initial allergen exposure. The allergen stimulates β-lymphocyte–mediated immunoglobulin E (IgE) production. Second is the early phase, occurring within minutes of subsequent allergen exposure. The early phase consists of rapid release of preformed mast cell mediators (e.g., histamine and proteases) as well as the production of additional mediators (e.g., prostaglandins, kinins, leukotrienes, neuropeptides). Figure 11-2 shows mediator-specific symptoms. The third phase is cellular recruitment. Circulating leukocytes, especially eosinophils, are attracted to the nasal mucosa and release more inflammatory mediators. Fourth is the late phase, which begins 2 to 4 hours after allergen exposure; symptoms include mucus hypersecretion secondary to submucosal gland hypertrophy and congestion. Continued persistent inflammation "primes" the tissue, resulting in a lower threshold for allergic- and nonallergic-mediated (e.g., cold air, strong odors) triggers.

## Signs and Symptoms of Allergic Rhinitis

Symptoms of allergic rhinitis include itching of the eyes, nose, and palate; bursts of repetitive sneezing; profuse watery rhinorrhea; postnasal drip; nasal congestion; and red, irritated eyes with conjunctival injection (prominent conjunctival blood vessels). Systemic symptoms include fatigue, irritability, malaise, and cognitive impairment. On physical examination of the patient's face, the practitioner may notice the signs listed Table 11-9.[42] Further physical examination of the chest and skin may aid in differentiating allergic rhinitis from other respiratory diseases such as asthma or chronic obstructive pulmonary disease (COPD).

## Complications of Allergic Rhinitis

Acute complications of allergic rhinitis include sinusitis and otitis media with effusion. Chronic complications include nasal polyps, sleep apnea, and hyposmia (diminished sense of smell).[43] Allergic rhinitis and asthma share

**TABLE 11-9 Possible Physical Findings in Patients with Allergic Rhinitis**

- Facial features
  - "Allergic shiners" (periorbital darkening secondary to venous congestion)
  - "Dennie's lines" (wrinkles beneath the lower eyelids)
  - "Allergic crease" (horizontal crease just about bulbar portion of the nose secondary to the "allergic salute")
  - "Allergic salute" (patient will rub the tip of the nose upward with the palm of the hand)
  - "Allergic gape" (open-mouth breathing secondary to nasal obstruction)
- Conjunctival pallor
- Engorged nasal mucosa
- Nonexudative cobblestone appearance of posterior oropharynx

*Source:* Adapted from reference 42.

a common pathology, and allergic rhinitis has been implicated in the development of asthma and exacerbations of preexisting asthma in children and adults. Depression, anxiety, delayed speech development, and facial or dental abnormalities also have been linked to allergic rhinitis.[41,43]

## Treatment of Allergic Rhinitis

Nonprescription allergy medications relieve and control symptoms of both SAR and PAR. Treatment of PAR is, by necessity, long term, whereas patients with SAR typically need medications only during peak pollen or mold seasons.

### *Treatment Goals*

Allergic rhinitis cannot be cured. The goals of therapy are to reduce symptoms and improve the patient's functional status and sense of well-being. Treatment is individualized to provide optimal symptomatic relief and control of symptoms.

### *General Treatment Approach*

Allergic rhinitis is treated in three steps: allergen avoidance, pharmacotherapy, and immunotherapy.[41] Clinicians should maximize each step before going on to the next intervention. Patient education is an important part of all three steps, especially regarding the administration of nonprescription medications (see Table 11-2 for intranasal preparations and Chapter 28 for ocular drugs). The algorithms in Figures 11-3 and 11-4 outline the self-treatment of SAR and PAR, respectively, and list exclusions for self-treatment.[44,45] Since allergen avoidance is usually not sufficient to provide complete relief of allergic rhinitis, targeted therapy with single-entity drugs usually is initiated. Nonprescription therapy with antihistamines or decongestants usually will treat most symptoms. Drugs with different mechanisms of action or delivery systems may be added if the single-drug therapy does not provide adequate relief or the symptoms are already moderately severe, particularly intense, or long lasting.

### *Nonpharmacologic Therapy*

Allergen avoidance is the primary nonpharmacologic measure for allergic rhinitis. Avoidance strategies depend on the specific allergen. House-dust mites (*Dermatophagoides* spp.), found in all but the driest regions of the United States, thrive in warm, humid household environments. The main allergen is a fecal glycoprotein, but other mite proteins and proteases are also allergenic. Avoidance strategies, targeted at reducing the mite population, include lowering the household humidity to less than 40%, application of acaricides, and reduction of mite-harboring dust by removing carpets, upholstered furniture, stuffed animals, and bookshelves from the patient's bedroom and other areas of the house if possible. Mite populations in bedding are reduced by encasing the mattress, box springs, and pillows with mite-impermeable materials. Bedding that cannot be encased should be washed at least weekly in hot (130°F [54.4°C]) water. Bedding that cannot be encased or laundered should be discarded.

Outdoor mold spores are prevalent in late summer and fall, especially on calm, clear, dry days. *Alternaria* and *Cladosporium* are common outdoor mold allergens; *Penicillium* and *Aspergillus* are common indoor molds. Avoiding activities that disturb decaying plant material (e.g., raking leaves) lessens exposure to outdoor mold. Indoor mold exposure is minimized by lowering household humidity, removing houseplants, venting food preparation areas and bathrooms, repairing damp basements or crawl spaces, and frequently applying fungicide to obviously moldy areas.

Cat-derived allergens (Fel d1; proteins secreted through sebaceous glands in the skin) are small and light and stay airborne for several hours. Cat allergens can be found in the house months after the cat is removed. Although unproven, weekly cat baths may reduce the allergen load.

Cockroaches are major urban allergens. To eliminate cockroaches, patients should be encouraged to keep areas clean, keep food stored tightly sealed, and treat infested areas with baits or pesticides. Infestations in multiple-family dwellings are difficult to eliminate.

Pollutants (e.g., ozone, diesel fumes) are an additional concern in urban environments. Pollutants such as diesel exhaust particles are especially irritating to the respiratory tract and have been shown to increase the severity of allergic rhinitis.[42] Patients whose allergies are triggered by air pollutants should be aware of the air quality index (AQI, a measure of five major air pollutants per 24 hours) and plan outdoor activities when the AQI is low.

Trees pollinate in March and April, grasses in May and June, and ragweed from mid-August to the first fall frost. Pollen counts (the number of pollen grains per cubic meter per 24 hours) help patients plan outdoor activities. Most patients are symptomatic when pollen counts are very high, and only very sensitive patients have symptoms when pollen counts are low. Pollen counts are highest early in the morning and in the evening and lowest after rainstorms clear the air. Avoiding outdoor activities when pollen counts are high plus closing house and car windows reduces pollen exposure.

Ventilation systems with high-efficiency particulate air (HEPA) filters remove pollen, mold spores, and cat allergens from household air but not house-dust mite fecal particles, which settle to the floor too quickly to be filtered. HEPA filtration systems are expensive and not effective for all patients. Patients should be encouraged to rent a HEPA filtration device before investing in freestanding or permanently installed systems. HEPA filters are also found in some vacuum cleaners. Weekly vacuuming of carpets, drapes, and upholstery may help reduce household allergens including dust mites.[46]

Nasal wetting agents (e.g., saline, propylene, polyethylene glycol sprays) may relieve nasal mucosal irritation and dryness, thus decreasing nasal stuffiness, rhinorrhea, and sneezing. These agents also aid in the removal of dried, encrusted, or thick mucus from the nose. Nasal wetting agents have no significant side effects.

### *Pharmacologic Therapy*

Pharmacotherapy is symptom-specific and depends on the severity of the illness. There is no single ideal medication, and combination drug regimens are commonly used. Nonprescription options include ocular and oral antihistamines, topical and oral decongestants, and mast cell stabilizers. Antihistamines and mast cell stabilizers should be used regularly rather than episodically. Patients with SAR should start taking antihistamines and/or mast cell stabilizers at least 1 week before symptoms typically appear. Patients with PAR should begin taking these medications before known allergen exposures, when possible.

#### Antihistamines

Antihistamines are one of the top choices for treating allergic rhinitis. The use of antihistamines in the United States has increased 35% since 1995.[1] These drugs are classified as sedating (first-generation, nonselective) or nonsedating (second-generation, peripherally selective). The role of sedating (first-generation) antihistamines in treating allergic rhinitis is controversial. Sedating antihistamines are effective, readily available without a prescription, and relatively inexpensive. However, these antihistamines expose patients to risks of sedation, impaired performance, and anticholinergic effects and should be used with caution.

*Mechanism of Action* Antihistamines compete with histamine at central and peripheral histamine$_1$-receptor sites, preventing the histamine-receptor interaction and subsequent mediator release. Second-generation antihistamines (e.g., loratadine) inhibit the release of mast cell mediators and may decrease cellular recruitment.

Differences among antihistamines relate to the rapidity and degree to which they penetrate the blood-brain barrier as well as to their receptor specificity. Sedating antihistamines are highly lipophilic molecules that readily cross the blood-brain barrier. Nonsedating antihistamines, large protein-bound lipophobic molecules with charged side chains, do not readily cross the blood-brain barrier. Both types of antihistamines are highly selective for histamine$_1$ receptors but have little effect on histamine$_2$ or histamine$_3$ receptors. The sedating antihistamines activate 5-hydroxytryptamine (serotonin) and α-adrenergic receptors and block cholinergic receptors.

Each antihistamine chemical class differs slightly in terms of its activity and side effect profile. For example, the alkylamines (chlorpheniramine, brompheniramine, pheniramine) are some of the most potent inhibitors of histamine$_1$ and, compared with other first-generation antihistamines, are more likely to cause paradoxical CNS stimulation than sedation. Chemical class differences make it reasonable to suggest switching to a different class of antihistamine if the patient has a less than optimal response to one class of antihistamine.

*Pharmacokinetics* The pharmacokinetics of the sedating antihistamines is not well characterized. However, most are well absorbed after oral administration with time to peak plasma concentrations in the 1.5- to 3-hour range for chlorpheniramine and diphenhydramine; protein binding is in the range of 78% to 99%. Antihistamines are metabolized by the hepatic microsomal mixed-function oxygenase system and undergo significant first-pass metabolism. Half-lives range from approximately 9 hours for diphenhydramine to 28 hours for chlorpheniramine.

Loratadine, the only nonprescription nonsedating antihistamine, is rapidly absorbed after oral administration and hepatically metabolized to descarboethoxyloratadine, an active metabolite. Time to peak concentrations for loratadine and descarboethoxyloratadine are 1.3 and 2.5 hours, respectively. The half-lives of loratadine and descarboethoxyloratadine are 8.4 and 28 hours, respectively. Loratadine and its metabolites are eliminated renally and in the feces.

*Indications* Antihistamines are indicated for relief of symptoms of allergic rhinitis (e.g., itching, sneezing, and rhinorrhea) and other types of immediate hypersensitivity reactions.

*Dosage and Dosage Formulations* FDA-approved dosages for antihistamines are listed in Table 11-10.[15] Nonprescription antihistamines are marketed as immediate- and sustained-release tablets and capsules, chewable tablets, oral disintegrating tablets and strips, solutions, and syrups. Alcohol-, sucrose-, and dye-free formulations are available.

*Overdosage* Sedating antihistamine overdoses are characterized by excessive histamine$_1$-receptor and cholinoreceptor blockade and by α-adrenergic and serotonergic activity. CNS symptoms (toxic psychosis, hallucinations, agitation, lethargy, tremor, insomnia, tonic-clonic seizures) predominate, with children being more sensitive to the CNS excitatory effects and adults more likely to experience CNS depression. Peripheral symptoms include tachycardia, hyperpyrexia, mydriasis, vasodilation, decreased exocrine secretion, urinary retention, decreased GI motility, dystonic reactions, rhabdomyolysis, and cardiac tachyarrhythmias and conduction abnormalities, including torsades de pointes (a dysrhythmia). Loratadine overdoses are characterized by headache, somnolence, and tachycardia. Extrapyramidal signs have been reported in children. Treatment is supportive for antihistamine overdoses.

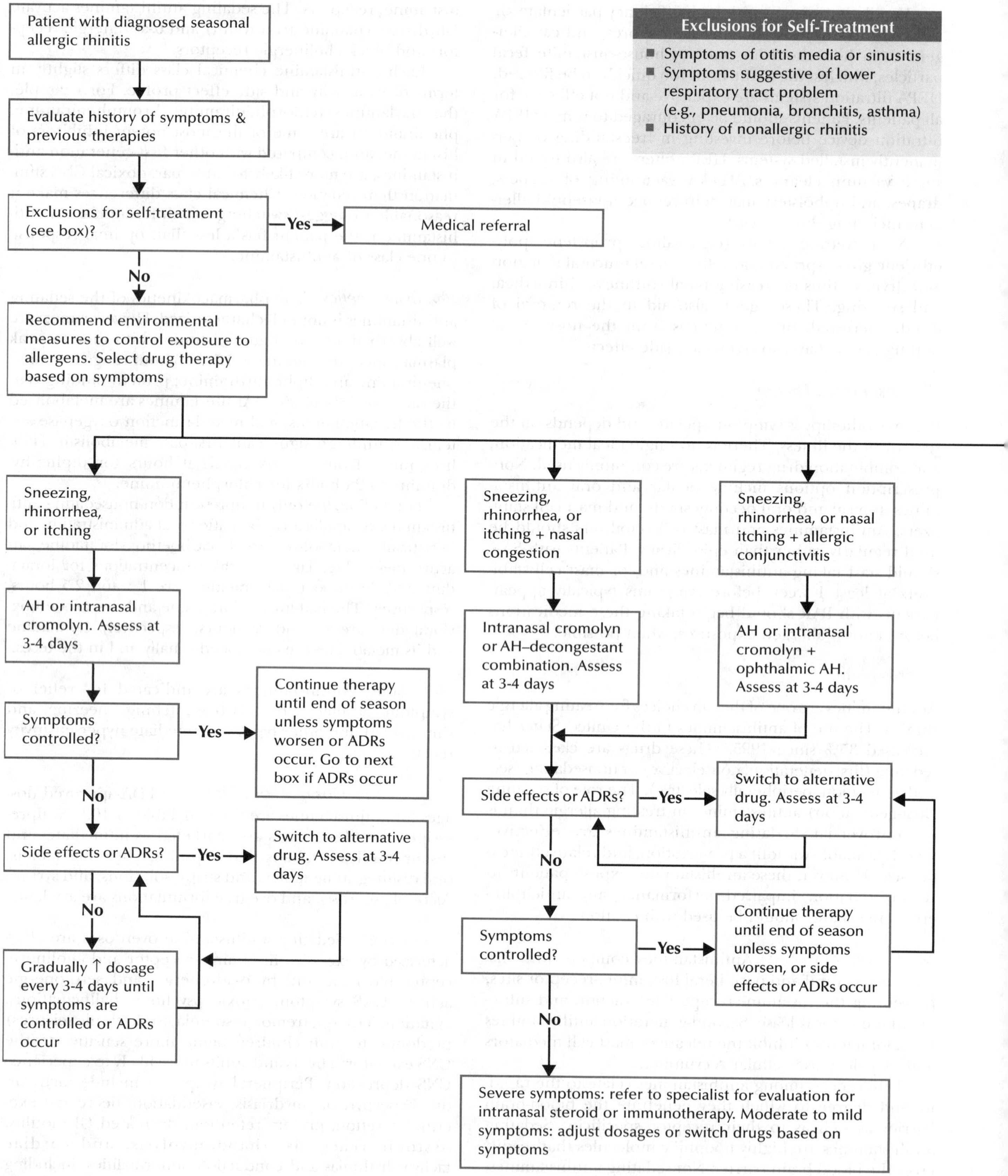


**Exclusions for Self-Treatment**

- Symptoms of otitis media or sinusitis
- Symptoms suggestive of lower respiratory tract problem (e.g., pneumonia, bronchitis, asthma)
- History of nonallergic rhinitis

**FIGURE 11-3** Self-care of seasonal allergic rhinitis. Key: ADR, adverse drug reaction; AH, antihistamine. (Adapted from reference 45.)

*Safety Considerations* The side effect profile of systemic antihistamines varies widely and depends on the receptor activity, chemical structure, and lipophilicity of the drug. The primary side effects are CNS effects (depression and stimulation) and anticholinergic effects. CNS effects are more likely to occur with first-generation antihistamines. CNS depressive effects include sedation and impaired performance (impaired driving performance, poor work performance, incoordination, reduced motor skills, and impaired information processing).[47] Performance may be impaired in the absence of sedation and may persist the morning after a nighttime dose. CNS stimulatory effects include anxiety, hallucinations, appetite stimulation, muscle dyskinesias, and activation of epileptogenic foci. High doses of first-generation antihistamines cause nervousness, tremor, insomnia, agitation, and irritability. Side effects associated with cholinergic blockage include dryness of the eyes and mucus membranes (mouth, nose, vagina); blurred vision; urinary hesitancy and retention; constipation; and tachycardia.

Side effects reported with ocular antihistamines include burning, stinging, itching, foreign body sensation, dry eye, hyperemia, and lid edema. Patients with a history of narrow-angle glaucoma may need to contact their eye care provider before choosing to self-treat with ocular antihistamines.

Antihistamines interact with numerous drugs (Table 11-6). All antihistamines decrease or prevent immediate dermal reactivity and should be discontinued at least 4 days before scheduled allergy skin testing.

The sedating antihistamines are contraindicated in newborns or premature infants, lactating women, patients with narrow-angle glaucoma, and patients with a history of hypersensitivity to the drug or those of similar chemical structure. Additional contraindications include acute

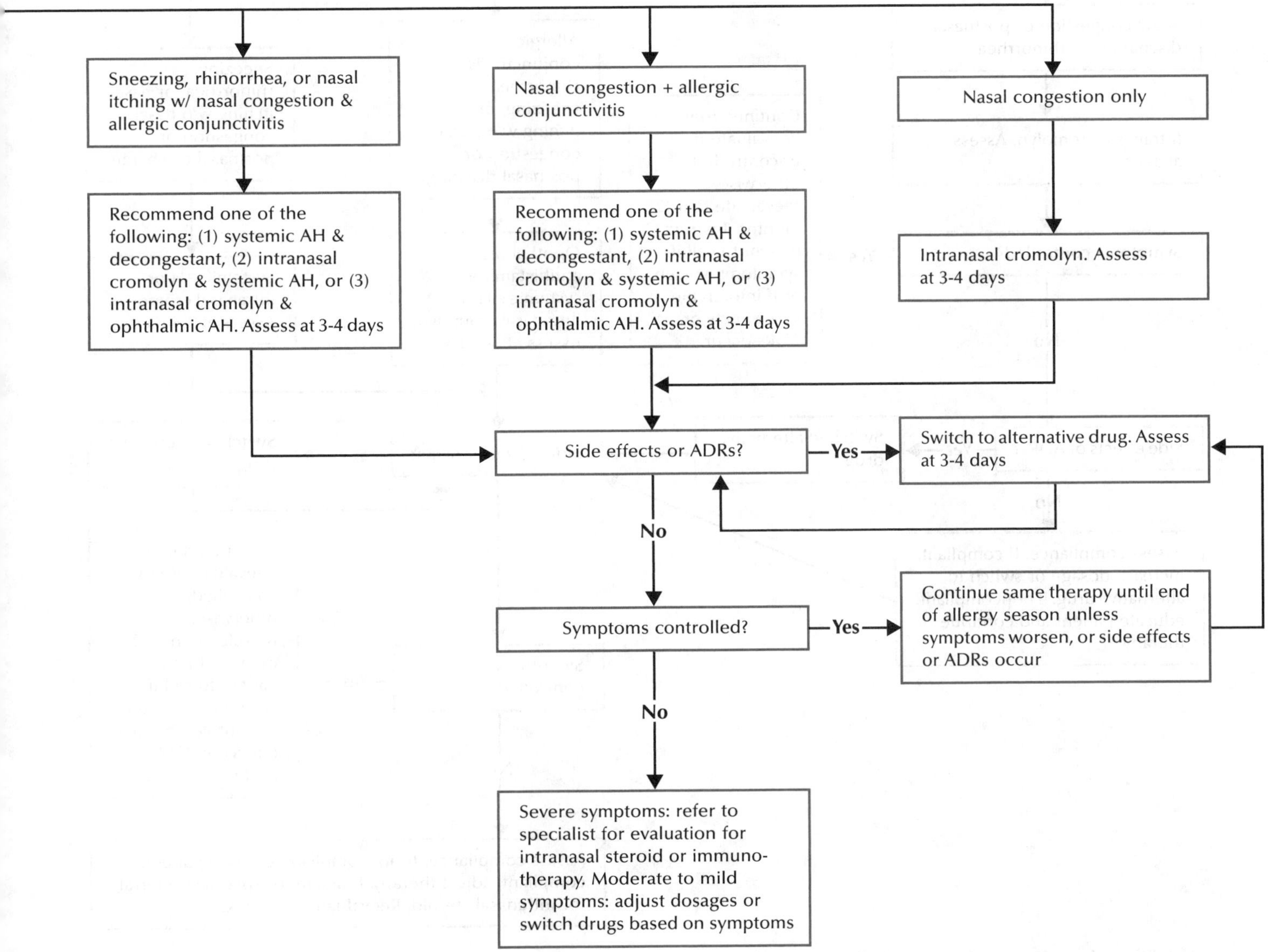


**FIGURE 11–3 (continued)**

### Exclusions for Self-Treatment

- Symptoms of otitis media or sinusitis
- Symptoms suggestive of lower respiratory tract problem (e.g., pneumonia, bronchitis, asthma)
- History of nonallergic rhinitis

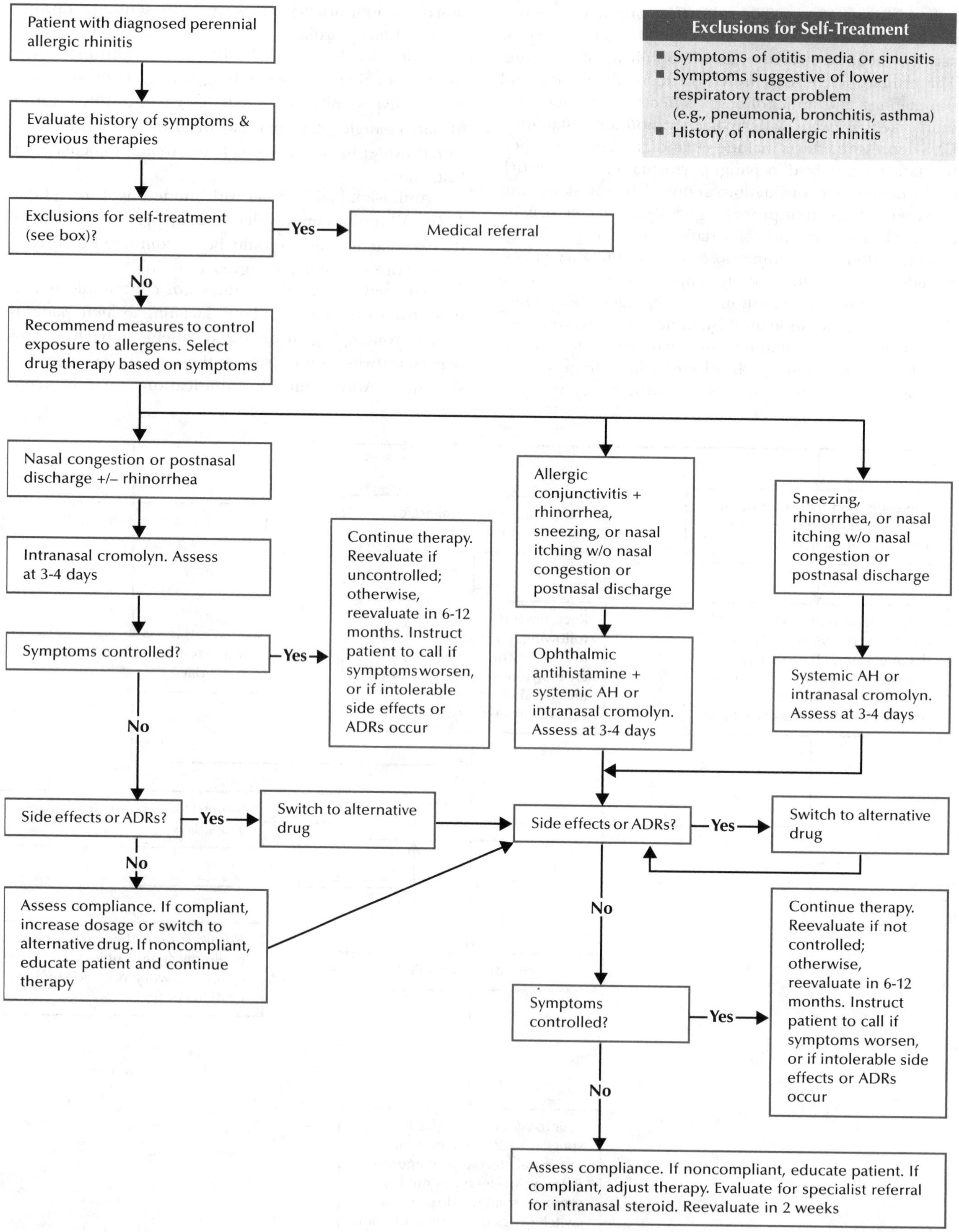


**FIGURE 11-4** Self-care of perennial allergic rhinitis. Key: ADR, adverse drug reaction; AH, antihistamine. (Adapted from reference 45.)

TABLE 11-10 Dosage Guidelines for Systemic Nonprescription Antihistamines[15]

| | Dosage (Maximum Daily Dosage) | | |
|---|---|---|---|
| Drug | Adults/Children ≥12 Years | Children 6-12 Years* | Children 2-6 Years* |
| Brompheniramine maleate | 4 mg q4-6h (24 mg) | 2 mg q4-6h (12 mg) | Not recommended for children <6 years except under advice of PCP |
| Chlorcyclizine HCl | 25 mg q6-8h (75 mg) | 12.5 mg q6-8h (37.5 mg) | 6.25 mg q6-8h (18.75 mg) |
| Chlorpheniramine maleate | 4 mg q4-6h (24 mg) | 2 mg q4-6h (12 mg) | 1 mg q4-6h (6 mg) |
| Dexbrompheniramine maleate | 2 mg q4-6h (12 mg) | 1 mg q4-6h (6 mg) | 0.5 mg q4-6h (3 mg) |
| Dexchlorpheniramine maleate | 2 mg q4-6h (12 mg) | 1 mg q4-6h (6 mg) | 0.5 mg q4-6h (3 mg) |
| Diphenhydramine citrate | 38-76 mg q4-6h (456 mg) | 19-38 mg q4-6h (228 mg) | 9.5 mg q4-6h (57 mg) |
| Diphenhydramine HCl | 25-50 mg q6-8h (300 mg) | 12.5-25 mg q4-6h (150 mg) | 6.25 mg q4-6h (37.5 mg) |
| Doxylamine succinate | 7.5-12.5 mg q4-6h (75 mg) | 3.75-6.25 mg q4-6h (37.5 mg) | 1.9-3.125 mg q4-6h (18.75 mg) |
| Loratadine | 10 mg q24h | 10 mg q24h | 5 mg q24h |
| Phenindamine tartrate | 25 mg q4-6h (150 mg) | 12.5 mg q4-6h (75 mg) | 6.25 mg q4-6h (37.5 mg) |
| Pheniramine | 12.5-25 mg q4-6h (150 mg) | 6.25-12.5 mg q4-6h (75 mg) | 3.125-6.25 mg q4-6h (37.5 mg) |
| Pyrilamine maleate | 25-50 mg q6-8h (200 mg) | 12.5-25 mg q6-8h (100 mg) | 6.25-12.5 mg q6-8h (50 mg) |
| Thonzylamine HCl | 50-100 mg q4-6h (600 mg) | 25-50 mg q4-6h (300 mg) | 12.5-25 mg q4-6h (150 mg) |
| Triprolidine HCl | 2.5 mg q4-6h (10 mg) | 1.25 mg q4-6h (5 mg) | Age 4-6 years: 0.938 mg q4-6h (3.744 mg)<br>Age 2-4 years: 0.625 mg q4-6h (2.5 mg)<br>Age 4 months to <2 years: 0.313 mg q4-6h (1.252 mg) |

Key: PCP, primary care provider.

* With the exception of triprolidine hydrochloride, these products are not recommended for children younger than 2 years, except with the advice and supervision of a PCP.

asthma exacerbation, stenosing peptic ulcer, symptomatic prostatic hypertrophy, bladder neck and pyloroduodenal obstruction, and concomitant use of MAOIs. Loratadine is contraindicated in patients with a history of hypersensitivity to the drug and in nursing mothers. The dosage formulations of 12- and 24-hour sustained-release loratadine–pseudoephedrine combination products are contraindicated in patients with esophageal narrowing, abnormal esophageal peristalsis, or a history of difficulty swallowing tablets.

Patients with lower respiratory tract diseases (e.g., emphysema, chronic bronchitis) should use sedating antihistamines with caution, as should any patient in a situation requiring mental alertness. Patients will be impaired even if they do not feel drowsy or if they have taken the dose the evening before. The sedating antihistamines are photosensitizing drugs. Patients should be advised to use sunscreens and wear protective clothing.

### Combination Products

Antihistamines are marketed in many combinations, including decongestant/antihistamine combinations and various combinations with analgesics, expectorants, and antitussives.

### Decongestants

Congestion is a common allergic rhinitis symptom controllable with systemic decongestants or short-term (fewer than 3 to 5 days) topical nasal decongestants. (See discussion of decongestants in the colds section of this chapter.)

### Cromolyn Sodium

Intranasal cromolyn is an anti-inflammatory drug indicated for preventing and treating the symptoms of allergic rhinitis. Cromolyn stabilizes mast cells, thereby preventing mediator release; the exact mechanism of action is not known. Cromolyn protects mast cells from immune-mediated (i.e., antigen-antibody) and nonimmune-mediated (e.g., cold air, hyperventilation, exercise) triggers. Less than 7% of an intranasal cromolyn dose is absorbed systemically, and what little is absorbed has no systemic activity. The absorbed drug is rapidly excreted unchanged in the urine and bile with a half-life of 1 to 2 hours. Swallowed cromolyn is excreted unchanged in the feces.

The recommended cromolyn dose is one spray in each nostril three to six times daily at regular intervals. Treatment is more effective if started before seasonal symptoms begin. It may take 3 to 7 days for its initial efficacy to become apparent and 2 to 4 weeks of continued therapy before maximal therapeutic benefit. Sneezing is the most common side effect reported for intranasal cromolyn. Other adverse effects include nasal stinging and burning. No drug interactions have been reported with intranasal cromolyn. Intranasal cromolyn is not indicated for children 5 years of age or younger or for anyone with a history of hypersensitivity to cromolyn or related drugs.

### Product Selection Guidelines

*Special Populations* Several treatment choices are available for pregnant women.[48] Because of its wide margin of safety, intranasal cromolyn is the initial drug of choice. Intranasal corticosteroids (prescription only) may be used if cromolyn is ineffective. Pregnancy Category B nonprescription antihistamines include chlorpheniramine, clemastine, diphenhydramine, and loratadine. Chlorpheniramine is the first-generation antihistamine of choice in pregnancy but, if possible, should be avoided during the last trimester because of increased reports of retrolental fibroplasia.[22] Loratadine is the preferred alternative if chlorpheniramine is not tolerated. Several large studies have shown that loratadine is safe to use during pregnancy despite initial reports of increased risk of hypospadias in male infants.[49] Although immunotherapy should not be initiated during pregnancy, maintenance therapy may be continued.[48]

Lactating women with allergic rhinitis have fewer options. Because of its limited systemic absorption, intranasal cromolyn is a good choice, and there are no reports of adverse effects on nursing infants.[22] Antihistamines are contraindicated during lactation because of their ability to pass into breast milk. There have been reports of drowsiness and irritability in infants after mothers took clemastine.[22,23] Short-acting chlorpheniramine or loratadine seem to be the best options if an oral antihistamine is needed but should be used with caution and under the supervision of a PCP. If an oral antihistamine is used during lactation, the mother should avoid long-acting and high-dose antihistamines and take the dose at bedtime after the last feeding of the day.[23] Several treatment choices are available for children.[51] Loratadine is the initial nonprescription drug of choice. Sedating antihistamines should be avoided in children because of paradoxical excitation. Intranasal mast cell stabilizers are safe for children 6 years of age and older but may be difficult for children to self-administer. Immunotherapy may be used in children older than 5 years of age.

Patients of advanced age may experience paradoxical excitation with sedating antihistamines and are more likely than younger adults to have CNS depressive side effects, including confusion, as well as hypotension. Loratadine and intranasal cromolyn are drugs of choice in the older population.

*Patient Factors and Preferences* The duration of treatment and the presence of concomitant disease will determine which product is selected. The side effects of and the patient's response to antihistamines determine which product to choose (Table 11-11). All first-generation antihistamines are sedating. The alkylamines (chlorpheniramine, brompheniramine, and pheniramine) are the least sedating, whereas the ethanolamines (diphenhydramine, doxylamine, and phenyltoloxamine) are the most sedating. Loratadine is a more expensive nonsedating antihistamine; the lack of sedation and impairment may justify the additional cost. Some patients report that antihistamines are less effective after prolonged use. This decline is most likely not true tolerance but rather stems from several factors, including patient nonadherence, an increase in antigen exposure, worsening of disease, the limited effectiveness of antihistamines in severe disease, or the development of similar symptoms from unrelated diseases. Although antihistamines induce their own metabolism, tolerance has not been clinically demonstrated. Nevertheless, some clinicians still recommend trying different structural classes of drugs when patients report a lack of response.

Systemic decongestants are preferred over topical decongestants. Many antihistamine–decongestant sustained-release products are marketed, allowing for convenient dosage regimens. However, these combination products should be used with caution because of the increased risk of side effects, especially insomnia, which compounds daytime fatigue already associated with this disease.

## *Immunotherapy*

Immunotherapy, a series of subcutaneous injections with patient-specific allergens, is indicated for refractory allergic rhinitis in patients with moderate to severe symptoms. The exact mechanism of action is not known, but many theories have been proposed, including reduced elevations in IgE, decreased circulating eosinophils, and reduced mast cells.[41] Immunotherapy is the only therapy shown to modify the immune system and therefore the disease process; it is most effective for pollen-related allergens. Under clinician supervision, injections are given weekly, increasing the concentrations of allergen gradually. The maintenance dose is generally reached within 4 to 8 months. Maintenance injections are repeated every 3 to 4 weeks for 3 to 5 years. Relative contraindications to immunotherapy include autoimmune disease, unstable coronary artery disease, unstable asthma, and concurrent therapy with β-adrenergic-blocking drugs.[50] Clinicians should have resuscitative equipment available in case of anaphylactic reaction.

## *Complementary Therapies*

Ephedra (ma-huang) and feverfew are commonly suggested herbal remedies for allergic rhinitis. Ephedra, a sympathomimetic decongestant, has been associated with serious adverse events (Table 11-8) and, as of April 2004, the FDA banned the sale of all nonprescription products containing ephedra (see Chapter 4). Parthenolide, feverfew's biologically active component, may have anti-inflammatory properties, but its safety and efficacy in allergic rhinitis are unproven. Feverfew's side effects include mouth ulcers and gastrointestinal upset. For a further discussion of these types of products, see Chapter 53. Homeopathic practitioners stress avoidance techniques but limit symptomatic treatment. Some homeopathic products actually contain known allergens (e.g., bioAllers

**TABLE 11-11 Selected Products for Allergic Rhinitis**

| Trade Name | Primary Ingredients |
|---|---|
| **Systemic First-generation Antihistamine Products** | |
| Benadryl Allergy Tablets | Diphenhydramine HCl 25 mg |
| Children's Benadryl Allergy Relief Syrup | Diphenhydramine HCl 12.5 mg/5 mL |
| Chlor-Trimeton Allergy (4, 8, or 12 Hour) Tablets | Chlorpheniramine 4 mg, 8 mg, or 12 mg |
| Nolahist Tablets | Phenindamine tartrate 25 mg |
| Tavist Allergy Tablets | Clemastine fumarate 1.34 mg |
| TheraFlu Thin Strips Multisymptom* | Diphenhydramine HCl 25 mg |
| Triaminic Thin Strips Cough & Runny Nose* | Diphenhydramine 12.5 mg |
| **Systemic Second-generation Antihistamine Products** | |
| Claritin Children's Formula Syrup† | Loratadine 5 mg/5 mL |
| Children's Dimetapp ND Allergy Syrup† | Loratadine 5 mg/5 mL |
| Claritin Non-Drowsy Tablets | Loratadine 10 mg |
| Alavert Orally Disintegrating Tablets | Loratadine 10 mg |
| Triaminic AllerChews Tablets | Loratadine 10 mg |
| **Combination Systemic Products** | |
| Actifed Allergy Nighttime Caplets | Diphenhydramine HCl 25 mg; pseudoephedrine HCl 30 mg |
| Advil Allergy Sinus Tablets | Chlorpheniramine 2 mg; pseudoephedrine HCl 30 mg;ibuprofen 200 mg |
| Allerest Maximum Strength Tablets | Chlorpheniramine 2 mg; pseudoephedrine HCl 30 mg |
| Claritin-D 24 Hour Tablets | Loratadine 10 mg; pseudoephedrine sulfate 240 mg |
| Tylenol Severe Allergy Tablets | Diphenhydramine HCl 12.5 mg; acetaminophen 500 mg |
| **Nasal Products** | |
| Entsol Nasal Gel | Propylene glycol; sodium chloride; aloe; vitamin E |
| NasalCrom Spray | Cromolyn sodium 5.2 mg/spray |
| Ocean Spray | Sodium chloride 0.65% |

*Contains alcohol; †contains sucrose.

Animal Hair and Dander Allergy Relief Liquid contains cat, cattle, dog, horse, and sheep wool extracts) and claim to induce long-term resistance by repeated exposure to controlled amounts of allergen. These products should be used with extreme caution. Symptom-specific homeopathic remedies include Sabadilla for nasal and ocular symptoms (red watery eyes) and Wyethia for itching. The effectiveness and value of homeopathic products are highly questionable. For a further discussion of these types of products, see Chapter 55.

## Assessment of Allergic Rhinitis: A Case-based Approach

Asking the patient for a detailed description of the symptoms is the first step in determining whether a patient has allergic rhinitis or rhinitis related to other causes. The patient's medical history and medication use (previous and current) may reveal nonallergic causes of rhinitis. The patient should be asked about the following:

- Recent use of topical nasal decongestants for longer than 3 to 5 days
- History of poor response to decongestant–antihistamine therapy
- Symptoms that began during pregnancy
- Unilateral symptoms
- Presence of anatomic abnormalities such as nasal polyps, deviated septum, or adenoid hypertrophy
- Patient's age
- Recent history of facial or head trauma
- History of cocaine abuse
- Use of medications that cause nasal congestion (e.g., β-adrenergic blockers, angiotensin-converting enzyme inhibitors, chlorpromazine, clonidine, reserpine, hydralazine, oral contraceptives, aspirin or other nonsteroidal anti-inflammatory drugs).

The medical history may uncover other respiratory illnesses that complicate treatment of allergic rhinitis. The patient's current medication use will also alert the practitioner to possible interactions with nonprescription allergy

## CASE 11-2

| Relevant Evaluation Criteria | Scenario/Model Outcome |
|---|---|
| **Information Gathering** | |
| 1. Gather essential information about the patient's symptoms, including: | |
| a. description of symptom(s) (i.e., nature, onset, duration, severity, associated symptoms) | Patient has been miserable since moving from Alaska to Georgia 6 months ago. His symptoms have been continuous and include red, itchy, and watery eyes; sneezing, mild nasal congestion, and daytime fatigue. |
| b. description of any factors that seem to precipitate, exacerbate, and/or relieve the patient's symptom(s) | His symptoms are worse after mowing his yard and visiting clients with pets. He feels best when working inside his air-conditioned office. |
| c. description of the patient's efforts to relieve the symptoms | Patient tried Breathe Right strips with no relief. |
| 2. Gather essential patient history information: | |
| a. patient's identity | Robert Johns |
| b. age, sex, height, and weight | 50 y/o M, 5'9", 200 lb |
| c. patient's occupation | Computer consultant |
| d. patient's dietary habits | Normal healthy diet |
| e. patient's sleep habits | Sleeps 5-6 hours a night; sleep is disturbed by symptoms. |
| f. concurrent medical conditions, prescription and nonprescription medications, and dietary supplements | Enalapril 5 mg 1 tablet twice daily for hypertension; Men's multivitamin 1 tablet daily |
| g. allergies | NKDA |
| h. history of other adverse reactions to medications | None |
| i. other (describe)_______ | Patient is concerned about lack of sleep and poor work performance. |
| **Assessment and Triage** | |
| 3. Differentiate the patient's signs/symptoms and correctly identify the patient's primary problem(s) (see Tables 11-1 and 11-9). | Perennial allergic rhinitis probably related to move to warmer, more humid climate and increased exposure to mold, pollen, and animals |
| 4. Identify exclusions for self-treatment (see Figure 11-4). | None |
| 5. Formulate a comprehensive list of therapeutic alternatives for the primary problem to determine if triage to a medical practitioner is required, and share this information with the patient. | Options include:<br>(1) Recommend a separate OTC product for each symptom; nonsedating or sedating antihistamine for red, itchy eyes and sneezing; a nasal or systemic decongestant for congestion.<br>(2) Refer Robert to his PCP for further evaluation and treatment.<br>(3) Recommend self-care until Robert can consult his primary provider.<br>(4) Take no action. |
| **Plan** | |
| 6. Select an optimal therapeutic alternative to address the patient's problem, taking into account patient preferences. | Recommend loratadine 10 mg. |
| 7. Describe the recommended therapeutic approach to the patient. | Take one tablet by mouth daily. |

**CASE 11-2 (continued)**

| Relevant Evaluation Criteria | Scenario/Model Outcome |
|---|---|
| 8. Explain to the patient the rationale for selecting the recommended therapeutic approach from the considered therapeutic alternatives. | Loratadine should not cause daytime drowsiness as other antihistamines do. It should not increase your blood pressure as decongestants will. |
| **Patient Education** | |
| 9. When recommending self-care with nonprescription medications and/or nondrug therapy, convey accurate information to the patient, including: | |
| a. appropriate dose and frequency of administration | Take this medication every day. |
| b. maximum number of days the therapy should be employed | Since you have perennial allergic rhinitis, you need to take this medication every day and may need to take it for years. |
| c. product administration procedures | Take with or without food. May want to take at bedtime in case it causes drowsiness. |
| d. expected time to onset of relief | You should start to feel some relief in 1-3 hours, but maximum benefit may not be apparent for several days. |
| e. degree of relief that can be reasonably expected | Antihistamines reduce but do not eliminate allergy symptoms. |
| f. most common side effects | The most common side effects include headache, dry mouth, and fatigue. |
| g. side effects that warrant medical intervention should they occur | Contact your primary care provider if you experience irregular or slow heart beat; chest tightness; trouble breathing; or severe drowsiness, nervousness, dizziness, or insomnia. |
| h. patient options in the event that condition worsens or persists | You may want to try intranasal cromolyn to prevent symptoms. You may try a different antihistamine. If symptoms are severe and do not respond to treatment, you need to see an allergist who may prescribe a short course of oral and/or nasal corticosteroids, a prescription antihistamine, or allergy shots. |
| i. product storage requirements | Store at room temperature. |
| j. specific nondrug measures | Avoidance strategies include staying in an air-conditioned environment, especially when pollen counts are high; hiring a lawn service to avoid freshly mowed grass; and asking pet-owning clients to visit you at your office. |
| 10. Solicit follow-up questions from patient. | May I take another loratadine tablet if the first dose does not control my symptoms? |
| 11. Answer patient's questions. | No. Doubling the dose would increase your risk for toxicity. If one tablet of loratadine does not control your symptoms on a regular basis, then consider switching to another drug (See 9h above). |

Key: NKDA, no known drug allergies; OTC, over-the-counter; PCP, primary care provider.

medications. The practitioner should also ask whether nonprescription products used to treat episodic or chronic rhinitis were effective and without adverse effects. Case 11-2 presents an example of the assessment of a patient with allergic rhinitis.

## Patient Counseling for Allergic Rhinitis

The practitioner should stress that the best method of treating allergic rhinitis is to avoid allergens. Many patients, however, have no control over their work environment or are unable to implement all the preventive measures at home. These patients usually rely on allergy medications for symptom control. The patient should be advised about proper use of the recommended medications and about the possible adverse effects, drug-drug and drug-disease interactions, and other precautions and warnings. Patients should also know the signs and symptoms that indicate the disorder has progressed to the point where medical care is needed. The box Patient Education for Allergic Rhinitis lists specific information to provide patients.

## Evaluation of Patient Outcomes for Allergic Rhinitis

Many patients achieve symptomatic relief with initial nonprescription drug therapy in 3 to 4 days. After this time frame the clinician should follow up with a telephone call

## PATIENT EDUCATION FOR ALLERGIC RHINITIS

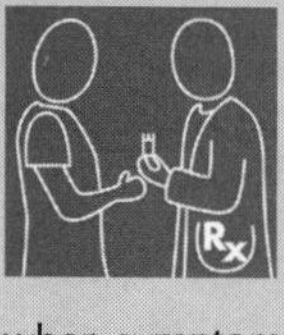

The primary objective of self-treatment is to prevent or reduce symptoms, which, in turn, will improve functioning and sense of well-being. For some patients, prescription therapy such as short-course oral corticosteroids may help control symptoms while other therapy is initiated or when symptoms are especially severe. For most patients, carefully following instructions for nonprescription allergy medications and the self-care measures listed here will help ensure optimal therapeutic outcomes.

### Nondrug Measures

- Avoidance of allergens is important regardless of whether allergy medications are being taken.
- For symptoms that develop mainly when outdoors:
  - Frequently check local pollen counts and air quality index (AQI).
  - Keep house and car windows shut on days with high levels of pollen (spring/summer), mold (late summer/fall), or pollution.
- Try not to do yard work or engage in outdoor sports.
- For symptoms that occur mainly when indoors:
  - Try to remove the symptom trigger(s) (e.g., cats, dust mites, tobacco smoke, molds) from the house.
  - Lower the humidity in the home to reduce molds. Use lower settings on humidifiers, repair damp basements and crawl spaces, vent kitchens and bathrooms, and remove houseplants.
  - Wash bedding in hot water (130°F [54.4°C]) every week and encase mattresses and pillows in dust mite resistant coverings.

### Nonprescription Medications

- Ask a clinician for help in selecting an allergy medication that treats the most bothersome symptoms. If needed, additional medications can be added for other symptoms:
  - Antihistamines are effective for itching, sneezing, and rhinorrhea but have little effect on nasal congestion.
  - Decongestants are effective for nasal congestion but have little effect on other symptoms.
  - Combination therapy with an antihistamine and a decongestant is common.
  - Intranasal and ocular medications reduce nasal and eye symptoms, respectively, but have little effect on other symptoms.
- Allergy medications are more effective if they are used regularly rather than episodically:
  - If you have seasonal allergies, start allergy medications at least 1 week before symptoms are expected to begin.
  - If you have perennial allergies, take allergy medications before exposure to allergens.

### *Nasal Congestion*

- See the box Patient Education for Colds for information about relieving nasal congestion.

Seek medical attention in the following situations:

- Your allergy symptoms do not improve while taking nonprescription medications.
- Your symptoms worsen while taking nonprescription medications.
- You develop signs or symptoms of secondary bacterial infections (i.e., thick nasal or respiratory secretions that are not clear, temperature higher than 101.5°F (38.6°C), shortness of breath, chest congestion, wheezing, significant ear pain, rash).

### *Rhinorrhea (Runny Nose) and Sneezing*

- Many factors cause a runny nose. Nonprescription antihistamines or prescription medications only partially treat this symptom. Because some nonprescription antihistamines may make you very drowsy, the potential benefits of the medication must be weighed against the potential risks.
- Sneezing may be reduced with nonprescription antihistamines. Sneezing is a common but rarely bothersome symptom. The potential benefits of using these medications must be weighed against the potential risks.
- Antihistamines are the preferred initial treatment for runny nose and sneezing in persons who are not pregnant.
- There are two types of antihistamines, sedating and nonsedating. Loratadine is a nonsedating antihistamine and usually does not cause significant drowsiness.
- Nasal saline solutions may relieve nasal irritation and dryness and aid in the removal of dried, encrusted, or thick mucus from the nose.
- Intranasal cromolyn is the preferred initial drug of choice during pregnancy. This medication is not absorbed into the body.
- The most common side effects include nasal stinging and burning.
- Note the following side effects for antihistamines:
  - The sedating antihistamines cause drowsiness and impair mental alertness. Mental alertness is impaired even if you do not feel drowsy or if you took the dose the prior evening. While taking these medications, do not drive a vehicle, operate machinery, or engage in other activities that require alertness.
  - Sedating antihistamines may cause sensitivity to sunlight. Use sunscreens and wear protective clothing when outdoors.
  - Use of sedating antihistamines may cause dryness in your mouth, nose, and other areas of your body.
  - Children and persons of advanced age may experience unexpected excitement with sedating antihistamines.
  - Persons of advanced age may need lower doses of antihistamines because they are more sensitive to the effects these medications have on the brain and heart.
- Do not use antihistamines:
  - If you are allergic to antihistamines or similar medications.
  - If you are breast-feeding.
- Do not give antihistamines to newborns or premature infants unless directed to do so by a PCP.
- Note the following precautions for use of nonprescription antihistamines:
  - Persons with narrow-angle glaucoma, stenosing peptic ulcer, symptomatic prostatic hypertrophy, bladder-neck obstruction, or pyloroduodenal obstruction should not use sedating (first-generation) antihistamines.
  - Persons with lower respiratory tract disease (e.g., emphysema, chronic bronchitis) should use sedating antihistamines with caution.
  - Persons with esophageal narrowing, abnormal esophageal peristalsis, or problems swallowing tablets should not take the 12- or 24-hour sustained-release dosage forms of loratadine combined with pseudoephedrine. There have been reports of esophageal obstruction and perforation with these sustained-release dosage forms.

**PATIENT EDUCATION FOR ALLERGIC RHINITIS (continued)**

- Sedating antihistamines interact with the following drugs:
  - Alcohol, sedatives, and other CNS depressants may cause additive depressive effects when taken with sedating antihistamines.
  - MAOIs (e.g., tranylcypromine, phenelzine), including the antibacterial furazolidone and the anticancer drug procarbazine, prolong and intensify some of the side effects of the sedating antihistamines.
  - Decreased blood pressure may occur when MAOIs are taken with dexchlorpheniramine.
  - Chlorpheniramine may increase the side effects of phenytoin.

or a scheduled appointment to determine whether symptom control has been achieved or the patient is encountering any side effects or problems. Patients who respond poorly to treatment should be assessed to determine if they are complying with allergen avoidance strategies and medication regimens. Options for patients who do not achieve relief include increasing current medications to maximally effective dosages or changing to a different medication or dosage formulation. Patients who do not respond to nonprescription therapy should be referred back to their PCP for prescription medications such as inhaled or systemic corticosteroids, leukotriene inhibitors, anticholinergics, or immunotherapy. Patients should also be reassessed, and the diagnosis of allergic rhinitis may need to be reconsidered. Patients who develop any of the warning signs or symptoms listed in the box Patient Education for Allergic Rhinitis should be referred to a PCP.

## Key Points for Disorders Related to Colds and Allergic Rhinitis

- Colds are self-limiting, viral infections characterized by initial sore throat followed by nasal symptoms and nonproductive cough.
- Medical referral is appropriate for patients with suspected colds who are immunocompromised, have underlying cardiopulmonary diseases, or have alarm symptoms (high fever, chest pain, shortness of breath, or wheezing).
- Treatment for colds is symptomatic and targeted at the most bothersome symptoms.
- Decongestants are the most common nonprescription treatment for congestion related to colds and allergic rhinitis but should be used cautiously in patients with hypertension, diabetes, and other chronic diseases.
- Medical referral is appropriate for patients with symptoms suggestive of nonallergic rhinitis, otitis media, sinusitis, or lower respiratory tract problems such as pneumonia, asthma, or bronchitis, and those who fail to respond to nonprescription medications.
- Therapy for allergic rhinitis is sequential and consists of allergen avoidance, pharmacotherapy, and allergen immunotherapy.
- No single medication is ideal for treating allergic rhinitis, but initial therapy should target the most dominant symptom.
- In treating allergic rhinitis, multiple drug formulations may be added or used initially if the patient presents with moderately severe, particularly intense, or long-lasting symptoms, or if the patient is at risk for exacerbation of an underlying disease.

## References


1. Woodwell DA and Cherry DK. *National Ambulatory Medical Care Survey: 2002 Summary.* Advance data from vital and health statistics; no. 346. Hyattsville, MD: National Center for Health Statistics. August 26, 2004.
2. National Institute of Allergy and Infectious Diseases. The common cold. National Institutes of Health. December 2004. Available at: www.niaid.nih.gov/factsheets/cold.htm Accessed January 1, 2005.
3. Can antiviral tissues prevent the spread of colds? *Consumer Reports.* 2004;69:56.
4. Fact sheet: the use of over-the-counter medicines. Consumer Healthcare Products Association. Available at: www.chpa-info.org/web/press_room/statistics/otc_sales.aspx. Accessed January 1, 2005.
5. Cohen S, Doyle WJ, Turner R, et al. Sociability and susceptibility to the common cold. *Psychological Science.* 2003;14:389-95.
6. Eccles R. Acute cooling of the body surface and the common cold. *Rhinology.* 2002;40(3):109-14.
7. Lee GM, Friedman JF, Ross-Degnan D, et al. Misconceptions about colds and predictors of health service utilization. *Pediatrics.* 2003;111:231-6.
8. Hendley JO. Clinical virology of rhinoviruses. *Adv Virus Res.* 1999; 54:453-66.
9. Gwaltney JM. Clinical significance and pathogenesis of viral respiratory infections. *Am J Med.* 2002;112 (suppl 6A):13-8S.
10. Self-care of the common cold. In: Albrant DH, ed. *Drug Treatment Protocols.* Washington, DC: American Pharmaceutical Association;2001:403-15.
11. Rennard BO, Ertl RF, Gossman GL, et al. Chicken soup inhibits neutrophil chemotaxis *in vitro. Chest.* 2000; 118(4):1150-7.
12. Ostberg B, Winther B, Borum P, et al. Common cold and high-dose ipratropium bromide: use of anticholinergic medication as an indicator of reflex-mediated hypersecretion. *Rhinology.* 1997; 35:58-62.
13. Turner RB, Sperber SJ, Sorrentino JV, et al. Effectiveness of clemastine fumarate for treatment of rhinorrhea and sneezing associated with the common cold. *Clin Infect Dis.* 1997;25:824-30.
14. Cold, cough, allergy, bronchodilator, and antiasthmatic drug products for over-the-counter human use; amendment of final monograph for over-the-counter nasal decongestant products. *Federal Register.* October 11, 2005;70:58974-7.
15. Cold, cough, allergy, bronchodilator, and antiasthmatic drug products for over-the counter human use. *Code of Federal Regulations.* Title 21, vol 5, pt 341. Revised April 1, 2004. Available at: http://www.fda.gov. Accessed January 1, 2005.

16. Graf P. Adverse effects of benzalkonium chloride on the nasal mucosa: allergic rhinitis and rhinitis medicamentosa. *Clin Ther.* 1999;21:1749-55.
17. Richard C. Off the shelf, out of reach: states limit access to pseudoephedrine products. *Pharmacy Today.* 2005;11:1, 22.
18. Bender BS. The scientific basis of folk remedies for colds and flu. *Chest.* 2000;118(4):887-8.
19. Freestone C, Eccles R. Assessment of the antitussive efficacy of codeine in cough associated with common cold. *J Pharm Pharmacol.* 1997;49:1045-9.
20. Lee PCL, Jawad MSM, Eccles R. Antitussive efficacy of dextromethorphan in cough associated with acute upper respiratory tract infections. *J Pharm Pharmacol.* 2000;52: 1137-42.
21. Kuhn JJ, Hendley JO, Adams KF, et al. Antitussive effect of guaifenesin in young adults with natural colds. *Chest.* 1982;82: 713-8.
22. Briggs GG, Freeman RK, Sumner JY. *Drugs in Pregnancy and Lactation.* 6th ed. Philadelphia: Lippincott Williams and Wilkins; 2002: 246, 285, 334, 384, 636, 1054, 1113, 1187.
23. Nice FJ, Snyder JL, Kotansky BC. Breastfeeding and over-the-counter medications. *J Hum Lact.* 2000;16:319-31.
24. Fleming T, ed. *PDR for Herbal Medications.* 2nd ed. Montvale, NJ: Medical Economics Co; 2000.
25. Fetrow CW, Avila JR. *The Complete Guide to Herbal Medicines.* New York: Simon & Shuster, Inc, 2000.
26. Marshall I. Zinc for the common cold (Cochrane Review). *The Cochrane Library.* 2003;1. Oxford: Update Software Ltd.
27. Douglas RM, Chalker EB, Treacy B. Vitamin C for preventing and treating the common cold (Cochrane Review). *The Cochrane Library.* 2003;1. Oxford: Update Software Ltd.
28. Melchart D, Linde K, Fischer P, et al. Echinacea for preventing and treating the common cold (Cochrane Review). *The Cochrane Library.* 2003;1. Oxford: Update Software Ltd.
29. Barnes PM, Powell-Griner E, McFann K, et al. *Complementary and Alternative Medicine Use Among Adults: United States, 2002.* Advance Data from Vital and Health Statistics; no 343. Hyattsville, MD: National Center for Health Statistics; May 27, 2004.
30. Barrett BP, Brown RL, Locken K, et al. Treatment of the common cold with unrefined echinacea: a randomized, double-blind, placebo-controlled trial. *Ann Intern Med.* 2002;137(12): 939-46.
31. Yale SH, Liu K. Echinacea purpurea therapy for the treatment of the common cold. *Arch Intern Med.* 2004;164:1237-41.
32. Jackson JL, Lesho E, Peterson C. Zinc and the common cold: a meta-analysis revisted. *J Nutr.* 2000;130:1512S-5S.
33. Mossad SB. Effect of zincum gluconicum nasal gel on the duration and symptom severity of the common cold in otherwise healthy adults. *Q J Med.* 2003;96:35-43.
34. Turner RB. Ineffectiveness of intranasal zinc gluconate for prevention of experimental rhinovirus colds. *CID.* 2001;33:1865-70.
35. Jafek BW, Linschoten MR, Murrow BW. Anosmia after intranasal zinc gluconate use. *Am J Rhinol.* 2004;18:137-41.
36. Hemila H. Vitamin C supplementation and common cold symptoms: factors affecting the magnitude of the benefit. *Med Hypotheses.* 1999;52:171-8.
37. Fineman SM. The burden of allergic rhinitis; beyond dollars and cents. *Ann Allergy Asthma Immunol.* 2002;88:S2-S7.
38. *Fastats—Allegies and Hay Fever.* Hyattsville, MD: National Center for Health Statistics; September 2004.
39. Reed SD, Lee TA, McCrory DC. The economic burden of allergic rhinitis: a critical evaluation of the literature. *Pharmacoeconomics.* 2004;22:345-61.
40. Lethbridge-Cejku M, Schiller JS, Bernadel L. Summary health statistics for U.S. adults: National Health Interview Survey, 2002. National Center for Health Statistics. *Vital Health Stat* 10; 2004: 222.
41. Quraishi SA, Davies MJ, Craig TJ. Inflammatory responses in allergic rhinitis: traditional approaches and novel treatment strategies. *JAOA.* 2004;104(suppl 5):S7-S15.
42. Marshall GD. Internal and external environmental influences in allergic diseases. *JAOA.* 2004;104:S1-6.
43. Skoner DP. Complications of allergic rhinitis. *J Allergy Clin Immunol.* 2000;105:S605-9.
44. Management of seasonal allergic rhinitis. In: Albrant DH, ed. *Drug Treatment Protocols.* Washington, DC: American Pharmaceutical Association; 2001:381-8.
45. Management of perennial allergic rhinitis. In: Albrant DH, ed. *Drug Treatment Protocols.* Washington, DC: American Pharmaceutical Association; 2001:373-80.
46. Public Education Committee. Tips to remember: indoor allergens. American Academy of Allergy, Asthma, and Immunology. 2003. Available at: http://www.aaaai.org/patients/publicedmat/tips/indoorallergens.stm. Accessed May 20, 2005.
47. Kay GG. The effects of antihistamines on cognition and performance. *J Allergy Clin Immunol.* 2000;105(suppl 1):S622-7.
48. The use of newer asthma and allergy medications during pregnancy. *Ann Allergy Asthma Immunol.* 2000; 84:475-80.
49. F-D-C Reports, Inc. Loratadine and birth defects. *The Tan Sheet.* March 22, 2004:10.
50. Huggins JL, Looney RJ. Allergen immunotherapy. *Am Fam Physician.* 2004;70:689-96.
51. Fireman P. Therapeutic approaches to allergic rhinitis: treating the child. *J Allergy Clin Immunol.* 2000;105(suppl 1): S616-21.

CHAPTER 12

# Cough

*Karen J. Tietze*

Cough is an important defensive respiratory reflex with potentially significant adverse physical and psychological consequences and economic impact. Therapy is symptomatic and is targeted at either suppressing the cough with antitussives or changing the volume and character of the respiratory secretions with protussives. Americans spend about $1 billion annually treating cough.[1] The eight cough products listed in the top 100 nonprescription medications by sales in 2003 accounted for more than $400 million in sales.[2]

## Epidemiology of Cough

Cough is the most common symptom for which patients seek medical care.[3] Approximately one in five ambulatory care visits to physician offices, hospital outpatient departments, and emergency departments is for diseases associated with cough (acute upper respiratory tract infections, allergic rhinitis, chronic rhinitis, asthma, chronic bronchitis).[4] Since many patients self-treat cough, the true incidence of cough is likely much higher.

## Physiology of Cough

Receptors located throughout the respiratory tract respond to a variety of chemical and mechanical (irritant) stimuli and inflammatory and immunologic mediators.[5] Cough is mediated by irritant receptors located in the airway mucosa.[6] Compared with the trachea and bronchi, the larynx is more sensitive to irritant stimuli.[7] Receptor density is greatest at the carina and bronchial branches and sparse in smaller bronchi; there are no cough receptors in the bronchioles or alveoli.[7] When activated, cough receptors send impulses through the brainstem reflex pathway, the voluntary cerebral cortex pathway, or both.[8,9] Afferents are primarily vagal, although nonvagal nerves innervating the upper airways and esophagus have a secondary role in cough.[10] The brainstem reflex pathway ends in the "cough center" of the medulla oblongata.[11] The voluntary pathway ends in the cerebral cortex.[9] Efferents are carried by the vagus, phrenicus, laryngeal, and spinal motor nerves.[8] A cough starts with a deep inspiration followed by closure of the glottis and forceful contraction of the chest wall, abdominal wall, and diaphragmatic muscles against the closed glottis; pressure in the thoracic cavity may reach 300 mm Hg with expiratory air velocities up to 500 mph. Mucus, cellular debris, and foreign material are propelled out of the respiratory system when the glottis opens.

## Etiology of Cough

Cough, classified as acute (i.e., duration of less than 3 weeks), subacute (i.e., duration of 3 to 8 weeks), or chronic (i.e., duration of longer than 8 weeks), is a symptom of diverse infectious and noninfectious disorders (Table 12-1).[12] Acute cough is most commonly caused by viral upper respiratory tract infection (URTI; e.g., the common cold). Subacute cough is commonly caused by infection, bacterial sinusitis, and asthma. The most common causes of chronic cough in adult nonsmokers are postnasal drip syndrome (PNDS), asthma, and gastroesophageal reflux disease (GERD). In children, cough may be a symptom of viral or bacterial respiratory infection, heart disease, foreign body aspiration, aspiration caused by poor coordination of sucking and swallowing, or esophageal motility disorders. Angiotensin-converting enzyme inhibitors cause dry cough in 20% or more of treated patients.[13] Systemic and ophthalmic β-adrenergic blockers may cause cough in patients with obstructive airway diseases (e.g., asthma or chronic obstructive pulmonary disease [COPD]).

## Signs and Symptoms of Cough

Coughs are described as productive or nonproductive. A productive cough (e.g., a wet or "chesty" cough) expels secretions from the lower respiratory tract that, if retained, could impair ventilation and the lungs' ability to resist infection. Productive coughs may be effective (secretions

**TABLE 12-1 Etiology of Cough[12]**

| Classification | Etiology |
|---|---|
| Acute | Viral URTI, pneumonia, acute left ventricular failure, asthma, foreign body aspiration |
| Subacute | Postinfectious cough, bacterial sinusitis, asthma |
| Chronic | PNDS, asthma, GERD, COPD (chronic bronchitis), ACEIs, bronchogenic carcinoma, carcinomatosis, sarcoidosis, left ventricular failure, aspiration secondary to pharyngeal dysfunction |

Key: ACEI, angiotensin-converting enzyme inhibitor; COPD, chronic obstructive pulmonary disease; GERD, gastroesophageal reflux disease; PNDS, postnasal drip syndrome; URTI, upper respiratory tract infection.

easily expelled) or ineffective (secretions present but difficult to expel). The secretions may be clear (e.g., bronchitis), purulent (e.g., bacterial infection), discolored (e.g., yellow with inflammatory disorders), or malodorous (e.g., anaerobic bacterial infection). A nonproductive cough (e.g., a dry or "hacking" cough) serves no useful physiologic purpose. Nonproductive coughs are caused by viral respiratory tract infections, atypical bacterial infections, GERD, cardiac disease, and some medications.

## Complications of Cough

Complications secondary to high intrathoracic pressures and expiratory velocities occur regardless of the cause or type of cough. Common complications include exhaustion, insomnia, musculoskeletal pain, hoarseness, excessive perspiration, and urinary incontinence. Less common complications include cardiac dysrhythmias, syncope, stroke, and rib fractures. Cough may cause prolonged absence from work or school, withdrawal from social activities, and fear that the cough is a symptom of a serious illness such as cancer or tuberculosis.

## Treatment of Cough

### *Treatment Goals*

The primary goal of self-treatment of cough is to reduce the number and severity of cough episodes. The second goal is to prevent complications. Cough treatment is symptomatic; the underlying disorder must be treated to stop the cause of the cough (e.g, antibiotics for bacterial pneumonia, acid-suppressive therapy and lifestyle modifications for GERD, decongestants for PNDS).

### *General Treatment Approach*

Selection of a medication for self-care of cough depends on the nature and etiology of the cough.[14] Figure 12-1 lists exclusions for self-care. Antitussives (cough suppressants) control or eliminate cough and are the drugs of choice for nonproductive coughs. Protussives (expectorants) change the consistency of mucus and increase the volume of expectorated sputum. Protussives are the drugs of choice for coughs that expel thick, tenacious secretions from the lungs with difficulty. Antitussives should not be taken by patients with productive coughs unless absolutely necessary (e.g., exhaustion from lack of sleep). Suppression of productive coughs may lead to retention of lower

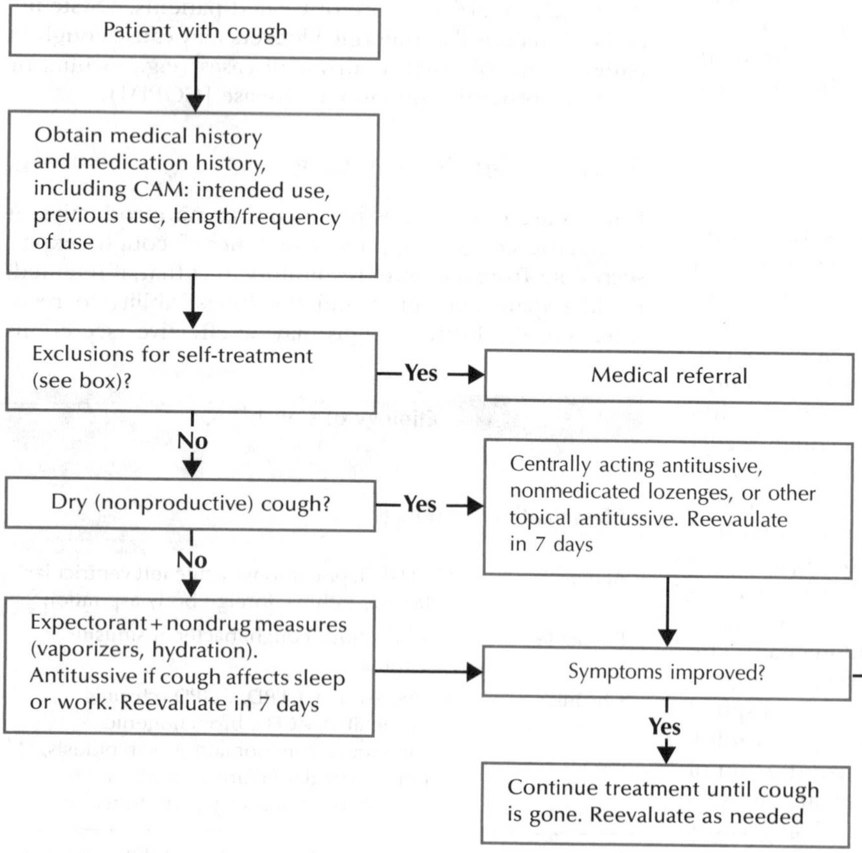


**Exclusions for Self-Treatment**

- Cough with thick yellow sputum or green phlegm
- Fever >101.5°F (38.6°C)
- Unintended weight loss
- Drenching nighttime sweats
- Hemoptysis
- History or symptoms of chronic underlying disease associated with cough (e.g., asthma, COPD, chronic bronchitis, CHF)
- Foreign object aspiration
- Suspected drug-associated cough
- Cough for >7 days
- Cough that worsens during self-treatment
- Development of new symptoms during self-treatment

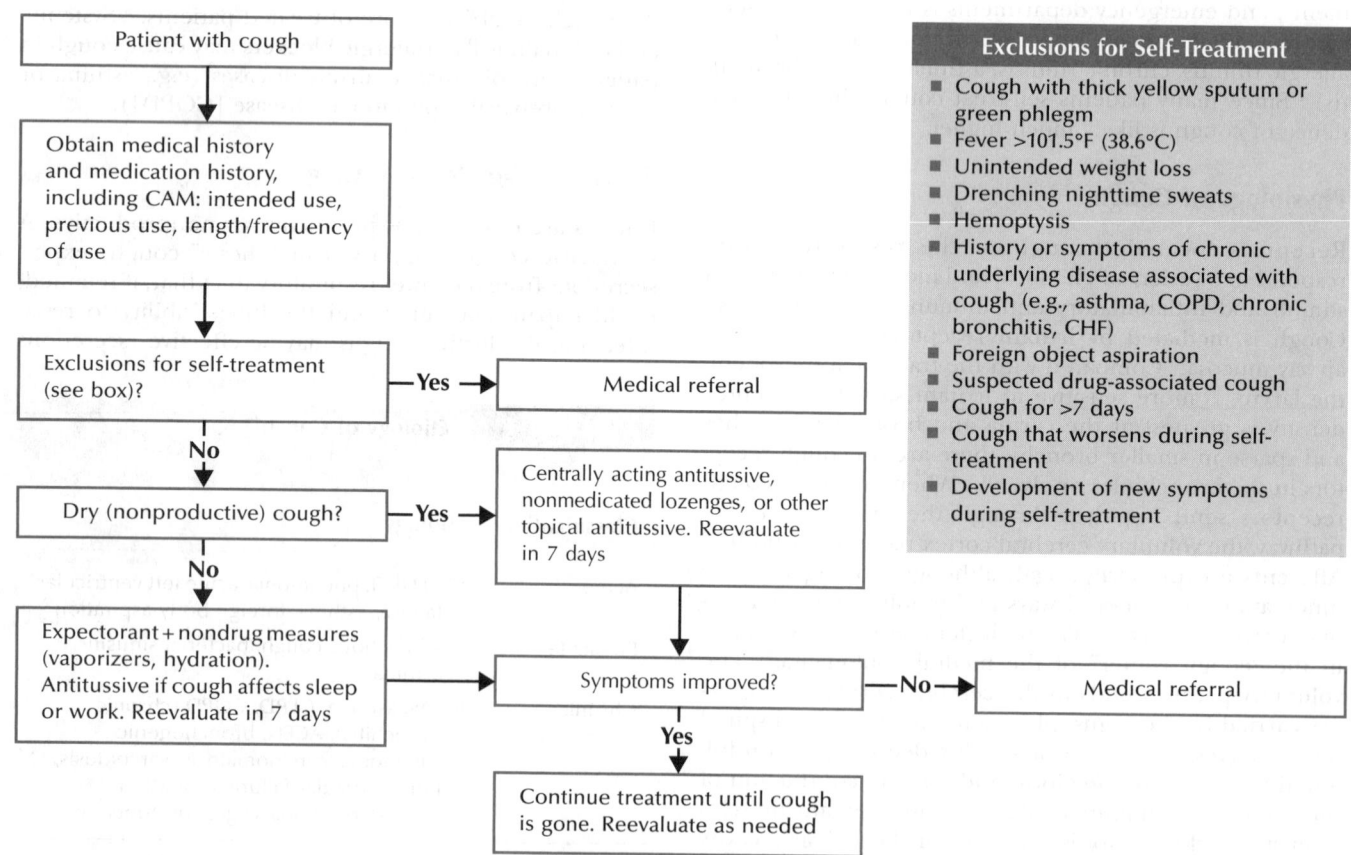

**FIGURE 12-1** Self-care of cough. Key: CAM, complementary and alternative medicine; CHF, congestive heart failure; COPD, chronic obstructive pulmonary disease. (Adapted from reference 14.)

respiratory tract secretions and potentially adverse consequences (e.g., secondary bacterial lower respiratory tract infection, airway obstruction).

Cough medications are marketed in a variety of dosage forms (syrups, liquids, tablets, capsules, lozenges, oral disintegrating strips, oral sprays, ointments and creams, and vaporizer solutions). In general, the newer convenience-oriented dosage forms (oral disintegrating strips, oral sprays, extended-release tablets) cost more per dose than older dosage forms. Products containing various combinations of antitussives, protussives, analgesics, decongestants, and antihistamines are available. Although convenient, cost per dose of combination products may be higher than single-entity products. In addition, products containing both an antitussive and a protussive are irrational and should be avoided.

## Nonpharmacologic Therapy

Nonpharmacologic therapy includes nonmedicated lozenges, humidification, and hydration. Hard candies and other nonmedicated lozenges reduce throat irritation and may decrease coughing. Humidifiers increase the amount of moisture in inspired air, which may soothe irritated airways. Moisture may be added to air by ultrasonic sound-wave vibration, high-speed rotating disk or fan (impeller), or evaporative mechanisms. However, high humidity may increase the amount of mold and dust mites in the house, thus worsening allergies. Humidifiers and vaporizers also disperse minerals and microorganisms into the air. Vaporizers are humidifiers with a medication well or cup for volatile inhalants that combine with the mist to produce a medicated vapor. Cool-mist humidifiers and vaporizers are preferred to warm-mist humidifiers and vaporizers because fewer bacteria grow at the cooler temperatures and there is less risk of scalding if they are tipped over. Humidifiers and vaporizers must be cleaned daily and disinfected weekly.

A clinical benefit of maintaining adequate hydration in patients with acute URTIs has not been proven. Theoretically, less viscous and thus easier-to-expel secretions are formed when a person is well hydrated. However, water cannot be incorporated into previously formed mucus, and there are theoretical risks of overhydration during respiratory infections. Excessive fluid intake may cause fluid overload and hyponatremia in patients with lower respiratory tract infections; it is not known whether this occurs with URTIs.[15] Most people need approximately eight 8-oz glasses of water daily. Cautious hydration is recommended for patients with lower respiratory tract infections, heart failure, renal failure, or other conditions potentially exacerbated by over hydration.

## Pharmacologic Therapy

Table 12-2 lists examples of products that contain oral antitussives, expectorants, and topical antitussives.

### Systemic Antitussives

Nonprescription systemic antitussives approved by the Food and Drug Administration (FDA) include codeine, dextromethorphan, and diphenhydramine.[16]

*Codeine* Codeine is the gold standard antitussive. At antitussive dosages, codeine is a Schedule C-V narcotic available without prescription in 29 states.[17] Codeine-containing Schedule C-V products must contain one or more noncodeine active ingredients and no more than 200 mg of codeine per 100 milliliters. Hydrocodone and hydromorphone have similar efficacy but are associated with a greater risk of dependency and are available only by prescription.

Mechanism of Action/Pharmacokinetics Codeine acts centrally on the medulla to increase the cough threshold. Codeine is the methyl ether of morphine; morphine may be the active antitussive. Codeine is well absorbed orally with a 15- to 30-minute onset of action and a 4- to 6-hour duration of effect. The elimination half-life is 2.5 to 3 hours. Ten percent of a codeine dose is demethylated in the liver to form morphine. Approximately 3% to 16% of codeine is eliminated unchanged in the urine.

Indications Codeine is indicated for the suppression of nonproductive cough caused by chemical or mechanical respiratory tract irritation. Though widely available, codeine's efficacy and safety as an antitussive drug in children have not been established.[18]

Dosage and Administration Guidelines Table 12-3 lists FDA-approved codeine dosages.[16] Pediatric dosage guidelines are extrapolated from the adult literature.[18] Reduced doses are appropriate for patients of advanced age and the debilitated. Codeine is available as oral solutions and syrups in combination with other active ingredients, including guaifenesin, antihistamines, and decongestants. Alcohol-, dye-, and sucrose-free formulations are available. The lethal dose of codeine in adults is 0.5 to 1 g, with death from marked respiratory depression and cardiopulmonary collapse.

Safety Considerations Usual antitussive codeine dosages have low toxicity and little risk of addiction. The most common side effects associated with antitussive codeine dosages are nausea, vomiting, sedation, dizziness, and constipation. Concomitant use of codeine and central nervous system (CNS) depressants (e.g., barbiturates, sedatives, alcohol) causes additive CNS depression. Codeine is contraindicated in patients with known codeine hypersensitivity and during labor when a premature birth is anticipated. Patients with impaired respiratory reserve (e.g., asthma or COPD) or preexisting respiratory depression, addicts, and those who take other respiratory depressants or sedatives, including alcohol, should use codeine with caution.

*Dextromethorphan* Considered approximately equipotent with codeine, dextromethorphan is a nonopioid with no analgesic, sedative, respiratory depressant, or addictive properties at usual antitussive doses.

Mechanism of Action/Pharmacokinetics Dextromethorphan is the methylated dextrorotatory analogue of levorphanol, a codeine analogue. Dextromethorphan acts centrally in the medulla to increase the cough threshold. It is

**TABLE 12-2 Selected Products for Cough**

| Trade Name | Primary Ingredients |
|---|---|
| **Single-entity Dextromethorphan Products** | |
| Benylin Adult Formula Cough Suppressant Solution[a-d] | Dextromethorphan hydrobromide 15 mg/5 mL |
| Delsym Extended Release Suspension[a,e] | Dextromethorphan polistirex equivalent to 30 mg dextromethorphan hydrobromide/5 mL |
| Hold DM Lozenges[a,f,g] | Dextromethorphan hydrobromide 5 mg/lozenge |
| Robitussin Pediatric Cough Syrup[a,d,h] | Dextromethorphan hydrobromide 7.5 mg/5 mL |
| Sucrets 8 Hour (cherry) Lozenges[a,d,f,i] | Dextromethorphan hydrobromide 10 mg/lozenge |
| Triaminic Thin Strips Long Acting Cough[d] | Dextromethorphan hydrobromide 7.5 mg/strip |
| Vicks 44 Cough Relief Liquid[a,i] | Dextromethorphan hydrobromide 30 mg/15 mL |
| Zicam Concentrated Cough Mist Spray for Kids[a,h] | Dextromethorphan hydrobromide 2.5 mg/spray |
| **Single-entity Guaifenesin Products** | |
| Diabetic Tussin EX Liquid[a,b,f,j,k] | Guaifenesin 100 mg/5 mL |
| Mucinex Extended Release Tablets[i] | Guaifenesin 600 mg |
| Robitussin Cough Syrup[a,d] | Guaifenesin 100 mg/5 mL |
| **Combination Products** | |
| Benylin Expectorant Liquid[a-d] | Dextromethorphan hydrobromide 5 mg/5 mL; guaifenesin 100 mg/5 mL |
| Cheracol Syrup | Codeine phosphate 10 mg/5 mL; guaifenesin 100 mg/5 mL |
| Robitussin Sugar Free Cough Syrup[a,b,j] | Dextromethorphan hydrobromide 10 mg/5 mL; guaifenesin 100 mg/5 mL |
| **Other Products** | |
| Silphen Cough Syrup[d] | Diphenhydramine HCl 12.5 mg/5 ml |
| Vicks Cough Drops (menthol)[a,f,j] | Menthol 3.3 mg/drop |
| Vicks VapoRub Ointment | Camphor 4.8%; menthol 2.6%; eucalyptus oil 1.2% |

[a]Alcohol-free; [b]sucrose-free; [c]contains FD&C red no. 33; [d]contains FD&C red no. 40; [e]contains FD&C yellow no. 6; [f]sodium-free; [g]contains FD& C yellow no. 10; [h]pediatric formula; [i]contains FD&C blue no. 1; [j]dye-free; [k]contains phenylalanine.

well absorbed orally with a 15- to 30-minute onset of action and a 3- to 6-hour duration of effect. Dextromethorphan exhibits polymorphic metabolism, with a usual elimination half-life of 1.2 to 2.2 hours. However, the half-life may be as long as 45 hours in people with a poor metabolism phenotype.

Indications Dextromethorphan is indicated for the suppression of nonproductive cough caused by chemical or mechanical respiratory tract irritation. As with codeine, the efficacy and safety of dextromethorphan as an antitussive drug in children have not been established.[18]

Dosage and Administration Guidelines Table 12-3 lists FDA-approved dextromethorphan dosages.[16] This agent is marketed in the form of syrups, liquids, extended-release oral suspensions, liquid-filled gelcaps, oral disintegrating strips, oral sprays, and lozenges. Alcohol-, sucrose-, and dye-free formulations are available. Dextromethorphan overdoses cause confusion, excitation, nervousness, irritability, restlessness, drowsiness, and severe nausea and vomiting; respiratory depression may occur with very high doses.

Safety Considerations Dextromethorphan has a wide margin of safety. Side effects with usual doses are uncommon but may include drowsiness, nausea or vomiting, stomach discomfort, or constipation. Dextromethorphan is sometimes abused for its phencyclidinelike euphoric effect;[19] abuse may be associated with psychosis and mania. Additive CNS depression occurs with alcohol, antihistamines, and psychotropic medications. Dextromethorphan blocks serotonin reuptake; the combination of monoamine oxidase inhibitors (MAOIs) and dextromethorphan may cause serotonergic syndrome (e.g., increased blood pressure, hyperpyrexia, arrhythmias, myoclonus). Patients who have known hypersensitivity to dextromethorphan or who have a prior history of dextromethorphan dependence should not take it. If the patient takes MAOIs, dextromethorphan should not be administered for at least 14 days after the MAOIs are halted.

*Diphenhydramine* Although diphenhydramine is an FDA-approved antitussive, it is not a first-line antitussive.

TABLE 12-3 Dosage Guidelines for Nonprescription Oral Antitussives and Expectorants[16]

| | Dosage (Maximum Daily Dosage) | | |
|---|---|---|---|
| Drug | Adults/Children ≥12 Years | Children 6 to <12 Years | Children 2 to <6 Years |
| Codeine*†‡ | 10-20 mg q4-6h (120 mg) | 5-10 mg q4-6h (60 mg) | 1 mg/kg/day in 4 equal divided dosages or by average body weight‡ |
| Dextromethorphan hydrobromide* | 10-20 mg q4h or 30 mg q6-8h (120 mg) | 5-10 mg q4h or 15 mg q6-8h (60 mg) | 2.5-5 mg q4h or 7.5 mg q6-8h (30 mg) |
| Diphenhydramine citrate*† | 38 mg q4h (228 mg) | 19 mg q4h (114 mg) | 9.5 mg q4h (57 mg) |
| Diphenhydramine HCl*† | 25 mg q4h (150 mg) | 12.5 mg q4h (75 mg) | 6.25 mg q4h (37.5 mg) |
| Guaifenesin* | 200-400 mg q4h (2.4 g) | 100-200 mg q4h (1.2 g) | 50-100 mg q4h (600 mg) |

* Not recommended for use in children younger than 2 years.

† FDA recommends that the labels on nonprescription products not provide dosage information for children younger than 6 years of age.

‡ Codeine may be dosed by average body weight: 2 years of age (average body weight of 12 kg) = 3 mg q4-6h (maximum in 24 hours: 12 mg); 3 years of age (average body weight of 14 kg) = 3.5 mg q4-6h (maximum in 24 hours: 14 mg); 4 years of age (average body weight of 16 kg) = 4 mg q4-6h (maximum in 24 hours: 16 mg); 5 years of age (average body weight of 18 kg) = 4.5 mg q4-6h (maximum in 24 hours: 18 mg). A dispensing device such as a dropper calibrated for age or weight should be dispensed along with the product when it is intended for use in children 2 to younger than 6 years, to prevent possible overdose from improperly measured dose.

Mechanism of Action/Pharmacokinetics Diphenhydramine is a nonselective (first-generation) antihistamine with significant sedating and anticholinergic properties. Diphenhydramine acts centrally in the medulla to increase the cough threshold. The antitussive effect is most likely related to anticholinergic activity and not competitive histamine antagonism; second-generation antihistamines (e.g., loratadine, fexofenadine) do not have antitussive activity.[20] Diphenhydramine is well absorbed following oral administration with a bioavailability of 40% to 70% and an onset of action of about 15 minutes. The volume of distribution, 3.3 to 4.5 L/kg in whites, is greater in Asians and in persons with chronic liver disease. Diphenhydramine is hepatically metabolized to n-dealkylated and acidic metabolites with a clearance of 0.4 to 0.7 L/kg per hour. Less than 4% is excreted unchanged in the urine.

Indications Diphenhydramine is indicated for the suppression of nonproductive cough caused by chemical or mechanical respiratory tract irritation. The American College of Chest Physicians recommends that first-generation antihistamines be used to treat PNDS-induced cough not mediated by histamine.[1]

Dosage and Administration Guidelines Table 12-3 lists FDA-approved diphenhydramine dosages.[16] Diphenhydramine's antitussive dose is lower than its antihistaminic dose. Antitussive diphenhydramine formulations include syrups, liquids, and oral disintegrating strips. Alcohol-, sucrose-, and dye-free formulations are available. Symptoms of diphenhydramine overdose include mild to severe CNS depression (e.g., mental confusion, sedation, respiratory depression), hypotension, and CNS stimulation (e.g., hallucinations, convulsions).

Safety Considerations Side effects of diphenhydramine include drowsiness, disturbed coordination, respiratory depression, blurred vision, urinary retention, dry mouth, and dry respiratory secretions. Uncommon side effects reported with diphenhydramine include acute dystonic reactions such as oculogyric crisis (rotation of the eyeballs), torticollis (contraction of neck muscles), and catatonialike states, as well as allergic and photoallergic reactions. Diphenhydramine may cause excitability, especially in children. Diphenhydramine potentiates the depressant effects of narcotics, nonnarcotic analgesics, benzodiazepines, tranquilizers, and alcohol on the CNS and intensifies the anticholinergic effect of MAOIs and other anticholinergics. Diphenhydramine is contraindicated in patients with known hypersensitivity to diphenhydramine or structurally similar antihistamines. Diphenhydramine should be used with caution in patients with a history of narrow-angle glaucoma, stenosing peptic ulcer, pyloroduodenal obstruction, symptomatic prostatic hypertrophy, bladder neck obstruction, asthma and other lower respiratory disease, elevated intraocular pressure, hyperthyroidism, cardiovascular disease, or hypertension. Because of the increased risk of toxicity, diphenhydramine-containing antitussives should not be used with any other diphenhydramine-containing product, including external products.

### Protussives (Expectorants)

Guaifenesin (glyceryl guaiacolate) is the only FDA-approved expectorant.[16] Historically, terpin hydrate, potassium iodide (saturated solution), iodinated glycerol and such diverse substances as systemic chloroform, iodides, ipecac fluid extract, ammonium chloride, benzoin preparations, camphor, eucalyptus oil, horehound, peppermint oil, menthol, pine tar preparations, and sodium citrate were used as expectorants, but these substances are now considered inactive ingredients.

*Mechanism of Action/Pharmacokinetics* Guaifenesin loosens and thins lower respiratory tract secretions, making minimally productive coughs more productive. However, few data support its efficacy, especially at nonprescription dosages.[21] The pharmacokinetics of guaifenesin are not well described.

*Indications* Guaifenesin is indicated for the symptomatic relief of acute, ineffective productive coughs.

*Dosage and Administration Guidelines* Table 12-3 lists FDA-approved dosages of guaifenesin.[16] Guaifenesin is marketed as oral liquids, syrups, and immediate-release and extended-release tablets. Alcohol-, sucrose-, and dye-free formulations are also available. Most reports of guaifenesin overdosages involve combinations of drugs and therefore are difficult to assess. However, signs and symptoms of overdosages appear to be extensions of the adverse effects.

*Safety Considerations* Guaifenesin is generally well tolerated, but its side effects may include nausea, vomiting, dizziness, headache, rash, diarrhea, drowsiness, and stomach pain. Guaifenesin may have a mild uricosuric effect and large dosages may cause urolithiasis. There are no reported drug interactions with guaifenesin. Guaifenesin is contraindicated in patients with a known hypersensitivity to guaifenesin.

### Topical Antitussives

Camphor and menthol are the only two FDA-approved topical antitussives.[16] Other volatile oils (e.g., eucalyptus), common in many cough and cold preparations, impart a strong medicinal odor to products, but are not FDA-approved antitussives.

*Mechanism of Action* Although the mechanism of action is not well described, inhaled vapors from topical ointments and creams, steam inhalation, topical patches, or oral lozenges stimulate sensory nerve endings within the nose and mucosa, creating a local anesthetic sensation and a sense of improved airflow. However, there is little objective evidence of clinical efficacy.

*Indications* Topical antitussives are approved cough suppressants.

*Dosage and Administration Guidelines* Topical antitussive ointments and creams contain camphor (4.7%-5.3%) or menthol (2.6%-2.8%). Steam inhalants contain 6.2% camphor or 3.2% menthol, patches contain 4.7% camphor and 2.6% menthol, and lozenges each contain 5 to 10 mg of menthol. Many lozenges and compressed tablet formulations contain one or more of the volatile oils. Table 12-4 provides administration guidelines for these agents. Table 12-2 lists selected trade-name products.

*Safety Considerations* Camphor- and menthol-containing products may splatter and cause serious burns if used near an open flame or placed in hot water or in a microwave oven. Ointments, solutions, and patches containing camphor or menthol are toxic if ingested. Toxicities include burning sensations in the mouth, nausea and vomiting, epigastric distress, restlessness, excitation, delirium, seizures, and death. Ingestion of as little as 4 teaspoons of products containing 5% camphor may be lethal for children.[22] Products with better risk–benefit ratios are preferred, especially for children.

## Product Selection Guidelines

*Efficacy* Antitussive efficacy depends on the etiology of the cough. Antitussives are effective in several models of experimentally induced cough and in chronic cough, but have not been shown to be effective for acute coughs associated with viral URTI.[23-26] Cough associated with URTIs involves the voluntary and brainstem reflex pathways,[27] which may partially explain the large placebo response (reported to be >80%)[25] and ineffectiveness of brainstem-active antitussives. Other factors such as taste, smell, color, viscosity, sugar content, and personal expectation may contribute to the placebo response.[25] The statements "There is no good evidence for or against the effectiveness of OTC medicines in acute cough,"[26] and "These OTC remedies should not be discarded unless there is good evidence that they do not work"[28] summarize the current dilemma. Efficacy will remain unproven until data are available from well-designed trials of subjects with natural disease assessed with standardized objective outcome parameters.

*Special Populations* Codeine is a Pregnancy Category C drug and should be used during pregnancy only if the potential benefits outweigh the risks. Nonteratogenic concerns include the risk of neonatal respiratory depression if codeine is taken close to the time of delivery and neonatal withdrawal if codeine is used regularly during the pregnancy. Although codeine is excreted in breast milk, the American Academy of Pediatrics lists codeine as a maternal medication usually compatible with breast-feeding.[29] There are no specific pharmacokinetic or pharmacodynamic studies of codeine as an antitussive in the persons of advanced age. Because they may be more susceptible to the sedating effects of codeine, the dose should be started at the lower end of the dosage range and titrated as tolerated with careful monitoring.

Although listed as a Pregnancy Category C drug, dextromethorphan is viewed by some clinicians as probably safe for use during pregnancy.[30] A study of 184 women who were exposed to dextromethorphan during pregnancy did not reveal an increase in the rate of major malformations.[31] It is not known whether dextromethorphan is excreted in breast milk. The American Academy of Pediatrics' current drugs and breast-feeding policy statement makes no recommendation regarding dextromethorphan and breast-feeding.[29] There are no specific pharmacokinetic or pharmacodynamic studies of

**TABLE 12-4 Administration Guidelines for Nonprescription Topical Antitussives (Adults and Children ≥2 Years*)[16]**

| Drug | Administration |
|---|---|
| Camphor ointment 4.7%-5.3% | Rub on the throat and chest as thick layer; application may be repeated up to 3 times daily or as directed by primary care provider; loosen clothing around throat and chest so vapors reach the nose and mouth; cover with a warm, dry cloth (optional). |
| Camphor 4.7%, menthol 2.6% patch | Open pouch; remove card and peel adhesive patch from card; apply patch to throat or chest; for repeated application, place new patch on a new area of skin; loosen clothing around throat and chest so vapors reach the nose and mouth; do not leave patch on more than 12 hours; moisten patch with water if difficult to remove. |
| Menthol ointment 2.6%-2.8% | Rub on the throat and chest as thick layer; application may be repeated up to 3 times daily or as directed by a primary care provider; loosen clothing around throat and chest so vapors reach the nose and mouth; cover with a warm, dry cloth (optional). |
| Menthol lozenges 5-10 mg | Allow lozenge to dissolve slowly in mouth; repeat hourly or as needed or directed by a primary care provider. |
| Camphor for steam inhalation 6.2% | For products to be added directly to cold water inside hot steam vaporizer: use 1 tablespoon solution for each quart of water; add solution directly to cold water in hot steam vaporizer; breathe in the medicated vapors up to 3 times daily.<br>For products to be placed in medication chamber of hot steam vaporizer: place water in vaporizer; place solution in medication chamber; breathe in the medicated vapors up to 3 times daily. |
| Menthol for steam inhalation 3.2% | For products to be added directly to cold water inside hot steam vaporizer: use 1 tablespoon solution for each quart of water; add solution directly to cold water in hot steam vaporizer; breathe in the medicated vapors up to 3 times daily.<br>For products to be placed in medication chamber of hot steam vaporizer: place water in vaporizer; place solution in medication chamber; breathe in the medicated vapors up to 3 times daily. |

* For children ages ≤2 years, consult a primary care provider.

**TABLE 12-5 Signs and Symptoms of Diseases Associated With Cough**

| Disease | Signs and Symptoms |
|---|---|
| Viral URTI | Sneezing, sore throat, rhinorrhea, low-grade oral temperature |
| Lower respiratory tract infection | Oral temperature >101.5°F (38.6°C); thick, purulent, discolored phlegm; drenching night sweats |
| PNDS | Mucus drainage from nose, frequent throat clearing |
| Asthma | Wheezing or chest tightness; coughing predominantly at night; cough in response to specific irritants such as dust, smoke, or pollen |
| COPD | Productive cough most days of the month at least 3 months of the year for at least 2 consecutive years |
| GERD | Heartburn, worsening of symptoms when supine, improvement with acid-lowering drugs |
| CHF | Fatigue, dependent edema, breathlessness |

Key: CHF, congestive heart failure; COPD, chronic obstructive pulmonary disease; GERD, gastroesophageal reflux disease; PNDS, postnasal drip syndrome; URTI, upper respiratory tract infection.

dextromethorphan in persons of advanced age. Because they may be more susceptible to the sedating effects of dextromethorphan, the dose should be started at the lower end of the dosage range and titrated as tolerated with careful monitoring.

Diphenhydramine is a Pregnancy Category B drug. It is excreted in breast milk and may cause unusual excitation and irritability in the infant; it may also decrease the flow of milk. Persons of advanced age are more likely to experience dizziness, excessive sedation, syncope, confusion, and hypotension with diphenhydramine compared with the general population. Children and persons of advanced age may experience paradoxical excitation, restlessness, and irritability with diphenhydramine. Dosing for the latter group should be started at the lower end of the dosage range and titrated as tolerated with careful monitoring.

*Patient Factors* Cough is a symptom of many acute and chronic diseases; self-treatment may delay effective treatment of the underlying disease. Patients with known, or signs and symptoms of, chronic diseases associated with cough (Table 12-5) should not attempt to self-treat cough, even cough caused by an acute viral URTI, because the acute infection may exacerbate the underlying disease. Patients with smoker's cough should be counseled regarding smoking cessation options (see Chapter 50). Guaifenesin is not indicated for chronic cough associated with chronic lower respiratory tract diseases such as asthma, chronic obstructive lung disease, emphysema, or smoker's cough. Guaifenesin should not be used to treat effectively productive coughs. Patients with identified exclusions for self-care (Figure 12-1) should be referred for further evaluation.

Codeine or dextromethorphan are the drugs of choice for nonproductive coughs. Neither dextromethorphan nor diphenhydramine should be taken by patients taking MAOIs. Diphenhydramine is a better choice for coughs associated with allergies but is highly sedating and should be avoided by patients at risk from the anticholinergic properties of the drug. Guaifenesin is the only marketed expectorant.

### *Complementary Therapies*

Hundreds of herbal and other complementary therapies are marketed for cough.[32,33] (See Chapters 53 and 55 for discussion of botanical and nonbotanical natural medicines.) Many products contain oropharyngeal demulcents.[34] Slippery elm (*Ulmus fulva*) and plantain (*Plantago lanceolata*), two popular though unproven complementary therapies, contain mucilage, which may soothe locally irritated oropharyngeal tissues. Systemic eucalyptus (dried leaf) may have expectorant properties. Numerous homeopathic cough products are available without prescription (e.g., Bryonia, Rumex, Ipecacuanha, Rhus toxicodendron, Kali carbonicum). (See Chapter 55 for a discussion of homeopathy.) Folk remedies include onion cough syrup, capsaicin-containing foods, and licorice. There is little evidence that any of these complementary therapies are effective; however, with the exception of licorice, there are no reported health hazards. Persons with diabetes, hypertension, liver or kidney disorders, or disorders associated with hypokalemia should not take licorice-containing products.

## Assessment of Cough: A Case-based Approach

Before recommending any treatment, the practitioner needs to know how long the patient has been coughing, whether the cough is productive, and whether it is associated with a chronic illness (Table 12-5). It is also important to obtain a list of all the patient's current medications to identify possible drug–drug or drug–disease interactions. In addition, the practitioner should find out how the patient has treated the current cough as well as previous coughs, and whether these treatments were satisfactory or effective. Cases 12-1 and 12-2 provide examples of the assessment of a patient with cough.

### CASE 12-1

| Relevant Evaluation Criteria | Scenario/Model Outcome |
|---|---|
| **Information Gathering** | |
| 1. Gather essential information about the patient's symptoms, including: | |
| a. description of symptom(s) (i.e., nature, onset, duration, severity, associated symptoms) | Patient has had a cold for the last few days. The rhinorrhea resolved in a couple of days but cough persists; it wakes him up at night and interferes with his work. Cough is dry and hacking. He has not taken his temperature, but he hasn't felt feverish. |
| b. description of any factors that seem to precipitate, exacerbate, and/or relieve the patient's symptom(s) | Cold, dry air precipitates cough. Nothing seems to make the cough better. |
| c. description of the patient's efforts to relieve the symptoms | Patient has been using nonmedicated cherry-flavored cough drops. |
| 2. Gather essential patient history information: | |
| a. patient's identity | Peter Lyver |
| b. age, sex, height, and weight | 31 y/o M, 5'10", 170 lb |
| c. patient's occupation | Small business owner |
| d. patient's dietary habits | Eats fast foods 5-10 times per week |
| e. patient's sleep habits | Usually sleeps 9 hours, but cough wakes him up several times. |
| f. concurrent medical conditions, prescription and nonprescription medications, and dietary supplements | Atypical depression for 15 years; currently taking Nardil 15 mg per day |
| g. allergies | Penicillin. He doesn't remember it, but his mother said it caused a rash. |

## CASE 12-1 (continued)

| Relevant Evaluation Criteria | Scenario/Model Outcome |
|---|---|
| h. history of other adverse reactions to medications | None |
| i. other (describe)_______ | None |
| **Assessment and Triage** | |
| 3. Differentiate the patient's signs/symptoms and correctly identify the patient's primary problem(s). | Peter has a cough related to an acute postviral URTI cough. Cough is nonproductive and interferes with his sleep. |
| 4. Identify exclusions for self-treatment (see Figure 12-1). | Peter has no signs or symptoms of chronic underlying diseases associated with cough (see Table 12-5) and no exclusions for self-care. |
| 5. Formulate a comprehensive list of therapeutic alternatives for the primary problem to determine if triage to a medical practitioner is required, and share this information with the patient. | Options include:<br>(1) Refer Peter for further evaluation.<br>(2) Recommend self-care with a nonprescription product containing an antitussive.<br>(3) Recommend a complementary therapy.<br>(4) Take no action. |
| **Plan** | |
| 6. Select an optimal therapeutic alternative to address the patient's problem, taking into account patient preferences. | Self-care with a nonprescription drug is appropriate. Postviral URTI cough is acute and usually resolves within a few days although it may last for several weeks. An antitussive drug is appropriate for his nonproductive cough although the efficacy of antitussive drugs in viral-associated cough is unproven. Dextromethorphan is contraindicated in patients taking MAOIs. Diphenhydramine intensifies the anticholinergic effects of MAOIs and should be avoided. Codeine is sedating and may interfere with his ability to drive or work and is not available in all states without a prescription. Complementary therapies for cough contain ingredients with unproven local demulcent/expectorant activity. |
| 7. Describe the recommended therapeutic approach to the patient. | I recommend cautious use of a single-entity nonprescription codeine cough syrup at bedtime. Combination products are not necessary because you have no other symptoms. The usual adult dose is 10-20 mg every 4-6 hours as needed. |
| 8. Explain to the patient the rationale for selecting the recommended therapeutic approach from the considered therapeutic alternatives. | You don't need to see a primary care provider at this time because your cough appears to be secondary to a viral upper respiratory tract infection and is self-limiting. You cannot take any cough medications that contain dextromethorphan or diphenhydramine because they interact with your Nardil. Codeine-containing cough syrups are available without a prescription in your state but must be used with caution. |
| **Patient Education** | |
| 9. When recommending self-care with nonprescription medications and/or nondrug therapy, convey accurate information to the patient, including: | |
| a. appropriate dose and frequency of administration | Take 10 mg codeine before bedtime to help control nighttime cough. |
| b. maximum number of days the therapy should be employed | See your primary care provider if the cough lasts for more than 7 days. |
| c. product administration procedures | Use a medication cup or clean teaspoon to measure the dose. |
| d. expected time to onset of relief | Benefit should be evident within an hour or so of taking the dose. |
| e. degree of relief that can be reasonably expected | Number and severity of cough episodes may be reduced. |

## CASE 12-1 (continued)

| Relevant Evaluation Criteria | Scenario/Model Outcome |
|---|---|
| f. most common side effects | Common codeine side effects include drowsiness, lightheadedness, dizziness, lack of coordination, constipation, and upset stomach. |
| g. side effects that warrant medical intervention should they occur | Contact your primary care provider if you have a rash, itching, problems breathing, abdominal pain, or a fast or slow heart beat. |
| h. patient options in the event that condition worsens or persists | Medical referral will be necessary if the cough lasts for more than 7 days or if you develop new symptoms. |
| i. product storage requirements | Store medication out of children's reach and at controlled room temperature with safety cap in place. |
| j. specific nondrug measures | Maintain normal fluid intake. Nonmedicated lozenges may reduce throat irritations. Increased humidity from steamy showers or cool-mist vaporizers may soothe irritated airways. |
| 10. Solicit follow-up questions from patient. | Can I get addicted to codeine? |
| 11. Answer patient's questions. | Codeine is addicting. However, limited use as an antitussive usually is not associated with addiction. |

Key: MAOI, monoamine oxidase inhibitor; URTI, upper respiratory tract infection.

## CASE 12-2

| Relevant Evaluation Criteria | Scenario/Model Outcome |
|---|---|
| **Information Gathering** | |
| 1. Gather essential information about the patient's symptoms, including: | |
| a. description of symptom(s) (i.e., nature, onset, duration, severity, associated symptoms) | Patient has an ineffective productive cough associated with a mild community-acquired pneumonia. The secretions are thick and difficult to cough up. Her physician recommended she try a nonprescription expectorant. |
| b. description of any factors that seem to precipitate, exacerbate, and/or relieve the patient's symptom(s) | None |
| c. description of the patient's efforts to relieve the symptoms | She started a course of antibiotics yesterday. |
| 2. Gather essential patient history information: | |
| a. patient's identity | Melissa Fraley |
| b. age, sex, height, and weight | 37 y/o F, 5'2", 114 lb |
| c. patient's occupation | Stay-at-home mom |
| d. patient's dietary habits | Low-carbohydrate diet |
| e. patient's sleep habits | Usually sleeps 6-8 hours a night. Cough is not interfering with sleep. |
| f. concurrent medical conditions, prescription and nonprescription medications, and dietary supplements | Viactiv 500 mg 3 times/day; Ortho Tri-Cyclen Lo 1 tablet once daily |
| g. allergies | NKDA |
| h. history of other adverse reactions to medications | None |
| i. other (describe)______ | None |

## CASE 12-2 (continued)

| Relevant Evaluation Criteria | Scenario/Model Outcome |
|---|---|
| **Assessment and Triage** | |
| 3. Differentiate the patient's signs/symptoms and correctly identify the patient's primary problem(s). | Melissa has an ineffective productive cough associated with a mild community-acquired pneumonia. She has been evaluated by her PCP for her lower respiratory tract infection and has no contraindications to self-care with an expectorant. |
| 4. Identify exclusions for self-treatment (see Figure 12-1). | Melissa has no signs or symptoms of chronic underlying diseases associated with cough (see Table 12-5). |
| 5. Formulate a comprehensive list of therapeutic alternatives for the primary problem to determine if triage to a medical practitioner is required, and share this information with the patient. | Options include:<br>(1) Recommend self-care with a nonprescription product containing an expectorant.<br>(2) Recommend a complementary therapy.<br>(3) Refer Melissa for further evaluation.<br>(4) Take no action. |
| **Plan** | |
| 6. Select an optimal therapeutic alternative to address the patient's problem, taking into account patient preferences. | Guaifenesin is the only FDA-approved expectorant. Systemic eucalyptus (dried leaf) may have expectorant properties although little evidence of efficacy exists. |
| 7. Describe the recommended therapeutic approach to the patient. | I recommend a single-entity nonprescription guaifenesin product. Combination products are not necessary because you have no other symptoms and you do not want to suppress the cough. The usual adult dose is 200-400 mg every 4 hours. Guaifenesin is available in syrups, liquids, immediate-release tablets, and extended-release tablets. |
| 8. Explain to the patient the rationale for selecting the recommended therapeutic approach from the considered therapeutic alternatives. | Guaifenesin is the only FDA-approved expectorant. |
| **Patient Education** | |
| 9. When recommending self-care with nonprescription medications and/or nondrug therapy, convey accurate information to the patient, including: | |
| a. appropriate dose and frequency of administration | The usual adult dose is 200-400 mg 4 times daily. |
| b. maximum number of days the therapy should be employed | Referral will be necessary if you develop new symptoms or if the cough lasts for more than 7 days. |
| c. product administration procedures | Use a medication cup or clean teaspoon to measure the dose of syrup or liquids. Do not crush or chew extended-release tablets. |
| d. expected time to onset of relief | Benefit should be evident within a few hours of taking the dose. |
| e. degree of relief that can be reasonably expected | The secretions should increase and become thinner and easier to cough out of the lungs. |
| f. most common side effects | Guaifenesin usually is well tolerated; however, dizziness, headache, rash, itching, and nausea and vomiting may occur. |
| g. side effects that warrant medical intervention should they occur | Stop taking the medication and tell your primary care provider if you develop a rash or itching while taking the medication. |
| h. patient options in the event that condition worsens or persists | Referral will be necessary if you continue to have difficulty coughing up your secretions. |
| i. product storage requirements | Store medication out of children's reach and at controlled room temperature with safety cap in place. |

**CASE 12-2 (continued)**

| Relevant Evaluation Criteria | Scenario/Model Outcome |
|---|---|
| j. specific nondrug measures | Drink at least eight 8-ounce glasses of water a day. You may produce less sticky secretions when you are well hydrated. |
| 10. Solicit follow-up questions from patient. | Will guaifenesin interfere with the antibiotic? |
| 11. Answer patient's questions. | There are no documented drug interactions for guaifenesin. |

Key: FDA, Food and Drug Administration; NKDA, no known drug allergies; PCP, primary care provider.

## Patient Counseling for Cough

The practitioner should explain the appropriate drug and nondrug measures for treating the patient's type of cough. After recommending a product, the dosage guidelines, drug administration techniques (for topical drugs), and possible side effects, drug–drug interactions, and precautions or warnings should be fully explained. The practitioner should ensure that the patient understands when self-care of cough should be discontinued and medical care sought. For patients with underlying medical disorders, the practitioner should explain which nonprescription medications are contraindicated and what symptoms indicate the need to seek medical care. The box Patient Education for Cough lists specific information for patients.

## Evaluation of Patient Outcomes for Cough

For most patients, 7 days of nonprescription drug therapy should relieve cough. If the cough persists but has improved at follow-up, the patient should continue the therapy until the cough is resolved. If the cough has worsened or the patient has developed other exclusions for self-treatment (Figure 12-1), the patient should be referred for further medical evaluation.

## Key Points for Cough

- Antitussives (cough suppressants) are the drugs of choice for nonproductive coughs.
- Protussives (expectorants) are the drugs of choice for coughs that expel thick, tenacious secretions from the lungs with difficulty.
- Patients with a history or symptoms of chronic underlying disease associated with cough should not self-treat cough.
- Counsel patients with cough on nondrug measures such as hydration (see box Patient Education for Cough).
- Efficacy of nonprescription antitussives for acute cough associated with viral URTIs remains unproven.
- Dextromethorphan is contraindicated in patients taking MAOIs.
- Refer patients with cough that persists for more than 7 days, worsens during self-treatment, or is associated with an oral temperature higher than 101.5°F (38.6°C) for further evaluation.

## References


1. Irwin RS, Boulet L-P, Cloutier MM, et al. Managing cough as a defense mechanism and as a symptom. A consensus panel report of the American College of Chest Physicians. *Chest.* 1998;114(2 suppl):133S-81S.
2. Levy S. Top 200 OTC/HBC brands in 2003. *Drug Topics.* 2004; 148:64.
3. Woodwell DA, Cherry DK. National Ambulatory Medical Care Survey: 2002 Summary. Advance data from vital and health statistics; no 346. Hyattsville, Md: National Center for Health Statistics. 2004.
4. Burt CW, Schappert SM. Ambulatory care visits to physician offices, hospital outpatient departments, and emergency departments: United States, 1999-2000. National Center for Health Statistics. *Vital Health Stat.* 2004:13(157):30.
5. Widdicombe J. Neuroregulation of cough: implications for drug therapy. *Curr Opin Pharmacol.* 2002;2:256-63.
6. Sant'Ambrogio G, Widdicombe J. Reflexes from airway rapidly adapting receptors. *Respir Physiol.* 2001;125:33-45.
7. Widdicombe J. Airway receptors. *Resp Physiol.* 2001;1259:3-15.
8. Karlsson J-A, Fuller RW. Pharmacological regulation of the cough reflex – from experimental models to antitussive effects in man. *Pulm Pharmacol Ther.* 1999;12:215-28.
9. Lee PCL, Cotterill-Jones C, Eccles R. Voluntary control of cough. *Pulm Pharmacol Ther.* 2002;15:317-20.
10. Canning BJ. Interactions between vagal afferent nerve subtypes mediating cough. *Pulm Pharmacol Ther.* 2002;15:187-92.
11. Pantaleo T, Bongianni F, Mutolo D. Central nervous mechanisms of cough. *Pulm Pharmacol Ther.* 2002;15:227-33.
12. Irwin RS, Madison JM. Primary care: the diagnosis and treatment of cough. *N Engl J Med.* 2000;343:1715-21.
13. Dykewicz MS. Cough and angioedema from angiotensin-converting enzyme inhibitors: new insights into mechanisms and management. *Curr Opin Allergy Clin Immunol.* 2004;4:267-70.
14. Self-care of coughing. In: Albrant DH, ed. *The American Pharmaceutical Association Drug Treatment Protocols.* Washington, DC: American Pharmaceutical Association; 2001:417-22.
15. Guppy MPB, Mickan SM, Del Mar CB. "Drink plenty of fluids": a systematic review of evidence for this recommendation in acute respiratory infections. *BMJ.* 2004;328:499-500.
16. Cold, cough, allergy, bronchodilator, and antiasthmatic drug products for over-the-counter human use. *CFR* [serial online]. 2004;Title 21, Vol 5, Pt 341. Available at: http://www.accessdata.fda.gov. Accessed January 4, 2005.
17. *2005 Survey of Pharmacy Law.* Mount Prospect, Ill: National Association of Boards of Pharmacy; 2005:69-73.
18. Use of codeine- and dextromethorphan-containing cough remedies in children. American Academy of Pediatrics. Committee on Drugs. *Pediatrics.* 1997;99:918-20.

## PATIENT EDUCATION FOR COUGH

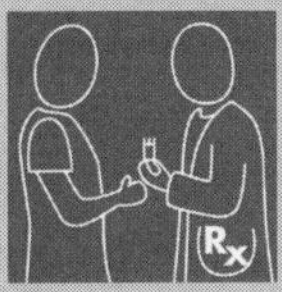

The goal of self-treatment is to reduce the number and severity of cough episodes and prevent complications. For most patients, carefully following product instructions and the self-care measures listed here will help ensure optimal therapeutic outcomes.

### Nondrug Measures

- Stay well hydrated. Most adults need about eight 8-ounce glasses of water per day.
- Reduce throat irritation by slowly dissolving nonmedicated lozenges and candies in mouth.
- Humidifiers and vaporizers increase the moisture in the air and may soothe irritated airways.
- Treat the underlying cause of cough (e.g., nasal congestion).

### Nonprescription Medications

- Cough is a symptom of an underlying disorder. Ask a clinician to help you select a cough medicine. Contact your primary care provider if you have any of the exclusions for self-care listed in Figure 12-1.
- Coughs are described as productive (wet or "chesty") or nonproductive (dry or "hacking").
- Slowly dissolve medicated lozenges in your mouth; do not chew.
- Swallow tablets and capsules whole; do not crush or chew.
- Slowly dissolve oral disintegrating strips on your tongue; do not chew.
- Hold the oral spray bottle close to your mouth. Depress the sprayer fully and swallow the medication. Do not inhale the mist.
- Store all these medications according to the manufacturer's recommendations. Do not use any expired drug.

### *Cough Suppressants (Antitussives)*

- Cough suppressants control or eliminate cough and are the drugs of choice for nonproductive coughs. Oral nonprescription cough suppressants include codeine (available without a prescription in some states), dextromethorphan, and diphenhydramine. (Dosages are listed in Table 12-3.) Topical nonprescription antitussives include camphor and menthol. (Dosages are listed in Table 12-4.)
- Codeine, dextromethorphan, and diphenhydramine are taken by mouth as needed.
- Camphor and menthol, available in lozenges, ointments, patches, and solutions for cool-mist or warm-mist vaporization, are used as needed. (Administration guidelines are listed in Table 12-4.) Do not heat, microwave, or add these products to hot water. Do not use these products near an open flame. Ointments, solutions, and patches containing camphor or menthol are toxic if ingested.
- Take the medications as recommended.
- The most common side effects of codeine include nausea, vomiting, sedation, dizziness, and constipation.
- Dextromethorphan's side effects are uncommon but may include drowsiness, nausea, vomiting, stomach discomfort, and constipation.
- The most common side effects of diphenhydramine include drowsiness, disturbed coordination, decreased respiration, blurred vision, difficult urination, and dry mouth.
- Codeine, dextromethorphan, and diphenhydramine interact with all drugs that cause drowsiness (e.g., narcotics, sedatives, some antihistamines, alcohol).
- Dextromethorphan also interacts with monoamine oxidase inhibitors (e.g., phenelzine, tranylcypromine, isocarboxazid). Do not take dextromethorphan within 14 days of taking one of these medications.
- Diphenhydramine also interacts with drugs that have anticholinergic activity, such as monoamine oxidase inhibitors.
- Patients with impaired respiratory reserve (e.g., asthma, chronic obstructive pulmonary disease) should use codeine and diphenhydramine with caution.
- Patients with narrow-angle glaucoma, stenosing peptic ulcer, pyloroduodenal obstruction, symptomatic prostatic hypertrophy, bladder neck obstruction, elevated intraocular pressure, hyperthyroidism, heart disease, or hypertension should use diphenhydramine with caution.
- Codeine and dextromethorphan should be used during pregnancy only if the potential benefits outweigh the risks.
- Codeine and diphenhydramine are excreted in breast milk and may cause side effects in the child.
- Older adults and children may have paradoxical excitation, restlessness, and irritability with diphenhydramine. Older adults are more likely than the general population to have side effects from diphenhydramine.

### *Expectorants (Protussives)*

- Expectorants make mucous more watery and increase the volume of sputum. Guaifenesin is the only available nonprescription protussive. (Dosages are listed in Table 12-3.)
- Take guaifenesin as recommended.
- Guaifenesin is generally well tolerated, but side effects may include nausea, vomiting, dizziness, headache, rash, diarrhea, drowsiness, and stomach pain.
- There are no reported drug interactions with guaifenesin.
- Guaifenesin is contraindicated in patients with a known hypersensitivity to the medication.
- Guaifenesin is not indicated for chronic cough associated with chronic lower respiratory tract diseases such as asthma, chronic obstructive lung disease, emphysema, or smoker's cough.


19. Banerji S, Anderson IB. Abuse of Coricidin HBP cough and cold tablets: episodes recorded by a poison center. *Am J Health Syst Pharm.* 2001;58:1811-14.
20. Dicpinigaitis PV, Gayle YE. Effect of the second-generation antihistamine, fexofenadine, on cough reflex sensitivity and pulmonary function. *Br J Clin Pharmacol.* 2003;56:501-4.
21. Over-the-counter (OTC) cough remedies. *Med Lett Drug Ther.* 2001;43:23-5.
22. American Academy of Pediatrics. Committee on Drugs. Camphor revisited: focus on toxicity. *Pediatrics.* 1994;94:127-8.
23. Schroeder K, Fahey T. Systematic review of randomised controlled trials of over-the-counter cough medicines for acute cough in adults. *BMJ.* 2002;324:329-34.
24. Schroeder K, Fahey T. Should we advise parents to administer over-the-counter cough medicines for acute cough? Systematic review of randomised controlled trials. *Arch Dis Child.* 2002;86:170-5.

25. Eccles R. The powerful placebo in cough studies? *Pulm Pharmacol Ther.* 2002;15:303-8.
26. Schroeder K, Fahey T. Over-the-counter medications for acute cough in children and adults in ambulatory settings. *Cochrane Database of Systematic Reviews;* 2004:3.
27. Lee PCL, Jawad MSN, Eccles R. Antitussive efficacy of dextromethorphan in cough associated with acute upper respiratory tract infection. *J Pharm Pharmacol.* 2000;52:1137-42.
28. Widdicombe J, Morice A. Over-the-counter cough medicines for acute cough: good quality research is needed. *BMJ.* 2002;324:1158.
29. American Academy of Pediatrics. Committee on Drugs. The transfer of drugs and other chemicals into human milk. *Pediatrics.* 2001;108:776-89.
30. Koren G, Pastuszak A, Ito S. Drug therapy: drugs in pregnancy. *N Engl J Med.* 1998;338:1128-37.
31. Einarson A, Lyszkiewicz D, Koren G. The safety of dextromethorphan in pregnancy. *Chest.* 2001;119:466-69.
32. LaGow B, ed. *PDR for Herbal Medications.* 3rd ed. Montvale, NJ: Medical Economics Company, Inc.; 2004.
33. Fetrow CW, Avila JR. *The Complete Guide to Herbal Medicines.* New York: Simon & Schuster, Inc; 2000.
34. Ziment I. Herbal antitussives. *Pulm Pharmacol Ther.* 2002;15:327-33.

# CHAPTER 13

# Asthma

*Suzanne G. Bollmeier and Theresa R. Prosser*

Asthma is the fourth most common chronic health condition in the United States[1] and is a common respiratory disease in both adults and children. Based on annual sales, an increasing number of people are using nonprescription products for breathing related problems (and presumably asthma). In 2003, almost 41,000 Primatene Mist inhalers were sold in pharmacies in the United States, which was an increase of 22.9% from 2002.[2]

Treatment of asthma places a significant burden on the health care system. In 2002, there were 13.9 million outpatient asthma visits to private physician offices and hospital outpatient departments.[3] Asthma is one of the 10 most common diagnoses seen in emergency departments and is responsible for 500,000 hospitalizations per year.[1] The direct medical care costs for asthma were estimated to be $3.64 billion in 1990, with over 50% of these costs related to emergent care in hospitals and emergency departments.

Untreated or inadequately treated asthma can have a significant impact on the quality of life of the patient and the family coping with asthma. An estimated 30% of children with asthma have an impairment of their physical activity, which is six times more than among children who do not have asthma. Children with asthma may also miss twice as many school days.[4] The resulting missed school or work time decreases productivity of patients, family members, and caregivers. Even mild symptoms from asthma can disrupt sleep and daytime activities and affect learning. The financial impact is also significant. In the United States, medical treatment for asthma is estimated to cost between 5.5% and 14.5% of a family's income.[4] Further indirect costs, such as missed work or school, transportation, disability, and premature death, may be 50% of the total cost of asthma.[1]

Although the number of deaths annually from asthma is low compared with those from other chronic diseases, asthma is a still a potentially serious disease. The death rate in the United States for children aged 5 to 14 years doubled during the period of 1979-80 to 1993-95, from 1.5 to 3.7 deaths per million children. During the same period, the death rate also doubled in persons 15-34 years old, from 2.8 to 6.3 deaths per million.[1] Many of these deaths are thought to result from inadequate long-term care or access to acute care and may be preventable. Healthy People 2010, which sets the national health goals in the United States, has several asthma care goals, including better prevention, detection, treatment, and educational efforts.[1]

Ideally, most treatment for asthma should take place in the ambulatory setting and focus on preventing asthma symptoms rather than treating serious asthma episodes. Patients with asthma need to know how to take their medications, monitor their asthma symptoms for severe episodes, manage environmental triggers, and recognize when to seek emergent medical care. Fortunately, asthma is usually responsive to appropriate, comprehensive treatment, and most patients with asthma have a normal life span and quality of life. But developing an optimal, comprehensive, and individualized asthma care plan requires a partnership between the individuals with asthma and their health care providers. Therefore, *self-care* is a critical part of asthma management.

Isolated, *self-treatment* of asthma or asthmalike symptoms outside of a broader treatment plan is potentially dangerous. Other serious conditions, such as chronic obstructive pulmonary disease and heart failure, can cause similar symptoms and require different therapy. Also, asthma itself is thought to be underdiagnosed. Perhaps because of the episodic and nonspecific nature of the symptoms, people may delay or not seek medical care. But permanent, fixed airway obstruction can develop long term without adequate asthma treatment. Once diagnosed, persistent asthma requires long-term control medications, which are available only by prescription. Recent data suggest that as many as 40% to 60% of patients with asthma are not on long-term control medications.[5] If unrecognized and inadequately treated, mild symptoms may potentially escalate quickly into serious, potentially life-threatening episodes. Therefore, it is critical that health care providers screen patients using nonprescription medications for asthmalike symptoms. Those who may need control asthma medications or do not have a confirmed diagnosis of asthma should be referred for further medical evaluation.

## Epidemiology of Asthma

An estimated 14.9 million people in the United States have asthma. The number of people with asthma increased over 100% between 1979-80 and 1993-94.[1] The asthma rate is increasing more rapidly in children than in adults.[1] Asthma is the second most common chronic disease in children.[6] A family history of asthma increases the risk of developing asthma, but those with atopy have an even greater risk of developing asthma.[6] Exposure to irritants

**Editor's Note:** This chapter is based, in part, on the 14th edition chapter with the same title, which was written by Dennis M. Williams and Timothy H. Self.

such as tobacco smoke and allergens early in life has also been shown to increase the incidence of asthma in children.[6]

Asthma more negatively affects some subsets of the population.[1] Children younger than than 5 years and women are more likely to be hospitalized for asthma. Nonwhite people are twice as likely to be hospitalized for or die from asthma despite similar asthma rates. Poverty also appears to be a factor in increasing disability and death rates, possibly because of inadequate access to health care, a greater exposure to environmental allergens and pollutants, and inadequate financial and other resources.[1]

## Anatomy and Physiology of the Respiratory System

The major role of the lungs is gas exchange; oxygen and carbon dioxide pass between the inspired air and the blood. The right lung has three lobes, and the left lung has two. The largest airway, the trachea, divides into bronchi for each lung. Progressive branching of the bronchi forms increasingly smaller bronchioles, terminal bronchioles, and finally the acinus, where gas exchange takes place.

Smooth muscle layers surround the airways, but as the diameter of the airways becomes smaller, the number of smooth muscle layers decreases. Stimulation of $\beta_2$-receptors in the smooth muscle results in bronchodilation and stimulation of cholinergic and $\alpha$-adrenergic receptors causes bronchoconstriction. Release of substance P and vasoactive intestinal peptide, (neuromediators from the noncholinergic, nonadrenergic nervous system) can also decrease airway diameter.

Numerous mucus-secreting goblet cells are intermixed throughout the pulmonary tree. Stimulation of the goblet cells by the vagal nerve increases mucus production. The purpose of mucus is to trap particulate matter from inhaled air. Small hairs lining the airways, called cilia, move the mucus toward the pharynx, thus keeping dust, bacteria, and other foreign matter out of the lower lungs.

The airflow and thus the relative diameter of the larger airways can be assessed by two spirometric tests: the forced expiratory volume at 1 second ($FEV_1$) and the peak expiratory flow (PEF). The $FEV_1$ measures the amount of air expired in the first second as the subject forcefully exhales from a maximum inspiration. More than one maneuver is usually performed to assess the consistency of the results. The PEF is similarly performed but it measures the amount of air expired in the first 10 milliseconds of the exhalation. As a result, it is less accurate and precise than the $FEV_1$, but the advantage of the PEF is that the equipment for the test is relatively inexpensive and portable. Also, less training is necessary to interpret the results. This makes PEF monitoring a suitable method for home assessment of asthma.

Values for PEF and $FEV_1$ are determined in part by the patient's age, gender, and height. A value greater than 80% of the predicted value is considered within normal limits. However, there is significant individual variation based on body type and ethnic background. Therefore, the optimal comparison measurement for the PEF and the one recommended for asthma self-care plans is the "personal best" PEF.[6] The personal best PEF is based on readings performed daily (in the early afternoon) over a 2-to-3-week period when a patient's asthma is well controlled. Variability in PEF is measured by comparing morning and afternoon readings.

## Etiology of Asthma

The exact etiology of asthma is unknown.[4] Asthma is commonly seen with concurrent atopy, which is a predisposition to produce abnormally high amounts of immunoglobulin E (IgE) after exposure to environmental allergens. There appears to be a genetic link to the risk of acquiring asthma, as a positive family history of asthma or atopy can increase the risk. The hygiene hypothesis proposes that the increased incidence of atopy in Western countries may be related to improvements in living conditions and general hygiene. The prevalence of atopy is noted to be greater in more affluent areas of developed countries and increases with smaller family sizes. A history of multiple respiratory infections early in life appears to decrease the risk of developing atopy and asthma later in life. Those with multiple siblings or who attend day care have a lower risk of developing asthma. The prevalence of atopy is also lower in populations who have contact with livestock and poultry (e.g., those who live on farms).

Atopy, however, may play a role in only 50% of those with asthma. There are also environmental risk factors. Smoking by the mother during pregnancy or exposure to secondhand smoke after birth increases the risk of asthma. It is unclear if smoking is a direct cause of asthma, but exposure to smoke can precipitate asthma symptoms, increase the rate of decline in lung function, and decrease the response to asthma therapy. A higher body mass index and obesity may also increase the risk of developing asthma. Severe viral respiratory infections in the first 3 years of life, and especially infections with respiratory syncytial viruses, may increase the risk of developing asthma and atopy.

Once asthma develops, various stimuli (often called "triggers"; Table 13-1) can precipitate asthma symptoms. There is considerable variability in triggers from person to person. Not all patients with asthma have the same triggers, and the response of an individual to a particular trigger can change over time. In addition to allergic rhinitis and tobacco smoking, gastroesophageal reflux disease (GERD), can cause airway hyperreactivity and therefore worsen asthma symptoms.

### *Allergic Rhinitis*

Because allergic rhinitis is an IgE-mediated atopic disease (see Chapter 11), it frequently is found in conjunction with asthma. Triggers for patients' allergy symptoms are often the same as for their asthma symptoms. Improving allergy symptoms may also improve upper airway hyperreactivity and asthma symptoms. Older nonprescription antihistamine labels (e.g., diphenhydramine) caution people with asthma against using these agents, because of their anticholinergic properties, which may thicken mucus and decrease mucociliary clearance. Newer antihistamines

**TABLE 13-1 Examples of Asthma Triggers**

| Environmental | Drugs/Chemicals | Conditions/Events |
|---|---|---|
| Cold air | β-Adrenergic blockers | Gastroesophageal reflux |
| House dust mites | Aspirin | Allergic rhinitis |
| Cockroaches | Nonsteroidal anti-inflammatory agents | Panic attacks |
| Animals (e.g., cats, dogs, rodents) | Food/drug preservatives (e.g., metabisulfite) | Menstruation/pregnancy |
| Indoor irritants (e.g., wood-burning stoves) | Seafood/shellfish | Viral respiratory infections |
| Outdoor air pollution (e.g., vehicle emissions, sulfur dioxide, ozone, nitrogen oxides) | Occupational exposure to dust/chemicals/irritants | Emotional stress/excitement |
| Indoor or outdoor molds/fungi | Household cleaning agents | Exercise |
| Tobacco smoke | Perfumes | |
| Pollens (e.g., grass, weeds, trees) | | |

(e.g., loratadine) do not have anticholinergic properties, and therefore no longer carry this labeling precaution.

### *Gastroesophageal Reflux Disease*

Gastroesophageal reflux disease is a potential trigger of asthma.[7] Approximately 77% of asthmatics report heartburn. The exact mechanism is unknown, but upper airway hyperreactivity can be increased in those with asthma and concurrent GERD. The risk of asthma-related hospitalization and the need for oral corticosteroid therapy is increased in patients with concurrent GERD. Studies have shown that more than half of patients with concomitant GERD and asthma respond well to proton pump inhibitor therapy. Pulmonary function has been shown to improve close to 30% in this population.[8] By using antacids and antisecretory medications to decrease GERD symptoms (see Chapter 14), asthma symptoms may improve significantly.

### *Tobacco Users*

Patients with asthma and their family members should be urged not to smoke. Environmental tobacco smoke not only directly irritates the lungs, it may also trigger asthma episodes. Studies have shown that lungs of smokers may be more reactive to triggers than those of nonsmokers. Mothers who smoke during pregnancy increase their children's risk of acquiring asthma.[9] Children exposed to tobacco smoke are more likely to develop asthma and have poorer control. Practitioners should educate all patients using tobacco products on options for cessation. Numerous options for nicotine replacement are available over the counter (see Chapter 50). All commercially available forms of nicotine replacement therapy (i.e., gum, transdermal patch, nasal spray, inhaler, and sublingual lozenges) may be effective as part of an overall tobacco cessation plan. However, prescription nicotine nasal spray and inhaler are not recommended for patients with asthma because inhaled nicotine could irritate the airway and trigger an episode.

### *Sensitivity to Nonsteroidal Anti-inflammatory Drugs*

Patients with asthma should be cautious about the use of nonprescription medications used to treat fever and/or pain and inflammation because of an increased risk of aspirin sensitivity (see Chapter 5). Symptoms from aspirin sensitivity can be severe and life-threatening and may include itchy or watery eyes, rash around the mouth, nasal congestion, hives, worsening asthma, cough or wheezing, anaphylaxis, and nasal polyps.[10] There is a significant potential for cross-sensitivity to other nonsteroidal anti-inflammatory agents (NSAIDs; e.g., ibuprofen, naproxen). If aspirin sensitivity is present, patients can usually tolerate acetaminophen. Aspirin is often a component of combination headache and pain relief nonprescription medications. Patients sensitive to aspirin should be cautioned about these "hidden sources" and to check the labels for all ingredients before using any product.

### *Food Allergies*

Some patients may insist that certain foods make them wheeze or experience shortness of breath. The confirmed incidence of adverse reactions to food is probably very small. Whether food allergies play a role in asthma is controversial.[11] Eggs and milk are the most common culprits, but others include wheat, soy, peanuts, fish, and shellfish. Some patients report an allergy to yellow dye and sulfite, an antioxidant sometimes used as a preservative. Questionnaires may help identify these triggers (see Nonpharmacologic Therapy). Even when the chemical or additive trigger is known, prospectively identifying and avoiding foods containing these compounds can be challenging. If patients need to avoid milk and other dairy products, they should be urged to take a calcium supplement to prevent osteoporosis later in life.

## Pathophysiology of Asthma

Asthma episodes were once thought to be caused mostly by airway bronchoconstriction. Now, it is recognized that while bronchoconstriction may be responsible for acute asthma symptoms, inflammation is largely responsible for severe and persistent asthma symptoms.[12]

Once a patient has been exposed to a trigger, an immediate or early asthmatic response occurs within minutes. The mechanism involves degranulation of mast cells to release histamine, eosinophil and neutrophil chemotactic factors, and leukotrienes, which cause smooth muscle constriction in the bronchioles. In atopic patients, IgE binding to the mast cells may cause the initial mediator release. As the airways narrow, the peak expiratory flow rate decreases. If clinically significant bronchoconstriction occurs, symptoms such as wheezing, chest tightness, and shortness of breath occur. Symptoms resolve spontaneously either with clearance of the mediators or after treatment with a bronchodilator.

If the mediators released recruit sufficient inflammatory cells, inflammation may occur several hours later. These inflammatory cells (eosinophils, neutrophils, and macrophages) release their own flood of mediators, causing microvascular leakage, airway edema, and increased mucus. This results in airway obstruction and the return of symptoms, decreasing the peak expiratory flow. If inflammation occurs, these symptoms often do not respond to treatment with bronchodilators and require anti-inflammatory medications.

Bronchial hyperresponsiveness (BHR) is an exaggerated airway bronchoconstriction and inflammation in response to triggers. BHR may develop with repeated trigger exposure in a susceptible person. Bronchial hyperresponsiveness can be expressed clinically as either frequent to continuous symptoms over a period of weeks (persistent asthma) or a significant worsening of asthma symptoms over several days (asthma exacerbations or episodes).

If untreated or undertreated, chronic inflammation can cause permanent airway remodeling. This process involves replacing injured tissue with scar tissue, an increase in smooth muscle, and increased mucus gland mass.[12] A fixed airway obstruction develops, and resulting symptoms are not responsive to treatment with either anti-inflammatory or bronchodilatory medications.[4,6]

Much is still not known about the pathophysiology of asthma. But what is known has affected the assessment of asthma episodes and approach to acute and chronic asthma treatment. Patients with persistent asthma can benefit by avoiding repeated trigger exposure or pretreating with medications before exposure to known triggers to prevent asthma episodes. Daily long-term control medications are used in persistent asthma to prevent chronic inflammation and airway remodeling. More severe symptoms, longer the duration of symptoms, and partial or poor response to bronchodilators imply that inflammation is likely present and anti-inflammatory medications are needed. As will be discussed in more detail later, only bronchodilator medications are available without a prescription. Therefore, a patient with asthma needs to recognize when significant airway inflammation is present and seek appropriate medical care.

## Signs and Symptoms of Asthma

Key features of asthma are recurrent bouts of wheezing, shortness of breath, chest tightness, and cough, especially at night and in the early morning hours. Asthma symptoms vary in duration, severity, and frequency (Table 13-2).

Other conditions can also present with wheezing and shortness of breath (Table 13-3). In assessing someone who presents with shortness of breath, it is important to inquire about the patient's past medical history for a prior diagnosis of asthma, tobacco use, and onset and duration of symptoms. It is also important to inquire about other associated signs (e.g., edema) or symptoms (e.g., feverishness). If the individual does not have a prior diagnosis of asthma or if the symptoms are different or more severe than usual, a medical referral is necessary for further evaluation.

## Complications of Asthma

Asthma is usually responsive to medications, however, complications can occur. Severe asthma episodes may require emergent care and systemic corticosteroids. Life-threatening episodes will require hospitalization, and possibly intubation, and mechanical ventilation. In very severe episodes, death can occur. Risk factors for death from asthma include a history of severe asthma episodes, previous intubation or admission to an intensive care unit for asthma, two or more hospitalizations or three or more emergency department visits for asthma within the past year, a hospitalization or emergency department visit within the past month, use or more than two canisters per month of inhaled short-acting $\beta_2$-agonist, a recent or current withdrawal from systemic corticosteroids, low socioeconomic status and urban residence, and illicit drug use.[6]

## Treatment of Asthma

Self-treatment of asthma is appropriate when a health care provider has made a prior diagnosis of mild, intermittent asthma, and the patient knows the warning symptoms indicating the need for urgent medical care (Figure 13-1). Nonprescription asthma medications are for short-term (<24 hours) treatment of moderate symptoms until the individual can be seen by a health care provider.

### *Treatment Goals*

Most patients realize that severe symptoms requiring the need for urgent medical care indicate uncontrolled asthma. Optimal therapy, however, implies that *all* goals allowing patients with asthma to live normal lives are met. Goals of successfully managing a patient's asthma include (1) achieving and maintaining control of the symptoms, a normal activity level, and pulmonary function as close to normal as possible; (2) preventing recurrent exacerbations and the need for urgent care visits; (3) providing optimal pharmacologic therapy with minimal or no adverse effects; (4) meeting the patient's and the family's expectations of asthma care; and (5) preventing mortality.[4,6]

Even relatively mild to moderate symptoms of asthma can significantly impair the quality of life not only of the

**TABLE 13-2 Classification Scheme for Asthma Exacerbations and Warning Symptoms[6]**

| | Mild | Moderate | Severe | Respiratory Arrest Imminent |
|---|---|---|---|---|
| **Symptoms** | | | | |
| Breathlessness | While walking; can lie down | While talking (infant: softer, shorter cry; difficulty feeding); sitting preferred | While at rest (infant: stops feeding); has to sit upright | |
| Talks in | Sentences | Phrases | Words | |
| Alertness | May be agitated | Usually agitated | Usually agitated | Drowsy or confused |
| **Signs** | | | | |
| Respiratory rate | Increased | Increased | Often >30/min | |
| Use of accessory muscles: suprasternal retractions | Usually not | Commonly | Usually | Paradoxical thoracoabdom inal movement |
| Wheeze | Moderate, often only end expiratory | Loud; throughout exhalation | Usually loud; throughout inhalation and exhalation | Absence of wheeze |
| Pulse/minute | <100 | 100-120 | >120 | Bradycardia |
| **Functional Assessment** | | | | |
| PEF | >80% | Approx. 50%-80% or response lasts <2 hours | <50% predicted or personal best | |

Key: PEF, peak expiratory flow.

**TABLE 13-3 Comparison of Selected Conditions That May Present with Shortness of Breath**

| | Asthma | Chronic Obstructive Pulmonary Disease | Respiratory Infection | Heart Failure |
|---|---|---|---|---|
| Signs | ↓ PEFR, ↑ heart rate, ↑ respiratory rate | Progressive decline in PEFR and $FEV_1$, polycythemia, signs of right heart failure, pulmonary hypertension, ↓ oxygen saturation, pursed lip breathing, ↑ heart rate, ↑ respiratory rate | ↑ Heart rate, ↑ respiratory rate, fever, ↑ white blood cell count | Ejection fraction <40%, lower extremity edema, $S_3$ heart sound, positive hepatojugular reflex, jugular venous distension |
| Symptoms | Wheezing, cough, chest tightness | Progressive dyspnea on exertion, productive cough, wheezing | Productive cough, nasal congestion, rhinorrhea | Dypsnea on exertion, orthopnea |
| Onset | Often occurs in childhood, but can develop in adults | Usually the forth or fifth decade of life, progressive, symptoms develop over years | Any age; symptoms acute, sudden | Older adults |
| Etiology | Often atopy | Most commonly tobacco smoking | Viruses, bacteria | Hypertension, coronary artery disease |
| Exacerbating factors | Trigger exposure | Continued smoking | | Heavy salt intake, myocardial infarction, nonadherence with medications |

Key: $FEV_1$, forced expiratory volume at 1 second; PEFR, peak expiratory flow rate.

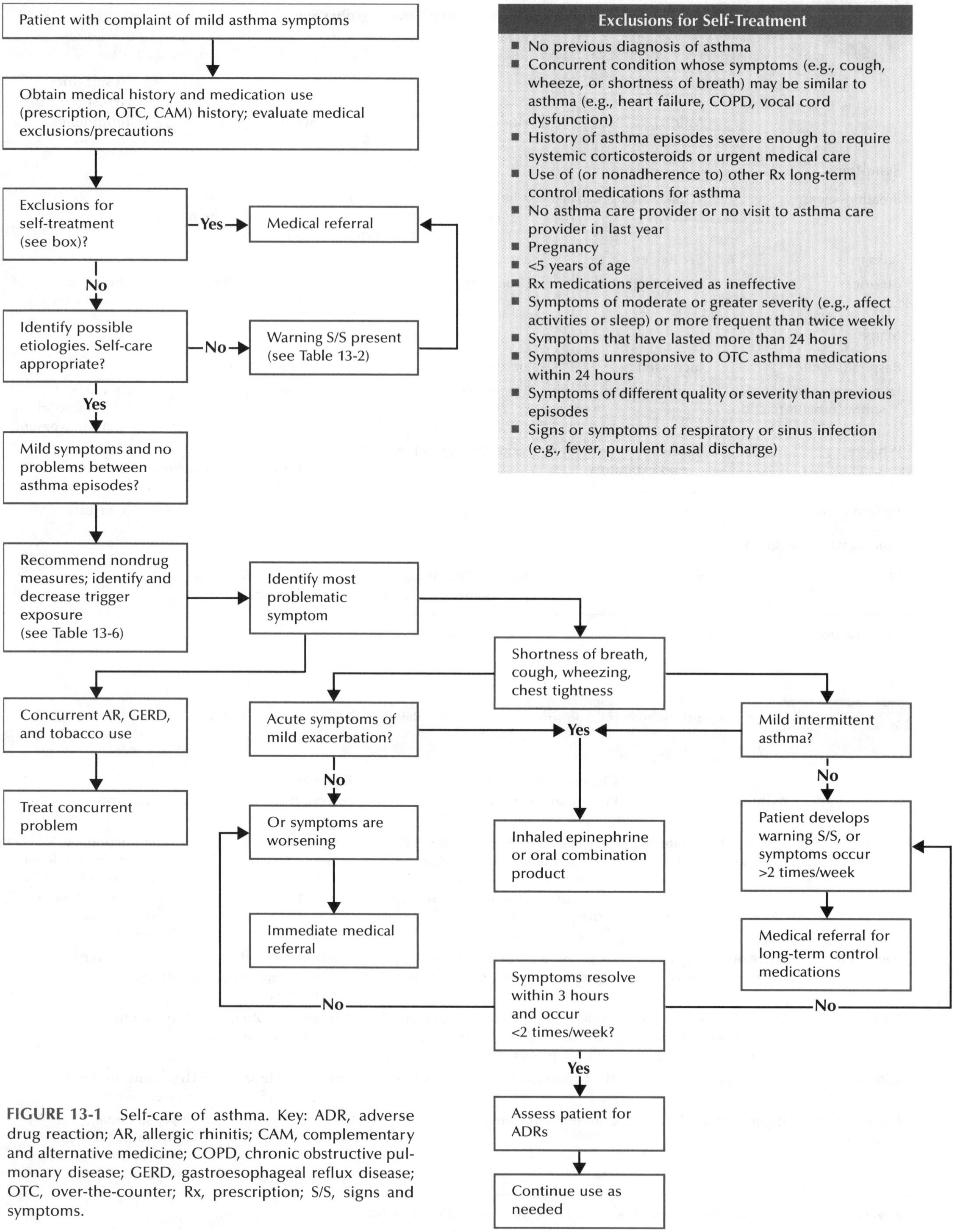


## Exclusions for Self-Treatment

- No previous diagnosis of asthma
- Concurrent condition whose symptoms (e.g., cough, wheeze, or shortness of breath) may be similar to asthma (e.g., heart failure, COPD, vocal cord dysfunction)
- History of asthma episodes severe enough to require systemic corticosteroids or urgent medical care
- Use of (or nonadherence to) other Rx long-term control medications for asthma
- No asthma care provider or no visit to asthma care provider in last year
- Pregnancy
- <5 years of age
- Rx medications perceived as ineffective
- Symptoms of moderate or greater severity (e.g., affect activities or sleep) or more frequent than twice weekly
- Symptoms that have lasted more than 24 hours
- Symptoms unresponsive to OTC asthma medications within 24 hours
- Symptoms of different quality or severity than previous episodes
- Signs or symptoms of respiratory or sinus infection (e.g., fever, purulent nasal discharge)

**FIGURE 13-1** Self-care of asthma. Key: ADR, adverse drug reaction; AR, allergic rhinitis; CAM, complementary and alternative medicine; COPD, chronic obstructive pulmonary disease; GERD, gastroesophageal reflux disease; OTC, over-the-counter; Rx, prescription; S/S, signs and symptoms.

patient, but also of the family and any caregivers. Unfortunately, because of common misperceptions about asthma and medications, a certain level of chronic symptoms may be accepted as part of having asthma. Patients may not consciously recognize that their awareness of asthma unnecessarily restricts their activities (e.g., not participating in competitive sports). Asthma episodes not only disrupt the lifestyle of the patient and family, but are potentially a source of significant stress. One major source of stress is deciding when and if asthma symptoms are severe enough to require emergent medical care. Some patients seek urgent care because they do not know how to treat asthma episodes effectively. In other cases, fatal asthma episodes could be prevented if care had been sought sooner. Because most patients' asthma is readily responsive to available medications, it is important to understand that frequent symptoms (even mild ones) can and should be prevented. Patients with asthma also need to be confident that when symptoms do occur, they can prevent escalation into significant asthma episodes.

### General Treatment Approach

The treatment of asthma is individualized on the basis of the patient's triggers and symptoms. A comprehensive, individualized *asthma self-care plan* would include when to use long-term control medications and quick-relief medications, how to use asthma devices to optimally deliver medications, how to avoid and minimize affects of asthma triggers, how to prevent the escalation of asthma symptoms into serious asthma episodes, and how to recognize warning signs of asthma that require emergent medical treatment (Figure 13-1). The plan also would include specific guidelines regarding when to use quick-relief medications (e.g., before exposure to known triggers) and how much to use (e.g., two puffs every 2 hours.) Figure 13-2 is an example of a symptom-based asthma self-care plan. Some self-care plans may also include recommendations for treatment based on the patient's personal best PEF value.

Inhaled medications are often used for asthma because of enhanced local effects, with fewer adverse reactions than if the medication was administered systemically. However, the effectiveness of inhaled medications can be severely limited when poor device technique decreases drug delivery to the lungs. Inhaled corticosteroids are the preferred long-term control agents because their anti-inflammatory properties are more effective in preventing asthma symptoms. Inhaled corticosteroids may also prevent long-term airway obstruction. Interested readers are referred to the guidelines from the Global Initiative for Asthma[4] and the National Asthma Education Prevention Program[6] for detailed discussions of the therapeutic options and rationale for the treatment of asthma in adults and children.

The severity of asthma episodes is assessed on the basis of symptom severity (Table 13-4).[13] It is important that patients with asthma know to monitor for worsening control of persistent asthma and identify the onset of acute asthma episodes. A drop in PEF can be the first sign of an impending episode and may precede the onset of significant symptoms. Patients with moderate to severe persistent asthma or a history of a severe asthma episode should have an asthma self-care plan, which provides guidance for treating their symptoms with medication and when to seek immediate medical attention. Early treatment with systemic anti-inflammatory agents may prevent the progression of asthma episodes and decrease the need for emergency department visits and hospitalizations for asthma.

### Nonpharmacologic Therapy

As exposure to triggers can lead to worsening asthma symptoms and each patient's asthma triggers are different, a comprehensive, individualized trigger management plan should be developed. If patients are unfamiliar with their specific triggers, a screening tool can be used to help identify them (Table 13-5). Once triggers are identified, suggestions are incorporated into the self-care plan to minimize exposure to them at home, work, or school (see Chapter 11).

### Pharmacologic Therapy

Asthma medications are categorized into two groups. *Quick-relief medications* are used as needed to treat symptoms. In this group, short-acting β-agonists and ipratropium or bronchodilators and systemic corticosteroids (e.g., prednisone) are used in moderate to severe asthma episodes to treat inflammation. *Long-term control medications* are used daily to prevent symptoms. These agents either interfere with the inflammatory cascade (e.g., inhaled corticosteroids [fluticasone] and leukotriene modifiers [montelukast]) or long-acting bronchodilators (e.g., salmeterol, formoterol.) In addition, β-agonists and mast cell stabilizers (e.g., cromolyn) can be used prior to exposure to a patient's known triggers (e.g., exercise, cigarette smoke) to prevent symptoms. All patients with asthma should have a quick-relief medication available. Those with persistent asthma, regardless of severity, should take a daily long-term control medication.

Few nonprescription medications have been approved to treat asthma. Because of its chronic and potentially serious nature, all patients with moderate to severe persistent asthma should be followed closely by a primary care practitioner. All nonprescription medications contain bronchodilators. None of these medications has anti-inflammatory activity. Therefore, nonprescription medications are generally indicated for mild intermittent symptoms only and are not appropriate for use as long-term control medications.

#### Bronchodilators

Two nonselective β-agonists, epinephrine and ephedrine, are available as nonprescription products. The dosage and administration guidelines for these agents are included in Table 13-6.[14-16] Because nonselective β-agonists also act on α-receptors, they can constrict blood vessels and increase blood pressure. By acting on $\beta_1$-receptors they can increase heart rate, presenting a potential for arrhythmias, nervousness, and palpitations. The duration of action of the nonprescription β-agonists is shorter than that of their

St.Louis Regional **Asthma Consortium**

Sponsored by the American Lung Association of Eastern Missouri

# ASTHMA ACTION PLAN

Name: ______________________

Provider: ______________________

Date: ______________________

Phone for doctor or clinic: ______________________

After office hours call: ______________________

## GREEN ZONE

- Breathing is good
- No cough or wheeze
- Can work and play

**YOU'RE OK! TAKE ALL OF THESE MEDICATIONS EVERY DAY!**

| Medicine | How much to take | When to take it |
|---|---|---|
| | | |
| | | |
| | | |
| | | |

20 minutes before physical activity, use this medicine: ______________________

## YELLOW ZONE

- You are feeling sick or it's harder to breathe

**CAUTION! TAKE 2 PUFFS (OR 1 NEBULIZER TREATMENT) OF YOUR QUICK RELIEVER MEDICINE NOW: ______________________**
**YOU MAY REPEAT THIS EVERY 20 MINUTES FOR 2 MORE TIMES.**
**IF YOU ARE NO BETTER CALL YOUR DOCTOR IMMEDIATELY AT ______________________!**

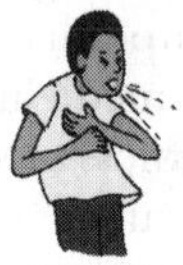

Cough

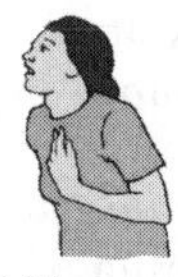

Wheeze

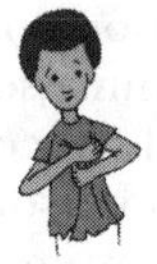

Tight chest

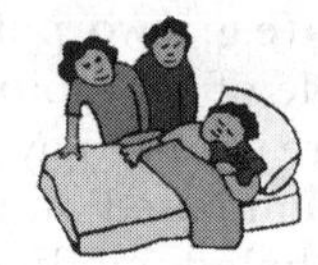

Wake up at night

| Medicine | How much to take | When to take it |
|---|---|---|
| | | |
| | | |

## RED ZONE

**DANGER!**
**TAKE 4 MORE PUFFS (OR 1 NEBULIZER TREATMENT) OF YOUR QUICK RELIEVER MEDICINE NOW.**
**CALL 9-1-1 OR GO DIRECTLY TO THE NEAREST HOSPITAL!**

- Medicine is not helping
- Breathing is hard and fast
- Nose opens wide
- Can't walk or talk well
- Ribs show

| Medicine | How much to take | When to take it |
|---|---|---|
| | | |
| | | |
| | | |

**FIGURE 13-2** Sample action plan for asthma. (Reprinted with the permission of the St. Louis Regional Asthma Consortium.)

TABLE 13-4 **Treatment Approach for Managing Asthma in Adults and Children Older than 5 Years of Age**[13]

| Classification | Symptoms | Lung Function | Preferred Therapy |
|---|---|---|---|
| Step 4<br>Severe persistent | Continual symptoms *or* limited physical activity *or*<br>frequent exacerbations *or* frequent nighttime symptoms | $FEV_1$ predicted *or* PEFR <60% personal best *or*<br>PEFR variability >30% | High-dose inhaled corticosteroid *and* long-acting β-agonist *and*, if needed, systemic corticosteroid<br>Short-acting bronchodilator: inhaled $\beta_2$-agonists as needed for symptoms |
| Step 3<br>Moderate persistent | Daily symptoms *or* daily use of inhaled short-acting β-agonists *or* that affect activity *or* exacerbations more than twice weekly; may last days *or* nighttime symptoms more than 1 time a week | $FEV_1$ predicted *or* PEFR 60%-80% personal best<br>*or*<br>PEFR variability >30% | Low- to medium-dose inhaled corticosteroids *and* long-acting β-agonist<br>Short-acting bronchodilator: inhaled $\beta_2$-agonists as needed for symptoms |
| Step 2<br>Mild persistent | Symptoms more than twice weekly but not daily *or* exacerbations may affect activity or nighttime symptoms more than twice monthly | $FEV_1$ predicted *or* PEFR >80% personal best *or*<br>PEFR variability 20%-30% | Low-dose inhaled corticosteroid<br>Short-acting bronchodilator: inhaled $\beta_2$-agonists as needed for symptoms |
| Step 1<br>Mild intermittent | Symptoms less than twice weekly *and* asymptomatic and normal PEF between exacerbations *and* exacerbations brief (from a few hours to a few days) intensity may vary *and* nighttime symptoms less than twice monthly | $FEV_1$ predicted *or*<br>PEFR is more than 80% personal best *and*<br>PEFR variability <20% | No daily control medication needed<br>Short-acting bronchodilator: inhaled $\beta_2$-agonists as needed for symptoms |

Key: $FEV_1$, forced expiratory volume at 1 second; PEF, peak expiratory flow; PEFR, peak expiratory flow rate.

*Notes:* Asthma severity is assigned to the most severe step in which *any* feature occurs. Sustained-release theophylline to serum concentration of 5-15 μg/mL may be used as an alternative therapy to inhaled corticosteroid in step 2 or replace the long-acting β-agonist in step 3.

prescription counterparts. Generally, nonprescription $\beta_2$-agonists have to be taken more frequently and have more potential side effects than similar prescription medications.

## Combination Bronchodilator Products

Because of the significant morbidity and mortality from asthma, effective treatment of persistent asthma requires prescription anti-inflammatory medications for long-term control. Thus, the role for nonprescription agents is very limited. Table 13-6 contains a description of selected nonprescription combination, oral bronchodilator products that are available. Systemic absorption of oral products gives them a greater potential for side effects than inhaled medications. The other agent often included in these combination products is guaifenesin, which is an expectorant (see Chapter 12). Because most patients with asthma do not have a productive cough, guaifenesin is usually unnecessary.

## Product Selection Guidelines

### *Special Populations*

Patients of Advanced Age Older patients should be strongly cautioned against self-treating with nonprescription asthma medications. This population is at increased risk of cardiovascular adverse effects of both inhaled and systemic bronchodilators. The older patient population may also have multiple concomitant problems that mimic some of the symptoms of asthma. If an elderly person complains of a new-onset breathing problem, a referral should be made for accurate diagnosis. These symptoms should be investigated in an effort to rule out other causes of shortness of breath such as congestive heart failure, pneumonia, and chronic obstructive pulmonary disease (Table 13-3). Arthritis and impaired vision may make it difficult for elderly people to use devices for delivering asthma medications. Only a small percentage of active drug is delivered even when these devices are used correctly, so poor administration technique may decrease drug delivery and effectiveness. A typical solution is to have these patients use nebulizers to deliver their medications.

Pregnant Patients Pregnant women with asthma should be urged not to use nonprescription medications. These women should be closely followed by a health care provider because poorly controlled asthma can worsen outcomes of the pregnancy. Ephedrine and epinephrine are both Pregnancy Category C drugs.[17,18] Epinephrine should be avoided during pregnancy because of its α-adrenergic effects. Inhaled prescription bronchodilators are preferred because localized delivery and selective $\beta_2$-adrenergic activity limits fetal drug exposure.

Children Not all children who wheeze or cough have asthma. Children who present with a chronic cough but do not have a diagnosis of asthma should be referred for further investigation.[19] Practitioners providing care for school-aged children should be familiar with local laws that may allow children to carry and administer asthma medications while

**TABLE 13-5 Sample Trigger-screening Tool***

Thinking about how you have felt in the past month, please answer the following questions:

- Do you ever have problems wheezing or catching your breath when exposed to cold air?
- Do you wheeze when dusting, vacuuming, or using cleaning solvents in the home?
- Do you wheeze, cough, sneeze, or become short of breath when around household pets such as cats or dogs?
- Do you have problems breathing when exposed to high levels of stress or excitement?
- Have you ever noticed wheezing or worsening shortness of breath before or during your menstrual period?
- Have you ever had a reaction such as shortness of breath, swollen throat, lips, or tongue after you took drugs such as aspirin or ibuprofen?
- Do you have breathing problems after eating shellfish or any other foods?
- Does it take you a long time to get over a viral cold?
- Do you have chronic heartburn?
- Do you have problems breathing at work, yet are fine during holidays or weekends spent at home? Does anyone else at work appear to have similar symptoms?
- Do you typically have a runny nose, watery eyes, and experience repetitive sneezing, during outdoor activities? Are these symptoms worse during
  - early spring?
  - late spring?
  - late summer to fall?
  - summer and fall?
- Do you experience shortness of breath during or after exercise?

If you answered yes to any of the above questions, please show this questionnaire to your health care provider.

* See Chapter 11 for further information on allergy triggers.

at school. Children old enough (commonly 8 to 10 years old) to understand how to use their quick-relief medications should be encouraged to carry them. This allows them to promptly respond to asthma symptoms and minimize asthma episodes when away from home. Written permission of the parents and practitioner may be required for children to carry their medications at school. The school nurse should also have a copy of each child's asthma self-care plan, enabling her or him to respond appropriately to acute asthma exacerbations that may develop. Student athletes should check with school administrators before self-administering nonprescription asthma medications. The ingredient ephedrine is banned from use by NCAA athletes,[20] and stimulants are banned from use by Olympic athletes.

*Patient Preferences* Patients with persistent asthma should be on a long-term control medication to prevent symptoms and long-term complications. Optimal therapy involves selecting the most effective medication and the best medication delivery system. Inhaled delivery systems are generally preferred to minimize systemic absorption and side effects such as increased heart rate, anxiety, and tremor. Administering medication by metered-dose inhaler is usually less expensive than by nebulizer and does not require special equipment. But metered-dose-inhalers are bulkier and can be cumbersome and difficult to use correctly compared with oral tablets (Table 13-7). Nebulizers do not require breath holding to deliver drugs and can be used with a facial mask to administer medications to even young children. Nebulizer treatments usually last 10 to 15 minutes, and the equipment should be meticulously cleaned to decrease the risk of infection. People may prefer oral medications (despite the risk of increased side effects) because tablets are more portable and do not require special equipment. Other patients (e.g., patients of advanced age, those with arthritis, or young children) may prefer oral medications because of relative ease of administration.

### Complementary and Alternative Therapies

People with chronic diseases often look for alternatives to recognized Western medicines. There are little data supporting the efficacy of complementary and alternative medicine (CAM) for asthma, but these modalities appear to be popular among patients with asthma and allergies. In a recent survey, the most popular modalities were herbalism, aroma therapy, homeopathy, acupuncture, acupressure, massage, and reflexology.[21] Other forms of CAM may include acupuncture and chiropractic manipulation.[22,23] The overall efficacy of CAM was evaluated as good to very good in 83% of people using them. Compared with the efficacy of conventional therapy, the effect of CAM was considered to be equal or greater by 62%.[21] Practitioners should therefore ask patients with asthma if they are using any form of CAM.

The use of herbal products is currently on the rise in the United States.[24] Populations along the United States–Mexico border show the highest rates of herbal product use. These agents can be classified into three groups based on their effects for asthma: agents that have minimal pharmacologic effect, agents that have potentially beneficial effects, and agents that should be avoided because of increased risk of harmful effects (Table 13-8). Vitamin A, vitamin E, vitamin C, selenium, magnesium, fish oil, and select omega-3 fatty acids have minimal documented physiologic effects for asthma and therefore should not be recommended. Of the herbal products, only ma huang has documented benefits,[25,26] but it also has significant potential for toxicity because of its nonselective activity at adrenergic receptors, and therefore should not be recommended.

## Assessment of Asthma: A Case-based Approach

To correctly assess whether a patient's breathing problems may be self-treatable, the practitioner needs to gather information from the patient regarding signs and symptoms and duration of the problem, and assess whether the patient meets criteria for self-treatment (Figure 13-1). Other disease states with signs and symptoms similar to those of asthma should be ruled out (Table 13-3). The

TABLE 13-6 Medications Included in Nonprescription Medications for the Treatment of Asthma[14-16]

| Drug | Mechanism | Dosage and Administration | Safety Considerations |
|---|---|---|---|
| Epinephrine (e.g., Primatene Mist Inhaler) | Bronchodilator | Adults and children >4 years of age: 1 puff at onset of symptoms, repeated in 1 minute if symptoms are not relieved; do not use again for 3 hours | Seek medical assistance if symptoms not relieved or worsen in 20 minutes<br>Adverse drug reactions: increased heart rate, arrhythmias, and nervousness<br>Do not use with concomitant MAOI therapy<br>Contraindications: pregnancy, cardiac arrhythmias, coronary insufficiency, poorly controlled hypertension, and uncontrolled hyperthyroidism, seizures, hypokalemia, angina, hyperglycemia |
| Racepinephrine (e.g., microNefrin) | Bronchodilator | Adults and children 4 years and older: microNefrin containing 2.25% racepinephrine HCl (1.125% epinephrine base)<br>Add 0.5 mL (10 drops) racepinephrine into nebulizer reservoir; add 3 mL diluent; administer for 15 minutes every 3-4 hours | Relative contraindications: pregnancy, hyperthyroid, hypertension, heart disease, "on other medications" (prescription, nonprescription, or herbal therapy)<br>Do not use if brown or cloudy |
| Ephedrine (e.g., Primatene tablets) | Bronchodilator | Not to exceed 150 mg in 24 hours | Palpitations, tachycardia, arrhythmias, seizures, hypokalemia, angina, hyperglycemia, hypotension, hypertension |
| Guaifenesin (e.g., Bronkaid Dual Action Formula) | Expectorant | Adults and children >12 years old: 1 tablet by mouth q4h as needed (max. daily dosage: 24 caplets) | Case reports have linked nephrolithiasis to guaifenesin alone and in combination with ephedrine |
| Ephedrine–guaifenesin combination products | Bronchodilator + expectorant | Bronkaid Dual Action Formula: ephedrine 25 mg; guaifenesin 400 mg; 1 tablet q4h as needed (max. daily dosage: 6 tablets)<br>Primatene tablets: ephedrine 12.5 mg; guaifenesin 200 mg; 2 tablets q4h as needed (max. daily dosage: 12 tablets)<br>Mini Two Way Action Tablets: ephedrine 12.5 mg, guaifenesin 200 mg; 1-2 tablets q4h as needed (max. daily dosage: 12 tablets)<br>Dynafed Asthma Relief Tablets: ephedrine 25 mg, guaifenesin 200 mg; 1/2-1 tablet q4h as needed (max. daily dosage: 6 tablets)<br>Mini Two Way Action Tablets: ephedrine 25 mg, guaifenesin 200 mg; 1/2-1 tablet q4h as needed (max. daily dosage: 6 tablets per day) | See above |

Key: MAOI, monoamine oxidase inhibitor.

practitioner should also inquire about the current use of prescription medications, nonprescription medications, and complementary therapies and dietary habits before recommending a nonprescription agent for asthma. Cases 13-1 and 13-2 give examples of assessment of patients with asthma.

## Patient Counseling for Asthma

The importance of educating patients with asthma cannot be stressed enough. Since even those with mild asthma can have moderate to severe asthma episodes, all patients with asthma must know how to self-monitor and recognize symptoms, and know the proper action to take if symptoms do not respond to quick-relief medications.[27] Practitioners should assess each patient's readiness to learn about asthma, and identify and understand misconceptions and any individualized goals patients with asthma may have. Any individual concerns or fears about asthma or asthma medications should be elicited and addressed.

### *Asthma Self-Care Plans*

Asthma self-care plans (Figure 13-2) are written instructions detailing how to manage both chronic and acute

## TABLE 13-7 Guidelines for Using MDIs

### Closed-mouth Technique

1. Remove dust cap from inhaler. Attach inhaler to spacer/holding chamber if you have one. Shake the inhaler well as shown in drawing A.
2. Blow out all the air in your lungs (see drawing B).
3. Seal lips tightly around the mouthpiece. As you breathe in slowly, press down on the inhaler to release the medicine until your lungs are full (see drawing C).
4. Hold your breath for 10 seconds to allow the medicine to reach deeply into your lungs (see drawing D).
5. Blow out the air in your lungs (see drawing E).

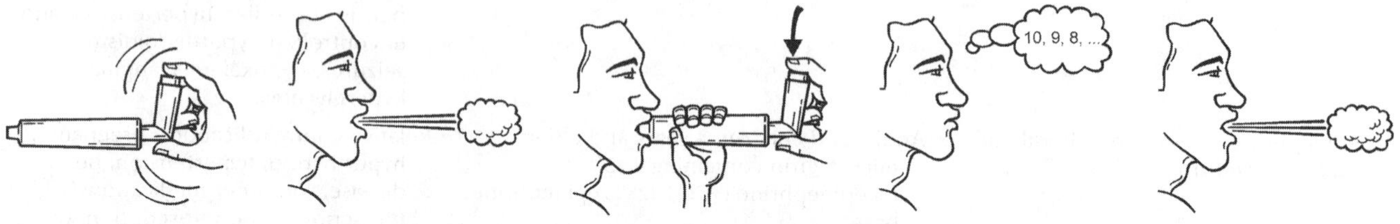


A B C D E

### Open-mouth Technique

1. Take off the cap. Shake the inhaler as shown in drawing F.
2. Stand up and tilt your head back a little (see drawing G).
3. Place your hand between your mouth and the inhaler as shown in drawing H to measure how far away the inhaler should be from your mouth.
4. Take a cleansing breath; in and out.
5. Open your mouth wide; start to breathe in slowly; push down on the inhaler; while continuing to breathe in (see drawing I).
6. Hold your breath; count to 10; then breathe out.
7. If your asthma care plan instructs you to use 2 puffs, wait 1 minute and repeat steps 1-6.

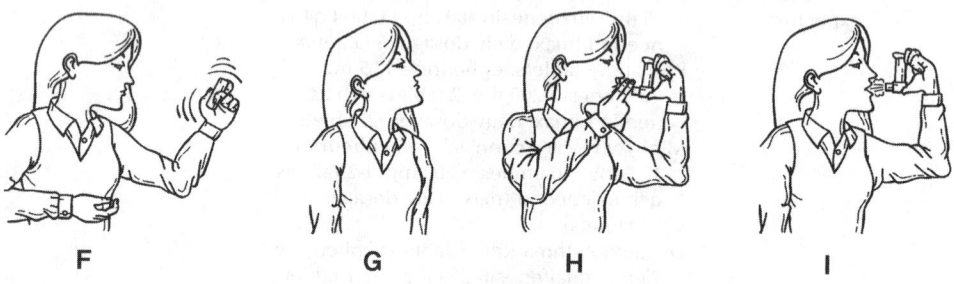

F G H I

## TABLE 13-8 Alternative Agents That May Worsen Asthma Symptoms or Cause Significant Harm[24]

| Agent | Risk |
|---|---|
| Coffee, black tea | Increased risk of hospitalization for acute asthma |
| Cinnamon, canela (tea), essential oil (from the bark) | Can be neurotoxic if ingested |
| Eucalyptus | Essential oil can be toxic if ingested, causing respiratory distress and neurologic symptoms |
| Oregano tea | May contain inhalant allergens |
| Cayenne, chile (active ingredient is capsaicin) | Single use may aggravate acute asthma episodes; bronchoconstriction possible if powder is inhaled |

## CASE 13-1

| Relevant Evaluation Criteria | Scenario/Model Outcome |
|---|---|
| **Information Gathering** | |
| 1. Gather essential information about the patient's symptoms, including: | |
| a. description of symptom(s) (i.e., nature, onset, duration, severity, associated symptoms) | Patient describes wheezing and chest tightness after playing soccer every Thursday afternoon with his friends on the college quadrangle. He states he has had these types of symptoms since he was a child, but hasn't experienced an episode since high school. The wheezing usually starts within 30 minutes of playing and lasts until he rests and goes indoors. He has never been hospitalized or needed an emergency department visit for these symptoms and has never taken oral corticosteroids. |
| b. description of any factors that seem to precipitate, exacerbate, and/or relieve the patient's symptom(s) | Patient's symptoms are always in conjunction with exercise, and are often relieved spontaneously on going indoors, drinking plenty of fluids, and resting. |
| c. description of the patient's efforts to relieve the symptoms | Rest; water; going indoors |
| 2. Gather essential patient history information: | |
| a. patient's identity | Josh Williams |
| b. age, sex, height, and weight | 19 y/o M, 6'1", 185 lb |
| c. patient's occupation | Full-time college student; has not missed any classes |
| d. patient's dietary habits | Eats in the college dormitory cafeteria three meals per day + one mid-day snack |
| e. patient's sleep habits | Sleeps 7 hours/night; reports feeling rested and denies daytime drowsiness |
| f. concurrent medical conditions, prescription and nonprescription medications, and dietary supplements | Elidel for eczema; Claritin OTC 10 mg daily as needed for allergic rhinitis; One A Day Men's multivitamin; no herbal products or alternative therapies |
| g. allergies | Penicillin (hives) |
| h. history of other adverse reactions to medications | N/A |
| i. other (describe)_______ | No runny nose or congestion if he takes his Claritin; no tobacco use |
| **Assessment and Triage** | |
| 3. Differentiate the patient's signs/symptoms and correctly identify the patient's primary problem(s) (see Tables 13-2 and 13-3). | Mild intermittent asthma triggered by exercise |
| 4. Identify exclusions for self-treatment (see Figure 13-1). | None |
| 5. Formulate a comprehensive list of therapeutic alternatives for the primary problem to determine if triage to a medical practitioner is required, and share this information with the patient. | Options include:<br>(1) Recommend nonprescription Primatene Mist inhaler before soccer.<br>(2) Recommend nonprescription Primatene Mist inhaler as needed for signs and symptoms of wheezing and chest tightness.<br>(3) Recommend oral nonprescription combination product as needed for wheezing and chest tightness.<br>(4) Refer Josh to his practitioner for follow-up or adequate diagnosis.<br>(5) Refer Josh to practitioner for prescription quick relief medication as an alternative to Primatene Mist.<br>(6) Refer Josh to his practitioner for a prescription agent to use prior to trigger exposure (e.g., cromolyn).<br>(7) Refer Josh to his practitioner for a prescription long-term control medication (e.g., inhaled corticosteroid).<br>(8) Take no action. |

CASE 13-1 (continued)

| Relevant Evaluation Criteria | Scenario/Model Outcome |
|---|---|
| **Plan** | |
| 6. Select an optimal therapeutic alternative to address the patient's problem, taking into account patient preferences. | The patient would prefer not to see a PCP at this time. His primary doctor is over 200 miles away from college and would prefer not to wait in line at the college's Student Health Services. Josh would prefer a nonprescription alternative. Primatene Mist inhaler can prevent symptoms if taken before activity and treat his symptoms of wheezing and chest tightness should they occur after soccer. |
| 7. Describe the recommended therapeutic approach to the patient. | Take Primatene Mist OTC inhaler, 1 puff as needed 15 minutes before soccer *and* 1 puff as needed for chest tightness and wheezing. You may repeat the dose once, but then do not use again for 3 hours. |
| 8. Explain to the patient the rationale for selecting the recommended therapeutic approach from the considered therapeutic alternatives. | Seeking a PCP, that is, primary care provider, may not be necessary if your mild symptoms can be controlled with this therapy. However, you should discuss your symptoms with your PCP at the next visit.<br>It usually takes less medication to prevent symptoms than to treat symptoms once they occur. It is better to use the inhaled route of medication than oral because of the decreased chance of side effects. |
| **Patient Education** | |
| 9. When recommending self-care with nonprescription medications and/or nondrug therapy, convey accurate information to the patient, including: | |
| a. appropriate dose and frequency of administration | 1 puff as needed 15 minutes before soccer *and* 1 puff as needed for chest tightness and wheezing. You may repeat dose once, but do not use again for 3 hours. |
| b. maximum number of days the therapy should be employed | You can use this medication long term as long as you don't need more than two doses per week. If symptoms increase in frequency, see PCP. |
| c. product administration procedures | See Figure 13-2. |
| d. expected time to onset of relief | Inhaler should adequately prevent symptoms for up to 1-2 hours (taken before exercise) and provide relief within 3-5 minutes if symptoms occur. |
| e. degree of relief that can reasonably be expected | Adequate prevention and relief from acute symptoms of wheezing and chest tightness are expected. |
| f. most common side effects | Increased heart rate, tremor, nervousness, insomnia |
| g. side effects that warrant medical intervention should they occur | Palpitations, irregular heart beat |
| h. patient options in the event that condition worsens or persists | Seek medical help if you experience an increase in frequency or severity of symptoms, or symptoms no longer respond to therapy. |
| i. product storage requirements | Store at room temperature 68°F to 77°F. Do not store near open flame or heat above 120°F. |
| j. specific nondrug measures | Warm up and cool down at least 15 minutes before and after exercise. |
| 10. Solicit follow-up questions from patient. | Should I continue to take my OTC Claritin tablet while using this inhaler? |
| 11. Answer patient's questions. | Yes. The Claritin may actually help prevent symptoms of wheezing, chest tightness because allergy symptoms may worsen asthma symptoms in some people. |

Key: N/A, no available; OTC, over-the-counter; PCP, primary care provider.

symptoms. Written self-care plans are recommended for all patients with moderate to severe persistent asthma and those with a history of severe exacerbations. Self-care plans are developed with a health care practitioner and help encourage communication and partnership between individuals and their providers. The self-care plans are concise and easily understandable written directions meant to empower the asthma patient to take charge of his or her own health.

Self-care plans allow patients to make decisions regarding when to seek medical care, whether or not attending work or school is appropriate, and when to seek immediate medical attention. Typically, self-care plans are divided into several "sections" or "zones." Typically the green zone

## CASE 13-2

| Relevant Evaluation Criteria | Scenario/Model Outcome |
|---|---|
| **Information Gathering** | |
| 1. Gather essential information about the patient's symptoms, including: | |
| a. description of symptom(s) (i.e., nature, onset, duration, severity, associated symptoms) | Patient complains of acute symptoms of wheezing, dyspnea, and cough. These episodes are making her anxious because they are occurring more and more frequently; currently 3 times a week. |
| b. description of any factors that seem to precipitate, exacerbate, and/or relieve the patient's symptom(s) | Episodes seem to be worse after work and while waiting for the bus. Symptoms in the past have been relieved with OTC inhaled epinephrine, but no longer respond with the same effectiveness; symptoms sometimes return the same day. No foods make it worse. |
| c. description of the patient's efforts to relieve the symptoms | OTC Primatene Mist Inhaler 3-4 puffs 3 times a week for 2 years |
| 2. Gather essential patient history information: | |
| a. patient's identity | Rosalyn Market |
| b. age, weight, sex, and height | 24 y/o F, 179 lb, 5'3" |
| c. patient's occupation | Works part-time at a local dry cleaning company |
| d. patient's dietary habits | Three meals a day; lunch consists of a "diet shake." |
| e. patient's sleep habits | Reports 8 hours sleep/night; for the past few months, reports waking up at night twice a week because of coughing fits |
| f. concurrent medical conditions, prescription and nonprescription medications, and dietary supplements | Sumatriptan 100 mg 1 tablet by mouth as needed at onset of migraine headache; OTC Primatene Mist inhaler 3-4 puffs 3 times a week; "diet shakes" (dietary supplement) for lunch |
| g. allergies | NKDA |
| h. history of other adverse reactions to medications | N/A |
| i. other (describe)_______ | (-) heartburn; (-) allergic rhinitis; (-) tobacco use; (-) pregnant |
| **Assessment and Triage** | |
| 3. Differentiate the patient's signs/symptoms and correctly identify the patient's primary problem(s) (see Tables 13-2 and 13-3). | Episodes of shortness of breath, wheezing, chest tightness, and cough could be consistent with asthma. The frequency of Rosalyn's symptoms is consistent with moderate persistent asthma, but she does not have a previous diagnosis. |
| 4. Identify exclusions for self-treatment (see Figure 13-1). | Possibly undiagnosed moderate persistent asthma; symptoms no longer responsive to OTC nonselective β-agonist |
| 5. Formulate a comprehensive list of therapeutic alternatives for the primary problem to determine if triage to a medical practitioner is required, and share this information with the patient. | Options include:<br>(1) Refer patient to health care provider for diagnosis and if asthma is present, patient will require a prescription long-term control medication.<br>(2) Continue OTC Primatene Mist Inhaler.<br>(3) Start nonprescription oral combination product.<br>(4) Take no action. |
| **Plan** | |
| 6. Select an optimal therapeutic alternative to address the patient's problem, taking into account patient preferences. | Refer patient to health care provider for accurate diagnosis and appropriate prescription therapy. |
| 7. Describe the recommended therapeutic approach to the patient. | You should see your primary care provider about this condition. |

| CASE 13-2 (continued) | |
|---|---|
| **Relevant Evaluation Criteria** | **Scenario/Model Outcome** |
| 8. Explain to the patient the rationale for selecting the recommended therapeutic approach from the considered therapeutic alternatives. | It is possible your symptoms are not asthma. If you do have asthma you may need prescription medications to adequately control your symptoms. |
| **Patient Education** | |
| 9. When recommending self-care with nonprescription medications and/or nondrug therapy, convey accurate information to the patient. | Criterion does not apply in this case. |
| 10. Solicit follow-up questions from patient. | Couldn't I just use more of the OTC inhaler instead? |
| 11. Answer patient's questions. | No. Increasing the amount or frequency of use of the inhaler will not be helpful and could increase your chance of experiencing adverse drug effects including heart palpitations, tremor, anxiety, insomnia, and nervousness to name a few. Asthma can be controlled so that symptoms do not interfere with your sleep and daily activities. Inadequately treated asthma is potentially dangerous. Severe episodes may require hospitalization. |

Key: N/A, not applicable; NKA, no known allergies; OTC, over-the-counter.

focuses on what to do when one feels well and lung function is normal. The green zone directions encourage adherence with long-term control medications. The yellow zone (caution) provides details to follow if PEF readings fall or symptoms begin or persist. Finally, the red zone section details instructions for an episode that is severe or does not resolve with initial treatment. Even patients with mild intermittent asthma can still experience significant asthma episodes, so they should learn how to recognize and manage severe symptoms.[27] Copies of self-care plans should be given to school nurses, teachers, and day care providers to ensure prompt treatment of asthma episodes that occur when children are away from the home.

### *Peak Flow Meters*

Peak flow meters are handheld devices, available by prescription. PEF measures the amount of airway obstruction, and a decrease in PEF can precede a significant asthma episode. Some patients with moderate to severe persistent asthma may monitor PEF daily as part of their asthma self-care plan. The green, yellow, and red zone method is often used (see preceding section). The green zone is a PEF reading of 80% of predicted or personal best, yellow zone is 50% to 80%, and the red zone is less than 50%. Readings may be recorded in a diary, which patients bring to each primary care visit, enabling a discussion with their provider about their asthma control. Table 13-9 provides step-by-step instructions for proper use of the meter.

### *Nonadherence to Prescription Asthma Medications*

Nonadherence to long-term control medications is a significant problem. Adherence ranges from 34% to 68%, depending on the medication.[28] Inhalers are the mainstay of therapy, but these items tend to be bulky for carrying to school or work. The most effective control medications are the inhaled corticosteroids, which possess anti-inflammatory properties. Because it may take up to several days to weeks to see the full anti-inflammatory effects and improvement of symptoms, patients often perceive long-term control medications as ineffective.[29] Confusion in the lay public between the potential toxicity of anabolic steroids used by athletes versus corticosteroids used for treatment of asthma and concerns about the long-term effects of medications can discourage adherence to long-term control medications for asthma. Compliance can usually be increased if the patient[4] (1) accepts the diagnosis of asthma, (2) believes that asthma may be dangerous or is a problem, (3) believes he or she is at risk, (4) believes the treatment is safe, (5) feels in control, and (6) feels that there is good communication with their health care provider. Education regarding asthma and asthma medications can therefore improve adherence with medications and self-care plans.

## Evaluation of Patient Outcomes for Asthma

Acute asthma symptoms should respond quickly (within 1 hour) to inhaled bronchodilators. Medical attention should be sought if symptoms worsen or persist for longer than 24 to 48 hours or if PEF readings remain in the yellow zone 2 days or more. If any symptoms of severe asthma episodes or imminent respiratory arrest develop, then immediate medical attention should be sought (Table 13-2).

Patients with persistent asthma should be scheduled for follow-up appointments at least every 6 months with

**TABLE 13-9 Guidelines for Using Peak Flow Meters**

1. Get your peak flow meter, a pencil, and your asthma care plan ready.
2. If your peak flow meter has a mouthpiece, put the mouthpiece on the meter as shown in drawing A.
3. Slide the button down as far as it will go to set the meter to zero as shown in drawing B).
4. Stand up. Keep the meter upright so the numbers run up and down. Do not cover the hole in the back of the meter or the numbers in the front with your fingers (see finger positions in drawing C). Take a deep breath.
5. Close your lips tightly around the mouthpiece as shown in drawing D. Do not put your tongue in the hole or your teeth on the mouthpiece. Blow one time as fast and as hard as you can.
6. Find your number. The button will go up and stay at the number you blew (see drawing E).
7. Repeat steps 1-6 two more times. Record the best of the three tries.
8. Check your asthma care plan (see Figure 13-2) for further instructions regarding the number you blew (e.g., red, yellow, and green zones).

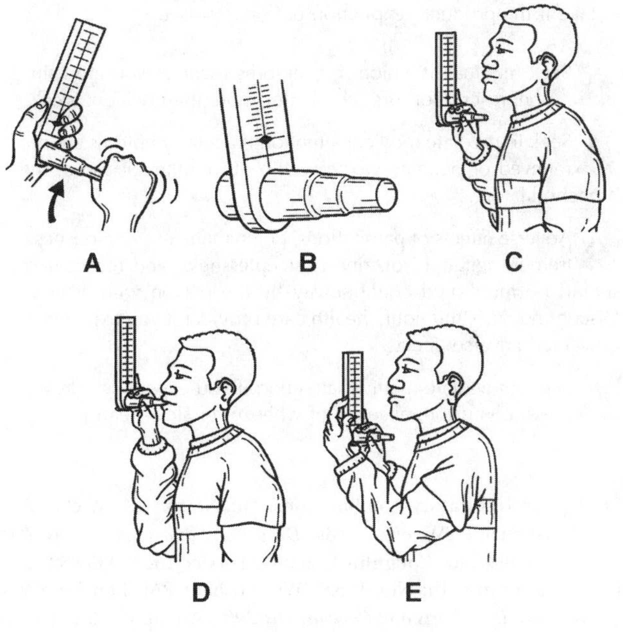


their primary medical provider to assess the adequacy of their self-care plan (Table 13-10). Patients with asthmalike symptoms who are not candidates for self-care should be referred to their health care practitioners (Figure 13-1).

## Key Points for Asthma

- Candidates for self-care of asthma are few. Those with concurrent diseases, without a prior diagnosis of asthma, or persistent asthma should be referred (Figure 13-1).
- Nonprescription medications should be used for mild intermittent symptoms or episodes lasting less than 2 days.

**TABLE 13-10 Goals and Monitoring of Asthma Therapy**

| Goal of Therapy | Monitoring Parameters |
|---|---|
| Control of symptoms | Wheezes 1-2 times/week; symptoms resolve within several minutes after bronchodilator |
| Normal pulmonary function | >80% personal best PEFR consistently every day; <20% variation of morning to evening PEFR readings |
| Normal activity levels | Few missed school/work days; able to do desired activities (playground, activities of daily living, etc.) |
| Prevent recurrent episodes of asthma (minimize the need for urgent care visits) | No hospitalizations or emergency department visits; regular follow-ups for asthma |
| Prevent adverse effects | No increased heart rate, insomnia, palpitations, nervousness, anxiety |
| Meet expectations of asthma care | Achieve patient's goals (e.g., desired activities): participates in care; comfortable asking questions; confident in dealing with symptoms and triggers |

- All patients with asthma need to know warning symptoms of severe asthma episodes to recognize when to seek urgent care.
- Education regarding asthma, medications, and self-monitoring is a crucial part of asthma self-care.
- Self-care plans should be developed in a partnership with health care practitioners. All patients with moderate to severe persistent asthma should have a written self-care plan.
- Environmental and trigger control can help reduce symptoms of asthma.
- Concomitant conditions (such as GERD, allergic rhinitis, and tobacco use) can worsen asthma symptoms and should be treated individually.

## References

1. *Healthy People 2010. Respiratory Diseases.* 2000; Chapter 24. Available at http://www.healthypeople.gov. Accessed January 15, 2005.
2. Levy S. Top 200 OTC/HBC brands in 2003. *Drug Topics.* June 7, 2004;148:64.
3. Centers for Disease Control. Asthma prevalence, health care use and mortality, 2002. Available at: http://www.cdc.gov/nchs/data/asthmahealthestat1.pdf. Accessed December 1, 2004.
4. *Global Initiative for Asthma. Global Strategy for Asthma Management and Prevention.* Bethesda, Md: US Department of Health and Human Services. Public Health Service. February 2002. NIH Publication No. 02-3659.
5. Moonie S, Strunk RC, Crocker S, et al. Community asthma program improves appropriate prescribing in moderate to severe asthma. *J Asthma.* 2005;42:281-9.

## PATIENT EDUCATION FOR ASTHMA

The objectives of self-treatment of asthma in patients identified as candidates for self-care (see Figure 13-1) are to (1) prevent acute asthma episodes with quick-relief medications, and (2) have tools available to manage acute episodes (see Figure 13-2). For most patients with mild, intermittent asthma, carefully following product instructions and the self-care measures listed here will help ensure optimal therapeutic outcomes.

### Nondrug Measures

- Identify and reduce exposures to relevant allergens and irritants that increase asthma symptoms (see Table 13-5).
- Stop smoking cigarettes.
- Control other conditions (e.g., concomitant diseases such as GERD and allergic rhinitis) and other factors that you know worsen your symptoms.
- Take the following precautions if you have exercise-induced bronchospasm:
  - Choose exercises, such as swimming, that are conducted in warm, humid areas.
  - Extend the warm-up period.
  - Increase your fitness level.
  - Eat at least 2 hours before exercise.
  - If needed, wear a face mask.
  - Use a peak flow meter to monitor your asthma (see Table 13-9).

### Nonprescription Medications

- See Table 13-6 for dosage information.
- If you are using a nonprescription asthma inhaler, check with your pharmacist or primary care provider periodically to ensure that you are using it correctly (see Table 13-7).
- If you are sensitive to aspirin, check the ingredients on nonprescription allergy, cough/cold, and analgesic (pain relieving) products. For relief of minor pain, take acetaminophen. Note that use of other nonprescription analgesics (ibuprofen, ketoprofen, and naproxen) may cause an asthma attack if you are sensitive to aspirin.
- If you exercise, take your asthma medication approximately 15 minutes before you begin exercising.
- Inhaled nonprescription asthma medications contain epinephrine and racepinephrine. Possible adverse drug effects include nervousness and rapid heart beat.
- Oral nonprescription asthma medications contain ephedrine or guaifenesin, or both ingredients. Possible adverse drug effects include nervousness, tremors, sleeplessness, nausea, and loss of appetite.
- Do not take oral or inhaled asthma medications if
  - you have not been diagnosed as having asthma.
  - you currently take a monoamine oxidase inhibitor.
  - you have heart disease, high blood pressure, thyroid disease, diabetes, or difficulty in urination caused by enlargement of the prostate gland unless directed to do so by a health care practitioner.
  - you have been hospitalized for asthma or are taking a prescription medication for asthma.
- Store oral combination products in a cool, dry place. Do not take if the product's expiration date has passed.

⚠ Seek medical attention if symptoms recur or you are using a nonprescription bronchodilator more than twice a week.

⚠ Seek immediate medical attention if acute symptoms are not relieved or become worse within 20 minutes of use of the bronchodilator.

⚠ Adverse effects of palpitations, angina, anxiety, nervousness, tremor, agitation, dizziness, sleeplessness, and restlessness should be monitored continuously by the person with asthma. Discontinue use and notify health care provider if you experience unwanted adverse effects.

⚠ Seek immediate medical attention if you experience drowsiness, confusion, absence of wheeze, or slow heart beat.

6. NHLBI, National Asthma Education and Prevention Program. *Clinical Practice Guidelines. Expert Panel Report 2. Guidelines for the Diagnosis and* Management *of Asthma.* Bethesda, Md: US Department of Health and Human Services; 1997. NIH Publication No. 97-4051.
7. Harding SM. Gastroesphageal reflux: a potential asthma trigger. *Immun Allergy Clin N Am.* 2005;25:131-48.
8. Kiljander, T. The role of proton pump inhibitors in the management of gastroesophageal reflux disease-related asthma and chronic cough. *Am J Med.* 2003;115(3A):65S-71S.
9. Hatch, GE. Asthma, inhaled oxidants, and dietary antioxidants. *Am J Clin Nutr.* 1995;61(suppl):625S-30S.
10. Parmet, S. Aspirin sensitivity. *JAMA.* 2004;292:3098.
11. Monteleone CA, Sherman AR. Nutrition and asthma. *Arch Intern Med.* 1997;157:23-33.
12. Bousquet Jean, Jeffery Peter K, Busse William W, et al. Asthma. From bronchoconstriction to airways inflammation and remodeling. *Am J Respir Crit Care Med.* 2000;161:1721-45.
13. NHLBI, National Asthma Education and Prevention Program. *Expert Panel Report Guidelines for the Diagnosis and Management of Asthma—Update on Selected Topics 2002.* Rockville, Md: US Department of Health and Human Services, National Heart, Lung, and Blood Institute; July 2002. NIH Publication 02-5075.
14. Upper respiratory combinations. In: Novak KK, Wickensham RM, Lenzini SW, et al., eds. *Drug Facts and Comparisons 2005.* Annapolis, Md: Coughlin Indexing Service Inc; 2005:882-3.
15. Expectorants. In: Novak KK, Wickensham RM, Lenzini SW, et al., eds. *Drug Facts and Comparisons 2005.* Annapolis, Md: Coughlin Indexing Service Incorporated; 2005:872.
16. Food and Drug Administration. Food and Drugs, subchapter D—Drugs for Human Use. 21CFR341.76. 2004; Title 21, Vol 5, pt 341. Available at: http://www.accessdata.fda.gov. Accessed March 11, 2005.
17. Briggs GG, Freeman RK, Yaffe SJ. Ephedrine. In: Mitchell CW, ed. *Drugs in Pregnancy and Lactation.* 5th ed. Baltimore: Williams and Wilkins; 1998:382-3.
18. Briggs GG, Freeman RK, Yaffe SJ. Epinephrine. In: Mitchell CW, ed. *Drugs in Pregnancy and Lactation.* 5th ed. Baltimore: Williams and Wilkins; 1998:383-4.
19. Gibson, PG, Simpson JL, Chalmers AN, et al. Airway eosinophilia is associated with wheeze but is uncommon in children with persistent cough and frequent chest colds. *Am J Respir Crit Care Med.* 2001;164:977-81.
20. NCAA Banned-Drug Classes 2004-2005. Available at: http://www.NCAA.org. Accessed May 11, 2005.

21. Schafer T. Epidemiology of complementary and alternative medicine for asthma and allergy in Europe and Germany. *Ann Allergy, Asthma, Immunol.* 2004;93(suppl 1):S5-S10.
22. Biernacki W, Peake D. Acupuncture in treatment of stable asthma. *Respir Med.* 1998; 92:1143-5.
23. Ziment I, Tashkin DP. Alternative medicine for allergy and asthma. *J Allergy Clin Immunol.* 2000;106:603-13
24. Rivera JO, Hughes HW, Stuart AG. Herbals and asthma: usage patterns among a border population. *Ann Pharm.* 2004;38:220-5.
25. Graham M, Blaiss M. Complementary/alternative medicine in the treatment of asthma. *Ann Allergy, Asthma, Immunol.* 2000;85:438-49.
26. Theoharides T, Bielory L. Mast cells and mast cell mediators as targets of dietary supplements. *Ann Allergy, Asthma, Immunol.* 2004;93:S24-S34.
27. Naureckas E, Solway J. Mild asthma. *N Engl J Med.* 2001;345:1257-62.
28. Jones C, Santanello JC, Boccuzzi SJ, et al. Adherence to prescribed treatment for asthma: evidence from pharmacy benefits data. *J Asthma.* 2003;40:93-101.
29. Farber HJ, Capra AM, Finkelstein JA, et al. Misunderstanding of asthma control medications: association with non-adherence. *J Asthma.* 2003;40:17-25.

SECTION V

# Gastrointestinal Disorders

CHAPTER 14

# Heartburn and Dyspepsia

*Ann Zweber and Rosemary R. Berardi*

Heartburn and dyspepsia are common symptoms that originate in the upper gastrointestinal (GI) tract and are frequently treated with nonprescription medications. Heartburn (pyrosis) is a burning sensation that usually arises from the substernal area (lower chest) and moves up toward the neck or throat.[1] Postprandial heartburn usually occurs within 2 hours after eating or when bending over or lying down. Nocturnal heartburn occurs during sleep and often awakens the individual. Most patients experience "simple" heartburn, which is typically mild, infrequent, episodic, and often associated with diet or lifestyle.[1] Others have more frequent heartburn that occurs 2 or more days a week. Heartburn that is frequent and persistent (3 or more months) is the most common symptom of gastroesophageal reflux disease (GERD). GERD is defined as symptoms, esophageal damage, or both resulting from the abnormal reflux of gastric contents into the esophagus.[2] About one half of all GERD cases are associated with endoscopic esophagitis.[3] However, patients with GERD may suffer heartburn even when esophageal injury is not present (nonerosive gastroesophageal reflux disease, NERD). Alhough it is not life-threatening, patients with frequent heartburn limit their food choices and often suffer from disruptions in sleep and work.[4,5] In 2000, the treatment of GERD ranked the highest in total direct and indirect costs (9.8 billion) among 17 selected GI diseases, with drug costs responsible for 63% of the direct costs.[6]

Dyspepsia (bad digestion) is a consistent or recurrent discomfort located primarily in the upper abdomen (epigastrium).[7] The discomfort is a subjective feeling that does not reach the level of pain and is usually characterized by bloating, belching, postprandial fullness, nausea, and early satiety, but is not necessarily restricted to meal-related symptoms. Patients with GERD, peptic ulcer disease (PUD), gastritis, delayed gastric emptying (e.g., gastroparesis), and irritable bowel syndrome often complain of dyspeptic symptoms.[7] The Rome II consensus definition and regulatory agencies in the United States have adopted definitions of dyspepsia for research purposes that exclude heartburn, while other definitions consider heartburn an accompanying symptom of dyspepsia.[8] Dyspepsia may be associated with an underlying cause such PUD and GERD or may not have any known cause.[7,9] Dyspeptic patients may have uninvestigated (no endoscopy has been performed) or investigated (endoscopy has been performed) dyspepsia. Nonulcer dyspepsia is a diagnosis that is made after endoscopy indicating that "ulcerlike" dyspeptic symptoms were not related to a peptic ulcer.[7] It is estimated that about 18 million adults in the United States take nonprescription medications for "indigestion."[2] The most widely used nonprescription medications include antacids, histamine$_2$-receptor antagonists ($H_2RA$), and proton pump inhibitors (PPI).

In clinical practice, it is not always possible to predict the cause of heartburn or dyspepsia on the basis of symptom assessment alone, as individuals may not describe adequately what they actually feel, and there is considerable overlap of symptoms. In addition, heartburn and dyspepsia may occur in association with other acid-related disorders, such as GERD and PUD. However, empirical treatment with nonprescription medications is appropriate and reasonable for most patients who have symptoms suggestive of heartburn and dyspepsia. Thus, assessment of the patient is most important in determining if the condition is self-treatable or if the individual should be referred for further evaluation. Medical referral is indicated if the patient is unresponsive to nonprescription medications, symptoms are severe, alarm symptoms are present, or symptoms suggest complicated disease.

This chapter focuses on the self-treatment and prevention of heartburn and dyspepsia. Emphasis is placed on distinguishing individuals who are appropriate candidates for self-treatment from those who require further medical evaluation. Specific recommendations for self-treatment, including dietary and lifestyle modifications and nonprescription medications, are provided.

## Epidemiology of Heartburn and Dyspepsia

The overall prevalence of heartburn in the United States is approximately 45% (about 110 million people) with an equal distribution between men and women of all age groups.[1] Among individuals who experience heartburn, 45% report heartburn 2 or more days a week, while 7% to 10% report heartburn daily.[10] Sixty-five percent of adults who experience heartburn at least once a week indicate that they have both daytime and nighttime heartburn.[4] Most women who are pregnant experience heartburn during the course of their pregnancy.[1] Approximately 25% of adults in the United States report having dyspeptic symptoms, with equal prevalence between men and women.[7] About 40% have dyspepsia associated with either PUD or GERD.[7] Gastric and esophageal cancer are less common causes, but may also be associated with dyspeptic symptoms.

**Editor's Note:** This chapter is based, in part, on the 14th edition chapter with the same title, which was written by Robert P. Henderson and Valerie T. Prince.

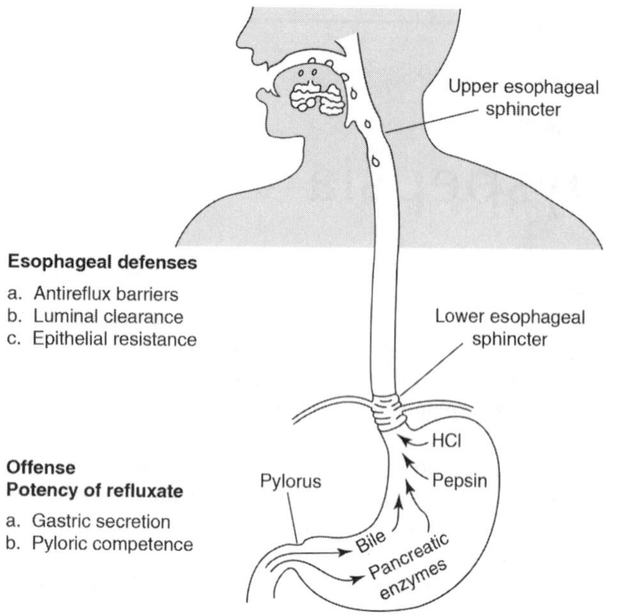


**FIGURE 14-1** Esophageal defense mechanisms and offensive factors associated with heartburn. (Reprinted with permission from Yamada T, Alpers DH, Laire L, et al., eds. *Textbook of Gastroenterology.* 3rd ed. Philadelphia: JB Lippincott; 1999:1236.)

Dyspepsia accounts for 20% to 70% of the GI complaints seen by general practitioners, and about 30% of these require referral to a gastroenterologist.[7]

## Anatomy and Physiology of the Esophagus and Stomach

### *Esophagus*

The esophagus is a tube that serves as a conduit between the pharynx and the stomach. The openings at both ends are guarded by specialized smooth muscle located where the pharynx meets the esophagus (upper esophageal sphincter) and at the lower end where the esophagus meets the stomach (lower esophageal sphincter, LES) (Figure 14-1). When the LES is functioning normally, it permits the passage of food into the stomach and serves as the primary antireflux barrier by preventing backflow of stomach contents upward into the esophagus. Although the LES is contracted at rest, healthy individuals experience relaxations of the LES throughout the day, often in association with swallowing.[1] When reflux occurs, the refluxate is cleared from the esophagus by peristaltic contractions brought on by swallowing, the neutralization of the refluxate by bicarbonate in the swallowed saliva and, when in the upright position, gravity. Esophageal mucosal resistance minimizes epithelial damage from noxious stomach contents. Thus, transient episodes of gastroesophageal reflux in healthy persons usually go unnoticed and do not damage the esophagus.

### *Stomach*

The stomach contains parietal cells that secrete hydrochloric acid and intrinsic factor (necessary for vitamin $B_{12}$ absorption), G cells that secrete gastrin, mucus-secreting cells, and chief cells that secrete pepsinogen.[11,12] Pepsinogen, an inactive precursor of pepsin, is converted to the proteolytic enzyme pepsin at an intragastric pH of 1.8 to 3.5, but is inactivated when the pH exceeds 5.[11] The parietal cells have receptors for histamine, acetylcholine, and gastrin, all of which stimulate hydrochloric acid secretion. When any of these substances comes into contact with its receptors on the parietal cell, intracellular calcium and cyclic adenosine monophosphate (cAMP) concentrations increase.[11] The increased levels of calcium and cAMP activate a unique proton pump, adenosine triphosphatase ($H^+/K^+/ATPase$), found only on the membranes of parietal cells. When stimulated, the proton pump secretes hydrogen ions in the stomach lumen in exchange for potassium. Thus, the proton pump is the final common pathway for gastric acid secretion.

The gastric mucosa withstands the acidic environment of the stomach through a combination of defense and repair mechanisms collectively called the gastric mucosal barrier.[11] Mucosal defense mechanisms include mucous and bicarbonate secretion, intrinsic epithelial cell defense, and mucosal blood flow.[11,12] The near neutral pH of the mucous-bicarbonate barrier protects the stomach from its acidic contents. Maintenance of mucosal integrity and repair is mediated by the production of endogenous prostaglandins.

## Etiology of Heartburn and Dyspepsia

Risk factors that may contribute to heartburn include diet, lifestyle, medications, and certain diseases (Table 14-1).[1,13-15] However, evidence to support each of the proposed risk factors is limited. Foods and beverages including coffee, tea, chocolate, and citrus, the regular use of aspirin and nonsteroidal anti-inflammatory drugs (NSAIDs), life stress, and tobacco smoking are widely recognized as precipitators of individual heartburn episodes.[11] Heartburn may also occur during certain types of exercise (e.g., weight lifting, cycling, or sit-ups). Obesity and pregnancy contribute to reflux by a direct physical effect (e.g., disrupting the intraabdominal pressure). Genetic factors may predispose to neurologic dysfunction of the LES.[14,15] Diseases such as gastroparesis and scleroderma increase intraabdominal pressure and lower LES pressure, respectively.

NSAIDs, including aspirin and cyclooxygenase-2 inhibitors, represent the most important cause of drug-induced dyspepsia.[7] Bisphosphonates, potassium or iron supplements, digoxin, theophylline, and certain antibiotics (e.g., erythromycin, ampicillin) are often associated with dyspeptic symptoms. Alcohol ingestion, tobacco, caffeine, and stress may contribute to dyspepsia.

## Pathophysiology of Heartburn and Dyspepsia

Heartburn arises from the sensory nerve endings in the esophageal epithelium and is most likely stimulated by spicy foods or by the reflux of acidic gastric contents into the esophagus.[1] The noxious quality of the refluxate (acid, pepsin) is central to the development of symptoms, esophageal damage, and complications (Figure 14-1). Individuals with an incompetent pylorus may reflux duodenal contents (bile, pancreatic enzymes) into the stomach, which

**TABLE 14-1 Risk Factors That May Contribute to Heartburn[1,13-15]**

| | |
|---|---|
| **Dietary** | **Medications** |
| Fatty foods | Bisphosphonates |
| Spicy foods | Aspirin/NSAIDs |
| Chocolate | Iron |
| Table salt | Potassium |
| Garlic or onions | Quinidine |
| Mint (e.g., spearmint, peppermint) | Tetracycline |
| Alcohol (ethanol) | Zidovudine |
| Caffeinated beverages | Anticholinergic agents |
| Carbonated beverages | α-Adrenergic antagonists |
| Citrus fruit or juices | Barbiturates |
| Tomatoes/juice | $\beta_2$-Adrenergic agonists |
| | Calcium channel blockers |
| **Lifestyle** | Benzodiazepines |
| Exercise | Dopamine |
| Smoking (tobacco) | Estrogen |
| Obesity | Narcotic analgesics |
| Stress | Nitrates |
| Supine body position | Progesterone |
| Tight-fitting clothing | Prostaglandins |
| Pregnancy | Theophylline |
| | TCAs |
| **Diseases** | Chemotherapy |
| Motility disorders (e.g., gastroparesis) | |
| | **Other** |
| Scleroderma | Genetics |
| PUD | |
| Zollinger-Ellison syndrome | |

Key: NSAID, nonsteroidal anti-inflammatory drug; PUD, peptic ulcer disease; TCA, tricyclic antidepressant.

increases the noxious quality of the gastric refluxate. Most patients with heartburn secrete normal amounts of gastric acid.[1] Esophageal tissue damage is caused primarily by gastric acid, pepsin, and bile salts. The esophageal epithelium is not as tolerant as that of the stomach to repetitive exposure of gastric acid.[1] What usually distinguishes individuals with heartburn from those with normal physiologic reflux is the increased frequency and duration of reflux episodes, which may result in esophageal tissue damage ranging from inflammation (esophagitis) to erosions and ulcers. However, there is no direct correlation between heartburn severity and underlying esophageal injury. The refluxed acidic contents also may damage the oropharynx, larynx, and respiratory system.[1]

Many patients with heartburn have transient LES relaxations.[1] In these patients, the higher pressure in the stomach creates enough force to overcome the LES pressure, allowing reflux of gastric contents into the lower esophagus (Figure 14-1). Hiatal hernia (a weakening in the diaphragmatic muscles resulting in the protrusion of the upper portion of the stomach into the thoracic cavity) may also contribute to heartburn by disrupting the gastroesophageal junction and lowering the LES pressure.[1] Delayed gastric emptying increases the volume of the noxious refluxate and increases intra-abdominal pressure. A sudden increase in intra-abdominal pressure such as when a person strains, coughs, or bends over, may also be associated with reflux. Impaired esophageal acid clearing mechanisms (peristalsis, saliva, gravity) prolong the duration of contact between the refluxate and the esophageal epithelium and are less operative during sleep or when the patient is lying down. Age-related decreases in saliva production or pH and esophageal motility may contribute to esophageal damage in older individuals.[16] Although controversial, *Helicobacter pylori* (*H. pylori*) infection does not appear to play a pathogenic role, but potentially may be protective.[1,17]

The pathophysiology of dyspepsia remains unclear. Dyspeptic symptoms may be associated with PUD, GERD, gastric cancer, *H. pylori*, or GI dysmotility, or may lack any identifiable cause.[7]

## Association of Heartburn With Other Acid-related Disorders

Heartburn may occur alone or be associated with acid-related disorders such as dyspepsia, GERD, and PUD (Table 14-2). Heartburn is highly specific for GERD and may suggest esophageal complications.[1] However, the frequency and severity of the heartburn do not predict esophageal injury, as patients with frequent and severe heartburn may not have esophageal damage (NERD). Upper endoscopy is the standard for determining the type and extent of esophageal mucosal damage. Patients with esophageal injury may have varying grades of severity as well as strictures (a narrowing of the esophageal lumen).[1] Symptomatic GERD is the strongest risk factor for the development of esophageal adenocarcinoma.[18] Barrett's esophagus, a precancerous condition, develops in the lower esophagus and is related to longstanding (greater than 5 years) moderate to severe erosive/ulcerative esophagitis.[1,19] This condition is more prevalent in men and increases with age. Barrett's esophagus is associated with an increased risk of esophageal adenocarcinoma with an annual incidence of less than 1%.[1,18,19]

Alarm symptoms result from complications associated with GERD (Table 14-2). Dysphagia (difficulty in swallowing) occurs initially with the ingestion of solid foods such as toast or crackers. It is evident in about 30% of patients with chronic GERD and may indicate severe erosive esophagitis, stricture, or cancer.[1] Odynophagia (painful swallowing) is less common, but may be reported with severe ulcerative esophagitis or esophageal cancer. However, its presence should raise questions about other causes of esophagitis including pill-induced (e.g., tetracycline, potassium chloride, quinine, vitamin C, aspirin, NSAIDs, bisphosphonates) and infections (e.g., herpes, fungal candidiasis).[1] Upper GI bleeding (e.g., hematemesis, melena, occult bleeding, anemia), may also result from esophageal complications.

Abnormal gastric reflux of stomach contents may also cause atypical (extraesophageal) manifestations of GERD (Table 14-2).[1] The atypical symptoms may or may not be accompanied by heartburn, making recognition of GERD difficult. GERD-related chest pain is usually substernal, but may mimic ischemic cardiac pain, radiating to the back, neck, jaw, or arms. It often worsens after meals, during periods of emotional stress, and may awaken the patient from sleep. Severe, crushing chest pain—especially if

**TABLE 14-2 Differentiation of Simple Heartburn from Other Acid-related Disorders**

| | Simple Heartburn | GERD | Dyspepsia | PUD |
|---|---|---|---|---|
| Etiology | See Table 14-1 | See Table 14-1 | Food, alcohol caffeine, stress, and medications contribute to dyspepsia; chronic dyspepsia associated with PUD, GERD, gastric cancer; or may lack an identifiable cause. | Gastric or duodenal ulcer caused most commonly by *H. pylori* infection and/or NSAIDs |
| Typical symptoms | Burning sensation behind the breastbone, which may move upward toward the neck or throat | Heartburn, acid regurgitation (acid taste in the mouth), hypersalivation | Primary: epigastric discomfort<br>Other: belching or burping, bloating, nausea, early satiety; may be accompanied by heartburn and acid regurgitation | Gnawing or burning epigastric pain, occurring during day and frequently at night; may be accompanied by heartburn and dyspepsia |
| Complications | | Erosive esophagitis, strictures, bleeding, Barrett's esophagus, esophageal cancer | | Perforation, obstruction, penetration, bleeding |
| Alarm symptoms | | Dysphagia; odynophagia; chest pain; upper GI bleeding; unexplained weight loss; continuous nauseau, vomiting, and diarrhea | | Upper GI bleeding; unexplained weight loss; continuous nauseau, vomiting, and diarrhea |
| Atypical symptoms | | Asthma, chronic laryngitis, hoarseness, cough, globus sensation (sensation of a lump in the throat), noncardiac chest pain, dental erosions | | |

Key: GERD, gastroesophageal reflux disease; GI, gastrointestinal; NSAID, nonsteroidal anti-inflammatory drug; PUD, peptic ulcer disease.

accompanied by nausea, vomiting, and sweating—suggests ischemic pain and possibly myocardial infarction. Other atypical symptoms result from the aspiration of refluxate into the upper airways and lungs.

## Treatment of Heartburn and Dyspepsia

### *Treatment Goals*

The goals of self-treatment of heartburn are to render the patient symptom-free, prevent meal- or exercise-related symptoms, improve quality of life, and prevent complications by using the most cost-effective therapy. The primary goal of self-treatment of dyspepsia is aimed at relieving abdominal discomfort.

### *General Treatment Approach*

The approach to self-treatment of heartburn and dyspepsia requires an initial assessment to determine whether the patient is a candidate for self-treatment (Figure 14-2). Individuals with exclusions to self-treatment should be referred for further medical evaluation. If the individual is a candidate for self-treatment (see box Patient Education for Heartburn and Dyspepsia), nondrug measures should be recommended and continued throughout treatment. If appropriate, a recommendation should also be made for a nonprescription medication. Antacids and nonprescription $H_2$RAs should be recommended for individuals with mild, infrequent heartburn and dyspepsia. Antacids are advantageous because they provide rapid relief of symptoms (Table 14-3). The use of antacids, however, is limited by their short duration when taken on an empty stomach. The duration of relief may be prolonged for several hours by taking the antacid after a meal. When used in recommended dosages, the antacids are interchangeable despite differences in antacid salts and potency. Products that contain antacids plus alginic acid are also effective in relieving heartburn, and may be superior to antacids alone.[2] Antacid/alginic acid products are usually more expensive than antacids and therefore are considered second-line agents for treating mild, occasional heartburn.

A nonprescription $H_2$RA is preferred to an antacid when individuals with mild to moderate, episodic heartburn require more prolonged relief of symptoms. Though $H_2$RAs do not relieve heartburn or dyspepsia as rapidly as an antacid (Table 14-3), this may not be a major factor for some individuals.[2] The $H_2$RAs may also be used to prevent

**Exclusions for Self-Treatment**

- Frequent heartburn for more than 3 months
- Heartburn while taking recommended dosages of nonprescription $H_2RA$ or PPI
- Heartburn that continues after 2 weeks of treatment with a nonprescription $H_2RA$ or PPI
- Heartburn and dyspepsia that occur when taking a prescription $H_2RA$ or PPI
- Severe heartburn and dyspepsia
- Nocturnal heartburn
- Difficulty or pain on swallowing solid foods
- Vomiting up blood or black material or black tarry stools
- Chronic hoarseness, wheezing, coughing, or choking
- Unexplained weight loss
- Continuous nausea, vomiting, or diarrhea
- Chest pain accompanied by sweating, pain radiating to shoulder, arm, neck, or jaw, and shortness of breath
- Pregnancy
- Nursing mothers
- Children younger than 12 years (for antacids, $H_2RAs$) or younger than 18 years (for omeprazole)

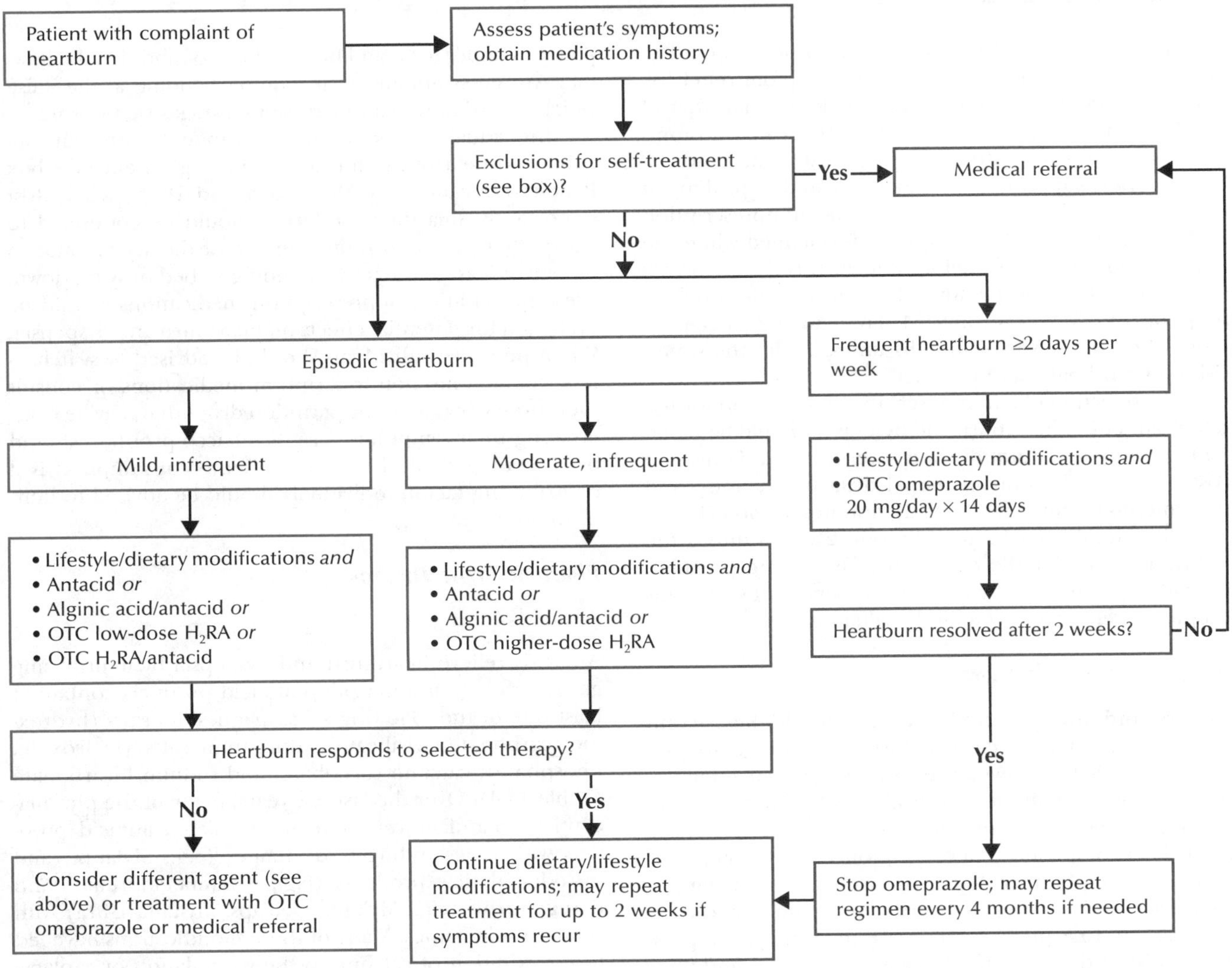


**FIGURE 14-2** Self-treatment of heartburn. Key: $H_2RA$, histamine$_2$-receptor antagonist; OTC, over-the-counter; PPI, proton pump inhibitor.

heartburn and acid indigestion when given 1 hour prior to a heavy or spicy meal and exercise. A combination product containing an $H_2RA$ plus an antacid may be recommended when rapid relief and longer duration are desirable (Table 14-3). Nonprescription $H_2RA$ products containing the lower doses (e.g., famotidine 10 mg twice daily) should be recommended for patients with mild, infrequent heartburn, while higher nonprescription dosages (e.g., famotidine 20 mg twice daily) should be reserved for moderate symptoms. When used in recommended and comparative dosages, the $H_2RAs$ are interchangeable despite minor differences in potency, onset, and duration of action. Patients taking continuous daily doses of a nonprescription $H_2RA$ should not exceed 14 days of self-treatment without consulting their primary care provider.

Nonprescription PPIs are the drugs of choice for treating individuals with frequent heartburn occurring 2 or

**TABLE 14-3 Effectiveness of Nonprescription Medications in Relieving Heartburn**

| Medication | Onset of Relief | Duration of Relief | Symptomatic Relief |
|---|---|---|---|
| Antacids | <5 minutes | 20-30 minutes* | Excellent |
| $H_2RAs$ | 30-45 minutes | 4-10 hours | Excellent |
| $H_2RA$ + antacid | <5 minutes | 8-10 hours | Excellent |
| PPIs | 2-3 hours | 12-24 hours | Superior |

Key: $H_2RAs$, histamine$_2$-receptor antagonist; PPI, proton pump inhibitor.

* Food prolongs duration of relief.

more days a week and for those who do not respond to nonprescription $H_2RAs$. The onset of symptom relief following an oral dose of omeprazole is slower than that of an $H_2RA$ (Table 14-3), and complete relief of symptoms may take 1 to 4 days after initiating treatment. However, PPIs provide superior symptom relief and a prolonged duration of action, compared with the nonprescription $H_2RAs$. Optimal relief of symptoms is obtained when the PPI is taken 30 minutes before a meal (preferably breakfast). Patients should be advised not to take the nonprescription PPI for more than 14 days and not to re-treat more often than every 4 months unless under the supervision of a primary care provider.

The selection of a nonprescription medication for the self-treatment of heartburn and dyspepsia should be based on the frequency, duration, and severity of symptoms, the cost of the medication, potential drug interactions, and the patient's preference. Antacids, nonprescription $H_2RAs$, and PPIs should not be used beyond 2 weeks unless the individual is under the care of a primary care provider. Individuals with severe, recurrent, or persistent symptoms should be referred for medical evaluation.

### *Nonpharmacologic Therapy*

Dietary and lifestyle modifications should be recommended for all patients with heartburn and dyspepsia despite the fact that evidence supporting their effectiveness is either lacking or equivocal.[2,14,15,20,21] These maneuvers may benefit many individuals, but changes alone are unlikely to completely relieve symptoms in the majority of patients.[2] Nonpharmacologic approaches to reducing the frequency and severity of heartburn include actions to increase the LES pressure, decrease the intragastric pressure, assist in the movement of gastric contents, and minimize exposure to triggering factors. A complete and accurate history will assist in identifying contributing factors. Recommendations should be tailored to the individual on the basis of specific dietary and lifestyle patterns.

Individuals should be asked to keep a diary to track dietary, lifestyle, and medication "triggers" (Table 14-1). Weight loss should be encouraged, although there is some controversy as to whether this will significantly decrease symptoms.[15,20-22] For nocturnal symptoms, some relief may be attained from elevating the head of the bed by placing 6-inch blocks underneath the legs of the head of the bed, or placing a foam wedge (e.g., GERD pillow) beneath the patient's upper torso and head.[22-24] Use of traditional pillows may worsen symptoms, as it requires bending at the waist, which contributes to an increase in intragastric pressure.

Individuals should be educated about factors that contribute to heartburn and how to manage them (see box Patient Education for Heartburn and Dyspepsia). Most importantly, heartburn sufferers should be counseled to eat smaller meals, to reduce intake of dietary fat, and to not eat at least 3 hours before going to bed or lying down. Prescription and nonprescription medications should be evaluated for potential effects on heartburn and dyspepsia. When possible, individuals should be advised to switch to less troublesome nonprescription medications or consult their prescriber about prescription drugs that may be exacerbating their symptoms. Use of tobacco products should be discouraged. If alcohol or caffeine consumption is a contributing factor, individuals should be advised to limit or discontinue use.

### *Pharmacologic Therapy*

#### Antacids

Antacids relieve heartburn and dyspepsia by neutralizing gastric acid. Nonprescription antacid products contain at least one of the following salts: magnesium salts (hydroxide, carbonate, trisilicate), aluminum salts (hydroxide, phosphate), calcium carbonate, and sodium bicarbonate (Table 14-4). Over the last few years, many of the pharmaceutical manufacturers have reformulated antacid products with longstanding trade names (e.g., Mylanta) and introduced new products (e.g., Mylanta Supreme) and dosage forms (e.g., Mylanta Gelcaps, Mylanta Ultra) with similar trade names. Many of these modifications have led to the addition of calcium to the formulation or replacement of another antacid salt with calcium (e.g., Maalox Total Stomach Relief Maximum Strength). Most antacids are relatively inexpensive, making them desirable products for the temporary relief of mild and infrequent heartburn and dyspepsia.

*Mechanism of Action/Pharmacokinetics* Antacids act as buffering agents in the lower esophagus, gastric lumen, and duodenal bulb. The cations react with chloride, whereas the anionic portion of the molecule reacts with hydrogen ions to form water and other compounds. As a result, a small, but noticeable increase in intragastric pH

TABLE 14-4 Selected Antacid and Bismuth Products and Dosage Regimens

| Trade Name | Primary Ingredients | Adult Dosage (Maximum Daily Dosage) |
|---|---|---|
| Alka-Mints Chewable Antacid | Calcium carbonate 850 mg | Chew 1 or 2 tablets q2h as needed (8 tablets) |
| Alka Seltzer Heartburn Relief | Sodium bicarbonate 1940 mg; citric acid 1000 mg | Dissolve 2 tablets in 4 oz of water every hour as needed (8 tablets) |
| Alka Seltzer Original | Sodium bicarbonate 1916 mg; citric acid 1000 mg; aspirin 325 mg | Dissolve 2 tablets in 4 oz of water every hour as needed (8 tablets) |
| Alternagel Liquid | Each 5 mL contains aluminum hydroxide 600 mg | 1-2 tsp between meals and at bedtime (18 tsp) |
| Gaviscon Extra Strength Liquid | Each 5 mL contains* aluminum hydroxide 254 mg; magnesium carbonate 237 mg | 2-4 tsp 4 times a day, after meals and at bedtime (16 tsp) |
| Gelusil Tablets | Aluminum hydroxide 200 mg; magnesium hydroxide 200 mg; simethicone 25 mg | Chew 2 to 4 tablets; repeat hourly if symptoms return (12 tablets) |
| Maalox Liquid Regular Strength Antacid/ Antigas | Each 5 mL contains aluminum hydroxide 200 mg; magnesium hydroxide 200 mg; simethicone 20 mg | 2-4 tsp 4 times a day (16 tsp) |
| Maalox Quick Dissolve Regular Strength Chewable Antacid Tablets | Calcium carbonate 600 mg | Chew 1-2 tablets as symptoms occur (12 tablets) |
| Maalox Total Stomach Relief Maximum Strength | Each 15 mL contains bismuth subsalicylate 500 mg | 2 tbsp q1/2-1h as required (up to 4 doses or 8 tbsp) |
| Mylanta Gelcaps | Calcium carbonate 550 mg; magnesium hydroxide 125 mg | Swallow 2-4 gelcaps as needed (12 gelcaps) |
| Mylanta Maximum Strength Liquid | Each 5 mL contains aluminum hydroxide 400 mg; magnesium hydroxide 400 mg; simethicone 40 mg | 2-4 tsp between meals and at bedtime (12 tsp) |
| Mylanta Regular Strength Liquid | Each 5 mL contains aluminum hydroxide 200 mg; magnesium hydroxide 200 mg; simethicone 20 mg | 2-4 tsp between meals and at bedtime (24 tsp) |
| Mylanta Supreme Liquid | Each 5 mL contains calcium carbonate 400 mg; magnesium hydroxide 135 mg | 2-4 tsp between meals and at bedtime (18 tsp) |
| Mylanta Ultra Chewable Tabs | Calcium carbonate 700 mg; magnesium hydroxide 300 mg | Chew 2-4 tablets between meals and at bedtime (10 tablets) |
| Pepto Bismol Maximum Strength Liquid | Each 15 mL contains bismuth subsalicylate 500 mg | 2 tbsp q1/2-1h as required (4 doses or 8 tbsp) |
| Pepto Bismol Original Liquid | Each 15 mL contains bismuth subsalicylate 262 mg | 2 tbsp q1/2-1h as required (8 doses or 16 tbsp) |
| Phillips Milk of Magnesia Original | Each 5 mL contains magnesium hydroxide 400 mg | 1-3 tsp q4h (4 times/day or 12 tbsp) |
| Rolaids Antacid Tablets | Calcium carbonate 550 mg; magnesium hydroxide 110 mg | Chew 2-4 tablets hourly as needed (12 tablets) |
| Tums E-X Extra Strength Tablets | Calcium carbonate 750 mg | Chew 2-4 tablets as needed symptoms (10 tablets) |
| Tums Regular Strength Tablets | Calcium carbonate 500 mg | Chew 2-4 tablets as needed symptoms (15 tablets) |

* Sodium alginate (alginic acid) is listed as an inactive ingredient.

occurs.[25] Increasing the intragastric pH above 5 blocks the conversion of pepsin to pepsinogen.[25] Antacids may also increase LES pressure.[1]

Sodium bicarbonate rapidly reacts with gastric acid to form sodium chloride, carbon dioxide, and water. Its duration of action is shortened by its quick elimination from the stomach.[25] Of the magnesium salts, magnesium hydroxide is used most often. Magnesium hydroxide rapidly reacts with gastric acid to form magnesium chloride and water. Its duration of action is shorter than that of calcium carbonate and aluminum hydroxide. Calcium carbonate is a potent antacid that dissolves slowly in gastric acid to form calcium chloride, carbon dioxide, and water. Its onset of action is slower, but its duration of effect is longer than magnesium hydroxide or sodium bicarbonate. Aluminum hydroxide reacts with hydrochloric acid to form aluminum chloride and water. It has a slower onset, but a longer duration than magnesium hydroxide.

Liquid antacids usually have a faster onset than tablets, because they are already dissolved or suspended and provide a maximal surface area for action. Of the tablet dosage forms, the quick-dissolve antacid tablets may provide the most rapid relief of symptoms. The duration of action for all antacids is transient, lasting only as long as the antacid remains in the stomach. The presence of food affects the duration of action of antacids. When administered within 1 hour after a meal, antacids may remain in the stomach for up to 3 hours.[25]

Differences in antacids are determined primarily on the cation, specific salt, and potency. Antacid potency is based on the number of milliequivalents of acid neutralizing capacity (ANC), which is defined as the amount of acid buffered per dose over a specified period of time. Factors that contribute to the ANC include product formulation, ingredients, and concentration.[25] As a result, ANC is product specific, which means equal volumes of liquid antacids or the same number of tablets are not necessarily equal in potency.

Most antacids are minimally absorbed into the systemic circulation. About 90% of calcium is converted to insoluble calcium salts, and the remaining 10% is absorbed systemically.[25] Approximately 15% to 30% of magnesium and 17% to 30% of aluminum may be absorbed and then excreted renally; therefore, accumulation may occur in patients with renal insufficiency.[25] In contrast, sodium bicarbonate is readily absorbed and eliminated.

*Indications* Antacids are indicated for the treatment of mild, infrequent heartburn, sour stomach, and acid indigestion. Combination products containing aspirin or acetaminophen are indicated for overindulgence in food and drink, and hangover. Individuals with mild dyspepsia may experience some relief with an antacids, but no studies demonstrate their effectiveness.[9,25]

*Dosage and Administration Guidelines* Antacids are administered orally. The effective dose of an antacid varies depending on product ingredients, milliequivalents of acid neutralizing capacity, formulation, and the frequency and severity of symptoms. Individuals should be instructed to take product-specific recommended dosages at the onset of symptoms. Dosing may be repeated in 1 to 2 hours, if needed, but should not exceed the maximum daily dosage for a particular product (Table 14-4). Individuals should be reevaluated if antacids are used more than twice a week or regularly for over 2 weeks. Frequent antacid users may need to be switched to a longer-acting product such as an $H_2RA$, an $H_2RA$ plus an antacid, or a PPI.

*Safety Considerations* Antacids are usually well tolerated. Side effects are generally associated with the cation. The most common side effect associated with magnesium-containing antacids is a dose-related diarrhea. Diarrhea may be reduced by combining magnesium-containing antacids with aluminum hydroxide. However, when higher dosages are used, the predominating effect is diarrhea. Magnesium excretion is impaired in patients with renal disease and may result in systemic accumulation of magnesium. Magnesium-containing antacids should not be used in patients with a creatinine clearance of less than 30 mL/minute.[25]

Aluminum-containing antacids are associated with dose-related constipation. Aluminum hydroxide binds dietary phosphate in the GI tract, increasing phosphate excretion in the feces. Frequent and prolonged use of aluminum hydroxide may lead to hypophosphatemia.[25] Chronic use of aluminum-containing antacids in renal failure may lead to aluminum toxicity and should be avoided.

Calcium carbonate may cause belching and flatulence as a result of carbon dioxide production. Patients may complain of constipation when taking calcium antacids, but there is little evidence to support this side effect.[25] Acid rebound with calcium-containing antacids has been reported. Although calcium stimulates gastric acid secretion, the clinical importance of this finding remains uncertain.[1,26] If renal elimination is impaired, hypercalcemia may occur and accumulation of calcium may result in the formation of renal calculi. Because many antacids have been reformulated to contain calcium, the risk of hypercalcemia exists when high and frequent dosages of calcium-containing antacids are taken with other calcium-containing medications such as prenatal vitamins or foods such as milk or orange juice with added calcium. Up to 2500 mg/day of elemental calcium can be ingested safely in individuals with normal renal function.[27]

Sodium bicarbonate frequently causes belching and flatulence resulting from the production of carbon dioxide.[25] The high sodium content (274 mg sodium/gram sodium bicarbonate) may cause fluid overload in patients with congestive heart failure, renal failure, cirrhosis, pregnancy, and those on sodium-restricted diets. In individuals with normal renal function, additional bicarbonate is excreted, whereas in patients with impaired renal function, retained bicarbonate may cause systemic alkalosis. A high intake of calcium along with an alkalinizing agent (such as sodium bicarbonate or calcium carbonate) may produce a condition referred to as milk-alkali syndrome. Signs and symptoms include hypercalcemia, alkalosis, irritability, headache, nausea, vomiting, weakness, and malaise.[25,26] Individuals who take additional calcium, such as pregnant and postmenopausal women should avoid using sodium bicarbonate as an antacid.

All antacids may potentially increase or decrease the absorption of other oral medications when given concomitantly, by adsorbing or chelating the other drug or increasing intragastric pH.[25,28] Medications such as tetracyclines, azithromycin, and fluoroquinolones bind to divalent and trivalent cations, potentially decreasing antibiotic absorption.[25,28] The absorption of medications such as itraconazole, ketoconazole, and iron, that depend on a low intragastric pH for disintegration, dissolution, or ionization, may also be decreased.[25,28] Specific antacids, such as aluminum hydroxide, may decrease the absorption of isoniazid. The absorption of enteric-coated products may be increased with concurrent administration of antacids.[28] The intraluminal interactions of antacids with other oral medications can

**TABLE 14-5 Nonprescription $H_2RA$ and PPI Products and Dosage Regimens**

| Trade Name | Primary Ingredients | Adult Dosage (Maximum Daily Dosage) |
|---|---|---|
| Tagamet HB | Cimetidine 200 mg | 1 tablet with a glass of water (2 tablets) |
| Axid AR | Nizatidine 75 mg | 1 tablet with a glass of water (2 tablets) |
| Pepcid AC | Famotidine 10 mg | 1 tablet with a glass of water (2 tablets) |
| Pepcid AC Maximum Strength | Famotidine 20 mg | 1 tablet with a glass of water (2 tablets) |
| Zantac 75 | Ranitidine 75 mg | 1 tablet with a glass of water (2 tablets) |
| Zantac 150 | Ranitidine 150 mg | 1 tablet with a glass of water (2 tablets) |
| Pepcid Complete | Famotidine 10 mg; calcium carbonate 800 mg; magnesium hydroxide 165 mg | Chew and swallow 1 tablet (2 tablets) |
| Prilosec OTC | Omeprazole 20 mg | 1 tablet with a glass of water 30 minutes before morning meal; take daily for 14 days (1 tablet) |

usually be avoided when potentially interacting drugs are separated by at least 2 hours. Antacid-induced alkalization of the urine may increase urinary excretion of salicylates and decrease blood concentrations.[28] In contrast, an increase in urine pH may decrease urinary excretion and increase blood concentrations of amphetamines and quinidine.[25]

*Additional Ingredients* Alginic acid reacts with sodium bicarbonate in saliva to form a viscous layer of sodium alginate that floats on the surface of gastric contents, theoretically forming a protective barrier against esophageal irritation.[1] Alginic acid by itself does not neutralize acid. Because there is insufficient evidence supporting its efficacy as a single agent, the Food and Drug Administration (FDA) has not granted alginic acid category I status. However, alginic acid may be found as an inactive ingredient in several antacid products (Table 14-4). Combination products of alginic several acid and an antacid may be superior to an antacid alone.[2] Several antacid products contain simethicone to decrease discomfort related to intestinal gas. See Chapter 15 (Intestinal Gas), for a more detailed description of simethicone.

## Histamine$_2$-Receptor Antagonists

The $H_2RAs$ relieve heartburn and dyspepsia by decreasing gastric acid secretion. The four $H_2RAs$ available for nonprescription use are cimetidine, ranitidine, famotidine, and nizatidine (Table 14-5). Initially, these medications were only available for nonprescription use at one half of the prescription dose. Today, nonprescription $H_2RAs$ also are available in the higher prescription dosages. For the most part, the four $H_2RAs$ are considered interchangeable, despite differences in onset and duration of symptom relief, side effects, and the potential for drug interactions. However, cimetidine does have the greatest potential for serious hepatic CYP 450 drug interactions and is associated with impotence in males.

*Mechanism of Action/Pharmacokinetics* $H_2RAs$ decrease gastric acid secretion by inhibiting the effect of histamine on the histamine$_2$ receptor of the parietal cell. In addition, $H_2RAs$ decrease the volume of secreted acid. Acid secretion is decreased regardless of the presence of food, which make these agents effective for fasting and nocturnal symptoms.[23] Their bioavailability is not affected by food, but may be reduced modestly by antacids. All of the $H_2RAs$ are eliminated by a combination of renal and hepatic metabolism, with renal elimination being the most important. Onset of symptom relief is not as quick as that of antacids, but their duration of effect is longer lasting (Table 14-3).[1,29] Cimetidine is the shortest-acting $H_2RA$, with a duration of action of 4 to 8 hours, while ranitidine, famotidine, and nizatidine have a somewhat longer duration. Tolerance to the gastric antisecretory effect may occur when $H_2RAs$ are taken daily (versus as needed) and may be responsible for diminished efficacy.[1]

*Indications* Nonprescription $H_2RAs$ are indicated for the treatment of mild to moderate infrequent, episodic heartburn and for the prevention of heartburn associated with acid indigestion and sour stomach. $H_2RAs$ have been shown to be more effective than placebo for relief of mild to moderate heartburn[2,4] and provide moderate improvement in patients with mild dyspeptic symptoms.[9,30] The combined antacid (magnesium hydroxide and calcium carbonate) and $H_2RA$ (famotidine) product is indicated for individuals with postprandial heartburn who have not premedicated with an $H_2RA$.

*Dosage and Administration Guidelines* $H_2RAs$ may be used at the onset of symptoms or 30 minutes to 1 hour prior to an event (meal or exercise) in which heartburn is anticipated. Self-treatment dosing should be limited to no more than two times a day. If the $H_2RA$ is used more than twice a week, or for more than 2 weeks, follow-up with a primary care provider is recommended. The combined antacid and $H_2RA$ product both provides immediate relief and prevents symptoms. Because tolerance to the antisecretory effect may develop, it is best to take an $H_2RA$ on an as-needed basis rather than by continuous daily dosing.[1] All four $H_2RAs$ require a dosage reduction in patients with reduced renal function.[12] Patients of advanced age, in particular, are at greatest risk for side effects when the $H_2RA$ daily dose is not reduced appropriately.[31]

*Safety Considerations* The four $H_2$RAs are well tolerated and have a low incidence of side effects.[11] The most common side effects occur with all four agents and include headache, diarrhea, constipation, dizziness, and drowsiness.[11,12] Cimetidine is associated with a weak antiandrogenic effect that may result in decreased libido, impotence, or gynecomastia in men.[12] Cimetidine binds to hepatic cytochrome P450 (3A4, 2D6, 1A2, and 2C9), inhibiting the metabolism of numerous drugs including phenytoin, warfarin, theophylline, tricyclic antidepressants, and amiodarone.[28,32] Ranitidine also binds to the cytochrome P450 system, but to a lesser extent, so interactions are uncommon at nonprescription doses. Famotidine and nizatidine do not interact with the cytochrome P450 system. Medications such as ketoconazole, itraconazole, and iron salts are dependent on an acidic environment for absorption.[11,28] When administered with an acid-reducing product, their absorption may be reduced. Cimetidine may inhibit the renal tubular secretion of drugs such as procainamide.[28]

### Proton Pump Inhibitors

PPIs are potent antisecretory drugs that relieve heartburn and dyspepsia by decreasing gastric acid secretion. Omeprazole was the first PPI to become available for nonprescription use in the United States at an oral dosage of 20 mg, which is identical to the prescription dosage.

*Mechanism of Action/Pharmacokinetics* The PPIs inhibit hydrogen potassium ATPase (the proton pump), irreversibly blocking the final step in gastric acid secretion.[33,34] PPIs have a more potent and prolonged antisecretory effect than do the $H_2$RAs (Table 14-3).[34] The relative bioavailability of the prescription dosage form (enteric-coated granules contained in a capsule) increases from 35% to 65% with continued daily dosing.[33] The nonprescription dosage form, available as a magnesium salt, is formulated as a tablet containing multiple enteric-coated pellets[36] and has a similar oral bioavailabilty.[10] Omeprazole is almost completely absorbed after oral administration, regardless of the presence of food.

The onset of symptom relief following an oral dose occurs in 2 to 3 hours, but complete relief may take 1 to 4 days.[33,35] However, the results of a recent study indicate that on day 1, the percentage of time the intragastric pH was greater than 4 with Prilosec OTC taken once daily was higher than with Pepcid AC taken twice a day and comparable to famotidine 20 mg twice daily.[36] In addition, the intragastric pH with Prilosec OTC was consistently higher than with both famotidine regimens on subsequent treatment days. Because the PPIs inhibit only those proton pumps that are actively secreting acid, they are most effective when taken 30 minutes before meals.[37]

*Indications* Nonprescription omeprazole is indicated for the treatment of frequent heartburn in patients who have symptoms 2 or more days a week. It is not intended for immediate relief of occasional or acute episodes of heartburn or for dyspepsia.

*Dosage and Administration Guidelines* Omeprazole should be taken 30 minutes before eating every morning for 14 days. Treatment of heartburn may be repeated after 4 months if symptoms recur.[35] If heartburn continues while taking omeprazole, persists for more than 2 weeks, or recurs within 4 months, follow-up with a primary care provider is recommended. The tablets should not be chewed or crushed, as this may decrease the effectiveness of the drug.

*Safety Considerations* The most common side effects of the PPIs are similar to those reported for the $H_2$RAs (e.g., diarrhea, constipation, and headache).[33] A recent retrospective review reported a higher incidence of community-acquired pneumonia in patients taking antisecretory drugs than in those who were not taking them.[38] The PPIs had a 1.89 and the $H_2$RAs had a 1.63 adjusted relative risk of pneumonia, compared with those who stopped PPIs and $H_2$RAs. The findings for PPIs were dose related. Possible increased risk of pneumonia may result from a decrease in the antibacterial action of gastric juice, which when aspirated may lead to an overgrowth of pathogens. Risk factors include asthma, chronic obstructive pulmonary disease, young or old age (e.g., children and elderly), and immunocompromised state. The clinical importance of these findings for ambulatory patients requiring PPI therapy is questionable.

Omeprazole may interact with other medications that depend on the hepatic CYP 2C19 for metabolism.[33,34] Although evidence for clinically important drug interactions is minimal given the widespread use of the omeprazole over the last decade, patients taking medications such as diazepam, phenytoin, and warfarin should be warned about the potential for a drug interaction.[35] Similar to antacids and $H_2$RAs, PPIs increase intragastric pH and may decrease the absorption of pH-dependent drugs[33] (see drug interaction section of antacids and $H_2$RAs). PPIs may increase the bioavailability of digoxin, but the clinical importance of this effect is unknown.

### Bismuth Subsalicylate

Bismuth subsalicylate (BSS) is indicated for heartburn, upset stomach, indigestion, nausea, and diarrhea. It is likely that BSS may eventually be approved by FDA for the relief of upset stomach associated with belching and gas resulting from overindulgence in food and drink. It is uncertain how BSS relieves heartburn, but for upset stomach, it is believed to act by a topical effect on the stomach mucosa. When used to treat acid-related symptoms, the adult dose of BSS is 262 to 500 mg every 1/2 to 1 hour as needed (Table 14-4). Recently, numerous nonprescription products have been reformulated to contain BSS. In the past, common trade name products, such as Maalox, contained only antacids. Today, product line extensions, such as Maalox Total Stomach Relief contain BSS and no antacid (Table 14-4). Thus, patients and health care providers are often confused and may not know what they are recommending or purchasing. Individuals taking these products need to know that bismuth salts may cause the stool and tongue to turn black. Dark-colored stools may be interpreted as an upper GI bleed, prompting a needless colonoscopy. For a complete discussion of BSS, see Chapter 17.

### Product Selection Guidelines

*Special Populations* Careful consideration should be given to the elderly before recommending self-treatment for new onset of heartburn or dyspepsia. Older patients are more likely to take medications that can contribute to heartburn and dyspepsia. In addition, they are at higher risk for developing complications and may have a more severe underlying disorder.[1,16] If self-treatment is appropriate, an assessment should be made to determine if the individual has renal impairment and to identify potentially interacting medications. Patients with decreased renal function should be cautioned about using aluminum- and magnesium-containing antacids. The daily $H_2RA$ dose should also be reduced, especially in those taking the higher nonprescription dosages. Omeprazole may be used in patients with renal impairment. Sodium bicarbonate should be avoided in patients taking cardiovascular medications.

Antacid selection for eligible patients should be based, in part, on potential side effects. For example, if a patient has a tendency toward constipation, a less constipating antacid, such as magnesium hydroxide, may be more appropriate, while constipating antacids, such as aluminum hydroxide, should be avoided.

Children under 12 years of age with heartburn or dyspepsia should be referred to their primary care provider for further evaluation.[39] Nonprescription antacids, such as calcium carbonate and magnesium hydroxide are labeled for children 12 years and older. If antacids are recommended, an assessment of the child's average daily intake of calcium may help guide the recommendation. The recommended daily intake of calcium for children 9 to 18 years old is 1300 mg.[27] Nonprescription $H_2RAs$ are labeled for patients age 12 or older, and nonprescription omeprazole is indicated for patients age 18 years and older.

Infrequent and mild heartburn in pregnant women should be treated initially with dietary and lifestyle modifications.[24] Calcium- and magnesium-containing antacids are pregnancy category B agents, and may be used safely if the recommended daily dosages are not exceeded.[40] Special attention should be given to the recommended intake of calcium during pregnancy (1300 mg/day), as with pediatric patients.[27] If a woman is meeting the recommendations, the addition of a calcium-containing antacid may cause her to exceed the upper limit of 2500 mg of calcium per day. Pregnant women with more frequent and severe heartburn should be referred to a primary care provider. Although cimetidine, famotidine, ranitidine, and nizatidine are listed as pregnancy category B and have been used during pregnancy, women should seek advice from their primary care provider prior to self-treating with an $H_2RA$. Omeprazole is a pregnancy category C drug and should not be used by pregnant women without the advice of their primary care provider.

Magnesium hydroxide and aluminum hydroxide are not secreted into breast milk in substantial amounts.[24] Therefore, these antacids may be safely recommended for self-treatment of heartburn in nursing mothers. The American Academy of Pediatrics considers cimetidine to be compatible with breast-feeding.[41] However, ranitidine and famotidine are less concentrated in the breast milk, and may be preferable. There is insufficient information regarding the use of omeprazole in women who are breast-feeding, so it cannot be recommended for nursing mothers at this time.[42]

*Patient Preferences* Antacids and antisecretory drugs are available in a wide range of prices, flavors, and dosage forms. Once the most appropriate nonprescription medication is determined, the individual should be involved in selecting a product that is affordable, palatable, and practical to administer. Other nonactive ingredients such as dyes, sodium, and sugar should be considered for individuals with allergies, sensitivities, or dietary restrictions.

### *Complementary Therapies*

A small number of herbal remedies have been used traditionally to treat heartburn and dyspepsia, but few have been well studied (Table 14-6; see also Chapter 53).[43-51] There is no evidence that herbal products increase intragastric pH and relieve heartburn. A few studies have shown an improvement in dyspeptic symptoms with combination herbal therapies. A product marketed as STW 5 contains iberis, peppermint, and chamomile and has been shown to be more effective than placebo, with no serious adverse effects.[46] Another product marketed as STW 5-II contains extracts of bitter candy tuft, matricaria flower, peppermint leaves, caraway, licorice root, and lemon balm. In patients with nonulcer dyspepsia, the combination relieved symptoms better than placebo.[47] A combination of peppermint oil and caraway oil was shown to be effective for dyspepsia.[51]

## Assessment of Heartburn and Dyspepsia: A Case-based Approach

Cases 14-1 and 14-2 illustrate the assessment of patients with heartburn and dyspepsia.

## Patient Counseling for Heartburn and Dyspepsia

Many cases of uncomplicated heartburn and dyspepsia are self-treatable. For optimal outcomes, individuals need to understand how to treat symptoms appropriately and when to seek additional care. This information is provided in the box Patient Education for Heartburn and Dyspepsia.

## Evaluation of Patient Outcomes for Heartburn and Dyspepsia

Individuals taking antacids or an $H_2RA$ for infrequent heartburn and dyspepsia should obtain symptom relief within 30 minutes to 1 hour. Patients taking omeprazole may require up to 4 days for complete relief of symptoms, but most individuals are asymptomatic within 1 or 2 days. Self-treating individuals should be encouraged to contact their health care provider to report on the effectiveness of therapy and problems, such as side effects, that may arise during treatment. In some cases, the clinician may

**TABLE 14-6 Botanical Medicines Used to Treat Heartburn and Dyspepsia[43-51]**

| Botanical Medicine (Scientific Name) | Risks | Effectiveness |
|---|---|---|
| Artichoke leaf (*Cynara scolymus*) | Likely safe in amounts found in foods; possible allergic reaction; artichoke extract: possible increased flatulence in some patients | Improvement in dyspepsia symptoms shown in small studies |
| Caraway oil (*Carum carvi*) | Likely safe in amounts found in foods; some reports of substernal burning, belching, and nausea when used with peppermint oil. | Possibly effective in when used combination with peppermint oil |
| Carrageenan (*Chondrus crispus*) | Likely safe in amounts found in foods; associated with intestinal ulcerations and neoplasms in animals | Insufficient evidence |
| Chamomile (*Matricaria recutita*) | Rare allergic reactions | Possibly effective when used in combination with iberis and peppermint oil |
| Coriander seed (*Coriandrum sativum*) | Likely safe in amounts found in foods; possible laxative effect | Insufficient evidence |
| Ginger (*Zingiber officinale*) | Likely safe in amounts found in foods; possible prolonged bleeding times in patients on oral anticoagulants | Insufficient evidence |
| Licorice (*Glycyrrhiza glabra*) and deglycyrrhizinated licorice | Possible pseudoaldosteronism with large doses (>50 g/day), resulting in hypokalemia, water retention, and hypertension; contraindicated in pregnancy, cholestatic liver, cirrhosis, hypokalemia, renal impairment | Insufficient evidence |
| Peppermint (*Mentha piperita*) | Likely safe in amounts found in foods; may decrease LES pressure | Possibly effective when used in combination with caraway oil |
| Sage (*Salvia officinalis*) | Likely safe in amounts found in foods; possibly unsafe in greater amounts; sage oil: possible CNS toxicity in higher doses | Insufficient evidence |
| Turmeric (*Curcuma longa*) | Likely safe in amounts found in foods; possible GI disturbances with overuse; contraindicated in patients with bile duct obstruction, gallstones, gastric ulcers, or hyperacidity disorders | Insufficient evidence |

Key: CNS, central nervous system; GI, gastrointestinal; LES, lower esophageal sphincter.

## CASE 14-1

| Relevant Evaluation Criteria | Scenario/Model Outcome |
|---|---|
| **Information Gathering** | |
| 1. Gather essential information about the patient's symptoms, including: | |
| a. description of symptom(s) (i.e., nature, onset, duration, severity, associated symptoms) | Patient experiences heartburn 3-4 times/week during the day and sometimes in the evening, occurring off and on for the past month. He rates discomfort as 3-5 on a scale of 1-10 (1 = no pain; 10 = worst pain imaginable), describes it as burning, accompanied by belching, and denies other symptoms. |
| b. description of any factors that seem to precipitate, exacerbate, and/or relieve the patient's symptom(s) | More noticeable when he eats larger meals later in the evening; lying down after eating makes it worse |
| c. description of the patient's efforts to relieve the symptoms | Has taken Tums in the past with temporary relief and tried Pepcid AC, but is looking for something less chalky tasting, more effective, and longer lasting |

## CASE 14-1 (continued)

| Relevant Evaluation Criteria | Scenario/Model Outcome |
|---|---|
| 2. Gather essential patient history information: | |
| a. patient's identity | Greg Samuels |
| b. age, sex, height, and weight | 38 yo M, 5'10", 195 lb |
| c. patient's occupation | Exterminator |
| d. patient's dietary habits | Primarily meat and potatoes–based meals; drinks one cup of coffee in the morning |
| e. patient's sleep habits | Stays up late when he experiences heartburn because it is uncomfortable to lie down; his sleep is not disrupted; rises for work at 6 AM |
| f. concurrent medical conditions, prescription and nonprescription medications, and dietary supplements | Tylenol 1000 mg 1-3 times a month for tension-type headaches; lovastatin 40 mg once daily for hyperlipidemia |
| g. allergies | Penicillin |
| h. history of other adverse reactions to medications | None |
| i. other (describe)_______ | Denies alcohol and tobacco use |
| **Assessment and Triage** | |
| 3. Differentiate the patient's signs/symptoms and correctly identify the patient's primary problem(s) (see Table 14-2). | Postprandial heartburn associated with large meals and recumbence. Evaluate specific dietary triggers associated with daytime symptoms. |
| 4. Identify exclusions for self-treatment (see Figure 14-2). | None. Alarm symptoms (see Table 14-2) and contraindications to self-treatment are absent. |
| 5. Formulate a comprehensive list of therapeutic alternatives for the primary problem to determine if triage to a medical practitioner is required, and share this information with the patient. | Options include:<br>(1) Recommend self-care with an appropriate nonprescription product and advise on nondrug measures.<br>(2) Recommend self-care with an appropriate nonprescription product and advise on nondrug measures until Greg can contact his PCP.<br>(3) Refer Greg to his PCP for medical evaluation of his symptoms.<br>(4) Take no action. |
| **Plan** | |
| 6. Select an optimal therapeutic alternative to address the patient's problem, taking into account patient preferences. | The patient meets the criteria for self-treatment with OTC omeprazole combined with nondrug measures. A swallowed tablet will avoid the "chalky taste" he dislikes. The PPI should be more effective in managing frequent symptoms. |
| 7. Describe the recommended therapeutic approach to the patient. | Take Prilosec OTC 20 mg once daily, 30 minutes before breakfast for 14 days. Avoid risk factors that may contribute to heartburn (see Table 14-1). |
| 8. Explain to the patient the rationale for selecting the recommended therapeutic approach from the considered therapeutic alternatives. | Seeing a PCP, that is, primary care provider, may not be necessary if adequate relief is obtained from appropriate use of omeprazole and if symptoms do not recur within 4 months. |
| **Patient Education** | |
| 9. When recommending self-care with nonprescription medications and/or nondrug therapy, convey accurate information to the patient, including: | |
| a. appropriate dose and frequency of administration | Take one tablet every morning. See the box Patient Education for Heartburn and Dyspepsia. |

## CASE 14-1 (continued)

| Relevant Evaluation Criteria | Scenario/Model Outcome |
|---|---|
| b. maximum number of days the therapy should be employed | 14 days; may repeat every 4 months if symptoms return |
| c. product administration procedures | Take with a glass of water 30 minutes before breakfast. |
| d. expected time to onset of relief | 2 to 3 hours; complete relief within 1 to 4 days |
| e. degree of relief that can be reasonably expected | Complete relief of symptoms |
| f. most common side effects | Headache, diarrhea, constipation |
| g. side effects that warrant medical intervention should they occur | Severe headache, diarrhea, constipation; allergic reaction to medication, e.g., rash, fever |
| h. patient options in the event that condition worsens or persists | A PCP should be consulted if the symptoms persist, worsen, or recur within 4 months, or if alarm symptoms develop. |
| i. product storage requirements | Store at 68°-77°F (20°-25°C); protect from heat and humidity. |
| j. specific nondrug measures | Eat dinner at least 3 hours prior to bedtime. Eat smaller meals. Consider starting a weight loss program. Elevate the head of the bed or use a foam wedge. |
| 10. Solicit patient's follow-up questions. | Could I take an antacid for immediate relief before omeprazole starts to work? |
| 11. Answer patient's questions. | Yes. It is safe to take Tums or another antacid initially until your symptoms are relieved. If a supplemental antacid continues to be necessary, contact your PCP. |

Key: OTC, over-the-counter; PCP, primary care provider; PPI, proton pump inhibitor.

## CASE 14-2

| Relevant Evaluation Criteria | Scenario/Model Outcome |
|---|---|
| **Information Gathering** | |
| 1. Gather essential information about the patient's symptoms, including: | |
| a. description of symptom(s) (i.e., nature, onset, duration, severity, associated symptoms) | Patient describes daily heartburn, bloating, and epigastric pain that occur during the day, often between meals, and sometimes awakens her at night. She rates discomfort as a 5-7 on a scale of 1-10 (1 = no pain; 10 = worst pain imaginable). Pain is diffuse and accompanied by nausea and sometimes vomiting. Pain started 3 months ago, and is increasing in frequency and severity. |
| b. description of any factors that seem to precipitate, exacerbate, and/or relieve the patient's symptom(s) | Food seems to diminish symptoms temporarily. |
| c. description of the patient's efforts to relieve the symptoms | She has taken Milk of Magnesia and Pepto Bismol in attempts to self-treat. They seemed to help early on, but she is not getting adequate relief with increasing doses. |
| 2. Gather essential patient history information: | |
| a. patient's identity | Ursula Alvarez |
| b. age, sex, height, and weight | 58 y/o F, 5'6"145 lb |
| c. patient's occupation | Homemaker |
| d. patient's dietary habits | Balanced diet; used to drink coffee in the mornings but quit when symptoms began |
| e. patient's sleep habits | Averages 7-8 hours per night |
| f. concurrent medical conditions, prescription and nonprescription medications, and dietary supplements | Diclofenac 75 mg 2 times/day for back pain for 5 years; Motrin Cold and Sinus 1 tablet 3 times/day for the last few weeks as she has been fighting a cold |

## CASE 14-2 (continued)

| Relevant Evaluation Criteria | Scenario/Model Outcome |
|---|---|
| g. allergies | NKA |
| h. history of other adverse reactions to medications | None |
| i. other (describe)_______ | Smokes half-pack of cigarettes/day for the past 30 years; quit drinking alcohol 4 years ago |
| **Assessment and Triage** | |
| 3. Differentiate the patient's signs/symptoms and correctly identify the patient's primary problem(s) (see Table 14-2). | Unable to identify primary problem without further medical evaluation. Symptoms are not consistent with self-treatable heartburn or dyspepsia. Relief of symptoms with food is not consistent with self-treatable heartburn. Alarm symptoms indicate referral. Use of multiple NSAIDs increases the risk of PUD. |
| 4. Identify exclusions for self-treatment (see Figure 14-2). | Symptoms increasing in frequency and severity for 3 months; nocturnal symptoms. Inadequate relief with self-treatment. |
| 5. Formulate a comprehensive list of therapeutic alternatives for the primary problem to determine if triage to a medical practitioner is required, and share this information with the patient. | Options include:<br>(1) Recommend self-care with an appropriate nonprescription product and advise on nondrug measures.<br>(2) Recommend self-care with an appropriate nonprescription product and advise on nondrug measures until Ursula can contact her PCP.<br>(3) Refer Ursula to her PCP for medical evaluation of her symptoms.<br>(4) Take no action. |
| **Plan** | |
| 6. Select an optimal therapeutic alternative to address the patient's problem, taking into account patient preferences. | Refer Ursula to her PCP for further medical evaluation. Recommend that she discontinue the Motrin Cold and Sinus, which contains ibuprofen 200 mg and pseudoephedrine 30 mg, since she is taking diclofenac. If needed, suggest taking only the pseudoephedrine for her cold.<br>If unable to see PCP within the next few days, recommend that Ursula take either Pepcid AC Max or Prilosec OTC. Instruct Ursula to tell her PCP what OTC medication she is taking until her appointment. Emphasize importance of seeing PCP as soon as possible. |
| 7. Describe the recommended therapeutic approach to the patient. | You should see your PCP, that is, primary care provider, for evaluation of your symptoms. |
| 8. Explain to the patient the rationale for selecting the recommended therapeutic approach from the considered therapeutic alternatives. | Seeing a PCP is necessary because your symptoms are not consistent with self-treatable conditions.<br>Pepcid-AC Max or Prilosec OTC may provide temporary relief until you can see your PCP. |
| **Patient Education** | |
| 9. When recommending self-care with nonprescription medications and/or nondrug therapy, convey accurate information to the patient, including: | Pepcid AC Max 20 mg: take 1 tablet twice daily for 14 days. Onset of symptom relief should occur within 30 to 45 minutes. See Case 14-1 for Prilosec OTC instructions. |
| 10. Solicit follow-up questions from patient. | What natural products are effective for these symptoms? |
| 11. Answer patient's questions. | There is insufficient information and evidence to support the use of natural products for your symptoms. |

Key: NKA, no known allergies; NSAID, nonsteroidal anti-inflammatory drug; OTC, over-the-counter; PCP, primary care provider; PUD, peptic ulcer disease.

## PATIENT EDUCATION FOR HEARTBURN AND DYSPEPSIA

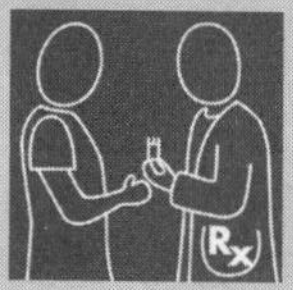

Heartburn and dyspepsia (indigestion) are often self-treatable conditions. Heartburn is characterized by a burning sensation in the chest, usually occurring after meals. Dyspepsia is characterized by discomfort in the upper abdomen. The objectives of self-treatment are to (1) provide complete relief of symptoms, (2) reduce frequency of intermittent episodes, (3) manage factors that contribute to the development of symptoms, (4) prevent and manage side effects of selected treatment, and (5) improve quality of life.

### Nondrug Measures

- Avoid food, beverages, and activities associated with an increased frequency and severity of symptoms.
- If possible, avoid the use of medications that may aggravate heartburn or dyspeptic symptoms.
- Avoid eating large meals.
- Stop or reduce smoking.
- Lose weight if overweight and not pregnant.
- Wear loose-fitting clothing.
- If nocturnal symptoms are present:
  - Avoid lying down within 3 hours of a meal.
  - Elevate the head of the bed using 6-inch blocks, or use a foam pillow wedge.

### Nonprescription Medications

- Store all medications at 68°F to 77°F (20°C to 25°C), and protect them from heat, humidity, and moisture. Discard after expiration date.

#### *Antacids*

- Antacids (sodium bicarbonate, calcium carbonate, magnesium hydroxide, aluminum hydroxide) are available alone and in combination with each other and other ingredients.
- Antacids work by neutralizing acid in the stomach.
- Antacids may be used for relief of mild, infrequent heartburn or dyspepsia (indigestion).
- Antacids are usually taken at the onset of symptoms. Onset of symptom relief usually occurs within 5 minutes.
- Because antacids come in a variety of strengths and concentrations, it is essential to consult the label of an individual product for correct dosing quantities and frequencies. Usually antacids should not be used more than four times a day, or regularly for more than 2 weeks.
- If symptoms are not relieved with recommended dosages, consult with a health care provider.
- Diarrhea may occur with magnesium- or magnesium/aluminum-containing antacids; constipation may occur with aluminum- or calcium-containing antacids. Consult with a heath care provider if these effects are severe or do not resolve in a few days.
- Patients with renal impairment should consult with their primary care provider prior to self-treatment with antacids.
- Patients taking tetracyclines, fluoroquinolones, azithromycin, digoxin, ketoconazole, itraconazole, and iron supplements should not take antacids within 2 hours of taking any of these medications.

#### *Histamine$_2$-Receptor Antagonists*

- $H_2$RAs (cimetidine, famotidine, nizatidine, ranitidine) work by decreasing acid production in the stomach.
- $H_2$RAs should be used for relief of mild to moderate, infrequent, and episodic heartburn and indigestion when a longer effect is needed; use the lower dosages for mild, infrequent heartburn; use the higher dosages for moderate infrequent symptoms.
- $H_2$RAs may be used to prevent heartburn and indigestion associated with meals.
- $H_2$RAs are usually taken at the onset of symptoms or 1 hour before symptoms are expected. Onset of symptom relief can be expected within 30 to 45 minutes. The combination product that contains both an antacid and an $H_2$RA provides more rapid symptom relief.
- $H_2$RAs generally provide symptom relief for 4 to 10 hours. $H_2$RAs can be taken when needed up to twice daily for 2 weeks.
- If symptoms are not relieved with recommended doses, or persist after 2 weeks of treatment, consult with a primary care provider.
- Side effects are uncommon. Consult with a health care provider if side effects are severe or do not resolve with a few days.
- Cimetidine may interact with certain prescription medications. Consult your health care provider if you are taking a blood thinner such as warfarin, an antifungal such as ketoconazole, antidepressants, anticonvulsants, theophylline, or amiodarone.

#### *Proton Pump Inhibitors*

- Proton pump inhibitors (omeprazole) work by decreasing acid production in the stomach.
- Omeprazole is indicated for mild to moderate frequent heartburn that occurs 2 or more days a week. It is not intended for the relief of mild, occasional heartburn.
- Omeprazole should be taken with a glass of water every morning 30 minutes before breakfast for 14 days. Make sure that you take the full 14-day course of treatment.
- Do not take more than 1 tablet a day.
- Complete resolution of symptoms should be noted within 4 days of initiating treatment.
- If symptoms persist, or are not adequately relieved after 2 weeks of treatment, or if symptoms recur before 4 months, consult your primary care provider.
- Do not crush or chew tablet, or crush tablet in food or beverage as this may decrease omeprazole's effectiveness.
- Side effects are uncommon. Consult with a health care provider if side effects are severe or do not resolve with a few days.
- Ask a health care provider if you are also taking blood thinners such as warfarin, antifungals such as ketoconazole, or antianxiety medications such as diazepam, or digoxin.

⚠ You should consult your primary care provider if any of the following symptoms occur:

- Heartburn or dyspepsia for over 3 months
- Heartburn or dyspepsia while taking recommended dosages of nonprescription medications
- Heartburn or dyspepsia after 2 weeks of continuous treatment with a nonprescription medication
- Heartburn that awakens you during the night
- Difficulty or pain on swallowing foods
- Lightheadedness, sweating, dizziness accompanied by vomiting blood or black material or black tarry bowel movements
- Chest pain or shoulder, arm, neck pain, with shortness of breath
- Chronic hoarseness, cough, choking, or wheezing
- Unexplained weight loss
- Continuous nausea, vomiting, or diarrhea
- Severe stomach pain

provide a follow-up phone call to assess therapeutic outcomes. Patients should be asked to describe the change in frequency and severity of symptoms since they initiated therapy. They should be questioned regarding side effects, and any new symptoms that may have developed. If an inadequate response is noted, the individual should be reevaluated to determine if a different product is suitable, or if referral to a primary care provider is necessary. Side effects may be managed by adjusting dosage or switching to another product. Development of atypical or alarm symptoms (Table 14-2) should be referred to a primary care provider.

## Key Points for Heartburn and Dyspepsia

- Limit the self-treatment of heartburn and dyspepsia to mild or moderate symptoms including postprandial burning in the upper abdomen or centralized abdominal discomfort.
- Refer patients with atypical or alarm symptoms (Table 14-2) for further evaluation.
- Refer children younger than 12 years with heartburn or dyspepsia to their primary care provider.
- Counsel patients with heartburn on nondrug measures such as dietary and lifestyle modifications (see box Patient Education for Heartburn and Dyspepsia).
- Advise self-treating individuals of the advantages and disadvantages of various antacids and acid-reducing products so they can select a product that is best suited for them.
- Antacids provide temporary relief for mild and infrequent heartburn and dyspepsia. Dosages are product specific because of variability in antacid ingredients and concentrations.
- $H_2$RAs are indicated for mild, infrequent heartburn or dyspepsia. They may be taken at the onset of symptoms or 1 hour prior to an event (meal or exercise) that causes symptoms.
- Combining an antacid with an $H_2$RA provides immediate relief of heartburn and is also effective in preventing further symptoms.
- The nonprescription PPI omeprazole is indicated for the treatment of frequent heartburn (heartburn that occurs 2 or more days a week) and is not intended for immediate relief of infrequent symptoms.
- Advise individuals with self-treatable symptoms that if symptoms worsen or do not improve after 14 days of effective self-treatment, they should contact their primary care provider.

## References


1. Richter JE. Gastroesophageal reflux disease. In: Yamada T, Alpers DH, Kaplowitz N, et al., eds. *Textbook of Gastroenterology.* 4th ed. Philadelphia: Lippincott Williams & Williams; 2003:1196-224.
2. DeVault KR, Castell DO. Updated guidelines for the diagnosis and treatment of gastroesophageal reflux disease. *Am J Gastroenterol.* 2005;100:190-200.
3. Sonnenberg A, El-Serag HHP. Clinical epidemiology and natural history of gastroesophageal reflux disease. *Yale J Biol Med.* 1999; 72:81-92.
4. Peterson WL, Berardi RR, El-Serag H, et al. American Gastroenterological Association Consensus Development Panel. In: *Improving the Management of GERD: Evidence-based Therapeutic Strategies.* Bethesda, Md: AGA Press; 2002:1-21.
5. Rivicki DA., Wood M, Maton PN, et al. The impact of gastroesophageal reflux disease on health-related quality of life. *Am J Med.* 1998;104:252-8.
6. Sandler RS, Everhart JE, Donowitz M, et al. The burden of selected digestive diseases in the United States. *Gastroenterology.* 2002;122:1500-11.
7. Talley NJ, Holtmann G. Approach to the patient with dyspepsia and related functional gastrointestinal complaints. In Yamada T, Alpers DH, Kaplowitz N, et al, eds. *Textbook of Gastroenterology.* 4th ed. Philadelphia: Lippincott Williams & Williams; 2003;655-77.
8. Vakil N. Dyspepsia and GERD: breaking the rules. *Am J Gastroenterol.* 2005;100:1489-90.
9. Erstad BL. Dyspepsia: initial evaluation and treatment. *J Am Pharm Assoc.* 2002;42:460-8.
10. Procter & Gamble. Data on file. Cincinnati, Ohio; 2002.
11. Del Valle J, Chey WD, Scheiman JM. Acid-peptic disorders. In: Yamada T, Alpers DH, Kaplowitz N, et al., eds. *Textbook of Gastroenterology.* 4th ed. Philadelphia: Lippincott Williams & Williams; 2003:1321-76.
12. Berardi RR, Welage LS. Peptic ulcer disease. In: DiPiro JT, Talbert RL, Yee GC, et al., eds. *Pharmacotherapy: A Pathophysiologic Approach.* 6th ed. McGraw-Hill, Inc; 2005;629-48.
13. Oliveria SA, Christos PJ, Talley NJ, et al. Heartburn risk factors, knowledge, and prevention strategies: a population-based survey of individuals with heartburn. *Arch Intern Med.* 1999;159:1592-8.
14. Nilsson M, Johnsen R, Ye W, et al. Lifestyle related risk factors in the aetiology of gastroesophageal reflux. *Gut.* 2004;53:1730-5.
15. Nandurkar S, Locke III GR, Fett S, et al. Relationship between body mass index, diet, exercise and gastro-oesophgeal reflux symptoms in a community. *Aliment Pharmacol Ther.* 2004;20:497-505.
16. Ferriolli E, Oliveira RB, Matsuda NM, et al. Aging, esophageal motility, and gastroesophageal reflux. *J Am Geriatr Soc.* 1998;46: 1534-7.
17. McColl KEL. Review article: Helicobacter pylori and gastro-oesophageal reflux disease—the European perspective. *Aliment Pharmacol Ther.* 2004;20(suppl 8):36-9.
18. Lagergren J, Bergstrom R, Lindgren A, et al. Symptomatic gastroesophageal reflux as a risk factor for esophageal adenocarcinoma. *N Engl J Med.* 1999;11:825-31.
19. Spechler SJ. Barrett's esophagus. *N Engl J Med.* 2002;346:836-42.
20. Dent J, Brun J, Fendrick AM, et al. An evidence-based appraisal of reflux disease management—the Genval Workshop Report. *Gut.* 1999;44:S1-16.
21. Dent J. Management of reflux disease. *Gut.* 2002;50: 67-71.
22. Howden CW, Chey WD. Gastroesophageal reflux disease. *J Family Practice.* 2003;52:240-7.
23. Scott M, Gelhot AR. Gastroesophageal reflux disease: diagnosis and management. *Am Family Physician.* 1999; 59:1161-9.
24. Broussard CN, Richter JE. Treating gastro-esophageal reflux disease during pregnancy and lactation: what are the safest therapy options? *Drug Safety.* 1998;19:325-37.
25. Maton PN, Burton ME. Antacids revisited: a review of their clinical pharmacology and recommended therapeutic use. *Drugs.* 1999;57:855-70.
26. Hade JE, Spiro HM. Calcium and acid rebound: a reappraisal. *J Clin Gastroenterol.* 1992;15:37-44.

27. Food and Nutrition Information Center Dietary Reference Intakes (DRI) and Recommended Dietary Allowances (RDA) National Agricultural; Library, United States Department of Agriculture. Available at: http://www.nal.usda.gov/fnic/etext/000105.html. Accessed July 15, 2005.
28. Welage LS, Berardi RR. Drug interactions with antiulcer agents: considerations in the treatment of acid-peptic disease. *J Pharm Pract.* 1994;7:177-95.
29. Marsh TD. Nonprescription $H_2$-receptor antagonists. *J Am Pharm Assoc.* 1997;37:552-6.
30. Bytzer P. H2 receptor antagonists and prokinetics in dyspepsia: a critical review. *Gut.* 2002;50(suppl IV):iv58-62.
31. Rodgers PT, Brengel GR. Famotidine-associated mental status changes. *Pharmacotherapy.* 1998;18:404-7.
32. Michalets EL. Update: clinically significant cytochrome P-450 drug interactions. Pharmacotherapy. 1998;18:84-112.
33. Berardi RR. Proton pump inhibitors: an effective, safe approach to GERD management. *Postgrad Med Special Report.* 2001;25-35.
34. Welage LS, Berardi RR. Evaluation of omeprazole, lansoprazole, pantoprazole, and rabeprazole in the treatment of acid-related diseases. *J Am Pharm Assoc.* 2000;40:52-62.
35. Proctor & Gamble. Prilosec OTC package insert. Cincinnati, Ohio; September 2003.
36. Miner PP, Graves MR, Grender JM, et al. Comparison of gastric acid pH with omeprazole magnesium 20.6 mg (Prilosec OTC) qd, famotidine 10 mg bid (Pepcid AC) and famotidine 20 mg bid over 14-days of treatment. *Am J Gastroenterol.* 2004;99(suppl): S8. abstract.
37. Hatlebakk JG, Katz PO, Camacho-Lobato L, et al. Proton pump inhibitors: better acid suppression when taken before a meal than without a meal. *Aliment Pharmacol Ther.* 2000;14:1267-72.
38. Laheij RJF, Sturkenboom MCJM, Hassing R, et al. Risk of community acquired pneumonia and use of gastric acid suppressive drugs. *JAMA.* 2004;292:1955-60.
39. Gremse DA. Gastroesophageal reflux disease in children: an overview of pathophysiology, diagnosis, and treatment. *J Ped Gastroenterol Nutr.* 2002;35:S297-9.
40. Baron TH, Ramirez B, Richter JE. Gastrointestinal motility disorders during pregnancy. *Ann Intern Med.* 1993;118:366-75.
41. American Academy of Pediatrics, Committee on Drugs. The transfer of drugs and other chemicals into human milk. *Pediatrics.* 2001;108:776-89.
42. Briggs GG, Freeman RK, Yaffe SJ. *Drugs in Pregnancy and Lactation.* 6th ed. Baltimore: Williams & Wilkins; 2002.
43. Indigestion—dyspepsia. In: Robbers JE, Tyler VE, eds. *Tyler's Herbs of Choice: The Therapeutic Use of Phytomedicinals.* New York: Haworth Press; 1999:65-88.
44. Murray WJ. Herbal medications for gastrointestinal problems. In: Miller LG, Murray WJ, eds. *Herbal Medicinals. A Clinician's Guide.* New York: Haworth Press; 1998:79-93.
45. Blumenthal M, Goldberg A, Brinkman J. Herbal Medicine: Expanded Commission E Monographs. Austin, Tex: American Botanical Council, 2000.
46. Thompson CJ, Ernst E. Systematic review: herbal medicinal products for non-ulcer dyspepsia. *Aliment Pharmacol Ther.* 2002;16: 1689-99.
47. Madisch A, Holtmann G, Mayr G, et al. Treatment of functional dyspepsia with a herbal preparation. A double-blind, randomized, placebo-controlled, multicenter trial. *Digestion.* 2004;69:45-52.
48. Melzer J, Rosch J, Reichling R, et al. Meta-analysis: phytotherapy of functional dyspepsia with the herbal drug preparation STW 5 (Iberogast). *Aliment Pharmacol Ther.* 2004;20:1279-87.
49. Bundy R, Walker AF, Middleton RW, et al. Artichoke leaf extract reduces symptoms of irritable bowel syndrome and improves quality of life in otherwise healthy volunteers suffering from concomitant dyspepsia: a subset analysis. *J Altern Complement Med.* 2004;10:667-9.
50. Holtmann G, Adams B, Haag S, et al. Efficacy of artichoke leaf extract in the treatment of patients with functional dyspepsia: a six-week placebo-controlled, double-blind, multicentre trial. *Aliment Pharmacol Ther.* 2003;18:1099-105.
51. May B, Kohler S, Schneider B. Efficacy and tolerability of a fixed combination of peppermint oil and caraway oil in patients suffering from functional dyspepsia. *Aliment Pharmacol Ther.* 2000; 14:1671-7.

CHAPTER 15

# Intestinal Gas

*Patrick D. Meek*

Symptoms attributed to intestinal gas are common. Eructation (belching of air) is a bothersome symptom related to the release of swallowed air through the esophagus. Bloating may be most uncomfortable after eating (particularly the evening meal) and is often perceived as the accumulation of intestinal gas. Flatulence (excessive air or other gas in the stomach and intestines) is most commonly associated with the passage of rectal gas and may be both uncomfortable and embarrassing. Patients may also complain of recurrent "gas pains" or abdominal discomfort that in some cases, may be related to another gastrointestinal (GI) problem, such as irritable bowel syndrome (IBS). Differentiation of healthy patients with intestinal gas symptoms from those with an underlying medical condition is important to optimize nonprescription treatment. Despite the frequency of intestinal gas complaints, the pathophysiology of symptoms is poorly understood and treatment is often unsatisfactory.

The primary categories of nonprescription pharmacologic therapies for intestinal gas symptoms are antiflatulent medications (simethicone, activated charcoal) and digestive enzymes (lactase replacement and α-galactosidase products). Sales of antiflatulent products account for a significant portion of the nonprescription drug market.[1] In 2001, a leading antiflatulent–antacid combination product ranked among the top 200 nonprescription medications, with annual sales of $40 million, a 5% increase over 2000 sales figures.[2] In the early 1990s, annual sales of two lactase replacement products each exceeded $10 million.[3]

Practitioners should be able to evaluate a patient's symptoms and determine whether self-treatment is appropriate. If the disorder is not amenable to self-care, the patient should be referred to his or her primary care provider. Practitioners also should understand the dietary aspects of intestinal gas formation, and the role of pharmacologic and nonpharmacologic options, to help patients develop an appropriate self-care strategy. If self-care is appropriate, the practitioner should provide dietary suggestions, advice on the selection of an antiflatulent or digestive enzyme, and information on the current use of medications for managing symptoms.

## Epidemiology of Intestinal Gas Complaints

A significant portion of the population of the United States is affected by conditions that may cause intestinal gas symptoms, such as lactose malabsorption (29% of the population), IBS (5% to 20%), and other less common medical conditions, such as celiac disease (0.4%).[4-6] However, the prevalence and incidence of intestinal gas symptoms are largely unknown because of the limited availability of published information on the frequency of these complaints in the general population. One survey of the U.S. population conducted in 1997 evaluated the prevalence and impact of abdominal pain, bloating, and other digestive complaints: 40.5% of survey respondents reported having one or more digestive symptoms in the past month, 21.8% reported that they experienced abdominal pain or discomfort (from any cause), and 15.9% reported having abdominal bloating or distention.[7] More than half of symptomatic respondents rated symptoms as moderate to severe, and most indicated that symptoms resulted in some limitation in their ability to conduct usual activities, with 10% reporting that their activities were reduced by half or more.

Ambulatory patients with intestinal gas symptoms frequently consult with primary care providers or take medications for these symptoms. In the year 2000, of the estimated 823.5 million visits by ambulatory patients to office-based community physicians' offices in the United States, 37.8 million were for digestive system symptoms. Approximately 3.2 million visits were made by patients with a complaint of "excessive belching," 8.8 million with gas pains, and 720,000 visits by patients with flatulence.[8] These findings suggest that intestinal gas symptoms and conditions that predispose patients to intestinal gas symptoms are common, and may cause considerable discomfort, lifestyle impairment, and health care resource consumption.

## Physiology of Intestinal Gas Formation

To help patients manage intestinal gas symptoms, practitioners and patients should have a general understanding of how the GI tract works. Each time food, liquid, and saliva are swallowed, a small amount of air from the atmosphere passes into the stomach. In the stomach, the swallowed food is mixed with gastric acid, pepsin, and other substances, churned into small fragments, and then emptied into the small intestine, where most of the absorption of vitamins, minerals, and calories occurs. The rate at which the stomach empties varies, but generally takes about 1 to 2 hours. Smooth muscle contractions in the small intestine move the liquid food fragments and air downstream toward the large intestine (colon) where the indigestible liquid waste is mixed with the bacterial flora of the colon. In the colon, most of the remaining liquid is absorbed from the mixture of liquid waste, bacteria, and intestinal gas as it is transported toward the rectum, and temporarily stored as stool prior to a bowel movement.

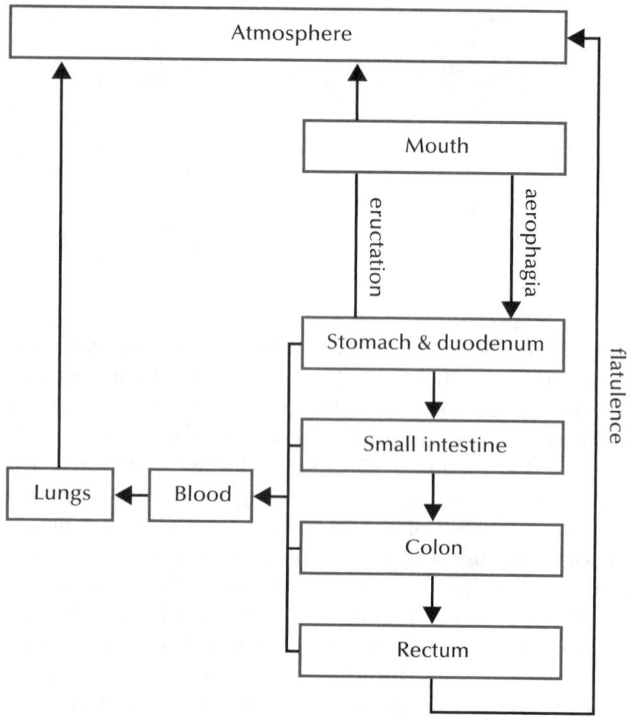


FIGURE 15-1 Pathways of intestinal gas elimination.

During a bowel movement, stool is eliminated and intestinal gas is expelled from the rectum as flatus.

Gas is produced and removed by various mechanical and biochemical processes during the transport, digestion, and elimination of food, nutrients, and waste from the GI tract (Figure 15-1). At any given time, approximately 200 mL of gas resides in the GI tract of most individuals, and is excreted at a rate ranging from 476 to 1491 mL/day. The primary gases present in the intestine are nitrogen ($N_2$ [11%-92%]), oxygen ($O_2$ [0%-11%]), carbon dioxide ($CO_2$ [3%-54%], hydrogen ($H_2$ [0%-86%]), and methane ($CH_4$ [0%-56%]), accounting for more than 99% of gas passed by the rectum (Figure 15-1).[9] None of these principal gases cause odor. The remaining 1% of colonic gas consists of volatile gases, such as hydrogen sulfide and other sulfur-based gases (e.g., sulfide acetate), which are produced by colon bacteria. These trace gases have an unpleasant smell and are noticeable in very small quantities (as low as a few parts per million).

The source and composition of intestinal gas varies throughout the GI tract. Gas in the upper GI tract (stomach, duodenum) arises from the swallowing of atmospheric air, which consists primarily of $N_2$ (78% by volume) and $O_2$ (20.8% by volume). Most swallowed air is subsequently eliminated through belching. In the first portion of the small intestine, carbon dioxide is produced when bicarbonate is secreted to neutralize gastric acid, and from metabolism of dietary substrates (such as fat and protein).[9] Most of the $CO_2$ formed in the upper GI tract subsequently diffuses rapidly from the small intestine into the blood, and does not contribute significantly to the volume of gas passed by rectum.

Compared with the gas composition of the upper GI tract, the lower GI tract (colon and rectum) contains less $O_2$, more $CH_4$, a similar amount of $N_2$, and variable amounts of $H_2$ and $CO_2$. Nitrogen from atmospheric air remains in the intestinal lumen while most of the $O_2$ diffuses into the bloodstream. In the colon, significant volumes of $H_2$, $CH_4$, and other trace gases result from the fermentation or bacterial metabolism of ingested materials by bacteria that reside naturally in the colon (Figure 15-1). Virtually all hydrogen production in the GI tract results from the fermentation of dietary carbohydrates (simple sugars, polysaccharides, and starches) that escape digestion earlier in the GI tract and enter the colon. Similarly, levels of $CO_2$ in flatus are believed to be produced almost entirely by bacterial fermentation of indigestible carbohydrates (such as those found in beans) in the colon. Since both result from the process of bacterial fermentation, the concentrations of $H_2$ and $CO_2$ are closely related. While the volume of flatus caused by $CO_2$ formed in the upper GI tract is insignificant, $CO_2$ formed in the lower GI tract may account for close to 60% of the volume of flatus. Like $H_2$, methane is also formed almost exclusively in the colon by bacterial metabolism. In the case of $CH_4$, anaerobic organisms (methanogens) utilize $H_2$ and $CO_2$ to form $CH_4$ (and water) in the colon through a process called methanogenesis. The rate of $CH_4$ production is only minimally influenced by food ingestion; however, some people consistently excrete large quantities of $CH_4$ while others excrete little or none.[10] Genetic factors appear to influence the level of $CH_4$ production and excretion, which may result from underlying differences in intestinal mucus composition and GI motility patterns.[11]

## Etiology/Pathophysiology of Intestinal Gas

Diet, underlying medical conditions, and drugs may precipitate or aggravate symptoms attributed to intestinal gas. Recent studies have revealed new theories of the pathophysiology of intestinal gas symptoms.[10,12-16] Although the exact mechanisms are not fully known, the origin of gas retention and symptoms appears to be affected by alterations in visceral perception and intestinal transit that varies at different physiologic locations along the GI tract.[12]

### *Diet*

Certain foods can increase intestinal gas production and lead to bothersome symptoms (Tables 15-1 and 15-2). Dietary sugars (e.g., lactose [dairy products], fructose [fruits, vegetables, candies, soft drinks], sucrose ["table sugar," sugar cane], and glucose ["dextrose," a breakdown product of starches]) may be incompletely absorbed in the healthy human small intestine.[17] These sugars are the principal substrates for $H_2$ production in the colon. Similarly, foods rich in complex carbohydrates (e.g., whole wheat, oats, potatoes, and corn), and indigestible oligosaccharides (e.g., raffinose, stachyose, and verbascose) are also malabsorbed. These substances remain in the intestinal lumen, are passed into the colon, and provide substrate for bacterial fermentation and colonic gas production ($H_2$ and $CO_2$).[10] Fermentation in the colon is the primary source of intestinal gas. The quantity of gas produced by

**TABLE 15-1 Gas-producing Foods[18,19]**

Foods that produce a normal amount of gas:

- Meat, fowl, fish
- Vegetables: asparagus, avocado, lettuce, okra, olives, peas, tomato, zucchini
- Fruit: cantaloupe (and other melons), grapes, berries
- Carbohydrates: rice, chips, popcorn, graham crackers
- All nuts, eggs, gelatin, fruit juice

Foods that cause moderate amounts of excessive gas:

- Root vegetables: potatoes, rutabaga, turnips
- Eggplant
- Vegetables: broccoli, cauliflower, cucumbers, peppers, radishes
- Citrus fruits, apples
- Carbohydrates: pastries, nonwheat breads (e.g., breads made from nonwheat flours, such as rice or potato flour)

Foods that cause major amounts of excessive gas:

- Vegetables: onions, celery, carrots, brussel sprouts, cabbage, kohlrabi, sauerkraut
- Legumes: most beans, especially dried beans and peas, baked beans, soy beans, lima beans
- Fruit: raisins, bananas, apricots, prunes
- Carbohydrates: all foods that contain wheat and wheat products, including cereals, breads, bagels, and pretzels
- Liquids: carbonated beverages, beer, red wine
- Dairy products: milk, ice cream, and cheese in people who have trouble digesting lactose
- Fatty foods: pan fried or deep fried foods, fatty meats; rich cream sauces and gravies (while fatty foods are not carbohydrates, these, too, can contribute to intestinal gas)
- Foods with high sugar content (e.g., soft drinks) and products containing sorbitol, and mannitol (e.g., diet foods and chewing gum)

**TABLE 15-2 Oligosaccharide-containing Foods That α-Galactosidase Might Affect[20]**

| Vegetables/ Legumes | Grains/Cereals/Seeds/ Nuts/Others |
|---|---|
| Beets | Barley |
| Broccoli | Breakfast cereals |
| Brussel sprouts | Granola |
| Cabbage | Oat bran |
| Carrots | Oat flour |
| Cauliflower | Pistachios |
| Corn | Rice bran |
| Cucumbers | Rye |
| Leeks | Sesame flour |
| Lettuce | Sorghum, grain |
| Onions | Sunflower flour |
| Parsley | Wheat bran |
| Peppers, sweet | Whole wheat flour |
| Black-eyed peas | Bagels |
| Bog beans | Baked beans |
| Broad beans | Bean salads |
| Chickpeas | Chili |
| Field beans | Lentil soup |
| Lentils | Pasta |
| Lima beans | Peanut butter |
| Mung beans | Soy milk |
| Peanuts | Split-pea soup |
| Peas | Stir-fried vegetables |
| Pinto beans | Stuffed cabbage |
| Red kidney beans | Tofu |
| Soybeans | Whole-grain breads |

fermentation of these substances in the colon is influenced by the quantity of foods ingested.

Diets high in roughage or dietary fiber (e.g., cellulose, lignin, pectin, and gums) may also lead to bloating and flatulence. Fiber is beneficial for reducing the risk of colorectal cancer (in the form of wheat bran) and cardiovascular disease, and is a valuable component of a balanced diet. According to the American Dietetic Association, most adults consume less than 15 g of fiber daily, although the recommended intake for optimum health is 20 to 35 g. There are two forms of fiber: insoluble and soluble. As the name implies, insoluble fiber does not dissolve in water, and is poorly fermentable. Foods naturally high in insoluble dietary fiber (e.g., bran, oatmeal, rice, barley, and the skin of raw fruits and vegetables) are effective for increasing stool frequency. The coarseness of insoluble fiber from dietary sources is a potential drawback and may trigger painful attacks in patients with bloating caused by IBS. In contrast, fiber available in the fleshy parts of raw fruits and vegetables (apples, bananas, oranges, carrots) and various commercial products (e.g., psyllium and calcium polycarbophil) is soluble in water and has a smooth texture. Soluble fiber absorbs water, increases stool mass, and stabilizes intestinal contractions, and may provide relief for constipation; however, studies have failed to show a benefit of soluble fiber supplementation in improving bloating, abdominal discomfort, and global symptoms in patients with IBS.[21-23] A soluble semisynthetic fiber supplement such as calcium polycarbophil may be preferred to natural fibers such as psyllium (see Chapter 16) for patients who experience gas-related symptoms (bloating, flatulence) from other fiber forms. However, in patients with IBS and slow intestinal transit, fiber may increase intestinal gas symptoms.[23]

Carbonated beverages, foods that contain artificial sweeteners (sorbitol), and fatty food, may also contribute to the formation of intestinal gases. The odor attributed to flatulence may be worsened by the ingestion of sulfate-containing foods (e.g., cruciferous vegetables such as broccoli and cabbage, sulfate additives contained in certain breads, beers, and sulfur-containing amino acids [e.g., methionine and cysteine] in proteins). Sulfur-based gases (e.g., hydrogen sulfide and sulfide acetate) are produced through the action of sulfate-reducing bacteria on sulfate.[15] Rating foods by their potential to cause intestinal gas symptoms is difficult, but clinical experience suggests that certain foods are generally more problematic than others (Table 15-1).

### *Swallowing and Other Contributory Factors*

Intestinal gas symptoms may also be related to the amount of air that enters the GI tract on swallowing. Smoking, chewing gum, sucking on hard candies, wearing poor-fitting dentures, and being overly anxious (and hyperventilating) may cause individuals to swallow larger amounts of air.[10,24] Poor eating habits such as gulping food or beverages too rapidly may also cause larger amounts of air to enter the stomach.

### *Medical Conditions*

A number of medical conditions cause or predispose patients to the formation of intestinal gas. Some conditions, such as carbohydrate malabsorption, lead to an increased amount of gas produced from bacterial fermentation in the colon. The most common cause of carbohydrate malabsorption is lactase deficiency. Lactase is the enzyme that normally breaks down lactose in the intestinal lumen so that it can be absorbed. Approximately 50 million people in the United States are lactose maldigesters, a number that is projected to reach 98 million by the year 2025.[25] The condition occurs more frequently in certain ethnic and racial groups; approximately 90% of Asian Americans, and 75% of African Americans are affected by the condition. Lactose maldigestion is least common in those who are of northern European descent (approximately 6%).[4] In patients with lactase deficiency, lactase enzyme is not available in sufficient quantities to break down lactose in dairy products before it reaches the colon.

In the colon, the malabsorbed lactose remains in the intestinal lumen where it is available to colonic bacteria for fermentation to $H_2$ and other substances. Individuals with lactase deficiency are intolerant to the lactose present in dairy products and experience GI symptoms such as gas pains, bloating, nausea, and diarrhea) on lactose ingestion. Bacterial fermentation in the small intestine resulting from bacterial overgrowth may also lead to excessive amounts of intestinal gas.

Other conditions such as IBS may predispose patients to intestinal gas symptoms. Gas pains and bloating are common complaints in patients with IBS.[26,27] These patients may experience symptoms attributed to intestinal gas caused by a heightened sensation of intestinal stretch (or visceral hypersensitivity), despite a normal degree of intraluminal distention. Some investigators have suggested that patients with IBS or functional bloating may have impaired transit of normal volumes of intestinal gas, suggesting that dysmotility also contributes to intestinal gas symptoms in these patients.[28]

Intestinal gas symptoms may also result from other less common medical conditions, such as celiac disease or diabetic gastroparesis (delayed stomach emptying). Patients with celiac disease have intolerance to gluten (a protein contained in wheat, rye, barley, and oats) and must follow a gluten-free diet. Intestinal gas symptoms may result from the inflammatory response that occurs in the GI tract after exposure to gluten. The most common sources of gluten are baked goods that contain the causative grains, wheat/oat cereals, noodles, and pastas; however, many other food products and some medications contain gluten. Successful adherence to a diet free of gluten requires rigorous label reading and close scrutiny of the gluten content of foods and nonprescription medications.

Intestinal gas symptoms may also result from certain medical procedures that cause abnormal release of intestinal gas. For instance, patients who undergo fundoplication (a procedure for the management of gastroesophageal reflux disease) may experience an inability to belch after the procedure.[29]

### *Drugs*

A variety of drugs may cause intestinal gas symptoms. These drugs can be broadly categorized by the mechanisms that cause symptoms: drugs that affect the intestinal flora (lactulose, antibiotics); drugs that affect the metabolism of glucose and other dietary substances ($\alpha$-glucosidase inhibitors [acarbose and miglitol], and the GI lipase inhibitor [orlistat]); drugs that affect GI motility (narcotics, anticholinergics, calcium channel blockers); drugs that are high in fiber (psyllium) or nonabsorbable polymers (cholestyramine); and drugs that contain or release gas (effervescent solutions such as Alka-Seltzer).

## Signs and Symptoms of Intestinal Gas

Patients with symptoms of intestinal gas complain most commonly of excessive belching, abdominal discomfort or cramping (gas pains), bloating, and flatulence. Gas pains and belching appear to be more common complaints than flatulence. Other less common symptoms associated with "gaseousness" include nausea, audible bowel sounds (borborygmi), and dyspepsia (indigestion).[8] Some patients may experience multiple symptoms concurrently.

### *Belching*

Everyone experiences belching, especially after eating. Belching is the easiest way for air to leave the stomach after it is swallowed. Some people have excessive belching, which may be annoying and embarrassing because of its frequency and/or unexpected occurrence. The more frequently a person swallows, the greater the potential for air to enter the stomach. Drinking carbonated beverages or eating food too quickly is an easy way to inadvertently increase the amount of air that is swallowed, which may then cause excessive belching.

### *Gas Pains*

Gas pains are often described as a generalized, crampy discomfort associated with gaseousness, which are relieved by passing gas. In some patients, symptoms may be brought on by stress or anxiety. In others the size of a meal may be associated with the onset and severity of gas pains, with larger meals (e.g., the evening meal) causing more bothersome symptoms. Patients who complain of chronic gas pains associated with a change in bowel function (either diarrhea or constipation) may have a form of IBS. Since gas pains can mimic other conditions, such as gallbladder or heart disease, a primary care provider should be consulted prior to initiating self-management.

### *Bloating*

Patients may characterize bloating as a sensation of tension in the abdominal area after eating, or a subjective sensation that the abdomen is larger than normal. Patients with bloating may observe that clothes fit more tightly or are difficult to fit into comfortably. The ingestion of certain foods (Tables 15-1 and 15-2), especially high-fiber foods, and eating too rapidly or too much may contribute to bloating. The onset of bloating may be associated with periods of stress and anxiety. For reasons that are unclear, complaints of abdominal bloating or distention are more common in women.[7] Similar to chronic gas pains, chronic bloating accompanied by a change in bowel function is suggestive of IBS. Patients with diabetes who complain that symptoms of bloating are accompanied by a sensation of early satiety or fullness after the ingestion of a small amount of food may be experiencing diabetic gastroparesis.

### Flatulence

Most patients who complain of flatulence are referring to the passage of intestinal gas through the rectum. Passing gas is normal and occurs either consciously or unconsciously about 14 times a day. Sometimes patients complain that flatulence occurs more frequently than expected or unexpectedly or uncontrollably. Certain foods (Tables 15-1 and 15-2), especially those that contain fiber, fructose (from fruits or artificially sweetened candies and beverages), lactose (from dairy products), sorbitol or mannitol (commonly used sweeteners in low-calorie foods and liquid medications), or oligosaccharides are more likely to cause gas and therefore can contribute to flatulence.

## Complications of Intestinal Gas

Intestinal gas symptoms are rarely a serious problem and can occasionally be treated with medications. However, intestinal gas complaints may be symptoms of an underlying chronic condition (inflammatory bowel disease, celiac disease, bacterial overgrowth, or IBS) or, in rare cases, a sign of a more serious problem (peptic ulcer disease, intestinal obstruction, or neoplastic disease). To avoid an unnecessary delay in initiating therapy, patients should be referred to a primary care provider for medical evaluation if any of the criteria for exclusion for self-management are met (Figure 15-2). Patients with lactose intolerance are at risk for developing low bone density (osteopenia or osteoporosis) because of reduced dietary intake and should be counseled to supplement their diets to achieve the recommended daily intake of 1000 to 1200 mg of elemental calcium per day.

## Treatment of Intestinal Gas

Most patients will be able to control symptoms by understanding how they occur, following steps to reduce predisposing factors, and making informed decisions regarding the use of nonprescription medications. Symptoms related to eating habits or diet will often subside quickly once the source of the problem is identified and the necessary changes are made. Self-treatment of intestinal gas symptoms (Figure 15-2) should begin with an assessment of the patient's history of symptoms, diet, eating habits, medication use, and relevant medical conditions. Patients who associate symptoms with specific food intolerance (i.e., to lactose or oligosaccharides) and who do not meet criteria for exclusion for self-treatment (Figure 15-2) may use digestive enzymes (lactase replacement and α-galactosidase products). Antiflatulents (activated charcoal and simethicone) may also be used, although evidence supporting the ability of these agents to reduce the amount of intestinal gas formation is contradictory. Referral to a primary care provider for further evaluation should be considered for patients with exclusions for self-treatment and in patients whose symptoms persist after simple treatment options such as dietary modification and nonprescription medications are initiated.

### Treatment Goals

The goals of therapy are to reduce (1) the frequency, intensity, and duration of intestinal gas symptoms and (2) the consequences of intestinal gas symptoms on the patient's lifestyle. Considering that a certain amount of intestinal gas production is normal and necessary for normal GI function, the complete elimination of intestinal gas is not a realistic goal.

### General Treatment Approach

Identification of the underlying cause of intestinal gas will guide treatment decisions (Figure 15-2). Inquiry into the patient's diet (including a review of eating habits and rate of food ingestion) can often lead to appropriate suggestions in attempting to reduce the problem. Although several nonprescription antiflatulent products are available, their use is largely empiric, and evidence supporting their benefit is limited. Exclusions for self-treatment (Figure 15-2) should be reviewed with the patient prior to recommending therapy.

### Nonpharmacologic Therapy

General information for controlling intestinal gas symptoms is provided in Table 15-3. Patients may benefit from changes in eating habits and dietary modification. Reducing the consumption of gas-producing foods (Tables 15-1 and 15-2) may be appropriate, depending on the patient's history. Some people are unable to tolerate gas-producing foods and need to completely avoid these foods in their diet. Patients with lactose intolerance should either avoid milk and dairy products or use lactase replacement products. Products with reduced lactose are also available and may be used as a substitute for milk or dairy products. Similarly, patients who are unable to tolerate foods with high oligosaccharide content should attempt to reduce or remove these foods from their diet.

### Pharmacologic Therapy

Simethicone and activated charcoal may relieve symptoms after intestinal gas has formed. α-Galactosidase and lactase enzymes are taken with foods to prevent gas from forming. Lactase replacement products may be beneficial for the treatment of intestinal gas and diarrhea associated with lactose intolerance, and are also used as digestive aids,

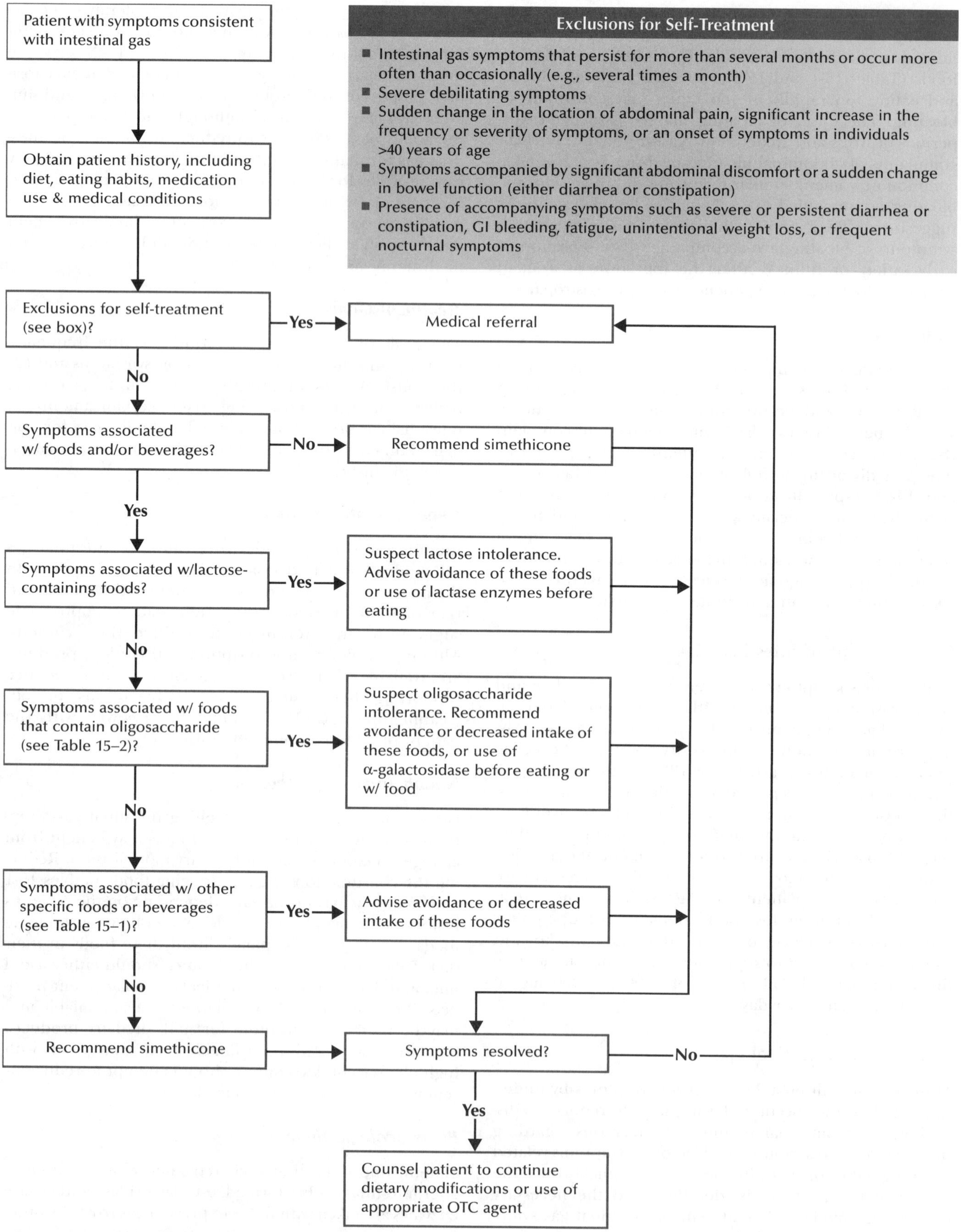


**FIGURE 15-2** Self-care of intestinal gas symptoms. Key: GI, gastrointestinal; OTC, over-the-counter.

**TABLE 15-3 Useful Information to Decrease Intestinal Gas Symptoms[30-32]**

**Eating Habits**

- Relax a bit before eating. Follow this simple breathing technique to enhance relaxation and release tension:
  - Sit straight in a comfortable position with your arms and legs uncrossed.
  - Breathe in comfortably, using your abdomen. Pause briefly before exhaling.
  - Each time you exhale, count silently to yourself, "one...two...three...four."
  - Repeat this cycle for 5 to 10 minutes.
  - Notice your breathing gradually slowing, your body relaxing, and your mind calming as you practice this breathing technique.
- Avoid the temptation to rush through a meal. Eat and drink slowly in a calm environment.
- Chew food thoroughly.
- Avoid washing solids down with a beverage.
- Avoid gulping and sipping liquids or drinking out of small-mouthed bottles, straws, or from water fountains.
- Eliminate pipe, cigar, and cigarette smoking.
- Avoid gum chewing and sucking hard candy (especially those that contain artificial sweeteners, such as sorbitol or mannitol).
- Check dentures for proper fit.
- Attempt to be aware of and avoid deep sighing.
- Do not attempt to induce belching or strain to pass gas.
- Do not overload the stomach at any one meal.

**Diet**

- Keep a dietary diary for a few days while tracking intestinal gas symptoms.
- Avoid foods that cause gas symptoms.
- Avoid gas-producing foods (Table 15-1).
- Avoid foods with air whipped into them, such as whipped cream, soufflés, sponge cake, and milk shakes.
- Avoid carbonated beverages, such as sodas and beer.

**Medication Use and Lifestyle Habits**

- Avoid long-term or frequent intermittent use of medications intended for relief of cold symptoms (e.g., anticholinergic antihistamines [brompheniramine, carbinoximine, chlorpheniramine, clemestine, diphenhydramine]).
- Avoid tight-fitting garments, girdles, and belts.
- Do not lie down or sit in a slumped position immediately after eating.
- Develop a regular routine of exercise and rest.

allowing individuals with lactose intolerance to incorporate dairy foods into their diet without producing intolerable symptoms. Most lactose maldigesters can tolerate up to 1 cup of milk, so these products should be used when more than that amount is ingested in one sitting. Osmotic laxatives may be used for patients with abdominal cramps, bloating, and gas associated with constipation (see Chapter 16).

### Simethicone

Simethicone, a mixture of inert silicon polymers, is used as a defoaming agent to relieve gas.

*Mechanism of Action* Simethicone acts in the stomach and intestine to reduce the surface tension of gas bubbles embedded in mucus in the GI tract. As surface tension changes, the gas bubbles are broken or coalesced and then eliminated more easily by belching or passing gas through the rectum.[33]

*Indications* FDA considers simethicone safe and effective as an antiflatulent agent. The ability of simethicone to reduce intestinal gas is questionable.[34] Nonetheless, the use of simethicone may be encouraged on a trial basis as some patients report benefit from it.

*Dosage and Administration Guidelines* The usual dosage for simethicone is 125 to 250 mg as needed after meals and at bedtime, not to exceed 500 mg/day. Many antacid products contain a combination of simethicone and antacids; therefore, patients should follow the label instructions for dosages. However, use of both agents is often unnecessary, and the efficacy of such combination products has not been well studied. Further, single-ingredient antiflatulent products (Table 15-4) usually contain a higher concentration of simethicone than that of the combination products.

*Safety Considerations* Because simethicone is not absorbed from the GI tract, it has no known systemic side effects and its safety has been well documented. Simethicone is contraindicated in patients with a known hypersensitivity to simethicone products or suspected intestinal perforation and obstruction.

### Activated Charcoal

The proposed antiflatulent properties of activated charcoal are related to the adsorbent effects of the substance, and the potential to facilitate the elimination of intestinal gas from the GI tract. Although activated charcoal is promoted for relief of intestinal gas, it is neither approved nor shown to be effective for this indication.[35] This substance also has poor palatability. Table 15-4 lists examples of commercially available products. Combination products containing simethicone and activated charcoal, which aim to provide relief from intestinal gas symptoms by combining the gas-reducing activity of each of the individual components, are available.

### α-Galactosidase

Another FDA-approved product for use as an antiflatulent is the enzyme α-galactosidase.

*Mechanism of Action* α-Galactosidase, which is derived from the *Aspergillus niger* mold and classified as a food, hydrolyzes oligosaccharides into their component parts before they can be metabolized by colonic bacteria.[33]

*Indications* Because high-fiber foods contain large amounts of oligosaccharides, α-galactosidase is recommended as a prophylactic treatment of intestinal gas symptoms produced by high-fiber diets or when eating foods

**TABLE 15-4 Selected Antiflatulent Products**

| Trade Name | Primary Ingredients |
|---|---|
| **Single-entity Simethicone Products** | |
| Alka-Seltzer Anti-Gas Gelcaps | Simethicone 125 mg |
| Gas-X Regular Strength Chewable Tablets | Simethicone 80 mg |
| Gas-X Extra Strength Chewable Tablets* | Simethicone 125 mg |
| Gas-X Extra Strength Oral Liquid | Simethicone 50 mg/5 mL |
| Gas-X Extra Strength Softgels† | Simethicone 125 mg |
| Gas-X Maximum Strength Softgels | Simethicone 166 mg |
| Maximum Strength GasAid Softgels | Simethicone 125 mg |
| Mylanta Gas Chewable Tablets | Simethicone 80 mg |
| Mylanta Gas Maximum Strength Chewable Tablets | Simethicone 125 mg |
| Mylanta Gas Maximum Strength Softgels | Simethicone 125 mg |
| Mylicon Infant's Drops‡ | Simethicone 40 mg/0.6 mL |
| Phazyme-125 mg Quick Dissolve Chewable Tablets | Simethicone 125 mg |
| Phazyme-180 mg Ultra Strength Softgels | Simethicone 180 mg |
| **Activated Charcoal Products** | |
| Activated Charcoal Tablets | Activated charcoal 250 mg |
| CharcoCaps Capsules*,†,§ | Activated charcoal 260 mg |
| **Combination Charcoal Product** | |
| Charcoal Plus | Activated charcoal 250 mg; simethicone 80 mg |
| **α-Galactosidase Replacement Products** | |
| Beano Tablets | 1 tablet = α-galactosidase 150 units |
| Beano Drops | 5 drops = α-galactosidase 150 units |
| Gaz Away Caplets | α-Galactosidase 150 units |
| **Lactase Replacement Products** | |
| Dairy Ease Tablets | Lactase 3000 units |
| Lactaid Extra Strength Caplets | Lactase 4500 units |
| Lactaid Original Strength Caplets | Lactase 3000 units |
| Lactaid Original Strength Drops (Canada) | Lactase 1250 units/drop |
| Lactaid Ultra Caplets | Lactase 9000 units |
| Lactrase Capsules | Lactase enzyme 250 mg |
| SureLac Tablets | Lactase 3000 units |

*Sodium-free; †sucrose-free; ‡pediatric-formulation; §dye-free.

that contain oligosaccharides (Table 15-2). A controlled trial of α-galactosidase demonstrated that the agent significantly reduced flatulence in patients fed oligosaccharide-containing foods.[36]

*Dosage and Administration Guidelines* The recommended dose is about 5 drops added to each serving of the problem food (usually two to three servings per meal) or 3 tablets per meal. A dose of 5 drops or 1 tablet contains α-galactosidase 150 units. The solution should be added after the food has cooled, because food temperatures higher than 130°F (54.4°C) may inactivate the enzyme.

*Safety Considerations* The safety of α-galactosidase also remains to be determined. Although this enzyme has been used in food processing for years and is regarded as safe by FDA, the amount contained in available products is probably much greater than that in processed foods. One patient developed an intestinal perforation after taking Beano for several weeks, but a causal relationship was not established and there have been no similar reports. Because the enzyme produces galactose, patients with galactosemia (an inherited metabolic disorder in which galactose accumulates in the blood as a result of deficiency of an enzyme catalyzing its conversion to glucose) should not use this product. Similarly, diabetic patients should be cautioned about the use of the enzyme, which may produce 2 to 6 g of carbohydrates per 100 g of food. Allergic reactions are also possible in patients allergic to molds.

### Lactase Replacement Products

Lactase replacement products are used in patients with lactose intolerance (see Chapter 17).

*Mechanism of Action* Lactase enzymes break down lactose, a disaccharide, into the monosaccharides glucose and galactose, which are absorbed.

*Indications* Lactase replacement products should be used in patients with lactose intolerance to aid in the digestion of dairy products.

*Dosage and Administration Guidelines* Lactase tablets or capsules should be taken at the time dairy products are ingested. The lowest recommended dose should be used and increased to a dosage that provides relief. Lactase drops (lactase 1250 units/drop) should be added to milk prior to ingesting. Usual ranges of these dosage forms are as follows: liquid, 5 (6250 lactase units) to 15 drops (18,750 lactase units) per 32 oz (or 1.25 to 3.75 drops per 8 oz) of milk (drops may be added up to 24 hours prior to ingestion); tablets, 1 to 3 tablets (3000 lactase units per tablet) with ingestion of dairy product (no more than 6 tablets at one time); and capsules, 1 to 2 capsules (4500 units per capsule) with ingestion of dairy product.

*Safety Considerations* No adverse effects are listed for lactase replacement products.

### Combination Products

Many antacid products contain a combination of simethicone and antacids; patients should follow the label instructions for dosages. However, use of both agents is often unnecessary, and the efficacy of such combination products is unknown. Combination products containing simethicone and activated charcoal are available that aim to provide relief from intestinal gas symptoms by combining the gas-reducing activity of each of the individual components.

### Product Selection Guidelines

*Patient Factors* Except for dairy products, α-galactosidase is intended for use as a preventive measure. Patients with symptoms of gas who need immediate relief or patients who cannot associate their symptoms with certain foods should receive with simethicone. If used on a regular basis, α-galactosidase is more cost-effective than simethicone. Because α-galactosidase produces carbohydrates, patients with galactosemia or diabetes mellitus should avoid this product and use simethicone instead. Lactase replacement products should be considered for patients with lactose intolerance when they ingest dairy products.

*Special Population Considerations* Several pediatric formulations of simethicone containing 40 mg of simethicone per 0.6 mL suspension are indicated for the relief of intestinal gas. These products are often promoted and used to relieve gas associated with colic, sometimes in infants. However, simethicone was not found to be superior to placebo for intestinal gas or infantile colic in a recent study.[37] Although its efficacy is questionable, simethicone is not absorbed from the GI tract and is considered safe for use in infants and children.[23] There are no reports linking simethicone to congenital defects.[23] Simethicone is a Pregnancy Category C drug and is considered to be safe for use by nursing mothers. For α-galactosidase products, safety and efficacy have not been evaluated in infants and children. Therefore, this product should not be used in pediatric patients until data are available to support such use. Manufacturers recommend that patients first consult with a primary care provider before using α-galactosidase if they are pregnant or nursing. No special population considerations are listed for lactase replacement products. Patients should consult a primary care provider if symptoms continue after using a product or if symptoms are unusual and seem unrelated to eating dairy.

## *Complementary Therapies*

A variety of complementary therapies (such as those listed in Table 15-5) are used to treat intestinal gas symptoms.[38,39] Carminatives, a term commonly used to describe herbs that relieve gas and colic, are used to ease gas discomfort (bloating and flatulence), dyspepsia, and intestinal cramping. Examples include fennel, caraway, peppermint, spearmint, and Japanese mint. Carminatives are among the foods that should be minimized or avoided by patients with gastroesophageal reflux disease (see Chapter 14);[40,41] however, their effect on lower esophageal sphincter tone in healthy individuals with intestinal gas symptoms may be less problematic.[42]

## Assessment of Intestinal Gas: A Case-based Approach

When a patient complains of intestinal gas, it is important to try to discern the causes, duration, and frequency of the symptoms (Table 15-6). Noting items that produce relief may provide clues as to the cause. A thorough review of dietary habits, medical problems, and use of prescription and nonprescription medications may provide other clues. Cases 15-1 and 15-2 give examples of assessment of patients with intestinal gas.

**TABLE 15-5 Selected Complementary/Alternative Medicines Used to Treat Intestinal Gas Symptoms[23,38,39,43]**

| Agent | Risks | Effectiveness |
|---|---|---|
| **Botanical Medicines (Scientific Name)** | | |
| Angelica root (*Angelica archangelica*) | Can cause photodermatitis (avoid excessive sunlight) | Not proven for digestive problems, including flatulence and fullness; GI effects attributed to antispasmodic and calcium-channel antagonist properties |
| Caraway seed (*Carum carvi*) | Avoid during pregnancy or lactation (lack of sufficient reliable safety information) | Not proven for digestive problems, including mild GI spasms, flatulence, and fullness; disagreement exists about caraway oil having antispasmodic effects |
| Dandelion root with herb (*Taraxacum herba*) | Can cause gastric hyperacidity, and dyspepsia; avoid in patients with gallbladder or biliary disease | Not proven for digestive problems, including indigestion, and flatulence; GI effects attributed to the substance taraxacin and its ability to increase bile flow (choleretic property) |
| Fennel (*Foeniculum vulgare*) | Can cause photodermatitis (avoid excessive sunlight); contraindicated during pregnancy; avoid use during lactation; coadministration with ciprofloxacin may reduce ciprofloxacin bioavailability (space doses appropriately) | Not proven as a stomach and bowel remedy for abdominal cramps and flatulence; GI effects attributed to promotility and antispasmodic properties |
| Gentian (*Gentiana lutea*) | Contraindicated in patients with PUD | Not proven for digestive problems, including fullness and flatulence; GI effects attributed to substances that appear to increase saliva and digestive juice secretion |
| Japanese mint (*Mentha canadensis*) | No significant toxicity reported; may reduce LES tone and cause/worsen gastroesophageal reflux symptoms | Not proven as remedy for flatulence; GI effects attributed to carminative properties |
| Spearmint (*Mentha spicata*) | No significant toxicity reported; may reduce LES tone and cause/worsen gastroesophageal reflux symptoms | Not proven as remedy for flatulence; GI effects attributed to carminative, local anesthetic, and antispasmodic properties |
| Peppermint (*Mentha piperita*) | No significant toxicity reported; may reduce LES tone and cause/worsen gastroesophageal reflux symptoms | Not proven as remedy for flatulence; GI effects attributed to carminative properties |
| Horehound herb (*Marrubii herba*) | No significant toxicity reported | Not proven for digestive problems, including indigestion and flatulence; GI effects attributed to choleretic properties |
| **Nonbotanical Natural Medicines** | | |
| ***Probiotics*** | | |
| *Lactobacillus* sp., *Bifidobacterium* sp. | No significant toxicity reported | Not proven for bloating, abdominal discomfort; possible improvement in patients with IBS; GI effects attributed to probiotic activity and reduced number of pathogenic organisms in GI tract |
| ***Behavioral Therapy*** | | |
| Hypnotherapy (including relaxation and breathing techniques, meditation, yoga) | Considered safe | May be useful for stress reduction (stress may increase GI symptoms by changing how the brain controls unwanted/painful sensation); evidence supports benefit of hypnotherapy and other behavioral interventions over placebo for reduction of symptoms in patients with IBS[23] |

Key: GI, gastrointestinal; IBS, irritable bowel syndrome; LES, lower esophageal sphincter; PUD, peptic ulcer disease.

## Patient Counseling for Intestinal Gas

Avoidance of foods or other substances that cause intestinal gas is the best advice to give patients suffering from this disorder. This advice is often difficult to follow, causing patients to resort to pharmacologic agents. The practitioner should explain the proper use of these medications and warn the patient of possible adverse effects. (See the box Patient Education for Intestinal Gas.)

TABLE 15-6 Differentiation of Intestinal Gas Discomfort and Irritable Bowel Syndrome

| Criterion | Intestinal Gas Discomfort | Irritable Bowel Syndrome |
|---|---|---|
| Location | Generalized discomfort in upper-, mid-, or lower-abdomen | Generalized discomfort (bloating and/or pain) in abdomen or colon |
| Signs | Eructation (upper abdomen): belching of air; bloating (mid-abdomen): perception of accumulated intestinal gas; flatulence (lower abdomen, colon): excessive air or other gas in stomach and intestines | Physical signs of disease may be absent; symptoms relieved with defecation or associated with change in frequency or consistency of stools |
| Symptoms | Physical discomfort may be minimal; negative psychosocial effects may be significant | Symptoms vary widely; typical symptoms: abdominal pain, accompanied by either diarrhea or constipation usually lasting at least 3 months |
| Onset | At any age | Early adulthood; rarely occurs after 60 years of age |
| Etiology | Primary causes: excessive amount of gas in stomach (eructation), bowel, and colon (bloating, flatulence); other causes: lactase deficiency, overgrowth of intestinal bacteria, and excessive air swallowing (aerophagia) | Cause unknown; altered GI motility and heightened visceral perception appear to contribute to condition |
| Exacerbating factors | Diet; underlying medical conditions; certain drugs (e.g., lactulose, antibiotics, $\alpha$-glucosidase inhibitors, orlistat, narcotics, anticholinergics, calcium channel blockers, psyllium or cholestyramine, and effervescent solutions) | Stress; overeating; problem foods (alcohol, chocolate, caffeinated beverages, dairy products, and sugar-free products [sorbitol or mannitol]); high-fat foods may aggravate symptoms |
| Modifying factors | Minimization of exacerbating factors | Minimization of exacerbating factors; physician evaluation; treatment |

## CASE 15-1

| Relevant Evaluation Criteria | Scenario/Model Outcome |
|---|---|
| **Information Gathering** | |
| 1. Gather essential information about the patient's symptoms, including: | |
| a. description of symptom(s) (i.e., nature, onset, duration, severity, associated symptoms) | Patient experiences gaseous bloating after eating dairy products. Her PCP recently told her she may be lactose intolerant. Her symptoms occur infrequently (about once a month) when she allows herself to indulge in certain foods. Her symptoms normally last less than a day and are mild, but she would like to try something that will reduce excessive intestinal gas on days when she knows her diet might cause problems. |
| b. description of any factors that seem to precipitate, exacerbate, and/or relieve the patient's symptom(s) | Symptoms are more noticeable after eating dairy products. Patient tries to avoid eating anything that contains milk. |
| c. description of the patient's efforts to relieve the symptoms | Dietary modification (see patient's dietary habits below) |
| 2. Gather essential patient history information: | |
| a. patient's identity | Stephanie Jones |
| b. patient's age, sex, height, and weight | 22 y/o F, 5'10", 138 lb |
| c. patient's occupation | College student, part-time sales clerk |
| d. patient's dietary habits | Minimizes dairy products. Otherwise diet is healthy and well rounded. She admits to "occasionally giving into" her sugar craving by indulging in artificially sweetened hard and soft candies. |
| e. patient's sleep habits | She enjoys sleeping and states that she gets about 7 or 8 hours of uninterrupted sleep each night. |

| CASE 15-1 (continued) | |
|---|---|
| **Relevant Evaluation Criteria** | **Scenario/Model Outcome** |
| f. concurrent medical conditions, prescription and nonprescription medications, and dietary supplements | Tums Ultra (400 mg of elemental calcium per tablet) 2 tablets by mouth 2 times/day (has been using for the past 3 months as a calcium supplement) |
| g. allergies | NKA |
| h. history of other adverse reactions to medications | None |
| i. other (describe)_______ | Patient experiences gaseous bloating after eating dairy products. Her PCP recently told her that she may be lactose intolerant. Her symptoms occur infrequently (about once a month) when she allows herself to indulge in certain foods. Her symptoms normally last less than a day and are mild, but she would like to try something that will reduce excessive intestinal gas on days when she knows her diet might cause problems. |
| **Assessment and Triage** | |
| 3. Differentiate the patient's signs/symptoms and correctly identify the patient's primary problem(s) (see Table 15-6). | Exacerbation of abdominal bloating appears to be a result of the ingestion of dairy products. Infrequent intake of foods artificially sweetened with sorbitol or mannitol may also be contributing to her symptoms. |
| 4. Identify exclusions for self-treatment (see Figure 15-2). | Stephanie denies having any symptoms that exclude self-treatment. |
| 5. Formulate a comprehensive list of therapeutic alternatives for the primary problem to determine if triage to a medical practitioner is required, and share this information with the patient. | Options include:<br>(1) Recommend dietary modification to minimize lactose exposure. Also, lactose-reduced milk and other products are available at many grocery stores, and may be used as milk substitutes.<br>(2) Avoid sorbitol- or mannitol-containing products (e.g., hard or soft candies, and other foods).<br>(3) Recommend an appropriate OTC product.<br>(4) Refer Stephanie to her PCP.<br>(5) Take no action. |
| **Plan** | |
| 6. Select an optimal therapeutic alternative to address the patient's problem, taking into account patient preferences. | OTC treatment with lactase tablets (3000 units) is appropriate. Reduce lactose exposure and continue calcium supplementation. |
| 7. Describe the recommended therapeutic approach to the patient. | Take a lactase replacement product when you eat lactose-containing foods. The lowest recommended dose should be used to start, and then increased to a dosage that provides relief. Make dietary modifications as listed in Table 15-1. |
| 8. Explain to the patient the rationale for selecting the recommended therapeutic approach from the considered therapeutic alternatives. | With the dietary modifications suggested, exacerbation of symptoms should be kept to a minimum. See your PCP, that is, primary care provider, if bloating worsens or persists beyond 1 week. |
| **Patient Education** | |
| 9. When recommending self-care with nonprescription medications and/or nondrug therapy, convey accurate information to the patient, including: | |
| a. appropriate dose and frequency of administration | Usual ranges of these dosage forms are as follows: liquid, 5 to 15 drops/qt of milk; tablets, 1 to 3 tablets with ingestion of dairy product (do not take more than 6 tablets [18,000 lactase units] at one time); and capsules, 1 to 2 capsules with ingestion of dairy product. |

## CASE 15-1 (continued)

| Relevant Evaluation Criteria | Scenario/Model Outcome |
|---|---|
| b. maximum number of days the therapy should be employed | If you continue to eat dairy foods, the product may be taken each day. Consult your PCP if symptoms continue after using the product, or appear to be unrelated to eating dairy. |
| c. product administration procedures | Lactase drops should be added to milk prior to ingesting it. (Treated milk can be stored in the refrigerator for up to 24 hours.) |
| d. expected time to onset of relief | Symptoms should be relieved quickly (within 1-4 hours) if the selected therapy is effective and the symptoms are caused by lactase deficiency. |
| e. degree of relief that can be reasonably expected | Complete elimination of bloating is possible. It is likely that symptoms will occasionally appear with dairy ingestion. |
| f. most common side effects | None |
| g. side effects that warrant medical intervention, should they occur | None |
| h. patient options in the event that condition worsens or persists | Consult your PCP if bloating is intolerable or persists after discontinuation of product. |
| i. product storage requirements | Keep in a tightly closed container in a clean, dry storage area. |
| j. specific nondrug measures | Dietary modification minimizes lactose exposure. |
| 10. Solicit follow-up questions from patient. | Can I double the dose of these products to get better more quickly? |
| 11. Answer patient's questions. | Doses may be gradually increased until an adequate response is obtained. Do not exceed 6 tablets or 15 drops (18,000 lactase units) at one time. |

Key: NKA, no known allergies; OTC, over-the-counter; PCP, primary care provider.

## CASE 15-2

| Relevant Evaluation Criteria | Scenario/Model Outcome |
|---|---|
| **Information Gathering** | |
| 1. Gather essential information about the patient's symptoms, including: | |
| a. description of symptom(s) (i.e., nature, onset, duration, severity, associated symptoms) | Patient has a 4- to 6-month history of bothersome GI symptoms. Her symptoms return every 2 to 3 weeks and last for 3 to 4 days. She experiences intense gas pains in her left lower abdomen every 2 to 3 weeks. Symptoms usually last for 3 to 4 days. She has made an appointment with her PCP to discuss her GI problems, but the appointment is 2 weeks from now. There is no evidence of fever, weight loss, or black or bloody stools. |
| b. description of any factors that seem to precipitate, exacerbate, and/or relieve the patient's symptom(s) | The pain usually occurs after 2 or 3 days of constipation and is more common during periods of stress. The pain and bloating are usually brief and are relieved after she passes gas through the rectum or has a bowel movement. |
| c. description of the patient's efforts to relieve the symptoms | Uses acetaminophen for pain and a fiber supplement for constipation. Patient has used various OTC laxatives (e.g., magnesium hydroxide and senna) during the past several months, none of which has provided lasting benefit. |
| 2. Gather essential patient history information: | |
| a. patient's identity | Candace Moore |
| b. patient's age, sex, height, and weight | 21 y/o F, 5'10", 106 lb |
| c. patient's occupation | Aerobics instructor and professional athlete/ triathlete |

## CASE 15-2 (continued)

| Relevant Evaluation Criteria | Scenario/Model Outcome |
|---|---|
| d. patient's dietary habits | Candace watches her diet closely to maintain her current weight. In general, she strives for a low-fat, high-fiber diet. Her busy lifestyle forces her to eat low-calorie frozen meals, which she heats in the microwave between aerobics classes. She states that she eats quickly and usually does not have time to sit down and relax during a meal. |
| e. patient's sleep habits | Strives to get about 8 hours of sleep each night; does not complain of nocturnal symptoms |
| f. concurrent medical conditions, prescription and nonprescription medications, and dietary supplements | Tylenol XS 1 or 2 tablets every 6 hours as needed for pain (usually uses 7-10 tablets each week); fiber supplement (orange-flavored Metamucil) 1 tbsp by mouth 3 times/day as needed for constipation (usually uses 2-3 days per week); denies current use of OTC laxatives |
| g. allergies | NKA |
| h. history of other adverse reactions to medications | Ibuprofen and other NSAIDs cause GI upset. |
| i. other (describe)______ | |
| **Assessment and Triage** | |
| 3. Differentiate the patient's signs/symptoms and correctly identify the patient's primary problem(s) (see Table 15-6). | Moderate to severe intestinal gas symptoms (gas pains and bloating) associated with a change in bowel pattern (constipation); symptoms occur frequently and are debilitating. |
| 4. Identify exclusions for self-treatment (see Figure 15-2). | Severe debilitating symptoms |
| 5. Formulate a comprehensive list of therapeutic alternatives for the primary problem to determine if triage to a medical practitioner is required, and share this information with the patient. | Options include:<br>(1) Recommend dietary modification to minimize ingestion of foods that increase intestinal gas.<br>(2) Refer patient to her PCP.<br>(3) Take no action. |
| **Plan** | |
| 6. Select an optimal therapeutic alternative to address the patient's problem, taking into account patient preferences. | The available OTC medications are unlikely to relieve Candace's symptoms. Medical evaluation for underlying GI disorders and subsequent treatment is warranted. |
| 7. Describe the recommended therapeutic approach to the patient. | You should consult your PCP, that is, primary care provider, as scheduled. Until then, you can try reducing intake of foods that increase intestinal gas; reducing your supplemental fiber intake or switch to an alternative product; and improving your eating habits (e.g., eating more slowly). |
| 8. Explain to the patient the rationale for selecting the recommended therapeutic approach from the considered therapeutic alternatives. | See a PCP or gastroenterologist as necessary because OTC products may not be appropriate. Your symptoms may be related to an underlying GI condition and are unlikely to be relieved by OTC remedies. Supplemental fiber may be contributing to intestinal gas production, which might be lessened at a lower dose (e.g., change your Metamucil dose to 1 tbsp each day), or by switching to an alternative supplement (e.g., calcium polycarbophil). Further evaluation and prescription therapy may provide relief of symptoms. |
| **Patient Education** | |
| 9. When recommending self-care with nonprescription medications and/or nondrug therapy, convey accurate information to the patient. | Criterion does not apply in this case. |
| 10. Solicit follow-up questions from patient. | Is there an OTC medication that might work? |

## CASE 15-2 (continued)

| Relevant Evaluation Criteria | Scenario/Model Outcome |
|---|---|
| 11. Answer patient's questions. | No OTC medications are approved and/or appropriate to recommend without a definite diagnosis from a PCP or gastroenterologist. |

Key: GI, gastrointestinal; NKA, no known allergies; NSAID, nonsteroidal anti-inflammatory drug; OTC, over-the-counter; PCP, primary care provider.

## PATIENT EDUCATION FOR INTESTINAL GAS

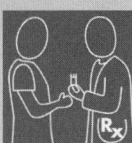

The objectives of self-treatment are to reduce (1) the symptoms of intestinal gas and (2) the chance of its recurrence. For most patients, carefully following product instructions and the self-care measures listed below will help ensure optimal therapeutic outcomes.

### Nondrug Measures

- If possible, avoid foods known to cause intestinal gas.
- Avoid activities known to introduce gas into the digestive system, such as drinking carbonated beverages.
- Nonprescription Medications
- Note that lactase replacement products and α-galactosidase should be taken with foods to prevent intestinal gas from forming.
- Note that simethicone is used to treat intestinal gas after it has occurred.

### Nonprescription Medications

#### *α-Galactosidase*

- If using drops, add 3 to 8 drops to the first bite of the offending food after if has cooled. High temperature (greater than 130°F [54.4°C]) may inactivate the enzyme.
- Do not cook with this product.
- If using tablets, swallow, chew, or crumble 2 to 3 tablets with the first bite of problem foods. If needed, use more tablets for larger meals. (One tablet is equivalent to 5 drops of α-galactosidase solution [α-galactosidase 150 units].)
- About 5 drops per food serving or 3 tablets per meal (1 tablet per 1/2 cup serving) of three servings of problem food is the manufacturer's recommended daily usage.

#### *Lactase Replacement Products*

- If using drops, add 3 to 4 drops (3750 to 5000 lactase units) to dairy products or take with milk at mealtimes.
- If using tablets, swallow or chew 1 or 2 tablets (3000 to 6000 lactase units) before eating dairy products.

#### *Simethicone*

- For adults, take 1 tablet (125 mg) after meals and at bedtime. Do not take more than 500 mg of simethicone within a 24-hour period.
- For infants younger than 2 years, give 0.3 mL (40 units/0.6 mL) four times daily after meals and at bedtime. To ease administration, mix the suspension with 1 oz of cool water, infant formula, or other liquid.
- For children older than 2 years, give 0.6 mL (40 units/0.6 mL) four times daily after meals and at bedtime.

## Evaluation of Patient Outcomes for Intestinal Gas

The practitioner should ask the patient to return or call after 1 week of self-treatment with dietary measures, nonprescription antiflatulents, or digestive enzymes. If symptoms persist or worsen, the patient should seek medical attention. Patients who achieve symptomatic relief should be advised to continue the self-care measures as needed.

## Key Points for Intestinal Gas Complaints

- Limit self-treatment of intestinal gas symptoms to minor symptoms and cases in which exclusions (Figure 15-2) do not exist.
- Counsel patients on dietary measures that may reduce the amount of intestinal gas. Certain foods (Tables 15-1 and 15-2) are more likely to cause gas and contribute to symptoms.
- Patients who associate symptoms with specific food intolerance (i.e., lactose or oligosaccharide intolerance) may use digestive enzymes (lactase replacement and α-galactosidase products).
- Antiflatulents (activated charcoal and simethicone) may also be used, although evidence supporting the ability of these agents to reduce intestinal gas formation is contradictory.
- Referral of the patient to a primary care provider for further evaluation should be considered for patients with exclusions for self-treatment or whose symptoms persist after simple treatment options, such as dietary modification and nonprescription medications are initiated.

## References


1. Levy S. The OTC/HBC market. *Drug Topics.* 1999;143:32.
2. The best new OTCs/HBCs of 2002. *Drug Topics.* 2003;147:45.
3. Hwang B. Makers of remedies breed a cash cow as they publicize lactose intolerance. *Wall Street Journal.* April 20, 1993:B1.
4. Jackson KA, Savaiano DA. Lactose maldigestion, calcium intake and osteoporosis in African-, Asian-, and Hispanic-Americans. *J Am Coll Nutr.* 2001;20(2 suppl):198S-207S.
5. Sandler RS, Everhart JE, Donowitz M, et al. The burden of selected digestive diseases in the United States. *Gastroenterology.* 2002;122:1500-11.
6. Nelsen DA, Jr. Gluten-sensitive enteropathy (celiac disease): more common than you think. *Am Fam Physician.* December 15, 2002;66:2259-66.
7. Sandler RS, Stewart WF, Liberman JN, et al. Abdominal pain, bloating, and diarrhea in the United States: prevalence and impact. *Dig Dis Sci.* June 2000;45:1166-71.
8. National Center for Health Statistics. National Ambulatory Medical Care Survey. 2002. Centers for Disease Control and Prevention. Available at: ftp://ftp.cdc.gov/pub/Health_Statistics/NCHS/Datasets/NAMCS. Accessed March 1, 2005.
9. Feldman M, Friedman LS, Sleisenger MH. Sleisenger & Fordtran's Gastrointestinal and Liver Disease: Pathophysiology, Diagnosis, Management. 7th ed. Philadelphia: Saunders; 2002.
10. Suarez FL. Intestinal gas. *Clin Perspect Gastroenterol.* 2000;Jul/Aug: 209-18.
11. Yamada T, Alpers DH. *Textbook of Gastroenterology.* 4th ed. Philadelphia: Lippincott Williams & Wilkins; 2003.
12. Salvioli B, Serra J, Azpiroz F, et al. Origin of gas retention and symptoms in patients with bloating. *Gastroenterology.* 2005;128: 574-9.
13. Harder H, Serra J, Azpiroz F, et al. Intestinal gas distribution determines abdominal symptoms. *Gut.* 2003;52:1708-13.
14. Serra J, Azpiroz F, Malagelada JR. Mechanisms of intestinal gas retention in humans: impaired propulsion versus obstructed evacuation. *Am J Physiol Gastrointest Liver Physiol.* 2001;281:G138-43.
15. Serra J, Azpiroz F, Malagelada JR. Intestinal gas dynamics and tolerance in humans. *Gastroenterology.* 1998;115:542-50.
16. Serra J, Azpiroz F, Malagelada JR. Perception and reflex responses to intestinal distention in humans are modified by simultaneous or previous stimulation. *Gastroenterology.* 1995;109: 1742-9.
17. Choi YK, Johlin FC Jr, Summers RW, et al. Fructose intolerance: an under-recognized problem. *Am J Gastroenterol.* 2003;98:1348-53.
18. Gas-producing foods and drinks. January 2002. Yale New Haven Health. Available at: http://yalenewhavenhealth.org/library/healthguide/en-us/support/topic.asp?hwid=tm6319. Accessed March 1, 2005.
19. Foods and flatus. January 2002. University of Michigan Health System. Available at: http://www.med.umich.edu/1libr/aha/umdigest24.htm. Accessed March 1, 2005.
20. Gassy food list. December 2002. GlaxoSmithKline. Available at: http://www.beanogas.com/foodlist.asp. Accessed March 1, 2005.
21. Toskes PP, Connery KL, Ritchey TW. Calcium polycarbophil compared with placebo in irritable bowel syndrome. *Aliment Pharmacol Ther.* 1993;7:87-92.
22. Longstreth GF, Fox DD, Youkeles L, et al. Psyllium therapy in the irritable bowel syndrome. A double-blind trial. *Ann Intern Med.* 1981;95:53-6.
23. Brandt LJ, Bjorkman D, Fennerty MB, et al. Systematic review on the management of irritable bowel syndrome in North America. *Am J Gastroenterol.* 2002;97(11 suppl):S7-26.
24. Dua K, Bardan E, Ren J, et al. Effect of chronic and acute cigarette smoking on the pharyngo-upper oesophageal sphincter contractile reflex and reflexive pharyngeal swallow. *Gut.* 1998; 43:537-41.
25. Srinivasan R, Minocha A. When to suspect lactose intolerance. Symptomatic, ethnic, and laboratory clues. *Postgrad Med.* 1998; 104:109-11, 115, 122. PMID: 9742907.
26. Zar S, Benson MJ, Kumar D. Review article: bloating in functional bowel disorders. *Aliment Pharmacol Ther.* 2002;16:1867-76.
27. Chang L, Lee OY, Naliboff B, et al. Sensation of bloating and visible abdominal distension in patients with irritable bowel syndrome. *Am J Gastroenterol.* 2001;96:3341-7.
28. Serra J, Azpiroz F, Malagelada JR. Impaired transit and tolerance of intestinal gas in the irritable bowel syndrome. *Gut.* 2001;48: 14-9.
29. Lundell L. Complications after anti-reflux surgery. *Best Pract Res Clin Gastroenterol.* 2004;18:935-45.
30. Gas and flatulence prevention diet. Jackson Gastroenterology. December 2002. Available at: http://www.gicare.com/pated/edtgs12.htm. Accessed March 1, 2005.
31. American College of Gastroenterology. Common gastrointestinal problems: intestinal gas problems. Available at: http://www.acg.gi.org/patientinfo/cgp/cgpvol3.html#gas. Accessed March 1, 2005.
32. Mayer EA. The neurobiology of stress and emotion. *Participate.* 2001;10:2-5.
33. American Society of Health-System Pharmacists. *American Hospital Formulary Service Drug Information.* Bethesda, Md: American Society of Health-System Pharmacists; 2003:56.
34. Friis H, Bode S, Rumessen JJ, et al. Effect of simethicone on lactulose-induced H2 production and gastrointestinal symptoms. *Digestion.* 1991;49:227-30.
35. Suarez FL, Furne J, Springfield J, et al. Failure of activated charcoal to reduce the release of gases produced by the colonic flora. *Am J Gastroenterol.* 1999;94:208-12.
36. Ganiats TG, Norcross WA, Halverson AL, et al. Does Beano prevent gas? A double-blind crossover study of oral alpha-galactosidase to treat dietary oligosaccharide intolerance. *J Fam Pract.* 1994;39:441-5.
37. Metcalf TJ, Irons TG, Sher LD, et al. Simethicone in the treatment of infant colic: a randomized, placebo-controlled, multicenter trial. *Pediatrics.* 1994;94:29-34.
38. Medical Economics Company. *PDR for Herbal Medicines.* Montvale, NJ: Medical Economics Co.; 2004:v.
39. Castell DO, Brunton S, Earnest D, et al. GERD: Management algorithms for the primary care physician and the specialist. *Pract Gastroenterol.* 1999(Feb 19):20-44.
40. Creamer B. Oesophageal reflux and the action of carminatives. *Lancet.* March 19 1955;268:590-2.
41. Bulat R, Fachnie E, Chauhan U, et al. Lack of effect of spearmint on lower oesophageal sphincter function and acid reflux in healthy volunteers. *Aliment Pharmacol Ther.* 1999;13:805-12.
42. Blumenthal M. *The Complete German Commission E Monographs: Therapeutic Guide to Herbal Medicines.* Boston: American Botanical Council, Integrative Medicine Communications;1998:685.
43. Zhu M, Wong PY, Li RC. Effect of oral administration of fennel (Foeniculum vulgare) on ciprofloxacin absorption and disposition in the rat. *J Pharm Pharmacol.* December 1999;51:1391-6.

CHAPTER 16

# Constipation

*Clarence E. Curry, Jr., and Demetris M. Butler*

Constipation is a common gastrointestinal complaint. However, the complaint is viewed differently by health care providers and patients. Physicians and other providers generally describe constipation as a decrease in the frequency of fecal elimination characterized by the difficult passage of hard, dry stools.[1] It usually results from the abnormally slow movement of feces through the colon with a resultant accumulation in the descending colon. Patients may describe constipation as (1) straining to have a stool, (2) the passage of hard, dry stool, (3) the passage of small stools, (4) feelings of incomplete bowel evacuation, or (5) bloating.

While constipation is a common reason for visiting a primary care provider, it also is a common reason for undertaking self-care. A laxative is often the layperson's treatment of choice for constipation. Laxative products are purchased in a variety of places. Laxative sales in the United States exceed $750 million and are projected to top $850 million by 2010.[2]

A laxative facilitates the passage and elimination of feces from the large intestine (colon) and rectum. Despite numerous recognized indications for when to use laxatives, many use them inappropriately to alleviate what they incorrectly consider to be constipation.

## Epidemiology of Constipation

Constipation is a heterogeneous disorder that occurs throughout the age continuum in both men and women. It is reported more often in women than in men.[3] The prevalence in the general population ranges from 2% to 28% and is higher in older adults (>65 years), possibly affecting over half of elderly residents in nursing homes.[4-7] Constipation is also a frequent complaint during pregnancy.

## Anatomy and Physiology of the Gastrointestinal Tract

All of the structures shown in Figure 16-1 contribute to the process of digestion. For example, the pharynx and esophagus serve as entryway to the system, the stomach serves as storage depot and digestive process initiator, the liver provides bile for fat emulsification, while nearly all absorption of solids (greater than 94%) occurs in the small intestine. The function of the colon is to allow for the orderly elimination from the body of nonabsorbed food products, desquamated cells from the gut lumen, and detoxified and metabolic end products. The colon functions to conserve fluid and electrolytes, so the quantity eliminated represents about 10% of what enters the colon in a 24-hour period. In addition, the colon has the capacity (as does the kidney) to absorb certain electrolytes because of differences in osmotic pressure.

Tonic contractions of the stomach churn and knead food, and large peristaltic waves start at the fundus and move food toward the duodenum. Autonomic reflexes and hormones influence the time it takes the stomach contents to empty into the duodenum. Carbohydrates are emptied from the stomach most rapidly, proteins more slowly, and fats the slowest.

The mixture and passage of the contents of the small and large intestines are the result of four muscular movements: pendular, segmental, peristaltic, and vermiform (wormlike). Pendular movements result from contractions of the longitudinal muscles of the intestine, which pass up and down small segments of the gut at the rate of about 10 contractions per minute. Pendular movements mix rather than propel the contents. Segmental movements resulting from contractions of the circular muscles occur at about the same rate as pendular movements. Their primary function is also mixing. Pendular and segmental movements are caused by the intrinsic contractility of smooth muscle and occur in the absence of innervation of intestinal tissue.

Peristaltic movements propel intestinal contents by circular contractions that form behind a point of stimulation and pass along the GI tract toward the rectum. The contraction rate ranges from 2 to 20 cm/second. These contractions require an intact myenteric (Auerbach's) nerve plexus, located in the muscularis propria of the intestine. Peristaltic waves move the intestinal contents through the small intestine in about 3.5 hours. Vermiform movements occur mainly in the large intestine and are caused by the contraction of several centimeters of the colonic smooth muscle at one time. In the cecum and ascending colon, the contents retain a fluid consistency. Peristaltic and antiperistaltic waves occur frequently, but, activity is very irregular in the transverse, descending, and sigmoid segments of the colon, where—through further water absorption—the contents become semisolid.

Three or four times a day, a strong peristaltic wave (mass movement) propels the contents about one third (38 cm) the length of the colon. When initiated by a meal, the mass movement is referred to as the gastrocolic reflex. This normal reflex seems to be associated with the entrance of food into the stomach and the subsequent distention of the stomach, and it is very strong in infants. The sigmoid colon serves as a storage place for fecal matter until defecation occurs.

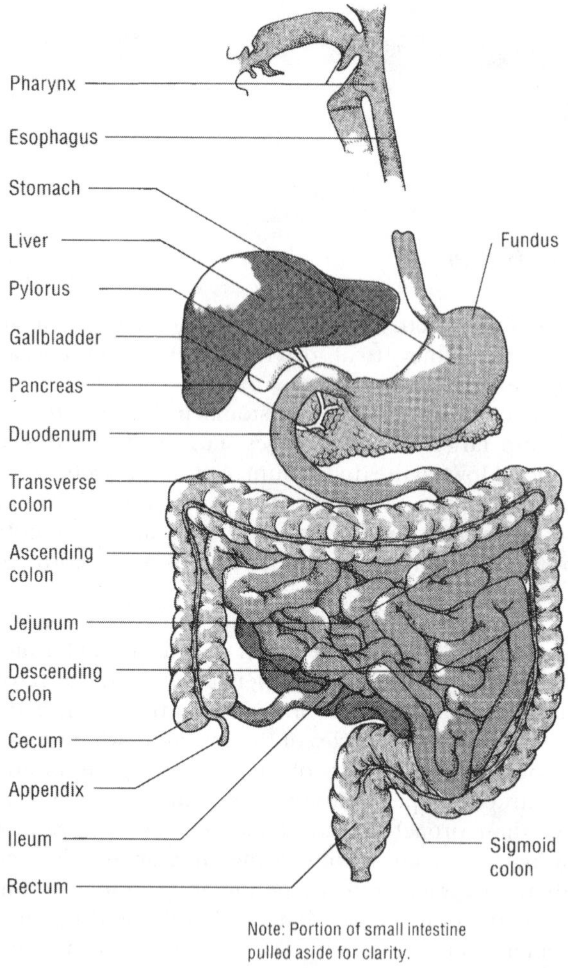


**FIGURE 16-1** Anatomy of the digestive system.

The act of defecation involves the rectal passage of accumulated fecal material. This material is propelled from the sigmoid colon into the rectum by a mass peristaltic movement. This movement results in a desire to defecate as somatic impulses are sent to the defecation center in the sacral spinal cord. The defecation center then sends impulses to the internal anal sphincter, causing it to relax and increasing intra-abdominal pressure as the muscles of the abdominal wall tighten; a Valsalva maneuver forces the stool down. Voluntary relaxation of the external anal sphincter occurs, followed by elevation of the pelvic diaphragm, which lifts the anal sphincter over the fecal mass, allowing the mass to be expelled. Defecation, a spinal reflex, is either voluntarily inhibited by keeping the external sphincter contracted or facilitated by relaxing the sphincter and contracting the abdominal muscles. Children usually defecate after meals; in adults, however, habits and cultural factors may determine the "proper" time for defecation.

## Etiology of Constipation

Causes of constipation are numerous and include various medical conditions and medications, psychologic and physiologic conditions (e.g., menopause or dehydration), and lifestyle characteristics. Some population groups are more susceptible to developing constipation as a result of one or more of the defined causes. Two distinct disorders of colorectal motility are characterized by constipation: slow-transit constipation (slower than normal movement of fecal contents) and pelvic floor dysfunction (storage of fecal contents for prolonged time in the rectum).[5]

### *Disease-induced Constipation*

Constipation of recent onset suggests a possible disease-related or drug-induced cause (Table 16-1).[5-7] In such situations, if a disease is the underlying cause, referral for proper diagnosis and medical treatment will be necessary.

Painful lesions of the anal canal such as ulcers, fissures, and thrombosed hemorrhoidal veins can lead to constipation if patients suppress defecation to avoid pain. Pain from various causes, including gallbladder disease, appendicitis, and regional ileitis, may inhibit GI reflexes, leading to functional and acute symptomatology.

### *Drug-induced Constipation*

Drugs with constipating side effects may counteract the therapeutic effects of laxatives or may require use of a laxative (Table 16-2).

A clinical condition known as the narcotic bowel syndrome is characterized by chronic abdominal pain, nausea and vomiting, abdominal distention, and constipation. Such a condition might occur in a cancer patient or in other patients who require chronic administration of large doses of narcotics. Typically, patients who use opiates chronically experience constipation and could be at risk for intestinal obstruction or impaction. Inhibition of peristalsis in the small and large intestine leads to prolongation of intestinal transit time along with increased electrolyte and water absorption. Other possible contributors to this form of constipation include impaired defecation response and increased anal sphincter tone.[10]

### *Psychogenic Causes*

Constipation can also be related to psychologic conditions. Depression, eating disorders such as anorexia nervosa, and conscious efforts to withhold stool are frequently responsible for the presence of constipation.

### *Lifestyle Factors*

A diet that is low in calories, carbohydrates (e.g., Atkins diet), and fiber can lead to diet-related constipation. Dietary fiber dissolves or swells in the intestinal fluid, which increases the bulk of fecal mass and, in turn, aids in stimulating peristalsis and eliminating stools. Increasing dietary fiber and reducing consumption of soft foods and foods that harden stools (e.g., processed cheese) help relieve constipation in many individuals. Some foods generally considered high in fiber could actually contribute to constipation because of the processed sugar they contain. Overcooked fruits and vegetables provide little roughage. Since vegetables are a major source of fiber in many

**TABLE 16-1 Selected Conditions Associated With Constipation[5-7]**

| | |
|---|---|
| **Metabolic Disorders** | **Disorders of the Large Intestine, Rectum, and Anus** |
| Amyloidosis | Anal fissure |
| Diabetic ketoacidosis | Chronic amebiasis |
| Diabetic neuropathy | Colonic inertia |
| Hypokalemia | Corrosive enemas |
| Hypomagnesemia | Diverticulitis |
| Porphyria | Hernias |
| Uremia | Internal rectal prolapse |
| **Endocrine Disorders** | Irritable bowel syndrome |
| Hypercalcemia: pseudohypoparathyroidism, hyperparathyroidism, milk alkali syndrome, carcinomatosis | Ischemic colitis |
| Hypothyroidism | Mucosal prolapse |
| Panhypopituitarism | Pelvic floor dysfunction and lesions |
| Pheochromocytoma | Rectocele |
| **Neurologic Disorders** | Stenotic obstruction |
| Aganglionosis, or Hirschsprung's disease | Strictures |
| Autonomic neuropathy: paraneoplastic, pseudo-obstruction | Surgical stricture (end-to-end anastomosis) |
| Dementia | Tumors |
| Cauda equina tumor | Ulcerative proctitis |
| Cerebrovascular accidents | **Muscular Disorders** |
| Chagas' disease | Dermatomyositis |
| Ganglioneuromatosis | Myotonic dystrophy |
| Multiple sclerosis | Segmental dilatation of the colon |
| Parkinson's disease | Systemic sclerosis |
| Shy Drager syndrome | |
| Tumors | |

low-carbohydrate diets, choice of vegetables should include those highest in fiber. Patients should be advised of these facts so that improper selection or preparation of foods does not cause them to abandon a healthful, high-fiber diet.

Inadequate intake of fluids may also contribute to the development of constipation. Intestinal fluids are essential for eliminating stools and must be replenished from dietary sources. Gravity and good abdominal muscle tone also aid in proper bowel function. Exercise increases muscle tone and promotes bowel motility. Immobility and sedentary lifestyles can contribute to the development of constipation as well.

Avoiding the urge to empty the bowel can eventually lead to constipation. When this stimulus is ignored or suppressed, rectal muscles can lose tonicity and become less effective in eliminating stool. Nerve pathways may degenerate and stop sending the signal to defecate. Bowel retraining will be necessary for most patients to establish a pattern of regular bowel movements.

### *Constipation in Older Adults*

Older adults frequently describe constipation as straining to move bowels and report fewer stools per week. The aging process is associated with physiologic changes that prolong the transit time through the colon, which decreases the perception of the urge to defecate. Constipation in older adults can be precipitated or aggravated by conditions such as neuromuscular disorders, confusion, dementia, and depression.[4-6] In addition, the older population tends to have multiple medical conditions and take multiple medications that may contribute to the development of constipation. Constipating medications commonly used by older adults include narcotic analgesics; sedatives; hypnotics; antidepressants; anticholinergics; some antacids and vitamins that contain calcium, aluminum, or iron; and calcium channel blockers.[7,8] Laxative use increases with age.[7] Abuse of stimulant laxatives, in an attempt to regulate bowel activity, was thought to lead paradoxically to worsening symptoms of constipation. However, lack of evidence supporting this view suggests otherwise.[11]

Lifestyle factors that can contribute to or worsen constipation in older adults include failure to establish a schedule for bowel movements; emotional stress; inadequate chewing of foods, which is often a result of poor dentition; a diet that is insufficient in calories and fiber; inadequate fluid intake; and limited exercise. Elderly patients who are confined to the bed or sedentary have an increased risk for developing constipation because walking has a positive impact on gut peristalsis.

If any of these factors exist, the health care provider should consider lifestyle modifications or an adjustment to current drug therapy before recommending a laxative.

### *Constipation in Children*

A number of factors can alter a child's bowel habits, including unavailable toilet facilities, emotional distress, febrile illness, chronic medical conditions (e.g., cystic fibrosis,

| TABLE 16-2 Drugs That May Induce Constipation[7-9] |
|---|
| Analgesics (including nonsteroidal anti-inflammatory drugs) |
| Antacids (e.g., calcium and aluminum compounds, bismuth) |
| Anticholinergics (e.g., benztropine) |
| Anticonvulsants (e.g., carbamazepine) |
| Antidepressants (specifically, tricyclics such as amitriptyline) |
| Antihistamines (e.g., diphenhydramine) |
| Antimotility (e.g., diphenoxylate, loperamide) |
| Barium sulfate |
| Benzodiazepines (especially alprazolam and estazolam) |
| Calcium-channel blockers (e.g., verapamil) |
| Calcium supplements |
| Diuretics (e.g., thiazide-type) |
| Ganglionic blockers (trimethaphan camsylate) |
| Hematinics (especially iron) |
| Hyperlipidemia agents (e.g., cholestyramine, pravastatin, simvastatin) |
| Hypotensives (e.g., angiotensin-converting enzyme inhibitors, β-blockers) |
| Memantine |
| Monoamine oxidase inhibitors (e.g., phenelzine) |
| Opiates (e.g., morphine, codeine) |
| Parasympatholytics (e.g., atropine) |
| Parkinsonism agents (e.g., bromocriptine) |
| Psychotherapeutic drugs (e.g., phenothiazines, butyrophenones) |
| Polystyrene sodium sulfonate |
| Sucralfate |
| Vinca alkaloids (e.g., vincristine) |

hypothyroidism), family conflict, dietary changes (e.g., switching from human to cow's milk), or a change in daily routine or environment.[12] Some children are poor or picky eaters, which may contribute to the development of constipation because of inadequate bulk and fluids in the diet. Constipation associated with an organic or pathologic etiology is uncommon in children.[13] Idiopathic constipation, the most common cause of constipation, often begins in early childhood but may be delayed until adolescence. Bowel movement patterns vary widely in children; therefore, constipation can be a complex problem that is often difficult to detect and manage. Infants and children appear to show a decreasing frequency of bowel movements with increasing age. Normally, neonates may pass more than four bowel movements a day during the first week of life. This number declines to approximately one to two bowel movements a day by 4 years of age.

Children typically describe constipation as a difficulty in passing stools. Straining to pass large or hard stools can be painful. The child may then avoid or withhold bowel movements, resulting in worsening symptoms and fear of toileting. If the symptoms last for even a short period of time, the child may experience a loss of appetite and become withdrawn or irritable. Constipation is a common complaint in the pediatric population, and health care providers must recognize the importance of taking a thorough history to establish a clear understanding of all contributing factors.

### *Constipation in Women*

Constipation is a more common complaint in women than in men.[7] Certain medical conditions (e.g., irritable bowel syndrome), hormonal changes, or slower gut transit times can be contributing factors in women who experience constipation.[13] Constipation is common during pregnancy and after childbirth or surgery. It is estimated that one in every three pregnant women experience constipation during the first and third trimesters.[14] The increasing size of the uterus compresses the colon, affecting the emptying of fecal material. In addition, reduced intestinal muscle tone, which can contribute to a decrease in peristalsis, is likely the primary reason.[15] Other contributing factors in pregnancy include the use of prenatal vitamin and mineral supplements that contain iron and calcium, a decease in dietary fiber and fluid, and a reduction in physical activity.[14] Constipation in pregnancy can lead to backaches, hemorrhoids, and fecal impaction.

## Pathophysiology of the Lower GI Tract Underlying Constipation

The pain from anal ulcers and fissures and thrombosed hemorrhoidal veins can induce spasms of the anal sphincter, which often result in reflexive suppression of defecation, leading to constipation. Pain from other causes, such as gallbladder disease, appendicitis, and regional ileitis, may inhibit GI reflexes. As a result, functional obstruction may occur in the small intestine, accompanied by symptoms of acute intestinal blockage.

Large masses of fecal material tend to accumulate in a greatly dilated rectum, especially in older patients. Ignoring or suppressing the urge to defecate may cause the loss of tonicity in the rectal musculature. Loss of tonicity may also be caused by degeneration of nerve pathways concerned with defecation reflexes.

The normal rectal mucosa is relatively insensitive to cutting or burning. However, when it is inflamed, it becomes highly sensitive to all stimuli, including those acting on the receptors mediating the stretch reflex.

A constant urge to defecate in the absence of appreciable material in the rectum may occur with an inflamed rectal mucosa.

## Signs and Symptoms of Constipation

If frequency of bowel movements decreases or difficult passage of hard stools occurs, other symptoms of varying degrees of severity may develop, including anorexia, dull headache, lassitude, low back pain, and abdominal distention. In addition, abdominal discomfort and an inadequate response to increasing varieties and dosages of laxatives are common complaints with constipation.

The frequency of bowel movements in humans is quite variable but generally ranges from three times a day to three times a week.[16] Those in the latter category can be symptom-free and do not have any specific abnormality related to their individual pattern of defecation. Therefore, constipation cannot be defined solely in terms of the number of bowel movements in any given period. Regularity is what is "regular" or typical for the individual who experiences none of the classic symptoms of constipation.

In some instances, self-care is inappropriate and medical referral is necessary, including all situations in which more than simple constipation is present, such as (1) recent weight loss, (2) presence of abdominal pain, (3) blood in the stool, (4) the likelihood of fecal impaction or obstruction, (5) persistence of symptoms for more than 1 or 2 weeks, (6) ineffectiveness of self-medication with nonprescription laxatives, and (7) presence of a disorder known to be accompanied by constipation.

Constipation can occur in infants who have one to two daily bowel movements and often is unrecognized. Infants whose frequency of bowel movements is less than average in the first weeks of life may be prone to developing chronic constipation in later years.[17,18]

## Complications of Constipation

Patients of advanced age often strain to pass hard stools, which may predispose them to complications, including cardiovascular problems and hemorrhoids. Because defecation has been found to alter hemodynamics, straining to defecate may result in blood pressure surges or cardiac rhythm disturbances. Occasionally, straining may lead to rectal prolapse.

## Treatment of Constipation

The patient should attempt nondrug measures initially to relieve constipation and help prevent recurrences. Constipation associated with an underlying medical condition or use of medications should be referred to a primary care provider to evaluate the need for medical treatment or adjust therapy with constipating medications.

At minimum, successful therapy for constipation should return the patient to the preconstipation frequency, consistency, and quantity of stool. Pharmacotherapy should restore usual function using the lowest effective dosage without producing adverse effects.

### *Treatment Goals*

The primary goals of treatment are to (1) relieve constipation and reestablish normal bowel function, (2) establish dietary and exercise habits that will aid in preventing recurrences, (3) promote the safe and effective use of laxative products, and (4) avoid the overuse of laxative products.

### *General Treatment Approach*

In general, constipation should be initially managed by adjusting the diet to include foods high in fiber and increasing fluid intake, accompanied by some form of exercise. Pharmacologic intervention can be used in conjunction with lifestyle modifications if more immediate relief is desired. Laxatives should be selected according to the age and health status of the patient as well as the mechanism of action of the individual product. The Food and Drug Administration (FDA) has long mandated labeling of laxatives to stress short-term (i.e., less than 1 week) use without the advice of a physician. Such use is thought to be sufficient for most cases of occasional simple or acute constipation. When constipation continues over several weeks to months, it can be referred to as chronic. Chronic constipation may require more sustained and aggressive physician-directed therapy.[19] Most patients who develop constipation will self-medicate and consult a health care provider only after a nonprescription preparation or dietary manipulation has failed. Treatment success is enhanced when likely causes of constipation have been identified and therapeutic modalities are tailored to the individual. The treatment algorithm in Figure 16-2 provides a systematic approach to the self-care of constipation[20] and lists exclusions for self-treatment.

### *Nonpharmacologic Therapy*

Constipation that does not have an organic etiology can often be alleviated with lifestyle modifications such as increased fiber in the diet, adequate fluid intake, and exercise. The American Dietetic Association recommends an adult daily dietary fiber intake of 20 to 35 g.[21] It is commonly believed that increasing dietary fiber enhances regularity; fiber improves bowel function by adding bulk and softening the stool. Both insoluble fiber (e.g., whole grain breads, prunes, raisins, and corn) and soluble fiber (e.g., beans, oat bran, barley, peas, carrots, citrus fruits, and apples) are believed to be instrumental in this regard (Table 16-3).[21,22] (For greater detail, see Chapter 16 and consult http://www.nal.usda.gov/fnic/foodcomp/Data/SR17/wtrank/sr17a291.pdf.) However, some people may not be able to consume sufficient amounts of fiber because of GI intolerance. The clinician should inform patients that increasing dietary bran may lead to erratic bowel habits, flatulence, and abdominal discomfort during the first few weeks. Excess bran should be avoided in patients with hypocalcemia or low serum iron, as the phytates found in bran may aggravate these conditions. Patients with slow-transit constipation or functional outlet obstruction may respond poorly to fiber supplementation.[23]An increase in dietary fiber and use of fiber supplements should be avoided in patients with fecal impaction, to avoid worsening the condition. Although increasing dietary fiber is generally recommended, its overall effectiveness remains controversial; therefore, its use is not a panacea for all cases of constipation.[6] When fiber is ineffective, natural remedies that include oat or wheat bran may help relieve symptoms. This approach may be preferred when constipation is related to a diet that is low in carbohydrates, such as the Atkins diet. Alternatively, a sugar-free bulk-forming fiber supplement containing psyllium may help minimize constipation associated with low-carbohydrate diets, but adequate fluid intake to avoid the development of paradoxical constipation is also required.[24]

In conjunction with fiber, an increase in the intake of fluids, especially water, helps alleviate constipation in most patients. Recommendations for daily fluid consumption vary widely, from 32 to 128 oz. This approach may be limited in patients who are fluid restricted or who have renal insufficiency. Most investigators generally believe the additional fluid expands and softens the fiber, although water-insoluble fiber is said to be primarily responsible for producing a laxative effect.[21]

As with adults, increasing both fluids and the bulk content of a child's diet may improve bowel habits and decrease frequency of constipation. Simply increasing the amount of fluid or sugar in the formula may be corrective during the first few months of life. Once solid foods are introduced, adding or increasing the amounts of high-fiber cereals, vegetables, and fruits to the diet may relieve symptoms of constipation. For children over 2 years of age, the recommended dietary fiber intake should equal or exceed their age plus 5 g/day.[21] Unbuttered popcorn is a good bulk-containing snack for children. Sugar-water solutions (e.g., fruit juice or soda) often diminish the child's appetite for solid foods and should be limited. The child should be encouraged to drink water. Although milk is the primary fluid consumed by most young children, milk intake should not be considered a substitute for water. In addition to dietary changes, some children may need to establish regular bowel habits including promptly responding to the urge to toilet as well as toileting in an unhurried manner.[12]

Because constipation often afflicts those with sedentary lifestyles, the importance to the body of exercise cannot be discounted. Although any concentrated regular exercise is good, aerobic exercise is best. Regular walking, running, or swimming, among other forms of exercise, may help alleviate constipation.

Finally, for people who achieve a beneficial effect from one of these measures, heeding the urge to pass the stool is paramount or the beneficial effect will be lost. When nondrug measures prove ineffective, a laxative may be indicated.

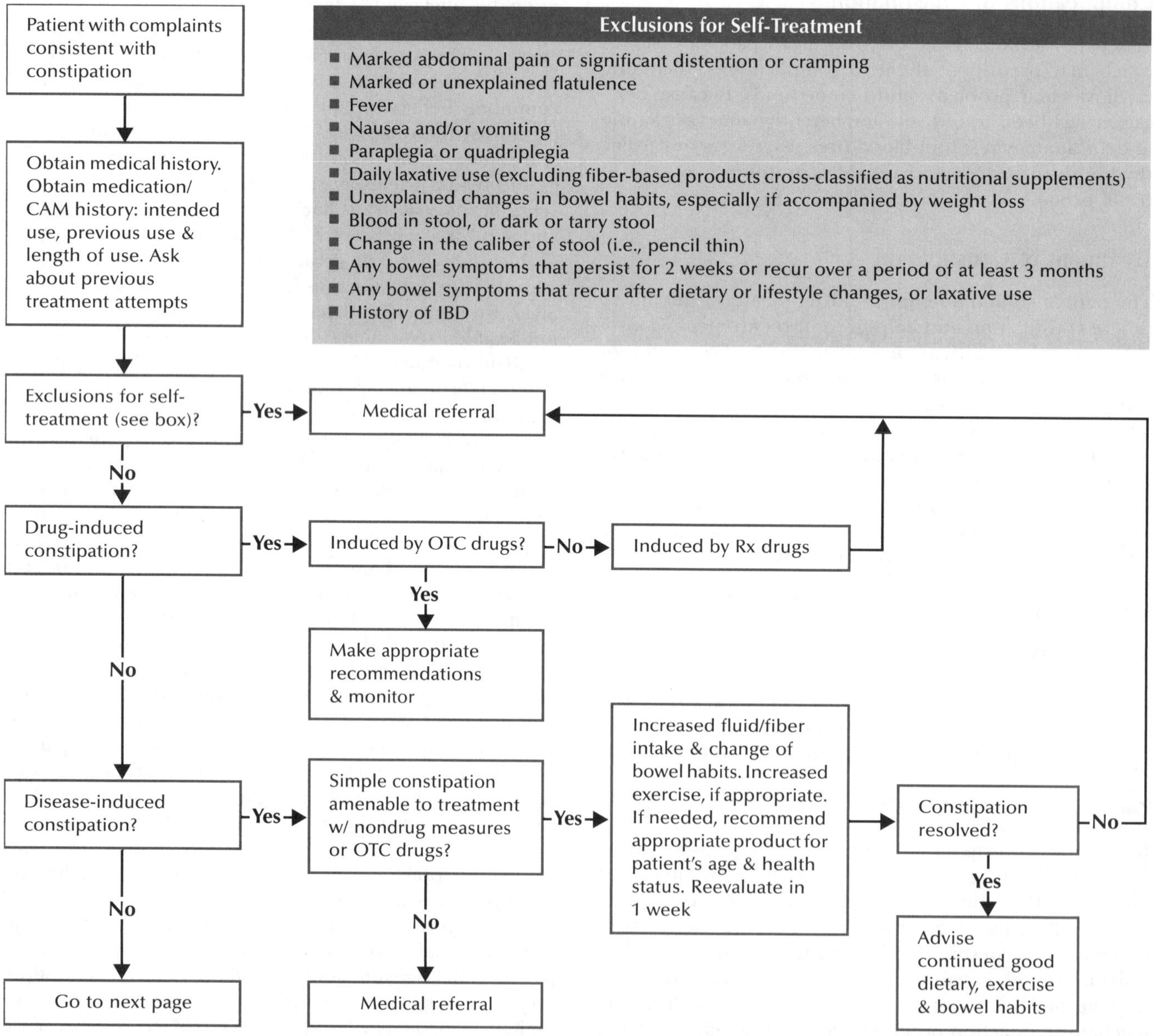


**FIGURE 16-2** Self-care of constipation. Key: CAM, complementary and alternative medicine; IBD, inflammatory bowel disease; OTC, over-the-counter; PCP, primary care provider; Rx, prescription.

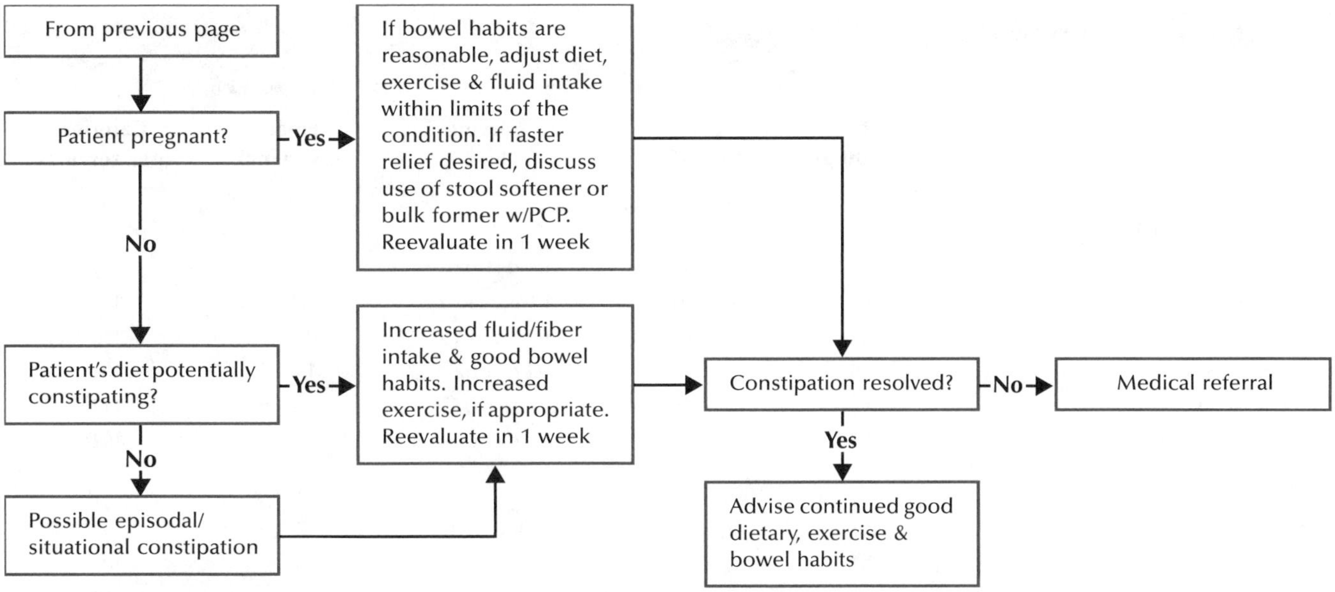


**FIGURE 16-2 (continued)**

### *Pharmacologic Therapy*

The ideal laxative would (1) be nonirritating and nontoxic, (2) act only on the descending and sigmoid colon, and (3) produce a normally formed stool within a few hours, after which its action would cease and normal bowel activity would resume. Because no currently available laxative precisely meets these criteria, proper selection of a laxative depends on the etiology of the constipation.

Agents used to treat constipation have been classified according to their chemical structure and site, intensity, or mechanism of action. The most meaningful classification is by mechanism of action, including bulk-forming, emollient, lubricant, saline, hyperosmotic, and stimulant agents (Table 16-4).

#### Bulk-forming Agents

Most bulk-forming laxatives are derived from natural sources such as agar, plantago (psyllium) seed, kelp (alginates), and plant gums (e.g., tragacanth, chondrus, karaya [*Sterculia*]). The synthetic cellulose derivatives—methylcellulose and carboxymethyl cellulose sodium—are also used, with methylcellulose products being more prominent. Another agent is calcium polycarbophil, the calcium salt of a synthetic polyacrylic resin. These synthetic colloidal materials have a high degree of uniformity and can be readily compressed into tablets. They are also less troublesome in that they tend to cause less "gas" than natural fiber. Guar gum is a natural product found in the bean cluster plant (*Cyamopsis tetragonolobus*), most useful today as partially hydrolyzed guar gum.[25]

*Mechanism of Action* Bulk-forming products are the recommended choice for the treatment of constipation, because they most closely approximate the physiologic mechanism in promoting evacuation. Among these agents are natural and semisynthetic hydrophilic polysaccharides and cellulose derivatives that dissolve or swell in the intestinal fluid, forming emollient gels that facilitate passage of the intestinal contents and stimulate peristalsis. Calcium polycarbophil has a marked capacity for binding water and is a quite useful agent of this class. Another bulk-forming agent, malt soup extract, is obtained from barley and contains maltose protein, potassium, and amylolytic enzymes. An interesting aspect of this agent is that it reduces fecal pH, which may contribute to its laxative activity.

*Pharmacokinetics* The hydrophilic colloid bulk-forming agents are not absorbed systemically and do not seem to interfere with the absorption of nutrients. The usual onset of action is from 12 to 24 hours but may be delayed as long as 72 hours.

*Indications* Bulk-forming agents are indicated as short-term therapy to relieve constipation, and they may be indicated for (1) patients on low-fiber (also referred to as low-residue) diets that cannot be corrected; (2) postpartum women; (3) older adult patients; and (4) patients with colostomies, irritable bowel syndrome (IBS), or diverticular disease. They are also indicated prophylactically in patients who should refrain from straining during a bowel movement.

***Dosage and Administration Guidelines*** Dosages vary according to the type of product. Table 16-4 lists dosing information for the various agents. Exceeding the recommended doses for a bulk-forming agent could lead to increased flatulence and obstruction if appropriate fluid intake is not maintained.

*Safety Considerations* Common adverse effects include abdominal cramping and flatulence. Esophageal obstruction has occurred in older adults, in patients who have difficulty swallowing, and in patients with strictures of the

**TABLE 16-3 Dietary Fiber[21,22]***

| Food | Fiber (g/100 g) | Calories (per 100 g) | Serving Size | Fiber (g/serving) | Calories (per serving) |
|---|---|---|---|---|---|
| **Breakfast Cereals** | | | | | |
| All-Bran | 29.9 | 249 | 1/3 c (1 oz) | 8.5 | 71 |
| Cheerios | 3.8 | 391 | 1 1/4 c (1 oz) | 1.1 | 111 |
| Cornflakes | 1.1 | 389 | 1 1/3 c (1 oz) | 0.3 | 110 |
| Grape-Nuts | 4.8 | 357 | 1/4 c (1 oz) | 1.4 | 101 |
| Rice Krispies | 0.2 | 395 | 1 c (1 oz) | 0.1 | 112 |
| Shredded Wheat | 9.3 | 359 | 2/3 c (1 oz) | 2.6 | 102 |
| **Fruits** | | | | | |
| Apple (w/skin) | 2.5 | 59 | 1 med | 3.5 | 81 |
| Banana | 2.1 | 92 | 1 med | 2.4 | 105 |
| Orange | 2.0 | 47 | 1 | 2.6 | 62 |
| Peach (with skin) | 2.1 | 43 | 1 | 1.9 | 37 |
| Pineapple | 1.4 | 49 | 1/2 c | 1.1 | 39 |
| Prunes | 11.9 | 239 | 3 | 3.0 | 60 |
| Strawberries | 2.0 | 30 | 1 c | 3.0 | 45 |
| **Juices** | | | | | |
| Apple | 0.3 | 47 | 1/2 c (4 oz) | 0.4 | 56 |
| Grape | 0.5 | 51 | 1/2 c (4 oz) | 0.6 | 64 |
| Orange | 0.4 | 45 | 1/2 c (4 oz) | 0.5 | 56 |
| **Vegetables, Cooked** | | | | | |
| Asparagus, cut | 1.5 | 20 | 1/2 c | 1.0 | 15 |
| Beans, string, green | 2.6 | 25 | 1/2 c | 1.6 | 16 |
| Kale, leaves | 2.6 | 34 | 1/2 c | 1.4 | 22 |
| Sweet potatoes | 2.4 | 141 | 1/2 med | 1.7 | 80 |
| **Vegetables, Raw** | | | | | |
| Onions, sliced | 1.3 | 23 | 1/2 c | 0.8 | 33 |
| Tomato | 1.5 | 22 | 1 med | 1.5 | 20 |
| **Legumes** | | | | | |
| Baked beans, tomato sauce | 7.3 | 121 | 1/2 c | 8.8 | 155 |
| Dried peas, cooked | 4.7 | 115 | 1/2 c | 4.7 | 115 |
| Lentils, cooked | 3.7 | 97 | 1/2 c | 3.7 | 97 |
| **Breads and Flours** | | | | | |
| Bran muffins | 6.3 | 263 | 1 muffin | 2.5 | 104 |
| Pita bread (5 in.) | 0.9 | 273 | 1 piece | 0.4 | 123 |
| White bread | 1.6 | 279 | 1 slice | 0.4 | 78 |
| **Pasta and Rice, Cooked** | | | | | |
| Macaroni | 0.8 | 111 | 1 c | 1.0 | 144 |
| Rice, brown | 1.2 | 119 | 1/2 c | 1.0 | 97 |
| Spaghetti (regular) | 0.8 | 111 | 1 c | 1.1 | 155 |

* The values are literature-derived averages. Also, cereals vary greatly in their fiber content, so consumers should read labels to determine fiber content per serving.

TABLE 16-4 Classification and Properties of Laxatives

| Agent | Dosage Form* | Daily Dosage Range | | Site of Action | Approximate Onset of Action | Systemic Absorption |
|---|---|---|---|---|---|---|
| | | Adults | Children | | | |
| **Bulk-forming** | | | | | | |
| Methylcellulose | Solid | 4-6 g | 1-1.5 g (>6 years) | Small and large intestines | 12-72 hours | No |
| Carboxymethyl cellulose sodium | Solid | 4-6 g | 1-1.5 g (>6 years) | Small and large intestines | 12-72 hours | No (laxative) Yes (sodium) |
| Malt soup extract | Solid, liquid, powder | 12-64 g | 6-32 mL (1 month to 2 years) | Small and large intestines | 12-72 hours | — |
| Partially hydrolyzed guar gum | Powder | 4 g | None identified | Small and large intestines | 12-72 hours | No |
| Polycarbophil | Solid | 1-6 g | 0.5-1.0 g (<2 years)<br>1-1.5 g (2-5 years)<br>1.5-3.0 g (6-12 years) | Small and large intestines | 12-72 hours | No |
| Plantago seeds | Solid | 2.5-30 g | 1.25-15 g (>6 years) | Small and large intestines | 12-72 hours | No |
| **Emollient** | | | | | | |
| Docusate calcium | Solid | 50-360 mg | 20-50 mg (<2 years)<br>50-150 mg (≥2 years) | Small and large intestines | 12-72 hours | Yes |
| Docusate sodium | Solid | 50-360 mg | 20-50 mg (<2 years)<br>50-150 mg (≥2 years) | Small and large intestines | 12-72 hours | Yes |
| | Liquid | 50-500 mg | 10-40 mg (<3 years)<br>20-60 mg (3-6 years)<br>40-150 mg (6-12 years) | Small and large intestines | — | — |
| Docusate potassium | Solid | 100-300 mg | 100 mg (≥6 years) | Small and large intestines | 12-72 hours | Yes |
| **Lubricant** | | | | | | |
| Mineral oil | Liquid | 14-45 mL | 10-15 mL (>6 years) | Colon | 6-8 hours | Yes, a minimal amount |
| **Saline** | | | | | | |
| Magnesium citrate | Liquid | 150-300 mL | 2-4 mL/kg given once or in divided doses (<6 years)<br>100-150 mL (6-12 years) | Small and large intestines | 0.5-3 hours | Yes |
| Magnesium hydroxide | Liquid | 30-60 mL | 0.5 mL/kg per dose (<2 years)<br>5-15 mL (2-5 years)<br>15-30 mL (6-12 years) | Small and large intestines | 0.5-3 hours | Yes |
| | Liquid (concentrate) | 15-30 mL | 2.5-7.5 mL (2-5 years)<br>7.5-15 mL (6-12 years) | Small and large intestines | 0.5-3 hours | Yes |
| | Solid | 6-8 tablets | 1-2 tablets (2-5 years)<br>3-4 tablets (6-11 years)<br>6-8 tablets (>12 years) | Small and large intestines | 0.5-3 hours | Yes |
| Magnesium sulfate | Solid | 10-30 g | 2.5-5.0 g (2-5 years)<br>5.0-10.0 g (≥6 years) | Small and large intestines | 0.5-3 hours | Yes |
| Dibasic sodium phosphate | Solid | 1.9-3.8 g | 1/4 adult dose (5-10 years)<br>1/2 adult dose (10 years) | Small and large intestines | 0.5-3 hours | Yes |

**TABLE 16-4 Classification and Properties of Laxatives (continued)**

| Agent | Dosage Form* | Daily Dosage Range | | Site of Action | Approximate Onset of Action | Systemic Absorption |
|---|---|---|---|---|---|---|
| | | Adults | Children | | | |
| | Solution (rectal) | 6.84-7.56 g once daily | 1/2 adult dose (2-11 years) | Colon | 2-15 minutes | Yes |
| Monobasic sodium phosphate | Solid | 8.3-16.6 g | 1/4 adult dose (5-10 years)<br>1/2 adult dose (10 years) | Small and large intestines | 0.5-3 hours | Yes |
| | Solution (rectal) | 18.24-20.16 g once daily | 1/2 adult dose (2-11 years) | Colon | 2-15 minutes | Yes |
| Sodium biphosphate | Solid | 9.6-19.2 g | 1/2 adult dose (5-10 years)<br>1/2 adult dose (10 years) | Small and large intestines | 0.5-3 hours | Yes |
| **Hyperosmotic** | | | | | | |
| Glycerin | Solid (rectal) | 3 g | 1-1.5 g (<6 years) | Colon | 0.25-1 hour | — |
| | Liquid (rectal) | 5-15 mL | 2-5 mL (<6 years) | — | — | — |
| **Stimulants (Anthraquinones)** | | | | | | |
| Senna | Solid | 187-374 mg standardized senna concentrate<br>8.6-17.2 mg sennosides | 187 mg standardized senna concentrate (BW >27 kg) | Colon | 6-10 hours | Yes |
| | Granules | 326 mg (1 tsp) standardized senna concentrate | 163 mg (1/2 tsp) standardized senna concentrate (BW >27 kg) | Colon | 6-10 hours | Yes |
| | Syrup | 436-654 mg standardized senna extract | 218-436 mg standardized senna extract (5-15 years)<br>109-218 mg standardized senna extract (1-5 years)<br>54.5-109 mg standardized senna extract (1 month to 1 year) | Colon | 6-10 hours | Yes |
| | Solid (rectal) | 652 mg standardized senna concentrate<br>30 mg sennosides | 326 mg standardized senna concentrate (BW >27 kg) | | | |
| **Stimulants (Diphenylmethane)** | | | | | | |
| Bisacodyl | Solid | 10-30 mg | 5-10 mg (>6 years)<br>10 mg (>11 years) | Colon | 6-10 hours | Yes |
| **Miscellaneous** | | | | | | |
| Castor oil | Liquid | 15-60 mL | 1-5 mL (>2 years)<br>5-15 mL (2-12 years) | Small intestine | 2-6 hours | Yes |

Key: BW, body weight.
*Note:* Em dash (—) indicates information could not be identified.
* All doses are oral unless indicated otherwise.

esophagus after they ingested a bulk laxative that had been chewed or taken in dry form. Symptoms of esophageal obstruction include chest pain, vomiting, excessive salivation, and an inhibited swallowing reflex that may precipitate choking. FDA previously announced its intent to amend the tentative final rule for nonprescription laxatives to reclassify psyllium granular products from category I (generally recognized as safe and effective) to category II (not generally recognized as safe and effective), because of its concern for the continued incidence of esophageal obstruction. Manufacturers were given the opportunity to submit appropriate data to FDA to justify maintaining category I status. No further action has been taken by FDA. Practitioners should advise patients to use extra care to observe administration guidelines regarding fluid use with such products.[26] There have also been reports of acute bronchospasm associated with the inhalation of dry hydrophilic mucilloid, as well as hypersensitivity reactions characterized by anaphylaxis.[27]

The use of oral tetracyclines with calcium polycarbophil may decrease absorption because of the possible formation of nonabsorbable calcium complexes. In general, concurrent use of bulk-forming agents with other medication may reduce the desired effect of the coadministered medications because of physical binding or other mechanisms, which hinder absorption. Caution should be exercised by advising patients not to take a bulking agent within 1 to 2 hours of taking other medication.

Because of the danger of fecal impaction or intestinal obstruction, individuals with intestinal ulcerations, stenosis, or disabling adhesions should not take bulk-forming products. Diarrhea, abdominal discomfort, flatulence, and excessive loss of fluid can also occur. However, when taken properly, these agents have few systemic side effects because they are not absorbed.

Bulk-forming products may be inappropriate for patients who must severely restrict their fluid intake, such as those with significant renal dysfunction or heart failure. Patients who have demonstrated a previous hypersensitivity or who may be susceptible to an allergic reaction should exercise caution when considering a bulk-forming laxatives, especially psyllium. Psyllium has a history of triggering hypersensitivity reactions.[23]

Caution should be exercised when recommending a bulk-forming agent for children younger than 6 years of age. Failure to consume sufficient fluid (at least 8 oz) with a bulk laxative decreases drug efficacy and may result in intestinal or esophageal obstruction. Intestinal obstruction is a particular risk for patients suffering from opiate-induced constipation who have inadequate fluid intake.

The maximum calcium content of calcium polycarbophil is approximately 150 mg (7.6 mEq) per tablet. Susceptible patients who ingest the recommended therapeutic doses of calcium polycarbophil may increase the risk of hypercalcemia, and should use caution. The U.S. recommended daily allowance of calcium for adults is 1000 to 1300 mg (see Chapter 23). Furthermore, a consensus development conference of the National Institutes of Health indicated that up to 2000 mg/day of calcium—from all sources—appears safe for most individuals.[28]

The dextrose content of some of the commercial products should be evaluated before use by diabetic patients and other patients on carbohydrate-restricted diets. Furthermore, sugar-free, bulk-forming agents that contain aspartame should be avoided by patients suffering from phenylketonuria.

### Emollients

Emollients include docusate sodium, docusate calcium, and docusate potassium.

*Mechanism of Action* Emollients are anionic surfactants. When administered orally, they increase the wetting efficiency of intestinal fluid and facilitate a mixture of aqueous and fatty substances to soften the fecal mass. These agents are commonly known as "stool softeners."

*Pharmacokinetics* Docusate has an onset of action after oral administration of between 24 and 72 hours, and the effect lasts about 72 hours. As a result, fecal-softening emollient laxatives are usually effective in 1 to 2 days but may take as long as 3 to 5 days in some patients. These agents are believed not to be appreciably absorbed from the GI tract. In addition, docusate does not retard absorption of nutrients from the intestinal tract.

*Indications* Orally administered emollients prevent constipation and are of little or no value in treating longstanding constipation, especially in older adults or patients who are debilitated. These agents may be used for up to 1 week without consulting a primary care provider. Emollients soften stool and prevent painful defecation when the patient has undergone or is about to undergo surgery for hemorrhoids or other anorectal disorders or when it is desirable for the patient to avoid straining at the stool (e.g., after abdominal surgery, immediately postpartum, or in patients with severe hypertension or cardiovascular disease). The patient should increase fluid intake to facilitate softening the stool. Because of the softening effect of docusate, it is frequently used along with a stimulant (senna or bisacodyl) as a long-term treatment for opiate-induced constipation. Stool softeners also are useful agents in colostomy patients requiring a laxative product (see Chapter 22).

*Dosage and Administration Guidelines* Table 16-4 lists dosing information for emollient agents. Children younger than 6 years old should not use emollients except as prescribed by a primary care provider. Doses above those recommended by the manufacturer may result in weakness, sweating, muscle cramps, and an irregular heartbeat in some patients.

*Safety Considerations* Docusate can potentially cause diarrhea and mild abdominal cramping.

Emollients facilitate the absorption of other poorly absorbed substances such as mineral oil and may increase the toxicity of these substances.[19] Docusate and its congeners are claimed to be nonabsorbable, relatively nontoxic, and pharmacologically inert. Caution should be exercised as the detergent (surfactant) properties of docusate are believed to facilitate transport of other substances across cell membranes. No additional drug interactions of clinical importance are noted.

Emollient use should be avoided if nausea and vomiting, symptoms of appendicitis (e.g., abdominal pain, nausea, vomiting), or undetermined abdominal pain exist.

### Lubricants

Mineral oil (liquid petrolatum) is the only nonprescription lubricant. Heavy mineral oil is used internally while light mineral oil is used to prepare topical products.

*Mechanism of Action* Mineral oil and certain digestible plant oils such as olive oil soften fecal contents by coating them, thus preventing colonic absorption of fecal water. Emulsified products are used to increase palatability. There is little difference in cathartic effect of these formulations, although emulsions of mineral oil penetrate and soften fecal matter more effectively than nonemulsified preparations.

*Pharmacokinetics* The onset of action of mineral oil is about 6 to 8 hours after oral administration and 5 to 15 minutes after rectal administration. Nonemulsified mineral oil is minimally absorbed after oral or rectal doses.

*Indications* Mineral oil is beneficial when used judiciously in cases requiring the maintenance of a soft stool to avoid straining (e.g., when there has been hernia, aneurysm, hypertension, myocardial infarction, or cerebrovascular accident, or after a hemorrhoidectomy or abdominal surgery). However, routine use of mineral oil in these cases is not indicated; instead, emollients such as docusate sodium are preferred for preventing constipation.

*Dosage and Administration Guidelines* Table 16-4 lists dosing information for mineral oil. This laxative should not be given to children younger than 6 years. Excessive dosage of mineral oil increases the possibility of loss of fat-soluble nutrients from the GI tract and enhances the likelihood of product aspiration and anal leakage.

*Safety Considerations* The adverse effects and toxicity of mineral oil are associated with its repeated and prolonged use. The oil droplets may reach the mesenteric lymph nodes and may also be present in the intestinal mucosa, liver, and spleen, where they elicit a typical foreign-body reaction.

Lipid pneumonia may result from the oral ingestion and subsequent aspiration of mineral oil, especially when the patient reclines. The pharynx may become coated with the oil, and droplets may reach the trachea and the posterior part of the lower lobes of the lungs. Because aspiration into the lungs is possible, mineral oil should not be administered at bedtime or to patients who are very young, of advanced age, or debilitated. When a patient takes large doses of mineral oil, the oil may leak through the anal sphincter and produce anal pruritus (pruritus ani), cryptitis, or other perianal conditions. The patient can avoid this leakage by reducing or dividing the dose, or by using a stable emulsion of mineral oil. Because surfactants tend to increase absorption of otherwise "nonabsorbable" drugs, the patient must not take mineral oil with emollients. The patient should also avoid prolonged use.

The role of mineral oil in impairing the absorption of fat-soluble nutrients is uncertain. Mineral oil may impair the absorption of vitamins A, D, E, and K; impaired vitamin D absorption may affect the absorption of calcium and phosphates. Patients should not take mineral oil with meals because it may delay gastric emptying. In addition, it should not be given to pregnant women because it can decrease the availability of vitamin K to the fetus. Patients taking oral anticoagulants should use mineral oil with caution because the potentially decreased absorption of vitamin K may increase the blood-thinning property of the anticoagulant. As indicated, mineral oil may reduce the absorption of oral anticoagulants, oral contraceptives, and digitalis glycosides. Its absorption may be enhanced when used concomitantly with docusate.

Mineral oil is contraindicated if a patient is bedridden and if any of the following are present: appendicitis or its symptoms, undiagnosed rectal bleeding, or dysphagia.

### Saline Laxatives

Saline laxative agents include magnesium citrate, magnesium hydroxide, magnesium sulfate, dibasic sodium phosphate, monobasic sodium phosphate, and sodium biphosphate.

*Mechanism of Action* The active constituents of saline laxatives (also referred to as osmotics) are relatively nonabsorbable cations and anions such as magnesium and sulfate ions. Sulfate salts are considered to be the most potent of this category of laxatives. The wall of the small intestine, which acts as a semipermeable membrane to the magnesium, sulfate, tartrate, phosphate, and citrate ions, retains the highly osmotic ions in the intestine. The presence of these ions draws water into the intestine, increasing intraluminal pressure. This increased pressure exerts a mechanical stimulus that increases intestinal motility.

However, different mechanisms that are independent of the osmotic effect may be partially responsible for the laxative properties of the salts. Saline laxatives produce a complex series of reactions, both secretory and motor, on the GI tract. For example, the action of magnesium sulfate on the GI tract is similar to that of cholecystokinin-pancreozymin. There is evidence that this hormone is released from the intestinal mucosa when saline laxatives are administered.[29] This release, in turn, favors accumulation of fluid and electrolytes within the intestinal lumen.

*Pharmacokinetics* Saline laxatives have an onset of action of between 30 minutes and 3 hours for oral doses and between 2 and 5 minutes for rectal doses. Up to 20% of an orally administered dose may be absorbed.

*Indications* Saline laxatives are indicated for use only when acute evacuation of the bowel is required, as when preparing for endoscopic examination or eliminating drugs in suspected poisonings. These agents have no place in the long-term management of constipation. In some cases of food or drug poisoning, saline laxatives are used in purging doses. Rectal phosphate products are used to prepare the bowel for a barium enema and eliminate fecal impaction.

*Dosage and Administration Guidelines* Table 16-4 lists dosing information for saline laxative agents. Rectal agents should not be used in children younger than 2 years. Oral products should not be used in children younger than 5 years. Any of the magnesium-containing products may lead to hypermagnesemia in both adults and children. Hypotension, muscle weakness, and electrocardiographic changes may indicate a toxic effect of magnesium. In addition, excessive levels of serum magnesium exert a depressant effect on the central nervous system and neuromuscular activity. Phosphate laxatives can be troublesome when dosed excessively. An overdose of a sodium phosphate enema led to a coma in one patient of advanced age as a result of hyperphosphatemia and hypocalcemia.[30] It is very important to monitor dosages of these products in any patient who has renal impairment.

*Safety Considerations* In some cases, the choice of a saline laxative may result in serious adverse effects. As much as 20% of the administered magnesium ion may be absorbed from magnesium salts. If renal function is normal, the absorbed ion can be eliminated without consequence. However, if renal function is markedly impaired, or if the patient is a newborn or older adult, concentrations of the magnesium ion could accumulate, resulting in toxicity.[29] Other adverse effects include abdominal cramping, excessive diuresis, nausea, vomiting, and dehydration. Although 90 mL oral sodium phosphate has been FDA-approved for several years, concern about adverse effects has prompted FDA to consider limiting package size to 45 mL or less.[31]

Saline laxatives can interact with oral anticoagulants, digitalis glycosides, and some phenothiazines (especially chlorpromazine). Magnesium-containing laxatives may interfere with the absorption of oral tetracycline products. If used concurrently with a magnesium salt, sodium polystyrene sulfonate may bind with magnesium and lead to systemic alkalosis.

Saline laxatives are contraindicated in patients with ileostomy or colostomy, dehydration syndromes, renal function impairment, or congestive heart failure.

Phosphate salts are available in oral and rectal dosage forms. The typical oral dose contains 96.5 mEq of sodium and, therefore, should be administered with caution to patients on sodium-restricted diets. When phosphate salts are given as an enema, up to 10% or more of the sodium content may be absorbed. FDA has issued a proposed rule to amend regulations regarding sodium labeling for nonprescription products, to include rectally administered drugs. This proposed rule would require sodium content labeling on products containing sodium phosphate and sodium bisphosphate. The action is being taken to protect patients who may be at risk for electrolyte imbalance while using such products.[32] Cathartics containing sodium may be toxic to individuals with edema, congestive heart disease, or renal failure; phosphates will accumulate with impaired renal function and should be avoided in such patients. Because dehydration may occur with the repeated use of hypertonic solutions of saline cathartics, patients who cannot tolerate fluid loss should not use phosphate salts. In patients who are not fluid restricted, oral phosphate salts should be followed by at least one full glass of water to prevent dehydration.

### Hyperosmotics

Glycerin is the primary example of a hyperosmotic agent. Other common agents in this class are prescription-only products and include lactulose, sorbitol, and polyethylene glycol (PEG) solutions with (e.g., Colyte) or without (e.g., MiraLax) electrolytes.

*Mechanism of Action* Glycerin's cathartic capability is caused by combining an osmotic effect with the local irritant effect of sodium stearate. The combination acts by drawing water into the rectum to stimulate a bowel movement. Lactulose and sorbitol are large nonabsorbable sugar molecules that, when hydrolyzed by gut bacteria, draw fluid into the colon by an osmotic effect. The result is an increase in colonic peristalsis. PEG solutions also consist of very large poorly absorbable ethylene glycol molecules that cause an osmotic effect, resulting in distension and catharsis.

*Pharmacokinetics* Glycerin is poorly absorbed after rectal administration. Use of glycerin suppositories in infants and adults usually produces a bowel movement within 30 minutes.

*Indications* Glycerin has been available for many years in suppository form to be used for lower bowel evacuation.

*Dosage and Administration Guidelines* Table 16-4 lists dosing information for glycerin. The customary rectal dose of glycerin considered safe and effective for adults and children older than 6 years is 3 g. Use of liquid glycerin as an enema is not recommended in adults and older children; such use may cause considerable rectal irritation. For infants and children younger than 6 years, the dose is 1 to 1.5 g as a suppository. Overdosage with glycerin might cause additional rectal irritation, but would not be expected to lead to serious sequelae.

*Safety Considerations* Adverse reactions and side effects from glycerin suppositories are minimal. Some rectal irritation may occur. The irritation can be attributed to the sodium stearate component of the suppository.

Interactions between glycerin and other drugs are not clinically important.

Use of glycerin may be inappropriate in patients with a previous condition involving rectal irritation. Chronic use or overuse may lead to reduced serum potassium concentrations.

### Stimulants

Stimulants are conveniently classified according to their chemical structure and pharmacologic activity. Anthraquinones include aloe, cascara sagrada, casanthranol, senna (including the sennosides, which are hydroanthracene glycosides derived from senna leaves), aloin, danthron, rhubarb, and frangula. The drugs of choice in this group are senna compounds. Recently, FDA reclassified several stimulants used as nonprescription laxatives as "misbranded," including cascara, casanthranol, and aloe products.[33] Manufacturers were invited to submit data to FDA, supporting the effectiveness of these agents, but declined. All products containing these ingredients were reformulated. Some of the affected products include Nature's Remedy (cascara sagrada and aloe), Peri-Colace (casanthranol), and Black Draught (casanthranol). The banned substances in these products have been replaced with sennosides, standardized senna, and senna, respectively. Patients should be informed that products containing the banned substances have not been proven to be unsafe, so the risk associated with taking products that may have already been purchased is minimal. Practitioners should not recommend rhubarb or aloin, which are very irritating, although these substances were not affected by the FDA ruling.

The most commonly used diphenylmethane laxatives have been bisacodyl and phenolphthalein. However, after a review of reports of the development of carcinogenic tumors and genetic damage in rats, FDA determined that phenolphthalein posed a risk, and subsequently placed it on the list of misbranded substances.[34] Phenolphthalein-containing products have been withdrawn from the marketplace.

Traditionally, castor oil has been classified as a third category of stimulant. However, it is viewed by some as an anionic surfactant.[35]

*Mechanism of Action* Stimulants are believed to increase the propulsive peristaltic activity of the intestine by local irritation of the mucosa or by a more selective action on the intramural nerve plexus of intestinal smooth muscle, thus increasing motility. It has been suggested that these laxative products stimulate secretion of water and electrolytes in either the small or large intestine or both, depending on the specific laxative.[7] Intensity of action is proportional to dosage, but individual effective doses vary.

The precise mechanism by which anthraquinones increase peristalsis is unknown. Senna and the sennosides appear to inhibit water and electrolyte absorption from the large intestine, resulting in increased intestinal volume and pressure that stimulates colonic motility. Bisacodyl acts in the colon on contact with the mucosal nerve plexus. Stimulation is segmented and axonal, producing contractions of the entire colon. Bisacodyl's action is independent of intestinal tone, and the drug is minimally absorbed systemically (approximately 5%).[35]

Castor oil's laxative action is produced by ricinoleic acid, which is produced when castor oil is hydrolyzed in the small intestine by pancreatic lipase. Its exact mechanism of action is unknown.

*Pharmacokinetics* The cathartic activity of anthraquinones is limited primarily to the colon. Anthraquinones usually produce their action 6 to 12 hours after administration, but may require up to 24 hours. The properties of each anthraquinone laxative varies somewhat, depending on the anthraquinone content and the speed with which the active principles are liberated. The anthraquinones are hydrolyzed by colonic bacteria into active compounds and are minimally absorbed. Senna's active constituents include sennosides A and B. Sennosides are metabolized to an active byproduct called rhein.

Bisacodyl is minimally absorbed whether given by oral or rectal administration. Action on the small intestine is negligible. A soft, formed stool is usually produced 6 to 10 hours after oral administration and 15 to 60 minutes after rectal administration.

Castor oil has an oral onset of action of about 2 to 6 hours. It is metabolized to ricinoleic acid, which is absorbed to a small extent. Castor oil, a glyceride, is probably metabolized like other fatty acids. Because the main site of action is the small intestine, its prolonged use may result in excessive loss of fluid, electrolytes, and nutrients. Castor oil is most effective when administered on an empty stomach.

*Indications* Stimulants such as bisacodyl are used before radiologic or endoscopic examination of the GI tract and GI surgery, when thorough evacuation of the bowel is crucial. Both bisacodyl and senna are finding wide use as treatment for chronic constipation induced by opiates.[10] Bisacodyl may be administered orally or rectally and may be used in combination with or instead of an enema or suppository for emptying the colon and rectum before proctologic or colonic examination or GI surgery. Because of its thoroughness in evacuating the bowel, bisacodyl is effective in patients with colostomies, and it may reduce or eliminate the need for irrigations.

*Dosage and Administration Guidelines* In general, stimulants may be used as initial drug therapy in patients with simple constipation, but they should not be used for more than 1 week unless ordered by a physician. The dose should be within the recommended dosage range listed in Table 16-4. However, listed doses and dosage ranges are only guides when determining the optimal individual dose. Overdoses of stimulants, especially anthraquinones, may lead to sudden vomiting, nausea, diarrhea, or severe abdominal cramping, requiring prompt medical attention.

*Safety Considerations* Major hazards of stimulant laxative use are severe cramping, electrolyte and fluid deficiencies, enteric loss of protein, malabsorption resulting from excessive hypermotility and catharsis, and hypokalemia. Stimulants are effective but should be recommended cautiously. Because the intensity of their activity is proportional to the dose used, a large enough dose of any stimulant laxative can produce unwanted and sometimes dangerous adverse effects. Nevertheless, these laxatives are frequently used by those who self-medicate for constipation. Because of their effectiveness, stimulant laxatives may be subject to overuse

## A WORD ABOUT
### Laxative Abuse

Routine, chronic use of most laxative preparations is considered laxative abuse, or at least laxative overuse, and should be avoided if at all possible. Some believe that the risk of abuse has been overemphasized. While the laxative abuser may commonly be thought of as an older adult, this is not an accurate view. Some adolescents, college students, and young adults (especially women) may misuse laxatives for weight control.[36,37] Such abuse is often part of a pattern of "purging behavior," which may also include self-induced vomiting. These individuals may suffer from bulimia nervosa or anorexia nervosa.[38]

Excessive use of laxatives can cause diarrhea and vomiting, leading to fluid and electrolyte losses, especially hypokalemia, which may result in a general loss of tone of smooth and striated muscle. Clinical features of laxative abuse may include (1) factitious diarrhea (a severe chronic watery diarrhea, frequently occurring at night and accompanied by abdominal pain, weight loss, nausea, and vomiting),[39] (2) electrolyte imbalance (e.g., hypokalemia, hypocalcemia, hypermagnesemia), (3) osteomalacia, (4) protein-losing enteropathy (intestinal disease), (5) steatorrhea, and (6) liver disease.

Cathartic colon, long thought to be associated with laxative abuse, is now largely dismissed for lack of evidence.[11] Although past literature offered a few case reports, the recent literature offers no support and it has been suggested that this is because currently used products are less capable of producing it than were older, out-of-favor products.[7]

Laxative abuse can usually be classified as either habitual or surreptitious. The habitual abuser often believes that a daily bowel movement is a necessity and uses a laxative to accomplish this end. Such patients may freely admit to this practice because they believe regular laxative use to be entirely correct and natural. Conversely, surreptitious abuse is similar to other illnesses. Surreptitious abusers tend to manifest various psychiatric disturbances. Confronting this type of abuser does not usually help resolve the problem, and psychiatric intervention should be encouraged. Practitioners should be alert to the possibility of laxative abuse when making a patient assessment. The diagnosis of laxative abuse may include a stool osmolarity test to detect salines and a colonoscopy to detect melanosis coli. Urine samples may be analyzed for the presence of the most commonly used laxatives.[40]

Once the abuse has been adequately substantiated, it may be possible to (1) wean the patient off the laxative before permanent bowel damage occurs and (2) regularize the patient's bowel habits with a high-fiber diet supplemented by bulk-forming laxatives as needed. After an abuser is withdrawn from one or more laxatives, several months may be required to retrain the bowel to work in regular, unaided function. Affected patients should be educated about laxative abuse. The information provided should describe types of laxatives and their harmful effects. Patients should be advised that constipation, weight gain, bloating, or abdominal distention may occur following the end of laxative abuse. These patients should be encouraged to exercise, increase dietary fiber, and maintain adequate fluid intake. The practitioner should also encourage them to discuss their attitudes about laxative abuse and be prepared to answer any questions that arise in such discussions.

(that is, indiscriminate or excessive routine use beyond accepted limits). Such use was once thought to contribute to "cathartic colon," described as a poorly functioning colon (see box A Word About Laxative Abuse). However, data seem unconvincing regarding stimulants ability to induce this alleged disorder.[4]

The prolonged use of anthraquinones can result in a harmless, reversible melanotic pigmentation of the colonic mucosa (melanosis coli), which is usually found on sigmoidoscopy, colonoscopy, or rectal biopsy.

Adverse effects of diphenylmethanes, which come with chronic, regular use (abuse), include metabolic acidosis or alkalosis, hypocalcemia, tetany, loss of enteric protein, and malabsorption. The suppository form may produce a burning sensation in the rectum. No systemic or adverse effects on the liver, kidney, or hematopoietic system have been observed following administration.

Senna may color urine pink to red, red to violet, or red to brown, thus affecting the accurate interpretation of the phenolsulfonphthalein test.

The administration of bisacodyl tablets within 1 hour of antacids, cimetidine, famotidine, ranitidine, or milk results in rapid erosion of the enteric coating, which may lead to gastric or duodenal irritation. Enteric-coated bisacodyl tablets prevent irritation of the gastric mucosa and, therefore, should not be broken, crushed, chewed, or administered with agents that increase gastric pH such as antacids, histamine$_2$-receptor antagonists, or proton pump inhibitors.

Stimulants should not be used for patients with undiagnosed rectal bleeding, signs of intestinal obstruction, or presence of appendicitis. Pregnant women should use stimulants under the direction of a physician, especially during the third trimester. All stimulants may produce griping, colic, increased mucus secretion and, in some people, excessive evacuation of fluid. Chrysophanic acid, a component of rhubarb and senna that is excreted in urine, colors acidic urine yellowish brown and colors alkaline urine reddish violet. The clinician should warn patients that a number of prescription and nonprescription medications, as well as some foods, will produce either alkaline or acidic urine and the use of senna may lead to urine discoloration. Because a laxative effect occurs quickly, castor oil should not be given at bedtime.

### Combination Products

Many combination laxative products are available (Table 16-5). Companies attempt to take advantage of multiple mechanisms of action and other factors to create a product that better meets the criteria for an ideal laxative. Several combination products contain a stimulant and a second entity. Emollients do not stimulate bowel movements when used alone but do achieve this purpose when combined with stimulant laxatives. A popular combination is docusate sodium with senna, which makes the best use of both cathartic action and stool softening effect.

**TABLE 16-5 Selected Laxative Products**

| Trade Name | Primary Ingredients |
|---|---|
| **Bulk-forming Laxatives** | |
| Citrucel Powder | Methylcellulose 2 g/tsp |
| Citrucel Sugar Free Powder* | Methylcellulose 2 g/tsp |
| FiberCon Tablets*†‡ | Calcium polycarbophil 625 mg |
| Konsyl Powder* | Psyllium mucilloid 6 g/tsp |
| Maltsupex Liquid | Barley malt extract 750 mg/tsp |
| Metamucil Fiber Wafer†‡ | Psyllium hydrophilic mucilloid 3.4 g/2 wafers |
| Metamucil Original Texture, Powder‡ | Psyllium hydrophilic mucilloid 3.4 g/tsp |
| Metamucil Original Texture, Regular Flavor Powder‡ | Psyllium hydrophilic mucilloid 3.4 g/tsp |
| Metamucil Smooth Texture, Orange Flavor Powder‡ | Psyllium hydrophilic mucilloid 3.4 g/tsp |
| Metamucil Smooth Texture, Sugar Free Orange Flavor Powder/Individual Packets*‡ | Psyllium hydrophilic mucilloid 3.4 g/tsp |
| Mitrolan Chewable Tablets§ | Calcium polycarbophil 500 mg |
| Serutan Granules | Psyllium hydrophilic mucilloid 2.5 mg/tsp |
| **Emollient Laxatives** | |
| Colace Liquid‡‖ | Docusate sodium 20 mg/5 mL |
| Colace Capsules | Docusate sodium 50 mg; 100 mg |
| Correctol Stool Softener Sofgels | Docusate sodium 100 mg |
| **Lubricant Laxatives** | |
| Fleet Mineral Oil Enema | Mineral oil 100% |
| Kondremul Emulsion§ | Mineral oil 55% |
| **Saline Laxatives** | |
| Citroma Solution | Magnesium citrate 1.745 g/oz |
| Fleet Ready-to-Use Enema | Monobasic sodium phosphate 19 g/133mL; dibasic sodium phosphate 7 g/133 mL |
| Fleet Ready-to-Use Enema for Children¶ | Monobasic sodium phosphate 9.5 g/59 mL; dibasic sodium phosphate 3.5 g/59 mL |
| Phillips' Milk of Magnesia Concentrate Suspension‡# | Magnesium hydroxide 800 mg/5 mL |
| Phillips' Milk of Magnesia Suspension‡# | Magnesium hydroxide 400 mg/5 mL |
| **Hyperosmotic Laxatives** | |
| Fleet Babylax Liquid | Glycerin 2.3 g |
| Fleet Glycerin Suppository (Adult/Child Size) | Glycerin 5.6 g |
| Fleet Glycerin Rectal Applicators Liquid | Glycerin 7.5 mL |
| **Stimulant Laxatives** | |
| Correctol Caplets/Tablets | Bisacodyl 5 mg |
| Dulcolax Tablets§ | Bisacodyl 5 mg |
| Ex-Lax Maximum Strength Tablets | Sennosides 25 mg |
| Ex-Lax Regular Strength Chocolate Tablets§ | Sennosides 15 mg |
| Feen-A-Mint Tablets | Bisacodyl 5 mg |
| Fleet Laxative Suppository | Bisacodyl 10 mg |
| Fleet Stimulant Laxative Tablets | Bisacodyl 5 mg |
| Purge Liquid*‡‖ | Castor oil 95% |
| Senokot Tablets | Standardized senna concentrate 8.6 mg sennosides |
| Senokot Children's Syrup#¶ | Extract of senna concentrate 8.8 mg/5 mL sennosides |
| X-Prep Liquid | Senna concentrate 3.7 g/75 mL standardized extract of senna fruit |

TABLE 16-5 Selected Laxative Products (continued)

| Trade Name | Primary Ingredients |
|---|---|
| **Combination Laxatives** | |
| Fleet Bisacodyl Enema | Bisacodyl 10 mg; glycerin |
| Phillips' M-O Flavored‡# | Mineral oil 1.25 mg/5 mL; magnesium hydroxide 300 mg/5 mL |
| Perdiem Granules | Senna (cassia pod concentrate) 0.74 g/tsp; psyllium 3.25 g/tsp |
| Senokot-S Tablets | Senna concentrate 8.6 mg sennosides; docusate sodium 50 mg |
| Surfak Liqui-gels‡§ | Docusate calcium 240 mg; glycerin |
| **Bowel Evacuant Kits** | |
| Evac-Q-Kwik System Liquid/Suppository/Tablets* | Tablets: bisacodyl 15 mg/3 tablets; suppository: bisacodyl 10 mg; liquid: magnesium citrate 25 mEq/30 mL |
| Fleet Prep Kit 1 | Tablets: bisacodyl 20 mg/4 tablets; suppository: bisacodyl 10 mg; liquid: sodium phosphate oral solution 45 mL (total sodium 495 mg/45 mL) |
| Fleet Prep Kit 2‖ | Tablets: bisacodyl 20 mg/4 tablets; liquid: sodium phosphate oral solution 45 mL; enema: Fleet Bagenema |
| Fleet Prep Kit 3 | Tablets: bisacodyl 20 mg/4 tablets; enema: bisacodyl 10 mg; liquid: sodium phosphate oral solution 45 mL |

*Sucrose-free; †dye-free; ‡lactose-free; §sodium-free; ‖sulfite-free; ¶pediatric formulation; #alcohol-free.

In many cases of fecal impaction, a solution of docusate is often added to the enema fluid. Mineral oil has been combined with stimulants to produce popular products. What may seem to be an unlikely combination—milk of magnesia and mineral oil—has been available for years in a popular formulation (Phillips' M-O). Some products incorporate senna with psyllium. The desired effect is for the senna to act quickly and the bulk-forming agents to continue to help the bowel function beyond the initial movement. Additional combination oral products exist and include various agents such as psyllium, bisacodyl, or docusate as the principal ingredient and glycerin as an adjunctive agent. It is unlikely that the contributing effect of glycerin is significant to the overall laxative action of the product. The amount of oral glycerin necessary to produce laxation would lead to appreciable glycerin absorption from the small intestine.

Because a common ingredient in most combination products is a stimulant, it is important to remember that combining laxative entities will have the potential for greater adverse impact if administration and dosing guidelines are not closely followed. If a stimulant and a stool softener are combined, the potential for adversity depends largely on the stimulant. However, if a stimulant and a saline are combined, a greater potential exists for adverse effects to occur because both agents have significant effects on the intestine.

Bowel evacuant kits are designed for use to prepare the bowel for endoscopic examination or surgery (Table 16-5). The kit usually contains separate dosages of the specific laxatives rather than a single dosage form containing all the ingredients. Although a patient may experience adverse effects from preparation kits, they are intended for a single use before a procedure, unlike the usual treatment for constipation.

## Pharmacotherapeutic Comparison

Head-to-head comparison studies solely among nonprescription laxatives are largely unavailable. Much of what is practiced has been gained through observation following laxative use. One study has suggested that psyllium is superior to docusate in treating chronic constipation. The multisite, randomized, and double-blind parallel design study of 170 subjects with chronic idiopathic constipation concluded that psyllium showed superior action to docusate for softening stools because it increased stool water content and exhibited greater overall laxative efficacy.[41] If used properly, a bulk-forming product should soften the stool by its normal action. Because both a traditional stool softener and a bulk-forming agent take about the same length of time to work, a bulk-forming agent may be the correct choice for some patients who require stool softening.

Very few new-entity laxative products have been introduced into the marketplace in recent years. Most principal ingredients were brought into being before the current era of rigorous comparative studies. Although stimulants and saline-type laxatives are widely used, it is important to recommend a product with the lowest likelihood of untoward effects.

## Product Selection Guidelines

When considering the use of any laxative to treat constipation, the clinician should remember that normal defecation empties only the rectum and the descending and sigmoid branches of the colon. The preparation chosen should duplicate the normal physiologic process as nearly as possible. Most stimulant products have the potential to promote catharsis, that is, a complete emptying of the entire colon. However, the laxative user who is unaware of this effect may take another laxative dose on the first or second postlaxative day, thereby maintaining a completely empty colon. Thus, when it is necessary to use a laxative to treat constipation, the recommended initial choice is most often a bulk-forming product. Mineral oil can cause malabsorption of fat-soluble vitamins or lipid pneumonia if it is aspirated, so its use should be avoided. (See Table 16-5 for selected trade-name laxative products.)

Acute constipation is the primary indication for self-treatment with a nonprescription laxative. However, nonprescription laxative products are also prescribed or indicated for patients preparing for diagnostic GI procedures and radiography. A primary care diagnostician should supervise the use of laxatives (1) during treatment for perianal disease (preoperatively or postoperatively), (2) with conditions in which straining is undesirable (e.g., postoperative or post–myocardial infarction), or (3) for chronic constipation. Although bulk-forming and emollient laxatives may be suitable for such problems, therapy in these situations is highly individualized.

*Guidelines for Use in Underlying Pathology* The practitioner should exercise caution when recommending magnesium-containing products to patients with renal failure because of the risk of hypermagnesemia. The practitioner should be similarly cautious when recommending sodium-containing products to patients with cardiovascular disease because of the potential for sodium overload. As a rule, laxative products whose maximum daily dose contains more than sodium 345 mg (15 mEq), potassium 975 mg (25 mEq), magnesium 600 mg (50 mEq), or calcium 1800 mg (90 mEq) should not be used in kidney or liver disease, heart failure, hypertension, or other conditions requiring sodium, potassium, magnesium, or calcium restriction.

Any product containing dextrose should be used with caution in labile diabetic patients because glycemic control may be lost. In addition, products containing aspartame should be avoided in patients with phenylketonuria.

*Guidelines for Use in Children* Normal frequency of bowel movements varies with the age of a child, therefore abnormal bowel habits may be difficult to recognize. Laxatives are often administered to children when the parent perceives that the child's normal bowel habits have been disrupted or have changed. As a result, indiscriminate use of laxatives may result if the child has a stooling pattern that is changing or when other constipating factors are present. Children should be encouraged to establish a regular pattern of bowel movements, and to avoid withholding of stools when the urge to have a bowel movement occurs. The clinician should always consider a child's age and any previous laxative use when recommending laxative products. The route of administration and the taste of oral products may be especially significant in children. Laxative use can be avoided in older children by encouraging them to adhere to suggested dietary guidelines to improve stool regularity.

If medications are indicated in children younger than 5 years, glycerin suppositories may initiate the defecation reflex with an onset usually within 15 to 60 minutes. Barley malt extract (malt soup extract) is relatively safe for infants younger than 2 months. Breast-fed infants may receive 6 to 10 mL in 2 to 4 oz of water or fruit juice twice daily. Bottle-fed infants may receive 7.5 to 32 mL in a day's total formula, or 5 to 10 mL every second feeding.

Dark corn syrup (1 to 2 tsp per feeding) or milk of magnesia (beginning with 1/2 tsp) may be useful for fecal impaction. Bisacodyl, magnesium citrate, and sorbitol may be used for moderate to severe constipation or fecal impaction.[12] Disimpaction can also be achieved by the use of enemas containing phosphate soda, saline, or mineral oil.[12] Enemas are not usually recommended for children younger than 2 years. Saline agents can lead to salt and water retention. Use in children younger than 2 years may lead to electrolyte abnormalities, such as hypocalcemia, tetany, hypernatremia, dehydration, and hyperphosphatemia. Electrolyte levels in these patients require careful monitoring.

In general, stimulants should be avoided, as should excessive use of enemas. Senna and mineral oil should be administered only on the advice of a primary care provider. Mineral oil can be chilled, given with ice cream or juice.[17]

When successful bowel evacuation cannot be achieved with oral supplementation or enemas, pediatricians may prescribe a prescription-only product such as a balanced PEG-electrolyte solution (e.g., Golytely or Colyte) for oral administration or a formulation without electrolytes (MiraLax).

*Guidelines for Use in Older Adults* Chronic laxative use is common among the aged population. The aging process can cause the colon to lack normal tone, resulting in an overreliance on oral laxatives or rectal enemas. However, because of the physiologic effects of chronic laxative use on the intestine, laxative dependency is often difficult to manage. Laxative preparations can also increase the rate at which other drugs pass through the GI tract by increasing GI motility, which then decreases absorption and the effectiveness of concurrently administered medications.

Older patients are particularly sensitive to shifts in fluid and electrolytes. Use of any laxative that alters the fluid and electrolyte balance, particularly saline-type laxatives, may be inappropriate in certain patients of advanced age. Such laxatives can place older patients, particularly those who are on diuretics or have decreased fluid intake, at risk for adverse effects.

It has been suggested that an acute episode of constipation be treated with plain water or saline enemas. Soapsuds enemas and enemas using detergents should be avoided because they can be irritating and can cause serious complications.[8,42] Sodium phosphate and biphosphate enemas are effective but can result in hyperphosphatemia in patients with renal disease. For patients with cardiac and renal disease, PEG-electrolyte solutions, commonly used as bowel preparations for GI procedures and available by prescription only, have been safely used for acute management of constipation because they are poorly absorbed.

Bulk-forming agents are generally preferred for older patients who are able to tolerate adequate fluid intake. The onset of effect is usually 12 to 72 hours. Sugar-free products are recommended for patients with diabetes. Adequate fluid intake is necessary to avoid worsening constipation from bulk-forming laxatives. Glycerin suppositories and the oral administration of lactulose or sorbitol (prescription-only products) are safe and have been used successfully in patients of advanced age. Although considerably more costly than sorbitol, lactulose may be of particular benefit to those who are bedridden, and it is preferred in patients with hepatic encephalopathy.[43]

Some health care providers may recommend chronic stimulant laxatives in certain situations, but these products should not be generally recommended for all older patients. The recommendation to use laxatives in this population should be patient specific. Older individuals can have complicating pathology, multiple medical complaints, and are vulnerable to the effects of medications. A complete and thorough history should aid in selecting the most appropriate product. Mineral oil must be used with care, if at all, by older adults. Bedridden older patients are especially prone to developing lipid pneumonia (see Lubricants, Safety Considerations).

*Guidelines for Use in Pregnancy* The main goal of treatment of constipation in pregnancy is to achieve soft stools without the use of laxatives. Dietary measures should be attempted as an initial measure in most patients. However, laxatives may be necessary postpartum in some women, to reestablish normal bowel function lost because of perineal pain. Other indications for laxative use may include ileus secondary to colonic dilatation in a decompressed abdomen, laxness of the anal sphincter and abdominal musculature, low fluid intake, hemorrhoids, and administration of enemas during labor. Consultation with a woman's health care provider is recommended prior to laxative use in more severe cases and when the safety of certain laxative products is questionable.

Because of the potential for adverse effects of several products, such as (1) decreased vitamin absorption caused by mineral oil, (2) premature labor brought on by the irritant effects of castor oil, or (3) possible dangerous electrolyte imbalances with osmotic agents, pregnant women should be very selective in choosing a laxative. Bulk-forming laxatives are the common first-line choice in pregnancy because of their safety and effectiveness.[7] These products require liberal amounts of fluid intake. Usual recommendations are at least 1500 mL/day. If bulk-forming laxatives are ineffective or intolerable, emollient laxatives, senna, or bisacodyl may relieve symptoms. Senna and bisacodyl have also been safely used during breast-feeding.[44] Although stimulant laxatives should generally be avoided during pregnancy, one source suggests that some stimulants may be acceptable for use during the lactation period.[45] Senna and bisacodyl have not been shown to be present in significant concentrations in breast milk, or no data are available suggesting any potential toxicity may result in infants. If these products are used, the infant should be carefully observed for diarrhea. Saline cathartics should be avoided during pregnancy and lactation because appreciable GI absorption can occur in the mother. Toxicity occurring from excessive use of a saline cathartic such as magnesium sulfate could be significant, resulting in diarrhea, drowsiness, respiratory difficulty, and hypotonia. Such products may promote sodium retention and edema. Patients who are pregnant and suspected of using these products should be monitored for serum sodium increases and weight gain.

*Guidelines for Selection of Dosage Forms* Laxative products are available in a wide array of dosage forms, most of them for oral use. This variety probably yields the most benefits for pediatric and geriatric patients. Many of the dosage forms enhance patient acceptability and perhaps make laxative use more pleasant. However, laxatives available as chewing gum, wafers, effervescent granules, and chocolate tablets may not be thought of as drug products, and thus are more likely to be misused and abused. Enemas and suppositories are popular nonoral dosage forms used for laxative administration.

Enemas Routine use of laxative enemas includes preparing patients for surgery, child delivery, and GI radiologic or endoscopic examinations as well as for treating certain cases of constipation. The enema fluid determines the mechanism by which evacuation is produced. Tap water and normal saline create bulk through an osmotic volume effect; vegetable oils lubricate, soften, and facilitate the passage of hardened fecal matter; and the irritant action of soapsuds produces defecation. However, prolonged rectal irritation may occur after soap enemas and may result in proctitis or colitis.[4,8] Therefore, soap enemas are not recommended.

The popular sodium phosphate/sodium biphosphate enemas (e.g., Fleet) fall into the category of saline laxatives. They are usually effective evacuants in preparing patients for surgical, diagnostic, or other procedures involving the bowel. These agents are more efficient and effective than tap water, soapsuds, or saline enemas. Because they can alter fluid and electrolyte balance significantly with prolonged use, chronic use of these products is not warranted for controlling constipation.

A properly administered enema cleans only the distal colon, most nearly approximating a normal bowel movement. Proper administration requires that the diagnosis, the enema fluid, and the technique of administration be correct. Improperly administered, an enema can produce fluid and electrolyte imbalances. Enema fluids have caused mucosal changes or spasm of the intestinal wall. Water intoxication has resulted from the use of tap water or soapsuds enemas in the presence of megacolon. A misdirected or inadequately lubricated nozzle may cause abrasion of the anal canal and rectal wall or may cause colonic perforation.

Patients should be advised to follow all directions carefully when using these products (Table 16-6). The patient should lie or be placed either on the left side with knees bent or in the knee-to-chest position. If the patient is in a sitting position, use of an enema clears only the rectum of fecal material. The solution should be allowed to flow into the rectum slowly; if the patient is uncomfortable, the flow

**TABLE 16-6 Administration of Rectal Suppositories or Enemas**

**Enemas**

1. If someone else is administering the enema, lie on your left side with knees bent or in the knee-to-chest position (see drawings A and B). Position A is preferred for children older than 2 years. If self-administering the enema, lie on your back with your knees bent and buttocks raised (see drawing C). A pillow may be placed under the buttocks.
2. If using a concentrated enema solution, dilute solution according to the product instructions. Prepare 1 pint (500 mL) for adults and 1/2 pint (250 mL) for children.
3. Lubricate the enema tip with petroleum jelly or other nonmedicated ointment/cream. Apply the lubricant to the anal area as well.
4. Gently insert the enema tip 2 (recommended depth for children) to 3 in. into the rectum.
5. Allow the solution to flow into the rectum slowly. If you experience discomfort, the flow is probably too fast.
6. Retain the enema solution until definite lower abdominal cramping is felt. The parent/caregiver may have to gently hold a child's buttocks closed to prevent the solution from being expelled too soon.

**Suppositories**

1. Gently squeeze the suppository to determine if it is firm enough to insert. Chill a soft suppository by placing it in the refrigerator for a few minutes or by running it under cool running water.
2. Remove the suppository from its wrapping.
3. Dip the suppository for a few seconds in lukewarm water to soften the exterior.
4. Lie on your left side with knees bent or in the knee-to-chest position (see drawings A and B). Position A is best for self-administration of a suppository. Small children can be held in a crawling position.
5. Relax the buttock just before inserting the suppository to ease insertion. Gently insert the tapered end of the suppository high into the rectum. If the suppository slips out, it was not inserted past the anal sphincter (the muscle that keeps the rectum closed).
6. Continue to lie down for a few minutes and hold the buttocks together to allow the suppository to dissolve in the rectum. The parent/caregiver may have to gently hold a child's buttocks closed.
7. Remember that the medication is most effective when the bowel is empty. Try to avoid a bowel movement after insertion of the suppository for up to 1 hour so that the intended action can occur.

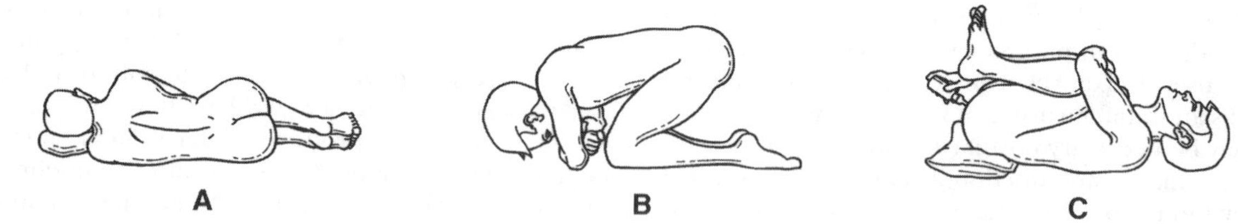


is probably too fast. One pint (500 mL) or less of properly introduced fluid usually produces adequate evacuation if it is retained until definite lower abdominal cramping is felt. As long as 1 hour may be needed for the entire procedure.

Suppositories Bisacodyl-containing suppositories are promoted as replacements for enemas when the distal colon requires cleaning. Suppositories that contain bisacodyl are used for postoperative, antepartum, and postpartum care, and are adequate in preparing for proctosigmoidoscopy. Although bisacodyl suppositories are prescribed and are used more often than other suppositories, some clinicians still prefer enemas as agents for cleaning the lower bowel. Glycerin suppositories are useful in initiating the defecation reflex in children and in promoting rectal emptying in adults (Table 16-6).

Liquids Liquid formulations of emollients may be made more palatable if mixed with juices or milk. The most commonly used products containing castor oil are the more palatable emulsions. When plain castor oil is used, it may be administered with fruit juice or a carbonated beverage to mask its unpleasant taste. Chilling the oral form of a sodium phosphate–type product or taking it with ice seems to make it more palatable. Palatability may also be improved by drinking the product with a citrus fruit juice or with a citrus-flavored carbonated beverage.

### *Complementary Therapies*

Patients frequently treat constipation with a botanical product (Table 16-7; see also Chapter 53).[20,32,45-48] Although many of the commercially available stimulant and bulk-forming laxatives are derived from plants, some consumers prefer to use a "more natural" version of these products. Consumers should be cautioned that FDA does not regulate these products and the manufacturers are not required to provide information on how to use the products safely and effectively. When FDA ruled that certain stimulant laxative ingredients found in many nonprescription products had not been shown to be safe or effective, they were ordered removed from the marketplace.[33] Nonprescription products that contained aloe, cascara sagrada, and casanthranol have been withdrawn from the market because of a lack of data supporting their safety and efficacy. However, the same ingredients are found in many dietary supplement formulations, which are unaffected by this ruling. Patients should consider alternative products that do not contain these ingredients whenever possible.

Although botanical products are considered dietary substances and not "medications," they can potentially interact with prescription medications. In addition, products

**TABLE 16-7 Selected Botanicals That May Act as Laxatives or Cathartics**

| Herb (Scientific Name) | Risks | Effectiveness in Constipation |
|---|---|---|
| Aloe (*Aloe vera*) | Use not recommended; FDA has classified OTC products containing aloe as generally not safe | FDA-classified as not generally effective; OTC products containing aloe have been removed from the market |
| Buckthorn (*Rhamnus catharticus*) | Significant adverse effects with chronic use or abuse, including abdominal pain, anxiety, decreased respirations, trembling, vomiting, and excessive diarrhea; contraindicated in children younger than 12 years, or during pregnancy or lactation | Harsh cathartic laxative that stimulates contraction of large intestine; contains anthraquinones, which are known to produce laxative effects; effectiveness appears to be dose related |
| Flaxseed (*Linum usitatissimum*) | Generally regarded as safe when taken orally; no known specific adverse reactions | Bulk-forming product used for chronic constipation; insufficient effectiveness data available |
| Licorice (*Glycyrrhiza glabra*) | Contraindicated during pregnancy or lactation, or in patients with renal or liver disease; significant drug interactions with warfarin, antiplatelets, digoxin, MAOIs | Mild laxative effect suggested, but limited research exists on use as a laxative |
| Plantago ovata seed (*Psyllium seed*) | See Chapter 53 | |
| Plant gums (*Sterculia*) | See Chapter 53 | |
| Plant seed mucilage (*Ispaghula*) | See Chapter 53 | |
| Rhubarb (*Rheum palmatum*) | Prolonged use not recommended; use during pregnancy not recommended; should be used only on the advice of PCP because of potential toxicity | Strong stimulant laxative properties; effectiveness appears to be dose related, but not sufficiently proven |
| Senna leaves (*Cassia* sp.) | Safe for short-term use; laxative dependence possible with prolonged use; medical supervision recommended in children, or during pregnancy or lactation | Stimulant laxative for constipation and as an adjunct to evacuation for diagnostic tests of the GI tract; short-term oral use generally recognized as effective |

Key: MAOI, monoamine oxidase inhibitor; OTC, over-the-counter; PCP, primary care provider.

can vary in quality, quantity, and dosage of active ingredients. Thus, users may experience inconsistent therapeutic effects or toxicity. A number of entities are offered for sale in the marketplace without sufficient evidence to support their use.[49] Among these are butternut, chicory, dandelion, dong quai, feverfew, fo-ti, manna, rhubarb, rose hips, sarsaparilla, and sunflower. Because the market is flooded with botanical products touted to relieve constipation, patients should seek out manufacturers that consistently provide quality products. They should also be cautioned against the use of botanical laxatives during pregnancy, while breastfeeding, and in children.[49] In general, patients should be encouraged to consult a primary care provider or pharmacist for advice on the safe use of these products, particularly if they are used concurrently with prescription medications.

## Assessment of Constipation: A Case-based Approach

The practitioner should obtain as much lifestyle and medical information as possible before making any recommendations for preventing or treating constipation. Appropriate information allows the practitioner to make rational recommendations based on knowledge of the patient, the problem, and the product, as well as on the practitioner's own judgment and experience. Evaluation of all drug use is critical in selecting appropriate laxatives. A patient who presents with constipation should initially be evaluated for any signs of significant gastrointestinal problems that may warrant medical evaluation, such as severe abdominal pain, nausea and vomiting, or rectal bleeding. The practitioner must recognize the situations in which laxative use is inappropriate. For example, laxatives are not recommended to treat constipation associated with intestinal pathology or secondary to laxative abuse unless bowel retraining has been successful. Laxatives also are not a cure for functional constipation and, therefore, are of only secondary importance in treating this condition. Attention should be directed first to questions relating to diet, fluid intake, physical activity, and any underlying pathology that may be producing constipation as a symptom.

Patients should then be questioned regarding the characteristics of bowel movements including the size, color, and texture of stools as well as the frequency of elimination. Additional assessment should include questions about use of medications, both prescription and nonprescription, as well as previous laxative use. Adequate patient assessment is essential to effective management of constipation. For older patients without a history of constipation, a thorough investigation should be conducted to determine whether acute cases of constipation have resulted from new or old diseases or from the use of medications. When information is insufficient to assess the cause of the symptoms or any doubt exists regarding the patient's disease status, medical referral is appropriate. Cases 16-1 and 16-2 give examples of the assessment of patients with constipation.

## Patient Counseling for Constipation

Because laxative products are both widely used and abused, clinicians can provide a valuable service by educating patients about the appropriate use of laxatives. Proper education about laxative products and wise advice on product selection and use are particularly crucial for children and older patients. Before recommending a laxative product, the clinician should first discuss the nondrug measures for treating constipation. Pregnant women and children, especially, should be counseled on proper diet, adequate fluid intake, and reasonable exercise. Individuals may not understand the importance of these factors in the development of constipation and how simple lifestyle changes can restore relatively normal bowel function without laxative use. If a laxative is needed, the health care provider should explain why a particular type of laxative is appropriate for the present situation, how to use the laxative, when to expect to see results, what adverse effects could occur, and what precautions to take. The box Patient Education for Constipation lists specific information to provide patients.

### CASE 16-1

| Relevant Evaluation Criteria | Scenario/Model Outcome |
|---|---|
| **Information Gathering** | |
| 1. Gather essential information about the patient's symptoms, including: | |
| a. description of symptom(s) (i.e., nature, onset, duration, severity, associated symptoms) | Patient indicates that she has experienced several bouts of constipation over the past 3 months since having her third child. During her periods of constipation, her stools have been difficult to pass. |
| b. description of any factors that seem to precipitate, exacerbate, and/or relieve the patient's symptom(s) | She has had problems with constipation in the past during her pregnancies. She cannot point to anything in particular associated with this series of occurrences. |
| c. description of the patient's efforts to relieve the symptoms | Patient has added more fresh fruit and vegetables to her diet during the past month with no discernible change. Her sister always drinks licorice tea to remain "regular," and she would like to try some because it is a "more natural" approach than drugs. |
| 2. Gather essential patient history information: | |
| a. patient's identity | Carlota |
| b. age, sex, height, and weight | 38 y/o F, 5'3", 135 lb |
| c. patient's occupation | Home-based financial services consultant |
| d. patient's dietary habits | Usual diet emphasizes grain and legumes. |
| e. patient's sleep habits | Naps during the day when the children are napping; sleeps about 6-7 hours nightly |
| f. concurrent medical conditions, prescription and nonprescription medications, and dietary supplements | Vitron-C 1 tablet once daily with lunch; history of IDA |
| g. allergies | NKA |
| h. history of other adverse reactions to medications | None |
| i. other (describe)______ | Pregnant in her third trimester |
| **Assessment and Triage** | |
| 3. Differentiate the patient's signs/symptoms and correctly identify the patient's primary problem(s). | Constipation during pregnancy and immediately after delivery is common. While her constipation may be associated with pregnancy, it could be related to her use of iron supplements or perhaps her expresso drinking. |
| 4. Identify exclusions for self-treatment (see Figure 16-2). | Symptoms have recurred over a period of at least 3 months and after dietary changes. |

## CASE 16-1 (continued)

| Relevant Evaluation Criteria | Scenario/Model Outcome |
|---|---|
| 5. Formulate a comprehensive list of therapeutic alternatives for the primary problem to determine if triage to a medical practitioner is required, and share this information with the patient. | Options include:<br>(1) Recommend new self-treatment with a stool softener or a bulk-forming agent or endorse Carlota's use of licorice tea.<br>(2) Recommend further lifestyle modifications: decreased coffee consumption and increased exercise.<br>(3) Refer Carlota to her PCP provider for evaluation.<br>(4) Take no action. |
| **Plan** | |
| 6. Select an optimal therapeutic alternative to address the patient's problem, taking into account patient preferences. | Carlota has had problems with constipation during prior pregnancies. Although the new occurrences are substantially beyond the time of her successful delivery, consideration must be given to whether a relationship exists. Carlota does use iron supplementation for IDA. There does not appear to be evidence of overuse of iron, but she might be especially sensitive to its constipating effect. Her routine intake of strong coffee (presumed to be caffeinated) may leave her somewhat dehydrated. However, the most powerful evidence might be her mention that constipation has been present off and on over a 3-month period of time. This extended experience coupled with her unsuccessful attempts at self-treatment suggest a referral is appropriate. |
| 7. Describe the recommended therapeutic approach to the patient. | You should continue your intake of fresh fruit and vegetables and dietary fiber but decrease consumption of expresso. Furthermore, you should obtain an appointment with your PCP, that is, primary care provider. |
| 8. Explain to the patient the rationale for selecting the recommended therapeutic approach from the considered therapeutic alternatives. | While the coffee consumption may be a minor contributor to the constipation episodes, the length of time over which they have occurred after delivery warrants medical evaluation. |
| **Patient Education** | |
| 9. When recommending self-care with nonprescription medications and/or nondrug therapy, convey accurate information to the patient, including: | |
| a. appropriate dose and frequency of administration | N/A |
| b. maximum number of days the therapy should be employed | N/A |
| c. product administration procedures | N/A |
| d. expected time to onset of relief | N/A |
| e. degree of relief that can be reasonably expected | The reduced coffee consumption might provide some relief, but may not be enough to resolve the current problem. |
| f. most common side effects | N/A |
| g. side effects that warrant medical intervention should they occur | N/A |
| h. patient options in the event that condition worsens or persists | If constipation worsens before your appointment, contact your PCP directly. |
| i. product storage requirements | N/A |
| j. specific nondrug measures | You must drink adequate fluid and continue to eat a diet rich in fruit, vegetables, whole grains, and legumes. |
| 10. Solicit follow-up questions from patient. | Should I take less iron until my constipation improves? |
| 11. Answer patient's questions. | No. Your PCP will evaluate your continued need for iron. |

Key: IDA, iron deficiency anemia; NKA, no known allergies; PCP, primary care provider.

## CASE 16-2

| Relevant Evaluation Criteria | Scenario/Model Outcome |
|---|---|
| **Information Gathering** | |
| 1. Gather essential information about the patient's symptoms, including: | |
| a. description of symptom(s) (i.e., nature, onset, duration, severity, associated symptoms) | Patient reports that he has had only one small bowel movement in 7 days. He also reports having had one or two similar episodes over the past year. Additionally, he reports having soiled underpants 2 days ago. |
| b. description of any factors that seem to precipitate, exacerbate, and/or relieve the patient's symptom(s) | Patient is unable to relate his symptoms to any recent event or activity. |
| c. description of the patient's efforts to relieve the symptoms | Although he tried to obtain relief by a recent purchase of an OTC sleep aid (diphenhydramine), he discovered that more sleep did not help him, so he stopped the medication after 2 nights use 2 days ago. He also reports on the day he began the sleep medicine, he ate 2 bowls of bran flakes for breakfast hoping that would help. |
| 2. Gather essential patient history information: | |
| a. patient's identity | Hobart |
| b. age, sex, height, and weight | 69 y/o M, 5'8", 205 lb |
| c. patient's occupation | Retired house painter |
| d. patient's dietary habits | Some fresh tropical fruit, occasional canned vegetables, but mostly meat-containing meals. Fluid intake consists principally of cola-type soft drinks and black tea. He admits to drinking very little water. |
| e. patient's sleep habits | Usually goes to bed late (watches television), but gets up around 6 AM every morning |
| f. concurrent medical conditions, prescription and nonprescription medications, and dietary supplements | Verapamil 240 mg sustained-release 1 capsule every morning, HTN for 7 years; HCTZ 25 mg 2 times/day for HTN for past 4 months; indomethacin 50 mg 3 times/day as needed for gouty arthritis for 2 years; pravastatin 10 mg 2 times/day for hyperlipidemia for 1 year |
| g. allergies | NKA |
| h. history of other adverse reactions to medications | None |
| i. other (describe)_______ | Hobart cannot remember being constipated as an adult prior to these recent episodes. He usually has a bowel movement every other day. When he was an adolescent, his mother would prepare a tea for him to drink if he became constipated. Recently, he stays around the house because he doesn't "feel much like doing anything." |
| **Assessment and Triage** | |
| 3. Differentiate the patient's signs/symptoms and correctly identify the patient's primary problem(s). | Hobart appears to be experiencing acute constipation that may have its roots in advancing age, reduced physical activity, a diet that seems low in fiber but high in protein, low fluid intake, and a constipating drug regimen. Additionally, his bran flakes breakfast, deficient fluid intake coupled with his complaint of soiling might suggest a developing fecal impaction. |
| 4. Identify exclusions for self-treatment (see Figure 16-2). | None |
| 5. Formulate a comprehensive list of therapeutic alternatives for the primary problem to determine if triage to a medical practitioner is required, and share this information with the patient. | Options include:<br>(1) Recommend self-care for constipation using lifestyle modifications and a stool softener.<br>(2) Call Hobart's PCP to discuss the impact of the constipation-inducing medication regimen, the possibility of impaction, and the potential use of an oil retention enema.<br>(3) Refer Hobart to his PCP for further evaluation.<br>(4) Take no action. |

## CASE 16-2 (continued)

| Relevant Evaluation Criteria | Scenario/Model Outcome |
|---|---|
| **Plan** | |
| 6. Select an optimal therapeutic alternative to address the patient's problem, taking into account patient preferences. | The best approach may involve a number of measures. First, recommend lifestyle changes, including an increase in exercise, a diet containing more fiber and less meat, and adequate fluid intake. Then, call the PCP to discuss Hobart's symptomatology. Where appropriate, offer alternative therapeutic agents that are less likely to induce constipation. Since the possibility exists that the patient may be developing an impaction, the patient's recent actions and symptoms should be discussed with the PCP. The potential use of a stool softener or an oil retention enema to resolve the current episode may need to be addressed. Subsequent to lessening the effect of constipating drugs and resolving the question of impaction, monitor Hobart for improvement. If Hobart has need of laxative therapy beyond successfully addressing these issues, a short-term resolution might employ bisacodyl (see Table 16-4). |
| 7. Describe the recommended therapeutic approach to the patient. | I will contact your PCP, that is, primary care provider, to discuss what changes can be made in your prescribed therapy. This will help determine the kind of additional medication needed to treat your constipation. Your breakfast of bran flakes along with your limited water consumption and your mention of underpants soiling compel me to speak with your PCP about the possibility of a developing stool blockage in your rectum. You may need to make an office visit for further examination pending our discussion. Lifestyle modifications will produce gradual improvement in the severity of your symptoms and may be curative particularly if the drug-induced concerns are resolved. In the short term beyond this current episode, bisacodyl may be appropriate for you, should a future need arise. |
| 8. Explain to the patient the rationale for selecting the recommended therapeutic approach from the considered therapeutic alternatives. | Drug-induced problems appear to be the main reason for your constipation. Lifestyle issues also contribute to the current problem. |
| **Patient Education** | |
| 9. When recommending self-care with nonprescription medications and/or nondrug therapy, convey accurate information to the patient, including: | |
| a. appropriate dose and frequency of administration | See Tables 16-4 and 16-5. |
| b. maximum number of days the therapy should be employed | Do not take this product for more than 1 week. |
| c. product administration procedures | Take each dose with a full glass of water. |
| d. expected time to onset of relief | See Table 16-4. |
| e. degree of relief that can be reasonably expected | You should expect to have a bowel movement and associated relief with this measure. Institution of the lifestyle changes should lead to long-term relief. |
| f. most common side effects | Upset stomach, nausea, diarrhea, and gas |
| g. side effects that warrant medical intervention should they occur | Confusion, irregular heartbeat, and muscle cramps |
| h. patient options in the event that condition worsens or persists | You should consult your PCP. |
| i. product storage requirements | Store bisacodyl at room temperature away from moisture and heat. |
| j. specific nondrug measures | Increasing dietary fiber through better meal choices will greatly assist in maintaining long-term bowel function. You must also maintain adequate fluid intake and exercise more frequently. |
| 10. Solicit follow-up questions from patient. | What happens if I take an overdose? |

## CASE 16-2 (continued)

| Relevant Evaluation Criteria | Scenario/Model Outcome |
|---|---|
| 11. Answer patient's questions. | You could experience mental confusion, erratic heartbeats, and severe muscle cramping. Seek emergency medical attention immediately. |

Key: HCTZ, hydrochlorothiazide; HTN, hypertension; NKA, no known allergies; OTC, over-the-counter; PCP, primary care provider.

## PATIENT EDUCATION FOR CONSTIPATION

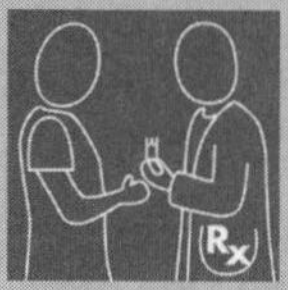


The objectives of self-treatment are to relieve constipation and restore "normal" bowel functioning by implementing (1) dietary and lifestyle measures and/or (2) the safe use of laxative products. For most patients, carefully following the product instructions and the self-care measures listed here will help ensure optimal therapeutic outcomes.

### Nondrug Measures

- Use natural methods such as a high-fiber diet, adequate fluid intake, and exercise to foster regular bowel movements.
- Increase dietary fiber by eating foods containing wheat grains, oats, fruits, and vegetables.
- Avoid constipating foods such as processed cheeses and concentrated sweets.
- Drink plenty of fluids (eight or more 8-oz glasses a day) to aid in stool softening and to facilitate fecal evacuation.
- Develop and maintain a routine exercise program. Walking can be beneficial if your cardiovascular system is healthy and if you have no other apparent health risks.
- Establish a regular pattern for bathroom visits. Do not delay responding to the urge to defecate; allow adequate time for elimination in a relaxed, unhurried atmosphere.
- Maintain general emotional well-being and avoid stressful situations.

### Nonprescription Medications

- Do not routinely take laxatives if your bowel habits are interrupted for a day or two, or to routinely "clean your system."
- Do not give laxatives to children younger than 6 years unless recommended by a primary care provider.
- If you have kidney or liver disease, heart failure, hypertension, or other conditions requiring sodium, potassium, magnesium, or calcium restriction, do not use laxative products whose maximum daily dose contains more than 345 mg (15 mEq) of sodium, 975 mg (25 mEq) of potassium, 600 mg (50 mEq) of magnesium, or 1800 mg (90 mEq) of calcium.
- Consult your primary care provider before using laxatives if you currently have or have a history of any of the following conditions: colectomy, ileostomy, diabetes, heart disease, kidney disease, or swallowing difficulties.
- Consult a primary care provider or pharmacist before using a laxative product if you are taking anticoagulants (blood thinners), digoxin (a heart medicine), sodium polystyrene sulfonate (a treatment for high potassium levels), or tetracycline antibiotics.
- Avoid taking laxatives within 2 hours of taking other medications.
- Do not take laxatives longer than 1 week. Consult a primary care provider if symptoms of constipation persist.
- Take most laxatives at bedtime, especially if more than 6 to 8 hours are required to produce results.
- Discard any medications that are outdated, that appear to have been tampered with, or that have an unusual appearance.

#### *Bulk-forming Laxatives*

- Unless a rapid effect, such as cleaning out the bowel for a diagnostic procedure or X-ray, is needed, take a bulk-forming laxative. Be sure to drink at least 8 oz of fluid with each dose to prevent intestinal obstruction.
- Use bulk-forming agents with caution if you have diabetes or are on a carbohydrate-restricted diet. These agents have a high caloric content per dose and contain sugar.
- Do not give sugar-free bulk-forming products to patients with phenylketonuria. Such products may contain aspartame, which contributes excessive levels of phenylalanine, an amino acid these patients cannot metabolize.

#### *Lubricants*

- Do not give mineral oil to children younger than 6 years of age, pregnant patients, older patients, or patients taking anticoagulants.
- Do not take mineral oil with emollient laxatives.
- To avoid delaying the absorption of foods, nutrients, and vitamins, do not take mineral oil within 2 hours of eating.

#### *Saline Laxatives*

- Take saline laxatives on an empty stomach; the presence of food will delay action.
- Do not take saline laxatives every day.
- Do not give these laxatives orally to children younger than 6 years of age or rectally to infants younger than 2 years of age.

#### *Stimulants*

- Do not use castor oil to treat constipation except under the advice of a primary care provider.

⚠ Do not take laxatives if you have any symptoms of appendicitis (i.e., abdominal pain, nausea, vomiting), rectal bleeding, painful anal or rectal conditions, bloating, or cramping. See a primary care provider immediately.

⚠ If symptoms are unrelieved by nondrug measures or by 1 week of laxative treatment, see a primary care provider. Chronic constipation may be a symptom of an underlying medical condition.

## Evaluation of Patient Outcomes for Constipation

Constipation often presents with a great degree of variability among individuals. Although a decrease in frequency of bowel movements is typically associated with constipation, difficulty in passing stools and a decrease in the amount passed are also common complaints. The type, severity, and chronicity of symptoms are important determinants in selecting the most appropriate treatment modality. Once therapy has been selected, effectiveness is determined by how rapidly constipation is relieved and to what degree normal bowel habits have been restored. For acute constipation, dietary changes and exercise or the use of bulk-forming laxatives may take several days to weeks to provide relief. Stimulant laxatives usually provide results within 24 hours; osmotic laxatives provide more immediate relief, usually within 15 minutes to 3 hours for oral preparations. Laxative enemas, often used when fecal impaction accompanies constipation, can produce evacuation within minutes. If initial treatment is ineffective, therapy should be repeated according to product-specific directions. If an adequate response is not achieved after a short period of time, usually within 1 week, chronic constipation should be considered. Follow-up should be attempted to assess whether the patient should receive further evaluation by a primary care provider.

Self-medication with laxatives can be safe and effective if used as directed and not excessively. Close monitoring of the frequency and duration of laxative use can be beneficial in determining whether normal bowel habits are actually reestablished between bouts of constipation or if a more severe condition exists. If a laxative must be continued for an extended period such as in chronic constipation, bulk-forming agents are preferred. However, the need for frequent laxative use should be discussed with a primary care provider, because this may be a sign of (1) a more severe form of constipation, (2) a side effect of a medication, or (3) an underlying medical problem. Overuse or extended use of some laxatives can alter the normal physiologic functioning of the gut and, in some persons, may lead to a dependence on laxatives for bowel function. Adhering to a diet high in fiber and drinking plenty of fluids can aid in preventing constipation and should be continued even during periods when bowel habits are normal.

Any signs of appendicitis, blood in the stool, severe abdominal pain, nausea and vomiting, or hypersensitivity reactions that occur during the course of treatment should be reported immediately to a primary care provider. An increase in dietary fiber or use of a bulk-forming laxative may cause an increase in flatulence or bloating that typically resolves after several days of continuous use and that is not usually a cause for concern.

## Key Points for Constipation

- Constipation is a decrease in frequency of fecal elimination characterized by the difficult passage of hard, dry stool.
- Successful treatment of constipation depends on careful identification of the cause.
- In determining whether self-treatment or medical referral is appropriate, the clinician also needs to know the case history and current symptoms as well as the patient's reason for desiring to purchase a laxative.
- If the case history discloses a sudden change in bowel habits that has persisted for 2 weeks, the patient should be immediately referred to a primary care provider.
- For most cases of simple constipation, proper diet, exercise, and adequate fluid intake should be helpful.
- In addition, patients should always be encouraged to establish a regular pattern for bathroom visits and never delay responding to the urge to defecate.
- Special circumstances and patient characteristics (i.e., pregnancy, age) should be considered when assessing the need for self-medication.
- Therapy with any laxative product should be limited, in most cases, to short-term use.
- Laxative treatment for constipation should not be recommended if the patient exhibits symptoms of appendicitis (i.e., abdominal pain, nausea, vomiting) rectal bleeding, painful anal or rectal conditions, bloating, or cramping.
- Patients should be advised to avoid taking laxatives within 2 hours of other medications to reduce the potential for drug interactions.
- The cost of laxative products is variable; however, concomitant use of nonpharmacologic measures may lead to lower cost of laxative products for the patient with simple constipation.

## References


1. Lembo A, Camilleri M. Chronic constipation. *N Engl J Med.* 2003; 349:1360-8.
2. Levy S. Drug outlets remain leader in laxative sales. *Drug Topics.* 2002;146:8.
3. Talley NJ. Definitions, epidemiology, and impact of chronic constipation. *Rev Gastroenterol Disord.* 2004;4(suppl 2):S3-S10.
4. Bossard W, Dreher R, Schnegg JF, et al. The treatment of chronic constipation in elderly people: an update. *Drugs Aging.* 2004;21: 911-30.
5. Locke GR III, Pemberton JH, Phillips SF. AGA medical position statement: guideline on constipation. *Gastroenterology.* 2000;119: 1761-6.
6. DeLillo AR, Rose S. Functional bowel disorders in the geriatric patient: constipation, fecal impaction and fecal incontinence. *Am J Gastroenterol.* 2000;95:901-5.
7. Lennard-Jones JE. Constipation. In: Feldman M, Scharschmidt BF, Sleisenger MH, eds. *Sleisenger & Fordtran's Gastrointestinal and Liver Disease: Pathophysiology, Diagnosis, Management.* 7th ed. Philadelphia: Elsevier Science; 2002:181-207.
8. Spruill WJ, Wade WE. Diarrhea, constipation, and irritable bowel syndrome. In: DiPiro JT, Talbert RL, Yee GC, et al., eds. *Pharmacotherapy: A Pathophysiologic Approach.* 6th ed. New York: McGraw-Hill, Inc; 2005:677-92.
9. Prather CM, Ortiz-Camacho CP. Evaluation and treatment of constipation and fecal impaction in adults. *Mayo Clin Proc.* 1998; 73:881-7.
10. Herndon CM, Jackson KC, Hallin PA. Management of opioid-induced gastrointestinal effects in patients receiving palliative care. *Pharmacotherapy.* 2002;22:240-50.

11. Muller-Lissner SA, Kamm MA, Scarpignato C, et al. Myths and misconceptions about chronic constipation. *Am J Gastroenterol.* 2005;100:232-42.
12. Baker SS, Liptak GS, Colletti RB, et al. Constipation in infants and children: evaluation and treatment. *J Pediatr Gastroenterol Nutr.* 2000;30:109.
13. Constipation. National Digestive Diseases Information Clearinghouse. June 2003. Available at: http://digestive.niddk.nih.gov/ddiseases/pubs/constipation/index.htm. Accessed February 26, 2005.
14. Bonapace ES Jr, Fisher RS. Constipation and diarrhea in pregnancy. *Gastroenterol Clin North Am.* 1998;27:197-211.
15. Riely CA, Davila R. Pregnancy-related Hepatic and Gastrointestinal Disorders. In: Feldman M, Scharschmidt BF, Sleisenger MH, eds. *Sleisenger & Fordtran's Gastrointestinal and Liver Disease: Pathophysiology, Diagnosis, Management.* 7th ed. Philadelphia: Elsevier Science; 2002:1457.
16. Locke GR III, Pemberton JH, Phillips SF. AGA technical review on constipation. *Gastroenterology.* 2000;119:1766-78.
17. Felt B, Wise CG, Olson A, et al. Guideline for the management of pediatric idiopathic constipation and soiling. *Arch Pediatr Adolesc Med.* 1999;153:380-5.
18. Murphy SM. Constipation. In: Walker WA, Durie PR, Hamilton JR, et al., eds. *Pediatric Gastrointestinal Disease: Pathophysiology, Diagnosis, Management.* 2nd ed. St. Louis: Mosby-Year Book; 1996: 293-321.
19. Berardi RR. Clinical update on the treatment of constipation in adults. *Pharmacy Times.* 2004;70(9):99-108.
20. Self-care for constipation. In: Albrant DH, ed. *The American Pharmaceutical Association Drug Treatment Protocols.* Washington, DC: American Pharmaceutical Association; 1999.
21. Marlett JA, McBurney MI, Slavin JL. Position of the American Dietetic Association: health implications of dietary fiber. *J Am Diet Assoc.* 2002;102:993-1000.
22. Nutritive Value of Food. USDA Agricultural Research Service *Home and Garden Bulletin.* 2002;72:20-95.
23. Schiller LR. Review article: the therapy of constipation. *Aliment Pharmacol Ther.* 2001;15:749-61.
24. Buff S. Atkins Nutritionals: How to Do Atkins: Overcoming Obstacles: Coping with constipation. Available at: http://atkins.com/Archive/2003/4/9-571070.html. Accessed February 27, 2005.
25. Patrick PG, Gohman SM, Marx SC et al. Effect of supplements of partially hydrolyzed guar gum on the occurrence of constipation and use of laxative agents. *J Am Diet Assoc.* 1998;98:912-4.
26. Laxative drug products for over-the-counter human use; proposed amendment to the tentative final monograph. *Federal Register.* 2003;68:46133-8.
27. Khalili B, Bardana EJ, Yunginger JW. Psyllium-associated anaphylaxis and death: a case report review of the literature. *Ann Allergy, Asthma, Immunol.* 2003;91:579-84.
28. National Institutes of Health. Optimal calcium intake [abstract]. Bethesda, Md: National Institutes of Health Consensus Development Conference Statement; September 1994.
29. Romero Y, Evans JM, Flemming FC, et al. Constipation and fecal incontinence in the elderly population. *Mayo Clin Proc.* 1996;71: 81-92.
30. Knobel B, Petechenko P. Hyperphosphatemic hypocalcemic coma caused by hypertonic sodium phosphate (fleet) enema intoxication. *J Clin Gastroenterol.* 1996;23:217-9.
31. Oral sodium phosphate laxative package limitations proffered again. *The Tan Sheet.* 2001;9:8.
32. Drug labeling: sodium labeling for over-the-counter drugs. *Federal Register.* 2004;69:69278-80.
33. Status of certain additional over-the-counter drug category II and III active ingredients. *Federal Register.* 2002;67:31125-7.
34. Laxative drug products for over-the-counter human use. Federal *Register.* 1999;64:4535-40.
35. Wald A. Is chronic use of stimulant laxatives harmful to the colon? *J Clin Gastro.* 2003;36:386-9.
36. Kovacs D. The associations between laxative abuse and other symptoms among adults with anorexia nervosa. *Int J Eat Disord.* 2004;36:224-8.
37. Denke MA. Anorexia nervosa, bulimia nervosa and obesity. In: Feldman M, Scharschmidt BF, Sleisenger MH, eds. *Sleisenger & Fordtran's Gastrointestinal and Liver Disease: Pathophysiology, Diagnosis, Management.* 7th ed. Philadelphia: Elsevier Science; 2002:310-36.
38. Favaro A, Santonastaso P. Self-injurious behavior in anorexia nervosa. *J Nerv Ment Dis.* 2000;188:537-42.
39. Powell DW. Approach to the patient with diarrhea. In: Goldman L, Bennett JC, eds. *Cecil Textbook of Medicine.* 21st ed. Philadelphia: WB Saunders; 2000.
40. Stolk LM, Hoogtanders K. Detection of laxative abuse by urine analysis with HPLC and diode array detection. *Pharm World Sci.* 1999;21:40-3.
41. McRorie JW, Daggy BP, Morel JG, et al. Psyllium is superior to docusate sodium for treatment of chronic constipation. Aliment *Pharmacol Ther.* 1998;12:491-7.
42. Wald A. Constipation. *Med Clin* North *Am.* 2000;84:1231-46.
43. Schaefer DC, Cheskin LJ. Constipation in the elderly. *Am Fam Physician.* 1998;58:7.
44. Briggs GG, Freeman RK, Yaffe SJ. *Drugs in Pregnancy and Lactation.* 6th ed. Baltimore: Williams & Wilkins; 2001.
45. Tyler VE, Foster S. *Tyler's Honest Herbal: A Sensible Guide to the Use of Herbs and Related Remedies.* 4th ed. New York: The Haworth Herbal Press; 1999:28, 115, 137, 141, 163, 233, 319, 335, 391.
46. *PDR for Herbal Medicines.* 2nd ed. Montvale, NJ: Medical Economics Company; 2000.
47. Blumenthal M. The Complete German Commission E Monographs: Therapeutic Guide to Herbal Medicine. Austin, Tex: American Botanical Council; 1998.
48. Gehrmann B, Koch WG, Tschirch CO et al. *Medicinal Herbs: A Compendium.* New York: The Haworth Herbal Press; 2005.

CHAPTER 17

# Diarrhea

*Paul C. Walker*

Diarrhea is a symptom characterized by an abnormal increase in stool frequency or liquidity. The normal frequency of bowel movements varies with each individual. Some healthy adults have as many as three well-formed stools a day, whereas others defecate only once every 2 or more days. More than three bowel movements per day are considered abnormal. Diarrhea may also be defined in terms of daily stool weight. The mean daily fecal weight loss is 100 to 150 g; an increase in stool weight above 200 g is interpreted as diarrhea. However, neither of these criteria should be stringently applied because some individuals, such as vegetarians and others who consume a fiber-rich diet, may produce daily stools of normal consistency that weigh more than 300 g.

Diarrhea may be acute, persistent, or chronic in nature. Acute diarrhea, defined as an episode of less than 14 days duration, can generally be managed with fluid/electrolyte replacement, dietary interventions, and nonprescription drug treatment. Persistent diarrhea is diarrhea of 14 days to 4 weeks duration. Chronic diarrhea, by definition, lasts more than 4 weeks. Chronic and persistent diarrheal illnesses need medical care and, therefore, are outside the scope of this book.

## Epidemiology of Diarrhea

Diarrhea is a common cause of morbidity. Between 200 million and 211 million episodes of diarrheal illness (diarrhea lasting more than 1 day or that impairs normal activities) occur in the United States annually.[1,2] The overall prevalence of acute gastroenteritis is estimated to be 11% of the general population, which results in an incidence rate ranging from 0.75 to 1.4 episodes per person per year. The prevalence of diarrheal disease is highest in children younger than 5 years and lowest in people 65 years of age and older; prevalence rates are estimated to be 10% for young children and 3% for persons of advanced age.[2] Most patients experience illness without seeking medical attention; however, approximately 774,000 cases result in hospitalization. Each year, acute gastroenteritis and its complications account for approximately 8200 deaths in the United States.[3] Risk factors for specific types of diarrheas are discussed in the Etiology section.

## Anatomy and Physiology of Small Intestine and Colon

The primary functions of the small intestine are digestion and absorption. Normally, about 9 L of digestive fluid enter the gastrointestinal (GI) tract daily. Most of this volume is absorbed; only about 150 mL are excreted in the stool each day.

Stool is approximately 75% water and 25% solid material; it contains unabsorbed food residue and minerals, bacteria, desquamated epithelial cells, and a small quantity of electrolytes. On average, a liter of stool contains 90 mEq potassium, 40 mEq sodium, 30 mEq bicarbonate, and 15 mEq chloride.

Colonic microorganisms produce enzymes needed to degrade waste products, synthesize certain vitamins, and generate ammonia. *Bacteroides* species and *Lactobacillus* species make up much of the bacterial flora although Enterobacteriaceae (e.g., *Escherichia coli*), enterococci, *Clostridium* species, and yeasts may comprise a small portion of the normal flora. Many factors, such as diet, intestinal pH, coexisting disease, and drugs, may influence the relative proportion of these organisms. If potential pathogens are allowed to overgrow or their normal balance is disrupted, serious symptoms and complications, including moderate to severe diarrhea, may result.

The functional organization of the intestinal mucosa is important to the absorption of substances from the GI tract. The luminal surface of the small intestine is covered by villi, which are numerous, minute, fingerlike projections that increase the absorptive surface area of the small intestine. The tips of the villi are lined by mature epithelial cells whose primary function is absorption of nutrients and electrolytes. In contrast to the small intestine, the colon is not lined with villi.

The plasma membranes of the epithelial cells that line the GI tract are impermeable to water; however, the cells are joined together by "tight junctions" that allow water to be absorbed between the cells. The paracellular spaces formed by these tight junctions serve as semipermeable membranes through which water is absorbed. Permeability of the paracellular spaces decreases from the base of the villus to its tip. Permeability also decreases along the length of the intestines; the colon is markedly less permeable to water than the proximal small intestine.

A balance between absorption and secretion is maintained during normal functioning of the small intestine and colon. Water absorption is passive and depends on the absorption of electrolytes and selected solutes (i.e., sodium, chloride, glucose, small peptides, and amino acids). As these substances are absorbed, water accompanies their movement to maintain an isotonic state. Generally, 1 L of water is absorbed with about 150 mEq of sodium chloride. Secretory mechanisms are also at work balancing isoosmotic pressure.

The enteric nervous system, a unique collection of intrinsic neurons located within the GI tract, controls and integrates the endocrine and exocrine functions, motility, and microcirculation of the GI tract. Various intracellular and extracellular regulators of the enteric nervous system (hormones, neurotransmitters, inflammatory mediators) modify the normal functioning of intestinal ion-transport processes, and thus can influence water and electrolyte absorption. More than 20 putative chemical mediators of the enteric nervous system have been identified (including vasoactive intestinal peptide, calmodulin, prostaglandins, acetylcholine, and secretin) although the functions of many have not yet been clearly elucidated. Immune cells (e.g., mast cells, neutrophils) and their inflammatory mediators are also important in regulation of fluid and electrolyte absorption, in both inflammatory and noninflammatory conditions. The enteric nervous system can be activated by enteric pathogens and, not surprisingly, is implicated in pathogenesis of secretory diarrhea associated with GI bacterial and viral infections.

## Etiology of Diarrhea

The specific causes of acute diarrhea differ between developing and developed countries. In the United States, viral and foodborne diarrheal illnesses are common. However, in the majority of cases, the causes cannot be determined. In developing countries, poor sanitation and poor hygiene lead to infectious diarrhea caused by parasites, bacteria, and viruses. Bacterial causes are as common as viral infections in these countries. Table 17-1 highlights some of the common viral, bacterial, and protozoal diarrheas and their treatment.[4-8]

**TABLE 17-1 Common Infectious Diarrheas and Their Treatment**

| Type | Epidemiologic/ Etiologic Factors | Symptoms | Treatment | Usual Prognosis |
|---|---|---|---|---|
| **Viral** | | | | |
| Rotaviruses | Infects infants; oral–fecal spread | Onset of 24-48 hours; vomiting, fever, nausea, acute watery diarrhea | Vigorous fluid and electrolyte replacement; no antibiotics | Self-limiting; usually lasts 5-8 days |
| Norovirus | Infects all ages; causes cruise ship outbreaks and "24-hour stomach flu" | Onset of 24-48 hours; sudden-onset vomiting, nausea, headache, myalgia, fever, watery diarrhea | Fluid and electrolytes; no antibiotics | Self-limiting; usually lasts 12-60 hours |
| **Bacterial** | | | | |
| *Campylobacter jejuni* | Ingestion of contaminated food or water; oral-fecal spread; immunocompromised host | Onset of 24-72 hours; nausea, vomiting, headache, malaise, fever, watery diarrhea | Fluid and electrolytes; in severe or persistent diarrhea, antibiotics may be required* | Self-limiting, usually <7 days |
| *Salmonella* | Ingestion of improperly cooked or refrigerated poultry and dairy products; immunocompromised host | Onset of 12-24 hours; diarrhea, fever, and chills | Fluid and electrolytes for mild cases; antibiotics reserved for complicated cases† | Self-limiting |
| *Shigella* | Ingestion of contaminated vegetables or water; immunocompromised host | Onset of 24-48 hours; nausea, vomiting, diarrhea | Fluid and electrolytes; antibiotics | Self-limiting |
| *Escherichia coli* Enterotoxigenic *E. coli* Enteroaggregative *E. coli* | Ingestion of contaminated food or water; recent travel outside the United States or to a U.S. border area | Onset of 8-72 hours; watery diarrhea, fever, abdominal cramps, bloating, malaise, occasional vomiting | Fluid and electrolytes; antibiotics‡ | Self-limiting, usually within 3-5 days |
| *Clostridium difficile* | Antibiotic-associated diarrhea leading to pseudomembranous colitis | Onset during or up to several weeks following antibiotic therapy; watery or mucoid diarrhea, high fever, cramping | Fluid and electrolytes; discontinuation of offending agent; antibiotics (metronidazole, vancomycin, bacitracin) | Self-limiting |
| *Staphylococcus aureus* | Ingestion of improperly cooked or stored food | Onset of 1-6 hours; nausea, vomiting, watery diarrhea | Fluid and electrolytes; no antibiotics | Self-limiting |

**TABLE 17-1 Common Infectious Diarrheas and Their Treatment (continued)**

| Type | Epidemiologic/ Etiologic Factors | Symptoms | Treatment | Usual Prognosis |
|---|---|---|---|---|
| *Yersinia enterocolitica* | Ingestion of contaminated food | Onset within 16-48 hours; fever, abdominal pain, diarrhea, vomiting | Fluid and electrolytes; antibiotics may be needed in severe cases | Self-limiting although diarrhea may persist for up to 3 weeks |
| *Bacillus cereus* | Ingestion of contaminated food | Onset within 10-12 hours; abdominal pain, watery diarrhea, tenesmus, nausea, vomiting | Fluid and electrolytes; no antibiotics | Self-limiting |
| **Protozoal** | | | | |
| *Giardia lamblia* | Ingestion of water contaminated with human or animal feces; travel outside the United States; immunocompromised host | Onset of 1-3 weeks; acute or chronic watery diarrhea, nausea, vomiting, anorexia, flatulence, abdominal bloating, epigastric pain | Fluids and electrolytes; antimicrobials[§‖] | Good, if treated |
| *Cryptosporidia* | Travel outside the United States; AIDS, immunocompromised host | Onset of 2-14 days; acute or chronic watery diarrhea; abdominal pain, flatulence, malaise | Fluid and electrolytes; antimicrobial therapy[‖¶] | Self-limiting, lasting up to 3 weeks, except in patients with AIDS or other immunosuppressi ve diseases |
| *Entamoeba histolytica* | Travel outside the United States; fecal-soiled food or water, immunocompromised host | Chronic watery diarrhea, abdominal pain, cramps | Fluid and electrolytes; antibiotics[#] | Good, except for immunocompro mised host |
| *Isospora belli* | Ingestion of contaminated food or water; immunocompromised host | Onset of approximately 1 week; profuse watery diarrhea, malaise, anorexia, weight loss, and abdominal cramps | Fluid and electrolytes; antibiotics | Self-limited, remitting in 2-3 weeks |

* Empirical antibiotic therapy should be considered for patients with febrile diarrheal illness, especially if moderate to severe invasive disease is suspected, and for patients in whom supportive therapy fails to manage symptoms. Azithromycin or erythromycin (both prescription antibiotics) may be used to eradicate the organism. Ciprofloxacin has been recommended; however, it is no longer considered a first-line agent because many *Campylobacter* strains are resistant to fluoroquinolones.

† Antibiotics are not indicated routinely for *Salmonella* gastroenteritis; antibiotic therapy is used in young infants and children who fail to respond to supportive treatment, who do not spontaneously remit, or who are at increased risk of disseminated disease. Antibiotic therapy is also indicated for suspected bacteremia in patients at high risk for this complication. These include patients who appear to be toxic with high fever (>102.2°F [39°C]); infants (<3 months); older adult patients (>65 years); patients with cancer, immunodeficiency (e.g., AIDS), or hemoglobinopathy (e.g., sickle cell disease); and those receiving corticosteroids or on hemodialysis. Duration of antimicrobial therapy is usually 7 to 10 days.

‡ Antibiotic treatment with fluoroquinolones, azithromycin, or rifaximin (prescription antibiotics) is given for traveler's diarrhea caused by *E. coli*. Trimethoprim-sulfamethoxazole is no longer an optimal choice because of increasing worldwide resistance. Antibiotic treatment is not recommended for gastroenteritis caused by *E. coli* 0157:H7 because it is likely to enhance toxin release and may increase risk for hemolytic uremic syndrome.

§ No nonprescription therapy is available for giardiasis; metronidazole, nitazoxanide, quinacrine, furazolidone, and paromomycin are effective alternatives.[4,7,8]

‖ Nitazoxanide is a broad-spectrum antiparasitic agent indicated for treatment of diarrhea caused by *Cryptosporidium parvum* in children 1 to 11 years of age and by *Giardia lamblia*. It is also effective for cryptosporidiosis in immunocompetent patients and may be added if needed; safety and effectiveness have not been established in immunocompromised patients, and its use in HIV-infected patients is controversial.[4,7]

¶ Symptomatic relief of cryptosporidiosis may be achieved in AIDS patients by adding paromomycin and azithromycin to their antiretroviral therapy.[4]

# Self-treatment of amebiasis is not appropriate; metronidazole followed by either paromycin or iodoquinol is the preferred treatment.[4]

*Source:* Adapted from references 4-8.

Epidemiologic factors increasing the risk for particular infectious diarrheal diseases or their spread include attendance or employment at day care centers, occupation as a food handler or caregiver, congregate living conditions (e.g., nursing homes, prisons, multifamily dwellings), consumption of unsafe foods (e.g., raw meat, eggs, shellfish), and presence of medical conditions predisposing to infectious diarrhea.[9] Diarrhea continues to be a significant problem for patients with acquired immunodeficiency syndrome (AIDS).

Acute diarrhea may also be caused by poisoning, medications, intolerance of certain foods, or various non-GI acute or chronic illnesses.

### *Viral Gastroenteritis*

Viruses may cause up to 80% to 85% of all episodes of acute gastroenteritis in the United States.[1] Noroviruses are the most common viral pathogens, accounting for approximately 70% to 75% of viral gastroenteritis. The symptoms and clinical course are described in Table 17-1. The virus is usually transmitted by contaminated water or food. Communitywide outbreaks may result when municipal water supplies become contaminated. Recent outbreaks of norovirus gastroenteritis on cruise ships have received attention although 60% to 80% of all outbreaks occur on land.[10] Contaminated food is the most frequently identified vehicle of infection in this setting; person-to-person transmission may also be important, and it has been suggested that infected cruise ship crew members may serve as reservoirs of infection for passengers.[10]

Rotaviruses account for about 12% of all acute gastroenteritis and up to 50% of infantile gastroenteritis, but the frequency differs by geographic location and season. Children ages 3 to 24 months have the highest incidence of rotavirus infection. Respiratory illnesses such as otitis media or tonsillitis may occur concurrently. The peak infectious period is during the winter months (November-February). Spread is by the fecal–oral route. Clinical features are presented in Table 17-1. Treatment is usually restricted to fluid and electrolyte therapy. Severe dehydration and electrolyte disturbances can occur, however, possibly resulting in death. In 1998, the Food and Drug Administration (FDA) licensed a rotavirus vaccine for routine use to prevent this illness in healthy infants, but it was quickly withdrawn in 1999 because of an association with intussusception.[11] Because of the significance of this illness, however, efforts to bring a safe, effective rotavirus vaccine to market continue.[12]

Other, less frequent viral causes of gastroenteritis include adenoviruses, astroviruses, and hepatitis A virus.

### *Bacterial Gastroenteritis*

Bacterial pathogens cause an estimated five million episodes of acute gastroenteritis in the United States each year.[1] Bacterial pathogens commonly responsible for producing diarrhea in the United States, in order of decreasing incidence, are *Campylobacter* sp., *Salmonella* sp., *Shigella* sp., *E. coli* (including O157:H7, non-O157:H7 Shigatoxin-producing *E. coli*, enterotoxigenic *E. coli*, and other diarrheagenic strains), *Staphylococcus* sp., *Clostridium* sp., *Yersinia enterocolitica*, and *Bacillus cereus*. *Aeromonas* sp. are being increasingly recognized as enteropathogens, particularly in food-borne disease.[9] In the United States, when all bacterial causes of bacterial gastroenteritis are considered, *Campylobacter* is found two to seven times more frequently than *Salmonella, Shigella,* or *E. coli.*[13] Some organisms cause diarrhea through an enterotoxin (toxigenic *E. coli* and *Staphylococcus aureus*). Others (*Shigella, Salmonella, Yersinia, Campylobacter jejuni,* and invasive *E. coli*) directly invade mucosal epithelial cells. Patients with diarrhea caused by toxin-producing agents have a watery diarrhea, which primarily involves the small intestine. If the large intestine is the site of attack, invasive organisms produce a dysenterylike (bloody diarrhea) syndrome. This syndrome is characterized by fever, abdominal cramps, tenesmus (straining), and frequent passage of small-volume stools that may contain blood and mucus. Table 17-1 presents clinical features of common bacterial diarrheas.

Foodborne transmission of pathogens accounts for 36% of acute gastroenteritis episodes in the United States; of these infections, 30% are due to bacteria, 67% to viruses, and 3% to protozoa.[1] Recent surveillance statistics on the incidence of foodborne illnesses in the United States document that *Salmonella* and *Campylobacter,* which caused 14.5 and 12.6 cases of illness per 100,000 population in 2003, respectively, are the most frequently diagnosed bacterial pathogens, followed by *Shigella* (7.3 cases per 100,000 population), *Yersinia* (4 cases per 100,000 population), *Vibrio* (3 cases per 100,000 population), *Listeria* (3.3 cases per 100,000 population), and *E. coli* O157:H7 (1.1 cases per 100,000 population).[14]

Outbreaks of foodborne bacterial infection have been traced to poor sanitary conditions in meat-processing plants and various retail outlets (e.g., grocery stores, restaurants). Outbreaks of infection have also been associated with specific foods, such as milk (*Campylobacter*), raw eggs (*Salmonella*), and raspberries (*Cyclospora*). Thus, an attentive and thorough history regarding food intake before onset of diarrhea is essential in identifying a probable cause. For example, *Staphylococcus aureus* grows rapidly in food (especially salads, custard, sausage, ham, dairy products, and poultry), producing a toxin. On ingestion, the enterotoxin provokes an attack of nausea and vomiting with diarrhea within 6 hours. In contrast, the incubation period for *Salmonella,* which is harbored on raw foods, particularly on eggs, is 12 to 24 hours. These microbes invade the mucosal layer to disrupt absorptive/secretory mechanisms. Fever, malaise, muscle aches, and profound epigastric or periumbilical discomfort with severe anorexia suggest an infectious, inflammatory disease of the large intestine. Abdominal pain, vomiting, and diarrhea suggest viral gastroenteritis, and symptoms usually persist for 2 to 3 days before gradually subsiding.

A major public health issue is contamination of food, especially undercooked hamburger and unpasteurized apple cider, with *E. coli* O157:H7 and other Shigatoxin-producing *E. coli.* The toxins produced by these organisms cause an acute bloody diarrhea, but may also be associated with serious, potentially fatal systemic complications, such as hemolytic uremic syndrome or thrombotic thrombocytopenic purpura.

Other pathogens of concern include *Listeria monocytogenes* and *Cyclospora cayetanensis.* Viruses also cause foodborne gastroenteritis. Noroviruses are responsible for more than two thirds of the foodborne illnesses caused by known pathogens.[1] Other enteric viruses, such as rotaviruses, have occasionally been implicated in foodborne disease.

Traveler's diarrhea is a secretory diarrhea acquired, for the most part, through ingestion of contaminated food or water. This acute diarrhea affects millions of tourists visiting foreign countries or U.S. border areas with poor sanitation, and is usually caused by bacterial enteropathogens. While *Salmonella, Shigella, Campylobacter, E. histolytica, Giardia,* and rotavirus have all been implicated in the disease, *E. coli* is the most common infecting organism in traveler's diarrhea. Two strains, enterotoxigenic *E. coli* (ETEC) and enteroaggregative *E. coli* (EAEC), are responsible for most cases. ETEC is found in up to 40% of travelers with diarrhea in various areas around the world; EAEC is almost as common, causing approximately 25% of cases of traveler's diarrhea.[14] The causative organisms are found most often on foods such as fruits, vegetables, raw meat, seafood, and even hot sauces; less commonly, pathogens are found in the local water, including ice cubes. After ingestion, ETEC produces two plasmid-mediated enterotoxins, known as heat-labile and heat-stable toxins. The pathogenic mechanisms underlying diarrhea caused by EAEC are not well understood; these organisms may produce disease through elaboration of heat-stable enterotoxin, a cytotoxin, or some other means.[15] The diarrheal disorder caused by these organisms is characterized in Table 17-1. Patients may experience between three and eight (or more) watery stools per day, and symptoms usually subside over 3 to 5 days.

Bacterial pathogens not only cause acute illness, but can also cause functional bowel disorders, including postinfectious irritable bowel syndrome (IBS), for 6 months or longer after a bout of acute gastroenteritis. Ten percent to 30% of patients report persistent bowel dysfunction 6 months after infectious diarrhea caused by *Campylobacter, Shigella, Salmonella* and diarrheagenic *E. coli* (ETEC and EAEC).[16,17] IBS is diagnosed in 4% to 10% of patients 1 to 2 years after an episode of acute bacterial gastroenteritis.[17,18]

### Protozoal Diarrhea

*Giardia lamblia* and *Entamoeba histolytica* are protozoa associated with acute diarrhea (Table 17-1). Giardiasis is an infection of the small intestine commonly affecting children, travelers, or institutionalized patients, as well as hikers who drink from streams or ponds. Diarrhea that occurs after travel to a mountainous or recreational water area is consistent with giardiasis. The prevalence of *Giardia* in day care centers ranges from 19% to 30%; these centers play an important role in disease transmission in urban areas. *Giardia* may also be transmitted sexually, particularly by intimate oral–anal contact. Many infected patients (25%-70%) will develop mild symptoms or be asymptomatic. *Giardia* should be suspected in patients not responding to empiric antibiotic therapy and in whom diarrhea persists longer than 14 days.

*E. histolytica* is an infrequent cause of traveler's diarrhea in developing countries. Amebiasis also occurs in areas with poor sanitation and among migrant workers and institutionalized patients.

Populations at risk for *Cryptosporidium* infection include immunosuppressed patients (such as AIDS patients), travelers, and children in developing countries. The organism is transmitted from person to person or from animal to person, and through contaminated food or water. Fluid management is the mainstay of therapy.

### Drug-induced Diarrhea

Drug-induced diarrhea is a frequent adverse outcome of therapy, comprising 7% of all adverse drug events.[19] Twenty-five percent of drug-induced diarrhea is caused by antibacterial agents. All antibiotics can produce diarrhea; however, the frequency of occurrence varies among agents and can be as high as 40%.[19] The frequency of diarrhea depends largely on the extent to which the drug disrupts the normal intestinal microflora. This is determined by the drug's spectrum of activity and its concentration in the intestinal lumen. Commonly prescribed antibiotics that have broad spectra of activity against aerobic and anaerobic organisms can produce diarrhea as a side effect (Table 17-2).[19,20] Antibiotics that achieve high intraluminal concentrations, either through biliary secretion or because they are incompletely or poorly absorbed, are associated with the highest frequency of diarrhea. Risk factors of lesser importance may include duration of antibacterial therapy, repeated courses of antibacterial therapy, and combination antibacterial therapy.[19]

Antibiotic-associated diarrhea (AAD) may be caused by an overgrowth of antibiotic-resistant bacteria, fungi, or

**TABLE 17-2 Comparison of the Propensities of Antibiotics to Cause Diarrhea**

| Drug | Frequency of Diarrhea (%) |
|---|---|
| Ampicillin | 5-10 |
| Amoxicillin | 5-10 |
| Amoxicillin/clavulanate | 10-25 |
| Cefixime | 15-20 |
| Cephalosporins, other | 2-5 |
| Clindamycin | 0.5-21 |
| Clotrimazole | <1 |
| Fluoroquinolones (ciprofloxacin, levofloxacin, norfloxacin) | 2-5 |
| Macrolides (azithromycin, clarithromycin, erythromycin) | 2-5 |
| Tetracycline | 2-5 |

*Source:* Adapted from references 19 and 20.

toxin-producing *C. difficile*. Intestinal microorganisms other than *C. difficile* that tend to proliferate during antibiotic therapy include *S. aureus, Pseudomonas aeruginosa, Streptococcus faecalis, Candida albicans,* and selected species of *Salmonella* and *Proteus*. Any antibiotic can cause AAD, and the disease can begin during or several weeks after treatment. AAD may be self-limiting with discontinuation of the antibiotic.

*C. difficile* is responsible for approximately 25% of all cases of AAD and causes more than 300,000 cases of AAD per year in the United States.[21] *C. difficile* AAD occurs most frequently in hospitalized patients or those in long-term care facilities; only about 20,000 cases occur in outpatients annually.[21] All antibiotics, including metronidazole and vancomycin, have been associated with *C. difficile* overgrowth and diarrhea; however, clindamycin, ampicillin, amoxicillin, and the cephalosporins are most frequently associated with the disorder. Although *C. difficile* produces at least two identified toxins (A and B), enterotoxin A is the primary cause of diarrhea. Both toxins are necessary for the full tissue damage that characterizes the disorder known as pseudomembranous colitis or *C. difficile* colitis.

Enteric isolation precautions are recommended for patients with AAD because these bacteria can be spread to other individuals. Diagnosis of pseudomembranous colitis is suggested by a test for toxins in the stool although toxins have been found in patients without AAD. The watery or greenish-mucoid diarrhea usually starts during antibiotic treatment, but it can begin up to 4 weeks after discontinuation of the antibiotic. To effectively manage this disorder, the offending antibiotic must be discontinued and *C. difficile* eradicated with appropriate antibiotic therapy. No nonprescription treatments are effective in eradicating *C. difficile*. Oral vancomycin or oral metronidazole is usually prescribed for adults. Treatment in children is less well defined although both metronidazole and vancomycin are used. Relapses and reinfections are common, occurring in 20% to 25% of patients.

Antibiotics may also cause diarrhea through direct effects on the intestine. Antibiotics exert prokinetic effects to increase GI motility (e.g., erythromycin) or may cause small-bowel enteropathy with malabsorption (e.g., clofazimine).[20,22] Antibiotic-induced alterations in colonic bile acid and carbohydrate metabolism have also been proposed, but their etiologic role in AAD is yet to be established.[22] Medications such as laxatives, misoprostol, olsalazine, anticancer agents, antihypertensive agents, quinidine, and colchicine may cause diarrhea through a variety of mechanisms. Drugs that cause retention of electrolytes and water in the intestinal lumen (e.g., mannitol, sorbitol, lactulose) may produce a hyperosmolar, osmotic diarrhea. Certain antacid laxative preparations containing magnesium may induce diarrhea, depending on the dose taken and the individual's susceptibility. Drugs that affect autonomic control of normal intestinal motility, such as certain antihypertensive agents with sympatholytic activity (e.g., guanethidine, methyldopa, reserpine), may also cause diarrhea. Generalized cramping and diarrhea may follow use of a prokinetic drug, such as bethanechol or metoclopramide, which also disrupts or alters intestinal motility. Drugs, such as digoxin, colchicines, or olsalazine, can also cause diarrhea by inhibiting the GI sodium-potassium ATPase pump, which disrupts water absorption.

Cytotoxic agents used in cancer chemotherapy may induce diarrhea through several mechanisms. By inhibiting mitosis in rapidly proliferating villus crypt cells, cytotoxic agents induce an imbalance between immature, secretory crypt cells and mature absorptive epithelial cells. An excessive number of immature cells produce an increase in intestinal fluid that results in diarrhea. Cytotoxic agents may also suppress normal GI flora, which enables microbial overgrowth and colonization of the intestines with pathogenic bacteria and fungi, such as *C. difficile* and *Cryptosporidium* sp., respectively.

### AIDS-associated Diarrhea

Patients with AIDS and individuals infected with human immunodeficiency virus (HIV) are known to be susceptible to many intestinal infections that produce diarrhea. An estimated 80% of AIDS patients will experience a diarrheal infection at some time in their illness. These immunocompromised patients may be infected with bacteria, fungi, parasites, viruses, and protozoal organisms. Common stool isolates are EAEC, *Cryptosporidium, Microsporidium, C. difficile, Isospora belli, Mycobacterium avium-intracellulare, G. lamblia,* and *E. histolytica.*

No nonprescription therapies are available to manage diarrhea in these patients and self-management is inappropriate; medical evaluation is required.

### Food-induced Diarrhea

Food intolerance can provoke diarrhea and may result from a food allergy or ingestion of foods that are excessively fatty or spicy or contain a high amount of roughage or many seeds. For patients with diverticulosis, avoiding food with seeds is the most effective measure.

Carbohydrates in the diet commonly include the disaccharides lactose and sucrose, which are normally hydrolyzed to monosaccharides by the enzyme lactase. When these disaccharides are not hydrolyzed, they pool in the lumen of the intestine, where they not only ferment but also produce an osmotic imbalance and pH change. The resultant hyperosmolarity draws fluid into the intestinal lumen, causing diarrhea. Lactase enzymatic activity may be reduced in intestinal disorders such as infectious diarrhea and GI allergy. Acute viral diarrhea may cause a temporary milk intolerance in patients of all ages. Infants born with a lactase deficiency and adults who develop one are intolerant of whole milk and milk-based products. Thus, milk and ice cream may be particularly problematic because of the lactose content. Lactase enzyme products are effective treatments for some patients (see Treatment of Diarrhea).

## Pathophysiology of Diarrhea

Variability in the causes of diarrhea makes identification of the pathophysiologic mechanisms difficult. The etiology, and subsequently the pathophysiology, can be determined by a thorough medical history in most cases. However, a complete medical assessment, including clinical

TABLE 17-3 Clinical Classification of Diarrhea

| Type | Mechanism | Common Causes |
|---|---|---|
| Osmotic | Unabsorbed solutes in intestines increase luminal osmotic load, retarding fluid absorption. Decreased fluid absorption of even a few hundred milliliters may cause diarrhea. Decreased absorption of solutes and fluid can be secondary to brush border damage caused by lactase deficiency or bacterial/viral infection. Viral-induced damage to epithelial cells accelerates migration of immature crypt cells to tip of the villus; altered epithelial turnover also decreases absorption. | Noroviruses, rotaviruses, E. *coli*, *C. jejuni*, lactase deficiency, magnesium antacid excess |
| Secretory | Stimulation of crypt cells produces net flow of electrolytes (most notably chloride) and fluids into intestinal lumen. Tumors can secrete GI hormones and peptides that act as secretagogues. | *C. jejuni, C. difficile, E. coli, Salmonella, Shigella, Vibrio,* rotaviruses, *G. lamblia, Cryptosporidium spp. Isospora,* ileal resection, thyroid cancer |
| Exudative | Impaired fluid absorption and leaking of mucus, blood, and pus into lumen caused by inflammation of intestinal mucosa (e.g., IBD) or bacterial infection (i.e., dysentery). | *C. jejuni, E. coli, Salmonella, Shigella, Yersinia, E. histolytica,* ulcerative colitis, Crohn disease |
| Motor | Abnormally rapid intestinal transit time reduces contact time between luminal contents and absorptive areas of intestinal wall. | IBS, diabetic neuropathy |

Key: GI, gastrointestinal ; IBD, inflammatory bowel disease ; IBS, irritable bowel syndrome.

laboratory evaluation, may be required to identify the cause in a subset of patients with severe or persistent diarrhea.

Diarrhea can be classified as osmotic, secretory, exudative, or motor, depending on the underlying pathophysiologic mechanisms that disrupt normal intestinal function. The common mechanisms of acute diarrhea are osmotic and secretory, whereas motor and exudative mechanisms commonly underlie chronic diarrheal illnesses. Table 17-3 correlates the clinical groups and mechanism with their most common causes.

Bacterial and viral enterotoxins play a role in the pathophysiology of secretory diarrheas. Enterotoxins elaborated by *E. coli* and *Vibrio cholera* produce secretory diarrhea by evoking the release of endogenous secretagogues that mediate secretory reflexes, including serotonin, substance P, and vasoactive intestinal peptide.[4,21] Some enterotoxins, such as cholera toxin, can directly stimulate GI secretomotor neurons to increase intestinal secretion. *C. difficile* enterotoxin A also injures enterocytes to evoke a necroinflammatory response that causes a secretory diarrhea. Rotavirus produces an enterotoxin that causes a calcium-mediated secretory diarrhea. In addition, inflammatory mediators (e.g., interleukins 1 and 6, prostaglandins, substance P, tissue necrosis factor α, platelet-activating factor) evoked by enteric infection stimulate a characteristic GI motility pattern that leads to the urgent defecation associated with diarrhea. This altered motility also causes abdominal cramps.

Stool characteristics give valuable information about the diarrhea's pathophysiology. For example, undigested food particles in the stool suggest disease of the small intestine. Black, tarry stools may indicate upper GI bleeding, and red stools suggest possible lower bowel or hemorrhoidal bleeding or simply recent ingestion of red food (e.g., beets) or drug products (e.g., rifampin). Diarrhea originating from the small intestine is characterized by a marked outpouring of fluid high in potassium and bicarbonate. Passage of many small-volume stools suggests diarrhea with a colonic disorder. Yellowish stools may suggest the presence of bilirubin and a potentially serious pathology of the liver. A whitish tint to the stool suggests a fat malabsorption disease. Patients who have stool containing blood or mucus need medical evaluation.

## Complications of Diarrhea

Fluid and electrolyte imbalance is the major complication of diarrheal illness. Therefore, assessment of the patient's risk for dehydration, as well as the degree of dehydration, is key in determining the appropriateness of self-care and the need for medical referral. The specific signs and symptoms of dehydration are associated with the severity of the diarrhea and related to the etiology and degree of fluid and electrolyte losses (Table 17-4). Previous management guidelines divided patients into three groups on the basis of the degree of fluid deficits: mild (3%-5%), moderate (6%-9%), and severe (>9%). Because it may be difficult to distinguish between mild and moderate dehydration on the basis of clinical signs alone, the current Centers for Disease Control (CDC) treatment recommendations for young children combine these patients into one group.[23]

Certain medical conditions can increase the risk for dehydration, and patients who have diabetes mellitus, severe cardiovascular or renal diseases, or multiple chronic medical conditions should be referred for medical care. Patients receiving cancer treatment, organ transplant recipients, patients with AIDS, or other immunocompromised patients also need medical evaluation. Self-care medication may also be inappropriate for diarrhea during pregnancy, and pregnant women should consult with a primary care provider before self-treating. Healthy patients with uncomplicated acute diarrhea usually improve clinically

**TABLE 17-4 Assessment of Dehydration and Severity of Acute Diarrhea**

| | Minimal or No Dehydration (self-treatable) | Mild to Moderate Dehydration/ Diarrhea (self-treatable) | Severe Dehydration/ Diarrhea (not self-treatable) |
|---|---|---|---|
| Degree of dehydration (loss of body weight) | <3% | 3%-9% | >9% |
| Signs of dehydration* | | | |
| Mental status | Well, alert | Normal, fatigued or restless, irritable | Apathetic, lethargic, unconscious |
| Thirst | Drinks normally; might refuse liquids | Thirsty, eager to drink | Drinks poorly, unable to drink |
| Heart rate | Normal | Normal to increased | Tachycardia; bradycardia in most severe cases |
| Quality of pulses | Normal | Normal to decreased | Weak, thready, impalpable |
| Breathing | Normal | Normal; fast | Deep |
| Eyes | Normal | Slight sunken† | Deeply sunken† |
| Tears | Present | Decreased† | Absent |
| Mouth and tongue | Moist | Dry | Parched |
| Skin fold | Instant recoil | Recoil in <2 seconds | Recoil in >2 seconds |
| Capillary refill | Normal | Prolonged | Prolonged; minimal |
| Extremities | Warm | Cool | Cold, mottled, cyanotic |
| Urine output | Normal to decreased | Decreased† | Minimal† |
| Number of unformed stools/day | <3 | ≤5 | 6-9 |
| Other signs/symptoms of diarrhea | Afebrile, normal blood pressure, no orthostatic changes in blood pressure/ pulse | May be afebrile or may develop fever >102.2°F (39°C); normal blood pressure; mild orthostatic blood pressure/pulse changes with or without mild orthostatic-related symptoms may be present; sunken fontanelle‡ | Fever >102.2°F (39°C), low blood pressure, dizziness, severe abdominal pain |

* If signs of dehydration are absent, rehydration therapy is not required. Maintenance therapy and replacement of stool losses should be undertaken.

† Signs and symptoms experienced especially by young children.

‡ Of particular concern for young infants.

*Source:* Adapted from reference 23.

within 24 to 48 hours. If the condition remains the same or worsens after 48 hours of onset, medical referral is necessary to prevent complications.

Children younger than 5 years and adults older than 65 years are at greater risk for complications than other age groups. In developed countries, most children experience complete recovery although some die of complications. In the United States, approximately 300 to 450 children die annually from acute gastroenteritis; most of these deaths occur in infants.[3,23] Children 2 years of age or younger are likely to suffer complications that require hospitalization. In newborns, water may comprise up to 75% of total body weight; severe diarrhea may cause water loss equal to 10% or more of body weight. After 8 to 10 bowel movements within a 24-hour period, a 2-month-old infant could lose enough fluid to cause circulatory collapse and renal failure. Moderate to severe diarrhea in infants requires evaluation by a primary care provider. Improved therapy for young children at risk for significant dehydration and better access to medical care have both helped lower the mortality rate.

In recent years, deaths from viral and bacterial GI infection have increased most sharply among people 65 years of age and older; diarrhea in this population is likely to be more severe than in other adult populations, and this population currently experiences the highest rate of death from enteric infections.[3]

In developing countries, an estimated 2.2 million people die annually from complications of acute diarrhea.[24] Diarrhea-associated morbidity also continues to be a significant concern in developing countries and, despite improved mortality rates, morbidity appears to be increasing. Evidence from developing countries suggests that persistent diarrhea in early childhood may be associated with long-term

**TABLE 17-5 Selected Oral Rehydration Products**

| Trade Name | Osmolarity | Calories | Carbohydrate | Electrolytes |
|---|---|---|---|---|
| WHO–ORS | 245 mOsm/L | 46 cal/L | Glucose 13.5 g/L | Sodium 75 mEq/L; chloride 65 mEq/L; citrate 30 mEq/L; potassium 20 mEq/L |
| CeraLyte 50 Powder Packets | <225 mOsm/L | 160 cal/L | Rice starch polymers, 40 g/L; sucrose 10 g/L | Sodium 50 mEq/L; chloride 40 mEq/L; citrate 30 mEq/L; potassium 20 mEq/L |
| CeraLyte 70 Powder Packets | 235 mOsm/L | 160 cal/L | Rice starch polymers, 40 g/L | Sodium 70 mEq/L; chloride 60 mEq/L; citrate 30 mEq/L; potassium 20 mEq/L |
| CeraLyte 90 Powder Packets | 260 mOsm/L | 160 Cal/L | Rice starch polymers, 40 g/L | Sodium 90 mEq/L; chloride 80 mEq/L; citrate 30 mEq/L; potassium 20 mEq/L |
| Enfalyte Solution*† | 200 mOsm/L | 126 cal/L | Rice syrup solids, 30 g/L | Sodium 50 mEq/L; chloride 45 mEq/L; citrate 34 mEq/L; potassium 25 mEq/L |
| Kaolectrolyte Packets†‡ | | 22 cal/L | Dextrose 5 g/L | Sodium 50 mEq/L; chloride 40 mEq/L; citrate 30 mEq/L; potassium 20 mEq/L |
| Pedialyte | 249 mOsm/L | 100 cal/L | Dextrose 20 g/L; fructose 5 g/L | Sodium 45 mEq/L; chloride 35 mEq/L; citrate 30 mEq/L; potassium 20 mEq/L |
| Pedialyte Freezer Pops§ | | 6.25 cal | Dextrose 25 g/L | Sodium 45 mEq/L; chloride 35 mEq/L; citrate 30 mEq/L; potassium 20 mEq/L |
| Rehydralyte Solution | 304 mOsm/L | 100 cal/L | Dextrose 25 g/L | Sodium 75 mEq/L; chloride 65 mEq/L; citrate 30 mEq/L; potassium 20 mEq/L |
| Revital Ice Freezer Pops | | 12 cal | Crystalline fructose 30 g/L | Sodium 45 mEq/L; chloride 35 mEq/L; citrate 30 mEq/L; potassium 20 mEq/L |

Key: WHO, World Health Organization; ORS, oral rehydration solution.

*Dye-free; †lactose-free; ‡product contains aspartame and phenylalanine; §product to be used with appropriate maintenance ORS.

adverse consequences on growth, physical and cognitive development, and school performance.[25]

## Treatment of Diarrhea

### *Treatment Goals*

The goals of self-treatment are to (1) prevent or correct fluid and electrolyte loss and acid–base disturbance, (2) relieve symptoms, (3) identify and treat the cause, and (4) prevent acute morbidity and mortality.

### *General Treatment Approach*

Infectious diarrhea is often self-limiting. Symptomatic relief and correction of fluid and electrolyte loss are generally adequate for mild to moderate, uncomplicated diarrhea. Initial self-management for adults and children should focus on fluid and electrolyte replacement by administering commercially available oral solutions (e.g., Pedialyte) in adequate doses (Table 17-5). Simultaneously, symptomatic relief can be achieved by using nonprescription antidiarrheal drugs, such as loperamide, in carefully selected patients. Attention should also be given to diet; dietary considerations are discussed in the following section. Normal function of the alimentary tract is often restored in 24 to 72 hours without additional treatment. Severe diarrhea constitutes a medical emergency, especially in young children, and requires immediate referral for medical evaluation and treatment. Initial management with intravenous (IV) fluid therapy is necessary until perfusion and mental status improve. Exclusions for self-treatment are listed in Figure 17-1.

### *Nonpharmacologic Therapy*

Simultaneous implementation of oral rehydration and specific dietary measures is appropriate for treating mild to moderate diarrheal illness.

#### Fluid and Electrolyte Management

Correction of fluid loss and electrolyte imbalances is important, and can be accomplished by oral or IV therapy. Oral rehydration therapy (ORT) is the preferred treatment for mild to moderate diarrhea.[9,23] ORT is as effective as IV therapy in managing fluid and electrolytes in children with mild to moderate dehydration secondary to diarrhea. The GI secretory and absorptive mechanisms appear to function independently of one another, and the glucose-sodium cotransport mechanism is not adversely affected by most diarrheal diseases. Therefore, an oral sugar/electrolyte solution can be absorbed during diarrhea, and can be useful in managing fluid and electrolyte balance. Oral rehydration solutions contain low concentrations of glucose or dextrose (2%-2.5%); the sugar molecules provide very little caloric support, but facilitate intestinal sodium and water absorption. Maximal sodium absorption occurs at a molar glucose-to-sodium ratio close to 1. In mild to

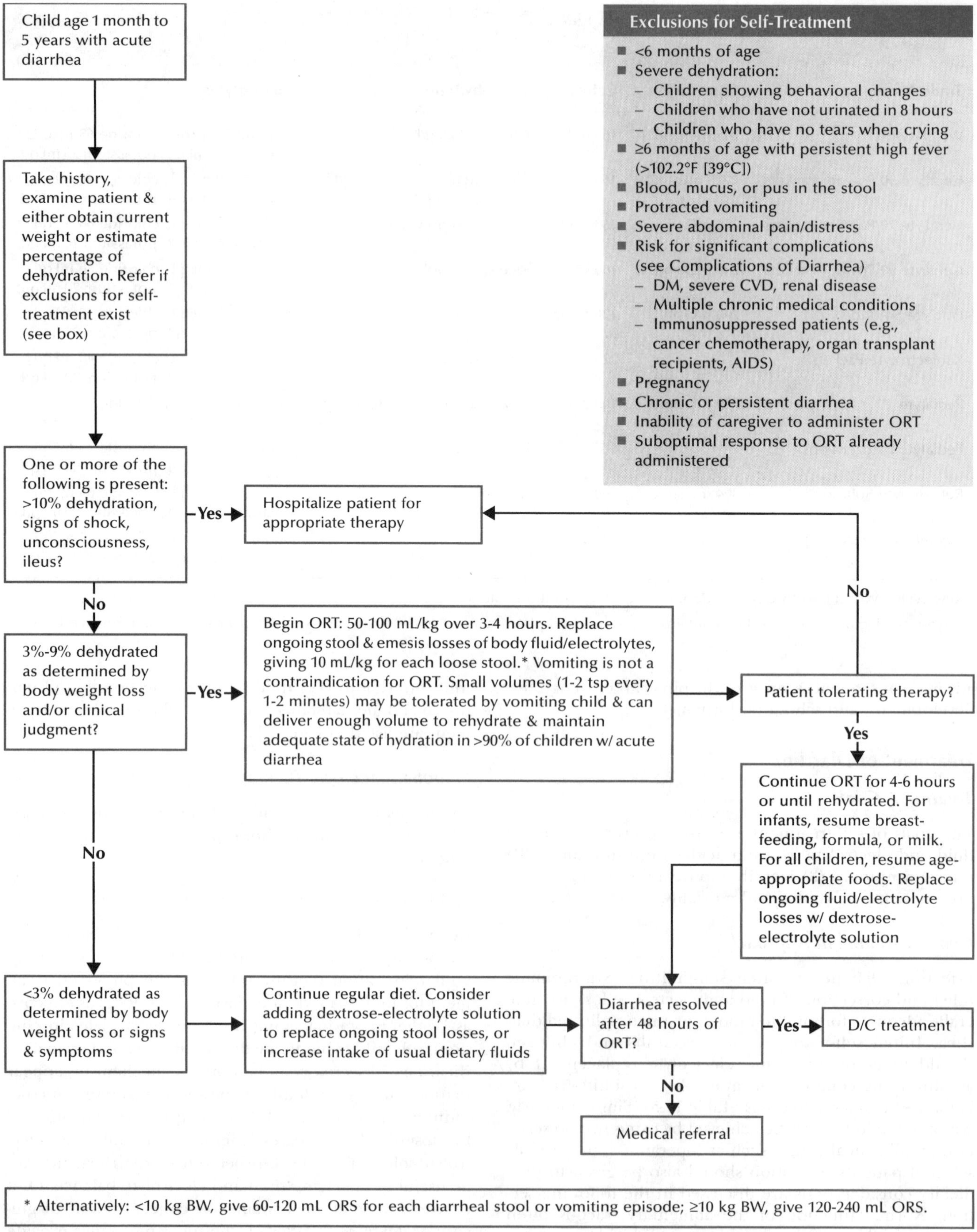


**FIGURE 17-1** Self-care of acute diarrhea in children 1 month to 5 years. Key: AIDS, acquired immunodeficiency syndrome; BW, body weight; CVD, cardiovascular disease; D/C, discontinue; DM, diabetes mellitus; ORT, oral rehydration therapy.

moderate diarrhea, practitioners can safely recommend an oral rehydration solution (ORS).

On the basis of the patient's fluid and electrolyte status, oral treatment may be carried out in two phases: rehydration and maintenance therapy. Rehydration over 3 to 4 hours quickly replaces water and electrolyte deficits to restore normal body composition. In the maintenance phase, electrolyte solutions are given to maintain normal body composition and adequate dietary intake is reestablished. Figures 17-1 and 17-2 outline rehydration and maintenance fluid and electrolyte therapy recommendations for children and adults. While ORSs generally are recommended for use in

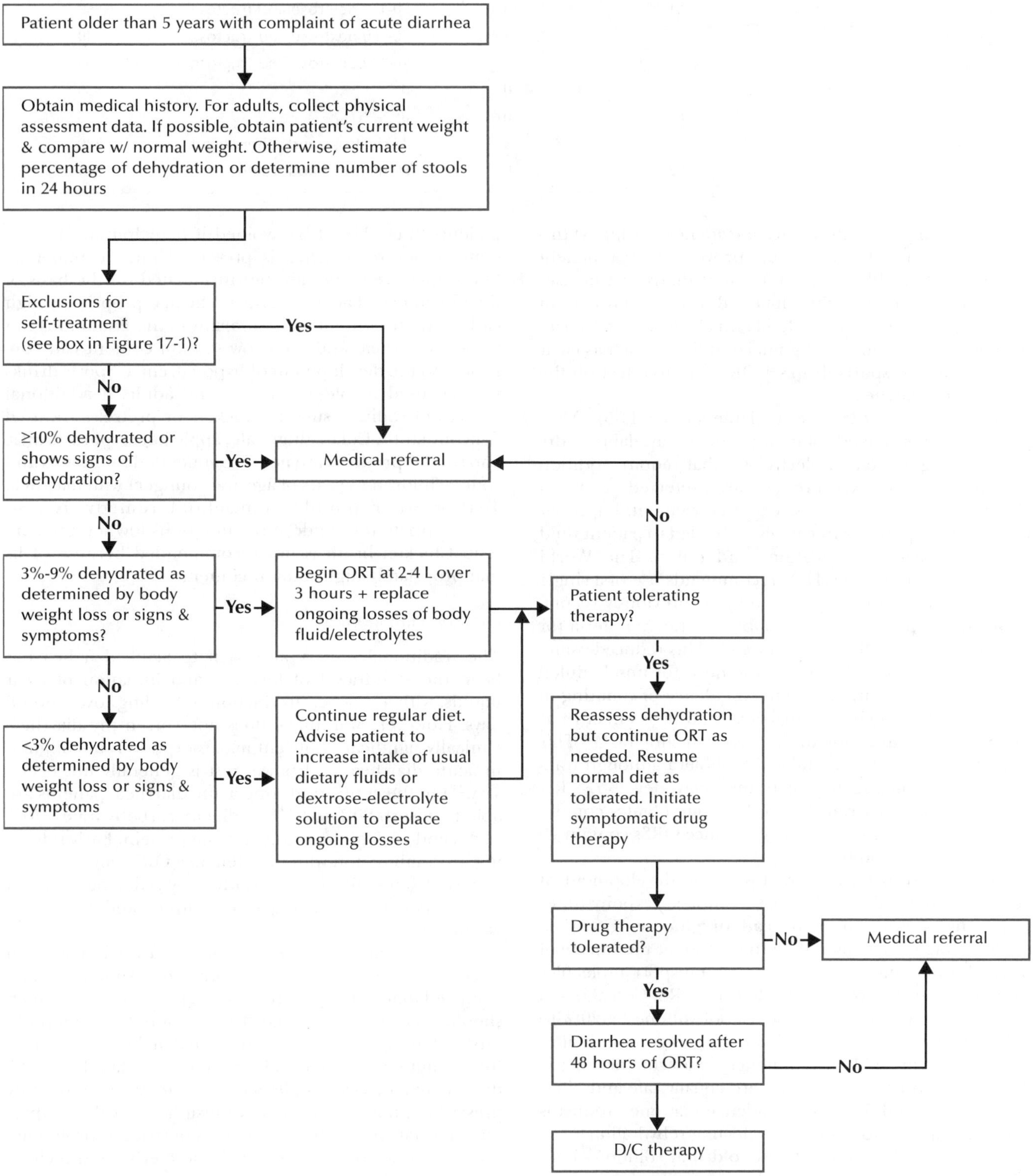


FIGURE 17-2 Self-care of acute diarrhea in children older than 5 years, adolescents, and adults. Key: D/C, discontinue; ORT, oral rehydration therapy.

TABLE 17-6 Comparison of Electrolyte-Dextrose Concentrations of Household Fluids

| Clear Liquids | Sodium (mEq/L) | Potassium (mEq/L) | Bicarbonate (mEq/L) | Dextrose (g/L) | Osmolarity (mOsm/L) |
|---|---|---|---|---|---|
| Cola | 2 | 0.1 | 13 | 50-150 dextrose and fructose | 550 |
| Ginger ale | 3 | 1 | 4 | 50-150 dextrose and fructose | 540 |
| Apple juice | 3 | 20 | 0 | 10-150 dextrose and fructose | 700 |
| Chicken broth | 250 | 5 | 0 | 0 | 450 |
| Tea | 0 | 0 | 0 | 0 | 5 |
| Gatorade | 20 | 3 | 3 | 45 dextrose and other sugars | 330 |
| Seven Up | 7.5 | 0.2 | 0 | 80 dextrose and fructose | 564 |

adults with diarrhea, there is scant evidence to support this recommendation. ORSs may not provide any real benefit to otherwise healthy adults with mild diarrhea who can maintain an adequate fluid intake during the episode of diarrhea; for these patients, fluid and electrolyte status can be maintained by increasing intake of fluids, such as clear juices, soups, or sports drinks.[26] ORT has no effect on the duration of diarrhea.

A variety of ORSs are available (Table 17-5). Most products are premixed solutions; a few are available as dry powders of glucose and electrolytes that require addition of water. The premixed products are preferred for use in children because they are safe and convenient; improper mixing of dry powders by caregivers has led to patient fluid and electrolyte complications and injury. The World Health Organization (WHO) recommends use of a single ORS containing 75 mEq/L of sodium (previously recommended 90 mEq/L), but has published range criteria for safe and effective ORS formulations.[27] This reduced-osmolarity ORS significantly reduces the need for unscheduled IV therapy, stool output, and the incidence of vomiting in children with noncholera diarrhea, and is as effective as the previous formulation in children with cholera.[27,28] This ORS is also effective in adults with cholera although transient, asymptomatic hyponatremia may develop.[29] Rehydration solutions available in the United States contain 75 to 90 mEq/L of sodium; maintenance ORSs contain 40 to 60 mEq/L of sodium.

ORSs have been improved with the development of cereal-based products that use complex carbohydrates (e.g., rice syrup solids) instead of glucose. Complex carbohydrates are converted into glucose at the intestinal brush border and provide more cotransport molecules while reducing the osmotic load of the ORS. Cereal-based ORS therapy potentially reduces stool volume by 20% to 30% in children with cholera, but may not significantly alter stool volume in children with noncholera acute diarrhea.[30] All available premixed solutions are equally safe and effective, however, and there is no evidence that one product is clinically superior to another in effecting rehydration.

A variety of common household oral solutions have also been used for oral rehydration and maintenance (Table 17-6). Although these home remedies may be sufficient to manage mild, self-limiting diarrhea in some patients, they should be avoided if dehydration or moderate to severe diarrhea is present. Unlike commercial ORSs, these remedies are not formulated on the basis of the physiology of acute diarrhea. The inappropriately high carbohydrate content and osmolality of these solutions can worsen diarrhea, and their low sodium content can contribute to the development of hyponatremia. Sports drinks may be used in older children and adults if additional sources of sodium, such as crackers or pretzels, are used concomitantly. Colas, ginger ale, apple juice, sports drinks, and similar products are not recommended for infants and young children (5 years of age and younger) with diarrhea. Tea, another popular household remedy, is also inappropriate for children because of its low sodium content. Chicken broth is not recommended because of its inappropriately high sodium content.

## Dietary Management

The traditional dietary approach to acute diarrhea has been the withdrawal of feedings and initiation of clear liquids, with a slow reintroduction of feedings over several days. However, oral intake does not worsen the diarrhea, clinically significant nutrient malabsorption is uncommon in acute diarrhea, and bowel rest is generally not necessary.[23] On the contrary, during acute diarrhea, patients are able to absorb 80% to 95% of dietary carbohydrates, 70% of fat, and 75% of the nitrogen from protein. Early refeeding, in combination with maintenance ORT, improves outcomes of acute diarrhea in children by reducing duration of the diarrhea, reducing stool output, and improving weight gain.

It is inappropriate to withhold food for longer than 24 hours.[23] A normal, age-appropriate diet should be reintroduced once the patient has been rehydrated, which should take no longer that 3 to 4 hours to accomplish. Most infants and children with acute diarrhea can tolerate full-strength breast milk and cow's milk. The familiar BRAT diet (bananas, rice, applesauce, and toast) is frequently prescribed; however, it provides insufficient calories, protein, and fat, especially in situations of strict or prolonged use, and is not recommended.[23] The diet should include complex carbohydrate-rich foods, yogurt, lean meats, fruits, and vegetables. Practitioners should advise patients (or their parents) to avoid fatty foods, foods rich in simple

**TABLE 17-7 Recommended Dosages of Antidiarrheal Agents for Acute Diarrhea**

| Medication | Dosage Forms | Adult Dosages (Maximum Daily Dosage) | Pediatric Dosages | Duration of Use |
|---|---|---|---|---|
| Loperamide | Caplets (2 mg), liquid (1 mg/5 mL) | 4 mg initially, then 2 mg after each loose stool (not to exceed 8 mg/day)* | Consult product instructions; not recommended for children <6 years except under medical supervision | 48 hours |
| Bismuth subsalicylate | Tablets (262 mg), caplets (262 mg), liquids (262 mg/ 15 mL, 525 mg/15 mL) | 525 mg every 30-60 up to 4200 mg /day; (8 doses/day) | Not recommended for children <12 years except under medical supervision | 48 hours |
| Digestive enzymes (lactase) | Chewable tablets, caplets, liquids | 5-15 drops placed in or taken with dairy product; 1-3 tablets or 1-2 capsules with first bite of dairy product | Same as adult dosage | Taken with each consumption of dairy product |

* For self-care, maximum dose is 8 mg/day. If patient is under medical supervision, up to 16 mg/day may be administered by prescription.

sugars that can cause osmotic diarrhea, and spicy foods that may cause GI upset. Caffeine-containing beverages should also be avoided because caffeine can increase cyclic adenosine monophosphate levels, which promotes fluid secretion and may worsen diarrhea. There is no evidence that fasting or dietary modification influences outcomes of acute diarrhea in adults; however, similar guidelines can be applied if a normal diet is not tolerated.[26]

### *Preventive Measures*

Infectious diarrhea, especially acute viral gastroenteritis, often occurs in congregate living conditions such as day care centers and nursing homes through person-to-person transmission. Isolating the individual with diarrhea, washing hands, and using sterile techniques are basic preventive measures that reduce the risk among such populations and their caregivers. Strict food handling, sanitation, and other hygienic practices help control transmission of bacteria and other infectious agents. Short-term bismuth subsalicylate (BSS) prophylaxis is frequently recommended to provide protection against traveler's diarrhea; however, FDA has deemed available data insufficient to support prophylactic use of BSS.[4,6,31] Antibiotics with reliable activity against enteropathogens in the region of travel provide effective prophylaxis; however, CDC does not recommend prophylactic antimicrobial agents to prevent traveler's diarrhea because the risk-to-benefit ratio of widespread use of these agents is uncertain.[32]

### *Pharmacologic Therapy*

Although most acute nonspecific diarrhea in the United States is self-limiting, nonprescription antidiarrheal products may provide relief and will usually do no harm when used according to label instructions. Table 17-7 lists dosage and administration guidelines for these agents. Some health care providers recommend loperamide or adsorbents for acute diarrhea. Scientific evidence that pharmacologic agents, with the exceptions of loperamide and BSS, reduce stool frequency or duration of disease in adults is lacking. Likewise, antidiarrheal drugs have not been shown to significantly improve clinical outcomes of acute nonspecific diarrhea in infants and children. Importantly, a change in stool consistency toward more formed stools does not necessarily indicate that antidiarrheal therapy has successfully treated the underlying problem. Formed stools can have a high water content, and substantial water losses may continue despite the change in consistency. Moreover, reliance on drugs shifts the focus away from fluid/electrolyte and dietary management and increases the risk for potentially dangerous side effects, such as toxic megacolon, without offering additional benefits. Because intestinal viruses are the leading cause of self-limiting acute gastroenteritis in children and infants, antibiotics are not routinely recommended.

#### Loperamide

Loperamide is a popular, effective, and safe nonprescription antidiarrheal agent used to provide symptomatic relief for acute, nonspecific diarrhea. Its therapeutic effects include reduction of daily fecal volume, increased viscosity, bulk volume, and reduced fluid and electrolyte loss.

*Mechanism of Action* Loperamide is a synthetic opioid agonist that produces antidiarrheal effects by stimulating μ-opioid receptors located on the intestinal circular muscles. This action slows intestinal motility, allowing absorption of electrolytes and water through the intestine. Stimulation of GI μ-opioid receptors also decreases GI secretion, which may contribute to the drug's antidiarrheal effects. Loperamide is approximately 50-fold more potent than morphine and two to three times more potent than diphenoxylate in its effects on GI motility, but it penetrates the central nervous system (CNS) poorly and thus has a lower risk for CNS side effects. Other pharmacologic mechanisms for loperamide's antidiarrheal effects may include disruption of cholinergic and noncholinergic mechanisms involved in the regulation of peristalsis, inhibition of calmodulin function, and inhibition of voltage-dependent calcium channels. The effects on calmodulin and calcium channels may contribute to loperamide's antisecretory effects.

*Indications* Loperamide is an effective antidiarrheal agent in traveler's diarrhea, nonspecific acute diarrhea, or chronic diarrhea associated with inflammatory bowel disease. It may be used when the patient is afebrile or has a low-grade fever and does not have bloody stools. Current product information provides directions for use in children as young as 2 years. However, its use in children younger than 6 years is not recommended because it produces only modest, clinically insignificant effects on stool volume and duration of illness, but an unacceptably high risk of side effects (including life-threatening side effects such as ileus and toxic megacolon).[23]

*Dosage and Administration Guidelines* See Table 17-7 for dosing information.

*Safety Considerations* At usual doses, loperamide has few side effects other than occasional dizziness and constipation. Other infrequently occurring adverse effects include abdominal pain, abdominal distention, nausea, vomiting, dry mouth, fatigue, and hypersensitivity reactions. Like all antiperistaltic drugs, it may worsen the effects of invasive (enteroinvasive *E. coli, Salmonella, Shigella, C. jejuni*) or inflammatory (*C. difficile*) bacterial infection and cause toxic megacolon in antibiotic-induced diarrhea or pseudomembranous colitis. If abdominal distention, constipation, or ileus occurs, loperamide should be discontinued.

No significant drug interactions are reported for loperamide.

Loperamide should not be used in patients with fecal leukocytes, high fever, or blood or mucus in the stool (dysentery). These signs suggest infection with invasive organisms or pseudomembranous colitis, both of which require evaluation by a primary care provider for proper management. Loperamide may cause paralytic ileus in patients with dysentery.

### Adsorbents

Nonprescription GI adsorbents (attapulgite, kaolin, and pectin) have been used to treat mild nonspecific acute diarrhea although little evidence supports their efficacy. Sufficient data support the effectiveness of kaolin in improving stool consistency within 24 to 48 hours although it does not reduce the number of stools passed, and it has been granted monograph status by the FDA.[31] There is no conclusive evidence that kaolin alters stool frequency, stool fluid losses, or duration of diarrhea in children, and it should not be used in children younger than 12 years without the specific recommendation of a physician.[23,31] Insufficient evidence is available to support use of attapulgite and pectin; therefore, products containing these adsorbents have either been reformulated or withdrawn from the market.

*Mechanism of Action* Adsorption by kaolin is not selective. When given orally, it may adsorb nutrients and digestive enzymes, as well as toxins, bacteria, and various noxious materials in the GI tract. It may also adsorb drugs in the GI tract.

*Dosage and Administration Guidelines* Although FDA has established labeling requirements, no single-ingredient kaolin products are currently available in the United States.[31]

### Bismuth Subsalicylate

BSS, another therapeutically versatile agent, is the only nonprescription bismuth compound available in the United States. It is effective in the treatment of acute diarrhea, including traveler's diarrhea, significantly reducing the number of diarrheal stools.[31,33]

*Mechanism of Action* BSS reacts with hydrochloric acid in the stomach to form bismuth oxychloride and salicylic acid. Bismuth oxychloride is insoluble and poorly absorbed from the GI tract; less than 1% of the administered dose is absorbed systemically. The salicylate is readily and efficiently absorbed. Both moieties are pharmacologically active; each produces effects that reduce frequency of unformed stools, increase stool consistency, relieve symptoms of abdominal cramping, and decrease nausea and vomiting in children and adults.

The therapeutic effects of BSS in traveler's diarrhea are attributed to direct antimicrobial effects of the bismuth moiety against enterotoxigenic and enteroaggregative *E. coli, C. jejuni*, and other diarrheal pathogens. The salicylate moiety exerts antisecretory effects that reduce fluid and electrolyte losses in acute diarrhea. These antisecretory effects may be mediated by several mechanisms, including inhibition of prostaglandin synthesis, inhibition of intestinal secretion through stimulation of sodium and chloride reabsorption, or disruption of calcium-mediated processes that regulate intestinal ion transport. BSS also directly binds to enterotoxins produced by *E. coli* and other diarrheal pathogens; however, the clinical significance of this effect in the treatment of diarrhea is not clear.

*Indications* BSS is FDA-approved for management of acute diarrhea, including traveler's diarrhea, in adults and children 12 years of age or older.[31,33] Although previously labeled for children as young as 3 years, it is not recommended for use in young children, and the product no longer carries labeling for children younger than 12 years. BSS is also indicated for indigestion and as an adjuvant to antibiotics for treating *Helicobacter pylori*–associated peptic ulcer disease (see Chapter 14).

*Dosage and Administration Guidelines* See Table 17-7 for dosing information.

*Safety Considerations* BSS dosage forms contain various amounts of salicylate. Methyl salicylate (oil of wintergreen) is used as a flavoring agent in the suspension dosage form and the original tablet formulation. The original suspension and cherry-flavored suspension dosage forms (262 mg/15 mL) contain 130 mg of salicylate, whereas the original tablets (262 mg) contain 102 mg of salicylate. The caplets (262 mg) and cherry-flavored tablets (262 mg) contain 99 mg of salicylate. If a patient is taking aspirin or other salicylate-containing drugs, toxic levels of salicylate may be reached even if the patient follows dosing directions on the label for each drug.

Mild tinnitus is a dose-related side effect that may be associated with moderate to severe salicylate toxicity. If tinnitus occurs, the product should be discontinued and the patient referred for medical evaluation.

Salicylates may cause adverse effects that are independent of the dose. Children and adolescents who have or are recovering from chicken pox or flu are at risk of Reye's syndrome, a rare but serious illness associated with salicylates, and they should not use BSS. In susceptible patients, salicylate-induced gout attacks have occurred. Patients who are sensitive to aspirin (resulting in asthmatic bronchospasm) should not use BSS.

Overdosage of bismuth products can cause neurotoxicity. Blood concentrations of bismuth greater than 50 mg/L have been associated with encephalopathy characterized by slow onset of tremors, postural instability, ataxia, myoclonus, and poor concentration. Confusion, memory impairment, seizures, visual and auditory hallucinations, psychosis, delirium, and depression may also develop. Most patients gradually recover after discontinuation of the bismuth preparation; however, some develop a permanent tremor, and the encephalopathy has resulted in fatality. AIDS patients with acute diarrhea may be at particular risk for bismuth encephalopathy, perhaps resulting from altered GI absorption.[34]

Harmless black staining of stool may occur, which should not be confused with melena; in addition, harmless darkening of the tongue may also occur. These frequent effects occur in more than 10% of patients treated with BSS. Bismuth salts react with hydrogen sulfide produced by bacteria in the mouth and colon. The resulting compound, bismuth sulfide, imparts the black discoloration.

BSS is contraindicated for nursing or pregnant women and should therefore not be used without medical advice. The salicylate moiety may exert antiplatelet effects. BSS should not be used in patients with AIDS because of the risk for neurotoxicity. Bismuth is radiopaque and may interfere with radiographic intestinal studies.

BSS may interact adversely with a number of other drugs, particularly those that potentially interact with aspirin. The salicylate moiety can increase the risk of toxicity with warfarin, valproic acid, and methotrexate by significantly decreasing plasma protein binding of these drugs in vivo. Salicylate can also increase the plasma concentration of methotrexate by decreasing its renal clearance. The uricosuric effects of probenecid may be inhibited by salicylate; the exact mechanism underlying this interaction is not known. The bismuth moiety is a trivalent cation and may decrease absorption of other medications, such as tetracycline and quinolone antibiotics, by forming complexes with them in the GI tract. When ciprofloxacin is used to treat traveler's diarrhea, the patient should be instructed to discontinue BSS. Solid dosage forms of BSS contain calcium carbonate and can also cause the cation complex interaction.

**TABLE 17-8 Selected Lactase Enzyme Products**

| Trade Name | Primary Ingredient |
|---|---|
| Lactaid Caplets* | Lactase enzyme 3000 FCC units/caplet |
| Lactaid Extra Strength Caplets* | Lactase enzyme 4500 FCC units/caplet |
| Lactaid Ultra Caplets* | Lactase enzyme 9000 FCC units/caplet |
| Lactrase Capsules | Lactase enzyme 250 mg/capsule |

* Dye-free.

### Digestive Enzymes

For patients with lactase GI enzyme deficiency, lactase enzyme preparations (Table 17-8) may be taken with milk at mealtimes to prevent osmotic diarrhea.

### Polycarbophil

Polycarbophil is a bulk laxative (see Chapter 16) that has been used to treat diarrhea. However, insufficient effectiveness data are available for polycarbophil and calcium polycarbophil (a simple salt of polycarbophil). This agent has been judged nonmonograph by FDA and should not be recommended for use in acute diarrhea.[31]

### Lactobacillus

The role of probiotics, defined as live organisms that, when ingested, confer a therapeutic or preventive health benefit, is controversial. *Lactobacillus* is a commercially prepared culture of *Lactobacillus acidophilus* often used to help manage or prevent acute, uncomplicated diarrhea; some preparations may contain *L. bulgaricus* or other species. A normal inhabitant of the human GI tract, *L. acidophilus* helps maintain normal GI flora by inhibiting bacterial overgrowth. The exact mechanisms underlying these effects are not clear; it is suggested *Lactobacillus* enhances immune responses, produces antimicrobial substances, and competes with bacteria for intestinal mucosal binding sites.[35]

Evidence demonstrates that probiotic therapy, especially with *Lactobacillus GG* (but also *L. rhamnosus, L. reuteri*), prevents or shortens the course of mild viral diarrhea in infants and young children.[36-38] *Lactobacillus GG* therapy can shorten duration of acute infectious diarrhea in children by an average of 0.7 days and reduce diarrhea frequency on day 2 of treatment by an average of 1.6 stools.[37] Probiotic therapy may also offer clinical benefit in antibiotic-associated diarrhea; a recent meta-analysis reported odds ratios favoring active treatment with live organisms (*Lactobacillus GG, L. acidophilus,* and *Saccharomyces boulardii,* another probiotic agent) over placebo in preventing this

**TABLE 17-9 Selected Antidiarrheal Products**

| | |
|---|---|
| **Loperamide Products** | |
| Imodium A-D Caplets* | Loperamide HCl 2 mg |
| Imodium Advanced Chewable Tablets | Loperamide HCl 2 mg; simethicone 125 mg |
| Imodium A-D Liquid* | Loperamide HCl 1 mg/5 mL |
| **Bismuth Subsalicylate Products** | |
| Kaopectate Liquid*† | Bismuth subsalicylate 262 mg/15 mL |
| Kaopectate Liquid*† | Bismuth subsalicylate 525 mg/15 mL |
| Kaopectate Children's Liquid*†‡ | Bismuth subsalicylate 87 mg/5 mL |
| Pepto-Bismol Caplets | Bismuth subsalicylate 262 mg |
| Pepto-Bismol Chewable Tablets* | Bismuth subsalicylate 262 mg |
| Pepto-Bismol Cherry Chewable Tablets* | Bismuth subsalicylate 262 mg |
| Pepto-Bismol Original Liquid*†§ | Bismuth subsalicylate 262 mg/15 mL |
| Pepto-Bismol Cherry Liquid*†§ | Bismuth subsalicylate 262 mg/15 mL |
| Pepto-Bismol Maximum Strength Liquid*†§ | Bismuth subsalicylate 525 mg/15 mL |

*Lactose-free; †sulfite-free; ‡pediatric formulation; §sucrose-free.

condition.[38] Probiotics appear to be safe; major side effects, such as *Lactobacillus* sepsis, have been reported only rarely.[39] The role of probiotics in bacterial gastroenteritis and moderate to severe diarrhea is not supported conclusively by available evidence. The Food and Agriculture Organization of the United Nations and the WHO have recognized the benefits of probiotics in the prevention and treatment of acute diarrhea.[40] However, *Lactobacillus* is not considered an effective antidiarrheal therapy by FDA; therefore, its use cannot be recommended to treat or prevent acute, uncomplicated diarrhea.

### Product Selection Guidelines

For young children (under 6 years of age), self-treatment is limited to treating dehydration with ORSs. If such solutions are ineffective, a primary care provider must be consulted. Selection of an antidiarrheal product for older children and adults should be based on patient factors such as the etiology of the diarrhea, if known, potential interactions with prescribed medications, and the applicable contraindications. A patient's preference for a particular dosage form or a product that requires fewer doses is another selection criterion. Table 17-7 provides a quick reference for recommended dosages and durations of therapy for selected antidiarrheal agents. Tables 17-8 and 17-9 list dosage forms and primary ingredients of selected trade-name products.

## *Emerging Treatments*

Recent investigations have focused on development of antisecretory agents that inhibit intestinal secretion without altering intestinal motility. Racecadotril, an enkephalinase inhibitor, blocks inactivation of endogenous enkephalins, prolonging their physiologic actions and reducing intestinal secretion of water and electrolytes. Racecadotril has been shown to promptly and significantly reduce total stool output in the 48 to 72 hours after initiation of treatment, significantly shorten the duration of acute diarrhea, and be well tolerated in adults and children as young as 30 months.[41,42] Zaldaride, another antisecretory agent, inhibits intestinal calmodulin to reduce the number of diarrheal stools by 35% to 45% and the duration of diarrhea by approximately 50% in adults with traveler's diarrhea.[43] Provir, a botanical preparation derived from the South American plant *Croton lechleri*, inhibits intestinal chloride ion secretion and effectively reduces the duration of acute diarrhea by 8 hours.[44] Provir is poorly absorbed from the GI tract and associated with a low occurrence of side effects, but is not widely available. These antisecretory agents are more physiologic in their effects than other antidiarrheal therapies and, when available, will likely become standard treatments for managing acute diarrheal symptoms.

Several large studies performed in developing countries have shown that zinc supplementation both prevents acute diarrhea and improves outcomes of acute diarrhea in young children.[45,46] As many as 33% to 45% of these children who are at risk for diarrheal disease are zinc deficient because of poor nutrition; in addition, diarrhea increases intestinal losses of zinc considerably, further compromising zinc status, even in those with normal plasma zinc concentrations.[45,47] Zinc deficiency is associated with impaired cellular and humoral immunity and with adverse GI effects such as impaired water and electrolyte absorption, increased secretion in response to bacterial endotoxin, and decreased brush border enzymes. Daily supplementation with 10 to 40 mg of elemental zinc during acute diarrhea reduces total stool output, frequency of watery stools, and duration and severity of diarrhea.[45,47] The role of zinc supplementation in young children with diarrhea in developed countries is not yet defined.

## *Complementary Therapies*

Many herbal and homeopathic therapies have been used to manage acute diarrhea (Table 17-10).[34,48-50] With the exception of *Lactobacillus* (as discussed previously), there is no evidence to substantiate the safety and effectiveness of these agents in the treatment of acute diarrheal diseases, and their use cannot be recommended.

## Assessment of Diarrhea: A Case-based Approach

To evaluate a patient with diarrhea, the practitioner differentiates symptoms and makes clinical judgments. This triage function is based on the patient's responses to questions designed to help determine the cause of the specific signs and symptoms, their characteristics, and their severity (Tables 17-1 and 17-4). The practitioner should therefore ask the patient about vomiting, high and/or prolonged fever, and other symptoms and determine the patient's susceptibility to complications. Persistent diarrhea, chronic diarrhea, or presence of high fever (greater than 102.2°F [39°C]), protracted vomiting, abdominal pain in patients older than 50 years, or blood or mucus in the stool precludes self-treatment and requires immediate medical referral. If none of these significant findings is present, the degree of dehydration is the next important assessment (Table 17-4); the practitioner should ask about the nature and amount of fluid intake. Severity of dehydration can be accurately assessed by evaluating changes in body weight. For example, in children, mild dehydration is associated with a 3% to 5% loss of body weight, whereas severe dehydration is associated with a loss of more than 9%. However, the patient (or the parent) seldom knows the exact premorbid weight for comparison and distinguishing between mild and moderate dehydration may be difficult.

The initial assessment of a pediatric patient should also seek to determine plausible causes of the symptoms. The common symptoms of acute gastroenteritis (e.g., vomiting, loose stools, and fever) are nonspecific findings associated with many other childhood diseases (e.g., acute otitis media, bacterial sepsis, meningitis, pneumonia, and urinary tract infections). This information is key to recommending a proper course of action, which may include self-treatment or referral to a primary care provider. A complete medication history must be assessed before a product is selected.

Physical assessment of a patient with complaints of diarrhea can provide information useful in assessing severity of the diarrhea (Table 17-4). Checking skin turgor and moistness of oral mucous membranes will help determine the degree of dehydration. Vital signs (e.g., pulse, temperature, respiration, and blood pressure) are important indicators of illness severity and should be routinely measured. Symptoms of moderate to severe dehydration may include postural (orthostatic) hypotension, defined as a drop in the systolic and/or diastolic pressure of greater than 15 to 20 mm Hg on moving from a supine to an upright position. Normally, the diastolic pressure remains the same or increases slightly, and the systolic pressure drops slightly on rising. If the blood pressure drops, the pulse should be checked simultaneously; the pulse rate should increase as blood pressure drops. Failure of the pulse to rise suggests the problem is neurogenic (e.g., diabetic patients with peripheral neuropathy) or the patient is taking a β-blocker. The presence of orthostatic hypotension suggests that the patient has lost 1 L or more of vascular volume and referral for medical care is necessary.

Cases 17-1 and 17-2 provide examples of assessment of patients with diarrhea.

## Patient Counseling for Diarrhea

Patients with diarrhea may focus on the need for a nonprescription medication to stop the frequent bowel movements. The practitioner should remind them that most episodes of acute diarrhea stop after 48 hours and preventing dehydration is the most important component of treating the problem. Counseling on the two-step treatment of dehydration and the need for dietary management should follow. For infants and children, educating parents and caregivers on the appropriate use of an ORS (including appropriate volumes to administer, rates of administration, and use in vomiting) and of dietary management is very important in preventive care. For patient safety reasons, premixed solutions are preferred. Importantly, if dry powder ORS is selected, the practitioner should give parents (or caregivers) explicit directions for mixing and verify that they understand the directions. For families with infants, the CDC recommends a home supply of ORS because early administration of an ORS at home is vital if hospitalization is to be avoided. If travelers are using ORS dry powder in developing countries, potable water should be used to reconstitute the powder.

If a nonspecific antidiarrheal is recommended, the practitioner should review label instructions with the patient. The practitioner should stress an appropriate dosage on the basis of the patient's age and weight, the maximum number of doses per 24 hours, and the auxiliary administration instructions. The practitioner should also explain potential drug interactions, side effects, contraindications, and the maximum duration of treatment before seeking medical help. The box Patient Education for Diarrhea specific information to provide patients.

## Evaluation of Patient Outcomes for Diarrhea

Many patients have mild to moderate diarrhea that is generally self-limiting within 48 hours. Mild to moderate diarrhea is managed with ORT, symptomatic drug therapy, and diet. The patient should be monitored for dehydration by measuring body weight, vital signs, and mental alertness. With effective symptomatic relief, the patient can expect reduced frequency and normal consistency of stools, as well as relief of generalized symptoms such as lethargy and abdominal pain. As the diarrheal episode clears, the appetite will return to normal and the diet can be advanced to a regular diet.

Medical referral is necessary if any of the following signs and symptoms occur before or during treatment: high fever, worsening illness, bloody or mucoid stools, diarrhea continuing beyond 48 hours, or signs of worsening dehydration (e.g., low blood pressure, rapid pulse, mental confusion). Also, medical referral is advised for infants, young children, frail patients of advanced age, and patients with chronic illness at risk from secondary complications (e.g., diabetes mellitus).

**TABLE 17-10 Complementary Therapies for Acute Diarrhea[34,48-50]**

| Agent | Risks | Effectiveness |
|---|---|---|
| **Botanical Medicines (Scientific Name)** | | |
| Acerola (*Malpighia glabra, M. emarginata*) | None reported | Not proven |
| Aletris (*Aletris farinose*) | None reported | Not proven |
| Barberry (*Berberis vulgaris*) | Contraindicated in pregnancy (stimulates uterine contraction) | Berberine alkaloids (berberine and berbamine) demonstrate antimicrobial activity against some enteric pathogens (e.g., *V. cholera, E. coli, G. lamblia*), but efficacy data lacking |
| Chamomile (*Matricaria chamomilla; Anthemis nobile*) | Contraindicated in pregnancy and lactation; suspected abortifacient; some components of chamomile possibly teratogenic; possible hypersensitivity reactions (anaphylaxis, urticaria, contact sensitivity) | Not proven |
| Chinese rhubarb (*Rheum palmatum*) | Contraindicated in pregnancy and lactation, ulcers, IBDs (e.g., colitis) | Not proven |
| Meadowsweet (*Filipendula ulmaria;* synonym *Spiraea ulmaria*) | Contraindicated in patients with salicylate sensitivity (active constituents include salicylates); safety in pregnancy and lactation not established | Not proven; no known adverse effects but classified by FDA as herb of undefined safety |
| Nutmeg (*Myristica fragrans*) | Toxic effects (hallucinations, confusion, tachycardia, nausea, vomiting, anticholinergic effects, seizures, acute psychosis, death); contraindicated in pregnancy and lactation | Not recommended because of toxicity risk |
| Oak bark (*Quercus robur, Q. petraea*) | None reported | Not proven |
| Pulsatilla (*Pulsatilla vulgaris, P. pratensis, P. patens*) | Fresh pulsatilla contains known toxin (protoanemonin, one main active constituent) and should not be consumed; documented allergic reactions have been documented; contraindicated in pregnancy | Not recommended for use because of toxicity |
| Quince (*Cydonia oblongata*) | None reported but contains a toxic, amygdalin; should not be consumed | Not recommended |
| Tormentil (*Potentilla erecta*) | None reported | Not proven; documentation of clinical benefit lacking |
| **Homeopathic Medicines** | | |
| Arsenicum album (common names: arsenic trioxide, white arsenic, white oxide of metallic arsenic, and arsenious acid) | None reported | Not proven |
| Mercurous corrosives | None reported | Not proven |
| Podophyllum (sources: *Podophyllum peltatum, P. hexandrum royale*) | Significant systemic toxicity: hypokalemia, neurologic effects ranging from confusion to coma, muscle paralysis with respiratory failure, renal failure, seizures and bone marrow suppression | Not recommended because of toxicity; efficacy not documented |
| Sulfur | None | Not proven |
| Veratrum (source: *Veratrum album*) | Considered toxic: cardiac arrhythmias, respiratory depression, GI distress | Not proven |

Key: GI, gastrointestinal; IBD, inflammatory bowel disease.

## CASE 17-1

| Relevant Evaluation Criteria | Scenario/Model Outcome |
|---|---|
| **Information Gathering** | |
| 1. Gather essential information about the patient's symptoms, including: | |
| a. description of symptom(s) (i.e., nature, onset, duration, severity, associated symptoms) | Mother reports that the patient has had multiple episodes of watery diarrhea, vomiting, and a fever of 100.8°F (38.2°C) for 24 hours. The patient has had 4 to 5 loose stools and 4 to 5 episodes of emesis. |
| b. description of any factors that seem to precipitate, exacerbate, and/or relieve the patient's symptoms. | No precipitating factors are present. Patient had previously been well. |
| c. description of the patient's efforts to relieve the symptoms | Mother has been giving the patient tea and apple juice and encouraged the patient to eat burnt toast and bananas. There has been no change in symptoms. |
| 2. Gather essential patient history information: | |
| a. patient's identity | Alex Wilson |
| b. age, sex, height, and weight | 4 y/o M, 3'1", 32 lb |
| c. patient's occupation | None |
| d. patient's dietary habits | Normal healthy diet. Since the onset of illness, Alex has not eaten much. Mother reports he has eaten some cereal, banana, and toast, and taken small amounts of tea and apple juice in the last 24 hours. |
| e. patient's sleep habits | Normal, averaging 9-10 hours/night |
| f. concurrent medical conditions, prescription and nonprescription medications, and dietary supplements | History of mild, persistent asthma; uses budesonide and albuterol by nebulization. Symptoms are under control. |
| g. allergies | Penicillin–hives |
| h. history of other adverse reactions to medications | None |
| i. other (describe)_______ | Mother states that Alex complains of thirst, dry mouth, and slight dizziness when he stands up. There is no blood or mucus in the stool or emesis. Mother also reports that Alex's 6-year-old sibling had similar symptoms a few days ago and recovered uneventfully. |
| **Assessment and Triage** | |
| 3. Differentiate the patient's signs/symptoms and correctly identify the patient's primary problem(s) (see Tables 17-1 and 17-4). | Alex has acute gastroenteritis, most likely of viral etiology, with mild to moderate dehydration. |
| 4. Identify exclusions for self-treatment (see Figure 17-1). | No exclusions for self-treatment |
| 5. Formulate a comprehensive list of therapeutic alternatives for the primary problem to determine if triage to a medical practitioner is required, and share this information with the caregiver. | Options include:<br>(1) Recommend self-care with an appropriate OTC product and nondrug therapies.<br>(2) Recommend self-care until a primary care provider can be consulted.<br>(3) Refer Alex for further evaluation and treatment.<br>(4) Take no action. |
| **Plan** | |
| 6. Select an optimal therapeutic alternative to address the patient's problem, taking into account patient preferences. | OTC treatment with an ORS is appropriate to manage mild to moderate dehydration. Vomiting is not a contraindication to use of ORS. (See Table 17-5 and the box Patient Education for Diarrhea.)<br>Pharmacologic intervention with OTC antidiarrheal products is not appropriate for children with acute diarrheal illness and should not be recommended. |

## CASE 17-1 (continued)

| Relevant Evaluation Criteria | Scenario/Model Outcome |
|---|---|
| 7. Describe the recommended therapeutic approach to the caregiver. | See Figure 17-1 and the box Patient Education for Diarrhea. |
| 8. Explain to the caregiver the rationale for selecting the recommended therapeutic approach from the considered therapeutic alternatives. | Treatment with ORS is appropriate for Alex because (1) acute gastroenteritis is usually self-limited; (2) mild to moderate dehydration can be effectively treated and ongoing fluid and electrolyte losses managed with ORS; and (3) no risk factors for significant complications are present. If the condition does not resolve in 48-72 hours or worsens, you should take Alex to his PCP for evaluation. |
| **Patient Education** | |
| 9. When recommending self-care with nonprescription medications and/or nondrug therapy, convey accurate information to the caregiver, including: | |
| a. appropriate dose and frequency of administration | See Figure 17-1 and the box Patient Education for Diarrhea. |
| b. maximum number of days the therapy should be employed | ORS may be used as a supplement to a normal diet and as maintenance fluids until the illness resolves. |
| c. product administration procedures | See Figure 17-1 and the box Patient Education for Diarrhea. If Alex continues to vomit, administer recommended amount of ORS in 5 mL portions every 1-2 minutes. |
| d. expected time to onset of relief | Mild to moderate dehydration should be corrected over 2-4 hours. |
| e. degree of relief that can be reasonably expected | ORS should completely relieve mild to moderate dehydration. |
| f. most common side effects | None |
| g. side effects that warrant medical intervention should they occur | None |
| h. patient options in the event that condition worsens or persists | Seek medication attention if the diarrhea or dehydration worsens, high fever develops, or blood or mucus appears in the stool. |
| i. product storage requirements | None |
| j. specific nondrug measures | Give Alex a normal diet as soon as possible. A diet of apple juice, tea, bananas, and toast is not appropriate because its nutrient content is inadequate. |
| 10. Solicit follow-up questions from caregiver. | May I give him anything for the fever? Is there anything I may give him to help stop the vomiting? |
| 11. Answer caregiver's questions. | Acetaminophen or ibuprofen would be appropriate if the fever needs to be reduced (see Chapter 6). However, the vomiting should resolve on its own, and, although it is uncomfortable for Alex, antiemetic drugs are not recommended. |

Key: OTC, over-the-counter; ORS, oral rehydration solution; PCP, primary care provider.

## CASE 17-2

| Relevant Evaluation Criteria | Scenario/Model Outcome |
|---|---|
| **Information Gathering** | |
| 1. Gather essential information about the patient's symptoms, including: | |
| a. description of symptom(s) (i.e., nature, onset, duration, severity, associated symptoms) | Patient complains of sudden onset of watery diarrhea, nausea, and vomiting that began 6 hours ago. Patient reports having 4 to 5 loose, watery stools and several episodes of emesis since the onset of illness. She is afebrile and there is no blood or mucus in the stool. She complains of mild, diffuse abdominal pain and cramping. |

## CASE 17-2 (continued)

| Relevant Evaluation Criteria | Scenario/Model Outcome |
|---|---|
| b. description of any factors that seem to precipitate, exacerbate, and/or relieve the patient's symptoms. | Patient reports having been well. She reports having had shellfish and salad for lunch (approximately 6 hours ago). |
| c. description of the patient's efforts to relieve the symptoms | Patient has not tried to treat GI symptoms. |
| 2. Gather essential patient history information: | |
| a. patient's identity | Martha Benson |
| b. age, sex, height, and weight | 44 y/o F, 5'6", 140 lb |
| c. patient's occupation | Computer analyst |
| d. patient's dietary habits | Normal healthy diet with no recent changes in diet noted |
| e. patient's sleep habits | Sleeps well, 7-8 hours/night on average |
| f. concurrent medical conditions, prescription and nonprescription medications, and dietary supplements | None |
| g. allergies | NKA |
| h. history of other adverse reactions to medications | None |
| i. other (describe)______ | Ms. Benson's buccal mucous membranes are moist. She has no symptoms to suggest mild to moderate dehydration is present. |
| **Assessment and Triage** | |
| 3. Differentiate the patient's signs/symptoms and correctly identify the patient's primary problem(s) (see Tables 17-1 and 17-4). | Acute uncomplicated gastroenteritis likely caused by foodborne illness, most likely of bacterial etiology. No signs or symptoms of dehydration are present. |
| 4. Identify exclusions for self-treatment (see Figure 17-1). | None |
| 5. Formulate a comprehensive list of therapeutic alternatives for the primary problem to determine if triage to a medical practitioner is required, and share this information with the patient. | Options include:<br>(1) Recommend self-care with an appropriate OTC product and nondrug therapies.<br>(2) Recommend self-care until a primary care provider can be consulted.<br>(3) Refer Ms. Benson for further evaluation and treatment.<br>(4) Take no action. |
| **Plan** | |
| 6. Select an optimal therapeutic alternative to address the patient's problem, taking into account patient preferences. | OTC treatment with loperamide is appropriate. BSS may be recommended as an alternative because of the vomiting although it is less effective than loperamide in most cases. (See Table 17-9 and the box Patient Education for Diarrhea.) |
| 7. Describe the recommended therapeutic approach to the patient. | See Table 17-7 and the box Patient Education for Diarrhea. |
| 8. Explain to the patient the rationale for selecting the recommended therapeutic approach from the considered therapeutic alternatives. | Treatment with loperamide or bismuth subsalicylate is appropriate because (1) acute uncomplicated gastroenteritis is usually self-limited; (2) you are well-hydrated with no evidence of dehydration; and (3) you have no risk factors that would place you at risk for significant complications. If the condition does not resolve in 48-72 hours, you should see your PCP. |
| **Patient Education** | |
| 9. When recommending self-care with nonprescription medications and/or nondrug therapy, convey accurate information to the patient, including: | |

**CASE 17-2 (continued)**

| Relevant Evaluation Criteria | Scenario/Model Outcome |
|---|---|
| a. appropriate dose and frequency of administration | See Table 17-7. |
| b. maximum number of days the therapy should be employed | Loperamide and BSS should not be used for more than 48 hours. |
| c. product administration procedures | For BSS, shake the liquid well before using. Chew the tablets or allow them to dissolve slowly in the mouth. |
| d. expected time to onset of relief | With loperamide, the onset of effect is 30-60 minutes; most patients experience relief (no occurrence of unformed stools) within 48-72 hours. The onset of effect of BSS is 4 hours, with significant relief in symptoms of diarrhea, nausea, and abdominal pain within 24 hours. |
| e. degree of relief that can be reasonably expected | Complete eradication of symptoms is expected. |
| f. most common side effects | Loperamide: occasional dizziness, constipation; BSS: black discoloration of tongue and stool |
| g. side effects that warrant medical intervention should they occur | Loperamide: bloating, severe constipation (see Chapter 16), loss of appetite, severe abdominal pain with nausea and vomiting, skin rash<br>BSS: tinnitus |
| h. patient options in the event that condition worsens or persists | Seek medical attention if diarrhea worsens, high fever develops, or blood or mucus appears in the stool. |
| i. product storage requirements | Keep both loperamide and BSS out of children's reach. Store away from heat, moisture, and direct light. |
| j. specific nondrug measures | You should maintain your fluid intake and eat your regular diet, but avoid fatty foods, sugar-rich foods, and spicy foods that might worsen your diarrhea. |
| 10. Solicit follow-up questions from patient. | What are the first signs of dehydration? |
| 11. Answer patient's questions. | Your mouth will feel slightly dry, and you will notice increased thirst. You may also experience a slight decrease in the volume of urine. |

Key: GI, gastrointestinal; NKA, no known allergies; OTC, over-the-counter; BSS, bismuth subsalicylate; PCP, primary care provider.

## Key Points for Diarrhea

- Limit the self-treatment of diarrhea to patients with acute diarrhea who have minimal, mild, or moderate dehydration. Patients who appear volume-depleted, weak, dizzy, or hypotensive should be referred for evaluation, as should all patients with severely acute, uncontrolled, or chronic complaints involving the GI tract.
- Oral rehydration solutions are the mainstay of therapy and should be used to rehydrate patients with minimal, mild, or moderate dehydration.
- Rehydration should be performed rapidly (i.e., within 3-4 hours; Figures 17-1 and 17-2).
- Additional ORS should be given to maintain hydration and replace ongoing fluid losses through diarrheal stools and/or vomiting (Figures 17-1 and 17-2).
- Instruct patients or their caregivers how to prepare and administer ORS.
- Older children and adults may use sports drinks instead of ORS, if additional sources of sodium (e.g., crackers, pretzels) are used concomitantly.
- An age-appropriate, unrestricted diet should be initiated as soon as the patient is rehydrated. Food should be withheld for no more than 24 hours.
- Loperamide and BSS may be used to help control acute diarrhea in carefully selected patients.
- Antibiotic therapy is generally not indicated for patients with acute diarrhea unless it is traveler's diarrhea.

## References


1. Mead PS, Slutsker L, Dietz V, et al. Food-related illness and death in the United States. *Emerg Infect Dis.* 1999;5:607-25.
2. Herikstad H, Yang S, Van Gilder TJ, et al. A population-based estimate of the burden of diarrhoeal illness in the United States: FoodNet, 1996-7. *Epidemiol Infect.* 2002;129:9-17.
3. Peterson CA, Calderon RL. Trends in enteric disease as a cause of death in the United States, 1989-1996. *Am J Epidemiol.* 2003; 157:58-65.
4. Gilbert DN, Moellering RC, Eliopoulos GM, et al. *The Sanford Guide to Antimicrobial Therapy.* 34th ed. Hyde Park, Vt: Antimicrobial Therapy; 2004:11-13, 93.
5. Campylobacter infections. In: *AAP 2003 Red Book: Report of the Committee on Infectious Diseases.* 26th ed. Elk Grove, Ill: American Academy of Pediatrics; 2003: 227-9, 702-12.
6. Ericsson CD. Travellers' diarrhoea. *Int J Antimicrob Agents.* 2003; 21:116-24.

## PATIENT EDUCATION FOR DIARRHEA

The primary objective of self-treatment is to prevent excessive fluid and electrolyte losses. For most patients, carefully following product instructions and the self-care measures listed here will help ensure optimal outcomes.

### Nondrug Measures

#### *Infants and Children 5 Years and Younger*

- For mild to moderate diarrhea, indicated by three to five unformed bowel movements per day, give the child or infant an oral rehydration solution (ORS) at a volume of 50 to 100 mL/kg of body weight over 2 to 4 hours to replace the fluid deficit. Give additional ORS to replace ongoing losses. Continue to give the solution for the next 4 to 6 hours or until the child is rehydrated.
- If the child is vomiting, give 1 teaspoon of ORS every few minutes.
- If the child is not dehydrated, give 10 mL/kg or 1/2 to 1 cup of the ORS for each bowel movement or 2 mL/kg for each episode of vomiting. As an alternative, to replace ongoing fluid losses, children weighing less than 10 kg should be given 60 to 120 mL of ORS for each episode of vomiting or diarrheal stool, and children weighing greater than 10 kg should be given 120 to 240 mL for each episode of vomiting or diarrheal stool.
- After the child is rehydrated, reintroduce food appropriate for the child's age while also administering oral solutions as maintenance therapy:
  - If breast-feeding an infant with diarrhea, continue the breast-feeding. If the infant is bottle-fed, consult your doctor or pediatrician about substituting a milk-based formula with a lactose-free formula.
  - Give children complex carbohydrate-rich foods, yogurt, lean meats, fruits, and vegetables. Do not give them fatty foods or sugary foods. Sugary foods can cause osmotic diarrhea.
  - Do not withhold food for more than 24 hours.

#### *Adults and Children Older Than 5 Years*

- For mild to moderate dehydration, indicated by a 3% to 9% drop in body weight or three to five unformed stools per day, drink 2 to 4 L of an ORS over 4 hours.
- If not dehydrated, drink 1/2 to 1 cup of ORS or fluids after each unformed bowel movement.
- If you have no medical conditions, you may consume sport drinks, diluted juices, salty crackers, soups, and broths until the diarrhea stops.
- Do not withhold food for more than 24 hours.

### Nonprescription Medications

- See Table 17-7 for dosages of loperamide and bismuth subsalicylate.

#### *Loperamide*

- Note that loperamide can cause dizziness and constipation.
- Do not take this agent if you are taking sedatives, antianxiety drugs, or other antidepressants.
- Do not give this agent to children 2 years of age or younger. Loperamide is not recommended for children younger than 6 years, except under the supervision of a primary care provider.
- If loperamide is not effective in treating your diarrhea (if no clinical improvement is observed in 48 hours), check with your primary care provider or pharmacist about using a different nonprescription medication. You may have a bacterial diarrhea or pseudomembranous colitis, conditions requiring specific antibiotic therapy that loperamide cannot treat.

#### *Bismuth Subsalicylate*

- Note that bismuth subsalicylate can cause a dark discoloration of the tongue and stool.
- Do not take this agent if you are taking tetracyclines, quinolones, or medicines for gout (uricosurics).
- Do not give this agent to children younger than 12 years of age.
- Do not give this agent to children or teenagers who have or are recovering from influenza or chicken pox. Reye's syndrome, a rare but serious condition, could occur.
- Do not give this agent to patients with AIDS.[29]
- Do not take this agent if you are sensitive to aspirin, have a history of GI bleeding, or have a history of problems with blood coagulation.

⚠ If the diarrhea has not resolved after 72 hours of initial treatment, see your primary care provider.

⚠ Monitor for excessive number of bowel movements, signs of dehydration, high fever, or blood in the stool. If any of these complications are present, discontinue bismuth subsalicylate and consult your primary care provider.


7. Bailey JM, Erramouspe J. Nitazoxanide treatment for giardiasis and cryptosporidiosis in children. *Ann Pharmacother.* 2004;38:634-40.
8. Vesy CJ, Peterson WL. Review article: the management of giardiasis. *Aliment Pharmacol Ther.* 1999;13:843-50.
9. Guerrant RL, Van Gilder T, Steiner TS, et al. Practice guidelines for the management of infectious diarrhea. *Clin Infect Dis.* 2001;32:331-50.
10. Centers for Disease Control and Prevention. Outbreaks of gastroenteritis associated with noroviruses on cruise ships–United States, 2002. *MMWR Morb Mortal Wkly Rep.* 2002;51:1112-5.
11. Centers for Disease Control and Prevention. Withdrawal of rotavirus vaccine recommendation. *MMWR Morb Mortal Wkly Rep.* 1999;48:1007-8.
12. Hopes and fears for rotavirus vaccines. *Lancet.* 2005.365(9455):190.
13. Allos BM. Campylobacter jejuni infections: update on emerging issues and trends. *Clin Infect Dis.* 2001;32:1201-6.
14. Preliminary FoodNet data on the incidence of infection with pathogens transmitted commonly through food selected sites, United States, 2003. *MMWR Morb Mortal Wkly Rep.* 2004;53:338-43.
15. Adachi JA, Zhi-Dong J, Mathewson JJ, et al. Enteroaggregative Escherichia coli as a major etiologic agent in traveler's diarrhea in 3 regions of the world. *Clin Infect Dis.* 2001;32:1706-9.
16. Neal KR, Hebden J, Spiller R. Prevalence of gastrointestinal symptoms six months after bacterial gastroenteritis and risk factors for development of the irritable bowel syndrome: postal survey. *BMJ.* 1997;314:779-82.

17. Wang LH, Fang XC, Pan GZ. Bacillary dysentery as a causative factor of irritable bowel syndrome and its pathogenesis. *Gut.* 2004;53:1096-101.
18. Garcia LA, Ruigomez A. Increased risk of irritable bowel syndrome after acute gastroenteritis: cohort study. *BMJ.* 1999;318:565-6.
19. Chassany O, Michaux A, Bergmann JF. Drug-induced diarrhea. *Drug Safety.* 2000;22:53-72.
20. Bartlett JG. Antibiotic-associated diarrhea. *N Engl J Med.* 2002; 346:334-9.
21. Mylonakis E, Ryan ET, Calderwood SB. Clostridium difficile-associated diarrhea. *Arch Intern Med.* 2001;161: 525-33.
22. Beaugerie L. Antibiotic-associated diarrhoea. *Best Practice Res Clin Gastroenterol.* 2004;18:337-52.
23. King CK, Glass R, Bresee JS, et al. Managing acute gastroenteritis among children: oral rehydration, maintenance, and nutritional therapy. *MMWR Morb Mortal Wkly Rep.* 2003;52(RR-16):1-16.
24. Davidson G, Barnes G, Bass D, et al. Infectious diarrhea in children: working group report of the First World Congress of Pediatric Gastroenterology, Hepatology, and Nutrition. *J Pediatr Gastroenterol Nutr.* 2002;35(suppl 2):S143-50.
25. Guerrant RL, Kosek M, Moore S, et al. Magnitude and impact of diarrheal diseases. *Arch Med Res.* 2002;33:351-5.
26. Wingate D, Phillips SF, Lewis SJ, et al. Guidelines for adults on self-medication for the treatment of acute diarrhea. *Aliment Pharmacol Ther.* 2001;15:773-82.
27. Oral rehydration salts (ORS): a new reduced osmolarity formulation. Available at: http://www.who.int/child-adolescent-health/NewPublications/NEWS/Statement.htm. Accessed August 31, 2004.
28. Hahn S, Kim Y, Garner P. Reduced osmolarity oral rehydration solution for treating dehydration due to diarrheoa in children: systematic review. *BMJ.* 2001;323:81-5.
29. Expert consultation on oral rehydration salts (ORS) formulation. WHO/Unicef. Available at: http://rehydrate.org/ors/expert-consultation.html. Accessed September 8, 2004.
30. Fontaine O, Gore SM, Pierce NF. Rice-based oral rehydration solution for treating diarrhoea. *Cochrane Database of Systematic Reviews* [database online]. Oxford: Update Software; 2001: 2000; 4(2):CD001264
31. Antidiarrheal drug products for over-the-counter human use: final monograph. *Federal Register.* 2003;68:18869-82.
32. Centers for Disease Control. Traveler's Diarrhea. Available at: http://www.cdc.gov/travel/diarrhea.htm. Accessed June 9, 2005.
33. Antidiarrheal drug products for over-the-counter human use; amendment of final monograph. *Fed Register.* 2004;69:26301-02.
34. MICROMEDEX® Healthcare Series. Greenwood, Colo: Thomson MICROMEDEX. (Edition expires 2005).
35. Isolauri E, Sutas Y, Kankaanpaa P, et al. Probiotics: effects on immunity. *Am J Clin Nutr.* 2001;73(suppl):444S-50S.
36. Guandalini S, Pensabene L, Zikri MA, et al. *Lactobacillus GG* administered in oral rehydration solution to children with acute diarrhea: a multicenter European trial. *J Pediatr Gastroenterol Nutr.* 2000;30:54-60.
37. Van Neil CW, Feudtner C, Garrison MM, et al. Lactobacillus therapy for acute infectious diarrhea in children: a meta analysis. *Pediatrics.* 2002;109:678-84.
38. D'Souza AL, Rajkumar C, Cooke J, et al. Probiotics in prevention of antibiotic associated diarrhea: meta-analysis. *BMJ.* 2002;324: 1361-6.
39. Land MH, Rouster-Stevens K, Woods, CR, et al. Lactobacillus sepsis associated with probiotic therapy. *Pediatrics.* 2005;115:178-81.
40. FAO/WHO. Health and nutritional properties of probiotics in food including milk with live lactic acid bacteria. Food and Agriculture Organization of the United Nations and the World Health Organization Expert Consultation Report. Available at: http://www.who.int/foodsafety/publications/fs_management/probiotics/en/. Accessed February 8, 2005.
41. Salazar-Lindo E, Santisteban-Ponce J, Chea-Woo E, et al. Racecadotril in the treatment of acute watery diarrhea in children. *N Engl J Med.* 2000;343:463-7.
42. Prado D. A multinational comparison of racecadotril and loperamide in the treatment of acute watery diarrhea. *Scand J Gastroenterol.* 2002;37:656-61.
43. DuPont HL, Ericsson CD, Mathewson JJ, et al. Zaldaride maleate, an intestinal calmodulin inhibitor, in the therapy of travelers' diarrhea. *Gastroenterology.* 1993;104:709-15.
44. DiCesare D, DuPont HL, Mathewson JJ, et al. A double blind, randomized, placebo-controlled study of SP-303 (Provir) in the symptomatic treatment of acute diarrhea among travelers to Jamaica and Mexico. *Am J Gastroenterol.* 2002;97:2585-8.
45. Bahl R, Bhandari N, Saksena M, et al. Efficacy of zinc-fortified oral rehydration solution in 6-to 35-month-old children with acute diarrhea. *J Pediatr.* 2002;141:677-82.
46. Strand TA, Chandyo RK, Bhal R, et al. Effectiveness and efficacy of zinc for the treatment of acute diarrhea in young children. *Pediatrics.* 2002;109:898-903.
47. Bhandari N, Bahl R, Taneja S, et al. Substantial reduction in severe diarrheal morbidity by daily zinc supplementation in young north Indian children. *Pediatrics.* 2002;109:e86.
48. Robbers JE, Tyler VE. *Tyler's Herbs of Choice: The Therapeutic Use of Phytomedicinals.* New York: Haworth Herbal Press; 1999:69-70.
49. Blumenthal M, Goldberg A, Brinckman J, eds. *Herbal Medicine: Expanded Commission E Monographs.* Newton, Mass: Integrative Medicine Communications; 2000:57-61, 253-6, 278-80.
50. DerMarderosian A, Beutler JA, eds. *The Review of Natural Products.* St. Louis: Facts and Comparisons; 2003.

CHAPTER 18

# Anorectal Disorders

*Juliana Chan and Rosemary R. Berardi*

Anorectal disorders involve the perianal area, the anal canal, and the lower rectum. Many signs and symptoms associated with hemorrhoids may also be related to nonhemorroidal anorectal disorders.[1] Hemorrhoids, also known as piles, can often be self-treated, whereas other anorectal disorders may require medical attention. This chapter focuses on the self-treatment of hemorrhoids and recognition of signs and symptoms requiring medical evaluation.[1]

A number of nonprescription products are available for the symptomatic treatment of anorectal disorders. An estimated two million prescriptions are written annually for anorectal products, and pharmacists recommend a hemorrhoidal preparation at least once every 30 days.[2] Total dollar sales for nonprescription hemorrhoidal remedies reached $83 million in 2001, up 18% from the previous year.[3,4]

## Epidemiology of Hemorrhoids

More than 10 million people in the United States complain of hemorrhoidal symptoms, a prevalence of about 5%.[2] However, the true prevalence of hemorrhoids is unknown as fewer than one third of individuals with hemorrhoids seek medical attention.[2] Hemorrhoids are more common in men than in women and increase with advancing age, peaking between the ages of 45 and 74 years.[2] In the United States, whites self-report hemorrhoidal symptoms 1.6 times more often than blacks.[2] Although epidemiologic data are lacking, the incidence of hemorrhoids is higher among pregnant women than nonpregnant women of similar childbearing age, particularly in the postpartum period.[5,6]

## Anatomy and Physiology of the Anorectal Area

Anorectal disorders occur in the perianal area, anal canal, and lower portion of the rectum (Figure 18-1). The perianal area is the portion of the skin and buttocks immediately surrounding the anus. The presence of sensory nerve endings makes this area very sensitive to pain. Perianal tissue differs from other skin tissue in that it is normally moister than exposed skin in other areas of the body.

The anal canal (about 4 cm long) is the channel connecting the end of the gastrointestinal (GI) tract (rectum) with the outside of the body.[7] The lower two thirds of the canal is covered by modified anal skin, which is structurally similar to the skin covering other parts of the body. Different types of epithelium line the anal canal and are defined by the dentate line, which is also referred to as the pectinate line. This dentate line divides the squamous epithelium from the columnar epithelium, and also delineates where sensory pain fibers occur in the anal canal. Thus, anorectal disorders that occur below the dentate line may be associated with pain, whereas those disorders above the line rarely cause any discomfort. The epithelium above the dentate line forms longitudinal folds known as the columns of Morgagni. In between and next to these columns are small pockets or crypts located at the lower end of the anal canal. These pockets are important because they may be obstructed by foreign material, possibly causing infections such as abscesses and fistulas. The external sphincter is a voluntary muscle located at the bottom of the anal canal that remains closed under normal conditions to prevent the involuntary passage of feces or discharges. The internal sphincter, which is innervated by the autonomic nervous system, is an involuntary muscle that is responsible for defecation.

In healthy individuals, the skin covering the anal canal serves as a barrier against absorption of substances into the body. Therefore, topical agents applied to this area may manifest primarily local effects. However, if there is a loss or break in the protective barrier, then the absorptive character of the anal canal skin may be altered, thereby diminishing the skin's protective capabilities.

The rectum is approximately 12 cm long and is the terminal portion of the large intestine that lies above the anal canal. It extends from the dentate line up to the sigmoid colon. The rectal mucosa is lined with a semipermeable membrane that is highly vascular and contains no sensory pain fibers. Similar to the anal canal, the rectum contains pressure receptors and a mucous membrane that protects the body from invasion by bacteria present in feces.

The most prominent parts of the vasculature in the region above and below the dentate line are three hemorrhoidal arteries and their accompanying veins. Arteries and veins lying above the dentate line are referred to as internal; those below are referred to as external. Because of the plexus of internal hemorrhoidal vessels located beneath the rectal mucosa, and the path followed by blood returning to the heart through the hemorrhoidal veins, rectally administered medications may be absorbed and enter the systemic circulation without passing through the liver.[7]

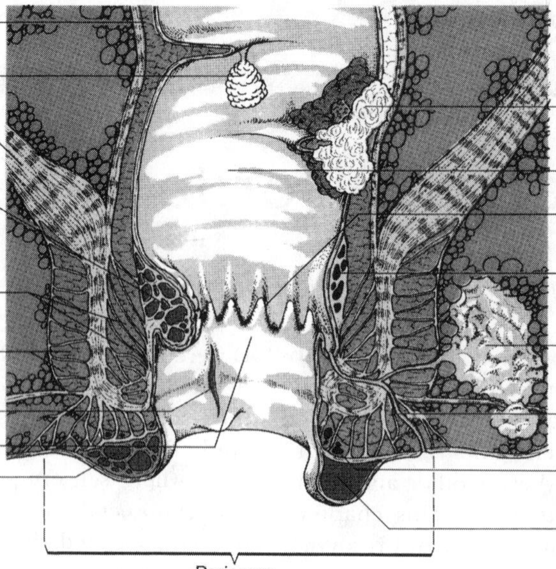


**FIGURE 18-1** Disorders of the anorectal canal.

## Etiology of Hemorrhoids

Hemorrhoids are abnormally large, bulging, symptomatic conglomerates of hemorrhoidal vessels, supporting tissues, and overlying mucous membranes or skin in the anorectal region. Many factors have been implicated in the etiology of hemorrhoids, including erect posture, pregnancy, prolonged standing or sitting, lack of dietary fiber, constipation, diarrhea, and heavy lifting with straining. Symptomatic hemorrhoids appear to develop in susceptible individuals. Although data are conflicting, heredity may play an important role. Socioeconomics, cultural factors (e.g., diet, number of meals a day, and lifestyle) and geographic location may be related to hemorrhoid formation.[2,8] Although there is insufficient evidence to support a relationship between dietary fiber intake and the development of hemorrhoids, increasing dietary fiber may reduce pain and bleeding associated with defecation in patients with hemorrhoids.[9] Bowel habits, such as straining at defecation or prolonged sitting on the toilet, may increase pressure within the hemorrhoidal vessels and precipitate the formation of hemorrhoids.[7] Alternatively, constipation may follow the onset of hemorrhoidal symptoms and improve with prolapse.[10,11] Hormonal changes and the gravid uterus may increase pressure in the hemorrhoidal veins, leading to the formation of hemorrhoids during pregnancy.[5,7]

## Pathophysiology of Anorectal Disorders

### *Hemorrhoids*

The most widely accepted pathophysiologic theory is that vascular cushions are part of the normal anatomy and are located circumferentially around the anal canal above the dentate line. The cushions are present at birth in three discrete masses and, by partially occluding the anus, contribute to continence. These cushions contain blood vessels, smooth muscle, and supportive connective tissue that project into the lumen, where they are subject to downward pressure during defecation. In younger individuals, the muscle fibers anchor the cushions and support the venous sinusoidal vessels. Hemorrhoids develop with increasing age, when the muscle fibers become weakened. The vascular cushions slide, become congested, bleed, and eventually protrude.[7] Downward pressure during defecation and a high resting anal pressure are both common denominators in developing hemorrhoids.[7] Hemorrhoids may originate either from the superior hemorrhoidal vein, producing internal hemorrhoids, or from the inferior hemorrhoidal vein, forming external hemorrhoids (Figure 18-1).[12]

#### Internal Hemorrhoids

Internal hemorrhoids occurring above the dentate line are covered with columnar epithelium and lack sensory fibers.[12] Internal hemorrhoids are graded by severity of prolapse into the anal canal using a degree system: first-degree hemorrhoids are enlarged but do not prolapse into the anal canal, second-degree hemorrhoids protrude into the anal canal and return spontaneously on defecation, third-degree hemorrhoids protrude into the anal canal on defecation but can be returned manually, and fourth-degree hemorrhoids are permanently prolapsed and cannot be reintroduced into the anus.[12]

#### External Hemorrhoids

External hemorrhoids develop below the dentate line and are covered with squamous epithelium; unlike internal hemorrhoids, they do have sensory fibers. External hemorrhoids are frequently visible as bluish lumps at the external or distal boundary of the anal canal (also known as the anal verge). The blue color may be caused by thrombosed blood vessels in the complex. Symptoms of thrombosed external hemorrhoids range from minimal discomfort to severe pain.[10,12]

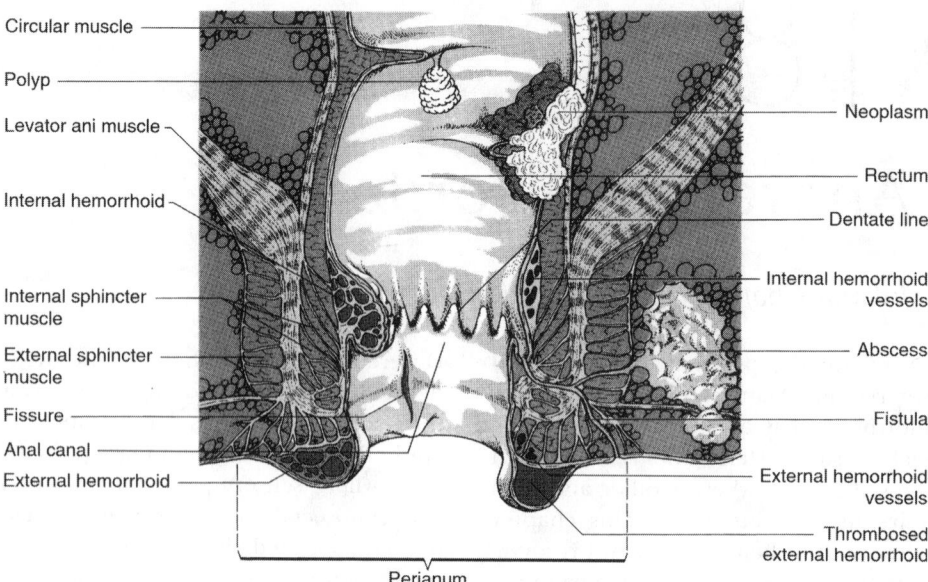

TABLE 18-1 Nonhemorrhoidal Anorectal Disorders[1,12-18]

| Disorder | Etiology/Pathophysiology | Common Signs and Symptoms | Comments |
|---|---|---|---|
| Anal abscess | Obstruction of anal glands, resulting in painful swelling in perianal or anal canal; usually leads to bacterial infection | Fever, local swelling, redness, tenderness, and a continuously painful bulge in the rectal or gluteal regions | Usually identified on history and physical examination; possible life-threatening sepsis if not identified and treated promptly |
| Anal fistula (or groove) | Unhealed or incomplete drainage of anorectal abscess located between internal and external opening of fistula tract, and manifested as hollow fibrous area lined with granulation tissue | Chronic, persistent drainage; pain; possible bleeding on defecation | Surgical repair required |
| Anal fissure | Slitlike ulcer in anal canal within or around anal verge | Pain during and after defecation, lasting several minutes to several hours; if bleeding is present, blood is usually seen on toilet tissue | Underlying disorders: IBD, tuberculosis, STIs, neoplasm, or HIV/AIDS |
| Anal neoplasms | | Bleeding, changes in bowel habits, constipation, diarrhea, anal discharge, an internal or external mass, pain, pruritus, or rash; asymptomatic in about 25% of patients | Relatively uncommon, accounting for 1%-2% of all GI malignancies; most are curable, but poor prognosis with anorectal melanomas (approx. 20% 5-year survival rate) |
| Polyps | Pedunculated growth that arises from GI mucosa and extends into lumen of body cavity; usually found in colon but may also be present in anal canal | Bleeding | May be benign or malignant |
| Pruritus ani | Usually associated with primary underlying condition (e.g., anorectal or dermatologic disorder); other causes: diet (e.g., caffeinated or dairy products), lifestyle preferences (e.g., dyed or scented toilet paper or soaps, tight clothing), or medications (e.g., mineral oil, antibiotics) | Persistent itching in perianal region; more bothersome at bedtime or when patient is not preoccupied | Affects men more often than women |

Key: AIDS, acquired immune deficiency syndrome; GI, gastrointestinal; HIV, human immunodeficiency virus; IBD, inflammatory bowel disease; STI, sexually transmitted infection.

### *Nonhemorrhoidal Anorectal Disorders*

Potentially serious nonhemorrhoidal anorectal disorders, including abscesses, fistulas, fissures, neoplasms, polyps, pruritus ani, and inflammatory bowel disease, may present with hemorrhoidlike symptoms and should not be self-treated (Table 18-1).[1,12-18] Patients should be referred for medical evaluation if any of the conditions are suspected.

## Signs and Symptoms of Anorectal Disorders

The Food and Drug Administration (FDA) Advisory Panel has identified specific signs and symptoms associated with hemorrhoidal complaints.[1] Itching, discomfort, irritation, burning, inflammation, and swelling are usually considered common signs and symptoms of minor anorectal disorders. In contrast, pain, bleeding, seepage, change in bowel patterns, prolapse, and thrombosis may indicate a more serious condition that requires medical referral (Table 18-2).[1,12,18]

## Treatment of Anorectal Disorders

### *Treatment Goals*

The goals of the treatment of patients with complaints of anorectal itching, irritation, burning, inflammation, discomfort, and swelling are to (1) alleviate and maintain remission of anorectal symptoms and (2) prevent complications leading to adverse consequences.

### *General Treatment Approach*

Figure 18-2 presents an algorithm for treating patients with minor anorectal signs and symptoms and lists exclusions to self-treatment. If self-treatable, the clinician should recommend appropriate nonpharmacologic measures and

**TABLE 18-2 Signs and Symptoms of Anorectal Disorders[1,12,18]**

| Sign/Symptom | Definition/Etiology |
|---|---|
| **Usually Self-Treatable** | |
| Itching (pruritus) | Mild stimulation of sensory nerve fibers in anorectal area; associated with many anorectal disorders, including hemorrhoids (typically with a mucoid discharge from prolapsing internal hemorrhoids)<br>Common causes: poor hygiene (including incomplete wiping or cleaning after defecation); diarrhea; parasitic diseases; fungal infections; allergies (including sensitivity to fabrics, soaps, laundry detergents, and dyes and perfumes in toilet tissue); anorectal lesions; moisture in anal area<br>May be secondary to swelling, diet (caffeinated beverages, chocolate, citrus fruits), and use of oral broad-spectrum drugs<br>Rare cause: psychogenic origins |
| Discomfort | May result from burning, itching, pain, irritation, inflammation, and swelling in anorectal area |
| Irritation | Uncomfortable feeling associated with stimulation of sensory nerve fibers in anorectal area |
| Burning | Greater degree of irritation of sensory nerve fibers than that seen in anal itching; common symptom of anorectal disorders; often associated with hemorrhoids; sensation of warmth or intense heat may be constant or occur only at defecation |
| Inflammation | Tissue reaction characterized by heat, redness or discoloration, pain, and swelling; often associated with trauma, allergy, or infection |
| Swelling | Temporary enlargement of cells and/or tissue resulting from excess fluid associated with hemorrhoids; may be accompanied by pain, burning, and itching |
| **Requires Medical Referral** | |
| Pain | Intense stimulation of sensory nerve fibers caused by inflammation or irritation; internal hemorrhoids usually painless; external hemorrhoids usually cause mild pain; acute, severe perianal pain may be from thrombosed external hemorrhoid; pain from anal fissure during bowel movement often described as "being cut with sharp glass"; abscess, fistula, or anorectal neoplasm may also cause pain |
| Bleeding | Hemorrhoids most common cause (from straining or passage of hard stool, or ulceration of perianal skin overlying thrombosed external hemorrhoid) of minor intermittent lower GI bleeding, but cannot be assumed as cause; appears as bright red spots or streaks on toilet tissue, or bright red blood around the stool or in toilet bowl<br>Other possible causes: anal fissures or other GI diseases including IBD, PUD, erosive esophagitis, esophageal or gastric varices, polyps, and malignant diseases of colon or rectum<br>Black or tarry stools (melena) or large amounts of red blood (hematochezia) in toilet bowl indication of possible upper GI bleeding (e.g., PUD)<br>Shortness of breath, dizziness, fatigue, or lightheadedness, especially on standing (orthostatic hypotension) with large volume of blood loss |
| Seepage | Involuntary passage of fecal material or mucus caused by an anal sphincter that does not close completely; may include discharge of pus or feces from a fistula that connects the rectum to the anal canal |
| Change in bowel pattern | Unexplained change in bowel frequency or in stool caliber; may signal serious underlying GI disorder (e.g., IBD), colorectal cancer |
| Prolapse (protrusion) | Protrusion of hemorrhoidal or rectal tissue of variable size into anal canal; usually appears after defecation, prolonged standing, unusual physical exertion, or swelling of hemorrhoidal tissue with loss of muscular support; painless except when accompanied by thrombosis, infection, or ulceration |
| Thrombosis | Strangulation of protruded (external) hemorrhoid by anal sphincter possibly leading to thrombosis; associated pain most acute during first 48-72 hours, but usually resolves after 7-10 days<br>Minimal pain associated with thrombosed internal hemorrhoids; patient likely to be unaware of condition unless sudden change in bowel habits occurs<br>If thrombosed hemorrhoid persists, ulcers or gangrene may develop on hemorrhoid's surface and cause bleeding, especially during defecation |

Key: GI, gastrointestinal; IBD, inflammatory bowel disease; PUD, peptic ulcer disease.

a nonprescription preparation containing a medication to treat that specific symptom (e.g., topical corticosteroids for the temporary relief of itching). The patient should be advised to maintain a well-balanced diet (preferably high in fiber and bulk) and good perianal hygiene, as well as to avoid prolonged sitting on the toilet. Table 18-3 outlines guidelines for applying anorectal products.

Women who are pregnant or breast-feeding should be restricted to the external use of anorectal products (except for certain protectants) because of the potential risk of

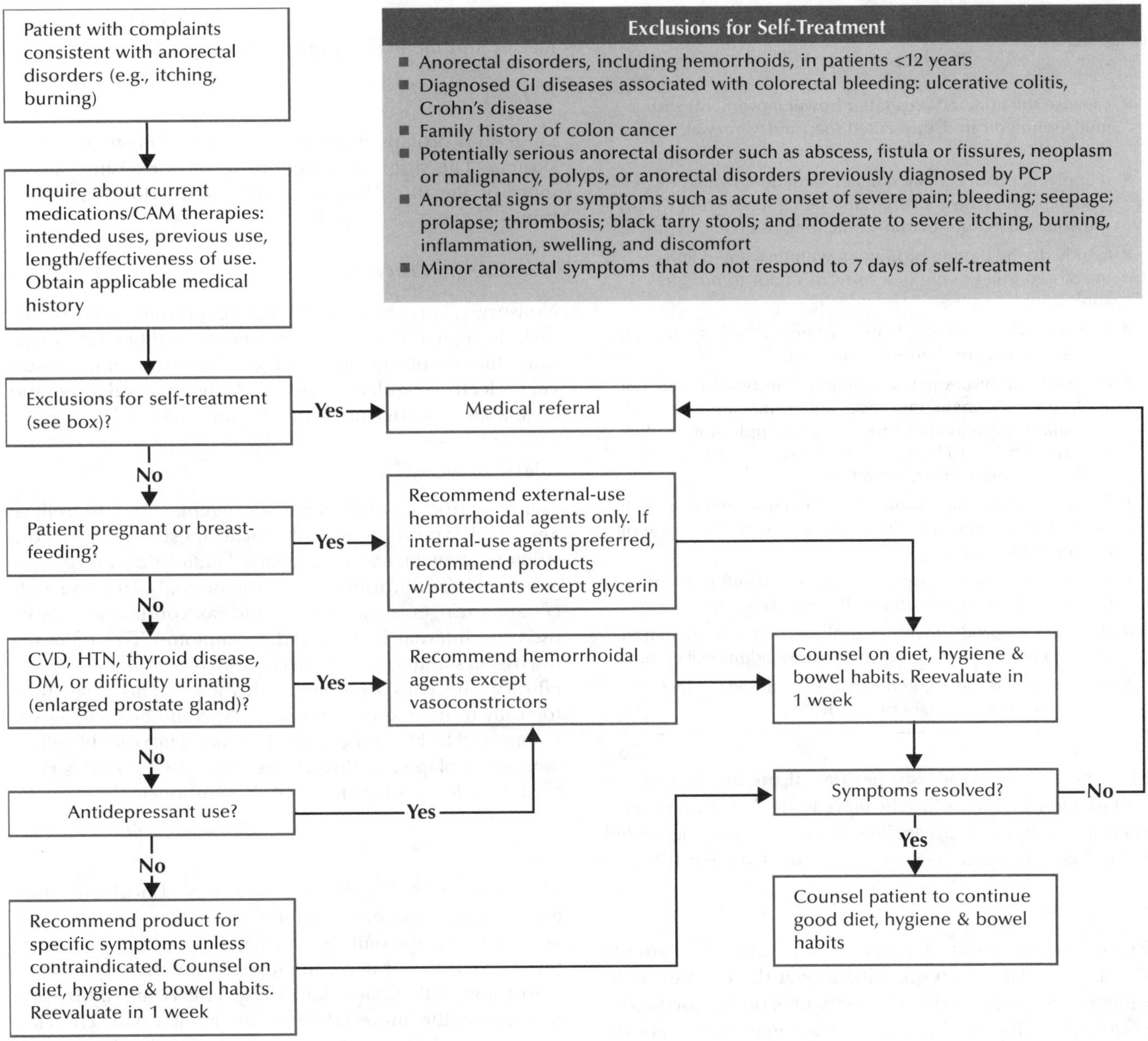


**FIGURE 18-2** Self-care of hemorrhoids. Key: CAM, complementary and alternative medicine; CVD, cardiovascular disease; DM, diabetes mellitus; GI, gastrointestinal; HTN, hypertension; PCP, primary care provider.

systemic drug absorption. Patients with high blood pressure, cardiac disease, diabetes, hyperthyroidism, or urination problems caused by enlargement of the prostate gland should not use anorectal products containing vasoconstrictors. In addition, patients taking monoamine oxidase inhibitors, tricyclic antidepressants, or antihypertensive agents should not use topical vasoconstrictors.[19]

## *Nonpharmacologic Therapy*

Nondrug measures for treating anorectal disorders such as hemorrhoids range from dietary measures to hygiene practices to surgical and nonsurgical methods for removing the hemorrhoids. In addition, patients diagnosed with or suspected of having hemorrhoids should be advised to (1) avoid lifting heavy objects, (2) avoid foods that may irritate or aggravate symptoms (e.g., caffeinated beverages), and (3) increase dietary fibers and exercise. If possible, nonsteroidal anti-inflammatory drugs or aspirin should be avoided as these medications may promote bleeding.

### Dietary Measures

Dietary fiber softens the stool and may prevent further irritation or formation of small symptomatic hemorrhoids. The addition of 25 to 30 g of fiber to a low-fiber diet, may permit the passage of softer stools, thus reducing or preventing irritation and straining at defecation.[7,9] Fiber should be introduced slowly and accompanied by an increase in fluid intake so that the patient drinks a total

**TABLE 18-3 Guidelines for Applying Anorectal Products[1,19]**

- Cleanse the affected area (after bowel movement) with a mild, nonmedicated, unscented soap and warm water; rinse thoroughly.
- If applying products that contain aluminum hydroxide gel or kaolin, clean the anorectal area, being sure to remove any previously used petrolatum-containing or greasy ointment.
- Gently dry by patting or blotting with unscented and uncolored toilet tissue or a soft cloth prior to product application.
- External application: Apply the ointment as a thin covering to the perianal area and the anal canal.
- Intrarectal application: Insert ointment using an intrarectal applicator or a finger. Intrarectal applicators are preferred to digital application because using the applicator enables the drug product to be applied to the rectal mucosa (which cannot be reached by using a finger).
- Intrarectal applicators should have lateral openings, as well as a hole in the tip, to facilitate application and coverage of the rectal mucosa.
- Intrarectal applicators should be lubricated before insertion by spreading ointment around the applicator tip.
- Do not use a product with an applicator if the introduction of the applicator into the rectum causes additional pain.
- Do not exceed the recommended daily dosage unless directed by your primary care provider.

of eight (8 ounces) glasses per day. If the amount of the dietary fiber intake cannot be increased, fiber supplements such as psyllium, methylcellulose, or guar may be added to the patient's treatment regimen (see Chapter 16).

### Defecation Time

Proper bowel habits should be encouraged. Patients should avoid sitting on the toilet longer than 5 minutes to reduce straining and decrease pressures on hemorrhoidal vessels. Avoiding the urge to defecate may lead to constipation and to the formation of hemorrhoids.[7]

### Anal Hygiene

Good anal hygiene may relieve anorectal symptoms and prevent the recurrence of perianal itching. The patient should clean the anorectal area regularly and after each bowel movement by using a mild, unscented soap and water or, more practically, by using commercially available hygienic and lubricated wipes or pads. Avoiding excessive scrubbing of the anorectal area may minimize aggravation to the sensitive anal region.[1]

### Sitz Baths

Sitz baths promote good hygiene and often relieve hemorrhoidal symptoms, especially after bowel movements. When possible, the patient should sit in warm water (110°F to 115°F [43.3°C to 46.1°C]) two to three times a day for about 15 minutes. Plastic sitz tubs that fit over the toilet rim are convenient, easily cleaned, and available at pharmacies and medical supply vendors.

## *Surgery*

Large and prolapsed hemorrhoids are often treated with surgery. The surgical procedure involves excising one or more of the three hemorrhoidal masses (hemorrhoidectomy).

## *Nonsurgical Procedures*

Nonsurgical procedures for treating internal hemorrhoids include injection of sclerosing agents, rubber band ligation, dilation of the anal canal and lower rectum, cryosurgery, electrocoagulation, infrared photocoagulation, and local anal hypothermia with a frozen finger.[7,20,21]

## *Pharmacologic Therapy*

Nonprescription pharmacologic agents used to relieve anorectal symptoms include local anesthetics, vasoconstrictors, protectants, astringents, keratolytics, analgesics/anesthetics/antipruritics, and corticosteroids. However, only certain astringents, protectants, and vasoconstrictors may be used for internal hemorrhoidal symptoms. The following discussion summarizes the mechanism of action, indications, efficacy, and risks associated with these agents when used topically to treat anorectal disorders. None of these agents is approved by FDA for the relief of anorectal pain, bleeding, seepage, prolapse, or thrombosis. Table 18-4 provides FDA-approved dosages for anorectal drug products.[19,22,23]

### Local Anesthetics

*Mechanism of Action/Pharmacokinetics* Local anesthetics, or topical anesthetics, temporarily relieve itching, irritation, burning, discomfort, and pain by reversibly blocking the transmission of nerve impulses. While there is minimal absorption with intact skin, these effects are more pronounced in the anorectal area with abraded skin. This class of drugs should be used with caution as the local anesthetic effects may mask the pain of a more severe anorectal disorders. Use of these products should be limited to the perianal region or in the area below the dentate line because the rectum is not innervated with sensory nerve fibers.[1]

*Indications* Local anesthetics listed in Table 18-4 are approved for external use in anorectal preparations for the temporary relief of external anal symptoms including discomfort, itching, pain, soreness, and burning associated with anorectal disorders.[1,19,22]

*Safety Considerations* Local anesthetics are composed of three distinct structure moieties: an aromatic portion, an intermediate chain, and an amine group.[24] Categories of local anesthetics are defined by the nature of the chemical linkage between the aromatic portion and the intermediate chain, ester, or amide.[25] The structural differences give rise to different allergenicity and absence of cross-reactivity among some agents.[26,27] Contact dermatitis may be more

TABLE 18-4 Dosage and Administration Guidelines for Anorectal Products[1,19]

| Ingredient | Concentration per Dosage Unit (%) | Frequency of Use (Maximum Daily Dosage) |
|---|---|---|
| **Local Anesthetics** | | |
| Benzocaine | 5-20 | Up to 6 times/day (2.4 g) |
| Benzyl alcohol | 1-4 | Up to 6 times/day (480 mg) |
| Dibucaine, dibucaine hydrochloride | 0.25-1 | Up to 3-4 times/day (80 mg) |
| Dyclonine hydrochloride | 0.5-1 | Up to 6 times/day (100 mg) |
| Lidocaine | 2-5 | Up to 6 times/day (500 mg) |
| Pramoxine hydrochloride* | 1 | Up to 5 times/day (100 mg) |
| Tetracaine, tetracaine hydrochloride | 0.5-1 | Up to 6 times/day (100 mg) |
| **Vasoconstrictors** | | |
| Ephedrine sulfate | 0.1-1.25 | Up to 4 times/day (100 mg) |
| Epinephrine hydrochloride/epinephrine | 0.005-0.01 | Up to 4 times/day (800 mg) |
| Phenylephrine hydrochloride | 0.25 | Up to 4 times/day (2 mg) |
| **Protectants** | | |
| Aluminum hydroxide gel, cocoa butter, glycerin, hard fat, kaolin, lanolin, mineral oil, white petrolatum, petrolatum, shark liver oil, zinc oxide, topical starch, calamine, cod liver oil | See footnote† | Petrolatum/white petrolatum: as often as needed; other protectants: up to 6 times/day or after each bowel movement |
| **Astringents** | | |
| Calamine‡ | 5-25 | Up to 6 times/day or after each bowel movement |
| Zinc oxide | 5-25 | Up to 6 times/day or after each bowel movement |
| Witch hazel | 10-50 | Up to 6 times/day or after each bowel movement |
| **Keratolytics** | | |
| Alcloxa | 0.2-2 | Up to 6 times/day |
| Resorcinol | 1-3 | Up to 6 times/day |
| **Analgesics/Anesthetics/Antipruritics** | | |
| Menthol | 0.1-1 | Up to 6 times/day |
| Juniper tar | 1-5 | Up to 6 times/day |
| Camphor | 0.1-3 | Up to 6 times/day |
| **Corticosteroids** | | |
| Hydrocortisone | 0.25-1 | Up to 3-4 times/day |

* External dosage forms may include aerosol foams, ointments, creams, and jellies (water-miscible base).

† If a single protectant ingredient is used, it must comprise at least 50% of the product. Aluminum hydroxide gel and kaolin may not be combined with other protectants when the combined percentage by weight of all protectants in the combination is at least 50% of the final product. Aqueous solutions of glycerin cannot contain less than 20% or more than 45% glycerin (weight-to-weight). (See Table 18-5 for concentrations of protectants used in combination products.)

‡ Concentration of calamine is not to exceed 25% by weight/dosage unit (based on zinc oxide content of calamine).

common with benzocaine than other topical anesthetics because of its chemical structure.[28] Thus, patients who have had an adverse reaction to benzocaine should use a different local anesthetic with a different chemical structure, for example, pramoxine.[28] These ingredients may also produce local allergic reactions (e.g., burning and itching), which are indistinguishable from the anorectal symptoms being treated. Anorectal preparations containing local anesthetics must carry a warning stating that allergic reactions may occur in some individuals.[1,19]

Local anesthetics may be rapidly absorbed through the rectal mucosa and may cause potentially toxic systemic effects. Absorption through the perianal skin is usually minimal unless the skin is abraded. However, systemic reactions including cardiovascular and central nervous system adverse effects may occur because of the abundant vasculature in the anal area. Accidental ingestion of dibucaine-containing anorectal products has been reported in children, resulting in lethargy, seizures, and cardiorespiratory arrest, and should be kept out of children's reach.[1] This caution also pertains to the other anorectal local anesthetic ingredients.[29]

### Vasoconstrictors

*Mechanism of Action/Pharmacokinetics* Vasoconstrictors are chemical agents structurally related to the naturally occurring catecholamines, epinephrine and norepinephrine. When ephedrine or epinephrine is applied topically to the anorectal area, stimulation of the α-adrenergic receptors in the vascular beds causes constriction of the arterioles thereby producing a modest and transient reduction of swelling. In addition, β-adrenergic receptors are stimulated simultaneously. This latter effect causes increased cardiac contractility, increased heart rate (tachycardia), and bronchodilation that may lead to adverse effects associated with its anorectal use. When used topically in the anal region, these agents relieve itching, discomfort, and irritation, in part because they produce a slight anesthetic effect by an unknown mechanism. Although studies have demonstrated locally applied vasoconstrictors alter mucosal blood supply promptly, FDA does not recognize or approve of the use of such agents to control minor anorectal bleeding.[1]

Phenylephrine hydrochloride is structurally related to norepinephrine and is a potent α-adrenergic stimulant with minimal effect on the central nervous system. In contrast to ephedrine and epinephrine, phenylephrine has minor effects on cardiac rhythm; thus, it does not cause significant bradycardia.[1]

*Indications* The vasoconstrictors listed in Table 18-4 are approved for external use for the temporary relief of discomfort, itching, swelling, and shrinkage of irritated hemorrhoidal tissue and other anorectal disorders. Ephedrine sulfate and phenylephrine hydrochloride may also be used for internal hemorrhoids.[19,22]

*Safety Considerations* Topical vasoconstrictors may be systemically absorbed and can cause nervousness, tremor, sleeplessness, nausea, and loss of appetite at recommended dosages.[1] Serious adverse effects such as elevation of blood pressure, aggravation of hyperthyroidism, cardiac arrhythmias, and irregular heart rate, are less likely to occur, but also may occur with recommended dosages.[1] Prolonged use may lead to anxiety or paranoia and, more commonly, rebound vasodilatation. Contact dermatitis may also occur. If these symptoms persist or become worse, the patient should be referred for medical evaluation.

Adverse effects may occur with concomitant administration of antihypertensive medications and vasoconstrictors. Vasoconstrictors attenuate the effects of antihypertensive agents and may increase blood pressure. Alternatively, the hypertensive effects of vasoconstrictors may be potentiated by monoamine oxidase inhibitors and tricyclic antidepressants. Concomitant use may lead to serious and even lethal outcomes including cerebral hemorrhage or stroke.[1,19] Patients with diabetes, thyroid disease, hypertension, angina pectoris, or an enlarged prostate and those taking antidepressants, antihypertensive agents, or cardiac medications should not use hemorrhoidal agents with vasoconstrictors without first consulting their primary care provider because of the possibility of serious systemic adverse effects.[1,19]

### Protectants

*Mechanism of Action* Protectants prevent irritation of the anorectal area and water loss from the stratum corneum by forming a physical barrier on the skin. In addition, these agents may act as a protective coat over the affected areas and soften the dry anal area by decreasing water loss. Perianal irritation by fecal matter may be reduced by applying protectants to minimize irritation, itching, burning, and discomfort in the affected anal area.[19]

*Indications* The protectant drug class includes absorbents, adsorbents, demulcents, and emollients. Protectants listed in Table 18-4 are approved for the temporary relief of discomfort, itching, irritation, and burning associated with external and internal hemorrhoids, with the exception of glycerin, which is for external use only.[22] They also prevent drying of the perianal. Products containing kaolin or aluminum hydroxide gel are indicated for the temporary relief of anorectal itching.

*Safety Considerations* Systemic absorption of protectants is minimal; therefore, adverse reactions to these agents as a class are uncommon. Lanolin is derived from wood alcohols, which are probably responsible for most cases of lanolin allergy. Preparations containing aluminum hydroxide gel and kaolin are required to contain a warning stating that petrolatum or greasy ointments should be removed before applying these agents because greasy substances interfere with the ability of aluminum hydroxide gel and kaolin to adhere properly to the skin.[19]

### Astringents

*Mechanism of Action* Astringents applied to the anorectal area promote coagulation of the skin cells, thereby protecting the underlying tissue while decreasing cell volume. In addition to coagulating the surface proteins, they form a thin layer to protect the underlying tissue from further irritation. Astringents cause contracting, wrinkling, blanching, of the affected area and also decrease secretions, making the region drier, which in turn decreases anal itching, burning, discomfort, and irritation.[19]

*Indications* Astringents listed in Table 18-4 are approved for the temporary relief of itching, irritation, and burning symptoms associated with anorectal disorders.[19] Witch hazel (hamamelis water, the original name prior to January

1, 1995) is indicated for external use, while calamine and zinc oxide may be used for both external and internal anorectal disorders.[19]

*Safety Considerations* Adverse effects associated with the topical use of calamine, zinc oxide, and witch hazel are uncommon. Witch hazel may cause a slight stinging sensation when applied because of the alcohol used to prepare the compound. Contact dermatitis may occur with witch hazel because it contains a small amount of volatile oil.[1] If calamine or zinc oxide is used for a prolonged period of time, especially for internal anorectal disorders, systemic zinc toxicity (nausea, vomiting, lethargy, and severe pain) may develop.

### Keratolytics

*Mechanism of Action* Keratolytics cause desquamation and debridement, or sloughing, of epidermal surface cells. By fostering cell turnover and loosening surface cells, keratolytics may help expose underlying tissue allowing local application of other medications. Keratolytics, when used externally in low concentrations, are somewhat useful in reducing itching and discomfort, but their exact mechanism of action is unknown. Because mucous membranes do not contain a keratin layer, intrarectal use of keratolytics is not justified and may be harmful.[19]

*Indications* The keratolytics approved for the temporary relief of external anorectal discomfort and itching in the perianal area associated with hemorrhoidal disease are listed in Table 18-4.[19]

*Safety Considerations* The absorption of resorcinol has led to methemoglobinemia, exfoliative dermatitis, and death in infants and myxedema in adults with repeated dosing.[1] Mild adverse effects of resorcinol include ringing in the ears, increased pulse rate, sweating, and shortness of breath. Severe adverse effects with resorcinol are methemoglobinemia, circulatory collapse, unconsciousness, and convulsions. Anorectal preparations containing resorcinol must list the following warnings: (1) "Certain persons can develop allergic reactions to ingredients in this product. If the symptoms being treated do not subside or if redness, irritation, swelling, pain or other symptoms develop or increase, discontinue use and consult a doctor." (2) "Do not use on open wounds near the anus" to minimize resorcinol absorption through abraded mucosal lining and decrease the potential for systemic toxicity.[19]

### Analgesics/Anesthetics/Antipruritics (Formerly Classified as "Counterirritants")

*Mechanism of Action* Menthol, juniper tar, and camphor are safe and effective when used externally in the perianal area. Such agents relieve pain, itching, burning, or discomfort by producing a local sensation that distracts from these complaints. The local sensation includes cool, warm, or tingling relief. The agents should not be used internally because the rectum has no identifiable nerve fibers.

*Indications* Approved products containing astringents/anesthetics/antipruritics are listed in Table 18-4. These agents are approved for the temporary relief of itching, discomfort, pain, and burning associated with perianal disorders or to provide a cooling sensation when applied to the involved area.[1,19,22]

*Safety Considerations* Menthol-containing products must bear the following warning: "Certain persons can develop allergic reactions to ingredients in this product. If the symptoms being treated do not subside or if redness, irritation, swelling, pain, or other symptoms develop or increase, discontinue use and consult a doctor."[19] In addition, extensive application of menthol to the trunk of the body has caused laryngospasm, dyspnea, and cyanosis; thus, it is important to use anorectal preparations with this ingredient sparingly.[1]

### Corticosteroids

*Mechanism of Action* Topical hydrocortisone acts as a vasoconstrictor and antipruritic. This agent has the potential to reduce itching and pain by producing lysosomal membrane stabilization and antimitotic activity. Its onset of action may require up to 12 hours, but its effect is of longer duration than most other agents (e.g., local anesthetics).

*Indications* Hydrocortisone is the only corticosteroid approved for nonprescription use in anorectal preparations. The maximum permitted concentration is 1%. Hydrocortisone is indicated for the temporary relief of minor external anal itching caused by minor irritation or rash.

*Safety Considerations* Hydrocortisone may mask the symptoms of bacterial and fungal infections.

### Combination Products

Federal regulations state that a nonprescription product may combine two or more safe and effective active ingredients and generally be recognized as safe and effective when (1) each active ingredient contributes to the claimed effect; (2) the combination of active ingredients does not decrease the safety or effectiveness of any individual active ingredient; and (3) the combination, when listing adequate directions for use and warning against unsafe use, provides rational, concurrent therapy for a significant proportion of the target population.[23] FDA placed the restrictions listed in Table 18-5 on nonprescription anorectal preparations containing combinations.[19]

Because some self-treatable anorectal disorders may have concurrent symptoms, combination preparations are reasonable. However, there is no evidence that an anorectal preparation with combined active ingredients is any more effective than a preparation with a therapeutic amount of a single ingredient. Theoretically, restricting the number of ingredients in the anorectal preparation should decrease the risk of interactions and adverse drug reactions and lessen the likelihood of altering the product's effectiveness.

**TABLE 18-5 FDA Restrictions for Combination Nonprescription Anorectal Preparations**

FDA allows the following combinations of ingredients in nonprescription anorectal preparations:

- 2, 3, or 4 protectants composing at least 50% of weight of final product*†‡§‖
- 1 local anesthetic or 1 vasoconstrictor or 1 astringent or 1 keratolytic or 1 analgesic/anesthetic/antipruritic ± 1 to 4 protectants
- 1 local anesthetic + 1 vasoconstrictor or 1 astringent or 1 keratolytic ± 1 to 4 protectants
- 1 local anesthetic + 1 vasoconstrictor + 1 astringent ± 1 to 4 protectants
- 1 local anesthetic + 1 astringent + 1 keratolytic ± 1 to 4 protectants
- 1 vasoconstrictor + 1 analgesic/anesthetic/antipruritic + 1 astringent ± 1 to 4 protectants
- 1 single analgesic/anesthetic/antipruritic + 1 keratolytic ± 1 astringent ± 1 to 4 protectants
- 1 astringent + 1 vasoconstrictor or 1 analgesic/anesthetic/antipruritic or 1 keratolytic ± 1 to 4 protectants

* Aluminum hydroxide gel and kaolin may not be combined with cocoa butter, cod liver oil, hard fat, lanolin, mineral oil, shark liver oil, petrolatum, or white petrolatum because these ingredients are greasy, which may prevent aluminum hydroxide gel and kaolin from adhering to the skin and providing protection.[1,19,22]

† Any protectant ingredient, except cod liver oil or shark liver oil, included in a combination must contribute at least 12.5% by weight.

‡ When included in a combination product, glycerin must constitute at least 10% of the product.

§ If calamine and zinc oxide are included in a combination product, their concentrations are limited to a maximum of 25% (weight-to-weight zinc oxide) per dosage units. When used as protectants in a combination product, these agents can be combined only with other protectant ingredients.

‖ When used as protectants in combination products, cod liver oil and shark liver oil can be combined only with other protectant ingredients. Cod liver oil and shark liver oil may be used as protectants if the product represents 10,000 USP units of vitamin A and 400 USP units of cholecalciferol (vitamin $D_3$) that is used in a 24-hour period.[1,19]

## Laxatives

To prevent straining during defecation, some patients may require the addition of a bulk-forming (e.g., psyllium) or emollient (e.g., docusate) laxative to a high-fiber diet and adequate fluid intake (see Chapter 16).[7,12] Patients with symptomatic hemorrhoids may experience a significant reduction in pain and bleeding within a few weeks after beginning regular use of a laxative. However, excessive dietary fiber and bulk-forming laxatives may cause diarrhea.

## Product Selection Guidelines

Table 18-6 contains examples of products that the clinician can recommend on the basis of the following patient factors or preferences.

Knowledge of a patient's present medical condition, medical history, medication profile, and relevant socioeconomic factors is necessary to determine how an individual may respond to self-treatment. The clinician should decide on a suitable anorectal product, if any, while taking into account the following: (1) the type, location, and severity of the anorectal disorder; (2) diseases or significant past medical history the patient may have; (3) medications the patient may be taking or allergies he or she may have; (4) the patient's ability to apply or insert the medication (physical, mental, and emotional limitations); and (5) any other factors, such as diet, daily activities, or cost of the product that may affect treatment. Pregnant and breast-feeding women should use only those products recommended for external use except for the recommended protectants, which may be used internally. Children younger than 12 years of age with hemorrhoids or any other anorectal disorder should be referred to a primary care provider.[1,19]

FDA does not require testing of anorectal products in the manufacturer's final dosage form. Thus, therapeutic differences among various dosage forms, if any, are not known. Products containing approved ingredients in appropriate dosages are probably therapeutically similar when used to treat indicated anorectal signs and symptoms. Whatever differences exist are most likely related to individual patient preference for a specific dosage form.

Medications used to treat symptomatic anorectal disorders are available in many dosage forms including ointments, creams, suppositories, and gels. Applicators, intrarectal applicators (pile pipes), or fingers are used to facilitate applying the preparations. Creams, ointments, gels, pastes, liquids, and foams are used externally. Although considerable pharmaceutical differences exist among ointments, creams, pastes, and gels, the therapeutic differences do not appear to be clinically important when treating patients with anorectal disorders. This discussion uses the term *ointment* to refer to all semisolid preparations designed for intrarectal or external use in the anorectal area. The primary function of an ointment is to provide a vehicle for the safe and efficient delivery of the active ingredients, yet some ointments also possess inherent protectant and emollient properties.

Suppositories also provide a lubricating effect, which may ease straining at defecation, thereby easing or alleviating hemorrhoidal symptoms. However, suppositories should not be recommended as an initial dosage form when treating anorectal disorders, because they may leave the affected anal region and ascend into the rectum and lower colon when the patient is in a prone (lying with the face downward) position. If the patient remains prone after inserting a suppository or an ointment, the active ingredients may not distribute evenly over the anal mucosa. Also, suppositories are relatively slow acting because they must melt to release the active ingredients (see Chapter 16).

Foam products should theoretically provide more rapid release of active ingredients than ointments. However, foam dosage forms are usually more expensive than ointments and do not offer any important advantage. In addition, the foam may not remain in the affected area,

**TABLE 18-6 Selected Products for Hemorrhoids**

| Trade Name | Primary Ingredients |
|---|---|
| **Local Anesthetics** | |
| Americaine Ointment | Benzocaine 20% |
| Anusol Ointment | Pramoxine HCl 1%; zinc oxide 12.5%; mineral oil 46.6%; cocoa butter; kaolin |
| Anusol Suppositories | Topical starch 51%; benzyl alcohol |
| Fleet Pain-Relief Pads | Pramoxine HCl 1%; glycerin 12% |
| Nupercainal Ointment | Dibucaine 1%; lanolin; white petrolatum; light mineral oil |
| Tronolane Cream | Pramoxine HCl 1%; zinc oxide 5%; glycerin |
| Tronothane Hydrochloride Cream | Pramoxine HCl 1%; glycerin |
| **Vasoconstrictors** | |
| Hemorid Creme | Phenylephrine HCl 0.25%; pramoxine HCl 1%; white petrolatum 30%; mineral oil 20% |
| Hemorid Ointment | Phenylephrine HCl 0.25%; pramoxine HCl 1%; white petrolatum 82.15%; light mineral oil 12.5% |
| Preparation H Cooling Gel | Witch hazel 50%; phenylephrine HCl 0.25% |
| Preparation H Cream | Phenylephrine HCl 0.25%; petrolatum 18%; glycerin 12%; shark liver oil 3%; lanolin |
| Preparation H Ointment | Phenylephrine HCl 0.25%; petrolatum 71.9%; mineral oil 14%; shark liver oil 3%; lanolin; glycerin |
| Preparation H Suppositories | Phenylephrine HCl 0.25%; cocoa butter 85.5%; shark liver oil 3%; starch |
| **Skin Protectants** | |
| Balneol Lotion | Mineral oil; lanolin oil |
| Rectacaine Ointment | Petrolatum 71.9%; mineral oil 14%; shark liver oil 3%; glycerin |
| Wyanoids Relief Factor Suppositories | Cocoa butter 79%; shark liver oil 3% |
| **Hydrocortisone Products** | |
| Anusol-HC-1 Ointment | Hydrocortisone acetate 1.12% (equivalent to hydrocortisone 1%); mineral oil; white petrolatum |
| Cortizone-10 External Anal Relief Cream | Hydrocortisone 1%; glycerin; light mineral oil; white petrolatum; white wax |
| Preparation H Hydrocortisone 1% Cream | Hydrocortisone 1%; glycerin; lanolin; petrolatum |
| **Miscellaneous Combination Products** | |
| Nupercainal Suppositories | Zinc oxide 0.25 g; cocoa butter 2.1 g |
| Preparation H Medicated Wipes | Witch hazel 50%; glycerin |
| Tronolane Suppositories | Zinc oxide 11%; hard fat 95% |
| Tucks Pads | Witch hazel 50%; glycerin |

and differences in the size of the foam bubbles may result in different concentrations of the active ingredient.

## *Complementary Therapies*

Complementary treatments for hemorrhoids include herbal and homeopathic products, as well as various home remedies.

### Herbal Remedies

Herbal remedies that have been used for anorectal disorders include aloe, bitter melon, black Culver's root, Bupleurum, cat's claw, comfrey, corn cockle, horse chestnut, indigo, marijuana, mullein, passion flower, Peru balsam, plantain, prickly pear, quinine, St. John's wort, storax, and witch hazel (see Chapter 53).[30-34] The combination of diosmin and hesperidin, a micronized purified flavonoid fraction, has been used to stop acute hemorrhoidal bleeding and decrease the intensity of hemorrhoidal symptoms.[35] The mechanism of action is still in question, but in animal models, it is thought to be associated with the inhibition of prostaglandin and thromboxane mediators, which decreases the inflammatory processes. The combination appears safe

**TABLE 18-7 Botanical Medicines Used to Treat Anorectal Disorders**

| Agent (Scientific Name) | Risks | Effectiveness |
|---|---|---|
| Aloe (*Aloe vera, A. perryi, A. barbadensis, A. vulgaris, A. ferox*) | Use not recommended, especially during pregnancy | Drastic laxative used when constipation suspected as cause of hemorrhoids; possible severe cramping and diarrhea; efficacy unproven |
| Bupleur um (*Bupleur um chinense)* | Adverse effects: flatulence, increase in bowel movements, sedation | Efficacy in treating hemorrhoids unproven |
| Cat's claw (*Uncaria tomentosa, U. guianensis*) | None reported | Efficacy of astringent and antidiarrheal properties in treating hemorrhoids unproven |
| Comfrey (*Symphytum officinale, S. asperum, S. tuberosum*) | Several reports of hepatic veno-occlusive disease when taken orally; on July 6, 2001, FDA removed products containing comfrey from the market | Claimed to heal hemorrhoids; not currently recommended for use |
| Corn cockle (*Agrostemma githago*) | Possible systemic poisoning from saponins githagin and agrostemmic acid; hogs have died from eating roots | Roots used to treat hemorrhoids; poisonous; do not use as a medication |
| Horse chestnut (*Aesculus hippocastanum, A. californica, A. glabra*) | Toxic; not recommended for internal use | Horse chestnut *(A. hippocastanum)* seed extracts used to treat hemorrhoids; however, classified by FDA as toxic and unsafe |
| Indigo (*Indigofera* spp.) | Some species possibly toxic; contraindicated during pregnancy | Efficacy in treating hemorrhoids unproven |
| Mullein (*Verbascum thapsus, V. phlomoides, V. thapsiforme*) | Long history of herbal use; no toxicity reported | Saponins, mucilage, tannins in leaves/flowers probably contribute to soothing topical effect; used to treat hemorrhoids; FDA Category II (generally not safe or effective) for treatment of anorectal disorders |
| Passion flower (*Passiflora* spp., primarily *P. incarnata*) | No significant toxicity reported; possible CNS depression with large doses of extract; possible vasculitis, increased respiratory rate, altered consciousness, depending on species | Efficacy of topical use on inflamed hemorrhoids unproven |
| Peru balsam (*Myroxylon pereirae*) | Contact dermatitis occurs frequently | Used topically to treat hemorrhoids (as a suppository); initially placed in Category III (as a wound-healing agent for anorectal disorders), but later removed from anorectal products because of insufficient data to establish effectiveness |
| Plantain (*Plantago lanceolata, P. major, P. psyllium, P. arenatia*) | At one time, digitalis found in psyllium preparations sold in health food stores; drug interactions reported between oral psyllium and oral lithium or carbamazepine; highly allergenic | Pulverized seeds mixed with oil and applied topically to inflamed sites or used orally as a bulk laxative; psyllium-containing preparations appear to reduce bleeding and pain of hemorrhoids during defecation |
| Prickly pear (*Opuntia tuna mill, O. ficus-indica*) | Dermatitis reported | Efficacy as astringent for healing hemorrhoids unproven |
| Quinine (*Cinchona succirubra*) | Possible cinchonism (severe headache, abdominal pain, convulsions, visual disturbances, blindness), paralysis, collapse, and auditory disturbances (tinnitus) with chronic ingestion/absorption; no significant toxicity with use as sclerosing agent; contraindicated during pregnancy and breast-feeding | Bark extracts used to treat hemorrhoids; quinine and urea hydrochloride mixture used as sclerosing agent in treating internal hemorrhoids; not recommended for hemorrhoids |
| St. John's wort (*Hypericum perforatum*) | Volatile oil of St. John's wort is an irritant; possible significant drug interactions if absorbed systemically | Efficacy of volatile oil extract of fresh flowers in topical treatment of hemorrhoids unproven |

**TABLE 18-7 Botanical Medicines Used to Treat Anorectal Disorders (continued)**

| Agent (Scientific Name) | Risks | Effectiveness |
|---|---|---|
| Storax (*Liquidamber orientalis, L. styraciflua*) | No significant toxicity reported | Efficacy of storax (one ingredient in compound tincture of benzoic) in treating hemorrhoids unproven |
| Witch hazel (*Hamamelis virginiana*) | No significant toxicity reported; avoid internal use | More than 30 traditional uses, including treatment of hemorrhoids; FDA-approved for treatment of external anorectal symptoms |

when both are taken orally for less than 6 months, with the most common adverse effects being abdominal pain, diarrhea, and gastritis. Table 18-7 summarizes the risks and effectiveness of the most common herbal remedies used in treating anorectal disorders.

Other herbs, including manna (*Fraxinus ornus*), senna leaf (*Cassia senna, C. angustifolia*), black psyllium seed (*Plantago psyllium, P. indica*), blonde psyllium seed (*Plantaginis ovata semen*), and blonde psyllium seed husk (*Plantaginis ovata testa*), have been approved by the German Commission E to prevent further irritation or the development of hemorrhoids because of their laxative effects (assuming that easier passage of stool is desirable).[30] In addition, butcher's broom (*Ruscus aculeatus*) and sweet clover (*Melilotus officinalis, M. altissimus*) are approved as supportive therapy for itching and burning associated with hemorrhoids.[30] Semisolid preparations made from poplar bud (*Populus canadensis*) are approved because they are believed to aid wound healing.

### Homeopathic Remedies

Homeopathic remedies used to treat anorectal disorders include Aesculus (Horse chestnut), aloe (Socotrina aloe), belladonna, collinsonia (stone root), graphites, hamamelis (witch hazel), Kali carbonicum (Potassium carbonate), Nux vomica (strychnine), Paeonia (Peony), Pulsatilla, Sepia, and basic remedies such as sulfur (see Chapter 55).[36-38] No comment can be made regarding the safety and effectiveness of such remedies. For example, bryonia (Bryonia root) has been recommended for its laxative properties for GI disorders such as hemorrhoids, but because of severe adverse effects, including dizziness, vomiting, kidney damage, and convulsion, its use is not warranted.[30,39] Calendula has been used as either an oral or topical homeopathic remedy, but this herbal ingredient has not been approved by the German Commission E for use in herbal preparations.[30,39]

### *Home Remedies*

One study involving African Americans showed they had used the following substances to treat hemorrhoids: butter, flour, kerosene, lard, olive oil, snuff, turpentine, and Vicks VapoRub.[40] Kerosene and turpentine are irritating and should not be used for this purpose. No data exist to support the efficacy of any of these home remedies.

## Assessment of Anorectal Disorders: A Case-based Approach

The clinician should obtain a thorough description of the patient's signs and symptoms to accurately assess whether the anorectal disorder is self-treatable. If the condition is self-treatable, targeted questions should be asked about the presence of specific diseases (e.g., hypertension, diabetes mellitus, benign prostatic hypertrophy), prescription and nonprescription medications, complementary and alternative medicines, as well as diet and lifestyle, before recommending self-treatment. Cases 18-1 and 18-2 illustrate assessment of patients with anorectal disorders.

**CASE 18-1**

| Relevant Evaluation Criteria | Scenario/Model Outcome |
|---|---|
| **Information Gathering** | |
| 1. Gather essential information about the patient's symptoms, including: | |
| a. description of symptom(s) (i.e., nature, onset, duration, severity, associated symptoms) | Patient complains of mild itching and irritation in the anal area for about a week. These symptoms occurred once before about a year ago, but resolved without treatment. A few days ago, she began to strain with each bowel movement and has noticed streaks of bright red blood on the toilet paper every time she wipes herself. |

## CASE 18-1 (continued)

| Relevant Evaluation Criteria | Scenario/Model Outcome |
|---|---|
| b. description of any factors that seem to precipitate, exacerbate, and/or relieve the patient's symptoms. | Discomfort, straining, and bleeding are associated with hard stools and difficult bowel movements |
| c. description of the patient's efforts to relieve the symptoms | Scratching the anal area seems to relieve the itching. Patient has not self-treated with any anorectal products, nor has she contacted her PCP about this condition. |
| 2. Gather essential patient history information: | |
| a. patient's identity | Wilma Thimby |
| b. age, sex, height, and weight | 47 y/o W, 5'9", 220 lb |
| c. patient's occupation | Computer programmer |
| d. patient's dietary habits | Wilma started the Atkins diet about 2 weeks ago in an attempt to lose weight quickly; she adheres strictly to the diet and eats mostly protein. |
| e. patient's sleep habits | Sleeps at least 7 to 8 hours a night |
| f. concurrent medical conditions, prescription and nonprescription medications, and dietary supplements | Calcium with vitamin D 3 times/day; Aleve 220 mg 2 times/day × 2 weeks for "twisted knee" (see Chapter 7); Benadryl 25 mg at bedtime as needed for sleep (see Chapter 48). |
| g. allergies | NKDA |
| h. history of other adverse reactions to medications | None |
| i. other (describe)_______ | None |
| **Assessment and Triage** | |
| 3. Differentiate the patient's signs/symptoms and correctly identify the patient's primary problem(s) (see Tables 18-1 and 18-2). | Wilma complains of mild itching and irritation recently accompanied by discomfort, straining, and bleeding. It is likely that the patient has hemorrhoids and that recent change in her diet and certain medications have contributed to her hard stools and difficult bowel movements. Straining and the passage of hard stools may have aggravated hemorrhoids and caused the bleeding. |
| 4. Identify exclusions for self-treatment (see Figure 18-2). | Patient noted streaks of bright red blood on the toilet paper. |
| 5. Formulate a comprehensive list of therapeutic alternatives for the primary problem to determine if triage to a medical practitioner is required, and share this information with the patient. | Options include:<br>(1) Recommend self-care with an appropriate nonprescription anorectal product and advise on nondrug measures.<br>(2) Recommend self-care with an appropriate anorectal product, and advise on nondrug measures until Wilma can contact her PCP.<br>(3) Refer Wilma to her PCP for medical evaluation of her symptoms.<br>(4) Take no action. |
| **Plan** | |
| 6. Select an optimal therapeutic alternative to address the patient's problem, taking into account patient preferences. | See Table 18-6 and Figure 18-2. Wilma should be referred for medical evaluation to rule out bleeding from other than a hemorrhoidal source. An appropriate anorectal product from Table 18-6 should be recommended to relieve the patient's itching, irritation, and discomfort until she can contact her PCP. Wilma prefers an anorectal ointment. |
| 7. Describe the recommended therapeutic approach to the patient. | You should contact your PCP as soon as possible so that he or she is aware of the bleeding. In the meantime, you can take some steps to relieve your itching, irritation, and discomfort. Apply an anorectal ointment listed in Table 18-6 as described in Tables 18-3 and 18-4. Because the Atkins diet does not contain adequate fiber, and may be a source of your hard stools, you may want to consider either altering your diet to include fiber and plenty of water, or take a fiber supplement or stool softener (see Chapter 16). You may also want to check with your PCP to see if you should continue taking the Benadryl and Advil, as both of these medications may contribute to hard stools. |

## CASE 18-1 (continued)

| Relevant Evaluation Criteria | Scenario/Model Outcome |
|---|---|
| 8. Explain to the patient the rationale for selecting the recommended therapeutic approach from the considered therapeutic alternatives. | Although your symptoms and the streaks of red blood on the toilet paper may be related to hemorrhoids, it is important for you to contact your PCP for further evaluation as other conditions may also cause similar symptoms and rectal bleeding. |
| **Patient Education** | |
| 9. When recommending self-care with nonprescription medications and/or nondrug therapy, convey accurate information to the patient, including: | |
| a. appropriate dose and frequency of administration | See Table 18-4. |
| b. maximum number of days the therapy should be employed | Contact your PCP, that is, primary care provider, as soon as possible even if your symptoms resolve with treatment. Be sure to let him or her know what self-care measures you have taken. Ask your PCP whether you should continue with your self-treatment program if your symptoms do not resolve after 7 days. |
| c. product administration procedures | See Table 18-3. |
| d. expected time to onset of relief | Itching, irritation, and discomfort may be relieved with a few days of applying the ointment as directed. Straining may be relieved with adequate fluids and a healthy diet or with a stool softener or fiber supplement. Although bleeding may stop with treatment, you should still contact your PCP. |
| e. degree of relief that can be reasonably expected | Complete relief of itching, irritation, discomfort is possible. |
| f. most common side effects | Most products, when applied to the anal area, are usually well tolerated. |
| g. side effects that warrant medical intervention should they occur | If you develop an allergic reaction (e.g., redness, swelling, increased irritation or pain) to the ointment, discontinue use and contact your PCP as soon as possible. |
| h. patient options in the event that condition worsens or persists | If your symptoms worsen, contact your PCP as soon as possible and let him or her know. |
| i. product storage requirements | Store medication out of the reach of children and at a controlled room temperature. |
| j. specific nondrug measures | Practice good anal hygiene, take sitz baths, and consider modifying your diet to increase fluids and fiber to soften stools and decrease straining (see Chapter 16). |
| 10. Solicit follow-up questions from patient. | Do you think that I have colon cancer? |
| 11. Answer patient's questions. | There are many conditions that cause bright red blood in the toilet or on the toilet paper. Although hemorrhoids are a common cause of bleeding, it is not possible to determine the source of the blood without further evaluation by your PCP. |

Key: NKDA, no known drug allergies; PCP, primary care provider.

## Patient Counseling for Anorectal Disorders

The clinician should explain the most appropriate drug and nondrug measures for treating the patient's specific anorectal signs and symptoms. Patient counseling should include information on dosage and frequency of administration, drug product administration techniques, possible adverse side effects, precautions or warnings, and product storage. In addition, the clinician should be sure that the patient understands when self-care of anorectal disorders should be discontinued and when to consult their primary care provider. The box Patient Education for Anorectal Disorders lists specific information to provide patients.

## Evaluation of Patient Outcomes for Anorectal Disorders

Self-treatment of anorectal disorders should be limited to minor symptoms. If serious or severe signs and symptoms are present or if symptoms worsen or alarm symptoms develop (e.g., blood in the stool, severe pain) or if symptoms persist or do not resolve after 7 days of self-treatment, the patient should be advised to contact the primary care provider.[19] If symptoms resolve, the patient should be encouraged to maintain a well-balanced diet, good personal hygiene, and good bowel habits.

## CASE 18-2

| Relevant Evaluation Criteria | Scenario/Model Outcome |
|---|---|
| **Information Gathering** | |
| 1. Gather essential information about the patient's symptoms, including: | |
| a. description of symptom(s) (i.e., nature, onset, duration, severity, associated symptoms) | Patient complains of mild to moderate itching, burning, and some discomfort in the anal area over the past few weeks. Symptoms have remained much the same over this period of time. Patient denies constipation or noticing any blood in the toilet or on the toilet paper. |
| b. description of any factors that seem to precipitate, exacerbate, and/or relieve the patient's symptoms. | Symptoms seem to get worse when he sits for prolonged periods of time. |
| c. description of the patient's efforts to relieve the symptoms | Taking a warm bath seems to relieve the symptoms at least for a short period of time. He tried several doses of acetaminophen, but it did not help the itching and burning. |
| 2. Gather essential patient history information: | |
| a. patient's identity | Jason Jimla |
| b. age, sex, height, and weight | 35 y/o WM, 5'11", 170 lb |
| c. patient's occupation | Used to work for the U.S. Postal Service as a letter carrier; promoted to a desk job several months ago |
| d. patient's dietary habits | Moderate carbohydrate and protein, low-fat, low-cholesterol diet |
| e. patient's sleep habits | Averages 8 hours per night |
| f. concurrent medical conditions, prescription and nonprescription medications, and dietary supplements | HTN × 5 years; HCTZ 25 mg/day; lisinopril 10 mg/day; simvastatin for high cholesterol and pantoprazole for acid reflux |
| g. allergies | NKA |
| h. history of other adverse reactions to medications | None |
| i. other (describe)_______ | |
| **Assessment and Triage** | |
| 3. Differentiate the patient's signs/symptoms and correctly identify the patient's primary problem(s) (see Tables 18-1 and 18-2). | Jason complains of mild to moderate anal itching, burning, and some discomfort, which is most likely associated with hemorrhoids. |
| 4. Identify exclusions for self-treatment (see Figure 18-2). | Jason does not appear to have any exclusions to self-care. No constipation or rectal bleeding was noted. |
| 5. Formulate a comprehensive list of therapeutic alternatives for the primary problem to determine if triage to a medical practitioner is required, and share this information with the patient. | Options include:<br>(1) Recommend self-care with an appropriate nonprescription anorectal product and advise on nondrug measures.<br>(2) Recommend self-care with an appropriate anorectal product and advise on nondrug measures until Jason can contact his PCP.<br>(3) Refer Jason to his PCP for medical evaluation of his symptoms.<br>(4) Take no action. |
| **Plan** | |
| 6. Select an optimal therapeutic alternative to address the patient's problem, taking into account patient preferences. | The optimal anorectal product should relieve the patient's itching, burning, and discomfort. Figure 18-2 lists appropriate therapeutic options. Table 18-6 lists specific products. Products that contain vasoconstrictors such as phenylephedrine should be avoided because the patient has hypertension. Jason states that he prefers an ointment that contains hydrocortisone. |

## CASE 18-2 (continued)

| Relevant Evaluation Criteria | Scenario/Model Outcome |
|---|---|
| 7. Describe the recommended therapeutic approach to the patient. | Apply the hydrocortisone 1% ointment to the external anal area up to three to four times a day, preferably after a bowel movement and at bedtime as described in Table 18-3. |
| 8. Explain to the patient the rationale for selecting the recommended therapeutic approach from the considered therapeutic alternatives. | You don't need to see your PCP, that is, primary care provider, at this time because your symptoms are relatively mild and may be related to hemorrhoids, which are usually treated with nonprescription products. Hydrocortisone 1% ointment, when applied to the anal area, should provide temporary relief of the itching, burning, and discomfort you describe. |
| **Patient Education** | |
| 9. When recommending self-care with nonprescription medications and/or nondrug therapy, convey accurate information to the patient, including: | |
| a. appropriate dose and frequency of administration | See Table 18-4. |
| b. maximum number of days the therapy should be employed | 7 days |
| c. product administration procedures | See Table 18-3. |
| d. expected time to onset of relief | Symptom relief should be evident within a few days of applying the ointment as directed. |
| e. degree of relief that can be reasonably expected | Complete relief of your itching, burning, and discomfort is possible. |
| f. most common side effects | Hydrocortisone ointment, when applied to the anal area, is usually well tolerated. |
| g. side effects that warrant medical intervention should they occur | Hydrocortisone ointment may mask the symptoms of an infection. If this occurs, you may notice worsening or recurrence of your symptoms when you discontinue this medication. |
| h. patient options in the event that condition worsens or persists | Contact your PCP if your symptoms worsen or persist beyond 7 days of self-treatment. See the box Patient Education for Anorectal Disorders. |
| i. product storage requirements | Store medication out of the reach of children and at a controlled room temperature. |
| j. specific nondrug measures | See the box Patient Education for Anorectal Disorders. |
| 10. Solicit follow-up questions from patient. | Are suppositories any more effective than ointments for my itching and burning? |
| 11. Answer patient's questions. | No. Both dosage forms are effective for your symptoms. However, an ointment is more likely to remain in the anal area. |

Key: HCTZ, hydrochlorothiazide; HTN, hypertension; NKA, no known allergies; PCP, primary care provider.

## Key Points for Anorectal Disorders

- Limit the self-treatment of anorectal disorders to minor signs and symptoms such as burning, itching, discomfort, swelling, and irritation.
- Advise patients with self-treatable symptoms that if the condition worsens, new symptoms develop, or symptoms do not improve after 7 days, they should contact their primary care provider.
- Use only products for external use (except for protectants) in pregnant and breast-feeding women.
- Refer children younger than 12 years and anyone with a family history of colon cancer to their primary care provider.
- Advise patients to select an anorectal product that contains the fewest number of ingredients necessary to treat specific symptoms to minimize undesirable effects.
- Instruct patients on how to use or apply specific anorectal products (Table 18-3).

## PATIENT EDUCATION FOR ANORECTAL DISORDERS

The objectives of self-treatment are to relieve specific signs and symptoms and prevent complications that may lead to more serious problems. For most patients, carefully following the product instructions and the self-care measures listed here will help ensure relief of symptoms.

### Nondrug Measures

- Maintain hydration and a healthy diet. If you experience hard stools, straining, or are constipated, increase the amount of fiber and fluids in your diet to reduce or prevent straining during bowel movements (see Chapter 16).
- If possible, avoid medications that cause constipation (see Chapter 16).
- Clean the anorectal area after each bowel movement with a moistened, unscented, white toilet tissue or a wipe.
- A sitz bath or soaking in the bathtub two to three times a day may help mild anal itching, burning, irritation, and discomfort.

### Nonprescription Medications

- Anorectal products contain local anesthetics, vasoconstrictors, protectants, analgesics/anesthetics/antipruritics, astringents, and keratolytics. Select products that contain only ingredients needed to relieve specific symptoms.
- See Table 18-3 for guidelines for applying anorectal products.
- See Table 18-4 for recommended dosages.
- Use only selected vasoconstrictors (ephedrine and phenylephrine), protectants (not glycerin), and astringents (calamine and zinc oxide) inside the rectum.
- Use only products approved for external use if the patient is pregnant. If internal use is required, then protectants, with the exception of glycerin, may be used.
- If you have a history of cardiovascular disease, diabetes, hypertension, hyperthyroidism, or difficulty urinating because of prostate problems, you should avoid topical anorectal products containing vasoconstrictors.
- If you are taking medications to treat hypertension or depression you should not use an anorectal product containing any vasoconstrictors without first consulting your primary care provider.
- Anorectal products containing ephedrine sulfate or phenylephrine may cause nervousness, tremor, sleeplessness, nausea, and loss of appetite.
- Appropriate use of anorectal products should reduce or relieve symptoms within a few days of self-treatment.
- Patient preferences should be considered especially when specific products may be used to treat the same symptoms, when there is a choice between an ointment and a suppository, and when generic products are available.

⚠ Stop using the anorectal product and contact a primary care provider as soon as possible if insertion of a product into the rectum causes pain.

⚠ Contact a primary care provider if symptoms worsen, new symptoms such as bleeding develop, or symptoms do not improve after 7 days of self-treatment.

⚠ Certain people may develop allergic or hypersensitivity reactions to anorectal products containing recommended concentrations of approved ingredients. Discontinue use of the product and contact a primary care provider as soon as possible if you develop signs or symptoms, such as a rash or increased itching, redness, burning or swelling in the anorectal area.

- Counsel patient on nondrug measures such as dietary measures and perianal hygiene (see box Patient Education for Anorectal Disorders).
- Do not use anorectal products that contain vasoconstrictors in patients with conditions such as diabetes, hypertension, and cardiac disease because of the possibility of systemic adverse effects.
- Advise patients of advantages and disadvantages of various anorectal dosage forms so they can select a product that is best suited for them.

## References


1. Anorectal drug products for over-the-counter human use: establishment of a monograph. *Federal Register.* 1980;45:35576-7.
2. Johanson JF. Hemorrhoids. In: Everhart JE, ed. *Digestive Diseases in the United States: Epidemiology and Impact.* US Department of Health and Human Services. Public Health Service, National Institutes of Health, National Institutes of Diabetes, Digestive and Kidney Diseases. Washington, DC: U.S. Government Printing Office; 1994: 271-98. NIH Publication No. 94-1447.
3. Fleming H. OTCs pharmacists recommend most. *Drug Topics.* 2000;14:24.
4. Levy S. Hemorrhoidal remedies category up across all outlets. *Drug Topics.* 2001;15. Available at: http://www.drugtopics.com/drugtopics/article/articleDetail.jsp?id=118857. Accessed February 2, 2005.
5. Madoff RD, Fleshman JW, Clinical Practice Committee, American Gastroenterological Association. American Gastroenterological Association technical review on the diagnosis and treatment of hemorrhoids. *Gastroenterology.* 2004;126:1463-73.
6. Abrameowitz L, Sobhani I, Benifla JL, et al. Anal fissure and thrombosed external hemorrhoids before and after delivery. *Dis Colon Rectum.* 2002;45:650-5.
7. Hull T. Examination and diseases of the anorectum. In: Feldman M, Friedman LS, Sleisenger MH, eds. *Sleisenger & Fordtran's Gastrointestinal and Liver Disease: Pathophysiology/Diagnosis/Management.* 7th ed. Philadelphia: WB Saunders; 2002:2277-93.
8. Ahmed SK, Thomson HJ. The effect of breakfast on minor anal complaints: a matched case-control study. *J R Coll Surg Edinb.* 1997;42:331-3.
9. Johanson JF. Nonsurgical treatment of hemorrhoids. *J Gastrointest Surg.* 2002;6:290-4.
10. Delco F, Sonnenberg A. Associations between hemorrhoids and other diagnoses. *Dis Colon Rectum.* 1998;41:1534-41.
11. Barnett JL. Anorectal diseases. In: Yamada T, Alpers DH, Powell DW, et al., eds. *Textbook of Gastroenterology.* 4th ed. Philadelphia: JB Lippincott; 2003:1990-2012.
12. Lunniss PJ, Mann CV. Classification of internal haemorrhoids: a discussion paper. *Colorectal Dis.* 2004;6:226-32.
13. Pfenninger JL, Zainea GG. Common anorectal conditions: part II, lesions. *Am Fam Physician.* 2001;64:77-88.
14. Hyman N. Anorectal abscess and fistula. *Prim Care.* 1999; 26:69-80.
15. Madoff RD, Fleshman JW. AGA technical review on the diagnosis and care of patients with anal fissure. *Gastroenterology.* 2003;124:235-45.

16. Moore HG, Guillem JG. Anal neoplasms. *Surg Clin North Am.* 2002;82:1233-51.
17. Vincent C. Anorectal pain and irritation—anal fissure, levator syndrome, proctalgia fugax, and pruritus ani. *Prim Care.* 1999; 26:53-68.
18. Pfenninger JL, Zainea GG. Common anorectal conditions: part I, symptoms and complaints. *Am Fam Physician.* 2001;63:2391-8.
19. Anorectal drug products for over-the-counter human use. *Federal Register.* 2002;5:265-70.
20. Hussain JN. Hemorrhoids. *Prim Care.* 1999;26:35-51.
21. El Ashaal Y, Chandran V, Prem V, et al. Short note: local anal hypothermia with a frozen finger: a treatment for acute painful prolapsed piles. *Br J Surg.* 1998;85:520-1.
22. Anorectal drug products for over-the-counter human use: tentative final monograph. *Federal Register.* 1988;53:30756-8.
23. Anorectal drug products for over-the-counter human use. CFR [serial online]. 2004; Title 21, Vol 5, Pt 346. Available at: http://www.accessdata.fda.gov. Accessed November 18, 2004.
24. Skidmore RA, Patterson JD, Tomsick RS. Local anesthetic. *Dermatol Surg.* 1996;22:511-22.
25. Eggleston ST, Lush LW. Understanding allergic reactions to local anesthetics. *Ann Pharmacother.* 1996;30:851-7.
26. Sanchez-Perez J, Cordoba S, Cortizas CF, et al. Allergic contact balanitis due to tetracaine (amethocaine) hydrochloride. *Contact Dermatitis.* 1998;39:268.
27. Young Lee AI. Allergic contact dermatitis from dibucaine in proctosedyl ointment without cross-sensitivity. *Contact Dermatitis.* 1998;39:261.
28. Lodi A, Ambonati M, Coassini A, et al. Contact allergy to 'caines' by anti-hemorrhoidal ointments. *Contact Dermatitis.* 1999;41:221-2.
29. Requirements for child-resistant packaging; requirements for products containing lidocaine or dibucaine. *Federal Register.* 1995; 60:17992-8005.
30. Blumenthal M. The Complete German Commission E Monographs—Therapeutic Guide to Herbal Medicines. Austin, Tex: American Botanical Council; 1998:190-2.
31. DerMarderosian A, Beutler JA., eds. *Facts and Comparisons—The Review of Natural Products.* 2nd ed. St. Louis: Facts and Comparisons; 2002.
32. Gruenwald J, Brendler T, Jaenicke C., eds. *PDR for Herbal Medicine.* 2nd ed. Montvale, NJ: Medical Economics Co; 2000.
33. Foster S, Tyler VE. *Tyler's Honest Herbal—A Sensible Guide to the Use of Herbs and Related Remedies.* 4th ed. New York: The Haworth Herbal Press; 1999:331-3.
34. Pittler MH, Ernst E. Horse-chestnut seed extract for chronic venous insufficiency: a criteria-based systemic review. *Arch Dermatol.* 1998;134:1356-60.
35. Misra MC, Parshad R. Randomized clinical trial of micronized flavonoids in the early control of bleeding from acute internal haemorrhoids. *Br J Surg.* 2000;87:868-72.
36. Downey P. *Homeopathy for the Primary Health Care Team.* 1st ed. Oxford, England: Butterworth-Heinemann; 1997:99-100.
37. Leckridge B. *Homeopathy in Primary Care.* 1st ed. New York: Churchill Livingstone; 1997:142, 191-2.
38. Skinner SE. *An Introduction to Homeopathic Medicine in Primary Care.* Gaithersburg, Md: Aspen Publishers, Inc; 2001:275-7.
39. Goldstein L. Ask the midwife. Prevention and care of hemorrhoids, including homeopathic remedies. *Birth Gaz.* 2000;16:13-6.
40. Boyd EL, Shimp LA, Hackney ML. *Home Remedies and the Black Elderly.* Ann Arbor: University of Michigan Press; 1984:19-22.

CHAPTER 19

# Pinworm Infection

*Jeffery A. Goad and Lawrence Neinstein*

Parasitic helminth (worms) infections cause significant morbidity and mortality worldwide.[1] This chapter will focus on the detection and management of pinworm (*Enterobius vermicularis*) infection because it is the most common worm infestation in the United States and is the only helminthic infection for which a nonprescription medication has been approved for treatment.[2,3] While pinworms are a nuisance, the infection presents little risk to the infected individual or the public.[4]

Worms that infect humans can be divided into the following phyla: (1) nematoda (roundworm), including pinworms, strongyloides, whipworms and hookworms; (2) cestoda (tapeworm), including beef and pork tapeworms; and (3) trematoda (fluke), including schistosomes. Table 19-1 shows the most common human nematode infections, their sources, common signs and symptoms, and treatment options.[2,5,6]

## Epidemiology of Pinworm Infection

Enterobiasis is commonly called "pinworm" or "seatworm infection." In the United States, pinworm infection is the most common of all worm infections, occurring in an estimated 42 million people, with the greatest infection rate in children ages 5 to 14 years.[3] *Enterobius vermicularis* infests only humans; pets cannot give children pinworms, contrary to what some parents believe. Unlike most other worm infections, pinworms do not live in the soil or water, but are transmitted person-to-person. Also, unlike many helminthic infections, enterobiasis is not limited to rural and poverty-stricken areas; it can occur in urban communities and infect individuals from all socioeconomic groups. *E. vermicularis* is found most commonly in congested districts, in institutionalized groups, and among family members.[3] Other roundworm infections, such as ascaris and hookworm, are found commonly in southeastern parts of the United States.

## Etiology of Pinworm Infection

The most common pinworm transmission route is probably person-to-person via the anus-to-mouth transfer of eggs when children use contaminated fingers or fomites to handle and ingest food.[7] Reinfection may occur readily because eggs often are found under fingernails of infected children who have scratched the anal area. Thumb sucking, nail biting, and nose picking, however, have not been associated with the initial infection, but can certainly contribute to reinfection.[4] Embryonated eggs also can be transferred from the perianal region to nightclothes, bedding, dust, and air. The eggs can remain infective for several days, especially under humid conditions, and can spread within a microcommunity, such as a household or school, partly by this route.[8] Sexual transmission may occur through oral–anal sex.[9]

## Pathophysiology of Pinworm Infection

The adult pinworm is small, white, and threadlike with a pin-shaped pointed tail (from which the name is derived; see Color Plates, photograph 1A.)[3,5] Adult male and female worms inhabit the first portion, or ileocecum, of the large intestine and seldom cause damage to the intestinal wall. The mature female, approximately 8 to 13 mm in length, usually stores approximately 11,000 eggs in her body (see Color Plates, photograph 1B). After migrating down the colon and out the anus, she deposits her sticky eggs in the perianal region, and dies shortly afterward. Males are smaller (2.5 mm), live only approximately 2 weeks, and do not migrate.[7] If eggs are not washed off, they hatch within a few hours, and larvae may return to the large intestine through the anus (retroinfection) or, rarely, in female patients, may mistakenly crawl into the urogenital tract.[5] Alternatively, eggs can be transferred to the mouth, most commonly on a child's fingers after scratching of the anal area. Within 2 to 6 weeks of egg ingestion, larvae are released and mature into gravid females, thus continuing the cycle, which can continue indefinitely unless appropriate behavioral and/or pharmacotherapeutic interventions are instituted.

## Signs and Symptoms of Pinworm Infection

Patients with minor pinworm infections are often asymptomatic. The most frequent symptom is usually an irritating perianal or perineal itch that typically occurs at night when the female deposits eggs. Major infections may produce symptoms ranging from abdominal discomfort to severe pain, insomnia, nervousness, inability to concentrate, loss of appetite (rather than an increase in hunger, as was commonly believed), nausea, diarrhea, and intractable localized itching.[5] Less common clinical features may include vaginitis, pelvic inflammatory disease, urethritis, dysuria, and hives.[4] Patients with these symptoms should be referred to a primary care provider for further evaluation.

Physical signs and symptoms are not the only misery-inducing effects of enterobiasis. Parents are often dismayed to find worms near a child's anus; this psychologic

TABLE 19-1 Common Nematode (Roundworm) Infections in the United States[2,5,6]

| Common Name (Scientific Name) | Source of Infection | Clinical Features | Treatment | Comments |
|---|---|---|---|---|
| Pinworm (*Enterobius vermicularis*) | Autoinoculation with eggs by anus to mouth transfer; retroinfection: larvae return to rectum; transmission: egg-contaminated fomites and aerosolized eggs | Minor infections asymptomatic; most frequent: irritating itch in perianal and perineal regions, usually at night; children: nervousness, inability to concentrate, lack of appetite | Drug of choice: pyrantel pamoate; adult/pediatric dose: 11 mg/kg or 5 mg/lb once (max: 1 g); repeat in 2 weeks if symptoms do not resolve; *alternative:* mebendazole (Vermox), adult/pediatric dose (>2 years): 100 mg once; repeat in 2 weeks if symptoms do not resolve | High rate of reinfection necessitates retreatment; pyrantel is OTC, available as liquid, caplets; mebendazole, available as chewable tablets |
| Giant roundworm (*Ascaris lumbricoides*) | Ingestion of soil containing mature eggs that hatch in the intestine; larvae penetrate lymphatics and travel to lungs, where they are coughed up and swallowed; larvae mature to adult worm and live for 12-18 months; female lays eggs, which are passed into the stool | Many patients asymptomatic; vague abdominal discomfort common; children: fever, weight loss, failure to grow; intestinal obstruction may lead to biliary colic, hepatitis, pancreatitis, or peritonitis; cough, substernal burning, wheezing, fever may occur during lung stage (1-2 wks long) | Drug of choice: albendazole (Albenza); adult/pediatric dose: 400 mg by mouth once; *alternatives:* pyrantel pamoate 11 mg/kg (1 g max) once, mebendazole 100 mg 2 times/day for 3 days or 500 mg once | FDA considers albendazole and pyrantel to be investigational drugs for ascariasis |
| Hookworm (*Ancylostoma duodenale* [Old World]; *Necator americanus* [New World]) | Penetration of intact skin by larvae living in contaminated soil; larvae travel to lungs, where they are coughed up and swallowed; maturation occurs in intestine; eggs are produced and passed into feces, where they develop into larvae | Erythematous maculopapular rash and edema with severe itching for several days; lesions commonly between toes (ground itch); pulmonary symptoms rare during lung stage; eosinophilia, 30%-70%; anemia common | Drug of choice: albendazole (Albenza); adult/pediatric dose: 400 mg by mouth once; *alternatives:* pyrantel pamoate 11 mg/kg (1 g max) once daily for 3 days, mebendazole 100 mg 2 times/day for 3 days or 500 mg once | FDA considers albendazole and pyrantel to be investigational drugs for hookworm; in addition to anthelminthic, need to treat anemia with iron; Old and New World treatment identical |

trauma or "pinworm neurosis" must be considered a harmful effect of enterobiasis. Patients and parents need to be assured that pinworms are common and curable, and that no social stigma is attached to their occurrence.[8]

## Complications of Pinworm Infection

Scratching to relieve itching from pinworm infection may lead to secondary bacterial infection of the perianal and perineal regions. Pinworms may cause vulvovaginitis and, rarely, enter the female genital tract, where they can become encapsulated within the uterus or fallopian tubules. Helminthic infections in the genital tract may lead to endometritis, salpingitis, tubo-ovarian abscess, pelvic inflammatory disease, and possibly infertility.[10] They may also migrate into the peritoneal cavity and form granulomas. Rarely, they may cause appendicitis in children.[11]

## Treatment of Pinworm Infection

### *Treatment Goals*

The goal of self-treatment is to eradicate pinworms from the patient and the household, thereby preventing reinfection.

**Exclusions for Self-Treatment**

- Liver disease
- Anemia
- Pregnancy
- Breast-feeding
- <2 years of age unless PCP has approved OTC treatment
- Weight <25 lb unless PCP has approved OTC treatment
- Vague symptoms and negative visual inspection
- Helminthic infections other than pinworms
- Hypersensitivity to pyrantel pamoate
- Need for repeat dosing

*Source:* Reference 2.

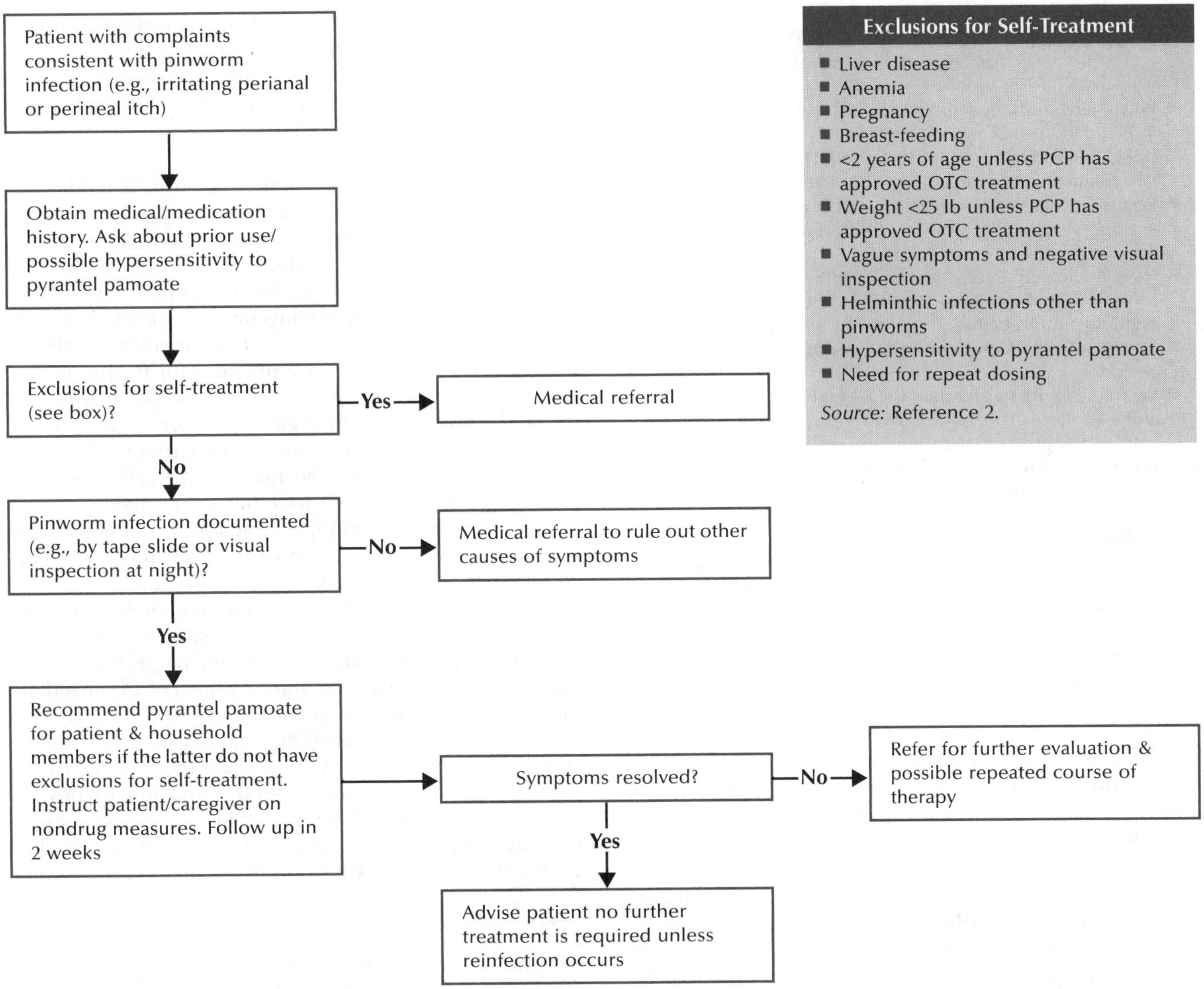


**FIGURE 19-1** Self-care of pinworm infection. Key: OTC, over-the-counter; PCP, primary care provider.

### General Treatment Approach

The management of pinworm infection includes drug treatment with pyrantel pamoate for the patient and for every household member, as well as prevention of reinfection. Strict hygiene (e.g., washing linens, disinfecting toilet seats) is an integral part of the treatment. Figure 19-1 outlines self-care of this infection and lists exclusions for self-treatment. Although pyrantel is not indicated for self-treatment of ascaris or hookworm, it can treat all three parasites at the same time (Table 19-1).

### Nonpharmacologic Therapy

Once pinworm infection is suspected, the patient or caregiver should follow the nondrug measures in Table 19-2[12,13] to minimize family and household infections and reinfections. Children can usually return to school after the first dose of an appropriate anthelminthic agent, and after their fingernails are cut and cleaned. Practitioners are in an ideal position to inform patients of behaviors that may increase their risk of helminthic infections.

### Pharmacologic Therapy

At one time, gentian violet was the only nonprescription medication available to treat pinworm infections. The Food and Drug Administration (FDA) has since declared gentian violet a "nonmonograph ingredient," and it can no longer be marketed as an anthelminthic. Pyrantel pamoate is the only nonprescription medication approved for pinworm infection.

#### Pyrantel Pamoate

Pyrantel pamoate was first used in veterinary practice as a broad-spectrum drug for pinworms, roundworms, and hookworms. Because of its effectiveness and lack of toxicity, it has become an important drug for treating certain helminthic infections in humans.[12]

**TABLE 19-2 Nondrug and Preventive Measures for Treating Pinworm Infection[12,13]**

- Wash bed linens, bedclothes, towels, and underwear of the infected individual and the entire family in hot water (131°F [55°C]) daily during treatment period. Do not shake these items; shaking can spread eggs into the air.
- Eggs are destroyed by sunlight, so ensure blinds or curtains are open in the affected room to enhance cleaning of the environment.
- Have the infected individual take daily morning showers to remove eggs deposited in the perianal region during the night (avoid tub baths).
- Use disinfectants on toilet seats daily during treatment period.
- Vacuum (do not sweep) daily the area around beds, curtains, and elsewhere in the bedroom where concentration of eggs is likely the greatest. Wet-mopping before or instead of vacuuming may limit spread of pinworm eggs into the air.
- Wear close-fitting shorts under one-piece pajamas at night to prevent migration of worms from the perianal and perineal regions.
- After an infected child uses the toilet, scrub the child's fingers with soap and a brush. Trim the child's nails regularly to prevent harboring of eggs and autoinoculation (hand-to-mouth reinfection). Wash hands frequently, especially before meals and after using the toilet.

The reported cure rate is 80% to 100% after one dose (Table 19-1).[14] Although this product is readily available, helminthic infections other than those caused by pinworms should be diagnosed and treated by a primary care provider.

*Mechanism of Action* Pyrantel pamoate is a depolarizing neuromuscular agent that paralyzes adult worms, causing them to loosen their hold on the intestinal wall and subsequently be passed out in the stool before they can lay eggs. It is poorly absorbed and 50% of the drug is excreted unchanged in the feces.

*Indications* Pyrantel pamoate is effective in treating pinworm infections without a primary care provider visit, but treatment of roundworm and hookworm infections require medical supervision (Table 19-1).[6]

*Dosage and Administration Guidelines* A single oral dose of pyrantel pamoate (liquid or caplet) is based on the body weight (5 mg/lb or 11 mg/kg) of adults and children. The maximum single dose is 1 g. The recommended dosage is the same for children younger than 2 years or weighing less than 25 lb; however, they should not be treated without first consulting a primary care provider. The product includes a schedule of recommended dosages based on body weight, which should not be exceeded. The dose may need to be repeated in 2 weeks if symptoms do not resolve since reinfection is common; however, the repeat dose should be administered only under the guidance of a primary care provider.[15] Reinfection may be due to the drug's lack of effect on eggs and larvae, and to the eggs being viable up to 20 days.[16]

Pyrantel pamoate may be taken at any time of the day with or without food. A special diet, fasting, or purging before or after administration is not necessary. The liquid formulation, containing 50 mg/mL, should be shaken well before the dose is measured.

*Safety Considerations* Side effects are usually mild, infrequent, and transient. The most common adverse effects involve the gastrointestinal (GI) tract and include nausea, vomiting, tenesmus, anorexia, diarrhea, and abdominal cramps.[17] However, a patient who experiences severe or persistent abdominal symptoms or other side effects after taking the first or second dose of this medication should be referred to a primary care provider for further evaluation. Less commonly, headache, dizziness, drowsiness, insomnia, rash, fever, and weakness may occur. In very rare circumstances, transient increases in aspartate aminotransferase, ototoxicity, optic neuritis, and hallucinations with confusion and paresthesia have been reported.[18]

The anthelminthics piperazine and pyrantel pamoate have antagonistic mechanisms of action; therefore, concomitant administration is not recommended.[2]

Pyrantel pamoate is contraindicated in patients with hypersensitivity to the drug. Patients with preexisting liver dysfunction, severe malnutrition, or anemia should not self-medicate without first consulting a primary care provider.[10] Pyrantel pamoate is a pregnancy Category C drug and has not been adequately studied in pregnant women; it should be used during pregnancy only when the benefits clearly outweigh the risks[2] and only under the direction of a primary care provider. Pyrantel pamoate should not be used in patients younger than 2 years or those weighing less than 25 lb unless under the direction of a primary care provider.

### Prescription Medications

Two prescription alternatives to pyrantel pamoate are mebendazole (Vermox) and albendazole (Albenza). Albendazole is approved to treat other helminthic infections, but FDA considers it an investigational drug when used to treat pinworms.[12] Mebendazole is considered equally effective, compared with pyrantel, but a primary care provider visit is required. Household members should be treated because they may also be infected and can act as a reservoir to reinfect others.[13,19]

### Product Selection Guidelines

Pyrantel pamoate is a safe and effective treatment for pinworms. The several brands listed in Table 19-3 are comparatively priced and generally less expensive than prescription treatment (e.g., Vermox). It should be noted that Antiminth is no longer produced by Pfizer in the United States.

## *Complementary Therapies*

Several herbal preparations boast, among other indications, that they can help expel worms. Some suggested ingredients include wormwood (*Artemisia absinthium* L.), rue (*Ruta graveolens* L.), and black walnut (*Juglans nigra*). Adequate scientific studies have not been conducted to allow recommendation of any of these products to treat

**TABLE 19-3 Selected Nonprescription Anthelminthic Products**

| Trade Name | Primary Ingredient |
|---|---|
| Pin-X Liquid | Pyrantel pamoate 50 mg/mL (base) |
| Pyrantel Pamoate Suspension | Pyrantel pamoate 50 mg/mL (base) |
| Reese's Pinworm Caplet | Pyrantel pamoate 180 mg (equals 62.5 mg pyrantel base) |
| Reese's Pinworm Liquid | Pyrantel pamoate 144 mg/mL (equals 50 mg pyrantel base) |

pinworms; in fact, evidence exists that the products may be dangerous. Wormwood is associated with a syndrome known as "absinthism," which is characterized by digestive problems, thirst, restlessness, vertigo, trembling of the limbs, numbness of the extremities, loss of intellect, delirium, paralysis, and death.[20] FDA considers wormwood an unsafe herb. Rue with antispasmodic properties can induce violent gastric pain and may be an abortifacient. Black walnut, used for everything from hair dye to an anthelminthic, is contraindicated in pregnancy and in patients with GI tract disease and is associated with severe allergic reactions.[20]

## Assessment of Pinworm Infection: A Case-based Approach

Before recommending treatment, the practitioner should explain how to confirm a pinworm infection by any of the following methods: (1) nighttime perianal or perineal itching in a child; (2) visual inspection of the perianal or perineal area for the adult worm; or (3) a cellophane tape test. Adult pinworms and eggs are seldom found in the feces; thus, looking for worms in the stool is not a reliable way to diagnose enterobiasis.[7] When symptoms of pinworms, such as nocturnal perianal or perineal itching, are present in children, nonprescription therapy may be initiated. However, since asymptomatic disease is common in enterobiasis, visual inspection may be necessary. To conduct a visual inspection, the parent should inspect the anal area during the night with a flashlight while the child is sleeping or in the very early morning before the child arises. White, threadlike, wriggling worms about the size of a staple may be seen. If pinworms are present, treatment should be initiated. Finally, if pinworms are suspected, but symptoms are vague and/or visual inspection is negative, a primary care provider may instruct the patient to obtain a cellophane tape ("Scotch tape") sample. The parent should apply the sticky side of the tape to the perianal area (usually with a tongue depressor) and affix it sticky side down on a glass slide. Commercially available kits use a sticky paddle instead of tape to affix to a slide (see Color Plates, photograph 1C). The sample should then be taken to a primary care provider for microscopic examination. Samples should be taken over 3 consecutive days upon the child's awakening, which may increase likelihood of detection to around 90%.[21] If this test is positive, treatment should be initiated. Cases 19-1 and 19-2 illustrate the assessment of patients with pinworm infections.

**CASE 19-1**

| Relevant Evaluation Criteria | Scenario/Model Outcome |
|---|---|
| **Information Gathering** | |
| 1. Gather essential information about the patient's symptoms, including: | |
| a. description of symptom(s) (i.e., nature, onset, duration, severity, associated symptoms) | Mother presents to the pharmacy with a prescription for mebendazole for her 3-year-old daughter, who was diagnosed on the basis of symptoms of perianal itching at night for the last few days. The PCP told the mother that her husband and 5-year-old son should also be treated, but that they would have to see their own PCP for a prescription. The parents and the son are not experiencing the same symptoms however. |
| b. description of any factors that seem to precipitate, exacerbate, and/or relieve the patient's symptom(s) | No precipitating factors |
| c. description of the patient's efforts to relieve the symptoms | Mother previously applied hydrocortisone to the daughter's perianal area with no relief. |
| 2. Gather essential patient history information: | |
| a. patient's identity | GP |
| b. age, sex, height, and weight | 3 y/o F, 30 lb (mother weighs 145 lb; 5-year-old son, 43 lb; father, 170 lb) |
| c. patient's occupation | None |
| d. patient's dietary habits | Normal |

## CASE 19-1 (continued)

| Relevant Evaluation Criteria | Scenario/Model Outcome |
|---|---|
| e. patient's sleep habits | Frequently wakes up at night with perianal itching |
| f. concurrent medical conditions, prescription and nonprescription medications, and dietary supplements | None |
| g. allergies | None |
| h. history of other adverse reactions to medications | None |
| i. other (describe)_______ | The family has recently emigrated from Mexico and does not have medical insurance. |
| **Assessment and Triage** | |
| 3. Differentiate the patient's signs/symptoms and correctly identify the patient's primary problem(s). | The PCP's diagnosis of pinworms is consistent with the reported symptoms and inconsistent with other helminthic infections (see Table 19-1). Pinworm infection is very contagious in household contacts, and its treatment is short and uncomplicated, making treatment of asymptomatic close contacts desirable. |
| 4. Identify exclusions for self-treatment (see Figure 19-1). | None |
| 5. Formulate a comprehensive list of therapeutic alternatives for the primary problem to determine if triage to a medical practitioner is required, and share this information with the caregiver. | Options include:<br>(1) Insist that the mother, husband, and male sibling see a PCP for a prescription for mebendazole.<br>(2) Recommend an appropriate OTC product such as pyrantel to treat the whole family.<br>(3) Recommend only environmental controls.<br>(4) Take no action. |
| **Plan** | |
| 6. Select an optimal therapeutic alternative to address the patient's problem, taking into account patient preferences. | See Figure 19-1. |
| 7. Describe the recommended therapeutic approach to the caregiver. | Mebendazole and pyrantel pamoate are equally effective in the treatment of pinworms. Since the mother needs a less expensive alternative to mebendazole and an office visit for her and her family, and her daughter has already been diagnosed with pinworms, pyrantel liquid would be a cost-effective alternative. The 60-mL size would treat her whole family.<br>Pyrantel pamoate is based on the weight of each family member. The 3-year-old would receive 3 mL (50 mg/mL), the 5-year-old, 4.3 mL, the mother, 15 mL, and the father, 17 mL. The total required volume for the initial dose is about 40 mL. |
| 8. Explain to the caregiver the rationale for selecting the recommended therapeutic approach from the considered therapeutic alternatives. | Pyrantel pamoate, a nonprescription antihelminthic, is available as a liquid and offers flexible dosing based on weight, whereas mebendazole does not. Pyrantel pamoate is also less expensive, and its use does not require the whole family to see a primary care provider. Pinworms are not life threatening and may resolve on their own if environmental and personal hygiene controls are enacted; however, treatment with pyrantel is more than 90% effective. |
| **Patient Education** | |
| 9. When recommending self-care with nonprescription medications and/or nondrug therapy, convey accurate information to the caregiver, including: | |
| a. appropriate dose and frequency of administration | The dose is 5 mg/lb or 11 mg/kg. GP should take one dose of 3 mL of a 50-mg/mL suspension of pyrantel pamoate. You may repeat this dose in 2 weeks if the PCP recommends retreatment. Other family members should also take the medication (see #7 for dosages for other family members). |

## CASE 19-1 (continued)

| Relevant Evaluation Criteria | Scenario/Model Outcome |
|---|---|
| b. maximum number of days the therapy should be employed | Single dose. Your primary care provider may recommend a repeat dose if symptoms do not subside in 2 weeks. |
| c. product administration procedures | Shake well. Administer the exact dose using an oral dosage syringe or dosing spoon. Take with or without food. |
| d. expected time to onset of relief | Several days |
| e. degree of relief that can be reasonably expected | Complete pinworm eradication with less perianal itching over successive days |
| f. most common side effects | Although side effects occur infrequently with this medication, GP may experience nausea, vomiting, spasms or straining during bowel movements, loss of appetite, diarrhea, or abdominal cramps after taking the medication. These side effects are usually mild and do not require evaluation by your primary care provider. |
| g. side effects that warrant medical intervention should they occur | Skin rash, any side effects listed in 8f that become severe, or persistence of pinworm-associated symptoms |
| h. patient options in the event that condition worsens or persists | Consult a health care provider if any of the severe side effects occur. |
| i. product storage requirements | Store at room temperature. Seal container tightly after use and protect from light. |
| j. specific nondrug measures | See Table 19-2. |

Key: N/A, not applicable; NKA, no known allergies; OTC, over-the-counter; PCP, primary care provider.

## CASE 19-2

| Relevant Evaluation Criteria | Scenario/Model Outcome |
|---|---|
| **Information Gathering** | |
| 1. Gather essential information about the patient's symptoms, including: | |
| a. description of symptom(s) (i.e., nature, onset, duration, severity, associated symptoms) | A mother asks for assistance in selecting a product to stop her daughter's itching. The mother explains that the child has intense perianal itching, especially at night, and has not been sleeping well. The child was diagnosed with *E. vermicularis* 10 days ago and treated with pyrantel at an appropriate dose. Her two other younger siblings were also treated, but the mother and father elected not to treat themselves. The PCP advised at that time that she could repeat the treatment if symptoms persisted. |
| b. description of any factors that seem to precipitate, exacerbate, and/or relieve the patient's symptom(s) | Itching gets worse at night. |
| c. description of the patient's efforts to relieve the symptoms | Mother has tried to discourage the child from scratching her perianal area. |
| 2. Gather essential patient history information: | |
| a. patient's identity | AG |
| b. age, sex, height, and weight | 5 y/o F, 43", 42 lb (mother weighs 150 lb; father, 220 lb; twin boys, 28 lb each) |
| c. patient's occupation | Student |
| d. patient's dietary habits | Normal diet; frequently eats with her hands |
| e. patient's sleep habits | Wakes up frequently during the night because of perianal itching |
| f. concurrent medical conditions, prescription and nonprescription medications, and dietary supplements | None |

## CASE 19-2 (continued)

| Relevant Evaluation Criteria | Scenario/Model Outcome |
|---|---|
| g. allergies | Ragweed |
| h. history of other adverse reactions to medications | None |
| i. other (describe)_______ | N/A |
| **Assessment and Triage** | |
| 3. Differentiate the patient's signs/symptoms and correctly identify the patient's primary problem(s). | Pinworm reinfestation is causing perianal itching and sleep disturbance. |
| 4. Identify exclusions for self-treatment (see Figure 19-1). | None |
| 5. Formulate a comprehensive list of therapeutic alternatives for the primary problem to determine if triage to a medical practitioner is required, and share this information with the patient. | Options include:<br>(1) Refer AG for medical evaluation and treatment.<br>(2) Recommend an appropriate OTC product for all family members and tell mother to inform their PCP of retreatment.<br>(3) Treat only AG with pyrantel pamoate.<br>(4) Take no action. |
| **Plan** | |
| 6. Select an optimal therapeutic alternative to address the patient's problem, taking into account patient preferences. | OTC treatment with pyrantel pamoate is appropriate at this time for AG, her mother and father, and their other two children. They should be instructed on environmental controls and behavioral modification (see Table 19-2). |
| 7. Describe the recommended therapeutic approach to the caregiver. | Give one dose (4.2 mL) of pyrantel pamoate 50 mg/mL suspension now to AG and a weight-appropriate dose to the other family members. |
| 8. Explain to the caregiver the rationale for selecting the recommended therapeutic approach from the considered therapeutic alternatives. | AG displays classic signs and symptoms of pinworm infection (nocturnal perianal itching and sleep loss) and is of the target age (5-14 years) for this infection. Since the mother and father were not treated and it is unclear whether environmental controls were enacted, it is likely AG has a reinfestation of pinworms. You could see your primary care provider for diagnosis and potential treatment with a prescription product (see Table 19-1), but that is probably unnecessary as OTC therapy is just as effective as prescription therapy and does not require an office visit. Treating only AG runs the risk of reinfestation by any of the other family members that may still be harboring the worm. |
| **Patient Education** | |
| 9. When recommending self-care with nonprescription medications and/or nondrug therapy, convey accurate information to the caregiver, including: | |
| a. appropriate dose and frequency of administration | The dose is 5 mg/lb or 11 mg/kg. AG should take 1 dose (4.2 mL) of a 50-mg/mL suspension of pyrantel pamoate. Other family members should receive the following weight-based doses: Mother weighs 150 lb, dose is 15 mL ($\frac{750\text{ mg}}{50\text{ mg/mL}}$ = 15 mL); father weighs 220 lb, dose is 20 mL (1 g = 20 mL; 1 g is maximum dose); twin 2-year-old boys weigh 28 lb each, dose is 2.8 mL each ($\frac{140\text{ mg}}{50\text{ mg/mL}}$ = 2.8 mL). Total volume required for entire family is 45 mL. |
| b. maximum number of days the therapy should be employed | Single dose |
| c. product administration procedures | Shake well. Administer the exact dose using an oral dosage syringe or dosing spoon. Take with or without food. |

CASE 19-2 (continued)

| Relevant Evaluation Criteria | Scenario/Model Outcome |
|---|---|
| d. expected time to onset of relief | Several days |
| e. degree of relief that can be reasonably expected | Complete pinworm eradication with less perianal itching over successive days |
| f. most common side effects | Although side effects occur infrequently with this medication, GP may experience nausea, vomiting, spasms or straining during bowel movements, loss of appetite, diarrhea, or abdominal cramps after taking the medication. These side effects are usually mild and do not require evaluation by your primary care provider. |
| g. side effects that warrant medical intervention should they occur | Skin rash, any side effects listed in 8f that become severe, or persistence of pinworm-associated symptoms |
| h. patient options in the event that condition worsens or persists | Consult a healthcare provider if any of the severe side effects occur. |
| i. product storage requirements | Store at room temperature. Seal container tightly after use and protect from light. |
| j. specific nondrug measures | See Table 19-2. |
| 10. Solicit follow-up questions from caregiver. | Should I give AG a higher dose of the pyrantel than the initial dose since the infestation has come back? |
| 11. Answer caregiver's questions. | No. A higher dose will not be more effective. All family members must take a weight-appropriate dose, and the child's environment must be cleaned as outlined in Table 19-2. |

Key: N/A, not applicable; NKA, no known allergies; OTC, over-the-counter; PCP, primary care provider.

## Patient Counseling for Pinworm Infection

After making the decision to treat a pinworm infection, the practitioner should review the package insert material for pyrantel pamoate with the patient/caregiver. This material explains the pinworm life cycle, symptoms of pinworm infection, and methods of transmitting the infection. The practitioner should calculate the doses for the patient and all family members, being sure to emphasize the need to treat the whole family. The patient/caregiver should be advised to implement strict hygienic measures to prevent reinfection or transmission of the infection to other family members (Table 19-2). The practitioner should explain that the side effects (see Case 19-1), of pyrantel pamoate are usually mild and infrequent, but if side effects are experienced, a primary care provider should be contacted before administering the repeat dose.[10] The most common adverse effects involve the GI tract and include nausea, vomiting, tenesmus, anorexia, diarrhea, and abdominal cramps.[17] Patients who experience severe or persistent abdominal cramps, nausea, vomiting, anorexia, diarrhea, headache, drowsiness, or dizziness after taking this medication should be referred for medical evaluation. Practitioners should also explain that the symptoms of pinworm infection (e.g., nocturnal perianal itching, etc.) should improve within 2 weeks with treatment. However, if symptoms persist or worsen to include systemic complaints (abdominal discomfort, insomnia, nervousness, etc.), patients should be instructed to see a primary care provider.

## Evaluation of Patient Outcomes for Pinworm Infection

The patient/caregiver should be instructed to contact a primary care provider if anal itching persists beyond 2 weeks or recurs, or if new symptoms develop. A second dose of pyrantel pamoate may then be given 2 weeks after the first dose while under medical care. If hygienic measures are not being followed, the practitioner should again stress their importance for preventing reinfection.

## Key Points for Pinworm Infection

- The practitioner should be familiar with common helminthic infections, their symptoms, and their treatment.
- Although pyrantel pamoate is used in treating other helminthic infections, only pinworm infection should be evaluated for self-treatment with a nonprescription drug.
- A primary care provider should be consulted when helminths other than pinworms are suspected.
- Pinworms are common in the United States and rarely cause significant morbidity.
- Practitioners can aid patients and caregivers in the self-diagnosis, counseling, and self-treatment with nonprescription anthelminthic medication.

## PATIENT EDUCATION FOR PINWORM INFECTION

The objectives of self-treatment are to (1) eradicate pinworms in the infected patient, (2) prevent reinfection, and (3) prevent transmission of the infection to others. For most patients, carefully following product instructions and the self-care measures listed here will help ensure optimal therapeutic outcomes.

### Nondrug Measures

- See Table 19-2 for nondrug/preventive measures.

### Nonprescription Medications

- Read package insert for pyrantel pamoate information carefully; this information will help prevent reinfection or transmission of the infection.
- Consult a primary care provider before giving the medication to a person with liver disease or anemia, to a child who is younger than 2 years and/or who weighs less than 25 lb, or to a woman who is pregnant or breast-feeding.
- Treat all household members to ensure elimination of the infection. Consult a primary care provider if household members meet criteria discussed above.
- Take only one dose as shown on the dosing schedule included with this product. For adults and children older than 2 years, dosing is the same: 11 mg/kg or 5 mg/lb, taken orally. The maximum dose is 1 g.
- Shake the liquid formulation well and use a measuring spoon to ensure an accurate dose.
- If desired, pyrantel pamoate may be taken with food, milk, or fruit juices on an empty stomach any time during the day. The liquid formulation may be mixed with milk or fruit juice.
- Note that fasting, laxatives, special diets, or purging is not necessary to aid treatment.

If abdominal cramps, nausea, vomiting, anorexia, rash, diarrhea, headache, drowsiness, or dizziness occurs and persists after taking the medication, consult a primary care provider.

If symptoms of the pinworm infection persist beyond 2 weeks, contact a primary care provider to determine whether a second dose is indicated.

## References


1. Liu, LX, Weller, PF. Antiparasitic drugs. *N Engl J Med.* 1996;334:1178-84.
2. *Drug Facts and Comparisons* Updated Monthly. St. Louis: Facts and Comparisons, a Wolters Kluwer Company; 2002.
3. Enterobiasis. In: Mandell GL, Bennett JE, Dolin J, eds. *Principles and Practice of Infectious Diseases.* 5th ed. Philadelphia: Churchill Livingstone; 2000:2939-40.
4. Jones, JE. Pinworms. *Am Fam Physician.* 1988;38:159-64.
5. Juckett, G. Common intestinal helminths. *Am Fam Physician.* 1995;52:2039-48, 2051-2.
6. Drugs for parasitic infections. *Med Lett Drugs Ther.* (serial online) 2002:1-12.
7. Liu, LX. Enterobiasis. In: Guerrant RL, Walker DH, Weller PF, eds. *Tropical Infectious Diseases :Principles, Pathogens & Practice.* Philadelphia: Churchill Livingstone; 1999:949-53.
8. Grencis, RK, Cooper, ES. Enterobius, trichuris, capillaria, and hookworm including ancylostoma caninum. *Gastroenterol Clin North Am.* 1996;25:579-97.
9. Verley, JR, Quin, C. Sexually transmitted intestinal syndromes. In: Holmes KK, ed. *Sexually Transmitted Diseases.* 3rd ed. New York: McGraw-Hill Health Professions Division, 1999;937-962.
10. Tandan, T, Pollard, AJ, Money, DM, et al. Pelvic inflammatory disease associated with Enterobius vermicularis. *Arch Dis Child.* 2002;86:439-40.
11. Arca MJ, Gates RL, Groner JI, et al. Clinical manifestations of appendiceal pinworms in children: an institutional experience and a review of the literature. *Pediatr Surg Int.* 2004;20:372-5.
12. Van Riper, G. Pyrantel pamoate for pinworm infestation. *Am Pharm.* 1993;NS33:43-5.
13. Chin, J. *Enterobiasis. Control of Communicable Diseases Manual.* 17th ed. Washington DC: American Public Health Association; 2000:187-8.
14. Abdi, YA. *Handbook of Drugs for Tropical Parasitic Infections.* 2nd ed. London; Bristol, Pa: Taylor & Francis; 1995.
15. *Anthelmintic Drug Products.* Rockville, Md: Food and Drug Administration. 1988;293-4.
16. Russell, LJ. The pinworm, Enterobius vermicularis. *Prim Care.* 1991;18:13-24.
17. Pyrantel Monograph (updated 7/1/02). *Clinical Pharmacology* (database online). Gold Standard Media. Last updated July 1, 2002.
18. American Society of Health-System Pharmacists. *AHFS Drug Handbook.* STAT!Ref Online Electronic Medical Library ed. Bethesda, Md: Lippincott Williams & Wilkins; 2003.
19. Mishriki, YY. Dealing with the unexpected nematode. Postgrad Med 1997;102:37-8.
20. *The Review of Natural Products* (database online). St. Louis: Facts and Comparisons; 2003.
21. Kucik, CJ, Martin, GL, Sortor, BV. Common intestinal parasites. *Am Fam Physician.* 2004;69:1161-8.

CHAPTER 20

# Nausea and Vomiting

*Laura Shane-McWhorter and Joli Fermo*

Nausea and vomiting (N/V) are two of the most abhorrent symptoms individuals may experience. Although these symptoms may occur in a variety of benign circumstances, they are also associated with several important medical disorders. Nonprescription antiemetics are used to prevent or control the symptoms of N/V that are primarily caused by motion sickness, pregnancy, and mild infectious diseases. Some nonprescription antiemetics are promoted for the relief of vague symptoms such as "upset stomach," indigestion, and distention associated with food overindulgence. Although accurate statistics are lacking, it is estimated that billions of dollars are spent on nonprescription products to treat N/V. In 2003, Dramamine Motion Sickness tablets generated $20 million in annual sales. Other products also generated large sales, such as Pepto-Bismol Stomach Remedy liquid/powder, and tablets, which accounted for $82 million in annual sales. Pepcid AC accounted for $81 million, and Zantac 75 for $76 million in annual sales.[1]

## Epidemiology of Nausea and Vomiting

N/V occur in both adults and children. Accurate statistics on the epidemiology of N/V are not available because these symptoms occur in many situations, and many persons do not report these disturbances to a health care provider. Three common situations that involve N/V are motion sickness, N/V of pregnancy (NVP), and viral gastroenteritis.

The severity of N/V related to motion sickness is difficult to quantify because there is interindividual variability and susceptibility to this malady. Motion sickness rarely occurs in infants but is more common in children 2 to 12 years of age, although the reason is not known.[2] Studies also confirm that women are more susceptible to motion sickness than men.[3]

Commonly called "morning sickness,"[4] NVP is more common during the first trimester with resolution of symptoms by the 20th week of pregnancy. However, some women may have NVP beyond this time. Nausea occurs in 70% to 85% of pregnant women, and half will vomit.[4,5] A very severe form of pregnancy-related vomiting, hyperemesis gravidarum, occurs in 1% of women. This is defined as intractable vomiting that causes dehydration, electrolyte disturbances, nutritional deficiencies, and weight loss.[6]

Acute transient attacks of vomiting in conjunction with diarrhea are frequently observed during viral gastroenteritis. This acute infectious disease may affect any age group and is usually self-limiting. However, pediatric patients may experience serious consequences. The two most common pathogens are rotavirus and norovirus.[7] According to the Centers for Disease Control and Prevention (CDC), it is difficult to quantify the epidemiology of gastroenteritis because of inaccurate reporting, especially underreporting of mild cases. The leading cause of gastroenteritis outbreaks is norovirus, resulting in 23 million cases each year, including 50,000 hospitalizations and 300 deaths.[7] In children, acute gastroenteritis causes diarrheal illness, accounting for more than 1.5 million outpatient visits, 200,000 hospitalizations, and an estimated 300 deaths per year.[8] The CDC reports that in children under 5 years of age, 5% to 10% of all diarrhea cases are caused by rotavirus, with more than 500,000 physician visits and approximately 50,000 hospitalizations each year. The costs exceed $250 million per year, and an estimated one in 200,000 children die from rotavirus complications.[9]

## Physiology of Vomiting Process[10,11]

Vomiting is a complex process involving both the central nervous system (CNS) and the gastrointestinal (GI) tract. Vomiting is coordinated by the lateral reticular formation of the medulla oblongata in the brain stem. This vomiting coordinating circuitry has been referred to as the vomiting center. Different areas provide input to the vomiting center. These include the chemotrigger receptor zone (CTZ), the vestibular apparatus, the cortex, and the GI tract.

The CTZ is located in the area postrema at the floor of the fourth ventricle. The neurons in the CTZ may be stimulated by many toxins, and only a slight barrier exists between the systemic circulation and these neurons. The CTZ also accepts several medullary neurons that may be responsible for inhibiting the action potential of these nerve cells, thus preventing them from firing more readily.

The vestibular apparatus also provides input to the vomiting center. It is located in the bony labyrinth of the temporal lobe. The vestibular apparatus detects changes in equilibrium. Direct input to the vomiting center is via cholinergic pathways.

The cortex provides direct input to the vomiting center through different neuroreceptors. Sensory input, including sight or smell or different toxins may elicit a strong sensation of nausea.

Finally, the vagus nerve and the GI tract also provide input to the vomiting center. Gut distention and decreased GI emptying may stimulate mechanoreceptors and may be responsible for eliciting nausea and emesis.

**TABLE 20-1 Primary Causes of Nausea and Vomiting[12-15]**

| Visceral Afferent Stimulation | CNS Disorders |
|---|---|
| *Mechanical Obstruction* | *Vestibular Disorders* |
| Gastric outlet obstruction (i.e., PUD, gastric carcinoma, pancreatic disease); small intestinal obstruction | Labyrinthitis; Ménière's syndrome; motion sickness |
| *Motility Disorders* | *Increased Intracranial Pressure* |
| Gastroparesis (i.e., DM, drug-induced, postviral); chronic intestinal pseudo-obstruction; IBS; anorexia nervosa; idiopathic gastric stasis | CNS tumor; subdural or subarachnoid hemorrhage |
| *Peritoneal Irritation* | *Infections* |
| Appendicitis; bacterial peritonitis | Meningitis; encephalitis |
| *Infections* | *Psychogenic* |
| Viral gastroenteritis (i.e., norovirus, rotavirus); food poisoning (i.e., toxins from *Bacillus cereus, Staphylococcus aureus, Clostridium perfringens*); Hepatitis A or B; acute systemic infections | Anticipatory vomiting; bulimia; psychiatric disorders |
| *Topical Gastrointestinal Irritants* | *Other CNS Disorders* |
| Alcohol; NSAIDs; antibiotics | Migraine headache |
| *Other* | **Irritation of CTZ** |
| Cardiac disease (i.e., MI, CHF); urologic disease (i.e., stones, pyelonephritis); overeating | *Initiated/Withdrawn Drugs* |
| | Cytotoxic chemotherapy; opiates; theophylline toxicity; digitalis toxicity; antibiotics; radiation therapy; drug withdrawal (i.e., opiates, BZDPs) |
| | *Systemic Disorders* |
| | DM (i.e., DKA); renal disease (i.e., uremia); adrenocortical crisis (i.e., Addison's disease); pregnancy |

Key: BZDP, benzodiazepenes; CHF, congestive heart failure; CNS, central nervous system; CTZ, chemotrigger receptor zone; DKA, diabetic ketoacidosis; DM, diabetes mellitus; IBS, irritable bowel syndrome; MI, myocardial infarction; NSAID, nonsteroidal anti-inflammatory drug; PUD, peptic ulcer disease.

The vomiting center receives different stimuli from these areas and sends impulses to the salivation center, vasomotor center, respiratory center, cranial nerves, then to the pharynx, and GI tract, and nausea and/or vomiting may occur.

## Etiology of Nausea and Vomiting

N/V may be caused by many stimuli: travel (i.e., motion sickness), pregnancy, drug therapy, stress, viral gastroenteritis, overeating, food poisoning, bulimia, abdominal distention, certain diseases, and other factors. Most occurrences of N/V are self-limiting and require minimal therapy. Table 20-1 lists the primary causes of N/V, however, many of these causes are not self-limiting and require extensive medical evaluation and treatment.[12-15] Some of these underlying causes are discussed in more detail in General Treatment Approach.

## Pathophysiology of Nausea and Vomiting

Mechanisms involved in vomiting include (1) psychogenic vomiting from the cerebral cortex and limbic system; (2) motion and space sickness from vestibular and visual afferents; (3) GI tract disturbance, including food poisoning, cancer chemotherapy, and radiation; (4) pregnancy; (5) postoperative vomiting; (6) miscellaneous problems, including vomiting from the heart, glossopharyngeal, and trigeminal afferents; and (7) blood poisoning involving the area postrema of the medulla (the chemoreceptor trigger zone).[10]

Major neurotransmitters and receptors involved in vomiting include dopamine $D_2$, histamine type 1, muscarinic ($M_1$) receptors[12] adrenergic type 2 receptors, and serotonin receptors.[10] The specific serotonin receptors are not known, although in cancer chemotherapy, serotonin $5\text{-}HT_3$ receptors are implicated in emesis,[12] while the cyclic vomiting syndrome may be affected by substance P and its receptor, neurokinin-1 ($NK_1$) as well as serotonin $5\text{-}HT_{1A}$ receptors.[10] Experimental drugs, such as the $NK_1$ receptor antagonists, and serotonin $5\text{-}HT_{1A}$ receptor agonists are being studied for cyclic vomiting syndrome.[10] Vomiting may also involve the μ-opioid receptor subtype.[10] One author has stated that in the GI tract, serotonin and $D_2$ receptors are associated with vomiting, while in motion sickness, acetylcholine, muscarinic, and histamine receptors are thought to mediate emesis.[13] However, the author did not specify which specific subtypes were associated with these receptors, except for dopamine.

N/V of motion sickness are produced by overstimulation of the labyrinth (inner ear) apparatus. The three semicircular canals in the labyrinth on each side of the head are responsible for maintaining equilibrium. Postural adjustments are made when the brain receives nerve impulses initiated by the movement of fluid in the canals. When the head is rotated on two axes simultaneously, unusual motion patterns may produce motion sickness. Other mechanisms are also important in eliciting motion sickness. Inaccurate interpretation of visual stimuli while standing or sitting still may produce motion sickness. For instance, a person may experience motion sickness when watching a film taken from a roller coaster or watching an airplane performing aerobatics, or when extending the head upward while standing on a rotating platform. Individuals differ in their response to motion sickness stimuli, such as flying and boating, but no one is immune. Regardless of the type of stimulus-producing event, motion sickness is easier to prevent than to treat.

## Signs and Symptoms of Nausea and Vomiting

Nausea is an unpleasant sensation associated with vague epigastric and abdominal symptoms, and usually precedes vomiting. Regurgitation is the reverse transit of stomach contents into the pharynx that stops short of oral expulsion. Retching is a strong, involuntary, and unsuccessful effort to vomit. Vomiting is the physical expulsion of stomach, esophageal, and oropharyngeal contents. Vomiting begins with a deep inspiration, the closing of the glottis, and depression of the soft palate. A forceful contraction of the diaphragm and abdominal musculature occurs, producing an increase in intrathoracic and intra-abdominal pressure that compresses the stomach and raises esophageal pressure. The stomach and esophageal musculature relax, and the positive intrathoracic and intra-abdominal pressure moves stomach contents into the esophagus and mouth. Several cycles of reflux into the esophagus occur before actual vomiting begins. Vomitus is expelled from the esophagus by a combination of increased intrathoracic pressure and reverse peristaltic waves. Normally, the glottis closes off the trachea and prevents the vomitus from entering the airway; however, aspiration of the vomitus may occur in patients with neurologic diseases, CNS depression, or an absent or impaired gag reflex.

## Complications of Nausea and Vomiting

Possible acute complications of vomiting include dehydration, aspiration, malnutrition, electrolyte and/or acid-base abnormalities, as well as Mallory-Weiss syndrome, which causes esophageal tears, typically at the gastroesophageal junction, that results in blood in the vomitus. Dehydration and electrolyte imbalances are the major concerns associated with vomiting. Signs and symptoms of dehydration include dry mouth, decreased skin turgor, excessive thirst, little or no urination, dizziness, lightheadedness, fainting, and reduced blood pressure.

## Treatment of Nausea and Vomiting

Use of nonprescription antiemetics is appropriate to prevent or relieve symptoms of occasional self-limiting N/V. Available products include antihistamines, antacids, histamine$_2$-receptor antagonists, and phosphorated carbohydrate solutions. Complementary products such as ginger, chamomile, peppermint, and other botanical products have also been used. Oral rehydration solutions (ORSs) are available for treating the dehydration that may result from prolonged vomiting.

### *Treatment Goals*

Treatment of N/V should focus on identifying and correcting the underlying cause. However, most acute vomiting cases are mild and self-limiting, resolve spontaneously, and require only symptomatic treatment. Acute vomiting that is severe necessitates further evaluation and may require hospitalization. Figures 20-1 and 20-2 list exclusions for self-care for adults[16-21] and children, respectively.[8,20,21] Causes and severity of the N/V determine the outcomes of pharmacologic or nonpharmacologic therapy. Symptomatic relief may not be possible until the underlying cause has been identified and corrected.

### *General Treatment Approach*

The algorithms in Figures 20-1 and 20-2 outline the self-care of N/V in adults and children, respectively. The following considerations of N/V associated with special population groups and certain etiologies are important in determining the appropriate use of an antiemetic product.

#### Nausea and Vomiting in Adults

Adults may experience N/V associated with viral gastroenteritis, food poisoning, or overeating. Females of childbearing age with N/V may suspect pregnancy and should seek medical evaluation if they have missed a period. Lactating women should also seek medical evaluation. (See Patient Counseling for Nausea and Vomiting.)

Certain situations involving N/V in adults may require referral for further evaluation (Figure 20-1).

#### Nausea and Vomiting in Children

In newborns, serious abnormalities may cause vomiting. These include GI tract obstruction, neurologic disorders, and neuromuscular control disorders. Vomiting may rapidly lead to acid-base disturbances and dehydration. Infants and young children may become dehydrated very quickly and, if not appropriately managed, dehydration may lead to death. Thus, referral for medical evaluation is always recommended.

Simple regurgitation or spitting up is common in infants and does not require medical attention. Esophageal sphincter blockage (pyloric stenosis) occurs when an infant forcefully vomits large amounts of fluid and requires medical referral.

Although N/V may occur secondary to head trauma, toxic ingestion, or CNS infection, the most common cause is acute viral gastroenteritis. Treatment is primarily directed at preventing and correcting dehydration and electrolyte disturbances. Fluid loss should generally be replaced within 24 hours. An ORS may be used to treat even minimal or mild to moderate cases. Recurrent or protracted N/V (with accompanying diarrhea) may lead to marked dehydration and electrolyte imbalance that cannot be ignored, especially in infants and small children. Parents should be educated to recognize signs and symptoms of dehydration such as dry mucous membranes, decreased skin turgor, irritability, altered mental status,

### Exclusions for Self-Treatment

- Urine ketones and/or high BG with signs of dehydration in patients with DM (may indicate DKA or HHS)
- Suspected food poisoning that is severe and/or does not clear up after 12 hours
- Severe abdominal pain in the middle or right lower quadrant (may indicate appendicitis or bowel obstruction)
- N/V with fever and/or diarrhea (may indicate infectious disease)
- Severe right upper quadrant pain, especially after eating fatty foods (may indicate cholecystitis or pancreatitis)
- Blood in the vomitus (may indicate ulcers, esophageal tears, or severe nosebleed)
- Yellow skin or eye discoloration and dark urine (may indicate hepatitis)
- Stiff neck with or without headache and sensitivity to brightness of normal light (may indicate meningitis)
- Head injury with N/V, blurry vision, or numbness and tingling
- Persons with glaucoma, BPH, chronic bronchitis, emphysema, or asthma (may react adversely to OTC antiemetics)
- Pregnancy (moderate to severe symptoms) or breast-feeding
- N/V caused by cancer chemotherapy; radiation therapy; serious metabolic disorders; CNS, GI, or endocrine disorders
- Drug-induced N/V: adverse effects of drugs used therapeutically (e.g., opioids, NSAIDs, antibiotics, estrogens); toxic doses of drugs used therapeutically (e.g., digoxin, theophylline, lithium); ethanol
- Psychogenic-induced N/V: bulimia, anorexia
- Chronic disease-induced N/V: gastroparesis with DM; DKA or HHS with DM; GERD

*Source:* References 16-21.

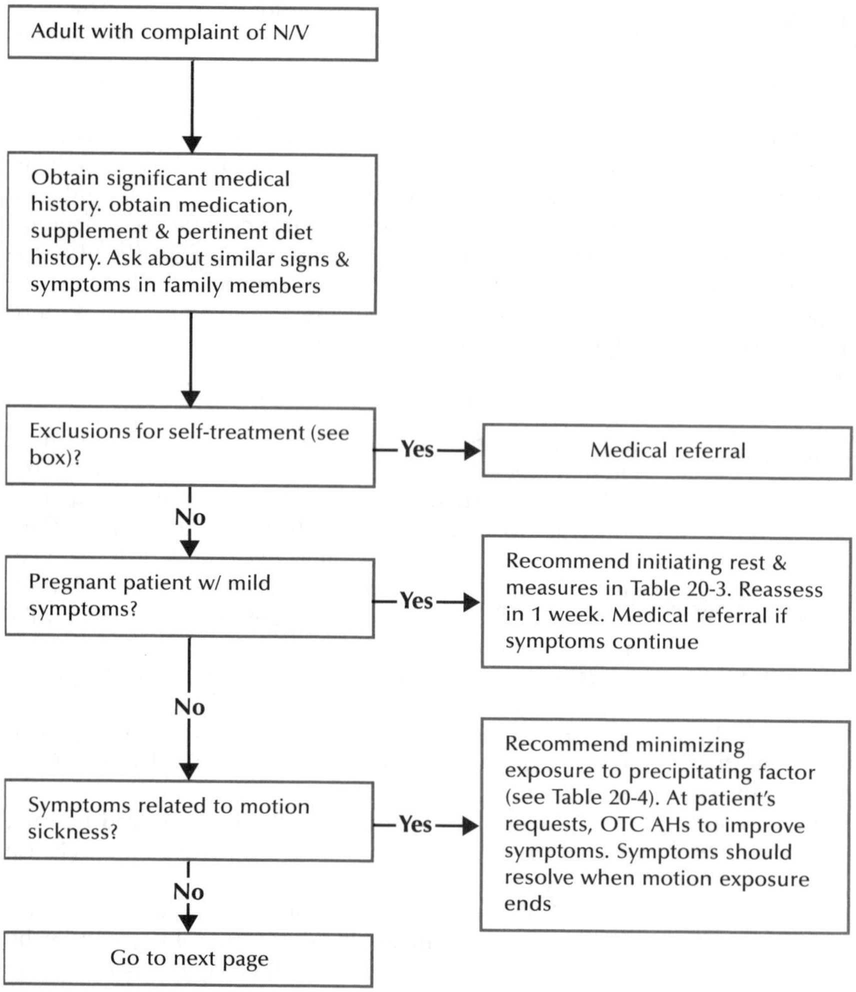


**FIGURE 20-1** Self-care of N/V in adults. Key: AH, antihistamine, BG, blood glucose; BPH, benign prostatic hyperplasia; CNS, central nervous system; DKA, diabetic ketoacidosis; GERD, gastroesophageal reflux disease; GI, gastrointestinal; HHS, hyperosmolar hyperglycemic syndrome; $H_2RA$, histamine$_2$-receptor antagonist; NSAID, nonsteroidal anti-inflammatory drug; OTC; over-the counter; PCP, primary care provider.

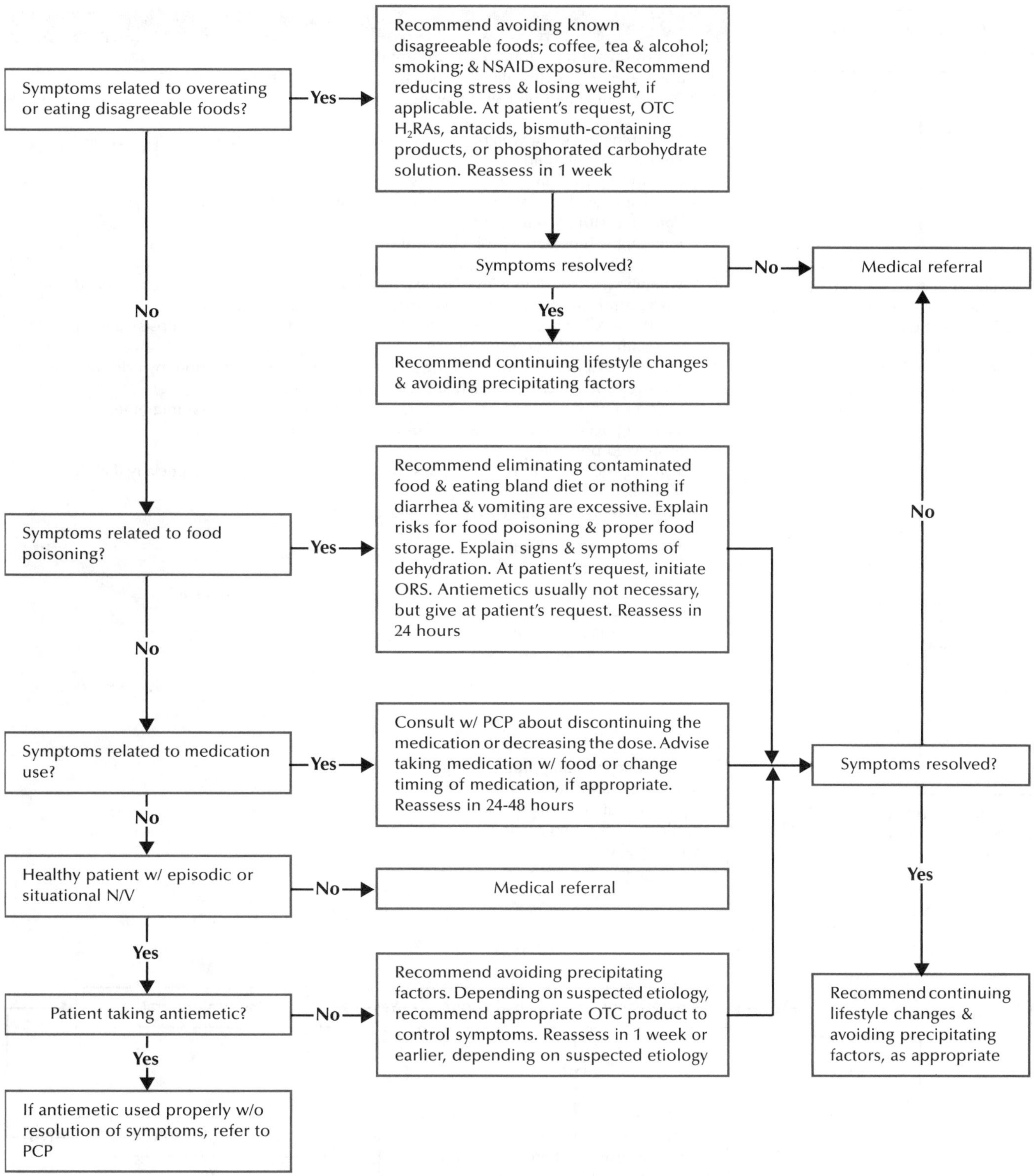


**FIGURE 20-1 (continued)**

and weight loss (Table 20-2).[8,20,21] Weight loss as an objective measure of dehydration should be emphasized, and an accurate infant weight scale is an essential tool to measure weight. The child should be referred for further evaluation when dehydration occurs (Table 20-2), if the child is under 6 months of age, weighs less than 8 kg, or has a fever greater than 100.4°F (38°C) if under 3 months of age or a fever greater than 102.2°F (39°C) if aged 3 to 36 months,[8] or if exclusions to self-treatment accompany N/V (Figure 20-2).[8,20,21]

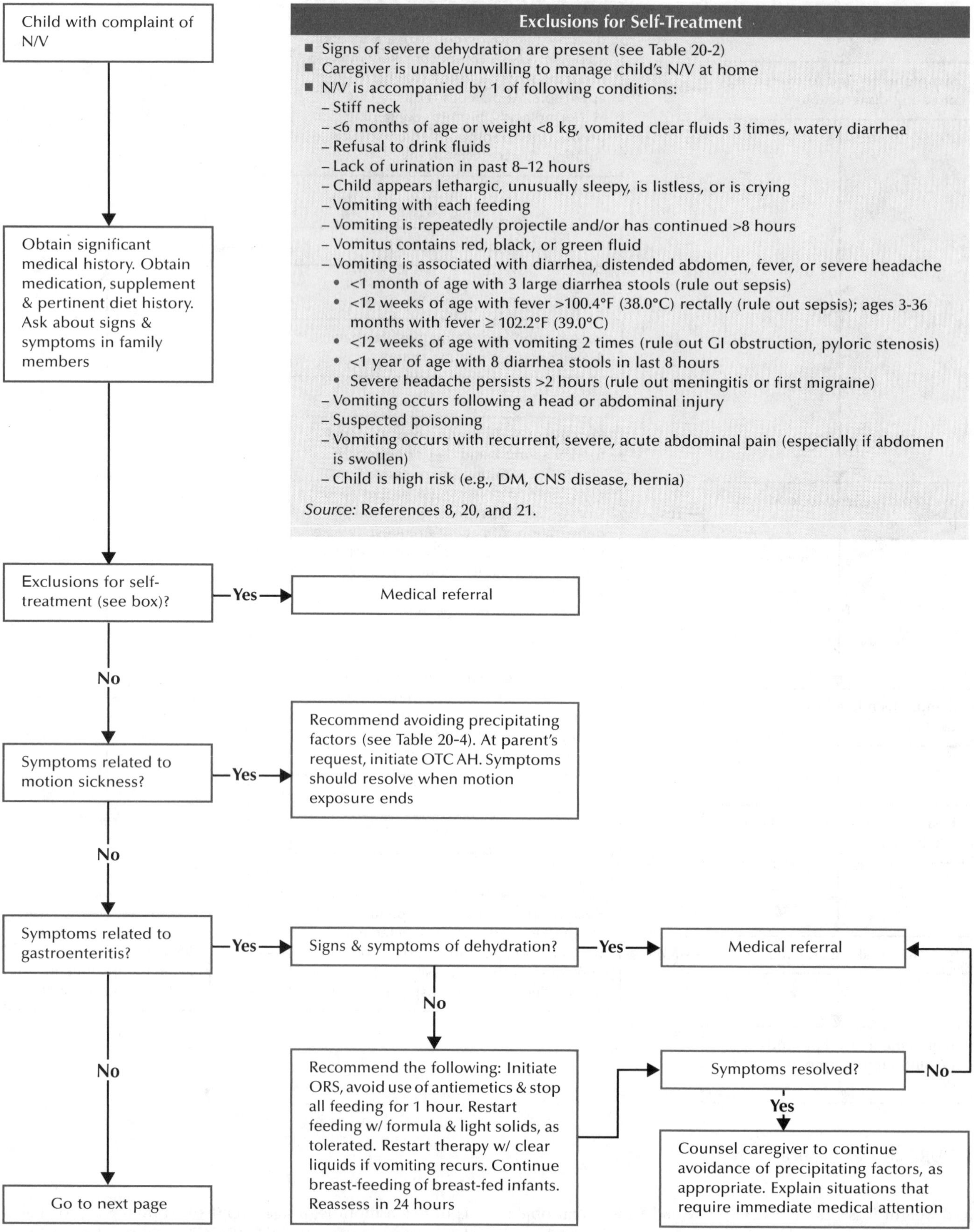


**FIGURE 20-2** Self-care of N/V in children. Key: AH, antihistamine; CNS, central nervous system; DM, diabetes mellitus; GI, gastrointestinal; ORS, oral rehydration solution; OTC, over-the counter.

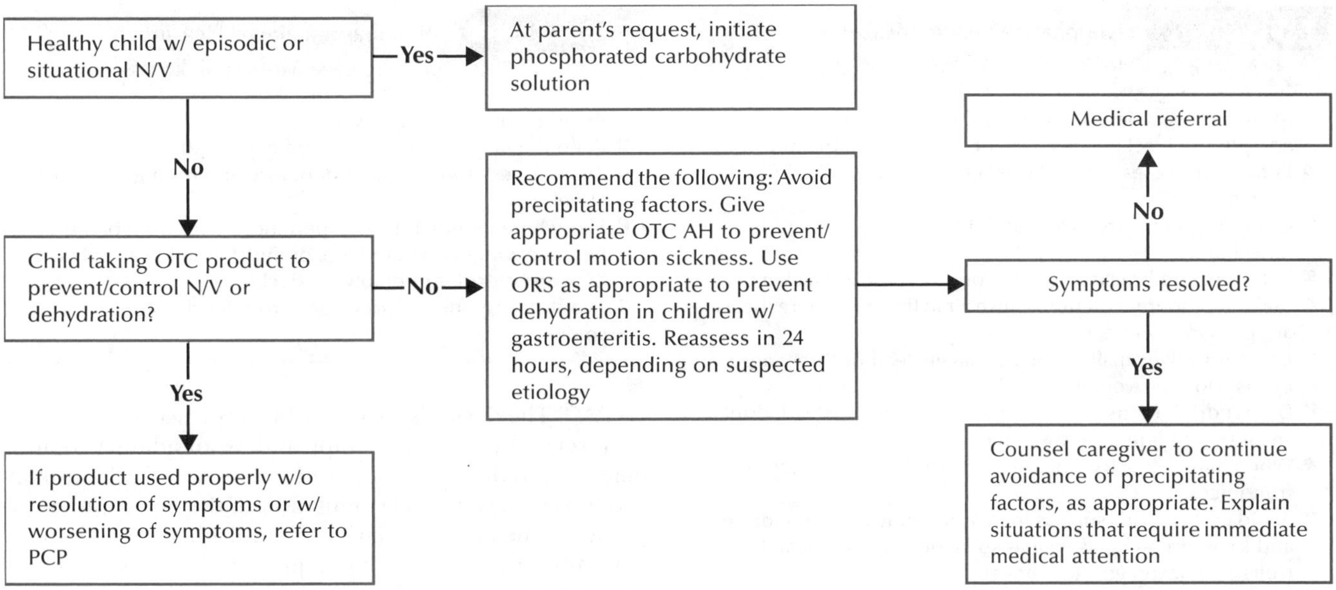


FIGURE 20-2 (continued)

**TABLE 20-2 Signs and Symptoms of Dehydration in Children[8,20,21]**

- Dry mouth and tongue
- Sunken and/or dry eyes
- Sunken fontanelle
- Decreased urine output (dry diapers for several hours)
- Dark urine
- Fast heartbeat
- Thirst (drinks extremely eagerly)
- Absence of tears when crying
- Decreased skin turgor
  - Increased axillary skinfolds
  - "Doughy" skin (may indicate hypernatremia)
  - When "pinched," skin returns to normal very slowly (prolonged skin tenting)
- Unusual listlessness, sleepiness, decreased alertness, or tiredness
  - Body is "floppy"
  - Lightheadedness when sitting or standing up (in older children)
  - Difficulty in waking up the child (may indicate severe dehydration)
- Weight loss
  - Noticeable decrease in abdominal ("tummy") size
  - Clothes or diaper fit loosely
  - <3% body weight loss indicates minimal or no dehydration
  - 3%-9% body weight loss indicates mild to moderate dehydration
  - >9% body weight loss indicates severe dehydration

Antiemetic use in children is controversial, and some clinicians question the value of using antiemetics to treat acute, self-limiting disorders.[18,21]

### Nausea and Vomiting During Pregnancy

Nausea, with or without vomiting, may be one of the earliest symptoms of pregnancy. A possible cause of NVP is rising levels of human chorionic gondadotropin.[5] A woman with N/V and a missed menstrual period should be referred for a pregnancy test and follow-up. It is important for clinicians to recognize that NVP may adversely affect a woman's well-being and activities.[4,22,23]

Because teratogenicity is a major consideration, most primary care providers are reluctant to prescribe any medication for a pregnant woman. Approved indications for nonprescription antiemetics do not include NVP. A number of nonpharmacologic approaches may be recommended, although they are not evidence-based (Table 20-3).[24-26]

### Nausea and Vomiting Related to Motion Sickness

Motion sickness occurs when there is a neural mismatch between visual and vestibular stimuli. Symptoms are varied and may include N/V. Some individuals are more susceptible. To minimize motion sickness, parents may seat a young child in a safe position that allows vision out of the car windows. Other nonpharmacologic measures are included in Table 20-4.[2] In some instances, antihistamines may be used to treat motion sickness.

### Nausea and Vomiting Related to Food Poisoning

Signs and symptoms of food poisoning may include vomiting, diarrhea, abdominal cramps, and fever.[18,19] Symptomatic treatment consists of fluid and electrolyte replacement, maintaining dietary intake, and antidiarrheal products when appropriate. Symptoms usually resolve

**TABLE 20-3 Nonpharmacologic Measures to Prevent NVP[24-26]**

- Make sure you have fresh air in the room where you sleep and put dry crackers beside your bed to eat in the morning.
- Before arising, eat several crackers and relax in bed for 10-15 minutes.
- Get out of bed very slowly and do not make any sudden movements.
- Before eating breakfast, nibble on dry toast or crackers.
- Make sure there is plenty of fresh air in the area where meals are prepared and eaten.
- Eat four to five small meals per day instead of three large meals. Do not overeat at meals.
- Do not drink fluids or eat soups at mealtime. Instead, drink small sips of liquid between meals.
- When nauseated, try small sips of carbonated beverages or fruit juices.
- Avoid greasy foods such as fried foods, gravies, mayonnaise, and salad dressing, as well as spicy or acidic foods (citrus fruits and beverages; tomatoes).
- If necessary, eat food that is chilled rather than warm or hot (tends to be less nauseating).

within 24 to 36 hours. If symptoms continue, referral for medical evaluation is recommended[7] (see Chapter 17).

### Other Causes of Nausea and Vomiting

N/V may be associated with medications used either therapeutically (e.g., cancer chemotherapeutic agents) or in toxic doses (e.g., theophylline). Psychiatric disorders (e.g., bulimia) may be a cause of N/V. Chronic medical conditions such as diabetes may result in complications such as gastroparesis and thus N/V. In all of these situations, the patient should be referred for medical evaluation and management (Figure 20-1).

## *Nonpharmacologic Therapy*

Acupressure wristbands are used to treat the symptoms of NVP, motion sickness, and overeating. Acupressure therapy to treat N/V is based on the ancient Eastern theory that the body is activated by the vital force, Chi. Chi energy travels along meridians known as "acu" points. For centuries, the Chinese have used stimulation of the Neiguan—or pericardium 6 (P6)—point, located bilaterally on the inner forearm three finger widths up from the first wrist crease, to relieve N/V symptoms. Acupressure wristbands such as SeaBands and Travel Aides are indicated to prevent motion sickness,[27] NVP,[28] and N/V associated with chemotherapy and anesthesia.[29] Acupressure wristbands offer an alternative and may be considered by patients who want to avoid the adverse effects of pharmacologic agents.[5] The manufacturer states that children as young as 2 years of age have used the wristbands.[29]

Another device that stimulates the P6 point became available in 1999. A battery-powered acustimulation band, ReliefBand NST (Nerve Stimulation Technology), is approved by the Food and Drug Administration (FDA) for nonprescription use in treating N/V related to motion sickness, as well as mild to moderate (but not severe) NVP.[30,31] The device is also available by prescription to treat N/V related to chemotherapy and as an adjunct to antiemetics in reducing postoperative nausea.[31] Mechanism of action is believed to be stimulation of the P6 acupuncture point by means of electricity.[31] Individuals may choose from five power settings. The prescription product has a higher power output than the device available for nonprescription use. The only reported adverse effect has been a mild, transient rash at the application site in a few patients following use of ReliefBand.[31] The wristband contains latex, which may cause allergic reactions. It is important for clinicians to advise patients that the device must be worn on the wrist to prevent interference with pacemakers. The manufacturer states that product use in children is not contraindicated.

**TABLE 20-4 Nonpharmacologic Measures to Decrease Motion Sickness[2]**

- Avoid reading during travel.
- Keep the line of vision fairly straight ahead.
- Avoid excess food or alcohol before and during extended travel.
- Stay where motion is least experienced (e.g., front of the car, near the wings of an airplane, or midship [midway between bow and stern], preferably on deck).
- Avoid strong odors, particularly from food or tobacco smoke.

The acupressure bands (SeaBands) and the acustimulation bands (ReliefBand) may both be used before the onset of anticipated motion sickness or when symptoms first occur. In contrast, nonprescription antiemetics such as dimenhydrinate must be taken at least 30 to 60 minutes before beginning the activity that causes motion sickness. Some antiemetic drugs may also cause drowsiness, which may not be acceptable to some travelers. Both devices may be used concomitantly with antiemetics.[29,31] The acupressure band is worn on both wrists, but the acustimulation device is worn on only one wrist. Cost may be a factor in selection of the products because the acustimulation device costs approximately eight times more than the acupressure band.

## *Pharmacologic Therapy*

Selection of a nonprescription medication is determined by the potential cause of N/V. Their myriad causes account for numerous medications used to treat these symptoms.

### Antihistamines

The antihistamines meclizine, cyclizine, dimenhydrinate, diphenhydramine, and doxylamine constitute the major class of nonprescription antiemetics.[32] Table 20-5 lists dosages for FDA-approved antiemetics. Although still used for N/V, doxylamine is not approved for antiemetic use.

*Mechanism of Action* Histamine levels increase in the hypothalamus, pons, and medulla oblongata in response to certain motions commonly associated with nausea and/or vomiting. Neural centers for salivation, vomiting, and

TABLE 20-5 Dosage Guidelines for Antiemetic Antihistamines[32,33]*

| Agent | Dosage (Maximum Daily Dosage) Adults | Children 6 to <12 years | Children 2 to <6 years |
|---|---|---|---|
| Meclizine | 25-50 mg 1 hour before travel (50 mg) | Not recommended | Not recommended |
| Cyclizine | 50 mg 30 minutes before travel then 60 mg q 4-6 h (200 mg) | 25 mg q6-8h (75 mg) | Not recommended |
| Diphenhydramine | 25-50 mg q4-6h (300 mg) | 12.5-25 mg q4-6h (150 mg) | 6.25 mg q4-6h (37.5 mg) |
| Dimenhydrinate | 50-100 mg q4-6h (400 mg) | 25-50 mg q6-8h (150 mg) | 12.5-25 mg q6-8h (75 mg) |

* Take antihistamines at least 30 to 60 minutes before travel; continue taking them during travel.

other symptoms associated with motion sickness contain histaminic neurons. Antihistamines that cross the blood-brain barrier depress labyrinth excitability and may prevent, as well as control, motion sickness in varying degrees.[34]

*Indications* Nonprescription antihistamines are classified as safe and effective for prevention and treatment of nausea, vomiting, or dizziness associated with motion sickness. However, there are age-specific limits. Dimenhydrinate and diphenhydramine should not be given to children younger than 2 years, cyclizine should not be given to children younger than 6 years, and meclizine should not be given to children younger than 12 years.[33]

*Dosage and Administration Guidelines* Because it is easier to prevent than treat motion sickness-related N/V, these agents are taken before boarding the vehicle that elicits motion sickness. Antihistamines should be taken at least 30 to 60 minutes before departure to allow ample time for onset of effect. Use should be continued during travel. Table 20-5 lists age-specific dosages and maximum daily limits for these agents.[32,33]

*Safety Considerations* Drowsiness is the most common side effect and may occur even with therapeutic doses. Patients should be cautioned not to combine antihistamines with alcohol-containing products, drive a vehicle, operate hazardous machinery, or engage in tasks requiring a high degree of physical dexterity or mental alertness. One study reported that 50 mg of diphenhydramine caused greater impairment than alcohol intoxication.[35] Anticholinergic adverse effects may occur, including blurred vision, dry mouth, urinary retention, and constipation. Paradoxical stimulatory reactions such as insomnia, nervousness, and irritability may also occur. In acute overdose, doxylamine and diphenhydramine have been reported to produce rhabdomyolysis.[36] Neuropsychiatric reactions have also been reported, including hallucinations and psychosis. Persons of advanced age may be particularly vulnerable to side effects of antihistamines.[37] Lactating women may have a reduced milk supply if antihistamines are used.[38]

When combined with other CNS depressants (e.g., alcohol, tranquilizers, hypnotics, sedatives), antihistamines may result in additive sedation. A small study[39] conducted in vitro and in vivo in 16 subjects found that diphenhydramine interfered with the biotransformation of metoprolol by inhibiting the polymorphic P-450 enzyme, CYP 2D6. Metoprolol clearance was decreased twofold in 10 of 16 subjects. The effects of metoprolol on decreasing heart rate and systolic blood pressure were also more pronounced.

A similar study[40] in 15 subjects found that diphenhydramine increased venlafaxine plasma concentration more than twofold. Diphenhydramine use warrants caution, particularly if a person is taking medications metabolized by CYP 2D6 isoenzymes (e.g., opiates, certain psychiatric medications, β-blockers, and certain antiarrhythmics).

Additive sedation or anticholinergic effects may occur when antihistamines are combined with tricyclic antidepressants.[32]

Specific warnings require that persons be advised not to use the product, unless directed by a primary care provider, if they have respiratory conditions (chronic bronchitis or emphysema) or glaucoma, or difficulty with urination because of prostate gland enlargement. Lactating women should also avoid antihistamines since milk supply may be affected.[38] These agents should be used with caution in children or elderly patients because of the increased possibility of side effects.[33,37]

FDA issued a final rule effective December 8, 2003, amending labeling for oral nonprescription antiemetics, antihistamines, antitussives, and nighttime sleep-aid drug products that contain diphenhydramine citrate or hydrochloride.[41] The label reads, "Do not use with any other product containing diphenhydramine, even one used on skin." Cases of toxic psychosis reported in children prompted this ruling.

A final precaution is that practitioners should be aware that nonprescription antihistamines such as cyclizine, diphenhydramine, or dimenhydrinate may be used and/or abused for psychiatric effects.[42,43]

**TABLE 20-6 Selected Antiemetic Products[32]**

| Trade Name | Primary Ingredients |
|---|---|
| Bonine Chewable Tablets | Meclizine HCl 25 mg |
| Dramamine Orange Chewable Tablets*†‡§‖ | Dimenhydrinate 50 mg |
| Marezine for Motion Sickness† | Cyclizine HCl 50 mg |
| Dramamine Less Drowsy Formula Tablets†¶ | Meclizine HCl 25 mg |
| Emetrol Cherry Flavor Liquid#**†† | Phosphoric acid 21.5 g/5 mL; dextrose 1.87 g/5 mL; fructose 1.87 g/5 mL |

*Lactose-free; †sodium-free: ‡contains 1.5 mg/tablet of phenylalanine: §contains FD&C yellow No. 5; ‖contains FD&C yellow No. 6: ¶contains FD&C yellow No. 10; #Alcohol-free; **Contains fructose: ††contains FD&C red No. 40.

### Agents Used to Treat Nausea Associated With Food or Beverages

Nausea and/or vomiting may be associated with excessive or disagreeable food or beverage intake. The exact prevalence of gastric upset associated with overindulgence is unknown, but symptoms may include heartburn, indigestion, and upset stomach. Antacids, histamine$_2$-receptor antagonists, bismuth subsalicylate, and phosphorated carbohydrate solution have been used to relieve the symptoms associated with dietary overindulgence.

*Antacids* Antacids contain various combinations of ingredients, including magnesium hydroxide, aluminum hydroxide, calcium carbonate, and magnesium carbonate. Antacids neutralize gastric acidity, increasing the pH of the stomach and duodenum.[32] Antacids are indicated for complaints of infrequent heartburn, dyspepsia, acid indigestion, and the symptomatic relief of upset stomach associated with gastric acidity.[32] The patient should take 15 mL of most antacids 30 minutes after meals and at bedtime. However, the efficacy of antacids for N/V associated with overeating has been marginal.[44] (See Chapter 14 for further discussion of antacids.)

*Histamine$_2$-Receptor Antagonists* Histamine$_2$-receptor antagonists include cimetidine, ranitidine, famotidine, and nizatidine. Histamine$_2$-receptor antagonists decrease acid secretion by competing with histamine for binding at $H_2$-receptor sites on parietal cells.[32] FDA has approved nonprescription use of these agents for infrequent heartburn and indigestion. However, the efficacy of histamine$_2$-receptor antagonists for N/V associated with overeating remains uncertain. (See Chapter 14 for further discussion of histamine$_2$-receptor antagonists.)

*Omeprazole* Omeprazole is a proton pump inhibitor (PPI) that decreases gastric acid by shutting down the acid (or proton) pumps in the stomach.[32] Omeprazole is not intended to provide immediate heartburn relief or provide protection before eating a spicy meal. Data are insufficient to support the use of omeprazole for treating N/V associated with overindulgence of food. (See Chapter 14 for further discussion of omeprazole.)

*Bismuth Products* Bismuth subsalicylate (Pepto-Bismol) has been used to treat various GI complaints, including nausea associated with indigestion, heartburn, and fullness (gas) caused by overindulgence in food and drink.[32] (See Chapter 17 for further discussion of bismuth products.)

*Phosphorated Carbohydrate Solution* Phosphorated carbohydrate solution is a mixture of levulose (fructose), dextrose (glucose), and phosphoric acid[32] (Table 20-6). Phosphoric acid is added to adjust the pH of the commercial product to between 1.5 and 1.6.

Mechanism of Action Hyperosmolar solutions with phosphoric acid are believed to relieve N/V by a direct local action on the GI tract wall that may decrease smooth muscle contraction and delay gastric emptying time. It is believed to have a dose-related effect.[32]

Indications Phosphorated carbohydrate solution is indicated for nausea associated with upset stomach caused by intestinal or stomach flu, and food or drink indiscretions. This hyperosmolar carbohydrate product has been used in attempts to alleviate NVP and for motion sickness.[32]

Dosage and Administration Guidelines The usual adult dosage of phosphorated carbohydrate solution is 15 to 30 mL (1 to 2 tbsp) at 15-minute intervals until vomiting ceases.[32] The dosage for children ages 2 to 12 years is 5 to 10 mL (1 to 2 tsp) every 15 minutes.[32] Patients should be told not to take this for more than 1 hour and not to exceed five doses. The solution should not be diluted, and the patient should not consume other liquids for 15 minutes after taking a dose. If symptoms do not cease after five doses, the patient should be referred for medical evaluation.[32] For NVP the dose is 15 to 30 mL on arising and repeated every 3 hours or if nausea threatens.[32] For regurgitation in infants, the dose is 5 to 10 mL administered 10 to 15 minutes before each feeding or for refractory cases, 10 to 15 mL 30 minutes before feeding.[32]

Safety Considerations Because of the product's high fructose and glucose content, phosphorated carbohydrate solution should not be used by individuals with hereditary fructose intolerance or diabetes.[32]

### Product Selection Guidelines

When considering use of certain products, several factors should be considered. These include whether the patient is a woman who is pregnant or lactating, the age of the patient (pediatric or elderly), and whether he or she has any limitations such as hepatic or renal impairment. Furthermore, the product should also be compatible with the patient's lifestyle, sensitivity to certain product ingredients such as dyes or fructose (Table 20-6), and frequency of dosing (Table 20-5). Hence, product selection guidelines should be compatible with special populations and patient factors, and should consider patient preferences, such as whether the product contains alcohol.

*Pregnancy* Many women experience NVP. Agents that have been used to treat NVP include antihistamines, pyridoxine, combinations of antihistamines and pyridoxine, acupressure or acustimulation devices, phosphorated carbohydrate solutions, and ginger (discussed in the Complementary Therapies section). Recently published evidence-based guidelines make recommendations for treating NVP.[45,46] The guidelines state that taking a multivitamin at conception may help decrease the severity of NVP.[45] Hence, the clinician may wish to suggest this in preconception counseling.

Antihistamines None of these agents has an FDA-approved indication for managing NVP, although all antihistamines appear to have a low risk of teratogenicity.[5,47] Meclizine, cyclizine, dimenhydrinate, and diphenhydramine are classified as pregnancy category B.[24] However, use should be reserved for pregnant women with severe N/V unresponsive to nonpharmacologic measures.[48] Pregnant women should always consult their primary care provider before taking any medication.

Pyridoxine Pyridoxine (vitamin $B_6$) is a water-soluble B complex essential vitamin. Uncontrolled studies in the 1940s suggested that pyridoxine might be effective in treating NVP. In 1979 the American Medical Association Council on Drugs found no conclusive evidence that pyridoxine was effective for treating NVP. Per the Cochrane Review, one controlled study of 25 mg of pyridoxine given orally every 8 hours produced significant improvement in women who complained of severe NVP.[5] Another study showed a lower dose, 30 mg/day, relieved nausea but not vomiting.[5] The specific mechanism of action of pyridoxine is unknown. Recent evidence-based guidelines suggest starting NVP treatment with pyridoxine 10 to 25 mg three or four times a day.[45] The Cochrane Review indicates that pyridoxine is the least likely product to result in adverse reactions.[5] Side effects are rare, but may include peripheral sensory neuropathic disturbances at high doses, although such disturbances have been reported with daily doses as low as 50 mg.[32] Extremely high doses (200 to 600 mg/day) have inhibited prolactin secretion.[32]

Doxylamine and Pyridoxine Doxylamine 10 mg was originally in the combination prescription product Bendectin, which also contained pyridoxine 10 mg (see Pyridoxine). Although FDA had approved this product for treating NVP, the manufacturer withdrew Bendectin from the market in 1983 because of the high cost of litigation regarding teratogenicity. Analysis of data describing Bendectin use in large numbers of women indicates there is no evidence of teratogenicity.[49,50] However, the ingredients—doxylamine and pyridoxine—remain available as nonprescription products, and primary care providers continue to recommend these agents, in combination, for NVP when nonpharmacologic measures do not work. Pyridoxine and doxylamine are both classified as pregnancy category A.[24] Recent evidence-based guidelines have suggested doxylamine 12.5 mg three or four times a day as second-line treatment for NVP.[45] In Canada, a sustained-release combination of 10 mg pyridoxine and 10 mg doxylamine is available under the trade name Diclectin.[46] Canadian guidelines suggest taking up to four tablets a day of this product (one in the morning, one in the afternoon, and two at bedtime) to treat NVP.[46]

Other Products Other agents that have been used in pregnancy include antacids, phosphorated carbohydrate solution, and ginger. Acupressure and acustimulation bands have also been used successfully[29,30] although results have been mixed.[5] Use of these devices should be considered only for cases of mild to moderate NVP. Histamine$_2$-receptor antagonists should not be used during pregnancy without consulting a primary care provider. Bismuth subsalicylate (BSS) is contraindicated during pregnancy.

*Lactating Women* Most antiemetic products may be used except for antihistamines, since they may adversely affect milk supply. However, BSS is contraindicated and there are no studies evaluating ginger in lactating women.

*Children* Agents used to treat N/V in children include antihistamines, phosphorated carbohydrate solution, and oral rehydration solutions. Antacids and histamine$_2$-receptor antagonists should be used only when recommended by primary care providers. BSS is not recommended for use in children, because of the possibility of Reye's syndrome.[32]

Antihistamines In children, antihistamines have been used to treat N/V associated with motion sickness and other causes. However, it is important for clinicians to counsel parents that these products may cause paradoxical stimulation and agitation.[33] There are certain age limitations regarding antihistamines (Table 20-5).

Phosphorated Carbohydrate Solution Children ages 2 to 12 years may use the same dose as adults. Infants may be given a smaller dose for regurgitation.[32]

Oral Rehydration Solutions Pediatric gastroenteritis is an important disorder that warrants close monitoring. Nausea, vomiting, diarrhea, and potentially dangerous dehydration account for $1 billion per year in direct costs for hospitalization and outpatient care.[8] In 1996, the American Academy of Pediatrics published practice parameters on acute gastroenteritis in children, but has recently endorsed and accepted guidelines from the CDC on managing gastroenteritis.[8] The treatment is supportive care while continuing diet and fluids. ORSs are the primary treatment for minimal or mild to moderate dehydration. The CDC guidelines recommend that parents have ORSs on hand in the home in case a child may be afflicted with diarrhea secondary to gastroenteritis.[8]

Dehydration secondary to vomiting and/or diarrhea is a result of a net loss of extracellular fluid, composed of sodium, chloride, potassium, water, and bicarbonate. Fluid replacement should mimic extracellular fluid losses. Because active glucose absorption in the small bowel promotes sodium absorption, oral rehydration therapy may thus increase sodium absorption and allow rapid replacement of extracellular fluid.[51] ORSs contain electrolyte mixtures. Some available solutions are Enfalyte, Pedialyte, and Rehydralyte (see Chapter 17).

Use of sports drinks, gelatin water, fruit juices, and carbonated beverages is discouraged since they are hyperosmolar and may worsen diarrhea; they are also deficient in electrolytes such as sodium, potassium, and chloride, which produce a rapid and significant therapeutic response to severe dehydration and electrolyte depletion.[8] Furthermore, use of homemade sugar-water or salt-water solutions should be discouraged because they may lack certain electrolytes, such as bicarbonate and potassium.[21]

Administration of an ORS is based on severity of dehydration, as measured by weight loss.[8] The child is considered to have minimal or no dehydration if body weight loss is less than 3%. In this case, if the child weighs less than 10 kg, administer 60 to 120 mL ORS for each diarrheal stool or vomiting episode and 120 to 240 mL ORS if weight is over 10 kg.[8] For mild to moderate dehydration (3% to 9% body weight loss) administer 50 to 100 mL/kg ORS over 2 to 4 hours.[8] Limited fluid volumes starting with 5 mL aliquots should be given every 1 to 2 minutes, increasing the amount gradually as tolerated. Severe dehydration (greater than 9% body weight loss) is a medical emergency and requires intravenous fluid replacement (see Chapter 17).[8] For all levels of dehydration, maintenance calories should be administered, such as breast-feeding or formula that is usually consumed; there is no need for special or diluted formula.[8] Certain situations are best handled on an in-patient basis, such as the caregiver being unable to provide adequate care at home, substantial difficulty with ORS administration or ORS refusal, intractable vomiting, or inadequate intake or failure of ORS treatment. In cases of severe dehydration, the child should also be admitted for in-patient care.[8]

*Patients of Advanced Age* Antiemetic use warrants caution in patients of advanced age, because they are at increased risk of adverse effects such as falls secondary to orthostasis or anticholinergic effects such as constipation, urinary retention, or dry eyes that may occur with antihistamine use. Many older patients take several medications, and there is an increased possibility of drug interactions with certain products such as antacids, certain histamine$_2$-receptor antagonists (cimetidine), PPIs, and BSS. For use of these agents, medical referral is always suggested. Phosphorated carbohydrate solution may be used safely if the patient does not have diabetes or hereditary fructose intolerance. Acupressure bands may be safely used, although acustimulation devices should not be used if the patient has a pacemaker.

Antihistamines are not an optimal treatment choice for older patients because of the possibility of anticholinergic effects, orthostasis, and drowsiness. Patients of advanced age may also experience confusion or cognitive dysfunction when taking antihistamines.[37]

What may be surmised regarding self-care products to treat N/V? Nonprescription antihistamines and phosphorated carbohydrate solutions are suitable to prevent or control self-limiting N/V, such as that associated with motion sickness or overindulgence in food and drink. Patients with hereditary fructose intolerance, however, should not take phosphorated carbohydrate solutions. Persons of advanced age and lactating women should avoid antihistamines.

Antacids, histamine$_2$-receptor antagonists, and BSS are appropriate for treating nausea related to overeating or eating disagreeable foods. Patients taking medications that may interact with salicylates should not take BSS. Children and teenagers recovering from chickenpox or viral influenza should also not take this agent, nor should pregnant or lactating women. Chapter 14 discusses possible drug interactions with antacids and histamine$_2$-receptor antagonists. Persons of advanced age and pregnant or lactating women may take either drug.

Vomiting related to food poisoning or other self-limiting causes should be treated with ORSs to prevent dehydration and electrolyte disturbances. Inability to eat or drink because of nausea may cause dehydration, which also may be treated with ORSs. All age groups, including pregnant or lactating women, may safely use ORSs.

The role of ginger, chamomile, peppermint, or other complementary therapies to treat N/V secondary to motion sickness, surgery, and/or pregnancy has not been clearly defined (see Chapter 53).

### Complementary Therapies

A variety of complementary products have been used to treat N/V.[52] The most popular products are ginger, chamomile, and peppermint, but other products include lemon balm and artichoke.

#### Ginger

Ginger (*Zingiber officinale*) is a botanical product that has been used to relieve nausea associated with motion sickness, pregnancy, and surgery (see Chapter 53). Ginger is used in different forms, including ginger ale, ginger root, and tablet extracts. It contains the chemical ingredients gingerols and shogaols, which may work at the level of the digestive tract to inhibit N/V.[52] Divided doses of 1000 mg/day have been used. One reason for the popularity of ginger is that, unlike antihistamines, it does not produce CNS depressant effects.

A systematic review of randomized trials evaluated the efficacy of ginger to treat N/V in a variety of situations including pregnancy-related illness, seasickness, and postoperative N/V.[53] Ginger was found superior to placebo and

**TABLE 20-7 Selected Botanical Medicines Used to Treat N/V[52]**

| Botanical Agent (Scientific Name) | Risks | Effectiveness |
|---|---|---|
| Artichoke (*Cynara scolymus*) | Possible allergic reactions and cross-reactions with members of Asteraceae (formerly Compositae) family (chrysanthemums, arnica pyrethrum) | Used for dyspeptic problems and prophylaxis against recurrent gallstones; efficacy not proven; use not recommended by German Commission E |
| Chamomile (*Matricaria recutita*) | Allergic reactions with members of Asteraceae family (arnica, yarrow, feverfew, tansy, artemesia) | Has spasmolytic properties and is used for gastric complaints; efficacy not proven |
| Ginger (*Zingiber officinale*) | Heartburn, worsening colic in persons with gallstones, possible bleeding reactions | Efficacy for N/V, NVP, and motion sickness shown in several trials; not recommended by German Commission E for NVP |
| Lemon balm (*Melissa officinalis*) | None known | Has spasmolytic and carminative effects for digestive disorders; used for different gastric complaints including vomiting; efficacy not proven; use not recommended by German Commission E |
| Peppermint (*Mentha piperita*) | Bronchial spasms in high doses; colic in persons with gallstones | Has spasmolytic properties and is used for dyspepsia; efficacy not proven; recommended by German Commission E |

Key: N/V, nausea and vomiting; NVP, nausea and vomiting of pregnancy.

as effective as metoclopramide for postoperative nausea.[53] Ginger has shown favorable effects for N/V caused by seasickness, and it has been evaluated in several trials for NVP.[54-58] A prospective study in 187 women indicated that ginger may be safely used during pregnancy[56] and another study found it was equivalent in efficacy to pyridoxine.[57] The only adverse effect that has occurred in treating NVP has been heartburn.[58] It is important for practitioners to tell patients that although ginger is listed as GRAS (generally recognized as safe) in the United States, it does not have FDA approval for treating N/V. Ginger may be safe when used as a food or spice, but higher doses may produce side effects, including antiplatelet effects that may lead to bleeding.[52] It may also interact with other antiplatelet agents such as warfarin or aspirin or with complementary therapies that have antiplatelet activity, and thus result in bleeding reactions.[52] The German Commission E warns that ginger should not be taken during pregnancy.[59] Doses used for NVP are 250 mg of powdered ginger root given before meals and at bedtime (1 g/day)[54] or ginger syrup 250 mg four times a day.[55] Ginger powder, ginger extracts, tea, and tinctures have also been used to treat N/V.[52,53,59]

### Other Herbal Remedies

Two other herbal products commonly used for GI disorders are chamomile and peppermint (see Chapter 53). Chamomile (*Matricaria recutita*) has been used for a variety of GI disorders.[52] Although it may exhibit various pharmacologic effects, in GI disorders it is thought to have antispasmodic and mild sedative activities.[52,59] Considered safe, chamomile has GRAS status in the United States, but may cause cross-sensitivity reactions in persons who are allergic to members of the Asteraceae/Compositae family, including ragweed, chrysanthemums, marigolds, and other members of the daisy family. One of the chemical constituents, apigenin, may decrease noradrenaline uptake and has produced an increase in atrial rate.[52] Since ingredients sometimes include coumarins, chamomile may have additive antiplatelet activity with medications or complementary therapies that also have antiplatelet properties. It may also cause additive sedation with medications or other products that possess intrinsic sedating effects.[52] Different dosage forms have included capsules, liquid, and oil. A typical dose is 3 g as an infusion.[52]

Peppermint oil (*Mentha piperita*) is another product whose many uses include treatment of N/V.[52] Peppermint is thought to have antispasmodic effects from direct action on digestive tract smooth muscle. Similar to chamomile in its safety profile, it has GRAS status, and is unsafe only when used in high doses or in very young children, since bronchospasm and respiratory arrest may occur. Colic may occur in patients with gallstones and should not be used in those with gastroesophageal reflux.[52] The average daily dose is 3 to 6 g and may also be prepared as a tincture or tea.[52] (Table 20-7 describes other herbs purported to treat N/V.)

## Assessment of Nausea and Vomiting: A Case-based Approach

Vomiting is a symptom produced not only by benign processes but also by serious illnesses. Vomiting may cause various complications. Physical assessment of the patient may help to determine whether some of the complications listed in Complications of Nausea and Vomiting have occurred. Physical assessment should include the patient's general appearance, mental status, and volume status and the presence of any abdominal pain. Evaluation of vital signs such as blood pressure, heart rate, temperature, and weight (to determine whether recent weight loss has occurred) is also pertinent.

A major concern with vomiting is the loss of fluids and the inability to eat or drink. This situation may result in dehydration and electrolyte disturbances. Self-care is inappropriate for patients with dehydration, severe anorexia, weight loss, or poor nutritional status. Medical evaluation for dehydration should be provided when severe vomiting or diarrhea persists for more than several hours in children or 48 hours in adults.[16-20]

Evaluation of concurrent signs and symptoms is useful in determining the potential cause of vomiting. Preexisting disease is also an important factor to rule out. Detailed information about the patient's medical history related to the GI tract is especially helpful in determining potential causes.

Practitioners should be aware that some patients might use nonprescription antiemetics to self-treat the early stages of a serious illness. Therefore, they should ask patients what they have used thus far to treat the symptoms, to avoid potential additive toxicity. Many patients choose to self-medicate N/V with various nonprescription products to avoid a medical office visit. However, the practitioner should be cautious about recommending self-medication for these symptoms and ask appropriate questions to determine whether referral to a primary care provider is indicated. Cases 20-1 and 20-2 give examples of the assessment of patients with vomiting.

## CASE 20-1

| Relevant Evaluation Criteria | Scenario/Model Outcome |
|---|---|
| **Information Gathering** | |
| 1. Gather essential information about the patient's symptoms, including: | |
| a. description of symptom(s) (i.e., nature, onset, duration, severity, associated symptoms) | Patient has suffered from several episodes of nausea and vomiting, usually in the morning, for the past 2 weeks. She is able to take small sips of liquids, but does not have an appetite. |
| b. description of any factors that seem to precipitate, exacerbate, and/or relieve the patient's symptoms. | Factors that precipitate or exacerbate the patient's symptoms include difficulty with cooking dinner since the sight and smell of raw meat nauseate her. No relief has been observed. |
| c. description of the patient's efforts to relieve the symptoms | The patient eats some soda crackers and takes small sips of soda or water. |
| 2. Gather essential patient history information: | |
| a. patient's identity | SB |
| b. age, sex, height, and weight | 29 y/o F, 5'7", 127 lb |
| c. patient's occupation | Fund-raiser for a children's organization |
| d. patient's dietary habits | Balanced diet; loves sushi and occasionally eats junk food |
| e. patient's sleep habits | Averages 7 hours per night |
| f. concurrent medical conditions, prescription and nonprescription medications, and dietary supplements | Just found out she is 9 weeks pregnant; taking a prenatal vitamin and does not want to take anything that "may hurt my baby" such as some of the "weird" supplements that persons reputedly take. SB also says she is supporting her husband in college, and finances are somewhat restricted. |
| g. allergies | NKA |
| h. history of other adverse reactions to medications | None |
| i. other (describe)_______ | N/A |
| **Assessment and Triage** | |
| 3. Differentiate the patient's signs/symptoms and correctly identify the patient's primary problem(s). | Nausea and vomiting in the morning over the past 2 weeks; unable to deal with certain odors; probably has NVP |
| 4. Identify exclusions for self-treatment (see Figure 20-1). | None |

## CASE 20-1 (continued)

| Relevant Evaluation Criteria | Scenario/Model Outcome |
|---|---|
| 5. Formulate a comprehensive list of therapeutic alternatives for the primary problem to determine if triage to a medical practitioner is required, and share this information with the patient. | Options include:<br>(1) Recommend self-care with:<br>– OTC pyridoxine<br>– OTC doxylamine<br>– OTC phosphorated carbohydrate solution<br>– Ginger<br>– Nondrug strategies (dietary and environmental changes; see Table 20-3)<br>– Acupressure or acustimulation bands<br>(2) Recommend self-care until PCP can be consulted.<br>(3) Refer for further evaluation.<br>(4) Take no action. |
| **Plan** | |
| 6. Select an optimal therapeutic alternative to address the patient's problem, taking into account patient preferences. | Since SB is not dehydrated and is able to drink small amounts of soda or water, you encourage her to continue the sips of liquid. You also advise SB of the signs/symptoms of dehydration such as fast heartbeat, no tears, decreased skin turgor, noticeable weight loss, or clothes fitting loosely. A therapeutic alternative is to start taking vitamin $B_6$ 10 to 25 mg 3-4 times/day. If symptoms of N/V persist, doxylamine 12.5 mg 3-4 times/day may be added. Nonpharmacologic suggestions in Table 20-3 should also be followed. If there is no relief, she may consult a PCP. |
| 7. Describe the recommended therapeutic approach to the patient. | You are probably suffering from nausea and vomiting related to your pregnancy, or NVP. Vitamin $B_6$ may be used to self-treat it. If the vitamin does not work, then you may add an antihistamine called doxylamine; take 12.5 mg 3-4 times/day.<br>You may also benefit from nonpharmacologic techniques (see Table 20-3) such as eating bland or dry foods and crackers in the morning before arising, sleeping in a well-ventilated room, and avoiding strong odors. If you do not have any relief, you may want to contact your PCP. |
| 8. Explain to the patient the rationale for selecting the recommended therapeutic approach from the considered therapeutic alternatives. | The American College of Obstetricians and Gynecologists (ACOG) has recently published guidelines for NVP. These include starting with vitamin $B_6$ and, if no relief, adding doxylamine. Since you are able to drink fluids and are not dehydrated, seeking medical care may not be necessary at this time. However, if nausea and/or vomiting worsen or persist, then a PCP should be consulted for further evaluation. |
| **Patient Education** | |
| 9. When recommending self-care with nonprescription medications and/or nondrug therapy, convey accurate information to the patient, including: | |
| a. appropriate dose and frequency of administration | Vitamin $B_6$ 10-25 mg 3 or 4 times/day |
| b. maximum number of days the therapy should be employed | No limitations |
| c. product administration procedures | Take 1 tablet with a small glass of water. |
| d. expected time to onset of relief | Variable |
| e. degree of relief that can be reasonably expected | Variable |
| f. most common side effects | Side effects are rare. Sensory neuropathy may occur with high doses although doses as small as 50 mg/day have resulted in this reversible effect. |
| g. side effects that warrant medical intervention should they occur | Numbness of the hands or feet (sensory neuropathic symptoms) |

## CASE 20-1 (continued)

| Relevant Evaluation Criteria | Scenario/Model Outcome |
|---|---|
| h. patient options in the event that condition worsens or persists | Add doxylamine, 12.5 mg (1/2 of a 25-mg tablet); take 1/2 tablet with a small glass of water 3 to 4 times/day. Doxylamine is available in the United States in an OTC sleep aid (Unisom Sleeptabs 25 mg) only. There are no limitations on the number of days the medication can be taken. Expected time to onset of relief and degree of relief are variable. Drowsiness is the most common side effect; it is important not to drive or operate machinery while taking the medication. Other possible effects include dry mouth, urinary retention, nasal congestion, dry eyes, and constipation. Side effects do not warrant medical attention unless they are severe. Consult your PCP if the condition does not improve or severe side effects from the OTC product occur. Store the product at 59°F-86°F (15°C-30°C). |
| i. product storage requirements | Store at 59°F-86°F (15°C-30°C) |
| j. specific nondrug measures | See Table 20-3 for dietary measures. |
| 10. Solicit follow-up questions from patient. | How do I know if these are safe to take during pregnancy? What other nonprescription products may be used? |
| 11. Answer patient's questions. | These products have been taken by other pregnant women and have not been shown to cause any problems with the baby. You should also ask your PCP about taking these products and obtain information from the information resources in Table 20-8.<br>Other products that have been used for NVP include phosphorated carbohydrate solution although it was not considered as an option in the evidence-based ACOG guidelines. Acupressure or acustimulation wristbands are also an option, but they are expensive and are therefore not an option because of financial constraints. Another option is ginger, but you prefer not to take any "weird supplements." |

Key: ACOG, American College of Obstetricians and Gynecologists; N/A, not applicable; NKA, no known allergies; NVP, nausea and vomiting during pregnancy; PCP, primary care provider.

## CASE 20-2

| Relevant Evaluation Criteria | Scenario/Model Outcome |
|---|---|
| **Information Gathering** | |
| 1. Gather essential information about the patient's symptoms, including: | |
| a. description of symptom(s) (i.e., nature, onset, duration, severity, associated symptoms) | Patient has experienced six episodes of N/V in the last 24 hours and has been unable to keep down any liquids or solids. |
| b. description of any factors that seem to precipitate, exacerbate, and/or relieve the patient's symptoms. | There are no precipitating or exacerbating factors. No relief has been observed. |
| c. description of the patient's efforts to relieve the symptoms | No attempt to relieve nausea and vomiting except to try to drink some ginger ale |
| 2. Gather essential patient history information: | |
| a. patient's identity | JM |
| b. age, sex, height, and weight | 71 y/o M, 5'11", 190 lb |
| c. patient's occupation | Retired from the steel industry |
| d. patient's dietary habits | Balanced diet; occasional junk food and alcohol |

| CASE 20-2 (continued) | |
|---|---|
| **Relevant Evaluation Criteria** | **Scenario/Model Outcome** |
| e. patient's sleep habits | Averages 6-7 hours/night |
| f. concurrent medical conditions, prescription and nonprescription medications, and dietary supplements | HTN, diabetes, osteoarthritis. glipizide 10 mg once daily, losartan 100 mg once daily, meloxicam 15 mg once daily, and acetaminophen 500 mg 4 times/day |
| g. allergies | NKA |
| h. history of other adverse reactions to medications | None |
| i. other (describe)_______ | JM had been babysitting his 3-year-old grandson Cody who had a mild 24-hour bout of diarrhea in the last week. He reports that his blood glucose was high this morning. This is unusual because it is usually about 130 mg/dL. Examination by the practitioner revealed JM's buccal mucous membranes are dry. In addition, his skin is tented and his capillary refill response is slow. He stays his clothes fit very loose today. He complains of dizziness when going from sitting to standing. Measurement of BP in the pharmacy is 82/60 sitting and 99/70 standing. His heart rate is 88 beats/minute. Temperature is 101°F (38.8°C). Measurement of JM's blood glucose is 400 mg/dL. |
| **Assessment and Triage** | |
| 3. Differentiate the patient's signs/symptoms and correctly identify the patient's primary problem(s). | Six episodes of N/V in the last 24 hours. Patient also appears to be dehydrated, has orthostasis, tachycardia, and has an elevated temperature and blood glucose. |
| 4. Identify exclusions for self-treatment (see Figure 20-1). | High blood glucose with signs of dehydration in patients with diabetes mellitus |
| 5. Formulate a comprehensive list of therapeutic alternatives for the primary problem to determine if triage to a medical practitioner is required, and share this information with the patient. | Options include:<br>(1) Recommend self-care with:<br>– OTC antihistamines<br>– OTC phosphorated carbohydrate solution<br>– Ginger<br>– Nondrug strategies: acupressure or acustimulation bands<br>(2) Recommend self-care until PCP can be consulted.<br>(3) Refer for further evaluation.<br>(4) Take no action. |
| **Plan** | |
| 6. Select an optimal therapeutic alternative to address the patient's problem, taking into account patient preferences. | The patient should be referred immediately to a PCP. |
| 7. Describe the recommended therapeutic approach to the patient. | Since your nausea and vomiting is accompanied by dehydration, an elevated temperature, dizziness, and high blood glucose and is possibly related to the grandson's recent diarrheal episode, you probably have gastroenteritis. Since you cannot tolerate liquids and have diabetes and elevated blood glucose, you should consult with a PCP for further evaluation as soon as possible. Taking a nonprescription antiemetic may not take care of the problem. |
| 8. Explain to the patient the rationale for selecting the recommended therapeutic approach from the considered therapeutic alternatives. | The nausea and vomiting you are experiencing is most likely situational and related to Cody's recent bout of diarrhea. Since you are not taking liquids and have signs of dehydration, as well as low blood pressure, an elevated temperature and high blood glucose, I think you should consult with a PCP as soon as possible for further evaluation. I am worried that you could have an acute complication of diabetes if you are not seen by a PCP. |

**CASE 20-2 (continued)**

| Relevant Evaluation Criteria | Scenario/Model Outcome |
|---|---|
| **Patient Education** | |
| 9. When recommending self-care with nonprescription medications and/or nondrug therapy, convey accurate information to the patient. | Criterion does not apply in this case. |
| 10. Solicit follow-up questions from patient. | Isn't there an OTC medication that might work so I don't have to go to the doctor? |
| 11. Answer patient's questions. | Although OTC antiemetics are available, since dehydration is a concern and you have diabetes, you need to consult with a PCP as soon as possible. |

Key: NKA, no known allergies; N/V, nausea and vomiting; OTC, over-the-counter; PCP, primary care provider.

## Patient Counseling for Nausea and Vomiting

The practitioner should stress that treatment of N/V must focus on identifying and, if possible, correcting the underlying cause. Patients prone to overeating, bulimia, or motion sickness should, when possible, avoid these behaviors or situations that cause N/V. The patient should be advised that acute vomiting requires only symptomatic treatment because it is usually self-limiting and will resolve spontaneously. If the cause of the symptoms is known and self-treatment is appropriate, the practitioner should explain the proper use of the recommended product. Patient education should include information about possible adverse effects, as well as signs and symptoms that indicate medical attention is warranted. The box Patient Education for Nausea and Vomiting lists specific information to provide patients.

Telling patients about information resources for N/V may help provide reassurance (Table 20-8).

## Evaluation of Patient Outcomes for Nausea and Vomiting

There are many causes of N/V including overeating, motion sickness, an acute illness, or pregnancy. In most cases N/V is self-limiting. Depending on the cause, various treatments or medications are used to treat N/V. After a clinician has provided information or suggestions for treatment of N/V, a follow-up assessment of the patient should occur within 24 hours of the initial encounter. Thus, the clinician may determine whether symptoms have improved, changed, or worsened. This may best be accomplished by a follow-up phone call and then a scheduled appointment if desired by the patient. The follow-up should include an assessment of whether the N/V has diminished or abated, whether there are any residual related symptoms such as signs or symptoms of dehydration,

**TABLE 20-8 Information Resources on Nausea and Vomiting**

- The American Academy of Family Physicians (AAFP) provides information on N/V in adults at www.familydoctor.org/flowcharts/529.html.
- The National Organization of Teratology Information Services refers patients to a Teratology Information Service in their area. Toll-free phone: 1-888-285-3410. Web site: www.otispregnancy.org.
- A help line for patients with NVP is available at 1-800-436-8477.
- Information on NVP is available at www.motherisk.org.
- The American Academy of Family Physicians (AAFP) provides tips about "morning sickness" is available at http://familydoctor.org.
- Tips on "morning sickness" are available at Nutritional Aids for Nausea and Vomiting in Pregnancy, WebMD Medical Reference, from "Nutrition & Pregnancy: A Guide from Preconception to Postdelivery," http://my.webmd.com.
- Evidence-based guidelines for NVP are at ACOG (American College of Obstetrics and Gynecology) Practice Bulletin: nausea and vomiting of pregnancy. Obstet Gynecol 2004;103:803-14.
- Evidence-based guidelines for NVP (Canada): Levichek Z, Atanackovic G, Oepkes D, et al. Nausea and vomiting of pregnancy. Evidence-based treatment algorithm. *Can Fam Physician*. 2002;48:267-8,2 77.
- Information on telephone triage for specific referral recommendations is available in Schmitt BD. *Pediatric Telephone Protocols: Office Version*. 9th ed. Elk Grove Park, Ill: American Academy of Pediatrics; 2002.
- King CB, Glass R, Bresee JS, Duggan C. Managing acute gastroenteritis among children: oral rehydration, maintenance, and nutritional therapy from the Centers for Disease Control and Prevention. *MMWR Morb Mortal Wkly Rep* Recomm Rep. 2003;52(RR-16):1-16. Available at: www.cdc.gov/mmwr/PDF/RR/RR5216.pdf.

Key: NVP, nausea and vomiting of pregnancy.

## PATIENT EDUCATION FOR NAUSEA AND VOMITING

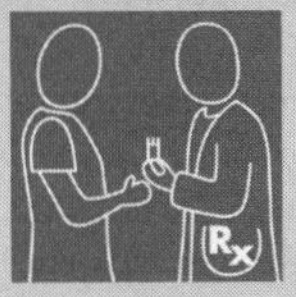

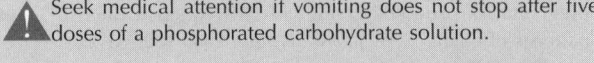

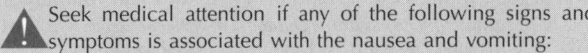

The objectives of self-treatment are to (1) prevent or control symptoms of occasional mild, self-limiting nausea and vomiting, (2) improve the symptoms and the patient's overall sense of well-being, and (3) avoid unnecessary emergency health care visits. For most patients, carefully following product instructions and the self-care measures listed here will help ensure optimal therapeutic outcomes.

### Nondrug Measures

- To prevent "morning sickness," eat small, frequent meals that are low in fat content. Sleep in a room with fresh air. Also, try eating crackers before getting up in the morning. Try lying down to relieve the symptoms once they occur. (See Tables 20-3 and 20-8.)
- To prevent motion sickness in young children, place them in a car seat that allows them to look out the windows (see Table 20-4.) Try acupressure wristbands to prevent motion sickness in adults or older children.
- To prevent nausea associated with overeating, avoid foods or beverages known to cause nausea; consume other foods and beverages in moderation.

### Nonprescription Medications

#### *Antacids, Histamine$_2$-Receptor Antagonists, or BSS*

- Take antacids, histamine$_2$-receptor antagonists (e.g., ranitidine, famotidine, cimetidine, or nizatidine), or BSS (Pepto-Bismol) for nausea caused by overeating. Follow product instructions for dosages. (See Chapters 14 and 17.)

#### *Phosphorated Carbohydrate Solution*

- Take phosphorated carbohydrate solutions for nausea and vomiting associated with upset stomach caused by viral gastroenteritis, food indiscretions, and emotional upset. (See Table 20-6 for selected brand-name products.)
- Give 1-2 tablespoonfuls (15–30 mL) of the solution to adults at 15-minute intervals until vomiting stops. For children ages 2-12 years old, give 1-2 teaspoonfuls (5-10 mL). Do not give more than five doses in 1 hour.
- Do not dilute the solution, and do not allow the patient to consume other liquids for 15 minutes after taking a dose.
- Do not take this product if you have hereditary fructose intolerance.
- If you have diabetes, consult your primary care provider before taking this product.

#### *Antihistamines*

- Take antihistamines for self-treatment of nausea and vomiting caused by motion sickness.
- To prevent motion sickness, take antihistamines at least 30 to 60 minutes before departure. Continue taking the medication during travel. Follow the dosage guidelines in Table 20-5.
- Avoid driving or operating hazardous machinery or engaging in tasks requiring a high degree of mental alertness while using antihistamines. Drowsiness is the most common adverse effect of these medications.
- If you have asthma, narrow-angle glaucoma, obstructive disease of the GI or genitourinary tract, or benign prostatic hypertrophy, consult a primary care provider before using antihistamines.
- Be aware that antihistamines may increase the sedative effects of alcohol, tranquilizers, hypnotics, and sedatives. Antihistamines may produce excitability in children or mental confusion in persons of advanced age.
- Do not take diphenhydramine oral products if you are using topical or external diphenhydramine preparations.

#### *Oral Rehydration Solutions*

- If needed, take an ORS to prevent dehydration secondary to vomiting and diarrhea.

⚠ Seek medical attention if vomiting does not stop after five doses of a phosphorated carbohydrate solution.

⚠ Seek medical attention if any of the following signs and symptoms is associated with the nausea and vomiting:

- Blood in the vomitus
- Abdominal pain or distention
- Projectile vomiting or prolonged nausea and vomiting (more than 24–48 hours), especially in children younger than 1 year
- Dehydration
- Weight loss of more than 9% of body weight
- Fever
- Severe headache
- Change in behavior or alertness
- Pregnancy
- Presence of diabetes or other medical conditions that may be affected by lack of nutritional intake or by missed doses of diabetes medications
- Recent trauma, particularly a significant head or abdominal injury
- Suspected poisoning

whether vital signs have returned to normal such as racing heart or delayed capillary refill or whether the patient is febrile. If the patient had prolonged N/V (longer than 24 to 48 hours) or if a change in or worsening of symptoms required immediate referral to a primary care provider, it is important for the clinician to follow up with the patient by telephone to determine whether the patient sought medical help and what type of treatment was administered. It is also important for the clinician to assess whether he or she needs to provide any further counseling or answer further patient questions. The clinician should also use this opportunity to provide reassurance and support.

## Key Points for Nausea and Vomiting

- N/V are symptoms of an underlying disorder, and treatment should focus on identifying and correcting the underlying cause.
- Nonprescription antiemetic medications are suitable for preventing and controlling the symptoms of occasional self-limiting N/V.
- Food overindulgence, food poisoning, and motion sickness may cause self-limiting cases of these symptoms.
- Food overindulgence may be treated with antacids, OTC histamine$_2$-blockers, or phosphorated carbohydrate solution.

- Agents of choice to treat N/V of motion sickness are antihistamines.
- Agents that may be used safely to treat N/V in all persons 2 years of age and older as well as NVP include acupressure/acustimulation devices as well as phosphorated carbohydrate solution.
- Uncomplicated NVP may be treated with pyridoxine, doxylamine, or acupressure/acustimulation devices.
- Loss of fluids and the inability to eat or drink because of N/V may result in dehydration and electrolyte disturbances. This primary complication of N/V should be treated with ORSs.
- A patient who presents with complicated issues relating to N/V may not be a candidate for self-treatment but instead should be referred.

## References


1. Information Resources, Inc., Chicago. Top 200 OTC/HBC brands in 2003. Drug Topics 2004. Available at: http://www.drugtopics.com. Accessed December10, 2004.
2. Farley D. Taming tummy turmoil. Available at: http://www.fda.gov/fdac/reprints/tummy.html. Accessed February 13, 2005.
3. Dobie T, McBride D, Dobie T Jr, et al. The effect of age and sex on susceptibility to motion sickness. *Aviat Space Environ Med* 2001; 72:13-20.
4. Lacroix R, Eason E, Melzack R. Nausea and vomiting during pregnancy: a prospective study of its frequency, intensity, and patterns of change. *Am J Obstet Gynecol* 2000;182:931-7.
5. Jewell MD, Young G. Interventions for nausea and vomiting in early pregnancy. *The Cochrane Database of Systemic Reviews* 2003;4. Art. No.: CD000145. DOI:10.1002/14651858.CD000145.
6. Goodwin TM. Hyperemesis gravidarum. *Clin Obstet Gynecol* 1998; 41:597-605.
7. Mead PS, Slutsker L, Dietz V, et al. Food-related illness and death in the United States. *Emerg Infect Dis* 1999;5:607-25.
8. King CB, Glass R, Bresee JS, et al. Managing acute gastroenteritis among children: oral rehydration, maintenance, and nutritional therapy from the Centers for Disease Control and Prevention. *MMWR Morb Mortal Wkly Rep* Recomm Rep 2003;52(RR-16):1-16. Available at: www.cdc.gov/mmwr/PDF/RR/RR5216.pdf. Accessed February 13, 2005.
9. Rotavirus diarrhea. Available at: http://www.cdc.gov/nip/diseases/rota/rotavirus.htm. Accessed June 15, 2005.
10. Miller AD. Central mechanisms of vomiting. *Dig Dis Sci* 1999;44: 39S-43S.
11. Herndon CM, Jackson II KC, Hallin PA: Management of opioid-induced gastrointestinal effects in patients receiving palliative care. *Pharmacotherapy* 2002;22:240-50.
12. Quigley EM, Hasler WL, Parkman HP. AGA technical review on nausea and vomiting. *Gastroenterology* 2001;120: 263-86.
13. Lindley C. Nausea and vomiting. In: Koda-Kimble MA, Young LY, Kradjan WA, et al., eds. *Applied Therapeutics: The Clinical Use of Drugs.* 8th ed. Baltimore: Lippincott Williams & Wilkins; 2004: 8-1–8-18.
14. McQuaid KR. Alimentary tract. In: Tierney LM, ed. *Current Medical Diagnosis and Treatment.* 42nd ed. New York: Lange Medical Books/McGraw-Hill; 2003:573-5.
15. Taylor AT. Nausea and vomiting. In: Dipiro JT, Talbert RL, Yee GC, et al., eds. *Pharmacotherapy: A Pathophysiologic Approach.* 5th ed. New York. McGraw-Hill, Inc; 2002: 641-53.
16. Davidson MB. Hyperglycemia. In: Franz MJ, ed. *A Core Curriculum for Diabetes Education: Diabetes and Complications.* 4th ed. Chicago: American Association of Diabetes Educators; 2001:19-42.
17. Kuver R, Sheffield JV, McDonald GB. Nausea and vomiting in adolescents and adults. Available at: http:// www.uwgi.org/cme/cmeCourseCD/ch_01/ch01txt.htm. Accessed February 14, 2005.
18. Carroll KC, Reimer L. Infectious diarrhea: pathogens and treatment. *J Med Liban* 2000;48:270-7.
19. Helton T, Rolston DD: What adults with acute diarrhea should be evaluated? What is the best diagnostic approach? *Cleve Clin J Med* 2004;71:778-9, 783-5.
20. Schmitt BD. *Pediatric Telephone Protocols: Office Version.* 9th ed. Elk Grove Park, Ill: American Academy of Pediatrics; 2002.
21. Armon K, Stephenson T, MacFaul R, et al. An evidence and consensus based guideline for acute diarrhoea management. *Arch Dis Child* 2001;85:132-42.
22. Smith C, Crowther C, Beilby J, et al. The impact of nausea and vomiting on women: a burden of early pregnancy. *Aust N Z J Obstet Gynaecol* 2000;40:397-401.
23. Mazzotta P, Gupta A, Maltepe C, et al. Pharmacologic treatment of nausea and vomiting during pregnancy. *Can Fam Physician* 1998;44:1455-7.
24. Quinlan JD, Hill DA. Nausea and vomiting of pregnancy. *Am Fam Physician* 2003;68:121-8.
25. Kaiser LL, Allen L. Position of the American Dietetic Association: nutrition and lifestyle for a healthy pregnancy outcome. *J Am Diet Assoc* 2002;102:1479-90.
26. Morning sickness. Available at: http://familydoctor.org/154.xml#4. Accessed February 13, 2005.
27. Stern RM, Jokerst MD, Muth ER, et al. Acupressure relieves the symptoms of motion sickness and reduces abnormal gastric activity. *Altern Ther Health Med* 2001;7: 91-4.
28. Steele NM, French J, Gatherer-Boyles J, et al. Effect of acupressure by sea-bands on nausea and vomiting of pregnancy. *J Obstet Gynecol Neonatal Nurs* 2001;30:61-70.
29. Sea-Band Acupressure Wrist Bands for Relief of Nausea & Vomiting. Available at: http://www.sea-band.com. Accessed February 26, 2005.
30. Rosen T, de Veciana M, Miller HS, et al. A randomized controlled trial of nerve stimulation for relief of nausea and vomiting in pregnancy. *Obstet Gynecol* 2003;102:129-35.
31. What is ReliefBand? ReliefBand Device. Available at: http://www.reliefband.com. Accessed February 14, 2005.
32. Wickersham RM, Novak KK, Schweain SL, eds. *Drug Facts & Comparisons.* St. Louis: Wolters Kluwer Health, Inc; 2005.
33. Taketomo CK, Hodding JH, Krause DM, eds. *Pediatric Dosage Handbook.* 9th ed. Hudson, Ohio: Lexi-Comp, Inc; 2002.
34. Pasricha PJ. Prokinetic agents, antiemetics, and agents used in irritable bowel syndrome. In: Hardman JG, Limbird LE, Gilman AG, eds. *The Pharmacological Basis of Therapeutics.* 10th ed. New York: McGraw-Hill, Inc; 2001:1021-36.
35. Weiler JM, Bloomfield JR, Woodworth GG, et al. Effects of fexofenadine, diphenhydramine, and alcohol on driving performance: a randomized, placebo-controlled trial in the Iowa driving simulator. *Ann Intern Med* 2000;132: 354-63.
36. Khosla U, Ruel KS, Hunt DB: Antihistamine-induced rhabdomyolysis. *South Med J* 2003;10:1023-6.
37. Fick DM, Cooper JW, Wade WE, et al. Updating the Beers criteria for potentially inappropriate medication use in older adults. *Arch Intern Med* 2003;163:2716-24.
38. Briggs GG, Freeman RK, Yaffe SJ, eds. *Drugs in Pregnancy and Lactation.* 6th ed. Philadelphia: Lippincott William & Wilkins; 2002.
39. Hamelin BA, Bouayad A, Methot J, et al. Significant interaction between the nonprescription antihistamine diphenhydramine and the CYP2D6 substrate metoprolol in healthy men with high or low CYP2D6 activity. *Clin Pharmacol Ther* 2000;67:466-77.
40. Lessard E, Yessine MA, Hamelin BA, et al. Diphenhydramine alters the disposition of venlafaxine through inhibition of CYP2D6 activity in humans. *J Clin Psychopharmacol* 2001;21:175-84.

41. Food and Drug Administration, Department of Health and Human Services. Labeling of diphenhydramine-containing drug products for over-the-counter human use: final rule. *Federal Register* 2002;67:72555-9.
42. Barsoum A, Kolivakis TT, Margolese HC, et al. Diphenhydramine (Unisom), a central anticholinergic and antihistaminic: abuse with massive ingestion in a patient with schizophrenia. *Can J Psychiatry* 2000;45: 846-7.
43. Halpert AG, Olmstead MC, Beninger RJ. Mechanisms and abuse liability of the antihistamine dimenhydrinate. *Neurosci Biobehav Rev* 2002;26:61-7.
44. Dickerson LM, King DE. Evaluation and management of nonulcer dyspepsia. *Am Fam Physician* 2004;70:107-14.
45. ACOG (American College of Obstetrics and Gynecology) Practice Bulletin: nausea and vomiting of pregnancy. *Obstet Gynecol* 2004;103:803-14.
46. Levichek Z, Atanackovic G, Oepkes D, et al. Nausea and vomiting of pregnancy. Evidence-based treatment algorithim. *Can Fam Physician* 2002;48:267-8, 277.
47. Mazzotta P, Magee LA. A risk–benefit assessment of pharmacological and nonpharmacological treatments for nausea and vomiting of pregnancy. *Drugs* 2000; 59:781-800.
48. Arsenault MY, Lane CA, MacKinnon CJ, et al. The management of nausea and vomiting of pregnancy. *J Obstet Gynaecol Can.* 2002; 24:817-31;832-3.
49. Brent R. Bendectin and birth defects: hopefully, the final chapter. *Birth Defects Res Part A Clin Mol Teratol* 2003;67:79-87.
50. Kutcher JS, Engle A, Firth J, et al. Bendectin and birth defects II: Ecological analyses. *Birth Defects Res Part A Clin Mol Teratol* 2003;67:88-97.
51. Gastanaduy AS, Begue RE: Acute gastroenteritis. *Clin Pediatr (Phil)* 1999;38:1-12.
52. Gruenwald J, Brendler T, Jaenicke C, eds. *PDR for Herbal Medicines.* 2nd ed. Montvale, NJ: Thomson Medical Economics; 2000.
53. Ernst E, Pittler MH. Efficacy of ginger for nausea and vomiting: a systematic review of randomized clinical trials. *Br J Anaesth* 2000;84:367-71.
54. Vutyavanich T, Kraisarin T, Ruangsri RA. Ginger for nausea and vomiting in pregnancy: randomized, double-masked, placebo-controlled trial. *Obstet Gynecol* 2001;97: 577-82.
55. Keating A, Chez RA. Ginger syrup as an antiemetic in early pregnancy. *Altern Ther Health Med* 2002;8:89-91.
56. Portnoi G, Chng L-A, Karimi-Tabesh L, et al. Prospective comparative study of the safety and effectiveness of ginger for the treatment of nausea and vomiting in pregnancy. *Am J Obstet Gynecol* 2003;189:1374-7.
57. Smith C, Crowther C, Willson K, et al. A randomized controlled trial of ginger to treat nausea and vomiting in pregnancy. *Obstet Gynecol* 2004;103:639-45.
58. Willetts KE, Ekangaki A, Eden JA. Effect of a ginger extract on pregnancy-induced nausea: a randomized controlled trial. *Aust N Z J Obstet Gynaecol* 2003;43:139-44.
59. Blumenthal M, Busse WR, Goldberg A, et al., eds. *The Complete German Commission E Monographs: Therapeutic Guide to Herbal Medicines.* Klein S, trans. Boston: American Botanical Council; 1998.

CHAPTER 21

# Poisoning

*Wendy Klein-Schwartz and Barbara Insley Crouch*

Poisoning is a common and potentially life-threatening injury. While unintentional poisoning is responsible for most toxic exposures in young children, poisonings in other age groups may be unintentional or intentional caused by suicide attempts, substance abuse, or drug misuse. The majority of poisonings are a result of ingestion of a substance, but poisonings may also occur after inhalation or contact with the skin and eyes. First aid for poisonings focuses on minimizing the extent of the exposure. For inhalation exposure, the person is removed to fresh air, and, for topical exposures, the skin or eye is irrigated to remove the toxic substance. Gastrointestinal (GI) decontamination reduces absorption of ingested toxins, thereby minimizing toxicity. Ipecac syrup, a nonprescription emetic, has been used to induce vomiting for some poisonings managed at home, but is no longer routinely recommended. Alternatively, activated charcoal may be used to adsorb substances in the GI tract, although it is not universally accepted as a self-treatment. A poison control center should be contacted for assessment and treatment of poisonings as well as for educational materials on poison prevention. Figure 21-1 shows the nationwide poison control center number and logo.

## Epidemiology of Poisoning

Unintentional poisonings are one of the leading causes of injury-related hospitalizations in preschool children, even though fatalities among preschoolers have declined significantly since the early 1970s. There were 46 deaths caused by unintentional poisoning in children younger than 5 years reported in the National Center for Health Statistics mortality data for 2001, of which 27 involved drugs.[1] Only 27 of the 1183 fatalities reported by poison control centers in 2004 involved children younger than 6 years.[2] Drugs (excluding ethanol) were the primary substances responsible for 940 (79.5%) fatalities and were involved in 32 additional deaths in which a nonpharmaceutical was the primary agent. In 2004, 62 poison control centers serving a population of 293.7 million reported 2,438,644 cases to the Toxic Exposure Surveillance System of the American Association of Poison Control Centers.[2]

The majority of poison exposures (51.3%) occur in children younger than 6 years.[2] Nonprescription and prescription medications are frequently responsible for potentially toxic exposures reported to poison control centers. Nonprescription products, such as analgesics and cough and cold preparations, are among the most common substances ingested by young children. The large number of nonprescription medications involved in pediatric exposures reflects their common use and availability of these products in the home.

Child-resistant closures help prevent unintentional poisonings. These closures have been responsible for a decline in mortality related to childhood poisoning with regulated substances such as aspirin, prescription drugs, and some household chemicals. Analysis of mortality rates from unintentional ingestion of oral prescription drugs found an annual reduction of 1.4 deaths per million children younger than 5 years attributed to the use of child-resistant packaging.[3] This reduction translates into approximately 460 fewer deaths from 1974 through 1992. A 34% reduction in the aspirin-related mortality rate in children younger than 5 years was associated with the use of child-resistant closures.[4] Similarly, the decline in iron poisonings from 2370 cases in 1996 to 790 cases in 1999 reported to the National Electronic Injury Surveillance System has been attributed to unit-dose packaging requirements for products containing 30 mg or more of elemental iron that were enacted by the Food and Drug Administration (FDA) in 1997.[5]

Nearly 74% of poison exposures reported to poison control centers are managed onsite, usually in a residence. Only 10.2% of children younger than 6 years are managed in a health care facility, and major effects or fatal outcomes occur in fewer than 1%.[2] However, unintentional childhood poisonings remain a common cause of injury-related morbidity, requiring significant expenditures of health care dollars for inpatient and outpatient care. Pediatric admissions to urban hospitals because of poisoning accounted for almost $1 million in hospital charges in 1995.[6] Alternatively, unnecessary economic costs are incurred when an emergency department is used as the initial means of intervention for unintentional pediatric ingestions, rather than a poison control center.[7] On the basis of a phone survey of poison control center callers and emergency department directors in the center's service area, a poison control center estimated the cost of unnecessary emergency department visits, if the poison control center was unavailable, at over $3.6 million with a burden of over $1 million to the state medical assistance program.[8] A benefit-cost analysis for poisonings in the United States found that poison control centers reduce medical spending by $355 million (1992 dollars) and cost $65 million (1992 dollars) for their operation.[9] A significant portion of the cost savings results from home observation and decontamination and the reduction of unnecessary emergency medical transport and treatment costs.

POISON Help™
1-800-222-1222

FIGURE 21-1 Nationwide toll-free telephone number to access a poison control center. (*Source:* Reprinted with permission from the American Association of Poison Control Centers, Washington, DC.)

## Etiology of Poisoning

Exposures to potentially harmful substances most commonly occur by ingestion; however, other routes include inhalation, dermal, ocular, and parenteral. While most poison exposures reported to poison control centers are unintentional, exposures also result from intentional or malicious behavior, contamination, and adverse reactions to drugs, food, and chemicals. Medications are the most common source of poison exposures, accounting for 50% of reports to poison control centers.[2] Other substances include cleaning substances, cosmetics and personal care products, plants, pesticides, food products/poisoning, alcohols, hydrocarbons (e.g., gasoline), and chemicals. Bites and envenomations are other potential sources of toxin exposures.

## Signs and Symptoms of Poisoning

Poisons can affect every organ system. Signs and symptoms of poisoning can range in severity from mild to life threatening. For some drugs, toxicity after overdose is similar to the drug's adverse effect profile with therapeutic use. For example, ibuprofen overdose is characterized primarily by nausea, vomiting, and abdominal pain. Patients with diphenhydramine overdose may exhibit sedation or stimulation (agitation, hallucinations), tachycardia, hypertension, dry mouth, and dilated pupils from its anticholinergic properties. Overdoses of other drugs, such as aspirin, result in multiorgan system effects including GI, central nervous system, metabolic, cardiovascular, pulmonary, and hematologic toxicity. A lack of symptoms immediately following a poison exposure does not preclude toxicity. Patients may be asymptomatic initially, but can develop severe toxicity hours later following ingestion of some sustained-released or enteric-coated products or products that delay gastric emptying and/or slow GI motility (e.g., diphenoxylate/atropine). For other drugs, such as levothyroxine and sulfasalazine, and some chemicals (e.g., methanol, acetonitrile), clinical effects are delayed while the substance is being metabolized to active or toxic metabolites. The time course of acetaminophen overdose is related to formation and covalent binding of a toxic metabolite to hepatic cells. As a result, a relatively mild initial clinical course characterized by nausea, vomiting, anorexia, and malaise can be followed by severe hepatic and renal toxicity 3 to 5 days later.

## Treatment of Poisoning

Most unintentional poison exposures in small children result in minimal, if any, effects, and require no other treatment than observation. Although self-treatment may be appropriate, practitioners, caregivers, and patients are encouraged to seek counsel from the nearest poison control center before attempting any treatment.

### *Treatment Goals*

The primary goal of therapy is to prevent absorption of toxins or stem the progression of toxicity, thus minimizing morbidity and mortality.

### *General Treatment Approach*

The first step in assessing a potential poison exposure is to determine whether the patient has symptoms and whether the exposure puts the patient at risk of toxicity. Many exposures are, in fact, nontoxic or minimally toxic because either the substance has a very low inherent toxicity or the amount consumed is too low to cause toxicity. A decision regarding the option for self-treatment depends on the nature of the poison exposure, toxicity of the agent, and general health status of the patient. Self-treatment should be considered only if the ingestion is unintentional and the potential for toxicity is assessed as minor. Any exposure to a toxin that can potentially result in moderate to severe toxicity should be referred immediately to a hospital, as well as all intentional exposures. If the patient exhibits potentially life-threatening clinical effects, such as coma, seizures, or syncope, transportation to an emergency department should be arranged immediately through the emergency 911 system. Additional exclusions for self-treatment can be found in Figure 21-2. Hospital care includes observing the patient, supporting vital functions (airway, breathing, and circulation), preventing absorption, enhancing elimination, and using antidotes.

The majority of individuals who do not require immediate hospital referral are managed with onsite observation only and no specific treatment.[2] In some instances, the approach is to attenuate the exposure by irrigating or preventing further absorption. The nonprescription drugs ipecac syrup and activated charcoal may prevent or reduce the absorption of some ingested substances. However, their routine use is not recommended without consultation with a poison control center. In the past, nonprescription cathartics have been recommended to decrease absorption of substances by facilitating their elimination through the GI tract. However, cathartics by themselves are not beneficial in the treatment of a poisoned patient. Figure 21-2 outlines an algorithm for self-care of exposure to poisons.

### *Nonpharmacologic Therapy*

Inhalation exposures are managed by removing the patient from the toxic fumes to fresh air. Irrigation may be beneficial to decrease the contact time of a chemical with the skin or mucosal surface. Skin surfaces should be washed with soap and water (usually twice) to decrease the contact time of a chemical exposure. Irrigation of the eye

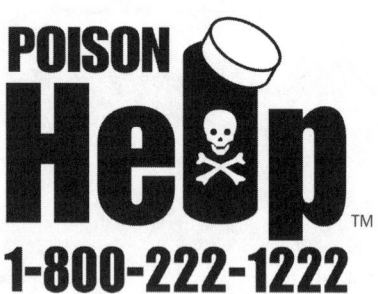

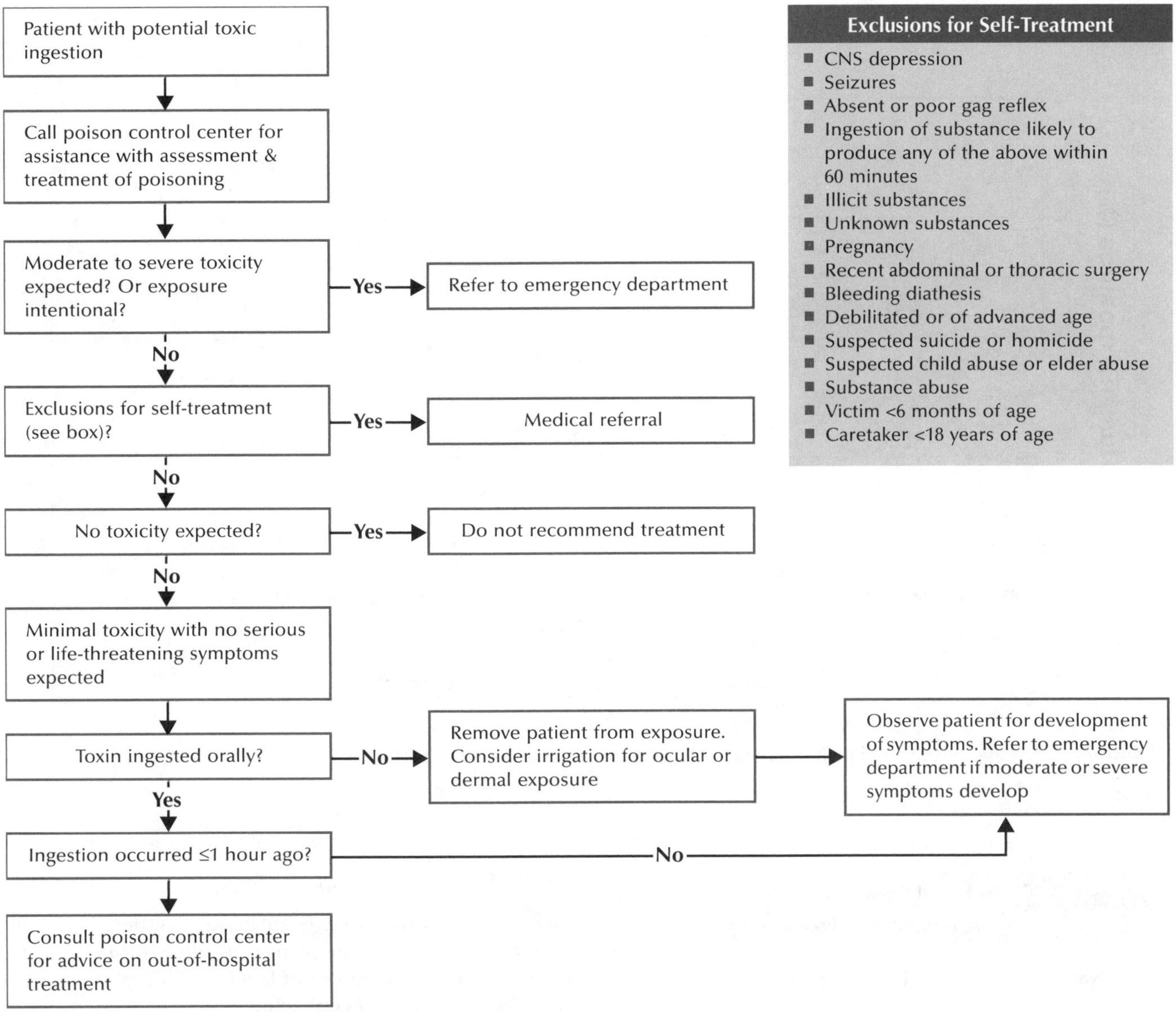


**FIGURE 21-2** Self-care for poisoning. Key: CNS, central nervous system.

with water should be initiated immediately after an ocular exposure to a chemical or drug not intended for ocular use (e.g., inadvertent ocular administration of an otic preparation). If an irritating chemical has been swallowed, the administration of a small amount of fluids may decrease the contact time of the chemical with the mucosal surface. The administration of a large amount of fluids should be discouraged as it is likely to result in spontaneous vomiting. The administration of oral fluids following an ingestion of a drug is not recommended, as the fluids theoretically may facilitate dissolution of a solid dosage form, thereby enhancing its absorption. Manually stimulating the gag reflex at the back of the throat with either a blunt object or a finger may induce vomiting but is not recommended and can lead to soft palate injury.

Gastric lavage, a procedure in which fluids are instilled into a tube placed into the stomach through the mouth or nose and then removed by suction or aspiration, is not an option for self-treatment. Improvement of patient outcome has not been definitively demonstrated and lavage is not without risks. Use of activated charcoal as the primary method of GI decontamination in health care facilities has further limited the role of lavage in the management of poisoning.

### *Pharmacologic Therapy*

Ipecac syrup, an emetic, and activated charcoal, an adsorbent, are the only approved self-treatments for ingested poisons. Table 21-1 lists selected trade-name products. Despite the availability of these agents for the self-treatment of poisoning, they are used only to a limited extent. In 2004, ipecac syrup was used in fewer than 1% of cases reported to poison control centers, and activated charcoal was used in just under 6% of cases (Figure 21-3).[2] Controversy surrounds the use of either treatment in the outpatient setting.

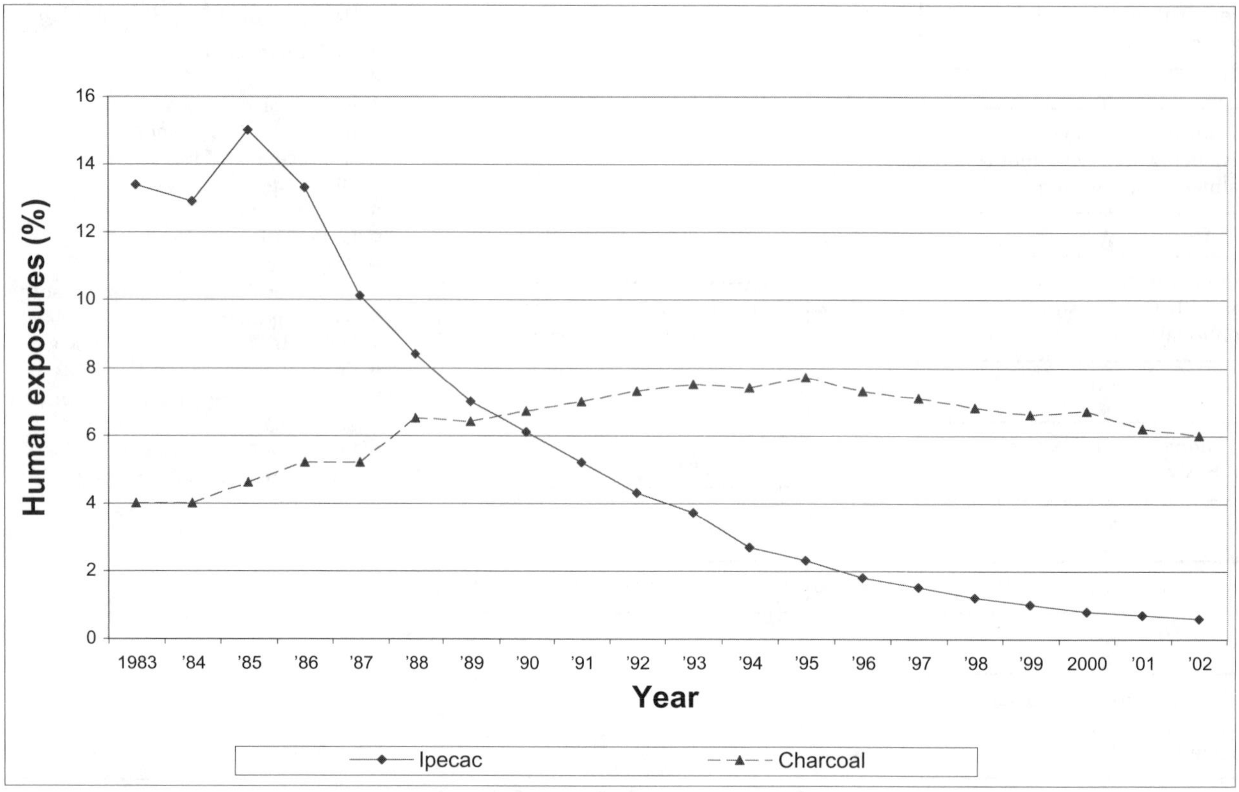


FIGURE 21-3 Use of ipecac and activated charcoal in poisoned patients, 1983-2004.

**TABLE 21-1 Selected Nonprescription Agents for Treatment of Poisoning***

| Trade Name | Primary Ingredients |
|---|---|
| **Emetics** | |
| Ipecac syrup | Emetine, cephaeline |
| **Activated Charcoal Products** | |
| Actidose-Aqua | Activated charcoal 25 g/120 mL, or 50 g/240 mL |
| Liqui Char | Activated charcoal 12.5 g/60 mL, 15 g/75 mL, 25 g/120 mL, 30 g/120 mL, or 50 g/240 mL |
| **Activated Charcoal Cathartic Products†** | |
| Actidose with Sorbitol | Activated charcoal 25 g/120 mL, or 50 g/240 mL; sorbitol |
| CharcoAid | Activated charcoal 15 g/120 mL, or 30g/150 mL with sorbitol |

* Ipecac is rarely recommended; activated charcoal is not universally accepted as a self-treatment (see text).

† Not for use in children younger than 1 year or when repeated doses are needed.

## Emetic Treatment with Ipecac Syrup

Ipecac syrup is prepared from ipecac powder, a natural product derived from the plant *Cephaelis ipecacuanha* or *C. acuminata*, and it contains not less than 90% of the ipecac alkaloids emetine and cephaeline.[10]

*Mechanism of Action* Ipecac syrup has a local irritant effect on the GI mucosa and also centrally stimulates the chemoreceptor trigger zone. Emetine and cephaeline probably produce the central effect (see Chapter 20).

*Indication* Ipecac syrup is FDA approved as an emetic for use in some poisonings.

*Dosage and Administration Guidelines* Ipecac syrup is no longer routinely recommended and should not be administered without consultation with a poison control center. The dose of ipecac syrup is 5 to 10 mL in children 6 months to 1 year of age, 15 mL in children 1 to 12 years of age, and 15 to 30 mL in adolescents and adults.[11]

*Safety Considerations* Serious toxicity following acute administration of ipecac syrup is rare. Following a therapeutic dose of ipecac syrup, diarrhea and drowsiness are common. Mild GI upset may last for several hours following emesis. Persistent vomiting is uncommon, but may lead

**TABLE 21-2 Contraindications to GI Decontamination as Self-treatment**

| Category | Inclusion Criteria | Recommendation |
|---|---|---|
| Patient condition | Coma, seizures, syncope, airway or breathing problems, blood pressure or pulse irregularities, hallucinations, and severe agitation | Refer to hospital for evaluation |
| Ingestion of low-viscosity hydrocarbons and terpenes | Gasoline; kerosene; mineral seal oil (furniture polish); naphtha (lighter fluid); pine oil (cleaners); turpentine (paint removers); mineral oil | Contact poison control center |
| Ingestion of caustic substances | Methacrylic acid (artificial nail primers); sodium silicate and carbonate (automatic dishwashing detergents); sulfuric acid (automotive battery, drain cleaners, toilet bowl cleaners); sodium hydroxide (Clinitest tablets, drain cleaners, oven cleaners, hair relaxers); hypochlorites (bleach, pool chlorine), thioglycolates (hair relaxers), hydrofluoric acid (rust removers), hydrochloric acid (toilet bowl cleaner) | Contact poison control center |
| Ingestion of substances not adsorbed by charcoal and/or too rapid absorption and onset for ipecac | Ethanol (alcoholic beverages, colognes, mouthwashes, aftershaves); isopropyl alcohol (rubbing alcohol); methanol (windshield washer fluid); ethylene glycol (antifreeze); ionized substances (potassium); heavy metals (lead, arsenic); cyanide (potassium cyanide, acetonitrile artificial nail remover, laetrile) | Contact poison control center |

Key: GI, gastrointestinal.

to dehydration. Aspiration of stomach contents may occur, especially if ipecac syrup is administered to patients with known contraindications to emesis. Clinical experience has shown that ingestion of 30 mL of ipecac syrup (the largest amount available without a prescription in a single unit of purchase) is safe in children older than 1 year. While serious and life-threatening effects are extremely rare, ipecac syrup has been associated with case reports of intracerebral hemorrhage, pneumomediastinum, Mallory-Weiss tear, diaphragmatic hernia, and gastric rupture.[11]

Chronic ipecac poisoning has been reported in patients who suffer from bulimia and following the intentional administration of ipecac to small children, also referred to as Münchhausen syndrome by proxy.[12-15] In addition to chronic vomiting and diarrhea, chronic exposure to ipecac syrup is associated with muscle weakness, cardiomyopathies, and electrolyte imbalances.[12] Pharmacists should question any person who frequently purchases ipecac syrup to ascertain if chronic misuse is occurring.

Ipecac-induced emesis is contraindicated in patients who have ingested a substance that may produce central nervous system depression or seizures within 60 minutes, even if the patient is currently not experiencing effects. In addition, the administration of ipecac syrup is contraindicated following the ingestion of low-viscosity hydrocarbons and terpenes, which have a high risk for aspiration, or of a corrosive substance (Table 21-2). The use of ipecac syrup is strongly discouraged in patients of advanced age, who are debilitated, or who have medical conditions that may be compromised by the induction of emesis. Ipecac syrup should not be used concurrently with activated charcoal. Patients who are given this combination are likely to vomit the activated charcoal, rendering it ineffective.

### Treatment With Activated Charcoal

Activated charcoal is a tasteless, gritty, fine, black insoluble powder made from the pyrolysis of various organic materials.[16] Wood or other carbon-containing compounds are "activated" by an oxidizing gas at high temperatures to produce a product with a very large surface area, resulting in a highly effective adsorbent for many drugs and chemicals. The surface area usually ranges from 950 to 2000 $m^2/g$.[16]

*Mechanism of Action* Activated charcoal has been shown to adsorb a large number of commonly ingested drugs as well as many other toxic agents. These substances are bound in the internal surface of the pores of the charcoal molecule, and thereby prevented from being absorbed. Activated charcoal is incapable of being digested, so is not absorbed from the GI tract. The higher the ratio of activated charcoal to toxin, the higher is the proportion of bound toxin.[16] Highly ionized substances, such as potassium and lithium, are poorly adsorbed by activated charcoal. Activated charcoal does not bind well to alcohols or glycols (e.g., ethanol, methanol, ethylene glycol), hydrocarbons, mineral acids and alkali, heavy metals (e.g., iron, lead, arsenic), or cyanide (Table 21-2). The presence of food in the GI tract may reduce the efficacy of activated charcoal.

*Indications* Activated charcoal is FDA approved for use as an emergency antidote in the treatment of an ingested poison.

*Dosage and Administration Guidelines* The usual dose of activated charcoal is 1 g/kg or 10 to 25 g in children up to 1 year of age, 25 to 50 g in children 1 to 12 years of age, and 25 to 100 g in adolescents and adults (Table 21-3).[16] Activated charcoal is available premixed with water, sorbitol

**TABLE 21-3 Activated Charcoal Dosing Information[16]**

| Age | Dose |
|---|---|
| 0-12 months* | 10-25 g |
| 10-12 years | 25-50 g |
| >12 years | 25-100 g |

* Do not use sorbitol-containing products.

(for catharsis), or water and carboxymethylcellulose (Table 21-1). Activated charcoal slurries are prone to settling, so these products should be vigorously shaken prior to administration. Activated charcoal is also available as a powder for reconstitution into an oral suspension just prior to use; this product should be stirred thoroughly or vigorously shaken after water is added. Flavoring agents have been used to try to increase the palatability of activated charcoal, but are generally avoided as they may reduce the adsorptive capacity of charcoal. Activated charcoal is most effective if given within 1 hour following ingestion. Repeat doses of activated charcoal (given in a health care facility setting only) may enhance the elimination of some drugs (e.g., phenobarbital, theophylline) after they are absorbed into the systemic circulation.

Activated charcoal is also available combined with sorbitol to improve palatability and act as a cathartic. The cathartic is intended to speed the transit of the activated charcoal complex through the GI tract and prevent constipation; however, the need for cathartics has been questioned.[17] Sorbitol-containing activated charcoal products are not recommended in children younger than 1 year or when multiple doses of activated charcoal are administered because of higher risk of fluid and electrolyte disturbances and hypotension. Most activated charcoal products marketed specifically for home use do not contain sorbitol.

Activated charcoal is used primarily for patients managed in a health care facility. While it is available as a nonprescription drug, it is not available in most homes. A study evaluating the administration of activated charcoal in the home to manage potentially toxic ingestions in children reported that 90% of parents did not have activated charcoal in their home, requiring them to obtain it from their local pharmacy for the poisoning incident.[18] Following a professional education program targeted at pharmacists, pediatricians, and family practice physicians in one state, a telephone survey found that 72% of 203 randomly selected pharmacies had activated charcoal on their shelves.[19] Practitioners should consult their poison control center to determine whether to promote routine availability of activated charcoal in the home.

*Safety Considerations* The most common adverse effects of activated charcoal are vomiting and black stools. Vomiting occurs in 12% to 20% of patients receiving activated charcoal.[16,20,21] One fifth of children younger than 18 years given activated charcoal for poisoning vomited a median time of 10 minutes after initiation of charcoal administration.[21] Previous vomiting was a significant risk factor for vomiting after activated charcoal administration. More serious complications, such as pulmonary aspiration and GI obstruction, are associated more often with administration of multiple doses of activated charcoal. In 878 patients who received two or more doses of activated charcoal, clinically significant complications were infrequent and included five pulmonary aspirations, eight electrolyte abnormalities, and one corneal abrasion.[22] Administration of a sorbitol-containing activated charcoal product increases the risk of vomiting, diarrhea, abdominal cramps, and electrolyte abnormalities. Hypernatremic dehydration has been reported with multiple-dose activated charcoal therapy with sorbitol-containing charcoal products.[20]

Activated charcoal is contraindicated in patients in whom the GI tract is not anatomically (e.g., following caustic injury) or functionally (e.g., ileus) intact. Activated charcoal is also contraindicated in patients at high risk for aspiration without airway protection (Table 21-2). Activated charcoal should not be administered following ingestion of substances that it does not adsorb, unless the presence of other ingestants that are adsorbed by charcoal is suspected.

### Pharmacotherapeutic Comparison of Ipecac Syrup and Activated Charcoal

Studies have demonstrated that the effectiveness of GI decontamination decreases significantly with increasing time interval since ingestion. For most overdoses, GI decontamination should be performed early, usually within an hour of the ingestion. Ipecac syrup is less effective at preventing absorption than activated charcoal for most poisons. Activated charcoal is the preferred agent for GI decontamination in health care facilities, where gastric emptying with ipecac syrup or lavage are no longer routinely recommended.[23-25] The action of either ipecac syrup or lavage is limited to emptying the stomach, while activated charcoal has the advantage of also adsorbing drug or toxin in the small intestine.

There is no convincing evidence that either ipecac or activated charcoal result in improved patient outcomes. The utility of gastric emptying (ipecac, lavage) or charcoal in adults with intentional overdoses has recently been questioned.[26] Some toxicologists question whether the risk–benefit ratio supports the administration of activated charcoal in the mild to moderately poisoned patient.[27,28] Position statements published by the American Academy of Clinical Toxicology and the European Association of Poison Control Centers and Clinical Toxicologists conclude that (1) there is no evidence that ipecac improves the outcome of poisoned patients, and thus it should not be routinely used to treat patients in an emergency department;[11] and (2) activated charcoal may be considered for a potentially toxic amount of a poison (adsorbed by charcoal) ingested up to 1 hour before treatment. There are insufficient data to support or exclude use of charcoal when poison ingestion occurred more than 1 hour previously.[16] Although most data reviewed for the ipecac position statement relate to home use of ipecac, the majority of studies regarding charcoal administration are conducted in a controlled research or hospital environment. Citing adverse effects and lack of efficacy as the primary reasons for a recent change in policy, the American Academy of Pediatrics (AAP) recommended that ipecac syrup not be used routinely as a poison prevention treatment in the home. AAP did not endorse the use of activated charcoal in lieu of ipecac syrup because of the lack of data demonstrating improved outcome with activated charcoal at this time. AAP encourages parents/caregivers to contact a poison control center as the first step in treating a child who may have ingested a toxic substance.[29] The American Association of Poison Control Centers Guideline Consensus Panel concluded that out-of-hospital use of ipecac syrup might have an acceptable risk–benefit ratio in rare situations.[30]

Poison control centers vary by region in recommending home use of ipecac syrup or activated charcoal for ingestions assessed as potentially toxic but not requiring health care facility management. A recent study documented that ipecac is recommended infrequently by poison control centers and, when recommended, it often is not available in the home. Emesis occurred in less than 60 minutes in only 36% of cases in which ipecac was recommended.[31] Another study failed to demonstrate that home ipecac syrup use decreased referral rates to health care facilities when poison control centers with low and high rates of home ipecac use were compared.[32]

Home use of activated charcoal is a more recent development not universally recommended by poison control centers. No clinical studies compare the use of ipecac syrup and activated charcoal in the home setting. Home administration of activated charcoal usually is intended for patient management outside a health care facility, but sometimes is given to provide early prehospital gastrointestinal decontamination in patients who subsequently are transported and treated in an emergency department. Data on prehospital administration of activated charcoal by emergency medical services or in-hospital administration by emergency department personnel provide insight into potential difficulty administering activated charcoal in the home setting. A study of prehospital administration of activated charcoal by emergency medical technicians or paramedics reported that charcoal was not given to 15.4% of patients in whom administration was attempted; in 71% of these cases the reason was patient refusal.[33] A pediatric emergency department found that 32% of young children offered oral-activated charcoal refused or were intolerant.[34] Of concern is the extent to which difficulty administering a therapeutic dose of activated charcoal to children at home impacts efficacy.[35,36] A study evaluating whether 15 children ages 13 to 30 months would consume a therapeutic dose of activated charcoal (1 g/kg) in a simulated home environment found that most children did not drink a full dose.[36] In contrast, in a study evaluating home management of poisoning with activated charcoal in 115 children (median age of 2 years; range, 1-14 years), parents reported administering a mean of 12.1 g of activated charcoal. Home use significantly reduced time to charcoal administration compared with its administration in the emergency department.[17]

### *Complementary Therapies*

The Natural Medicines Comprehensive Database lists over 40 herbs with emetic properties. For the majority of these herbs, either sufficient information about safety was unavailable, or the herb was deemed unsafe; no reliable data existed on the efficacy of any herbs with potential emetic properties.[37]

## Assessment of Poisoning: A Case-based Approach

Assessment of airway, breathing, and circulation is the primary concern in a poisoned patient.

- Determine whether the airway is open.
- Determine whether the patient is breathing.
- Determine cardiovascular status by assessing blood pressure and pulse.
- Determine whether the patient's mental status is altered. Specifically, determine whether the patient is experiencing:
  - Coma or stupor
  - Seizures
  - Agitation, disorientation, or hallucinations

After obtaining the history regarding the exposure and performing an initial assessment of the patient's condition, it must be decided whether to refer the patient directly to an emergency treatment facility, manage him or her at home, or not provide any specific treatment. Involving the poison control center in this triage and treatment decision is important since poison control centers have specialized resources not usually available to practitioners as well as considerable experience managing poisoned patients. The nationwide toll-free poison control center number is 1-800-222-1222, which connects callers to the center in their geographic area (Figure 21-1). In most states, the poison control center can also be reached by dialing 911.

Obtaining a reliable history, identifying the drug or toxin, and accurately assessing the patient's condition are critical steps in determining appropriate treatment for a poisoned patient. Self-treatment at home is primarily intended for unintentional poison exposures in children younger than 6 years in whom no or at most minimal toxicity is expected. In addition, unintentional inhalation or skin or eye exposures in any age group, with possible minimal toxicity, can often be self-treated.

If an individual inquires about purchasing ipecac syrup or activated charcoal, the pharmacist must determine whether these drugs are being purchased for an acute situation in which case the poison control center should be contacted to assess the appropriateness of self-treatment. The poison control center will need information about the patient (age, weight, past medical history, whether the patient is currently experiencing clinical effects), the toxin (name of the toxin, dose, route of exposure, time since exposure), and what treatment, if any, has already been administered. Cases 21-1 and 21-2 provide examples of assessment of patients who have been poisoned.

## CASE 21-1

| Relevant Evaluation Criteria | Scenario/Model Outcome |
|---|---|
| **Information Gathering** | |
| 1. Gather essential information about the patient's symptoms, including: | |
| a. description of symptom(s) (i.e., nature, onset, duration, severity, associated symptoms) | Patient used enzyme cleaner on contact lens and put lens in left eye. She immediately experienced pain, and her eye is red and tearing. |
| b. description of any factors that seem to precipitate, exacerbate, and/or relieve the patient's symptom(s) | N/A |
| c. description of the patient's efforts to relieve the symptoms | She removed the contact lens and placed a damp washcloth over her eye. |
| 2. Gather essential patient history information: | |
| a. patient's identity | Lisa Smith |
| b. patient's age, sex, height, and weight | 42 y/o F, 5'1", 115 lb |
| c. patient's occupation | N/A |
| d. patient's dietary habits | N/A |
| e. patient's sleep habits | N/A |
| f. concurrent medical conditions, prescription and nonprescription medications, and dietary supplements | N/A |
| g. allergies | NKA |
| h. history of other adverse reactions to medications | None |
| i. other (describe)_______ | N/A |
| **Assessment and Triage** | |
| 3. Differentiate the patient's signs/symptoms and correctly identify the patient's primary problem(s). | Lisa did not rinse enzyme cleaner off contact lens prior to inserting it. She has not adequately terminated the exposure and is experiencing ocular toxicity from the cleaner. |
| 4. Identify exclusions for self-treatment (see Figure 21-2). | None |
| 5. Formulate a comprehensive list of therapeutic alternatives for the primary problem to determine if triage to a medical practitioner is required, and share this information with the patient. | Options include:<br>(1) Recommend irrigation of the eye with an OTC eyewash (e.g., Collyrium).<br>(2) Recommend irrigation of the eye with water at home and contact the poison control center for consultation regarding whether referral for additional irrigation and ophthalmic examination for burns is needed.<br>(3) Refer Lisa to her ophthalmologist or the emergency department for irrigation and ophthalmic examination for burns.<br>(4) Take no action. |
| **Plan** | |
| 6. Select an optimal therapeutic alternative to address the patient's problem, taking into account patient preferences. | Irrigate the eye with tap water for 10-15 minutes and then assess symptoms. Contact the poison control center for advice after irrigating. |
| 7. Describe the recommended therapeutic approach to the patient. | Place your head under a faucet with left eye lower down. Run water at low pressure and comfortable temperature. Let water hit bridge of nose and then flow into eye. Following irrigation, wait 15-30 minutes and reassess how the eye feels. |

## CASE 21-1 (continued)

| Relevant Evaluation Criteria | Scenario/Model Outcome |
|---|---|
| 8. Explain to the patient the rationale for selecting the recommended therapeutic approach from the considered therapeutic alternatives. | Seeking medical attention is not immediately necessary. You should first irrigate the eye to terminate the exposure. Placing a damp washcloth over the eye is an inappropriate technique for treating eye exposures. Irrigation with small volumes of nonprescription eyewashes is inadequate for potentially toxic eye exposures. After irrigation, the poison control center may recommend a medical or emergency department referral if redness and pain persist or if additional clinical effects such as blurred vision or foreign body sensation develop. |
| **Patient Education** | |
| 9. When recommending self-care with nonprescription medications and/or nondrug therapy, convey accurate information to the patient, including: | |
| a. appropriate dose and frequency of administration | Irrigate eye with water for 10-15 minutes. |
| b. maximum number of days the therapy should be employed | N/A |
| c. product administration procedures | N/A |
| d. expected time to onset of relief | Your eye should feel better within 15-30 minutes after irrigation. If not, medical referral is appropriate and the poison control center can help facilitate the referral. |
| e. degree of relief that can be reasonably expected | Complete relief is possible, although irrigation may be insufficient if burns have occurred. |
| f. most common side effects | N/A |
| g. side effects that warrant medical intervention should they occur | N/A |
| h. patient options in the event that condition worsens or persists | You should see an ophthalmologist or emergency department physician immediately if clinical effects do not resolve with irrigation. |
| i. product storage requirements | N/A |
| j. specific nondrug measures | Irrigation of eye with water |
| 10. Solicit patient's follow-up questions. | May I put nonprescription drops in my eye to "get the red out"? |
| 11. Answer patient's questions. | No. Topical vasoconstrictors, such as tetrahydrozoline, are not recommended. Vasoconstrictors improve the eye's appearance but have no therapeutic effect. They can mask one of the clinical effects that should be monitored to help determine the need for referral. |

Key: N/A, not applicable; NKA, no known allergies; OTC, over-the-counter.

## CASE 21-2

| Relevant Evaluation Criteria | Scenario/Model Outcome |
|---|---|
| **Information Gathering** | |
| 1. Gather essential information about the patient's symptoms, including: | |

## CASE 21-2 (continued)

| Relevant Evaluation Criteria | Scenario/Model Outcome |
|---|---|
| a. description of symptom(s) (i.e., nature, onset, duration, severity, associated symptoms) | Father asks about treatment for his 3-year-old son, who ingested 15 ferrous sulfate 325 mg tablets 15 minutes earlier. The iron tablets were in a container with a child-resistant closure that had not been properly closed. |
| b. description of any factors that seem to precipitate, exacerbate, and/or relieve the patient's symptom(s) | The child is currently asymptomatic. |
| c. description of the patient's efforts to relieve the symptoms | Father gave the child approximately 6 oz of juice. |
| 2. Gather essential patient history information: | |
| a. patient's identity | Sammy Williams |
| b. patient's age, sex, height, and weight | 3 y/o M, 3'1", 33 lb |
| c. patient's occupation | N/A |
| d. patient's dietary habits | N/A |
| e. patient's sleep habits | N/A |
| f. concurrent medical conditions, prescription and nonprescription medications, and dietary supplements | None |
| g. allergies | NKA |
| h. history of other adverse reactions to medications | None |
| i. other (describe)_______ | N/A |
| **Assessment and Triage** | |
| 3. Differentiate the patient's signs/symptoms and correctly identify the patient's primary problem(s). | Acute overdose of iron. Sammy has ingested 65 mg/kg of elemental iron. This dose is well beyond the normal therapeutic dose. |
| 4. Identify exclusions for self-treatment (see Figure 21-2). | None |
| 5. Formulate a comprehensive list of therapeutic alternatives for the primary problem to determine if triage to a medical practitioner is required, and share this information with the caregiver. | Options include:<br>(1) Contact the poison control center for recommendations regarding whether to refer Sammy to an emergency department for GI decontamination and evaluation.<br>(2) Have father administer an OTC treatment to decrease absorption at home.<br>(3) Have father administer oral fluids such as milk to dilute and minimize GI irritation.<br>(4) Take no action. |
| **Plan** | |
| 6. Select an optimal therapeutic alternative to address the patient's problem, taking into account patient preferences. | Father should contact a poison control center immediately. The poison control center will determine if this dose of iron can be treated at home or is too large for self-treatment and requires medical evaluation and treatment. |
| 7. Describe the recommended therapeutic approach to the caregiver. | No treatment should be provided at home. You should call the poison control center immediately and follow staff instructions. |
| 8. Explain to the caregiver the rationale for selecting the recommended therapeutic approach from the considered therapeutic alternatives. | Sammy has ingested a very large dose of iron; the poison center will assess if he needs medical treatment immediately. An antidote for iron is available but must be given in a hospital setting. The poison control center can refer you to the appropriate health care facility and will provide treatment recommendations to the health care practitioners at that facility. |

## CASE 21-2 (continued)

| Relevant Evaluation Criteria | Scenario/Model Outcome |
|---|---|
| **Patient Education** | |
| 9. When recommending self-care with nonprescription medications and/or nondrug therapy, convey accurate information to the caregiver. | Criterion does not apply in this case. |
| 10. Solicit caregiver's follow-up questions. | The poison control center recommends that Sammy be treated in the hospital. We are 10 minutes from an emergency department. May I drive to the hospital, or should I call 911 for an ambulance? |
| 11. Answer caregiver's questions. | It is not necessary to call 911. You can drive Sammy to the hospital. |

Key: GI, gastrointestinal; N/A, not applicable; NKA, no known allergies; OTC, over-the-counter.

## PATIENT EDUCATION FOR TOXIC EXPOSURES

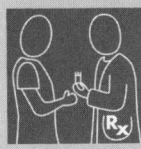

The objectives of self-treatment are to (1) minimize exposure by removing the patient to fresh air, irrigating the skin or eyes or preventing absorption of potentially toxic agents in the GI tract, and (2) treat patients with minimally toxic ingestions at home under supervision of a poison control center. For most patients, carefully following the self-care measures listed here will help ensure optimal therapeutic outcomes.

### Treatment

- For eye exposures immediately irrigate with water for 10 to 15 minutes.
- For skin exposures, immediately wash with soap and water.
- For inhalation exposures, immediately remove the patient to fresh air.
- Contact the poison control center to obtain a consultation, or refer the patient to the poison control center (see Figure 21-1 for toll-free number) for advice on the appropriateness of self-treatment of the toxic exposure, including ingested toxins.

⚠ Refer the patient to a health care facility via 911 if the patient

- is lethargic or comatose or is having seizures
- has decreased respirations or is having difficulty breathing
- has abnormal blood pressure or pulse
- has taken medications that may produce a rapid decline in consciousness or seizures

## Patient Counseling for Poisoning

After removal from toxic fumes, patients should be counseled about when to seek medical attention (e.g., difficulty breathing, worsening or persistent symptoms). In the home or nonindustry setting, fumes are often soluble, irritant gases (e.g., chlorine), so clinical effects are evident immediately and usually resolve soon after exposure stops. Patients also should be counseled about ventilating the room to facilitate dispersion of the vapor. If the exposure resulted from mixing products such as bleach and ammonia, the patient should be warned not to mix household products in the future. If carbon monoxide is suspected, the patient should be instructed to have the source turned off or removed (e.g., malfunctioning furnace, stove, vehicle). The poison control center should be contacted to assess severity and expected duration of clinical effects in symptomatic patients and the possibility of delayed onset in asymptomatic patients.

Patients with eye exposures should be counseled on how to irrigate the eye at home under the faucet (Case 21-1). Patients with skin exposures should be counseled to remove clothing, if necessary, and wash affected areas thoroughly. For eye and skin exposures, counseling should stress the importance of immediate irrigation or washing. If the poison control center in a region is recommending either ipecac syrup or activated charcoal for home use, pharmacies in that area should stock the appropriate product and practitioners should educate parents that these agents should never be used without first consulting a poison control center staff member or a primary care provider. Patients who purchase ipecac syrup or activated charcoal for immediate use following the recommendation of a poison control center should be counseled to ensure appropriate drug use. The practitioner should also explain the specific agent's potential adverse effects, as well as signs and symptoms that indicate medical attention should be sought. The box Patient Education for Poisoning lists specific information to provide parents, caregivers, or patients.

Counseling should include providing the nationwide toll-free number for the poison control center (Figure 21-1) and promoting poison prevention practices, including purchase of nonprescription drugs and household products with child-resistant packaging. If parents or caregivers choose to purchase a product without a child-resistant closure, the practitioner should advise them to place the container in a locked cabinet or store the container out of sight and out of reach of young children to avoid an unintentional poisoning.

## Evaluation of Patient Outcomes for Poisoning

Patients who have inhaled potentially toxic fumes, or spilled or splashed a substance on their skin or in their eye, should be reassessed for symptoms after removal to fresh air or irrigation. If clinical effects are minimal and resolve within a relatively short period of time (e.g., under 30 minutes) the patient may be observed at home. If symptoms persist or worsen, the patient should be referred to a health care provider or the emergency department, depending on the severity of symptoms and immediacy of need for medical evaluation. The poison control center can facilitate referral to the appropriate health care facility and provide treatment recommendations to the health care provider.

Patients who vomit after ipecac syrup is given or who receive activated charcoal should be contacted at least once to determine whether any symptoms related to the exposure develop. The time of the call depends on the substance ingested, how rapidly it is absorbed, and when symptoms would be anticipated. If clinical effects develop and are minor, the patient may be observed at home. If more significant effects develop, the patient should be referred to an emergency department for treatment. Assuming the poison control center recommended self-treatment with ipecac syrup or activated charcoal, the center staff should remain involved in subsequent decisions regarding the appropriateness of continued home treatment of these patients.

## Key Points for Poisoning

- Poison exposures are a common pediatric injury.
- There are no data demonstrating that self-treatment for poisoning with ipecac or activated charcoal improves patient outcomes.
- Self-treatment should be considered only for unintentional poison exposures that are likely to cause no or minimal toxicity (i.e., no serious or life-threatening symptoms; Figure 21-2).
- Practitioners should consult with the poison control center for input regarding patient assessment and decisions regarding the appropriateness of self-treatment.
- All patients who exhibit potentially life-threatening clinical effects (e.g., convulsions, coma) should be referred to an emergency department through the emergency 911 system.
- Since poison control centers vary by region regarding when to recommend self-treatment and what options are available for self-treatment, health care practitioners should contact their poison control center to discuss regional preferences for self-treatment as well as to obtain patient education materials.

## References


1. CDC Wonder Mortality Query. February 2005. Available at: http://wonder.cdc.gov. Accessed February 2, 2005.
2. Watson WA, Litovitz TL, Rodgers GC, et al. 2004 Annual Report of the American Association of Poison Control Centers Toxic Exposure Surveillance System. *Am J Emerg Med.* 2005;23:589-666.
3. Rodgers GB. The safety of child-resistant packaging for oral prescription drugs: two decades of experience. *JAMA.* 1996;275:1661-5.
4. Rodgers GB. The effectiveness of child-resistant packaging for aspirin. *Arch Pediatr Adolesc Med.* 2002;156:929-33.
5. Morris CC. Recent trends in pediatric iron poisonings. *South Med J.* 2000;93:1229.
6. Woolf A, Wieler J, Greenes D. Costs of poison-related hospitalizations at an urban teaching hospital for children. *Arch Pediatr Adolesc Med.* 1997;151:719-23.
7. Stremski ES. Accidental pediatric ingestion, hospital charges and failure to utilize a poison control center. *West J Med.* 1999;98:29-33.
8. Darwin J, Seger D. Reaffirmed cost-effectiveness of poison centers. *Ann Emerg Med.* 2003;41:159-60.
9. Miller T, Lestina DC. Costs of poisoning in the United States and savings from poison control centers: a benefit–cost analysis. *Ann Emerg Med.* 1997;29:239-45.
10. Ipecac syrup. In: McEvoy GK, ed. *AHFS Drug Information 2005.* Bethesda, Md: American Society of Health-System Pharmacists; 2005:2795-8.
11. American Academy of Clinical Toxicology and the European Association of Poison Control Centers and Clinical Toxicologists. Position statement: ipecac syrup. *J Toxicol Clin Toxicol.* 2004;42:133-43.
12. Ho PC, Dweik R, Cohen MC. Rapidly reversible cardiomyopathy associated with chronic ipecac ingestion. *Clin Cardiol.* 1998;21:780-3.
13. Cooper CP, Kamath KR. A toddler with persistent vomiting and diarrhoea. *Eur J Pediatr.* 1998;157:775-6.
14. Schneider DJ, Perez A, Knilans TE, et al. Clinical and pathologic aspects of cardiomyopathy from ipecac administration in Munchausen's syndrome by proxy. *Pediatrics.* 1996;97:902-6.
15. Bader AA, Kerzner B. Ipecac toxicity in "Munchausen syndrome by proxy." *Ther Drug Monit.* 1999;21:259-60.
16. American Academy of Clinical Toxicology and the European Association of Poison Control Centers and Clinical Toxicologists. Position statement: single dose activated charcoal. *J Toxicol Clin Toxicol.* 1997;35:721-41.
17. American Academy of Clinical Toxicology and the European Association of Poison Control Centers and Clinical Toxicologists. Position statement: cathartics. *J Toxicol Clin Toxicol.* 1997;35:743-52.
18. Spiller HA, Rodgers GC. Evaluation of administration of activated charcoal in the home. *Pediatrics.* 2001;108:E100.
19. Spiller HA, Revolinski DH, Rodgers GC. Evaluation of professional education program to have activated charcoal available in local pharmacies [abstract]. *J Toxicol Clin Toxicol.* 1997;35:485.
20. McFarland AK, Chyka PA. Selection of activated charcoal products for the treatment of poisonings. *Ann Pharmacother.* 1993;27:358-61.
21. Osterhoudt KC, Durbin D, Alpern ER, et al. Risk factors for emesis after therapeutic use of activated charcoal in acutely poisoned children. *Pediatrics.* 2004;113:806-10.
22. Dorrington CL, Johnson DW, Brant R, et al. The frequency of complications associated with the use of multiple-dose activated charcoal. *Ann Emerg Med.* 2003;41:370-7.
23. Shannon M. Ingestion of toxic substances by children. *N Engl J Med.* 2000;342:186-91.

24. Pond SM, Lewis-Driver DJ, Williams GM, et al. Gastric emptying in acute overdose: a prospective randomised controlled trial. *Med J Aust.* 1995;163:345-9.
25. Ardagh MW. Gastrointestinal decontamination after poisoning. *N Z Med J.* 1998:111:397-9.
26. Merigian KS, Blaho KE. Single-dose oral activated charcoal in the treatment of the self-poisoned patient: a prospective, randomized, controlled trial. *Am J Ther.* 2002;9:301-8.
27. Seger D. Single-dose activated charcoal-backup and reassess. *J Toxicol Clin Toxicol.* 2004;42:101-10.
28. Bond GR. Activated charcoal in the home: helpful and important or simply a distraction? *Pediatrics.* 2002;109:145-6.
29. American Academy of Pediatrics Committee on Injury, Violence, and Poison Prevention. Poison treatment in the home. *Pediatrics.* 2003;112:1182-5.
30. Manoguerra AS, Cobaugh DJ, Guidelines for the Management of Poisonings Consensus Panel. Guideline on the use of ipecac syrup in the out-of-hospital management of ingested poisons. *J Toxicol Clin Toxicol.* 2005;43:1-10.
31. Garrison J, Shepherd G, Huddleston WL, et al. Evaluation of the time frame for home ipecac syrup use when not kept in the home. *J Tox Clin Toxicol.* 2003; 41: 217-21.
32. Bond GR. Home syrup of ipecac use does not reduce emergency department use or improve outcome. *Pediatrics.* 2003;112:1061-4.
33. Alaspaa AO, Kuisma MJ, Hoppu K, et al. Out-of-hospital administration of activated charcoal by emergency medical services. *Ann Emerg Med.* 2005;45:207-12.
34. Osterhoudt KC, Alpern ER, Durbin D, et al. Activated charcoal administration in a pediatric emergency department. *Pediatr Emerg Care.* 2004;20:493-8.
35. Grbcich PA, Lacouture PG, Woolf A. Administration of charcoal in the home. *Vet Hum Toxicol.* 1987;29:458.
36. Scharman EJ, Cloonan HA, Durback-Morris LF. Home administration of charcoal: can mothers administer a therapeutic dose? *J Emerg Med.* 2001;21:357-61.
37. Natural Medicines Comprehensive Database. Available at: http: //naturaldatabase.com. Accessed January 31, 2005.

CHAPTER 22

# Ostomy Care and Supplies

*Joan Lerner Selekof and Sharon Wilson*

An *ostomy* is an opening or outlet through the abdominal wall created surgically for the purpose of eliminating waste. It is usually made by bringing a portion of the bladder, colon, small intestine, or ureters through the abdominal wall. The opening of the ostomy is called the stoma (from the Latin word for mouth).

The creation of an ostomy may be a dramatic life-changing event. Thus, it is important for clinicians to provide reassurance, support, and education for the patient and family. An understanding of improvements in surgical procedures, ostomy supplies, and outcomes can allay much of a patient's fear and anxiety. The goal in ostomy care is to enable the individual to resume his or her lifestyle—to be a person, not a patient. A person with an ostomy carefully notes the reactions of health care professionals to the disorder; any negative response may reinforce the patient's negative feelings about the ostomy.

## Prevalence of Ostomies

It is estimated that 750,000 Americans are currently living with an ostomy, and 75,000 new surgeries are performed annually.[1] Ostomy surgery is performed in individuals of all ages and for many reasons, both acquired and congenital.

## Indications for Ostomies

Ostomies may be permanent or temporary, and they are performed in individuals ranging from neonates to persons of advanced age. Reasons for performing ostomies include congenital anomalies (e.g., imperforate anus, Hirschsprung's disease), inflammatory bowel disease, familial polyposis, cancer, radiation damage, pressure ulcers, trauma, and any other reason to divert the urinary or fecal stream.[2,3] The type of ostomy depends on the condition being treated.

The two most common disorders leading to ileostomy surgery are (1) ulcerative colitis, which affects the large intestine and rectum, and (2) Crohn's disease, which may involve any part of the gastrointestinal (GI) tract. Other conditions that may require an ileostomy include traumatic injury, cancer, familial polyposis, and necrotizing enterocolitis.

The most common reasons for colostomy surgery are (1) cancer of the colon or rectum, (2) diverticulitis, and (3) trauma. Other indications include obstruction of the colon or rectum, genetic malformation, radiation colitis, and loss of anal muscular control. In some cases, a temporary colostomy may be performed to protect areas of the colon that have been surgically repaired. Healing of a diseased or damaged bowel may take several weeks, months, or years, but eventually the colon and rectum are reconnected and bowel continuity is restored. Figure 22-1 shows the location of various types of colostomies.

Urinary diversions are created to correct bladder loss or dysfunction, which can be caused by cancer, neurogenic bladder, genetic malformation, or interstitial cystitis.

## Types of Ostomies

The three basic types of ostomies are (1) ileostomy, (2) colostomy (the most common type), and (3) urinary diversion (see Color Plates, photographs 2A-I). Each type of ostomy has several variations, depending on the location of the stoma, reason for surgical procedure, or whether the procedure renders a patient continent.

### *Ileostomy*

An ileostomy is surgically created by bringing a portion of the ileum through the abdominal wall (see Color Plates, photograph 2A.) Initially, the discharge is liquid, but as the ileum adapts, it assumes some of the absorptive functions of the colon and the discharge may become semisoft. The discharge is continuous and contains intestinal enzymes that may irritate the peristomal skin.

#### Continent Ileostomy

Several types of continent ileostomies exist. An internal pouch is created from the ileum, and an intussusception (a slipping of a length of intestine into an adjacent portion) of the bowel is used to create a "nipple" that renders the patient continent for stool and flatus. The pouch is periodically emptied by inserting a catheter through the nipple into the pouch. At first, the pouch holds about 75 mL, but it stretches with use so that at 6 months postoperatively it may hold 600 to 800 mL and can be drained three to five times daily. Patients do not need to wear an external pouching system, but often wear a gauze pad or stoma cap (see Color Plates, photograph 2B).

#### Ileoanal Reservoir

The restorative proctocolectomy (S pouch or J pouch) ileoanal reservoir spares the rectum of patients with ulcerative colitis or familial polyposis. Diseased mucosa is stripped from the rectum, and an internal pouch is created from the ileum. The distal end is pulled through the rectum and attached. Thus, the sphincter is preserved, and ostomy appliances are unnecessary. Patients will have more frequent bowel movements and may experience perianal skin irritation (see Color Plates, photograph 2B).

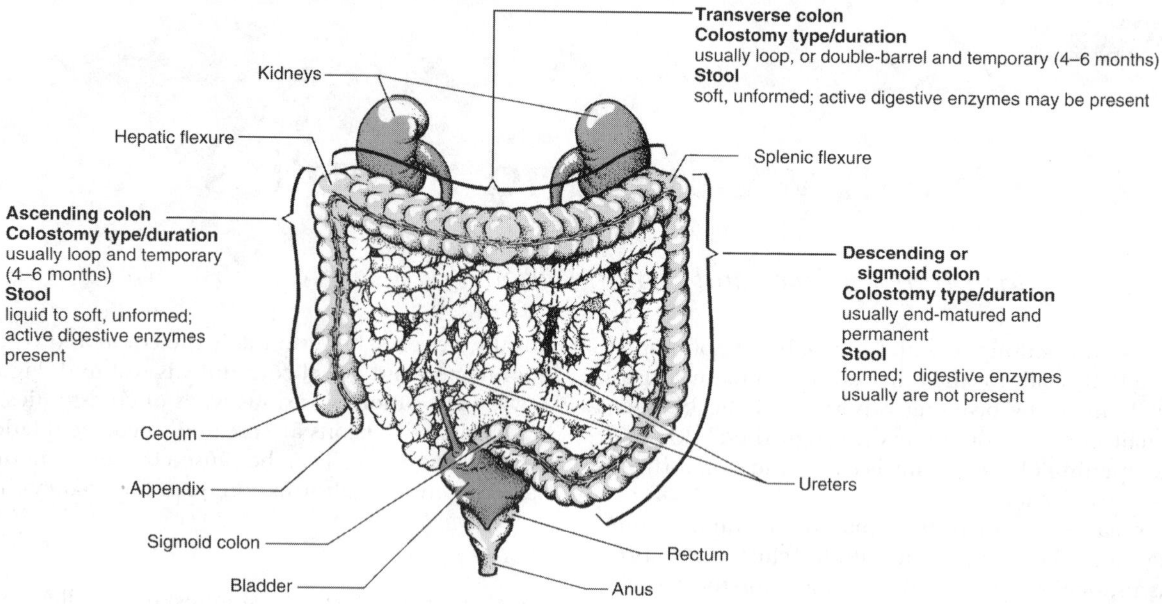


**FIGURE 22-1** Anatomic drawing of the lower digestive and urinary tracts, which depicts the location and permanence of colostomies. (Adapted with permission from *Am J Nurs*. 1977;77:443.)

## *Colostomy*

A colostomy is created by bringing a portion of the large bowel (colon) through the abdominal wall. The discharge may be semisoft, pastelike, or formed depending on the portion of bowel used (Figure 22-1).

### Ascending Colostomy

This type of colostomy is uncommon. The ascending colon is retained, but the rest of the large bowel is removed or bypassed (see Color Plates, photograph 2C). The stoma is usually on the right side of the abdomen. The discharge is semisoft, and a pouch must be worn at all times.

### Transverse Colostomy

The transverse colon is the site of most temporary colostomies (Figure 22-1). A loop of the transverse colon is lifted through the abdominal incision, and a rod or bridge (which is removed within 1-2 weeks) is placed under the loop to give it support while it heals. The discharge is usually semiliquid or very soft.

### Loop Colostomy

Loop colostomies have one large opening, but two tracts (see Color Plates, photograph 2D). The proximal tract discharges fecal material, and the distal tract secretes small amounts of mucus. An appliance must be worn at all times. A patient with a loop colostomy may also pass a minimal amount of stool or mucus via the rectum. This is a normal occurrence.

### Double-barrel Transverse Colostomy

When a double-barrel transverse colostomy is performed, the bowel is completely divided by bringing both the proximal end and the distal end through the abdominal wall and suturing it to the skin. The distal stoma may also be called the mucous fistula (see Color Plates, photograph 2E).

### Descending and Sigmoid Colostomies

Descending and sigmoid colostomies are fairly common, and generally the stoma is on the left side of the abdomen (see Color Plates, photograph 2F). The fecal discharge has a pastelike consistency and at times may consist of formed stool. This type of colostomy may be regulated by irrigation; therefore, a pouching system may not be needed. However, many patients prefer a pouch to irrigation; not everyone with a descending or sigmoid colostomy is a good candidate for irrigation or prefers irrigation. Factors to consider in making the decision to irrigate include the presence or absence of stomal complications as well as the patient's normal stooling pattern, psychomotor ability, and willingness to commit the time required to be successful.

## *Urinary Diversions*

Urinary diversion surgery diverts the urine through an opening in the abdominal wall. Urinary stomas should function immediately following surgery.

### Ileal and Colon Conduits

The ileal conduit is the most common type of urinary diversion (see Color Plates, photograph 2G). After the bladder is removed, ileal and colon conduits are created by implanting the ureters into an isolated loop of bowel, the distal end of which is brought to the surface of the abdomen. The stoma looks like an ileostomy or colostomy. A pouching system must be worn continuously. Mucous shreds will be present in the urine if the bowel is used to create the diversion (see Color Plates, photograph 2H). Because the ileum is used to create an ileal conduit, some people incorrectly refer to the ileal conduit as an ileostomy.

Clarification of the type of effluent (stool or urine) will help in selecting the correct type of pouch.

#### Ureterostomy

In this procedure, one or both ureters are detached from the bladder and brought to the outside of the abdominal wall, where a stoma is created. This procedure is used less frequently because the ureters tend to narrow unless they have been dilated permanently by previous disease (see Color Plates, photograph 2I).

#### Cystostomy

A cystostomy is performed when blockage or narrowing of the urethra occurs. Urine is diverted from the bladder to the abdominal wall. A pouch must be worn continuously. An infant may use diapers instead of a pouch.

#### Continent Urostomy

The continent urinary diversion is available for selected patients, but requires certain criteria. An Indiana pouch is a type of continent urostomy in which a pouch is created from part of the cecum and a portion of the ileum and is brought through the abdominal wall. The ureters are attached to the cecum pouch. The remaining ileum is reattached to the colon for normal digestive flow. The ileocecal valve is left intact and becomes part of the continence mechanism. The pouch is emptied by inserting a catheter into the stoma to drain the urine. Patients are usually placed on a strict schedule and will eventually catheterize the stoma often enough to avoid leakage. The new pouch may hold up to 600 mL of urine. An external pouching system is not necessary. Most patients wear a gauze pad or stoma cap. The orthotopic neobladder procedure includes connecting the newly created bladder to the urethra, which allows the patient to void through the urethra. The neobladder is an internal urinary reservoir (pouch) usually constructed of a detubularized segment of the ileum to which the ureters and urethra are sewn.

## Complications of Ostomies

Patients with ostomies may experience both psychologic and physical complications. The clinician should be prepared to address these complications or to refer patients to their primary care provider or a wound ostomy continence nurse (WOCN). WOCNs are often based in hospitals or home health care agencies. The United Ostomy Association is an organization that provides peer support for patients. To alleviate any anxiety, patients should receive a thorough explanation before surgery that describes what procedure will be performed, what to expect during the postsurgical recovery period, and what appliances and supplies the patient will use. The clinician can use the following information on potential complications to assist patients seeking advice after their surgery.

### *Psychologic Complications*

Some patients fear they will not be able to continue their former job, participate in sports, perform sexually, or have children. These patients need reassurance that an ostomy will not impair their ability to carry out such activities. Calling the local United Ostomy Association is of utmost importance in assisting with the rehabilitation of these patients; both clinicians and patients may call this organization. Patients may also want to find a local WOCN. Patient Counseling for Ostomy Care provides information on support groups and available literature.

### *Physiologic Complications*

The major physiologic consequence of a GI ostomy is fluid and electrolyte imbalance, which is most problematic in patients with a liquid or semisoft stoma discharge, such as ileostomies or ascending and transverse colostomies. Patients with these types of ostomies must maintain adequate fluid intake to compensate for loss of the absorptive function of the colon and loss of ileocecal valve function. Patients with ileostomies lose about 500 to 1000 mL of fluid daily through the stoma, compared with a loss of 100 to 200 mL daily by individuals with a normally functioning colon.[3] During illnesses, patients with ileostomies, especially infants, are particularly vulnerable to fluid and electrolyte imbalance caused by vomiting and diarrhea. They should be counseled regarding common signs and symptoms of imbalance (Table 22-1).[3-5]

**TABLE 22-1 Signs and Symptoms of Fluid and Electrolyte Imbalance[3-5]**

| Adults | Infants |
|---|---|
| Increased thirst | Depressed fontanelle |
| Dry mouth and mucous membranes | Lethargy |
| Orthostatic hypotension | Sunken eyes |
| Decreased urine volume | Weak cry |
| Increased urine concentration (dark in color) | Decreased frequency of wet diaper |
| Sunken eyes | Increased urine concentration (dark in color) |
| Extreme weakness | |
| Flaccid muscles | |
| Diminished reflexes | |
| Muscle cramps (abdominal and leg) | |
| Lethargy | |
| Tingling or cramping in feet and hands | |
| Confusion | |
| Nausea and vomiting | |
| Shortness of breath | |

**TABLE 22-2 Effects of Food on Stoma Output[3,5,14,15]**

**Foods That Thicken Stool**
Applesauce; bananas; bread; buttermilk; cheese; marshmallows; milk, boiled; pasta; peanut butter, creamy; potatoes; pretzels; rice; tapioca; toast; yogurt

**Foods That Loosen Stool**
Beer and other alcoholic beverages; chocolate; dried or string beans; fried foods; greasy foods; highly spiced foods; leafy green vegetables (lettuce, broccoli, spinach); prune or grape juice; raw fruits (except bananas); raw vegetables

**Foods That Cause Stool Odor**
Asparagus; beans; cabbage-family vegetables (onions, cabbage, brussels sprouts, broccoli, cauliflower); cheese; eggs; fish; garlic; some spices; turnips

**Foods That Cause Urine Odor**
Asparagus; seafood; some spices

**Foods That Combat Urine Odor**
Buttermilk; cranberry juice; yogurt

**Foods That Cause Gas**
Beans (dried, string, or baked); beer; cabbage-family vegetables (onions, cabbage, brussels sprouts, broccoli, cauliflower); carbonated beverages; corn; cucumbers; dairy products; mushrooms; peas; radishes; spinach

**Foods That Color Stool**
Beets; berries; chocolate; fats; fish; meat (large amounts of red); milk; red gelatin; vegetables

Because the GI tract is the site of nutrient absorption, some patients with ostomies may experience deficiencies. For example, iron and vitamins $D_2$ and $D_3$ are absorbed in the small intestine; riboflavin is absorbed in the upper GI tract; vitamin $B_{12}$ is absorbed in the terminal ileum; phytonadione is absorbed in the proximal small intestine; menadione is absorbed in the distal small intestine; and calcium, pyridoxine, pantothenic acid, biotin, choline, inositol, carnitine, vitamins C and E, and thiamin are absorbed in various sites within the intestinal tract (specific sites not identified). Vitamin A deficiency may be seen in individuals with disease of the terminal ileum (e.g., Crohn's disease). Hypophosphatemia and hypomagnesemia are present in individuals with calcium deficiency caused by malabsorption. In addition, copper deficiency, which interferes with the absorption of iron, has been reported in individuals who have undergone intestinal bypass surgery. Folic acid absorption requires interaction with enzymes present in the upper part of the jejunum; therefore, most absorption of folic acid takes place in the proximal part of the small intestine.[6-9] The effect of ostomy surgery on absorption of vitamins and minerals has not been well studied; patients with ileostomies or colostomies should be monitored for signs and symptoms of deficiencies.

Patients with urostomy, ileostomy, or ascending colostomy must include an adequate amount of fluid in their diets to prevent the precipitation of crystals or kidney stones in the urine. They also may have an increased incidence of gallbladder stone formation. Patients with urostomies should adjust their diet to produce an acidic urine, thus reducing the risk of infection and crystal formation around the stoma. These patients are at risk of urine reflux onto the stoma, which increases the risk of infection and skin breakdown. Some evidence suggests that cranberries in the form of juice or tablets may assist in maintaining a healthy urinary tract. However, more data are needed to provide evidence of cranberry's role in urinary health.[10-13]

### *Systemic Complications*

#### Constipation

Constipation is caused by the regular use of constipating analgesics or other medications or by a patient's eating habits. Patients should be encouraged to avoid the foods listed in Table 22-2 that can thicken the stool.[3,5,11,12] Constipation may be a problem in patients with descending and sigmoid colostomies. Treatment depends on the cause and may include dietary changes or medication adjustment.

#### Diarrhea

Certain foods can cause diarrhea in ostomy patients (Table 22-2).[3,5,14,15] Gut pathology (ulcerative colitis, Crohn's disease, *Clostridium difficile* colitis) or obstruction caused by a food bolus can also cause diarrhea. Medications, influenza, and food poisoning are other potential causes. Diarrhea is a special problem in patients with ileostomies and ascending colostomies, which cause impaired fluid and electrolyte reabsorption. Patients with chronically loose stools may want to use an absorptive agent (Ileosorb and Par-Sorb) designed for use in the pouch. Absorptive agents do not correct the problem, but assist with coping. Increased fiber (e.g., Metamucil, Citracel) may be used to help correct the diarrhea. Also, an unexpected high output in a patient with an ileostomy may represent a partial small-bowel obstruction. In this case, the patient needs to seek emergency medical attention.

#### Odor or Intestinal Gas

Intestinal gas may be related to food. Eliminating foods that cause gas from the diet may solve the problem (Table 22-2). Odor is not normal except when the pouching system is changed or emptied. Otherwise, odor may be an indication of poor hygiene or leakage, failure to properly connect the pouch to the skin barrier, or use of a pouch with small holes that allow gas to escape. The clinician should review proper care and connection of the pouching system with patients who are concerned about odor. Oral deodorants are also available that will act in the digestive system to eliminate odors from digested foods.

### *Local Complications*

The normal stoma is shiny, moist, and either pink or red. The stoma does not contain nerve fibers, so it does not transmit pain or other sensations. In an adult, the stoma size is approximately 1/8 to 3 in., depending on the portion of the bowel or urinary tract used. The stoma gradually shrinks after surgery and reaches its permanent size within 6 weeks.

### Skin Irritation

Output from the intestines or kidneys can irritate the skin around the stoma. Ostomy pouching systems and accessories can also irritate skin, because of materials used in their composition or poor fit. The peristomal skin may look weepy or erythematous and have papules and macules. The patient may use karaya powder, pectin base powder, ostomy creams, or barriers to protect the skin, although a properly fitting appliance should be the first priority.

### Excoriation

Excoriation is caused by erosion of the epidermis by digestive enzymes. The eroded or denuded epidermis may bleed, and is painful when touched and when applying the pouch. Excoriation occurs when an improper pouch is worn, when the pouch opening is too big or too small, or when the pouch has leaked and not been promptly replaced. These problems can allow the output to come in contact with the skin. The output produced by patients with ileostomies is particularly irritating. The patient should be referred to a WOCN or primary care provider for treatment. A karaya- or pectin-based powder may be applied to the peristomal skin before the pouch is applied. The pouch should be changed more often to reduce the risk of further irritation. Treatment should be continued until the skin is clear.

### Contact Dermatitis

Contact dermatitis is characterized by burning, stinging, itching, and red or denuded skin. This complication usually results from an allergic reaction to the appliance or an accessory. A patch test in patients who have a history of allergy, reaction to adhesive tape, eczema, or psoriasis, as well as those who have very fair skin, will identify the allergen. Patients exhibiting a sensitivity may need to change products. A fabric pouch cover may be helpful if the allergy is to the pouch itself. Special precautions are necessary in patients with a latex allergy. On request, a manufacturer will provide written information regarding the natural latex rubber content of its products and packaging (check the manufacturer's Web site). In some cases, the latex source is a dry, natural latex rubber, which is used to seal blister packs that contain nonlatex products.

### Alkaline Dermatitis (Encrustations)

Alkaline dermatitis (encrustation) may occur in patients with urinary diversions because of the alkaline nature of the output. The skin around the stoma may feel gritty, like sandpaper. Alkaline dermatitis is a common cause of blood in the pouch because it renders the stoma extremely friable. A cloth soaked with a solution of one third white vinegar to two thirds water should be applied to the stoma for 5 to 10 minutes at least once weekly before putting on the appliance. Patients who use a two-piece system can apply the solution as often as three to four times daily. The vinegar may cause the stoma to blanch, but blanching is not indicative of damage.

Treatment for alkaline dermatitis is acidification of the urine. Patients should avoid alkaline ash foods, such as citrus fruits and juices, which, although acidic when consumed, are excreted in alkaline form. Increasing fluid intake to between 2 and 3 qt daily may reduce alkalinity. Use of a urinary appliance with an antireflux feature is recommended.

### Hyperplasia

Hyperplasia (an overgrowth of skin) occurs when the pouch opening is too large. There is no pain in the early stages, but later the affected skin cells multiply and cause agonizing pain. The condition resembles a mucosal polyp and may also be called hyperkeratosis or pseudoverrucous lesion. Treatment entails ensuring that the pouch has the correct size opening and the seal is secure. The seal is achieved with paste, paste strips, or an Eakin seal that will mold into the irregular surfaces. Other management approaches include cauterization using silver nitrate sticks and/or surgical removal.

### Mechanical Irritation

Mechanical irritation is caused by a poorly fitting appliance, a skin barrier, a stoma that is difficult to access, or tight-fitting clothing. Poorly fitting appliances can be corrected by measuring the stoma before each purchase of supplies, selecting a skin barrier of the proper size, and adjusting the size of the skin barrier opening, if necessary. Patients experiencing mechanical irritation should be encouraged to contact a WOCN.

### Skin Stripping

Skin stripping refers to inadvertent sloughing or removal of the top layer of skin around the stoma. The skin around the stoma may be irritated by using too strong an adhesive or by removing the skin barrier in a rough manner. The skin barrier should be removed by pushing the skin away from the barrier, not by pulling the barrier away from the skin. Adhesive removers are useful in preventing skin damage if the stoma is new or the peristomal skin is fragile. After use of adhesive removers, the peristomal skin must be cleaned to remove all the adhesive remover residue as blistering, irritation, or ineffective adhesion of a new pouching system may occur.

### Stenosis

Stenosis of the stoma results from the formation of scar tissue. Excessive scar tissue is usually caused by improper surgical construction, postoperative ischemia, active disease, or alkaline stomatitis or dermatitis. Although dilation of the stoma is often advocated to prevent or palliate this problem, the only cure is revision of the stoma.

### Excessive Sweating

Sweating under the pouch can decrease wearing time and cause monilial infection. A skin sealant or cement plus a belt may be necessary to hold the appliance in place. Purchasing or making a cover or bib to keep the pouch material from touching the skin can alleviate discomfort from perspiration underneath the collection pouch.

### Folliculitis

Folliculitis, an inflammation of the hair follicles, is characterized by redness at the base of the hair follicles around the stoma. Aggressive removal of any adhesive around the stoma can remove hairs, resulting in irritation and infection. Using an electric razor to shave the areas on which adhesive will be applied can prevent folliculitis.

### Infection

With the possible exception of patients with Crohn's disease or ruptured diverticulitis, or those undergoing radiation, patients with ostomies do not have more frequent infections than patients without ostomies. In some cases, however, infections under the appliance can be problematic. Candidal infection may be a problem in patients who wear an appliance continuously. A dark, warm, moist environment promotes the growth of *Candida* species. The primary symptom is itching and rash. If the infection is allowed to continue unchecked, the skin will become denuded, the appliance will not stick, and additional skin irritation will result from the output.

If the skin is indurated, swollen, and red, it may need incision and draining. Culture and susceptibility testing should be performed and an appropriate antibiotic should be prescribed for topical use, systemic use, or both. Patients should be encouraged to contact a WOCN for assistance. Minor candidal infections may be treated with nystatin powder or miconazole 2% powder. Excess powder should be brushed off before the pouch is applied. Antifungal preparations are generally used every other day for 1 week after the skin has become clear. When treating candidal infections, it is important to ascertain whether the patient is taking antibiotics. Any antibiotic, but especially a broad-spectrum agent, changes the flora of the skin, and the entrenched *Candida* can become difficult to eradicate. Thus, it is often helpful to continue using nystatin powder or 2% miconazole powder for 1 month after all signs of candidal infection are gone in ostomy patients being treated with antibiotics.[16,17]

### Peristomal Hernia

A peristomal hernia is a protrusion of the colon or ileum into the subcutaneous layers of the skin around the stoma. It usually occurs if the abdominal wall is weak or the stoma was placed lateral to the rectus muscle. The patient may complain of a bulge when standing or sitting. Modification of the pouching system or technique, clothing, or diet may help alleviate a peristomal hernia. An ostomy support belt/binder may be used to provide comfort and prevent further herniation. The patient should be referred to the WOCN for a plan of care. Surgery may be required if the patient has increased pain at the site or increased herniation.

### Fistula

A fistula is a formation of an opening between two internal organs or from inside the body to the skin. Enterocutaneous fistulas can occur in patients with or without an ostomy. This complication is most often a manifestation of inflammatory bowel disease. Other causes include cancer, abscess formation, foreign body retention, radiation, tuberculosis, and trauma. If a fistula has excessive drainage, an ostomy appliance may be applied to contain the drainage and prevent the skin from becoming denuded.

### Prolapse

Prolapse is a telescoping of the bowel through the stoma. This problem results when the opening in the abdominal wall is too large. Women with ileostomies may experience prolapse of the ileostomy during pregnancy. Other causes include inadequate fixation of the bowel to the abdominal wall, poorly developed fascial support, or increased abdominal pressure associated with tumors, coughing, or crying (the latter being of special concern in infants). The danger of prolapse is the resultant decrease in blood supply to the bowel outside the abdominal cavity.

A prolapse may be reduced by having the patient lie on his or her back and apply continuous pressure on the most distal part of the stoma. Once the prolapse is reduced, a rigid pouching system should be avoided because of the risk of strangulation. The patient should apply a flexible pouch with resized opening, while lying on his or her back. A support belt may also be used. Surgical correction may be required if the stoma becomes purple, ecchymotic, or continues to prolapse.

### Retraction

Retraction, a recession of the stoma to a subnormal length at or below skin level, is caused by several factors. Active Crohn's disease and weight gain may lead to this damage of the skin surface. If it is not severe, a convex pouching system and use of an elastic belt may be adequate. In other cases, treatment may require surgical correction.

### Organic Impotence

Organic impotence results from a radical resection of the rectum or bladder caused by disruption of nerves and vascular supply. Male patients who are impotent should be referred to a urologist for assistance in regaining erectile function.

## Management of Ostomies

### *Management Goals*

The ideal ostomy system should be leak-proof, odor-proof, comfortable, easily manipulated, inconspicuous, safe, and as inexpensive as possible. The clinician, in conjunction with other clinicians such as a WOCN or primary care provider, can help the patient achieve these outcomes.

## General Management Approach

Patients are most likely to achieve optimal outcomes if a pouching system is properly fitted (Figure 22-2), and the stoma is cared for appropriately. The clinician should always be aware of the sensitive nature of the topic and ensure that privacy is respected during all discussions. Failure to provide a comfortable environment in which to discuss problems, concerns, and alternatives may cause patients to avoid such discussions and result in less than optimal outcomes. Follow-up assessment and care may be via telephone, scheduled appointment, or during routine visits to purchase supplies or medications.

Frequent changes in the pouching system and accessories should signal a potential problem, as should the use of multiple products intended for the same purpose. In many cases, patients may be referred to a primary care provider or WOCN for follow-up of problems identified by the clinician. Complications such as impotence, peristomal hernia, and stenosis, prolapse, retraction, or excoriation of the stoma require medical referral. In some cases, however, self-care is appropriate, particularly by experienced ostomy patients.

The presence of an ostomy and its location should always be noted on the patient's profile to minimize medication-related risks. It is helpful to maintain a record of current and past ostomy products the patient used and of any problems the patient has experienced. This information can be useful in making future recommendations.

## Ostomy Pouching System

The ostomy pouching system is an extremely important aspect of the ostomy patient's well-being. The ostomy industry is highly specialized and rapidly changing in an effort to improve designs, resulting in a wide range of choices. Pouch selection is highly personal, based on the patient's specific needs, abilities, and cost.

The patient has lost a normal body function; the pouching system takes over that lost function and becomes almost a part of the body. It is common for patients and their families to find discussing ostomy needs difficult or embarrassing, especially during the first several weeks or months after surgery.

Adult and adolescent patients must be taught self-care skills to maintain the stoma, including (1) sizing the stoma, (2) cutting a pouch or skin barrier to fit the stoma, (3) cleaning the skin, (4) applying paste or powder if necessary, (5) applying the pouch, (6) removing the pouch, and (7) emptying the pouch. Patients must be prepared for effluent from the stoma at any time during the pouch-changing procedure. One- and two-piece pouching systems are available for the younger child. The Hollister, Convatec, and Coloplast companies have excellent teaching booklets for children. The Hollister Company will also provide ostomy dolls for children with ostomies. Table 22-3 lists contact information for these companies.

### Types of Pouches

The surgical technique used to create the stoma influences the pouching equipment required, the complexity of the pouching procedure, and the risks of stomal and peristomal complications (e.g., necrosis, stenosis, or hernia). In the past, most ostomy pouches were reusable. The advantages of reusable pouching systems were their durability, availability in numerous configurations, and relatively low cost. Their disadvantages were that they required cleaning before each use, and they were heavy, tended to retain odor, and often required a separate skin barrier.

Most ostomy patients are now fitted with odor-proof, lightweight, disposable pouching systems. Most pouches incorporate a skin barrier in each flange or one-piece pouch, which eliminates the need for a separate skin barrier. Disposable equipment is available in one- and two-piece systems (Figure 22-3). The one-piece system is easy to apply, especially for patients with impaired manual dexterity. The two-piece system allows patients to center the flange easily and change the pouch, if desired, without having to remove the flange from the skin. It is easy to apply and is generally more pliable and adaptable to different abdominal contours.

Although pouches are available for infants, some ostomies are managed with a diaper instead. If a diaper is used, care must be taken to avoid skin irritation from a caustic effluent. Barriers and creams are required for neonates and infants that are only diapered. The decision to diaper or pouch is based on the location of the stoma, type and amount of effluent, and the child's activity. Once a child is crawling or exploring, it is difficult to keep stool contained in a diaper.

Both one- and two-piece pouch systems are available in drainable, closed-end, and urostomy styles. Drainable styles are used when bowel regulation cannot be established, and they allow for easy and frequent emptying. Closed-end systems are used by patients who have regulated colostomies and routinely irrigate the ostomy to remove output. No output from the stoma occurs between irrigations. Urostomy systems allow a constant output of urine and easy emptying throughout the day through a narrow valve opening.

### Fitting and Application

Reusable and disposable pouches are available in transparent and opaque styles and various sizes. The pouch opening may be cut to fit or presized. If it is cut to fit, the stoma pattern is traced onto the skin barrier/wafer surface of the pouch and then cut out before being applied. Newer, one-piece convexity pouches are available with oval openings that fit flush with the skin, allowing the contents to flow into the pouch without leaking onto the skin.

Measuring the stoma to determine the proper fit of a pouch is an important part of ostomy care. The diameter of the round stoma is measured at the base, where the mucosa meets the skin, which is considered the widest measurement. Oval stomas should be measured at both their widest and narrowest diameters. A stoma may swell if the pouch fits too tightly or slips, or if the patient falls or experiences a hard blow to the stoma. It is important to reassess the size for proper fitting.

Other considerations in fitting the pouch include body contour, stoma location, skin creases and scars, and

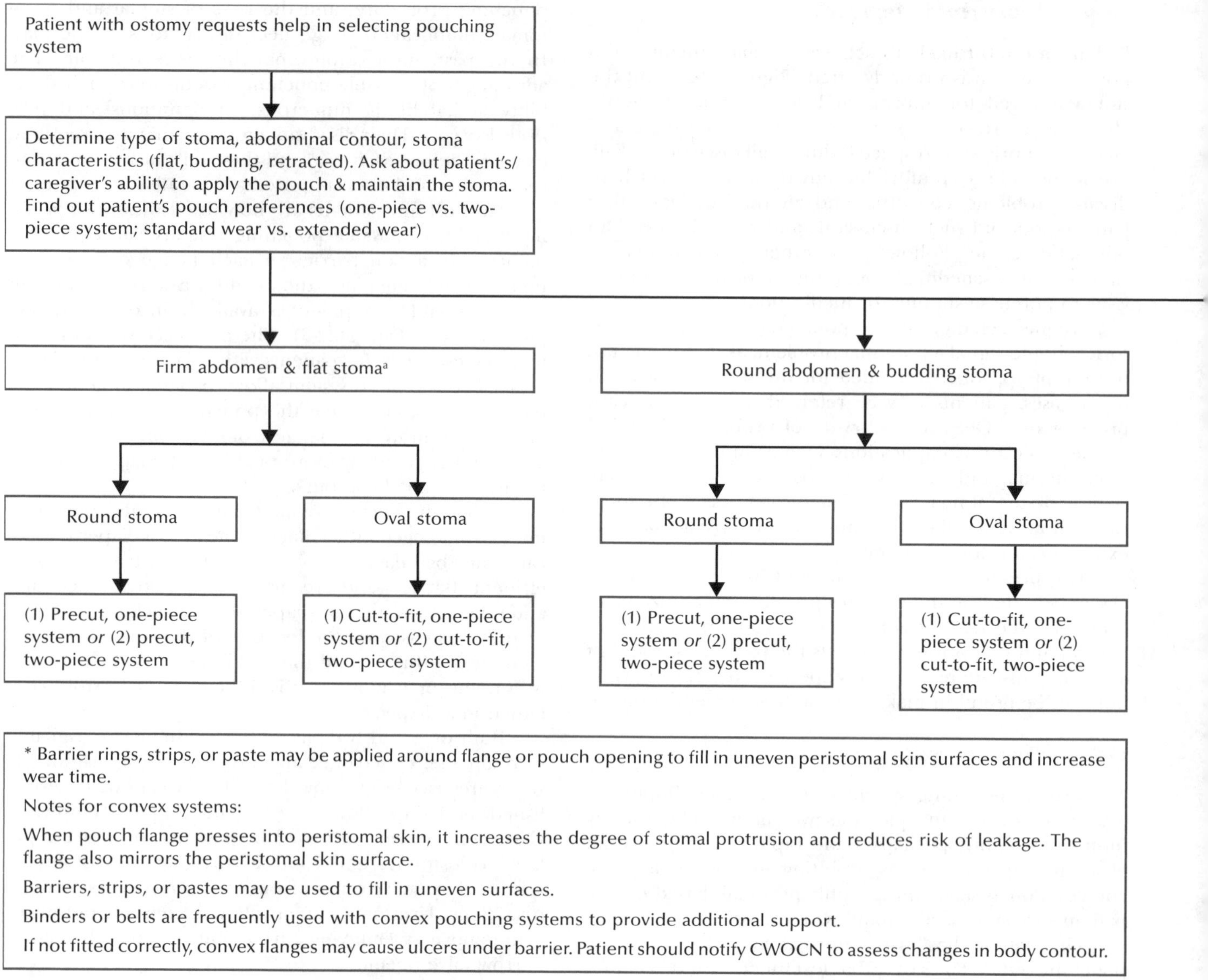

Patient with ostomy requests help in selecting pouching system
Determine type of stoma, abdominal contour, stoma characteristics (flat, budding, retracted). Ask about patient's/caregiver's ability to apply the pouch & maintain the stoma. Find out patient's pouch preferences (one-piece vs. two-piece system; standard wear vs. extended wear)
Firm abdomen & flat stoma[a]
Round abdomen & budding stoma
Round stoma
Oval stoma
Round stoma
Oval stoma
(1) Precut, one-piece system *or* (2) precut, two-piece system
(1) Cut-to-fit, one-piece system *or* (2) cut-to-fit, two-piece system
(1) Precut, one-piece system *or* (2) precut, two-piece system
(1) Cut-to-fit, one-piece system *or* (2) cut-to-fit, two-piece system
* Barrier rings, strips, or paste may be applied around flange or pouch opening to fill in uneven peristomal skin surfaces and increase wear time.
Notes for convex systems:
When pouch flange presses into peristomal skin, it increases the degree of stomal protrusion and reduces risk of leakage. The flange also mirrors the peristomal skin surface.
Barriers, strips, or pastes may be used to fill in uneven surfaces.
Binders or belts are frequently used with convex pouching systems to provide additional support.
If not fitted correctly, convex flanges may cause ulcers under barrier. Patient should notify CWOCN to assess changes in body contour.


**FIGURE 22-2** Selection of ostomy pouching system. Key: WOCN, Wound ostomy and continence nurse.

type of ostomy. The lack of uniformity in types of ostomies and ostomy equipment makes it difficult to give standard instructions for application. Also, the stoma and the contour of the area surrounding it change over time, necessitating continuous adjustments to pouches and accessories. In general, when a rigid barrier is used, the opening should provide a clearance of 1/16 to 1/8 in. around the stoma. Less clearance (0-1 mm) is required with a flexible barrier. A WOCN is an excellent source of assistance in custom fitting these appliances.

## Wearing Time

The pouch should be emptied when it is one-third to one-half full to prevent leakage. With a two-piece system, the closed-end pouch is simply removed from the flange and thrown away. Patients who want to save on pouch costs may use the two-piece drainable system and alternate the use of two pouches. The full pouch is removed, replaced by a second pouch, emptied, washed, and then reused when the second pouch is changed. One-piece, closed-end systems are removed and disposed of once or twice daily; those that can be drained can be left in place as long as they are comfortable and there is no leakage. The flange and skin barrier may be left in place for 3 to 7 days, depending on the condition of the skin and skin barrier. Although activities such as swimming or playing tennis may decrease the wear time of the pouch, this decreased time should not discourage participation in physical activities. New pouch adhesives can effectively keep the system in place during such activities. Because water will not enter the stoma, it is not necessary to cover it while swimming, bathing, or showering. However, the pouching system can be secured with waterproof tape (e.g., Hy-Tape, Pink Tape) to prevent leakage of output from the stoma, by taping around the edges of the wafer/flange.

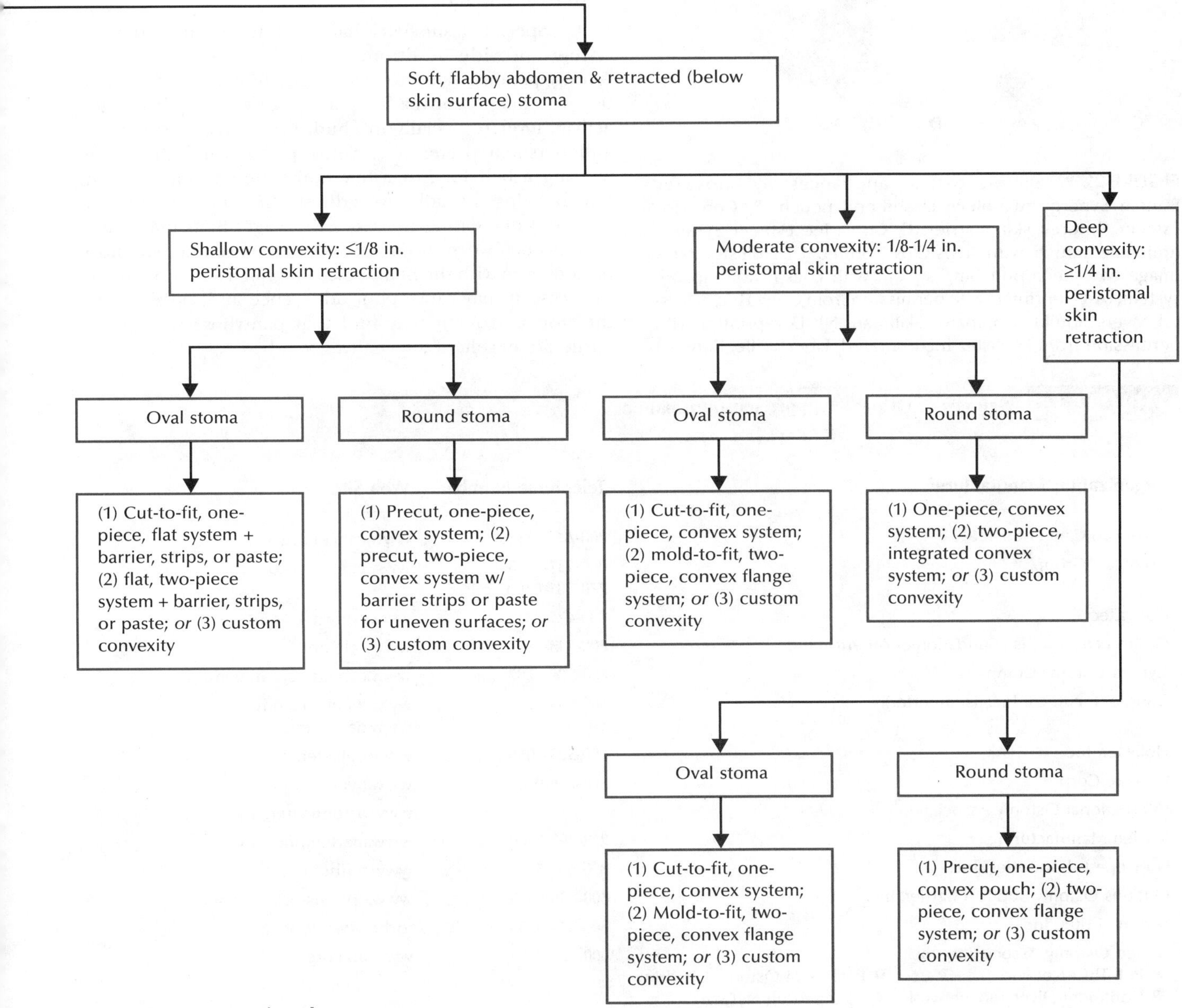


**FIGURE 22-2 (continued)**

## Product Selection Guidelines

The selection of products must be tailored to the patient's activity level and, if present, specific disabilities. Some systems require manipulation that a patient with arthritis may not be able to perform. Special products are also available to assist patients who have poor vision. In general, patients with visual or physical impairments will do best with one-piece systems because they are precut or prefitted and require minimal manipulation. Other options include the

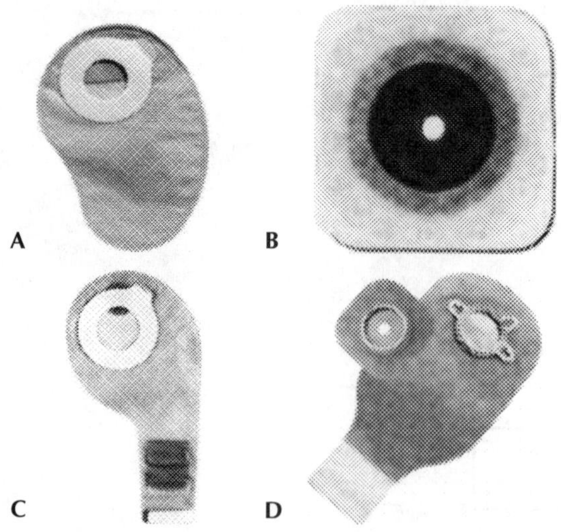


**FIGURE 22-3** Sample ostomy appliances: **A,** ConvaTec Esteem Synergy two-piece closed-end pouch; **B,** ConvaTec Esteem Synergy skin barrier; **C,** ConvaTec Esteem Synergy drainable pouch with InvisiClose outlet; **D,** Hollister New Image two piece pouching system with Lock'n Roll closure system. (A-C reprinted with permission from ConvaTec, A Bristol Myers Squibb Company, Skillman, NJ; D reprinted with permission from Hollister Incorporated, Libertyville, Illinois.)

use of waterproof materials or a stoma cover. Selection of these and other options depends on how the stoma functions. Table 22-4 lists examples of commercially available pouching systems. No particular device will prevent patients who are confused (e.g., with Alzheimer's disease) from reaching and dislodging it. It may be helpful to dress such patients in garments that make it difficult for the patient to reach the pouch. With infants, dressing them in one-piece clothing will help prevent them from exploring and pulling off their pouches.

### Ostomy Accessories

*Belts* Special elastic belts that attach to various pouching systems provide additional support. However, not all ostomy patients need to wear belts. Indications for their use are a deeply convex faceplate, poor wearing time, high activity level (especially in children), heavy perspiration, and personal preference. Some patients may find that wearing a belt for just a few hours after changing their pouch helps the adhesive adhere, thus increasing wear time and decreasing the risk of leakage. Belts may cause skin ulcers if worn too tight. To be effective, the belt must be kept even with the belt hooks. If the belt slips up around the waist, it may cause poor adherence and, possibly, cut the stoma. Women may find that pantyhose or a panty girdle are excellent alternatives to a belt.

**TABLE 22-3 Sources of Ostomy Support and Information**

| Organization/Manufacturer | Telephone Number | Web Site* |
|---|---|---|
| American Cancer Society | 800-ACS-2345 | www.cancer.org |
| Coloplast Group | 800-237-4555<br>770-281-8400 | www.coloplast.com |
| ConvaTec | 800-422-8811 | www.convatec.com |
| Crohn's and Colitis Foundation of America, Inc. | 800-343-3637 | www.ccfa.org |
| Cymed Ostomy Company | 800-582-0707 | www.cymed-ostomy.com |
| Dansac (Incutech, Inc., is importer) | 800-699-4232 | www.incutech.com<br>www.dansac.dk |
| Hollister, Inc. | 800-323-4060 | www.hollister.com |
| Hy-Tape Corp. | 800-248-0101 | www.hytape.com |
| International Ostomy Association | | www.ostomyinternational.org |
| Marlen Manufacturing | 212-292-7060 | www.marlenmfg.com |
| Nu-Hope Laboratories, Inc. | 800-899-5017 | www.nu-hope.com |
| Options Ostomy Support Barrier, Inc. | 800-736-6555 | www.options-ostomy.com |
| Torbot Group, Inc. | 800-545-4254 | torbot@worldnet.att.net |
| United Ostomy Association, Inc.<br>■ Pull-Thru Network ■ Parents of Ostomy Children<br>■ Continent Diversion Network ■ Young Adult Network<br>■ Gay and Lesbian Ostomates ■ Youth Rally | 800-826-0826 | www.uoa.org |
| United Ostomy Association of Canada, Inc. | 416-595-5452<br>888-969-9698 | www3.ns.sympatico.ca/canada.ostomy |
| EHOB/VPI | 800-966-EHOB | |
| Wound Ostomy Continence Nurses Society (WOCN) | 888-224-WOCN | www.wocn.org |

* Some Web sites may copyright their information. People who access a site should read and follow the instructions in the copyright statement, if one is given.

**TABLE 22-4 Selected Ostomy Pouching Systems***

| Trade Name | Product Features |
|---|---|
| **Two-piece Ileostomy and/or Colostomy Pouching Systems** | |
| Coloplast Assura AC Drainable/Closed/Mini/Caps Pouches | EasiClose wide outlet closure (clampless, easy to use); range of sizes (3/8-2 3/4 in.), color coded according to size; easy to close integrated system; no clamp needed; pediatric sizes available |
| Coloplast Assura AC Two-Piece Flange (Flat/Convex) | Adhesive coupling system; range of sizes:(small: 3/8-1 15/18 in.; medium: 3/8-1 7/8 in.; large: 3/8-2 3/4 in.), color coded according to size; highly absorbent flexible spiral barrier; extended-wear adhesive |
| Convatec Esteem synergy Drainable/Closed/Mini Pouches | Range of sizes (1 3/8-3 1/2 in.); straight, right-, and left-sided pouch; minimal dexterity needed; may be repositioned easily; no pressure needed; adjustable gas filter system; new InvisiClose Outlet (clampless, easy to use) |
| Convatec Esteem synergy Durahesive Moldable Convex Skin Barrier Flange | Range of sizes (small: 1/2-7/8 in. stoma; medium: 7/8-1 1/4 in. stoma; large1: 1/4-1 3/4 in.); moldable for oval or round convex stomas |
| Convatec Esteem synergy Skin Barriers with Landing Zone Flange | Innovative Adhesive Coupling Technology provides discretion of one-piece and versatility of two-piece system; low profile, conforms easily to body contour; range of sizes (1 3/8-3 1/2 in.); precut and cut-to-fit |
| Convatec Sur-Fit Natura Drainable/High Output/Closed End Pouch/Cap/Mini Pouch | Range of sizes (1 3/4-2 3/4 in.); pediatric and 10-14 in. drainable pouches; gas filters available; can be worn with belt for support; new InvisiClose Outlet (clampless, easy to use) |
| Convatec Sur-Fit Natura Durahesive "Moldable" Convex Skin Barrier Flange | Range of sizes (1 3/4-2 1/4 in.); moldable for oval or round convex stomas |
| Convatec Sur-Fit Natura Flange | Range of sizes (1 3/4-2 3/4 in.); available in flexible and convex barrier |
| Cymed Two-Piece System with Microskin and MicroDerm Barrier Drainable/Closed and mini Pouch | Range of sizes (7/8-1 1/2 in.); very moldable barrier; waterproof system; barrier supports pouch without belt |
| EHOB/VPI Non-Adhesive Colostomy/Ileostomy System | No adhesive needed to adhere pouch; O-ring with belt used to adhere pouch; available in drainable and closed pouches |
| Hollister New Image Skin Barriers with Floating Flange† | Range of sizes(1 3/4-2 3/4 in.) and cut-to-fit; Flextend (extended wear) or FlexWear (standard wear) barrier; tape and tapeless skin barrier options; convex skin barrier also available |
| Hollister New Image Drainable/Closed and Mini Pouch | Range of sizes (1 3/4-2 1/4 in.); new drainable pouch with integrated filter and Lock'n Roll (clampless, easy to use) closure system; closed pouches with integrated filters; can be worn with belt for support |
| Hollister New Image Skin Barriers with Stationary Flange | Range of sizes(1 3/4-2 1/4 in.) and cut-to-fit; lies flat against the skin, providing a low profile; Flextend (extended wear) or FlexWear (standard wear) barrier; tape and tapeless skin barrier options; convex skin barrier also available |
| **Two-piece Urostomy Pouching Systems** | |
| Coloplast Assura Urostomy Pouches | Adheres to Assura flange; unique microurostomy pouch; easy to use spout |
| Convatec Esteem synergy Urostomy Pouches | Adheres to same flanges used for ileostomy and colostomy pouches |
| Convatec Sur-Fit Natura Urostomy Pouches | Adheres to same flanges used for ileostomy and colostomy pouches; Accuseal tap closure for ease of use; night drainage container set available; Little Ones pediatric pouches also available |
| Cymed Urostomy Pouch | Range of sizes (3/4-1 3/4 in.) |
| EHOB/VPI Non-Adherent Urostomy Pouch | No adhesive needed to adhere pouch; excellent for someone allergic to adhesives; O-ring with belt used to adhere pouch |
| Hollister New Image Urostomy Pouch | Adheres to same flanges used for ileostomy and colostomy pouches; easy to use spout; pediatric sizes available |
| **One-piece Ileostomy/Colostomy Pouch** | |
| Coloplast Assura and Assura AC Small/Standard Drainable/Closed Pouch/Caps | Precut and cut-to-fit pouches; easy to use integral closure for drainable pouch |
| Convatec Active Life Drainable/Closed Pouch with Durahesive | Range of sizes (3/4-2 1/2 in.) precut and cut-to-fit; extended wear; easy to use by patients with poor manual dexterity; convexity available |

**TABLE 22-4 Selected Ostomy Pouching Systems* (continued)**

| Trade Name | Product Features |
|---|---|
| Convatec Active Life Drainable/Closed Pouch with Stomahesive | Range of sizes (3/4-2 1/2 in.) and cut-to-fit; easy to use by patients with poor manual dexterity; pediatric sizes available |
| Convatec Active Life Stoma Cap | Range of sizes (3/4-2 in.); for patients who irrigate |
| Convatec Little Ones Drainable Pouch | Range of sizes (5/16-2 in.); cut-to-fit barrier with no tape collar |
| Cymed Drainable Pouch with Microskin and MicroDerm Barrier | Cut-to-fit opening with integrated barrier; molds easily into creases |
| Hollister First Choice Closed Pouch | Standard wear; filter integrated into pouch; belt tabs for support |
| Hollister First Choice Convex Closed Pouch | Pouch opening up to 2 1/2 in.; standard wear; filter integrated into pouch; belt tabs for support |
| Hollister PouchkinsOne Piece Pediatric Ostomy System | SoftFlex (standard wear) drainable pouches; cut-to-fit up to 1 3/8 in. |
| Hollister Premier Drainable/Mini/Closed Pouches with Flextend Barrier | Lock'n Roll closure system available on drainable pouch; range of sizes (3/4-2 1/2 in.) precut and cut-to-fit; extended-wear barrier; easy to use; convexity available with cut-to-fit convexity options |
| Marlen One-Piece Convex/Flat Pouches | Flat and convex integrated barrier; easy to use Kwick-Klose pouch closure; choice of AquaTack or Skin Shield barrier; choice of 3 convexities |
| Nu-Hope Nu-Flex Adult Drainable/Closed End Pouches | Precut and cut-to-fit pouches; custom pouching: regular to deep convexity, oval to round stomas |
| **One-piece Urostomy Pouch** | |
| Austin Medical Stoma Caps | Waterproof, one-piece, latex-free, low profile; collects drainage from continent ileostomy, continent urostomy, regulated colostomies, or mucous fistulas; oval and rectangular sizes available |
| Coloplast Assura Urostomy Pouch | Spiral adhesive for longer wear; range of sizes (5/8-2 1/8 in.); precut and cut-to-fit; convexity available; easy urostomy closure |
| Convatec Active Life Urostomy Pouch with Durahesive | Range of sizes (3/4-2 1/2 in.) and cut-to-fit; extended wear; easy to use by patients with poor manual dexterity; deep convexity available |
| Cymed Urostomy Pouch with Microskin and MicroDerm Barrier | Cut-to-fit opening with integrated barrier; molds easily into creases |
| Hollister Premier Urostomy Pouch with Flextend Barrier | Range of sizes (1/2-2 in.); precut and cut-to-fit; extended-wear barrier; easy to use; convexity available with cut-to-fit convexity options; pediatric sizes available |
| Marlen Ultralite Urostomy Pouch | Flat and convex integrated barrier; easy to use snap lock pouch closure; choice of AquaTack or Skin Shield barrier; choice of 3 convexities |
| Nu-Hope Nu-Flex Urostomy Pouches | Precut and cut-to-fit pouches; custom pouching: regular to deep convexity, oval to round stomas |

* Both transparent and opaque pouches are available.

† Hollister recommends placing flanges on body as a diamond shape to prevent edges from rolling. Fingertips can be placed under flange for support while pouch is attached to barrier. Skin wipes should not be used with Flextend flanges.

Many belts contain latex, so the patient should be asked about latex allergy before recommending a belt.

*Skin Barriers/Powders/Pastes* Skin barriers, powders, and pastes are available for special skin problems (Table 22-5). Skin barriers are intended to protect the skin immediately adjacent to the stoma from stoma discharge and serve as a means of attaching a pouching system. They correct imperfections in skin surface, allowing the pouching system to fit securely. Powders are used on weeping skin. Pastes (which are not a glue but have a pastelike consistency) are used to seal the area around the stoma and fill creases in the skin. Pastes produce a flat surface for application of other skin barriers.

Solid skin barriers are preattached to the pouch (one-piece system) or provided separately (two-piece system) and may be custom cut (sizable) or precut (presized). Some manufacturers will custom cut the barriers; however, in most cases, the patient or WOCN modifies the barrier to fit the stoma. The opening in the skin barrier should match the size and shape of the patient's stoma. To create a skin barrier, the patient should apply a bead of skin barrier paste around the stoma or directly to the inside edge of the skin barrier, apply the skin barrier to wrinkle-free skin, and then press the skin barrier around the stoma to

**TABLE 22-5 Selected Ostomy Skin Barriers, Adhesives, Adhesive Removers, Belts, Powders, Cleaners, and Air Vent System**

| | |
|---|---|
| Adapt Lubricating Deodorant | Available in 8 oz bottle or 8 mL packs |
| Coloplast Strip Paste | Moldable strips to fill in uneven surfaces |
| Convatec Allkare Protective BarrierWipes | Thin film protects against skin stripping; excellent barrier for adhesives, tapes, and self-adhesive dressings |
| Convatec AllKare Adhesive Remover Wipes | Helps prevent skin damage by easing removal of all adhesives; has oily residue; skin should be washed after use |
| Convatec Eakin Cohesive Seals | Moldable, double-sided adhesive seals designed to help prevent skin damage; absorbs moisture and forms a gel to further protect skin; adheres to moist, sore skin; suitable for all types of ostomies (especially hard to fit stomas); can be used with pastes and all skin barriers and pouching systems |
| Convatec Stomahesive Paste | Pectin product; helps prevent leakage and skin irritation by filling in uneven surfaces; new easy-to-squeeze tube |
| Convatec Stomahesive Powder | Pectin base; light dusting applied to excoriated skin to promote healing |
| Hollister Adapt Barrier Rings, Strips, Paste | Custom (mold, bend, shape, and stack) convex barrier rings; barrier strips can mold and stack; paste in easy-to-squeeze tube |
| Hollister Medical Adhesive | Improves adhesive contact between skin and barrier |
| Hollister M9 Cleaner/Decrystallizer | Cleans urinary drainage systems; pH balanced and nonacidic |
| Hollister M9 Odor Eliminator | Available in spray or drops, scented or unscented |
| Hollister Premium Powder | Light dusting applied to excoriated skin to promote healing |
| Hollister Universal Remover Wipes | Removes adhesives and barriers; available as spray and wipes |
| KEM Air VENT System (OSTO-EZ-VENT) | Quickly and easily releases gas buildup in ostomy pouches |
| Nu-Hope Barrier Rings and Strips | Karaya/pectin; moldable rings and strips |
| Nu-Hope Cement | Natural rubber; hexane; excellent adherence for the difficult pouching |
| Nu-Hope Support Belt | Standard 2 3/8 in. opening; 3-9 in. widths; customized belts available; provides excellent support to prevent parastomal herniation; prolapse overbelt and custom openings available |
| Skin Bond Cement | 4 oz can; natural rubber; hexane; excellent adherence for difficult pouching |
| Smith & Nephew Adhesive Remover | Helps prevent skin damage by easing removal of all adhesives |
| 3M No Sting Wipes | Does not contain alcohol; thin film protects against skin stripping; excellent barrier for adhesives, tapes, and self-adhesive dressings |

improve adherence. Newer moldable seals are now available from major manufacturers.

Solid skin barriers may melt if exposed to high temperatures. Therefore, during the summer, and especially when traveling, the solid skin barrier should be put in an insulated box (ice is not required) to minimize the risk of melting.

*Absorbent Gel Packets/Flakes* These packets (e.g., Ileosorb and Par-Sorb) dissolve as the pouch fills, turning the liquid into gel. They reduce noise caused by sloshing of stomal fluids, control odor, prevent peristomal skin irritation, and prevent leakage, especially at night while the patient sleeps.

## Cleansing and Special Skin Care Products

The stoma and surrounding skin are best cleansed with plain water. If soap is used, it should be rinsed off thoroughly and the skin dried before a new pouching system is applied. Use of moisturizers and products containing lanolin, petrolatum, or oils should be avoided because they prevent the pouching system from adhering to the skin.

*Adhesives* Adhesives, in the form of cements or tapes, are used to keep the pouch in place. Hypoallergenic tape may be used to support the pouch. A strip may be applied across the top, bottom, and sides of the flange, with half on the flange and half on the skin. Waterproof tape may be used during swimming or bathing. Solvents are available to remove adhesive residue.

*Irrigating Sets* In patients who are candidates for irrigation, control can be maintained without a pouch. Irrigation is similar to performing an enema at the site of the stoma. Approximately 1000 mL of lukewarm tap water is instilled via a cone into the bowel through the stoma. The bowel then expands, causing peristalsis and elimination of waste through the stoma. A good candidate for irrigation is an adult patient who has a colostomy distal to the splenic flexure and does not have a history of irritable bowel syndrome, is not undergoing chemotherapy, and does not have a disability. For the process to be safe and effective, the patient should use a colostomy irrigation set, rather than a standard enema set.

Frequency of irrigation depends somewhat on a patient's normal bowel habits. It is recommended to irrigate

**TABLE 22-6 High-Fiber Foods[3-5]***

| | |
|---|---|
| Apple skins | Hot dogs |
| Apricots | Mushrooms |
| Asparagus | Nuts |
| Beans and lentils | Oranges and orange rinds |
| Bologna | Pineapples |
| Bran | Popcorn |
| Celery | Potato peels |
| Chinese vegetables | Raisins |
| Coconut | Raw vegetables |
| Corn | Sausage |
| Dried figs | Seeds |
| Grapefruits | Shrimp |
| Grapes | Tomatoes |

* To be consumed cautiously by persons with ileostomies.

**TABLE 22-7 Signs and Symptoms of Intestinal Obstruction[3,4]**

| Partial Obstruction | Complete Obstruction |
|---|---|
| Cramping abdominal pain | Absence of output (urine and fecal) |
| Watery output with foul odor | Severe cramping pain |
| Abdominal distention (possible) | Abdominal distention |
| Stomal swelling (possible) | Stomal swelling |
| Nausea and vomiting (possible) | Nausea and vomiting |
| | Decreased pulse rate |
| | Fever (possible) |

**TABLE 22-8 Conservative Management of Food Blockage[3]**

1. Sit in warm tub bath to relax abdominal muscles.
2. Massage the peristomal area while in the knee-to-chest position to attempt dislodgement of fibrous mass.
3. If stoma is swollen, remove pouch and replace with a pouch that has a larger stoma opening.
4. If able to tolerate fluids (i.e., not vomiting) and passing stool, increase intake of fluid and electrolytes, but avoid solid foods. Drink one glass of liquid each time pouch is emptied. Juices such as grape juice exert a mild cathartic effect.
5. If vomiting, not passing stool, or both, do not take liquids or solid food orally.
6. Notify a primary care provider or WOCN if any of the following develops:
   - Stool output stops (complete blockage)
   - Conservative measures (listed above) fail to resolve symptoms
   - Signs of partial obstruction persist (see Table 22-7)
   - Inability to tolerate fluids or replace fluids and electrolytes
   - Signs and symptoms of fluid and electrolyte imbalance (see Table 22-1)

at the same time every day and eventually regulate to every other day. It takes approximately 6 weeks to become regulated. After achieving control, the patient may wear a security pouch or a piece of gauze, a stoma cover, or a cap over the stoma. Irrigation is not necessary for health; it is merely one method of colostomy management. Patients should use this procedure only if instructed to do so by a WOCN or primary care provider.

*Deodorizers* Regular emptying/changing of the pouch is all that is needed to prevent odor. However, liquid concentrates are available as companion products to most ostomy pouches, and can be placed directly into the pouch to neutralize odor. DevKo external tablets may also be placed into the pouch to decrease odor. Derifil internal deodorant tablets (active ingredient is 100 mg chlorophyllin copper complex sodium) may also be used.

In addition to local methods of odor control, many pouches have charcoal filters built into the pouch devices that fit directly on the pouch to control gas and odor (Osto-EZ-vent).

### Changes in Diet

Diet does not generally play an important role in ostomy management. Most patients can eat their usual diet, including all the food they ate before surgery, if they chew their food well. However, it is wise to remain on a diet low in fiber for the first 6 weeks after surgery to allow the intestine to heal and swelling to resolve. Their usual diet can be resumed after that time.

The effects of various foods on ostomy output are summarized in Table 22-2. Patients with a urostomy may want to avoid foods that cause odor. Patients with colostomies, especially those who irrigate, should avoid foods that cause loose stools. (This problem varies among individuals.) Because patients have no control over gas passage, patients with fecal ostomies may prefer to reduce their intake of gas-forming foods. Products such as α-D-galactosidase may be used to control gas (see Chapter 15). Patients with ileostomies are more prone to intestinal obstruction from high-fiber foods eaten in large quantities or exclusive of other foods (Table 22-6). Chewing high-fiber foods well and eating them in small amounts and with other types of food will help prevent food blockage. The patient should be instructed how to manage food blockage, if it occurs. Table 22-7 lists signs and symptoms of blockage; Table 22-8 describes its management.[3]

### Precautions for Medication Use

Because part or all of the colon has been removed and intestinal transit time may be altered, the patient may experience adverse effects from taking prescription or nonprescription medications, or the medications may be ineffective. Table 22-9 lists a broad selection of medications

TABLE 22-9 Potential Effects of Selected Prescription Drugs in Patients with Ostomies[19-35]

| Class | Type of Ostomy | Potential Effects |
|---|---|---|
| Histamine$_1$-receptor antagonists | Ileostomy, colostomy, urostomy | No reported problems with cetirizine, loratadine, and fexofenadine |
| Anti-inflammatories | Ileostomy | NSAIDs associated with GI irritation and bleeding: use with caution if history of GI ulceration or bleeding exists (COX-2 inhibitors may have lower risk profile); no reported problems with Celecoxib |
| Opiates | Colostomy | Tramadol's opiate agonist activity can cause constipation, similar to opiates such as oxycodone; liquids, immediate-release products, or patches preferred to avoid erratic absorption associated with ER products |
| Selective serotonin reuptake inhibitors | Ileostomy | No reported problems with sertraline, citalopram, or fluoxetine; hyponatremia and diarrhea reported with paroxetine, requiring close monitoring of fluid and electrolyte status |
| Antipsychotics | Colostomy, ileal conduit | Constipation reported with olanzapine, caused primarily by drug's anticholinergic effect; constipation possible with all anticholinergic drugs; reported delayed lithium toxicity requires close monitoring of serum levels in patients with ileal conduits |
| Antidiabetic | Ileostomy | Possible dose-related GI effects related to variable absorption of metformin, a weak base primarily absorbed in the small intestine; no reported problems with other antidiabetic agents |
| Anticonvulsants | Ileostomy | Erratic absorption reported with enteric-coated and sustained-release products; use of liquids or immediate-release products generally recommended |
| Antilipidemics | Ileostomy, colostomy, urostomy | No reported problems with use of HMG-CoA reductase inhibitors |
| Cardiac/antihypertensive drugs | Ileostomy | Fluid and electrolyte abnormalities common; careful monitoring recommended during use of ACE inhibitors; hyperkalemia may be a particular problem |
| GI medications | Ileostomy, colostomy | Diarrhea associated with all PPIs, requiring careful monitoring of fluid and electrolyte status; no reported problems with H$_2$RAs |
| Antimicrobial agents | Ileostomy, urostomy, colostomy | Altered normal bowel flora and diarrhea related to broad-spectrum antibiotics can be a significant problem for patients with ileostomies; high doses of ciprofloxacin associated with alkaline urine (if used, urinary acidification to avoid bacterial overgrowth in urostomy patients requires close monitoring) |
| Other drugs | End jejunostomy, ileostomy | Some reports of drug failure associated with malabsorption of warfarin in patients with short-bowel syndrome; length of functionally intact proximal small bowel important in cyclosporine dosing (if liquid formulation or IV is required, more frequent monitoring is recommended); variable volume of distribution and increased clearance of gentamicin reported in patients with ileostomies, possibly requiring more frequent monitoring; highly variable bioavailability of digoxin (depends on length of remaining bowel) requires monitoring for drug failure |

Key: ACE inhibitors, angiotensin-converting enzyme inhibitors; COX-2, cyclooxygenase-2; ER, extended-release; GI, gastrointestinal; HMG-CoA, human menopausal gonadotropin coenzyme A; H$_2$RAs, histamine$_2$-receptor antagonists; NSAID, nonsteroidal anti-inflammatory drug; PPI, proton pump inhibitor.

and their potential to cause adverse effects, which vary with different dosage forms.[16-29] Ostomy patients should be instructed to check the pouch for undissolved tablets or tablet fragments whenever they take solid oral medications. Coated or sustained-release preparations may pass through the intestinal tract without being absorbed; thus, patients may receive a subtherapeutic dose. Liquid preparations or preparations that are crushed or chewed before swallowing are preferred. Some medications are contained on a wax matrix (e.g., Slow K). The active medication is leached out as the tablet moves through the GI tract. Although inactive fragments normally pass through the intestines, the medication is fully absorbed.

Patients must be careful when taking antibiotics, diuretics, and laxatives. Antibiotics may alter the normal flora of the intestinal tract, causing diarrhea or fungal infection of the skin surrounding the stoma. Antidiarrheal and antimotility drugs may reduce ileal output. Sulfa drugs should be used with caution because crystallization in the kidney may occur more often in patients who have difficulty with fluid balance. To minimize this problem, patients should increase fluid intake and not acidify the urine. Because fluid and electrolyte balance is more difficult to maintain in patients who have had an ileostomy, diuretics should be given with care.

**TABLE 22-10 Selected Drugs That Discolor Feces and Urine**

**Drugs That Discolor Feces**

*Black*
Acetazolamide
Aluminum hydroxide
Aminophylline
Amphetamine
Amphotericin B*
Anticoagulants*
Aspirin*
Barium
Bismuth
Chloramphenicol
Chlorpropamide
Cholestyramine
Corticosteroids
Cyclophosphamide
Cytarabine
Ethacrynic acid
Fluorouracil
Hydralazine
Iodide-containing drugs
Iron
Levodopa
Melphalan
Methotrexate
Nitrates
Nonsteroidal anti-inflammatory drugs*
Phenylephrine
Potassium salts*
Procarbazine
Sulfonamides
Tetracycline
Thallium
Theophylline
Thiotepa*

*Blue*
Manganese dioxide
Chloramphenicol

*Gray*
Colchicine

*Green*
Indomethacin
Iron
Medroxyprogesterone

*Green-gray*
Oral antibiotics

*Orange-red*
Phenazopyridine
Rifampin
Rifapentine

*Orange-brown*
Rifabutin

*Pink-red*
Anticoagulants*
Aspirin
Barium
Cefdinir†
Nonsteroidal anti-inflammatory drugs*
Tetracycline syrup
Clofazimine

*White or speckled*
Aluminum hydroxide
Barium
Oral antibiotics

*Yellow or yellow-green*
Senna

**Drugs That Discolor Urine**

*Black*
Ferrous salts
Phenacetin

*Blue or Green*
Amitriptyline
Cimetidine (injection)
Flutamide
Methocarbamol
Mitoxantrone
Promethazine (injection)
Propofol (injection)
Triamterene

*Dark*
Aminosalicylic acid
Metronidazole
Phenacetin

*Orange*
Chlorzoxazone
Warfarin

*Orange-red*
Phenazopyridine
Rifampin

*Pink-red*
Phenothiazines
Phenytoin

*Purplish Red*
Chlorzoxazone

*Red*
Carbidopa/levodopa
Daunorubicin
Dimethylsulfoxide
Doxorubicin
Idarubicin

*Red-brown*
Aloe
Levodopa
Phenytoin
Warfarin

*Violet*
Senna

*Yellow*
Aloe
Riboflavin
Vitamin $B_{12}$

*Yellow-brown*
Cascara
Nitrofurantoin
Senna
Sulfonamides

*Yellow-orange*
Vitamin A

*Yellow-pink*
Cascara

* Discoloration may be caused by bleeding.

† Discoloration caused by nonabsorbable complex between cefdinir or metabolites and iron in the GI tract.

Patients with colostomies may use laxatives, but only under close supervision. Ileostomy patients should never use laxatives unless ordered by their primary care provider, because of the risk of electrolyte imbalance and dehydration. If the patient is constipated, the clinician may recommend a stool softener. Prokinetic agents (e.g., metoclopramide, erythromycin) and certain antacids should be taken with caution. Products that contain calcium may cause calcium stones in patients with a urostomy, products containing magnesium may cause diarrhea in patients with an ileostomy, and aluminum products may cause constipation in patients with a colostomy.

To alleviate anxiety, the clinician should counsel the patient about medications that may discolor the feces. Some of these medications and the discoloration they cause are listed in Table 22-10.[30-35]

## Assessment of Patients with Ostomies: A Case-based Approach

In most cases, ostomy surgery necessitates the use of a pouching system designed to collect the waste material normally eliminated through the bowel or bladder. Because each ostomy patient is different, one patient may benefit from a particular type of pouch, accessory, or procedure, whereas another may develop problems with it. Moreover, pouch needs may change over time. An appliance, accessory, or procedure that previously produced ideal outcomes may no longer be appropriate because of changes in body contour caused by aging, pregnancy, weight change, or concurrent medical conditions. As the obesity epidemic continues, so do the challenges in caring for that ostomy population.

Patients who have an ostomy are often apprehensive about how the surgery will proceed, how to manage the ostomy, and how they will be perceived by others. A patient's self-esteem may also be affected. Therefore, a special effort should be made to ensure the patient's privacy and to gain the patient's confidence during the assessment encounter. Cases 22-1 and 22-2 illustrate assessment of patients with ostomies.

| CASE 22-1 | |
|---|---|
| **Relevant Evaluation Criteria** | **Scenario/Model Outcome** |
| **Information Gathering** | |
| 1. Gather essential information about the patient's symptoms, including: | |
| a. description of symptom(s) (i.e., nature, onset, duration, severity, associated symptoms) | Symptoms began during a vacation at the beach, when he was perspiring a lot. |
| b. description of any factors that seem to precipitate, exacerbate, and/or relieve the patient's symptom(s) | Patient applied pectin-based powder prior to appliance changes, but symptoms have not resolved. |
| c. description of the patient's efforts to relieve the symptoms | Patient has experienced itching and rash underneath his urostomy for the past week and is now becoming denuded. His pouch has started to leak more often. He usually wears his appliances for 1 week but can keep it on for only 24 hours. |
| 2. Gather essential patient history information: | |
| a. patient's identity | Joel S. |
| b. patient's age, sex, height, and weight | 58 y/o M, 5'10", 220 lb |
| c. patient's occupation | Computer analyst |
| d. patient's dietary habits | Diabetic diet |
| e. patient's sleep habits | N/A |
| f. concurrent medical conditions, prescription and nonprescription medications, and dietary supplements | Glucophage 500 mg 2 times/day, Flovent 220 mg 2 puffs 2 times/day, albuterol 2 puffs q6h as needed; underwent ileal loop for bladder cancer 2 years ago |
| g. allergies | Aspirin |
| h. history of other adverse reactions to medications | None |
| i. other (describe)______ | N/A |
| **Assessment and Triage** | |
| 3. Differentiate the patient's signs/symptoms and correctly identify the patient's primary problem(s). | Since going to the beach, Joel has developed a rash and itching. This rash appears to be caused by *Candida*, which thrives in dark, damp areas (caused by Joel's leaking appliance, perspiration, and denuded skin). Joel's diabetes is another related factor. |
| 4. Identify exclusions for self-treatment. | None |
| 5. Formulate a comprehensive list of therapeutic alternatives for the primary problem to determine if triage to a medical practitioner is required, and share this information with the patient. | Options include:<br>(1) Refer Joel to a WOCN.<br>(2) Recommend application of miconazole 2% powder to affected area with each pouch change.<br>(3) Have Joel see his PCP for a prescription for nystatin powder to apply to the affected area with each pouch change if 2% miconazole is not effective.<br>(4) Take no action. |
| **Plan** | |
| 6. Select an optimal therapeutic alternative to address the patient's problem, taking into account patient preferences. | OTC treatment with a powder containing 2% miconazole is appropriate for Joel. He should also change his appliance more frequently. |

## CASE 22-1 (continued)

| Relevant Evaluation Criteria | Scenario/Model Outcome |
|---|---|
| 7. Describe the recommended therapeutic approach to the patient. | You can use an OTC powder to get rid of the rash and itching. You should change your appliance more often and apply the powder at each change to prevent these symptoms from occurring again. |
| 8. Explain to the patient the rationale for selecting the recommended therapeutic approach from the considered therapeutic alternatives. | Seeing a WOCN, that is, wound ostomy and continence nurse, or your PCP, that is, primary care provider, will not be necessary because rash and itching are quite common in this situation. A referral is necessary only if the symptoms do not resolve. |
| **Patient Education** | |
| 9. When recommending self-care with nonprescription medications and/or nondrug therapy, convey accurate information to the patient. | Wash peristomal skin per your usual routine. Apply 2% miconazole powder sparingly and massage into peristomal skin. Dust off excess. A sealant (3M No Sting, etc.) may be applied to enhance the pouch seal.<br>Apply pouch. Use the miconazole powder with each pouch change until 1 week after rash has resolved. You should change the appliance every other day until the rash clears, then return to once-a-week appliance changes. If rash and itching continue, consult a WOCN or your PCP. |
| 10. Solicit patient's follow-up questions. | How long should I continue using the 2% miconazole or the Nystatin powder? |
| 11. Answer patient's questions. | Use for 1 week after rash has resolved. May use as needed if it develops again. |

Key: N/A, not applicable; OTC, over-the-counter; WOCN, wound ostomy and continence nurse.

## CASE 22-2

| Relevant Evaluation Criteria | Scenario/Model Outcome |
|---|---|
| **Information Gathering** | |
| 1. Gather essential information about the patient's symptoms, including: | |
| a. description of symptom(s) (i.e., nature, onset, duration, severity, associated symptoms) | Patient has developed leakage from her ileostomy appliance in the past few weeks. She also noticed redness and denuded skin around her ileostomy. Pain at site is also frustrating patient. |
| b. description of any factors that seem to precipitate, exacerbate, and/or relieve the patient's symptom(s) | Since surgery 6 months ago, patient has gained 30 lb. She usually changes her pouch once a week but now she has to change it every 48 hours and continues to have leakage and redness. |
| c. description of the patient's efforts to relieve the symptoms | Patient applied karaya powder and skin sealant to protect skin but continues to have skin irritation and leakage. |
| 2. Gather essential patient history information: | |
| a. patient's identity | Kara Michelle |
| b. patient's age, sex, height, and weight | 22 y/o F, 5'4", 160 lb |
| c. patient's occupation | Sales consultant |
| d. patient's dietary habits | High-fiber diet with junk food |
| e. patient's sleep habits | N/A |
| f. concurrent medical conditions, prescription and nonprescription medications, and dietary supplements | Nasonex 2 sprays once daily or 1 spray in each nostril once daily; Imodium A-D 2 mg taken after each unformed stool, not to exceed 16 mg/day.<br>Kara developed ulcerative colitis 5 years ago. Following a major bleeding episode and failure of medical management, she underwent total colectomy and ileostomy. |

## CASE 22-2 (continued)

| Relevant Evaluation Criteria | Scenario/Model Outcome |
|---|---|
| g. allergies | Latex |
| h. history of other adverse reactions to medications | None |
| i. other (describe)_______ | Patient has been nervous about her job and has been constantly eating, which has increased her weight. |
| **Assessment and Triage** | |
| 3. Differentiate the patient's signs/symptoms and correctly identify the patient's primary problem(s). | Leakage, burning sensation, and denuded skin around her ileostomy is caused by abdominal creases from increased weight. |
| 4. Identify exclusions for self-treatment. | None |
| 5. Formulate a comprehensive list of therapeutic alternatives for the primary problem to determine if triage to a medical practitioner is required, and share this information with the patient. | Options include:<br>(1) Refer Kara to a WOCN for further assessment and treatment.<br>(2) Recommend use of pectin or karaya powder to improve peristomal skin followed by application of skin sealant.<br>(3) Recommend use of pouch convexity and belt for support. |
| **Plan** | |
| 6. Select an optimal therapeutic alternative to address the patient's problem, taking into account patient preferences. | Assessment of the stoma and skin indicates a convex pouch with a belt for support is needed. Upon further discussion, Kara says she prefers a one-piece convex pouch with belt versus a two-piece pouch. |
| 7. Describe the recommended therapeutic approach to the patient. | Since your stoma has retracted to skin level, you will need a convex pouch with a belt for support. Treat skin around the stoma with a pectin-based powder, such as Stomahesive powder, and a skin sealant, such as 3M No Sting, before applying the pouch. Change pouch twice a week until peristomal skin is free of burning and denuded skin, then return to once a week.<br>Losing some weight will also decrease the retraction of the stoma. |
| 8. Explain to the patient the rationale for selecting the recommended therapeutic approach from the considered therapeutic alternatives. | Pouch leakage, denuded skin, and pain will decrease with proper follow-up with your WOCN, or wound ostomy and continence nurse, to modify pouching technique.<br>Refer to the United Ostomy Association in local area for peer support to improve self-esteem and body image. |
| **Patient Education** | |
| 9. When recommending self-care with nonprescription medications and/or nondrug therapy, convey accurate information to the patient, including: | |
| a. appropriate dose and frequency of administration | See Figure 22-2 for proper assessment of convexity and Figures 22-3 and 22-4 for proper pouching and skin accessories. |
| b. maximum number of days the therapy should be employed | Change twice a week. |
| c. product administration procedures | Wash peristomal skin as usual. Apply thin layer of powder. Massage in well and dust off excess. Apply skin sealant prior to pouch application. |
| d. expected time to onset of relief | With proper convexity and powder application, leakage and excoriation should decrease within 24 hours. You will notice a decrease in the burning sensation. |
| e. degree of relief that can be reasonably expected | Deceased intensity of symptoms within 24-48 hours |
| f. most common side effects | Allergic reaction to the powder or pouch adhesive |

**CASE 22-2 (continued)**

| Relevant Evaluation Criteria | Scenario/Model Outcome |
|---|---|
| g. side effects that warrant medical intervention should they occur | Burning, stinging, local irritation |
| h. patient options in the event that condition worsens or persists | Consult a WOCN or your PCP, that is, primary care provider, if leakage or burning continues after 1 week of treatment. |
| i. product storage requirements | Store away from heat. |
| j. specific nondrug measures | Change pouch twice a week until peristomal skin is clear. |
| 10. Solicit patient's follow-up questions. | What happens if I can't lose weight and I have more creases and my stoma retracts more. |
| 11. Answer patient's questions. | Consult a WOCN or your PCP; you may need another type of pouching system. Obesity is now epidemic; consult nutritionist for proper diet program. |

Key: N/A, not available; WOCN, wound ostomy and continence nurse.

## Patient Counseling for Ostomy Care

The pharmaceutical care needs of a patient with an ostomy include procurement and distribution of ostomy supplies and selection of appropriate products. Monitoring a patient's management of the ostomy and counseling on special needs (e.g., skin care, diet, fluid intake, drug therapy) are other important components of pharmaceutical care for these patients.

When counseling an ostomy patient, the clinician should provide services in a sensitive and caring manner. An ostomy patient's self-esteem is often damaged; therefore, when assisting a patient with ostomy needs, the clinician must take special care to avoid verbal or facial expressions that might convey negative feelings regarding the procedure. Peer support can be especially helpful to such patients; therefore, the clinician should consider providing patients with a list of local and national ostomy associations, as well as a list of product manufacturers who can supply information about product use (Table 22-3). Patients who want to contact a WOCN in their area should be advised to check the Web site at www.wocn.org. The following "self-help" books should also be recommended to patients with ostomies:

- Barrie B. *Second Act.* New York: Scribner; 1997.
- Benirschke R. *Alive & Kicking.* San Diego: Rolf Benirschke Enterprises, Inc; 1999.
- Benirschke R. *Great Comebacks.* San Diego: Rolf Benirschke Enterprises, Inc; 2002.
- Kupfer B, Foley-Bolch K, Kasouf MF, et al. *Yes We Can.* Worchester, Mass: Chandler House Press; 2000.

The patient should be encouraged to express problems and concerns so the clinician can better assess the patient's ability to achieve self-treatment objectives. Moreover, the clinician must maintain an awareness of the patient's special needs when managing conditions unrelated to the ostomy. The box Patient Education for Ostomy Care lists specific information to provide to a patient with an ostomy.

## Key Points for Ostomy Care

- Patients with ostomies may experience both psychologic and physical complications after ostomy surgery. It is the obligation of the clinician to address these issues and refer patients to their primary care provider, WOCN, and/or United Ostomy Association.
- The objectives of self-care of an ostomy are to understand how the stoma functions and how to manage it; to understand proper use of the pouching system and accessories, and to avoid complications that result from improper use; and to reduce the risks of other complications.
- Patients should be advised about the effects of food on stomal output and the need to monitor for signs and symptoms of dehydration.
- The selection of appropriate pouching depends on the patient's body contour, manual dexterity, and type of ostomy.
- The ideal ostomy pouching system should be leak-proof, odor-proof, comfortable, and easy to use. The clinician as well as the WOCN can assist the patient in achieving these outcomes.
- Patients should be counseled on the effects of medications: liquid, crushed, or chewed medications are the preferred; coated or sustained-release medications should be used with caution because most of these should not be crushed or chewed. Use caution when taking antibiotics and diuretics. Antibiotics can cause diarrhea or fungal infections of the skin around the stoma. Diuretics can cause dehydration or electrolyte imbalance in patients with ileostomies. Use caution when taking laxatives, antidiarrheals, or other medications that alter GI motility. Laxatives can increase fecal output in patients with ileostomies, whereas antidiarrheals decrease the fecal output.

## PATIENT EDUCATION FOR OSTOMY CARE

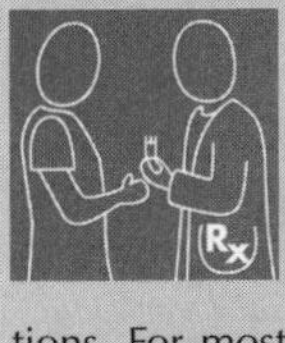

The objectives of self-care of ostomies are to: (1) understand how the stoma functions and how to manage it; (2) understand the proper use of the pouching system and accessories, and avoid complications that result from improper use; and (3) reduce the risk of other types of complications. For most patients, carefully following the product instructions and the self-care measures listed here will help to ensure optimal therapeutic outcomes.

### Appliance Selection and Use

- Use only the type of pouching system recommended for your type of ostomy.
- If is system no longer fits well, consult your WOCN or clinician before changing to a different type of pouching system.
- Do not consider skin irritation to be inevitable; identify the cause and treat it as soon as it occurs.
- If possible, identify the cause for leakage around the pouching system and correct immediately. Consult your WOCN or primary care provider if you cannot determine the cause.
- Establish a routine for ostomy care. Keep the routine simple; use as few accessories as possible.

### Effects of Medication Use

- Sustained- or extended-release medicines may undergo erratic absorption, thus making their effect unpredictable. These medications should be used with caution. Coated medications, as well as sustained- or extended-release medications should not be crushed or chewed.
- Use caution when taking antibiotics and diuretics. Antibiotics can cause diarrhea or fungal infections of the skin around the stoma. Diuretics can cause dehydration or electrolyte imbalance in individuals with ileostomies.
- Use caution when taking laxatives, antidiarrheals, or other medications that alter GI motility. Laxatives can increase fecal output in individuals with ileostomies, whereas antidiarrheals decrease the fecal output.
- Know which medications will discolor the urine or feces (see Table 22-10).

### Complications

- Patients with a urostomy/ileal conduit, to prevent urine crystals from forming and causing skin irritation, apply a cloth soaked with a solution of one third white vinegar to two thirds water for 5 to 10 minutes to the stoma at least once weekly before putting on the pouching system. If you use a two-piece system, apply the solution as often as three to four times daily. The vinegar may cause the stoma to turn white, but this effect does not indicate the stoma is being harmed.
- Consult your clinician about using nonprescription medications to treat diarrhea or constipation. Return for reevaluation of the problem after 1 week of treatment.

See your WOCN if you experience any of the following complications:

- Depression and anxiety
- Sexual dysfunction
- Abdominal pain
- Narrowing of the stoma
- A bulge near the stoma
- An extension of the bowel through the stoma
- Recession of the stoma to a subnormal length
- Bleeding from or around the stoma
- Pain when touching the skin around the stoma or when applying the appliance
- Overgrowth of the skin around the stoma

## References


1. United Ostomy Association Fact Sheet. Available at: www.uoa.org. Accessed April 28, 2003.
2. Wise B, McKenna, Gavin G, et al. *APSNA Nursing Care of the General Pediatric Surgical Patient.* Gathersburg, Md: Aspen Publishers; 2000.
3. Colwell JC, Goldberg MT, Carmel JE. *Fecal & Urinary Diversions Management Principles.* St. Louis: Mosby, Inc; 2004:224.
4. Colwell JC, Goldberg MT, Carmel JE. *Fecal & Urinary Diversions Management Principles.* St. Louis: Mosby, Inc; 2004.
5. Krenta KS. Living *with Confidence after Ileostomy Surgery.* Princeton, NJ: ConvaTec, a Bristol Myers Squibb Co; 2003.
6. Hillman RS. Hematopoietic agents: growth factors, minerals, and vitamins. In: Hardman JG, Limbird LE, eds. *Goodman and Gilman's The Pharmacological Basis of Therapeutics.* 10th ed. New York: McGraw-Hill, Inc; 2001:1487-517.
7. Marcus R. Agents affecting calcification and bone turnover: calcium, phosphate, parathyroid hormone, vitamin D, calcitonin, and other compounds. In: Hardman JG, Limbird LE, eds. *Goodman and Gilman's The Pharmacological Basis of Therapeutics.* 10th ed. New York: McGraw-Hill, Inc; 2001:1715-43.
8. Marcus R, Coulston AM. Water-soluble vitamins: the vitamin B complex and ascorbic acid. In: Hardman JG, Limbird LE, eds. *Goodman and Gilman's The Pharmacological Basis of Therapeutics.* 10th ed. New York: McGraw-Hill, Inc; 2001:1753-71.
9. Marcus R, Coulston AM. Fat-soluble vitamins: vitamins A, K, and E. In: Hardman JG, Limbird LE, eds. *Goodman and Gilman's The Pharmacological Basis of Therapeutics.* 10th ed. New York: McGraw-Hill, Inc; 2001:1773-91.
10. Gray M. Are cranberry juice or cranberry products effective in the prevention or management of urinary tract infection? *J WOCN.* 2002;29:122-6.
11. Raz R, Chazan B, Dan M. *Cranberry Juice and Urinary Tract Infection.* CID 2004;38:1413-9.
12. Jepson RG, Mihaljevicl, Craig J. Cranberries for treating urinary tract infections. *Cochrane Database Syst Rev.* 2002;2:CD001322.
13. Jepson RG, Mihaljevicl, Craig J. Cranberries for preventing urinary tract infections. *Cochrane Database Syst Rev.* 2004;2: CD001321.pub3.
14. Patient Education Series: What's right for me?. Libertyville, Ill: Hollister, Inc; 2003.
15. Krenta KS. *Living with Confidence after Urostomy Surgery.* Princeton, NJ: ConvaTec, a Bristol-Myers Squibb Co; 2003.
16. Aly R, Forney R, Bayes C. Treatment for common superficial fungal infections. *Dermatol Nurs.* 2001;13:91-9.

17. Erwin-Toth P. Caring for a stoma. *Nursing 2001.* 2001;31(5):36-40.
18. Colwell JC, Goldberg MT, Carmel JE. *Fecal & Urinary Diversions Management Principles.* St. Louis: Mosby, Inc; 2004:345-8.
19. *AHFS Drug Information.* Bethesda, Md: American Society of Health-System Pharmacists; 2003.
20. Colwell JC, Goldberg MT, Carmel JE. *Fecal & Urinary Diversions Management Principles.* St. Louis: Mosby, Inc; 2004:345-8.
21. Severijnen R, Bayat N, Bakker H, et al. Enteral drug absorption in patients with short small bowel—a review. *Clin Pharmacokinet.* 2004;43:951-62.
22. Tewari A, Ward RG, Sells RA, et al. Reduced bioavailability of cyclosporine A capsules in a renal transplant patient with partial gastrectomy and ileal resection. *Ann Clin Biochem.* 1993;30:587-9.
23. Gaskin TL, Duffull SB. Enhanced gentamicin clearance associated with ileostomy fluid loss. *Aust N Z J Med.* 1997;27:196-7.
24. Ritchie HA, Duggull SB. Another case of high gentamicin clearance and volume of distribution in a patient with high output ileostomy. *Aust N Z J Med.* 1998;28:212-3.
25. Al-Habet S, Kinsella HC, Rogers HJ, et al. Malabsorption of prednisolone from enteric-coated tablets after ileostomy. *BMJ.* 1980;281:843-4.
26. Owens JP, Mirtallo JM, Murphy CC. Oral anticoagulation in patients with short-bowel syndrome. *DICP.* 1990;24:585-9.
27. Lutomski DM, LaFrance RJ, Bower RH, et al. Warfarin absorption after massive small bowel resection. *Am J Gastroenterol.* 1985; 80:99-102.
28. Brophy DF, Ford SL, Crouch MA. Warfarin resistance in a patient with short bowel syndrome. *Pharmacotherapy.* 1998;18:1375-6.
29. Roberts R, Sketris IS, Abraham I, et al. Cyclosporine absorption in two patients with short-bowel syndrome. *DICP.* 1988;22:570-2.
30. Knoben JE, Anderson PO. Handbook *of Clinical Drug Data.* 7th ed. Hamilton, Ill: Drug Intelligence Publications, Inc; 1998.
31. Allen J, Burson SC. Drug discoloration of the urine. Document 150907. Stockton, Calif: *Pharmacist's Letter,* September 1999.
32. *Physicians' Desk Reference* Electronic *Library.* Montvale, NJ: Medical Economics Company; 2003.
33. Fecal discoloration induced by drugs, chemicals, and disease states. In: Gelman CR, Rumack BH, Hutchison TA, eds. *DRUGDEX System.* Englewood, NJ: Micromedex, Inc; 2003.
34. Alhasso A, Bryden AA, Neilson D. Lithium toxicity after urinary diversion with ileal conduit. BMJ. 2000;320:1037.
35. Urinary discoloration—drug and disease induced. In: *DRUGDEX System.* Englewood, NJ: Micromedex, Inc; 2003.

SECTION VI

# Nutrition and Nutritional Supplementation

CHAPTER 23

# Essential and Conditionally Essential Nutrients

*Yvonne Huckleberry and Carol J. Rollins*

Approximately 40% to 50% of Americans consume a vitamin, dietary, or mineral supplement daily, accounting for estimated annual sales in excess of $7.5 billion.[1] Nutrition experts agree that foods are the preferred source of vitamins and minerals and that most individuals can easily meet their requirements by eating a balanced diet. There is less agreement, however, about the extent to which the U.S. population consumes a balanced diet. Many believe that most Americans receive adequate levels of vitamins and minerals from their diet; the lack of deficiency symptoms in this country supports this position. However, there is growing concern that subclinical deficiencies may be contributing to chronic diseases such as arteriosclerosis, osteoporosis, and cancer.[2-4] This finding suggests primary attention should be directed toward improving the selection of nutrient-dense foods. Despite such attention, some individuals are unlikely to consume adequate amounts of vitamins and minerals; therefore, a multivitamin supplement may be appropriate.

The issue of who will benefit from or be harmed by oral supplements is complex. For example, one study evaluated the role of dietary supplements in improving the overall nutrient intake of adults.[5] These authors found that regular use of dietary supplements helps patients meet dietary requirements. However, many supplement users exceeded the tolerable upper intake levels (ULs) of some nutrients, thereby increasing the risk of adverse effects.

One of the greatest dangers of food fads, multiple supplements, and large doses of single vitamins is that they are sometimes used in place of sound medical care. The lure of superior health or freedom from disease may attract desperate or uninformed patients who have cancer, heart disease, arthritis, or other serious illnesses. This may place them at greater risk by causing a delay in seeking and receiving appropriate medical attention.

## Epidemiology/Etiology of Nutritional Deficiencies

Although overt nutrient deficiency is rare in the United States, the prevalence of subclinical deficiencies is unknown. Specific patient populations may be at higher risk of deficient nutrient intakes because of the following pathophysiologic, physiologic, behavioral, or economic situations:

- *Inadequate dietary intake:* patients who are alcoholics, impoverished, or on severe calorie-restricted or fad diets, or those who have eating disorders
- *Increased metabolic requirements:* pregnant and breast-feeding women, infants, children undergoing periods of accelerated growth, postsurgical patients, and patients with cancer, severe injury, infection, or trauma
- *Poor absorption:* patients of advanced age or those with conditions such as prolonged diarrhea, severe gastrointestinal (GI) disorders or malignancy, surgical removal of a section of the GI tract, celiac disease, obstructive jaundice, or cystic fibrosis
- *Iatrogenic situations:* patients taking prolonged broad-spectrum antibiotics, those with drug–nutrient interactions, or those who are receiving parenteral nutrition

Although several factors increase the risk of malnutrition in patients of advanced age (Table 23-1), vitamin and mineral deficiency among noninstitutionalized older patients is uncommon. This has been attributed to an increasing number of healthy, active individuals older than 65 years, better nutrition, and an increase in self-treatment with vitamin and mineral supplements.[6,7] While clinical deficiency is rare, dietary intakes for some older patients may still be below optimum levels.[8] Since foods contain numerous other compounds that are important for health maintenance and disease prevention, health care professionals play an important role in educating these patients on nutrient-dense food choices before vitamin and/or mineral supplementation is recommended.

## Pathophysiology of Nutritional Deficiencies

A comprehensive discussion of the pathophysiology of vitamin and mineral deficiencies is outside the scope of this chapter. The reader is referred to standard medical and nutrition textbooks for such information.

## Signs and Symptoms of Nutritional Deficiencies

A vitamin deficiency may evolve in several stages (Table 23-2).[9] Signs and symptoms of vitamin and mineral deficiencies are discussed in the individual micronutrient sections.

**TABLE 23-1 Factors Contributing to Nutritional Deficiency in Patients of Advanced Age[6,7]**

- Mastication or swallowing difficulty, or xerostomia
- Loss of taste, smell, or sight perception
- Constipation or diarrhea
- Decreased absorption of some nutrients such as lactose
- Gastric hypochlorhydria or atrophic gastritis
- Inability to buy or prepare meals because of tremor, fatigue, or arthritic pain
- Anorexia caused by reduced physical activity, social isolation, pain, or depression
- Dementia
- Lack of knowledge about balanced nutrition
- Poverty
- Substance abuse
- Inadequate exposure to sunlight
- Medications affecting judgment, coordination, memory, appetite, nutrient absorption, or GI tract function

**TABLE 23-2 Stages in Evolution of Vitamin Deficiency[9]**

1. Inadequate nutrient delivery, synthesis, or absorption
2. Depletion of nutrient stores
3. Biochemical changes
4. Physical manifestations of deficiency
5. Morbidity and mortality

## Complications of Malnutrition

Poor nutrition increases the risks of chronic disease, infection, and complications from surgery and chemotherapy. In addition, wound-healing time and mortality may be increased. The conditions associated with severe malnutrition include marasmus, kwashiorkor, and mixed malnutrition. Marasmus, also referred to as energy malnutrition, is caused by inadequate caloric intake and presents as decreased fat deposits, decreased muscle mass, and cachexia. Serum protein status is maintained. Kwashiorkor, or protein malnutrition, is caused by inadequate dietary intake of protein, and is characterized by edema with decreased serum protein levels, including hypoalbuminemia. Mixed malnutrition is caused by inadequate dietary intake of calories and protein; it exhibits features of both marasmus and kwashiorkor. This form of malnutrition is commonly referred to as protein-energy malnutrition. Vitamin and mineral deficiencies can accompany all three forms of malnutrition.

## Nutrient Supplementation

Nutritional supplements should be used as adjuncts to a balanced diet and not as substitutes for nutritious food. Nutritional supplements are often self-prescribed. Although nutritional supplements can be obtained without a prescription, they are complex agents with specific indications. Medical assessment should precede their use, especially if intakes exceed the dietary reference intakes (DRIs) for vitamins and/or minerals. Furthermore, the patient should be reminded that vitamins and minerals are often better absorbed from food sources than supplements. The practitioner may refer patients to a Registered Dietitian for personalized counseling on diet modification as well as nutritional supplementation.

### *Intent of Use*

Nutritional supplement use is intended to prevent nutritional deficiencies, replenish compromised stores, or maintain the present nutritional status. Over-the-counter nutritional supplements are not intended for the self-treatment of vitamin deficiencies.

### *General Approach to Use*

If a patient's diet is not providing the required levels of micronutrients, supplementation with vitamins and minerals is appropriate, as long as the patient has no underlying pathology and is not taking megadoses of micronutrients. A once-daily multivitamin providing no more than 100% of the DRIs should suffice in most cases. Patients should be reminded that there is no established benefit for healthy individuals to supplement nutrients in doses above the DRI.[10]

Practitioners should also counsel patients regarding the potential disparity of product contents versus the label. Several studies have reported significant discrepancies when supplements were analyzed for the labeled dietary ingredient.[11-13] This potential for labeling inaccuracy exists because dietary supplements are not assessed for compliance by any government agency. Unlike prescription drugs, dietary supplements do not need proof of safety, efficacy, or production under good manufacturing practices at this time. However, the U.S. Pharmacopeia (USP) provides a Dietary Supplement Verification Program that allows product labeling with the USP mark if the tested product meets specific requirements. These requirements include verification of product ingredients and amounts, effective disintegration and dissolution for absorption, absence of harmful contaminants, and safe, sanitary, well-controlled manufacturing.[14] Practitioners should advise patients to look for this USP mark on vitamin and mineral supplement labels.

Some patients need supplemental macronutrients (e.g., fat, protein, carbohydrate) because they are unable to consume all the nutrients they need. Liquid nutritional supplements (e.g., Ensure, Boost) are discussed in Chapter 24.

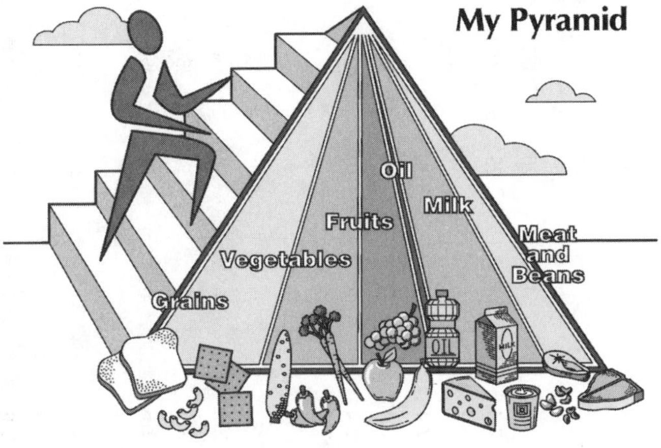


FIGURE 23-1 The Food Guide Pyramid. (Image from Mini-Poster Download at mypyramid.gov.)

### *Nonpharmacologic Therapy*

The best method to avoid nutritional deficiencies is to eat a balanced diet that includes foods from sources high in several essential nutrients each day. To guide consumers in selection of a balanced diet while allowing for individual preferences, the U.S. Department of Health and Human Services recently released Dietary Guidelines for Americans 2005.[15] In these guidelines, consumers are advised to regularly choose a variety of nutrient-dense foods, as exemplified in the Food Guide Pyramid (Figure 23-1). Each food group in the pyramid represents a significant source of one or more essential and conditionally essential nutrients. For example, the milk group is a major source of calcium, while the fruits and vegetables groups are sources of fiber and the primary sources of antioxidant vitamins. By selecting a variety of foods within the various groups and eating the appropriate number of servings from each food group daily, consumers can "balance" their diet relative to essential and conditionally essential nutrients. In terms of portion size, approximately 1/2 cup of fruit, vegetable, rice, pasta, or cereal; 3 ounces of meat, fish, or poultry; or 1 cup of milk typically count as one serving. Avoidance of "hidden" servings (e.g., the fat and bread servings in addition to the poultry serving of a batter-coated fried chicken breast) is a key to calorie control (see Chapter 27). Several alternative food pyramids and various other plans, such as food selection by color, are reported in the popular press, but few of these plans have been adequately evaluated for the balance of nutrients they provide. Thus, the Food Guide Pyramid remains the most appropriate tool for assessing the need for nutrient supplementation, and practitioners should inquire about the patient's intake from these food groups.[10]

### *Pharmacologic Therapy*

Although there are situations in which high doses of specific vitamins and minerals are reported to be of therapeutic benefit, the claims of megavitamin enthusiasts have not been objectively confirmed. Those vitamins and minerals that have therapeutic value in the treatment of medical conditions (e.g., niacin therapy for hyperlipidemia) are actually being used as drugs rather than supplements for disease prevention or health maintenance. Deficiency states should be treated under medical supervision. Furthermore, prolonged ingestion of vitamin and mineral supplements has not been tested for safety. Some vitamins, such as A, D, niacin, and pyridoxine, and minerals such as iron and fluoride, are known to be toxic in high doses. Thus, patients should be cautioned against initiating high-dose self-medication with vitamins and minerals. Practitioners should discourage chronic, high-dose ingestion of any nutrient without proper medical supervision.

#### Vitamins

Vitamins are used as both dietary supplements and therapeutic agents to treat deficiencies or other pathologic conditions. DRIs have replaced the traditional recommended dietary allowances (RDAs) as reference values of daily nutrient intake recommended by the Food and Nutrition Board of the Institute of Medicine, National Academy of Science[16,17] (Tables 23-3 and 23-4). The DRIs include four reference categories: estimated average requirements (EARs), RDAs, adequate intakes (AIs), and ULs. EARs are values obtained after a careful review of the literature on specific nutrients. The EARs provide nutrient intake values that are estimated to meet the requirements of half of the healthy individuals in a specific gender and age group. An RDA value is set at 2 standard deviations above the EAR as an estimate of daily nutrient intake sufficient to meet requirements of nearly all individuals of a specified age group and gender. AIs are used as recommended intakes for nutrients when adequate scientific data are lacking and an EAR cannot be established with confidence. Finally, the ULs are the highest dose of nutrient intake that may be consumed daily without risk of adverse effects in the general population. Like EARs, these are based on current literature. ULs are not available for all nutrients (Table 23-5).[16-20] DRIs should be used as guidelines for nutritional assessment. The application of DRIs to individuals may require adjustment according to strenuous physical activity or the presence of disease.

The Food and Drug Administration (FDA) has published a less comprehensive set of values to be used for food and dietary supplement labeling.[21] Nutrients are listed as a percentage of daily value (%DV). The vitamin or mineral supplement label includes a box with the heading Supplement Facts. In addition to information on serving size and servings per container, the label lists all required nutrients that are present in the dietary supplement in significant amounts and the %DV where a reference has been established. It also lists all other dietary ingredients present in the product, including botanicals and amino acids, for which no %DV has been established. The %DV is based on DRI values for adults and for children age 4 years or older, unless the product is designed for children younger than 4 years, for pregnant women, or for lactating women.

Frequently, "natural" vitamin products are supplemented with synthetic vitamins. For example, because the

**TABLE 23-3 Recommended Intakes for Individuals: Vitamins Food and Nutrition Board, Institute of Medicine, National Academies**

| Life Stage Group | Vitamin A (μg/day)* | Vitamin C (mg/day) | Vitamin D (μg/day)†‡ | Vitamin E (mg/day)§ | Vitamin K (μg/ day) | Thiamin (mg/day) | Riboflavin (mg/day) | Niacin (mg/day)‖ | Vitamin $B_6$ (mg/day) | Folate (μg/day)¶ | Vitamin $B_{12}$ (μg/day) | Pantothenic Acid (mg/day) | Biotin (μg/ day) | Choline# (mg/day) |
|---|---|---|---|---|---|---|---|---|---|---|---|---|---|---|
| **Infants** | | | | | | | | | | | | | | |
| 0-6 months | 400* | 40* | 5* | 4* | 2.0* | 0.2* | 0.3* | 2* | 0.1* | 65* | 0.4* | 1.7* | 5* | 125* |
| 1-12 months | 500* | 50* | 5* | 5* | 2.5* | 0.3* | 0.4* | 4* | 0.3* | 80* | 0.5* | 1.8* | 6* | 150* |
| **Children** | | | | | | | | | | | | | | |
| 1-3 years | 300 | 15 | 5* | 6 | 30* | 0.5 | 0.5 | 6 | 0.5 | 150 | 0.9 | 2* | 8* | 200* |
| 4-8 years | 400 | 25 | 5* | 7 | 55* | 0.6 | 0.6 | 8 | 0.6 | 200 | 1.2 | 3* | 12* | 250* |
| **Males** | | | | | | | | | | | | | | |
| 9-13 years | 600 | 45 | 5* | 11 | 60* | 0.9 | 0.9 | 12 | 1.0 | 300 | 1.8 | 4* | 20* | 375* |
| 14-18 years | 900 | 75 | 5* | 15 | 75* | 1.2 | 1.3 | 16 | 1.3 | 400 | 2.4 | 5* | 25* | 550* |
| 19-30 years | 900 | 90 | 5* | 15 | 120* | 1.2 | 1.3 | 16 | 1.3 | 400 | 2.4 | 5* | 30* | 550* |
| 31-50 years | 900 | 90 | 5* | 15 | 120* | 1.2 | 1.3 | 16 | 1.3 | 400 | 2.4 | 5* | 30* | 550* |
| 51-70 years | 900 | 90 | 10* | 15 | 120* | 1.2 | 1.3 | 16 | 1.7 | 400 | 2.4** | 5* | 30* | 550* |
| >70 years | 900 | 90 | 15* | 15 | 120* | 1.2 | 1.3 | 16 | 1.7 | 400 | 2.4** | 5* | 30* | 550* |
| **Females** | | | | | | | | | | | | | | |
| 9-13 years | 600 | 45 | 5* | 11 | 60* | 0.9 | 0.9 | 12 | 1.0 | 300 | 1.8 | 4* | 20* | 375* |
| 14-18 years | 700 | 65 | 5* | 15 | 75* | 1.0 | 1.0 | 14 | 1.2 | 400†† | 2.4 | 5* | 25* | 400* |
| 19-30 years | 700 | 75 | 5* | 15 | 90* | 1.1 | 1.1 | 14 | 1.3 | 400†† | 2.4 | 5* | 30* | 425* |
| 31-50 years | 700 | 75 | 5* | 15 | 90* | 1.1 | 1.1 | 14 | 1.3 | 400†† | 2.4 | 5* | 30* | 425* |
| 51-70 years | 700 | 75 | 10* | 15 | 90* | 1.1 | 1.1 | 14 | 1.5 | 400 | 2.4** | 5* | 30* | 425* |
| >70 years | 700 | 75 | 15* | 15 | 90* | 1.1 | 1.1 | 14 | 1.5 | 400 | 2.4** | 5* | 30* | 425* |
| **Pregnancy** | | | | | | | | | | | | | | |
| ≤ 18 years | 750 | 80 | 5* | 15 | 75* | 1.4 | 1.4 | 18 | 1.9 | 600‡‡ | 2.6 | 6* | 30* | 450* |
| 19-30 years | 770 | 85 | 5* | 15 | 90* | 1.4 | 1.4 | 18 | 1.9 | 600‡‡ | 2.6 | 6* | 30* | 450* |
| 31-50 years | 770 | 85 | 5* | 15 | 90* | 1.4 | 1.4 | 18 | 1.9 | 600‡‡ | 2.6 | 6* | 30* | 450* |
| Lactation | | | | | | | | | | | | | | |
| ≤ 18 years | 1200 | 115 | 5* | 19 | 75* | 1.4 | 1.6 | 17 | 2.0 | 500 | 2.8 | 7* | 35* | 550* |
| 19-30 years | 1300 | 120 | 5* | 19 | 90* | 1.4 | 1.6 | 17 | 2.0 | 500 | 2.8 | 7* | 35* | 550* |
| 31-50 years | 1300 | 120 | 5* | 19 | 90* | 1.4 | 1.6 | 17 | 2.0 | 500 | 2.8 | 7* | 35* | 550* |

*Note:* This table (taken from the DRI reports; see www.nap.edu) presents recommended dietary allowances (RDAs) in **bold type** and adequate intakes (AIs) in ordinary type followed by a *single* asterisk (*). RDAs and AIs may both be used as goals for individual intake. RDAs are set to meet the needs of almost all (97%-98%) individuals in a group. For healthy breast-fed infants, AI is the mean intake. AI for other life stage and gender groups is believed to cover needs of all individuals in the group, but lack of data or uncertainty in the data prevents being able to specify with confidence the percentage of individuals covered by this intake.

* As retinol activity equivalents (RAEs). 1 RAE = retinol 1 μg, β-carotene 12 μg, α-carotene 24 μg, or β-cryptoxanthin 24 μg. To calculate RAEs from REs of provitamin A carotenoids in foods, divide REs by 2. For preformed vitamin A in foods or supplements and for provitamin A carotenoids in supplements, 1 RE = 1 RAE.

† As cholecalciferol. Cholecalciferol 1 μg = vitamin D 40 IU.

‡ In the absence of adequate exposure to sunlight.

§ As α-tocopherol. α-Tocopherol includes *RRR*-α-tocopherol, the only form of α-tocopherol that occurs naturally in foods, and the *2R*-stereoisomeric forms of α-tocopherol (*RRR*-, *RSR*-, *RRS*-, and *RSS*-α-tocopherol) that occur in fortified foods and supplements. It does not include the *2S*-stereoisomeric forms of α-tocopherol (*SRR*-, *SSR*-, *SRS*-, and *SSS*-α-tocopherol), also found in fortified foods and supplements.

‖ As niacin equivalents (NE). Niacin 1 mg = tryptophan 60 mg ; 06 months = preformed niacin (not NE).

¶ As dietary folate equivalents (DFE). 1 DFE = food folate 1 μg = folic acid 0.6 μg from fortified food or as a supplement consumed with food = supplement 0.5 μg taken on an empty stomach.

# Although AIs have been set for choline, there are few data to assess whether a dietary supply of choline is needed at all stages of the life cycle; the choline requirement may be met by endogenous synthesis at some of these stages.

** Because 10% to 30% of people of advanced age may malabsorb food-bound $B_{12}$, it is advisable for those older than 50 years to meet their RDA mainly by consuming foods fortified with $B_{12}$ or a supplement containing $B_{12}$.

†† In view of evidence linking folate intake with neural tube defects in the fetus, it is recommended that all women capable of becoming pregnant consume folate 400 μg from supplements or fortified foods in addition to intake of food folate from a varied diet.

‡‡ It is assumed that women will continue consuming folic acid 400 μg from supplements or fortified food until their pregnancy is confirmed and they enter prenatal care, which ordinarily occurs after the end of the periconceptional period the critical time for formation of the neural tube.

*Source*: Reprinted with permission from references 16-19. 

**TABLE 23-4** Recommended Intakes for Individuals: Elements Food and Nutrition Board, Institute of Medicine, National Academies

| Life Stage Group | Calcium (mg/day) | Chromium (μg/day) | Copper (μg/ day) | Fluoride (mg/day) | Iodine (μg/day) | Iron (mg /day) | Magnesium (mg/day) | Manganese (mg/day) | Molybdenum (μg/day) | Phosphorus (mg/day) | Selenium (μg/day) | Zinc (mg /day) |
|---|---|---|---|---|---|---|---|---|---|---|---|---|
| **Infants** | | | | | | | | | | | | |
| 0-6 months | 210* | 0.2* | 200* | 0.01* | 110* | 0.27* | 30* | 0.003* | 2* | 100* | 15* | 2* |
| 7-12 months | 270* | 5.5* | 220* | 0.5 | 130* | 11 | 75* | 0.6* | 3* | 275* | 20* | 3 |
| **Children** | | | | | | | | | | | | |
| 1-3 years | 500* | 11* | 340 | 0.7* | 90 | 7 | 80 | 1.2* | 17 | 460 | 20 | 3 |
| 4-8 years | 800* | 15* | 440 | 1* | 90 | 10 | 130 | 1.5* | 22 | 500 | 30 | 5 |
| **Males** | | | | | | | | | | | | |
| 9-13 years | 1300* | 25* | 700 | 2* | 120 | 8 | 240 | 1.9* | 34 | 1250 | 40 | 8 |
| 14-18 years | 1300* | 35* | 890 | 3* | 150 | 11 | 410 | 2.2* | 43 | 1250 | 55 | 11 |
| 19-30 years | 1000* | 35* | 900 | 4* | 150 | 8 | 400 | 2.3* | 45 | 700 | 55 | 11 |
| 31-50 years | 1000* | 35* | 900 | 4* | 150 | 8 | 420 | 2.3* | 45 | 700 | 55 | 11 |
| 51-70 years | 1200* | 30* | 900 | 4* | 150 | 8 | 420 | 2.3* | 45 | 700 | 55 | 11 |
| >70 years | 1200* | 30* | 900 | 4* | 150 | 8 | 420 | 2.3* | 45 | 700 | 55 | 11 |
| **Females** | | | | | | | | | | | | |
| 9-13 years | 1300* | 21* | 700 | 2* | 120 | 8 | 240 | 1.6* | 34 | 1250 | 40 | 8 |
| 14-18 years | 1300* | 24* | 890 | 3* | 150 | 15 | 360 | 1.6* | 43 | 1250 | 55 | 9 |
| 19-30 years | 1000* | 25* | 900 | 3* | 150 | 18 | 310 | 1.8* | 45 | 700 | 55 | 8 |
| 31-50 years | 1000* | 25* | 900 | 3* | 150 | 18 | 320 | 1.8* | 45 | 700 | 55 | 8 |
| 51-70 years | 1200* | 20* | 900 | 3* | 150 | 8 | 320 | 1.8* | 45 | 700 | 55 | 8 |
| >70 years | 1200* | 20* | 900 | 3* | 150 | 8 | 320 | 1.8* | 45 | 700 | 55 | 8 |
| **Pregnancy** | | | | | | | | | | | | |
| ≤18 years | 1300* | 29* | 1000 | 3* | 220 | 27 | 400 | 2.0* | 50 | 1250 | 60 | 13 |
| 19-30 years | 1000* | 30* | 1000 | 3* | 220 | 27 | 350 | 2.0* | 50 | 700 | 60 | 11 |
| 31-50 years | 1000* | 30* | 1000 | 3* | 220 | 27 | 360 | 2.0* | 50 | 700 | 60 | 11 |
| **Lactation** | | | | | | | | | | | | |
| ≤18 years | 1300* | 44 | 1300 | 3* | 290 | 10 | 360 | 2.6* | 50 | 1250 | 70 | 14 |
| 19-30 years | 1000* | 45* | 1300 | 3* | 290 | 9 | 310 | 2.6* | 50 | 700 | 70 | 12 |
| 31-50 years | 1000* | 45* | 1300 | 3* | 290 | 9 | 320 | 2.6* | 50 | 700 | 70 | 12 |

*Note:* This table presents recommended dietary allowances (RDAs) in **bold type** and adequate intakes (AIs) in ordinary type followed by a *single* asterisk (*). RDAs and AIs may both be used as goals for individual intake. RDAs are set to meet the needs of almost all (97%-98%) individuals in a group. For healthy breast-fed infants, AI is the mean intake. AI for other life stage, and gender groups is believed to cover needs of all individuals in the group, but lack of data or uncertainty in the data prevents ability to specify with confidence the percentage of individuals covered by this intake.

*Source:* Reprinted with permission from references 16-19. Copyright 2001 by the National Academy of Sciences.

**TABLE 23-5 Adult Tolerable Upper Intake Levels of Selected Nutrients[16-19]**

| | |
|---|---|
| Vitamin A | 3 |
| Vitamin D | 0.05 |
| Vitamin E | 1000 |
| Vitamin C | 2000 |
| Folate | 1 |
| Niacin | 35 |
| Vitamin $B_6$ | 100 |
| Choline | 3500 |
| Calcium | 2500 |
| Iron | 45 |
| Magnesium | 350 |
| Phosphorus | 4000 |
| Copper | 10 |
| Fluoride | 10 |
| Iodine | 1.1 |
| Manganese | 11 |
| Molybdenum | 2 |
| Selenium | 0.4 |
| Vanadium | 1.8 |
| Zinc | 40 |

amount of vitamin C that can be acquired from rose hips (the fleshy fruit of a rose) is relatively small, synthetic vitamin C is added to prevent too large a tablet size. However, this addition may not be noted on the label, and the price of the partially natural product is often considerably higher than that for the completely synthetic, but equally effective, product. Patients should be informed that the body cannot distinguish between a vitamin molecule derived from a synthetic source and one derived from a natural source, and that most synthetic vitamins are equal to the more expensive "natural" vitamins. One exception may be vitamin E, in which the natural RRR-α-tocopherol form of the vitamin appears to have improved biological activity compared with synthetic forms of the vitamin.[22]

Vitamins are grouped in two broad classifications: fat soluble and water soluble. Vitamins A, D, E, and K are fat-soluble vitamins. They are soluble in lipids and are usually absorbed into the lymphatic system of the small intestine, and subsequently pass into the general circulation. Their absorption is facilitated by bile. These vitamins are stored in body tissues and ingestion of excessive quantities may be toxic. Deficiencies occur when fat intake is limited or fat absorption is compromised. Examples of disease states that may cause malabsorption of fat-soluble vitamins include celiac disease, cystic fibrosis, obstructive jaundice, cirrhosis of the liver, and short bowel syndrome. Drugs that affect lipid absorption, such as cholestyramine (which binds bile acids, thereby hindering lipid emulsification), orlistat (which inhibits gastric and pancreatic lipases in the intestinal lumen), and mineral oil (which is an unabsorbed oil that increases the fecal loss of fat-soluble vitamins), may precipitate such a deficiency. Consumption of snack foods that contain olestra, a fat substitute that is neither digested nor absorbed, has been associated with a decreased absorption of fat-soluble vitamins. However, this effect may be offset by the supplementation of fat-soluble vitamins in olestra-containing foods.[23] A daily multivitamin supplement is recommended by the manufacturer for those taking orlistat.

Vitamin C and the B-complex vitamins (riboflavin, thiamin, $B_6$, $B_{12}$, niacin, pantothenic acid, biotin, and folic acid) are water-soluble vitamins. These vitamins are generally not stored in the body, and excessive quantities tend to be excreted in the urine. Therefore, daily intake of these vitamins is desirable for optimal health.

As nutritional supplements, vitamins are usually dosed at 50% to 150% of the DRI values. Practitioners should advise caution with high-dose supplements that provide greater than 200% of the DRI. As therapeutic agents, vitamins should be recommended only for specific evidence-based medical indications.

*Vitamin A* The designation vitamin A refers to a group of compounds that includes the retinoids (e.g., retinol) and the carotenoids (e.g., α-carotene, β-carotene). The term *retinoid* is also used to refer to this very large group of compounds, some of which lack vitamin A activity. Biochemical changes occur in the retinoids and carotenoids during absorption in the intestine to form active compounds.

In healthy adults, more than 90% of the body's supply of vitamin A is stored in the liver. Because of this generous reserve, there is minimal risk of deficiency with short-term periods of inadequate intake or fat malabsorption. Infants and young children, however, are more susceptible to vitamin A deficiency because they have not established the necessary reserves.

Function Vitamin A is essential for normal growth and reproduction, normal skeletal and tooth development, and proper functioning of most organs of the body, notably the specialized functions involving the conjunctiva, retina, and cornea of the eye. It is thus indicated in preventing and treating symptoms of vitamin A deficiency, such as xerophthalmia (dry eye) and nyctalopia (night blindness). The synthesis of the glycoproteins necessary to maintain normal epithelial cell mucous secretions also requires vitamin A. This barrier is vital to the body's defense against bacterial infections in the upper respiratory system.

One of the most encouraging developments in vitamin research has been the discovery that vitamin A analogues may be useful in preventing and treating certain cancers and skin disorders. For example, all-trans-retinoic acid is being used to induce remission in patients with acute promyelocytic leukemia. Topical retinoic acid (Retin-A) and systemic isotretinoin (Accutane) are being used to treat acne vulgaris and severe recalcitrant cystic acne, respectively.[24] However, there is no evidence that high doses of vitamin A itself have any beneficial effect in these conditions and self-treatment is not indicated.

Dietary Sources See Table 23-6.

**TABLE 23-6 Food Sources Rich in Selected Nutrients[25]**

| Vitamin | Food Sources |
|---|---|
| Vitamin A | Liver, milk fat, egg yolk, yellow and dark green leafy vegetables, apricots, cantaloupe, peaches |
| Vitamin D | Vitamin D supplemented milk, egg yolk, liver, salmon, tuna, sardines, milk fat |
| Vitamin E | Wheat germ, vegetable oils, margarine, green leafy vegetables, milk fat, egg yolks, nuts |
| Vitamin K | Liver, vegetable oil, spinach, kale, cabbage, cauliflower |
| Vitamin C | Green and red peppers, broccoli, spinach, tomatoes, potatoes, strawberries, citrus fruit, kiwi |
| Vitamin $B_{12}$ | Liver, meat, poultry, oysters, clams, dairy products |
| Folate | Liver, lean beef, wheat, whole-grain cereals, eggs, fish, dry beans, lentils, green leafy vegetables |
| Niacin | Lean meats, fish, liver, poultry, many grains, eggs, peanuts, milk, legumes |
| Pantothenic acid | Eggs, kidney, liver, salmon, yeast, some present in all foods |
| Vitamin $B_6$ | Meats, cereals, lentils, legumes, nuts, egg yolk, milk |
| Riboflavin | Meats, poultry, fish, dairy products, green leafy vegetables, enriched cereals and breads, eggs |
| Thiamin | Legumes, whole-grain and enriched cereals and breads, wheat germ, pork, beef |
| Biotin | Liver, egg yolk, mushrooms, peanuts, milk, most vegetables, bananas, yeast |
| l-Carnitine | Dairy products, meat |
| Choline | Egg yolks, cereal, fish, meats |
| Calcium | Dairy products, sardines, clams, oysters, turnip greens, mustard greens |
| Iron | Liver, meat, egg yolk, legumes, whole or enriched grains, dark green vegetables, shrimp |
| Magnesium | Whole-grain cereals, tofu, nuts, legumes, green vegetables |
| Phosphorus | Milk, meat, poultry, fish, seeds, nuts, egg yolk |
| Chromium | Liver, fish, clams, meats, whole-grain cereals, milk, corn oil |
| Cobalt | Organ meats, oysters, clams, poultry, milk, cream, cheese |
| Copper | Liver, shellfish, whole grains, cherries, legumes, poultry, oysters, chocolate |
| Manganese | Vegetables, fruits, nuts, legumes, whole-grain cereals |
| Molybdenum | Legumes, cereals, dark green leafy vegetables, organ meats, milk |
| Selenium | Meat, grains, onions, milk |
| Silicon | Cereal products, root vegetables |
| Vanadium | Shellfish, mushrooms, parsley, dill seed, black pepper |
| Zinc | Oysters, shellfish, liver, beef, lamb, pork, legumes, milk, wheat bran |

Deficiency Vitamin A deficiency is rare in well-nourished populations. However, approximately 500,000 children worldwide develop blindness each year because of vitamin A deficiency.[26] Conditions such as cancer, tuberculosis, pneumonia, chronic nephritis, urinary tract infections, and prostate disease, as well as therapy with corticosteroids, may cause excessive excretion of vitamin A. Fat malabsorption may impair vitamin A absorption. Neomycin, cholestyramine, or orlistat may cause significant malabsorption of vitamin A and other fat-soluble vitamins and precipitate deficiencies with long-term use. In the United States, vitamin A deficiency occurs more often from diseases of fat malabsorption than from malnutrition.

One of the earliest symptoms of vitamin A deficiency is night blindness.[25,26] Other characteristic clinical findings include follicular hyperkeratosis, loss of appetite, impaired taste and smell, and impaired equilibrium. Some of these findings may be masked by concurrent deficiencies of other nutrients. Notable, however, is the drying and hyperkeratinization of the skin, since disruption of vitamin A–dependent epithelial integrity predisposes patients to infections.

Dose/DRI Vitamin A is FDA approved for use in the treatment and prevention of vitamin A deficiency.[27] To avoid toxicity, the patient's dietary intake of vitamin A should be estimated when determining a dose for supplementation.

The DRI values for vitamin A are measured in micrograms of retinol activity equivalents (RAEs). The Food and Nutrition Board recommended RAEs as a way to determine the amount of absorption of the carotenoids, as well as their degree of conversion to vitamin A in the body. RAEs replace the former designation of retinol equivalents (REs) used to calculate total vitamin A values from various dietary sources. These RAEs are listed in Table 23-7.

The DRI values for vitamin A are listed in Table 23-3. A UL of 3 mg has been established for vitamin A, on the basis of risks of physical birth defects in the young and liver abnormalities in adults associated with vitamin A toxicity.[19]

**TABLE 23-7 Retinol Activity Equivalents**

| | |
|---|---|
| 1 retinol activity equivalent | = 1 retinol equivalent |
| | = 1 μg retinol |
| | = 12 μg β-carotene |
| | = 24 μg α-carotene |
| | = 24 μg β-cryptoxanthin |
| | = 3.33 IU vitamin A activity from retinol |
| | = 10 IU vitamin A activity from β-carotene |

Recent evidence suggests that vitamin A intake below the established UL may be associated with an increased risk of bone fractures.[28]

Clearly, if the practitioner determines that a vitamin A supplement is appropriate, the recommendation should be a nonprescription multivitamin that contains no more than the DRI value of vitamin A. Preferably, a significant percentage of total vitamin A content should be contributed by β-carotene since β-carotene intake is not associated with the risk of fractures or vitamin A toxicity. The improved safety profile of β-carotene may be related to limitations in absorption and conversion to retinol.[28] High-dose vitamin A therapy should never be undertaken without close medical supervision.

Safety Considerations Because vitamin A is stored in the body, high doses of it can lead to a toxic syndrome known as hypervitaminosis A. The incidence of hypervitaminosis A is increasing because of publicity regarding the potential therapeutic benefits of vitamin A in cancer, skin disorders, and wound healing. A single megadose of retinol (25,000 IU/kg; 7507 RAE/kg) may precipitate acute toxicity 4 to 8 hours after ingestion. Chronic daily ingestion of 4000 IU/kg (approximately 1200 RAE/kg) has resulted in toxicity in adults.[24] Headache is a predominant symptom, but it may be accompanied by diplopia (double vision), nausea, vomiting, vertigo, fatigue, or drowsiness. Treatment consists of discontinuing vitamin A supplementation and the prognosis is good. Although β-carotene toxicity is not likely, eating large amounts of carrots daily may result in carotenemia, which can produce a yellow skin hue. Pregnant women or women of childbearing age should avoid vitamin A doses above the DRI because of the teratogenic risk. For this reason, women of childbearing age should carefully evaluate the total vitamin A content of all dietary supplements and fortified foods regularly consumed. These patients should be reminded not to take other dietary supplements when a prescription prenatal vitamin is dispensed.

Potential drug–nutrient interactions are listed in Table 23-8.

*Vitamin D (Calciferol)* A number of chemicals are associated with vitamin D activity. Cholecalciferol (vitamin $D_3$) is the naturally occurring form of vitamin D. It is synthesized in the skin from endogenous or dietary cholesterol on exposure to ultraviolet radiation (sunlight). Ergocalciferol, which differs structurally only slightly from cholecalciferol, is used as a food additive. Ergocalciferol and cholecalciferol are equipotent.

Activation of vitamin D requires both the liver and the kidney. One metabolite, 25-hydroxycholecalciferol (available as calcifediol), is formed by the liver and then hydroxylated by the kidney to its active form, 1,25-dihydroxycholecalciferol. Thus, both renal and hepatic dysfunction may result in clinical manifestations of vitamin D deficiency. In patients with renal failure, impaired vitamin D hydroxylation may cause hypocalcemia that persists despite massive doses of vitamin D. Administration of 1,25-dihydroxycholecalciferol (available as calcitriol) to these patients has been successful. Similarly, supplementation with 25-hydroxycholecalciferol is sufficient to prevent or treat vitamin D deficiency in patients with hepatic failure.

Function Vitamin D, which has properties of both a hormone and a vitamin, is necessary for the proper formation of bone and for mineral homeostasis. It is closely involved with parathyroid hormone, phosphate, and calcitonin in the homeostasis of serum calcium. Adequate vitamin D intake reportedly reduces the risk of bone fractures, heart disease, and some cancers. However, data supporting these claims have been inconclusive.[29-31]

Dietary Sources Milk and milk products are the major sources of preformed vitamin D in the United States because milk is routinely supplemented with 100 IU (30 RAE) of vitamin D per cup. Other sources of vitamin D are listed in Table 23-6. Vitamin D is stable, and normal food processing does not appear to alter its activity.

Deficiency Vitamin D deficiency may result from inadequate intake, GI disease (hepatobiliary disease, malabsorption, or chronic pancreatitis), chronic renal failure, inadequate sunlight exposure, hereditary disorders of vitamin D metabolism, or long-term phenytoin therapy.

The signs and symptoms of vitamin D deficiency are reflected as calcium abnormalities, specifically those involved with bone formation. The classic deficiency state is rickets. Vitamin D increases calcium and phosphate absorption from the small intestine, mobilizes calcium from bone, permits normal bone mineralization, improves renal reabsorption of calcium, and maintains serum calcium and phosphorus levels. As serum calcium decreases, compensatory mechanisms attempt to increase calcium levels. Parathyroid hormone secretion increases, possibly leading to secondary hyperparathyroidism. If physiologic mechanisms fail to make the appropriate adjustments in levels of calcium and phosphorus, demineralization of bone will ensue to maintain essential plasma calcium levels. During growth, this leads to a failure of bone matrix mineralization. The epiphyseal plate may widen because of the weight load on softened bone structures during growth. As a result, rickets is manifested by soft bones and deformed joints. In adults, such demineralization may lead to severe osteomalacia.

The incidence of rickets in the United States is low, but the increasing popularity of vegetarian diets has led to

**TABLE 23-8 Micronutrient–Drug and Micronutrient–Micronutrient Interactions**

| Micronutrient | Drug/Micronutrient | Effect | Precautionary Measures |
|---|---|---|---|
| **Vitamins** | | | |
| Vitamins A, E (large doses) | Warfarin | ↑ Anticoagulation | Take only recommended U.S. DRIs. |
| Vitamins A, E, D, K, C | Cholestyramine, colestipol, or mineral oil (unabsorbed) | Possible ↓ vitamin absorption | Avoid prolonged use of cholestyramine, colestipol, or mineral oil. |
| Vitamin D | Phenytoin or barbiturates | Possible ↓ half-life of vitamin D | Ensure adequate dietary intake of vitamin D. |
| Vitamin K | Broad-spectrum antibiotics (long-term therapy) | Vitamin K deficiency induced by ↓ gut flora | Ensure adequate dietary intake of vitamin K. |
| | Warfarin | ↓ Anticoagulation | Keep daily intake of vitamin K consistent. |
| | Vitamin E (large doses) | Antagonizes function of vitamin K | Avoid chronic supplementation with high-dose vitamin E. |
| Vitamin $B_{12}$ | Metformin, colchicine, anticonvulsants, ascorbic acid supplements, antiulcer agents, and antibiotics | Potential ↓ absorption of cyanocobalamin | Clinical significance unknown. |
| Folic acid | Phenytoin and possibly other related anticonvulsants (chronic use) | Possibly inhibit folic acid absorption, leading to megaloblastic anemia. Subsequent ↑ folic acid supplementation may decrease serum phenytoin levels and complicate seizure control. | Monitor for megaloblastic anemia. Consult with neurologist regarding supplementation, if possible. |
| | Trimethoprim | Weak folic acid antagonism; ↓ activity/effectiveness. Rarely, megaloblastic anemia may occur in patients with low folic acid level at onset of trimethoprim therapy. | Monitor for megaloblastic anemia. |
| | Pyrimethamine (large doses) | Possible megaloblastic anemia | Monitor for megaloblastic anemia. |
| | Methotrexate | Folic acid antagonism; ↓ activity/effectiveness | Monitor use of folic acid in patients on maintenance regimens for psoriasis or rheumatoid arthritis. |
| | Sulfasalazine | ↓ Folic acid absorption when these agents are administered together | Separate dosing of these agents. |
| Niacin | Oral hypoglycemics | ↓ Hypoglycemic effects | Monitor blood glucose with regular finger sticks. |
| | Sulfinpyrazone and probenecid | Possible inhibited uricosuric effects | |
| Vitamin $B_6$ | Isoniazid, hydralazine | Pyridoxine antagonism, manifested as perioral numbness resulting from peripheral neuropathy | Routinely take 50 mg/day of pyridoxine hydrochloride with isoniazid or 10 mg of pyridoxine for each 100 mg of isoniazid. |
| | Phenobarbital and phenytoin | ↓ Serum levels of the drugs | Consider monitoring levels in patients taking high-dose pyridoxine. |
| | Levodopa | Levodopa antagonism ↓ effectiveness | Avoid supplemental pyridoxine or, if possible, substitute levodopa carbidopa for levodopa. |
| **Minerals** | | | |
| Calcium | Iron, zinc, other essential minerals | Inhibited mineral absorption caused by high calcium intake | Separate dosing by at least 2 hours. |
| | Corticosteroids | Inhibited calcium absorption from gut; ↑ bone fractures and osteoporosis | Consider calcium supplementation. |

TABLE 23-8 Micronutrient–Drug and Micronutrient–Micronutrient Interactions (continued)

| Micronutrient | Drug/Micronutrient | Effect | Precautionary Measures |
|---|---|---|---|
| | Aluminum-containing antacids, phosphates, magnesium, cholestyramine | ↓ Calcium serum levels | Separate dosing by at least 2 hours. |
| | Tetracyclines, fluoroquinolones | ↓ Antibiotic absorption | Separate dosing by 2 hours before or 6 hours after the antibiotic. |
| Magnesium | Tetracyclines, fluoroquinolones | ↓ Antibiotic absorption | Separate dosing by 2 hours before or 6 hours after the antibiotic. |
| Phosphorus | Sucralfate or antacids containing magnesium, calcium, or aluminum | ↓ Absorption of phosphorus | Ensure adequate intake of dietary phosphorus. |
| Iron | Antacids | ↓ Iron solubility and absorption | Separate dosing by at least 2 hours. |
| | Tetracyclines, fluoroquinolones | ↓ Antibiotic and iron absorption | If concurrent administration is medically necessary, take tetracycline or fluoroquinolone 2 hours before or 6 hours after taking iron. |
| **Trace Elements** | | | |
| Copper | Zinc, high-dose vitamin C | Copper antagonism | May compete for absorption and utilization. |
| Fluoride | Magnesium, aluminum, calcium | ↓ Effect and absorption of fluoride | Separate supplementation by at least 2 hours. |
| Iodine (potassium iodide) | Lithium salts | Possible additive hypothyroid effects | Monitor thyroid function tests. |
| Zinc | Copper | Possible ↓ copper levels | May require copper supplementation if high-dose, prolonged zinc supplementation. |
| | Tetracyclines, fluoroquinolones | Possible ↓ antibiotic absorption | Separate dosing by 2 hours before or 6 hours after the antibiotic. |

Key: DRI, dietary reference intake.

rickets in some children who abstain from milk and infants breast-fed by mothers who do not drink milk, who fail to take prenatal vitamins, who have inadequate exposure to sunlight, or who otherwise receive inadequate intake of vitamin D.[32]

Dose/DRI Most people obtain the AI for vitamin D from dietary sources and exposure to sunlight (Table 23-3). People regularly exposed to sunlight will generally have no dietary requirement for vitamin D. However, a substantial part of the U.S. population is exposed to very little sunlight, especially during the winter.

Vitamin D is FDA approved for treating refractory rickets, hypophosphatemia, and hypoparathyroidism. Calcifediol and calcitriol are FDA approved for managing hypocalcemia in patients with chronic renal failure undergoing hemodialysis.[27]

If the practitioner determines that vitamin D supplementation is appropriate on the basis of poor dietary intake or inadequate exposure to sunlight, a multivitamin supplement containing no more than cholecalciferol 5 to 10 μg (200 to 400 IU) should be recommended. Liquid preparations that contain vitamin D should be measured carefully, particularly when given to infants. The UL for vitamin D is 50 μg daily.

Vitamin D is included in most multivitamin preparations. Calcifediol and calcitriol are available by prescription for use in patients with hypocalcemia associated with renal failure. The former compound has a longer half-life but is less potent.

Large daily doses of vitamin D (250 to 1500 μg) are prescribed for the treatment of rickets. Calcitriol capsules or solution (0.25 to 1 μg/day) are often prescribed for adults with osteomalacia caused by renal disease.[16]

Safety Considerations Taking more than the UL of vitamin D daily may lead to adverse effects, including anorexia, hypercalcemia, soft-tissue calcification, kidney stones, and renal failure.[3,20] Patients receiving treatment for rickets should be closely monitored for these adverse effects.

Phenytoin may decrease the half-life of vitamin D, resulting in osteomalacia. Vitamin D and calcium supplementation for patients on phenytoin may be warranted, especially if therapy is prolonged or high doses are required.[28] Other potential drug interactions with vitamin D are listed in Table 23-8.

*Vitamin E (Tocopherol)* The term vitamin E refers to the tocopherols and the tocotrienols, which are naturally occurring compounds in plants.

Function Vitamin E functions primarily as an antioxidant, protecting cellular membranes from oxidative damage or destruction. This process may be aided by selenium and vitamin C. Vitamin E may also have a role in heme biosynthesis, steroid metabolism, and collagen formation.

Vitamin E supplements have been used for treatment of claudication, atherosclerosis, diabetes, cancer, Parkinson's disease, and Alzheimer's disease with inconclusive results. Moderate consumption of dietary sources of vitamin E may reduce the risk of diseases such as Parkinson's disease and diabetes.[33,34]

Dietary Sources See Table 23-6.

Deficiency Vitamin E deficiency is extremely rare but may occur in two groups: premature, very-low-birth-weight infants and patients who do not absorb fat normally. For example, neurologic abnormalities responsive to supplemental vitamin E have been reported in some patients with biliary disease and cystic fibrosis. Vitamin E deficiency has also been associated with symptoms of peripheral neuropathy, intermittent claudication, muscle weakness, and hemolytic anemia.

Dose/DRI The average diet contains approximately 3 to 15 mg of vitamin E daily; therefore, large doses (i.e., in excess of the DRI) are not necessary unless the patient is experiencing fat malabsorption. The FDA-approved use of vitamin E is for prevention and treatment of hemolytic anemia associated with deficiency.[27]

Vitamin E requirements may vary in proportion to the amount of polyunsaturated fatty acids in the diet. The polyunsaturated fatty acid content of the U.S. diet has increased, and the plant oils responsible for the increase are rich in tocopherol. Concern over the increasing oxidant insult in the form of atmospheric pollutants has led to the theory that all individuals should increase their intake of vitamin E. However, the lack of evidence of deficiency at the present intake supports the current adult DRI of 15 mg/day. The UL for vitamin E is 1000 mg daily.

Adverse Effects Vitamin E is relatively nontoxic. Most adults tolerate 100 to 800 mg daily without adverse effects, but the hazards of long-term, high-dose therapy are unknown.

Drug–Nutrient Interactions Vitamin E has been reported to enhance warfarin anticoagulation, possibly by inducing vitamin K deficiency.[27] This and other potential drug–nutrient interactions are listed in Table 23-8.

*Vitamin K* Phytonadione (vitamin $K_1$) is present in many vegetables. Menaquinone (vitamin $K_2$) is a product of bacterial metabolism, and the colonic bacteria may be able to synthesize about 2 μg/kg of body weight per day of the vitamin. Menadione (vitamin $K_3$) is a synthetic compound that is two to three times as potent as the natural vitamin K. Several proteins in the body depend on vitamin K for hepatic synthesis, including factors II (prothrombin), VII, IX, and X of the plasma-clotting cascade.

Function Vitamin K has two roles in normal physiology. First, it promotes the synthesis of clotting factors II, VII, IX, and X in the liver. Second, it activates these factors, along with the anticoagulation proteins C and S. The clotting factors remain inactive in the liver in the presence of warfarin or in the absence of vitamin K. When vitamin K is administered, normal activity of the clotting factors resumes.

Dietary Sources See Table 23-6.

Deficiency The mean dietary intake of vitamin K is approximately 90 μg daily.[35] Moreover, microbiologic flora of the normal gut synthesize enough menaquinone to supply a significant part of the body's requirement for vitamin K. Thus, there is a low incidence of deficiency among healthy, well-nourished individuals. Interference with bile production or secretion may contribute to a vitamin K deficiency because the absorption of vitamin K requires bile in the small intestine. Malabsorption syndromes and bowel resections may decrease vitamin K absorption. Liver disease may also cause symptoms of vitamin K deficiency if hepatic production of the prothrombin-clotting factor is decreased. Other potential causes of deficiency include intestinal disease or resection; and chronic, broad-spectrum antibiotic therapy. A deficiency may be evidenced by unusual bleeding and demonstrated by a prolonged prothrombin time (PT).

Dose/DRI The 2001 DRI values for vitamin K are listed in Table 23-3. Vitamin $K_1$ (phytonadione) is FDA approved for use in neonates at birth (one dose of 1 mg) to prevent hemorrhaging. This dose is necessary because placental transport of vitamin K is low and the neonate has yet to acquire the intestinal microflora that produce the vitamin. Other approved uses include the prevention and treatment of hypoprothrombinemia caused by drug-induced deficiency and the treatment of hemorrhage.[27] A UL for vitamin K has not been established.

Safety Considerations Even in large amounts over an extended period, vitamin K does not produce toxic manifestations.

Consistent dietary intake of vitamin K (70 to 140 μg daily) does not usually interfere with warfarin anticoagulant activity. However, sudden changes in the dietary intake of vitamin K can significantly alter the patient's PT and INR.[28] Other potential drug interactions with this vitamin are listed in Table 23-8.

*Vitamin C (Ascorbic Acid)* Vitamin C is the most easily destroyed of all the vitamins as it is sensitive to heat, oxygen, and alkaline environments. Although a relatively simple compound, it is a powerful reducing agent that serves to protect the capillary basement membrane.

Function Vitamin C is necessary for the biosynthesis of hydroxyproline, a precursor of collagen, osteoid, and dentin. It also assists in the absorption of nonheme iron from food by reducing the ferric iron in the stomach. However, use of vitamin C supplementation with iron is generally not necessary for patients taking adequate iron supplementation.

Large doses of vitamin C (500 to 1000 mg daily) have been promoted to prevent the common cold. However, such claims are largely unsupported by well-designed controlled clinical studies.[18,26] Consumption of five servings or more of fruits and vegetables daily (≥200 mg vitamin C) has been associated with a lower incidence of cancer, including cancer of the oral cavity, esophagus, stomach, colon, and lung. In contrast, similar doses of vitamin C taken as a supplement have not shown reduced risk of colorectal and stomach cancer.[36]

Dietary Sources Vitamin C has been called the "fresh-food" vitamin, and most of the daily intake is derived from vegetables and fruit sources (Table 23-6).

Deficiency Characteristics of vitamin C deficiency include fatigue, capillary hemorrhages and petechiae, swollen hemorrhagic gums, and bone changes. A deficiency may also impair wound healing. A profound dietary deficiency can eventually lead to scurvy, producing widespread capillary hemorrhaging and a weakening of collagenous structures.

Scurvy is rare in the United States. It develops only with chronically inadequate consumption of vitamin C. Infants who are fed artificial formulas without vitamin supplements may develop symptoms of scurvy. In adults, however, scurvy occurs only after 3 to 5 months on a diet free of vitamin C.

Dose/DRI Practitioners are rarely confronted with overt symptoms of vitamin C deficiency. Only 10 mg/day of vitamin C prevents scurvy; a normal diet containing fresh fruits and vegetables contains many times this amount. The DRI values for vitamin C are listed in Table 23-3. Supplementation of 100 to 125 mg daily is recommended for smokers, on the basis of higher daily ascorbic acid losses observed in these individuals.[18,36] The UL for vitamin C is 2 g/day.

Most adult multivitamin supplements contain vitamin C 60 to 100 mg, an appropriate level to consume if supplements are required. A dose greater than 200 mg/day is rarely indicated because the body will excrete most of a dose above this level. In patients with a severe vitamin C deficiency, as evidenced by clinical signs of scurvy, vitamin C 100 to 300 mg daily for at least 2 weeks is recommended to replenish body stores.[27] Infants who do not have vitamin C supplements in their formula should receive 40 to 50 mg/day; those who are breast-fed by well-nourished mothers will receive a sufficient amount. If a supplement is warranted, the practitioner may recommend a multivitamin product containing vitamin C 60 to 200 mg to be taken once a day. Vitamin C is FDA approved for use in the prevention and treatment of scurvy and to acidify the urine.[27]

Safety Considerations The practitioner is urged to weigh the relative risks and benefits of ascorbic acid therapy. Short-term use to promote healing in potentially deficient patients may warrant a trial of ascorbic acid with medical supervision. Megadoses, however, may cause nausea, stomach cramps, diarrhea, and nephrolithiasis. Ascorbic acid toxicity can also lead to hemolysis in patients deficient in glucose 6-phosphate dehydrogenase. Rebound scurvy has occurred on sudden withdrawal of ascorbic acid in infants whose mothers took megadoses of vitamin C during pregnancy. Patients with diabetes mellitus, recurrent renal calculi, or renal dysfunction should avoid prolonged use of high-dose vitamin C supplementation.

Vitamin C therapy causes acidification of the urine, resulting in enhanced reabsorption of acidic drugs from the renal tubules and higher, more prolonged blood levels of these agents. Conversely, basic drugs such as tricyclic antidepressants and amphetamines may be excreted more rapidly from acidified urine, and their effect may be reduced by ascorbic acid therapy. The clinical significance of the effects of ascorbic acid on the reabsorption and elimination of acidic and basic drugs is controversial because the ascorbic acid–induced decrease in urine pH has been shown to be small. Nevertheless, patients should be monitored if they are on medications eliminated by renal excretion if megadose ascorbic acid therapy is initiated.

*Vitamin $B_{12}$ (Cyanocobalamin)* Cyanocobalamin contains a single atom of cobalt and is the most complex vitamin molecule. The term vitamin $B_{12}$ refers to all cobalamins that have vitamin activity in humans. Cyanocobalamin, the common pharmaceutical form of the vitamin, is also the most stable of the cobalamins.

Function Vitamin $B_{12}$ is active in all cells, especially those in the bone marrow, the central nervous system (CNS), and the GI tract. It is also involved in fat, protein, and carbohydrate metabolism. A cobalamin coenzyme functions in the synthesis of DNA, and in the synthesis and transfer of single-carbon units (e.g., the methyl group in the synthesis of methionine and choline). Vitamin $B_{12}$ participates in methylation reactions and cell division, usually in concert with folic acid. It is necessary for the metabolism of folates; therefore, a folate deficiency may be observed as a feature of vitamin $B_{12}$ deficiency. Vitamin $B_{12}$ is also necessary for the metabolism of lipids and formation of myelin.

Vitamin $B_{12}$ has been studied in relation to elevated levels of homocysteine, an amino acid that requires vitamins $B_{12}$, $B_6$, and folate as cofactors for metabolism. Hyperhomocysteinanemia has been identified as an independent risk factor for Alzheimer's disease (promoted by cerebrovascular disease) as well as cardiovascular disease.[37] Although vitamin $B_{12}$ supplementation has not shown a significant effect on homocysteine levels in healthy volunteers, it may be effective in some patients with low vitamin $B_{12}$ levels.[38]

Dietary Sources Vitamin B12 is found almost exclusively in animal protein (Table 23-6).

Deficiency In healthy individuals who have not restricted their diets, cyanocobalamin deficiency is rare. Vitamin $B_{12}$ deficiency may be caused by poor absorption or utilization, or by an increased requirement or excretion of this vitamin. Because the body conserves vitamin $B_{12}$, approximately 3 years is required for the deficiency to develop. In patients with malabsorption (e.g., those with ileal diseases, intestinal resection, or gastrectomy), the reabsorption phase of the enterohepatic cycle is affected, and the deficiency may occur much earlier. Patients with atrophic gastritis, a condition that occurs in 10% to 30% of those 50 years or older, are at increased risk of pernicious anemia caused by inadequate production of intrinsic factor, which is essential for vitamin $B_{12}$ absorption. A more common cause of $B_{12}$ deficiency in older adults is the inability to absorb food-bound $B_{12}$. In addition, reduced intestinal motility, achlorhydria, and gastric acid-lowering agents contribute to bacterial overgrowth in the small intestine, and these microorganisms utilize available vitamin $B_{12}$.[38] For these reasons, vitamin $B_{12}$ supplementation is recommended from either fortified foods or a dietary supplement for this age group.[10,16]

Vegetarians who do not consume any animal products are also at risk for developing a vitamin $B_{12}$ deficiency, including infants breast-fed by vegetarian mothers. Vitamin $B_{12}$ supplementation should be encouraged for these patients.

The symptoms of a vitamin $B_{12}$ deficiency mimic those of a folate deficiency and are manifested in organ systems with rapidly duplicating cells. Thus, one effect of such a deficiency on the hematopoietic system is macrocytic anemia. The GI tract is also affected, with glossitis and epithelial changes occurring along the entire digestive tract. Some people lack the glycoprotein (intrinsic factor) necessary for absorbing vitamin $B_{12}$, resulting in pernicious anemia. Because vitamin $B_{12}$ is necessary for the maintenance of myelin, deficiency states produce many neurologic symptoms: paresthesia, peripheral neuropathy, unsteadiness, poor muscular coordination, mental confusion, agitation, hallucinations, and overt psychosis.

The practitioner should caution patients that an accurate diagnosis of the causes of a suspected anemia is essential in selecting effective treatment. For example, anemia resulting from a folic acid deficiency should be treated with folic acid, pernicious anemia should be treated with vitamin $B_{12}$, and iron-deficiency anemia should be treated with iron. Practitioners should avoid use of a "shotgun" antianemia preparation that contains multiple hematinic factors.

Dose/DRI The DRI values for vitamin $B_{12}$ are listed in Table 23-3. Oral forms can be used if the deficiency is caused by inadequate intake; intramuscular or deep subcutaneous administration is often necessary for deficiencies caused by malabsorption. Vitamin $B_{12}$ is FDA approved for use in the treatment of pernicious anemia and vitamin $B_{12}$ deficiency. Other approved uses include supplementation during periods of increased requirements such as pregnancy, thyrotoxicosis, hemorrhage, malignancy, liver disease, or kidney disease.[27] A UL has not been established for cyanocobalamin.

Hydroxocobalamin is a longer-acting form equal in hematopoietic effect to cyanocobalamin. Because it is more extensively bound to proteins at the site of injection and in plasma, renal excretion is slower, and the vitamin remains in the body for a longer period.

Safety Considerations Excessive doses have not resulted in toxicity, nor has any benefit been reported from nondeficient patients taking large quantities of the vitamin. Certain drugs may impair absorption of vitamin $B_{12}$ (Table 23-8). In fact, vitamin $B_{12}$ deficiency has been reported after 3 months of metformin therapy.[39]

*Folic Acid (Pteroylglutamic Acid, Folate)* Function Folates are reduced in vivo to the bioactive form, tetrahydrofolic acid, and are involved in the biosynthesis of purines and pyrimidines. Folic acid is further biotransformed in the body, and is involved in DNA synthesis and red blood cell maturation. The function of folic acid is closely related to that of vitamin $B_{12}$. A folic acid deficiency can occur as a consequence of vitamin $B_{12}$ deficiency. Low plasma levels of folate, vitamin $B_6$, and vitamin $B_{12}$ have been linked with elevated levels of homocysteine, which may increase the risk of coronary artery disease and Alzheimer's disease.[37] Folate supplementation in particular has been shown to reduce homocysteine levels.[26,38] More studies evaluating the relationship between homocysteine levels and vascular disease are currently underway.

Dietary Sources Folates are present in nearly all natural foods. Primary food sources are listed in Table 23-6. Folates are heat labile and the folic acid content of food depends on how the food is processed. Canning, long exposure to heat, and extensive refining may destroy 50% to 100% of naturally occurring folic acid in a given food. Many commercially prepared carbohydrate foods (e.g., breads, pasta) are now fortified with folic acid.

Deficiency The requirements for folic acid are related to metabolic rate and cell turnover, and increased amounts of folic acid are needed during pregnancy, lactation, and infancy. Infection, hemolytic anemias, and blood loss (in which red blood cell production must be increased to replenish blood supply), and hypermetabolic states such as hyperthyroidism also increase folic acid requirements. Because folic acid deficiency has been associated with an increased risk of neural tube defects in newborns, supplementation for all women anticipating a pregnancy is recommended.

Causes of folic acid deficiency include alcoholism, malabsorption, food faddism, and liver disease. Iatrogenic causes are associated with the administration of various therapeutic agents such as dihydrofolate reductase inhibitors (e.g., methotrexate, trimethoprim), anticonvulsants, and sulfasalazine.[27]

A deficiency of folic acid results in impaired cell division and protein synthesis. Symptoms of folic acid deficiency are similar to those of vitamin $B_{12}$ deficiency, including sore mouth, diarrhea, and CNS symptoms such as irritability and forgetfulness. The most common laboratory-identified feature of folic acid deficiency is megaloblastic anemia, an anemia characterized by large erythroblasts circulating in the blood.

Because vitamin $B_{12}$ is essential for the metabolism of folates, a megaloblastic anemia responsive to folic acid administration is a feature of pernicious anemia. Folic acid given without vitamin $B_{12}$ to patients with pernicious anemia will correct the anemia but will have no effect on the more insidious damage to the CNS, characterized by lack of coordination, impaired sense of position, and various behavioral disturbances. Because of the potential for folic acid to mask the signs, but not the progression, of pernicious anemia (which is caused by a vitamin $B_{12}$ deficiency), products containing more than 0.4 mg of folic acid per dose are available only by prescription. Patients with suspected anemia should receive an appropriate medical evaluation for the cause of anemia rather than an empiric combination antianemia preparation.

Dose/DRI The DRI values for folic acid are listed in Table 23-3. Folate is FDA approved for use in the treatment of megaloblastic anemias caused by folate deficiency associated with tropical and nontropical sprue, nutritional anemias, pregnancy, infancy, or lactation. Folate is also approved for prophylactic use against neural tube defects of the newborn.[27]

The absorption of folate from food is significantly lower than that of synthetic folic acid.[10,20] Recommendations for women of childbearing age are synthetic folic acid 400 μg daily from fortified foods and/or dietary supplementation in addition to the folate obtained from food.[20]

The supplemental dose of folic acid for correction of a deficiency is usually 1 mg/day, particularly if the deficiency occurs with conditions that may increase the folate requirement or suppress red blood cell formation (e.g., pregnancy, hypermetabolic states, alcoholism, or hemolytic anemia). Doses larger than the UL of 1 mg/day are not necessary except in some life-threatening hematologic diseases. Maintenance therapy for deficiencies may be stopped after 1 to 4 months if the diet contains at least one fresh fruit or vegetable daily. For chronic malabsorption diseases, folic acid treatment may be lifelong and parenteral doses may be required.

Safety Considerations Folic acid toxicity is virtually nonexistent because of its water solubility and rapid excretion. Doses up to 15 mg have been given daily without toxic effect. Several drugs taken chronically may increase the need for folic acid (Table 23-8).

*Niacin (Nicotinic Acid)* The physiologically active form of niacin is niacinamide. Niacin and niacinamide are constituents of the coenzymes nicotinamide adenine dinucleotide and nicotinamide adenine dinucleotide phosphate.

Function The niacin coenzymes are electron transfer agents; that is, they accept or donate hydrogen in the aerobic respiration of all body cells. Niacin is unusual as a vitamin in that humans can synthesize it from dietary tryptophan, with about 60 mg of tryptophan being equivalent to 1 mg of niacin. Most individuals receive about 50% of their niacin requirement from tryptophan-containing proteins and the rest as preformed niacin or niacinamide. In therapeutic doses, niacin will lower triglycerides and low-density lipoprotein cholesterol by mechanisms unrelated to its function as an essential micronutrient.

Dietary Sources See Table 23-6.

Deficiency The classic and only described niacin deficiency state is pellagra. Pellagra is rare, occurring most often in alcoholics, poorly nourished persons of advanced age, and individuals on bizarre diets that restrict sources of niacin. It may occur in areas where much corn is eaten because niacin in corn may be bound to undigestible constituents, making it unavailable. Other causes of pellagra include isoniazid therapy and decreased tryptophan conversion, as in Hartnup disease and carcinoid tumors.

Clinical findings of niacin deficiency include the "three Ds" of *d*ermatitis, *d*iarrhea, and *d*ementia, often accompanied by neuropathy, glossitis, stomatitis, and proctitis. Patients manifest a characteristic rash. The skin over the face and on pressure points may become thickened or hyperpigmented, or it may appear burned. Secondary infections may occur in such lesions. The entire GI tract is generally affected, with angular fissures around the mouth and atrophy of the epithelium. Inflammation of the small intestine may be associated with episodes of occult bleeding and/or diarrhea.

Dose/DRI The DRI values for niacin are listed in Table 23-3. The recommended UL for this vitamin is 35 mg/day.[11]

Niacin requirements are increased when the patient has an acute illness; when the patient is convalescing after a severe injury, infection, or burn; when the patient has substantially increased caloric expenditure or dietary caloric intake; or when the patient has a low tryptophan intake (e.g., a low-protein diet or a high intake of corn as a staple in the diet). The FDA-approved use of niacin, but not niacinamide, is for adjunctive treatment of hyperlipidemia and hypercholesterolemia. Both niacin and niacinamide are approved for the prevention and treatment of pellagra.[27]

Treatment of pellagra involves the ingestion of niacinamide or niacin 150 to 500 mg daily in divided doses. Niacin has been used in daily dosages of 1 to 2 g three times per day, up to 8 g/day, to treat hypercholesterolemia and hyperlipidemias. Niacin treatment increases beneficial high-density lipoprotein cholesterol and decreases levels of potentially harmful triglycerides, total cholesterol, and low-density lipoprotein cholesterol. Niacin treatment of hyperlipidemias requires close medical supervision for evidence of effectiveness and manifestations of drug-induced toxicity.

Safety Considerations Niacin toxicity can involve GI symptoms (e.g., nausea, vomiting, diarrhea), hepatotoxicity, skin lesions, tachycardia, and hypertension. Patients should be forewarned that therapeutic doses of niacin may cause flushing and a sensation of warmth, especially around the face, neck, and ears. This reaction, which many people experience especially on initiation of therapy, may be diminished if they take aspirin 325 mg or ibuprofen 200 mg 30 minutes before the niacin dose, provided there are no contraindications. Itching or tingling and headache may also occur. All these effects will usually subside or decrease in intensity within 2 weeks of continued therapy. If niacin causes GI upset, it should be taken with meals. Niacinamide does not produce the discomforting side effects associated with therapeutic doses of niacin; however, it does not have a beneficial lowering effect on plasma lipids.

Potential drug–nutrient interactions with niacin are listed in Table 23-8.

Because of the adverse effects on the GI tract, high doses of niacin are contraindicated in patients with gastritis or peptic ulcer disease. Niacin can provoke the release of histamine, so its use in patients with asthma should be undertaken carefully. Niacin may also impair liver function, disturb glucose tolerance, and cause hyperuricemia. Patients prescribed therapeutic doses of this nutrient must be monitored regularly for potential adverse effects.

*Pantothenic Acid* Pantothenic acid is a water-soluble vitamin of the B-complex family.

Function Pantothenic acid is a precursor of coenzyme A (CoA), a product that is active in many biological reactions and plays a primary role in cholesterol, steroid, and fatty acid synthesis. Pantothenic acid is important for acetylation reactions and the formation of citric acid for the Krebs cycle, and it is crucial in the intraneuronal synthesis of acetylcholine. It is also important in gluconeogenesis; in the synthesis and degradation of fatty acids; in the synthesis of sterols, steroid hormones, and porphyrins; and in the release of energy from carbohydrates.

Dietary Sources Pantothenic acid is widely distributed in foods (Table 23-6).

Deficiency Because pantothenic acid is contained in many foods, deficiency states are rare and hard to detect. In malabsorption syndromes, it is difficult to separate pantothenic acid deficiency symptoms from those of other deficiencies. Symptoms of pantothenic acid deficiency include the following: somnolence, fatigue, cardiovascular instability, GI complaints, and paresthesia of hands and/or feet followed by hyperreflexia and muscular weakness in the legs. Administration of pharmacologic doses of pantothenic acid reverses these symptoms and has even been used to eliminate burning feet syndrome.

Dose/DRI AI values for this vitamin are listed in Table 23-3. There is no established UL for pantothenic acid.

Safety Considerations Pantothenic acid is generally considered nontoxic, even in large doses. Doses as high as 10 g of calcium pantothenate daily have been given to young men for 6 weeks with no toxic symptoms. However, ingestion of more than 20 g has been reported to result in diarrhea and water retention.

Significant drug–nutrient interactions with pantothenic acid have not been reported.

*Vitamin $B_6$ (Pyridoxine)* This water-soluble vitamin exists in three forms: pyridoxine (vitamin $B_6$), pyridoxal, and pyridoxamine. Although all three forms are equally effective in nutrition, pyridoxine hydrochloride is the form most often used in vitamin formulations.

Function Vitamin $B_6$ serves as a cofactor for more than 60 enzymes, including decarboxylases, synthetases, transaminases, and hydroxylases. It is important in heme production and in the metabolism of homocysteine. As previously stated, hyperhomocysteinemia is a potential risk factor for coronary artery and cerebrovascular disease, and it has been shown to respond particularly to folic acid supplementation but also to vitamin $B_6$. Whether or not the impact of these nutrients on homocysteine levels results in improved outcomes has yet to be determined.[37] Vitamin $B_6$ has also been suggested as a potential treatment of carpal tunnel syndrome, premenstrual syndrome (PMS), depression, and migraine. Unfortunately, no clinical research evidence supports use of vitamin $B_6$ for these ailments.[40]

Dietary Sources See Table 23-6 for food sources; cooking destroys some vitamin $B_6$.

Deficiency Causes of vitamin $B_6$ deficiency include alcoholism, severe diarrheal syndromes, food faddism, malabsorption syndromes, drugs (isoniazid, hydralazine, penicillamine, and cycloserine), and genetic diseases (cystathioninuria and xanthinuric aciduria).

The symptoms of severe vitamin $B_6$ deficiency in infants include irritability and convulsive disorders. Treatment with vitamin $B_6$ hydrochloride (2 mg/day for infants) generally normalizes the electroencephalogram and resolves clinical symptoms. Symptoms in adults whose diets are deficient in vitamin $B_6$ or who have been given a vitamin $B_6$ antagonist are difficult to distinguish from symptoms of niacin and riboflavin deficiencies. These symptoms include pellagralike dermatitis; oral lesions; peripheral neuropathy; scaliness around the nose, mouth, and eyes; and dulling of mentation. Serious deficiency symptoms include convulsions, peripheral neuritis, and sideroblastic anemia.

Dose/DRI DRI values for vitamin $B_6$ are listed in Table 23-3. The FDA-approved use of this vitamin is for treatment of vitamin $B_6$ deficiency, including drug-induced deficiency as seen with isoniazid.[27] Daily doses up to 250 mg of vitamin $B_6$ have been used in the treatment of hyperhomocysteinemia.[38] However, the UL for this vitamin is 100 mg/day for adults and patients of advanced age.[20]

Treatment of sideroblastic anemia requires 50 to 200 mg/day of pyridoxine hydrochloride to aid production of hemoglobin and erythrocytes. At least five vitamin $B_6$– dependent inborn errors of metabolism have been shown to respond to large doses of vitamin $B_6$.

Safety Considerations Vitamin $B_6$ may be toxic in high doses. A severe sensory neuropathy, similar to that observed with the deficiency state, has been reported when gram quantities were taken to relieve symptoms of PMS. Similar symptoms have been reported in women taking doses as small as 50 mg/day for PMS. Recovery occurred on withdrawal of vitamin $B_6$ but it was slow.

High daily doses of vitamin $B_6$ (200 to 600 mg) inhibit prolactin. Prenatal vitamins, which contain 1 to 10 mg per dosage unit, do not appear to have a significant antiprolactin effect.

Potential drug–nutrient interactions are listed in Table 23-8.

*Riboflavin (Vitamin $B_2$)* Riboflavin is a water-soluble vitamin essential for cellular growth and maintenance of vision, mucous membranes, skin, nails, and hair.

Function Riboflavin is a constituent of two coenzymes: flavin adenine dinucleotide and flavin mononucleotide. It is involved in numerous oxidation and reduction reactions, including the cytochrome P-450 reductase enzyme system involved in drug metabolism.

Dietary Sources See Table 23-6.

Deficiency Riboflavin deficiency, although rare, may be caused by inadequate intake, alcoholism, or malabsorption syndromes. Deficiency of this vitamin may occur in association with other vitamin B-complex deficiency states (e.g., pellagra) or during pregnancy. Early signs of riboflavin deficiency may involve ocular symptoms as the eyes become light sensitive and easily fatigued. The patient may develop blurred vision; itching, watering, sore eyes, and corneal vascularization, which causes a bloodshot appearance of the eye. Clinical findings of more advanced deficiency include stomatitis, seborrheic dermatitis, and magenta tongue.

Dose/DRI The DRI values for riboflavin are listed in Table 23-3. The need for riboflavin appears to increase during periods of increased cell growth, such as during pregnancy and wound healing. Absorption is enhanced when taken with food. Alternatively, riboflavin may be injected intramuscularly or given intravenously as a component of an injectable multivitamin. The FDA-approved use of riboflavin is in the prevention of riboflavin deficiency and the treatment of ariboflavinosis.[27] No UL has been determined for this vitamin.

High-dose riboflavin (400 mg daily) may be effective in the prevention of migraine. One randomized controlled trial in 55 adult patients showed significantly reduced incidence and duration of migraine attacks compared with placebo after 3 months of prophylactic therapy.[41] Another small study suggested this same high-dose riboflavin therapy was equal to β-blockers in reducing the frequency of migraines.[42] Further study on riboflavin therapy for migraine prevention is warranted.

Safety Considerations The use of riboflavin may cause a yellow-orange fluorescence or discoloration of the urine. Patients who report this effect should be reassured that this color is normal. There is no known toxicity level, and no significant drug interactions have been reported for riboflavin.

*Thiamin (Vitamin $B_1$)* Thiamin is a water-soluble, B-complex vitamin available in oral tablet and injectable dosage forms.

Function Thiamin's active form, thiamin pyrophosphate (formerly known as cocarboxylase), plays a vital role in the oxidative decarboxylation of pyruvic acid; in the formation of acetyl CoA, which enters the Krebs cycle; and in other important biochemical conversion cycles. Thiamin is necessary for myocardial function, nerve cell function, and carbohydrate metabolism. The amount of thiamin required increases with increased carbohydrate consumption.

Dietary Sources Dietary sources highest in thiamin are listed in Table 23-6. The thiamin content of food can be destroyed by heat, oxidation, and an alkaline environment but is stable through frozen storage.

Deficiency The primary causes of thiamin deficiency are generally inadequate diet, alcoholism, malabsorption syndromes, prolonged diarrhea, increased requirements (pregnancy), or food faddism.

Thiamin deficiency in the United States is found primarily in alcoholics. Not only is their diet often nutritionally deficient, but alcohol ingestion also impairs thiamin absorption and transport across the intestine, and increases the rate of destruction of thiamin diphosphate. Thiamin deficiency, also known as beriberi, may present with neuromuscular symptoms such as peripheral neuritis, weakness, and Wernicke's encephalopathy. Cardiac dysfunction may also be observed, possibly accompanied by edema, tachycardia on minimal exertion, enlarged heart, and electrocardiographic abnormalities. Because of these risks, a vitamin supplement containing thiamin should be prescribed for the alcoholic patient.

Dose/DRI The DRI values for thiamin are listed in Table 23-3. To treat the symptoms of heart failure caused by a thiamin deficiency, the patient should take thiamin 5 to 10 mg three times daily. At this dosage, the failure is rapidly corrected, but the neurologic signs correct much more slowly. The FDA-approved use of thiamin is for the treatment of thiamin deficiency.[27]

Safety Considerations The kidney easily clears excessive thiamin intake, and oral doses of 500 mg have been found to be nontoxic.

Diuretics have been shown to increase the urinary excretion of thiamin. Therefore, patients on chronic diuretic therapy, such as those with congestive heart failure or hypertension, may be at risk of subclinical thiamin deficiency and its associated cardiovascular complications. While the effect of thiamin supplementation in this patient population has yet to be evaluated, recommending supplementation with 100% of the DRI for this vitamin would be reasonable.[43]

*Biotin (Vitamin H)* Biotin is included in several multivitamin preparations.

Function Biotin, a member of the B-complex group of vitamins, is required for various metabolic functions, including carbohydrate, fat, and amino acid metabolism. Several biotin-dependent enzymes are now known to exist.

Dietary Sources Food sources of biotin are listed in Table 23-6. In addition to food sources, colonic flora probably synthesize a considerable amount of biotin, which is then absorbed from the large intestine into the bloodstream.

Deficiency Deficiency states of biotin are rare but appear to result in symptoms of nausea, vomiting, lassitude, muscle pain, anorexia, anemia, and depression. Dermatitis, a grayish color of the skin, and glossitis may be among the physical findings; hypercholesterolemia and cardiac abnormalities may also occur.

Biotin deficiency in humans can be caused by ingesting a large number of raw egg whites. Raw egg white contains avidin, a protein that binds biotin, thereby preventing its absorption. Individuals undergoing a rapid weight-loss program with intense caloric restriction or those with chronic malabsorption may not be obtaining adequate biotin and should receive supplementation.

Dose/DRI See Table 23-3.

Safety Considerations Adverse effects have not been reported with biotin therapy.

### Vitaminlike Compounds and Pseudovitamins

Vitaminlike compounds, or pseudovitamins, are substances that have a chemical structure very similar to that of vitamins but lack the usual physiologic or biochemical actions. That is, they are not essential for specific body functions of growth, maintenance, and reproduction.

*L-Carnitine* Carnitine, a vitaminlike molecule, can be synthesized from lysine and methionine in the liver and kidney. Thus, it is considered an essential nutrient but not necessarily a vitamin.

Function L-Carnitine is required to transport long-chain fatty acids into mitochondria, which is prerequisite to their β-oxidation and maintenance of energy production. Although carnitine is biosynthesized adequately by adults, newborns have a low capacity for carnitine synthesis from lysine and methionine. Newborns may be further compromised if fed soy formulas or maintained on total parenteral nutrition without supplemental carnitine.

Dietary Sources Dietary sources and synthesis in the liver and kidney satisfy the primary need for carnitine. Food sources are listed in Table 23-6.

Deficiency Carnitine deficiency may be evidenced by muscle weakness, cardiomyopathy, abnormal hepatic function, decreased ketogenesis, hypertriglyceridemia, and hypoglycemia during fasting. Lipids may accumulate between muscle fibers and in the liver. Rarely, valproic acid can induce carnitine deficiency; thus, carnitine is sometimes given with valproic acid, particularly if there are liver function abnormalities. Carnitine deficiency has been reported in adults with liver disease and in preterm infants fed formulas low in carnitine. Also, a deficiency state may be seen in patients with end-stage renal disease as carnitine may be removed by hemodialysis.[26]

Dose/DRI Human carnitine deficiency has been documented, but a DRI has not been established. Oral levocarnitine (L-carnitine) is FDA-approved for use in carnitine deficiency.[20]

Safety Considerations L-Carnitine is without appreciable adverse effects in healthy adults, and oral doses of 15 g/day have been well tolerated. However, new-onset and increased frequency of seizures has been observed with oral and intravenous L-carnitine administration in patients at risk.[27] No drug interactions have been reported for this pseudovitamin.

*Choline* Choline is contained in most living cells and in foods. It is usually present in the form of phosphatidylcholine, commonly known as lecithin, and in several other phospholipids found in cell membranes. Intestinal mucosal cells and pancreatic secretions contain enzymes capable of splitting phospholipids to release choline. Choline is also found in sphingomyelin and is highly concentrated in nervous tissue.

Function Choline, a precursor in the biosynthesis of acetylcholine, is an important donor of methyl groups used in the biochemical formation of other substances in vivo. It can be biosynthesized in humans. Furthermore, choline and inositol are considered to be lipotropic agents (i.e., agents involved in the mobilization of lipids). They have been used to treat fatty liver and abnormal fat metabolism, but their efficacy has not been established.

Dietary Sources Although choline is found in food sources, it is also synthesized in the body. Therefore, it is doubtful that choline is a vitamin. Choline is obtained from the diet as either choline or lecithin. Food sources are listed in Table 23-6.

Deficiency A deficiency state has not been identified in humans, possibly because choline is readily available in the diet and synthesized in the body.

Dose/DRI See Table 23-3 for DRI values. An average diet furnishes 400 to 900 mg of choline daily. The recommended UL for choline is 3.5 g/day.[17,20]

Safety Considerations The administration of large doses of lecithin has been associated with sweating, GI distress, vomiting, and diarrhea. No drug interactions have been reported.

**TABLE 23-9 Selected Calcium Supplements**

| Trade Name | Primary Ingredients |
|---|---|
| Caltrate 600 + D High Potency Tablets | Elemental calcium 600 mg (as carbonate); vitamin D 200 IU |
| Citracal + D Caplets | Elemental calcium 315 mg (as citrate); vitamin D 200 IU |
| Os-Cal 500 + D Tablets | Elemental calcium 500 mg (as carbonate); vitamin D 125 IU |
| Posture Tablets | Elemental calcium 600 mg (as tribasic phosphate) |
| Tums 500 Chewable Tablets | Elemental calcium 500 mg (as carbonate) |

*Taurine (Aminoethanesulfonate)* Along with carnitine and choline, taurine has been referred to as a vitaminlike compound. The most common dietary source of taurine is human breast milk. It is now considered important enough to be included in human infant formulas, enteral products, and parenteral nutritional solutions for pediatric or neonatal patients (see Chapter 26).

## Minerals

Minerals constitute about 4% of body weight. These micronutrients are present in the body in a diverse array of organic compounds (e.g., phosphoproteins, phospholipids, hemoglobin, and thyroxine). They function as constituents of many enzymes, hormones, vitamins, and inorganic compounds (e.g., sodium chloride, potassium chloride, calcium, and phosphorus), which are present as free ions. Different body tissues contain various quantities of different minerals. For example, bone has a high content of calcium, phosphorus, and magnesium; soft tissue has a high quantity of potassium. Minerals are involved in regulating cell membrane permeability, osmotic pressure, and acid-base and water balance. In addition, certain ions act as the mediators of action potential conduction and neurotransmitter action.

A well-balanced diet is required to maintain proper mineral balance. Optimal mineral intake values for humans are still imprecise; only AIs are available for trace element minerals such as chromium, fluoride, and manganese. Similarly, the possible adverse effects of long-term ingestion of high-dose mineral supplements are often unknown, and high doses of one mineral can decrease the bioavailability of other minerals and vitamins.

*Calcium* The most abundant cation in the body is calcium (about 1200 g). Approximately 99% of calcium is present in the skeleton, and the remaining 1% is present in the extracellular fluid, intracellular structures, and cell membranes. Calcium is a major component of bones and teeth. The calcium content in bone is continuously undergoing a process of resorption and formation. In people of advanced age, the resorption process predominates over formation, and a decrease in calcium absorption efficiency results in a gradual loss of bone density that leads to osteoporosis. This effect can be minimized by encouraging optimal calcium intake throughout the life cycle as well as regular participation in weight-bearing exercise.

Function Calcium is important for several reasons. It activates a number of enzymes and is required for acetylcholine synthesis. Calcium increases cell membrane permeability, aids in vitamin $B_{12}$ absorption, regulates muscle contraction and relaxation, and catalyzes several steps in the activation of plasma-clotting factors. Calcium is also necessary for the functional integrity of many cells, especially those of the neuromuscular and cardiovascular system.

The small intestine controls calcium absorption. Patients ingesting relatively low amounts of calcium absorb proportionately more, and patients taking large amounts of calcium excrete more as fecal calcium.

Dietary Sources Dietary sources of calcium are listed in Table 23-6. Teenagers experiencing rapid growth and bone maturation need to consume adequate calcium through dairy products, especially milk, or through a nutritional supplement. Adults can easily meet calcium AI levels by incorporating dairy products into their diets daily. Nonfat milk contains about 300 mg of calcium per 8 oz. As an alternative, calcium supplements are usually well tolerated in daily doses of less than 2 g. Table 23-9 lists selected tradename calcium supplements.

Practitioners should evaluate the dietary intake of calcium, including calcium-fortified foods, before recommending daily calcium supplementation. Calcium fortification is found in numerous nontraditional sources such as juices, breads, and breakfast bars. Dietary factors that increase calcium absorption from supplements or foods include avoiding intake with bran, whole-grain cereals, or high oxalate foods (e.g., cocoa, soybeans, spinach) and obtaining adequate vitamin D.

Deficiency Decreased calcium levels may have profound and diverse consequences, including convulsions, tetany, behavioral and personality disorders, mental and growth retardation, and bone deformities (the most common being rickets in children and osteomalacia in adults). Changes that occur in osteomalacia include softening of bones, rheumatic-type pain in the bones of the legs and lower back, general weakness with difficulty walking, and spontaneous fractures. Common causes of hypocalcemia and associated skeletal disorders are as follows: malabsorption syndromes; hypoparathyroidism; vitamin D deficiency; renal failure with impaired activation of vitamin D; long-term anticonvulsant therapy (with increased breakdown of vitamin D); and decreased dietary intake of calcium, particularly during periods of growth, pregnancy, and lactation and among people of advanced age.

Dose/DRI The AIs for calcium are listed in Table 23-4. Oral calcium supplements are FDA approved for use in the treatment and prevention of calcium deficiency, which may result in rickets, osteomalacia, or osteoporosis. Other FDA-approved uses include treatment of acid indigestion and hyperphosphatemia associated with end-stage renal disease.[27] The recommended UL for calcium is 2.5 g/day for all individuals older than 1 year.[20]

Calcium supplementation may be effective in the prevention of PMS. One randomized controlled multicenter trial showed that supplementation of elemental calcium 1200 mg daily for three menstrual cycles resulted in a significant reduction in PMS symptoms.[44] The American College of Obstetrics and Gynecology recommends regular calcium supplementation for women with PMS.[45]

Numerous studies have evaluated the relationship between calcium intake and the risk of colon cancer; however, the results of these studies have been inconsistent.[46] Further research to better define this relationship is currently underway.

Practitioners should counsel patients regarding potential constipation associated with calcium supplementation and the importance of adequate hydration, dietary fiber, and physical activity. In addition, calcium absorption is improved by dividing the dose into 500 mg doses to be taken two to three times daily with meals.

Recommendations for calcium intake are based on elemental calcium and not the calcium salt. Since labels can be misleading, practitioners should be familiar with the many salt forms and the different percentages of calcium in each, including carbonate (40%), citrate (21%), lactate (18%), gluconate (9%), and phosphate salts (23% to 39%). Calcium carbonate and calcium phosphate salts are insoluble, and should be taken with meals to enhance absorption, which is optimal in a low pH. Patients requiring supplementation who have achlorhydria or who are on histamine$_2$ antagonists or proton pump inhibitors may need to take a soluble salt (e.g., calcium citrate, calcium lactate, calcium gluconate). In conjunction with adequate calcium and vitamin D, weight-bearing exercise is essential in maintaining bone mass.

Safety Considerations Calcium in doses greater than 2 g/day can be harmful. Large amounts taken as dietary supplements or antacids can lead to high levels of calcium in the urine and to renal stones; the latter development may result in renal damage. Hypercalcemia—with associated anorexia, nausea, vomiting, constipation, and polyuria—is also possible, particularly in patients taking high-dose vitamin D preparations. Hypercalcemia can also result in an increased deposition of calcium in soft tissue.

Calcium supplementation and calcium-fortified foods may alter the absorption of several drugs. Examples of drug–nutrient interactions with calcium are listed in Table 23-8.

*Iron* Iron is widely available in the U.S. diet. Iron absorption from the intestinal tract is controlled by the body's need for iron, the intestinal lumen conditions, the food source of iron, and the food components of the meal, such as the vitamin C content.

Function Iron plays an important role in oxygen and electron transport. In the body, it is either functional or stored. Functional iron is found in hemoglobin, myoglobin, heme-containing enzymes, and transferrin, which is the transport form of iron. Stored iron is primarily found in the hemoglobin of red blood cells, which contains 60% to 70% of total body iron. The rest is stored primarily in the form of ferritin and hemosiderin in the intestinal mucosa, liver, spleen, and bone marrow.

Dietary Sources Dietary iron is available in two forms. Heme iron is found in meats and is reasonably well absorbed. Nonheme iron, such as that found in enriched grains and dark green vegetables, constitutes most of dietary iron but is poorly absorbed. Therefore, the published values of iron content in foods are misleading, as the amount absorbed depends on the nature of the iron. Although there are specific ways to calculate the iron absorption from a given meal, the available iron content of foods is often estimated by assuming that about 10% of the total iron (heme plus nonheme) is absorbed if no iron deficiency exists. In the iron-deficient state, iron absorption improves, so as much as 20% may be absorbed and used from an average diet. However, this estimate would not be valid in the absence of heme iron.

Ingested nonheme iron, which is mostly in the form of ferric hydroxide, is solubilized in gastric juice to ferric chloride, then reduced to the ferrous form and chelated to substances such as ascorbic acid, sugars, and amino acids. Chelates have a low molecular weight and can be solubilized and absorbed before they reach the alkaline medium of the distal small intestine, where precipitation may occur. In intestinal mucosal cells, iron is stored in a protein-bound form known as ferritin. As needed, it is released into the plasma, where it is oxidized to the ferric state and bound to a β-globulin to form transferrin. When released at the spleen, liver, bone marrow, intestinal mucosa, and other iron storage sites, the iron is combined with apoferritin to form ferritin or hemosiderin. Iron is used in all cells of the body; however, most of it is incorporated into the hemoglobin of red blood cells. The major source of iron loss is through blood loss (e.g., hemorrhagic loss and menstruation). Iron is also lost from the body by the sloughing of skin cells and GI mucosal cells and by excretion of urine, sweat, and feces.

Deficiency Early symptoms of iron deficiency are vague. Pallor and easy fatigability cannot in themselves be easily related to iron deficiency. Other signs and symptoms of iron-deficiency anemia include split or "spoon-shaped" nails, sore tongue, angular stomatitis, and dyspnea on exertion. Coldness and numbness of the extremities may be reported. Hypochromic microcytosis, as evidenced by a decreased mean corpuscular volume and low hemoglobin concentrations (decreased mean corpuscular hemoglobin concentration), characterizes iron deficiency.

Iron-deficiency anemia is a widespread clinical problem and the most common form of anemia in the United States. Although it causes few deaths, it does contribute to the poor health and suboptimal performance of many people. Iron deficiency results from inadequate diet, malabsorption, pregnancy and lactation, or blood loss. Treatment with epoetin alfa combined with inadequate iron supplementation can also cause iron deficiency. Because normal iron losses through the urine, feces, and skin are minimal, and the majority of total body iron is efficiently stored and conserved (recycled), iron deficiency caused by poor diet or malabsorption develops very slowly over the course of several months.

Despite fortification of flour and educational efforts regarding proper nutrition, iron deficiency remains a problem, especially during the following four life periods:

- *During childhood under 2 years of age:* Children obtain low iron content from cow's milk.
- *During adolescence:* In addition to blood loss during menses, young women experience rapid growth, which entails an expanding red cell mass and the need for iron in myoglobin.
- *During and after pregnancy:* Women face the expanding blood volume of pregnancy, the demands of the fetus and placenta, and the blood loss of childbirth.
- *During later years:* Persons of advanced age often consume inadequate dietary iron, demonstrate compromised absorption caused by achlorhydria, and experience an increased incidence of GI tract blood loss resulting from malignancy, gastric ulceration, or use of nonsteroidal anti-inflammatory drugs.[7] However, the prevalence of elevated iron stores may be significantly greater than iron deficiency in this age group.[47] It has been suggested that high iron stores may contribute to chronic diseases such as cancer and heart disease, although research to date has been inconclusive.[3] In the absence of a confirmed diagnosis of iron-deficiency anemia, routine supplementation for this age group is not recommended.

Supplemental iron may be warranted for women with heavy and/or prolonged menstrual blood loss or patients who frequently donate blood. In addition, iron may be indicated during recovery from disease- and injury-associated blood loss. Examples include peptic ulcer disease, esophageal varices, cancer, and traumatic injury such as motor vehicle accidents.

Chronic use of drugs such as salicylates, nonsteroidal anti-inflammatory drugs, corticosteroids, or anticoagulants may cause drug-induced blood loss. This may be the result of direct irritation of the gastric mucosa or the increased bleeding tendency these medications cause. Iron supplementation should be used cautiously, if at all, with patients at high risk of GI bleeding.

Medications such as aspirin or ibuprofen may not be included on a medication record. Thus, the practitioner should routinely question the patient regarding the use of nonprescription drugs and ascertain whether the patient's problem is chronic, whether self-treatment has been tried, and whether medical evaluation for anemia or conditions that could contribute to anemia has been sought or received. Anemia in patients who are not pregnant, lactating, or menstruating or not on a meat-restricted diet may be a symptom of a more serious medical disorder. Such patients require further evaluation to determine the cause of anemia and should not simply be treated empirically. Patients who report bleeding should be immediately referred to a primary care provider. Abnormal blood loss may be indicated by (1) hematemesis or "coffee-ground" vomitus; (2) bright red blood in the stool or black, tarry stools; (3) large clots or an abnormally heavy flow during the menstrual period; or (4) cloudy or pink-red urine (if the use of drugs that may cause urine discoloration has been ruled out).

Blood loss, particularly through the stool, is not always obvious. Even when abnormal blood loss occurs, the patient may not notice or report it. Periodic testing using home occult blood test kits may be considered for certain high-risk patients.

Dose/DRI The DRI values for iron are listed in Table 23-4. Because of the GI side effects associated with oral iron supplementation, the UL for elemental iron has been set at 45 mg/day.[19] Oral iron supplements are FDA approved for the prevention and treatment of iron-deficiency anemia.[27]

In a ferrous sulfate 325 mg tablet, 20% (about 60 mg) is elemental iron. In patients with iron deficiency, 20% of the elemental iron (12 mg) may be absorbed. Because iron 36 to 48 mg daily is enough to support maximum incorporation into red blood cells and replace iron stores, the usual therapeutic dose of two to four tablets daily for 3 months is probably reasonable in treating a deficiency. If the patient has an inadequate response or if symptoms worsen during this time, the patient should consult a primary care provider. In cases of severe or chronic iron deficiency, when serious medical conditions have been ruled out, continuous maintenance doses of three to four tablets daily for approximately 3 to 6 months should normalize hemoglobin and replace iron stores, in the absence of ongoing bleeding.

If iron supplementation is appropriate, the practitioner will need to evaluate which iron product is best. The choice should be based on how well the iron preparation is absorbed and tolerated, on the amount of elemental iron per dose, and on its price. Because ferrous salts are more efficiently absorbed than ferric salts, an iron product of the ferrous group is usually appropriate. Ferrous sulfate is the standard against which other iron salts are compared. Table 23-10 lists selected trade-name iron products.

Ferrous salts may be given in combination with ascorbic acid to improve iron absorption. The practitioner can encourage the consumption of fruit or juice high in ascorbic acid or a vitamin C supplement to be taken with the iron, if necessary. Combination products with iron and ascorbic acid are also available, but these can be expensive. Chemicals that may decrease iron absorption include phosphates in eggs and milk, phytates in cereals, carbonates, oxalates, and tannins.

**TABLE 23-10 Selected Iron Supplements**

| Trade Name | Primary Ingredients |
|---|---|
| Femiron Daily Iron Supplement Tablets | Elemental iron 20 mg (as fumarate) |
| Feosol Tablets | Elemental iron 65 mg (as sulfate) |
| Fer-In-Sol Drops*†‡§ | Elemental iron 15 mg/0.6 mL (as sulfate) |
| Fer-In-Sol Syrup*†‡§ | Elemental iron 18 mg/5 mL (as sulfate) |
| Fergon Tablets | Elemental iron 27 mg (as gluconate) |
| Slow Fe Tablets¶ | Elemental iron 50 mg (as sulfate) |

*Dye-free; †lactose-free; ‡sulfite-free; §pediatric formulation; ¶sodium-free.

Iron is available in numerous salt forms and as immediate- and controlled-release products. The enteric-coated and delayed-release products are generally more expensive but may cause fewer symptoms of gastric irritation. However, since progressively less iron is absorbed as it is passed from the duodenum (the site of maximum absorption) to the ileum of the small intestine, overall iron absorption is decreased by delaying the time of release.

Safety Considerations All iron products tend to irritate the GI mucosa and may produce nausea, abdominal pain, and diarrhea. These adverse effects may be minimized by reducing the dose or by giving iron with meals; however, food may decrease the amount of iron absorbed by as much as 50%. Practitioners may want to recommend iron be initiated on an empty stomach, instructing the patient to change this routine and take the iron with food if GI side effects occur.

A frequent side effect of iron therapy is constipation. This adverse effect has prompted the formulation of iron products that also contain a stool softener (e.g., docusate). During iron therapy, stools commonly have a black, tarry appearance because of the presence of unabsorbed iron in the feces. Unfortunately, this symptom may also indicate GI blood loss and a serious medical problem. Medical evaluation is indicated if an underlying GI condition is suspected or if there is a history of GI disease. If the stool does not darken somewhat during iron therapy, however, the iron product may not have disintegrated properly or released the iron.

Iron must be dispensed and stored in a child-resistant container. Accidental poisoning with iron occurs most often in children, who are attracted to the sugar-coated, colored tablets. It can also occur from an overdose of chewable multivitamins containing iron. Such poisoning is considered a medical emergency. As few as 15 tablets of ferrous sulfate 325 mg have been lethal to children; however, recovery has followed the ingestion of as many as 70 such tablets. The clinical outcome depends on the speed and adequacy of treatment.

Symptoms of acute iron poisoning include abdominal pain, vomiting, diarrhea, electrolyte imbalances, and shock. In later stages, cardiovascular collapse may occur, especially if the cause has not been properly recognized and treated as a medical emergency. Treatment of iron toxicity may begin immediately at home after consultation with a poison control center or local emergency room.

Iron is chelated, or its solubility is altered, by many substances. Examples of drug interactions with iron are listed in Table 23-8.

*Magnesium* Magnesium, which is essential for all living cells, is the second most plentiful cation of the intracellular fluids and the fourth most abundant cation in the body. About 2000 mEq of magnesium are present in an average 70 kg adult, with about 50% of this in bone, about 45% as an intracellular cation, and about 1% to 5% in the extracellular fluid.

Function Magnesium is required for normal bone structure formation and the proper function of more than 300 enzymes, including those involved with ATP (adenosine triphosphatase)-dependent phosphorylation, protein synthesis, and carbohydrate metabolism. Extracellular magnesium is critical to both the maintenance of nerve and muscle electrical potentials and the transmission of impulses across neuromuscular junctions.

Magnesium tends to mimic calcium in its effects on the CNS and skeletal muscle. Magnesium deficiency blunts the normal response of the parathyroid glands to hypocalcemia. Thus, tetany, caused by a lack of calcium, cannot be corrected with calcium unless the hypomagnesemia is also corrected. Similarly, magnesium deficiency impairs the renal conservation of potassium, and hypokalemia cannot be corrected in the presence of magnesium deficiency.

Dietary Sources Individuals consuming fresh foods regularly should not develop magnesium deficiency because all unprocessed foods contain magnesium, albeit in widely varying amounts. Food sources highest in magnesium are listed in Table 23-6. Processing, which leads to removal of the germ and outer layers of cereal grains, results in a loss of more than 80% of the magnesium available.

Deficiency Deficiency states are usually caused by malabsorption syndromes, general malnutrition, alcoholism, and iatrogenic causes. In addition, hypomagnesemia may result from prolonged total parenteral nutrition therapy with magnesium-free formulations, hemodialysis, diabetes mellitus, pancreatitis, diuretic-induced electrolyte imbalance, and primary aldosteronism, a condition characterized by loss of body potassium, muscular weakness, and elevated blood pressure.

Symptoms of magnesium deficiency may include neuromuscular irritability, increased CNS stimulation, delirium, and convulsions.

Dose/DRI The DRI values for magnesium are listed in Table 23-4. Oral magnesium supplements are FDA approved for use in treatment and prevention of hypomagnesemia.[27] The recommended UL for this nutrient is 350 mg/day.[16,20]

Controversial uses of magnesium supplements include prophylaxis of premenstrual syndrome, migraine, and atherosclerosis as well as the treatment of asthma and hypertension.[45,48,49] Magnesium deficiency may potentially contribute to these ailments, but there is insufficient data to support oral magnesium supplementation for therapeutic use in a generally well-nourished population.

Safety Considerations No evidence is available to suggest that oral intake of magnesium is harmful to individuals with normal renal function although diarrhea may occur with large doses. Hypermagnesemia can occur with overzealous use of magnesium sulfate (Epsom salts) or magnesium hydroxide (milk of magnesia) as a laxative, or even with use of magnesium-containing antacids in patients with severe renal failure. Hypermagnesemia may cause diminished deep tendon reflexes and varying degrees of muscle weakness, lethargy, and sedation. This may progress to stupor and coma, especially at high serum concentrations. Cardiovascular symptoms may include hypotension and dysrhythmia potentially progressing to cardiac arrest.

Potential drug–nutrient interactions are listed in Table 23-8.

*Phosphorus* Phosphorus is present throughout the body, but approximately 85% of the body's store is located in bone.

Function Phosphorus is essential for many metabolic processes. As calcium phosphate, it serves as an integral structural component of the bone matrix and as a functional component of phospholipids, carbohydrates, nucleoproteins, and high-energy nucleotides. Plasma phosphate levels are under tight biological control, involving parathyroid hormone, calcitonin, and vitamin D. DNA and RNA structures contain sugar-phosphate linkages. Cell membranes contain phospholipids, which regulate the transport of solutes into and out of the cell. Many metabolic processes depend on phosphorylation. The adenosine diphosphate–ATP system, which provides a mechanism for storage and release of energy for use in all of the body's metabolic processes, involves phosphorus compounds. An important buffer system of the body consists of inorganic phosphates.

There is a reciprocal relationship between calcium and phosphorus. Both minerals are regulated partially by parathyroid hormone. Secretion of parathyroid hormone stimulates an increase in serum calcium levels through increased bone resorption, gut absorption, and reabsorption in renal tubules. Parathyroid hormone also causes a decrease in the resorption of phosphate by the kidney. Thus, when serum calcium is high, serum phosphate is generally low, and vice versa.

Dietary Sources Phosphorus is present in nearly all foods, especially protein-rich foods and cereal grains (Table 23-6).

Deficiency Because nearly all foods contain phosphorus, deficiency states do not usually occur unless induced. For example, patients receiving aluminum hydroxide as an antacid for prolonged periods may exhibit weakness, anorexia, malaise, pain, and bone loss. The aluminum hydroxide binds phosphorus, making it unavailable for GI absorption through formation of insoluble and poorly absorbed complexes.

Dose/DRI The DRI values for phosphorus are listed in Table 23-4. The FDA-approved use for phosphorus is to alleviate the deficiency state. In addition, phosphates have been used to decrease serum calcium levels in hypercalcemia. The recommended UL for phosphorus is 4 g/day.[16,20]

Safety Considerations Gastrointestinal side effects such as diarrhea and stomach pain have been reported with oral supplementation of phosphate salts. Potential drug–nutrient interactions with phosphorus are listed in Table 23-8.

### Trace Elements

Trace elements, which are present in minute quantities in plant and animal tissue, are considered essential for numerous physiologic processes. Zinc and manganese are trace elements. "Ultratrace" minerals have been defined as those elements with an estimated dietary requirement of less than 1 mg/day. The essential ultratrace minerals include arsenic, boron, cobalt, copper, chromium, iodine, molybdenum, nickel, selenium, and silicon. Lithium and vanadium are considered probably essential minerals, but further study is required. Bromine, cadmium, fluorine, lead, and tin are not considered essential.

*Chromium* About 5 mg of chromium is present in the normal adult, and levels decline with age.

Function Chromium is a component of glucose tolerance factor. This dietary organic chromium complex potentiates the activity of insulin.

Chromium combines with picolinic acid (a metabolite of tryptophan) to form chromium picolinate (a form of chromium with enhanced bioavailability). Chromium picolinate, in doses of 200 μg/day, has been promoted for the general population as an aid in controlling diabetes, lowering cholesterol, producing weight loss, and increasing muscle mass. However, reliable data are insufficient to support any therapeutic value of chromium supplementation in the absence of a diagnosed deficiency.

Dietary Sources See Table 23-6.

Deficiency Deficiency of trivalent chromium (the chemical form present in diets) is manifested by glucose intolerance, elevated circulating insulin, glycosuria, fasting hyperglycemia, elevated serum cholesterol and triglycerides, neuropathy, and encephalopathy.

Dose/DRI Chromium intake in the United States is low (about 50 μg/day) compared with that of other countries. The estimated DRI values for chromium are listed in Table 23-4. Oral administration of trivalent chromium has a relatively high margin of safety, and there is no UL for chromium.[19]

Safety Considerations Oral chromium has not been reported to be toxic. However, the hexavalent forms of chromium can be toxic and carcinogenic. These forms, which are encountered through industrial exposure, may enter the body through inhalation or cutaneous absorption.

Drug interactions have not been reported for chromium.

*Cobalt* Cobalt is an essential component of vitamin $B_{12}$, but ingested cyanocobalamin is metabolized in vivo to form the $B_{12}$ coenzymes.

Function Cobalt's nutritional functions are the same as those for cyanocobalamin (see Cyanocobalamin [Vitamin $B_{12}$]).

Dietary Sources Cobalt is an integral part of vitamin $B_{12}$ and, therefore, the normal dietary sources of cobalt are the same as for vitamin $B_{12}$ (Table 23-6).

Deficiency No deficiency state for cobalt is reported to exist in humans.

Dose/DRI No DRI values exist for cobalt.

Safety Considerations Large doses of cobalt may result in goiter, congestive heart failure, and myxedema. Cardiomyopathy has also been described. Cyanosis and coma may result from accidental ingestion by children. There are no known drug–nutrient interactions with cobalt.

*Copper* Copper ions exist in two states: the cuprous and the cupric (a potent oxidizing agent). Copper is similar to zinc in the complexes it forms with a number of the same chelating agents. Copper is found in virtually all tissues of the body, but concentrations are highest in the liver, brain, heart, and kidney.

Function Copper is essential for the proper structure and function of the CNS, and it plays a major role in iron metabolism. Ceruloplasmin, one of the copper metalloenzymes, is especially important in converting absorbed ferrous iron to transported ferric iron. Other copper-containing enzymes are cytochrome oxidase, dopamine β-hydroxylase, and superoxide dismutase.

Dietary Sources See Table 23-6.

Deficiency Copper deficiency is uncommon in humans, even though many individuals may have lower than recommended intake. Contemporary diets provide about 1.2 mg/day for men and 0.9 mg/day for women, and these amounts approximate the suggested AI for this nutrient. Deficiencies have been observed in premature infants; in severely malnourished infants fed milk-based, low-copper diets; and in patients receiving parenteral nutrition with inadequate copper.

One of the prominent features of copper deficiency is impaired iron absorption, which results in hypochromic anemia. In copper-deficient animals, bone cortices are fragile and thin, resulting from the failure of collagen cross-linking. Spontaneous rupture of major vessels may also be observed in deficiency states.

Dose/DRI The DRI values for copper are listed in Table 23-4. To protect against possible hepatoxicity, the recommended UL for this nutrient is 10 mg/day.[19]

Safety Considerations Copper sulfate doses in excess of 250 mg produce vomiting. However, copper salts should not be used for this purpose.

Wilson's disease is an inborn error of metabolism causing a failure to eliminate copper. These individuals must avoid any copper supplementation. Wilson's disease results in CNS, kidney, and liver damage. Acute symptoms of copper toxicity include nausea, vomiting, diarrhea, hemolysis, convulsions, and GI bleeding. Symptoms respond to treatment with penicillamine.

Supplementation should be avoided in patients with severe hepatic dysfunction or cholestasis caused by compromised biliary clearance of copper.

Potential drug–nutrient interactions are listed in Table 23-8.

*Fluoride* Available therapeutic forms of fluoride include sodium fluoride, acidulated phosphate fluoride, and stannous fluoride. Sodium fluoride contains about 45% fluoride ion, whereas stannous fluoride contains about 24% fluoride ion.

Function Fluoride occurs normally in bones and tooth enamel as a calcium salt. Intake of small amounts has been shown to markedly reduce tooth decay, presumably by making the enamel more resistant to the erosive action of acids produced by bacteria in the oral cavity.

Dietary Sources Fluoride is present in soil and water, but the content varies widely from region to region. Most municipal water supplies are fluoridated to 1 ppm of fluoride, a level that has been shown to be safe and to reduce caries in children by about 50%. Estimates of fluoride intake from food, beverages, and water vary greatly, depending on the presence of fluoridated drinking water.

Deficiency Fluoride deficiency states in humans, other than potential dental decay, have not been described.

Dose/DRI The DRI values for fluoride are listed in Table 23-4. The recommended UL for this trace element is 10 mg/day for adults.[16,20]

Fluoride is FDA approved for use in the prevention of dental caries.[20] Fluoride is a normal constituent of the diet, given that it occurs in soils, water supplies, plants, and animals. All sources of fluoride should be evaluated before supplementation is recommended for children whose home water supply is low in fluoride. Children may obtain fluoride from other water sources (e.g., day care, school) or from other beverages such as soft drinks, juices, and bottled water that may contain varying amounts of fluoride.[50]

Sodium fluoride is available by prescription as oral tablets and solutions, topical solutions, and gels, as well as in combination products. Nonprescription topical rinses containing fluoride 0.01% to 0.02%, such as sodium fluoride, and gels containing 0.4% stannous fluoride (e.g., Gel-Kam) are brushed onto the teeth to reduce sensitivity and prevent dental cavities.

Safety Considerations Excessive fluoride can be toxic. Acute toxicity should not result from the low levels present in drinking water but may result from the administration of excessive doses of fluoride supplements. Because acute toxicity affects the GI system and the CNS, it can be life threatening. Symptoms include salivation, GI distress, muscle weakness, tremors, and (rarely) seizures. Because of the calcium-binding effect of fluoride, symptoms of calcium deficiency, including tetany, may be seen. Eventually, respiratory and cardiac failure may occur. The dose that causes acute toxicity in adults is approximately 5 g. Death has occurred after ingestion of 2 g in adults, but much larger overdoses have been treated successfully. In children, 0.5 g of sodium fluoride may be fatal. Treatment includes precipitation of the fluoride by using gastric lavage with calcium hydroxide 0.15% solution, intravenous dextrose and saline for hydration, and treatment with calcium to prevent tetany.

Chronic fluoride toxicity is manifested as changes in the structure of bones and teeth. Tooth enamel, if still under development, acquires a mottled appearance consisting of white, patchy plaques occurring with pitting brown stains. Prolonged ingestion of water that contains more than 2 ppm of fluoride has resulted in a significant incidence of mottling. Extremely large doses (e.g., 20 to 80 mg/day) have resulted in chalky, brittle bones that tend to fracture easily, a condition known as crippling skeletal fluorosis.

Potential drug–nutrient interactions are listed in Table 23-8.

*Iodine* The thyroid gland contains about one third of the iodine in the body, stored in the form of a complex glycoprotein, thyroglobulin. The only known function of thyroglobulin is to provide thyroxine and triiodothyronine, which are hormones that regulate the metabolic rate of cells and, therefore, influence physical and mental growth, nervous and muscle tissue function, circulatory activity, and use of nutrients.

Function Iodine is an essential micronutrient required to synthesize thyroxine and triiodothyronine. High concentrations of iodine inhibit the release of these hormones. In the absence of iodine, thyroid hypertrophy occurs, resulting in goiter. The iodine content of produce reflects that of the soil in which it is grown. The consumption of foods from diverse locations and the addition of iodide to table salt have essentially eliminated goiter as a health problem in the United States.

Dietary Sources The primary dietary source of iodine is iodized salt, which contains 1 part of sodium or potassium iodide per 10,000 parts (0.01%) of salt. A dose of about 95 μg of iodine can be obtained from about 1/4 tsp of salt (1.25 g). In the United States, most of the table salt sold is iodized; however, salt used in food processing and for institutional use is not. Additional dietary sources of iodine include saltwater fish and shellfish.

Deficiency A moderate deficiency of iodine can result in goiter; severe deficiency results in hypothyroidism.

Dose/DRI Because of the fortification of salt, the iodine content of typical diets in the United States is still well above the DRI values for adults (Table 23-4). Iodine supplements are unwarranted for most individuals. Potassium iodide is available as a tablet, syrup, and solution, and is included in various combination products.

Safety Considerations Some individuals are allergic to iodide or organic preparations containing iodine and may develop a rash. Symptoms of chronic iodism (iodide intoxication) may include an unpleasant taste and burning in the mouth or throat, along with soreness of the teeth or gums. Increased salivation, sneezing, irritation of the eyes, and swelling of the eyelids commonly occur. In addition, prolonged use of iodine supplementation can result in hypothyroidism.[26] A UL of iodine 1.1 mg/day has been recommended.[19]

Potential drug–nutrient interactions are listed in Table 23-8.

*Manganese* The body concentrates its stores of manganese in the liver, pancreas, kidney, muscle, and bone.

Function Manganese is required for the utilization of glucose; the synthesis of mucopolysaccharides of cartilage; the biosynthesis of steroids, cholesterol, and fatty acids; and the biological activity of pyruvate carboxylase.

Dietary Sources Manganese is widely available in foods; primary dietary sources are listed in Table 23-6.

Deficiency Manganese deficiency is extremely rare, and the only theorized method of manganese deficiency is insufficient dietary intake.

Dose/DRI Even though manganese is poorly absorbed after oral administration (3%), sufficient quantities are present in the average diet to maintain appropriate levels. A dose or dietary intake of 2 to 5 mg/day is considered safe and adequate. The estimated AIs for manganese are listed in Table 23-4. The recommended UL of 11 mg/day is based on data that showed no adverse effects with long-term consumption at this level.[19]

Safety Considerations Toxicity is rare for orally administered manganese. It has been observed, however, from inhalation of dust and industrial fumes containing manganese. Manganese supplementation should be avoided in patients with severe liver dysfunction or cholestasis caused by reduced biliary clearance of this trace element.

Significant drug interactions with manganese have not been reported.

*Molybdenum* Molybdenum is an ultratrace mineral that has only rarely been associated with deficiency. Practitioners monitoring patients on long-term parenteral nutrition must be aware of the potential for deficiency in this population.

Function Molybdenum readily changes its oxidation state and acts as an electron transfer agent in oxidation-reduction reactions. It may also function as an enzyme cofactor and is involved in the metabolism of sulfur and purines.

Dietary Sources The molybdenum content of food varies, depending on the growth environment. Dietary sources of molybdenum are listed in Table 23-6.

Deficiency Molybdenum is a cofactor for several flavoprotein enzymes and is found in xanthine oxidase. Because xanthine oxidase is involved in the oxidation of xanthine to uric acid, high molybdenum intake has been associated with goutlike symptoms. Parenteral nutrition without molybdenum has resulted in an acquired molybdenum deficiency, which has been treated with ammonium molybdate. Symptoms of molybdenum deficiency may include tachycardia, tachypnea, headache, lethargy, and disorientation. Congenital deficiency of specific molybdenum cofactors results in severe neurologic dysfunction and mental retardation.

Dose/DRI/Safety Considerations The human molybdenum requirement is low and is easily furnished by the average diet (Table 23-4). Supplements are rarely warranted.

On the basis of animal studies showing impaired reproduction and growth with prolonged intake of excessive molybdenum, a UL of 2 mg/day is recommended.[19]

No significant drug interactions have been reported with molybdenum.

*Selenium* Selenium is present in all tissues, and is generally incorporated into organic compounds involving amino acids such as methionine or cysteine. Selenium compounds are about 80% absorbed. The highest concentrations are in the kidneys and liver; the lowest are in the lungs and brain. The kidney is the primary route of excretion although losses can also occur through the gastrointestinal tract.

Function Selenium is an antioxidant that serves as part of glutathione peroxidase. This enzyme protects cells from the peroxidase-induced oxidative damage that occurs with cellular metabolism.

The antioxidant properties of selenium have prompted evaluation for its use in cancer prevention. For example, a recent randomized controlled trial evaluated the effect of 200 µg selenium daily on the risk of various types of cancer. Selenium was found to significantly reduce the incidence of prostate cancer but not of lung or colorectal cancer.[51] Additional trials evaluating the role of selenium in cancer risk reduction are warranted.

Dietary Sources See Table 23-6. The selenium content of foods depends on the soils in which the plants are grown.

Deficiency Selenium is an essential trace element in humans, but deficiencies are not common in the general population. Selenium deficiency has been reported in patients with alcoholic cirrhosis, probably because of an insufficient diet or the altered metabolism of selenium. It has been reported rarely in patients on long-term parenteral nutrition. Limited evidence in humans suggests that deficiency results in cardiomyopathy, musculoskeletal pain, bleaching of the hair and skin, and abnormal nail beds. Epidemiologic studies suggest that cancer and heart disease may be common in areas of low selenium availability. Keshan disease, a cardiomyopathy that occurs almost exclusively in children, has been shown to respond to selenium.

Dose/DRI The DRI values for selenium are listed in Table 23-4. The UL for this mineral is 400 µg/day.[18]

Safety Considerations Toxic effects of selenium may include loss of hair and nails, skin lesions, muscular weakness, fatigue, and CNS abnormalities. No significant drug interactions with selenium have been reported.

*Silicon* Little is known about the absorption, distribution, metabolism, and excretion of silicon.

Function Silicon apparently functions in the development and maintenance of connective tissue. It is required for collagen biosynthesis and the mineralization process in bone calcification.

Dietary Sources See Table 23-6. The role of silicon in human nutrition, if any, is unknown at present.

Deficiency Silicon deficiency states in humans have not been described.

Dose/DRI The daily requirement of silicon has not been established, and the best product form for silicon administration has not been determined. There is no established UL for silicon.[19]

Safety Considerations When taken orally, silicon is essentially nontoxic. This lack of toxicity is evidenced by the administration of silicon-containing magnesium trisilicate (a nonprescription antacid that has been available for many years without apparent toxic effects) and by the ingestion of simethicone (a common antigas ingredient in many nonprescription antacids).

Potential drug–nutrient interactions are listed in Table 23-8.

*Vanadium* The most important forms of vanadium in biological systems are the tetravalent and pentavalent states. The tetravalent form easily complexes with other substances, such as transferrin or hemoglobin, to stabilize it against oxidation.

Function Vanadium may be involved in functions related to growth and reproduction; however, the evidence of its necessity is not well established.

Dietary Sources Food sources highest in vanadium are listed in Table 23-6.

Deficiency Vanadium is presumed essential, but a deficiency state has not been confirmed. It is obtained in sufficient quantities in the diet.

Dose/DRI There are no established DRI values for vanadium. However, a UL of vanadium 1.8 mg/day has been recommended on the basis of adverse effects reported in animal studies.[10]

Safety Considerations Toxicity can occur through excessive dietary intake. Symptoms of toxicity include diarrhea, anorexia, depressed growth, and neurotoxicity. Vanadium toxicity may be diminished by administration of ascorbic acid, ethylenediaminetetraacetic acid (EDTA), chromium, protein, ferrous iron, chloride, and possibly aluminum hydroxide.

No drug interactions have been reported for vanadium.

*Zinc* Zinc is an integral part of at least 70 metalloenzymes, including carbonic anhydrase, lactic dehydrogenase, alkaline phosphatase, carboxypeptidase, aminopeptidase, and alcohol dehydrogenase.

Function Zinc is a cofactor in the synthesis of DNA and RNA. It is involved in the mobilization of vitamin A from the liver, and in the enhancement of follicle-stimulating hormone and luteinizing hormone. Zinc is essential for normal cellular immune functions and for spermatogenesis and normal testicular function. It is important in the stabilization of membrane structure.

The divalent ion is most commonly found and used in the body. Zinc has a relatively rapid turnover rate. The balance between zinc absorption from the small intestine and excretion via the feces is efficiently regulated by the body. Vegetarians may require higher amounts of zinc because diets high in fiber and phytates hinder zinc absorption.[19]

Dietary Sources Most dietary zinc (about 70%) is derived from animal products (Table 23-6).

Deficiency Although zinc deficiencies are not widespread in the United States, marginally low zinc values have been associated with growth retardation in children, slow wound healing in adults, and birth defects. Additional symptoms include immunologic abnormalities, impaired taste and smell, delayed sexual maturation, hypogonadism, hypospermia, and dermatitis.

Malabsorption syndromes, infection, major surgery, alcoholism, pregnancy, lactation, and high-fiber diets rich in phytate predispose an individual to a suboptimal zinc status. Zinc depletion is relatively rare but may be seen in patients on long-term parenteral nutrition and in patients with GI tract abnormalities, such as fistulas and prolonged, severe diarrhea.

Zinc deficiencies adversely affect DNA, RNA, carbohydrate, and protein metabolism. Iron supplements decrease zinc absorption just as zinc supplements decrease iron absorption, probably resulting from competition for the same transport system. If these minerals are taken with a meal, the adverse interaction is less pronounced. In patients with impaired wound healing, zinc supplementation may be marginally beneficial.

Dose/DRI The DRI values for zinc are listed in Table 23-4. Typical Western diets supply 10 to 15 mg of zinc per day. Because zinc is only 10% to 40% absorbed from the GI tract, ingestion of zinc sulfate 220 mg (50 mg of elemental zinc) will supply 5 to 20 mg of zinc. Treatment of suspected deficiencies usually involves short-term administration of elemental zinc 150 mg in three divided doses daily. Patients with large GI losses through fistulas, ostomies, or stool require larger supplemental doses of zinc. At doses above 40 mg elemental zinc per day, copper deficiency may be induced. On the basis of this interaction, the UL for elemental zinc is 40 mg daily if therapy with zinc is going to be long term.[19] Absorption of zinc supplements may be reduced if taken with foods high in calcium or phosphorus.[27]

Zinc has been evaluated in numerous studies as a potential treatment for the common cold. However, zinc formulations and doses have varied and trial results have been conflicting.[52] A meta-analysis on the use of zinc lozenges concluded that insufficient evidence exists for routine use of these products in the treatment of the cold.[53]

Safety Considerations Because ingestion of zinc sulfate 2 g or more has resulted in GI irritation and vomiting, zinc should be taken with food. Zinc is also toxic, although the emetic effect that occurs after consumption of large amounts may minimize problems with accidental overdose. Reported signs of zinc toxicity in humans include vomiting, dehydration, muscle incoordination, dizziness, and abdominal pain.

Potential drug–nutrient interactions are listed in Table 23-8.

## Assessment of Nutritional Adequacy: A Case-based Approach

Assessing a patient's nutritional status is difficult in the ambulatory environment. Clinical impressions are often erroneous because the stages between well-nourished and poorly nourished states are not readily evident. There are guidelines, however, that may help provide a more objective assessment of a patient's nutritional status. Practitioners should exercise good observational skills, know which questions yield helpful information, and know which population groups tend to be poorly nourished. By asking key questions, the practitioner may detect cultural, physical, environmental, and social conditions that suggest inadequate vitamin intake. The more specific the information obtained from the patient, the more helpful the practitioner can be in determining the need for nutritional supplementation. Questions about food generally not included in the diet and about previous treatment of similar symptoms may also be important.

Although most nutritional assessment measures are beyond the scope of routine pharmacy practice, the pharmacist can observe the physical status of the patient. For example, a patient's fingernails may indicate malnutrition if they are not lustrous and are dark at the upper ends. The texture, amount, and appearance of hair may indicate the patient's nutritional status. The eyes, particularly the conjunctiva, may indicate vitamin A and iron deficiencies. The mouth may show stomatitis, glossitis, or hypertrophic or pale gums. Poor dentition may limit the foods a patient is able to eat, thus compromising intake from certain food groups such as protein. Visible goiter, poor skin color and texture, obesity or thinness relative to bone structure, and the presence of edema may also indicate malnutrition. The pharmacist should be able to recognize overt but nonspecific symptoms of vitamin and mineral deficiencies for which prompt referral to a primary care provider may be crucial.

Checking a patient's medication history is important because of the number of potential drug–micronutrient interactions (Table 23-8). It is also the practitioner's responsibility to refer patients with a suspected serious illness to a primary care provider. Just as nutritional deficiencies may lead to disease, disease may lead to nutritional deficiencies. Patients may present with one or more deficiencies, which may be very difficult to identify. Rarely in the United States do practitioners encounter patients with severe deficiencies resulting in diseases such as scurvy, pellagra, or kwashiorkor. However, milder forms of malnutrition may be seen. Cases 23-1 and 23-2 illustrate the assessment of patients with nutritional inadequacy.

## CASE 23-1

| Relevant Evaluation Criteria | Scenario/Model Outcome |
|---|---|
| **Information Gathering** | |
| 1. Gather essential information about the patient's symptoms, including: | |
| a. description of symptom(s) (i.e., nature, onset, duration, severity, associated symptoms) | Patient does not have any complaints. However, on inquiry of supplements taken at home, patient says she regularly takes a multivitamin, an antioxidant supplement plus extra β-carotene once daily for vision, and generic calcium carbonate with 500 mg elemental calcium 2 times/day for osteoporosis prevention. |
| b. description of any factors that seem to precipitate, exacerbate, and/or relieve the patient's symptom(s) | N/A |
| c. description of the patient's efforts to relieve the symptoms | N/A |
| 2. Gather essential patient history information: | |
| a. patient's identity | Sophia Chase |
| b. patient's age, sex, weight, and height | 50 y/o F, 5'4", 180 lb |
| c. patient's occupation | Florist |
| d. patient's dietary habits | Cereal or toast for breakfast; takeout meals for lunch, makes "anything easy" for dinner—typically a protein, a starch, and a vegetable. |
| e. patient's sleep habits | N/A |
| f. concurrent medical conditions, prescription and nonprescription medications, and dietary supplements | Lisinopril 10 mg once daily for 2 years for hypertension; atorvastatin 10 mg once daily; 2 fish oil tablets once daily; and 300 mg garlic 3 times/day for hyperlipidemia |
| g. allergies | Penicillin |
| h. history of other adverse reactions to medications | N/A |
| i. other (describe)______ | |

## CASE 23-1 (continued)

| Relevant Evaluation Criteria | Scenario/Model Outcome |
|---|---|
| **Assessment and Triage** | |
| 3. Differentiate the patient's signs/symptoms and correctly identify the patient's primary problem(s). | Taking multiple supplements can increase the risk of exceeding the UL for various nutrients. No evidence exists that this practice is beneficial, and concern exists that it is potentially harmful. Of greatest concern is an excessive intake of fat-soluble vitamins such as vitamin A. |
| 4. Identify exclusions for self-treatment. | None |
| 5. Formulate a comprehensive list of therapeutic alternatives for the primary problem to determine if triage to a medical practitioner is required, and share this information with the patient. | Options include:<br>(1) Assess the client's perceived need for the nutrient supplements.<br>(2) Compare the vitamin and mineral content of the three supplements, noting excessive intake of any vitamin or mineral.<br>(3) Encourage the patient to work toward a more balanced diet.<br>(4) Take no action. |
| **Plan** | |
| 6. Select an optimal therapeutic alternative to address the patient's problem, taking into account patient preferences. | If the multivitamin provides 3500 IU of vitamin A, the antioxidant supplement provides 1000 IU of β-carotene, and the third product contains 25,000 IU of β-carotene, the patient intake of vitamin A likely is excessive. The DRI for this client is 700 μg as RAE with a UL of 3 mg daily.<br>To convert the client's supplemented intake to micrograms of RAE per day, you note that 1 μg as RAE = 10 IU vitamin A activity as β-carotene = 3.33 IU vitamin A activity as retinol. This calculates to 3651 μg as RAE daily in supplements alone.<br>Discontinue the β-carotene supplement and consider sticking with a USP-approved multivitamin with no more than 100% of DRI for vitamins and minerals, including antioxidants. |
| 7. Describe the recommended therapeutic approach to the patient. | Unless specifically recommended by your primary care provider or ophthalmologist, reconsider taking the supplement for vision if you are taking a USP-approved multivitamin with minerals and antioxidants. Separate the multivitamin from the calcium supplement (see Table 23-9). |
| 8. Explain to the patient the rationale for selecting the recommended therapeutic approach from the considered therapeutic alternatives. | Your current supplemental intake for vitamin A exceeds the level that is known to be safe. To improve your intake of nutrients good for vision and disease prevention, consider a gradual change to a diet rich in fruits and vegetables. These provide lutein, a carotenoid associated with reduced risk of age-related macular degeneration when consumed regularly. Also include low-fat dairy products, lean protein sources, and whole grains. A daily multivitamin with minerals and antioxidants could be included to ensure adequate intake. Overall, a commitment to better nutrition, portion control, and daily exercise would support weight maintenance, lower blood pressure, improve the serum lipid profile, and help maintain bone strength. |
| **Patient Education** | |
| 9. When recommending self-care with nonprescription medications and/or nondrug therapy, convey accurate information to the patient, including: | |
| a. appropriate dose and frequency of administration | Consider one USP-approved multivitamin daily that contains no more than 100% of DRI for nutrients, including antioxidants. |
| b. maximum number of days the therapy should be employed | N/A |
| c. product administration procedures | You may need to take your supplements separately from certain medications. Check with your pharmacist on all new prescriptions. |
| d. expected time to onset of relief | N/A |
| e. degree of relief that can be reasonably expected | N/A |

## CASE 23-1 (continued)

| Relevant Evaluation Criteria | Scenario/Model Outcome |
|---|---|
| f. most common side effects | N/A |
| g. side effects that warrant medical intervention should they occur | N/A |
| h. patient options in the event that condition worsens or persists | N/A |
| i. product storage requirements | N/A |
| j. specific nondrug measures | N/A |
| 10. Solicit follow-up questions from patient. | Which fruits and vegetables are highest in lutein? |
| 11. Answer patient's questions. | Dark green leafy vegetables are the richest sources of lutein. However, lutein can also be found in orange and yellow produce such as corn, squash, and tomatoes. |

Key: DRI, dietary reference intake N/A, not applicable; RAE, retinol activity equivalent; UL, upper intake level.

## CASE 23-2

| Relevant Evaluation Criteria | Scenario/Model Outcome |
|---|---|
| **Information Gathering** | |
| 1. Gather essential information about the patient's symptoms, including: | |
| a. description of symptom(s) (i.e., nature, onset, duration, severity, associated symptoms) | Patient does not complain of any symptoms but inquires about nutrient supplementation for optimal health and the prevention of skin cancer. |
| b. description of any factors that seem to precipitate, exacerbate, and/or relieve the patient's symptom(s) | N/A |
| c. description of the patient's efforts to relieve the symptoms | N/A |
| 2. Gather essential patient history information: | |
| a. patient's identity | Lyle Osler |
| b. patient's age, sex, weight, and height | 69 y/o M, 5'11", 190 lb |
| c. patient's occupation | Recently retired geologist |
| d. patient's dietary habits | Intake from food groups is inconsistent, particularly from meat products; loves fruits and vegetables; drinks one glass of red wine with dinner |
| e. patient's sleep habits | Recent insomnia |
| f. concurrent medical conditions, prescription and nonprescription medications, and dietary supplements | Does not take any medications; uncle has had malignant melanoma detected and removed; lives with a smoker |
| g. allergies | NKA |
| h. history of other adverse reactions to medications | None |
| i. other (describe)______ | N/A |
| **Assessment and Triage** | |
| 3. Differentiate the patient's signs/symptoms and correctly identify the patient's primary problem(s). | Advanced age, risk of melanoma, regular exposure to secondhand smoke |

## CASE 23-2 (continued)

| Relevant Evaluation Criteria | Scenario/Model Outcome |
| --- | --- |
| 4. Identify exclusions for self-treatment. | None |
| 5. Formulate a comprehensive list of therapeutic alternatives for the primary problem to determine if triage to a medical practitioner is required, and share this information with the patient. | Options include:<br>(1) Assess Lyle's dietary intake in comparison to the Food Guide Pyramid. Modify food choices to meet dietary requirements.<br>(2) Evaluate the potential for suboptimal intake of vitamin $B_{12}$.<br>(3) Select a USP-approved multivitamin supplement with no more than 100% of the DRI for the nutrients.<br>(4) Recommend calcium supplement, if warranted.<br>(5) Take no action. |
| **Plan** | |
| 6. Select an optimal therapeutic alternative to address the patient's problem, taking into account patient preferences. | Recommend a multivitamin product with no more than 100% of the DRI for vitamins and minerals. If Lyle's intake from dairy products falls short of at least 3 servings daily, a separate calcium supplement may also be warranted. The calcium supplement should be taken separately (see Table 23-9). Since Lyle regularly consumes fruits and vegetables, he likely is meeting the slightly increased requirement for vitamin C recommended for smokers. Additional intake from the multivitamin ensures this. |
| 7. Describe the recommended therapeutic approach to the patient. | If your diet remains primarily vegetarian, supplementation with a multivitamin plus minerals would be reasonable. There is no evidence to suggest you would need any more than 100% of the DRI for these micronutrients. |
| 8. Explain to the patient the rationale for selecting the recommended therapeutic approach from the considered therapeutic alternatives. | The multivitamin will ensure you are receiving adequate amounts of vitamin $B_{12}$, which is found almost exclusively in animal products such as meat and dairy products. The multivitamin will also ensure you are receiving enough vitamin C to combat the effects of living with a smoker. If your current intake of dairy products is lower than that recommended by the USDA, the calcium supplement will help meet your requirements. |
| **Patient Education** | |
| 9. When recommending self-care with nonprescription medications and/or nondrug therapy, convey accurate information to the patient, including: | |
| a. appropriate dose and frequency of administration | Take the multivitamin on a regular basis, preferably at the same time each day. If you take a calcium supplement, it should be taken at least a few hours later. |
| b. maximum number of days the therapy should be employed | N/A |
| c. product administration procedures | Vitamins and minerals may interact with certain medications. Be sure to discuss this with your pharmacist when prescribed new medications. |
| d. expected time to onset of relief | N/A |
| e. degree of relief that can be reasonably expected | N/A |
| f. most common side effects | N/A |
| g. side effects that warrant medical intervention should they occur | N/A |
| h. patient options in the event that condition worsens or persists | N/A |
| i. product storage requirements | N/A |
| j. specific nondrug measures | N/A |
| 10. Solicit follow-up questions from patient. | I've heard antioxidants can help prevent skin cancer. |

## CASE 23-2 (continued)

| Relevant Evaluation Criteria | Scenario/Model Outcome |
|---|---|
| 11. Answer patient's questions. | There are no data supporting supplementation of antioxidant combinations for the prevention or treatment of cancer. Furthermore, supplementation of β-carotene has been found to increase the risk of lung cancer. While single antioxidants may play a role in the prevention of specific cancers, dosing above the DRI cannot be recommended at this time. |

Key: DRI, dietary reference intake; N/A, not applicable; NKA, no known allergies.

## PATIENT EDUCATION FOR NUTRITIONAL DEFICIENCIES

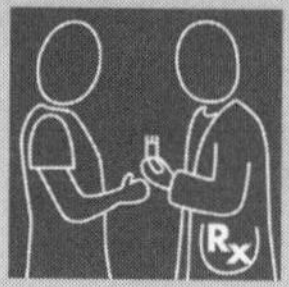

The objective of self-treatment is to prevent nutritional deficiencies or maintain present nutritional status. For most patients, carefully following product instructions and the self-care measures listed here will help ensure optimal therapeutic outcomes.

### Vitamins, Minerals, and Trace Elements

- To ensure proper nutrition, eat a varied diet as recommended in the Food Guide Pyramid (see Figure 23-1). Vitamin supplements are not a substitute for a well-balanced diet.
- Read labels on all vitamin and mineral preparations carefully before taking them. Note the quantity of vitamins and minerals required to meet the DRI values.
- Do not take doses of vitamins and minerals higher than the recommended DRIs. High doses of vitamins or minerals may be dangerous and should not be taken indiscriminately.
- Take vitamins and mineral supplements with meals if you experience GI symptoms.
- Women of childbearing age should take 400 μg supplemental folic acid in addition to a well-balanced diet. This has been shown to reduce the risk of neural tube defects in the fetus.
- Be aware that iron supplements or vitamins with iron may turn the stool black. This occurrence is not a cause for alarm, unless it is associated with other symptoms involving the digestive system.
- As with any medicine, store vitamin and combination vitamin and mineral supplements out of the reach of children, especially if the product contains iron. Teach children that vitamins are drugs and potential poisons, and that vitamins cannot be taken indiscriminately.
- Be aware that therapeutic use of niacin-containing products may cause a flushing, itching, or tingling sensation, which should decrease in intensity with continued therapy. Taking an aspirin or nonsteroidal anti-inflammatory agent 30 to 60 minutes before niacin may help decrease these effects.

⚠ Do not self-medicate if you suspect a vitamin deficiency; consult a health care practitioner instead.

## Patient Counseling for Nutrient Supplementation

The public is often exposed to exaggerated and fraudulent claims concerning vitamin products. The practitioner can help expose such claims by keeping up with medical and pharmaceutical literature and not supporting or appearing to support the claims until they are substantiated by reliable clinical studies. Patients inquiring about such claims should be educated about the increased potential risk of the nontraditional use of vitamins. They should be told, for example, about adverse drug reactions that might occur with such products when used in alternative doses or in combination with prescription and nonprescription drug products. This advice, however, becomes difficult to give when patients purchase nutritional supplements from health food stores or from online and mail-order vendors.

Patients purchasing a nonprescription liquid dietary supplement should be instructed on its proper use and storage, including dilution and preparation techniques. In addition, the practitioner should offer to discuss with the patient possible adverse effects such as diarrhea.

The box Patient Education for Nutritional Deficiencies lists specific information to provide patients. The practitioner could also refer the consumer to Web sites and printed literature with evidence-based recommendations for vitamin and mineral supplementation, such as those listed in the reference section of this chapter.

## Evaluation of Patient Outcomes for Nutritional Adequacy

Nutritional therapy should involve a diet based on the Food Guide Pyramid and possibly the use of nutritional supplements. The practitioner should advise patients to return after 30 days of implementing nutritional therapy, or sooner if the symptoms worsen. Patients whose symptoms have worsened should be referred to a primary care provider. Patients whose symptoms have improved while taking nutritional supplements should be encouraged to eat a healthful diet and not to rely on supplements as the primary source for vitamins and minerals.

## Key Points for Nutritional Adequacy

- The benefits of a varied, balanced diet in terms of health maintenance and disease prevention have been demonstrated repeatedly. However, the same benefits have not been observed when suboptimal dietary intake is augmented with vitamin and mineral supplementation.
- Practitioners can assess the variety of food choices by comparing the patient's typical food pattern to that recommended in the Food Guide Pyramid. The practitioner may refer patients to a Registered Dietitian for personalized and/or more complete counseling on diet modification as well as nutritional supplementation.
- Overt vitamin or mineral deficiencies are rare in this country; however, subclinical deficiencies may be contributing to chronic disease.
- Vitamin and/or mineral supplementation may be appropriate on the basis of the practitioner's assessment of the patient's dietary intake, metabolic requirements, absorptive capability, and potential drug–nutrient interactions.

## References


1. Chavis LM. Pharmacy-based consulting on dietary supplements. *J Am Pharm Assoc.* 2001;41:181-91.
2. Fairfield KM, Fletcher RH. Vitamins for chronic disease prevention in adults: scientific review. *JAMA.* 2002;287:3116-26.
3. Fairfield KM, Fletcher RH. Vitamins for chronic disease prevention in adults: clinical applications. *JAMA.* 2002;287:3127-9.
4. Ames BN, Wakimoto P. Are vitamin and mineral deficiencies a major cancer risk? *Nat Reviews Cancer.* 2002;2:694-704.
5. Troppmann L, Gray-Donald K, Johns T. Supplement use: is there any nutritional benefit? *J Am Diet Assoc.* 2002;102:818-25.
6. Zawada, ET. Malnutrition in the elderly: is it simply a matter of not eating enough? *Postgrad Med.* 1996;100:207-8, 211-4, 220-2.
7. Harris NG. Nutrition in aging. In: Mahan LK, Escott-Stump S, eds. *Krause's Food, Nutrition, and Diet Therapy.* 10th ed. Philadelphia: WB Saunders; 2000:290-9.
8. Foote JA, Giuliano AR, Harris RB. Older adults need guidance to meet nutritional recommendations. *J Am Coll Nutr.* 2000;19:628-40.
9. Fuhrman, MP. Identifying your patient's risk for a vitamin deficiency. *Nutr Clin Pract.* 2001;16:S8-S11.
10. American Dietetic Association. Position of the American Dietetic Association: food fortification and dietary supplements. *J Am Diet Assoc.* 2001;101:115-25.
11. Cooperman T, Obermeyer W. Do all supplements contain what their labels say they contain? *US Pharmacist.* Oct 2002;68, 71-2, 74.
12. Massey PB. Dietary supplements. *Med Clin North Am.* 2002;86:127-8.
13 Feifer AH, Fleshner NE, Klotz L. Analytical accuracy and reliability of commonly used nutritional supplements in prostate disease. *J Urol.* 2002;168:150-4.
14. U.S. Pharmacopeia Dietary Supplement Program. The United States Pharmacopeial Convention, Inc. 1997-2003. Available at: http://www.wsp-dsvp.org. Accessed May 7, 2003.
15. *Dietary Guidelines for Americans 2005.* Washington, DC: US Department of Health and Human Services, U.S. Department of Agriculture. January 12, 2005. HHS Publication HHS-ODPHP-2005-01-DGA-A.
16. Food and Nutrition Board, Institute of Medicine. *Dietary Reference Intakes for Calcium, Phosphorus, Magnesium, Vitamin D, and Fluoride.* Washington, DC: National Academy Press; 1997.
17. Food and Nutrition Board, Institute of Medicine. Dietary Reference Intakes for Thiamin, Riboflavin, Niacin, Vitamin B6, Folate, Vitamin B12, Pantothenic Acid, Biotin, and Choline. Washington, DC: National Academy Press; 2000.
18. Food and Nutrition Board, Institute of Medicine. *Dietary Reference Intakes for Vitamin C, Vitamin E, Selenium, and Carotenoids.* Washington, DC: National Academy Press; 2000.
19. Food and Nutrition, Board Institute of Medicine. Dietary Reference Intakes for Vitamin A, Vitamin K, Arsenic, Boron, Chromium, Copper, Iodine, Iron, Manganese, Molybdenum, Nickel, Silicon, Vanadium, and Zinc. Washington, DC: National Academy Press; 2002.
20. Yates AA, Schlicker SA, Suitor CW. Dietary reference intakes: the new basis for recommendations for calcium and related nutrients, B vitamins, and choline. *J Am Diet Assoc.* 1998;98:699-708.
21. Hathcock J. Dietary supplements: how they are used and regulated. *J Nutr.* 2001;131:1114S-7S.
22. Stone WL, LeClair I, Ponder T, et al. Infants discriminate between natural and synthetic vitamin E. *Am J Clin Nutr.* 2003;77:899-906.
23. Thomson AB, Hunt RH, Zorich NL. Review article: olestra and its gastrointestinal safety. *Aliment Pharm Ther.* 1998;12:1185-200.
24. *American Hospital Formulary Service Drug Information 2001.* Bethesda, Md: American Society of Health-System Pharmacists; 2001.
25. Combs GF. Vitamins. In: Mahan LK, Escott-Stump S, eds. *Krause's Food, Nutrition, and Diet Therapy.* 10th ed. Philadelphia: WB Saunders; 2000:168-9.
26. Balint JP. Physical findings in nutritional deficiencies. *Ped Clin North Am.* 1998;45:245-60.
27. Lacy CF, Armstrong LL, Goldman MP, et al. *Drug Information Handbook.* 10th ed. Hudson, Ohio: Lexi-Comp; 2002.
28. Feskanich D, Singh V, Willett W, et al. Vitamin A intake and hip fractures among postmenopausal women. *JAMA.* 2002;287:47-54.
29. Papadimitropoulos E, Wells G, Shea B, et al. VIII: Meta-analysis of the efficacy of vitamin D treatment in preventing osteoporosis in postmenopausal women. *Endocr Rev.* 2002;23:560-9.
30. Osborne JE, Hutchinson PE. Vitamin D and systemic cancer: is this relevant to malignant melanoma? *Br J Dermatol.* 2002;147:197-213.
31. Zittermann A, Schleithoff SS, Tenderich G, et al. Low vitamin D status: a contributing factor in the pathogenesis of congestive heart failure? *J Am Coll Cardiol.* 2003;41:105-12.
32. Hartman JJ. Vitamin D deficiency rickets in children: prevalence and need for community education. *Orthoped Nurs.* 2000;19:63-7.
33. Zhang SM et al. Intakes of vitamins E and C, carotenoids, vitamin supplements, and PD risk. *Neurology.* 2002;59:1161-9.
34. Jiang R, Manson JE, Stampler MJ, et al. Nut and peanut butter consumption and risk of type 2 diabetes in women. *JAMA.* 2002;288:2554-60.
35. Vitamin K intake in micrograms by sex, age, and income level: United States, 1988-94. The National Academy of Sciences, 2002. Available at: www.cdc.gov/nchs/data/series/sr_11/sr11/245.pdf. Accessed July 31, 2005.
36. Levine M, Rumsey SC, Daruwala R, et al. Criteria and recommendations for vitamin C intake. *JAMA.* 1999; 281:1415-23, 1460.
37. LeBoeuf R. Homocysteine and Alzheimer's disease. *J Am Diet Assoc.* 2003;103:304-7.
38. Desouza C, Keebler M, McNamara, et al. Drugs affecting homocysteine metabolism: impact on cardiovascular risk. *Drugs.* 2002; 62:605-16.
39. Dharmarajan TS, Adiga GU, Norkus EP. Vitamin $B_{12}$ deficiency: recognizing subtle symptoms in older adults. *Geriatrics.* 2003;58:30-38.

40. Bender DA. Non-nutritional uses of vitamin B6. *Br J Nutr.* 1999; 81:7-20.
41. Schoenen J, Jacquy J, Lenaerts M. Effectiveness of high-dose riboflavin in migraine prophylaxis: a randomized controlled trial. *Neurology.* 1998;50:466-70.
42. Sandor PS, Afra J, Ambrosini A, et al. Prophylactic treatment of migraine with beta-blockers and riboflavin: differential effects on the intensity dependence of auditory evoked cortical potentials. *Headache.* 2000;40:30-5.
43. Suter PM, Vetter W. Diuretics and vitamin $B_1$: are diuretics a risk factor for thiamin malnutrition? *Nutr Rev.* 2001;58:319-23.
44. Thys-Jacobs S, Starkey P, Bernstein D, et al. Calcium carbonate and the premenstrual syndrome: effects on premenstrual and menstrual symptoms. Premenstrual Syndrome Study Group. *Am J Obstet Gynecol.* 1998;179:444-52.
45. Dickerson LM, Mazyck PJ, Hunter MH. Premenstrual syndrome. *Am Fam Physician.* 2003;67:1743-52.
46. Wu K, Willett WC, Fuchs CS, et al. Calcium intake and risk of colon cancer in women and men. *J Natl Cancer Inst.* 2002;94:437-46.
47. Fleming DJ, Jacques PF, Tucker KL, et al. Iron status of the free-living, elderly Framingham Heart Study cohort: an iron-replete population with a high prevalence of elevated iron stores. *Am J Clin Nutr.* 2001;73:638-46.
48. Bigal ME, Rapoport AM, Sheftell FD, et al. New migraine preventative options: an update with pathophysiological considerations. *Rev Hosp Clin Fac Med S Paulo.* 2002;57:293-8.
49. Saris NL, Mervaala E, Karppanen H, et al. Magnesium: an update on physiological, clinical and analytical aspects. *Clin Chem Acta.* 2000;294:1-26.
50. Levy SM. An update on fluorides and fluorosis. *J Can Dent Assoc.* 2003;69):286-91.
51. Duffield-Lillico AJ, Reid ME, Turnbull BW, et al. Baseline characteristics and the effect of selenium supplementation on cancer incidence in a randomized clinical trial: a summary report of the Nutritional Prevention of Cancer Trial. *Cancer Epidemiol Biomarkers Prev.* 2003;11:630-9.
52. Mossad SB. Effect of zincum gluconicum nasal gel on the duration and symptoms severity of the common cold in otherwise healthy adults. *QJM.* 2003;96:35-43.
53. Jackson JL, Lesho E, Peterson C. Zinc and the common cold: a meta-analysis revisited. *J Nutr.* 2000;130:1512S-5S.

CHAPTER 24

# Functional and Meal Replacement Foods

*Carol J. Rollins*

Nutrition serves many purposes in our lives. Foremost is its role in survival, providing us with the sustenance needed to maintain metabolism and be physically active. Our lives have changed significantly from the days when activity was focused primarily on obtaining the next meal; many of us now live in an abundant society in which nutritional excess is common. Knowledge of both good and bad effects of diet on health is rapidly expanding and there is an increased interest in wellness and preventive medicine, particularly among the aging baby-boom generation. At the same time our lives are frenzied, leaving little time to plan and prepare meals. Convenience rules in this environment and health-conscious consumers seek convenient methods to optimize nutrition for wellness and health promotion, including fast yet healthy alternatives to traditional "sit-down" meals. In addition, more individuals with conditions or impairments that affect their ability to obtain adequate nutrients through a regular diet are living independently and may seek convenient methods to supplement or replace conventional meals. Although dietitians are the recognized food and nutrition experts, it is important for all health care practitioners to be aware of the role foods may play in an overall plan to improve or maintain health, especially foods that may have benefits beyond those of their basic nutrients (see Chapter 23 for a discussion of basic nutrition) or that may help patients reach nutrient goals when healthy meals are not readily available or cannot be ingested. This chapter provides an introduction to foods used for their potential health benefits (functional foods) as well as foods intended to replace regular meals (meal replacement foods).

### Drugs, Dietary Supplements, and Foods

The Food and Drug Administration (FDA) is charged with regulation of drugs, dietary supplements, and foods. The intended use of a product determines its classification for purposes of FDA oversight and regulations define each category of product.[1] Drugs are used to diagnose, treat, or cure a disease, and dietary supplements are intended to maintain healthy structure or function of the body (calcium builds strong bones) rather than address a disease or health-related condition (see Chapters 53 and 54 for a discussion of dietary supplements). Foods are defined as articles used for food or drink or components of any such article, or substances providing taste, aroma, or nutritive value. Specific FDA regulations pertain to food safety and labeling. FDA requires all regulated foods provide assurance in advance (premarket) that ingredients are safe and claims are substantiated, truthful, and not misleading. Particular forms or uses of foods, such as infant formulas (see Chapter 26) and medical foods, are further required to meet specific criteria.

## FUNCTIONAL FOODS

Functional foods blur the distinction between drugs, dietary supplements, and foods established by FDA definitions. The term *functional food* is not sanctioned officially by FDA, and there is no legal definition to determine if a foodstuff is a functional food.[1] This lack of validation makes it difficult to determine which foods should be included in the sales figures and market estimates for functional foods. Nonetheless, the Government Accounting Office estimated that sales of functional foods increased from $11.3 billion in 1995 to $16.2 billion in 1999 and expects it will reach $49 billion by 2010.[2]

Several organizations include "health benefits beyond those of basic nutrition" as a major component of functional foods.[3-5] Such definitions encompass unmodified whole foods (fruits, vegetables, and whole-grain products). Examples include tomatoes for their lycopene content and soybeans, which provide isoflavones. The Institute of Medicine (IOM) Food and Nutrition Board, defines functional food as those in which the concentration of one or more ingredients has been altered to enhance the food's contribution to a healthful diet.[3] This definition includes foods enriched or fortified with nutrients, phytochemicals, or botanical products. Examples include calcium added to orange juice and kava kava added to potato chips. Elements isolated from nontraditional food sources and added to traditional foods, such as stanol esters added to margarine-type spreads or orange juice, also fit this definition of functional foods. The European consensus regarding unique features of functional foods includes both whole foods and foods altered to increase the concentration of or added components not normally present in a food.[4]

### Categories of Foods Classified as Functional Foods

Functional foods typically fit into one of five categories on the basis of statutory definitions and regulatory guidelines for label claims on foods. Foods associated with health claims recognized by FDA are commonly acknowledged as functional foods, as are foods that carry structure or function claims. Foods for special dietary use and medical foods may be categorized as functional foods. In addition, many conventional foods are sometimes defined as functional. Practitioners should have a basic understanding of these food categories since the degree of scientific evidence supporting a "functional" status and the need for medical supervision vary from one category to another.

### Foods With Health Claims

Health claims are statements describing an association between a food, food component, dietary ingredient, or dietary supplement and risk of a disease or health-related condition;[6] dietary supplements are not discussed here (see Chapters 53 and 54). Three types of health claims can be made for conventional foods: authorized, authoritative, and qualified. Each type of claim is associated with specific levels of supportive data and specified labeling criteria. *Authorized* health claims require publication of an FDA regulation after an extensive review of the scientific literature along with significant scientific agreement that the food/nutrient and disease relationship is well established. Of the health claims allowed for foods, authorized claims undergo the most thorough FDA review. The exact wording of the claim statement is not specified although the statement appearing on the food label must meet specific criteria.

Statements for authorized health claims cannot quantify the degree of risk reduction, and the terms *may* or *might* must be used to qualify the relationship between a food or dietary component and disease. The label must state that the disease or health-related condition depends on many factors, implying that diet is not the only consideration in disease management. It also must indicate that the benefit related to a disease or health-related condition is as part of a total dietary pattern; thus, the need for an overall healthy diet is enforced. Health claims cannot be made for foods containing more than a specified amount of a component associated with negative health risks. This amount includes content at or above 13 to 26 g of fat, 4 to 8 g of saturated fat, 60 to 120 mg of cholesterol, or 480 to 960 mg of sodium per reference amount (RA), depending on the product category (food, main dish, or meal product).[6] The RA is typically one serving as defined on the product label. Health claims cannot be indicated for infants or toddlers younger than 2 years. Table 24-1 lists authorized health claims and requirements for foods listing these health claims in addition to sample statements that might be used on a food label. Table 24-2 shows amounts of soy in various foods although not all of the foods listed meet all qualifications for a health claim related to soy protein and risk of coronary heart disease (CHD).[7,8]

Certain health claims for foods, food components, or dietary ingredients (but not dietary supplements) can be made through notification of FDA after a statement from an authoritative scientific body of the U.S. government with responsibility to protect public health or conduct research related to human nutrition (an "*authoritative* claim").[6] The National Institutes of Health, the Centers for Disease Control and Prevention, and the National Academy of Sciences are sources for authoritative claims. Significant scientific evidence supports such health claims although FDA itself does not complete an extensive review of the data. Specific wording is required on the claims statement. Authoritative health claims currently recognized by FDA and the required label statement are included in Table 24-1.

The third type of health claims is a *qualified* claim. When evidence of health benefits for a food, food component, or dietary supplement is still emerging, scientific research supporting the claim tends to be limited or preliminary, and the "significant scientific agreement" level of evidence required for authorized and authoritative health claims seldom is met. FDA-issued health claims for such products require specific wording that includes "qualifying" terms to indicate evidence for the claim is limited.[6] To some extent, the specific wording required in the claim reflects the level of scientific evidence available. Qualified health claims currently are allowed for three conventional foods: walnuts, omega-3 fatty acids, and olive oil (Table 24-3). These three claims are all related to reduced risk of coronary heart disease; however, no regulation limits qualified claims to a specific disease or condition. The claims for walnuts and omega-3 fatty acids are based on a moderate level of scientific evidence; the level of evidence for olive oil is low. Table 24-4 outlines the levels of scientific evidence and proposed language for qualified claims.

Structure and function claims are commonly associated with dietary supplements, but can also appear on food labels. These claims indicate the effect of consuming the product on a body structure or function, such as building strong bones or supporting the immune system. They differ from health claims in that FDA validation or authorization is not required prior to use and the claims can make no reference regarding reduced risk of disease.[6] Foods that carry a structure or function claim are considered functional foods; they are not dietary supplements when they are represented as a conventional food. For instance, margarine-type spreads with added stanol esters are a food. A product sold as a soup is a food despite the addition of a "dietary supplement" such as echinacea or gingko, which would be considered a food additive. FDA requires substances added to foods to be generally recognized as safe (GRAS) by qualified experts or they must undergo FDA review and approval process as a food additive.[2] However, dietary supplements in food form (drinks, bars) that are labeled and marketed as dietary supplements are regulated as dietary supplements. Distinguishing functional foods from dietary supplements can therefore be confusing.

### Foods for Special Dietary Use

Foods for special dietary use, as defined by FDA, include foods used to supply *particular dietary needs* or to supplement or fortify the usual diet and are marketed as such; they do not meet general dietary needs (see Chapter 23).[9] Particular dietary needs may exist because of physical, physiologic, pathologic, or other conditions, such as disease, convalescence, pregnancy, lactation, underweight,

TABLE 24-1 Authorized and Authoritative Health Claims

| Health Claim | Requirements for Foods | Sample Claim Statement Containing Required Components | Selected Foods Meeting Claim Requirements |
|---|---|---|---|
| Calcium and osteoporosis* | High in calcium<br>Bioavailable<br>Phosphorus content no more than calcium content | Regular exercise and healthy diet with enough calcium helps teens, and white and Asian women maintain good bone health and may reduce their high risk of osteoporosis later in life. | Milk<br>Orange juice with added calcium |
| Sodium and hypertension* | Low sodium content | Diets low in sodium may reduce the risk of high blood pressure, a disease associated with many risk factors. | Fresh fruits and vegetables<br>Canned or frozen fruits and vegetables with no added salt |
| Dietary fat and cancer* | Low fat<br>"Extra lean" fish and game meat | Development of cancer depends on many factors. A diet low in total fat may reduce the risk of some cancers. | Fruits and vegetables, fresh, frozen, or canned<br>Most cereals<br>Nonfat and low-fat milk and dairy products |
| Dietary saturated fat and cholesterol and risk of coronary heart disease* | Low saturated fat<br>Low cholesterol<br>Low fat<br>"Extra lean" fish and game meat | While many factors affect heart disease, diets low in saturated fat and cholesterol may reduce the risk. | Fruits and vegetables, fresh, frozen, or canned<br>Most cereals<br>Nonfat and low-fat milk and dairy products |
| Fiber-containing grain products, fruits, and vegetables and cancer* | Grain product, fruit, or vegetable containing dietary fiber<br>Low fat<br>Good source of fiber without fortification | Low-fat diets rich in fiber-containing grain products, fruits, and vegetables may reduce the risk of some types of cancer, a disease associated with many factors. | Fruits and vegetables, fresh, frozen, or canned<br>Whole-grain breads, cereals, and pasta<br>Brown rice |
| Fruits, vegetables, and grain products that contain fiber (particularly soluble fiber) and risk of coronary heart disease* | Fruit, vegetable, or grain product containing fiber<br>Low saturated fat<br>Low cholesterol<br>Low fat<br>Minimum of 0.6 g soluble fiber per RA without fortification | Diets low in saturated fat and cholesterol and rich in fruits, vegetables, and grain products that contain some types of dietary fiber, particularly soluble fiber, may reduce the risk of heart disease, a disease associated with many factors. | Fruits and vegetables, fresh, frozen, or canned<br>Whole-grain breads, cereals, and pasta<br>Brown rice |
| Fruits and vegetables and cancer* | Fruit or vegetable<br>Low fat<br>Good source of vitamin A or C, or dietary fiber without fortification | Low-fat diets rich in fruits and vegetables (foods that are low in fat and may contain dietary fiber, vitamin A, or vitamin C) may reduce the risk of some types of cancer, a disease associated with many factors. [X food is high in vitamin A, vitamin C, and/or is a good source of fiber.] | Broccoli<br>Berries<br>Green beans<br>Carrots<br>Cantaloupe<br>Citrus fruit<br>Most dark green leafy vegetables |
| Folate and neural tube defects* | Contains at least 40 μg folate per serving<br>Good source without fortification<br>Contains not more than the RDI for vitamin A as retinol or preformed vitamin A or D | Healthful diets with adequate folate may reduce a woman's risk of having a child with a brain or spinal cord defect. | Most dark green leafy vegetables (see Chapter 23) |
| Dietary sugar alcohol and dental caries* | Sugar-free<br>Acceptable sugar alcohols: xylitol, sorbitol, mannitol, maltitol, isomalt, lactitol, hydrogenated starch hydrolysate, hydrogenated glucose syrup, erythritol, or a combination<br>Does not lower plaque pH below 5.7 when fermentable carbohydrate is present | Frequent between-meal consumption of foods high in sugars and starches promotes tooth decay. Sugar alcohols in [name of food] do not promote tooth decay.<br>Short claim for small packages: Does not promote tooth decay | Many "dietetic" sugar-free products marketed for people with diabetes.<br>Many low-calorie products marketed for weight loss |

**TABLE 24-1 Authorized and Authoritative Health Claims (continued)**

| Health Claim | Requirements for Foods | Sample Claim Statement Containing Required Components | Selected Foods Meeting Claim Requirements |
|---|---|---|---|
| Soluble fiber from certain foods and risk of coronary heart disease* | Low saturated fat<br>Low cholesterol<br>Low fat<br>Includes either: (1) an eligible source of whole oats with ≥0.75 g whole oat soluble fiber (β-glucan) per RA<br>(2) psyllium containing ≥1.7 g psyllium husk soluble fiber per RA | Soluble fiber from foods such as [name of soluble fiber source (optional - name of food product)], as part of a diet low in saturated fat and cholesterol, may reduce the risk of heart disease. A serving of [name of food product] supplies [X] grams of the soluble fiber from [name of soluble fiber source] necessary per day to have his effect. | Rolled oats<br>Oatmeal<br>Whole oats cold cereals<br>Cereals with added psyllium |
| Soy protein and risk of coronary heart disease* | Contains ≥6.25 g soy protein per RA<br>Low saturated fat<br>Low cholesterol<br>Low fat, unless fat is from whole soybeans | Example 1: 25 g of soy protein a day, as part of a diet low in saturated fat and cholesterol, may reduce the risk of heart disease. A serving of [name of food] supplies [X] grams of soy protein.<br>Example 2: Diets low in saturated fat and cholesterol that include 25 g of soy protein a day may reduce the risk of heart disease. One serving of [name of food] provides [X] grams of soy protein. | See Table 24-2 for soy protein content of some foods |
| Plant sterol/stanol esters and risk of coronary heart disease* | Spreads and salad dressings must contain ≥0.65 g plant sterol esters per RA<br>Spreads, salad dressings, and snack bars must contain ≥1.7 g plant stanol esters per RA<br>Low saturated fat<br>Low cholesterol | Example 1: Foods containing at least 0.65 g per serving of vegetable oil sterol esters, eaten twice a day with meals for a total intake of at least 1.3 g, as part of a diet low in saturated fat and cholesterol, may reduce the risk of heart disease. A serving of [name of food] supplies [X] grams of vegetable oil serol esters.<br>Example 2: Diets low in saturated fat and cholesterol that include two servings of foods that provide a daily total of at least 3.4 g of plant stanol esters in two meals may reduce the risk of heart disease. A serving of [name of food] supplies [X] grams of plant stanol esters. | Margarine spreads with added sterol/stanol esters<br>Orange juice with added sterol/stanol esters |
| Whole-grain foods and risk of heart disease and certain cancers† | Must contain 51% or more whole-grain ingredients by weight<br>Low fat<br>Must meet specified dietary fiber content: 3 g/RA of 55 g; 2.8 g/RA of 50 g; 2.5 g/RA of 45 g; 1.7 g/RA of 35 g | Diets rich in whole-grain foods and other plant foods and low in total fat, saturated fat, and cholesterol may reduce the risk of heart disease and some types of cancer. | Low-fat whole-grain breads and cereals<br>Whole-grain cereals and pasta<br>Brown rice |
| Potassium and the risk of high blood pressure and stroke† | Good source of potassium<br>Low sodium<br>Low fat<br>Low saturated fat<br>Low cholesterol | Diets containing foods that are a good source of potassium and that are low in sodium may reduce the risk of high blood pressure and stroke. | Many fruits and vegetables (see Chapter 23) |

Key: RA, reference amount (usually one serving as listed on label); RDI, recommended dietary intake.

* Authorized health claim.

† Authoritative health claim; wording in sample claim statement is required by FDA.

**TABLE 24-5 Examples of Conventional Foods Classified as Functional Foods**

| Food | Functional Component | Potential Health Benefit | Comments |
|---|---|---|---|
| Apples | Flavonols, phenols, proanthocyanidins, soluble fiber (pectin) | Reduce risk of certain types of cancer; improve glucose and cholesterol; may contribute to maintenance of heart health | Recommend one/day but amount for health benefit not defined |
| Banana, ripe | Prebiotics, fructooligosaccharides | Reduce hypertension and hypercholesterolemia | Weak evidence for 3-10 g/day |
| Berries | Anthocyanidins | Antioxidant functions; may contribute to healthy immune system | Recommend 1/2-1 cup/day but amount for health benefit not defined |
| Cherries | Anthocyanidins | Antioxidant functions; may contribute to healthy immune system | Recommend 1/2-1 cup/day but amount for health benefit not defined |
| Cinnamon | Proanthocyanidins | May contribute to maintenance of urinary tract and heart health | Weak evidence; amount for health benefit not well researched |
| Citrus fruits | Lutein, zeaxanthin, limonene | Reduce risk of age-related macular degeneration; reduced cancer risk | Weak to moderate evidence for macular degeneration with 6 mg/day as lutein; rodent studies with limonene and cancer |
| Cocoa, chocolate (especially dark chocolate) | Flavonols | Antioxidant functions, reduce risk of coronary heart disease | |
| Corn | Lutein, zeaxanthin, free stanols/sterols | Reduce risk of age-related macular degeneration; may reduce risk of CHD | Weak to moderate evidence for 6 mg/day as lutein; health claim for stanol/sterol esters added to foods |
| Cranberry juice | Proanthocyanidins | Reduce UTI by reducing adherence of bacteria to cell walls; may also prevent adhesion of plaque-forming bacteria in the mouth | Moderate evidence for 300 mL/day to reduce UTI (58% reduction in bacteruria in 150 elderly women in the first randomized controlled trial [1994]) |
| Cruciferous vegetables: broccoli, brussels sprouts, cauliflower, cabbage | Glucosinolates, indoles, isothiocyanates (sulphoraphane); organosulfur compounds, thiols | Reduce risk of certain types of cancer | Weak to moderate evidence for greater than 1/2 cup/day |
| Dairy products, including some cheese | Conjugated linoleic acid | Reduce risk of breast cancer; possible role in improved body composition | Weak evidence for breast cancer link; animal studies suggest role in reducing body fat; necessary amount not determined for health effects |
| Dairy products, fermented (acidophilus milk, buttermilk, kefir, yogurt) | Probiotic organisms (lactobacilli, bifidobacteria) | Maintain GI tract health; reduce colon cancer risk; reduce cholesterol | Moderate evidence for 1-2 billion CFU/day to maintain GI tract health; weak to moderate evidence for colon cancer risk; results for cholesterol effect are equivocal |
| Eggs (yolk) | Lutein, zeaxanthin | Reduce risk of age-related macular degeneration | Weak to moderate evidence for 6 mg/day as lutein |
| Eggs, enriched with DHA | DHA | Reduce risk of CHD, increased HDL-cholesterol | Chickens are fed fish oils or algae as a source of DHA |
| Fatty fish (wild salmon, herring) | Omega-3 fatty acids | Reduce triglycerides and risk of heart disease, including fatal and nonfatal MI | Recommend 2 meals/week with fatty fish |

**TABLE 24-5 Examples of Conventional Foods Classified as Functional Foods (continued)**

| Food | Functional Component | Potential Health Benefit | Comments |
|---|---|---|---|
| Flax | Phytoestrogens (lignans); α-linoleic acid | Reduce risk of CHD by decreasing cholesterol and platelet aggregation; weak estrogenic activity may decrease hormone-related cancers; maintenance of a healthy immune system; α-linoleic acid may contribute to maintenance of visual function | Weak evidence for CHD association; very weak evidence for cancer risk; amounts necessary for health benefit from flax is not defined |
| Garlic | Organosulfur compounds, thiols | Reduce total and LDL cholesterol; may reduce the risk of cancer | Weak to moderate evidence for about one fresh clove daily for cholesterol; epidemiologic evidence for reduced cancer is equivocal; considerable variation exists in the amount of active compounds for available products |
| Grapes, red and black | Anthocyanidins; phenolic compounds | Antioxidant functions; cardiovascular risk reduction | Epidemiologic evidence suggests inverse association with cardiovascular disease risk |
| Grape juice | Resvertrol | Reduce risk of MI caused by reduced platelet aggregation | Moderate to strong evidence for 8-16 oz/day |
| Greens: spinach, kale, collards | Lutein, zeaxanthin | Reduce risk of age-related macular degeneration | Weak to moderate evidence for 6 mg/day as lutein |
| Jerusalem artichoke | Prebiotics, fructooligosaccharides | Reduce hypertension; reduce hypercholesterolemia | Weak evidence for 3-10 g/day |
| Meat (beef, lamb, turkey) | Conjugated linoleic acid | Antitumor effect; possible role in improved body composition | Effect suppression of cancer cell growth in rat studies; animal studies suggest role in reducing body fat; necessary amount not determined for health effects |
| Onions, leeks, scallions | Organosulfur compounds, thiols | Reduce total and LDL cholesterol | Weak to moderate evidence |
| Onion powder | Prebiotics, fructooligosaccharides | Reduce hypertension; reduce hypercholesterolemia | Weak evidence for 3-10 g/day |
| Rye | Phytoestrogens (ligans) | May contribute to maintenance of heart health and healthy immune system | |
| Tea, black | Polyphenols; flavonoids | Reduce risk of coronary heart disease | Evidence is not conclusive |
| Tea, green | Catechins (epigallocatechin-3-gallate, epigallocatechin, epicatechin-3-gallate, epicatechin) | Reduce risk of certain types of cancer | Moderate evidence for 4-6 cups/day |
| Tomatoes and processed tomato products | Lycopene | Antioxidant that efficiently reduced singlet oxygen in biologic systems; reduce risk of prostate cancer; possibly reduce risk of other cancers (breast, cervix, bladder, GI tract, skin) and MI | Moderate evidence for 1/2 cup/day or 10 servings/week for prostate cancer; weak evidence for other functions based on inverse associations of tissue lycopene and cancers or MI |
| Tree nuts | Monounsaturated fatty acids, vitamin E | Reduce risk of CHD | Moderate evidence for 1-2 oz/day; qualified health claim for walnuts only |

Key: CFU, colony-forming units; CHD, coronary heart disease; DHA, docosahexaenoic acid; GI, gastrointestinal; MI, myocardial infarction (heart attack); UTI, urinary tract infection.

**TABLE 24-6 Adequate Intakes and Actual Intakes for Fiber (g/day)[15-18]**

| | Younger Age* | Older Age† | Data Source |
|---|---|---|---|
| **Men** | | | |
| AI: total fiber | 38 | 30 | IOM[17] |
| Actual intake | | | |
| Total fiber—mean | 20 | 19 | NHANES III[16] |
| Total fiber—median | 17 | 16 | NHANES III[16] |
| Soluble fiber | 7.1 | 6.5 | NHANES III[16] |
| Insoluble fiber | 13.1 | 12.7 | NHANES III[16] |
| Mean intake (50th percentile) | 17.4-17.9 | 17.5-16.5 | CSFII[15] |
| Median intake | 18.8-20.3 | 17.7 | NHIS[18] |
| **Women** | | | |
| AI: total fiber | 25 | 21 | IOM[17] |
| Actual intake | | | |
| Total fiber—mean | 14 | 15 | NHANES III[16] |
| Total fiber—median | 13 | 13 | NHANES III[16] |
| Soluble fiber | 4.9 | 5.3 | NHANES III[16] |
| Insoluble fiber | 9.4 | 10.3 | NHANES III[16] |
| Mean intake (50th percentile) | 12.1-13.1 | 13.3-13.8 | CSFII[15] |
| Median intake | 14.1-14.8 | 14.1 | NHIS[18] |
| **Pregnancy/Lactation** | | | |
| AI | 28/29 | N/A | IOM[17] |
| Actual intake | ND | N/A | |

Key: AI, adequate intake; CSFII, Continuing Survey of Food Intakes by Individuals; IOM, Institute of Medicine; N/A, not applicable; ND, no data available; NHANES III, third National Health and Nutrition Survey; NHIS, 2000 National Health Interview Survey.

* Younger age (years) = 19 to 50 for AI and CSFII; 18 to 59 for NHIS; 20 to 59 for NHANES III.

† Older age (years) = 51 and older for AI and CSFII; 60 and older for NHIS and NHANES III.

soluble or insoluble. The changing definition of dietary fiber is important to consider when evaluating studies on the health effects of fiber because different fiber components may have different health effects. In addition, because extraction of fiber from cell walls may alter its chemical and physical properties, extracted fiber may have different effects than in situ fiber. These factors likely contribute to the conflicting results sometimes reported for studies related to health benefits of fiber.

The terms *dietary fiber* and *functional fiber*, related to dietary reference intakes (DRI; see Chapter 23), distinguish sources of fiber.[15] Total fiber is the sum of dietary and functional fiber. Dietary fiber is defined as nondigestible carbohydrates and lignin that are naturally occurring (intrinsic and intact) in plants. Functional fiber is defined as isolated nondigestible carbohydrates that have beneficial physiologic effects in humans. Fiber extracted or modified from plants or animal sources, including chitin and chitosan from the shells of crustaceans, is included as functional fiber. The third National Health and Nutrition Survey (NHANES III) uses the terms *total fiber*, *soluble fiber*, and *insoluble fiber*.[16] Because of their current widespread use in both professional and nonprofessional literature, the terms *soluble fiber* and *insoluble fiber* are used here. However, gradual replacement of these terms by the specific fibers has been recommended because viscosity and fermentability may be more important correlates with health effects.[14]

*Recommended and Actual Intake* Adequate intakes (AI) have been published by the IOM for total fiber (see Chapter 23 for general information on AI), as shown in Table 24-6.[17] The AI is based on usual caloric intake in each age group and 14 g dietary fiber per 1000 calories, which appears to be the amount needed to promote heart health.[15] Unfortunately, as Table 24-6 shows, actual mean and median intake of adults in the United States falls considerably below the AI, as determined from national surveys of dietary intake for several thousand participants. The surveys include NHANES III,[16] the Continuing Survey of Food Intakes by Individuals (CSFII),[15] and the 2000 National Health Interview Survey (NHIS).[18] Data from CSFII indicate that mean fiber intake did not reach the AI

**TABLE 24-7 Components and Sources of Soluble and Insoluble Fiber**

| | Soluble Fiber | Insoluble Fiber |
|---|---|---|
| Food component | Pectins, gums, mucilages, algal substances, and some hemicellulose | Cellulose, lignin, and most hemicellulose |
| Food with ≥2.5 g of total fiber per serving* | Cereals: oat bran (uncooked, 2/3 cup), oatmeal (cooked, 1 cup)<br>Fruits: apples and pears with skin on, oranges (1 medium size), figs and prunes (3 small size)<br>Vegetables: broccoli, carrots, cauliflower, corn, kale and other greens, dark green or loose leaf lettuce, peas, squash, zucchini (cooked, 3/4-1 cup) | Bran and whole grain (corn, rye, wheat) products: bran cereals (dry cereal, 1/3-1 cup), brown rice (cooked, 1 cup), whole-wheat bread (2 slices)<br>Dried beans: lima, kidney, pinto, white (cooked, 1/4-1/2 cup)<br>Dried peas: green, split (cooked, 1/4-1/2 cup) |
| Functional fiber sources | Beet fiber, fructooligosaccharides (FOS), guar gum (galactomannan; Benefiber), inulin, karaya gum, konjac mannan, locust bean gum, pectin, psyllium (ispaghula seed husk), soy polysaccharide | Calcium polycarbophil, methylcellulose, powdered cellulose |

* Serving size shown in parentheses.

in younger adults (ages 19-50 years) until the 99th percentile for usual daily intake of dietary fiber; among those 51 years of age and older, men reached the AI at the 95th percentile and women at the 90th percentile.[15] Only 38.5% of men and 16.2% of women met recommended intakes for fiber among the NHIS participants older than 18 years.[18] Other estimates suggest 15 to 25 g/day of polysaccharides, including resistant starches, reach the colon daily in Americans.[19] Nonstarch polysaccharides are the major component of fiber intake excluding lignan, a relatively small contributor to insoluble fiber.

Despite potentially different health benefits from soluble versus insoluble fiber, the AI do not specify amounts of fiber on the basis of solubility. Different methods can be used to determine solubility; thus, different amounts of soluble and insoluble fiber are reported for the same foods. In addition, there was heavy reliance on epidemiologic data correlating fiber intake from foods to health benefits when determining the AI. Foods nearly always provide a mixture of soluble and insoluble fiber along with other potentially beneficial ingredients; however, the ratios differ among foods and health effects may vary from those associated with both types of fiber to those associated with either soluble or insoluble fiber. Examples of the ratios of soluble and insoluble fiber include 15% soluble/85% insoluble for whole wheat flour and brown rice; 35% soluble/65% insoluble in broccoli, spinach, and tomatoes; 50% soluble/50% insoluble in dried fruit and oatmeal; and 60% soluble/40% insoluble in oranges.[8] The NHANES III data suggest fiber intake is about one third soluble, two thirds insoluble for people in the United States, as shown in Table 24-6.[16]

*Soluble and Insoluble Fibers* Soluble fibers typically undergo substantial degradation and fermentation in the colon; negligible degradation and fermentation occur with most insoluble fibers.[13] Table 24-7 outlines the components and sources typically attributed to soluble and insoluble fibers. The food sources listed are good to excellent sources of total dietary fiber and are listed under the heading that exemplifies their predominant health effects. Terms indicating the fiber content of foods are defined by FDA.[20] Excellent sources of fiber are classified as "high fiber," and one serving provides 5 g or more of fiber. Foods providing 2.5 to 4.9 g of fiber per serving are considered a "good source" of fiber.

*Methods of Increasing Fiber Intake* Table 24-8 lists ideas for increasing fiber content in the diet. It is advisable to increase fiber intake gradually because a sudden increase can cause GI distress, including bloating, gas, and occasionally diarrhea. A reasonable approach is to add one or two servings of foods that are an abundant source of fiber, as listed in Table 24-7, to the diet every few days until the AI or other goal for fiber intake is reached. Reading ingredient labels is essential to ensure adequate fiber content, especially for breads and cereals in which a *whole* grain should be the first ingredient listed.

*Benefits of Fiber* The generally accepted benefits of fiber are laxation effects, normalization of blood lipid concentrations, and attenuation of blood glucose response. These are the accepted measures of efficacy for fiber sources as required for label claims of fiber content in Canada. Other possible benefits of fiber are not as well-defined in humans. Furthermore, conflicting or controversial study results are often found, or no studies of adequate size and duration are available to draw strong conclusions regarding the effect of fiber. However, there is considerable interest in some of the other potential benefits of fiber, especially effects on GI diseases.

Laxation Stool characteristics associated with laxation, or improved bowel function include increased stool bulk, weight, and water content; decreased stool transit time to 2 to 4 days and normalization of stool frequency to once daily; reduced symptoms of constipation (see Chapter 16); and an overall improvement in ease of defecation. Epidemiologic studies strongly support the positive role of fiber

**TABLE 24-8 Ideas for Increasing Fiber in the Diet**

- Eat breads containing whole wheat, whole-wheat flour, or other whole grains as the first ingredient on the label. These products should replace breads from refined flours that do not include whole grains.
- Replace part of other cereals with whole-wheat cereal for persons who prefer other cereals.
- Eat oatmeal as a hot breakfast cereal, or select a cold cereal with oats or whole wheat listed as the primary ingredient.
- Sprinkle bran on cereal, yogurt, or other foods.
- Eat brown rice, whole-wheat pasta, and whole-wheat crackers rather than white rice and products from refined grains.
- Add fruit to breakfast cereals.
- Select recipes that use whole-grain flours, and/or add rolled oats for baked goods.
- Select recipes for baked goods that include apples, applesauce, carrots, pumpkins, or other fruits or vegetables as a significant ingredient.
- Add kidney, garbanzo, navy, or other beans to salads and soups, including canned soups. Rinse and drain canned beans to reduce components prone to cause gas.
- Serve fruit and/or vegetable salads with picnic lunches rather than potato chips.
- Serve baked beans as an alternative protein source.
- Eat fresh or dried fruit for snacks and desserts; frozen and canned fruits can also be used.
- Use a low-fat refried bean dip or humus with baked tortilla chips for snacks.
- Include "finger food" vegetables (carrots, celery, cauliflower pieces, broccoli flowerets) in lunch boxes and as snacks.
- For children, make animal or other fun shapes from vegetables pieces.

from whole grains, fruits, and vegetables in laxation. Most studies show strong correlations between dietary fiber intake and increased stool weight and decreased transit time. In a meta-analysis including approximately 100 studies, stool weight increased by 5.4 g/gram of wheat bran fiber, compared with 4.9 g/gram of fruits and vegetables, 3 g/gram of cellulose, and only 1.3 g/gram of pectin.[15] The first three sources of fiber are associated with improved laxation, whereas the highly fermentable and soluble fiber, pectin, is not. Caution must be used in interpreting stool weight alone, however, since an increase in bacteria within the stool could increase weight without affecting transit time.

A Cochrane review of constipation in pregnancy supports the role of fiber in laxation, concluding that bran and wheat fiber increased frequency of defecation and resulted in softer stools.[21] However, in a systematic review of treatment for *chronic* constipation, the American College of Gastroenterology found insufficient evidence to make a recommendation on the efficacy of bran.[22] Only one placebo-controlled randomized trial of wheat bran was included in the systematic review. Unfortunately, this crossover study appeared to suffer from a "placebo run-in effect" since, compared with the baseline, wheat bran increased stool frequency, but the overall effect did not differ from that of placebo when fiber was given before placebo.[22] Whether increased fiber intake is effective for chronic constipation or not, a recommendation by practitioners to increase whole grain, fruits, and vegetables in the diet is reasonable for people without major GI pathology on the basis of general guidelines for a healthy diet (see Chapter 23).

The role of functional fibers in laxation is well accepted, and adequate scientific evidence exists to support FDA approval of psyllium (Metamucil), methylcellulose (Citrucel), and calcium polycarbophil (Perdiem Fiber Therapy, Fibercon) as nonprescription bulking agents for treatment of *occasional* constipation (see Chapter 16). However, studies supporting the efficacy of bulk-forming fibers in *chronic* constipation tend to be of intermediate to low quality because of their short duration (14 days or less) and/or small sample sizes. In a systematic review of treatment for chronic constipation, the American College of Gastroenterology concluded that psyllium increased stool frequency, but noted that studies were only of intermediate quality.[22] They found insufficient evidence to recommend methylcellulose and calcium polycarbophil as efficacious for chronic constipation.

**Normalization of Blood Lipid Concentrations** Lowering of total and LDL cholesterol is associated with reduced risk of CHD and serves as a surrogate marker for CHD. Data on reduced risk of CHD are strong enough for certain fibers to support an FDA-authorized health claim, including claims for psyllium and β-glucan in whole oats and oat bran (Table 24-1 lists health claims).

Multiple epidemiologic studies have reported a reduced risk of CHD with consumption of high amounts of dietary fiber and/or fiber-rich foods. Table 24-9 summarizes data related to risk of CHD from various studies including some very large, well-designed prospective epidemiologic studies with longer-term follow-up.[3,14,15,23,24] The overall conclusion from these studies is that a strong inverse relationship exists between risk of CHD and intake of cereal fiber, in particular, high-viscosity soluble fiber sources including oats, barley, and rye.

A large number of relatively small intervention studies have reported cholesterol-lowering effects with fiber intake, including trials with oats, beans, guar gum, pectin, and psyllium. A meta-analysis also supports the role of "practical" quantities (2-10 g/day) of fiber from guar gum, oat bran, pectin, or psyllium to significantly reduce both total and LDL-cholesterol concentrations.[23]

The key to fiber's ability to lower cholesterol and reduce CHD risk appears to be consuming an adequate quantity of highly viscous fiber. Foods most likely to provide a positive effect include cereal grains such as oats, barley, or rye, and beans (legumes). Highly viscous functional fibers associated with lower cholesterol and/or reduced risk of CHD include guar gum, pectin, and psyllium.

**Attenuation of Blood Glucose Response** Multiple, large, well-designed prospective epidemiologic studies with longer-term follow-up have reported an association between consumption of fiber and attenuation of blood glucose, improved insulin response, and/or reduced risk of diabetes, as summarized in Table 24-9.[3,14,15,25-31] The overall

**TABLE 24-9 Summary of Studies Related to Fiber and Risk of CHD and Improved Glucose Control**

| Study | Number and Gender* | Age Range (years) | Follow-up Time (years) | Results/Conclusions |
|---|---|---|---|---|
| Nurse's Health Study[15,24,25] | >65,000 women | 37-64 | 10 | *CHD:* An inverse relationship between dietary fiber intake and risk of CHD evident only for dietary fiber from cereal sources, not fruits and vegetables; cereal fiber intake averaging 7.7 g/day reduced risk of CHD by 34%, compared with average intake of 2.2 g/day; RR 0.77 with higher fiber intake; 19% decrease in risk for CHD events per 10 g/day increase in dietary fiber and a 37% decrease per 5 g increase in cereal fiber<br>*Glucose:* RR type 2 DM 2.5 for high-GL/low-cereal-fiber diet (< 2.5 g/day), compared with low-GL/high-cereal-fiber diet (>5.8 g/day); more frequent intake of dark breads, whole-grain breakfast cereals, and brown rice associated with decreased likelihood of developing diabetes |
| Health Professionals' Follow-up Study[15,25] | >42,000 men | 40-75 | 6-12 | *CHD:* RR fatal CHD 0.45 and RR total MI 0.59 in those averaging 28.9 g dietary fiber/day, compared with those averaging 12.5 g/day; stronger association with cereal fiber than with fruits and vegetables; 19% decrease in risk of MI per 10 g/day increase in dietary fiber and a 29% decrease per 10 g/day increase in cereal fiber<br>*Glucose:* RR type 2 DM 2.17 for high-GL/low-cereal-fiber diet (<2.5 g/day), compared with low-GL/high-cereal-fiber diet (>5.8 g/day) |
| Iowa Women's Health Study[3,15,25] | Nearly 36,000 women | Post-meno-pause | 6 | *CHD:* Approximately one-third decrease in risk of fatal CHD in women with ≥1 serving/day of whole grains, compared with those with little whole-grain intake; risk decreased with fiber from cereals, not fruits and vegetables; decreased likelihood of mortality from ischemic heart disease with more frequent intake of dark (whole-grain) bread and whole-grain breakfast cereals<br>*Glucose:* Inverse relationship of insoluble fiber intake from cereals and risk of DM; no relationship to fruit, vegetable, legume intake; RR diabetes 0.79 for median intake of 20.5 servings/week of whole-grain products, compared with median of 1 serving/week |
| Mediterranean-type diet, intervention[27] | 54 for intent to treat; 46 compliant to diet | Adults, type 1 DM | 24 weeks, controlled study | *CHD:* No significant changes found in total cholesterol, HDL cholesterol, or triglyceride concentration between high- and low-fiber intake<br>*Glucose:* Those compliant to a high-fiber diet (average 39 g/day) significantly decreased glycosylated hemoglobin (from 9.1% to 8.6%) and mean daily glucose (23.8%) with the effect most pronounced after lunch, compared with low-fiber intake (average 15 g/day); based on intent to treat, only mean daily glucose decreased significantly (18.6%) with high-fiber intake; high-fiber intake >30 g/day, low-fiber intake <20 g/day for compliance to high- and low-fiber diet, respectively |
| Very-high-fiber diet, intervention[28] | | Adults, type 1 DM | 6 weeks, controlled study | *CHD:* Very-high-fiber diet (50 g/day total fiber, 25 g/day soluble) reduced total cholesterol 6.7%, triglycerides 10.2%, and VLDL cholesterol 12.5%, compared with a moderate fiber diet (24 g/day total fiber, 8 g/day soluble)<br>*Glucose:* Very-high-fiber diet decreased mean daily preprandial glucose, lowered the 24 hour plasma glucose area under the curve by 10% and the insulin concentration by 12%, compared with moderate fiber intake |

**TABLE 24-9 Summary of Studies Related to Fiber and Risk of CHD and Improved Glucose Control (continued)**

| Study | Number and Gender* | Age Range (years) | Follow-up Time (years) | Results/Conclusions |
|---|---|---|---|---|
| α-Tocopherol, β-carotene cancer prevention study[15] | Nearly 22,000 men | 50-69 | 6 | *CHD:* RR CHD 0.84 for those averaging 34.5 g dietary fiber/day, compared with those averaging 16.1 g/day with fiber intake adjusted to 2000 calories; high-fiber intake: 12.9 g/1000 cal; low-fiber intake: 5.9 g/1000 cal |
| Meta-analysis, diets high in soluble fibers[23] | 67 controlled trials | | | *CHD:* Small but significant decrease in total and LDL cholesterol with intake of 2-10 g/day of viscous fibers including guar gum, oat bran, pectin, or psyllium |
| Atherosclerosis Risk in Communities (ARIC) Study[25] | 12,251; White and African-Americans | 45-64 | 9 | *Glucose:* Inverse relationship of cereal fiber intake and risk of DM in both African American and white subgroups, but statistically significant only in whites; no relationship to fruit and legume intake in either subgroup |
| Finnish Mobile Clinic Health Examination Survey[25,29] | 2286 men and 2030 women | 40-69 | 10 | *Glucose:* Inverse relationship of cereal fiber intake and risk of DM (cereal fiber predominantly from rye; little wheat) |
| U.S. population[25] | 9665 | Adults | 18 | *Glucose:* Inverse relationship of vegetable intake with risk of DM |
| Seven Countries Study[25] | 338, Finnish and Dutch cohorts | Adults | 20 | *Glucose:* Inverse relationship of legume and vegetable intake with risk of DM |
| Danish Inter99 Study[30] | 5675 | 30-60 | Baseline data | *Glucose:* Inverse relationship between dietary fiber, fruit, and vegetable intake and insulin resistance |
| Insulin Resistance Atherosclerosis Study (IRAS)[31] | 978 | 40-69, normal (67%) and impaired (33%) glucose tolerance | Data from interview and 1-year, semiquantitative food-frequency questionnaire | *Glucose:* High-fiber bran or granola cereals and shredded wheat showed a strong positive association with insulin sensitivity and a strong inverse relationship with fasting insulin; the associations for whole-wheat, rye, pumpernickel, and other high-fiber bread was evident, but not as strong; no associations noted for cooked oatmeal, cream of wheat, or grits |
| Meta-analysis[26] | 24 studies, average of 13-16 subjects | Adults, DM | Averaged under 45 days | *Glucose:* Significant decreases of 13%-14% in fasting, postprandial, and average daily glucose with a high-CHO/high-fiber diet, compared with a low-fiber diet; significant decrease (21%) in postprandial glucose with moderate CHO-high fiber intake; high-fiber intake: 20 g or more/1000 cal |

Key: CHD, coronary heart disease; CHO, carbohydrate; DM, diabetes mellitus; GL, glycemic load; HDL, high-density lipoprotein; LDL, low-density lipoprotein; MI, myocardial infarction; RR, relative risk; VLDL, very-low-density lipoprotein.

* Number of participants included in the analysis is not always the entire study population; number of trials included in meta-analysis.

conclusion from these studies is that an inverse relationship exists between risk of diabetes and intake of dietary fiber. Intake of cereal fiber appears to be most frequently related to improved glucose control and/or reduced risk of diabetes although intake of legumes (beans), fruit, and vegetables has also shown an association in some studies. High viscosity is likely the consistent characteristic among these fiber sources. Evidence suggests that nonviscous fibers, such as wheat bran, have little effect on glycemic control.

Many small, short-term interventional studies have reported an association between fiber intake and improvement in glucose control, insulin sensitivity, and/or insulin resistance. Studies have been conducted with types 1 and 2 diabetes. A meta-analysis supports significant improvement in glucose control, especially with a high carbohydrate (55% to 65% of calories) and very high fiber intake, as shown in Table 24-9.[26] This effect does appear to be sustainable longer term, at least in patients with type 1 diabetes who comply with the high-fiber diet.[27]

Adequate intake of highly viscous fiber appears to be key to improving glucose control and reducing diabetes risk, with total fiber intake at the AI or higher (up to 20 g/1000 calories). Carbohydrate intake may also influence the effect of fiber on glucose control; most parameters improve with a high-carbohydrate diet. Foods most likely to provide a positive effect include cereal grains such as oats, barley, and rye. Some legumes (beans), fruits, and vegetables also may have a beneficial effect on glucose control. Functional fibers considered highly viscous and associated with improved glucose control and/or reduced risk of diabetes include guar gum and pectin.

Weight Loss and Maintenance Epidemiologic studies show lower body mass in men and women who eat a high-fiber diet and greater incidence of obesity in those with low intake of dietary fiber.[15] Interventional studies show mixed results with diets high in fiber and weight loss (see Chapter 27). At this time, there is no significant evidence to support a role for dietary fiber in satiety or weight maintenance.

GI Disorders The role of fiber in colorectal cancer, irritable bowel syndrome (IBS), and diverticular disease remains controversial. These conditions may require medical intervention; however, practitioners should be familiar with general guidelines for fiber use in these conditions.

Colorectal Cancer Epidemiologic evidence from the European Prospective Investigation into Cancer and Nutrition (EPIC) found an inverse relationship between fiber intake from foods and the risk of colorectal cancer.[32] The relative risk was 0.75 for the highest quintile, compared with the lowest quintile. Data from 520,000 participants from 10 European countries were included in this study, and a wide range of fiber intake was reported (12.7 to 35.6 g/day in men and 12.6 to 31.9 g/day for women). Most other epidemiologic studies also have reported a protective effect of dietary fiber against colorectal cancer, with up to 25% less likelihood of developing colorectal cancer.[20,33] Important exceptions are the Nurse's Health Study and the Health Professionals Follow-up Study, which reported no relationship between fiber intake and the incidence of colorectal cancer and adenomas.[15,34] In addition, some interventional studies have failed to show a relationship between a diet rich in fruits and vegetables or wheat bran supplements and formation of new colon tumors, specifically adenomas.[15] A systematic review also concluded that no evidence from randomized controlled trials supported a role for increased dietary fiber intake in prevention of adenomatous polyps within a 2- to 4-year period.[35] Although adenomas can progress to colorectal cancer, their etiology appears to differ significantly from that of cancer based on distribution within the colon, male to female ratios, different prevalence in the same population, and the effects of alcohol and tobacco as risk factors; thus, failure to prevent adenoma recurrence may not be an appropriate indicator of colorectal cancer prevention.[36]

A medical position statement issued by The American Gastroenterological Association (AGA) noted that support for a protective role of fiber against development of colorectal cancer was not unequivocal.[19] However, on the basis of critical analysis of the whole body of evidence, the AGA considered it reasonable to recommend an intake of 30 to 35 g/day of dietary fiber from all sources. Whole-grain cereals, fruits, vegetables, and other fiber-rich foods were suggested since these foods appear to better demonstrate a protective effect against colorectal cancer than dietary fiber alone.[19] Although this position statement and technical review were published before the EPIC and recent intervention trial results were available, the balance of evidence still appears to support the position statement.[15,19]

Irritable Bowel Syndrome Guidelines for primary care (outpatient) management of IBS recommend increased fiber intake for patients with constipation. A systematic review that included 1363 referred patients (nonprimary care) also noted an overall favorable effect of fiber on IBS-related constipation, with a relative risk of 1.56% and 95% confidence interval (CI) of 1.21 to 2.02.[37] Wheat bran showed favorable results for constipation (relative risk 1.54; 95% CI, 1.1-2.14), as did ispaghula (psyllium). Of the 17 studies included in the systematic review, 12 reported improvement in global symptoms of IBS with fiber (relative risk 1.33; 95% CI, 1.19-1.5), but no improvement in abdominal pain. Soluble fiber also improved global symptoms of IBS (relative risk 1.55; 95% CI, 1.35-1.78), but did not improve abdominal pain or bloating. None of the studies showed bran (wheat, corn, or millet) to be better than placebo for improvement in global symptoms, and some global symptoms become worse with both bran and placebo, indicating no protective effect of bran on the disease process.

Diverticular Disease The Health Professionals Follow-up Study reported a strong negative association between dietary fiber intake and the incidence of symptomatic diverticular disease.[15] The strongest inverse relationship appears to be with nonviscous dietary fiber, especially cellulose. Case control studies also find lower dietary fiber intake among people with diverticula.[15] Recommendations for fiber intake in people with diverticular disease depend on the stage of disease.[38] Intake of 25 to 35 g/day of fiber is recommended for those with asymptomatic disease and no complications; limited intake (5 to 15 g/day) is suggested with mild disease and no evidence of infection (normal temperature and white blood cell count [WBC] and negative computed tomographic [CT] scan). Patients with evidence of infection, obstruction, or perforation (increased temperature or WBC, positive CT scan, significant abdominal pain) should be referred to a physician immediately and should follow provided dietary advice, usually including avoidance of fiber intake.

### Prebiotics

Food components that act as prebiotics move through the small bowel without being digested or absorbed and reach the colon where bacteria ferment them; thus, they are classified as fiber. To be considered a prebiotic, fiber must "selectively stimulate the growth and/or activity of one or a limited number of bacteria in the colon" and benefit the host.[4,5] These bacteria are the beneficial or "friendly" commensal bacteria found naturally in the colon, such as bifidobacteria and lactobacilli.

*Sources and Intake* Inulin and fructose oligosaccharides (FOS) are the most common prebiotic food components. They are found in many edible plants including artichoke, asparagus, bananas, chicory, onion, and wheat, and are added to foods to provide a source of fiber and to provide a creamy, fatlike mouth-feel in certain foods. The average intake for adults in the United States is estimated to be 2.6 g/day of inulin and 2.5 g/day of FOS, but intake varies from 1 to 12 g/day depending on the diet.[4,5]

*Pharmacology* Prebiotic food components, such as inulin and FOS, contain fructose polymers (fructans) or chains of fructose monosaccharide linked together by β2-1 glycosidic bonds that cannot be digested by enzymes produced in the human GI tract.[39] Most bifidobacteria contain relatively high amounts of a β-fructosidase with selectivity for β2-1 glycosidic bonds; thus, bifidobacteria are thought to be a major contributor to production of fructose in the colon from prebiotics. Fructose is fermented, and the acid environment created by fermentation products is thought to favor the beneficial bacteria while inhibiting growth of pathogenic bacteria, such as enterococci and enterobacteria.[39,40] The bacteria receive energy for growth from the fermentation products, which include short-chain fatty acids (acetate, butyrate, and propionate) and lactate. Short-chain fatty acids also can be absorbed by the host and are estimated to provide 1.5 to 2.5 cal/g of ingested prebiotic.[15]

*Health Effects* Studies assessing the prebiotic effect of FOS in humans have shown significant increases in bifidobacteria. Most studies are small, a few are double-blind, placebo-controlled studies, but most are not. Although 7 g/day of FOS increased bifidobacteria in one study, the optimal dose for increasing bifidobacteria without developing GI side effects in a 7-day study involving 40 healthy subjects was 10 g/day.[40] Larger doses of prebiotics appear to significantly increase side effects. In a double-blind crossover study with 64 women, 14 g/day of insulin resulted in significantly increased GI side effects and 12% of participants considered the flatulence to be unacceptable.[41] The likely cause of GI side effects (flatulence, rumbling, cramps, and bloating) reported in many human studies of prebiotics is hydrogen, carbon dioxide, and a small amount of methane produced by fermentation.

Beneficial effects related to prebiotics may include improved glucose control, reduced risk of colon cancer, improved laxation, and better absorption of minerals from the diet. Short-chain fatty acids from prebiotic fermentation appear to contribute to the first two beneficial effects.[15] Propionate may play a role in improving glucose control since it inhibits gluconeogenesis from lactate and enhances glycolysis.[39] In a small double-blind crossover study with healthy subjects, 20 g/day of FOS was shown to significantly decrease hepatic glucose production. Another small study demonstrated improved fasting glucose with 8 g/day of FOS. Many studies have evaluated the role of butyrate in the colon. Butyrate is acknowledged as the major energy source for colon cells and appears to play a role in reducing the risk of colon cancer although studies concerning this effect are not conclusive.[39] Improved laxation has been reported in several studies, including increased stool frequency and bulk. In a group of 25 people of advanced age with constipation, inulin had a better laxative effect than laculose.[40] The effect of inulin and FOS on mineral absorption, particularly calcium, has been extensively studied in animals. The limited human studies conducted thus far have shown significant increases in apparent calcium absorption or equivocal results.[4,5] Positive effects on apparent calcium absorption were reported in two studies with a 26% increase reported from 15 g/day of FOS and a 58% increase from 40 g/day of inulin.[4] Several small studies also indicate increased magnesium absorption with inulin and FOS.[42] Improved absorption of iron and zinc also have been reported in animal studies, but these effects have not been confirmed in humans.[5] Other potential benefits shown in animals that have not been confirmed in humans include inhibition of hepatic lipogenesis resulting in a hypotriglyceride effect and an anti-inflammatory effect in enterocolitis.

### Probiotics

Probiotics are nonpathogenic, living microorganisms that appear to improve the balance of microflora in the GI tract and have a beneficial effect on the host when consumed in adequate amounts.[5,43] Lactobacilli, bifidobacteria, and streptococci species, and *Saccharomyces boulardii* typically are used as probiotics in studies. These microorganisms do not permanently colonize the GI tract and must be taken regularly in sufficient quantity to maintain their presence in the colon. When a sufficient number of these bacteria are present, they appear to reduce colonization by pathogenic bacteria and enhance mucosal defenses in the colon.[5] Mechanisms by which this occurs are not clear, but may include enhanced production of immune globulin A (IgA), stimulation of the immune response, competition with pathogenic bacteria for nutrients and/or binding sites on the intestinal mucosa, production of inhibitory substances (organic acids, hydrogen peroxide, bacteriocins), degradation of toxin receptors (such as those for *Clostridium difficile*), increased mucous secretion, and reduction of leakage across intestinal tight junctions.[5,43]

*Health Effects* Interest in probiotics has been mainly in prevention or treatment of diarrhea (see Chapter 17) and various GI disorders. Many studies have been published, but most are of poor quality because of small size, imprecise endpoints, or inadequate specification of the species and number of microorganisms used. Despite these study limitations, it does appear that *S. boulardii, Enterococcus faecium,* and *Lactobacillus* have a beneficial effect on antibiotic-associated diarrhea. In double-blind, placebo-controlled trials, these three organisms have shown significant effects on reducing diarrhea.[44] In addition, multiple studies have demonstrated that *Lactobacillus* GG can prevent or reduce the duration of rotavirus-induced diarrhea. There is also evidence, although not conclusive, that probiotics may improve *C. difficile*-induced diarrhea, traveler's diarrhea, IBD and colitis, food allergy and atopic eczema, lactose intolerance, and vaginitis. However, most studies have used isolated bacteria (classified as nutritional supplements) rather than foods that naturally contain the beneficial bacteria (functional foods). This approach makes it difficult to interpret the role of functional foods containing beneficial bacteria, compared with dietary supplements of the bacteria.[5,43,44]

*Sources* Many traditional foods are fermented by bacteria and contain high concentrations of lactobacilli. Corn, cassava, millet, leafy vegetables (cabbage), and beans commonly serve as the basic food for fermentation. The vast majority of these foods are eaten primarily in developing countries and only rarely in industrialized countries. A few fermented foods are occasionally eaten in the United States, such as brined olives, kim chi (Korean form of fermented cabbage), miso, sauerkraut, and tempeh; however, the major food source of probiotic bacteria is dairy foods. Many major brands of yogurt contain probiotic bacteria although viable cultures are not required for yogurt in the United States and labels do not list the number of viable probiotic organisms. The "Live Active Culture" seal of the National Yogurt Association is allowed on products containing $10^8$ viable organisms per gram at the time of manufacture.[43] Unfortunately, the seal's value is limited because starter cultures for acid production are not distinguished from probiotic bacteria. Liquid yogurt drinks (kefir) and cultured fluid milk, such as sweet acidophilus milk and buttermilk, can contain variable amounts of viable organisms; however, most provide adequate amounts ($10^8$ viable organisms per gram). A few brands of cottage cheese contain active cultures, but most do not.

## Assessment of Functional Food Use: A Case-based Approach

Functional foods play a role in preventing disease and optimizing health. For patients at risk of CHD or with mild signs of CHD, functional foods may provide a viable option to pharmacotherapy. Case 24-1 illustrates use of functional foods for a patient with mild hypercholesterolemia who does not wish to start statin therapy.

### CASE 24-1

| Relevant Evaluation Criteria | Scenario/Model Outcome |
|---|---|
| **Information Gathering** | |
| 1. Gather essential information about the patient's symptoms, including: | |
| a. description of symptom(s) (i.e., nature, onset, duration, severity, associated symptoms) | Cholesterol is "borderline" on the basis of laboratory tests; patient does not remember the numbers, only that it was borderline and his PCP told him if it did not improve within a few month he would want to start a "statin" drug. |
| b. description of any factors that seem to precipitate, exacerbate, and/or relieve the patient's symptom(s) | Patient is asymptomatic; visit to PCP was prompted by a friend the same age having a heart attack about 3 months ago. No other cholesterol values in the past 5 years for comparison. |
| c. description of the patient's efforts to relieve the symptoms | Patient has lost about 15 lb since his friend's heart attack. He has been parking at the back of a large parking lot and walking out to the car again for his lunch. His office is on the third floor and he now takes the stairs most days. He is trying to eat healthier and limit saturated fat by changing from butter to margarine, changing to "light" mayonnaise, and using ground sirloin rather than regular ground beef. Most days he brings his lunch now rather than going to the fast food places three to four times per week as he previously did. He tried skim milk but did not like it. |
| 2. Gather essential patient history information: | |
| a. patient's identity | Richard Grubber |
| b. patient's age, sex, height, and weight | 58 y/o M, 5'10", 172 lb |
| c. patient's occupation | High school science teacher |
| d. patient's dietary habits | Eats breakfast every morning: usually a couple slices of toast (white bread) and cornflakes with 2% milk on work days; bagels, cream cheese and lox most of the time on Sunday.<br>Lunches: For the past 3 months patient has been taking a sandwich, commonly ham and cheese, bologna with mustard, or chicken salad, and also potato chips and soda; although he acknowledged the chips probably need to be replaced by something more healthy, he really likes to have something crunchy with his sandwich.<br>Afternoon snack: typically a candy bar or 3-4 small cookies<br>Dinner: meat (ham, beef, or chicken) with white rice or potatoes, canned or frozen vegetable, 2% milk during the weekdays, a glass of red wine on Friday and Saturday nights, sweet dessert (cake, pie, baked goods) at least 4-5 nights/week |
| e. patient's sleep habits | He usually sleeps 7.5-8 hours each night, but only about 5-6 hours when he has tests or term papers to grade. |

## CASE 24-1 (continued)

| Relevant Evaluation Criteria | Scenario/Model Outcome |
|---|---|
| f. concurrent medical conditions, prescription and nonprescription medications, and dietary supplements | Ibuprofen 200 mg as needed for muscle soreness, averages 1-2 days/week (usually weekends); one baby aspirin daily (self-initiated after his friend's heart attack); multivitamin for men daily; stool softener for constipation |
| g. allergies | NKA |
| h. history of other adverse reactions to medications | Erythromycin gives him a "terrible stomach ache." |
| i. other (describe)_______ | No family history of heart attacks. His father was 80 and his mother was 77 years of age when they died in a car crash. Both had taken blood pressure medicine for about 10 years; otherwise they were healthy. Richard is the youngest of five brothers; all are healthy except the twins have some mild pulmonary disease and high blood pressure. |
| **Assessment and Triage** | |
| 3. Differentiate the patient's signs/symptoms and correctly identify the patient's primary problem(s). | Richard has "borderline" high cholesterol for which his PCP has suggested "statin" therapy if it does not improve. Richard has reviewed information about statins and cholesterol on the Internet and wants to try lifestyle changes first. |
| 4. Identify exclusions for self-treatment. | None |
| 5. Formulate a comprehensive list of therapeutic alternatives for the primary problem to determine if triage to a medical practitioner is required, and share this information with the patient. | Options include:<br>(1) Take no action. Richard has already lost weight, is walking more, and has made limited dietary changes.<br>(2) Recommend he start the statin therapy suggested by his PCP.<br>(3) Recommend consultation with a registered dietitian to help him make further dietary changes.<br>(4) Recommend additional lifestyle changes including replacement of some of his current foods with functional foods associated with reduced risk of CHD, specifically lower total and LDL cholesterol. |
| **Plan** | |
| 6. Select an optimal therapeutic alternative to address the patient's problem, taking into account patient preferences. | Richard does not want to start statin therapy at this time but to control his "borderline" elevated cholesterol by lifestyle changes. There are multiple functional foods associated with reduced risk of CHD. Five FDA-authorized health claims are related to lower cholesterol and reduced risk of CHD. There is one applicable authoritative health claim for whole-grain foods and reduced risk of heart disease. In addition, there are qualified health claims for reduced risk of CHD with walnuts, omega-3 fatty acids, and monounsaturated fats from olive oil; however, these do not have the same volume and strength of data supporting the claim as do authorized and authoritative claims. |
| 7. Describe the recommended therapeutic approach to the patient. | On the basis of the description of your diet, it sounds like using certain functional foods in place of your current foods could help lower your cholesterol. FDA allows a number of health claims on foods that relate to decreased risk of CHD, which translates into decreased risk of events such as heart attack. Foods that meet specific criteria can have the claim on their package. You want to lower cholesterol to reduce the risk of CHD. |
| 8. Explain to the patient the rationale for selecting the recommended therapeutic approach from the considered therapeutic alternatives. | The statin drugs are very effective in lowering cholesterol and decreasing the risk of CHD; however, as you are aware, they do have some serious side effects. Since your cholesterol is only borderline elevated and you do not have a family history of significant heart disease, it is reasonable to try lifestyle changes before starting a statin. For lifestyle changes to work, you must be committed to making necessary changes and sticking with those changes. It sounds like you have already made some very positive changes and you appear to be committed to a nondrug approach to control your cholesterol. Foods with FDA-approved health claims related to decreased risk of CHD can provide significant reductions in cholesterol, especially when accompanied by lifestyle changes you have already started, such as weight loss and increased exercise. Many foods with these claims are readily available in the grocery store and most are no more expensive than foods you purchase already. |

## CASE 24-1 (continued)

| Relevant Evaluation Criteria | Scenario/Model Outcome |
|---|---|
| **Patient Education** | |
| 9. When recommending self-care with nonprescription medications and/or nondrug therapy, convey accurate information to the patient, including: | |
| a. appropriate dose and frequency of administration | To decrease dietary saturated fat and cholesterol, you should at least limit intake to the recommended not more than 10% of calories from saturated fat and not more than 300 mg cholesterol per day, but less is better. Most people find 1% milk to be more acceptable than nonfat (skim) milk so you might want to try it in place of 2% milk, or you could try soymilk.<br>You should eat fruits, vegetables, and grain products that contain fiber, particularly soluble fiber, and replace white breads, pasta, and rice with whole grain. Total dietary fiber should be at least 30 g/day (AI for men 51 years of age and older). Look for breads and cereals with heart health claim.<br>You can incorporate soluble fiber from oat bran, rolled oats, or whole-oat flour in certain foods into the diet as replacement for non–whole-grain breads and cereals. Look for cereals with ≥5 g of fiber per serving.<br>As for soy protein, 25 g/day is required in conjunction with a diet low in saturated fat and cholesterol.<br>As for plant sterol and stanol esters, total intake of at least 1.3 g/day of sterol esters or 3.4 g/day of stanol esters is recommended as part of a diet low in saturated fat and cholesterol; you usually need to eat the products at least twice a day to get the recommended amount; some margarines and orange juice have added plant sterols/stanol esters. These products should replace your regular margarine or orange juice.<br>As for whole-grain foods, this health claim overlaps somewhat with that for "grain products that contain fiber" (second one listed), but does not specify "particularly soluble fiber." Insoluble fibers also are important in health. Look for a whole grain, such as whole wheat, as the first ingredient on labels.<br>To make these health claims, foods must generally contain a certain amount of the component. Check food labels for these claims and for ingredient amounts.<br>There are also three health claims with less vigorous supporting data; therefore, these foods may not be as effective or the claim might be changed if new studies are reported. Since they are otherwise healthful foods when used in moderation, they can still be safely incorporated into your diet:<br>– Walnuts; 1.5 oz/day; remember that nuts are a concentrated source of calories, so use judiciously.<br>– Omega-3 fatty acids; FDA recommends that intake not exceed 3 g/day of these fats, specifically eicosapentaenoic acid (EPA) and docosahexaenoic acid (DHA); two meals per week containing salmon, lake trout, herring, and other oily fish are recommended.<br>– Monounsaturated fats from olive oil; 23 g (2 tbsp)/day in place of a similar amount of saturated fat. A number of salad dressings and a few soft margarines now include olive oil. |
| b. maximum number of days the therapy should be employed | No limit; preferably, these foods will be incorporated as part of an ongoing healthful diet for life. |
| c. product administration procedures | These are foods that can replace other foods in your diet so that total calories do not increase. You will need to read food labels carefully to be sure you are getting whole grains, low saturated fats and low cholesterol, and sterol/stanol esters in the product. Also look for the amount of soy or soluble fiber. |
| d. expected time to onset of relief | A few weeks |
| e. degree of relief that can be reasonably expected | Mild to moderate decrease in total and LDL cholesterol. You should be able to decrease "borderline" high cholesterol to within an acceptable range, but these foods alone probably would not be enough if you had significantly elevated cholesterol and a strong history of heart disease in the family. |

**CASE 24-1 (continued)**

| Scenario/Model Outcome | Scenario/Model Outcome |
|---|---|
| f. most common side effects | Rapid increases in fiber content of the diet can cause gas and bloating, so it is best to gradually increase the fiber in your diet. Replace 1-2 servings of white bread and rice with whole-grain bread and brown rice every few days until totally replaced. Also add extra fiber by gradually replacing the cornflakes with a whole-grain cereal. Fruits and vegetables can be increased gradually as well to replace snacks and desserts. Be sure to take plenty of water with a high-fiber diet. |
| g. side effects that warrant medical intervention should they occur | Moderate to severe abdominal pain, nausea, and vomiting may be signs of bowel obstruction or diverticulitis. |
| h. patient options in the event that condition worsens or persists | Cholesterol levels should be monitored periodically; if cholesterol worsens, it may be necessary to start statin therapy. |
| i. product storage requirements | See food label. |
| j. specific nondrug measures | N/A |
| 10. Solicit patient's follow-up questions. | (1) What if I want more in-depth information on dietary changes and diet plans? I have not seen much specific information on the Internet except advertising for dietary supplements.<br>(2) Are the supplements as good as the functional foods? |
| 11. Answer patient's questions. | (1) The FDA Web site (www.fda.gov) includes information on health claims and food labels that you might find helpful. You could consider making an appointment with a registered dietitian who could help develop some menus that incorporate foods you like and provide more specific plans for substituting healthier foods; your health plan from school may contract with a dietitian. If not, the American Dietetic Association can provide the name(s) of private consultants and the contact information for a dietitian. The phone number for referrals is on their Web site (www.eatright.org).<br>(2) In general, foods are better than supplements. Many studies have shown beneficial effects from a diet containing fiber-rich foods and whole grains but not with isolated supplements. Psyllium, found in products such as Metamucil, fits criteria for a health claim related to soluble fiber and risk of CHD, and could be used to increase soluble fiber. It also has the added benefit of reducing constipation, as do fibers from whole grains. |

Key: CHD, coronary heart disease; FDA, Food and Drug Administration; LDL, low-density lipoprotein; N/A, not applicable; NKA, no known allergies; PCP, primary care provider.

## MEDICAL FOODS AND MEAL REPLACEMENT FOODS

Medical foods are typically semisynthetic liquid formulas intended for oral consumption or administration through a feeding tube; these products are commonly known as enteral formulas. In addition, certain liquid diets designed for use in medically supervised very-low-calorie diets or bariatric programs (Resource Optisource, Optifast) are classified as medical foods. Various puddings, shakes, and other solid or semisolid food forms specially formulated and processed to meet *distinctive* nutritional requirements of the disease or condition for which they are intended can also be classified as medical foods. Both liquid and solid medical foods replace regular meals or enhance nutrient intake to meet the distinctive nutritional requirements of patients. However, many enteral formulas frequently are used to meet general nutritional needs. Practitioners involved with self-care counseling should determine when a product is used as a medical food to meet truly *distinctive* nutritional requirements, as determined by scientific studies, and when it is used for meal replacement or enhancement to meet general nutritional requirements. Foods intended to meet general nutritional requirements (see Chapter 23) do not need medical oversight and can be used safely for self-care. In contrast, FDA regulations state that medical foods require recommendation or prescription by a physician and ongoing medical supervision.[9] When enteral formulas are used to meet general nutritional requirements, however, third-party providers may refuse to cover them under insurance benefits, classifying them as a food that replaces regular meals and leaving patients with self-care responsibility. Thus, it is useful for practitioners involved in self-care counseling to be familiar with the basics of enteral formulas.

### Enteral Formula Uses

#### *Tube Feeding*

Enteral formulas are best known as complete nutritional replacements for patients requiring a feeding tube to meet their nutritional needs, such as stroke patients with severe dysphagia.

Patients who cannot, should not, or will not take adequate nutrients by mouth are candidates for tube feeding. Advances in products specifically designed for enteral use and the availability of sophisticated formulas, small-core nasogastric tubes, and constant-infusion delivery systems have led to a resurgence of interest in enteral nutrition in the hospital, home, and long-term care settings in recent years. Feeding via the GI tract is preferred over intravenous (parenteral) nutrition because enteral feeding helps preserve the structure and function of the GI tract, improve immunity, decrease the incidence of infection, and reduce metabolic complications such as hyperglycemia compared with parenteral nutrition. Enteral nutrition also is less expensive, requires less monitoring, and is easier to implement in self-care settings. The knowledgeable practitioner can assist patients and caregivers in selecting the appropriate formula on the basis of underlying pathology, tolerance to the product, and cost. A complete discussion of enteral nutrition is beyond the scope of this text; therefore, for in-depth information on this topic, the practitioner is referred to one of the many specialized references available on enteral nutrition or to the American Society for Parenteral and Enteral Nutrition (ASPEN), the national organization that focuses on specialized nutrition support. Only basic information related to formulas and administration is included here, with an emphasis on formulas that can be used in self-care.

More than 100 commercial preparations currently are available for enteral feeding. The majority of formulas are marketed to provide nutrition for patients with impaired ingestion or digestion. Those intended for patients with impaired ingestion typically follow general dietary guidelines and are safe for use in self-care. Formulas intended for patients with impaired digestion and those designed for specific metabolic or clinical conditions generally are best used with physician oversight. Common formula characteristics that are likely to result in its use as a true medical food requiring medical supervision are listed in Table 24-10 along with a few representative products.

### Supplementation of Nutrition Intake

A second use of these products is to supplement normal or impaired nutrition intake; an example is a paraplegic patient with skin breakdown who consumes a high-protein enteral formula three times a day to boost protein intake and accelerate wound healing. Finally, enteral formulas have been increasingly marketed as "meal replacements." Marketing targets healthy individuals who perceive a meal replacement product as a healthier alternative to fast foods or skipping a meal, such as a 35-year-old, slightly overweight man who replaces a meal with a prepackaged, low-carbohydrate protein bar to be compliant with a low-carbohydrate diet.

## Classification of Enteral Nutrition Products

Enteral feeding products can be classified as polymeric formulas, oligomeric formulas, and modular components.

**TABLE 24-10 Enteral Formula Characteristics Consistent with Need for Medical Supervision**

| Characteristic | Examples |
|---|---|
| Protein as peptides and/or free amino acids | Peptamen, Crucial, Vivonex |
| Alteration of the amino acid content by addition of individual amino acids, such as glutamine, arginine, or branch-chain amino acids (leucine, valine, isoleucine) | Impact, HepatAmine |
| Addition of specific fatty acids to alter the inflammatory response | Oxepa |
| Addition of significant amounts of medium-chain triglycerides to alter absorption | Portagen |
| High percentage (>50%) of calories from fat | Pulmocare |
| Very-high-protein content (≥25% of calories as protein) | Peptamen VHP |
| Intended for patients with organ failure | Nepro, NutriRenal, NutriHep |

In addition, a growing segment of meal supplement and meal replacement products, including beverages, bars, and puddings, are designed to assist in meeting nutritional goals.

### Polymeric Formulas

Polymeric formulas are the most commonly used formulas. These formulas are designed for patients with normal digestive capability and contain macronutrients in the form of intact proteins, carbohydrates, and fatty acids or oils. Most patients who require alternative nutrition support will tolerate and do well with standard, polymeric formulas. The standard formulas usually (1) are 1.0 kcal/mL unless concentrated to provide less free water, (2) contain a macronutrient composition typical of the American diet (carbohydrate 45%-70%, protein 10%-18%, and fat 20%-40%), and (3) are isotonic to slightly hypertonic (300-450 mOsm/kg) to reduce the risk of osmotic diarrhea; however, flavored products are often in the range of 500 to 700 mOsm/kg. These formulas are generally safe for self-care when taken orally or administered via a feeding tube. Patients with a feeding tube should inform their primary care provider of the type and amount of formula they are taking. The formulas listed in Table 24-11 as generally safe for self-care are polymeric formulas.

### Oligomeric Formulas

Oligomeric products are referred to as elemental or predigested because they require minimal digestion. They contain hydrolyzed or partially hydrolyzed protein and less complex carbohydrates, and frequently alter the fat content to improve absorption in patients with impaired absorption. These formulas rarely are consumed orally because of very poor palatability. In general, oligomeric formulas should be used under medical supervision rather than for self-care.

### *Modular Products*

Modular products are designed to supplement a single macronutrient content of an enteral formula or food. Examples include protein powder, medium-chain triglyceride oil, emulsified oils, and powdered flavorless glucose polymers. These products can be incorporated into food to increase the protein and calories consumed by the patient. They are used in enteral formulas to provide a more appropriate balance between macronutrient calorie sources for an individual patient. For example, a protein powder may be useful in a person of advanced age who has a decubitus ulcer and is having difficulty meeting the protein requirement with their usual oral diet. If a routine polymeric enteral supplement were provided and dosed to meet the protein goals for the patient, it likely would provide excessive calories if the oral diet was adequate except for protein. In this case, a modular protein powder added to provide appropriate protein intake would allow the person to continue the oral diet without an excessive increase in calorie consumption.

### *Specialty Formulas*

Specialty formulas may be either polymeric or oligomeric. They are designed to optimize the nutrient intake and improve disease management for patients with specific disease states such as renal insufficiency, diabetes mellitus, hepatic dysfunction, and carbon dioxide-retaining pulmonary dysfunction. The use of specialty formulas is controversial because data supporting improved outcomes are minimal. In general, specialty formulas should be used with medical supervision, not for self-treatment. Consultation with a registered dietitian or board-certified nutrition support pharmacist may be warranted.

Some "specialty" formulas, such as certain pulmonary and diabetic formulas, alter the ratio of fat and carbohydrate, but contain no special dietary components that are not available in regular foods. While technically such products are medical foods, there would be little concern for most patients who used them to replace a few meals per week. However, patients must be encouraged to limit use of these products unless otherwise advised by their primary care provider or practitioner specializing in nutritional management of their condition. They should advise their primary care provider when they use these products because management of the underlying disease itself requires medical oversight. Table 24-11 includes examples of pulmonary and diabetic formulas.[45-48]

## Product Use for Self-Care

All products recommended for self-care should contain basic nutrition labeling including serving size, calories, protein, fat, and other components consistent with food labeling so that nutrient intake can be determined in the same manner as with regular foods. Many formulas are available in a variety of flavors to reduce taste fatigue; slight differences in nutrient content may be noted among the flavors. As a rule, flavors include vanilla, chocolate, and strawberry; less common flavors include black walnut, butter pecan, chocolate malt, chocolate mocha, coffee, coffee latte, eggnog, and orange creme.

### *Administration and Monitoring Guidelines for Enteral Nutrition*

If the preparations are taken orally, the practitioner should encourage the patient to chill the product, vary the flavors to avoid taste fatigue, and consume the product after an attempt to eat a well-balanced meal or a between-meal snack. Once opened, the container should be kept cold to prevent bacterial growth, and all prepared products should be discarded after 24 hours. In tube feeding, formulas may be infused continuously around the clock, infused continuously during the night only to allow daytime freedom from the pump, or, for gastrostomy tubes only, given as a bolus several times daily to mimic the natural meal process. Unopened tube-feeding products should be stored at room temperature, and the expiration date should be checked before use. Generally, the tube should be flushed frequently to prevent occlusion. If the tube feeding is continuous, the tube should be flushed several times daily with about 10 to 30 mL of water, but the amount may be increased, depending on the patient's fluid requirements and fluid needs not met by the formula or oral intake.[49] When checking for gastric residuals, the tube should be flushed with 30 mL of water before and after each residual check. Medications should be given orally whenever possible, but, if a feeding tube is used, each medication should be given separately, with a minimum of 5 mL of water flushed between each medication and 10 to 30 mL before and after the medications. It is important to note that not all medications are water soluble, and water might precipitate clogging.

If diarrhea, nausea, or abdominal distention occurs, feedings may be withheld for up to 24 hours and then resumed gradually. Tube feeding-related diarrhea is an osmotic diarrhea that usually stops within 24 hours of discontinuing the formula; diarrhea persisting for longer is unlikely to be caused by the formula per se. Lactose intolerance is seldom an issue with enteral formulas because most formulas are lactose-free except powders prepared with milk. Elevating the head of the bed 30 to 45 degrees is advisable during administration via a feeding tube to avoid aspiration, especially for persons of advanced age or those who are unconscious. High-fat products can delay gastric emptying but have not been associated with aspiration risk. Tube placement into the small bowel, if possible, may provide a reduction in risk, but this action remains unproven.[45]

Tube-fed patients must be monitored for biochemical abnormalities as well as adequate nutrition and hydration.[45,49] Blood glucose concentrations should be monitored initially. Patients with diabetes may require increased insulin doses, although some patients may improve glycemic control with the predictability of the caloric source

**TABLE 24-11 Meal Replacement Products/Tube-feeding Formulas Suitable for Self-Care[46-48]**

| Product Name | Energy kcal/mL | Protein g/L (%) | CHO g/L (%) | Fat g/L (%) | Fiber g/L | Comments |
|---|---|---|---|---|---|---|
| **Routine** | | | | | | |
| Boost Drink | 1.01 | 42 (17) | 173 (67) | 17.8 (16) | None | |
| Boost with Benefiber and FOS | 1.01 | 42 (17) | 180 (67) | 17 (16) | 13 | Fiber from guar gum and FOS |
| Ensure | 1.06 | 37 (14) | 143 (64) | 37 (22) | None | Also available as Ensure Fiber with FOS and as Ensure High Calcium; similar nutrient content |
| Jevity 1 Cal | 1.06 | 44 (17) | 155 (54) | 35 (29) | 14.4 | Fiber from soy |
| **Routine with Extra Protein** | | | | | | |
| Boost High Protein Drink | 1.01 | 61 (24) | 139 (55) | 23 (21) | None | |
| Ensure High Protein | 0.95 | 50 (21) | 129 (55) | 25 (24) | None | |
| **Routine Concentrated** | | | | | | |
| Boost Plus | 1.52 | 59 (16) | 200 (50) | 58 (34) | <4 | |
| Ensure Plus | 1.50 | 54 (15) | 208 (56) | 46 (29) | None | |
| Jevity 1.2 Cal | 1.2 | 56 (18.5) | 172 (52.5) | 39 (29) | 22 | 75% insoluble/25% soluble fiber from soy fiber, oat fiber, gum arabic, and carboxymethylcellulose; includes 10 g/L FOS |
| Jevity 1.5 Cal | 1.5 | 64 (17) | 216 (54) | 50 (29) | 22 | 75% insoluble/25% soluble fiber from soy fiber, oat fiber, gum arabic, and carboxymethylcellulose; includes 10 g/L FOS |
| **Diabetic*** | | | | | | |
| Choice DM Beverage | 0.93 | 39 (17) | 101 (40) | 41 (43) | 11 | Fiber from soy polysaccharide, acacia, and microcrystalline cellulose; use sparingly if used for self-care because of high fat |
| Glucerna Select | 1.0 | 50 (20) | 96 (31) | 54 (49) | 6.7 | Fiber from FOS; use sparingly if used for self-care because of high fat |
| Glytrol | 1.0 | 45 (18) | 100 (40) | 48 (42) | 15.2 | Fiber from soluble sources; use sparingly if used for self-care because of high fat |
| RESOURCE Diabetic | 1.06 | 64 (24) | 100 (36) | 47 (40) | 12.8 | Fiber from soy and soluble sources; use sparingly if used for self-care because of high fat and high protein |
| **Pulmonary†** | | | | | | |
| Pulmocare | 1.5 | 63 (17) | 106 (28) | 93 (55) | None | Use sparingly if used for self-care because of high fat |
| Respalor | 1.5 | 75 (20) | 146 (40) | 68 (40) | None | Use sparingly if used for self-care because of high fat |
| **Other Meal Replacements and Supplements** | | | | | | |
| Boost Breeze | 0.68 | 34 (20) | 131 (80) | None | | Clear liquid; not intended as sole source of nutrition |
| Boost Pudding | 1.69 | 7 (11) | 33 (55) | 9 (34) | | Content per 5 oz serving |

**TABLE 24-11 Meal Replacement Products/Tube-feeding Formulas Suitable for Self-Care[46-48] (continued)**

| Product Name | Energy kcal/mL | Protein g/L (%) | CHO g/L (%) | Fat g/L (%) | Fiber g/L | Comments |
|---|---|---|---|---|---|---|
| Carnation Instant Breakfast | 0.92 | 13 (25) | 39 (13) | 2.5 (4) | | 1 packet in 1 cup skim milk; mixing with 2% or whole milk would increase calories as fat |
| Ensure Pudding | 1.67 | 4 (27) | 27 (64) | 5 (27) | | Content per 5 oz serving |
| Ensure Healthy Mom Shake | 0.84 | 42 (20) | 138 (66) | 12.5 (14) | | Intended for pregnant and nursing women; available in 8-oz bottles |
| Forta Shake | 1.20 | 17 (24) | 35 (50) | 8 (26) | | 1.4 oz mix with 1 cup whole milk |
| Glucerna Shake | 0.92 | 42 (18) | 121 (47) | 33 (35) | 12.5 | FOS and soy polysaccharide; for oral use, not tube feeding |
| Glucerna Weight Loss Shake | 0.88 | 39 (18) | 118 (48) | 33 (34) | 12 | Corn and soy fiber plus FOS; CHO modified for slow absorption; for oral use only, not tube feeding; available in 11-oz cans |
| Microlipid | 4.5 | 0 | 0 | 500 (100) | | Modular component composed of safflower oil; add to enteral formula or foods to increase calories as fat; available in 89 mL bottle |
| Moducal Powder | 30/tsp | 0 | 8/tsp (100) | 0 | | Modular component composed of maltodextrin; add to enteral formula or foods to increase calories |
| ProMod Powder | 28 | 5 (71) | 0.67 (10) | 0.60 (19) | | Modular component; add to enteral formula or foods to increase protein; amounts listed are per 6.6 g scoop |
| RESOURCE Benecalorie | 7 | 16 (9) | 0 | 71 (91) | None | Modular component; add to enteral formula or foods to increase calories |
| RESOURCE Benefiber | | 3 per serving (100) | | | 3 per serving | Soluble fiber; available in individual serving packets and 3.5-oz bottles; amounts listed are per serving |
| RESOURCE Benefiber Juice Drink | 0.58 | 0 | 25 | 0 | 25 | Soluble fiber from guar gum and pectin; apple and orange juices in 4-oz containers |
| RESOURCE Fruit Beverage | 1.18 | 67 (12) | 255 (88) | 0 | 0 | Classified as clear liquid; available in apple, cranberry, orange, and golden tropical |
| RESOURCE Shake Plus | 2.0 | 62 (13) | 288 (57) | 66 (30) | | Low lactose; available in 8-oz cartons |

Key: CHO, carbohydrate; FOS, fructose oligosaccharides.

* Data supporting improved glycemic control is lacking; therefore, ASPEN does not recommend the routine use of diabetic specialty formulas.[45] Fat content is higher than recommended by general dietary guidelines and the American Diabetes Association.

† Data supporting excessive carbon dioxide production with appropriate caloric intake and decreased hospitalizations with use of pulmonary formulas is lacking; therefore, ASPEN does not recommend the routine use of pulmonary-specific formulas.[45] Fat content is higher than recommended by general dietary guidelines.

from continuous tube feeding. Monitoring albumin and prealbumin serially assesses response to enteral feeding and visceral protein status. Frequency of monitoring depends on the patient's current status and volatility. Prealbumin has a shorter half-life than albumin and can be beneficial in monitoring short-term changes in visceral protein status.

### *Food–Medication Interactions*

Interactions between medications and enteral feeding often are complex and poorly understood. The practitioner is advised to consult specialty references for a more complete listing and explanation of such interactions. The general practice for certain medications (including phenytoin, carbamazepine, and warfarin) is to hold the tube feeding for an hour or 2 before and after administering the medication through the feeding tube, especially when therapeutic levels are not achieved with reasonable doses. Vitamin K content of the formula should also be checked for patients on warfarin. Although most formulas provide no more vitamin K than a typical diet, a few contain amounts that could interfere with anticoagulation. Manufacturers' Web sites provide up-to-date information on the nutrient content of formulas.[46-48]

## Other Medical Foods and Meal Replacement Food

Foods designed for use in weight loss and bariatric programs are medical foods that require medical supervision when used as intended because of the significant medical risks associated with rapid weight loss. These foods include liquid diets (Resource Optisource High Protein Drink, Optifast 800 Ready to Drink) and various nutrition bars (Resource Optisource Mini Nutrition Bar, Optitrim, Optifast Nutrition Bar). Although it is stated that the low-calorie diet requires physician monitoring to maximize weight loss, Medifast food supplements, including shakes, bars, soups, oatmeal, chili, and various other foods, are available on the Internet as part of the Take Shape for Life program.[50] Medifast Plus foods also are offered for joint health, women's health, and coronary health although it is unclear if these products are functional foods or dietary supplements. Meal replacement foods such as Slim Fast, Weight Watchers, and Jenny Craig products can be used safely without medical supervision; however, they should be used as part of an overall weight loss plan (see Chapter 27).

## Assessment of Enteral Nutrition and Meal Replacements: A Case-based Approach

The first step in assessing what type of meal replacement (or supplement) to recommend is asking the patient/caregiver what medical condition, if any, the patient has and whether a primary care provider has prescribed a particular product. Any product, prescribed or recommended, should be evaluated to ensure that the product is appropriate for the patient's digestive capability, meets the patient's specific nutritional needs, and does not contain excessive or contraindicated macronutrients and micronutrients for the patient's health status.

Meal replacement products can address many separate issues. Traditionally, meal replacement has been considered a therapeutic intervention needed to maintain adequate nutrition in malnourished patients, to completely replace nutritional intake in patients with a physical limitation interfering with nutritional intake such as dysphagia, or to precisely control intake of specific dietary components (calories for obesity, phenylalanine in phenylketonuria). Increasingly, nutrition products are used as lifestyle choices of self-directed therapy. This is particularly true of the meal replacement products used by working individuals who are too busy to prepare or eat a proper meal or who perceive these products to offer a healthier alternative to a meal. Case 24-2 illustrates the assessment of patients needing additional nutrition to supplement inadequate oral intake.

### CASE 24-2

| Relevant Evaluation Criteria | Scenario/Model Outcome |
|---|---|
| **Information Gathering** | |
| 1. Gather essential information about the patient's symptoms, including: | |
| a. description of symptom(s) (i.e., nature, onset, duration, severity, associated symptoms) | The patient is an older woman who complains of no appetite and feeling full very quickly when she does eat; it hurts to swallow. She also complains of feeling weak. Her daughter is with her and reports the patient had lost 15 lb over 6 or 7 months before surgery for a noncancerous esophageal stricture and has lost another 5 lb in the 2 weeks since she was discharged from the hospital. The patient refused discharge home with tube feeding as had been suggested by the dietitian at the hospital. The surgeon thought her appetite would return fairly quickly and said the pain on swallowing also should go away within a couple weeks. The surgeon suggested just getting some enteral formula to drink and said any of them will do. |
| b. description of any factors that seem to precipitate, exacerbate, and/or relieve the patient's symptom(s) | It hurts mostly when she tries to swallow solid foods although really thick foods like pudding also seem to stick and take a long time to get down. |
| c. description of the patient's efforts to relieve the symptoms | Patient tried an instant breakfast drink mixed with lactose-free milk, but it was too sweet and the chocolate flavor did not taste right to her. Her daughter has made chicken broth for her, but she drinks only about 3/4 of a cup before feeling full. |
| 2. Gather essential patient history information: | |
| a. patient's identity | Metheya King |

## CASE 24-2 (continued)

| Relevant Evaluation Criteria | Scenario/Model Outcome |
|---|---|
| b. patient's age, sex, height, and weight | 64 y/o F, 5'6", 120 lb |
| c. patient's occupation | Sales clerk at a shoe store |
| d. patient's dietary habits | Prior to 7 months ago she ate a "healthy diet" except for snacking when she watched TV at night. Starting about 7 months ago she noticed difficulty swallowing some foods and gradually reached the point where she was taking only soups and liquids. While in the hospital she received tube feeding. Since hospital discharge, she is eating primarily liquids and very small amounts. |
| e. patient's sleep habits | When healthy, 8 hours; since hospital discharge, about 9 hours |
| f. concurrent medical conditions, prescription and nonprescription medications, and dietary supplements | Immediately postoperative for a benign esophageal stricture; acetaminophen with codeine for surgery-related pain; HCTZ for high blood pressure; acetaminophen for knee pain after working for more than half a day; carbidopa/levodopa for restless leg syndrome |
| g. allergies | Sulfa (rash, edema) |
| h. history of other adverse reactions to medications | Hallucinations with morphine. She has no other adverse reactions to medications; however, she does have lactose intolerance. |
| i. other (describe)_______ | Metheya waited until she could swallow very little before seeing a physician because she was afraid it was cancer and did not want any chemotherapy. She thought if it was not cancer it would get better on its own. The daughter says her mother does not like seeing the doctor and does not like taking pills. |
| **Assessment and Triage** | |
| 3. Differentiate the patient's signs/symptoms and correctly identify the patient's primary problem(s). | Significant weight loss over 6 months related to nonmalignant esophageal stricture; now with postoperative anorexia, early satiety, and further weight loss |
| 4. Identify exclusions for self-treatment. | The patient is under medical supervision, and the surgeon recommended she drink an enteral formula, with no exclusions for use of a formula. |
| 5. Formulate a comprehensive list of therapeutic alternatives for the primary problem to determine if triage to a medical practitioner is required, and share this information with the patient. | Options include:<br>(1) Take no action.<br>(2) Start tube feedings as a home patient. The patient had refused continuation of the tube feeding at home when she was discharged from the hospital.<br>(3) Start an appetite stimulant and possibly an antidepressant if symptoms of depression are present.<br>(4) Try an enteral formula by mouth. |
| **Plan** | |
| 6. Select an optimal therapeutic alternative to address the patient's problem, taking into account patient preferences. | Taking no action is not appropriate given the significant weight loss. Trying an enteral formula by mouth appears to be more acceptable to the patient than tube feeding because she had tried an instant breakfast drink. Metheya should be assessed for depression before recommending an antidepressant, especially since she does not like taking pills.<br>An appetite stimulant could be considered, but she does not like taking pills. |
| 7. Describe the recommended therapeutic approach to the patient. | There are several ready-to-use formulas that do not contain lactose you can drink. They contain all the nutrients you need if you take enough. A concentrated formula that gives you more calories per cup would be good for you since you are having trouble taking enough volume. |
| 8. Explain to the patient the rationale for selecting the recommended therapeutic approach from the considered therapeutic alternatives. | Tube feeding would be easier for you since you would not have to swallow to get the nutrition you need and you would probably feel stronger with it. However, since you can swallow liquids it is possible to get adequate nutrition by drinking an enteral formula. It will take some effort on your part since you will need to take formula several times per day even if you do not feel hungry. The formula is better than soups right now because most soups make you feel full without giving you a lot of calories or protein. You need the protein for the surgical cut to heal. |

## CASE 24-2 (continued)

| Relevant Evaluation Criteria | Scenario/Model Outcome |
|---|---|
| **Patient Education** | |
| 9. When recommending self-care with nonprescription medications and/or nondrug therapy, convey accurate information to the patient, including: | |
| a. appropriate dose and frequency of administration | To get the required calories and protein, you will need to drink 3-4 cans (8 oz) per day of a 2 cal/mL formula. You can try taking 1/2 can (4 oz) five times during the day to start; then increase the amount to 3/4 can (6 oz) five times per day. |
| b. maximum number of days the therapy should be employed | Most enteral formulas provide complete nutrition and can be used safely for years. You should need the formula for only a couple weeks until your throat pain improves. |
| c. product administration procedures | You will be drinking the formula. Most people prefer the formula chilled; it also can be frozen and made into a slushy-type drink. Sometimes cold helps numb the pain. |
| d. expected time to onset of relief | You should begin to feel somewhat stronger within a few days if you are taking between 3 and 4 cans of formula a day. |
| e. degree of relief that can be reasonably expected | Taking the formula stop your weight loss and may help you gain back a pound or two before you see the surgeon again in 2 weeks. |
| f. most common side effects | Loose stools (stools are less formed with a liquid diet than with solid foods) |
| g. side effects that warrant medical intervention should they occur | You should see the surgeon immediately if the pain associated with swallowing worsens, you notice blood when you cough, or you develop diarrhea that does not end within a day of stopping the formula (may be an infectious diarrhea). |
| h. patient options in the event that condition worsens or persists | Placement of a feeding tube and initiation of tube feeding |
| i. product storage requirements | Unopened cans can be stored at room temperature. Opened cans should be stored covered in the refrigerator and used within 24 hours of opening. |
| j. specific nondrug measures | N/A |
| 10. Solicit patient's follow-up questions. | (1) What if I do not like the formula?<br>(2) What is the cost? |
| 11. Answer patient's questions. | (1) Several flavors of formula are available, so you might want to buy one or two of a couple different flavors. The vanilla-flavored formulas often taste less sweet, or you could buy an unflavored formula and add a flavor like vanilla or maple. If you do that, try a small sample first, as some flavorings might curdle the formula.<br>(2) The cost is about $1 to $1.50 per can, depending on the brand and the store where you buy it. |

Key: HCTZ, hydrochlorothiazide; N/A, not available.

## Patient Counseling for Enteral Nutrition and Meal Replacements

Advancements in enteral nutrition products and home infusion therapy are allowing more people with serious, even terminal, illnesses to be cared for at home. These products also are appropriate for ambulatory patients with metabolic or digestive diseases and for persons who want to ensure adequate nutrition for their life stage. Practitioners serve a pivotal role in helping patients use the product best suited for their nutritional needs and use it under medical supervision when appropriate. The box Patient Education for Enteral Nutrition Products lists specific information to provide patients and caregivers.

## KEY POINTS FOR FUNCTIONAL AND MEAL REPLACEMENT FOODS

- The definition of functional foods typically includes "health benefits beyond those of basic nutrition."
- Health claims are statements describing an association between a food, food component, dietary ingredient, or dietary supplement and risk of a disease or health-related condition.

## PATIENT EDUCATION FOR MEAL REPLACEMENT PRODUCTS

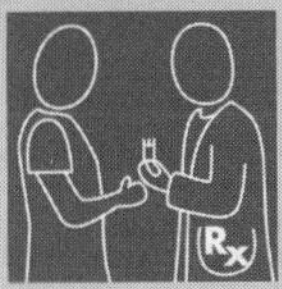

The objective of self-treatment is to provide the appropriate amount and types of specific micronutrients and macronutrients to meet the patient's nutritional needs. For most patients, carefully after product instructions and the self-care measures listed here will help ensure optimal therapeutic outcomes.

- Most preparations provide 1 cal/mL; however, 1.5 cal/mL formulas are also readily available in supermarkets and drugstores.
- For preparations taken orally, take 100 to 240 mL at one time. The formula can be taken at room temperature, chilled, or semifrozen as a slush-type drink.
- For preparations administered by tube, the product should be at room temperature.
- Bolus administration of 100 to 240 mL at one time can be used with gastric tubes, if tolerated. Small bowel feeding generally requires an infusion control device with formula administered over several hours (usually overnight) or continuously.
- Keep opened containers appropriately stored (refrigerated and covered) to prevent bacterial growth; discard all remaining prepared products after 24 hours. Unopened product can be stored at room temperature.
- To maintain feeding tube patency and meet fluid needs, flush water through the tubing at least three times a day.
- If diarrhea, nausea, or abdominal distention occurs, withhold the preparation for 2 hours and then gradually resume feeding after consulting with the patient's primary care provider.
- When persons of advanced age, unconscious people, or patients who have recently had surgery are being fed by tube, elevate the head of the bed 30 to 45 degrees during feeding to avoid aspiration.
- Be sure patients on long-term enteral nutrition are monitored for biochemical abnormalities, electrolyte values, and adequate nutrition and hydration.
- Monitor urine and blood glucose concentrations in patients with diabetes. They may require increased insulin doses.

---

- Authorized and authoritative health claims meet the significant scientific agreement level of evidence.
- Qualified health claims do not meet the significant scientific agreement level of evidence; claims statements must include language indicating the "qualified" nature of the health claim.
- Structure and function claims lack the significant scientific agreement level of evidence and make no association between the product and risk of a disease or health-related condition; they do not require validation or authorization by FDA.
- Foods for special dietary use meet *particular dietary needs* related to physical, physiologic, pathologic, or other conditions, such as disease, convalescence, pregnancy, lactation, underweight, overweight, infancy, or need for sodium restriction, or they supplement or fortify the usual diet; they are subject to general labeling requirements for foods and do not require use under medical supervision.
- Medical foods are specially formulated and processed to meet *distinctive nutritional requirements* (established by medical evaluation based on recognized scientific principles) of the disease or condition for which they are intended and are to be recommended and used under medical supervision.
- Conventional foods classified as functional foods are typically associated with health benefits in epidemiologic studies, and the evidence supporting a functional role for these foods is weak to moderate with clinical trials often lacking.
- Epidemiologic studies strongly support the positive role of fiber from whole grains, fruits, and vegetables in laxation.
- Adequate intake of highly viscous fiber, including cereal grains, guar gum, pectin, and psyllium, are associated with reduced cholesterol and CHD risk.
- Improved glucose control and diabetes risk reduction are associated with highly viscous fiber, including cereal grains, legumes, fruits, vegetables, guar gum, and pectin.
- Prebiotics are fermentable fibers that selectively stimulate the growth and/or activity of one or a limited number of bacteria in the colon (bifidobacteria and lactobacilli) and benefit the host.
- Probiotics are nonpathogenic, living microorganisms that appear to improve the balance of microflora in the GI tract and have a beneficial effect on the host when consumed regularly in adequate amounts. They are often present in fermented products from milk (yogurt, kefir) or plants (sauerkraut, miso).
- Enteral nutrition products are classified as medical foods; however, many polymeric enteral formulas are readily available without enforcement of the provision for medical supervision and can often be used safely as a meal replacement product.
- Specialty enteral formulas should generally be used with medical supervision, not for self-treatment.
- Tube-fed patients should be monitored for appropriate response to the formula and biochemical abnormalities.

## References


1. Ross S. Functional foods: the Food and Drug Administration perspective. *Am J Clin Nutr.* 2000;71(suppl):1735S-8S.
2. US General Accounting Office. Food safety: improvements needed in overseeing the safety of dietary supplements and "functional foods." Report to congressional committees, GAO/RCED-00-156, July 2000.
3. Hasler CM, Bloch AS, Thomson CA, et al. Position of the American Dietetic Association: functional foods. *J Am Diet Assoc.* 2004;104:814-26.
4. Roberfroid M. Functional food concept and its application to prebiotics. *Digest Liver Dis.* 2002;34(suppl.2):S105-10.
5. Duggan C, Gannon J, Walker WA. Protective nutrients and functional foods for the gastrointestinal tract. *Am J Clin Nutr.* 2002;75:789-808.
6. Claims that can be made for conventional foods and dietary supplements. Available at: www.cfsan.fda.gov/~dms/hclaims.html. Accessed March 10, 2005.

7. Henkel J. Soy: health claims for soy protein, questions about other components. *FDA Consumer Magazine.* May-June 2000. Available at: www.fda.gov/fdac/features/2000/300_soy.html. Accessed July 28, 2005.
8. Agriculture Research Service, US Department of Agriculture (USDA). Nutrient data laboratory. Search the USDA National Nutrient Database for standard reference. Available at: www.nal.usda.gov/fnic/foodcomp/search. Accessed June 3, 2005.
9. FDA/CFSAN Federal Reg. 61 FR 60661, November 29, 1996. Available at: http://vm.cfsan.fda.gov/~Ind/fr961129.html. Accessed April 20, 2005.
10. International Food Information Council Foundation. Functional foods. May 2004. Available at: www.ific.org/nutrition/functional/index.cfm. Accessed June 4, 2005.
11. Hasler CM. Functional foods: their role in disease prevention and health promotion. *Food Tech.* 1998;52(2):57-62. Available at: www.nutriwatch.org/04Foods/ff.html. Accessed June 17, 2005.
12. Jones PJ. Clinical nutrition:7. functional foods—more than just nutrition. *CMAJ.* 2002;166:1555-63.
13. Ferguson LR, Chavan RR, Harris PJ. Changing concepts of dietary fiber: implications for carcinogenesis. *Nutr Cancer.* 2001; 39:155-69.
14. Marlett JA, McBurney MI, Slavin JL. Position of the American Dietetic Association: health implications of dietary fiber. *J Am Diet Assoc.* 2002;102:993-1000.
15. Dietary Reference Intakes for Energy, Carbohydrates, Fiber, Fat, Protein and Amino Acids (Macronutrients), 2002. Dietary, functional, and total fiber. Available at: www.nap.edu/openbook/0309085373/html/285-333.html. Accessed March 29, 2005.
16. Bialostosky K, Wright JD, Kennedy-Stephenson J, et al. Dietary intake of macronutrients, micronutrients and other dietary constituents: United States 1988-94. *National Center for Health Statistics Vital Health Stat.* 11(245);2002. Available at: www.cdc.gov/nchs/data/series/sr_11/sr11/245.pdf. Accessed March 27, 2005.
17. Food and Nutrition Board, Institute of Medicine, National Academy of Sciences. Dietary Reference Intakes for Energy, Carbohydrates, Fiber, Fat, Protein and Amino Acids, 2002. Dietary reference intakes: recommended intakes for individuals, macronutrients. Available at: www.iom.edu/object.file/Master/21/372/0.pdf. Accessed March 20, 2005.
18. Thompson FE, Midthune D, Subar AF, et al. Dietary intake estimates in the National Health Interview Survey, 2000: methodology, results, and interpretation. *J Am Diet Assoc.* 2005;105:352-63.
19. Kim Y-I. AGA technical review: impact of dietary fiber on colon cancer occurrence. *Gastroenterology.* 2000;118:1235-57.
20. International Food Information Council Foundation. Focus on fiber: why roughage still warrants our attention. *Food Insights.* July/August 2004. Available at: www.ific.org/foodinsight. Accessed July 25, 2005.
21. Jewell DJ, Young G. Interventions for treating constipation in pregnancy. *Cochrane Database Syst Rev.* 2001;2:CD001142.
22. Brandt LJ, Prather CM, Quigley EMM, et al. Systematic review on the management of chronic constipation in North America. *Am J Gastroenterol.* 2005;100(suppl 1):S5-S22.
23. Brown L, Rosner B, Willett WW, et al. Cholesterol-lowering effects of dietary fiber: a meta-analysis. *Am J Clin Nutr.* 1999;69:30-42.
24. Lui S, Stampfer MJ, Hu FB, et al. Whole-grain consumption and risk of coronary heart disease: results from the Nurses' Health Study. *Am J Clin Nutr.* 1999;70:412-9.
25. Parillo M, Riccardi G. Diet composition and the risk of type 2 diabetes: epidemiological and clinical evidence. *Br J Nutr.* 2004; 92:7-19.
26. Anderson JW, Randles KM, Kendall CWC, et al. Carbohydrate and fiber recommendations for individuals with diabetes: a quantitative assessment and meta-analysis of the evidence. *Am Coll Nutr.* 2004;23:5-17.
27. Giacco R, Parillo M, Rivellese AA, et al. Long-term dietary treatment with increased amounts of fiber-rich low-glycemic index natural foods improves blood glucose control and reduces the number of hypoglycemic events in type 1 diabetic patients. *Diabetes Care.* 2000;23:1461-6.
28. Chandalia M, Garg A, Lutjohann D, et al. Beneficial effects of high dietary fiber intake in patients with type 2 diabetes mellitus. *N Engl J Med.* 2000;342:1392-8.
29. Montonen J, Kneki P, Jaarvinen R, et al. Whole-grain and fiber intake and the incidence of type 2 diabetes. *Am J Clin Nutr.* 2003; 77:622-9.
30. Lau C, Faerch K, Glumer C, et al. Dietary glycemic index, glycemic load, fiber, simple sugars, and insulin resistance: the Inter99 study. *Diabetes Care.* 2005;28:1397-404.
31. Liese AD, Roach AK, Sparks KC, et al. Whole-grain intake and insulin sensitivity: the Insulin Resistance Atherosclerosis Study. *Am J Clin Nutr.* 2003;78:965-71.
32. Bingham SA, Day NE, Luben R, et al. Dietary fiber in food and protection against colorectal cancer in the European Prospective Investigation into Cancer and Nutrition (EPIC): an observational study. *Lancet.* 2003;361:1496-501.
33. Reddy B. Role of dietary fiber in colon cancer: an overview. *Am J Med.* 1999;106(suppl 1):16S-26S.
34. Fuchs C, Giovannucci E, Colditz G, et al. Dietary fiber and the risk of colorectal cancer and adenoma in women. *N Engl J Med.* 1999;340:169-71.
35. Asano T, McLeod RS. Dietary fibre (fiber) for the prevention of colorectal adenomas and carcinomas. *Cochrane Database of Syst Rev.* 2002;2:CD003430.
36. Hill MJ. Cereals, cereal fibre and colorectal cancer risk: a review of the epidemiological literature. *Eur J Cancer Prev.* 1997;6:219-25.
37. Bijkerk CJ, Muris JWM, Knottnerus JA, et al. Systematic review: the role of different types of fibre in the treatment of irritable bowel syndrome. *Aliment Pharmacol Ther.* 2004;19:245-51.
38. Floch MH, Bina I. The natural history of diverticulitis: fact and theory. *J Clin Gastroenterol.* 2004;38(5 suppl):S2-7.
39. Bornet FRJ, Brouns F, Tashiro Y, et al. Nutritional aspects of short-chain fructooligosaccharides: natural occurrence, chemistry, physiology, and health implications. Digest *Liver Dis.* 2002; 34(suppl 2):S111-20.
40. Kolida S, Tuohy K, Gibson GR. Prebiotic effects of inulin and oligofructose. *Br J Nutr.* 2002;87(suppl 2):S193-7.
41. Cummings JH, Macfarlane GT. Gastrointestinal effects of prebiotics. *Br J Nutr.* 2002;87(suppl 2):S145-51.
42. Coudray C, Demigne C, Rayssiguier Y. Effects of dietary fibers on magnesium absorption in animals and humans. *J Nutr.* 2003; 133:1-4.
43. Sanders ME. Considerations for use of probiotic bacteria to modulate human health. *J Nutr.* 2000;130:384S-90S.
44. Rolf RD. The role of probiotic cultures in the control of gastrointestinal health. *J Nutr.* 2000;130:396S-402S.
45. August D, Chair. ASPEN Board of Directors and the Clinical Guideline Task Force. Guidelines for the Use of Parenteral and Enteral Nutrition in Adult and Pediatric Patients. *JPEN J Parenter Enteral Nutr.* 2002;26(suppl):78SA-80SA.
46. Ross Clinical Nutrition. Product handbook, adult. Available at: www.ross.com. Accessed July 3, 2005.
47. Nestle Clinical Nutrition. Enteral products reference guide. Available at: www.nestleclinicalnutrition.com. Accessed July 3, 2005.
48. Novartis Medical Nutrition. Product list, United States. Available at: www.novartisnutrition.com.html. Accessed July 3, 2005.
49. Lord L, Trumbore L, Zaloga G. Enteral nutrition implementation and management. In: Kohn-Keeth C, ed. *The ASPEN Nutrition Support Practice Manual.* Silver Spring, Md: American Society for Parenteral and Enteral Nutrition; 1998:5.1-5.16.
50. Take Shape for Life program. Medifast and Medfast Plus foods. Available at: www.thinnerwinners.tsfl.com. Accessed July 30, 2005.

CHAPTER 25

# Sports Nutrition and Performance-enhancing Nutrients

*Mark Newnham*

It is not unusual for individuals to spend their leisure time pursuing a physically active hobby such as weight lifting, yoga, aerobics, or endurance events such as marathon running or triathlon. Active individuals may spend 5 to 10 hours per week in physical activity and require a specific nutritional intake to maintain or enhance their performance. This chapter reviews macronutrient and food supplement products and their effect on these leisure activities. Food supplements and natural products have been marketed to athletes with two primary purposes: as ergogenic aids that improve strength and power, and as endurance aids to prolong the duration of exercise by providing fuel for continued effort and replacing electrolytes lost from sweat to promote normal muscle contractions. Readers are referred to a joint statement of the American Dietetic Association (ADA) and the Canadian Dietetic Association for guidelines and detailed discussion of this topic.[1]

## Consumers of Sports Nutrition Products

Sports nutrition products and performance-enhancing supplements have gained wide acceptance in both athletes and mildly to moderately active individuals. Electrolyte- and carbohydrate-containing sports beverages are so popular that almost all marathon and triathlon participants report experience with them, and local 5 km charity run provide participants with a cup of a sports beverage for participating.

While historical sales of these products have been driven by serious athletes who choose to exercise regularly, emerging marketing trends show that sales to nonathletes are far outweighing sales to athletes. Recent data suggest that only 28% of sales are driven by physically active adults.[2] Increasing numbers of consumers are not athletic club devotees yet are choosing sports nutrition products as lifestyle alternatives to traditional beverages and snacks. The market has responded with advertising aimed at wellness benefits and active lifestyles as well as focused marketing to performance driven athletes. Women, children, and the increasing Hispanic population are also emerging as sales targets.

Retail sales for sports nutrition products in 2003 are reported at over $3 billion, with the market share driven by the sports beverage market, followed by supplements, and then energy bars and gels. The beverage market includes energy drinks, isotonic recovery drinks, and other nutrient-enhanced soft drinks, juices, and waters. The supplement market includes tablets, capsules, and powders that are both macronutrient-based and herbal supplement–based.

**Editor's Note:** This chapter is based, in part, on the 14th edition chapter "Meal Replacement and Performance-enhancing Foods," written by Mark Newnham.

## Macronutrient Aids for Athletic Performance

Clinical trials of athletic supplements use resistance training as a measure of strength, power, and muscle mass, or exercise time on a treadmill or bicycle ergometer as a measure of endurance. Largely anaerobic, resistance training is quantified either as total weight lifted over a series of exercises or the maximum weight lifted by the athlete in one repetition, referred to as 1-Repmax. Endurance training is generally quantified by the total time of exercise, also known as time to exhaustion, or time to complete a predetermined distance. Endurance testing must be controlled for the athlete's level of aerobic versus anaerobic effort by measuring the athlete's ability to extract oxygen ($O_2$) from inspired air. This measure is known as the $VO_2$, or volume of $O_2$ consumed in liters per minute, and allows for a control when comparing exercise efforts between two separate athletes or even comparing one athlete's effort with a previous baseline effort. For an endurance study, the athlete might be asked to run continuously on a treadmill until exhaustion while drinking a carbohydrate-containing sports drink and then return a week later to run the same trial receiving only water. The speed of the treadmill would be adjusted to the athlete's effort, as measured by oxygen extraction, to ensure that both efforts are similar. In this case, the athlete might be asked to exercise at 50% of $VO_{2max}$, which would represent an aerobic effort.

The lactate threshold is an invisible barrier representing the point at which an athlete begins to exercise in a relative state of oxygen deprivation. The muscles' ability to produce energy in the form of adenosine triphosphate (ATP) is determined by the relative amount of oxygen available for metabolism. When oxygen is relatively deficient, the anaerobic utilization of glucose and production of ATP also leads to production of lactic acid. The balance between aerobic and anaerobic metabolism is referred to as the lactate threshold. There is no credible evidence that any herbal supplement or ergogenic aid can improve an athlete's $VO_2$ or lactate threshold. The only known influence on lactate threshold is physical activity.[3-5]

Endurance athletes rely on both fat and carbohydrates for athletic performance.[3] At low-intensity "aerobic" efforts, fat metabolism will make up 70% to 80% or more of ATP production with carbohydrate providing as little as 20% of ATP needs.[3] The human adaptation is to preserve glycogen for high-intensity efforts such as hunting or "fight or flight" reflex energy. As effort increases, the total amount of ATP contributed by fat remains relatively constant, since fatty acid metabolism is both a rate-limited and an oxygen-dependent process. Carbohydrates act as a second type of "fuel" for high-intensity activity.[3] Carbohydrate utilization is added to the baseline fat oxidation to improve total ATP production and therefore provide more energy for a more intense effort.[3,4] Training can influence this process, making athletes more efficient at fat metabolism, and thus allowing longer and/or more intense efforts before accessing vital stores of carbohydrate.[4]

The body stores carbohydrate as glycogen in the muscles and the liver. Athletes rely on muscle glycogen to provide substrate for ATP production via the Krebs cycle.[3-5] The rate of glycogen depletion depends on the intensity and duration of exercise. In aerobic efforts, carbohydrate utilization makes up only 20% of energy needs. As intensity increases, this percentage increases to 50% for 10 km running races and 80% to 90% for sprint events (100 m).[4]

Glycogen depletion depends on duration and rate of use. Intensity and rapid glycogen utilization can lead a football or soccer athlete to deplete muscle glycogen in as little as 30 minutes. By comparison, glycogen depletion in marathon runners is relatively slow and occurs several hours into the race, since these athletes have adapted to more efficient fatty acid metabolism. Despite the slow use of glycogen, any endurance athlete will experience muscle glycogen depletion as a sudden and dramatic decrease in performance that is often referred to as "hitting the wall." For most long-distance runners, this experience is relatively predictable, occurring about 2 hours, or 18 to 22 miles, into a marathon. Early marathon runners applied the concept of carbohydrate loading in an attempt to increase muscle glycogen stores and therefore prolong their effort before hitting the wall. Carbohydrate loading involved two phases, starting 3 to 5 days prior to the event. First the athlete restricts dietary carbohydrate severely while continuing to exercise at a high-intensity, glycogen-depleting effort. The goal of this glycogen depletion is to stimulate adaptation to more efficient fat utilization and enhance natural signals for carbohydrate storage. The second phase involves oral carbohydrate loading 12 to 24 hours prior to the event to maximize glycogen stores at the start of the race.

The sports nutrition market was initially aimed at high-intensity athletes with the goal of replacing muscle glycogen, along with electrolytes and fluids, during short breaks in competition. The market then evolved toward endurance sports by replacing pre-event carbohydrate loading with provision of small amounts of carbohydrates to athletes frequently during an event, so as to preserve muscle glycogen and maintain performance. There is no reason for these products to be marketed to sedentary individuals.

### *Carbohydrate-based Products*

Carbohydrate-based products can be categorized by their glycemic index. Products that contain sucrose or dextrose provide a rapid absorption and availability of carbohydrate. These products also stimulate a larger release of insulin, which can cause hypoglycemia if the athletic effort continues without further supplementation of carbohydrate. High glycemic index products are optimized for intermediate sprint effort sports such as soccer and football. Moderate glycemic products use maltodextrin and fructose to provide carbohydrate energy with a less significant release of insulin. There is essentially no difference in the effectiveness of the different forms of carbohydrates (i.e., drinks, gels, and bars) other than the amount of water and electrolytes in the products and the glycemic index of the carbohydrate. One advantage of bars and gels is that they are lighter and easier to carry than an equivalent amount of calories in the form of a sports' drink. The primary disadvantage is that bars and gels require a water source for proper dissolution, absorption, and gastrointestinal (GI) tolerance. Also, sports bars tend to contain other macronutrients such as fats and proteins that are often not part of a sports drink, making them more applicable to after-exercise recovery than for glycogen preservation during an event.

While the original intent of these products was to provide fuel on the go, the market has evolved to provide meal replacements for active people in a hurry, and they are frequently perceived by the public as healthier than soft drinks, candy bars, or even regular meals. It is not uncommon to see someone skip a meal and eat a prepackaged sports nutrition bar because it is convenient and perceived as a healthful alternative. Clinicians should be aware of the caloric density and glycemic index of these sports drinks and meal replacement bars. The clinician should be prepared to read and interpret the nutrition label with patients and to calculate total calories if the package offers multiple servings. Examples of these bars, gels, and drinks are presented in Table 25-1.

### *Triglyceride-containing Products*

Medium-chain triglycerides (MCTs) have been packaged into sports drinks and powders to provide an alternative fuel to glucose and reduce muscle glycogen utilization.[5,6] The moderate length (8-12 carbons) of MCTs allow them to be absorbed from the GI tract directly into the bloodstream. This allows for much more rapid utilization than occurs with long-chain triglycerides (LCTs) and accounts for the marketing claim that MCTs can spare muscle glycogen. Clinical data in athletes suggest that MCTs are absorbed and can be utilized metabolically within 30 minutes of ingestion, but no data show these products can improve performance.[6] MCTs and LCTs should be avoided in exercise sports nutrition products used before and during exercise because they tend to slow gastric emptying and may cause discomfort and bloating during intense exercise. Meals containing fat should be consumed 2 hours before exercise because of delayed gastric emptying and the risk of GI intolerance.

**TABLE 25-1 Sports Nutrition Products***

| | Carbohydrate (g) | Sugars (g) | Protein (g) | Fat (g) | Sodium (mg) | Potassium (mg) | Energy (kcal) | Serving Size | Comments |
|---|---|---|---|---|---|---|---|---|---|
| **Electrolyte Drinks, Capsules, and Wafers (Low-calorie)** | | | | | | | | | |
| Nuun Active Hydration (wafer) | 0 | 0 | 0 | 0 | 175 | 50 | 5 | 1 wafer | Calcium 12.5 mg; magnesium 12.5 mg |
| Powerade Option | 2 | 2 | 0 | 0 | 50 | 35 | 10 | 8 oz | Vitamins $B_6$, $B_{12}$, C, E, niacin ($B_3$), and pantothenic acid ($B_5$) |
| Propel Fitness Water | 3 | 2 | 0 | 0 | 35 | 40 | 10 | 8 oz | Vitamins $B_6$, $B_{12}$, C, E, niacin ($B_3$), and pantothenic acid ($B_5$) |
| Ultima Replenisher | 2 | 0 | 0 | 0 | 25 | 50 | 8 | 1/3 scoop | Calcium 23 mg; magnesium 8 mg; 13 vitamins and minerals |
| Endurolytes (capsules) | 0 | 0 | 0 | 0 | 100 | 25 | 0 | 1-3 caps | Calcium 50 mg; magnesium 25 mg |
| Thermolyte (capsules) | 0 | 0 | 0 | 0 | 300 | 85.2 | 0 | 2 caps | Calcium 25 mg; magnesium 12 mg |
| **Energy Drinks (Calories and Electrolytes)** | | | | | | | | | |
| Accelerade | 21 | 20 | 5 | 1 | 190 | 64 | 140 | 1 scoop | 37 g/scoop/12 oz |
| Cytomax | 20 | 11 | 0 | 0 | 100 | 110 | 95 | 1 scoop | 25 g/scoop/16 oz |
| E Fuel | 18 | 6 | 0 | 0 | 130 | 50 | 70 | | 1/3 pack /8 oz |
| Gatorade | 14 | 14 | 0 | 0 | 110 | 30 | 50 | | |
| Gatorade Endurance | 15 | 14 | 0 | 0 | 200 | 90 | 60 | 8 oz | |
| $Gu_2O$ | 26 | 4 | 0 | 0 | 240 | 40 | 100 | 2 scoop | 2 scoops/16 oz; contains maltodextrin, fructose |
| **Recovery Drinks** | | | | | | | | | |
| Endurox R4 | 53 | 30 | 14 | 1.5 | 230 | 140 | 280 | 74 g/12 oz | Glutamine |
| Gatorade Shake | 54 | 28 | 20 | 6 | 280 | 560 | 370 | 11 oz | |
| GNC Distance | 38 | 13 | 7 | 1 | 140 | 35 | 190 | 53 g/14 oz | |
| MetRx Protein Shake | 19 | 1 | 25 | 2.5 | 110 | 190 | 200 | 1 packet | |
| Power Dream | 43 | 23 | 10 | 5 | 160 | 370 | 240 | 11 oz | Soy milk |
| IsoPure Endurance | 60 | 40 | 20 | 0 | 210 | 120 | 320 | 20 oz | |
| IsoPure ZeroCarb | 0 | 0 | 40 | 0 | 80 | 45 | 160 | 20 oz | |
| **Energy Gels** | | | | | | | | | |
| Accel Gel | 20 | 10 | 5 | 0 | 95 | 40 | 90 | 1 packet | |
| CarbBoom | 26-27 | 2-4 | 0 | 0 | 50 | 50-75 | 110 | 1 packet | |
| Clif Shot | 24-25 | 7-8 | 0 | 0-0.5 | 40 | 25-50 | 100 | 1 packet | |
| E Gel | 37 | 7 | 0 | 0 | 230 | 85 | 150 | 1 pack | Contains maltodextrin, fructose |
| Gu | 20-25 | 3-4 | 0 | 0–2 | 40-55 | 30-40 | 100 | 1 packet | |
| Hammer Gel | 22-23 | 2 | 0 | 0 | 18-27 | No data | 86-93 | 1 packet | 2 tbsp |
| Power Bar/PowerGel | 28 | 5 | 0 | 0 | 50 | 40 | 110 | 41 g | |

**TABLE 25-1 Sports Nutrition Products* (continued)**

| | Carbo-hydrate (g) | Sugars (g) | Protein (g) | Fat (g) | Sodium (mg) | Potassium (mg) | Energy (kcal) | Serving Size | Comments |
|---|---|---|---|---|---|---|---|---|---|
| **Energy Bars** | | | | | | | | | |
| Bakers Breakfast Cookie | 52-59 | 19-26 | 6-8 | 4-11 | 180-260 | | 270-320 | 1 cookie | |
| Balance Bar Gold | 22-24 | 17-20 | 14-15 | 6 | 90-230 | 85-220 | 200 | 1 bar | |
| Cliff Bar | 43-46 | 20-23 | 10-11 | 3-6 | 90-200 | 210-270 | 230-250 | 1 bar | |
| Luna Bar | 24-28 | 8-12 | 10 | 3-5 | 125-200 | 90-160 | 170-180 | 1 bar | |
| Power Bar Performance | 45 | 18-20 | 9-10 | 2-3.5 | 90-120 | 105-200 | 230-240 | 1 bar | |
| **Protein Bars** | | | | | | | | | |
| Balance Outdoor | 21 | 12 | 15 | 6 | 140 | 260 | 200 | 1 bar | |
| PowerBar Protein Plus | 36 | 19 | 24 | 5 | 140 | n/a | 110 | 1 bar | |
| Pure Fit | 28 | 14 | 18 | 6 | 180 | n/a | 240 | 1 bar | |

* Composition per serving.

### *Protein Products*

Body-building athletes ingest large quantities of protein in an effort to build muscle, and the resulting bigger, stronger body. The source of protein can vary from athlete to athlete, and includes dietary intake of meat, vegetarian sources of protein such as legumes, beans, and nuts and prepackaged protein sources such as protein powders, amino acid supplements, and various protein containing bars, gels, and drinks. Most adults need to consume 0.8 to 1 g of protein per kilogram of body weight per day to maintain their muscle mass.[7,8] When initiating exercise, the body will require a greater proportion of protein to maintain a neutral nitrogen balance, so the ADA recommends a protein intake of 1.2 to 1.4 g/kg/day in highly active adults who participate in endurance excercise.[1] An active athlete who exercises for 5 to 10 hours per week will have an increased protein requirement, compared with the general population. The ADA suggests that athlete's protein needs are increased to assist in the repair of exercise-induced muscle damage, to build and maintain increased lean body mass and to provide some calorie source for energy.

Body builders have an even larger increase in lean body mass than most athletes; thus, the ADA recommends that 1.5 g/kg/day of protein may be required for those who are attempting to increase body mass. Anecdotal evidence of athletes ingesting protein in the quantities of 1.7 to 2.5 g/kg/day has been reported despite a lack of data supporting its effectiveness. A large number of protein supplement products exist in the marketplace, and they have proven quite popular with the serious body builders. Despite the large market demand, the ADA indicates that simple adjustments to the athlete's diet can provide sufficient protein to meet goal dietary intake for increasing muscle mass. There is no evidence that packaged protein supplements are more effective at increasing body mass, compared with ingested whole foods with equal amounts of protein. The use of branch-chain amino acids for endurance performance is discussed later in this chapter.

#### Clinical Evidence for Effectiveness of Protein and Building Muscle

There is little clinical research on the subject of high-protein diets and muscle accumulation. Radiolabeled carbon studies could be used to quantify the amount of dietary carbon that is incorporated into muscle; however, test subjects would be required to undergo painful muscle biopsies. One small study (N = 13) used radiolabeled $C^{13}$-leucine to measure nitrogen balance.[9] Participants received a 13-day diet of protein 0.86, 1.4, or 2.4 g/kg/day prior to a nitrogen balance study and then were crossed over between groups after 14 days. The athletes achieved a zero nitrogen balance with the moderate protein intake of 1.4 g/kg/day. The high-protein diet did not affect nitrogen balance, but leucine oxidation was significantly increased, indicating that the extra protein was utilized for ATP production.

Another important consideration of high-protein diets is the lack of rapid weight gain observed in studies.[8,9] Skeletal muscle mass is approximately 70% water; thus, incorporation of protein into muscle should also result in accumulation of water weight. Many high-protein diet studies have focused on a protein intake of 2 to 2.5 g/kg/day in an attempt to build muscle mass. Evidence shown previously suggests that athletes need protein in quantities of 1.5 g/kg/day to maintain a zero nitrogen balance.[1,9] If an assumption is made that all additional protein intake (0.5 g/kg/day) is incorporated into skeletal muscle, then a 75 kg athlete should gain at least 3 kg of body weight over a 12-week trial. The 3 kg weight gain from protein increases to 6 kg (13 lb) or 1 lb per week when the additional water weight is considered. Well-designed studies of high protein intake have not resulted in consistent weight gain, compared with the control groups.[1,8,9] Muscle mass building is not simply a matter of increasing protein intake or adding a protein supplement to an athlete's diet. An athlete who desires an increase in muscle mass will need to train, provide adequate calories from nonprotein calorie sources to meet maintenance energy needs as well as the increased energy requirement of exercise and still meet target protein intake goals.

The manufacturers of amino acid supplements claim that athletes should use specific amino acid–enriched products, because building muscle will require increased amounts of specific amino acids, the essential amino acids, or the branch-chain amino acids. No clinical research supports these marketing claims, and the ADA does not make particular recommendations regarding supplemental amino acid intake since most athletes seeking to build muscle can obtain the necessary protein goals with complete proteins from their diet. Available data on high-protein diets fail to show a true benefit in terms of increased strength or muscle mass. Many athletes choose to use expensive protein supplements to reach a high protein intake goal. Available data would imply that this expense is of no value to the athlete, compared with a normal diet or a food-based high-protein diet. At this time, it is not appropriate to recommend a protein intake for athletes that is greater than the ADA-recommended level of 1.5 g/kg/day.[1]

### Adverse Effect of High-protein Diets

Proteins are complex structures composed of hundreds of amino acids held together by chemical bonds. Free amino acids are separated, or in a single state, from their original protein source, while peptide-bonded amino acids are in short chains of amino acids still bonded together but lacking the complex structure of intact proteins. There is no advantage to the consumption of whole-source complete proteins or manufactured, packaged individual amino acids, when evaluated by muscle incorporation. However, free amino acids result in a higher osmotic effect, and that can cause diarrhea. Incomplete proteins can be deficient in one or more of the essential amino acids, which may adversely affect growth and development.

Athletes seeking a high-protein diet or diet supplementation should be cautioned to closely evaluate the effects of high protein intake on kidney function over time. Unfortunately, most of the available data are either anecdotal or limited in study duration.[10,11] Several short-duration comparisons of high-protein diets on creatinine clearance estimates have not shown a negative effect after 4 to 12 weeks of supplementation. However, the conclusions in these studies should be questioned because of poor methodology, including the use of creatinine clearance as an estimate of glomerular filtration, because creatinine is a breakdown product of creatine. A high-protein diet, which is high in red meat, will result in an increased dietary intake of creatine. The elevated creatine intake from the diet can result in increased creatinine in the blood and therefore affect the accuracy of the creatinine clearance measurement. This study methodology is not sufficient to prove that high-protein diets over many years are either safe or unsafe.

High protein intake may also affect hydration status or increase the risk of dehydration, since the increased protein load can lead to an increase in nitrogenous wastes that must be eliminated. The elimination of this nitrogen can cause the urine to look very dark yellow to orange, and alter its smell. At one time the tested method for predicting dehydration risk was to evaluate urine color, with pale or light yellow urine considered a good sign of adequate hydration. An athlete may mistakenly assume that dark-colored urine is related to a protein supplement or to a multivitamin product, and not take the proper precaution to increase hydration. A second simple method to monitor for dehydration is for athletes to weigh themselves before and after exercise as any significant weight loss from a short duration of exercise is likely to be a reflection of dehydration.

## Water and Electrolytes

### Free Water

For athletes, water and electrolytes are essential to performance. A 2% decrease in total body water can affect performance, although these laboratory-based studies occurred on stationary treadmills in climate-controlled rooms with little to no convective air flow to help sweat evaporation.[1,12] Because of such studies, athletes have been taught that they need to drink as much as possible to prevent dehydration. This position has been called into question following recent clinical observations of weight gain, severe hyponatremia, cerebral edema, and death from athletes who consumed free water without electrolytes during intense athletic events.[13-15] For example, increased water availability has not resulted in a decrease in athletes seeking medical care after marathon races. Clinical hyponatremia is more likely to occur in nonelite athletes who require more than 4 hours to finish a marathon, and in long-course triathletes who require 13 to 17 hours to complete their events.[13,16] Providing pre-event athlete education, and electrolyte-containing sports drinks during the event, resulted in a reduction in hyponatremia cases in triathletes, but did not appear to impact the risk of hyponatremia in experienced marathon runners.[13,16]

The result of these observations is an advisory statement from the International Marathon Medical Directors Association.[17] This advisory statement suggests that heat production by an athlete is significantly affected by the effort; therefore, a 10-km race effort will generate more heat than a marathon effort (42.2 km). Since an average athlete runs slower than an elite athlete, the average athlete is at less risk of heat illness than the elite athlete, and has more time to consume water at aid stations. Average athletes exercising for more than 4 hours can consume excess free water resulting in an increased risk of hyponatremia. The recommendations suggest that athletes should choose an electrolyte replacement drink instead of free water to avoid the risk of hyponatremia when competing is events of 4 hour and longer.[17] Most important, dehydration during endurance events is still a significant concern, therefore, it is important for the clinician to recognize the risks associated with dehydration, including event duration, and educate the athlete on the difference between drinking pure water and water with electrolytes.

A second paradigm shift is that an athlete who collapses immediately after crossing the finishing line may be suffering from postural hypotension, rather than heat-related illness or dehydration. When an athlete crosses the finish line, the sudden decrease in leg muscle contractions allows for pooling of blood in the legs and a decrease in venous return. The resulting decrease in cardiac output may leave the brain underperfused with oxygenated blood, causing the athlete to black out.[17] One of the most important recommendations of this guideline is to ensure that athletes continue walking past the finish line to prevent this reaction. Only athlete's demonstrating a rectal temperature higher than 104°F (40°C) should be treated for heat illness.[17]

### Carbonated, Oxygen-enhanced, and Clustered Water

Carbonation of water is not beneficial to athletes and may be detrimental. Dissolved gases can accumulate and cause GI distress and bloating, resulting in a decrease in total fluid consumption.[18] Oxygenated water is distilled water to which pressure has been applied to increase the percentage of dissolved oxygen to a claimed rate of 30% or greater. Marketing claims have suggested that oxygenated water improves muscle endurance, benefits athletes competing in anaerobic events such as weight lifting, and assists athletes with asthma by reducing shortness of breath. Research does not substantiate these effects in humans.[19] The results are predictable since oxygen-enhanced water, packaged in plastic bottles, may have no more dissolved oxygen than tap water, and the amount of dissolved oxygen in a 12-oz bottle packed in glass is less than that contained in a single breath of room air.[19] Similarly, one brand of bottled water, sold under the brand Penta®, has claimed to improve hydration and physical performance in athletes by altering the structure of water to form microclusters. No published data support this claim of improved hydration and performance in humans who use microclustered water.

### Electrolytes and Water Without Added Carbohydrates

For events lasting longer than 4 hours, there is a clear indication for water and electrolyte replacement to maintain homeostasis of electrolyte losses from sweat.[1,12] Sodium and potassium are commonly added to electrolyte replacement drinks. The absorption rate of water is improved with the addition of small amounts of electrolytes, particularly sodium, and the volume of fluid consumed improves with a small amount of added sodium.[1] Electrolyte replacement may be important in shorter events (1 to 2 hours) that occur in hot and humid conditions, particularly for athletes who produce very high volumes of sweat, and athletes who work out several times daily, such as high-school football players doing two-a-day workouts in early preseason training.[1] The ADA does not recommend electrolyte replacement during an event lasting less than 1 hour, as long as the athlete consumes a salty meal or snack before or after the event.[1]

One market segment increasing in popularity is low-calorie carbohydrate-containing sports drinks, which are formulated to provide hydration and smaller amounts of electrolytes without the carbohydrate and caloric load of typical sports drinks. Some of these low-calorie sports drinks provide as little as 3 g of carbohydrates per serving, or just 10 kcal. This is in contrast to the 14 to 26 g of carbohydrates and 100 to 190 kcal per serving contained in most carbohydrate-containing sports drinks. While electrolyte-containing sports drinks can be used after exercise of any duration, there is no evidence that they are superior to food sources of electrolytes a normal postexercise meal provides.

### Electrolytes, Carbohydrates, and Water

Sports nutrition drinks containing water, electrolytes, and carbohydrates were invented at the University of Florida as a means of replacing electrolytes and glycogen in football players. Gatorade, the market leader in sales, was named after the school's mascot. Addition of carbohydrates to sports drinks is beneficial to athletes competing longer than an hour, replacing muscle glycogen lost during periods of intense effort. The ADA does not recommend sports drinks containing carbohydrates for any event lasting less than an hour, but they do support use of carbohydrate supplementation during events as a method of glycogen preservation. As exercise duration increases, muscle glycogen will be converted to carbohydrates as a source of energy. Carbohydrate supplementation during exercise provides the exercising muscle with fuel for energy while allowing the muscle to maintain its stored carbohydrate energy as glycogen. This strategy of providing fuel during exercise has been shown to prolong the time to exhaustion in long-distance runners and cyclists.[1]

Athletes should be familiar with the glycemic index of the carbohydrate drink they are using for muscle glycogen preservation. Glucose is a high glycemic index sugar that is rapidly absorbed and promotes significant insulin release. Carbohydrate calories not immediately consumed in ATP generation, or stored as glycogen, will likely be converted to fat for storage. Many insulin-sensitive athletes will need to consume repeated doses of glucose at regular intervals to prevent hypoglycemia, since insulin circulates longer than available glucose, particularly in the face of rapid glucose utilization in high-intensity efforts. Many sports drinks use complex carbohydrates that have a lower glycemic index and are better suited to events lasting many hours. For these reasons, athletes should be familiar with the specific carbohydrate in their sports drinks and the relative glycemic index of that carbohydrate.

### Electrolytes, Carbohydrates, Protein, and Water

The latest trend in sports nutrition products is to introduce protein, in the form of amino acids, to the existing carbohydrate- and electrolyte-containing drinks. Amino acids are added to provide an additional metabolic fuel for ATP production via the Krebs cycle. These products are marketed to long-distance endurance athletes competing at aerobic intensities for long durations, including marathon runners (2.5 to 5 hours), long-distance triathletes (2 to 17 hours), and adventure racers (12 hours to 5 days). Several studies have supported a benefit to the alternative calorie source when measured by time to exhaustion at a fixed effort.[20,21] In these studies, carbohydrate and water outperform water alone, and protein-carbohydrate-water outperforms carbohydrate alone. The protein sources have two limitations. These protein-containing drinks come in a powder, and can release a significant amount of gas when mixed with water. Bubbles and foam appear on the top layer of the hydrated powder and can influence GI tolerance in athletes. This intolerance can be significant when the athlete is unfamiliar with the product; therefore, protein-containing sports drinks should be introduced as part of the training regimen so that the athlete can gain tolerance before the drinks are used to improve performance. Because hydrolysis can affect stability of some proteins once mixed with water, optimal effect may require that the athlete carry the powder unmixed and add water during the event. This can introduce a safety variable in triathlon events, for example, if athletes try mixing the powder while riding a bicycle. Glutamine, which has been added to sports drink powders, is an unstable compound and will rapidly break down into glutamate and ammonia since its half-life is 1 hour. Athletes should know not to mix their carbohydrate-protein drink bottles the night before the event as they have with carbohydrate-only sports drinks. Once mixed, all sports drinks should be consumed or stored in the refrigerator within 2 hours.

### *Postexercise Nutrition and Recovery Drinks*

The goal of postexercise nutrition is to replace muscle glycogen, repair muscle damage, and prepare for the next activity. The addition of protein to a carbohydrate sports drink has been proposed to improve muscle glycogen restoration and has led to subsequent performance gains, compared with carbohydrate-only drinks.[22] Others have found that the addition of protein to isocaloric carbohydrates has no effect on muscle glycogen levels.[23,24] This evidence needs to be critically considered because of the difficulty in providing true isocaloric comparator groups since the protein provides additional calories. Recreational athletes are likely to benefit equally by consuming an isocaloric, isonitrogenous meal versus a specific "recovery" sports drink.

### *Specific Ergogenic Supplements*

#### Antioxidants and Exercise

Many sports nutrition products include antioxidants which claim to be able to reduce oxidative stress during exercise or speed recovery following exercise. The antioxidants used include α-lipoic acid, carotenoids, glutathione, *n*-acetylcysteine, the ubiquinones including coenzyme Q-10, and vitamins E and C. Several clinical trials have assessed the efficacy of *n*-acetylcysteine and vitamins E and C without proof of benefit.[25]

*Arginine* Administration of arginine has been promoted to improve muscle building and cardiovascular functioning through the production of nitrous oxide, which causes cardiac vasodilatation and increased oxygen delivery to the heart. Limited data support these claims. In patients with stable angina pectoris, supplementation with arginine 6 g/day has been shown to improve exercise tolerance until measured ischemia appears on an electrocardiogram.[26] In a randomized, double-blind, crossover study, the arginine-treated exercise times were increased by 2.5 to 3 minutes in patients with stable angina pectoris. A recent randomized, double-blind study compared a supplement containing arginine 5 g/day, β-hydroxy-β-methylbutyrate 2 g/day, lysine 1.5 g/day and ascorbic acid 500 mg/day to an isocaloric, isonitrogenous control that did not contain these four products.[27] Subjects consisted of 29 female nursing home residents, who were between 62 and 85 years of age. The supplement or the control was taken daily for 12 weeks. The subjects were tested for their ability to "get up and go," a measure of daily activity that consisted of rising from a seated position, ambulating 40 m, and returning to the seat. The supplemented group was able to decrease their time by 2.3 seconds, a 15% decrease from baseline, compared with the control group time, which was unchanged.

*β-Hydroxy-β-methylbutyrate* One of the metabolites of leucine metabolism is β-hydroxy-β-methylbutyrate (HMB). HMB is claimed to decrease muscle protein breakdown following a workout, thereby improving the likelihood of increased muscle mass. HMB has also been proposed to improve aerobic performance. Clinical studies to date have been poorly designed, with the control groups receiving a diet containing fewer total calories and less protein than the experimental groups, who received a high-protein diet supplemented with HMB 3 g daily.[28,29] One study showed an increase in muscle mass and greater total weight lifted in the experimental arm, but the lack of an isocaloric, isonitrogenous control group prevents concluding that the benefits were gained from HMB alone.[28] A second study failed to show aerobic benefits of HMB in endurance cyclists.[29] There is insufficient evidence to support an ergogenic benefit to HMB.

*Branch-chain Amino Acids* Skeletal muscle cells are adapted to use branch-chain amino acids (BCAA) to supply limited amounts of energy during exercise. In addition, supplementation of BCAAs may reduce fatigue and increase exercise time to exhaustion by reducing serum levels of L-tryptophan and its effect on serotonin levels in the brain.[30] The BCAAs are isoleucine, leucine, and valine. Their catabolism increases during intense exercise, particularly in very hot conditions when muscle glycogen has been depleted. BCAAs are frequently added to sports nutrition bars and gels as a source of energy in addition to glucose, and as a source of protein for muscle building. Two recent studies failed to identify improvements in aerobic endurance performance or in time to fatigue with BCAA supplementation.[30,31]

In the first study, seven male subjects completed two separate 2-day exercise tests.[30] The randomized, crossover design had each subject serve as his own control. On day 1 of each test, the subjects completed a series of cycle ergometer and treadmill running tests designed to create a glycogen-depleted, dehydrated state (a 4% loss of body mass). Subjects remained in a controlled facility where rehydration and carbohydrate calorie consumption were controlled to prevent rebuilding of glycogen stores. On the next day (24 hours later) the subjects began with a 60-minute cycle ergometer test followed immediately by a 30-minute cycle ergometer time trial for distance in a climate-controlled room set at 104°F (40°C) and 20% humidity. Isocaloric fluids were provided as a carbohydrate or a carbohydrate/BCAA-supplemented drink with a total of 1.5 L over the 90-minute test period. Distance traveled in the 30-minute time trial was not significantly different whether the subjects were supplemented with carbohydrate or carbohydrate and BCAA.

In the second study, eight male subjects consumed one of three hydration drinks before and during intermittent shuttle running until exhaustion.[31] The mixed protocol of sprinting, running, and walking was designed to mimic on-field activities seen in soccer, basketball, and hockey. Participants were given one of three beverages to drink during the exercise: a flavored placebo drink, a carbohydrate-only drink, or an isocaloric carbohydrate/BCAA-supplemented drink. There was no difference in total exercise time between the carbohydrate and the carbohydrate/BCAA drink. Both supplemented drinks improved exercise time over the no-calorie placebo.

*Carnitine* Carnitine is an essential cofactor for the transport of long-chain fatty acids into the mitochondria. It is supplied in the diet but is not classified as an essential dietary component since the liver can make carnitine from lysine and methionine. Although carnitine deficiency has not been reported in athletes, carnitine supplementation has been proposed to improve fatty acid oxidation and oxygen absorption, or $VO_2$, in athletes, and therefore reduce lactic acid accumulation. Clinical studies of carnitine supplementation up to 5 g a day have not consistently demonstrated an improvement in $VO_2$.[31] Similarly, there is no evidence to support marketing claims that carnitine supplementation can result in increased metabolic rates or fat burning in active adults seeking weight loss.[32]

*Chromium* Chromium has been marketed to athletes and diabetic patients as a natural product to enhance carbohydrate utilization in the body, thereby improving glycemic control, endurance, and strength. It is frequently included in protein supplements based on the premise that enhanced glucose utilization will allow for the protein to be metabolically spared and utilized for building muscle mass. Several studies in humans have failed to demonstrate a benefit for glycemic control in diabetics. Supplementation has also not been proven to benefit strength or reduce body fat percentage in resistance-trained athletes.[33,34]

*Conjugated Linoleic Acid* Conjugated linoleic acid (CLA) has been promoted as a thermogenic aid, body fat reducer, and ergogenic aid for endurance athletes that enhances fat metabolism. No data support CLA's ability to induce a clinically relevant amount of weight loss or body fat reduction in humans, despite risks associated with lower high-density lipoprotein and increased lipoprotein(a) concentrations in treated subjects.[35] CLA does not improve endurance or increase muscle strength,[36] and should not be recommended as a performance-enhancing supplement or body fat reducer.

*Cordyceps sinensis* *Cordyceps sinensis* is used in Chinese medicine to treat lung disease and fatigue. The mushroom grows primarily in China and Tibet on plateaus above 12,000 foot of elevation. Chinese and Russian literature implies that use of the mushroom can decrease oxygen consumption and improve mortality in mice raised in a hypoxic environment. This literature also implies that the Tibetan Sherpas drink a tea that provides them with *Cordyceps* and *Rhodiola,* which may play a role in their increased endurance at high altitudes. There is limited human research on *Cordyceps* published in English literature. In one study, 22 male cyclists were given 3 g/day of a proprietary product that includes *Cordyceps.* Compared with placebo results, the cyclists experienced no change in $V0_{2max}$, or time trial performance.[37] Currently available English literature is inadequate to make a conclusion on the effectiveness of *Cordyceps* as a performance-enhancing supplement.

*Creatine* Creatine is a naturally occurring substance that is found in all skeletal muscle as free creatine or high-energy phosphorylated creatine. Creatine is synthesized by the body or absorbed intact following ingestion of red meats and fish. Phosphorylated creatine functions as an energy buffer, transferring its phosphate group to adenosine diphosphate, thus rapidly regenerating ATP during periods of exercise. Research has indicated that as many as 50% of high school and college football players use creatine for performance. Supplementation with creatine for 5 to 7 days can attenuate the normal decrease in force associated with repeated work applications such as lifting weights.[38] A normal weightlifter may be able to move a set amount of weight 10 times, then eight times following 30 seconds of rest, and then only six times in the third set of lifts following an additional rest period. Creatine can statistically and clinically improve the athletes' strength so that they can complete more lifts in each subsequent repetition (e.g., 10, 10, and 8 repetitions rather than 10, 8, and 6).[38] Creatine is also useful for athletic events that require repeated, short, explosive bursts of power such football and track and field events. There does not appear to be a benefit to creatine in sports that require more than 20 to 30 seconds of high-intensity activity.

Available data indicate that an athlete can load on creatine at 20 g/day for 5 days (or 0.3 g/kg/day) and then maintain steady-state levels of creatine by taking 5 g/day. GI tolerance has been an issue, and the daily dosage is usually divided into four doses. When supplementation is stopped, there is a rapid return to normal muscle creatine concentrations, although missing one or two doses is unlikely to affect performance. Strength, speed, and recovery time can be improved by creatine supplementation during training, but there is no evidence that the benefits gained during creatine supplementation can be maintained after it is stopped. Athletes will need to consume maintenance doses of creatine to maintain the increased strength.

Adverse effects reported with creatine include GI upset and nausea. Muscle cramping has also been reported, leading to concerns of increased risk of heat-related illness when using creatine. Also, similar to high-protein diets, little is known about the adverse effects of long-term creatine supplementation on renal function. Two reports have followed college football players while taking creatine supplements for as long as 3 years. Athletes were followed for reports of muscle cramping, heat illness, dehydration, muscle strains, total injury reports, and missed practices and were compared with their teammates who were not taking creatine.[39,40] The authors concluded that there was no difference between the groups in occurrence of adverse effects.

The clinician can assist athletes by recommending that creatine be used only as long as necessary. For example, an athlete can consider loading creatine just prior to a specific event to maximize performance. Alternatively, an athlete may maintain creatine intake for 1 to 2 months of a sports season, and then maintain a creatine-free period until the next season. The clinician should also recommend appropriate hydration during creatine exposure because creatine is a protein that is filtered through the kidneys. If an athlete becomes significantly dehydrated, it is best to temporarily hold creatine until a proper fluid balance is established.

*Ephedra and Pseudoephedrine* The Food and Drug Administration (FDA) determined in 2004 that ephedra was unsafe for consumption and removed it from the market. This was partly a result of safety data on ephedra use published by the poison centers from Texas[41] and data supplied to the FDA via MedWatch.[42] Among the reported adverse events subjectively determined to be definitely, probably, or possibly associated with ephedra use were 17 cases of hypertension, 13 cases of palpitations or tachycardia, 10 cases of stroke, and 7 cases of seizures. Ten of these events resulted in death. Many of these adverse events occurred in active, healthy young adults who were not considered at risk based on appropriate prior health screening.

The ephedra alkaloids, which include ephedrine, pseudoephedrine, and phenylpropanolamine, are still available in many foreign markets. Pseudoephedrine is still available as an OTC decongestant in the United States, therefore, data are still included in this text. There is considerable controversy around the subject of ephedra supplementation for athletes seeking enhanced athletic performance. The authors of a recent meta-analysis screened 530 articles and reviewed 52 controlled trials of ephedra use for weight loss and athletic performance.[43] The report included eight controlled studies of ephedra, seven of which used ephedra combined with caffeine. The authors concluded that there are no data to support that ephedra alone is useful for athletic performance and that the combination of ephedra and caffeine is unproven at this time.

There is no evidence that pseudoephedrine is performance enhancing when used at labeled OTC doses.[44] Despite this evidence, pseudoephedrine is considered a sympathomimetic chemical and remains a banned substance by the U.S. antidoping agency. This has been a problem for elite athletes who are subject to random drug testing as the product can appear in their urine for an unpredictable amount of time even when used temporarily for symptomatic improvement of nasal congestion. At this time it would be inappropriate to recommend the ephedra alkaloids for any use without direct consultation with a primary care provider.

*Rhodiola rosea* *Rhodiola rosea* is a Chinese herb used to stimulate the nervous system, affect depression symptoms, improve aerobic work performance, and eliminate fatigue. Similar to *Cordyceps*, *Rhodiola* is reported in Chinese and Russian literature to improve oxygenation at high altitudes and is therefore thought to be helpful for endurance athletes. Limited human research on *Rhodiola* is published in English-language literature. In one double-blind, placebo-controlled, randomized study, 24 men were tested at baseline and then given 200 mg of *Rhodiola rosea*.[45] The subjects were retested at 24 hours. Compared with their baseline, 1-Repmax knee extention and $VO_{2max}$ were statistically improved by *Rhodiola*. Time to exhaustion on a cycle ergometer was improved by less than 30 seconds in a 17-minute test, which was statistically significant but does not appear to be clinically significant. The same subjects were then washed out and given *Rhodiola* 200 mg/day for 4 weeks and retested, showing similar improvements. In a second, small study, 14 well-trained cyclists were given either placebo or a propriety blend of *Rhodiola rosea* for 14 days.[46] The propriety blend included *Rhodiola rosea* 300 mg/day, *Cordyceps sinensis* 1000 mg/day, chromium chelate 200 μg/day, and 800 mg of a blend of pyruvate, sodium phosphate, potassium phosphate, ribose, and adenosine (Optygen). This small study failed to affect $VO_{2max}$, watts of power output, or time to exhaustion on a cycle ergometer in a 40-minute test. Currently available English literature is inadequate to conclude on the effectiveness of *Rhodiola* as a performance-enhancing supplement.

*Steroidal Precursors* Dehydroepiandrosterone (DHEA) and androstenedione are precursors to testosterone. These agents have been promoted as ergogenic aids that elevate an athlete's natural testosterone levels. They have been touted as natural and safe anabolic steroids. Well-designed studies in humans have proven that supplementation does not lead to elevations in serum testosterone levels.[47-50] These studies have actually demonstrated significant elevations in estradiol and estrone in men who take the supplement because the enzyme aromatase converts these products to estrogenic hormones. There is also no credibility to the claim that other herbal products can be added to the steroidal precursors to inhibit the aromatase enzyme and result in increased testosterone levels. Well-designed trials, using daily doses of androstenedione 300 mg and DHEA 150 mg, alone or in combination, have failed to show a performance benefit, compared with placebo in resistance-trained athletes and nonathletes beginning a training program.[47-50] There is no evidence that DHEA supplementation can improve muscle strength; therefore, these products should not be recommended as performance-enhancing supplements. Clinicians should also be aware of recent findings in which androstenedione supplementation resulted in 2 mg/dL decreases in high-density lipoprotein concentrations, which may increase cardiovascular risk.[47-50]

*Stacking* It is important to point out that marketing and sales of sports nutrition products are often complicated by the combination of several agents into a single product, a process known as "stacking." A good example is the commercial product Optygen, which contains a blend of eight ingredients. In the past, androstenedione and DHEA have been combined with other compounds referred to as "natural" aromatization inhibitors designed to prevent the conversion of testosterone to estrone and estradiol. Stacking also results in other products being added for "general health," such as ginseng, ginkgo biloba, and vitamin C. The products frequently claim that the additives will prevent fatigue-related decreases in performance, although no data support this claim. Other products are included to reduce or prevent side effects, such as milk thistle to provide detoxification properties for the liver when athletes use steroids or herbal substances intended to affect hormone levels.

## Assessment of Performance-enhancing Nutrients: A Case-based Approach

Performance enhancers run the gamut from electrolyte solutions to energy bars to hormone precursor supplements. When a person needs help in selecting a product, the practitioner should find out the type of exercise or physical activity in which the person engages. The intensity and duration of the activity are also important information. The patient should also be asked if he or she has experienced any ill effects after the physical activity or after using a performance enhancer. (See Cases 25-1 and 25-2.)

Sales of sports nutrition products designed to enhance or improve performance are increasing every year. The most common self-treatment is carbohydrate administration during exercise to preserve muscle glycogen and prolong endurance. Other products, such as the recovery drinks, are designed to achieve rapid muscle glycogen replenishment when used after exercise. Several herbal supplements, such as carnitine, *Cordyceps,* and *Rhodiola,* claim to enhance performance, but evidence to support these claims is currently lacking. Although these natural herbal products are touted as safe, there is evidence that some, including androstenedione and DHEA, may have detrimental effects on long-term health by altering natural, sex-determined hormone levels.

### CASE 25-1

| Relevant Evaluation Criteria | Scenario/Model Outcome |
|---|---|
| **Information Gathering** | |
| 1. Gather essential information about the patient's symptoms, including: | The patient reports that he has experienced dehydration and fatigue after 90-120 minutes of exercise while training for his first marathon. The fatigue is sufficient to decrease his intensity from a slow run to a walk. |
| a. description of symptom(s) (i.e., nature, onset, duration, severity, associated symptoms) | The fatigue sets in earlier if he runs quickly. Once the fatigue sets in, he is reduced to a slow run or walk. If he attempts to run faster, he experiences muscle cramping in his legs. |
| b. description of any factors that seem to precipitate, exacerbate, and/or relieve the patient's symptom(s) | Patient saw his PCP for a health checkup and lab tests prior to starting his marathon training. The patient is running to raise money for a charity, and for his own personal health and weight control. His PCP advised that he perform most of his long runs on cool weekend mornings at a local park with a water fountain. |
| c. description of the patient's efforts to relieve the symptoms | The patient reports that he has experienced dehydration and fatigue after 90-120 minutes of exercise while training for his first marathon. The fatigue is sufficient to decrease his intensity from a slow run to a walk. |
| 2. Gather essential patient history information: | |
| a. patient's identity | Michael Smith |
| b. patient's age, sex, height, and weight | 37 y/o M, 5'7", 185 lb |
| c. patient's occupation | Accountant |
| d. patient's dietary habits | He usually eats a healthy diet consistent with the Food Guide Pyramid (see Chapter 23) with occasional takeout and junk food lunches. |
| e. patient's sleep habits | He sleeps 7.5-8 hours each night and states that the quality of his sleep is improved by exercise. |

## CASE 25-1 (continued)

| Relevant Evaluation Criteria | Scenario/Model Outcome |
|---|---|
| f. concurrent medical conditions, prescription and nonprescription medications, and dietary supplements | Ibuprofen 200 mg as needed for muscle soreness |
| g. allergies | NKA |
| h. history of other adverse reactions to medications | NONE |
| i. other (describe)_______ | Michael comments that white lines of salt are visible on his clothing when it dries. |
| **Assessment and Triage** | |
| 3. Differentiate the patient's signs/symptoms and correctly identify the patient's primary problem(s). | Michael is drinking only free water to prevent dehydration, but is not replacing the sodium lost through sweating. In addition, after 90 minutes of exercise, Michael may be experiencing muscle glycogen depletion, contributing to his fatigue. |
| 4. Identify exclusions for self-treatment. | None |
| 5. Formulate a comprehensive list of therapeutic alternatives for the primary problem to determine if triage to a medical practitioner is required, and share this information with the patient. | Options include:<br>(1) Recommend increased dietary salt intake before and after weekend runs.<br>(2) Recommend use of a sports drink containing electrolytes, especially sodium, and glucose during his weekend runs for glycogen sparing. Michael should consider training with the same sports drink that will be provided during the marathon race.<br>(3) Recommend use of an inexpensive food containing carbohydrates and salt supplemented with water from the fountain during his training runs. Examples include pretzels, fig newtons, and natural granola bars.<br>(4) Take no action. Symptoms may improve with further training. |
| **Plan** | |
| 6. Select an optimal therapeutic alternative to address the patient's problem, taking into account patient preferences. | Several sports drinks that contain carbohydrates and electrolytes are readily available and beneficial for this purpose (see Table 25-1). Clinically, there is little to justify one product over another except for price and convenience, although, powdered forms cost less than ready-to-drink versions. Pretzels, saltine crackers, and candy corn also provide convenient sources of carbohydrates and sodium. |
| 7. Describe the recommended therapeutic approach to the patient. | Since you don't have high blood pressure, you can increase your salt intake in meals before and after long runs. Initially, for long (>90 minutes) periods of exercise, you should drink 8 oz of Gatorade every 30 minutes, starting 30 minutes after exercise begins. You can use a powdered version of the product and mix it with water at the park to decrease expenses. |
| 8. Explain to the patient the rationale for selecting the recommended therapeutic approach from the considered therapeutic alternatives. | Taking 8 oz of Gatorade will provide you with glucose during exercise, which should help to maintain muscle glycogen and prolong your endurance. Sodium and potassium replacement during exercise should decrease muscle cramping. The marathon training newsletter indicated that Gatorade brand sports drink will be provided at each hydration station, so training with Gatorade is logical to ensure GI tolerance during the marathon itself. |
| **Patient Education** | |
| 9. When recommending self-care with nonprescription medications and/or nondrug therapy, convey accurate information to the patient, including: | |
| a. appropriate dose and frequency of administration | Since GI intolerance to sports drinks while running is common, you can start by taking smaller amounts more frequently (3-4 oz every 15 minutes) until your tolerance is established. This may require running a short 1-2 mile loop, setting out bottles in advance along the run course, or carrying a hydration pack. |

## CASE 25-1 (continued)

| Relevant Evaluation Criteria | Scenario/Model Outcome |
|---|---|
| b. maximum number of days the therapy should be employed | Glycogen sparing during runs should be necessary only during long runs lasting more than 90 minutes. This means you need a carbohydrate-containing product only once each week if you are following the typical pattern of these long runs once each week while training for a marathon. Sports drinks are a significant source of carbohydrate calories and should be avoided after shorter runs (<60 minutes) since muscle glycogen preservation is not required for this duration of effort and the high glycemic index of the sports drink may stimulate a spike in insulin release. High insulin levels may hamper your weight control efforts by inhibiting fatty acid metabolism and may stimulate the storage of carbohydrate calories as fat. |
| c. product administration procedures | N/A |
| d. expected time to onset of relief | Glucose absorption is rapid. If your symptoms are caused by muscle glycogen depletion, then you should experience some relief of your fatigue within a few minutes of consuming more carbohydrates. |
| e. degree of relief that can be reasonably expected | With experience, you should be able to maintain muscle glycogen supplies and, therefore, your training pace for a longer period of time and/or longer distance prior to experiencing fatigue. The addition of electrolytes should significantly reduce or eliminate muscle spasm. |
| f. most common side effects | Stomach upset, gas, and bloating may occur if you consume water or a sports drink while exercising. Research indicates that athletes experienced with a sports drink will drink more of that sports drink if it is flavored, and that the addition of electrolytes speeds the absorption of that fluid, compared with water alone. However, your personal preference for a particular flavor, or preference for saltiness or sweetness of an electrolyte sports drinks can limit the total volume you consume and therefore affect your performance. These side effects tend to decrease with training and experience. |
| g. side effects that warrant medical intervention, should they occur | You should see your PCP, that is, primary care provider, if muscle cramping is persistent despite the use of the sports drink. The PCP can test for electrolyte deficiencies, including sodium, potassium, and magnesium. You should bring your current and oldest running shoes with you to the doctor, since a review of running shoe breakdown and biomechanics can assist in identifying potential injuries and additional strains on muscle groups caused by equipment failure. Your PCP should be familiar with the basics of screening for biomechanical issues, or should refer you to a specialist in sports medicine. |
| h. patient options in the event that condition worsens or persists | A full 26.2-mile marathon is a lofty, but obtainable goal for a new runner. You may want to consider setting intermediate goals, such as completing one or two half-marathon (13.1 mile) events before the full marathon. This strategy will allow you to experience the training and nutritional considerations of marathoning before pursuing the full event. You can also set intermediate body weight goals prior to the full marathon event. Your training should address the fatigue symptoms with continued forward motion, including a mix of walking and slow running while refueling with carbohydrates. Also, training with another runner or a group of runners will provide valuable camaraderie and a degree of safety when the training plan calls for the long runs. |
| i. product storage requirements | Powdered drinks can be stored at room temperature until mixed with water. Unopened containers of ready-to-drink products can also be stored at room temperature. Opened containers and mixed powders should be consumed within 2 hours or refrigerated immediately. |
| j. specific nondrug measures | N/A |
| 10. Solicit follow-up questions from patient. | I don't like the taste of Gatorade. Can I use water and salt tablets instead? |
| 11. Answer patient's questions. | Since you appear to have significant sodium loss from sweat, you can consider increasing the amount of sodium in your postexercise meal. Salt tablets (sodium chloride) and electrolyte capsules can be used as alternatives for sodium replacement from sports drinks. This can be a useful alternative to provide sodium without the carbohydrate. A 1000 mg tablet of sodium chloride contains approximately 400 mg of sodium, which is equivalent to the sodium load from two 8-oz doses of sports drink. |

Key: GI, gastrointestinal; N/A, not applicable; NKA, no known allergies; PCP, primary care provider.

## CASE 25-2

| Relevant Evaluation Criteria | Scenario/Model Outcome |
|---|---|
| **Information Gathering** | |
| 1. Gather essential information about the patient's symptoms, including: | |
| a. description of symptom(s) (i.e., nature, onset, duration, severity, associated symptoms) | The patient is a high-school-age male athlete who is small for his age and trying out for the football team. He states that he performs well in practices on the field that emphasize agility, endurance, and leg strength, but that he performs poorly in the weight room, where he experiences significant decreases in weight lifted between repetition sets. He can usually lift a set weight for 10 lifts the first set, but cannot do even 5 lifts of the second set. His coach expects the weight to be lifted 10 times for three sets. |
| b. description of any factors that seem to precipitate, exacerbate, and/or relieve the patient's symptom(s) | The decreased performance in weight lifting is most evident with upper body muscles for the larger muscle groups. The fatigue progresses through the workout, with the later "set" being even more difficult to complete. |
| c. description of the patient's efforts to relieve the symptoms | He has tried consuming carbohydrate- and caffeine-containing sports beverages to improve performance. When this failed to improve performance, his friends recommended that he find a protein powder supplement that includes ephedra, androstenedione, or DHEA. |
| 2. Gather essential patient history information: | |
| a. patient's identity | Duante Jones |
| b. patient's age, sex, weight, and height | 16 y/o M, 5'5", 138 lb |
| c. patient's occupation | Student |
| d. patient's dietary habits | Normal healthy diet when his parents prepare meals. Typical teenage junk food diet at school. Duante seldom eats breakfast, avoids milk products because of lactose intolerance, and rarely eats fruits and vegetables. |
| e. patient's sleep habits | Poor sleep habits. Stays up late, seldom sleeping more than 5-6 hours per night during the week, and falls asleep in class. Sleeps in on weekends. |
| f. concurrent medical conditions, prescription and nonprescription medications, and dietary supplements | None |
| g. allergies | Penicillin rash as a child |
| h. history of other adverse reactions to medications | N/A |
| i. other (describe)_______ | He is a high-school junior and is feeling peer pressure to make the Varsity football team. In the weight room, he attempts to move the same weight as his best friend, who is larger, stronger, and has little trouble moving the weight the prescribed number of lifts and sets. He is embarrassed to change the weight between sets, thus slowing down his partners. |
| **Assessment and Triage** | |
| 3. Differentiate the patient's signs/symptoms and correctly identify the patient's primary problem(s). | Duante is experiencing a common effect of resistance training. Resistance training involves lifting a weight repeatedly 10-15 times for one "set," resting for 60 seconds, and then attempting to repeat the set by lifting the weight 10-15 times again. Decreased performance is expected and even desired, since the stress stimulates the muscle repair and growth process, empirically referred to as "no pain, no gain." Completion of three full sets at a desired weight is an indication to increase the weight. There is a point at which overstress can increase the risk of injury. He is also smaller than his friend and may not be capable of lifting the same weight at this point of his training. This type of fatigue will not be overcome by carbohydrate supplementation. |
| 4. Identify exclusions for self-treatment. | Duante's motivation and level of desire should be carefully investigated, since he provides clues to a risk pattern for anabolic steroid use and/or inappropriate use of herbal performance products. Undersized high school athletes attempting to compete against their peers are at risk for this type of behavior. If risk patterns are identified, a parent, coach, PCP, or possibly all three should be alerted. |

## CASE 25-2 (continued)

| Relevant Evaluation Criteria | Scenario/Model Outcome |
|---|---|
| 5. Formulate a comprehensive list of therapeutic alternatives for the primary problem to determine if triage to a medical practitioner is required, and share this information with the patient. | Options include:<br>(1) Work with the strength and conditioning coach to identify the appropriate initial weight to ensure that he can complete the prescribed workout without risk of injury. This will likely require that the weights be lowered to a more appropriate starting point. This option may also require that Duante lift with a different partner who is more evenly matched for strength.<br>(2) Duante should be educated on lack of evidence supporting the use of "natural" steroidal precursors as well as the possible adverse reactions, including androgenic effects (acne) and the effects on estrogenic hormone levels. Duante should also be carefully educated to the risk of anabolic steroid use in growing adolescents and be referred to his PCP for follow-up questions regarding growth and puberty.<br>(3) Creatine supplementation for the duration of football season may improve Duante's performance by attenuating the reduced strength of contraction that follows repeated sets of weight lifting.<br>(4) Take no action. His experience and performance are a natural effect of early training and may improve in time with experience and additional training. This is an appropriate action. |
| **Plan** | |
| 6. Select an optimal therapeutic alternative to address the patient's problem, taking into account patient preferences. | Duante needs to decrease the pressure to perform against others and concentrate on improving his performance against himself. Working with the strength and conditioning coach or teaming with an ability-matched partner are appropriate first steps. Duante also wants the extra assurance of a nutritional plan involving an appropriate high-protein diet with creatine supplementation. |
| 7. Describe the recommended therapeutic approach to the patient. | Conservative management is appropriate for a 16-year-old who may be small because of late puberty. Additional protein is appropriate for any athlete seeking gains in muscle mass, but only as part of a training plan that emphasizes proper training and nutrition, including adequate calories. This can be accomplished with proper diet selection at lunch and possibly a high-protein sports bar as a snack, 60-90 minutes prior to afternoon football practice. Experience with creatine has indicated that it can improve his specific symptoms of strength attenuation from repeated lifts. |
| 8. Explain to the patient the rationale for selecting the recommended therapeutic approach from the considered therapeutic alternatives. | You should target a daily protein intake of 95-100 g (approximately 1.5 g/kg/day of protein). Experience with creatine has indicated that it can improve the loss of strength that occurs with repeated lifts like you describe, and this is considered part of the daily protein intake. An adequate amount of calories is also needed to prevent the protein from being used for energy rather than muscle mass. A high-protein snack bar or other "high-protein, high-energy" snack, such as a nuts and dried fruit mix, in the afternoon may help you meet your protein and calorie goals. It is important to include fruits and vegetables in your diet and healthy food choices more frequently since you need healthy food to make a strong, healthy body. You may want to look at the Food Guide Pyramid on the Internet (www.mypyramid.com) to see recommendations for a healthy diet, although this is not specific to athletes. |
| **Patient Education** | |
| 9. When recommending self-care with nonprescription medications and/or nondrug therapy, convey accurate information to the patient, including: | |
| a. appropriate dose and frequency of administration | Creatine powder can be started at 20 g/day (0.3 g/kg/day) for 5 days as a loading dose, followed by 5 g/day as a maintenance dose. |

## CASE 25-2 (continued)

| Relevant Evaluation Criteria | Scenario/Model Outcome |
|---|---|
| b. maximum number of days the therapy should be employed | Performance benefits are related to an increased supply of creatine and creatine-phosphate bonds, therefore, the benefits are present only while creatine maintenance doses are provided. Creatine should be stopped after the football season (typically 3-4 months) because long-term use could damage the kidneys. Creatine is not needed during the off-season when the pressure to compete is reduced. You can continue to perform strength training in the off-season when the pressures of performance are reduced. You will need to use a new set of weight-lifting goals while not supplemented with creatine for fair comparison of week to week changes in performance. |
| c. product administration procedures | N/A |
| d. expected time to onset of relief | Strength gains from creatine supplementation are subjectively felt within 1-2 days. |
| e. degree of relief that can be reasonably expected | The relative increase in strength has been shown to be 8%-15% in 1-Repmax studies, a measure of the maximum amount of weight that can be lifted in a single lift. However, the benefits of strength attenuation prevention are more difficult to measure. Total weight lifted during a single workout (the sum of all weight lifted for all sets over a single workout) can increase by 10%-20% with creatine supplementation in young adults. Data for adolescents less than 18 years of age are unavailable. |
| f. most common side effects | Side effects are not commonly reported by clinical research. Anecdotal evidence suggests increased rates of heat illness, muscle cramping, and GI intolerance, but clinical studies up to 3 years have not shown this effect in college-age athletes. Hydration should be part of the plan regardless of the use of creatine. |
| g. side effects that warrant medical intervention should they occur | Side effects warranting medical care usually do not occur; however, Duante should routinely describe any sensations that are "unusual" to his coaches and family as the season progresses. Referral to the PCP is based largely on the athlete's total experience and impressions. |
| h. patient options in the event that condition worsens or persists | N/A |
| i. product storage requirements | Creatine is available in tablets that can be stored at room temperature, and as powdered drinks that can be stored at room temperature until mixed with water. Mixed powders should be consumed within 2 hours or refrigerated immediately. |
| j. specific nondrug measures | N/A |
| 10. Solicit follow-up questions from patient. | Are the tablets or the powder better? |
| 11. Answer patient's questions. | Some people find the tablets more convenient but others like the powder better. It really doesn't matter which you use as long as you take an equal amount of creatine. |

Key: DHEA, dehydroepiandrosterone; N/A, not applicable; PCP, primary care provider.

## Patient Counseling for Performance-enhancing Nutrients

The quest for enhanced physical performance has resulted in serious health consequences for some athletes. Excessive intake of micronutrients can cause problems in otherwise healthy individuals. Clinical studies of some of the botanical and hormonal dietary supplements touted as performance enhancers reveal significant adverse effects and little or no enhancement in physical performance. Practitioners should be prepared to steer patients asking for advice on these products to the safest and most appropriate product. The box Patient Education for Performance Enhancers lists specific information to provide patients.

## Key Points for Sports Nutrition and Performance-enhancing Nutrients

- Despite marketing claims, most "performance-enhancing" nutritional products and ergogenic aids are unproven, and several may be unsafe. By comparison, "training" regularly, and eating a well-balanced diet have consistently been shown to benefit most sports and activities.
- Most sports nutrition drinks, gels, and bars are significant sources of carbohydrate calories and should be avoided unless indicated by duration of physical activity and risk of glycogen depletion.

## PATIENT EDUCATION FOR PERFORMANCE-ENHANCING NUTRIENTS

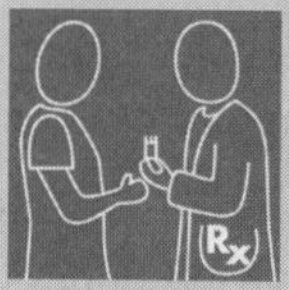

The objective in selecting a performance enhancer is to choose a product that is safe and appropriate for the type, intensity, and duration of the physical activity. Following the recommendations of a primary care provider and other clinicians, as well as carefully following product instructions and the self-care measures listed here, will help to ensure optimal therapeutic outcomes.

### Muscle Glycogen Preservation

- High glycemic index products, including most carbohydrate-containing sports drinks, contain sucrose. They are optimal for intermediate sprint activities, such as soccer and football, and for endurance events that last longer than 45 minutes but less than 3 hours. Small doses repeated every 15 to 30 minutes may be necessary for sustained energy over longer events since the insulin effect will outlast a single dose of sucrose.
- Moderate glycemic index products contain maltodextrin, galactose, and fructose. They are optimal for athletic events that last longer than 4 hours.
- Diabetic athletes should seek the advice of a primary care provider before beginning an exercise program, and be prepared to address the symptoms of hypoglycemia while exercising.
- Diabetic athletes should exercise with a friend or in a public setting such as a gym or athletic center due to the risk of exercise-induced hypoglycemia.
- Diabetic athletes who exercise for long durations (greater than 1 hour) may require repeated doses of glucose at regular intervals to prevent hypoglycemia. There is no preferred glucose source provided that the athlete is experienced with the products, their effect on insulin requirements, and the effect of exercise intensity and duration on their monitoring plan.
- See Table 25-2 for specific products. Note that the sports bars often contain other macronutrients such as fats and proteins. Many of these bars are more appropriate for after-exercise recovery than for use during athletic events. Sports bars also contain more than twice the calories of a regular chocolate bar.
- Long-chain triglycerides can cause discomfort and bloating during intense exercise; therefore, consume meals containing fat 2 hours before exercise.

### Enhancement of Muscle Mass

- Athletes should not exceed the American Dietetic Association's recommended daily intake of 1.5 grams of protein per kilogram of body weight to increase body mass. Available data do not show that higher intakes produce more muscle mass or additional strength.
- Athletes who ingest high amounts of protein either through their foods or protein supplements should monitor the effects of high protein intake on their kidney function.
- Little clinical evidence is available to support the claims that arginine and β-hydroxy-β-methylbutrate help to increase muscle mass.

### Hydration and Electrolytes

- Athletes exercising for less than 90 minutes usually can complete their exercise with water alone, although the addition of small amounts of carbohydrates and/or electrolytes may be performance enhancing.
- Athletes exercising for longer than 90 minutes should incorporate a carbohydrate and electrolyte containing sports drink into the exercise program for optimal performance.
- Athletes exercising for 4 hours and longer are discouraged from drinking free (regular) water due to the risk of dilutional hyponatremia. Exercise of this duration (e.g., marathon running and long distance triathlons) will require electrolyte and carbohydrate replacement for optimal performance.
- Athletes should consume 400 to 800 mL of water per hour during exercise. Slower runners/walkers exercising in cool conditions can consume water at the lower rate, while faster/heavier athletes and those exercising in heat and humidity should target the higher end for their goal consumption.
- Carbonated water may case gastrointestinal distress and bloating; avoid drinking carbonated water before or during an athletic event.
- There is little clinical information to support the premise that oxygen-enhanced water affects athletic performance.

### Ergogenic Supplements

- Little clinical evidence is available to support claims that antioxidants (vitamins A, $B_1$, $B_6$, $B_{12}$, E, and C) and coenzyme Q-10 reduce oxidative stress during exercise or speed recovery after exercise.
- Little clinical evidence is available to support the performance-enhancing claims for carnitine (improved oxygen absorption and fatty acid absorption), chromium (improved glycemic control, endurance, and strength), and dehydroepiandrosterone (DHEA) and androstenedione (ANDRO) (improved muscle strength).
- Do not use conjugated linoleic acid to reduce body fat or increase endurance and strength. Little clinical evidence is available to support these claims.
- Consult your primary care provider before using ephedra. Use of ephedra has been linked with an increased risk of psychiatric reactions, autonomic symptoms, gastrointestinal distress, and heart palpitations as well as more severe adverse effects.
- Creatine may increase muscle strength while it is being used, but gastrointestinal discomfort may occur. Take the daily dose (5 mg) in four separate doses to avoid this problem and maintain proper hydration to assist in the elimination of metabolic waste. There is no known benefit to long-term use of creatine.

---

- Dehydration can significantly affect performance. However, there is no evidence that sports nutrition drinks are beneficial when used during events lasting 60 minutes or less.
- Sports nutrition drinks that contain electrolytes and carbohydrates can prolong the time until glycogen depletion in events lasting 120 minutes or longer and therefore may improve performance. Adding protein to a carbohydrate sports drink may result in additional performance benefits.
- Average athletes exercising for very long periods of time should use a sports drink that contains electrolytes and carbohydrates as an alternative to plain water to minimize the risk of hyponatremia caused by the intake of

salt-free fluids. An example would be a recreational runner completing a slow marathon over 5 to 6 hours.

- All athletes should be encouraged to continue moving or walking for several minutes at the completion of a race, since the continued muscle contraction of the legs may reduce the risk of orthostasis. Athletes who stop moving or lie down in a prone position immediately after crossing the finish line are at risk of orthostatic hypotension caused by blood pooling in their legs.
- Creatine supplementation can increase muscle phosphocreatine concentrations, thus increasing the amount of stored energy in the muscle. Phosphocreatine can lend its high-energy phosphate bond to ADP to rapidly restore ATP, allowing for increased strength and power for single and repeated activities for 30 seconds or less.
- Athletes engaging in intense weight training and activities requiring repeated sprints with short recovery times may benefit from creatine supplementation; however, the strength benefits associated with creatine "wash out" when the supplementation stops.
- Pseudoephedrine is banned by the U.S. antidoping agency, and athletes subject to testing for banned substances should be warned of any product containing pseudoephedrine. A similar warning should be given for any cough and cold product that includes a sympathomimetic amine as a decongestant, such as Afrin nasal spray.

## References


1. Manore MM, Barr SI, Butterfield GE. Position of the American Dietetic Association, Dieticians of Canada, and the American College of Sports Medicine: Nutrition and athletic performance. *J Am Diet Assoc.* 2000;100:1543-56.
2. Available at: www.packagedfacts.com. Accessed February 26, 2005.
3. Coyle EF. Substrate utilization during exercise in active people. *Am J Clin Nutr.* 1995;61(suppl):968S-79S.
4. Spencer MR, Gastin PB. Energy system contribution during 200-1500 meter running in highly trained athletes. *Med Sci Sport Excer.* 2001;33:157-62.
5. Turcotte LP. Role of fats in exercise. *Clin Sports Med.* 1999;18:485-97.
6. Vistisen B, Nybo L, Xu X, et al. Minor amounts of plasma medium-chain fatty acids and no improved time trial performance after consuming lipids. *J Appl Physiol.* 2003;95:2434-43.
7. Lemon PW. Beyond the zone: protein needs of active individuals. *J Am Coll Nutr.* 2000;19:513S-21S.
8. Wolfe RR. Protein supplements and exercise. *Am J Clin Nutr.* 2000;72(suppl):551S-7S.
9. Tarnopolsky MA, Atkinson SA, MacDougal JD, et al. Evaluation of protein requirements for trained strength athletes. *J Appl Physiol.* 1992;73:1986-95.
10. Brandle E, Sieberth HG, Hautmann RE. Effect of chronic dietary protein intake on the renal function of healthy subjects. *Eur J Clin Nutr.* 1996;50:734-40.
11. Poortmans JR, Dellalieux O. Do regular high protein diets have potential health risks on kidney function in athletes? *Int J Sport Nutr Exerc Metab.* 2000;10:28-38.
12. Murray D. Fluid replacement: the American College of Sports Medicine position stand. Available at: http://www.gssiweb.com/reflib/refs/135/d00000002000002c2.cfm?pid=38. Accessed February 26, 2005.
13. Speedy DB, Noakes TD, Rogers IR, et al. Hyponatremia in ultradistance triathletes. *Med Sci Sports Exer.* 1999;31:809-15.
14. Davis DP, Videen JS, Marino A, et al. Exercise-associated hyponatremia in marathon runners: a two-year experience. *J Emerg Med.* 2001;21:47-57.
15. Ayus JC, Varon J, Arieff AI. Hyponatremia, cerebral edema, and non-cardiogenic pulmonary edema in marathon runners. *Ann Intern Med.* 2000;132:711-4.
16. Almond CS, Shin AY, Fortescue EB, et al. Hyponatremia among runners in the boston marathon. *N Engl J Med.* 2005;325:1550-6.
17. Noakes T, Martin DE. IMMDA-AIMS Advisory statement on guidelines for fluid replacement during marathon running. March 2002, IAAF. Available at: http://www.aims-association.org/guidelines_for_fluid_replacement.htm. Accessed Feb 26, 2005.
18. Passe DH, Horn M, Murray R. The effects of beverage carbonation on sensory responses and voluntary fluid intake following exercise. *Int J Sport Nutr.* 1997;7:286-97.
19. Hampsom NB, Pollock NW, Piantadosi CA. Oxygenated water and athletic performance. *JAMA.* 2003;290;2408-9.
20. Saunders MJ, Kane MD, Todd, MK. Effects of a carbohydrate-protein beverage on cycling endurance and muscle damage. *Med Sci Sport Excerc.* 2004;36:1233-8.
21. Ivy JL, Res PT, Sprague RC, et al. Effects of a carbohydrate-protein beverage on endurance performance during exercise of varying intensity. *Int J Sport Nutr Exerc Metab.* 2003;382-95.
22. Williams MB, Raven PB, Fogt Dl, et al. Effects of recovery beverages on glycogen restoration and endurance exercise performance. *J Strength Cond Res.* 2003;17:12-9.
23. Carrithers JA, Williamson JA, Gallagher PM, et al. Effects of postexercise carbohydrate-protein feedings on muscle glycogen restoration. *J Appl Physiol.* 2000;88:1976-82.
24. Jentjens RL, Addition of protein and amino acids to carbohydrates does not enhance postexercise muscle glycogen synthesis. *J Appl Physiol.* 2001;91:839-46.
25. Powers SK, Hamilton K. Antioxidants and exercise. *Clin Sports Med.* 1999;18:525-35.
26. Ceremuzynski L, Chamiec T, Herbaczynska-Cedro K. Effect of supplemental oral l-arginine on exercise capacity in patients with stable angina pectoris. *Am J Cardiol.* 1997;80:331-3.
27. Flakoll P, Sharp R, Baier S, et al. Effect of β-hydroxy-β-methylbutyrate, arginine and lysine supplementation on strength, functionality, body composition and protein metabolism in elderly women. *Nutrition.* 2004;20:445-51.
28. Nissen S, Sharp R, Ray M, et al. Effect of leucine metabolite beta-hydroxy-beta-methylbutyrate on muscle metabolism during resistance exercise training. *J Appl Physiol.* 1996;81:2095-104.
29. Vokovich MD, Dreifort GD. Effect of beta-hydroxy-beta-methylbutyrate on the onset of blood lactate accumulation and V02 peak in endurance-trained cyclists. *J Strength Cond Res.* 2001;15:491-7.
30. Cheuvront SN, Carter R, Kolka MA, et al. Branched-chain amino acid supplementation and human performance when hypohydrated in the heat. *J Appl Physiol.* 2004;97:1275-82.
31. Davis JM, Welsh RS, De Volve KL, et al. Effects of branched-chain amino acids and carbohydrate on fatigue during intermittent, high-intensity running. *Int J Sports Med.* 1999;20(5):309-14.
32. Karlic H, Lohninger A. Supplementation of L-carnitine in athletes: does it make sense? *Nutrition.* 2004;20:709-15.
33. Campbell WW, Joseph LJ, Davey SL, et al. Effects of resistance training and chromium picolinate on body composition and skeletal muscle in older men. *J Appl Physiol.* 1999;86:29-39.
34. Walker LS, Bemben MG, Bemben DA, et al. Chromium picolinate effects on body performance and muscular function in wrestlers. *Med Sci Sport Exerc.* 1998;30:1730-7.

35. Kreider RB, Ferreira MP, Greenwood M, et al. Effects of conjugated linoleic acid supplementation during resistance training on body composition, bone density, strength, and selected hematological markers. *J Strength Cond Res.* 2002;16:325-34.
36. Gaullier JM, Halse J, Hoye K, et al. Conjugated linoleic acid supplementation for 1 year reduces body fat mass in healthy overweigh humans. *Am J Clin Nutr.* 2004;79:1118-25.
37. Parcell AC, Smith JM, Schulthies SS, et al. Cordyceps sinensis (CordyMax Cs-4) supplementation does not improve endurance exercise performance. *Int J Sport Nutr Exerc Metab.* April 2004; 14(2):236-42.
38. Kraemer WJ, Volek JW. Creatine supplementation. Its role in human performance. *Clin Sports Med.* 1999;18:651-66.
39. Greenwood M, Kreider RB, Greenwood L, et al. Cramping and injury incidence in collegiate football players are reduced by creatine supplementation. *J Athlet Train.* 2004;38:216-9.
40. Greenwood M, Kreider RB, Melton C, et al. Creatine supplementation during college football training does not increase the incidence of cramping or injury. *Mol Cell Biochem.* 2003;244:83-8.
41. Centers for Disease Control and Prevention. Adverse events associated with ephedrine containing products–Texas, December 1993-September 1995. *MMWR Morb Mortal Wkly Rep.* 1996;45:689-93.
42. Haller CA, Benowitz NL. Adverse cardiovascular and central nervous system events associated with dietary supplements containing ephedra alkaloids. *N Engl J Med.* 2000;343:1833-8.
43. Shekelle PG, Hardy ML, Morton SC, et al. Efficacy and safety of ephedra and ephedrine for weight loss and athletic performance: a meta analysis. *JAMA.* 2003;289:1537-45.
44. Hodges AN, Lynn BM, Bula JE, et al. Effects of pseudoephedrine on maximal cycling power and submaximal cycling efficiency. *Med Sci Sports Exerc.* Aug 2003;35(8):1316-9.
45. De Bock K, Eijnde BO, Ramaekers M, et al. Acute Rhodiola rosea intake can improve endurance exercise performance. *Int J Sport Nutr Exerc Metab.* June 2004;14(3):298-307.
46. Earnest CP, Morss GM. Effects of a commercial herbal-based formula on exercise performance in cyclists. *Med Sci Sports Exerc.* March 2004;36(3):504-9.
47. Broeder C, Quindrey J, Brittingham K, et.al. The androstenedione project. The physiological and hormonal influences of androstenedione supplementation in men 35-65 years old participating in a high-intensity resistance-training program. *Arch Intern Med.* 2000;160:3039-104.
48. Brown GA, Vukovich MD, Sharp RL, et al. Effect of oral DHEA on serum testosterone and adaptations to resistance training in young men. *J Appl Physiol.* 1999;87:2274-83.
49. King DS, Sharp RL, Vukovich MD, et al. Effect of oral androstenedione on serum testosterone and adaptations to resistance training in young men: a randomized controlled trial. *JAMA.* 1999;281:2020-8.
50. Leder BZ, Longcope C, Catlin DH, et al. Oral androstenedione administration and serum testosterone concentrations in young men. *JAMA.* 2000;283:779-82.

CHAPTER 26

# Infant Nutrition and Special Nutritional Needs of Children

*Katherine H. Chessman*

Human milk is most physiologically suited to infants and is the optimal milk source for feeding infants during the first year of life. The American Academy of Pediatrics (AAP) recommends that human milk be used as the sole source of nutrition for infants during the first 6 months of life. For infants whose mothers cannot or will not breast-feed, the nutritional quality, safety, and convenience of infant formulas make them an appropriate alternative. Variations among formulas allow for product selection that will meet a specific infant's nutritional requirements while offering differences in palatability, digestibility, nutrient sources, convenience, and cost.

A health care practitioner should be able to provide information to parents or other caregivers to encourage successful breast-feeding. Additionally, in consultation with the child's parents and primary care provider, the clinician should be able to evaluate indications, advise on the selection of a formula, and help ensure its appropriate use. This service requires knowledge of infant and child nutrition needs, breast-feeding, and commercially prepared infant and pediatric formulas, including differences in formula composition and specific uses for therapeutic formulas.

Some children will require enteral formulas after the age of 1 year because of various disease states and conditions. The clinician needs to be knowledgeable of these products and their appropriate use to be able to answer caregiver questions regarding them, facilitate their procurement, and successfully triage complications associated with these products.

## Gastrointestinal Maturation and Infant Growth

Knowledge of the development of the gastrointestinal (GI) tract and the kidney is crucial to understanding infant nutrition. Comparison of an individual infant's or child's growth with their own previous growth rate or to the Centers for Disease Control (CDC) age- and gender-specific standardized growth charts for infants and children is the method most often used to confirm whether nutrition needs are being met.

### *Maturation*

By the end of the second trimester of pregnancy, all segments of the fetus' GI tract are formed and display some physiologic function. The third trimester, however, is the period of maximal GI tract growth and differentiation. Thus premature infants (those born before 38 weeks gestation) often have reduced GI tract function, especially those born prior to 32 weeks gestation. Transition from intrauterine nutrition via the maternal-fetal unit (i.e., the placenta) to extrauterine nutrition via milk requires the maturation of many physiologic processes. These processes include effective sucking, swallowing, gastric emptying, intestinal peristalsis, and defecation; salivary, gastric, pancreatic, and hepatobiliary secretions; and, intestinal brush border enzymes and transport systems.[1]

Nutritive sucking develops at approximately 34 weeks gestation. In term infants, a mature, efficient pattern of sucking is seen within a few days after birth. In premature infants, an immature, inefficient pattern may persist for a month or more. Infants born before 34 weeks gestation cannot coordinate sucking, swallowing, and breathing, and thus require tube feedings for several months until these reflexes mature. Liquid nutrition is appropriate for all infants until complex tongue movements and swallowing reflexes mature. This maturation of reflexes typically occurs at 4 to 6 months of age, and it is at this time that solid foods can be safely added to an infant's diet.[1]

Early in life, frequent feedings (every 2 to 3 hours) are necessary because the stomach capacity of a term newborn with a birth weight greater than 2500 g (5 lb 8 oz) is only 20 to 90 mL. Gastric capacity increases to 90 to 150 mL by 1 month of age, at which time longer periods between feedings are possible. Human milk empties more rapidly from the stomach than does infant formula, thus human milk–fed infants will typically eat more often than their formula-fed peers.

In term infants, gastric acid and pepsin secretion peak in the first 10 days of life, decrease between days 10 and 30 of life, and then increase to adult levels by 3 months of age. In premature infants, basal acid output is lower than that of a term infant but increases with postnatal age. Milk in the stomach causes a sharp increase in the pH of the gastric contents and a slower return to lower pH values than in older children and adults. Gastric acidity in the newborn is unsuitable for optimal pepsin action. Therefore, little protein digestion occurs in the stomach because of low pepsin activity. The extent of protein absorption, however, is similar to that seen in children and adults. Amino acids and peptides produced by protein digestion are absorbed passively or by active transport mechanisms that reach adult levels by the age of 14 weeks.

Premature and full-term infants can digest most carbohydrates because the production of intestinal enzymes such as sucrase, maltase, isomaltase, and glucoamylase is sufficiently mature at birth. Lactase activity rises relatively late in fetal life and begins to decline after the age of 3 years, especially in African-American and Asian children. By adulthood, approximately 15% of Caucasians, 40% of Asians, and 85% of African Americans are deficient in intestinal lactase.[2] Pancreatic amylase secretion does not reach adult levels until approximately 1 year of age. Salivary amylase may help compensate for this relative lactase and amylase deficiency in early infancy and in premature infants. Despite this relative lactase deficiency, most term and preterm infants tolerate lactose-containing formulas with negligible unabsorbed carbohydrate output in their stools. Unabsorbed lactose that enters the colon undergoes bacterial fermentation (colonic salvage) to short-chain fatty acids, which creates an acidic environment favoring growth of acidophilic bacterial flora (Lactobacilli) and suppressing growth of more pathogenic organisms. This acidity also promotes water absorption and prevents osmotic diarrhea. Because of the relative abundance of glucoamylase to lactase in the premature infant's intestine, glucose polymers are digested and absorbed better than lactose.[1]

Newborns exhibit low pancreatic lipase concentrations and slower rates of bile acid synthesis, both of which are important for fat absorption. The rate of bile acid synthesis increases throughout gestation and with increasing postnatal age. The bile acid pool in a premature infant is one sixth that of an adult, whereas a term infant's is one half that of an adult. However, fat malabsorption is not a major problem in preterm or term infants because lingual and gastric lipase are present. Infants born earlier than 34 weeks gestation, however, may exhibit steatorrhea.

Intestinal length may also affect nutrient absorption. At birth, a term infant's small intestine is approximately 270 cm in length. During the third trimester, the intestinal length approximately doubles. Therefore, infants born prematurely will have less small intestine and, therefore, decreased surface area for absorption. Adult intestinal length of 4 to 5 meters is reached by about 4 years of age.

Maturation of the kidney is also important in nutrition, as it determines the ability of the kidney to excrete a solute load. Glomerular filtration begins around the ninth week of fetal life; however, kidney function does not appear to be necessary for normal intrauterine homeostasis, the placenta serving as the major excretory organ. After birth, the rate of glomerular filtration increases until growth stops, toward the end of the second decade of life. Even after correction for body surface area, the glomerular filtration rate of a child does not approximate adult values until the third year of life.

### Growth

Birth weight is determined primarily by maternal pre-pregnancy weight and pregnancy weight changes. The average birth weight for a term infant is approximately 3500 g (7 lb 8 oz). Premature infants are categorized based on birth weight: low birth weight (LBW) infants weigh less than 2500 g (5 lb 8 oz); very low birth weight (VLBW) infants weigh less than 1500 g (3 lb 4 oz); extremely low birth weight (ELBW) infants weigh less than 1000 g (2 lb 3 oz); and micropremies weigh less than 750 g (1 lb 10 oz).

Water weight loss (6% to 10% of body weight) occurs immediately after birth over a period of 1 to 2 weeks and is followed by an average weight gain of 1% to 2% of birth weight daily (25 to 35 g/day in term infants) during the first 4 months and 15 g/day over the next 8 months. Most term infants can be expected to double their birth weight by 4 months of age and triple it by 12 months of age. Premature infants may reach these milestones sooner. From 2 years to approximately 10 years of age, the growth rate is fairly constant at about 2.3 kg (5 lb) each year. Growth velocity increases and a major growth spurt occurs during adolescence. Height shows a growth pattern similar to that of weight; most infants increase their length by 50% in the first year, 100% in the first 4 years, and 300% by 13 years of age. Changes in body composition accompany height and weight changes. Most notably, total body water decreases as adipose tissue increases. Total body water accounts for approximately 90% of total body weight at 24 weeks gestation, 70% at term, and 60% by 1 year of age.

Normal values of weight, length/height, and head circumference (until 3 years of age) for infants and children are generally expressed in terms of percentile-for-age; the reference standards most commonly used are the CDC growth charts developed by the National Center for Health Statistics (NCHS). The 1977 growth charts were significantly revised in 2000 using an expanded data set more representative of the diverse ethnicity and combined breast- and bottle-feeding of infants in the United States.[3] Twenty age-, and gender-specific charts can be downloaded free of charge at www.cdc.gov/growthcharts (accessed November 6, 2005). The infant charts are intended for use in term infants. Once premature infants reach 40 weeks gestational age, their growth parameters can be plotted on these charts, but their age must be corrected for gestational age (i.e., chronological age in weeks minus number of weeks premature) until 24 months of age. Charts for premature infants less than 40 weeks gestation and children with specific conditions (e.g., Down syndrome, cerebral palsy, Turner syndrome) are available and should be used when appropriate. Most infants' growth parameters will fall between the 3rd and 97th percentiles on the gender-specific weight-for-age, length/height-for-age, weight-for-length, and head circumference-for-age charts. Most children grow along a percentile established shortly after birth, but spurts and plateaus are common. Failure-to-thrive is defined as a fall of two or more growth percentiles from a previously established percentile in 6 months or less. If growth is not progressing as expected, particularly in the first year of life when growth should be rapid, the infant's diet and other potential contributory factors (e.g., environment, diseases, syndromes) should be evaluated. Satisfactory growth, therefore, is the most sensitive indicator of whether energy needs are being met.

For children over 2 years of age, body mass index (BMI)-for-age charts can be useful in assessing obesity risk. BMI is calculated as weight in kilograms divided by height in meters squared. Per CDC guidelines, a child with a BMI

**TABLE 26-1 Dietary Reference Intakes for Full-term Infants and Children*†**

| Nutrient | 0-6 Months | 7-12 Months | 1-3 Years | 4-8 Years | 9-13 Years |
|---|---|---|---|---|---|
| Energy‡ (kcal/day) | M: 570<br>F: 520 | M: 743<br>F: 676 | M: 1046<br>F: 992 | M: 1742<br>F: 1642 | M: 2279<br>F: 2071 |
| Protein (g/kg/day) | 1.52 | 1.5 | 1.1 | 0.95 | 0.95 |
| Carbohydrate (g/day) | 60 | 95 | 130§ | 130§ | 130§ |
| Water (L/day)‖ | 0.7 | 0.8 | 1.3 | 1.7 | M: 24<br>F: 21 |
| Fat (g/day) | 31 | 30 | ND | ND | ND |
| α-Linolenic acid (g/day) | 0.5 | 0.5 | 0.7 | 0.9 | M: 12<br>F: 10 |
| Linoleic acid (g/day) | 4.4 | 4.6 | 7 | 10 | M: 12<br>F: 10 |
| Fiber (g/day) | ND | ND | 19 | 25 | M: 31<br>F: 26 |

Key: AI, Adequate Intake; DRI, Dietary Reference Intakes; F, female; M, male; ND, not determined; RDA, Recommended Dietary Intakes.

* Expressed as AIs unless otherwise noted.

† DRIs have not been established for premature infants.

‡ Estimated energy requirement, includes needs associated with growth (i.e., energy deposition). Reference age and weight are 0 to 6 months—3 months, 6 kg; 7 to 12 months—9 months, 9 kg; 1 to 3 years—24 months, 12 kg; 4 to 8 years—6 years, 20 kg; and 9 to 13 years—11 years, 36 kg for males, 37 kg for females.

§ Expressed as RDA.

‖ Water from all sources including foods, formula, and human milk.

*Source:* Reference 4.

greater than the 85th percentile on the gender-specific, BMI-for-age NCHS chart is considered at risk of overweight, and a child with a BMI greater than the 95th percentile is overweight. Nearly 25% of all children in the United States now fall into the "at risk for overweight" category. A BMI less than the 5th percentile is indicative of underweight. However, the clinician should realize that because of the way the growth charts were developed, 5% of normally growing and healthy children will fall either below the 5th or above the 95th percentile on the weight-for-age or height-for-age charts. These children should not be branded as "malnourished" or "obese."

## Infant Nutritional Standards

Acceptable growth is achievable only with adequate intake, absorption, and utilization of energy, protein, carbohydrates, minerals, and vitamins. The Food and Nutrition Board of the National Research Council has established Dietary Reference Intakes (DRIs) as reference values for nutrient intake sufficiency and safety. The DRIs for micronutrients are discussed in detail in Chapter 23, and tables in that chapter list the current established Recommended Dietary Allowances (RDAs) and Adequate Intakes (AIs) for healthy infants and children. Table 26-1 provides the DRIs for macronutrients for healthy infants and children.[4] Children with various diseases and syndromes may have different needs. One example is the need for "catch-up" calories in infants and children recovering from failure-to-thrive. Calorie requirements for catch-up growth are often 1.5 times or more those of age-matched peers depending on the degree of catch-up growth needed.

An amendment to the Federal Food, Drug, and Cosmetic Act (Infant Formula Act of 1980; amended 1986) gives the Food and Drug Administration (FDA) the authority to revise nutrient levels for infant formulas, establish quality control, and require adequate labeling. FDA sets specifications for minimum amounts of 29 nutrients and maximum amounts of nine of those nutrients. All formulas marketed in the United States must meet these requirements. Parents should be cautioned against using any infant formula not manufactured in the United States. A recent FDA alert warned of the dangers of using an infant formula from China, Guan Wei Yuan, sold in New York, whose contents were found to fall well below FDA standards. Formulas granted exemption from FDA-established nutrient specifications must be labeled for use by infants who have inborn errors of metabolism, had a low birth weight, or otherwise have unusual medical or dietary problems. These formulas require a prescription for use and cannot be sold retail. They can be ordered for patients through a pharmacy or directly from the company. A list of exempt formulas can be obtained at www.cfsan.fda.gov/~dms/inf-exmp.html (accessed November 6, 2005).

Energy requirements vary with age and clinical condition. Total energy expenditure is a combination of basal energy needs, the energy required to digest food (thermic effect of feeding, also called "specific dynamic action of food" in some references), thermoregulation, and activity. Estimates of energy requirements for infants and children are based on meeting total energy expenditure plus promoting growth. The infant's energy requirement is higher in relation to body mass than an adult or older child because of the rapid growth experienced during infancy. Estimated energy requirements for term infants and children are shown in Table 26-1. Although no RDA has been established, premature infants generally require 120 to 150 kcal/kg/day for adequate growth.

## Components of a Healthy Diet

Infants require the same dietary components as adults: fluid, carbohydrates, proteins, fats, and micronutrients. However, the desired proportion of these components in the infant diet differs.

### *Fluid*

Water is an important part of an infant's diet because it makes up a larger proportion of the infant's body weight than in older children or adults. The Holliday-Segar method is most often used to estimate maintenance water needs: 100 mL/kg/day for the first 10 kg of body weight plus 50 mL/kg/day for each kilogram between 10 and 20 kg and 20 mL/kg/day for each kilogram over 20 kg. Body surface area may also be used to estimate daily fluid requirements; fluid requirements are approximately 1500 mL/m$^2$/day. Adequate water intake in the first 6 months of life can be derived from human milk or formula. Both contain sufficient amounts of water that the normal, healthy infant does not need supplemental water. From 6 to 12 months of age, when solid foods are introduced, water intake remains high because most infant foods contain at least 60% to 70% more water than other foods, and formula or human milk intake should still be high.

Renal excretion, evaporation from the skin and lungs, and, to a lesser extent, feces are the major routes of fluid loss. Increases in water loss caused by diarrhea, fever, or unusually rapid breathing, particularly in concert with decreased water intake, may result in significant dehydration and electrolyte imbalance and must be offset by fluid intake in excess of maintenance needs.

Carbohydrates

An AI for carbohydrates has been established for infants (Table 26-1). Under normal circumstances, an infant can efficiently use 40% to 50% of total calories from a carbohydrate source. Carbohydrate intake should be balanced with adequate fat intake to allow proper neurologic development. A carbohydrate-free diet is not desirable because it leads to metabolic modifications favoring fatty acid breakdown, dehydration, and tissue protein and cation loss. Lactose, the primary carbohydrate source in human milk and most milk-based formulas, is hydrolyzed to its monosaccharide components, glucose and galactose, by gastric acid and lactase. Congenital lactase deficiency is a rare type of lactose intolerance that results from an inborn error of metabolism. Infants born prematurely, prior to the maturation of significant lactase activity (before approximately 36 weeks gestation), are relatively lactase deficient. Secondary lactase deficiency is a temporary reduction in intestinal lactase caused by gastroenteritis or significant malnutrition. Because of low lactase activity, infants with congenital lactase deficiency, premature infants, and infants recovering from diarrhea or severe malnutrition may be unable to completely metabolize the quantity of lactose found in human milk or milk-based infant formulas and may develop lactose intolerance resulting in diarrhea, abdominal pain or distention, bloating, gas, and cramping.

Fiber intake is of considerable interest because, in adults, high-fiber diets have been associated with the prevention of diverticular disease, colon cancer, and coronary heart disease. The American Health Foundation has recommended a daily fiber intake calculated by using the equation: fiber (grams/day) = age (in years) plus 5. Age plus 10 g/day is also felt to be a safe intake.[5] An AI for fiber for infants 0 to 12 months of age has not been established. Infants rarely require fiber during the first year of life to maintain normal bowel function. However, from age 6 to 12 months, whole cereals, green vegetables, and legumes provide a source of fiber in the infant's diet. The fiber AI for older children is shown in Table 26-1. Adult values are reached by the teens.

### *Protein and Amino Acids*

The most recent revision of the DRIs established new AIs for protein in term infants and children (Table 26-1).[4] Total body protein increases by an average of 3.5 g/day in the first 4 months of life and by 3.1 g/day over the next 8 months, representing an overall increase in body protein composition from 11% to 15% of total body weight.

The protein's amino acid composition (i.e., chemical value) is also important. Amino acids are classified as essential, nonessential, or conditionally essential. Isoleucine, leucine, lysine, methionine, phenylalanine, threonine, tryptophan, and valine are considered essential amino acids because the human body cannot synthesize them from precursors. Histidine, tyrosine, cysteine, and taurine are considered conditionally essential amino acids during infancy because immature biochemical pathways for synthesis or interconversion prevent adequate synthesis for normal growth and development.

Taurine is an especially important amino acid in infancy. Quantities in human milk are high, but amounts found in unsupplemented cow milk– and soy protein–based formulas are low. Taurine is not an energy source nor is it used for protein synthesis, but it serves as a cell membrane protector by attenuating toxic substances (e.g., oxidants, secondary bile acids, and excess retinoids) and acting as an osmoregulator. Taurine deficiency can result in retinal dysfunction, slow development of auditory brain stem–evoked response in preterm infants, and poor fat absorption in preterm infants and children with cystic fibrosis. These conditions can be improved with taurine supplements. Although disagreement still exists as to the necessity of taurine supplementation, taurine is now added to infant formulas to provide the same margin of physiologic safety that is provided by human milk.[6]

Despite similar amino acid densities and milk intakes, serum concentrations of some amino acids seen in formula–fed infants tend to exceed those measured in human milk–fed infants; however, growth of these infants is equivalent. Although the protein content of human milk adjusts to a growing infant's needs, the high protein needs of preterm infants are not completely met by early human milk. Fortification is required to achieve reasonable amino acid profiles and for the infant to meet expected growth rates. In evaluating the adequacy of an infant's protein intake, one must consider not only the absolute amount of protein ingested but also the growth rate, the quantity of nonprotein calories and other nutrients necessary for protein synthesis, and the quality of the protein itself. Some authors have suggested that amino acid and protein requirements are more meaningful when expressed in terms of calorie intake; therefore, requirements or supplementation levels may be reported as grams of protein per 100 kcal.

### Fat and Essential Fatty Acids

Fat is the most calorically dense component in the diet, providing 9 kcal/g compared with 4 kcal/g for both protein and carbohydrates. Fat accounts for approximately 50% of the nonprotein energy in both human milk and infant formula. Although concern exists that adult dietary fat intake and infant feeding practices are risk factors for obesity and others diseases (e.g., diabetes, cardiovascular disease) in adulthood, AAP recommends that children younger than 2 years of age (the time of most rapid growth and development requiring high-energy intakes) not receive a fat- or cholesterol-restricted diet because of the need for adequate fatty acid intake for normal neurologic development and adequate calories for growth.[7,8] Between 2 and 5 years of age, children should be encouraged to adopt a diet that contains 20% to 30% of total calories from fat with less than 10% of calories from saturated fats.[7]

The diet must also contain small amounts of the essential polyunsaturated fatty acids (PUFAs), linoleic and α-linolenic acid. Linoleic acid deficiency is rare in the United States and manifests as increased metabolic rate, hair loss, dry, flaky skin, and impaired wound healing. Because of substantial fat stores, clinical manifestations of essential fatty acid deficiency are generally delayed for months in older children and adults; however, rapid onset (within days to weeks) may occur in premature infants with inadequate linoleic acid in their diets. Linoleic acid represents the bulk of PUFAs in infant formulas. Generally, an intake of linoleic acid equal to 1% to 2% of total dietary calories is adequate to prevent biochemical and clinical evidence of deficiency; 3% to 7% is the amount found in human milk. The AI for the essential PUFAs is shown in Table 26-1.

A recent change in most infant formulas was the addition of docosahexanoic acid (DHA) and arachidonic acid (ARA). These PUFAs, which are abundant in human milk but not in cow milk, are not considered essential but thought to provide extra benefit. DHA is known to be important in both brain and eye development. The role of ARA is less clear. AAP has not taken an official stand on whether or not infant formulas should be supplemented with DHA and ARA. Some studies have shown benefits to an infant's visual function, cognitive and behavioral development, and growth with DHA and ARA supplementation.[9-15] However, other studies have shown no differences in supplemented versus nonsupplemented infants.[16,17] No adverse effects have been noted in infants receiving DHA- and AHA-supplemented formulas. FDA has issued a "generally recognized as safe" (GRAS) notification to Martek Biosciences Corporation for its patented plant-based fatty acid blends, DHASCO and ARASCO, which are currently used to supplement infant formulas. Over 60 countries permit the addition of fatty acids to infant formula. There is also growing evidence that maternal diet can affect fatty acid concentrations in the infant both in utero and during lactation for human milk–fed infants. Expecta LIPIL, softgel capsules that contain 200 mg DHA, have recently been marketed as a supplement for pregnant and lactating women to increase maternal dietary DHA, and thus increase DHA concentrations in their infants. More information is needed before this therapy is routinely recommended.

### Micronutrients

DRIs for term infants (given as AIs if defined, or as RDAs if AIs are not yet defined) for vitamins and minerals, including trace elements, are shown in tables in Chapter 23. Precise needs are difficult to define and depend on energy, protein, and fat intakes as well as absorption and nutrient stores. Infant formulas are supplemented with adequate amounts of vitamins and minerals to meet the needs of most term and premature infants. As with protein, human milk must be fortified to meet the micronutrient needs of most premature infants. Appropriate supplementation is included later in this chapter with the discussion of specific milks and formulas.

## Infant Food Sources

Human and cow milk–based formulas are the primary food sources for most infants in the United States. Soy protein–based formulas and goat milk are alternative food sources. A variety of formulas are available to feed infants with special nutritional needs including those unable to consume a regular oral diet, those with inborn errors of metabolism, and those with various malabsorptive conditions. Most infants and children receive either human milk or an enteral formula orally; however, some children will receive these through feeding tubes such as naso- or orogastric, gastrostomy, or jejunostomy tubes. A discussion of these feeding techniques is beyond the scope of this chapter.

### Human Milk

Breast-feeding initiation rates have increased steadily since 1990 with the rate at hospital discharge increasing from a low of 24.7% in 1971 to 70% in 2001. At 6 months of age, however, the rate of any breast-feeding is only 33%, not much higher than the 1971 rate of 29.5%. Infants of black women are less likely than those of white or Hispanic women to be breast-fed. In 2001, approximately 53% of black women were breast-feeding at hospital discharge and 22% when their infants were 6 months of age compared with 72% and 34% for white women and 73% and 33% for Hispanic women, respectively, at hospital discharge and 6 months of age. At 1 year of age, rates were still different, though less so, with only 18% of white and Hispanic women compared with 12% of black women still breast-feeding at that time.[18,19] Poor and poorly educated women are also less likely to breast-feed their infants.

Because breast-feeding is a major public health concern, breast-feeding goals were included in *Healthy People 2000: National Health Promotion and Disease Prevention Objectives,* the national plan to improve the health of the American people.[20] One objective of *Healthy People 2000* was to have 75% of all infants in the United States breast-fed at birth, with 50% receiving human milk at 6 months of age. This objective was not reached by 2000, and it was included, along with the objective of having 25% of infants breast-fed at 1 year of age, in *Healthy People 2010*.[21] However, from 1994 to 1996, only 13.7% ($5.6 million) of the research grants awarded in areas related to breast-feeding went to projects with either a direct or indirect impact on achieving these goals.[22] AAP has recently updated its policy statement on breast-feeding to include recommendations to increase breast-feeding and to address reasons women were not breast-feeding (e.g., insufficient prenatal breast-feeding education, hospital policies disruptive to breast-feeding, early hospital discharge, physician apathy and misinformation, lack of broad societal support, media portrayal of bottle-feeding as the norm, and promotion of formula through hospital discharge packs, coupons, and television and magazine advertising).[19]

Breast-feeding not only offers an optimal source of nutrition for the infant, it provides other benefits, such as improved mother-child bonding. There are advantages to the infant's general health, growth, and development. Strong evidence indicates that human milk decreases the incidence and/or severity of various infections (e.g., diarrhea, respiratory tract infections, otitis media, bacteremia, bacterial meningitis, necrotizing enterocolitis, urinary tract infections, and late-onset sepsis) in premature infants.[19] Other proposed benefits of human milk include decreased rates of sudden infant death syndrome, types 1 and 2 diabetes mellitus, lymphoma, leukemia, Hodgkin disease, overweight, obesity, hypercholesterolemia, and asthma. Breast-feeding has also been associated with slightly enhanced performance on tests of cognitive development; however, the effect of genetic and socioenvironmental factors on intelligence is hard to measure separately from breast-feeding.[19,23]

Besides enhanced mother-child bonding, maternal benefits of breast-feeding include decreased postpartum bleeding, more rapid uterine involution, decreased menstrual blood loss, increased spacing between children, earlier return to pre-pregnancy weight, decreased risk of breast and ovarian cancer, and decreased hip fracture and osteoporosis in the postmenopausal period.

A potential $3.6 billion decrease in annual health care costs has been estimated with improved rates of breast-feeding.[19] An economic analysis of estimated direct health care costs for diarrhea, lower respiratory tract infections, and otitis media in the first year of life found that costs for infants never breast-fed were $300 more than for infants exclusively breast-fed for at least 3 months.[24]

Questions remain about the apparent protective effects of breast-feeding. What is the duration of protection after breast-feeding is discontinued? What influence does maternal age have on the protective effect? How great is the interactive effect of social and demographic variables? How does the addition of solid foods to the diet of a human milk–fed infant influence the protective effect? What consequence does partial formula-feeding have on the protective effect of human milk–feeding? Better-designed studies are needed to answer these questions.

There are very few contraindications to human milk. In developed countries, such as the United States, one reason for women not breast-feeding is the maternal diagnosis of human immunodeficiency virus (HIV) infection, which can be transmitted via human milk. Women with HIV in underdeveloped countries, however, are encouraged to breast-feed because the risk of infant morbidity and mortality with formula use (from inadequate sanitation, refrigeration, and illiteracy) is greater than the risk of HIV transmission.[19] Other reasons women in developed countries may not be able to breast-feed either temporarily or permanently are classic galactosemia; active, untreated tuberculosis; human T-cell lymphotropic virus types I or II; herpes simplex lesion on the breast (may use other breast); and the use of contraindicated drugs (Table 26-2). Several excellent texts provide information regarding the use of drugs during lactation (and pregnancy).[25,26]

In the United States and other countries, human milk donor banks have been established. In 1999, approximately 322,700 oz of human milk were processed and distributed by the seven member banks of the Human Milk Banking Association of North America (NMBANA).[27] In 2002, 300 infants and young children and 15 adults received donor human milk from the seven member banks (six in the United States, one in Canada).[28] In the early 1980s, there were 30 active milk banks in the United States; however, currently there are nine, with three in various stages of development. These banks take human milk donations from carefully screened, unpaid donors. The milk undergoes Holder pasteurization to eliminate potential viral and bacterial contaminants while maintaining most of the milk's unique immunologic factors. It has been estimated that about 50% of the immunoglobulin A (IgA) is lost in processing; however, because cow milk contains no IgA, infants who receive donor human milk still benefit from its presence. Donor human milk has been used for many sick and premature infants in neonatal intensive care units (NICUs) across the United States. It has also been used for older children and adults with a variety of conditions including short bowel syndrome, metabolic disorders, severe food allergies, cancer, and immune deficiency disorders. Adopted infants with no medical problems have also received donor human milk. More information about donor human milk banks including how to be a donor and receive donor human milk can be obtained at HMBANA's Web site at www.hmbana.org (accessed November 6, 2005).

**TABLE 26-2 Selected Drugs Contraindicated or to Be Used Cautiously While Breast-feeding**

| Prescription Drugs | Drugs of Abuse | Radiopharmaceuticals (Time to Wait After Exposure) |
|---|---|---|
| **Contraindicated Drugs** | | |
| Cyclophosphamide | Amphetamine | Copper 64 (50 hours) |
| Cyclosporine | Cocaine | Gallium 67 (2 weeks) |
| Doxorubicin | Heroin | Indium 111 (20 hours) |
| Leflunomide | Marijuana | Iodine 123 (36 hours) |
| Methotrexate | Phencyclidine | Iodine 125 (12 days) |
| | | Iodine 131 (2-14 days) |
| | | Radioactive sodium (96 hours) |
| | | Technetium 99m (15 hours to 3 days) |
| **Drugs to Be Used Cautiously Owing to Significant Potential Adverse Effects** | | |
| Acebutolol | Bromocriptine | Phenindione |
| 5-Aminosalicylic acid | Clemastine | Phenobarbital |
| Atenolol | Ergotamine | Primidone |
| Aspirin | Lithium | Sulfasalazine |

*Source:* Reference 19 and American Academy of Pediatrics, Committee on Drugs. Transfer of drugs and other chemicals into human milk. *Pediatrics.* 2001;108:776-89.

### *Cow Milk*

Cow milk is the primary nutrient source for commercially prepared milk-based infant formulas. Both human and cow milk contain more than 200 ingredients in the fat- and water-soluble fractions. Estimates of the nutrients contained in pooled mature human milk and cow milk are listed in Table 26-3.

### *Whole Cow Milk*

Whole cow milk is not suitable for providing nutrition to infants less than 1 year of age. Because of its low concentration of and poor bioavailability of iron, whole cow milk has been associated with iron-deficiency anemia.[29,30] Sensitivity to dietary proteins, most commonly cow or soy milk proteins, can manifest as occult GI bleeding, further increasing the risk of anemia. In the past decade, convincing evidence has accumulated to indicate that iron deficiency impairs psychomotor development and cognitive function in infants, even with relatively mild anemia. Milk-protein intolerance and/or allergy can also result in rash, wheezing, diarrhea, vomiting, colic, and anaphylaxis when whole cow milk is used. When whole cow milk is fed with solid food, infants receive unnecessarily high intakes of protein and electrolytes, resulting in a high renal solute load (RSL). The implications of a high RSL will be discussed later in this chapter. The current position of AAP's Committee on Nutrition (CON) is that iron-fortified infant formula is the only acceptable alternative to human milk. The use of whole cow milk is not recommended during the first year of life.[29]

### *Reduced-fat Cow Milk*

Reduced-fat cow milk, such as skim milk (0.1% fat), low-fat milk (1% fat), and reduced-fat milk (2% fat), has been advocated to prevent obesity and atherosclerosis as part of a "healthy diet." However, when the low-fat diet recommended for adults is imposed on children younger than 2 years, it puts them at risk for failure-to-thrive and impaired neurologic development. Infants who receive a major percentage of their caloric intake from reduced-fat milk may receive an exceedingly high protein intake and an inadequate intake of essential fatty acids. The maximum protein concentration allowed by the FDA in infant formulas is 4.5 g/100 kcal, but skim milk provides approximately 8 to 10 g/100 kcal, and 2% milk provides 7 to 10 g/100 kcal. Thus, using reduced-fat milk for infant nutrition provides an unbalanced percentage of calories supplied from protein, fat, and carbohydrates.

It is also important to recognize that, per unit volume, skim milk has a slightly higher RSL than does whole cow milk (Table 26-4). The solute concentration is further increased by water loss during processing. Reduced-fat milk is not recommended during episodes of diarrhea because of the possibility of hypertonic dehydration. As stated previously, AAP does not recommend the use of low-fat diets during the first 2 years of life.

### *Evaporated Milk*

Between 1930 and 1960, evaporated milk was frequently used in preparing infant formula, but by 1978 few infants received evaporated milk formulas. Evaporated milk is a sterile, convenient source of cow milk that has standardized concentrations of protein, fat, and carbohydrate.

**TABLE 26-3 Average Composition of Mature Human Milk and Whole Cow Milk**

| Component | Human Milk | Cow Milk |
|---|---|---|
| Water (mL/100 mL) | 87.1 | 87.2 |
| Energy | | |
| (kcal/100 mL) | 69 | 66 |
| (kcal/oz) | 20 | 19 |
| Protein (g/100 mL) | 0.9 | 3.3 |
| Whey:casein ratio | 60:40 | 18:82 |
| α-Lactalbumin (g/100 mL) | 0.3 | 0.1 |
| α-Lactoglobulin (g/100 mL) | — | 0.4 |
| Lactoferrin (g/100 mL) | 0.2 | trace |
| Secretory IgA (g/100 mL) | 0.1 | trace |
| Albumin (g/100 mL) | 0.04 | 0.04 |
| Fat (g/100 mL) | 3.9 | 3.4 |
| Carbohydrate (g/100 mL) | 6.7* | 4.8† |
| **Minerals** | | |
| Calcium (mg/L) | 200-250 | 1230 |
| Phosphorus (mg/L) | 120-140 | 960 |
| Calcium: phosphorus ratio | 2:1 | 1.3:1 |
| Sodium (mg/L) | 120-250 | 500 |
| Potassium (mg/L) | 400-550 | 1560 |
| Chloride (mg/L) | 400-450 | 1028-1060 |
| Magnesium (mg/L) | 30-35 | 120 |
| Sulfur (mg/L) | 140 | 300 |
| **Vitamins** | | |
| Vitamin A (IU/L) | 1898 | 1025 |
| Thiamin (μg/L) | 200 | 370 |
| Riboflavin (μg/L) | 400-600 | 1700 |
| Niacin (mg/L) | 1.8-6 | 0.9 |
| Pyridoxine (mg/L) | 0.09-0.31 | 0.46 |
| Pantothenate (mg/L) | 2-2.5 | 3.6 |
| Folic acid (μg/L) | 80-140 | 68 |
| Biotin (μg/L) | 5-9 | 35 |
| Vitamin $B_{12}$ (μg/L) | 0.5-1 | 4 |
| Vitamin C (mg/L) | 100 | 17 |
| Vitamin D (μg/L) | 0.33 | 14 |
| Vitamin E (IU/L) | 3-8 | 0.4 |
| Vitamin K (μg/L) | 2-3 | 17 |
| **Trace Minerals** | | |
| Chromium (μg/L) | 45-55 | 20 |
| Manganese (μg/L) | 3 | 20-40 |
| Copper (mg/L) | 0.2-0.4 | 110 |
| Zinc (mg/L) | 1-3 | 3-5 |
| Iodine (μg/L) | 150 | 80 |
| Selenium (μg/L) | 7-33 | 5-50 |
| Iron (mg/L) | trace | trace |

* As lactose, glucose, oligosaccharides.

† As lactose.

*Sources:* Picciano MF. Representative values for constituents of human milk. In: Schanler RJ, ed. Breastfeeding 2001, Part 1: The evidence for breastfeeding. *Ped Clin N Amer.* 2001:48:263-4; Committee on Nutrition, American Academy of Pediatrics. Appendix A. In: Kleinman RE, ed. *Pediatric Nutrition Handbook.* 4th ed. Elk Grove Village, Ill: American Academy of Pediatrics; 1998, 631-2; and reference 19.

**TABLE 26-4 Potential Renal Solute Loads (PRSLs) of Selected Milks and Infant Formulas**

| | PRSL | |
|---|---|---|
| | mOsm/L | mOsm/100 kcal |
| Human milk | 93 | 14 |
| Milk–based formula | 135 | 20 |
| Soy protein–based formula | 160 | 24 |
| Whole cow milk | 308 | 46 |
| Skim cow milk | 326 | 93 |
| FDA upper limit | 277 | 41 |

When ingested, evaporated milk produces a smaller, softer curd than that formed from boiled whole cow milk. Vitamin D is typically added to evaporated milk during processing, but evaporated milk formulas fail to meet vitamin E recommendations for premature infants, and ascorbic acid and essential fatty acid requirements for full-term infants. Therefore, evaporated milk is not recommended for infant feeding.

### *Goat Milk*

While goat milk is the primary milk source for more than 50% of the world's population, it is used rarely in the United States for infants intolerant to cow milk. Goat milk is commercially available in powdered and evaporated forms. It contains primarily medium- and short-chain fatty acids and thus the fat is more readily digested than the fat in cow milk. Unfortified goat milk is deficient in folate and is low in iron and vitamin D and is, therefore, not recommended during infancy. The evaporated form of Meyenberg goat milk, however, is supplemented with vitamin D and folic acid. Powdered Meyenberg goat milk is supplemented with folic acid only and is recommended only for children older than 1 year. Because the powder formulation is not a complete formula for infants, if it is used in infants, vitamin supplementation is required.

### Commercial Infant Formulas

When provision of human milk to an infant is not possible or not desired by the mother, then commercially supplied infant formulas are an acceptable alternative (Table 26-5). Differences in palatability, digestibility, sources of nutrients, convenience of administration, and cost among these formulas allow for individualization to the infant's special nutrient needs and the family's resources.

#### Formula Properties

An infant formula must be pathogen-free and its constituents must meet certain concentrations to ensure optimum nutrition. Guidelines have been established to ensure safety and efficacy of infant formulas.

*Microbiologic Safety* Guidelines of the Infant Formula Council (a voluntary, nonprofit trade association composed of companies that manufacture and market infant formulas) require liquid formulations to be free of all viable pathogens, their spores, and other organisms that may cause product degradation. To ensure that this requirement is met, manufacturers usually sterilize liquid formulas using heat treatment. Samples of the sterilized formulas are incubated and analyzed for guideline compliance. Quality control measures help to ensure the production of a sterile product that is free of microbes as long as the container remains intact. Powdered formulas, however, are not required or guaranteed to be sterile. Heat sterilization of the powder would destroy some of the nutrients. Manufacturers do culture powdered formulas to ensure that coliforms and other pathogens are absent and that contamination with other microorganisms is below the acceptable government standards. The heating required during the final preparation of the infant formula (as indicated on label directions) destroys most microorganisms. If microbiologic contamination occurs, the infant ingesting such a formula could develop diarrhea with subsequent fluid and electrolyte losses. Recently, FDA issued an alert after the death of an infant in an NICU because of contamination of powdered formula with *Enterobacter sakazakii* at the manufacturing site.[31]

Risk for infection after exposure to contaminated formulas likely depends on a number of factors including immune status. For this reason, to minimize risk for premature infants, ready-to-feed or liquid concentrates are recommended unless there is no suitable alternative to a powdered formula. The initial FDA response to the *Enterobacter* contamination incident recommended reconstituting powdered formulas with boiling water; however, this recommendation was withdrawn. Use of boiling water results in loss of some nutrients, including vitamins and protein, causes the formula to clump, may not kill bacteria that are present, and is potentially dangerous for those preparing the formula.[32] These recommendations were meant to apply only to infants in NICUs; however, these infants may be discharged early and need to be cared for at home. It is best to avoid using powdered formulas for feeding premature or immunocompromised infants if at all possible; however, there is currently no alternative to the powdered, human milk fortifiers discussed later in this chapter.

*Physical Characteristics* Infant formulas are emulsions of edible oils in aqueous solutions, but fat separation rarely occurs. If it does, shaking the container will usually redisperse the fat. Redispersion may not happen if stabilizers are lacking or if the formula was stored beyond its shelf life. Liquid infant formulas may contain thickening agents, stabilizers, and emulsifiers to provide uniform consistency and prolong stability. Protein agglomeration may occur, however, if storage time is excessive. This agglomeration ranges from a slight, grainy development through increased viscosity and gel formation to eventual protein precipitation. Agglomeration and separation do not affect a formula's safety or nutritional value; however, the formula's appearance may deter caregivers from using it.

*Caloric Density* The standard caloric density for infant formulas is 20 kcal/oz or 67 kcal/100 mL, which mimics the average caloric density of human milk. A healthy, term infant should have no difficulty in consuming enough formula to meet both calorie and fluid needs with this caloric density. Premature, malnourished, or severely ill infants who require more calories (130 to 150 kcal/kg/day) or infants who are volume restricted may require formulas with higher caloric densities (e.g., 22, 24, or 27 kcal/oz or higher) to meet their caloric needs. Infant formulas with caloric densities significantly lower or higher than 20 kcal/oz are regarded as therapeutic formulas to be used in managing special clinical conditions (Tables 26-5 and 26-6). These formulas should be used only under close medical supervision.

*Osmolarity and Osmolality* The osmolarity of an infant formula may be expressed as the concentration of solute per unit of total volume of solution or as the number of milliosmoles of solute per liter of solution (mOsm/L). The osmolarity of human milk is approximately 273 mOsm/L. AAP/CON recommends that formulas for infants have osmolarities no higher than 400 mOsm/L; formulas with higher osmolarities should have a warning statement on the label. Infant formulas with 20 or 24 kcal/oz that are routinely used to feed premature infants have osmolarities less than or equal to 300 mOsm/L and pose no apparent increased risk of GI mucosal injury.

Osmolality may be expressed as the number of milliosmoles of solute per kilogram of solvent (mOsm/kg). Osmolality is directly related to the concentration of

**TABLE 26-5 Selected Formulas for Infants and Children**

| Trade Name [Form] (Mfr) | Kcal* (per oz) | Protein* (g/L) (C:W ratio) | Carbohydrate* (g/L) | Fat* (g/L) | MCTs (% fat kcal) | Iron *† (mg/L) |
|---|---|---|---|---|---|---|
| **Infant Formulas** | | | | | | |
| ***Milk-based Formulas*** | | | | | | |
| Nestlé Good Start Supreme<br>Nestlé Good Start Supreme DHA&ARA [C,P,R] (Nes) | 20 | 14.7 (0:100) | 75 | 34.2 | — | 10.1 |
| Nestlé Good Start Essentials [C,P,R] (Nes) | 20 | 14.7 (60:40) | 75 | 34.2 | — | 10.1 |
| Enfamil LIPIL<br>Enfamil LIPIL with Iron<br>Enfamil with Iron<br>Enfamil LIPIL Low Iron [C,P,R] (MJ) | 20 | 14 (40:60) | 72.7 | 35.3 | — | 12.2 (4.7) |
| Enfamil 24 [R] (MJ) | 24 | 17.4 (40:60) | 88 | 43 | — | 14.6 (5.7) |
| Similac Advance with Iron<br>Similac with Iron<br>Similac Low Iron [C,P,R] (Ro) | 20 | 14 (52:48) | 73 | 36.5 | — | 12.2 (4.7) |
| Store Brand Milk-based Formula [C,P,R] (Wy) | 20 | 15 (40:60) | 72 | 36 | — | 12 |
| ***Soy Protein–based Therapeutic Formulas*** | | | | | | |
| Nestlé Good Start Supreme Soy DHA & ARA [C,P,R] (Nes) | 20 | 16.8 | 75 | 34.2 | — | 10.1 |
| Similac Isomil [C,P,R] (Ro)<br>Similac Isomil Advance [P,R] (Ro) | 20 | 16.6 | 69.7 | 36.9 | — | 12.2 |
| Similac Isomil DF [R] (Ro) | 20 | 18 | 68.3<br>(6 g fiber) | 36.9 | — | 12.2 |
| Enfamil ProSobee LIPIL [C,P,R] (MJ) | 20 | 16.7 | 70.7 | 35.3 | — | 12 |
| Store Brand Soy Infant Formula [C,P,R] (Wy) | 20 | 18 | 69 | 36 | — | 12 |
| ***Other Therapeutic Infant Formulas*** | | | | | | |
| Enfamil A.R. LIPIL [P,R] (MJ) | 20 | 16.7 (82:18) | 73.3 | 34 | — | 12 |
| Enfamil Lactofree LIPIL [C,P,R] (MJ) | 20 | 14 (82:18) | 72.7 | 35.3 | — | 12 |
| Similac Lactose Free Advance [C,P,R] (Ro) | 20 | 14.5 (18:82) | 72.4 | 36.5 | — | 12.2 |
| Similac PM 60/40* [P] (Ro) | 20 | 15 (40:60) | 69 | 37.8 | — | 4.7 |
| Enfamil Nutramigen LIPIL [C,P,R] (MJ) | 20 | 18.7 | 68.7 | 35.3 | — | 12 |
| Enfamil Pregestimil [P,R] (MJ) | 20 | 18.7 | 68 | 37.3 | 55 | 12.5 |
| Enfamil Pregestimil [R] (MJ) | 24 | 22.2 | 81 | 44.4 | 55 | 14.9 |
| Similac Alimentum Advance [R, P] (Ro) | 20 | 18.6 | 69 | 37.5 | 33 | 12.2 |
| Neocate [P] (SHS) | 20 | 20.7 | 78 | 30 | 5 | 12.3 |
| Portagen [P] (MJ) | 20 | 25.2 | 65.9 | 34 | 87 | 13.3 |
| RCF‡ [C] (Ro) | 20 | 20 | 68.3 | 36.1 | — | 12.2 |
| Product 3232A [P] (MJ) | 12.7 | 18.9 | 91 | 28 | 85 | 12.5 |
| Product 3232A‡ [P] (MJ) | 20 | 18.9 | 91 | 28 | 85 | 12.5 |
| ***Formulas for Premature Infants: Initial Feeding*** | | | | | | |
| Enfamil Premature LIPIL Iron Fortified/<br>Enfamil Premature LIPIL Low Iron [R] (MJ) | 20 | 20 | 73.3 | 34 | 40 | 12 (3.3) |
| Enfamil Premature LIPIL Iron Fortified/<br>Enfamil Premature LIPIL Low Iron [R] (MJ) | 24 | 23.8 | 87.3 | 40.5 | 40 | 14.3 (4) |
| Similac Special Care Advance 20<br>Similac Special Care Advance 20 with Iron [R] (Ro) | 20 | 20.3 | 69.7 | 36.7 | 50 | 12.2 (2.5) |
| Similac Special Care Advance 24<br>Similac Special Care Advance 24 with Iron [R] (Ro) | 24 | 24.4 | 83.6 | 44.1 | 50 | 14.6 (3) |

**TABLE 26-5 Selected Formulas for Infants and Children (continued)**

| Trade Name [Form] (Mfr) | Kcal* (per oz) | Protein* (g/L) (C:W ratio) | Carbohydrate* (g/L) | Fat* (g/L) | MCTs (% fat kcal) | Iron *† (mg/L) |
|---|---|---|---|---|---|---|
| ***Formulas for Premature Infants: Transition or Postdischarge*** | | | | | | |
| Similac NeoSure Advance [P, R] (Ro) | 22 | 20.8 | 75.1 | 40.9 | 25 | 13.4 |
| Enfamil EnfaCare LIPIL [P,R] (MJ) | 22 | 20.7 | 77 | 39.3 | 20 | 13.3 |
| **Infant/Toddler or Children's Formulas** | | | | | | |
| Nestlé Good Start 2 Supreme DHA&ARA [C,P,R] (Nes) | 20 | 14.7 (0:100) | 75 | 34.2 | — | 10.1 |
| Nestlé Good Start 2 Essentials [C,P,R] (Nes) | 20 | 17.4 (82:18) | 88.4 | 27.5 | — | 12.1 |
| Similac 2 Advance [P] (Ro) | 20 | 14 | 71.7 | 37.1 | — | 12.2 |
| Store Brand Formula for Older Infants [P] (Wy) | 20 | 18 (50:50) | 69 | 36 | — | 12 |
| Enfamil NEXT STEP LIPIL [P] (MJ) | 20 | 17.3 (82:18) | 70 | 35.3 | — | 13.3 |
| Enfamil Kindercal | 31.8 | 30 | 135 | 44 | 12 | 10.6 |
| Enfamil Kindercal TF<br>Enfamil Kindercal TF with Fiber [R] (MJ) | 31.8 | 30 | 138<br>(6.3 g fiber) | 44 | 12 | 10.6 |
| PediaSure<br>PediaSure Enteral Formula§ [R] (Ro) | 30 | 30 | 132.5 | 39.7 | 16 | 14 |
| PediaSure With Fiber<br>PediaSure With Fiber Enteral Formula§ [R] (Ro) | 30 | 30 | 138<br>(5g/8 g fiber) | 39.7 | 16 | 14 |
| Nutren Junior<br>Nutren Junior With Fiber [R] (Nes) | 30 | 30 | 110<br>(6 g fiber; PreBio[1]) | 49.6 | 22 | 14 |
| RESOURCE Just For Kids 1.5<br>RESOURCE Just For Kids with Fiber [R] (Nov) | 30 | 30 | 110<br>(6 g fiber) | 50 | 20 | 14 |
| RESOURCE Just For Kids 1.5 CAL<br>RESOURCE Just For Kids with Fiber 1.5 CAL [R] (Nov) | 45 | 42 | 165<br>(9 g fiber) | 75 | 20 | 14 |
| Compleat Pediatric [R] (Nov) | 30 | 38 | 130<br>(6.8 g fiber) | 39 | 20 | 13 |
| Carnation Instant Breakfast Junior [R] (Nes) | 30 | 32 | 108<br>(7.2 g fiber as Prebio[1]) | 48 | — | 14 |
| **Therapeutic Infant/Toddler or Children's Formulas** | | | | | | |
| Nestlé Good Start 2 Essentials Soy [P] (Nes) | 20 | 20.8 | 80.4 | 29.5 | — | 12.1 |
| Enfamil NEXT STEP Prosobee LIPIL [P] (MJ) | 20 | 22 | 78.7 | 29.3 | — | 13.3 |
| Similac Isomil 2 Advance [P] (Ro) | 20 | 16.6 | 69.7 | 36.9 | — | 12.2 |
| Neocate Junior [P] (SHS) | 30 | 32 | 109 | 49 | 35 | 14 |
| Neocate One + [P] (SHS) | 30 | 25 | 146 | 35 | 35 | 7.7 |
| Pediatric E028 [R] (SHS) | 30 | 25 | 146 | 35 | 35 | 7.7 |
| Vivonex Pediatric* [P] (Nov) | 24 | 24 | 130 | 24 | 68 | 10 |
| Peptamen Junior [P,R] (Nes) | 30 | 30 | 137.6 | 38.5 | 60 | 14 |
| Peptamen Junior with Prebio[1] [R] (Nes) | 30 | 30 | 137.6<br>(3.6 g fiber) | 38.4 | 60 | 14 |
| EleCare [P] (Ro) | 20 | 20.4 | 72.8 | 32.2 | 33 | 12 |
| EleCare [P] (Ro) | 30 | 30 | 108.5 | 48.3 | 33 | 18 |
| Pediatric Peptinex DT<br>Pediatric Peptinex DT with Fiber [R] (Nov) | 30 | 30 | 138<br>(6 g fiber) | 39 | 50 | 14 |
| Pepdite One + [R] (SHS) | 30 | 31 | 106 | 50 | 35 | 14 |

**TABLE 26-5 Selected Formulas for Infants and Children (continued)**

Key: C, concentrate; MCTs, medium-chain triglycerides; MJ, Mead Johnson Nutritionals; Nes, Nestlé; Nov, Novartis Nutritionals; P, powder; R, ready to feed; Ro, Ross Nutritionals; SHS, SHS International; Wy, Wyeth Nutritionals.

* When powder is prepared to the stated caloric density.

† Values in parentheses pertain to low-iron version of formula.

‡ When carbohydrate is added as directed to make a 20 kcal/oz concentration.

§ Enteral formula contains less sucrose and has a lower osmolality.

Prebio[1] is a unique blend of fructooligosaccharides (FOS) and inulin. These compounds may increase colonic mucosal integrity and permeability, promote potentially beneficial bacteria, and improve colonic absorption of water and electrolytes.

*Source:* Mead Johnson Nutritionals at http://www.meadjohnson.com; Ross Products Division, Abbott Laboratories at http://www.ross.com; Nestlé Infant and Clinical Nutrition at http://www.nestleusa.com; Novartis Medical Nutrition at http://www.novartismedicalnutrition.com; and, SHS North America at http://www.shsna.com. All Web sites accessed on June 22, 2005.

molecular or ionic particles in the solution and inversely proportional to the concentration of water in the formula. The osmolality of human milk is approximately 290 mOsm/kg. Osmolality is related to the formula's carbohydrate and mineral content. For dilute solutions, there is little difference between osmolality and osmolarity. However, because infant formulas are relatively concentrated solutions, osmolarity may be approximately 80% of the osmolality. Osmolality is the preferred term for reporting the osmotic activities of infant formulas because osmotic activity is a function of a solute-solvent relationship. Manufacturers report both osmolality and osmolarity.

The osmolality of a formula increases with increasing caloric content. The relationship between osmolality and caloric density is reasonably linear within the range of caloric concentrations that are usually fed to infants. If the osmolality of a 20 kcal/oz formula is known, that of a formula with any other caloric density can be calculated, assuming a direct proportion between osmolality and caloric density. For example, if a 20 kcal/oz formula has an osmolality of 283 mOsm/kg, then the same formula concentrated to 24 kcal/oz would have an osmolality of approximately 340 mOsm/kg.

No clinically meaningful difference exists in the osmolalities of the commonly used 20 kcal/oz, ready-to-use formulas. Additionally, when concentrated products are diluted to provide a formula with 20 kcal/oz, there are no meaningful differences in osmolalities compared with the similar ready-to-use product. However, directions for diluting concentrated and powdered formulas must be followed exactly. Soy protein–based formulas have somewhat lower osmolalities than milk-based formulas because of the difference in carbohydrate source.

*Renal Solute Load* The potential RSL (PRSL) is the solute load that would be derived from the diet and require excretion by the kidney if the amino acids from protein digestion were not used for growth or eliminated by nonrenal routes. The PRSL can be calculated with the following equation: PRSL (mOsm) = N/28 + sodium + chloride + potassium + $\text{phosphorus}_{\text{(available)}}$, where N is the total nitrogen in milligrams, and sodium, chloride, potassium, and $\text{phosphorus}_{\text{(available)}}$ ($P_a$) are expressed as millimoles (or milliosmoles). The $P_a$ is assumed to be the total phosphorus content except in soy-based formulas, in which it is only two thirds of the total phosphorus. Table 26-4 lists PRSLs for various milks and infant formulas compared with the FDA-recommended upper PRSL limit.[33] Under usual conditions, 20 kcal/oz infant formulas supply approximately 1.5 mL of water per kilocalories ingested, an adequate amount of water to cover usual losses, including urinary excretion. During health, the PRSL is not a factor. However, during illness associated with water loss such as vomiting, diarrhea, and fever, or in infants with compromised renal function or diabetes insipidus, the PRSL of the infant's formula becomes a factor in maintaining fluid balance. Feeding a formula with a high PRSL (i.e., high protein content or concentrated to more than 24 kcal/oz) may produce a hypertonic urine leading to increased renal water losses and dehydration.

## Types, Uses, and Selection of Commercial Infant Formulas

Formulas for term infants are milk-based or milk-based with added whey protein (whey predominant). Other formulas are available for infants and children with specific needs and should be used only under medical supervision.

*Milk-based Formulas* Milk-based formulas (Table 26-5) are prepared from nonfat cow milk, vegetable oils, and added carbohydrate (lactose). The added carbohydrate is necessary because the ratio of carbohydrate to protein in nonfat cow milk solids is less than desirable for infant formulas. Protein provides approximately 9% to 11% of calories, and fat provides 48% to 50% of calories. The most widely used vegetable oils are corn, coconut, safflower, sunflower, palm olein, and soy. Replacement of the butterfat with vegetable oils allows for better fat absorption. Vitamins and minerals are added to meet FDA guidelines. Some milk-based formulas are available both as iron-fortified and low-iron, but there are few indications for low-iron formulas. AAP has stated that there are no known contraindications to the use of iron-fortified formulas and has advocated that low-iron formulas be removed from the market. Despite AAP's position, 8% to 30% of formula sold in the United States is low-iron formula because of unproven concerns that iron-fortified formulas contribute to colic, constipation, fussiness, cramping, and gastroesophageal

**TABLE 26-6 Indications for Therapeutic Infant Formulas**

| Problem | Suggested Therapeutic Formula | Comments |
|---|---|---|
| Allergy or sensitivity to cow milk or soy protein | Enfamil Nutramigen LIPIL, Similac, Alimentum Advance, Enfamil Pregestimil, Neocate | Protein hydrolysate or free amino acid formula best; up to 50% cross-sensitivity between cow milk and soy protein allergies |
| Biliary atresia, cholestatic liver disease | Enfamil Pregestimil, Similac Alimentum Advance, EleCare Portagen | Impaired digestion and absorption of long-chain fats; higher percentage of MCTs may improve absorption; monitor for linoleic acid deficiency, if Portagen used |
| Carbohydrate intolerance (severe) | RCF, Product 3232A | Carbohydrate-free formulas; patient-tolerated carbohydrate source is added gradually |
| Cardiac disease | Similac PM 60/40 | Low electrolyte content, may require supplementation in patients receiving diuretics; calorically dense, standard formulas often used owing to failure-to-thrive and volume restriction |
| Celiac disease | Enfamil Pregestimil, Enfamil Nutramigen LIPIL, Enfamil LactoFree LIPIL, EleCare, Neocate, Isomil DF | Advance to standard formulas as intestinal epithelium returns to normal; diet must be gluten-free |
| Chylothorax | Portagen | High MCT intake decreases flow through the lymphatic system |
| Constipation | No therapeutic formula necessary | Continue routine formula; increase water; refer severe constipation |
| Cystic fibrosis | Enfamil Pregestimil, Similac Alimentum Advance | Impaired digestion and absorption of long-chain fats; cow milk–based formula or human milk may be used with appropriate pancreatic enzyme supplementation; supplementation may be required even with predigested therapeutic formulas; soy protein–based formulas contraindicated |
| Diarrhea | | |
| Chronic nonspecific | Enfamil Lactofree LIPIL, Similac Lactose Free Advance, Enfamil Prosobee LIPIL, Similac Isomil Advance, Enfamil Nutramigen LIPIL | Trial of lactose-free cow milk or soy protein–based formula may be needed; avoid fruit juices |
| Intractable | Enfamil Pregestimil, Similac Alimentum Advance, EleCare, RCF, Product 3232A | Hydrolyzed protein needed owing to impaired digestion of intact protein, long-chain fats, and disaccharides; Alimentum contains sucrose and may not be appropriate for all cases |
| Failure-to-thrive | Enfamil Pregestimil, Similac Alimentum Advance | Most cases related to inadequate intake; start with standard formula, may need more calorically dense formula for catch-up growth; change to predigested formula only if malabsorption present |
| Galactosemia | Similac Isomil Advance, Enfamil Prosobee LIPIL | Soy protein–based formula initially; cow and human milk contraindicated |
| Gastroesophageal reflux | Enfamil A.R. LIPIL | Start with standard formula thickened with rice cereal (1 tbsp/oz of formula); attempt small, frequent feedings; avoid using products like Thick-It and SimplyThick to thicken formula (products are intended for patients with dysphagia or swallowing difficulties); use more calorically dense formula if decreased volume or catch-up growth needed |
| Hepatitis | | |
| Without liver failure | No therapeutic formula necessary | Impaired digestion and absorption of long-chain fats is uncommon |
| With liver failure | Enfamil Pregestimil, EleCare, Similac Alimentum Advance Portagen | Impaired digestion and absorption of long-chain fats |
| Lactose intolerance (primary or secondary) | Enfamil Lactofree LIPIL, Similac Lactose Free Advance, Enfamil Prosobee LIPIL, Similac Isomil Advance | Remove lactose from diet; use lactose-free formula |

**TABLE 26-6 Indications for Therapeutic Infant Formulas (continued)**

| Problem | Suggested Therapeutic Formula | Comments |
|---|---|---|
| Necrotizing enterocolitis (during recovery or postresection) | Enfamil Pregestimil, Similac Alimentum Advance, Neocate, EleCare | Impaired digestion and absorption requires a hydrolysate or free amino acid formula |
| Prematurity | Fortified human milk, premature (Similac Special Care Advance, Enfamil Premature LIPIL) or transition infant formula (Similac NeoSure Advance, Enfamil EnfaCare LIPIL) | Transition formula (Enfamil EnfaCare LIPIL, Similac NeoSure Advance) can be added to human milk to increase caloric density after discharge (1 tsp/90 mL human milk makes 24 kcal/oz) |
| Renal insufficiency | Similac PM 60/40 | Low phosphate, low PRSL |

Key: MCT, medium-chain triglyceride; PRSL, potential renal solute load.

*Source:* Mead Johnson Nutritionals at http://www.meadjohnson.com; Ross Products Division, Abbott Laboratories at http://www.ross.com; Nestlé Infant and Clinical Nutrition at http://www.nestleusa.com; Novartis Medical Nutrition at http://www.novartismedicalnutrition.com; and, SHS North America at http://www.shsna.com. All Web sites accessed on November 2, 2005.

reflux.[29,30] Although Enfamil Lactofree LIPIL and Similac Lactose Free Advance are milk-based formulas, they contain corn syrup solids or corn syrup solids with sucrose rather than lactose as the carbohydrate source and may be used for infants with lactose intolerance.

*Therapeutic Formulas* Therapeutic infant formulas are used for infants with conditions that require dietary adjustment and should be used with medical supervision rather than being self-selected by parents. Table 26-6 lists indications for various therapeutic formulas including soy protein–based, casein-based, casein or whey hydrolysate–based, and low-electrolyte and -mineral formulas. Formulas intended for use by premature infants and those formulated specifically for children from 1 to 10 years of age are also considered therapeutic formulas.

Prethickened Milk-based Formula Enfamil A.R. LIPIL was developed specifically for infants with gastroesophageal reflux. This iron-fortified formula contains a carbohydrate blend of lactose (57%), rice starch (30%), and maltodextrin (13%), as well as a high amylopectin rice starch for thickening. Before ingestion, Enfamil A.R. LIPIL with Iron has a viscosity 10 times that of ready-to-use Enfamil LIPIL with Iron. In contrast, Enfamil LIPIL thickened with rice cereal (1 tbsp/oz) has a viscosity 30 times that of Enfamil LIPIL. Therefore, Enfamil A.R. LIPIL flows better through the nipple than standard formula thickened with rice cereal. Once ingested, however, the viscosity increases dramatically in the acidic pH of the stomach, reaching a viscosity equal to the Enfamil LIPIL plus rice cereal combination. This effect may be minimized in infants receiving a histamine$_2$-receptor antagonist (e.g., ranitidine, famotidine) or proton pump inhibitor (e.g., omeprazole, lansoprazole) for treatment of their gastroesophageal reflux if the gastric pH is greater than 5.4. Enfamil A.R. LIPIL is not recommended for use in premature infants as it will not adequately meet nutrient needs, especially protein, calcium, and phosphorus.

Soy Protein–based Formulas Despite relatively few true indications for soy protein–based formulas, approximately 25% of formulas sold in the United States are soy protein–based, suggesting that these formulas are being selected by parents rather than being prescribed by health care practitioners.[29,34] Soy protein–based formulas (Table 26-5) contain a soy isolate fortified with L-methionine. Vegetable oils, including palm olein, soy, coconut, high-oleic safflower, and sunflower provide the fat content. Corn maltodextrin, corn syrup solids, and sucrose supply the carbohydrate in these formulas; none contains lactose. Soy formulas are a safe and nutritionally sound alternative for normal growth and development in infants who are not fed human milk, do not tolerate cow milk–based formula, or whose parents choose them for other reasons.

Food allergy occurs in infants because the immature digestive and metabolic processes may not be completely effective in converting dietary proteins into nonallergenic amino acids. Cow milk protein allergy occurs in 2% to 3% of infants and is defined as symptomatology involving the respiratory tract (wheezing), skin (rash), or GI tract (diarrhea, bloody stools) that disappears when cow milk is removed from the diet and reappears on two separate challenges when cow milk is reintroduced during a symptom-free period. Cow milk protein intolerance symptoms regress within 3 to 4 years in most children.

Soy protein–based formulas are appropriate for infants with lactose intolerance because of lactase deficiency and with documented immunoglobulin E (IgE)-mediated allergy to cow milk protein. Infants with cow milk protein–induced enteropathy or enterocolitis are also frequently sensitive to soy protein (up to 50% cross-sensitivity); AAP/CON recommends protein hydrolysate formulas for these infants.[35] Most infants suspected of having adverse reactions to milk-based formulas have not experienced life-threatening manifestations. These infants appear to tolerate soy protein–based formulas that are less expensive and better tasting than the protein hydrolysate formulas. Routine use of soy protein–based formulas has no proven value in prevention of atopic disease.[34] Some infants with gastroenteritis develop intolerance to lactose and sucrose because of a temporary lactase and sucrase deficiency. However, after rehydration most infants with diarrhea can be managed by continuing their usual nutrition regimen whether milk-based or soy protein–based. Soy protein–based formulas also provide an alternative nutritional source for infants whose parents are vegetarians and do not wish to use animal protein–based formulas.

The high protein and manganese content of soy protein–based formulas is a concern because PRSL is increased. In addition, manganese absorption is enhanced in children who are iron deficient, which may result in manganese accumulation and neurologic symptoms in children whose biliary manganese excretion is compromised (e.g., those with biliary atresia or cholestasis). On the positive side, exposure to phytoestrogens early in life may have long-term health benefits for hormone-dependent diseases.[36] More studies are needed in this area.

RCF (previously known as Ross Carbohydrate Free) is a soy protein–based formula that contains no carbohydrates. This formula is used only in the dietary management of infants unable to tolerate the type or amount of carbohydrates in human milk or infant formulas. A carbohydrate source (sucrose, dextrose, fructose, or glucose polymers) is added gradually in increasing amounts to slowly increase carbohydrate tolerance.

Similac Isomil DF is a formula that contains added dietary fiber from soy and was specifically formulated for infants with diarrhea secondary to antibiotics. It is best used short term until diarrhea resolves. It may also help increase the consistency of ileostomy or colostomy output in those infants requiring these devices for conditions such as Hirschsprung's disease, imperforate anus, necrotizing enterocolitis, or intestinal atresias.

Soy protein–based formulas are not recommended for the routine feeding of preterm infants because of reduced calcium, phosphorus, and vitamin D bioavailability, which predisposes these infants, especially those weighing less than 1500 g, to developing rickets.[34] In addition, soy protein–based formulas are not recommended for infants with cystic fibrosis because these children do not use soy protein adequately, will lose substantial nitrogen in their stools, and develop hypoproteinemia or even anasarca (generalized infiltration of fluid into subcutaneous connective tissue). Formula-fed infants with cystic fibrosis do well nutritionally when given an easily digested formula that contains elemental protein and medium-chain triglycerides (MCTs) (e.g., a casein hydrolysate–based formula). However, recent studies have shown that they do equally well on a regular cow milk–based formula or human milk as long as adequate pancreatic enzyme replacement is given.[37]

**Casein Hydrolysate–based Formulas** Protein is supplied by enzymatically hydrolyzed, charcoal-treated casein rather than by whole protein in casein hydrolysate–based formulas, which include Enfamil Pregestimil, Enfamil Nutramigen LIPIL, and Similac Alimentum Advance (Table 26-7). They contain nonantigenic polypeptides with molecular weights less than 1200 daltons; therefore, they can be fed to infants who are sensitive to intact milk protein. Casein hydrolysate formulas are supplemented with L-cysteine, L-tyrosine, and L-tryptophan (Similac Alimentum Advance also contains L-methionine) because the concentrations of these amino acids are reduced during the charcoal treatment.

Carbohydrate sources in casein hydrolysate–based formulas include corn syrup solids, modified corn and tapioca starch, sucrose, and dextrose; however, sources vary for specific formulas (Table 26-7). Glucose polymers found in corn syrup solids or modified corn starch are particularly useful in infants who have malabsorption disorders and are frequently intolerant to lactose, sucrose, and glucose. In addition, glucose polymers contribute little to the total osmolar load. Low osmolarity is an advantage in intestinal disorders in which the osmolar load of disaccharide- or glucose-containing elemental diets may not be tolerated.

These formulas also contain modified fat sources: MCTs from fractionated coconut and palm olein oils; corn, soy, and high-oleic safflower oils. MCTs do not require emulsification with bile and are more easily digested and absorbed than long-chain fats. Shorter-chain fatty acids and MCTs are directly absorbed into the portal system, not into the lacteals of the lymphatic system. In addition, MCTs enhance the absorption of long-chain triglycerides and do not require carnitine for transport into the mitochondria, where oxidation and energy production occur. However, MCTs cannot be the sole source of fat in the diet as they do not provide essential fatty acids, increasing the risk of essential fatty acid deficiency. Diarrhea can result from MCT malabsorption caused by overfeeding or intestinal mucosal disease.

Enfamil Pregestimil is often used for infants with massive small bowel resection (short bowel syndrome), severe intractable diarrhea, steatorrhea, protein-calorie malnutrition, or cystic fibrosis. Enfamil Nutramigen LIPIL is used for infants with severe diarrhea or GI disturbances and for infants with severe or multiple food allergies. In cases of galactosemia, a relatively rare disorder resulting from a galactose-*1*-phosphate uridyltransferase or galactokinase deficiency, dietary lactose must be eliminated from the diet so the body may convert glucose to the amount of galactose it requires. Infants with galactosemia must be fed formulas without lactose or sucrose (Enfamil Nutramigen LIPIL, Enfamil Pregestimil, or Enfamil ProSobee LIPIL). Similac Alimentum Advance contains sucrose and modified tapioca starch. These carbohydrates are digested and absorbed by separate mechanisms (principally glucoamylase and sucrase-$\alpha$-dextrinase). This formula can be used for infants with protein sensitivity, pancreatic insufficiency (e.g., cystic fibrosis), or intractable diarrhea.

Use of these casein hydrolysate–based formulas for allergy prophylaxis is controversial. AAP's policy statement on hypoallergenic formulas states that infants with a high risk for developing allergy identified by a strong family history (both parents or one parent and a sibling) may benefit from a hypoallergenic formula, but studies are not conclusive.[35] Currently, no evidence exists to support the use of hydrolysate formulas for treating colic or irritability. Though these symptoms are common in infants, they are rarely a result of an IgE-mediated allergic reaction to cow milk protein.

**TABLE 26-7 Composition of Selected Hydrolysate and Amino Acid-based Formulas**

| Formula (Mfr) | Carbohydrate | Protein | Fat |
|---|---|---|---|
| Enfamil Pregestimil (MJ) | Corn syrup solids; tapioca starch | Casein hydrolysates | MCT 55%; corn oil |
| Similac Alimentum Advance (Ro) | Sucrose; tapioca starch | Casein hydrolysates, L-cystine, L-tyrosine, L-tryptophan, L-methionine | MCT 33%; safflower and soy oils |
| Enfamil Nutramigen LIPIL (MJ) | Corn syrup solids; modified corn starch | Casein hydrolysates | Corn oil |
| Product 3232A (MJ) | Modified tapioca starch | Casein hydrolysates, L-cystine, L-tyrosine, L-tryptophan | MCT 85%; corn oil |
| Pepdite One + (SHS) | Corn syrup solids | Hydrolyzed pork and soy proteins | MCT 35%; fractionated coconut, canola and high-oleic safflower oils |
| Neocate (SHS) | Corn syrup solids | Free amino acids | MCT 5%; safflower, coconut, and soy oils |
| Neocate One + (SHS) | Corn syrup solids | Free amino acids | MCT 35%; fractionated coconut, canola, and high-oleic safflower oils |
| Pediatric E028 (SHS) | Maltodextrin, sucrose | Free amino acids | MCT 35%; fractionated coconut, canola, and high-oleic safflower oils |
| Neocate Junior (SHS) | Corn syrup solids | Free amino acids | MCT 35%; fractionated coconut, canola, and high-oleic safflower oils |
| EleCare (Ro) | Corn syrup solids | Free amino acids | MCT 33%; high-oleic safflower, fractionated coconut, and soy oils |
| Peptamen Junior (Nes) | Maltodextrin; corn starch | Hydrolyzed whey protein | MCT 60%; fractionated coconut and palm kernel, soybean, and canola oils |
| Peptamen Junior with Prebio[1]* (Nes) | Maltodextrin; corn starch; sucrose (flavored) | Hydrolyzed whey protein | MCT 60%; fractionated coconut and palm kernel, soybean, and canola oils |

Key: MCT, medium-chain triglycerides; MJ, Mead Johnson; Nes, Nestlé Clinical Nutrition; Nov, Novartis Nutrition; Ro, Ross Products; SHS, SHS Nutritionals.

* Prebio[1] is a unique blend of fructooligosaccharides (FOS) and inulin. These compounds may increase colonic mucosal integrity and permeability, promote potentially beneficial bacteria, and improve colonic absorption of water and electrolytes.

*Source:* Mead Johnson Nutritionals at http://www.meadjohnson.com; Ross Products Division, Abbott Laboratories at http://www.ross.com; Nestlé Infant and Clinical Nutrition at http://www.nestleusa.com; Novartis Medical Nutrition at http://www.novartismedicalnutrition.com; and, SHS North America at http://www.shsna.com. All Web sites accessed on November 2, 2005.

Extensively hydrolyzed casein makes formulas less palatable. If the formula is rejected when first offered, it should be tried again after a few hours. These products are designed to provide a sole source of nutrition for infants up to 4 to 6 months of age and a primary source of nutrition through 12 months of age, when indicated. Extended use of hydrolysate formulas as a sole source of nutrition in children older than 6 months requires close medical supervision and monitoring.

Whey Hydrolysate–based Formula Enzymatically hydrolyzed whey protein is another protein source used in infant formulas (Nestlé Good Start Supreme). The effectiveness of whey hydrolysate formula in infants who have GI intolerance to cow milk but are not allergic to it suggests that this formula may be an acceptable alternative to other cow milk– and soy protein–based formulas. This product is promoted as having a pleasant taste, smell, and appearance. It may be better accepted than casein hydrolysate–based formulas, which parents and infants find noticeably different from cow milk– and soy protein–based formulas in appearance and taste.

Amino Acid–based Formulas Occasionally, some infants are intolerant to even hydrolyzed casein and require a free amino acid–based formula. Neocate and EleCare contain 100% free amino acids and are considered hypoallergenic. They are used for infants with cow milk–protein allergy, multiple food protein allergies or intolerance to casein hydrolysate formulas.

High MCT Formula Portagen is unique because of its high MCT content (i.e., 87% of the fat). It also contains higher concentrations of both lipid- and water-soluble vitamins than are found in casein hydrolysate–based formulas. The higher concentrations of MCTs and vitamins in Portagen help compensate for the impaired digestion and absorption of long-chain fats in patients with pancreatic insufficiency (e.g., cystic fibrosis), bile acid deficiency (e.g., biliary atresia, cholestatic jaundice), and intestinal resection. Another use for Portagen is to decrease flow through the lymphatic system in patient with lymphatic anomalies such as chylothorax and chylous ascites. It can be used as the sole dietary source for both infants and older children or as a beverage to be consumed with each meal. Mead Johnson Nutritionals no longer recommends Portagen as an infant formula because of the concerns with bacterial contamination of powdered formulas leading to a recall of one batch in March 2002. Since there is no good alternative for infants, including premature infants, with certain medical conditions such as chylothorax and chylous ascites, such infants will require it. These infants should be monitored carefully for signs of GI infection such as diarrhea and abdominal distention.

Premature Infant Formulas Because of their increased nutrient needs and somewhat decreased ability to consume an adequate volume, premature infants (especially those less than 34 weeks gestation) often need formulas that provide a higher caloric density, as well as increased protein, calcium, phosphorus, and other nutrients. Inadequate nutrient intake can occur in human milk–fed premature infants because human milk does not meet the needs of this population. The nutritional goal for a preterm infant is to achieve a postnatal growth rate that approximates the intrauterine growth rate of a normal fetus of the same postconceptional age.

No commercially available formula is completely satisfactory for premature infants. Formulas for premature infants (Table 26-5) share features, such as whey-predominant proteins, carbohydrate mixtures of lactose and corn syrup solids, and fat mixtures containing both medium- and long-chain triglycerides. They differ in electrolyte, vitamin, mineral, protein, and caloric content. When given in sufficient volume, these formulas promote adequate growth in preterm infants. An isotonic osmolality (approximately 300 mOsm/kg of water) is maintained at a caloric density of 24 kcal/oz or 80 kcal/100 mL.

Calcium and phosphorus are crucial to the development and maintenance of the human skeleton. In addition, calcium and phosphorus are integral components of many biochemical reactions. Calcium requirements are affected by protein and phosphorus intake because these nutrients interact with the renal tubular reabsorption of calcium. Calcium-to-phosphorus weight ratios vary significantly for human milk (2:1) and cow milk (1.2:1). This ratio varies in commercial infant formulas. Formulas designed for term infants will not meet the calcium and phosphorus needs of premature infants. For these infants, the additional calcium and phosphorus found in premature infant formulas is necessary for normal bone growth and mineralization. Human milk fed to premature infants also requires calcium and phosphorus supplementation.

Nutrient-enriched transition or postdischarge formulas are designed specifically to provide for continued catch-up growth in premature infants after hospital discharge. Similac NeoSure Advance and Enfamil EnfaCare LIPIL (both milk-based formulas) contain MCTs as part of the fat source. The caloric (22 kcal/oz), protein, vitamin, and mineral content of these formulas exceeds that of standard term formulas but is less than that of premature infant formulas. Use of these formulas in preterm infants until 9 months postnatal age results in greater linear growth, weight gain, and bone mineral content than is seen with the use of standard, term infant formulas.[38] Similac PM 60/40 is often included in this category and, because of its lower mineral content, may be used in premature or term infants with decreased ability to excrete an RSL, especially those with renal insufficiency.

Human Milk Fortifiers Mothers who deliver prematurely produce milk that is higher in protein, sodium, potassium, and possibly other nutrients than the milk of mothers who deliver at full term. However, these nutrients decline to the amounts found in mature human milk by 4 to 8 weeks after delivery. During the third trimester, the fetus receives 125 to 150 mg of calcium and 65 to 80 mg of phosphorus daily, most of which is deposited in bone. Human milk, whether preterm or mature, cannot supply this amount of calcium and phosphorus, which is needed to prevent osteopenia of prematurity.

Commercial products have been developed to supplement the nutrient content of human milk so that it meets the needs of most preterm infants. Enfamil Human Milk Fortifier and Similac Human Milk Fortifier are powders that add nutrients to human milk without displacing a significant amount of volume. Similac Natural Care Advance is a liquid that may be given alternately with human milk or mixed in various ratios with human milk to augment the nutrients provided. All three products are made from cow milk supplemented with whey protein to provide a whey-casein ratio of 60:40, and a fat mixture that provides MCTs. When added to human milk they increase the osmolality by 10 to 35 mOsm/kg. Table 26-8 lists the composition of the three available human milk fortifiers. Studies support adequate weight gain and nutrient retention in infants when either fortified human milk or commercial preterm formulas are ingested. Although both groups gained weight at rates equivalent to intrauterine growth rates (15 g/kg/day), as recommended by AAP, time to reach a weight of 1800 g was reduced by 7 days in a group of premature infants receiving Similac Human Milk Fortifier compared with those receiving Enfamil Human Milk Fortifier.[39,40] This improved weight gain has the potential to shorten length of hospital stay, but this has not been evaluated. Linear growth was also consistent with goals (1 cm/week) in both groups, but higher in the Similac Human Milk Fortifier group, an effect likely resulting from the increased calcium and phosphorus found in the Similac product. The use of either product will result in weight gain equivalent to intrauterine growth rates in most premature infants. Product selection will, therefore, be dictated by cost and clinical preference. These products are expensive, costing about $1 per packet, and one packet is generally added to each 25 mL of human milk to yield a 24 kcal/oz concentration. Once the infant is ready for discharge from the hospital or has reached a weight of 2.5 kg, one of the transition or postdischarge formulas can be

**TABLE 26-8 Human Milk Fortifiers**

| Component | Similac Human Milk Fortifier* | Enfamil Human Milk Fortifier* | Similac Natural Care Advance (per 123 mL) |
|---|---|---|---|
| Calories | 14 | 14 | 100 |
| Protein (g) | 1 | 1.1 | 2.71 |
| Fat (g) | 0.36 | 1 | 5.43 |
| Carbohydrates (g) | 1.8 | <0.4 | 10.3 |
| Vitamin A (IU) | 620 | 950 | 1250 |
| Vitamin D (IU) | 120 | 150 | 150 |
| Vitamin E (IU) | 3.2 | 4.6 | 4.0 |
| Vitamin K (μg) | 8 | 4.4 | 12 |
| Thiamin (μg) | 233 | 150 | 250 |
| Riboflavin (μg) | 417 | 220 | 620 |
| Vitamin $B_6$ (μg) | 211 | 115 | 250 |
| Vitamin $B_{12}$ (μg) | 0.64 | 0.18 | 0.55 |
| Niacin (μg) | 3570 | 3000 | 5000 |
| Folic acid (μg) | 23 | 25 | 37 |
| Pantothenic acid (μg) | 1500 | 730 | 1900 |
| Biotin (μg) | 26 | 2.7 | 37 |
| Vitamin C (mg) | 25 | 12 | 37 |
| Calcium (mg) | 117 | 90 | 210 |
| Phosphorus (mg) | 67 | 50 | 116 |
| Magnesium (mg) | 7 | 1 | 12 |
| Iron (mg) | 0.4 | 1.44 | 0.4 |
| Zinc (mg) | 1 | 0.72 | 1.5 |
| Manganese (μg) | 7 | 10 | 12 |
| Copper (μg) | 170 | 44 | 250 |
| Selenium (μg) | 0.5 | — | 1.8 |
| Sodium (mg) | 15 | 16 | 43 |
| Potassium (mg) | 63 | 29 | 129 |
| Chloride (mg) | 38 | 13 | 81 |

* Amount per 4 packets; generally mixed with 100 mL human milk to yield 120 mL at a caloric density of 24 kcal/oz.

*Source:* www.ross.com/productHandbook; www.meadjohnson.com/products. Both Web sites accessed November 6, 2005.

added to human milk to increase the caloric density (1 tsp powder added to 90 mL formula yields 24 kcal/oz) and delivery of other nutrients.

Metabolic Formulas Infants with various inherited inborn errors of metabolism require specific formulas tailored to their particular condition and must be under the care of a specialist, usually a pediatric endocrinologist or geneticist. Information about these formulas is available on the manufacturers' Web sites at www.meadjohnson.com, www.ross.com, and www.shs.com (accessed November 6, 2005). These formulas are classified by the FDA as "exempt formulas," which means, as stated previously, that they are exempt from FDA nutrient content and labeling requirements, require a prescription for use, and cannot be sold retail.

Concentrated Formulas A child with special nutritional needs exceeding normal requirements may be given concentrated formula under medical supervision. Some ready-to-use formulas made from cow milk are available in a caloric density of 24 kcal/oz (Table 26-5). Various concentrations can be prepared from liquid concentrates or powders by varying the amount of water added (Tables 26-9 and 26-10). Concentrating formulas by adding less water to increase caloric density also results in increased delivery of protein and electrolytes as well as a decrease in fluid delivery. Though this is often desired, increased concentrations of protein and electrolytes (i.e., PRSL) in conjunction with decreased fluid intake may result in dehydration and electrolyte imbalances. Careful monitoring of the infant's fluid intake and output, weight, serum electrolytes, blood urea nitrogen, and specific gravity and osmolality of

**TABLE 26-9 Dilution of Concentrated Liquid Infant Formulas***

| Caloric Concentration Desired (kcal/oz) | Liquid Formula Concentrate (oz) | Added Water (oz) |
|---|---|---|
| 20 | 1 | 1 |
| 22 (actual 21.8) | 3 | 2.5 |
| 24 | 3 | 2 |
| 26-27 (actual 26.7) | 3 | 1.5 |
| 28-29 (actual 28.6) | 5 | 2 |

* Commercial concentrates of infant formula contain 40 kcal/oz before dilution with water.

**TABLE 26-10 Dilution of Powdered Term Infant Formulas***

| Caloric Concentration Desired (kcal/oz) | Formula Powder (tbsp)† | Added Water (oz) |
|---|---|---|
| 20 | 1 | 2 |
| 24 | 3 | 5 |
| 28 | 4 | 5.5 |
| 28 | 7 | 10 |

* Powdered infant formulas contain 40 kcal per level, packed tablespoonful before dilution. If a large volume of formula is to be prepared, add powder necessary to supply desired calories, then add water to the final volume desired.

† 1 tbsp = 1 scoop.

urine is recommended, especially on initiation of the concentrated formula.

Modular macronutrient components (Table 26-11) that can be added to either human milk or infant formula are available as an alternative to concentrating formulas. Adding carbohydrates as glucose can result in diarrhea. Protein supplementation may increase the PRSL. Fat may be added as MCTs (MCT Oil) or Microlipid for infants with fat malabsorption or intolerance. Microlipid is an emulsion made from safflower oil that provides long-chain fatty acids and mixes well with formula. Addition of fat can lead to diarrhea, steatorrhea, delayed gastric emptying, and vomiting or gastroesophageal reflux. Adding modular components is more expensive and time-consuming than simply concentrating the formula and should be reserved for situations in which a single nutrient is needed or concentrating the formula further is not appropriate.

Follow-up Formulas "Follow-up," "follow-on," or toddler formulas (Table 26-5) are designed for infants 4 to 12 months of age. AAP/CON, however, has stated that these formulas offer no nutritional advantages; standard formulas are appropriate for infants up to 12 months of age.[29]

Formulas for Children 1 to 10 Years of Age Nutritionally complete, isotonic, virtually lactose-free enteral formulas designed for young children who cannot tolerate a normal diet or eat solid food are available (Table 26-5). Flavored products contain sucrose, have a pleasant taste, and can be used as oral supplements to increase caloric intake. These formulas are also appropriate to use as tube feedings regardless of tube tip placement. They contain adequate

**TABLE 26-11 Modular Additives**

| Additive* (Mfr) | Nutrient Provided | Primary Nutrient | Calories |
|---|---|---|---|
| ProMod (Ro) | Whey protein | Protein 5 g/scoop | 28 kcal/scoop |
| Casec (Nov) | Casein protein | Protein 4 g/tbsp | 17 kcal/tbsp |
| Beneprotein (Nov) | Whey protein | Protein 6 g/scoop | 25 kcal/scoop |
| Polycose (Ro) (liquid) | Carbohydrate | Carbohydrate 0.5 g/mL | 2 kcal/mL |
| Polycose (Ro) | Carbohydrate | Carbohydrate 6 g/tbsp | 23 kcal/tbsp |
| Moducal (Nov) | Carbohydrate | Carbohydrate 6 g/tbsp | 30 kcal/tbsp |
| Microlipid (Nov) | Long-chain fats | Fat 0.5 g/mL | 4.5 kcal/mL |
| MCT oil (Nov) | MCTs | Fat 0.9 g/mL | 7.7 kcal/mL |
| Super Soluble Duocal (SHS) | Carbohydrate and fat | Carbohydrate 6 g/tbsp; fat 2 g/tbsp | 42 kcal/tbsp (scoop) |
| Additions (Nes) | Protein, carbohydrate, and fat | Protein 6 g/scoop; carbohydrate 9 g/scoop; fat 5 g/scoop (35% MCT) | 100 kcal/scoop |
| Benecalorie (Nov) (liquid) | Protein and fat | Fat 33 g/1.5 oz; protein 7 g/1.5 oz | 7 kcal/mL |

Key: MCT, medium chain triglycerides; Nes, Nestlé Infant and Clinical Nutrition; Nov, Novartis Medical Nutrition; Ro, Ross Products Division, Abbott Laboratories; SHS, SHS North America.

* Products listed are powders unless otherwise specified.

amounts of calcium, phosphorus, iron, and vitamin D for this age group; the amounts contained in adult enteral products are typically inadequate.

Several therapeutic formulas have also been developed for children 1 to 10 years of age (Table 26–5). Peptamen Junior and Pepdite One+ are peptide-based, semi-elemental formulas. Vivonex Pediatric, Neocate One+, Neocate Junior, Pediatric E028 (a liquid, flavored version of Neocate One+), and EleCare are amino acid–based, elemental formulas. These products are intended for use in children with altered digestion and/or absorptive capabilities caused by a number of conditions (Table 26-6).

### Potential Problems with Infant Formulas

As with any food, GI problems, especially diarrhea, can occur with the use of infant formulas as well as human milk. Tooth decay and nutritional deficiencies are other potential problems.

*Diarrhea* Infants are particularly susceptible to dehydration because of their high metabolic rate and ratio of surface area to weight and height. Fluid depletion by diarrhea or vomiting may quickly (within 24 hours) produce severe dehydration with fluid and electrolyte imbalances, shock, and possible death. A potential cause of diarrhea and vomiting is the improper dilution of a concentrated liquid or powdered formula or the incorrect addition of a modular product.

If diarrhea develops, the clinician should ascertain the severity and duration of the diarrhea, stool frequency, and formula preparation method. If the diarrhea appears severe (i.e., many more stools per day than normal) or has continued for more than 48 hours, or if the infant is clinically ill (fever, lethargy, anorexia, irritability, dry mucous membranes, decreased urine output, or weight loss), the infant should be referred for medical attention (see Chapter 17).

Mild diarrhea will usually resolve without the need for medical intervention, but the infant should be observed closely for signs of dehydration. Temporarily discontinuing usual dietary intake is no longer recommended except during a 4- to 6-hour period of oral rehydration with a rehydrating solution (e.g., Rehydralyte) in the presence of dehydration. Oral electrolyte replacement solutions especially manufactured for infants (e.g., Pedialyte) may be used for short-term replacement of fluid and electrolyte losses in mild to moderate dehydration to augment fluid intake, but should not replace formula or human milk intake.[41] Prevention of dehydration by replacement of ongoing losses with a glucose/electrolyte solution in liquid or frozen form is the best intervention for diarrhea in infants and children.

Lactose-free formulas or a lactose-free diet may be considered for those infants and children with severe diarrheal illness, but full-strength lactose-containing formulas, human milk, or a regular diet can be used in most. Parents should be advised that diarrhea is likely to continue for 3 to 7 days regardless of type of formula, and seeking medical consultation is advised if a sudden increase in stool output occurs with resumption of feeding.[41]

*Other GI Issues* Adverse GI effects of formula include mechanical obstruction (inspissated milk curds) and hypersensitivity to specific milk protein. Cow milk intolerance is associated most often with an inability to digest lactose or milk proteins. Hyperosmolar formulas may adversely affect premature infants during the early neonatal period and may be a contributing factor to the development of necrotizing enterocolitis, a severe inflammation of the intestinal mucous membranes. For this reason, initiation of feedings in these infants is most often done with human milk or a 20 kcal/oz formula. The caloric density can be advanced as needed once tolerance is demonstrated.

*Tooth Decay* Baby bottle tooth decay can occur in children who are bottle-fed beyond the typical weaning period and who go to sleep with their bottles. It can also occur if the infant is allowed to sip on a bottle or training cup frequently during the day. Caries are seen in children younger than 2 years and may involve the maxillary incisors, maxillary and mandibular first molars, or maxillary and mandibular canines. Restorative dentistry is often required, leading to the potential for difficulty in speech development. Methods for prevention once teeth start to erupt include substituting plain water for carbohydrate-containing formula or other drinks given in a bottle until the infant is weaned from the bottle, ensuring adequate fluoride intake, cleaning the baby's mouth at least once daily, and weaning from breast or bottle by 10 to 12 months of age.[42] Sleeping with a bottle should be actively discouraged in all infants.

*Nutritional Deficiencies or Toxicities* Generally, age- and condition-appropriate commercial infant formulas are nutritionally adequate and safe for most infants and children. Nutritional deficiencies reported historically with commercial infant formulas have been corrected with appropriate supplementation procedures and technologic advances in processing.

Because of concern about possible aluminum contamination of infant formulas, the Food and Agricultural Organization of the United Nations has set a provisional tolerable aluminum intake of 1 mg/kg per day. Aluminum toxicity can interfere with cellular and metabolic processes in the nervous system as well as negatively affect bone and liver tissues.[43] This is primarily a concern in patients with decreased or immature renal function, such as occurs in premature infants. If an infant were to ingest as much as 200 mL/kg per day of a formula known to have the highest aluminum concentration, the amount of aluminum received per day would still be less than 0.5 mg/kg per day. The highest aluminum concentrations in infant formulas (500 to 2400 mg/L) have been reported in soy protein–based formulas because plants readily absorb aluminum from soil.

### Infant Formula Preparation

Most formulas are available as a liquid ready-to-use or liquid concentrate or as a powder for reconstitution that is mixed with water. Concentrated liquids typically require the mixing of equal amounts of water and concentrated liquid (e.g., 13 oz can of formula with 13 oz can of water) to prepare a 20 kcal/oz formula (Table 26-9). Powdered term and preterm transition or postdischarge formulas provide a measuring scoop in the can and require addition of 1 packed level scoop (1 tbsp) of powder to each 2 oz of water for a 20 kcal/oz formula and 22 kcal/oz formula, respectively. Directions for preparation vary and should always be compared with the manufacturer's or health care professional's directions. For example, mixing directions for Neocate vary substantially from those for other formulas. Additionally, if the family is given alternative directions from those printed on the can, these should be in writing and explained thoroughly to the caregiver. Directions should be provided in Spanish or other appropriate language for non-English-speaking patients. At least one infant formula, NAN, now has bilingual (Spanish and English) labeling. Before use, infant formula containers should be inspected for expiration dates and damage. Unopened formula containers, cans or bottles, can be stored at room temperature, but must not be subjected to extreme temperature changes.

*Preparation Techniques* Each infant formula has specific instructions for preparation, and most formulas have symbols on the containers that can be used as guidelines in preparing formula. Because infants may be more susceptible to infection, various sterilization methods have been recommended for infant formula preparation. Table 26-12 reviews sterilization methods for different types of formulas. Studies have shown that the clean method of preparing formula (not boiling the water) is as safe as terminal sterilization (boiling the water), and some practitioners do not recommend boiling water. AAP currently recommends that all water for formula preparation be boiled because of reports of municipal water supply contamination in some areas. If well or pond water is used or if the area is prone to flooding, the water must be boiled. If tap water is used, cold water should be run for at least 2 minutes before using, to decrease lead exposure by clearing any lead that might be in the pipes. For the same reason, water from the hot water tap should never be used for formula preparation or for drinking. Tap water should not be boiled for more than 5 minutes because excessive boiling may concentrate lead and other impurities in the water. If bottled water is used in infant formula preparation, it should be treated the same as tap or well water (i.e., boil and cool it prior to use) unless the water is labeled as sterile.

Using a microwave oven to warm infant formula or expressed human milk or to thaw frozen human milk can cause scald injuries, palatal burns, and exploding containers. In addition, glass bottles can get hotter than plastic bottles, and the temperature of the milk may not be evenly distributed. Patient Counseling for Infant Nutrition provides specific guidelines on using a microwave oven for formula preparation.

Table 26-12 provides handling instructions and recommendations for storage of infant formulas once the original container has been opened. Human milk that is expressed should be stored in appropriate containers, refrigerated, and used within 24 to 72 hours. Human milk can be frozen for up to 1 month (3 to 6 months if in a 0°F freezer). Milk should always be used within 24 hours of thawing.

*Adverse Effects of Improperly Prepared and/or Administered Formulas* As stated previously, the failure to properly dilute a concentrated infant formula can result in a hypertonic solution that could result in diarrhea and dehydration. In extreme cases, the ingestion of an overly concentrated formula can lead to hypernatremic dehydration (induced by water deficit), metabolic acidosis, and renal failure. Excessive formula dilution can lead to water intoxication that can result in irritability, hyponatremia, coma, or brain damage. Such a situation may occur when a caregiver misunderstands the instructions for preparing a concentrated formula, dilutes a ready-to-use formula, or tries to make the baby's formula last longer by diluting it.

Parents or other caregivers may have questions about how much infant formula their child should receive. Typically, a health care provider at the hospital will have given parents feeding instructions prior to discharge. However, when a formula change is made after hospital discharge, adequate information may not be provided in some health care settings. Generally, the required daily formula intake depends on an infant's age, weight, and individual considerations such as the need for catch-up growth (Table 26-13). During the first year of life, a normal healthy formula-fed term infant usually eats every 3 to 5 hours (average 4 hours). Small or weak infants may eat every 2 to 3 hours because they have smaller stomach capacities, shorter gastric emptying times, or tire easily during feedings. Breast-fed infants or those receiving human milk from a bottle also will nurse or eat more often because human milk empties from the stomach more rapidly than formula. Most term infants will lengthen the interval between feedings to 4 hours by the age of 3 to 4 weeks. Premature infants may continue to require frequent feedings past 6 to 8 weeks of age, depending on the infant's birth weight and growth. Typically, infants begin to stop nighttime feedings after 1 to 2 months of age or when they reach 8 to 10 lb.

The amount of formula offered to a bottle-fed infant should be consistent with the DRI for energy according to age and weight (Table 26-1). Table 26-13 lists typical quantities of feedings for various age groups. The infant should be fed on demand and not forced to take more formula than is desired at any one feeding. If the infant finishes a bottle and still seems hungry, more formula should be offered. Parents should also be aware that an infant typically loses weight during the first week of life, but by 2 weeks of age, the child should be gaining weight. Appropriate weight gain usually indicates that an infant is receiving an appropriate amount of formula. The NCHS standardized growth curves are used to determine whether an infant is growing appropriately. Weight, length/height, and head circumference should be plotted at each medical visit.

Both underfeeding and overfeeding are potential problems. Breast-fed infants who like to "graze" all day can take in too much milk and gain too much weight. Other

**TABLE 26-12 Sterilization Method for Infant Formula Preparation**

### General Preparation

- Always wash hands before preparing the formula or handling bottles and nipples, and repeat washing if interrupted.
- Sterilize bottles and other equipment (e.g., glass measuring cup, spoons, nipples, rings, and disks) separately from the formula.*
  - Using tongs, place all equipment in a deep pan or sterilizer, cover all equipment with cold tap water, bring to a boil and continue boiling for 5 minutes.
  - Using tongs, remove all items from the pan or sterilizer, and place on a clean towel. Place bottles and nipples on the towel with their open ends facing down.
- Tap water and bottled water should be heated until it reaches a rolling boil, allowed to continue to boil for 1 to 2 minutes, and then allowed to cool to room temperature.† Boiling for a longer period of time may concentrate impurities (e.g., lead) in the water.

### Concentrated Liquid Formula

- Wash top of can with hot water and detergent, rinse in hot running water, and dry.
- Shake can, open it with a clean punch-type can opener.
- Mix appropriate amounts of concentrated liquid and sterilized water (according to product label or health care practitioner instructions). For accuracy, use a measuring cup for all measurements of formula and water.
- Pour formula into sterilized bottles. Place nipples, rings, and disks on bottles.
- Tightly cover any unused formula and store in refrigerator. Use formula within 48 hours of preparation or discard.

### Powdered Formula

- Wash top of can with hot water and detergent, rinse in hot running water, and dry.
- Open can, and mix appropriate amounts of powder and sterilized water (according to product label or health care practitioner instructions). For accuracy, use the scoop provided or a dry measuring cup for all measurements.
- Pour formula into sterilized bottles. Place nipples, rings, and disks on the bottles.
- Tightly cover any unused formula, and store in the refrigerator. Use formula within 48 hours of preparation.
- Cover any formula remaining in the can with the plastic top. Store in a cool, dry place for up to 1 month.

### Ready-to-Use Formula

*Cans*

- Wash top of can with hot water and detergent, rinse in hot running water, and dry.
- Shake can well to mix the formula, and open it with a clean punch-type can opener.
- Add the amount of formula needed for a single feeding to one sterilized bottle or to the number of bottles needed for a full day's feedings.
- *Do not add water.*
- Place nipple and ring on bottle.
- Prepared bottles and any formula left in the can should be tightly covered and refrigerated for up to 48 hours after the can was opened.

*Bottles*

- The protective cap must be removed, and a sterile nipple screwed onto the bottle before feeding.
- Shake each bottle well to ensure mixing of formula.

### All Types of Formulas

- Warm bottle to desired temperature by immersing in hot water bath or running under hot water.
- Heating bottles in the microwave is not recommended.
- Never boil or overheat formula.
- Test formula temperature before feeding infant.
- Shake each bottle well before feeding infant.
- After feeding, discard any formula left in bottle, and immediately rinse bottle and nipple in cool water.

* If disposable bottle liners are used, only nipples, rings, and screw tops of bottles need to be sterilized. The manufacturer has sterilized the bottle liners.

† Not all health care practitioners recommend boiling water; however, AAP recommends boiling municipal water. They do not have a recommendation on bottled waters, but these are not guaranteed to be sterile.

**TABLE 26-13 Average Age-appropriate Number of Daily Feedings and Average Volume per Feeding**

| Age | Average No. of Daily Feedings | Average Volume per Feeding (oz) |
|---|---|---|
| Birth-2 weeks | 6-10 | 2-3 |
| 2 weeks-1 month | 6-8 | 4-5 |
| 1-3 months | 5-6 | 5-6 |
| 3-4 months | 4-5 | 6-7 |
| 4-12 months | 3-4 | 7-8 |

problems associated with overfeeding are regurgitation, gastroesophageal reflux, vomiting, loose stools, constipation, and colic. Spitting up a small amount of formula, even if it is after every feeding, is usually not a cause for concern. If an infant is regurgitating or vomiting significant amounts, a primary care provider should be consulted. Bilious (green) emesis is always a reason to consult the child's primary care practitioner.

Loose stools can be normal for some infants, especially those receiving human milk or hydrolyzed formulas. They may also be caused by an improperly concentrated formula, overfeeding, or administration of contaminated formula. Human milk–fed infants may have only one stool every 1 to 3 days. However, some human milk–fed infants will have 10 to 12 stools each day. Formula-fed infants usually have 1 to 3 stools per day. Diarrhea, defined as increased stool volume and frequency from the usual volume and frequency, warrants medical attention. Constipation is rare in human milk–fed or formula-fed infants. It is most often a result of inadequate formula intake. Severe or prolonged constipation with straining and streaks of blood on the stool warrant a visit to the primary care provider.

### Product Selection Guidelines

For healthy, term infants who do not need a therapeutic formula, a milk-based formula or a milk-based formula with added whey protein is indicated. When recommending a formula, the clinician should consider preparation methods, the caregiver's ability to follow directions, the parents' attitudes and preferences, sanitary conditions and refrigeration facilities available, and cost. Before assisting parents in selecting a therapeutic formula, the clinician should determine whether a primary care provider recommended the formula.

For many parents, cost may be a critical factor in formula selection. Concentrated liquids and powders are typically less expensive than ready-to-use products. Convenience is also a consideration. The preparation of powdered and concentrated liquid formulas requires more manipulative functions and more attention to clean technique. The formula selected should be one that is well tolerated by the infant, convenient for the parents, and priced to fit the family's budget. To simplify formula preparation away from home, parents can select products that are available in unit-of-use packaging for ready-to-use liquids and powder packets.

The federally funded Special Supplemental Nutrition Program for Women, Infants, and Children (WIC) helps ensure that all infants, children (up to 5 years of age), and pregnant, postpartum, and breast-feeding women have access to adequate nutrition. State health departments and other agencies administer the federal grant program (i.e., a specific amount—$5.2 billion in 2005—is allocated for the program each year, and distributed to the states). Formula and other preventive services are free to eligible participants. More than 7.6 million people received WIC benefits each month in 2003, most of them infants and children.[44]

## Vitamin and Mineral Supplementation

Routine multivitamin and mineral supplementation is unnecessary for most formula-fed, term infants or for normal, human milk–fed infants of well-nourished mothers. However, some healthy infants may be at risk and require supplementation. Cases of vitamin D–deficiency rickets continue to be reported in the United States, and iron-deficiency anemia is still a problem despite routine use of iron-fortified formulas and infant foods. Recent information suggests that the prevalence of iron deficiency in children 1 to 2 years of age is high and particular care should be given to ensure that children in this age group get adequate dietary iron. AAP does not endorse routine iron supplementation in this age group at this time.

Vitamin and mineral supplementation may be needed for preterm and human milk–fed infants whose mothers are inadequately nourished (Table 26-14). These infants and those with other nutritional deficiencies, malabsorptive and other chronic diseases, rare vitamin-dependent conditions, inborn errors of vitamin or mineral metabolism, or deficiencies related to the intake of certain medications will need medically supervised vitamin and mineral supplementation.

### *Human Milk–fed, Full-term Infants*

In routine circumstances, the healthy, full-term human milk–fed infant requires little to no special supplementation for the first 4 to 6 months of life except for vitamin D and iron. AAP recommends vitamin D supplementation (200 IU/day; cholecalciferol 5 mg/day) for all human milk–fed infants unless they are weaned to at least 500 mL/day of vitamin D–fortified formula. Risk factors for vitamin D deficiency include increased birth order (third child or later), dark skin, cultural factors that minimize maternal skin exposure to sunlight, and delayed intake of dairy products in the infant or mother because of intolerance or other factors.[45] Mothers should be encouraged to maintain a balanced diet and to drink three to five 8 oz glasses of milk each day while breast-feeding. If the mother cannot tolerate milk because of lactose intolerance, lactose digestion aids (e.g., Lactaid, Dairy Aid, Lactogest, or Dairy Ease) or lactose-free milk are available. Mothers who do not drink milk should be encouraged to increase vitamin D and calcium intake through other dietary sources or by taking supplements.

Human milk–fed infants rarely develop iron-deficiency anemia before 4 to 6 months of age. Iron concentration in human milk averages only 0.3 to 0.5 mg/L, but the form of iron is well absorbed. At 4 to 6 months of age and beyond, the iron stores in infants exclusively human milk–fed may become exhausted, requiring a supplemental source. The addition of iron-enriched foods such as fortified infant cereals will usually meet needs, or alternatively, an iron supplement (elemental iron 2 mg as ferrous sulfate/kilogram per day) can be given. Term infants who are small-for-gestational age are likely to have higher requirements, but the necessity of supplementation in this population is unclear.[46]

The first iron-enriched food introduced into the infant's diet is typically infant cereal. Bioavailability of the large-particle, electrolytic iron powder used to fortify dry infant cereals is substantially less than that of the ferrous sulfate iron used in milk- or soy protein–based formulas. Cereals also contain potent inhibitors of iron absorption and are unreliable in preventing iron deficiency when infants receive minimal iron from other sources. Iron-fortified, wet-packed cereal and fruit combinations marketed in jars offer no exposure of the iron sulfate to oxygen until the jar is opened; therefore, iron absorption is improved. Consuming fruit juices and other products containing ascorbic acid along with iron-fortified cereals has been shown to enhance iron absorption.[47]

**TABLE 26-14 Guidelines for Use of Vitamin and Mineral Supplements in Healthy Infants***

| | Multivitamin/Mineral | Vitamin D† | Vitamin E‡ | Folate | Iron§ |
|---|---|---|---|---|---|
| **Full-term Infants** | | | | | |
| Human milk–fed | 0 | + | 0 | 0 | ± |
| Formula-fed | 0 | ±‖ | 0 | 0 | 0 |
| **Preterm Infants** | | | | | |
| Human milk–fed¶ | + | + | 0 | 0 | + |
| Formula-fed¶ | + | + | 0 | 0 | + |
| **Older Infants (>6 Months)** | | | | | |
| Normal | 0 | 0 | 0 | 0 | ± |
| High-risk# | + | 0 | 0 | 0 | ± |

Key: +, supplement usually indicated; ±, supplement possibly or sometimes indicated; 0, supplement not usually indicated.

* Not shown is vitamin K for newborn infants and fluoride in areas where there is insufficient fluoride in the water.

† All infants should have a minimal intake of 200 IU vitamin D per day beginning during the first 2 months of life; this intake should be continued throughout childhood and adolescence.

‡ Vitamin E should be in a form that is well absorbed by small, preterm infants. If this form of vitamin E is present in formulas, it need not be given separately to formula-fed infants. Infants fed human milk are less susceptible to vitamin E deficiency.

§ Iron-fortified formula and/or infant cereal is a more convenient and reliable source of iron than a supplement.

‖ If receiving less than 500 mL/day of infant formula.

¶ Multivitamin supplements (plus added folate) are needed primarily when calorie intake is below approximately 300 kcal/day or when the infant weighs less than 2.5 kg; vitamin D should be supplied at least until 6 months of age in human milk–fed infants. Iron should be started by 2 months of age.

# Multivitamin/mineral preparations including iron are preferred to supplements containing iron alone.

*Source:* Adapted from Committee on Nutrition American Academy of Pediatrics. Vitamins. In: Kleinman RE, ed. *Pediatric Nutrition Handbook*. 5th edition. Elk Grove Village, Ill: American Academy of Pediatrics; 2004: 339-65; and reference 5.

### *Formula-fed, Full-term Infants*

Full-term infants who consume adequate amounts of an iron-fortified, milk-based formula do not need vitamin and mineral supplementation in the first 6 months of life. An iron-fortified formula is preferred to ensure adequate iron stores for growing infants. Infants fed iron-fortified formulas do not demonstrate a difference in stool consistency, fussiness, colic, or regurgitation compared with infants fed low-iron formulas. Vitamin and mineral supplements are not needed for infants older than 6 months who receive a diet of formula and increasing amounts of infant and table foods. A multivitamin with minerals may be needed, however, if the infant is at special nutritional risk.

### *Preterm Infants*

Preterm infants, either human milk–fed or formula-fed, need vitamin and mineral supplementation. Their nutrient needs are greater than those of full-term infants because of their more rapid growth rate, inability to ingest an adequate volume of formula or human milk, decreased intestinal absorption, and decreased body stores. Until these infants can consume about 300 kcal/day or until they reach a body weight of 2.5 kg, a multivitamin supplement should be administered to provide the equivalent of the recommended intakes for full-term infants.

Premature infants are especially susceptible to iron-deficiency anemia because of marginal iron stores at birth. Without supplementation (e.g., blood transfusions), iron stores will be depleted by 2 months of age, in contrast to depletion at 4 to 6 months of age in full-term infants. AAP/CON recommends iron supplementation at a dosage of 2 mg elemental iron per kilogram daily for premature infants with birth weights between 1500 and 2500 g once they are 2 months old or have doubled their birth weight.[30,37] Preterm infants weighing less than 1500 g should receive 4 mg elemental iron per kilogram daily and those receiving erythropoietin should receive 6 mg elemental iron per kilogram daily. To minimize the possibility of hemolytic anemia in infants with insufficient vitamin E absorption, iron supplements should be withheld until the preterm infant is several weeks old. However, with adequate vitamin E supplementation in formula, the risk of hemolytic anemia is minimal.

Supplementation of calcium, phosphorus, and vitamin D in preterm infant formulas is necessary to ensure adequate bone mineralization and to prevent osteopenia and rickets. The prevention of severe bone disease in preterm infants appears to depend on both high oral intakes of calcium and phosphorus and the intake of at least vitamin D 400 IU (12.5 mg) per day.[37] Therefore, preterm infants should receive a special preterm infant formula containing appropriate amounts of calcium, phosphorus, and vitamin D.

### *Fluoride Supplementation*

When used appropriately, fluoride is both safe and effective in preventing and controlling dental caries. Fluoride reduces dental decay by reducing the solubility of enamel, reducing the ability of bacteria to produce acid, and promoting remineralization. Systemic fluoride, such as that obtained from fluoridated water, primarily provides a topical benefit to teeth as fluoride is secreted from the salivary glands. Slightly less than two thirds of the municipalities in the United States optimally fluoridate water at a cost of $0.50 per person per year.[48]

Fluoride supplementation is currently not recommended from birth to 6 months of age. Furthermore, the recommended supplementation for children 6 months to 6 years of age whose drinking water is inadequately fluoridated and who do not receive adequate fluoride from other sources has been decreased from previous recommendations because of an increased incidence of fluorosis.[49] Fluorosis, which affects approximately 22% of children, is a cosmetic change in the appearance of the teeth ranging from minor white lines running across the teeth to a very chalky appearance resulting from too much fluoride. If a powdered or concentrated formula is used, fluoride supplements should be administered only if the community's drinking water contains less than fluoride 0.3 ppm. Table 26-15 can be used to determine the proper fluoride supplementation for a child, depending on the level of fluoride in the drinking water. Ready-to-use formulas are manufactured with defluoridated water and contain less than fluoride 0.3 ppm. If an infant fed ready-to-use formula does not drink water, the primary care provider may recommend a fluoride supplement.

**TABLE 26-15 Recommended Fluoride Supplementation (mg/day)***

| | Fluoride Concentration of Drinking Water (ppm) | | |
|---|---|---|---|
| **Age** | **<0.3** | **0.3-0.6** | **>0.6** |
| Birth-6 months | 0 | 0 | 0 |
| 6 months-3 years | 0.25 | 0 | 0 |
| 3-6 years | 0.50 | 0.25 | 0 |
| 6-16 years | 1.00 | 0.50 | 0 |

* Sodium fluoride 2.2 mg contains fluoride 1 mg.

*Sources*: References 48 and 49.

## Assessment of Infant Nutrition: A Case-based Approach

Body weight, length, and head circumference are the growth standards for determining whether infants are receiving the appropriate nutrients, are properly using ingested nutrients, or both. If an infant appears to be underweight or underdeveloped, the clinician should advise the parent to take the infant to a primary care provider for evaluation.

The practitioner's primary role is to provide information about breast-feeding and infant formula products, including assistance with product selection and preparation instructions. Cases 26-1 and 26-2 illustrate assessment of infant nutrition.

**CASE 26-1**

| Relevant Evaluation Criteria | Scenario/Model Outcome |
|---|---|
| **Information Gathering** | |
| 1. Gather essential information about the patient's symptoms, including: | |
| a. description of symptom(s) (i.e., nature, onset, duration, severity, associated symptoms) | Infant is spitting up formula after every feeding; sometimes forcefully vomits formula after a feeding. Some emesis has occurred since birth, but the amount and frequency has increased over the last week since weaning from human milk to exclusively formula. Infant has also developed a significant problem with gas; often cries in association with the gas. |
| b. description of any factors that seem to precipitate, exacerbate, and/or relieve the patient's symptoms. | Emesis occurs only following feedings. Infant seems to be less irritable after emesis episodes. Gas is often relieved by the use of simethicone. |
| c. description of the patient's efforts to relieve the symptoms | Simethicone has been used intermittently to treat gas pains. |

## CASE 26-1 (continued)

| Relevant Evaluation Criteria | Scenario/Model Outcome |
|---|---|
| 2. Gather essential patient history information including: | |
| a. patient's identity | Johnny Jones (JJ) |
| b. patient's age, sex, height, and weight | 7-week-old M, 22", 8 lb 2 oz; weight, length, and head circumference have grown appropriately since birth, as measured at his 6-week well-baby check-up |
| c. patient's occupation | Mom is a receptionist in a medical office. Dad is a medical equipment salesman. |
| d. patient's dietary habits | JJ was breast-fed until 1 week ago when his mother went back to work and weaned him from the breast. He now receives a cow milk–based formula. He is taking 150 mL (5 oz) every 4 hours. No extra water or juice is given during the day. |
| e. patient's sleep habits | He is not sleeping through the night. |
| f. concurrent medical conditions, prescription and nonprescription medications, and dietary supplements | No other medical conditions; otherwise healthy infant |
| g. allergies | NKA |
| h. history of other adverse reactions to medications | None |
| i. other (describe)_______ | Powdered formula is used. Parents are mixing 1 scoop with 2 oz water. They use well water and boil it as instructed by their primary care provider. Otherwise they follow the directions on the can. |
| **Assessment and Triage** | |
| 3. Differentiate the patient's signs/symptoms and correctly identify the patient's primary problem(s). | Primary problem: emesis with feedings; secondary problem: increased intestinal gas production |
| 4. Identify exclusions for self-treatment. | Self-treatment is not recommended if the infant has significant vomiting after every feeding, appears dehydrated, or has bilious (green) or blood-tinged emesis. |
| 5. Formulate a comprehensive list of therapeutic alternatives for the primary problem to determine if triage to a medical practitioner is required, and share this information with the caregiver. | Options include:<br>(1) Recommend changes in feeding amount and schedule.<br>(2) Recommend change in type of formula.<br>(3) Refer JJ to his PCP for evaluation.<br>(4) Take no action. |
| **Plan** | |
| 6. Select an optimal therapeutic alternative to address the patient's problem, taking into account patient/caregiver preferences. | According to the DRI for calories at his age (see Table 26-1), JJ should be receiving 100 mL every 4 hours of a 20 kcal/oz formula. He is receiving 150 mL every 4 hours, 50% more than needed. |
| 7. Describe the recommended therapeutic approach to the caregiver. | The best initial option is to decrease amount of formula to 3.5 oz (105 mL) every 4 hours. If JJ seems to be hungry on that schedule, he can receive 2.5 oz (75 mL) every 3 hours instead. If symptoms continue after 3 to 5 days on this schedule, another formula such as a lactose-free cow milk–based or soy protein–based formula (see Table 26-6) might be appropriate for JJ. You should discuss this with JJ's PCP, that is, primary care provider, before making any change.<br>If symptoms worsen, especially if you see blood in his stools, he may have a cow milk–protein allergy, and JJ should be seen by his PCP to decide if a special hydrolysate formula (see Table 26-6) is indicated.<br>If the vomiting worsens or if JJ fails to gain weight or has other complications (e.g., pneumonia, trouble breathing), he should be seen by his primary care provider to evaluate for gastroesophageal reflux disease, pyloric stenosis, or other conditions. |

**CASE 26-1 (continued)**

| Relevant Evaluation Criteria | Scenario/Model Outcome |
|---|---|
| 8. Explain to the caregiver the rationale for selecting the recommended therapeutic approach from the considered therapeutic alternatives. | Because the symptoms started (or worsened) with the change to bottle feedings, and the volume of the bottle feedings is more than the amount usually required by an infant of JJ's weight and age, overfeeding is the most likely cause of his problems. Reducing JJ's intake of formula will have almost immediate results if overfeeding is the cause of his symptoms. |
| **Patient Education** | |
| 9. When recommending self-care with nonprescription medications and/or nondrug therapy, convey accurate information to the caregiver, including: | |
| a. appropriate dose and frequency of administration | New feeding regimen: 3.5 oz every 4 hours or 2.5 oz every 3 hours |
| b. maximum number of days the therapy should be employed | If no improvement has occurred in 3 to 5 days, JJ will need to be seen by his PCP to determine if another feeding or formula change is appropriate. |
| c. product administration procedures | The formula should be mixed per product instructions (i.e., 1 scoop per 2 oz water). See the box Patient Education for Infant Nutrition. |
| d. expected time to onset of relief | Significant improvement may be seen almost immediately. |
| e. degree of relief that can be reasonably expected | Emesis will not likely be completely eliminated. All infants have some gastroesophageal reflux and will spit up or vomit from time to time. |
| f. most common side effects | N/A |
| g. side effects that warrant medical intervention should they occur | JJ should be evaluated by his PCP if he has any of the following symptoms: persistent severe vomiting, weight loss, dehydration, recurrent respiratory illnesses, or bloody stools. |
| h. caregiver options in the event that condition worsens or persists | Contact JJ's PCP to evaluate for cow milk–protein allergy, gastroesophageal reflux disease, or other conditions. |
| i. product storage requirements | See product label information and Table 26-12. |
| j. specific nondrug measures | (1) Burp JJ several times during each feeding.<br>(2) Keep JJ in an upright position and do not bounce him immediately after feedings.<br>(3) Avoid forcing JJ's legs into a flexed position (e.g., sitting in a car seat, changing his diaper) immediately after feedings, if possible. |
| 10. Solicit follow-up questions from caregiver. | (1) What if JJ does not seem satisfied with the smaller amount of formula?<br>(2) What if JJ continues to throw up after every feeding? |
| 11. Answer caregiver's questions. | (1) JJ has been vomiting the additional formula that he has received because his stomach was distended by each feeding. The new volume should still adequately fill his stomach, and he should be satisfied. Try other soothing techniques after feedings to calm him if he is fussy. If he still seems hungry, you may try to feed him an additional 1/2 oz (15 mL) after waiting 15 to 20 minutes.<br>(2) If vomiting occurs for more than 3 to 5 days after the change in feeding volume, call JJ's PCP. |

Key: N/A, not applicable; NKA, no known allergies; PCP, primary care provider.

## Patient Counseling for Infant Nutrition

The number and variety of infant formulas available may bewilder some parents. Once the formula type recommended or prescribed by the baby's primary care provider is known, the clinician can direct parents to the appropriate products. If parents need further assistance with product selection, the practitioner can recommend a product to match the parents' preferences. At these encounters, the parents should be questioned to make sure they know how to properly prepare their baby's formula and how much formula to give at each feeding. The box Patient Education for Infant Nutrition lists specific information to provide parents. Additionally, families who may qualify for WIC but are not enrolled can be advised of its availability and benefits.

## CASE 26-2

| Relevant Evaluation Criteria | Scenario/Model Outcome |
|---|---|
| **Information Gathering** | |
| 1. Gather essential information about the patient's symptoms, including: | |
| a. description of symptom(s) (i.e., nature, onset, duration, severity, associated symptoms) | Infant cries constantly. She always seems to be hungry and wants to eat all day. She rarely goes more than 2 hours between feedings. She has lots of wet diapers and only 1 bowel movement each day. She doesn't seem to have gained any weight in the last 2 weeks. |
| b. description of any factors that seem to precipitate, exacerbate, and/or relieve the patient's symptoms. | Crying is relieved by giving a bottle, but only for a short period of time. |
| c. description of the patient's efforts to relieve the symptoms | Mother has tried simethicone, acetaminophen, frequent diaper changes, and different pacifiers. Nothing works but giving a bottle. |
| 2. Gather essential patient history information, including: | |
| a. patient's identity | Maria Sanchez |
| b. patient's age, sex, height, and weight | 7-week-old F, 19", 5 lb 6 oz; born at 28 weeks gestational age |
| c. patient's occupation | Mom works at a hotel as a housekeeper. Dad is currently between jobs. Both parents speak Spanish and a little English. |
| d. patient's dietary habits | Maria is receiving a transition formula for premature infants (see Table 26-6). She has been taking 75 mL (2.5 oz) every 2 to 3 hours since she was discharged from the hospital last week. |
| e. patient's sleep habits | MS rarely sleeps more than 2 hours at a time. She is not sleeping through the night. |
| f. concurrent medical conditions, prescription and nonprescription medications, and dietary supplements | MS was diagnosed with gastroesophageal reflux and is on metoclopramide 0.3 mg by mouth 4 times/day and ranitidine 7.5 mg by mouth 2 times/day. |
| g. allergies | NKA |
| h. history of other adverse reactions to medications | None |
| i. other (describe)______ | Mom is mixing 1 scoop powder with 4 oz water.<br>Mom lost the instruction sheet she was given at discharge. She says that it was written in English, and she could not read it. Mom states that they have had a hard time buying the amount of formula that Maria needs. |
| **Assessment and Triage** | |
| 3. Differentiate the patient's signs/symptoms and correctly identify the patient's primary problem(s). | Primary problem: persistent crying, likely resulting from hunger. Most likely etiology: improper preparation of formula. Administration of dilute formula results in increased intake by the infant to try to take in enough calories. Could be other causes such as otitis media, but in the absence of fever, infection is unlikely. |
| 4. Identify exclusions for self-treatment. | Self-treatment is not recommended if the infant has significant vomiting or diarrhea, appears dehydrated or otherwise clinically ill, or has bilious (green) or blood-tinged emesis or bloody stools. |
| 5. Formulate a comprehensive list of therapeutic alternatives for the primary problem to determine if triage to a medical practitioner is required, and share this information with the caregiver. | Options include:<br>(1) Give Mom appropriate instructions in Spanish for preparing formula at the correct strength. Contact PCP to follow-up and reinforce information at the next visit.<br>(2) Have Mom take Maria to her PCP for evaluation.<br>(3) Take no action. |

## CASE 26-2 (continued)

| Relevant Evaluation Criteria | Scenario/Model Outcome |
|---|---|
| **Plan** | |
| 6. Select an optimal therapeutic alternative to address the patient's problem, taking into account patient/caregiver preferences. | Because mixing the formula correctly will result in almost immediate response from the infant, Mom will be given directions on how to appropriately mix the formula. |
| 7. Describe the recommended therapeutic approach to the caregiver. | You should mix formula as directed on the can: 1 scoop with every 2 oz of water. Give Maria 1.5-2 oz (45-60 mL) formula every 3 hours. The county health department can give you information on the WIC program, which helps families buy formula and food for infants and children.<br>Request follow-up the next 1 to 2 days. If mixing formula correctly doesn't stop Maria's constant hunger and provide good weight gain, you should talk with MS's PCP, that is, primary care provider, to determine if there are other reasons for the problem. |
| 8. Explain to the caregiver the rationale for selecting the recommended therapeutic approach from the considered therapeutic alternatives. | Because the formula is too weak, Maria is not getting enough calories with each feeding. She is hungry most of the time, which is the most likely reason for her symptoms. Let's see how she does with this change before looking for other causes for her crying. |
| **Patient Education** | |
| 9. When recommending self-care with nonprescription medications and/or nondrug therapy, convey accurate information to the caregiver, including: | |
| a. appropriate dose and frequency of administration | Maria should eat 1.5-2 oz (45-60 mL) of properly prepared formula approximately every 3 hours. |
| b. maximum number of days the therapy should be employed | Crying should be reduced and satisfaction should improve within 1 to 2 days. Feedings volume should then increase gradually as the baby grows. |
| c. product administration procedures | Formula should be mixed per product instructions. (Practitioner should provide written instructions in Spanish, available from manufacturers' Web sites, and review the instructions verbally with the parents.) |
| d. expected time to onset of relief | Within days |
| e. degree of relief that can be reasonably expected | All infants will cry. Crying will not be eliminated, but the infant should seem better satisfied between feedings. |
| f. most common side effects | N/A |
| g. side effects that warrant medical intervention should they occur | Maria has gastroesophageal reflux, and as medication dosages are outgrown, vomiting or spitting up may recur. Symptoms could be more evident once formula is made correctly, but this is unlikely as the volume consumed will likely decrease. |
| h. caregiver options in the event that condition worsens or persists | Call the child's PCP. |
| i. product storage requirements | Per product labeling |
| j. specific nondrug measures | (1) Burp Maria several times during each feeding.<br>(2) Keep Maria in an upright position and do not bounce her immediately after feedings.<br>(3) Avoid forcing Maria's legs into a flexed position (e.g., sitting in a car seat, changing her diaper) immediately after feedings, if possible. |
| 10. Solicit follow-up questions from caregiver. | (1) What if my baby doesn't stop eating so much?<br>(2) What if my baby is not gaining weight? |

## CASE 26-2 (continued)

| Relevant Evaluation Criteria | Scenario/Model Outcome |
|---|---|
| 11. Answer caregiver's questions. | (1) Once you start mixing the formula correctly, Maria should be satisfied with less formula. You may need to give an additional small amount if she does not seem satisfied after a feeding.<br>(2) If Maria does not start gaining weight with this change, you should take her to the PCP, who will look for other causes of poor weight gain. |

## PATIENT EDUCATION FOR INFANT NUTRITION

Optimal nutrition is critical in infants and children to ensure normal growth and development. Parents who carefully follow product instructions and the measures listed here will help ensure optimal nutrition-related outcomes.

- Check unopened formula containers for damage. Do not use products if they are significantly dented or if the expiration date has passed.
- When preparing formula from powder or liquid concentrate, carefully follow instructions for diluting the formula to the desired caloric density (see Tables 26-9 and 26-10). If the formula is too concentrated, the baby may have diarrhea or become dehydrated. If it is too dilute, the baby can become water intoxicated, which might lead to irritability, seizures, coma, or brain damage.
- When preparing formula from powder or liquid concentrate, follow the technique for aseptic sterilization. Be sure to sterilize the bottles (or use sterile liners) and other equipment, and boil the water used to make the formula (see Table 26-12).
- When preparing ready-to-use formulas, do not add water to the formula. Follow the instructions in Table 26-12. Be sure to sterilize the bottles (or use sterile liners) and other equipment.
- Use prepared or opened ready-to-use formula within 48 hours. Keep refrigerated.
- Feed your baby according to the frequency and quantities listed in Table 26-13 unless instructed otherwise by the baby's primary care provider.
- Heating formula in a microwave is not recommended. However, if formula or human milk is warmed in a microwave, follow the instructions below to prevent exploding containers, scalds, or burns to the baby's mouth:
  - Remove the bottle cover to allow heat to escape.
  - Heat only 4 oz or more of refrigerated milk; do not thaw frozen human milk in a microwave. Place frozen human milk in a warm water bath to thaw.
  - Heat 4 oz of refrigerated formula on full power for no longer than 30 seconds; heat 8 oz of refrigerated formula for 45 seconds.
  - After heating the formula, replace the nipple assembly and invert the bottle a minimum of 10 times.
  - Test the formula's temperature by putting a few drops on your tongue or the top part of your hand or the back of the wrist. Do not feed the baby any formula unless it feels cool to the touch.

Seek medical attention if:

- Your baby is regurgitating or vomiting significant amounts of formula. A small amount of spitting up is normal. Projectile vomiting or bilious vomiting (i.e., green) always requires immediate medical attention.
- Your baby has severe diarrhea or diarrhea that persists for more than 3 to 5 days.
- Your baby appears dehydrated (e.g., decreased number of wet diapers, dark urine, limp, no tears, or lethargic).
- Your baby's bowel movements have blood in them.

## Key Points for Infant Nutrition and Special Nutritional Needs of Children

- Human milk is the optimal food for infants under 12 months of age, and its use should be encouraged for nearly all infants. When breast-feeding or provision of human milk is not possible or desired, commercial infant formulas provide a safe, nutritionally adequate substitute.
- Commercial formulas are available in a variety of types to meet the needs of most infants and children with special nutritional needs, including premature infants and those with alterations in nutrition needs caused by disease or other conditions. Therapeutic formulas vary in content and are not generally generically equivalent.
- Accurate preparation of formula is critical to ensure optimal nutrition outcomes. Patients should be counseled on proper preparation techniques.
- Some infants will require vitamin and/or mineral supplementation when needs are not adequately met by their formula intake.
- Parents should be referred to their child's primary care provider if their infant or child has persistent vomiting or at any time the emesis is bilious (green).
- Parents should be referred to their child's primary care provider if their infant or child has diarrhea lasting more than 3 to 5 days, especially if dehydration develops, if the child looks clinically ill, or if there is blood in the bowel movements.

## References


1. Committee on Nutrition, American Academy of Pediatrics. Infant nutrition and the development of gastrointestinal function. In: Kleinman RE, ed. *Pediatric Nutrition Handbook.* 5th ed. Elk Grove Village, Ill: American Academy of Pediatrics; 2004:3-22.
2. Garcia-Careagg M, Kerner JA. Malabsorptive disorders. In: Behrman RE, Kliegman RM, Jenson HB, eds. *Nelson Textbook of Pediatrics.* 17th ed. Philadelphia: Elsevier Science; 2004:1258-72.
3. Kuczmarski RJ, Ogden CL, Grummer-Strawn LM, et al. *CDC Growth Charts: United States.* Advance data from vital and health statistics no. 314. Hyattsville, Md: National Center for Health Statistics; 2000. DHHS Pub No. PHS 2000–1250. Available at: www.cdc.gov/growth_charts. Accessed November 6, 2005.
4. Institute of Medicine, Food and Nutrition Board, Standing Committee on the Scientific Evaluation of Dietary Reference Intakes. *Reference Intakes for Energy, Carbohydrate, Fiber, Fat, Fatty Acids, Cholesterol, Protein, and Amino Acids.* Washington, DC: National Academy Press; 2002. Available at: www.nal.usda.gov/fnic/etext/000105.html. Accessed November 6, 2005.
5. Committee on Nutrition, American Academy of Pediatrics. Carbohydrate and dietary fiber. In: Kleinman RE, ed. *Pediatric Nutrition Handbook.* 5th ed. Elk Grove Village, Ill: American Academy of Pediatrics; 2004:247-59.
6. Chesney RW, Helms RA, Christensen M, et al. An updated view of the value of taurine in infant nutrition. *Adv Pediatr.* 1998;45:179-200.
7. Committee on Nutrition, American Academy of Pediatrics. Cholesterol in childhood. *Pediatrics.* 1998:101:141-7. Guideline reaffirmed by AAP in April 2001.
8. Bier DM, Brosnan JT, Flatt RW, et al. Report of the IDECG Working Group in lower and upper limits of carbohydrate and fat intake. *Eur J Clin Nutr.* 1999;53:S177-8.
9. O'Connor DL, Hall R, Adamkin D, et al. Growth and development in preterm infants fed long-chain polyunsaturated fatty acids: a prospective, randomized controlled trial. *Pediatrics.* 2001;108:359-71.
10. Birch EE, Hoffman DR, Castañeda YS, et al. A randomized controlled trial of long-chain polyunsaturated fatty acid supplementation of formula in term infants after weaning at 6 weeks of age. *Am J Clin Nutr.* 2002;75:570-80.
11. Lucas A, Stafford M, Morley R, et al. Efficacy and safety of long-chain polyunsaturated fatty acid supplementation of infant-formula milk: a randomised trial. *Lancet.* 1999; 354:1948-54.
12. Innis SM, Adamkin DH, Hall RT, et al. Docosahexaenoic acid and arachidonic acid enhance growth with no adverse effects in preterm infants fed formula. *J Pediatr.* 2002;140:547-54.
13. SanGiovanni JP, Parra-Cabrera S, Colditz GA, et al. Meta-analysis of dietary essential fatty acids and long-chain polyunsaturated fatty acids as they relate to visual resolution acuity in healthy preterm infants. *Pediatrics.* 2000;105:1292-8.
14. Birch EE, Castañeda YS, Wheaton DH, et al. Visual maturation of term infants fed long-chain polyunsaturated fatty acid-supplemented or control formula for 12 mo. *Am J Clin Nutr.* 2005;81:871-9.
15. Clandinin MT, Van Aerde JE, Merkel KL, et al. Growth and development of preterm infants fed infant formulas containing docosahexaenoic acid and arachidonic acid. *J Pediatr.* 2005:146:461-8.
16. Makrides M, Neumann MA, Simmer K, et al. A critical appraisal of the role of dietary long-chain polyunsaturated fatty acids on neural indices of term infants: a randomized, controlled trial. *Pediatrics.* 2000;105:32-8.
17. Auestad N, Halter R, Halla RT, et al. Growth and development in term infants fed long-chain polyunsaturated fatty acids: a double-masked, randomized, parallel, prospective, multivariate study. *Pediatrics.* 2001;108:372-81.
18. Newton ER. The epidemiology of breastfeeding. *Clin Obstet Gynecol.* 2004;47:613-23.
19. Section on Breastfeeding, American Academy of Pediatrics. Breastfeeding and the use of human milk. *Pediatrics.* 2005;115:496-506. Also available at: http://www.pediatrics.org/cgi/content/full/115/2/496. Accessed November 6, 2005.
20. U.S. Department of Health and Human Services. *Healthy People 2000: National Health Promotion and Disease Prevention Objectives.* Washington, DC: U.S. Government Printing Office; 1990. Publication no. PHS 9450212.
21. U.S. Department of Health and Human Services. *Healthy People 2010.* Washington, DC: U.S. Government Printing Office; 2000.
22. Brown LP, Bair AH, Meier PP. Does federal funding for breastfeeding research target our national health objectives? *Pediatrics.* 2003;111:e360-4.
23. Jacobson SW, Chiodo LM, Jacobson JL. Breastfeeding effects on intelligence quotient in 4- and 11-year old children. *Pediatrics.* 1999;103:e71.
24. Ball TM, Bennett DM. The economic impact of breastfeeding. *Pediatr Clin North Am.* 2001;48:253-62.
25. Briggs GG, Freeman RK, Yaffee SJ, ed. Drugs in Pregnancy and Lactation, 7th ed. Philadelphia: Lippincott Williams & Wilkins; 2005.
26. Hale TW. *Medications & Mothers' Milk 2004.* 11th ed. Amarillo, Tex: Pharmasoft Publishing, L.P.; 2004.
27. Tully MR. A year of remarkable growth for donor milk banking in North America. *J Hum Lact.* 2000;16:235-6.
28. Tully MR, Lockhart-Borman L, Updegrove K. Stories of success: the use of donor breast milk is increasing in North American. *J Hum Lact.* 2004;20:75-7.
29. Committee on Nutrition, American Academy of Pediatrics. Formula feeding of term infants. In: Kleinman RE, ed. *Pediatric Nutrition Handbook.* 5th ed. Elk Grove Village, Ill: American Academy of Pediatrics; 2004:87-97.
30. Committee on Nutrition, American Academy of Pediatrics. Iron fortification of infant formulas. *Pediatrics.*1999;104:119-23. Guideline reaffirmed by AAP in November 2002.
31. Centers for Disease Control and Prevention. Enterobacter sakazakii infections associated with the use of powdered infant formula—Tennessee, 2001. *MMWR Morb Mortal Wkly Rep.* 2002;51:297-300.
32. Baker RD. Infant formula safety. *Pediatrics.* 2002;110: 833-5.
33. Fomon SJ, Ziegler EE. Renal solute load and potential renal solute load in infancy. *J Pediatr.* 1999;134:11-4.
34. Committee on Nutrition, American Academy of Pediatrics. Soy protein-based formulas: recommendations for use in infant feeding. *Pediatrics.* 1998;101:148-53. Guideline reaffirmed by AAP in April 2001.
35. Committee on Nutrition, American Academy of Pediatrics. Hypoallergenic infant formulas. *Pediatrics.* 2000;106:346-9.
36. Setchell KD, Zimmer-Nechemias L, Cai J, et al. Isoflavone content of infant formula and the metabolic fate of these phytoestrogens in early life. *Am J Clin Nutr.* 1998;68(6 suppl):1453-61S.
37. Ellis L, Kalnias D, Corey M, et al. Do infants with cystic fibrosis need a protein hydrolysate formula? A prospective, randomized, comparative study. *J Pediatr.* 1998;132:270-6.
38. Committee on Nutrition, American Academy of Pediatrics. Nutritional needs of preterm infants. In: Kleinman RE, ed. *Pediatric Nutrition Handbook.* 5th ed. Elk Grove Village, Ill: American Academy of Pediatrics; 2004:23-54.
39. Reis BB, Hall RT, Schanler RJ, et al. Enhanced growth of preterm infants fed a new powdered human milk fortifier: a randomized, controlled trial. *Pediatrics.* 2000;106:581-8.

40. Porcelli P, Schanler R, Greer F, et al. Growth in human milk-fed very low birth weight infants receiving a new human milk fortifier. *Ann Nutr Metab.* 2000;44:2-10.
41. Centers for Disease Control and Prevention. Managing acute gastroenteritis among children: oral rehydration, maintenance, and nutritional therapy. *MMWR Morb Mortal Wkly Rep.* 2003;52 (No. RR-16):1-20. Available at: http://www.cdc.gov/mmwr/PDF/RR/RR5216.pdf. Accessed November 6, 2005.
42. Caufield PW, Griffen AL. Dental caries: an infectious and transmissible disease. *Pediatr Clin North Am.* 2000;47:1001-20.
43. Committee on Nutrition, American Academy of Pediatrics. Aluminum toxicity in infants and children. *Pediatrics.* 1996;97:413-6. Guideline reaffirmed by AAP in April 1999.
44. U.S. Department of Agriculture, Food and Nutrition Service. WIC: the special supplemental nutrition program for women, infants and children. Available at: http://www.fns.usda.gov/wic. Accessed November 6, 2005.
45. Gartner LM, Greer FR, Section on Breastfeeding and Committee on Nutrition, American Academy of Pediatrics. Clinical report: Prevention of rickets and vitamin D deficiency: new guidelines for vitamin D intake. *Pediatrics.* 2003;111:908-10.
46. Griffin IJ, Abrams SA. Iron and breastfeeding. *Pediatr Clin North Am.* 2001;48(2):401-13.
47. Lynch SR, Stoltzfus RJ. Iron and ascorbic acid: proposed fortification levels and recommended iron compounds. *J Nutr.* 2003; 133:2978S-84S.
48. Committee on Nutrition, American Academy of Pediatrics. Nutrition and oral health. In: Kleinman RE, ed. *Pediatric Nutrition Handbook.* 5th ed. Elk Grove Village, Ill: American Academy of Pediatrics; 2004:789-800.
49. Centers for Disease Control and Prevention. Recommendations for using fluoride to prevent and control dental caries in the United States. *MMWR Morb Mortal Wkly Rep.* 2001;50 (N0. RR-14): 1-59. Available at: http://www.cdc.gov/mmwr/PDF/RR/RR5014.pdf. Accessed November 6, 2005.

CHAPTER 27

# Overweight and Obesity

Sarah J. Miller and Cathy L. Bartels

Overweight and obesity are increasing in both the United States and worldwide. The percentage of obese individuals in economies in transition and in developed countries far outnumbers the percentage that are underweight, whereas malnutrition and underweight remain much more common than overweight in undeveloped countries. In the United States, increasing concern centers on the developing epidemic of overweight and obesity in children and adolescents. Overweight and obesity are conditions of considerable significance because they are associated with increased morbidity from various conditions, including cardiovascular diseases, Type 2 diabetes mellitus (DM), gallbladder disease, osteoarthritis, respiratory problems, and several cancers.[1] Despite the well-recognized risks of obesity, primary care providers frequently fail to encourage their obese patients to lose weight. Discussing obesity and weight loss–related health benefits should be encouraged since patients who report receiving advice from their primary care providers to lose weight are more likely to report trying to lose weight than those who do not receive such advice.

The economic impact of overweight and obesity is substantial. For 2003, the estimated direct cost of obesity in the United States was $75 billion; this does not include indirect costs associated with lost productivity and mortality.[2] Quantitation of indirect costs is difficult as many of the comorbidities of obesity listed above may have etiologies other than obesity. One study in a health maintenance organization demonstrated that patients with obesity experienced more hospitalizations, took more prescription drugs, made more professional health care claims, and made more outpatient visits than patients who were not obese.[3] Americans spend tens of billions of dollars on weight control products and services annually.

The Behavioral Risk Factor Surveillance System (BRFSS) found in a 2000 survey conducted by state health departments that about 39% of U.S. adults were trying to lose weight.[4] Because of the lack of proven, available nonprescription products for weight loss, the practitioner should be knowledgeable in discussing the limitations and potential harm of weight loss products and gimmicks and comfortable in recommending nonpharmacologic therapies including diet and exercise. In addition, since evidence for available prescription drug therapies exists, the practitioner may also refer patients failing nonpharmacologic therapies for medical evaluation and consideration for prescription weight loss therapies.

## Clinical Indicators of Overweight and Obesity

The 1998 National Heart, Lung, and Blood Institute (NHLBI) expert report, entitled *Clinical Guidelines on the Identification, Evaluation, and Treatment of Overweight and Obesity in Adults,* defines overweight and obesity in terms of the body mass index (BMI), a reliable parameter that takes into account both height and weight.[5] Table 27-1 illustrates BMI values for persons of various heights and weights and gives equations for calculation of the BMI value. Overweight is defined in adults as a BMI of 25 to 29.9 and obesity as a BMI of 30 or greater. The World Health Organization (WHO) has adopted the same BMI cutoffs as an international standard. The NHLBI report also addresses the possible importance of the distribution of body fat to risk of morbidity and mortality from various diseases. Abdominal fat may be associated with greater health risk than fat in the buttock or thigh region. NHLBI classifies men with waist circumference greater than 40 inches and women with waist circumference greater than 35 inches as being at increased relative risk of Type 2 DM and cardiovascular disease (Table 27-2). In children and adolescents, the Centers for Disease Control and Prevention discourage the use of the term obesity because of its negative connotations. They define a BMI percentile for age between the 85th and 95th percentiles as "at risk for overweight" and a BMI percentile of 95 or greater as "overweight."[6] Measurement of height and weight to calculate BMI and measurement of waist circumference are physical assessment techniques easily accomplished even in a busy clinical setting.

A syndrome characterized by the presence of certain metabolic risk factors has been associated with increased risk of coronary artery disease, other vascular diseases, and diabetes. Patients with three or more of the following are said to have the metabolic syndrome: waist circumference greater than 40 inches in men or 35 inches in women; serum triglycerides 150 mg/dL or greater; high-density lipoprotein (HDL) cholesterol less than 40 mg/dL in men or less than 50 mg/dL in women; blood pressure level 130/85 mm Hg or higher; and fasting serum glucose of 100 mg/dL or greater. These persons are likely to demonstrate insulin resistance and may benefit more from weight loss in terms of reduced morbidity and mortality compared with overweight or obese persons who are not insulin resistant. Persons with metabolic syndrome are at especially high risk of morbidity and mortality from cardiovascular disease.

**TABLE 27-1 BMI Corresponding to Height and Body Weights***

| Height (in.) | BMI (kg/m²)† 19 | 20 | 21 | 22 | 23 | 24 | 25 | 26 | 27 | 28 | 29 | 30 | 35 | 40 |
|---|---|---|---|---|---|---|---|---|---|---|---|---|---|---|
| | Body Weight (lb) | | | | | | | | | | | | | |
| 58 | 91 | 96 | 100 | 105 | 110 | 115 | 119 | 124 | 129 | 134 | 138 | 143 | 167 | 191 |
| 59 | 94 | 99 | 104 | 109 | 114 | 119 | 124 | 128 | 133 | 138 | 143 | 148 | 173 | 198 |
| 60 | 97 | 102 | 107 | 112 | 118 | 123 | 128 | 133 | 138 | 143 | 148 | 153 | 179 | 204 |
| 61 | 100 | 106 | 111 | 116 | 122 | 127 | 132 | 137 | 143 | 148 | 153 | 158 | 185 | 211 |
| 62 | 104 | 109 | 115 | 120 | 126 | 131 | 136 | 142 | 147 | 153 | 158 | 164 | 191 | 218 |
| 63 | 107 | 113 | 118 | 124 | 130 | 135 | 141 | 146 | 152 | 158 | 163 | 169 | 197 | 225 |
| 64 | 110 | 116 | 122 | 128 | 134 | 140 | 145 | 151 | 157 | 163 | 169 | 174 | 204 | 232 |
| 65 | 114 | 120 | 126 | 132 | 138 | 144 | 150 | 156 | 162 | 168 | 174 | 180 | 210 | 240 |
| 66 | 118 | 124 | 130 | 136 | 142 | 148 | 155 | 161 | 167 | 173 | 179 | 186 | 216 | 247 |
| 67 | 121 | 127 | 134 | 140 | 146 | 153 | 159 | 166 | 172 | 178 | 185 | 191 | 223 | 255 |
| 68 | 125 | 131 | 138 | 144 | 151 | 158 | 164 | 171 | 177 | 184 | 190 | 197 | 230 | 262 |
| 69 | 128 | 135 | 142 | 149 | 155 | 162 | 169 | 176 | 182 | 189 | 196 | 203 | 236 | 270 |
| 70 | 132 | 139 | 146 | 153 | 160 | 167 | 172 | 181 | 188 | 195 | 202 | 207 | 243 | 278 |
| 71 | 136 | 143 | 150 | 157 | 165 | 172 | 179 | 186 | 193 | 200 | 208 | 215 | 250 | 286 |
| 72 | 140 | 147 | 154 | 162 | 169 | 177 | 184 | 191 | 199 | 206 | 213 | 221 | 258 | 294 |
| 73 | 144 | 151 | 159 | 166 | 174 | 182 | 189 | 197 | 204 | 212 | 219 | 227 | 265 | 302 |
| 74 | 148 | 155 | 163 | 171 | 179 | 186 | 194 | 202 | 210 | 218 | 225 | 233 | 272 | 311 |
| 75 | 152 | 160 | 168 | 176 | 184 | 192 | 200 | 208 | 216 | 224 | 232 | 240 | 279 | 319 |
| 76 | 156 | 164 | 172 | 180 | 189 | 197 | 205 | 213 | 221 | 230 | 238 | 246 | 287 | 328 |

* To determine BMI, find the height in the left-hand column; then move across the row to a given weight. The number above the weight column is the BMI for that height and weight.

† BMI calculations: weight (kg)/height ($m^2$) or (weight [lb]/height [$in^2$]) × 703.

*Source:* Reprinted with permission from reference 1.

Some studies have challenged the concept that persons with a BMI of 25 to 29.9 have an increased risk of mortality compared with those with a BMI less than 25.[7] These researchers warn that the NHLBI guidelines stigmatize too many people as being overweight, minimizing the risks associated with low weight. This concept is of particular concern in older persons, where some studies have not shown mortality benefit with lower versus higher BMI values. There is some evidence to support that cardiorespiratory fitness is an independent determinant of mortality in overweight and obese persons (i.e., the concept that being fat but fit carries significantly lower risk than being fat and unfit).[1]

## Epidemiology of Overweight and Obesity

The National Health and Nutrition Examination Surveys (NHANES) of the U.S. population have tracked prevalence of overweight and obesity in adults from 1960 to 2002. These surveys have demonstrated a marked increase in obesity (as defined by the 1998 NHLBI guidelines) in both men and women across all age and ethnic groups (Figure 27-1).[1,8] Extreme obesity (defined as BMI ≥40) is most common in non-Hispanic black women with a prevalence of 13.5% in NHANES 2001-2002 data. Also illustrated in Figure 27-1 are the changes in prevalence of overweight across the various NHANES surveys. These have remained fairly stable, with the possible exception of the 2001-2002 data among women.

Of equal or even greater concern is the rising prevalence of overweight and obesity during childhood and adolescence, as tracked by the NHANES data.[8,9] Overweight children often become overweight adults. For children, overweight is defined as a BMI value at or above the 95th percentile of the sex-specific BMI growth chart. In addition to the increased prevalence charted in Figure 27-2 for children from 6 to 19 years of age, prevalence of overweight in preschool children has increased from 5% to 10.3% in 2- to 5-year-olds from 1971-74 to 2001-2002.[9] The increases in overweight children have been particularly striking in non-Hispanic black and Mexican-American adolescents, of whom 20.5% and 22.1% were overweight, respectively, in 2001-2002.[9]

TABLE 27-2 Classification of Overweight and Obesity by BMI, Waist Circumference, and Associated Disease Risk[1]

| | BMI (kg/m²) | Disease Risk* Relative to Normal Weight and Waist Circumference† Men ≤40 in. Women ≤35 in. | Men >40 in. Women >35 in. |
|---|---|---|---|
| Underweight | <18.5 | | |
| Normal | 18.5-24.9 | | |
| Overweight | 25.0-29.9 | Increased | High |
| **Obesity, Class** | | | |
| I | 30.0-34.9 | High | Very high |
| II | 35.0-39.9 | Very high | Very high |
| III (Extreme obesity) | ≥40 | Extremely high | Extremely high |

* Disease risk for Type 2 DM, hypertension, and cardiovascular disease.

† Increased waist circumference can also be a marker for increased risk even in patients of normal weight.

*Note:* Risk factors as defined by the NHLBI include established coronary heart disease, presence of other atherosclerotic disease, Type 2 DM, cigarette smoking, hypertension, low-density lipoprotein cholesterol >160 mg/dL, high-density lipoprotein cholesterol <35 mg/dL, impaired fasting glucose, family history of premature coronary heart disease, age (male >45 years, female >55 years), physical inactivity, and high triglycerides (undefined number).

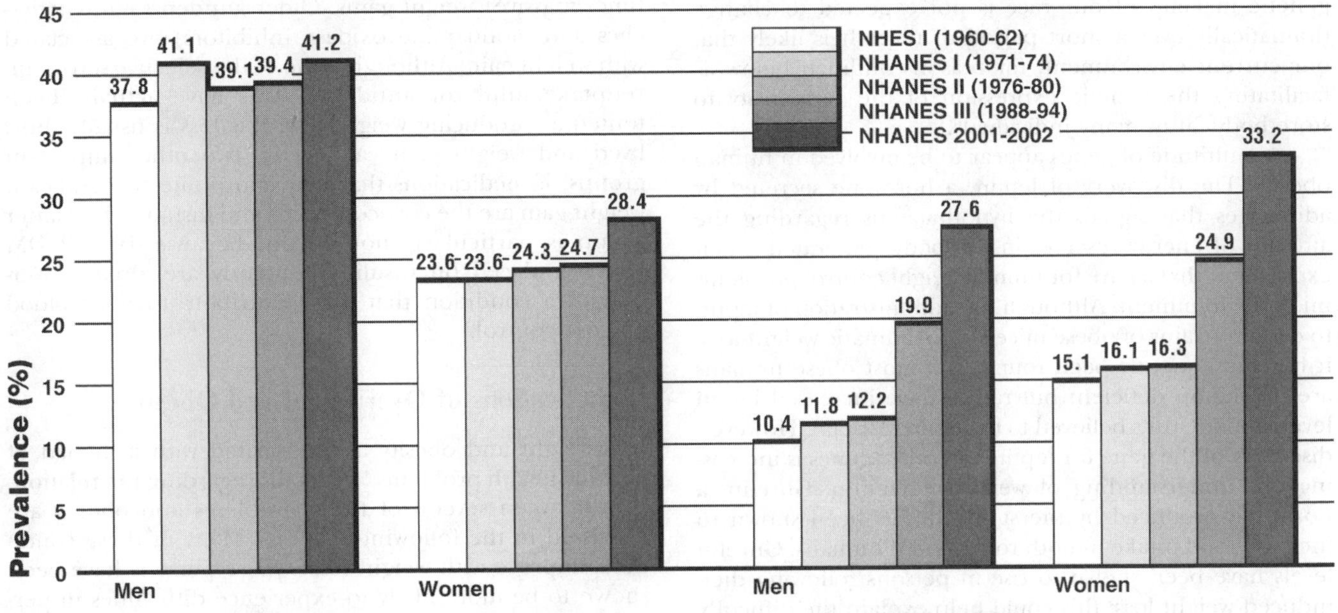


FIGURE 27-1 Age-adjusted prevalence of overweight (BMI 25-29.9) and obesity (BMI ≥30). Key: NHES, National Health Examination Survey; NHANES, National Health and Nutrition Examination Survey. (Adapted from references 1 and 8.)

## Etiology of Overweight and Obesity

Simply put, weight gain is a reflection of energy intake exceeding energy expenditure. A pound of adipose tissue represents about 3500 calories (kcal) of energy. An excess intake of only 10 kcal per day over the level of energy expenditure should thus result in a gain of approximately 1 lb of fat in a year's time. The physiology of energy intake and expenditure is complex and involves numerous body systems, including the hypothalamic-pituitary axis, the

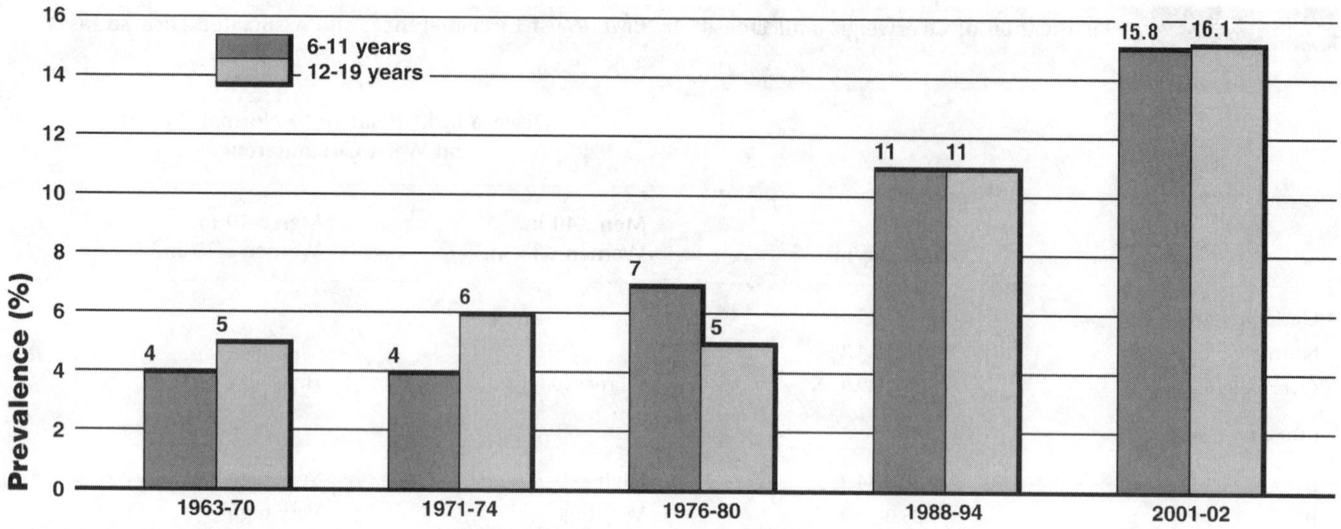


FIGURE 27-2 Prevalence of overweight among children and adolescents ages 6 to 19 years. (*Sources:* References 8 and 9.)

autonomic nervous system, the central nervous system, the endocrine system, the gastrointestinal (GI) tract, and adipose tissue.

Both genetic and environmental factors are important in the etiology of overweight and obesity, and there is a complex interplay between these factors. The rapid increase in overweight individuals over the past few decades argues for a strong environmental role, since the genetic makeup of our race is not expected to change dramatically over a short period of time. It is likely that our current environment, for reasons outlined below, is facilitating the genetic expression of the propensity to store body fat in many individuals.

A multitude of genes appear to be involved in human obesity. The discovery of leptin, a hormone secreted by adipocytes that signals the hypothalamus regarding the amount of energy reserves in the body, generated much excitement that a cure for human weight control problems might be imminent. Although the administration of leptin to certain strains of obese mice led to dramatic weight loss, it has subsequently been found that most obese humans are not leptin deficient but rather have increased leptin levels and are thus believed to be leptin resistant. However, discovery of the gene for leptin and other genes is increasing our understanding of weight regulation. Ghrelin, a hormone produced by the stomach, has been shown to increase food intake in both rodents and humans. Ghrelin levels have been shown to rise in persons following diet-induced weight loss; this could help explain the difficulty people have in trying to keep from regaining weight. Peptide $YY_{3\text{-}36}$ and α-melanocyte–stimulating hormone are other endogenous compounds whose roles in the etiology of obesity are being studied.

Environmental factors that appear to be fueling the recent increase in overweight and obesity in the United States as well as many other parts of the world include decreases in physical activity coupled with increases in food availability, especially calorie-dense foods.[10] Fewer than half of Americans meet guidelines for regular moderate physical activity. Significant increases in portion sizes of food, as well as increased working hours leading to less time to prepare food at home, may be other environmental factors contributing to excessive energy intake relative to energy expenditure. See Chapter 23 for a discussion of a healthy diet and the Food Guide Pyramid.

Medications are a potential etiology of weight gain. Many of the newer atypical antipsychotics, especially clozapine and olanzapine, can contribute to significant (sometimes massive) weight gains. Older antidepressants (tricyclics and monoamine oxidase inhibitors) are associated with weight gain. Although some of the selective serotonin reuptake inhibitor antidepressants have actually been touted as producing weight loss, this loss is usually short lived and weight gain can occur. Two other important groups of medications that may contribute to significant weight gain are the corticosteroids and insulins. This latter group is particularly noteworthy, because Type 2 DM patients placed on insulin frequently are already overweight, a condition that may contribute to poor blood glucose control.

## Complications of Overweight and Obesity

Overweight and obesity are associated with a myriad of chronic health problems.[1,11] Details regarding the relationship between several of these problems and obesity are discussed in the following sections. Many of these conditions improve with weight loss. Obese persons have been shown to be more likely to experience difficulties in performing activities of daily living such as walking several flights of stairs or bending and kneeling. The Centers for Disease Control and Prevention (CDC) estimates that poor diet and physical inactivity were associated with more than 100,000 deaths in 2000.[12]

### *Cardiovascular Disease*

Obesity is associated with coronary heart disease (CHD) through its impact on risk factors such as hypertension, dyslipidemia, and Type 2 DM. Overweight and obesity have been linked to increased risk for congestive heart failure

(CHF) and stroke. The American Heart Association has classified obesity as a major, modifiable risk factor for CHD.

Prevalence of hypertension begins to increase at relatively low levels of overweight (i.e., BMI of 26-27).[11] Patients with a BMI of 30 and higher are about twice as likely to have hypertension than those with a BMI of 25 or lower.[1] The pathophysiology of obesity-related hypertension appears to involve a combination of increased sodium retention, increased sympathetic nervous system activity, alteration of the renin-angiotensin system, and insulin resistance.[1] The NHLBI guidelines conclude that weight loss produced by lifestyle modification reduces blood pressure in both overweight hypertensive and overweight nonhypertensive individuals.[1]

The relationship between CHD and obesity has not been consistent across all studies. This may be because of poor control of confounding factors such as other risk factors (e.g., blood lipid levels, blood pressure, DM, and smoking) in these studies. Smokers often weigh less than nonsmokers but have higher rates of CHD.[1] Several studies that have carefully controlled for these confounders have been able to show a significant association between BMI and risk of CHD in both men and women.[1]

Overweight and obesity are established independent risk factors for CHF.[1] However, to gain an understanding of the role of obesity itself, clinical trials must be designed to account for other risk factors for CHF often present in the obese patient (e.g., hypertension or Type 2 DM). Recent data from the Framingham Heart Study indicate a doubling of the risk of heart failure in obese subjects (BMI $\geq$30) compared with subjects of normal weight (BMI 18.5-24.9).[13] Framingham data also recently revealed an increased risk of atrial fibrillation associated with obesity, an effect that appears to be mediated by enlargement of the left atrium in obesity.[14]

The relationship between overweight and obesity and the risk of stroke has not been consistent across studies, perhaps partially because investigators do not distinguish between ischemic and hemorrhagic stroke, and partially because of the lack of control for concomitant hypertension and DM. Data from the Physicians' Health Study showed approximately a twofold increase in risk of either ischemic or hemorrhagic stroke in subjects with a BMI of 30 and higher compared with those with a BMI of 23 or less.[15] This effect was apparently independent of the presence of hypertension, DM, or dyslipidemia. The BMI may affect stroke risk through an increase in prothrombotic factors found in obese persons.[15]

### Dyslipidemia

There is a strong correlation between BMI and triglyceride levels in both men and women in all adult age groups.[1] Beneficial HDL cholesterol levels are lower in both men and women with higher BMI values.[1] On the other hand, low-density lipoprotein (LDL) cholesterol tends to increase as BMI increases.[1] The beneficial impact of even modest weight loss on blood lipid levels has been well documented.[1] These changes in lipid levels would be expected to positively impact cardiovascular risk.

### Diabetes Mellitus

The relationship between overweight and obesity and DM is well documented (see Chapter 47). Data from NHANES III indicate that 67% of patients with Type 2 DM have a BMI of at least 27.[11] Data from the Behavioral Risk Factor Surveillance System in 2001 indicated approximately a 1.6-fold increase in DM in patients with a BMI of 25 to 29.9 compared with those with a BMI of 18.5 to 24.9.[16] The corresponding number for patients with a BMI of 30 to 39.9 was a 3.4-fold increase, and there was a 7.4-fold increase in DM for those with a BMI of 40 or greater.[16] Modest weight gains after 18 years of age, as well as visceral adiposity (high waist circumference), have been shown to be risk factors for development of Type 2 DM.[11] Persons who are initially insulin resistant, typically evidenced by high plasma triglycerides and low HDL cholesterol, are most likely to benefit from weight loss in terms of reduced morbidity and mortality not only from type 2 DM but also from hypertension and CHD.[17] Modest weight loss has been shown to be effective in improving blood glucose control in patients with Type 2 DM and preventing development of Type 2 DM in those at risk.[1,18]

### Psychosocial Consequences

Negative attitudes toward obese people, leading to social stigmatization and discrimination, have been reported in the United States and other developed societies, particularly among Caucasians.[1] Studies relating to whether obesity has significant psychologic and emotional impacts have yielded disparate results.[1] Obese patients who seek treatment in clinic settings seem to demonstrate more psychopathology than obese patients who do not seek treatment.[1] Overweight children may develop psychosocial difficulties stemming from compromised peer relationships and being teased about their weight.[19]

### Other Complications of Obesity

Obesity appears to increase the risk for a number of other diseases as well, including gallbladder disease, osteoarthritis, sleep apnea, certain types of cancer, and disorders of female reproduction.[1,11,20] The risk for gallstones and cholecystectomy increases with obesity; rapid weight loss may also precipitate gallstones. Osteoarthritis and pain in weight-bearing joints is increased in obese patients. Obesity is also a risk factor for hyperuricemia and gout. The risk of sleep apnea increases with upper body obesity but not excess fat in the lower body.

Obesity may account for 14% to 20% of cancer deaths in the United States. Of particular concern are cancers with a hormonal basis such as cancers of the breast, prostate, endometrium, colon, and gallbladder. In addition, female reproduction disorders are associated with obesity, including menstrual irregularities and infertility. Polycystic ovary syndrome is associated with abdominal obesity. Hypertension and gestational diabetes are more likely to develop in obese women who become pregnant, and labor and delivery complications are more common. Babies of obese women may be more likely to have a neural tube defect.

## Management of Overweight and Obesity

### Management Goals and General Management Approach

For many individuals, losing weight or maintaining a weight loss is a lifelong challenge. Lifestyle changes, dietary modification, and increased exercise are the preferred weight-loss therapies. Successful weight loss and especially maintenance of weight loss typically require significant behavioral modification. Pharmacologic therapy using nonprescription agents should be only a short-term measure unless a primary care provider supervises the therapy. Long-term use of prescription therapies under the care of a primary care provider is emerging as an option for patients with a BMI of 30 or higher or a BMI of 27 or higher with comorbid conditions.[1] Bariatric surgery may be considered for patients with a BMI of 40 or higher or a BMI of 35 or higher with comorbid conditions.[1]

Weight-loss goals set by many individuals are unrealistic and based more on desired cosmetic effect than on health benefit. Weight loss (and maintenance of that loss) of 5% to 10% of initial weight has been shown to have positive benefits in individuals with hypertension and DM. The NHLBI guidelines state that the initial goal of weight loss is to reduce body weight by about 10% over 6 months.[1] If this goal is achieved and further weight loss is indicated, it can be attempted. However, the first 10% loss probably carries the most health benefit and is also easiest to attain, since weight often plateaus after 6 months because of a decreased basal metabolic rate at the lower weight. It is probably more important to maintain the 10% weight loss than to pursue further weight loss in many patients. Another often overlooked approach may be to simply prevent further weight gain in persons who have been slowly but steadily gaining weight over a period of years or decades; this would be particularly appropriate for persons who are still in the overweight (not yet obese) category.[10] Figure 27-3 is a useful guide for the practitioner recommending weight-loss measures.

Weight loss is indicated for individuals with health problems (e.g., sleep apnea, hypertension, osteoarthritis, or Type 2 DM) that can be lessened by weight loss. Unsupervised weight loss should be discouraged in individuals outlined in Figure 27-3.

### Nonpharmacologic Therapy

Dietary modification or restriction is the mainstay of weight-loss therapy. Although physical activity alone produces less weight loss than caloric restriction, such activity is an important component of maintaining weight-loss and improving overall fitness. The American Dietetic Association, in their position statement on weight management, stresses that successful weight management requires a lifelong commitment to behaviors emphasizing "sustainable and enjoyable eating practices and daily physical activity."[10]

#### Dietary Change

Dietary change is the most commonly used weight-loss strategy. Methods range from caloric restriction to changes in dietary proportions of fat, protein, and carbohydrate or use of macronutrient substitutes (i.e., sugar and fat substitutes). Short-term success for many of these methods has been documented; however, information on effectiveness and safety in the longer term is limited. Weight loss at the end of relatively short-term programs can exceed 10% of initial body weight. However, there is a strong tendency to regain weight—as much as two thirds of it within 1 year after completing a program and almost all of it after 5 years. Nonetheless, a small percentage of participants do maintain their weight loss over more extended periods. The National Weight Control Registry tracks individuals who have maintained a weight loss of at least 30 pounds for at least 1 year.[21] Persons in this registry used a variety of methods, from self-directed diet programs to liquid formula diets, to initially lose weight. Most of these individuals report maintaining their weight loss through a combination of a low-calorie, low-fat diet and exercise. Surprisingly, this group generally reports that weight maintenance becomes easier the further out in time they get from their initial weight loss, perhaps as a result of behavioral changes becoming more ingrained.

Even small changes in dietary patterns can have a positive effect over time. Cutting portion sizes (e.g., two pieces of pizza instead of the usual three), eating fast food one fewer time per week, switching to water or diet soda rather than soda sweetened with sugar, and keeping healthy snacks such as fruits and vegetables on hand are useful, sustainable strategies for decreasing calories. Again, the reader is referred to Chapter 23 for more details regarding healthy diets.

#### Caloric Restriction

Daily caloric allowances for moderately active individuals vary with age, gender, and body weight. As a general rule, an intake of 3500 kcal over expenditure will produce a weight gain of approximately 1 lb, whereas an expenditure of 3500 kcal over intake will result in a loss of 1 lb of body fat. Daily caloric intake allowances for an average 30-year-old man (BMI, 18.5 to 25; height, 5 ft 11 in.) in a temperate climate range from 2200 to 3000 kcal/day, depending on activity level. Corresponding figures for an average 30-year-old woman (BMI, 18.5 to 25; height, 5 ft 5 in.) are 1800 to 2800 kcal/day.[22] These figures decrease for older persons, whereas they increase for younger adults. Caloric requirements for women increase during pregnancy and lactation (see Chapter 23).[22] Self-initiated weight loss during pregnancy is not recommended and should be discussed with a primary care provider, even for severely overweight women, because of possible risk to the developing baby.

A diet that is individually planned and takes into account the patient's overweight status to create a deficit of 300 to 1000 kcal/day should be an integral part of any weight-loss program.[1,10] Two levels of caloric restriction are commonly used. A low-calorie diet (LCD) of about 800 to 1500 kcal/day may involve a structured commercial program with formulated and calorically defined food products, or it may involve guidelines for selecting conventional foods, including careful attention to portion sizes. Weight loss on an LCD is typically 1 to 2 lb/week. A very-low-calorie

**Exclusions for Self-Treatment**

- Severe obesity (BMI ≥40)
- Pregnancy or breast-feeding
- <18 years of age or >65 years of age
- Cardiovascular disease, dyslipidemia, DM, or HTN
- Eating disorders

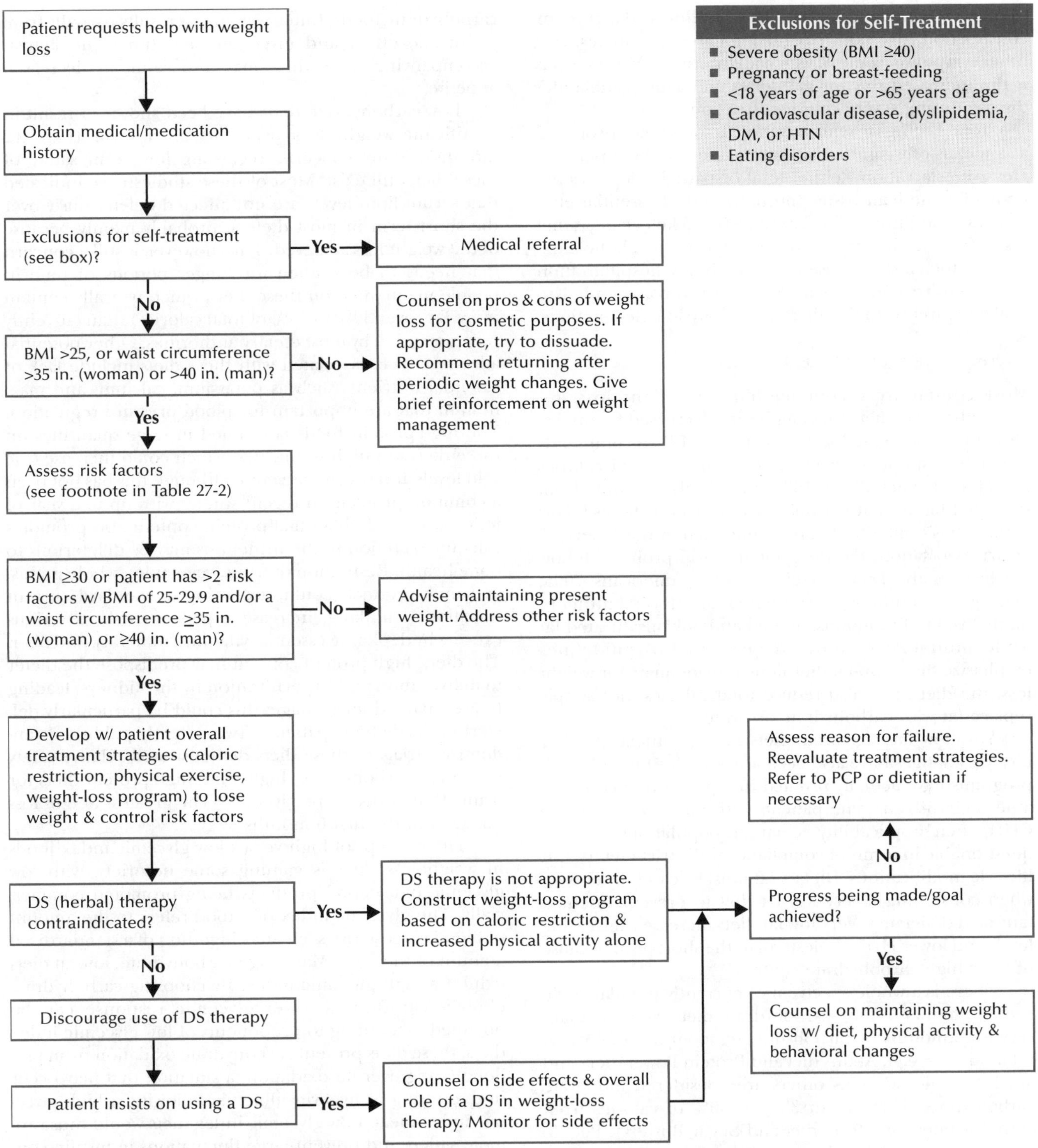


**FIGURE 27-3** Self-care of overweight and obesity. Key: BMI, body mass index; DM, diabetes mellitus; DS, dietary supplement; HTN, hypertension; PCP, primary care provider.

diet (VLCD) of 800 or fewer calories per day should be conducted under the supervision and monitoring of a primary care provider, and it should be restricted to patients with a BMI higher than 30.[10] A VLCD should contain at least 1 g/kg of ideal body weight per day of protein. VLCDs are frequently administered as liquid formulas (shakes) given several times a day. Although weight loss with VLCDs may be faster than with LCDs, long-term results are generally no better with VLCDs than with LCDs. A multivitamin/multimineral preparation should be recommended to patients consuming fewer than 1200 kcal/day for prolonged periods.

VLCDs and fasting are associated with numerous short-term adverse effects. Rapid weight loss is frequently associated with fatigue, hair loss, dizziness, diarrhea or constipation, dry skin, irregular menses in females, and other symptoms, some of which are transient. More serious is the increased risk for gallstones and acute gallbladder disease during severe caloric restriction.

Total fasting or semistarvation is sometimes proposed as a means of weight reduction in severely obese persons. However, starvation—either total or partial—depletes the body of some lean tissue (protein) and of essential electrolytes in addition to fat. The ketosis and ketoacidosis that result from fasting represent a significant metabolic alteration. If total fasting is used to treat obesity, hospitalization and intensive medical supervision are recommended to deal effectively with the alteration of physiologic functions.

### Altered Proportions of Food Groups

Most commonly recommended for weight loss are reduced-calorie diets that emphasize decreased fat intake, particularly decreased saturated fat. NHLBI recommends a diet that supplies no more than 30% of total calories from fat, of which 8% to 10% of total calories come from saturated fat, and at least 55% from carbohydrates.[1] This approach is similar to that recommended by the American Heart Association. Future guidelines will probably follow the lead of the Dietary Guidelines for Americans 2005, placing less emphasis on restricting fat calories and more on inclusion of monounsaturated and polyunsaturated fat while minimizing saturated fat.[23] NHLBI guidelines emphasize that a low-fat diet alone is inadequate for weight loss; the diet must also reduce total calories, not simply replace fat with carbohydrate or protein.

Very low fat vegetarian diets in the context of other lifestyle changes have also been advocated. Although such programs have actually resulted in regression of coronary atherosclerosis in some patients with moderate to severe CHD, their applicability to larger populations remains questionable in terms of compliance with strict dietary and lifestyle modifications. Dietary fat must be carefully chosen when consuming a very low fat diet to prevent essential fatty acid deficiency. Very low fat diets increase triglyceride levels and lower HDL cholesterol in the short term because of their high carbohydrate content.

There is a whole spectrum of currently popular high-protein, higher-fat, low-carbohydrate diets. Some contain very low amounts of carbohydrates (about 5% to 15% of total calories; e.g., Atkins diet and Protein Power diet) and are ketogenic, whereas others are considered moderate carbohydrate diets (about 35% to 50% of calories from carbohydrate; e.g., Zone diet and Sugar Busters). People often start out on the ultra-low form of the diet and transition to a more moderate form; despite the popular initial impression that eating high-protein and high-fat foods will be enjoyable, many persons get tired of a regimen in which consumption of items such as bread, pasta, fruits, and vegetables is severely curtailed.

The theory behind the very low carbohydrate diets is that they prevent the elevated insulin levels that promote storage of body fat seen with higher-carbohydrate diets. In reality, much of the weight loss seen with these diets is a result of decreased caloric intake from avoidance of high-carbohydrate foods. Initial weight loss results partially from a diuretic effect and glycogen depletion. The ketosis accompanying these diets may also result in decreased appetite.

Low-carbohydrate diets have been shown to result in significant weight loss over the short term (6 to 12 months). Many concerns regarding long-term safety of these diets still exist. Most of these studies have indicated that serum lipid levels are not affected deleteriously over the short term in most dieters, probably mainly because of the weight loss achieved. This, however, is still a concern that needs to be studied for longer periods of time in people maintained on these diets, which typically contain more fat (over 30% to 35% of total calories) than currently recommended by most dietary authorities. Other potential adverse effects associated with these diets include lack of essential nutrients such as potassium, calcium, and magnesium that are important for blood pressure regulation. The high-protein foods consumed in large quantities on these diets are high in purines, which could increase uric acid levels and precipitate gout, although this has not been a common problem in recent studies with up to a year of follow-up.[24,25] High animal protein content also promotes calcium excretion in the urine; this may be deleterious to bone health. Restriction of fruits, vegetables, whole grains, and milk products could, according to standard current nutritional thinking, increase a person's risk of various cancers by depleting essential vitamins, minerals, and fiber. The diets' high protein content may predispose the dieter to dehydration and hyperfiltration by the kidneys, leading to eventual kidney damage; this could be particularly deleterious in diabetic patients. Two recently published randomized trials of these diets demonstrated relative safety of the low-carbohydrate, higher-fat, high-protein diets for 6 and 12 months, respectively.[24,25] The greatest weight loss was seen in the first 6 months.

The concept of high versus low glycemic index foods in weight-loss diets is gaining some notoriety, with low glycemic index food products being promoted commercially. The glycemic index of a food refers to the amount of blood glucose rise seen after ingestion of a standardized amount of the food. Many high-carbohydrate, low-fat diets exhibit a high glycemic index. By choosing carbohydrate choices carefully, a lower glycemic response can be obtained. According to proponents of low glycemic index diets, these diets prevent carbohydrate oxidation from predominating over fat oxidation, a situation that may occur in the setting of hyperinsulinemia following a high glycemic index meal. Low glycemic index diets would thus promote satiety and prevent large fluctuations in insulin concentrations and might help maintain insulin sensitivity. Studies have not consistently supported the usefulness of low-glycemic diets in weight control, although this topic deserves further research attention.

### Use of Food Additives

Some patients may use food additives such as artificial sweeteners and fat substitutes as adjunct measures to reduce caloric intake. Although theoretically their use should help decrease caloric intake, data showing that use

**TABLE 27-3 Sugar and Fat Substitutes**

| Substitute (Sample Trade Name) | Comments |
|---|---|
| **Sugar Substitutes** | |
| Saccharin (Sweet 'n Low) | Has bitter taste; has been replaced largely by newer sweeteners |
| Aspartame (Nutra Sweet) | See text; contains phenylalanine, thus, contraindicated in patients with phenylketonuria; not for use in cooking or baking as heat breaks it down into free amino acids, which impart a bitter taste |
| Fructose | Nutritive sweetener and should not be viewed as "sugar-free"; insulin not required for fructose utilization in the body |
| Sorbitol | Nutritive sweetener and should not be viewed as "sugar-free"; does not cause tooth decay, but can cause osmotic diarrhea when ingested in large quantities |
| Xylitol | Nutritive sweetener and should not be viewed as "sugar-free"; does not cause tooth decay |
| Acesulfame-potassium (Sunette, Sweet One) | May be substituted for sucrose in cooking; may be combined with aspartame as some people detect a metallic aftertaste with acesulfame-potassium alone |
| Sucralose (Splenda) | May be used in cooking |
| Neotame | May be used in cooking |
| Cyclamates | Banned by FDA in 1969 because of association with cancer in animals; applicability of this finding to humans has been challenged, but petition before FDA for reapproval is pending |
| **Fat Substitutes** | |
| Microparticulated protein (Simplesse) | Used in frozen desserts |
| Soluble fiber (Oatrim) | Derived from oats and designed to replace fat in meats, cheeses, baked goods, and frozen desserts |
| Sucrose polyester (Olean) | Also known as olestra; is not absorbed; can cause malabsorption of fat-soluble vitamins; manufacturers must supply specified amounts of fat-soluble vitamins A, D, E, and K to foods containing olestra; GI side effects can be seen with ingestion of large quantities; can be used for cooking and frying |

of these substances is associated with significant weight loss or better weight maintenance are conflicting. Saccharin and aspartame are the most widely used artificial sweeteners, but others are available. Table 27-3 outlines pertinent information related to sugar and fat substitutes. Patients who have phenylketonuria (i.e., cannot metabolize a metabolic product of phenylalanine) must be alerted that aspartame contains phenylalanine. Products containing aspartame must carry the warning: "Phenylketonurics: Contains Phenylalanine."

### Meal Replacement Therapy

These commercial products are typically geared toward replacing up to two meals a day with a liquid drink, a snack bar, or a measured frozen meal, with the dieter encouraged to eat a "reasonable" third meal each day. The main advantage to this approach is portion control. These products might typically contain about 200 kcal per serving, consisting of 50% to 60% carbohydrate, up to 30% protein, and 10% fat. Early weight loss with these products, part of which may be a result of low sodium content that leads to water loss, can give a psychologic boost to the dieter to adhere to the program. When used properly, Slim-Fast and similar products can be efficacious for weight loss and maintenance.[26] Meal replacement products are discussed further in Chapter 24.

### Commercial Weight-loss Programs

Structured commercial weight-loss programs such as Weight Watchers, Jenny Craig, and Take Off Pounds Sensibly (TOPS) are very popular in the United States. Women tend to gravitate to these programs more than men. Several articles in the mainstream medical literature have examined the results of the Weight Watchers programs; most of these articles were coauthored by representatives of Weight Watchers International. A recent systematic review of commercial weight-loss programs concluded that data supporting the use of these programs are suboptimal and controlled trials are necessary before their efficacy and cost-effectiveness can be touted.[27]

Participation in some of the structured commercial programs may be expensive, as participants are required to purchase specially packaged meals that are available only from the company. A large component of the success of these programs for many participants is likely the social support aspect that develops with periodic meetings of groups of dieters engaged in the program.

### Physical Activity

Encouragement of physical activity as a method of preventing overweight and obesity is an important public health strategy for all age groups, including children. The Dietary Guidelines for Americans 2005 outline several physical activity recommendations.[23] According to these recommendations, children and adolescents should be physically active for at least 60 minutes on most (preferably all) days of the week. For the general population, engaging in at least 30 minutes of moderate intensity exercise (such as brisk walking) on most days of the week is suggested to reduce the risk of chronic disease. For body weight management to prevent gradual body weight gain, 60 minutes of moderate to vigorous activity on most days of the week are recommended. Sixty to 90 minutes of moderate intensity exercise daily may be necessary to sustain weight loss over a long period of time. For older adults, participation in regular exercise can help reduce functional declines of aging.

Increased physical activity is an important component of weight-loss therapy, and perhaps even more important in weight maintenance after weight loss. Patients who regularly exercise may, in general, be more committed to a healthy lifestyle regime. Exercise may also build muscle that has a higher metabolic rate than a corresponding amount of fat. The amount of weight loss that can be achieved by exercise programs alone is modest; combining a reduced-calorie diet with increased physical activity produces greater weight loss and reduction in abdominal fat than either approach alone. Some patients may have underlying medical conditions such as heart disease or severe arthritis that make some types of exercise ill advised. These patients are advised to have a medical evaluation before starting an exercise regimen. Also, regardless of concomitant disease states, current recommendations call for all men over age 40 years and women over age 50 years to undergo a medical evaluation before starting an exercise program.

For sedentary patients, a walking program is often a good place to begin exercise. Patients can start by walking 30 minutes each day for 3 days a week, building up to at least 60 minutes of moderate intensity physical activity on most days of the week.[22] The 60-minute activity periods can be accrued in multiple smaller increments throughout the day with similar benefit. Table 27-4 lists the calories expended during 1 hour of various types of exercise for an average-size male. These values vary with gender, weight, and body composition. Patients should be encouraged to participate in activities that they enjoy and are thus more likely to continue for the long-term.

**TABLE 27-4 Caloric Expenditure Rates**

| Activity (1 hour) | Calories Expended |
|---|---|
| Bicycling (6 mph) | 240 |
| Bicycling (12 mph) | 410 |
| Cross-country skiing | 700 |
| Jogging (5.5 mph) | 740 |
| Jogging (7 mph) | 920 |
| Jumping rope | 720 |
| Running in place | 650 |
| Swimming (50 yd/minute) | 500 |
| Tennis (singles) | 400 |
| Walking (2 mph) | 240 |
| Walking (3 mph) | 320 |
| Walking (4.5 mph) | 440 |

### Behavioral Therapy

Behavioral therapy can improve the outcome of weight-loss programs when used in combination with other strategies such as diet and exercise. The benefit of behavioral therapy is most evident during the active stage of the treatment, with little benefit seen in the long term in the absence of continued intervention. Behavioral therapy may be administered in either an individual or group setting by professionals or lay leaders. Controlled trial data comparing the various potential combinations for delivery of behavioral therapy in weight loss program (e.g., lay leaders in a group setting, profession counseling in an individual setting) have not yet accumulated.

Behavioral techniques include the following:[28]

- *Self-monitoring:* keeping daily records of time and place of eating and what was eaten along with a log of physical activity
- *Stimulus control:* identifying and avoiding triggers for overeating and underexercising
- *Social support:* identifying and building a network of family and friends to help modify lifestyle
- *Cognitive restructuring:* replacing negative thoughts, beliefs, and attitudes with positive ones
- *Problem-solving skills:* learning to analyze problems and find solutions
- *Relapse prevention:* teaching methods to recover from episodes of overeating

### Pharmacologic Therapy

Pharmacologic therapy is generally not recommended for most individuals seeking to lose weight, as exemplified by the fact that more weight-loss products have been removed from the market than approved in recent years because of safety concerns. The ideal drug, namely, one that would provide fast and permanent weight loss with no adverse effects, simply does not exist despite the billions of dollars spent on these products by consumers.

The most current federal guidelines for treatment of overweight and obesity recommend that prescription weight-loss medications approved by FDA for long-term use be reserved as an adjunct to diet and physical activity for patients with a BMI of 30 or higher, or for patients with a BMI of 27 or higher with concomitant diseases or risk factors. They also recommend these drugs be used singly (not in combination) and at the lowest effective dose to reduce the likelihood of adverse events.[1] The same guidelines for use should apply to all weight-loss products, whether prescription or over-the-counter (OTC) drugs or dietary supplements. Any of these medications or supplements should be used with concomitant lifestyle modification and continuous assessment for efficacy, safety, and tolerance. Only in situations in which the drug is efficacious in weight loss and maintenance, and has minimal adverse effects should pharmacotherapy be continued.

### Status of Nonprescription Weight-loss Products

Because of the lack of safety and efficacy data, FDA banned 111 weight-control ingredients in nonprescription drug products in 1991.[29] In 2000, FDA requested all drug companies discontinue marketing phenylpropanolamine-containing products because of safety issues.[30] In addition, OTC drugs containing ephedrine and related alkaloids in combination with a stimulant or analgesic can no longer be marketed as of 2001,[31] and the stimulant laxative ingredients aloe and cascara sagrada were banned as ingredients in OTC drugs in 2002.[32] However, many of these ingredients may still be marketed in dietary supplements and are often found as components of weight-loss products.

Dietary supplements are distinct entities from OTC drugs. They include herbal and other products meant to supplement the diet, and are regulated under DSHEA (refer to Chapter 53) and generally recognized as safe unless FDA proves otherwise. OTC drugs, conversely, are regulated as drugs by FDA and must adhere to much more stringent regulations of safety, efficacy, and quality.

The only drugs currently considered safe and efficacious for weight loss are restricted to prescription-only status and include benzphetamine (Didrex), diethylpropion (Tenuate), mazindol (Sanorex), methamphetamine (Desoxyn), orlistat (Xenical), phendimetrazine (Bontril), phentermine (Ionamin), and sibutramine (Meridia). The reader is directed to standard references for more information about these drugs. Also, on January 23, 2006, two FDA advisory committees jointly recommended approval of a nonprescription, 60 mg dose of orlistat.[33] At press time, the agency had not acted on the recommendation.

### Phenylpropanolamine's Removal from the Market

Phenylpropanolamine (PPA) was generally recognized as safe and effective for weight control by expert panels in 1982. However, because of concerns regarding occasional reports of hemorrhagic stroke associated with its use, FDA asked the pharmaceutical industry to conduct a study evaluating this risk. In 2000, FDA's Nonprescription Drugs Advisory Committee (NDAC) recommended that PPA not be considered generally recognized as safe for OTC use for weight control or as a nasal decongestant. Although the risk of hemorrhagic stroke is extremely low, FDA voiced concerns regarding the serious irreversible nature of this adverse event and the inability to accurately predict who is at risk. Because of this, FDA agreed with NDAC's recommendation and issued a letter later in 2000 to manufacturers asking for a voluntary discontinuation of marketing of PPA-containing products.[30]

### The Ephedra Debate

Until recently, ephedra, or ma-huang, was the most widely used weight-loss dietary supplement in the United States. Ephedrine alkaloids are the active ingredients in ephedra; these are compounds with nervous and cardiovascular system stimulant activity.[34] While some studies suggest that synthetic ephedrine, previously found in many OTC allergy and cold preparations, may be beneficial for weight loss when used alone or in combination with caffeine, it is not approved as an OTC weight-loss ingredient. Many manufacturers of dietary supplement products incorporated the natural product ma-huang as a source of ephedra, and guarana or cola nut as sources of caffeine.[35] Although a limited number of clinical studies report modest weight losses with these products, safety issues are of particular concern, especially when they are used together.

The results of a RAND Corporation study commissioned by the National Institutes of Health provided additional evidence of health risks associated with ephedra together with limited evidence of a beneficial effect on weight loss. The RAND study reviewed over 16,000 adverse events reported after ephedra use and found approximately 20 "sentinel events," including heart attack, stroke, and death, that occurred in the absence of other contributing factors.[36] Based on this and other medical evidence, FDA published the final rule on dietary supplements containing ephedrine alkaloids on February 11, 2004, declaring these supplements adulterated because they present an unreasonable risk of illness or injury. The final rule applies to dietary supplements containing ephedrine alkaloids from various botanical species such as *Ephedra* sp., *Sida cordifolia* L., and *Pinellia ternata* (Thunb.) Makino. Common names used for the various botanicals that contain the ephedrine alkaloids include sea grape, yellow horse, joint fir, popotillo, ma huang, and country mallow.[37] The rule went into effect on April 12, 2004. On April 15, 2005, a federal judge in Utah limited the scope of this ban, stating the FDA's methods in banning ephedra violated DSHEA (see Chapter 53) by shifting the burden of proof of safety from FDA to the manufacturers. This ruling applies only to products containing a maximum of 10 mg of ephedrine alkaloids per daily serving, and it has no effect on those states that have already banned all sales of dietary supplements containing ephedrine alkaloids.[38] At present, the ruling has limited effects, as the FDA served a notice of appeal to the U.S. District Court of Utah on June 13, 2005.[39] The American Herbal Products Association (AHPA) recommends that none of its members sell dietary supplements containing ephedra until the legal arguments are resolved.[38]

### Reformulated Weight-loss Products

Since the FDA ruling on ephedra-containing dietary supplements, many manufacturers are including bitter orange (*Citrus aurantium*) in weight-loss medications, often in combination with sources of caffeine such as cola nut (*Cola acuminata* or *C. nitida*), guarana (*Paullinia cupana* or *P. sorbilis*), or maté (*Ilex paraguariensis*). Bitter orange contains synephrine, which is structurally similar to epinephrine, and octopamine, which is similar to norepinephrine. It is being touted as a safe alternative to ephedra in many herbal weight-loss products. Although adrenergic effects of synephrine and octopamine have the potential for appetite suppression and lipolysis, these products also carry the same potential health risks as ephedra. A recent randomized, double-blind, placebo-controlled study of single doses of *C. aurantium* in healthy adults reported significant increases in heart rate and blood pressure, compared with placebo. The authors state that the effects likely are due to a combination of *C. aurantium*, caffeine, and other stimulants contained in the multicomponent preparation.[40] The only clinical trial of *C. aurantium* for weight loss used a combination product containing 975 mg *C. aurantium* extract, 528 mg caffeine, and 900 mg St. John's wort (3% hypericum), and found that the herbal product was not superior to placebo for weight loss.[41] Many OTC weight-loss products list multiple ingredients, many of which are herbal extracts with varying active ingredients, together with vitamins and minerals. Many of these ingredients lack any scientific evidence for usefulness in weight loss. To confuse matters even more, many of the herbal extracts are listed by their common or not-so-common names (e.g., bitter orange, Seville orange, and sour orange are all common names for *C. aurantium*), and many do not list the botanical name, making it difficult to determine exactly what the herbal product contains.

Chattem, Inc., has launched a line of OTC products named Dexatrim Natural that exemplify the lack of botanical names. Their Green Tea Formula contains calcium, chromium, green tea leaf, and Asian ginseng root. Their Ephedrine Free Formula contains chromium, bitter orange peel powder extract, eleuthero extract, green tea leaf with added caffeine, fenugreek seed extract, guarana seed extract with added caffeine, cola nut extract with added caffeine, ginger root, licorice root, and vanadium amino acid chelate. Their No Caffeine Formula contains calcium, chromium, garcinia fruit extract, bitter orange fruit extract, and Asian ginseng root.[42]

The majority of these products have not been clearly demonstrated to be effective or safe, and many have been associated with serious adverse effects. Practitioners are advised to carefully review the labels of all dietary supplement weight-loss products to determine the risk for adverse reactions and drug-herb interactions.

### Benzocaine

Benzocaine is thought to produce appetite suppression and weight loss by local anesthetic effects on the oral cavity and GI mucosa, altering the taste of food. It is currently undergoing review by the FDA Advisory Panel on OTC Miscellaneous Internal Drug Products as an anorectic.[43] A randomized placebo-controlled trial comparing phenylpropanolamine with and without benzocaine gum reported an increase in adverse effects with no increase in weight loss in the combination treatment arm.[44] It should be noted, however, that certain OTC products continue to include benzocaine as the active ingredient (e.g., ZoCal lozenges).

### Use of Inappropriate Medications for Weight Loss

Individuals seeking to lose weight will sometimes turn to inappropriate, potentially dangerous methods to induce weight loss, such as laxatives or diuretics. The risks associated with laxatives and diuretics are discussed in Chapters 16 and 9, respectively.

## Complementary Therapies

Overweight or obese patients often use complementary therapies to stabilize blood sugars, customize exercise plans, and promote emotional well-being. Mind-body techniques and behavioral modification can help the patient align weight-loss goals with the goal of overall good health. Homeopathic remedies specifically designed for a given patient may be combined with lifestyle modification to assist with weight loss. Acupuncture may be used to help balance the various systems of the body and relieve stress. Massage may also be beneficial to relieve stress.

Dietary supplement weight-loss products are often used for assistance in losing weight. While proponents of these supplements correlate the term "natural" with safe, many have been associated with serious side effects, and the majority have not been clearly demonstrated to be effective. In fact, Chapter 53 does not list any herbal product as a safe and effective treatment for weight loss. Many of these supplements lack standards for potency and purity of ingredients, and reliable dosing guidelines, safety information, and monitoring advice are generally not available.

### Herbal Products

A summary of botanicals commonly used in weight-loss supplements is provided in Table 27-5. Many of these supplements also contain vitamins and minerals, presumably to ensure adequate intake of these essential nutrients by patients on low-caloric diets. In addition, the majority of these supplements contain multiple ingredients with several purported actions, although the advertising claims frequently focus on one solitary ingredient and/or action. To further complicate the problem, many of the supplements contain "proprietary blends." Ingredients of proprietary blends must be listed, but the amounts of the ingredients do not have to be specified. It is important to note, however, that many of these ingredients lack any scientific evidence for usefulness in weight loss. Broadly speaking, the ingredients of weight-loss supplements can be categorized as follows:

- *Stimulants and energy boosters and thermogenic aids* claim to increase basal metabolism, increase energy, and counteract fatigue (e.g., caffeine, bitter orange)
- *Fat and carbohydrate modulators* claim to alter fat and/or carbohydrate metabolism, resulting in decreased body fat mass and increased lean muscle mass (e.g., green tea, chromium, garcinia)
- *Appetite suppressants and satiety promoters* claim to decrease caloric intake by suppressing appetite or promoting satiety (e.g., guar gum, glucomannan, psyllium)
- *Fat absorption blockers* claim to block intestinal absorption of dietary fat (e.g., chitosan, derived from exoskeletons of marine organisms)
- *Carbohydrate absorption blockers* claim to block intestinal absorption of dietary carbohydrates (e.g., kidney bean extract, mung bean extract).

**TABLE 27-5 Complementary Therapies Commonly Used for Weight Loss[34,35,40,41,44-49]**

| Agent | Risks | Effectiveness for Weight Loss |
|---|---|---|
| **Botanical Medicines (Scientific Name)** | | |
| Bitter orange (*Citrus aurantium*) | Hypertension, cardiovascular toxicity, myocardial infarction, stroke, seizure | Synephrine source; acts as a stimulant; effectiveness not proven; use not recommended |
| Cascara sagrada (*Rhamnus purshiana*) | Abdominal pain, cramps, diarrhea; chronic use can lead to potassium depletion, disturbed heart function, and muscle weakness; avoid in patients taking digoxin or potassium-depleting diuretics | Acts as a laxative; effectiveness not proven |
| Cola nut (*Cola acuminata, C. nitida*) | GI distress, nausea, dehydration, headaches, insomnia, nervousness, anxiety, muscle tension, heart palpitations, hypertension, addiction, and possible genetic damage; avoid in patients with gastric ulcers | Caffeine source; acts as a stimulant and a diuretic; effectiveness not proven; use not recommended |
| Dandelion (*Taraxacum officinale*) | Avoid in patients with allergies to ragweed, marigolds, etc. (Asteraceae/Compositae family); contraindicated in patients with gallbladder or bile duct obstruction, or with bowel obstruction or pus in the pleural cavity | Acts as a diuretic; effectiveness not proven |
| Garcinia or brindleberry (*Garcinia cambogia*) | GI distress with high doses; not recommended in patients with DM or dementia | Hydroxycitric acid source; purported to inhibit fat synthesis; effectiveness not proven |
| Ginseng (*Panax* sp.) | Nervousness, excitation, inability to concentrate, estrogenic effects, Stevens-Johnson syndrome, allergy, hypoglycemic effects; may interact with several drugs including warfarin, digoxin, alcohol, and phenelzine | Claimed to boost performance and endurance and increase vitality; effectiveness not proven |
| Glucomannan (*Amorphophallus konjac*) | Similar to those of plantain | Insoluble fiber source claimed to increase satiety; effectiveness not demonstrated clearly |
| Green tea (*Camellia sinensis*) | GI distress, decreased appetite, insomnia, nervousness, hyperactivity, hypertension, increased heart rate, and gastric irritation; high doses associated with headache, heart palpitations, and vertigo; use with caution in patients with renal disease, panic disorder, hyperthyroidism, anxiety, or susceptibility to spasm; use only under medical supervision in patients with peptic ulcers, cardiovascular disease, or blood-clotting abnormalities; discontinue use at least 24 hours before surgery; may alter effects of anticoagulant medications | Caffeine and catechin source; stimulant; fat metabolism modifier; effectiveness not demonstrated clearly |
| Guarana (*Paullinia cupana, P. sorbilis*) | Similar to cola nut | Caffeine source; stimulant; poorly studied; use not recommended |
| Guar gum (*Cyamopsis tetragonolobus*) | Similar to those of plantain | Insoluble fiber source claimed to increase satiety; effectiveness not demonstrated clearly |
| Guggul (*Commiphora mukul*) | GI distress, diarrhea, nausea, skin rash; use only under medical supervision in patients with hyperthyroidism; may alter effects of thyroid medications, cholesterol-lowering medications, anticoagulants, antiplatelet medications, propranolol, and diltiazem | Claimed to release endogenous thyroid hormone; effectiveness not proven |
| Maté (*Ilex paraguariensis*) | Similar to those of cola nut | Caffeine source; stimulant; diuretic; poorly studied; use not recommended |
| Plantain or psyllium (*Plantago lanceolata, P. major, P. psyllium, P. arenatia*) | Flatulence, GI distress, nausea, and vomiting; may interact with lithium or carbamazepine | Laxation; effectiveness not proven |

**TABLE 27-5 Complementary Therapies Commonly Used for Weight Loss[34,35,40,41,44-49] (continued)**

| Agent | Risks | Effectiveness for Weight Loss |
|---|---|---|
| St. John's wort (*Hypericum perforatum*) | GI distress, nausea, loss of appetite, constipation, dry mouth, photosensitivity, allergic reactions, skin rash, hives, tiredness, fatigue, insomnia, restlessness, dizziness, confusion, and fast or irregular breathing; avoid in patients who are attempting to become pregnant, have received organ transplants, or are taking immunosuppressants; use only under medical supervision in patients with severe depression; may alter effects of oral contraceptives, anti-HIV medications, digoxin, immunosuppressants, anticoagulants, chemotherapy, asthma medications, and MAOIs | Component of herbal fen-phen (together with bitter orange); effectiveness not proven |
| Willow bark (*Salix alba*) | None reported when taken orally | Salicin source; claimed to have additive thermogenic effects with bitter orange and caffeine; poorly studied; use not recommended |
| **Nonbotanical Dietary Supplements** | | |
| Calcium | Constipation, nausea, vomiting | May increase lipolysis and preserve thermogenesis; possibly effective when ingested as naturally occurring calcium in foods; calcium supplements not proven to be effective for weight loss |
| Chromium | Rhabdomyolysis, renal failure with large doses | May increase lean body mass and decrease fat mass; effectiveness not proven; use not recommended |
| Conjugated linoleic acid | GI upset | May increase fat oxidation and decrease triglyceride uptake in adipose cells; effectiveness not proven |
| Pyruvate | None reported | May increase fat oxidation and decrease carbohydrate oxidation; effectiveness not proven |

Key: BPH, benign prostatic hyperplasia; DM, diabetes mellitus; GI, gastrointestinal; HIV, human immunodeficiency virus; MAOIs, monoamine oxidase inhibitors.

- *Cortisol blockers* claim to block stress-induced release of cortisol, which is claimed to cause increased appetite and fat storage (e.g., beta-sitosterol, phosphatidylserine, theanine)
- *Laxatives* (e.g., cascara sagrada, psyllium)
- *Diuretics* (e.g., dandelion, caffeine)

Herbal laxatives and diuretics are often included in multiple-ingredient dietary supplements marketed for weight loss. For example, "dieter's" or "slimming" teas contain a variety of botanical laxatives and diuretics. Diuretics, whether herbal or drug, may result in an initial transient weight loss, but this effect lasts only a few days. Herbal or drug laxatives typically act in the colon and, therefore, will not decrease caloric absorption in the small intestine, which is the primary site of food absorption. Many of these botanicals are stimulant laxatives that should be used for only 1 to 2 weeks at a time. Prolonged use may lead to electrolyte imbalances and dependence on the laxative for regular bowel movements (cathartic colon), as discussed in Chapter 16.

Herbal sources of caffeine have often been used in combination with ephedra and willow bark (as a source of salicin) for weight loss because of purported synergistic effects. This combination is often referred to as a "fat-burning stack" or "ECA" (ephedrine-caffeine-aspirin), with claims of additive thermogenic or heat-producing effects.[35,50] However, adverse reactions to these products, either alone or in combination, range from relatively mild symptoms such as headache, nervousness, and hypertension, to more severe reactions such as stroke, myocardial infarction, and sudden death. In several cases, significant adverse events occurred in otherwise healthy young or middle-aged adults, and many occurred following consumption of relatively low doses for short periods.[50]

So-called herbal fen-phen combinations have been marketed in response to the recall of the prescription medication fenfluramine, which was often prescribed in combination with phentermine. These products contained ephedra in combination with St. John's wort (*Hypericum perforatum*). Proponents claim the combination increases energy and metabolism while suppressing appetite, yet scientific evidence supporting this claim is lacking. Although FDA's ban on sales of products containing ephedra has removed ECA products from the market, bitter orange is now often combined with caffeine, willow bark, and St. John's wort in its place (see The Ephedra Debate).

### Calcium

Some evidence suggests that increasing calcium intake from dairy products results in increased weight loss in patients on a calorie-restricted diet. Data suggest that an increased calcium intake of approximately two dairy servings per day is associated with a weight loss ranging from 0.11 to 4.9 kg/year.[49] However, a similar effect was not demonstrated using calcium supplementation with 1000 mg/day in conjunction with moderate dietary restriction.[48]

### Chromium

Chromium is an essential nutrient with adequate intake set at 20 to 35 μg/day. It is promoted for weight loss either alone or as a component of multi-ingredient weight-loss supplements. There is some evidence that chromium picolinate can increase lean body mass and decrease fat mass, although this remains controversial and some studies have shown no benefit.[46,47] Chromium is known to increase insulin sensitivity and is often referred to as a glucose tolerance factor. The picolinate salt of chromium is a naturally occurring derivative of the amino acid tryptophan and may be responsible for the changes in mood and sleep, headaches, and cognitive and perception dysfunction that have been reported with chromium picolinate.[44] Perhaps of even greater concern are several recent cases of rhabdomyolysis and/or renal failure in patients taking megadoses of chromium.[47]

## Assessment of Overweight and Obesity: A Case-based Approach

When practitioners are asked to recommend a weight-loss method or product, they should find out why the patient wants to lose weight. The reason may be immediately obvious for some patients; others may want to lose a few pounds to improve their appearance or to enhance their perception of their own good health. The practitioner should calculate the patient's BMI to determine if the patient is, in fact, overweight or obese. The practitioner should also review the patient's current prescription and nonprescription drug history, and ask about use of herbal products and other dietary supplements. Anyone with significant diseases superimposed on obesity should be discouraged from using dietary supplements. The practitioner should also find out what type of weight-loss methods were used previously and whether the attempts were successful so other methods or adjunctive products may be considered, if needed. Whether the patient received dietary counseling or was seeing a registered dietitian should also be determined.

A dieter needs support from family and friends to succeed at losing weight. It may be difficult to change eating and other behavioral habits if family members are not willing to support the dieter. Cultural differences and food preferences in different parts of the country may complicate weight-loss efforts. The practitioner must explore the family dynamic before recommending weight-loss measures. Still, such factors should not be seen as insurmountable obstacles to weight loss.

Individuals who are within the normal height/weight range but want to lose weight for other reasons (e.g., improved appearance or sense of well-being) should be advised about the difficulty of the task and the potential adverse physical and psychologic effects.

Coupled with other information obtained during the assessment, the practitioner can decide whether weight loss is appropriate and, if warranted, can help select the type, intensity, and length of a weight-loss program. Cases 27-1 and 27-2 illustrate assessment of patients who seek assistance with weight control.

### CASE 27-1

| Relevant Evaluation Criteria | Scenario/Model Outcome |
|---|---|
| **Information Gathering** | |
| 1. Gather essential information about the patient's symptoms, including: | |
| a. description of symptom(s) (i.e., nature, onset, duration, severity, associated symptoms) | Patient has been overweight since early in elementary school. She has experienced a 10-lb weight gain over the past year, with a concomitant gain in height of 1 inch. Patient is self-conscious about her weight and her energy level is low. |
| b. description of any factors that seem to precipitate, exacerbate, and/or relieve the patient's symptoms. | Patient often seeks "comfort foods" to make her feel better, especially in the evenings and on weekends when she is watching television. She rarely participates in outdoor activities; physical education is not required in her school. |

## CASE 27-1 (continued)

| Relevant Evaluation Criteria | Scenario/Model Outcome |
|---|---|
| c. description of the patient's efforts to relieve the symptoms | Patient's mother has been attempting to fix dinners with lower fat content, but both the mother and her daughter enjoy high-fat snacks. |
| 2. Gather essential patient history information: | |
| a. patient's identity | Jan Stafford |
| b. age, sex, height, and weight | 14 y/o F, 5'2", 145 lb |
| c. patient's occupation | High school freshman |
| d. patient's dietary habits | Eats light breakfast, eats school cafeteria "fast food" for lunch, often eats dinner and high-fat snacks while watching television in the evening. |
| e. patient's sleep habits | Usually gets 8 hours of sleep on school nights, often sleeps until noon on weekends. |
| f. concurrent medical conditions, prescription and nonprescription medications, and dietary supplements | None |
| g. allergies | NKA |
| h. history of other adverse reactions to medications | None |
| i. other (describe)_______ | Patient's mother and father are both overweight. Patient has recently visited her primary care provider who recommended diet and exercise for weight control. |
| **Assessment and Triage** | |
| 3. Differentiate the patient's signs/symptoms and correctly identify the patient's primary problem(s). | Jan's BMI is [145 lb/2.2 kg/lb]/[(62 in.)(2.54 cm/in.)(1 m/100 cm)]$^2$ = 27 (see Table 27-1), and she is above the 85th percentile of BMI for her age, classifying her as at risk for overweight. Overweight in adolescents increases risk for Type 2 DM, high cholesterol, hypertension, sleep apnea, and orthopedic problems during both adolescence and adulthood if weight is not normalized. Her consumption of fast food at lunch and high-fat snack foods in the evening, along with her inactivity, are contributing to her weight problem. |
| 4. Identify exclusions for self-treatment (see Figure 27-3). | Age less than 18 years is an exclusion for self-treatment. However, the patient has recently been cleared by her primary care provider to begin a diet and exercise program. |
| 5. Formulate a comprehensive list of therapeutic alternatives for the primary problem to determine if triage to a medical practitioner is required, and share this information with the patient. | Options include:<br>(1) Recommend lifestyle modification alone.<br>(2) Refer Jan to a dietitian and/or personal trainer to design a diet/exercise plan.<br>(3) Take no action. |
| **Plan** | |
| 6. Select an optimal therapeutic alternative to address the patient's problem, taking into account patient preferences. | Lifestyle modification is in order. Because the patient is eager to lose weight, she is willing to entertain suggestions. |
| 7. Describe the recommended therapeutic approach to the patient. | Eating a healthy, but substantial breakfast may be helpful in preventing overeating at lunch. Packing a low-fat lunch or choosing low-fat alternatives in the school cafeteria (e.g., lean meat sandwiches, fruit) will help cut calorie consumption. Keeping low-fat, healthy foods (e.g., fruit, carrots, pretzels) available for evening snacks should also curb calories. Engaging in an enjoyable activity for 30 to 60 minutes most days of the week is desirable (see Table 27-4). |
| 8. Explain to the patient the rationale for selecting the recommended therapeutic approach from the considered therapeutic alternatives. | Eating lower-calorie, lower-fat foods, and engaging in physical activity should help achieve a neutral or negative calorie balance and facilitate weight loss or at least weight maintenance. (See the box Patient Education for Overweight and Obesity.) |

## CASE 27-1 (continued)

| Relevant Evaluation Criteria | Scenario/Model Outcome |
|---|---|
| **Patient Education** | |
| 9. When recommending self-care with nonprescription medications and/or nondrug therapy, convey accurate information to the patient, including: | |
| a. appropriate dose and frequency of administration | N/A |
| b. maximum number of days the therapy should be employed | Healthy eating habits and exercise should be a lifelong goal. |
| c. product administration procedures | N/A |
| d. expected time to onset of relief | N/A |
| e. degree of relief that can be reasonably expected | A realistic weight-loss goal is 10% of initial weight over a 6-month period, or about 0.5-1 lb/week. |
| f. most common side effects | N/A |
| g. side effects that warrant medical intervention should they occur | N/A |
| h. patient options in the event that condition worsens or persists | Visiting a dietitian or personal trainer may provide further motivation. |
| i. product storage requirements | N/A |
| j. specific nondrug measures | See the box Patient Education for Overweight and Obesity. |
| 10. Solicit follow-up questions from patient. | Isn't there a pill I can use to help curb my appetite? |
| 11. Answer patient's questions. | None of the OTC drugs or supplements marketed for weight loss has been shown to be effective. These products should not be used because of potential safety issues. Prescription products for weight loss are not recommended for patients of your age and weight. |

Key: BMI, body mass index; DM, diabetes mellitus; N/A, not applicable; NKA, no known allergies; OTC, over-the-counter.

## CASE 27-2

| Relevant Evaluation Criteria | Scenario/Model Outcome |
|---|---|
| **Information Gathering** | |
| 1. Gather essential information about the patient's symptoms, including: | Patient has been overweight or obese since adolescence. Over the past 10 years, his weight has increased roughly 5 lb/year, which he attributes to stress on the job and marriage to a good cook (who is also overweight). His obesity has contributed to several health problems, including Type 2 DM and hyperlipidemia. |
| a. description of symptom(s) (i.e., nature, onset, duration, severity, associated symptoms) | He gets winded when walking and climbing stairs (which he tries to avoid), and his major exercises are playing with his infant son and walking from his couch to the refrigerator for his beer while watching television. |
| b. description of any factors that seem to precipitate, exacerbate, and/or relieve the patient's symptoms. | Patient states he's tried low-fat and low-carbohydrate diets in the past as well as phenylpropanolamine when it was still available with little success. Two weeks ago he sought help from his physician, who recommended a comprehensive program combining diet, exercise, drug therapy, and monthly visits for at least 1 year. |
| c. description of the patient's efforts to relieve the symptoms | N/A |

## CASE 27-2 (continued)

| Relevant Evaluation Criteria | Scenario/Model Outcome |
|---|---|
| 2. Gather essential patient history information: | |
| a. patient's identity | Brad Sharp |
| b. age, sex, height, and weight | 34 y/o M, 5'10", 243 lb, waist circumference 41" |
| c. patient's occupation | High school math teacher |
| d. patient's dietary habits | Brad has changed his diet and increased his physical activity over the course of the past 2 weeks, but has cravings for sweet and salty foods that are hard to control. |
| e. patient's sleep habits | Brad has trouble sleeping through the night, but this has been a chronic problem for him. |
| f. concurrent medical conditions, prescription and nonprescription medications, and dietary supplements | Xenical 120 mg 3 times/day for obesity; Glucovance 2.5/500 2 times/day for Type 2 DM; Lipitor 20 mg daily for hyperlipidemia |
| g. allergies | NKA |
| h. history of other adverse reactions to medications | None |
| i. other (describe)_______ | With the above medications, patient's blood pressure is 128/78; glucose 108 mg/dL; total cholesterol 160 mg/dL; HDL 35 mg/dL; LDL 111 mg/dL; and triglycerides 160 mg/dL |
| **Assessment and Triage** | |
| 3. Differentiate the patient's signs/symptoms and correctly identify the patient's primary problem(s). | Patient's BMI is [243 lb/2.2 lb/kg]/[(70 in.)(2.54 cm/in)(1 m/100 cm)]$^2$ = 35 (see Table 27-1), classifying patient as class II obesity with comorbid conditions of Type 2 DM and hyperlipidemia. He has metabolic syndrome based on his waist circumference, triglycerides, HDL cholesterol, and fasting glucose. |
| 4. Identify exclusions for self-treatment (see Figure 27-3). | DM and dyslipidemia usually are exclusions to self-treatment; however, in this case, the patient states that his physician has already recommended that he start a weight loss regimen as an adjunct to his orlistat therapy. |
| 5. Formulate a comprehensive list of therapeutic alternatives for the primary problem to determine if triage to a medical practitioner is required, and share this information with the patient. | Options include:<br>(1) Reiterate lifestyle modification begun 2 weeks ago.<br>(2) Refer Brad to a dietitian or personal trainer for additional counseling and advice.<br>(3) Take no action. |
| **Plan** | |
| 6. Select an optimal therapeutic alternative to address the patient's problem, taking into account patient preferences. | Brad should be encouraged to adhere to his current diet and exercise program and continue taking his prescribed medications. A low-fat diet would be preferred to improve tolerance to the prescribed weight-loss medication, taking into account the patient's preferences. Depending on his beer consumption, counseling regarding cutting back may be appropriate, as this beverage could be adding significant caloric intake. Lifestyle modifications should be reviewed (see Figure 27-3). Motivation for this patient could include appealing to his desire to be healthy for the sake of his family. Patient should discuss his sleep issues with his PCP. See Chapter 48 for discussion of treatment options/advice for insomnia. |
| 7. Describe the recommended therapeutic approach to the patient. | See the box Patient Education for Overweight and Obesity. |
| 8. Explain to the patient the rationale for selecting the recommended therapeutic approach from the considered therapeutic alternatives. | Your PCP, that is, primary care provider, should rule out any potential underlying causes for your sleep disturbances, such as sleep apnea. By continuing with a comprehensive weight-loss program, your cravings should become less bothersome. When cravings occur, consider a diversion technique such as taking a walk or doing simple stretches; also keeping on hand low-calorie snacks such as carrots or celery could be helpful. |

CASE 27-2 (continued)

| Relevant Evaluation Criteria | Scenario/Model Outcome |
|---|---|
| **Patient Education** | |
| 9. When recommending self-care with nonprescription medications and/or nondrug therapy, convey accurate information to the patient, including: | |
| a. appropriate dose and frequency of administration | N/A |
| b. maximum number of days the therapy should be employed | Healthy eating habits and exercise (30 to 90 minutes on most days–can be cumulative throughout day) should be a lifelong goal. |
| c. product administration procedures | N/A |
| d. expected time to onset of relief | You should start experiencing weight loss within the first month after starting your weight loss and exercise program. You should start noticing a higher energy level and less shortness of breath when walking or climbing stairs as you continue with the program. |
| e. degree of relief that can be reasonably expected | See 9d. |
| f. most common side effects | N/A |
| g. side effects that warrant medical intervention should they occur | N/A |
| h. patient options in the event that condition worsens or persists | Your PCP may switch you to an alternative prescription weight-loss medication. Bariatric surgery would only be an option if you continue with a BMI greater than 35 with comorbid conditions. |
| i. product storage requirements | N/A |
| j. specific nondrug measures | See the box Patient Education for Overweight and Obesity. |
| 10. Solicit follow-up questions from patient. | I've heard that chromium might reduce my food cravings and help control my blood sugars. Is it safe for me to take this product? |
| 11. Answer patient's questions. | While some studies suggest that chromium picolinate can increase muscle mass and decrease fat mass, other studies show no benefit. Chromium does increase insulin sensitivity. However, large doses have potential additive effects with your atorvastatin for causing muscle deterioration or rhabdomyolysis. I don't recommend using this product. |

Key: BMI, body mass index; DM, diabetes mellitus; HDL, high-density lipoprotein; LDL, low-density lipoprotein; N/A, not applicable; PCP, primary care provider.

## Patient Counseling for Overweight and Obesity

The objectives for counseling patients who want to lose weight are to foster realistic goals for weight loss together with a healthy restricted-calorie diet and increased physical activity. The ultimate goal is to achieve a healthy weight and maintain that weight over the long term. For those patients unable to lose weight, the objective is to prevent further weight gain.

## Evaluation of Patient Outcomes for Overweight and Obesity

Successful weight loss generally requires a lifelong approach combining healthy eating and exercise patterns. Realistic weight-loss goals of 10% of the initial weight over 6 months, or 1 to 2 lb/week, should be encouraged. During any weight-loss program, the patient should be monitored for healthy eating and exercise patterns, and, at a minimum, blood pressure should be routinely measured. More extensive physical examinations and laboratory measures may be indicated, particularly in those patients with comorbid conditions such as hypertension or DM. Follow-up with patients attempting weight loss should be encouraged, preferably on a monthly basis. In addition to measuring weight at monthly follow-ups, the practitioner should explore eating habits and exercise patterns with the patient, especially if weight loss is not being achieved. Referral to a dietitian or personal trainer may be helpful in such cases. Referral to a primary care provider for pharmacologic therapy may be an option for patients with more significant obesity who fail to lose weight through lifestyle modifications.

## PATIENT EDUCATION FOR OVERWEIGHT AND OBESITY

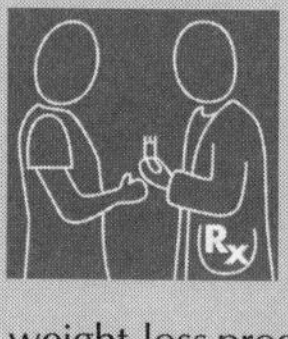

The objectives of self-treatment are to (1) foster realistic weight-loss and exercise goals, (2) maintain a healthy weight, and (3) prevent further weight gain. For most patients, carefully following the self-care measures listed here, together with continued adherence to a safe and effective weight-loss program, will help ensure optimal therapeutic outcomes.

### Health Risks of Obesity

- Health risks related to overweight and obesity include:
  - Coronary heart disease
  - Type 2 diabetes mellitus
  - Sleep apnea
  - Elevated serum triglycerides and dyslipidemia
  - Hypertension
  - Stroke
  - Gallbladder disease
  - Osteoarthritis
  - Certain types of cancers

### Nondrug Treatment Guidelines

- Focus on small, gradual changes in eating and exercise patterns.
- Maintain realistic goals for weight loss and increased activity levels.
- Eat a low-calorie balanced diet.
- Eat meals at the table, and do nothing else while eating (no television, etc.).
- Set a regular eating schedule, and avoid skipping meals.
- Eat slowly and enjoy the food.
- Put your fork or spoon down between bites.
- Try to leave some food on your plate each time you eat.
- Wait 5 minutes before going back for extra helpings of food.
- Remove serving dishes from the table after the first servings have been made.
- Leave the table after eating.
- Use smaller plates so moderate servings don't appear too small.
- Start a meal with a broth-based soup (low-salt) to help you feel more full.
- Strive to consume at least five servings a day of fruits and vegetables.
- Keep on hand healthful snacks such as fruits and vegetables, low-fat cheese and yogurt, and frozen fruit juice bars.
- Drink at least eight glasses of noncaloric beverages each day to help you feel full.
- When you experience a craving, try doing something else, such as going for a walk; cravings generally pass within minutes.
- Shop for food immediately after a meal, and use a prepared list.
- Gradually increase your activity level, with the goal of engaging in 60 minutes of moderate-intensity physical activity most days of the week.
- Increase your lifestyle activity: walk more, climb stairs, park further away.
- Limit the amount of time spent watching television, playing video games, or surfing the Internet.
- Keep a diary of your weight, physical activity, and caloric intake so you can see your progress and success.

### Drug Management Guidelines

- Avoid taking OTC drugs and supplements marketed for weight loss. They are not proven to work, and they can cause significant side effects.
- If you do decide to take one of these products, make sure to notify your primary care provider and pharmacist so you can be adequately followed for potential side effects and interactions with drugs.

## Key Points for Overweight and Obesity

- A reasonable goal for weight loss in most overweight and obese subjects is a 10% loss over 6 months.
- Even though this amount of weight loss may not result in the cosmetic effect desired by the dieter, it is associated with a reduction in risk for chronic disease.
- The safest approach to losing weight entails combining a reduced-calorie diet with increased physical activity.
- Physical activity typically needs to be something the person enjoys if it is to be sustained over long periods of time.
- A key to sustained weight loss is modification of behavior related to eating and exercise.
- If OTC or dietary supplement products for weight loss are used, they should be continuously assessed for efficacy, safety, and tolerance.
- Labels of OTC or dietary supplement weight-loss products should be carefully reviewed to determine the risk for adverse reactions and drug-herb interactions.

## References


1. National Heart, Lung, and Blood Institute of the National Institutes of Health. Clinical guidelines on the identification, evaluation, and treatment of overweight and obesity in adults. The evidence report. 1998. Available at: http://www.nhlbi.nih.gov/guidelines/obesity/ob_gdlns.pdf. Accessed July 5, 2005.
2. Finkelstein EA, Fiebelkorn IC, Wang G. State-level estimates of annual medical expenditures attributable to obesity. *Obes Res.* 2004;12:18-24.
3. Raebel MA, Malone DC, Conner DA, et al. Health services use and health care costs of obese and nonobese individuals. *Arch Intern Med.* 2004;164:2135-40.
4. Mokdad AH, Bowman BA, Ford ES, et al. The continuing epidemics of obesity and diabetes in the United States. *JAMA.* 2001; 286:1195-200.
5. National Heart, Lung, and Blood Institute of the National Institutes of Health and North American Association for the Study of Obesity. The practical guide. Identification, evaluation, and treatment of overweight and obesity in adults. 2000. Available at: http://www.nhlbi.nih.gov/guidelines/obesity/prctgd_c.pdf. Accessed July 5, 2005.
6. National Center for Health Statistics. Centers for Disease Control and Prevention Growth Charts: United States. Available at: http://www.cdc.gov/nchs/about/major/nhanes/growthcharts/charts.htm. Accessed June 22, 2005.
7. Strawbridge WJ, Wallhagen MI, Shema SJ. New NHLBI clinical guidelines for obesity and overweight: will they promote health? *Am J Public Health.* 2000;90:340-3.
8. Hedley AA, Ogden CL, Johnson CL, et al. Prevalence of overweight and obesity among US children, adolescents, and adults, 1999-2002. *JAMA.* 2004;291:2847-50.

9. National Center for Health Statistics. Prevalence of overweight among children and adolescents ages 6-19 years [Reviewed December 16, 2004]. Available at: http://www.cdc.gov/nchs/products/pubs/pubd/hestats/overwght99.htm. Accessed July 5, 2005.
10. Cummings S, Parham ES, Strain GW. Position of the American Dietetic Association: weight management. *J Am Diet Assoc.* 2002;102:1145-55.
11. Overweight, obesity, and health risk. National Task Force on the Prevention and Treatment of Obesity. *Arch Intern Med.* 2000;160:898-904.
12. Flegal KM, Graubard BI, Williamson DF, Gail MH. Excess deaths associated with underweight, overweight, and obesity. *JAMA.* 2005;293:1861-7.
13. Kenchaiah S, Evans JC, Levy D, et al. Obesity and the risk of heart failure. *N Engl J Med.* 2004;347:305-13.
14. Wang TJ, Parise H, Levy D, et al. Obesity and the risk of new-onset atrial fibrillation. *JAMA.* 2004;292:2471-7.
15. Kurth T, Gaziano JM, Berger K, et al. Body mass index and the risk of stroke in men. *Arch Intern Med.* 2002;162:2557-62.
16. Mokdad AH, Ford ES, Bowman BA, et al. Prevalence of obesity, diabetes, and obesity-related health risk factors, 2001. *JAMA.* 2003;289:76-79.
17. Reaven GM. Importance of identifying the overweight patient who will benefit the most by losing weight. *Ann Intern Med.* 2003;138:420-3.
18. Knowler WC, Barrett-Conner E, Fowler SE, et al. Reduction in the incidence of type 2 diabetes with lifestyle intervention or metformin. *N Engl J Med.* 2002;346: 393-403.
19. Daniels SR, Arnett DK, Eckel RH, et al. Overweight in children and adolescents. *Circulation.* 2005;111:1999-2012.
20. Calle EE, Rodriguez C, Walker-Thurmond K, et al. Overweight, obesity, and mortality from cancer in a prospectively studied cohort of US adults. *N Engl J Med.* 2003;348:1725-38.
21. The National Weight Control Registry. Available at: http://www.lifespan.org/services/bmed/wt_loss/nwcr/. Accessed July 5, 2005.
22. Dietary Reference Intakes for Energy, Carbohydrate, Fiber, Fat, Fatty Acids, Cholesterol, Protein, and Amino Acids (Macronutrients). Washington, DC: National Academy Press; 2002. Available at: http://www.nap.edu/books/0309085373/html/. Accessed July 5, 2005.
23. US Department of Health and Human Services and US Department of Agriculture. Dietary guidelines for Americans 2005. Available at: www.healthierus.gov/dietaryguidelines. Accessed July 5, 2005.
24. Yancy WS, Olsen MK, Guyton JR, et al. A low-carbohydrate, ketogenic diet versus a low-fat diet to treat obesity and hyperlipidemia. *Ann Intern Med.* 2004;140:769-77.
25. Stern L, Iqbal N, Seshadri P, et al. The effects of low-carbohydrate versus conventional weight loss diets in severely obese adults: one-year follow-up of a randomized trial. *Ann Intern Med.* 2004;140:778-85.
26. Noakes M, Foster PR, Keogh JB, et al. Meal replacements are as effective as structured weight-loss diets for treating obesity in adults with features of metabolic syndrome. *J Nutr.* 2004;134:1894-9.
27. Tsai AG, Wadden TA. Systematic review: an evaluation of major commercial weight loss programs in the United States. *Ann Intern Med.* 2005;143:56-66.
28. Klein S, Wadden T, Sugerman HJ. AGA technical review on obesity. *Gastroenterology.* 2002;123:882-932.
29. Aikman B. FDA to ban 111 diet product ingredients. August 7, 1991. Available at: http://www.fda.gov/bbs/topics/NEWS/NEW00003.html. Accessed July 5, 2005.
30. Woodcock J. FDA letter to manufacturers of drug products containing phenylpropanolamine (PPA). November 3, 2000. Available at: http://www.fda.gov/cder/drug/infopage/ppa/default.htm. Accessed July 5, 2005.
31. Dotzel MM. Cold, cough, allergy, bronchodilator, and antiasthmatic drug products for over-the-counter human use; partial final rule for combination drug products containing a bronchodilator. Department of Health and Human Services. Food and Drug Administration. 21 CFR Part 341 [Docket No. 76N-052G] RIN 0910-AA01. September 20, 2001. Available at: http://www.fda.gov/ohrms/dockets/98fr/cdotc998.pdf. Accessed July 5, 2005.
32. Dotzel MM. Status of certain additional over-the-counter drug category II and III active ingredients. Department of Health and Human Services. Food and Drug Administration. 21 CFR Part 310 [Docket No. 78N-0366] RIN 0910-AA01. April 29, 2002. Available at: http://www.fda.gov/OHRMS/DOCKETS/98fr/050902a.htm. Accessed July 5, 2005.
33. Panel supports offering diet pill orlistat over the counter. *Washington Post.* January 24, 2006;A02.
34. Hebel SK, Burnham TH, Short RM, et al. *The Lawrence Review of Natural Products.* St. Louis: Facts and Comparisons; 1999.
35. Boozer CN, Daly PA, Homel P, et al. Herbal ephedra/caffeine for weight loss: a 6-month safety and efficacy trial. *Int J Obes Relat Metab Disord.* 2002;26:593-604.
36. Food and Drug Administration. HHS acts to reduce potential risks of dietary supplements containing ephedra. February 28, 2003. Available at: http://www.fda.gov/bbs/topics/NEWS/2003/NEW00875.html. Accessed July 5, 2005.
37. McClellan MB. Final rule declaring dietary supplements containing ephedrine alkaloids adulterated because they present an unreasonable risk. Department of Health and Human Services. Food and Drug Administration. 21 CFR Part 119 [Docket No. 1995N-0304] RIN 0910-AA59. February 11, 2004. Available at: http://www.fda.gov/OHRMS/DOCKETS/98fr/1995n-0304-nfr0001.pdf. Accessed July 5, 2005.
38. Amin RM, Blumenthal M. Federal court overturns FDA ban on ephedra at low doses. *HerbalGram.* 2005;64:52-3.
39. FDA appeals Utah ephedra ruling (6-15-05). Available at: http://www.ahpa.org/update_05_0615.htm. Accessed June 30, 2005.
40. Haller CA, Benowitz NF, Jacob P III. Hemodynamic effects of ephedra-free weight-loss supplements in humans. *Am J Med.* 2005;118:998-1003.
41. Colker CM, Kalman DS, Torina GC, et al. Effects of *Citrus aurantium* extract, caffeine, and St. John's wort on body fat loss, lipid levels, and mood states in overweight healthy adults. *Curr Ther Res.* 1999;60:145-53.
42. Dexatrim dietary supplements product information. Available at: http://www.dexatrim.com/product.asp. Accessed July 5, 2005.
43. OTC ingredient list. Updated July 2003. Available at: http://www.fda.gov/cder/offices/otc/Ingredient_List_A-C.pdf. Accessed July 5, 2005.
44. Greenway F, Herber D, Raum W, et al. Double-blind, randomized, placebo-controlled trials with non-prescription medications for the treatment of obesity. *Obes Res.* 1999;7:370-8.
45. Blumenthal M, Busse WR, Goldberg A, et al., eds. *The Complete German Commission E Monographs. Therapeutic Guide to Herbal Medicines.* Austin, Tex: American Botanical Council; 1998.
46. Pittler MH, Ernst E. Dietary supplements for body-weight reduction: a systematic review. *Am J Clin Nutr.* 2004;79:529-36.
47. Saper RB, Eisenberg DM, Phillips RS. Common dietary supplements for weight loss. *Am Fam Physician.* 2004;70:1731-8.
48. Heaney RP, Davies M, Barger-Lux J. Calcium and weight: clinical studies. *J Am Coll Nutr.* 2002;21:152S-5S.
49. Shapses SA, Heshka S, Heymsfield SB. Effect of calcium supplementation on weight and fat loss in women. *J Clin Endocrinol Metab.* 2004;89:632-7.
50. Shekelle PG, Hardy ML, Morton SC, et al. Efficacy and safety of ephedra and ephedrine for weight loss and athletic performance: a meta-analysis. *JAMA.* 2003;289:1537-45.

SECTION VII

# Ophthalmic, Otic, and Oral Disorders

CHAPTER 28

# Ophthalmic Disorders

Richard G. Fiscella and Michael Kirk Jensen

The nonprescription ophthalmic market consists of products that treat a wide range of disorders. Little population-based data are available on the epidemiology of these disorders. People with ocular conditions are commonly seen in the primary care provider's office, the emergency department, the eye care practitioner's office, or the pharmacy. Ocular discomfort associated with dry eye may be the most common condition for which nonprescription ophthalmic products can be used. It may affect as many as 4.3 million people in the United States and 20% of persons of advanced age.[1]

Many common conditions causing ocular discomfort are minor and self-limiting. In some instances, however, relatively minor symptoms may be associated with severe, potentially vision-threatening conditions. Practitioners should be well versed in eye anatomy and physiology as well as in common ocular conditions so they can provide the best possible guidance for patients who want help in choosing between self-treatment and professional medical care.

Self-treatable ophthalmic disorders occur primarily on the eyelids; however, a few disorders of the eye surface may be amenable to self-treatment. They include dry eyes, allergic conjunctivitis, viral conjunctivitis, diagnosed corneal edema, presence of loose foreign debris, minor ocular irritation, diagnosed age-related macular degeneration, and the cleaning or lubricating of artificial eyes. Disorders of the eyelid and adjacent areas that are amenable to self-care include contact dermatitis, lice infestations, hordeolum, chalazion, and blepharitis. Obviously, careful assessment is important, especially with ongoing symptoms, to rule out more complicated manifestations that may require specialized eye care.

## EYE ANATOMY AND PHYSIOLOGY

The external location and exposure of the eye make it susceptible to environmental and microbiologic contamination. However, the eye has many natural defense mechanisms to protect it against contamination, and the eyelid is one of its major protective elements (Figure 28-1).

The eyelids are a multilayer tissue covered externally by the skin and internally by a thin, mucocutaneous epithelial layer called the palpebral conjunctiva. The middle portion of the eyelid contains glandular tissue and muscles for lid movement. The five main types of glandular tissue found within the eyelid, along with conjunctival goblet cells, secrete the bulk of nonstimulated tears.

The eyelids primarily protect the anterior surface of the eye and spread the tears produced by the glandular tissue over the ocular surface. The lids force the flow of tears toward the nose, where drainage canals are located in the upper and lower eyelids. The drainage canals converge, forming the lacrimal sac between the inner eyelid and nose. The lacrimal sac is drained by a canal opening just below the inferior turbinate of the nasal cavity. A highly vascularized epithelium lines the lacrimal drainage system, and absorption into the systemic circulation along this pathway gives rise to potential systemic effects of topically administered eye medications.[2]

The tear layer keeps the ocular surface lubricated, provides a mechanism for removing debris that touches the ocular surface, and has a potent antimicrobial action provided by specific enzymes and a number of immunoglobulins, most notably immunoglobulin A. The tear layer is a complex multilayer film. The outer lipid layer maintains the eyes' optical properties and reduces evaporation. The middle aqueous layer is largely responsible for the wetting properties of the tear film. The inner mucinous layer allows the aqueous and lipid layers to maintain constant adhesion across the cornea and conjunctiva. Abnormalities within any one of the tear layers can result in ocular discomfort.

Tears are produced at a rate of 1 to 2 μL/minute, with a turnover of approximately 16% of the total volume per minute.[3,4] As much as 25% of the total tear volume is lost to evaporation.[3] An ambient tear volume of approximately 7 to 10 μL is found on the ocular surface at any point in time.[3] During episodes of ocular irritation, reflex tearing is stimulated by the lacrimal gland found underneath the outer portion of the upper eyelid, and tear production increases to greater than 300% of the nonstimulated production rate.[5] Reflex tearing occurs immediately on instillation of a drug into the eye, diluting the drug's concentration. Drug penetration into the eye is reduced because of increased lacrimal drainage and tearing that falls down the cheek. Studies have shown that as much as 90% of an instilled dose of a drug administered to the eye may be lost.[6]

The visible external portion of the eye is composed of the cornea and sclera; the former is innervated, whereas the latter is not. The sclera is a tough, collagenous layer that gives the eye rigidity and encases the internal eye structures. The visible sclera is covered by two epithelial layers: the episclera and the bulbar conjunctiva. The bulbar conjunctiva is contiguous with the palpebral conjunctiva at the junction between the eyelid and the ocular

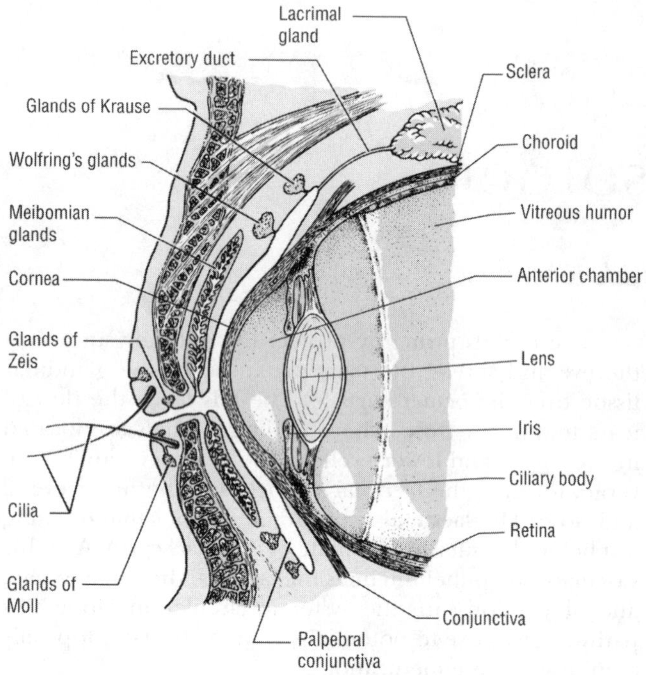


**FIGURE 28-1** Anatomy of the eyelid and eye surface.

surface (the fornix). The episcleral and bulbar conjunctival layers contain the vascular and lymphatic systems of the anterior eye surface and are the sources of visible eye redness in ocular irritation or inflammation.

The cornea is an aspherical, avascular tissue that is the principal refractive element of the eye. It is approximately 12 mm wide and 0.5 mm thick and consists of five distinct layers. Of the five corneal layers, the outermost epithelium layer, the middle and most abundant stromal layer, and the innermost endothelial layer affect the pharmacokinetics of ocularly administered drugs. The corneal epithelium is lipophilic and facilitates the passage of fat-soluble drugs. The epithelium is often the rate-limiting step in absorption of medication into the anterior chamber. The corneal stroma is hydrophilic and allows the passage of water-soluble drugs. Damage to the corneal epithelium may often increase drug absorption rates. Comparative studies with intact and compromised epithelium have shown that drug penetration into the aqueous humor may be increased by as much as threefold in corneas with compromised epithelium.[7] Corneal epithelium can be compromised by trauma, routine contact lens wear, topical ocular anesthetics, and thermal or ultraviolet (UV) light exposure.

Directly behind the cornea is the anterior chamber, a cavity filled with aqueous humor. The aqueous humor maintains the normal intraocular pressure (IOP) and provides nutritional support for the cornea and crystalline lens. It is produced by the ciliary body and drained from the anterior chamber through the uveoscleral tract and the trabecular meshwork. The trabecular meshwork, which is located at the junction of the cornea and iris, accounts for approximately 80% to 90% of aqueous drainage from the anterior chamber. The uveoscleral tract, located posteriorly to the iris and comprising the sclera, ciliary body, and choroid areas, accounts for approximately 10% to 20% of aqueous drainage, although this may vary with age and disease state. During episodes of internal eye inflammation, inflammatory cells may block the drainage system, causing the IOP to rise. Increased IOP is one of the most significant risk factors for primary open-angle glaucoma. Similarly, during episodes of angle-closure glaucoma, the iris physically blocks the trabecular meshwork, thereby also resulting in an increase in IOP. Dilating the pupil with mydriatic drugs may precipitate an angle-closure attack. Such attacks often occur as the pupil is returning to its normal state several hours after the mydriatic drug has been instilled. Any agent with anticholinergic or dilating effect has the potential to cause angle closure. The most common symptoms are brow ache or headache, often accompanied by nausea and vomiting. These symptoms are typically severe enough to cause an individual to visit an eye care practitioner.

The visible, colored portion of the eye, the iris is located in the anterior segment of the eye, behind the cornea. It functions in much the same way as an aperture on a camera by regulating the amount of light striking the retina. The central opening in the iris is the pupil. The pupillary diameter is controlled by two opposing muscles within the iris: the sphincter and the dilator. Sphincter muscles are circular at the pupillary border and cause a miotic effect through parasympathetic stimulation. Dilator muscles are radial from the pupillary border and cause a mydriatic effect through sympathetic stimulation. Prostaglandins released by the iris during episodes of inflammation may affect the sphincter muscle, resulting in constriction of the pupil. Interestingly, patients with light-colored irides exhibit greater drug absorption than patients with dark-color irides.

The ciliary body is bordered anteriorly by the iris and is continuous posteriorly with the choroid. Besides aqueous humor production, it participates in focusing the optical mechanism (lens) for near viewing, a process known as accommodation. During episodes of ocular inflammation, the ciliary muscle may go into spasm, resulting in fluctuating vision and pain. Thus, inhibition of the ciliary muscle (cycloplegia) with anticholinergic agents is a frequent treatment for internal ocular inflammation.

The vitreous cavity, located in the posterior segment of the eye, is the largest portion of the eye and is filled with vitreous humor. Floating spots in the visual field ("floaters") are related to this area. Problems in this area are not amenable to self-treatment and require professional evaluation because of the possibility of concurrent retinal problems.

The retina is responsible for the initial processing and transmission of light signals. A number of inflammatory conditions of the retina can occur, and most have prominent symptoms. Some, however, have relatively mild symptoms, mimicking common irritative conditions. Trauma, even minor, may cause the retina to separate from its underlying layer (the pigment epithelium), resulting in retinal detachment. The retinal pigment epithelium provides vital "electrical" support to the retina. Macular degeneration, the leading cause of blindness in the United States, is directly related to atrophy in the pigment epithelium.

## DRY EYE

### Etiology/Signs and Symptoms of Dry Eye

Dry eye is among the most common disorders affecting the anterior eye. Most often associated with the aging process (especially with postmenopausal women), dry eye can also be caused by lid defects, corneal defects, loss of lid tissue turgor, Sjögren's syndrome, Bell's palsy, various collagen diseases such as rheumatoid arthritis, and systemic medications. Refractive surgery patients may complain of transient dry eyes for weeks to months after the procedure. Generally, this is mild if it does occur but can be more pronounced in some patients. Drugs with anticholinergic properties (e.g., antihistamines and antidepressants), diuretics, and β-blockers are some of the more common pharmacologic causes of dry eye. The condition may be exacerbated by allergens or other environmental conditions such as dry, dusty working situations, or by heating and air conditioning systems that reduce relative humidity, thereby increasing the evaporation of tears.

Dry eye is characterized by a white or mildly red eye, and patients may complain of a sandy, gritty feeling or a sensation that something is in the eye. Contrary to what the name suggests, dry eye may often initially present with excessive tearing. Abnormalities in the tear layer cause less-than-optimal lubrication of the ocular surface, thus producing more inadequate tears and beginning a vicious cycle. Failure to properly diagnose and treat dry eye syndromes can result in severe damage to eye tissue, particularly to the corneal surface (see Color Plates, photograph 3). Recent evidence demonstrates that dry eye disease can be linked to a T cell–mediated inflammatory process, which can respond to immunomodulatory agents such as cyclosporine.[8]

### Treatment of Dry Eye

#### *Treatment Goals*

The goal in treating dry eye is to alleviate and control the dryness of the ocular surface, thereby relieving the symptoms of irritation and preventing possible tissue and corneal damage.

#### *General Treatment Approach*

The primary self-treatment for dry eye is the use of ocular lubricants. The availability of synthetic chemicals suitable for topical application to the eye has resulted in the development of various solutions (artificial tears) to help alleviate dryness of the ocular surface. Artificial tear products vary by viscosity according to the ingredients used in their preparation. Increasing the viscosity of the product results in a more prolonged ocular contact time and greater resistance to tear dilution. Mild cases of dry eye may be treated with less viscous products, whereas more severe cases may require more viscous products. Bland (nonmedicated; e.g., petrolatum) ophthalmic ointment is another type of ocular lubricant. Ointment preparations are typically reserved for use at bedtime or for severe cases of dry eye because of their tendency to cause blurred vision. As with ointments, the greater the viscosity of tear drops, the greater the blurring effect. Vitamin A preparations are also available for treating dry eye. Nonpharmacologic measures, such as lid scrubs with warm compresses, may also increase eye comfort for patients with this disorder.

Eye care practitioners treat the most severe cases of dry eye with ocular inserts or sodium hyaluronate, or by occlusion of the lacrimal drainage system with plugs to increase the available tear pool. As mentioned previously, recent advances in the underlying pathophysiology of dry eye suggest that patients may benefit from treatment with topical cyclosporine.[8] However, minor dry eye disease may require only relief of ocular surface dryness, while more moderate to severe dry eye disease may benefit from a combined approach of immunomodulating agents, such as topical cyclosporine, in conjunction with ocular surface lubrication.

#### *Nonpharmacologic Therapy*

The primary nondrug measure is avoiding environments that increase evaporation of the tear film. If possible, the patient should avoid dry or dusty places. Using humidifiers or repositioning workstations away from heating and air conditioning vents may help alleviate dry eyes. Also, avoiding prolonged viewing of computer screens and avoiding windy, outdoor environments without eye protection (e.g., sunglasses, goggles) may further help alleviate dry eye problems.

#### *Pharmacologic Therapy*

Nonmedicated ointments are a mainstay of treating minor ophthalmic disorders, including dry eye. Because ointments can cause blurred vision, resulting in severe vision limitations, combination therapy using artificial tears and nonmedicated ointments is usually recommended. Gels offer some advantage to patients in that they do not disturb vision as much as ointments and are better tolerated. The effectiveness of retinol solutions for treating dry eye is still speculative.

##### Artificial Tear Solutions

Although many advances have been made in understanding the mechanisms involved in tear film formation, the role of tears in maintaining a normal conjunctival and corneal surface is still not completely understood. Lubricants that are formulated as artificial tear solutions consist of preservatives, inorganic electrolytes to achieve tonicity and maintain pH, and water-soluble polymeric systems. The lubricating agents in artificial tear products are similar, but buffering agents, preservatives, pH, and other formulation components may vary (Table 28-1).

One class of ophthalmic vehicles is the substituted cellulose ethers, which include hydroxypropyl methylcellulose (HPMC), hydroxyethylcellulose, hydroxypropylcellulose, methylcellulose, and carboxymethylcellulose (CMC). These solutions are colorless and vary in viscosity, depending on the grade and concentration of cellulose ether. Polyvinyl alcohol (PVA) and povidone are two other

**TABLE 28-1 Selected Ophthalmic Lubricants**

| | |
|---|---|
| **Artificial Tear Solutions** | |
| Akwa Tears | PVA 1.4%; BAK 0.01% |
| AquaSite | Dextran 70, 0.1%; polycarbophil; sorbic acid 0.2% |
| AquaSite Preservative Free* | Dextran 70, 0.1%; PEG 400, 0.2% |
| Bion Tears* | Hydroxypropyl methylcellulose 0.3%; dextran 70, 0.1% |
| Celluvisc* | CMC sodium 1% |
| Comfort Tears | Hydroxyethylcellulose; BAK 0.005%; EDTA |
| Computer Eye Drops | Glycerin 1%; NaCl; BAK 0.01%; boric acid; EDTA |
| Dry Eyes | PVA 1.4% ; sodium phosphate; NaCl; BAK 0.01%; EDTA |
| Dwelle | PVA 2.7%; povidone 2%; NPX 0.001% |
| GenTeal Tears† | Hydroxypropyl methylcellulose; boric acid; phosphonic acid; NaCl; sodium perborate |
| Hypo Tears | PVA 1%; PEG 400; BAK 0.01% |
| Hypo Tears Preservative Free* | PVA 1%; PEG 400 |
| Isopto Plain<br>Isopto Tears | Hydroxypropyl methylcellulose 2910, 0.5%; BAK 0.01% ; NaCl; sodium citrate; sodium phosphate |
| Just Tears | BAK; EDTA; PVA 1.4%; NaCl; potassium chloride |
| Liquifilm Tears | PVA 1.4%; chlorobutanol 0.5% |
| Moisture Eyes | Propylene glycol 1%; glycerin 0.3%; BAK 0.01% |
| Moisture Eyes Preservative Free* | Propylene glycol 0.95% |
| Murine Tears Lubricant | Povidone 0.6%; PVA 0.5%; BAK |
| Murocel Lubricant Ophthalmic | Methylcellulose 1%; propylene glycol; methylparaben 0.023%; propylparaben 0.01% |
| Nature's Tears | Hydroxypropyl methylcellulose 2906 0.4%; potassium chloride; NaCl; sodium phosphate; BAK 0.01%; EDTA |
| Nature's Tears Spray | Pure water mist |
| Nu-Tears | PVA 1.4%; EDTA; NaCl; BAK; potassium chloride |
| Nu-Tears II | PVA 1.4%; PEG-400; EDTA; BAK |
| Ocucoat Lubricating | Hydroxypropyl methylcellulose 0.8%; dextran 70, 0.1%; BAK 0.01% |
| Ocucoat PF Lubricating* | Hydroxypropyl methylcellulose 0.8%; dextran 70, 0.1% |
| OptiZen | 0.5% Polysorbent 80; EDTA, NaCl; sodium phosphate; sorbic acid |
| Preservative Free Moisture Eyes* | 0.95% Propylene glycol; boric acid; NaCl; KCl; sodium borate; EDTA |
| Puralube Tears | PVA 1%; PEG-400 1%; EDTA; BAK |
| Refresh | PVA 1.4%; povidone 0.6% |
| Refresh Endura Emulsion | Glycerin 1.0%; polysorbate 80 1.0% (polymer matrix, emulsifying agent; carbomer; castor oil) |
| Refresh Liquigel | CMC sodium 1%; Purite (stabilized oxychloro complex) |
| Refresh Plus* | CMC sodium 0.5% |
| Refresh Tears | CMC sodium 0.5%; Purite (stabilized oxychloro complex) |
| Soothe | Restoryl (Drakeol-15 1.0% and Drakeol-35 4.5%); Polysorbate 80 0.4%; octoxynol 40 ; NaCl; sodium phosphate; EDTA; polyhexamethylene biguanide preservative |
| Systane | PEG-400, 0.4%; propylene glycol 0.3%; boric acid; calcium chloride; hydroxypropyl guar; magnesium chloride; polyquaternium preservative; potassium chloride; NaCl; zinc chloride; water |
| TearGard | Sorbic acid 0.25%; EDTA 0.1%; hydroxyethyl cellulose |
| Teargen | BAK 0.01%; EDTA; NaCl; PVA |
| Teargen II | Hydroxypropyl methylcellulose 2910, 4 mg; dextran 70, 0.1%; NaCl; potassium chloride; sodium borate |
| Tearisol | Hydroxypropyl methylcellulose 0.5%; BAK 0.01% |
| Tears Again Liposome Lid Spray | Purified water; lecithin; ethanol 1%; NaCl; vitamin A; vitamin E; phenoxyethanol 0.5% |
| Tears Naturale | Hydroxypropyl methylcellulose 0.3%; dextran 70, 0.1%; BAK 0.01% |
| Tears Naturale Forte | 0.1% Dextran 70; 0.3% hydroxypropyl methylcellulose; 0.2% glycerin; 0.001% polyquaternium 1; NaCl; KCl; sodium borate |

**TABLE 28-1 Selected Ophthalmic Lubricants (continued)**

| | |
|---|---|
| Tears Naturale Free* | Hydroxypropyl methylcellulose 0.3%; dextran 70, 0.1% |
| Tears Naturale II | Hydroxypropyl methylcellulose 0.3%; dextran 70, 0.1%; Polyquad 0.001% |
| Tears Plus | PVA 1.4%; povidone 0.6%; chlorobutanol 0.5% |
| Tears Renewed | BAK 0.01%; EDTA; dextran 70, 0.1%; NaCl; hydroxypropyl methylcellulose 2906, 0.3% |
| Theratears PF* | Carboxymethylcellulose 0.25% |
| Ultra Tears | 1% hydroxypropyl methylcellulose BAK 0.01%; NaCl |
| 20/20 Tears | 1.4% polyvinyl alcohol, NaCl; 0.05% EDTA ; 0.01% BAK |
| Viva-Drops | Polysorbate 80; NaCl; EDTA; retinyl palmitate; mannitol; sodium citrate; pyruvate |
| **Nonmedicated Ointments** | |
| Akwa Tears* | White petrolatum; mineral oil; lanolin |
| Artificial Tears PF* | White petrolatum; anhydrous liquid lanolin; mineral oil |
| Dry Eyesa | White petrolatum; mineral oil, lanolin |
| DuraTears Naturale* | Petrolatum; mineral oil; lanolin |
| Hypo Tears | White petrolatum; light mineral oil |
| Lacri-Lube N.P.* | White petrolatum 57.3%; mineral oil 42.5%; lanolin alcohols |
| Lacri-Lube S.O.P. | White petrolatum 56.8%; mineral oil 42.5%; lanolin alcohols; chlorobutanol 0.5% |
| Moisture Eyes PM* | White petrolatum 80%; mineral oil 20% |
| Puralube | White petrolatum; light mineral oil |
| Refresh P.M.* | White petrolatum 56.8%; mineral oil 41.5%; lanolin alcohols |
| Stye | White petrolatum 55%; mineral oil 32%; boric acid; stearic acid; wheat germ oil |
| Tears Renewed* | White petrolatum; light mineral oil |
| **Nonmedicated Gels** | |
| GenTeal Lubricant Eye Gel† | Hydroxypropyl methylcellulose 0.3%; sodium perborate 0.028%; carbopol 980; phosphoric acid; sorbitol |
| Tears Again Gel | CMC 1.5% (stabilized oxyborate complex) |
| Theratears Gel | Carboxymethylcellulose 1%, KCl, sodium bicarbonate; NaCl, sodium phosphate |

Key: BAK, benzalkonium chloride; CMC, carboxymethylcellulose; EDTA, ethylenediamine tetraacetic acid; PEG, polyethylene glycol; PVA, polyvinyl alcohol.

* Preservative-free.

† Available in formulations for mild, moderate, and severe ocular discomfort.

commonly used vehicles. Formulation Considerations for Ocular Lubricants and Other Ophthalmic Products discusses ophthalmic vehicles, preservatives, and excipients in greater detail.

*Indications/Mechanism of Action* Perhaps the most important property of the cellulose ethers in artificial tear formulations is their ability to stabilize the tear film, which retards tear evaporation. Both effects are beneficial for patients with dry eye.[9] Combining drugs with these vehicles increases the vehicles' viscosity, thereby enhancing the drug's action. The increased viscosity retards drainage of the active ingredient from the eye, thus increasing the retention time of the active drug and enhancing bioavailability at the external ocular tissues. These effects generally occur without irritation or toxicity to the ocular tissues. Like the cellulose ethers, PVA also enhances stability of the tear film without causing ocular irritation or toxicity.

Povidone has surface-active properties similar to those of cellulose ethers. This compound is believed to form a hydrophilic layer on the corneal surface, mimicking natural conjunctival mucin. This "mucomimetic" property has firmly established the role of povidone as an artificial tear formulation. Because this agent promotes wetting of the ocular surface, both mucin- and aqueous-deficient dry eyes appear to benefit from its use.

Refresh Endura contains glycerin 1%, polysorbate 80, 1%, and castor oil, and is believed to supplement the lipid component of the tear film. It provides lubrication for a more prolonged period (it is dosed two or three times daily) and may be supplemented with aqueous artificial tears. It is the vehicle of the prescription product Restasis (cyclosporine 0.05%). Soothe is a new artificial tear that contains a lipid restorative layer, which provides a barrier to prevent loss of the aqueous component of the tears.

Systane is a lubricant eye drop that contains a gelling and polymer system. HP Guar binds to the hydrophobic corneal surface forming a glycocalyx, or gel-like, environment that keeps the demulcent system in contact with the ocular surface for a longer period of time. Systane is said to create an ocular shield, allowing for epithelial repair that promotes patient comfort and relief of symptoms.

Studies have shown that formulations of artificial tears without preservatives are less likely to irritate the ocular surface than those with preservatives.[10] Both practitioners and patients should be aware, however, that nonpreserved products may have limited stability and require specialized storage conditions (e.g., refrigeration) once they are opened.

*Dosage and Administration Guidelines* Most patients with mild cases of dry eye instill drops of artificial tears once or twice per day, typically on arising in the morning and/or before bedtime (Table 28-2).[11] Recommending drops at least twice per day is a good starting point. The viscosity of the drops and amount used can then be adjusted based on the patient's response. For more severe cases, the dosage can be increased to three to four times daily. If the patient's clinical needs and response to therapy indicate more frequent use, these solutions may be given as often as hourly. Preservative-free products or those with less-toxic preservatives (e.g., Purite or sodium perborate; see Ophthalmic Preservatives) are preferred in patients with moderate to severe disease.

*Safety Considerations* Use of ocular lubricants requires balancing the number of drops per day, the viscosity of the recommended solution, and the presence of a preservative. As the number of drops per day increases, toxicity from preservatives becomes more likely.[12]

Although PVA is compatible with many commonly used drugs and preservatives, certain compounds (including sodium bicarbonate, sodium borate, and the sulfates of sodium, potassium, and zinc) can thicken or gel solutions. For example, sodium borate is found in some extraocular irrigating solutions or irrigants, and may react with contact lens wetting solutions containing PVA.[13] Thus, it is important to be cautious when using solutions that contain PVA.

## Nonmedicated Ophthalmic Ointments

The primary ingredients in commercial nonprescription ophthalmic ointments (Table 28-1) are white petrolatum (a lubricant and ointment base), mineral oil (which helps the ointment melt at body temperature), and lanolin (which facilitates incorporation of water-soluble medications and also prevents evaporation).

*Mechanism of Action/Indications* The principal advantage of nonmedicated (bland) ointments is their enhanced retention time in the eye, which appears to enhance the integrity of the tear film. Thus, both mucin- and aqueous-deficient eyes can benefit from the application of lubricating ointments.

*Dosage and Administration Guidelines* Ointment formulations are usually administered twice daily (Table 28-3). However, depending on the patient's clinical needs

**TABLE 28-2 Administration Guidelines for Eye Drops**

1. If you have difficulty telling whether eye drops touch the eye surface, refrigerate the solution before instilling it. Do not refrigerate suspensions.
2. Wash hands thoroughly. Wash areas of the face around the eyes. Contact lenses should be removed unless the product is designed specifically for use with contact lenses.
3. Tilt head back.
4. Gently grasp lower outer eyelid below lashes, and pull eyelid away from eye to create a pouch.
5. Place dropper over eye by looking directly at it as shown in the drawing.
6. Just before applying a single drop, look up.
7. As soon as the drop is applied, release the eyelid slowly. Close eyes gently for 3 minutes by placing your head down as though looking at the floor (using gravity to pull the drop onto the cornea). Minimize blinking or squeezing the eyelid.
8. Use a finger to put gentle pressure over the opening of the tear duct.
9. Blot excessive solution from around the eye.
10. If multiple drop therapy is indicated, wait at least 5 minutes before instilling the next drop. This pause helps ensure that the first drop is not flushed away by the second, or that the second drop is not diluted by the first.
11. If using a suspension, place that drop in last.
12. If both drop and ointment therapy are indicated, instill the drops at least 10 minutes before the ointment so the ointment does not become a barrier to the drops' penetrating the tear film or cornea.

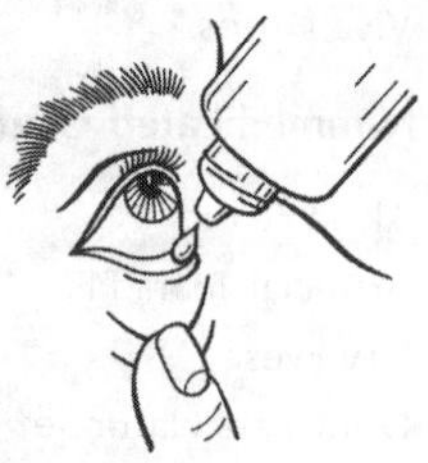

**TABLE 28-3 Administration Guidelines for Eye Ointments**

1. Wash hands thoroughly. Wash areas of the face around the eyes.
2. If both drop and ointment therapy are indicated, instill the drops at least 10 minutes before the ointment so that the ointment does not become a barrier to the drops' penetrating the tear film or cornea.
3. Tilt head back.
4. Gently grasp lower outer eyelid below lashes, and pull eyelid away from eye as shown in the drawing.
5. Place ointment tube over eye by looking directly at it.
6. With a sweeping motion, place 1/4 to 1/2 in. of ointment inside the lower eyelid by gently squeezing the tube, but avoid touching the tube tip to any tissue surface.
7. Release the eyelid slowly.
8. Close eyes gently for 1 to 2 minutes.
9. Blot excessive ointment from around the eye.
10. Vision may be temporarily blurred. Avoid activities requiring good visual ability until vision clears.

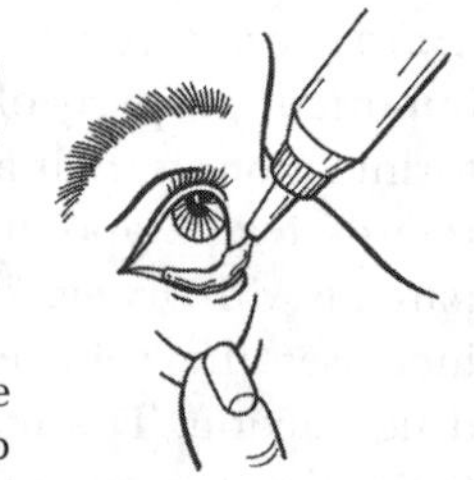

and therapeutic response, ointments may be administered as often as every few hours or only occasionally, as needed. Many patients prefer to instill the ointment at bedtime to keep the eyes moist during sleep and improve morning symptoms of dry eye.

*Safety Considerations* Because of the viscosity of the melted ointment base in the tear film, many patients complain of blurred vision when using ointments. This can usually be managed by decreasing the amount of ointment instilled or by administering the ointment at bedtime. The practitioner should routinely counsel the patient about the blurred vision associated with eye ointments.

Ointment preparations are generally nonirritating, but preservatives can be toxic to ocular tissues. Some patients develop hypersensitivity reactions, which may prompt them to discontinue therapy. Changing to preservative-free formulations (e.g., Duratears Naturale, HypoTears, Lacri-Lube NP, Refresh PM) can often eliminate symptoms associated with ointment products containing preservatives; preservative-free products are particularly helpful in long-term treatment. As a rule, it is better to recommend nonmedicated ointments without preservatives for the treatment of dry eye, to avoid the potential problems associated with preservatives.

### Formulation Considerations for Ocular Lubricants and Other Ophthalmic Products

Ocular lubricants and other nonprescription ophthalmic drugs are formulated to reduce the stinging, burning, and other side effects common with some ophthalmic drugs. Carefully controlling the pH, as well as the use of buffers, tonicity adjusters, and preservative systems produces a product that is comfortable to use and will, therefore, encourage patients to adhere to self-treatment. Drug vehicle and preservative systems are among the most important inactive ingredients of these products. Various other ingredients are often included as excipients.

*Ophthalmic Vehicles* Ophthalmic vehicles enhance drug action by providing increased viscosity. The greater viscosity of ophthalmic vehicles compared with aqueous solution vehicles increases the retention time of the active drug, thus enhancing its bioavailability at the external ocular tissues. These polymers are generally of high molecular weight. Some of the molecules can even bind to the corneal surface to increase drug retention and stabilize the tear film.

The most commonly used ophthalmic vehicles are CMC, povidone, PVA, HPMC, and poloxamer 407. Ointments are also used as vehicles. PVA is a water-soluble viscosity enhancer commonly used in a concentration of 1.4%.[14] PVA is generally nonirritating to the eye. PVA has been shown to facilitate healing of abraded corneal epithelium.[15] Similar to PVA, HPMC is available in several molecular weights; however, HPMC 0.5% has been shown to exhibit twice the ocular retention time of PVA 1.4%.[16] CMC in concentrations of 0.5% and 1% is also frequently used.

Povidone is not bound to membrane surfaces, and thus does not provide long-lasting viscosity enhancement beyond its normal residence time in the tears. Its viscosity does not change until near pH 1.0, at which point it doubles. Thus, the povidone molecule has no appreciable ionic character at pharmaceutical or physiologic pH ranges.

The first polyionic vehicle to be evaluated in the eye was poloxamer 407, a surfactant with a hydrophobic nucleus, hydrophilic end groups, and surfactant properties. Polyionic vehicles such as poloxamer 407 produce an artificial microenvironment in the tear film that can greatly enhance the bioavailability of certain ocular drugs.[17]

Ophthalmic ointments, which are semisolids at room temperature, are produced by mixing white petrolatum and mineral oil with or without a water-miscible agent such as lanolin. The mineral oil in the vehicle allows the ointment to melt at body temperature, whereas the lanolin absorbs water. This formulation allows for the incorporation of water and water-soluble drugs into the delivery system. Commercial ophthalmic ointments are generally derivatives of a mixture of petrolatum 60% USP and mineral oil 40% USP. In general, ointments are well tolerated by the ocular tissues. The primary clinical purpose for an ophthalmic ointment is to increase the ocular contact time of the instilled product. The ocular contact time of an ointment vehicle is about twice as long in the blinking eye and four times as long in the nonblinking or patched eye as that of a saline vehicle. Other commonly used vehicles are dextran 70, gelatin, glycerin, hydroxyethylcellulose, methylcellulose, polyethylene glycol, and propylene glycol.

*Ophthalmic Preservatives* Preservatives are incorporated into multidose ophthalmic products. These components are intended to destroy or limit the growth of microorganisms inadvertently introduced into the product. Surfactants, one of two distinct groups of preservatives, are usually bactericidal. These molecules disrupt the bacterial plasma membrane. The other group includes the metals mercury and iodine, their derivatives, and alcohols. Of the quaternary surfactants, benzalkonium chloride (BAK) and benzethonium chloride are preferred by many manufacturers because of their stability, excellent antimicrobial activity, and long shelf life. Unfortunately, these agents have toxic effects on both the tear film and the corneal epithelium.[18] A single drop of BAK 0.01% can break the superficial lipid layer of the tear film into numerous oil droplets. This preservative can reduce the tear film breakup time and thus may represent a poor choice for an antimicrobial preservative in artificial tear products.[19] The inclusion of BAK in artificial tear formulations does not provide protection to the corneal epithelium or promote a stable oily tear surface. BAK can be retained in ocular tissues for up to 7 days, and repeat doses may produce a cumulative toxic effect. Long-term use of topical products containing BAK can damage conjunctival and corneal epithelial cells. High concentrations of BAK have been associated with necrosis, whereas low concentrations have been associated with an apoptotic effect. Complications associated with BAK include allergy, fibrosis, dry eye syndrome, and increased risk of glaucoma surgery failure.[20]

In actual patient use, these disadvantages may become problematic only for those using multiple doses per day. Polyquad, a large-molecular-weight quaternary compound, does not bind to contact lenses and is less toxic than BAK.

Chlorhexidine is useful as an antimicrobial agent in the same range of concentrations as BAK, yet it is used at lower concentrations in commercial ophthalmic formulations. Because it does not alter corneal permeability to the same extent as BAK, chlorhexidine is not as toxic to the eye.

Of the mercurial preservatives, thimerosal is less likely to degrade into mercury than either phenylmercuric acetate or phenylmercuric nitrate. Compared with BAK, which undermines tear film stability, thimerosal has no known effects on the tear film. However, some patients who become sensitized to thimerosal develop contact blepharitis or conjunctivitis after several weeks of exposure and must discontinue the use of products that contain it. These products are rapidly disappearing from the marketplace.

Chlorobutanol is less effective than BAK as an antimicrobial preservative and, in fact, tends to disappear from bottles during prolonged storage.[14] However, prolonged use of chlorobutanol does not appear to produce allergic reactions.

Methylparaben and propylparaben have a long history of use in some ophthalmic medications, especially artificial tears and nonmedicated ointments. However, these preservatives are unstable at high pH and can sometimes induce allergic reactions.

Ethylenediamine tetraacetic acid (EDTA) is a chelating agent that preferentially binds and sequesters divalent cations. EDTA assists the action of thimerosal, BAK, and other agents. EDTA can sometimes induce contact allergic reactions.[21]

Sodium perborate, which has been used extensively as a tooth-bleaching agent, has found a new use as an ophthalmic preservative. One of two so-called disappearing preservatives, sodium perborate dissociates on contact with the eye to form hydrogen peroxide, which, in turn, rapidly dissociates to oxygen and water. The amount of hydrogen peroxide formed is so small that it does not produce eye irritation. Purite (oxychloro complex) is also designed to dissociate on contact with the eye. After exposure to long-wavelength UV light, Purite breaks down quickly to water and sodium chloride. The disappearing preservatives have the advantage of microbial protection while potentially limiting preservative toxicity.

Other, less common ophthalmic preservatives include cetylpyridinium chloride, phenylethyl alcohol, sodium propionate, and sorbic acid.

*Ophthalmic Excipients* Other useful excipients are antioxidants, wetting agents, buffers, and tonicity adjusters. Antioxidants prevent or delay deterioration of products that are exposed to oxygen. Wetting agents reduce surface tension, allowing the drug solution to spread more easily over the ocular surface. Buffers are added to help maintain a pH range of 6.0 to 8.0, thus preventing ocular discomfort on product instillation. Tonicity adjusters allow the medication to be isotonic with the physiologic tear film. Products in the sodium chloride equivalence range of 0.9% to 1.2% are considered isotonic and help reduce ocular irritation and tissue damage. Solutions in the tonicity range of 0.6% to 1.8% are usually comfortable when placed on the human eye. Hypertonic solutions used for corneal edema are not well tolerated.

### Retinol Solution

Vitamin A deficiency can affect many epithelial-lined organs, including the eye; therefore, topical administration of retinol (the alcohol form of vitamin A) has been advocated for treating various dry eye disorders. Unfortunately, few controlled clinical trials have been conducted to substantiate the usefulness of retinol solution in dry eye syndromes. Until more definitive data become available, however, the specific benefits of topically applied vitamin A solution for treating dry eye will remain speculative. Retinol is available in nonprescription formulations, usually containing vitamin A 5000 IU and polysorbate 80.

### Product Selection Guidelines

In recent years, artificial tear preparations have been introduced in preservative-free formulations and, more recently, in so-called disappearing preservative formulations. These preparations are beneficial for patients who are sensitive to preservatives such as BAK and thimerosal, those who use drops frequently, and/or those with compromised corneas. Three solution products, Genteal (mild-moderate-severe), Refresh Liquigel, and Refresh Tears, and two lubricant gels, Genteal Gel (mild-moderate-severe) and Tears Again Gel, are uniquely formulated to allow the preservative to rapidly dissociate into nontoxic components on the ocular surface. True preservative-free artificial tear preparations (e.g., Bion Tears, Celluvisc, HypoTearsPF, Refresh Plus) are available in a variety of unit-dose dispensers, and some of these products are formulated to provide electrolyte support to the damaged surface epithelium of the eye. In general, however, preservative-free formulations are more expensive than preserved artificial tear solutions, and they are easily contaminated by the patient during use. Thus, patients must follow strict hygienic procedures for self-administration and should discard any unused solution according to the manufacturer's guidelines.

Although a benefit of ophthalmic lubricant therapy is to increase the viscosity of existing tears, high viscosity alone does not necessarily provide relief for all dry eye conditions. Methylcellulose, in a concentration of 0.25% to 1.0%, was the primary cellulose ether in the first artificial tear solutions. Most contemporary artificial tear solutions incorporate other less viscous substituted cellulose ethers, especially CMC, hydroxyethylcellulose, and hydroxypropylcellulose. The latter ethers, which have emollient properties equal or superior to those of methylcellulose, can also be combined with other polymers such as PVA or povidone for use as artificial tears. PVA is generally used in a 1.4% concentration and is considerably less viscous than methylcellulose.

Clinical results and patient acceptance remain the final criteria for determining a product's efficacy in the treatment of patients with dry eye. Importantly, no single formulation has yet been identified that will universally improve clinical signs and symptoms while maintaining patient comfort and acceptance.[12,13] If the patient fails to respond to initial nonprescription therapy with artificial tears or other lubricants, the appropriate strategy is to change to a different lubricant (especially one with a different polymer or preservative system), to increase the number of drops used per day, or to add an ointment at bedtime. A few sprays are also available (i.e., Nature's Tears, Tears Again Liposome Spray), but it is unknown if these products offer patients any improved outcomes. If there is still no response, the patient should be encouraged to seek professional assessment and care from an ophthalmic practitioner.

## ALLERGIC CONJUNCTIVITIS

### Etiology/Signs and Symptoms of Allergic Conjunctivitis

The list of antigens that can cause ocular allergy is virtually endless, but the most common allergens include pollen, animal dander, and topical eye preparations. Patients with ocular allergy will often report seasonal allergic rhinitis as well. Allergic conjunctivitis is characterized by a red eye with watery discharge (see Color Plates, photograph 4). The hallmark symptom accompanying ocular allergy is itching. Vision is usually not impaired but may be blurred because of excessive tearing. Contact lenses should not be used until the condition resolves.[22]

### Treatment of Allergic Conjunctivitis

#### *Treatment Goals*

The goals in treating allergic conjunctivitis are to (1) remove or avoid the allergen, (2) limit or reduce the severity of the allergic reaction, (3) provide symptomatic relief, and (4) protect the ocular surface.

#### *General Treatment Approach*

Questioning the patient about exposure to allergens may help identify the offending substance. Removal or avoidance of the responsible allergen is the best treatment, but ocular lubricants, ocular decongestants, ocular decongestant-antihistamine preparations, nonprescription oral antihistamines, and cold compresses will help relieve symptoms.

#### *Nonpharmacologic Therapy*

In addition to removing and/or avoiding exposure to the offending allergen, applying cold compresses to the eyes three to four times per day will help reduce redness and itching.

#### *Pharmacologic Therapy*

The first-line treatment of allergic conjunctivitis is to instill artificial tears as needed (see Treatment of Dry Eye). If symptoms persist, the patient should switch to an ophthalmic antihistamine-decongestant product. An oral antihistamine can be added to the second regimen if needed. Medical referral is indicated if symptoms do not resolve.

Nonprescription ophthalmic products designated specifically for treatment of allergic conjunctivitis include decongestants, antihistamines, or combinations of the two agents (see Chapter 11 for discussion of systemic nonprescription antihistamines).

##### Ophthalmic Decongestants

Four decongestants are available in nonprescription strength for topical application to the eye: phenylephrine, naphazoline, tetrahydrozoline, and oxymetazoline (Table 28-4). In nonprescription ophthalmic products, phenylephrine is available in a concentration of 0.12%. Naphazoline, tetrahydrozoline, and oxymetazoline are chemically classified as imidazoles. As Table 28-4 shows, these agents are available as solutions in a variety of concentrations.

*Mechanism of Action/Indications* Phenylephrine acts primarily on α-adrenergic receptors of the ophthalmic vasculature to constrict conjunctival vessels, thereby reducing eye redness. The higher concentration, prescription-only products that contain this agent are generally reserved for the short-term dilation needed for eye examinations. Like phenylephrine, the imidazoles have greater α- than β-receptor activity and are, therefore, clinically useful in constricting conjunctival blood vessels. These agents have only minimal effect on the underlying vessels of the episclera and sclera. Naphazoline has been shown to be effective in constricting conjunctival vessels as well as in reducing tearing and pain associated with superficial ocular inflammation.23 Satisfactory results have also been obtained with tetrahydrozoline in most patients with allergic or chronic conjunctivitis. Topical treatment with oxymetazoline will improve most symptoms associated with allergic or noninfectious conjunctivitis, including burning, itching, tearing, and foreign body sensation.

*Dosage and Administration Guidelines* See Table 28-5 for dosages of ophthalmic decongestants.

*Safety Considerations* When used as directed, ocular decongestants generally do not induce ocular or systemic side effects. In fact, systemic adverse effects are extremely rare after topical instillation of nonprescription phenylephrine for ocular decongestion. However, their availability to and use in children should be carefully monitored. Ingestion of these products can result in coronary emergencies and death. The most important and common side effect following chronic use of phenylephrine and the imidazoles for ocular decongestion is rebound congestion of the conjunctiva, in which the conjunctival vessels become progressively more dilated with continued use of the drug. This phenomenon can create a vicious cycle in

**TABLE 28-4 Selected Ophthalmic Products Containing Decongestants, Antihistamines, and/or Astringents**

| Trade Name | Primary Ingredients |
|---|---|
| **Decongestant Eye Drop Products** | |
| AK-Con | Naphazoline 0.1%; BAK 0.01%; EDTA |
| AK-Nefrin | Phenylephrine HCl 0.12%; BAK 0.005%; EDTA; PVA 1.4% |
| Albalon | Naphazoline 0.1%; BAK 0.004%; EDTA; 1.4% polyvinyl alcohol |
| 20/20 Eye | Naphazoline 0.012% ; BAK; EDTA; glycerin 0.2% |
| All Clear | Naphazoline 0.012% ; PEG 300, 0.2%; BAK 0.01%; EDTA |
| All Clear AR | Naphazoline 0.03%; BAK 0.01%; hydroxypropyl methylcellulose 0.5%; EDTA |
| Allerest | Naphazoline 0.012%; BAK; EDTA |
| Clear Eyes | Naphazoline HCl 0.012%; glycerin 0.2%; BAK |
| Clear Eyes ACR | Naphazoline 0.012%; BAK; EDTA; zinc sulfate 0.25%; glycerin 0.2% |
| Collyrium Fresh | Tetrahydrozoline HCl 0.05%; BAK 0.01%; EDTA |
| Comfort Eye Drops | Naphazoline 0.03%; BAK 0.005%; EDTA 0.02% |
| Eyesine | Tetrahydrozoline 0.05% |
| Geneye | Tetrahydrozoline 0.05%; BAK; EDTA |
| Maximum Strength Allergy | Naphazoline 0.03%; BAK 0.01%; hydroxypropyl methylcellulose 0.5%; EDTA |
| Murine Tears Plus | Tetrahydrozoline HCl 0.05%; povidone 0.6%; PVA 0.5%; BAK |
| Nafazair | Naphazoline 0.1%; BAK 0.01%; EDTA |
| Nafazair A | Naphazoline 0.025%; pheniramine maleate 0.3%; BAK 0.01%; EDTA; boric acid; sodium borate |
| Naphcon | Naphazoline HCl 0.012%; BAK 0.01% |
| Ocu Clear | Oxymetazoline HCl 0.025%; BAK 0.01% |
| Optigene 3 | Tetrahydrozoline HCl 0.05%; BAK; EDTA |
| Prefin Liquifilm | Phenylephrine HCl 0.12%; PVA 1.4%; BAK 0.005% |
| Relief* | Phenylephrine, PVA 1.4%; EDTA |
| Tetrasine | Tetrahydrozoline 0.05% |
| Tetrasine Extra | Tetrahydrozoline 0.05%; 1% polyethylene glycol 400; EDTA; BAK |
| VasoClear | Naphazoline 0.02%; BAK 0.01%; PVA 0.25%; PEG 400, 1%; EDTA |
| Vasocon | Naphazoline HCl 0.1%; BAK; PVA; EDTA; polyethylene glycol 8000 |
| Visine Allergy Relief | Tetrahydrozoline HCl 0.05%; PEG 400, 1.0%; povidone 1.0%; BAK 0.01%; dextran 70, 1.0% |
| Visine L.R. | Oxymetazoline HCl 0.025%; BAK 0.01% |
| Visine Moisturizing | Tetrahydrozoline HCl 0.05%; BAK 0.01%; EDTA; hydroxypropyl methylcellulose 0.5% |
| Visine Original | Tetrahydrozoline HCl 0.05%; BAK 0.01% |
| **Antihistamine–Decongestant Eye Drop Products** | |
| Naphcon A | Pheniramine maleate 0.3%; naphazoline HCl 0.025%; BAK 0.01% |
| Naphazoline HCl & Pheniramine Maleate Solution | Pheniramine maleate 0.3%; naphazoline HCl 0.025%; BAK 0.01% |
| Opcon-A | Pheniramine maleate 0.315%; naphazoline HCl 0.02675%; hydroxypropyl methylcellulose 0.5%; BAK 0.01% |
| Vasocon A | Antazoline phosphate 0.5%; naphazoline HCl 0.05%; BAK 0.01% |
| Visine-A | Pheniramine maleate 0.3%; naphazoline HCl 0.025%; BAK 0.01% |
| **Decongestant–Astringent Eye Drop Products** | |
| Clear Eyes ACR | Naphazoline HCl 0.012%; zinc sulfate 0.25%; glycerin 0.2%; BAK |
| VasoClear A | Naphazoline HCl 0.02%; zinc sulfate 0.25%; PVA 0.25%; BAK 0.05% |
| Visine Allergy Relief | Tetrahydrozoline HCl 0.05%; zinc sulfate 0.25%; BAK 0.01% |
| Zincfrin | Phenylephrine HCl 0.12%; zinc sulfate 0.25%; BAK 0.01% |

Key: BAK, benzalkonium chloride; EDTA, ethylenediamine tetraacetic acid; PEG, polyethylene glycol; PVA, polyvinyl alcohol.

* Preservative-free.

TABLE 28-5 Dosage Guidelines for Ophthalmic Decongestants and Antihistamines

| Agent | Nonprescription Concentration (%) | Dosage | Duration of Action (hours) | Duration of Use |
|---|---|---|---|---|
| **Decongestant Products** | | | | |
| Phenylephrine | 0.12 | 1-2 drops up to 4 times/day | 0.5-1.5 | 72 hours |
| Naphazoline | 0.1, 0.12, 0.02, 0.03 | 1-2 drops up to 4 times/day | 3-4 | 72 hours |
| Oxymetazoline | 0.025 | 1-2 drops q6h | 4-6 | 72 hours |
| Tetrahydrozoline | 0.05 | 1-2 drops q4h | 1-4 | 72 hours |
| **Decongestant–Antihistamine Products** | | | | |
| Naphazoline–pheniramine | 0.025 (naphazoline) 0.3 (pheniramine) | 1-2 drops 3-4 times/day | 3-4 | 72 hours |
| Naphazoline–antazoline | 0.05 (naphazoline) 0.5 (antazoline) | 1-2 drops 3-4 times/day | | 72 hours |

which phenylephrine is instilled to quiet an inflamed conjunctiva, which then becomes progressively more congested because of repeated instillation of the medication. Patients with apparent rebound congestion should be referred to an eye care practitioner for differential diagnosis and management.

Ocular decongestants have the potential for producing rebound conjunctival hyperemia, allergic conjunctivitis, and allergic blepharitis when used excessively or long term.[24] Rebound congestion appears to be less likely with topical ocular use of naphazoline or tetrahydrozoline than with oxymetazoline.

The low concentrations of phenylephrine used in nonprescription topical decongestants may dilate the pupil if enough of it penetrates the corneal epithelium. Pupillary dilation is not uncommon in persons who wear contact lenses and who may instill the medication following lens wear. Indiscriminate use of phenylephrine to quiet an irritated eye can induce pupillary dilation and precipitate angle-closure glaucoma in eyes that have narrow anterior chamber angles. This adverse effect is more likely if the cornea is damaged or diseased, thereby allowing increased corneal drug penetration. Naphazoline can also alter pupil size; patients with lightly pigmented irides (e.g., blue or green eyes) appear to be more sensitive to the mydriatic effect of naphazoline. Use of these products in angle-closure glaucoma is contraindicated, and practitioners should counsel patients with angle-closure glaucoma against using these products in treating allergic conjunctivitis. In addition, patients should be cautioned against instilling these agents too often because of concerns for rebound phenomena.

Certain patients may experience mild, transient stinging immediately following instillation of tetrahydrozoline drops. Furthermore, some patients may experience epithelial xerosis (abnormal dryness) from prolonged topical instillation of ocular decongestants, which may exacerbate the symptoms of irritation, pain, and dryness associated with allergic conjunctivitis.

Although not reported in the literature, certain drug-drug interactions involving low concentrations of phenylephrine and the imidazoles are theoretically possible. The pressor effects of these agents may be enhanced in patients taking atropine, tricyclic antidepressants, monoamine oxidase inhibitors, reserpine, guanethidine, or methyldopa. Ocular decongestants should, therefore, be used cautiously by patients with systemic hypertension, arteriosclerosis, other cardiovascular diseases, or diabetes. Adverse cardiovascular events are also possible when these agents are used in patients with hyperthyroidism.[25] Because of these possible adverse reactions, patients should not use phenylephrine and other ocular decongestants as ocular irrigants.

Women should use ocular decongestants sparingly, if at all, during pregnancy. To ensure that a subpotent product is not being used, patients should check expiration dates because loss of pharmacologic activity may occur without visible changes in solution color. In addition, products should be stored at manufacturer-recommended temperatures. Storage of solutions at high temperatures may cause ocular reactions and severe mydriatic responses to instillation. Because phenylephrine is highly susceptible to oxidation, manufacturers often add sodium bisulfite, an antioxidant, to products containing phenylephrine to prolong the product's shelf life. If offending ophthalmic signs or symptoms do not resolve within 72 hours, the patient should see an eye care practitioner.

### Ophthalmic Antihistamines

Two nonprescription antihistamines are available for topical ophthalmic use: pheniramine maleate and antazoline phosphate. Although these antihistamines are effective by themselves, nonprescription products containing them also contain a decongestant. The two combinations are pheniramine–naphazoline and antazoline–naphazoline (Table 28-4).

*Mechanism of Action/Indications* Pheniramine and antazoline are in different antihistamine classes, but both act as specific histamine$_1$-receptor antagonists.[26] They do, however, differ somewhat in their pharmacologic actions, both systemically and on the ocular surface. Antazoline has been shown to have anesthetic properties, but these properties are insufficient to produce clinical effects when antazoline is used topically.[27] Pheniramine has been shown to have little effect on intraocular pressure, whereas antazoline can increase it slightly.[27] This effect is not clinically significant during typical usage.

Topical antihistamines are used for rapid relief of symptoms associated with seasonal or atopic conjunctivitis. Using a decongestant with the topical antihistamines has been shown to be more effective than using either agent alone.[23,28] The Food and Drug Administration (FDA) has classified topical antihistamines as less than effective, primarily because clinical trial data on effectiveness are lacking.

*Dosage and Administration Guidelines* See Table 28-5 for dosages of the antihistamine combination products.

*Safety Considerations* Burning, stinging, and discomfort on instillation are the most common side effects of ophthalmic antihistamines. Although both pheniramine and antazoline may produce stinging, pheniramine may cause somewhat less stinging than antazoline. Severe side effects (death, thrombocytopenia, and allergic pneumonitis) that have been associated with systemic antihistamine use have not been reported with topical ophthalmic preparations.[29-33]

Ophthalmic antihistamines have anticholinergic properties and may cause pupil dilation. This effect is most commonly seen in people with light-colored irides or compromised corneas, such as contact lens wearers.[34] In susceptible patients, pupil dilation can lead to angle-closure glaucoma. Therefore, these drugs are contraindicated in people with a known risk of angle-closure glaucoma.[35] Sensitivity to one of the components is another contraindication to the use of products containing topical antihistamines.

#### Product Selection Guidelines

Although decongestants and antihistamines are the only nonprescription ophthalmic products for which product-to-product comparisons have been done, it is difficult to reach definitive conclusions regarding clinical comparisons of the available nonprescription ocular decongestants. Most of the tested preparations produce blanching of conjunctival vessels, but naphazoline 0.02% seems to produce greater blanching compared with other nonprescription decongestants containing tetrahydrozoline 0.05% or phenylephrine 0.12%.[36] Investigators have observed no significant differences in conjunctival blanching with preparations containing naphazoline in concentrations of 0.02%, 0.05%, and 0.1%.[36] Thus, naphazoline 0.02% is an excellent choice for nonprescription therapy of mild to moderate conjunctivitis of environmental, viral, or noninfectious origin.

Because rebound congestion appears to be less likely following topical ocular use of naphazoline or tetrahydrozoline, these agents should generally be recommended over phenylephrine or oxymetazoline.

#### Complementary Therapies

The homeopathic product known as Similasan Eye Drops #2 is indicated for relief from itching and burning caused by allergic reactions. The active homeopathic ingredients are Apis, Euphrasia, and Sabadilla. (See Chapter 55 for further discussion of these types of products.) The efficacy of this formulation has not been established in controlled clinical trials.

## VIRAL CONJUNCTIVITIS

### Etiology/Signs and Symptoms of Viral Conjunctivitis

Viral conjunctivitis ("pink eye") is the most common form of conjunctivitis. This condition is highly contagious and poses a significant health problem in schools and workplaces where touch contamination is poorly controlled. A recent cold, sore throat, or exposure to someone with viral conjunctivitis is a common precursor of this condition. Patients with viral conjunctivitis will usually have a pink eye with a copious amount of watery discharge (see Color Plates, photograph 5). Symptoms include nonspecific ocular discomfort and a mild to moderate sensation of a foreign object in the eye; vision may occasionally be blurred. Low-grade fever may be present, and swollen preauricular or submandibular lymph nodes may be found. If the etiology of the conjunctivitis is not clear, the patient should be referred to an eye care practitioner. Intense eye pain probably indicates trauma to the cornea and requires immediate referral to an eye care practitioner to rule out a corneal abrasion.

### Treatment of Viral Conjunctivitis

#### Treatment Goals

The goal in treating viral conjunctivitis is to relieve symptoms while the infection runs its course.

#### General Treatment Approach

Viral conjunctivitis is usually self-limiting, with symptoms resolving within 1 to 3 weeks. Artificial tear preparations and ocular decongestants may be used to relieve symptoms of blurred vision. Because certain forms of viral conjunctivitis can be extremely contagious, strict adherence to proper hygienic measures are also important.

#### Nonpharmacologic Therapy

Patients with viral conjunctivitis should wash their hands after touching an infected eye and properly dispose of tissues used to blot an infected eye. They should also avoid sharing towels or other objects that might come in contact with the infected eye.

#### Pharmacologic Therapy

See Treatment of Dry Eye for a discussion of artificial tear preparations, as well as Treatment of Allergic Conjunctivitis for a discussion of ocular decongestants.

## CORNEAL EDEMA

### Etiology/Signs and Symptoms of Corneal Edema

Corneal edema may occur from a variety of conditions, including overwear of contact lenses, surgical damage to the cornea, and inherited corneal dystrophies. The edematous area of the cornea is often confined to the epithelium. Because fluid accumulation distorts the optical properties of the cornea, halos or starbursts around lights (with or without reduced vision) are a hallmark symptom of corneal edema. An eye care practitioner must diagnose this disorder.

### Treatment of Corneal Edema

#### *Treatment Goals*

The goal in treating corneal edema is to draw fluid from the cornea, thereby relieving the associated symptoms.

#### *General Treatment Approach*

Once the initial diagnosis is established, patients can use topical hyperosmotic formulations to treat corneal edema. Of the topical ophthalmic hyperosmotic agents available, only sodium chloride can be obtained without a prescription in both solution and ointment formulations (Table 28-6). Sodium chloride is available as a 2% or 5% solution, and as a 5% ointment. First-line treatment is instillation of a 2% solution four times per day. If symptoms persist, nighttime use of a 5% hyperosmotic ointment should be added to the regimen. If symptoms do not respond to the augmented treatment, the patient should switch to a 5% hyperosmotic solution and continue nighttime use of the ointment. If symptoms still persist, medical referral is necessary.

#### *Pharmacologic Therapy*

##### Hyperosmotics

*Mechanism of Action* Hyperosmotic agents increase the tonicity of the tear film, promoting movement of fluid from the cornea to the more highly osmotic tear film. Normal tear flow mechanisms then eliminate the excess fluid. Many patients with mild to moderate corneal epithelial edema may experience improved subjective comfort and vision following appropriate use of these medications.

*Dosage and Administration Guidelines* Usually, the patient instills one or two drops of the solution every 3 to 4 hours (see Table 28-2). The ointment formulation, however, requires less frequent instillation and is usually reserved for use at bedtime to minimize symptoms of blurred vision (see Table 28-3). Because vision associated with edematous corneas is often worse on awakening, several instillations of the solution during the first few waking hours may be helpful.

*Safety Considerations* In general, sodium chloride 5% in ointment form is the most effective in reducing corneal edema and improving vision, but it tends to cause stinging and burning. For that reason, patients often prefer the 2% solution for long-term therapy. Hypertonic saline, however, is nontoxic to the external ocular tissues, and allergic reactions are rare.

Perhaps the most important contraindication to topical hyperosmotic sodium chloride is its use to clear edematous corneas with traumatized epithelium. The intact corneal epithelium permits only limited permeability to inorganic ions; therefore, an absent or compromised corneal epithelium will result in increased corneal penetration of the hyperosmotic product, reducing its osmotic effect. Consequently, the management of corneal edema associated with traumatized epithelium requires the use of organic hyperosmotic agents that are available only by prescription.[37] Patients whose history or physical appearance suggests a damaged corneal epithelium should be referred to an eye care practitioner immediately. Patients must be informed never to prepare homemade saline solutions for use in the eye because of the risk of infection.

## LOOSE FOREIGN SUBSTANCES IN THE EYE

### Etiology/Signs and Symptoms of Loose Foreign Substances in the Eye

Despite the protective effect of the lids, foreign substances often contact the ocular surface. The immediate response of the eye is watering (tearing). If the substance causes only minor irritation and does not abrade the eye surface, self-treatment is appropriate.

### Treatment of Loose Foreign Substances in the Eye

#### *Treatment Goals*

The goal in treating loose foreign substances in the eye is to remove the irritant by irrigating the eye. Known foreign substances from wood or metal fragments (such as hammering incidents) should be treated automatically as possible penetrating injuries and examined by an eye care practitioner.

#### *General Treatment Approach*

If reflex tearing does not remove the foreign substance, the eye may need to be flushed. Lint, dust, and similar materials can usually be removed by rinsing the eye with sterile saline or specific eyewash preparations (irrigants). Outside of a medical setting, in the case of loose particles and chemical exposures to the eyes, the eyes should be flushed with copious amounts of water from a sink faucet or a garden hose.

#### *Pharmacologic Therapy*

##### Ocular Irrigants

*Indications/Mechanism of Action* An ocular irrigant is used to cleanse ocular tissues while maintaining their moisture; these solutions must be physiologically balanced with respect to pH and osmolality. Because the tissues with

**TABLE 28-6 Selected Miscellaneous Ophthalmic Products**

| Trade Name | Primary Ingredients |
|---|---|
| **Irrigant Solutions** | |
| Accu-Wash | NaCl; sodium phosphate; BAK |
| AK-Rinse | NaCl; sodium phosphate; EDTA; BAK |
| Collyrium for Fresh Eyes | Boric acid; sodium borate; BAK |
| Dacriose | Sodium phosphate; NaCl; BAK 0.1%; EDTA 0.3% |
| Bausch and Lomb Eye Wash | Sodium borate; boric acid; NaCl; sorbic acid 0.1%; EDTA 0.025% |
| Eye Stream | Sodium acetate 0.39%; sodium citrate 0.17%; sodium hydroxide and/or hydrochloric acid; BAK |
| Irrigate Eye Wash | NaCl; mono and dibasic sodium phosphate; EDTA; BAK |
| Lavoptik Eye Wash | Sodium phosphate; NaCl 0.49%; BAK 0.005% |
| Optigene | NaCl; mono and dibasic sodium phosphate; EDTA; BAK |
| Visual-Eyes | NaCl; mono and dibasic sodium phosphate; BAK; EDTA |
| **Hyperosmotics** | |
| Adsorbonac Solution* | NaCl 2% and 5%; thimerosal 0.04% |
| AK-NaCl Solution | NaCl 5%; methylparaben 0.023%; propylparaben 0.017% |
| AK-NaCl Ointment† | NaCl 5%; lanolin oil; mineral oil; white petrolatum |
| Muro 128 Solution 2% | NaCl 2%; hydroxypropyl methylcellulose 2906; methylparaben 0.046%; propylparaben 0.02%; propylene glycol; boric acid |
| Muro 128 Solution 5% | NaCl 5%; boric acid; hydroxypropyl methylcellulose 2910; propylene glycol; methylparaben 0.023%; propylparaben 0.01% |
| Muro 128 Ointment† | Mineral oil; white petrolatum; lanolin |
| **Eyelid Scrubs** | |
| Eye Scrub Solution | Polyethylene glycol 200 glyceryl monotallowate; disodium laureth sulfosuccinate; cocoamidopropylamine oxide; polyethylene glycol 78 glyceryl monococoate; benzyl alcohol; EDTA |
| Lid Wipes-SPF Pads | Polyethylene glycol 200 glyceryl monotallowate; polyethylene glycol 80 glyceryl cocoate; laureth-23; cocoamidopropylamine oxide; NaCl; glycerin |
| OcuSoft Solution and Pads | Polyethylene glycol 80 sorbitan laureth; sodium trideceth sulfate; cocoamidopropyl hydroxysulftaine; polyethylene glycol 150 distearate; lauroamphocarboxyglycinate; sodium laureth-13 carboxylate; polyethylene glycol 15 tallow polyamine; quaternium-15 |
| **Prosthesis Lubricant/Cleaner** | |
| Enuclene Solution | Tyloxapol 0.25%; hydroxypropyl methylcellulose 0.85%; BAK 0.02% |

Key: BAK, benzalkonium chloride; EDTA, ethylenediamine tetraacetic acid.

*Contains thimerosal; †preservative free.

which they come in contact obtain nutrients elsewhere, the role of irrigants is primarily to clear away unwanted materials or debris from the ocular surface. Patients should use ocular irrigants on a short-term basis only. All ophthalmic irrigating solutions are available without a prescription (Table 28-6).

In the ophthalmic practitioner's office, irrigating solutions come in handy following certain clinical procedures, and they are often used to wash away mucous or purulent exudates from the eye. They are also administered in the hospital to clean out eyes between changes of ocular dressings.

*Dosage and Administration Guidelines* See Table 28-7 for instructions on how to use ophthalmic irrigants.

*Safety Considerations* Ocular irrigants should not be used for open wounds in or near the eyes. These agents should also not be applied with contact lenses in place because the solutions cause contact lens irritation by reducing the mucin component of the tear film. In the case of rigid gas-permeable lenses, the solutions reduce the hydrophilicity of the lens surface.[38] Furthermore, soft lens absorption of the preservatives BAK and phenylmercuric acetate can have a deleterious effect on the corneal epithelium. Although irrigating solutions may be used to wash out the eyes after contact lens wear, they have no particular value as contact lens wetting, cleansing, or cushioning solutions.

**TABLE 28-7 Administration Guidelines for Ophthalmic Irrigants**

1. Discard the eyecup that comes with the irrigant, if one is provided. Preventing viral, fungal, or bacterial contamination of the cup is very difficult.
2. Bend over a sink or bathtub, and tilt the ear next to the affected eye downward slightly.
3. Hold the bottle next to the nose near the corner of the affected eye, being careful not to touch the eye.
4. Squeeze the bottle, and allow the irrigant to flow across the entire eye surface.
5. If necessary, adjust the angle of the head during instillation of the irrigant to ensure that the entire eye surface is flushed.
6. Blot excessive solution from around the eye.
7. If both eyes are affected, repeat the procedure for the other eye.

In cases in which the patient experiences continuous eye pain, changes in vision, or continued redness or irritation of the eye or the ocular condition persists or worsens, evaluation by an eye care practitioner should be strongly encouraged. Commercial irrigating products that use an eyecup should generally be avoided because of difficulties in cleaning the eyecup, with the resultant risk of bacterial or fungal contamination.

## MINOR EYE IRRITATION

### Etiology/Signs and Symptoms of Minor Eye Irritation

Nonallergic, minor eye irritation can be caused by a loose foreign substance in the eye, contact lens wear, or exposure of the eye to wind, sun (e.g., snow skiing without protective eye goggles), smog, chemical fumes, or chlorine. Redness of the eye is the common sign of minor irritation. In cases of snow blindness, other UV burns, or arc welder's burns, additional common signs are pain and the feeling of "sand in the eyes."

### Treatment of Minor Eye Irritation

Minor irritation often responds well to artificial tear solutions or nonmedicated ointments (see Treatment of Dry Eye).

Zinc sulfate, a mild astringent, may be recommended for temporary relief of minor ocular irritation. The dosage is 1 to 2 drops up to four times daily.

The homeopathic product known as Similasan Eye Drops #1 is marketed to relieve dryness and redness caused by smog, contact lenses, and other causes. The active homeopathic ingredients are Belladonna, Euphrasia, and Mercurius sublimatus (see Chapter 55 for further discussion of these types of products). Controlled clinical trials have not demonstrated the efficacy of this formulation in the treatment of this condition.

## CHEMICAL BURN

### Etiology/Signs and Symptoms of Chemical Burn

Chemical burns may occur from exposure to alkali (e.g., oven cleaners, cement, or lye), acids (e.g., battery acid or vinegar), detergents, and various solvents and irritants (e.g., tear gas or mace). Burns may range from mild to severe depending on the inciting agent and/or exposure time. Patients complain of pain, irritation, photophobia, and tearing. Signs vary depending on the severity. Less severe signs include superficial punctate keratitis (small pinpoint loss of epithelial cells in the cornea), perilimbal ischemia, chemosis, hyperemia, eyelid edema, hemorrhages, and first- or second-degree burns of the lid and outer skin. More severe signs include corneal edema and opacification, anterior chamber inflammation, increased IOP, and retinal toxicity from scleral penetration. Alkali burns are more penetrating and potentially more damaging to eye tissues than acid burns. They are often more resistant to irrigation and have greater tissue destruction when they penetrate into the deeper (stromal) layers of the cornea. If the burns are more superficial and just several layers of the corneal epithelium are affected, the cells should be replenished within approximately 24 hours. If signs and symptoms persist past 24 hours, an eye care practitioner should be seen.

### Treatment of Chemical Burn

Emergent treatment includes immediate copious irrigation with sterile saline or even tap water if nothing else is available. It cannot be stressed enough that irrigation must be continued until an eye care practitioner can be seen. If irrigation is stopped prematurely, the pH of the tear film may revert back to either acidic or alkaline because of residual material that may still be under the lid or in the inferior cul-de-sac. Further treatment after irrigation may include the use of cycloplegic agents, topical antibiotics, and analgesics. In more severe cases, topical steroids are sometimes employed if significant inflammation of the anterior chamber or cornea is present. Antiglaucoma medications are also used if the IOP is elevated. Follow-up by the eye care practitioner is required to prevent conjunctival adhesions and corneal complications. Chemical burns are considered ophthalmic emergencies and should be immediately referred to an eye care practitioner or emergency department.

## ARTIFICIAL EYES

Besides the obvious esthetic benefits, clearing dried mucus or fluid secretions from the surfaces of artificial eyes eliminates a potential medium for bacterial growth. A sterile isotonic buffered solution containing tyloxapol 0.25% and BAK 0.02% is available especially for cleaning and lubricating ophthalmic prostheses. The primary method of preventing bacterial growth is routine hygiene with mild, nonallergenic soap and water.

Tyloxapol is a surfactant that softens solid matter on the prosthesis, and BAK aids tyloxapol in wetting the artificial eye. The solution is used in the same manner as ordinary artificial tears. With the artificial eye in place, 1 or 2 drops of solution should be applied three or four times daily. In addition, the solution can be used as a cleaner to remove oily or mucus deposits; in this case, the artificial eye is then rubbed between the fingers and rinsed with tap water before reinsertion.

## MACULAR DEGENERATION

Age-related macular degeneration (AMD) is the leading cause of blindness in the United States. It takes two forms: neovascular (wet or bleeding) and atrophic (dry). Presently, there is no definitive "cure" for AMD, and research into the etiology and possible cure of the disease is being pursued vigorously. Until a cure is found, the treatments used are aimed at slowing the rate of progression and extent of visual loss. Treatment of the neovascular form is limited, requiring continual follow-up care and medical treatment by an ophthalmologist. Currently, it is believed antioxidants plus zinc therapy may provide some benefit in the atrophic form of the disease. Side effects and the number of people who develop the hemorrhagic form of macular degeneration limit this treatment. Animal models have shown that oxidative mechanisms play a role in the development of both forms of this disorder. Human studies have indicated a general inverse association with antioxidant levels.[39]

β-Carotene (a specific vitamin A analogue), ascorbic acid (vitamin C), and tocopherol (vitamin E), as well as the trace elements zinc and selenium, have been implicated as possibly helpful in reducing progression of the disorder.[39,40] The most definitive results on antioxidant therapy to date came from the Age-Related Eye Disease Study (AREDS) report of 2001. In it, researchers concluded that patients older than 55 years with moderate or advanced AMD, or vision loss caused by AMD in one eye, and without contraindications (e.g., smoking history) would benefit from taking antioxidants plus zinc. The recommended doses of these antioxidants were vitamin C 500 mg, vitamin E 400 IU, β-carotene 15 mg, zinc oxide 80 mg, and cupric oxide 2 mg.[41] Additionally, dietary factors lutein and zeaxanthin (related to β-carotene) are factors that may potentially be associated with a reduced risk of advanced AMD.[42] These two factors were not part of the AREDS study, and further definitive studies are underway to confirm their beneficial effects.

The possible benefit of antioxidants in treating this disorder has led to the development of numerous nonprescription oral ophthalmic preparations containing these vitamins. No specific product recommendation can be made at this time. However, a product containing the ingredients is recommended by the AREDS study (Ocuvite PreserVision). Because other treatment options are limited and side effects are rare, eye care practitioners frequently recommend these products to their patients diagnosed with AMD.

These products are generally taken twice daily and are usually well tolerated, with gastrointestinal side effects rarely reported (see Chapter 23). Practitioners should make sure that ophthalmic vitamin products are not taken in conjunction with other multivitamin supplements, which could possibly lead to hypervitaminosis.

## CONTACT DERMATITIS

### Etiology/Signs and Symptoms of Contact Dermatitis

Contact dermatitis of the eyelid can be a reaction to either an allergen or an irritant. A change in cosmetics or soap or exposure to eye medication or another foreign substance is usually the cause. The involvement of both eyelids suggests allergy because both eyes are often exposed. Swelling, scaling, or redness of the eyelid along with profuse itching are common. Sunburns of the eyelids and ultraviolet burns to the cornea (e.g., recent sun exposure without eye protection from beach or ski outings) should be ruled out.

### Treatment of Contact Dermatitis

Questioning the patient about use of eye medications or new products (e.g., eyeliner, eye shadow) may quickly identify the offending substance. Discontinuing use of the suspected products is the best treatment. If swelling of the eyelid is marked, nonprescription oral antihistamines along with cold compresses applied three to four times per day will help reduce the inflammation and itching.

## LICE INFESTATION OF THE EYELID

### Etiology/Signs and Symptoms of Lice Infestation of the Eyelid

Infestation of the eyelids with the organisms *Phthirus pubis* (crab louse) or *Pediculus humanus capitis* (head louse) may cause symptoms similar to blepharitis (i.e., red, scaly, thickened eyelids). These organisms are also responsible for sexually transmitted lice infestation. Children are rarely affected by the crab louse but are commonly affected by the head louse.

### Treatment of Lice Infestation of the Eyelid

Frequent (4-5 times daily) cleaning with a mild soap and water and the use of a bland (nonmedicated) ophthalmic ointment (e.g., petrolatum) for 10 days is the recommended self-treatment. The ointment suffocates the louse and deprives its eggs of adequate oxygen to hatch. Practitioners should carefully instruct patients about the need to take appropriate hygienic measures, such as washing clothing and bedding that may contain unhatched eggs. Lice shampoo products cannot be used on the eyelids.

## BLEPHARITIS

### Etiology/Signs and Symptoms of Blepharitis

Blepharitis is an extremely common inflammatory condition of the eyelid margins. The most commonly associated factors are *Staphylococcus epidermidis, S. aureus,* and seborrheic dermatitis or a combination of these.[43] Red, scaly, thickened eyelids (often with loss of the eyelashes) are typical signs of blepharitis. Itching and burning are the most common complaints. All forms of blepharitis tend to be chronic, and individuals are often aware of their diagnosis.

### Treatment of Blepharitis

#### *Treatment Goals*

The goals in treating blepharitis are to (1) control the disorder with good eyelid hygiene and (2) provide symptomatic relief.

#### *General Treatment Approach*

Careful and diligent eyelid hygiene is the mainstay of therapy for the many forms of blepharitis. The chronic nature of blepharitis makes the use of careful eyelid hygiene preferable to the long-term use of topical antibiotics. Ocular lubricants can be used if eye irritation is also present (see Treatment of Dry Eye).

Good eyelid hygiene involves the use of hot compresses for 15 to 20 minutes, 2 to 4 times daily. Each application of a compress should be followed by lid scrubs, using a mild detergent cleanser compatible with the ocular tissues.

#### *Pharmacologic Therapy*

##### Lid Scrubs

Lid scrub procedures are usually effective and well tolerated. Table 28-8 provides instructions on how to perform lid scrubs. This procedure can also be used for hygienic eyelid cleansing in people who wear contact lenses. Eyelid cleansers are commercially available. However, cleansers for lid scrubs can be made from various brands of "no more tears" baby shampoos (e.g., Johnson and Johnson's). This involves mixing 1/4 teaspoonful of shampoo in 1 cup of tepid warm water, mixed to a bubbly froth, and scrubbing the lids using a clean, cotton-tipped applicator. Lids should be rinsed thoroughly after each cleaning. Although this approach is acceptable, the commercially available cleansers are equally effective, and patients may experience less ocular stinging and burning with their use.[44]

Commercial lid scrub products are specifically intended for the removal of oils, debris, or desquamated skin associated with the inflamed eyelid (see Table 28-6). Some commercial products are packaged with gauze pads, which provide an abrasive action to augment the cleansing properties of the detergent solution.

Eyelid scrubs using commercially available detergents are most effective in patients with noninfectious blepharitis. If the patient's signs or symptoms fail to improve, the patient should be referred to an eye care practitioner.

**TABLE 28-8 Administration Guidelines for Eyelid Scrubs**

1. Wash hands thoroughly.
2. Apply 3 to 4 drops of baby shampoo or eyelid cleanser to cotton-tipped applicator or gauze pad.
3. Close one eye, and clean the upper eyelid and eyelashes using side-to-side strokes, being careful not to touch eyeball with applicator or fingers.
4. Open eye, look up, and clean lower eyelid and eyelashes using side-to-side strokes.
5. Repeat the procedures on the other eye using a clean applicator or gauze pad.
6. Rinse eyelids and eyelashes with clean, warm water.

## HORDEOLUM/CHALAZION

### Etiology/Signs and Symptoms of Hordeolum/Chalazion

By definition, a hordeolum (stye) is an infection of one of the glands of the eyelid. An internal hordeolum is an infection of the meibomian gland, whereas an external hordeolum is an infection of the glands of Zeis and Moll (Figure 28-1). A palpable, tender nodule is always present. Swelling of the eyelid, almost to the point of closure, can occur with a severe internal hordeolum. The cause is invariably one of the staphylococcal species associated with blepharitis.

By definition, chalazion is not infectious and may involve one of the lid glands or may be located near (but not on) the eyelid (see Color Plates, photograph 6). A chalazion, which is a sterile granuloma, is very similar in appearance to an internal hordeolum. However, a chalazion is not tender to gentle touching, whereas a hordeolum is typically quite tender.

It is important to be aware that basal cell carcinoma on the eyelid may present as a nodule with a white, pearl-like appearance, and carcinoma of a sebaceous gland may be black in appearance, with loss of cilia (eyelashes), neovascularization, and/or bleeding. Patients who have an ocular nodule with these symptoms should see an eye care practitioner for evaluation.

### Treatment of Hordeolum/Chalazion

A hordeolum typically responds well to hot compresses applied 3 to 4 times daily for 5 to 10 minutes. Gentle pressure, applied by rolling the compress gently around the affected area, is recommended. A fresh, clean compress should be used with each treatment. Clearing usually occurs within 1 week. An external hordeolum may be treated with a topical antibiotic; however, an internal hordeolum does not respond well to such treatment and is best treated with a course of oral antibiotics. Surgical drainage may be required in recalcitrant cases.

Hot compresses applied in the same manner are usually sufficient to drain a chalazion. If either type of nodule does not drain within 1 week or has been present chronically, medical referral is appropriate. Periodic use of lid scrubs may reduce the recurrences of chalazion and hordeolum (Table 28-8). Chalazia may or may not resolve and are often a cosmetic problem, but they have been associated with changes in visual acuity if they occur on the eyelid margin.

## ASSESSMENT OF OPHTHALMIC DISORDERS: A CASE-BASED APPROACH

For patients who have not seen an eye care practitioner, the pharmacist or primary care practitioner must determine whether the ophthalmic disorder is self-treatable or requires medical referral. The practitioner must also take great care in assessing a patient with a new, acute problem. Ocular inflammation and irritation can be caused by many conditions, some of which can be treated safely and effectively with nonprescription ophthalmic products. These products are used primarily to relieve minor symptoms of burning, stinging, itching, and watering. FDA has suggested that self-treatment may be indicated for tear insufficiency, corneal edema, and external inflammation or irritation. Self-treatment may also be effective in managing hordeolum (stye), blepharitis, and allergic and viral conjunctivitis. Cases 28-1 and 28-2 give examples of the assessment of patients with ophthalmic disorders.

### CASE 28-1

| Relevant Evaluation Criteria | Scenario/Model Outcome |
|---|---|
| **Information Gathering** | |
| 1. Gather essential information about the patient's symptoms, including: | |
| a. description of symptom(s) (i.e., nature, onset, duration, severity, associated symptoms) | Patient has redness, burning, and watering in both eyes. No itching or other eye discharge is noted. For the last several years, symptoms have been more severe in the morning. |
| b. description of any factors that seem to precipitate, exacerbate, and/or relieve the patient's symptom(s) | Symptoms appear to be getting worse in the last few years. She has recently tried artificial tears and RefreshPM ointment and Visine to relieve her symptoms. Little relief has been observed. |
| c. description of the patient's efforts to relieve the symptoms | Patient has applied ocular lubricants and a topical decongestant to lessen her symptoms and to make her eye less red. |
| 2. Gather essential patient history information: | |
| a. patient's identity | Lola |
| b. patient's age, sex, height, and weight | 67 y/o F |
| c. patient's occupation | N/A |
| d. patient's dietary habits | N/A |
| e. patient's sleep habits | N/A |
| f. concurrent medical conditions, prescription and nonprescription medications, and dietary supplements | Monopril 20 mg once daily for hypertension; Premarin 1.25 mg once daily for 21 days, then off 7 days; Os-Cal 500 once daily for mild osteoporosis; Advil 200 mg 2 tablets as needed for osteoarthritis, headache, etc. |
| g. allergies | NKA, although she does have a history of seasonal allergic rhinitis |
| h. history of other adverse reactions to medications | None |
| i. other (describe)______ | |
| **Assessment and Triage** | |
| 3. Differentiate the patient's signs/symptoms and correctly identify the patient's primary problem(s). | Red, burning, and watering eyes |
| 4. Identify exclusions for self-treatment (see Figure 28-2). | Red, burning, and watering eyes |

## CASE 28-1 (continued)

| Relevant Evaluation Criteria | Scenario/Model Outcome |
|---|---|
| 5. Formulate a comprehensive list of therapeutic alternatives for the primary problem to determine if triage to a medical practitioner is required, and share this information with the patient. | Options include:<br>(1) Recommend continuing with the RefreshPM at bedtime.<br>(2) Change to Refresh Tears during the day.<br>(3) Discontinue Visine.<br>(4) Refer Lola for medical evaluation if no response.<br>(5) Take no action. |
| **Plan** | |
| 6. Select an optimal therapeutic alternative to address the patient's problem, taking into account patient preferences. | Any preservative-free or rapidly dissolving artificial tears could be used during the day. Topical vasoconstrictors (i.e., Visine) may potentiate the red eye and cause more eye irritation. Lola should be instructed on proper eye drop and ointment administration. |
| 7. Describe the recommended therapeutic approach to the patient. | You should switch to artificial tears (e.g., Refresh Tears, Hypotears) during the day and discontinue the Visine. Refer to the box Patient Education for Ophthalmic Disorders for proper nondrug and drug use. |
| 8. Explain to the patient the rationale for selecting the recommended therapeutic approach from the considered therapeutic alternatives. | You may need to see an eye care practitioner if you do not get relief. A new prescription treatment has become available for the treatment of moderate to severe dry eye (cyclosporine 0.05%). |
| **Patient Education** | |
| 9. When recommending self-care with nonprescription medications and/or nondrug therapy, convey accurate information to the patient, including: | |
| a. appropriate dose and frequency of administration | Artificial tears may be used as often as needed. |
| b. maximum number of days the therapy should be employed | Topical decongestants are not recommended for more than 3 days use (see Table 28-5). |
| c. product administration procedures | See the box Patient Education for Ophthalmic Disorders, and Tables 28-2 and 28-3. |
| d. expected time to onset of relief | With discontinuation of Visine and usage of eye lubricant drops/ointments, noticeable improvement could be observed within a few days. |
| e. degree of relief that can be reasonably expected | Relief of symptoms should occur almost immediately with use of the drops during the day and ointment at bedtime. However, this is most likely a lifelong situation that requires careful monitoring to prevent ocular complications. |
| f. most common side effects | Stinging, burning with drops; blurred vision with an ointment |
| g. side effects that warrant medical intervention should they occur | Continued or worsening of burning, itching, pain, or ocular redness |
| h. patient options in the event that condition worsens or persists | An eye care practitioner should be consulted if symptoms do not improve. |
| i. product storage requirements | Keep tightly closed in a cool, dry area. Always replace tops on eye medications when not in use. Be careful not to contaminate eye drops and ointments. If you use preservative-free eye drops be sure to discard as indicated. |
| j. specific nondrug measures | You should use lid scrubs (see Table 28-8) and warm compresses 2-4 times daily to keep the eyelid glands from being plugged and to get vascular supply back to the lids. Good lid hygiene is often beneficial in patients with dry eye disease since they may often have blepharitis (eyelid inflammation). See also the box Patient Education for Ophthalmic Disorders. |
| 10. Solicit patient's follow-up questions. | Is there anything I can do to prevent or lessen some of the dry eye symptoms? |
| 11. Answer patient's questions. | Yes. Avoid dry windy environments. Protect your eyes from sunlight and undue exposure by wearing sunglasses or goggles when appropriate. Continue with the lids scrubs and warm compresses as described above. |

Key: N/A, not applicable; NKA, no known allergies.

## CASE 28-2

| Relevant Evaluation Criteria | Scenario/Model Outcome |
|---|---|
| **Information Gathering** | |
| 1. Gather essential information about the patient's symptoms, including: | |
| a. description of symptom(s) (i.e., nature, onset, duration, severity, associated symptoms) | Patient is experiencing itching and burning of his eyelids as well as itching of the scalp and genitals. He has reddened eyelid margins. |
| b. description of any factors that seem to precipitate, exacerbate, and/or relieve the patient's symptom(s) | |
| c. description of the patient's efforts to relieve the symptoms | Patient has been prescribed oral tetracycline 250 mg 4 times/day for 30 days, and told to use Eye-Scrub solution, Lacrilube ophthalmic ointment, and Nix 1% cream rinse. |
| 2. Gather essential patient history information: | |
| a. patient's identity | Craig |
| b. patient's age, sex, height, and weight | 37 y/o M |
| c. patient's occupation | N/A |
| d. patient's dietary habits | N/A |
| e. patient's sleep habits | N/A |
| f. concurrent medical conditions, prescription and nonprescription medications, and dietary supplements | Nix 1% cream rinse and Lacrilube ophthalmic ointment for lice infestation |
| g. allergies | NKA |
| h. history of other adverse reactions to medications | None |
| i. other (describe)_______ | |
| **Assessment and Triage** | |
| 3. Differentiate the patient's signs/symptoms and correctly identify the patient's primary problem(s). | Itching and burning of eyelids, and itching of scalp and genitals caused by lice. |
| 4. Identify exclusions for self-treatment (see Figure 28-3). | None |
| 5. Formulate a comprehensive list of therapeutic alternatives for the primary problem to determine if triage to a medical practitioner is required, and share this information with the patient. | Options include:<br>(1) Recommend continuing with Eye-Scrub.<br>(2) Recommend that Craig apply Lacrilube on the eyelids.<br>(3) Remind Craig that Nix is not to be used on the lids or near the eye.<br>(4) Remind Craig of importance of not reinfecting himself.<br>(5) Take no action. |
| **Plan** | |
| 6. Select an optimal therapeutic alternative to address the patient's problem, taking into account patient preferences. | Any ophthalmic lubricant ointment would be reasonable. Some patients may use baby shampoo diluted 50:50 instead of Eye-Scrub to save money, although this may cause additional irritation. Instruct patient on proper eyelid scrub technique (see Table 28-8). |
| 7. Describe the recommended therapeutic approach to the patient. | Lacrilube is to be applied to the lid itself (not in the lid as is the case for dry eye patients) after the eyelid scrub. The ointment is believed to "suffocate" the lice and help to prevent their spread. |

**CASE 28-2 (continued)**

| Relevant Evaluation Criteria | Scenario/Model Outcome |
|---|---|
| 8. Explain to the patient the rationale for selecting the recommended therapeutic approach from the considered therapeutic alternatives. | Seeking an eye care practitioner may not be necessary at this time if you follow the proper order of administration and do not allow Nix to be used near the eye. |
| **Patient Education** | |
| 9. When recommending self-care with nonprescription medications and/or nondrug therapy, convey accurate information to the patient, including: | |
| a. appropriate dose and frequency of administration | Nix should be used as described on the directions in the box (see Chapter 37). Ophthalmic ointment is applied 4-5 times daily. |
| b. maximum number of days the therapy should be employed | Eye-Scrub and Lacrilube should be used for 10 days. Nix has specific recommendations for local use (see Chapter 37). |
| c. product administration procedures | See the box Patient Education for Ophthalmic Disorders and Table 28-8. |
| d. expected time to onset of relief | Reasonable response should occur within a few days to a week. |
| e. degree of relief that can be reasonably expected | Relief of itching and burning should occur within a few days if Nix is not used close to the eye. |
| f. most common side effects | Blurred vision, eye irritation |
| g. side effects that warrant medical intervention should they occur | Continued burning or itching, or recurrence of symptoms after a period of relief |
| h. patient options in the event that condition worsens or persists | An eye care practitioner should be consulted if symptoms do not improve. |
| i. product storage requirements | Keep tightly closed in a cool, dry area. Always replace eye ointment tops to prevent contamination. |
| j. specific nondrug measures | You should clean all bed linens, towels, etc. at the time of your Nix application. You can reinfect yourself when you reuse contaminated items. |
| 10. Solicit patient's follow-up questions. | Is there anything I can do to prevent recurrence of the scabies? |
| 11. Answer patient's questions. | Yes. As mentioned earlier, all auxiliary items must be cleaned and disinfected at the same time to prevent reinfection. Continue with the lid scrubs as described. |

Key: N/A, not applicable; NKA, no known allergies.

Table 28-9 describes the major features of disorders that require medical referral. Any self-treated condition that does not resolve within a reasonably short time should also be referred to an eye care practitioner for care.

## PATIENT COUNSELING FOR OPHTHALMIC DISORDERS

Before counseling a patient, the practitioner should carefully consider the nature and extent of ocular involvement. It is important that patients with acute ocular disease receive a prompt, definitive diagnosis, including baseline visual acuity, before the practitioner considers the appropriateness of nonprescription therapy. Some acute conditions, which may or may not involve ocular pain or blurred vision, can be appropriately treated with nonprescription agents, but a recent diagnosis from an ophthalmic practitioner can give additional reassurance and confidence in recommending such treatment. Although the cost-effectiveness of ophthalmic care can be greatly improved through the use of nonprescription agents, severe visual impairment, including blindness, can be a serious clinical and medicolegal complication if the practitioner delays referral for definitive diagnosis and treatment. After careful consideration of the history, the practitioner should always counsel patients on the indications for and limitations of self-treatment. The algorithms in Figures 28-2 and 28-3 can assist the practitioner in recommending the appropriate treatment for disorders of the eye surface and eyelid, respectively.

Numerous nonprescription ophthalmic products for treating minor ocular irritations are available for self-administration by the patient with minimal or no supervision. Such products are also adequate for treating certain clinical conditions diagnosed by primary care providers or eye care practitioners. First-line therapy should always include counseling on nonpharmacologic treatment.

**TABLE 28-9 Differentiation of Ophthalmic Disorders That Require Medical Referral**

| Disorder | Potential Signs/Symptoms | Complications | Treatment Approach |
|---|---|---|---|
| Blunt trauma | Ruptured blood vessels, bleeding into eyelid tissue space, swelling, ocular discomfort, facial drooping | Internal eye bleeding, secondary glaucoma, detached retina, periorbital bone fracture (blowout fracture) | Medical referral |
| Foreign particles trapped/embedded in the eye | Reddened eyes, profuse tearing, ocular discomfort | Corneal abrasions/ scarring, chronic red eye, interocular penetration from metal striking metal at high speeds | Medical referral for removal of particles |
| Ocular abrasions | Partial/total loss of corneal epithelium, blurred vision, profuse tearing, difficulty opening the eye | Risk of bacterial/fungal infection if eye exposed to organic material, corneal scarring, anterior chamber rupture | Medical referral |
| Infections of eyelid/eye surface | Red, thickened lids; scaling | Scarring of lids, dry eye, corneal abrasion or scarring, loss of vision | Medical referral |
| Eye exposure to chemical splash, solid chemical, or chemical fumes | Reddened eyes, watering, difficulty opening eye | Scarring of eyelids and eye surface, loss of vision | To prevent/reduce scarring of eyelids from chemical burns, flush eye immediately for at least 10 minutes, preferably with sterile saline/water. If neither is available, flush with tap water. After flushing eye, arrange immediate transportation to an emergency facility. No recommendation for acid-base balance |
| Thermal injury to eye (welder's arc) | Reddened eyes, pain, sensitivity to light | Corneal scarring, secondary infection | Medical referral for definitive care, including possible eye patching |
| Bacterial conjunctivitis | Reddened eyes with purulent (mucus) discharge, ocular discomfort, eyelids stuck together on awakening | Typically self-limiting in 2 weeks | Medical referral for treatment with topical antibiotics to clear infection more quickly; some require systemic antibiotic treatment |
| Chlamydial conjunctivitis | Watery or mucus discharge, ocular discomfort, low-grade fever, possible blurred vision | Scarring | If infection with *Chlamydia* sp. is known or suspected, or if symptoms are too vague to rule in viral or allergic conjunctivitis, medical referral mandatory |

These treatments alone are frequently sufficient to relieve the ocular symptoms or are necessary as an adjunct to the ophthalmic drug therapy. Proper drug instillation technique is critical if the target tissue (the eye) is to receive the maximum benefit from the medication. Ophthalmic solutions and ointments, as well as eyelid scrubs, are often used incorrectly. By carefully instructing patients in the proper self-administration procedures, the practitioner can help ensure maximum safety and effectiveness of these agents. Appropriate patient education and counseling must accompany dispensing of any ophthalmic product.

Although drug side effects and interactions are rare with topically applied ophthalmic products, the potential for such effects does exist. Therefore, the practitioner should advise the patient of possible adverse effects, including the clinical signs of drug toxicity or allergy.

The practitioner must actively assist patients in selecting the appropriate product that will enhance compliance, minimize or avoid side effects, and reduce the attendant costs of therapy. The other major considerations in making therapeutic recommendations are whether the person has a sensitivity to one of the product constituents, the product can be used with contact lenses, and the product has the potential to wash out prescription ophthalmic drugs the patient may be using. With the exception of ophthalmic antihistamines and decongestants, little product-to-product comparative research has been done for nonprescription ophthalmic preparations. The practitioner must, therefore, make therapy recommendations based on the patient's diagnosis and the products the patient is currently using. The box Patient Education for Ophthalmic Disorders lists specific information to provide patients.

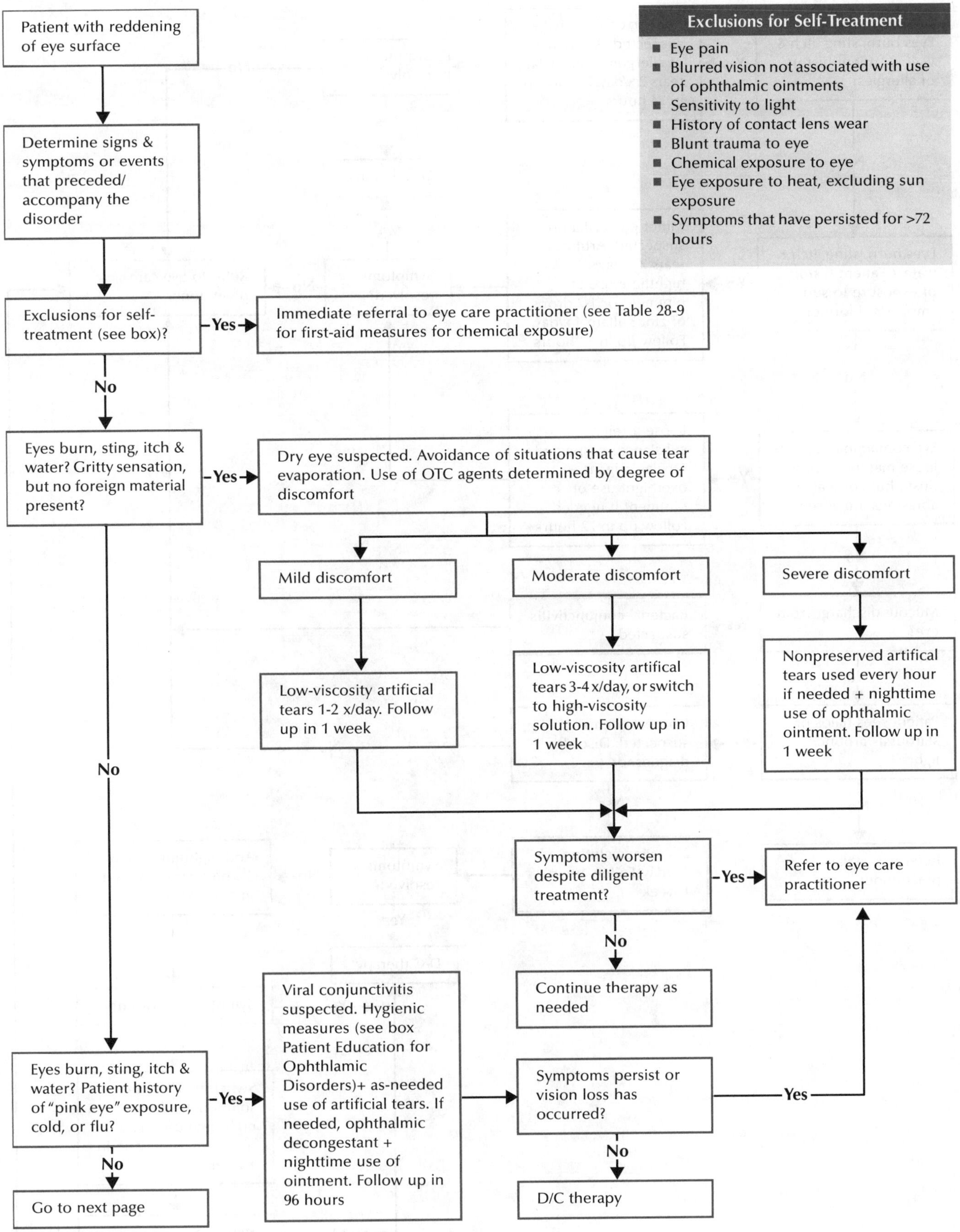


**FIGURE 28-2** Self-care of eye surface disorders. Key: AH, antihistamine; D/C, discontinue; OTC, over-the-counter.

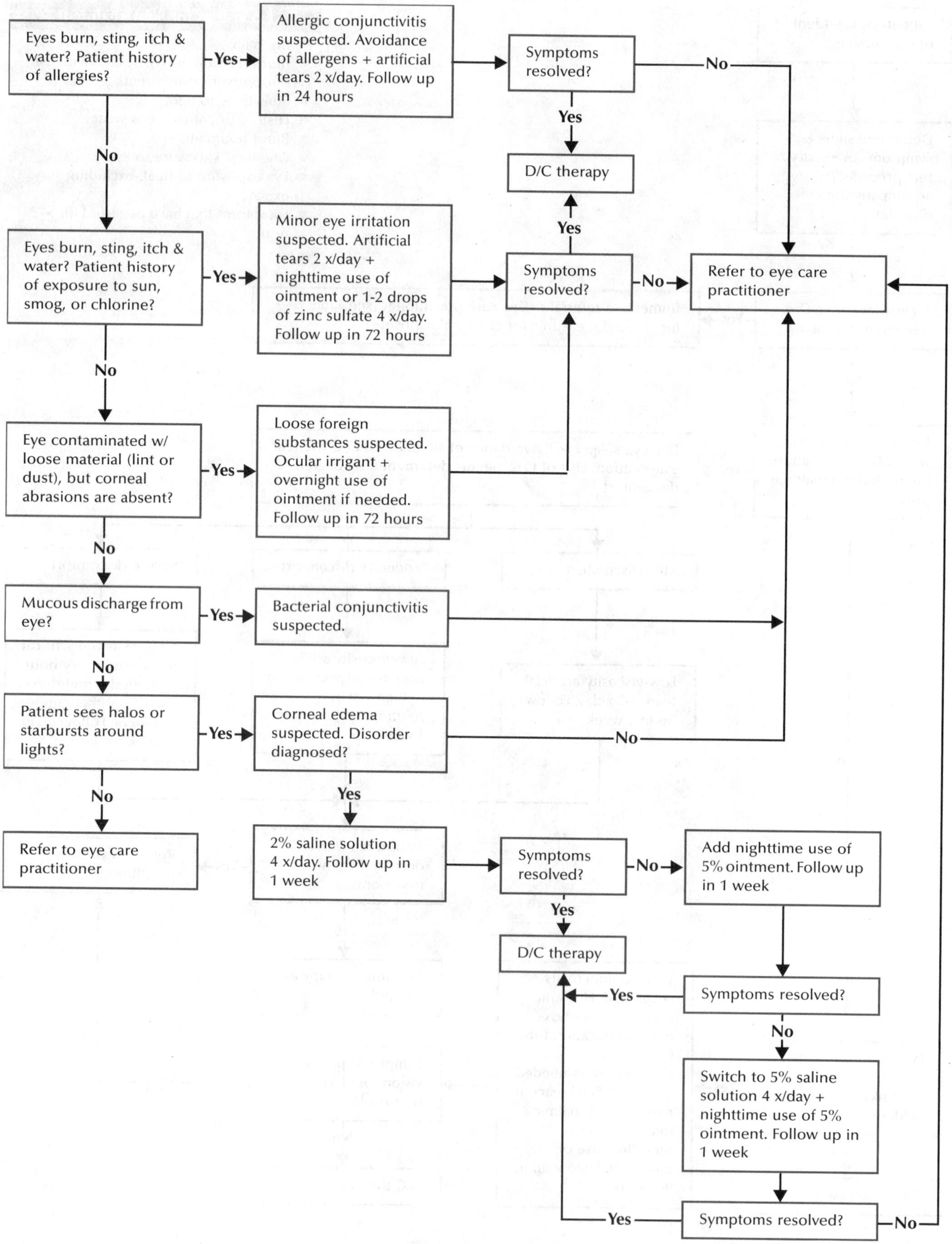


**FIGURE 28-2 (continued)** Self-care of eye surface disorders. Key: AH, antihistamine; D/C, discontinue; OTC, over-the-counter.

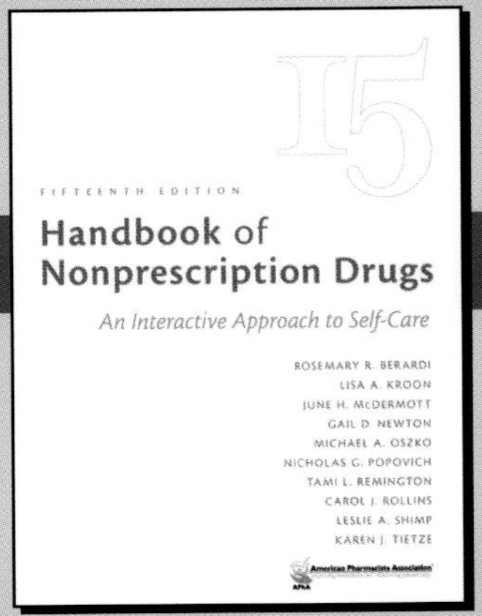


# HANDBOOK OF NONPRESCRIPTION DRUGS

## E-Book Version

## Welcome!

As a free bonus, purchasers of the 15th edition of the *Handbook of Nonprescription Drugs* get . . .

- ONE free download to ONE computer
- Fast access to the complete content of the book from your laptop or desktop computer. It is completely searchable and can be annotated with your comments.
- Technical support information is available at **http://www.OTCHandbook.com** by clicking on "Download eBook."

## How to Get Started

1. Open your browser and visit **http://www.OTCHandbook.com**
2. Click on "Download eBook."
3. Complete the registration form.
4. Enter the unique download code on this card EXACTLY as it appears.
5. Click "Submit."

E-Book Download Code:

2c1a24b8

06-057

**Exclusions for Self-Treatment**

- Signs and symptoms of infection of eyelids (e.g., red, thickened eyelids; scaling)
- Blunt trauma to eye
- Exposure of eye to chemicals

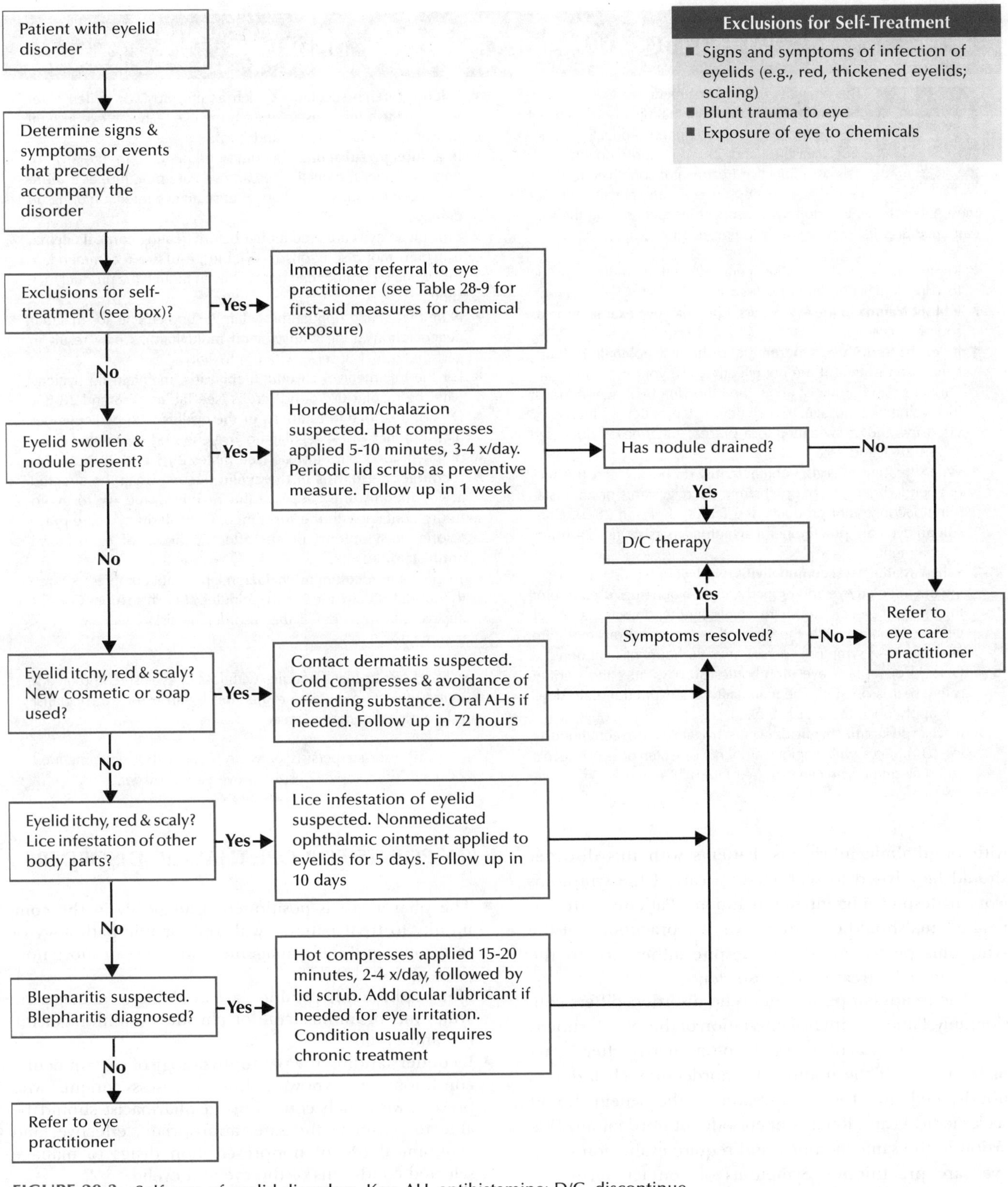


FIGURE 28-3 Self-care of eyelid disorders. Key: AH, antihistamine; D/C, discontinue.

## EVALUATION OF PATIENT OUTCOMES FOR OPHTHALMIC DISORDERS

Patients who self-treat allergic conjunctivitis, loose foreign substances in the eye, or minor eye irritation should see an eye care practitioner if the symptoms persist after 24 hours of treatment. Those who are self-treating viral conjunctivitis should seek medical care if vision loss occurs or symptoms persist after 96 hours of treatment. Dry eye is often a chronic disorder, requiring continuous treatment

## PATIENT EDUCATION FOR OPHTHALMIC DISORDERS

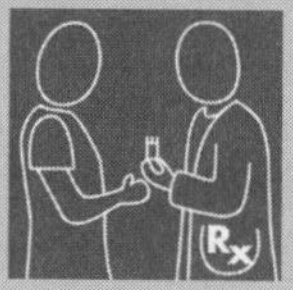

The objectives of self-treatment are to (1) relieve the symptoms of minor ophthalmic disorders using the appropriate nonprescription products or nondrug measures, and (2) use nonprescription products as adjunctive treatment of ophthalmic disorders diagnosed by an eye care practitioner. For most patients, carefully following product instructions and the self-care measures listed here will help ensure good outcomes.

- Remove the causative ocular agent/irritant that predisposes you to your ocular condition or disease.
- If **blunt trauma** to the eye occurs, obtain an eye examination as soon as possible.
- If you have **dry eye syndrome** and the first ophthalmic lubricants used to treat it are not effective, ask your eye care practitioner or a pharmacist about the following treatment options: increasing the dosage, switching to a product of increased viscosity, and/or switching to a preservative-free product (see Tables 28-1 and 28-2).
- When treating **allergic conjunctivitis**, do not exceed the recommended dosages of ophthalmic decongestants or antihistamine-decongestant products (see Tables 28-4 and 28-5). Consult an eye care practitioner if symptoms persist after 24 hours of treatment.
- When treating **viral conjunctivitis**, wash your hands after touching the infected eye and properly dispose of tissues used to blot the infected eye. Do not share towels or other objects that might come in contact with the infected eye. Consult an eye care practitioner if symptoms persist after 96 hours of treatment.
- Discard or replace eye drop bottles 30 days after the sterility safety seal is opened. The manufacturer's expiration date does not apply once the seal is broken.
- If **eye exposure to chemicals** occurs, irrigate the eye continuously for 10 minutes with copious amounts of water or eye irrigants and seek immediate eye care (see Tables 28-6 and 28-7).
- If **loose foreign substances** such as lint, dust, or pollen enter the eye, flush the substance from the eye using an eye irrigant or water (see Tables 28-6 and 28-7).
- If a **foreign substance** becomes embedded in the eye or trapped under the eyelid, see an eye care practitioner. Failure to remove the substance could cause an eye infection or tissue damage.
- Consult an eye care practitioner before treating **corneal edema**. If hyperosmotic solutions (see Table 28-6) are recommended, follow the recommended dosages even though the product may sting.
- Note that taking ophthalmic vitamin supplements for macular degeneration along with general multivitamins may result in gastrointestinal upset or vitamin toxicity.
- For the treatment of **chronic blepharitis**, maintain lid hygiene with the regular use of lid scrubs (see Tables 28-6 and 28-8).
- Do not treat **lice infestations of the eyelids** with pediculicides (lice products); use regular lid hygiene and a nonmedicated ointment for 5 days instead (see Tables 28-1 and 28-3).
- If **contact dermatitis of the eyelid** occurs, wash the affected areas, identify the cause of the reaction, and try to avoid future contact with the substance. Consult an eye care practitioner if symptoms persist after 72 hours of use of oral antihistamines.
- To clear a **hordeolum or chalazion**, apply hot compresses three to four times daily for 5 to 10 minutes at each session. Consult an eye care provider if the disorder persists after 1 week of treatment.

⚠ Pearl-like or black nodules with loss of eyelashes and bleeding require immediate evaluation by an eye care specialist to rule out carcinoma (cancer).

⚠ If the disorder persists or worsens after the recommended length of therapy, consult an eye care provider.

with ophthalmic lubricants. Patients with this disorder should be advised to seek medical care if the symptoms worsen despite diligent self-treatment. Patients with corneal edema should consult an eye care practitioner if the symptoms persist or worsen despite adherence to the instructions for treating the disorder.

The treatment period for eyelid disorders differs considerably. Patients with lice infestation of the eyelids should see an eye care practitioner if symptoms persist after 5 days of treatment. If the nodule of a hordeolum/chalazion is not drained after 1 week of treatment, the patient should seek medical care. Recurrent episodes of hordeolum/chalazion in the same area or gland require evaluation by an eye care practitioner. Symptoms of contact dermatitis should resolve quickly once the offending substance is removed. If symptoms persist after 72 hours of antihistamine use, the patient should see an eye care practitioner. Blepharitis usually requires chronic treatment. Patients with diagnosed blepharitis should self-treat the disorder daily as described in Treatment of Blepharitis, but if symptoms worsen, the patient should seek medical care.

## KEY POINTS FOR OPHTHALMIC DISORDERS

- The pharmacist is positioned strategically in the community to treat patients with ophthalmic pathology or to recommend self-management with one or more nonprescription drugs.
- Many ophthalmic products are available to manage the symptoms of minor acute or chronic conditions of the eye and eyelid.
- By understanding the pathophysiology of certain ocular conditions and knowing how to assess patients who present with such conditions, a pharmacist should be able to optimize the safe, appropriate, effective, and economical use of nonprescription drugs to manage selected conditions of the eye and eyelid.
- Nonprescription ophthalmic products should be used only in cases of minor pain or discomfort. If doubt exists concerning the nature of the problem, the practitioner should refer the patient for professional care.
- Nonprescription ocular medications should not be recommended to patients who have demonstrated an allergy to any of the active ingredients, preservatives, or other excipients in the product.

- Patients who already are using a prescription ophthalmic product should use nonprescription products only after consulting with an ophthalmic practitioner or pharmacist.
- Patients with narrow anterior chamber angles or narrow-angle glaucoma should not use topical ocular decongestants because of the risk of angle-closure glaucoma.
- Drug application should be conservative in patients with hyperemic conjunctiva because of the potential for increased systemic drug absorption and the risk of adverse effects.
- The lowest concentration and conservative dosage frequencies should be used, especially for ocular decongestants and overuse should be avoided.
- Ophthalmic products frequently are used incorrectly; therefore, counseling on appropriate application of products is crucial.

## References


1. Schein OD, Munoz B, Tielsch JM, et al. Prevalence of dry eye among the elderly. *Am J Ophthalmol.* 1997;124:723-8.
2. Warwick R. In: *Anatomy of the Eye and Orbit.* 7th ed. Philadelphia: WB Saunders; 1975:195-219.
3. Milder B. The lacrimal apparatus. In: Moses RA, Hart WM, eds. *Adler's Physiology of the Eye.* 8th ed. St. Louis: Mosby; 1987:15-35.
4. Mishima S, Gasset A, Klyce SO, et al. Determination of tear volume and tear flow. *Invest Ophthalmol.* 1966;3: 264-76.
5. Jordan A, Baum J. Basic tear flow. Does it exist? *Ophthalmology.* 1980;9:920-30.
6. Harris LS, Galin MA. Dose response analysis of pilocarpine-induced ocular hypotension. *Arch Ophthalmol.* 1970;1:605-8.
7. Pfister RR, Burstein N. The effects of ophthalmic drugs, vehicles, and preservatives on corneal epithelium; a scanning electron microscope study. *Invest Ophthalmol.* 1976; 15:246-59.
8. Stern ME, Beurman RW, Fox RI, et al. The pathology of dry eye: the interaction between the ocular surface and lacrimal glands. *Cornea.* 1998;17:584-9.
9. Norn MS. Desiccation of the precorneal film, I: corneal wetting time. *Acta Ophthalmol.* 1969;47:865-80.
10. Lopez-Bernal D, Ubels JL. Quantitative evaluation of the corneal epithelial barrier effect: effect of artificial tears and preservatives. *Curr Eye Res.* 1991;7:645-66.
11. Swanson M. Compliance with and typical usage of artificial tears in dry eye conditions. *J Am Optom Assoc.* 1998;69: 649-55.
12. Berdy GJ, Abelson MB, Smith LM, et al. Preservative free artificial tear solutions. *Arch Ophthalmol.* 1992;110:528-32.
13. Pensyl CD. Lubricants and other preparations for ocular surface disease. In: Bartlett JD, Jaanus SD, eds. *Clinical Ocular Pharmacology.* 4th ed. Boston: Butterworth-Heinemann; 2001:315-32.
14. Schilling H, Koch JM, Waubke TN, et al. Treatment of dry eye with vitamin A acid: an impression cytology controlled study. *Fortschr Ophthalmol.* 1989;5:530-4.
15. Mullen W, Sheppard W, Leibowitz J. Ophthalmic preservatives and vehicles. *Surv Ophthalmol.* 1973;17:469-83.
16. Sabiston DW. The dry eye. *Trans Ophthalmol Soc N Z.* 1969; 21: 96-100.
17. Linn ML, Jones LT. Rate of lacrimal excretion of ophthalmic vehicles. *Am J Ophthalmol.* 1968;65:76-8.
18. Fiscella R, Burstein NL. Ophthalmic drug formulations. In: Bartlett JD, Jaanus SD, eds. *Clinical Ocular Pharmacology.* Boston: Butterworth-Heinemann; 2001:19-40.
19. Burstein NL. Preservative cytotoxic threshold for benzalkonium chloride and chlorhexidine digluconate in cat and rabbit corneas. *Invest Ophthalmol Vis Sci.* 1980;19:308-13.
20. Debbasch C, Brignole F, Pisella P-J, et al. Quarternary ammoniums and other preservatives, contribution in oxidative stress and apoptosis on chang conjunctival cells. *Invest Ophthalmol Vis Sci.* 2001;42:642-52.
21. Wilson WS, Duncan AJ, Jay JL. Effect of benzalkonium chloride on the stability of the precorneal tear film in rabbit and man. *Br J Ophthalmol.* 1975;59:667-9.
22. Mondino BJ, Salamon SM, Zaidman GW. Allergic and toxic reactions in soft contact lens wearers. *Surv Ophthalmol.* 1982;26:337-44.
23. Miller J, Wolf EM. Antazoline phosphate and naphazoline hydrochloride, singly and in combination for the treatment of allergic conjunctivitis—a controlled double-blind clinical trial. *Ann Allergy.* 1975;35:81-6.
24. Soparkar CN, Wilhelmus KR, Koch DD, et al. Acute and chronic conjunctivitis due to over-the-counter ophthalmic decongestants. *Arch Ophthalmol.* 1997;115:34-8.
25. Portello JK, Jaanus SD. Mydriatics and mydriolytics. In: Bartlett JD, Jaanus SD, eds. *Clinical Ocular Pharmacology.* 4th ed. Boston: Butterworth-Heinemann; 2001:135-48.
26. Jaanus SD. Antiallergy drugs and decongestants. In: Bartlett JD, Jaanus SD, eds. *Clinical Ocular Pharmacology.* 4th ed. Boston: Butterworth-Heinemann; 2001:299-314.
27. Krupin T, Silverstein B, Faitt M, et al. The effect of H1 blocking antihistamines on intraocular pressure in rabbits. *Ophthalmology.* 1980;87:1167-72.
28. Abelson MB, Allansmith MR, Freidlaender MH. Effects of topically applied ocular decongestant and antihistamine. *Am J Ophthalmol.* 1980;90:254-7.
29. Petrusewicz J, Kalizan R. Blood platelet adrenoreceptor: aggregatory and antiaggregatory activity of imidazole drugs. *Pharmacology.* 1986;33:249-55.
30. Pahissa A, Guardia J, Botil JM, et al. Antazoline induced allergic pneumonitis. *BMJ.* 1979;2:1328.
31. Bengtsson U, Larsson O, Lindstedt G, et al. Antazoline induced immune hemolytic anemia, hemoglobulinuria, and acute renal failure. *Acta Med Scand.* 1975;198:223-7.
32. Neilsen JL, Dahl R, Kissmeyer-Neilsen F. Immune thrombocytopenia due to antazoline. *Allergy.* 1981;36:517-9.
33. Ogbuihi S, Audick W, Bohn G. Sudden infant death-fatal intoxication with pheniramine. *Z Rechtsmed.* 1990;103:221-5.
34. Berdy GJ, Abelson MB, George MA, et al. Allergic conjunctivitis—a survey of new antihistamines. *J Ocul Pharmacol.* 1991;7:313-24.
35. Gelmi C, Occuzzi R. Mydriatic effect of ocular decongestants studied by pupillography. *Ophthalmologica.* 1994;208:243-6.
36. Abelson MB, Yamamoto GK, Allansmith MR. Effects of ocular decongestants. *Arch Ophthalmol.* 1980;98:856-8.
37. Lamberts DW. Topical hyperosmotic agents and secretory stimulants. *Int Ophthalmol Clin.* 1980;20:163-9.
38. Hales RH. Contact lens solutions. In: *Contact Lenses: A Clinical Approach to Fitting.* Baltimore: Williams & Wilkins; 1978:32-50.
39. Christen WG. Antioxidant vitamins and age-related eye disease. *Proc Assoc Amer Phys.* 1999;111:16-21.
40. Sperduto RD, Ferris FL, Kurinij N. Do we have a nutritional treatment for age-related cataract or macular degeneration? *Arch Ophthalmol.* 1990;108:1403-5.
41. Age-Related Eye Disease Study Research Group. A randomized, placebo-controlled, clinical trial of high-dose supplementation with vitamins C and E, beta carotene, and zinc for age-related macular degeneration and vision loss. *Arch Ophthalmol.* 2001;119: 1417-36.
42. Marse-Perlman JA, Fisher AI, Klein R, et al. Lutein and zeaxanthin in the diet and serum and their relation to age-related maculopathy in the Third National Health and Nutrition Examination Survey. *Am J Epidem.* 2001;153:424-32.
43. Jones DB, Liesegang TJ, Robinson NM. Laboratory diagnosis of ocular infections. Paper presented at: Annual Meeting of the American Society for Microbiology, Washington, DC; May 26-30, 1981.
44. Polack FM, Goodman DF. Experience with a new detergent lid scrub in the management of chronic blepharitis. *Arch Ophthalmol.* 1988;106:719-20.

CHAPTER 29

# Prevention of Contact Lens–related Disorders

Janet P. Engle

The greatly enhanced comfort of soft contact lenses, introduced in the 1970s, led to a significant expansion of the contact lens market. Similarly, improvements in rigid gas-permeable (RGP) hard lenses provide the comfort of soft lenses and the enhanced optical qualities of hard lenses. Continuous-wear lenses, toric lenses for astigmatism, tinted lenses, bifocal contact lenses, and disposable lenses have also greatly expanded the patient population who can wear contact lenses.

Although much of the motivation to wear contact lenses may be cosmetic, properly fitted lenses can provide significant vision advantages over eyeglasses. Of the 38 million Americans currently wearing contact lenses, nearly 90% use the lenses to correct the vision of an otherwise healthy eye. Contact lenses reduce size distortion and prismatic effects, and improve peripheral vision. Elimination of spectacle fogging, dirt accumulation, and frame distraction are also significant advantages to many users. Most soft contact lens wearers say their lenses are more comfortable than eyeglasses. However, it is important to note that approximately 2.7 million contact lens patients stop wearing their lenses every year. The most commonly cited reason is lens discomfort. Proper care of lenses can help eliminate discomfort and encourage patients to continue wearing their lenses.

It has been well established that contact lenses, even when expertly fitted, somewhat alter ocular tissues and change the corneal metabolism. Thus, it is imperative that both the user and the health care professional understand the proper care, maintenance, and safe use of these products. Failure to do so can greatly increase the chance of corneal infection, corneal ulcers, and other ocular conditions that may result in permanent eye damage. Fortunately, however, most side effects of contact lens use are reversible if attended to promptly.

More than 100 nonprescription contact lens care products are available, and consumers are likely to be overwhelmed by the variety. Other than the lens prescriber, pharmacists are the most accessible health care professionals to counsel contact lens wearers as to which products to choose. Product selection depends on the products' compatibility with each other as well as with the specific contact lens. Therefore, the pharmacist's responsibility is to understand this area of professional practice and provide effective, up-to-date information when consulting with the contact lens wearer.

## Use of Contact Lenses

Most people can wear one or more types of contact lenses without problems if certain precautions are taken. In a few cases, use of contact lenses is contraindicated.

### *Indications for Contact Lenses*

Some patients wear contact lenses because eyeglasses cannot provide satisfactory vision. Others wear them for cosmetic reasons or because they find eyeglasses a hindrance during sports or other activities. However, most patients with vision problems can use either eyeglasses or contact lenses for purely visual reasons.

#### Therapeutic Necessity

The decision to wear contact lenses rather than eyeglasses is sometimes based on therapeutic necessity. For example, in patients with keratoconus, a gradual protrusion of the central cornea, satisfactory vision is usually unattainable with ordinary eyeglasses but can be obtained with rigid contact lenses. Other examples of therapeutic necessity are lenses used as collagen shields and soft contact lenses saturated with antibiotic agents.

Aphakic patients characteristically see better with contact lenses than with spectacles. Continuous-wear contacts are particularly beneficial for such patients because their poor vision makes it difficult for them to insert and remove lenses.

Visual aberrations caused by corneal scarring are also often better corrected with rigid contact lenses. Whereas eyeglasses simply correct refractive error by changing the focus of light incident on the cornea, the proximity of the rigid contact lens actually masks irregularities in corneal topography. Prosthetic lenses may also make corneal scarring cosmetically unnoticeable.

#### Refractive Examination

Other indications for the use of contacts include refractive errors such as myopia (nearsightedness), hyperopia (farsightedness), astigmatism, and presbyopia.

Astigmatism occurs when an unequal curvature of the refractive surfaces of the eye results in a fuzzy image. RGP lenses, hard lenses, and toric soft lenses, to a lesser extent, can be used to correct an astigmatism.

Presbyopia (old vision) is a condition caused by aging, in which the crystalline lens cannot properly focus on near objects. More than 50% of visually corrected patients are presbyopic. Contact lenses have not been overly successful in improving vision for these patients. Because vision correction is needed for both near vision and far vision, two optical corrections are required in each bifocal contact lens.

To correct presbyopia with eyeglasses, bifocal or trifocal lenses (often called multifocal lenses) are needed. If properly selected and indoctrinated, patients trying bifocal contact lenses can achieve adequate vision 60% to 70% of the time. Monovision is one method of presbyopic contact lens correction that has been successful in some cases; the dominant eye is fitted with a lens for far vision, and the other eye is fitted with a lens that corrects for close-up objects and reading. In most individuals, the eyes adjust in a relatively short time; reading is done with the nondominant eye, and distant objects are viewed with the dominant one.

#### Other Benefits

Perhaps the main reason for choosing contact lenses is the perceived improvement in personal appearance. Other strongly influencing factors include (1) no obstruction of vision from eyeglass frames, (2) greater clarity in peripheral vision, (3) no fogging of lenses caused by sudden temperature changes, and (4) more freedom of motion during vigorous activity (e.g., sports). A number of factors, such as increased sensitivity to light and improved quality of the retinal image, contribute to the subjective perception of vision improvement by the contact lens wearer. With eyeglasses, the myopic individual sees a smaller-than-normal image and the hyperopic individual sees a larger-than-normal image. With contacts, both myopic and hyperopic individuals see objects in nearly their true sizes; for highly myopic persons, the image size increase with contact lenses is significant and decidedly beneficial.

### *Contraindications for Contact Lenses*

Some individuals who require vision correction cannot or should not wear contact lenses. Contraindications are often based on lifestyle as well as on medical history.

#### Occupational Hazards

Occupational conditions that may prohibit the wearing of contact lenses include exposure to wind, glare, molten metals, irritants, dust and particulate matter, tobacco smoke, chemicals, and chemical fumes. Certain chemical fumes have been suggested as being particularly hazardous because of the potential concentration of irritants under a hard lens or inside a soft lens. The lens theoretically prolongs contact of such substances with the cornea and can lead to corneal toxicity. However, these theoretical occupational contraindications have not been proven.

#### Medical Conditions

Contact lenses should not be used if a patient has active pathologic intraocular or corneal conditions. Medical contraindications to wearing contact lenses include (1) chronic conjunctivitis; (2) blepharitis; (3) recurrent viral, bacterial, or fungal infections; and (4) poor blink rate or incomplete blink. Patients who have insufficient tear production, a deficiency or excess of mucin, excessive lipid production, or need to spend time in excessively dry environments may also be unable to use contact lenses successfully.

Diabetic patients are often advised against continuous-wear contact lenses because of retarded healing processes and the tendency toward prolonged corneal abrasion with such use. This precaution is probably unnecessary for daily wear of lenses unless problems occur.

Chronic common colds or allergic conditions such as hay fever and asthma may also make contact lens wear extremely uncomfortable or impossible.

In women, the corneal topography may be altered by pregnancy or the use of oral contraceptives. The fluid-retaining properties of estrogen may lead to edema of the cornea and eyelids as well as to decreased tear production. Dry spots on the cornea, often found in postmenopausal women, may also preclude successful contact lens wear. These spots, possibly caused by the absence of the precorneal film, are often identified with lacrimal insufficiency.

Contact lenses can be used with care by persons of advanced age; care is needed because of possible lacrimal insufficiency and loose lid tissues, which create a sagging conjunctival cul-de-sac and therefore make lens retention difficult. Contact lenses should be used with caution by patients with severe arthritis. Individuals with arthritis (as well as other conditions such as stroke) may lack the dexterity needed to insert lenses.

Lens wearers moving from a low to a high altitude may encounter hypoxia (low oxygen content of the cornea) or metabolic deficiency, resulting in irritation and corneal abrasions.

During the period needed for adapting to rigid contact lenses, the eyelids may become hyperemic (congested with excessive blood); this condition may lead to blepharitis (inflammation of the eyelids), especially in the upper lid. Short pseudoblinks, by new wearers of hard lenses, may irritate the conjunctiva of the upper eyelid. Chin elevation and squinting may result from the patient's efforts to minimize the irritation.

## Characteristics of Contact Lenses

Contact lenses are often broadly classified into three distinct groups based on their chemical makeup and physical properties (Table 29-1). Lenses that are relatively inflexible, do not appreciably absorb water (less than 10%), and retain their shape when removed from the eye are commonly called rigid lenses. Rigid lenses made of polymethylmethacrylate (PMMA) are not permeable to oxygen and are called hard contact lenses. Rigid lenses made of more flexible polymers are permeable to oxygen and thus are called rigid gas-permeable (RGP) lenses. Hard lenses are now seldom prescribed but may be replaced for individuals

**TABLE 29-1 Comparison of Contact Lens Characteristics**

| | Hard Lenses | Soft Lenses | RGP Lenses |
|---|---|---|---|
| **Lens Characteristics** | | | |
| Rigidity | +++ | 0 | +++ |
| Durability | +++ | + | ++ |
| Oxygen transmission | 0 | ++ | +++ |
| Chemical adsorption | 0 | +++ | 0 |
| **Optical Quality** | | | |
| Visual acuity | +++ | + | +++ |
| Correction of astigmatism | Yes | Toric | Yes |
| Photophobia | +++ | + | ++ |
| Spectacle blur | +++ | 0 | ++ |
| **Convenience** | | | |
| Comfort | + | +++ | ++ |
| Adaptation period | Weeks | Days | Days |
| Continuous wear | No | Yes | Yes |
| Intermittent wear | No | Yes | No |

Key: + indicates the degree to which the characteristic is present; 0 means the characteristic is not present.

who successfully wore them before the advent of RGP lenses. Contact lenses that are moderately to highly flexible, absorb a high percentage of water (greater than 10%), and conform to the shape of a supporting structure are commonly called soft lenses. Although the overwhelming majority of contact lenses fall into these three categories, a few do not. Those few are called flexible nonhydrogel lenses.

Subgroups of contact lenses are continuous-wear lenses and disposable lenses. Continuous-wear lenses can be either soft or, occasionally, RGP lenses that are designed to be worn for an extended time before removal. Disposable lenses are designed to be worn for 1 to 14 days and then discarded.

Contact lenses are manufactured from polymers that vary widely in their chemical and physical properties. Each material has physical and surface characteristics that correlate with the specific problems that the patient may encounter.

Physical characteristics of contact lenses include dimensional stability, physical breakage, and polymer stability. Generally, hard lenses are dimensionally stable and tend to hold their parameters with little change. Soft lenses, however, are much less stable physically; water content, to a large extent, dictates their physical strength. RGP lenses generally have a high degree of dimensional stability. As they dehydrate, however, curvature of the plastic surfaces may be altered slightly.

Physical characteristics of the different contact lenses account for most of the problems that patients encounter. Unfortunately, many patients do not know which type of lens they are wearing. This underscores the importance of the pharmacist establishing an excellent relationship with contact lens practitioners in the area.

To maintain a healthy cornea, an adequate amount of oxygen is needed. The more oxygen that passes through the contact lens, the more adequately normal corneal metabolism can be maintained. Oxygen permeability describes the ability of a specific material to permit the passage of oxygen. Oxygen permeability is expressed as the *Dk* value of the material, where *D* is the diffusion coefficient, and *k* is the solubility coefficient. The higher the *Dk* value, the higher the oxygen permeability. The *Dk/L* value, in which *L* corresponds to the thickness of the material, is a measure of oxygen transmissibility (i.e., the amount of oxygen that can be transmitted through a contact lens of specific thickness) and is the value to which most practitioners and manufacturers refer. Because the lens thickness varies depending on the power of the lens, many manufacturers report the *Dk/L* value for a lens with a 23.00D (diopter) prescription. For example, a lens that corrects a large myopia (minus lens) will be thinner in the center than a lens that corrects hyperopia (plus lens), which will be thicker in the center than on the periphery.

Oxygen transmission depends primarily on the water content of the soft lens. The higher the water content, the more oxygen is transmitted through the lens. However, as water content increases, durability decreases, and the lens must be made thicker, which in turn hinders oxygen permeability. Thus, a thick lens with a high water content may transmit the same amount of oxygen as a thin lens with a lower water content.[1] Another problem is that, as water content increases, the lenses tend to attract tear deposits such as lipids, proteins, and polysaccharides. Further, and especially if large pores or many pores are present, lenses with a high water content tend to be more susceptible to the growth of bacteria and fungi on the surface than lenses with a lower water content.[2]

The majority (87%) of patients who wear contact lenses are fitted with soft (hydrophilic) lenses. Rigid (primarily RGP) lenses are prescribed for 13% of patients. Continuous-wear lenses (soft or RGP) are worn by 25% of patients wearing contact lenses. Approximately 76% of patients wearing contact lenses wear some type of disposable or planned replacement lenses.[3]

## Formulation Considerations for Lens Care Products

Lens care products include surface-active cleaners, enzymatic cleaners, disinfecting solutions, wetting and rewetting solutions, and multipurpose solutions that combine several steps into one. Each type of contact lens has specific care procedures.

The manufacturing and marketing of contact lenses are regulated by the ophthalmic devices division of the Food and Drug Administration (FDA). Even though contact lens solutions are not considered drug products, formulation considerations still are applicable. Contact lens wearers should use only lens care products that have been approved by FDA for use with their specific contact lens.

The basic considerations for a well-formulated contact lens solution include pH, viscosity, isotonicity with tears, stability, sterility, and provision for maintenance of sterility (bactericidal action). The pH range of comfort is not well defined because, although normal tear pH is 7.4, tear pH varies among individuals. It is best to have a weakly buffered solution that can readily adjust to any tear pH, given that highly buffered solutions can cause significant discomfort, even ocular damage, when they are instilled. However, as with therapeutic ophthalmic solutions, the stability of the solution components takes precedence over comfort. For this reason, many contact lens solutions are formulated with pH values above or below 7.4. These systems are weakly buffered and are usually well tolerated by the eye.

Solutions from different manufacturers should not be mixed because a precipitate may form. For instance, a product containing alkaline borate buffers forms a gummy, gel-like precipitate on lenses if mixed with a wetting solution containing polyvinyl alcohol. Furthermore, solutions containing a cationic preservative, such as chlorhexidine, polyquaternium-1 (Polyquad), or polyaminopropyl biguanide (Dymed), should not be mixed with solutions containing an anionic preservative such as sorbic acid because this, too, will cause a precipitate to form.[4]

### *Preservatives*

Routine daily use of any contact lens solution increases the risk of bacterial contamination. Depending on specific lens care procedures, a single container may last for a month or more. The solution must therefore contain a bactericidal agent that is both effective over the long term and nonirritating to the eye with daily use. Few preservatives fulfill these criteria. Commonly used agents are benzalkonium chloride, thimerosal, and sorbic acid products, all of which can cause irritation, depending on concentration and patient sensitivity.

Several preservatives are used in contact lens products. Older types of preservatives used include benzalkonium chloride, thimerosal, sorbic acid, chlorhexidine, and ethylenediaminetetraacetic acid (EDTA) (see Chapter 28). Several newer preservatives (polyquaternium-1 and polyaminopropyl biguanide) have been recently introduced. These preservatives are believed to cause fewer adverse effects than some of the older preservatives.

#### Polyquaternium-1

Polyquaternium-1 (Polyquad) is a quaternary ammonium preservative shown to be effective against certain bacteria, fungi, and yeast. To date, few toxicity or sensitivity problems have been noted with this preservative. When it was introduced to the market, formulations containing polyquaternium-1 were not compatible with lenses that had a high water content because the methacrylic acid component of the lens had the ability to adsorb the preservative in toxic levels. However, recent formulations do not seem to have this problem.

#### Polyhexamethylene Biguanide

Polyhexamethylene biguanide (PHMB), also known as polyaminopropyl biguanide, Dymed, or polyhexanide, is a cationic polymeric biguanide that is effective against certain bacteria and yeast, although its activity against *Acanthamoeba* and fungi does not appear to be optimal. No significant adverse effects to polyaminopropyl biguanide have been reported in lens wearers.

## Hard Contact Lenses

Hard contact lenses were the first lenses to be used in the United States. Hard lenses are polymerized products of esters of acrylic acid or methacrylic acid. The most common plastic found in hard lenses is PMMA, known commercially as Lucite or Plexiglas.

PMMA is not significantly permeable to oxygen; therefore, for the cornea to remain healthy, the lens must be able to slide and rock over the corneal surface in response to a blink so oxygenation can occur. As the hard lens moves, a layer of tears forms under it and is continually recirculated by the sliding and rocking motion of the tear fluid–pumping phenomenon. To allow this movement over the eye, hard lenses are relatively small in diameter (8.0 to 9.5 mm) and thus may pop out of the wearer's eye.

Contact lenses made of PMMA are hydrophobic, and PMMA is now rarely used for new contact lens fittings because of its negligible permeability to oxygen. However, PMMA possesses characteristics, such as a refractive index similar to glass, that make it suitable for a corrective lens in contact with the ocular surface. One phenomenon associated primarily with hard lenses is spectacle blur. A hard lens, while in place on the cornea, alters the surface topography of the eye and creates hypoxic edema. As a result, the patient may not see well with glasses immediately after removing the lens. Generally, spectacle blur abates in 20 to 30 minutes. The hardness of these lenses is lower than that of glass but higher than that of RGP or soft lenses. Thus, reasonable care must be exercised with hard lenses to avoid scratching or chipping them. Inadequate care or neglect of hard lenses may lead to corneal problems or wearer discomfort, but the lens will still maintain its optical qualities.

### *Care of Hard Lenses*

Hard contact lens care products help minimize the stress on the eye. These products aid the wearer, providing comfort and safety. Hard lens care involves three important steps: cleaning, soaking, and wetting (Figure 29-1). For optimal lens care, all three steps should be performed each time the lenses are removed from the eye.

#### Cleaning Solutions

Normal tears are composed of secretions from many specialized glands lining the lacrimal apparatus, conjunctiva, and lids. Many components are somewhat hydrophobic and tend to adhere to the surface of a hard lens during normal daily wear. This residue, primarily proteinaceous debris and oils, acts as a growth medium for bacteria. If it

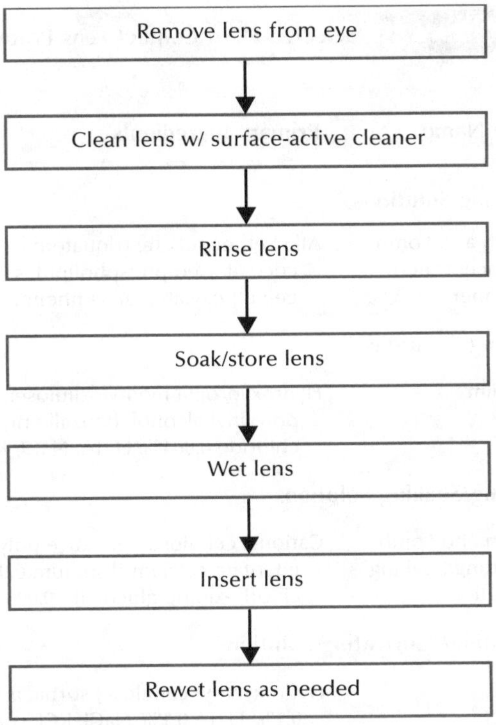


**FIGURE 29–1** Self-care of hard lenses.

is not routinely removed by daily cleaning, the residue may harden to form coatings or tenacious deposits that create an irregular surface on the lens. This residue will eventually irritate the eyelids and corneal epithelium, and it may progress to infection or another pathology. Decreased visual acuity and lens wear time are likely consequences of a cloudy lens or allergenic reactions to the residue.

Contact lens cleaning solutions typically contain nonionic or amphoteric surfactants that emulsify oils and aid in solubilizing other debris. Proteins and lipids are soluble in highly alkaline media, but high pH can cause lens decomposition. Weak alkaline solutions may dislodge deposits from the lens in conjunction with the surface tension–lowering properties of the surfactants. Homemade cleaning solutions such as baking soda mixed with distilled water or cleaning solution may scratch lenses and may not rinse off easily.[5] Use of household cleansers and homemade solutions (including salt tablet solutions) of any kind should be strongly discouraged to prevent lens damage, contamination leading to infection, and ocular irritation. Tables 29-2 and 29-3 provide instructions for properly cleaning hard lenses.

**TABLE 29-2 General Cleaning Procedures for All Lens Types**

- Wash hands with noncosmetic soap and rinse thoroughly before handling lenses.
- Clean contact lenses only with agents specifically made for that purpose. Homemade cleansers can scratch the lenses or cause eye irritation or injury.
- Care for each type of lens with only commercially manufactured products made specifically for that type of lens.
- Do not mix contact lens care products from different manufacturers unless an eye care practitioner says they are compatible.
- When handling lenses over a sink, cover or close the drain to prevent loss of a lens.
- During cleaning, check lenses for scratches, chips, or tears, and the presence of foreign particles, warpage, or discoloration. Also, check that lenses are clean and thoroughly rinsed of cleaner. These factors could cause eye discomfort.
- When cleaning a lens, rub it in a back-and-forth rather than in a circular direction.
- Clean the second lens as thoroughly as the first to prevent "left lens syndrome," in which the left lens has more deposits than the right lens because the right lens is often removed first and cleaned more thoroughly.
- Discard cleansers and other lens care products if the labeled expiration date has passed.

**TABLE 29-3 Specific Cleaning Procedures for Hard Lenses**

- Apply appropriate cleaning solution to both surfaces of the lenses; rub the lens between thumb and forefinger or between forefinger and palm of opposite hand for approximately 20 seconds.
- Do not wipe lenses dry with tissue as this may scratch the lenses.
- Avoid overvigorous cleaning of lenses, as this may cause scratches or warpage.
- Always clean hard lenses before storing them.

## Soaking Solutions

A soaking solution is used to store hard contact lenses whenever they are removed from the eyes. The solution maintains the lens in a constant state of hydration for maximum comfort and visual acuity. It also aids in removing deposits that accumulate on the lens during wear.

A rigid lens absorbs between 1% and 3% moisture by weight. On exposure to air, the lens dehydrates; it subsequently rehydrates when it comes in contact with a soaking solution or the lacrimal fluid. Placing a dehydrated lens into the eye causes discomfort as the lens absorbs tears from the precorneal area. In addition, a dehydrated lens is flatter than a hydrated lens; this factor causes problems with both comfort and visual acuity.

If lenses are allowed to dry out during overnight storage, accumulated deposits are more difficult to remove by normal cleaning. Storage in a soaking solution reduces the likelihood of deposits forming.

To maintain sterility, storage solutions use essentially the same preservatives as wetting solutions. The main difference is that the concentration can be somewhat higher in a soaking solution because the solution is rinsed from the lens before insertion. However, preservative levels are carefully selected because higher levels do not necessarily result in increased effectiveness and may lead to impaired wetting or corneal irritation because of the adsorption of preservatives onto the lens.

### Wetting Solutions

An ideal wetting solution performs the following functions: (1) converts the hydrophobic lens surface to a hydrophilic surface by means of a uniform film that does not easily wash away; (2) increases comfort by providing cushioning and lubrication between the corneal surface and the inner surface of the lens, and between the lens and the inner surface of the eyelid; (3) places a viscous coating on the lens to protect it from oil on the fingers during insertion; and (4) stabilizes the lens on the fingertip to ease insertion, particularly for individuals with poor manual dexterity or unsteady hands.

If the lens is thoroughly cleaned before insertion, lacrimal fluid can adequately wet the lens. Indeed, the wetting action of popular wetting solutions is sometimes not significantly better than that of saline. Furthermore, patients whose tears are capable of wetting a lens almost immediately upon insertion often do not use these solutions.

The basic wetting solution comprises components from the following main categories: (1) cushioning agents (e.g., viscosity-inducing additives such as methylcellulose or hydroxypropyl methylcellulose); (2) wetting agents (e.g., polyvinyl alcohol or other surfactants); (3) preservatives (e.g., benzalkonium chloride, thimerosal, polyquaternium-1, sorbic acid, or polyaminopropyl biguanide); and (4) buffering agents and salts added to adjust the pH and tonicity.

The cushioning effect of a wetting solution is achieved by hydrophilic polymers that lubricate the interface between the lens and the surfaces of the cornea and eyelid. Cellulose gum derivatives are often used. Although compounds such as methylcellulose possess a degree of surfactant activity, they do not promote uniform wetting of a rigid lens. For this reason, polyvinyl alcohol is also often used to decrease surface tension.

The concentration of the cushioning polymer in wetting solutions affects both eye comfort and the quality of vision immediately following insertion. In some individuals, a concentration that is too low causes discomfort after only a short time. In other wearers, a high polymer concentration results in blurred vision because the viscous solution mixes poorly with tears. Overspill of solution onto the lids and eyelashes causes crusting as the solution dries; this crusty residue can be a source of foreign material falling into the eye. Saliva should never be used to wet contact lenses because it can lead to infection by *Acanthamoeba, Pseudomonas aeruginosa,* or other pathogens.

### Rewetting Solutions

Rewetting solutions are intended to clean and rewet the contact lens while it is in the eye. These solutions depend on the use of surfactants to loosen deposits; removal is assisted by the natural cleaning action of blinking. Although these products function well to recondition the lens, the cornea benefits more if the lens is actually removed, cleaned, and rewetted. Removing the lens for even a brief time allows the cornea to be resurfaced with a new proteinaceous or mucinaceous layer.

**TABLE 29-4 Selected Hard Contact Lens Products**

| Trade Name | Primary Ingredients |
|---|---|
| **Cleaning Solutions** | |
| Bausch and Lomb Concentrated Cleaner | Alkyl ether sulfate; triquaternary cocoa-based phospholipid; silica gel; ethoxylated alkyl phenol |
| **Wetting Solutions** | |
| Liquifilm | Hydroxypropyl methylcellulose; polyvinyl alcohol; benzalkonium chloride 0.004%; EDTA; NaCl; KCl |
| **Wetting/Soaking Solutions** | |
| Bausch and Lomb Wetting/Soaking Solution | Cationic cellulose derivative polymer; edentate calcium disodium 0.05%; chlorhexidine gluconate 0.006% |
| **Rewetting/Lubricating Solutions** | |
| Clerz 2 | Hydroxyethyl cellulose; sorbic acid 0.1%; EDTA 0.1%; NaCl; KCl; sodium borate; boric acid |

Key: EDTA, ethylenediamine tetraacetic acid; KCl, potassium chloride; NaCl, sodium chloride.

### Other Products

Other ophthalmic products are available to the hard lens wearer for occasional use. Some, such as artificial tears and ocular decongestants, are not recommended for use with the lenses in place. Because of their emollient and lubricating effect, artificial tears can be used to soothe the eye. Ocular decongestants reduce mild conjunctival hyperemia associated with prolonged lens wear. However, these topical decongestants can induce conjunctival hypoxia, which may harm the patient. Thus, routine use of these products should be avoided. If symptoms requiring their use persist, a visit to an eye care practitioner is advised.

### Product Selection Guidelines

The variety of lens care solutions available to hard lens wearers poses a selection problem (Table 29-4). The availability of single- and multipurpose products within the same product line can further frustrate and confuse some wearers. Thus, product selection is an area in which pharmacists can perform a much-needed role as a consultant. Unfortunately, information at hand is not always sufficient to provide a complete foundation for patient consultation. One factor that could help determine which products to recommend is the adequacy of the labeling. Product labeling is often incomplete or limited to general information. The specific agents and concentrations of preservatives are usually adequately listed, but concentrations of cushioning and lubricating polymers are often absent. Other ingredients are often listed simply as cleaning agents or buffers, making alternative selections a random process. A surfactant

**TABLE 29-5 Insertion of Hard and RGP Lenses**

- After washing hands, remove one lens from the lens storage case, rinse it with fresh conditioning/soaking solution, and inspect it for cleanliness and signs of damage (cracks or chips).
- If a wetting or conditioning solution is being used, place a few drops on the lens.
- Place the lens on the top of the index finger (see drawing A).
- Place the middle finger of the same hand on the lower lid and pull it down (see drawing B).
- With the other hand, use a finger to lift the upper lid and then place the lens on the eye (see drawing C).
- Release the lids and blink.
- Check vision immediately to see if the lens is in the proper position.
- If vision is blurred, blink three to four times. If vision is still blurred, the lens may be off center, on the wrong eye, or dirty.
- Instill one to three drops of rewetting or reconditioning drops into the eye.
- If vision is not improved, remove the lens, place several drops of wetting/conditioning solution onto both surfaces, and reinsert.
- Repeat all steps with the other lens.

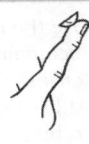

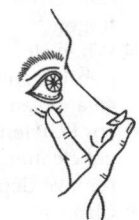
A

B

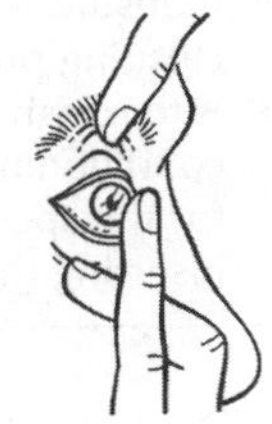
C

cleaner, a soaking solution, a wetting solution, and a rewetting solution should be recommended.

### *Insertion and Removal*

See Tables 29-5 and 29-6 for instructions on inserting and removing hard lenses.

## RGP Contact Lenses

The new generation of RGP lenses combines the optical qualities of PMMA and the oxygen permeability of soft lenses. Generally, RGP lenses can deliver two to three times more oxygen to the cornea than soft lenses of the same thickness. However, to maintain rigidity (which is important for the proper lens fit and correction of astigmatism), RGP lenses are generally thicker than soft lenses. Newer RGP lenses still transmit much more oxygen to the cornea than do most soft lenses, while covering only the central 75% of the cornea. RGP lenses, unlike soft lenses, also exchange up to 20% of the postlens tear volume per blink.

RGP lenses have been investigated for continuous-wear use, and some have been approved for 1 to 30 days of extended wear. The use of continuous-wear lenses is somewhat controversial as these lenses have been implicated in causing corneal ulcers (eruptions on the corneal surface), which, in rare instances, can lead to partial or complete blindness.

RGP lenses are available in several types of materials. One type of RGP lens is composed of silicone acrylates that combine silicone with methyl methacrylate and methacrylic

**TABLE 29-6 Removal of Hard and RGP Lenses**

- Before removing the lens, fill the storage cases with soaking/conditioning solution.
- Remove the top from the cleaning solution.
- Place a hand (or a towel) under the eye.
- Use one of the following methods to remove the lens from the eye.

**Two-finger Method of Removing Lenses**

- Place the tip of the forefinger of one hand on the middle of the upper eyelid by the lashes as shown in drawing A.
- Place the forefinger of the other hand on the middle lower lid margin (see drawing A).
- Push the lids inward and then together (see drawing B). The lens should pop out.
- If the lens becomes decentered onto only the white part of the eye, recenter the lens and try again.

**Temporal Pull/Blink Method of Removing Lenses**

- Place an index finger on the temporal edge of the lower and upper lids. Initially, widen the eyelids a little as shown in drawing C.
- Stretch the skin outward and slightly upward without allowing the lid to slide over the lens. Blink briskly (see drawing D). The lens will pop out because of the pressure of the eyelids at the top and bottom of the lens. Blinking facilitates removal after the lids have been tightened around the lens.

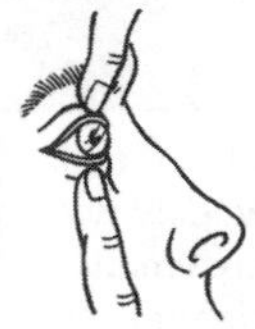
A

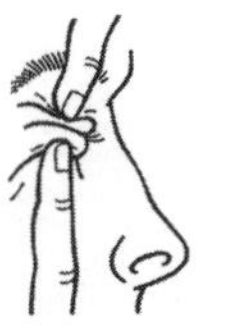
B

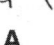

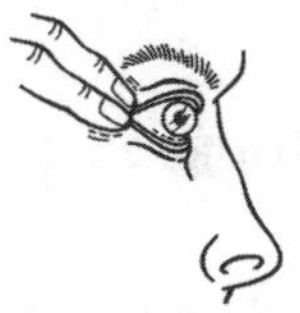
C

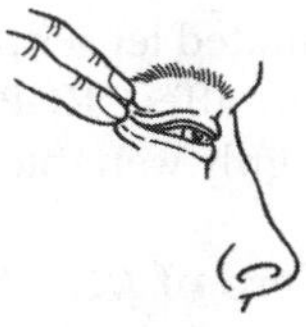
D

acid and/or hydroxyethyl methacrylate (HEMA) in varying amounts. This material is relatively stable and fairly inflexible. Examples of this type of lens include Polycon II and Paraperm $O_2$.

Fluorine may also be a component of RGP lenses, in the form of either fluorosilicone acrylate or fluoropolymer lenses. An example of this type of lens is the Boston Equalens.

Of the many RGP materials available, the fluorosilicone acrylates are the most commonly used.[6]

### *Advantages*

Advantages of RGP lenses vary depending on the type of materials used. Fluorinated lenses offer the advantages of increased oxygen transmissibility and reduced lipophilicity problems. These lenses also have less surface reactivity, thereby decreasing tear deposits.

### *Disadvantages*

Disadvantages of RGP lenses also vary depending on the type of materials used. Silicone acrylate lenses have less

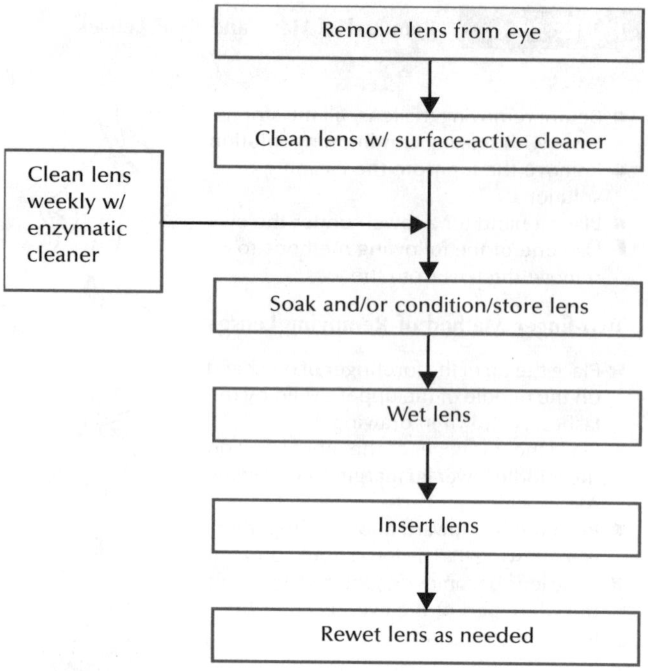


**FIGURE 29–2** Self-care of RGP lenses.

**TABLE 29-7 Specific Cleaning Procedures for RGP Lenses**

- Use the cleansing, soaking, and conditioning products recommended by your eye care practitioner to clean your lenses.
- At least once a day, apply an appropriate cleaning solution to both surfaces of the lenses; rub the lens between forefinger and palm of opposite hand to avoid chipping an edge, which may occur if lenses are cleaned between the fingers.
- When cleaning the lens, do not apply too much pressure. If debris is still on the lens, soak a cotton swab in the surfactant cleaner, and use the swab to clean the lens.
- For RGP lenses with high silicone content only, use a silica gel cleaner (i.e., Boston Advance) if other cleaners do not remove deposits.
- Clean silicone acrylate RGP lenses once a week with an enzymatic cleaner to avoid the need for professional polishing or replacement of lenses.
- If unsure of lens type, ask the eye practitioner about proper cleaning procedures.
- After cleaning RGP lenses, soak them in a soaking or a conditioning solution recommended by the eye practitioner for the specified amount of time. Rewet lenses before inserting them in the eyes.

surface wettability than PMMA because silicone has relatively higher hydrophobicity. Silicone acrylates also tend to have a negative surface charge, which can attract lysozymes and other positively charged deposits. Fluorinated lenses have the disadvantage of greater mass, which can affect RGP lens fit. These lenses also tend not to be highly wettable.

### *Care of RGP Lenses*

The diversity and variation in materials used in RGP lenses preclude generalizations. Lens wearers should be advised by their eye care practitioners about the products and regimens recommended for their particular lenses. The labeling on contact lens products also indicates the lenses for which they are approved; however, patients must know what type of lens they are wearing to be able to use this information.

#### Procedures

The care of an RGP lens is similar to that of a hard contact lens (Figure 29-2). Unlike hard lenses, however, RGP lenses should be cleaned in the palm of the hand, not between fingertips, to reduce the risk of chipping an edge. (See Tables 29-2 and 29-7 for the proper cleaning procedures.)

Some RGP lenses have a high silicone content and thus have decreased surface wettability. As previously noted, the lens surface tends to have a negative charge, which promotes the binding of positively charged tear constituents. Cleaners designed for conventional hard or RGP lenses may not effectively remove the more tenacious deposits. Other cleaners formulated for this type of lens (e.g., Boston Advance Cleaner, Original Formula Boston Cleaner) contain silica gel, which acts to mechanically break the adhesive bonds that have formed between the lens and the deposits. Patients should be counseled to discard these solutions 90 days after opening the product. There is a space on the label to record the date that the product is opened.

Because high-silicone lenses have decreased surface wettability, conditioning solutions are generally used instead of soaking solutions to aid the formation of a cushioning tear layer. A conditioning solution is essentially a specially formulated wetting solution. The conditioner system enhances wettability of the lens, increases comfort, and disinfects the lens. The lenses must be soaked at least 4 hours in this solution before they are reinserted into the eyes. It is important to counsel the patient that the Boston Advance Conditioning solution must be discarded 90 days after opening. There is a space on the label to record the date that the product is opened.

Reconditioning and rewetting drops may also be used while the lens is on the eye to rewet the lens as necessary. Boston Rewetting Drops must be discarded 90 days after opening. Heat disinfection cannot be used with RGP lenses.

As the silicone content of RGP lenses increases, so does the amount of protein adherence. Silicone acrylate lenses have an active surface that promotes the binding of tear constituents. Protein deposits on a lens will decrease the oxygen permeability, and the patient may experience discomfort. Lenses of this type should be cleaned with an enzymatic product once weekly.[7] Failure to comply with this cleaning step may result in the need for professional polishing or replacement of the lens.

Products containing chlorhexidine gluconate should not be used with silicone or styrene lenses because this agent will make the lens surface more difficult to wet and may also cause surface clouding. Fluorosilicone acrylate

**TABLE 29-8 Selected Products for RGP Lenses**

| Trade Name | Primary Ingredients |
|---|---|
| **Cleaning Solutions** | |
| Boston Advance Cleaner* | Silica gel; alkyl ether sulfate; ethoxylated alkyl phenol; triquaternary cocoa-based phospholipid |
| Boston Cleaner | Silica gel; alkyl ether sulfate; titanium dioxide; NaCl |
| Opti-Clean II Daily Cleaner | Cleaning agent; polysorbate 21; hydroxyethyl cellulose; EDTA 0.1%; Polyquad 0.001%, boric acid; sodium borate; NaCl; sodium hydroxide |
| Opti-Free Daily Cleaner | Nylon 11; polysorbate 21; hydroxyethyl cellulose; polyquaternium-1; EDTA; boric acid; sodium borate; hydrochloric acid and/or sodium hydroxide |
| **Enzymatic Cleaning Products** | |
| Boston One Step Liquid Enzymatic Cleaner | Subtilisin; glycerol |
| Opti-Zyme Weekly Enzymatic Cleaner* | Pancreatin |
| Pro Free/GP Weekly Enzymatic Cleaner | Papain; EDTA; NaCl; sodium carbonate; sodium borate |
| **Wetting/Soaking/Disinfecting Solutions** | |
| Boston Advance Comfort Formula Conditioning Solution | Cellulosic viscosifier; polyvinyl alcohol; cationic cellulose derivative polymer; derivatized PEG; chlorhexidine gluconate 0.003%; polyaminopropyl biguanide 0.0005%; EDTA 0.05% |
| Boston Conditioning Solution | Hydroxyethyl cellulose; polyvinyl alcohol; cationic cellulose derivatives; poloxamer 407; chlorhexidine gluconate 0.006%; EDTA 0.05% |
| Wet-N-Soak Plus | Polyvinyl alcohol; benzalkonium chloride 0.003%; EDTA |
| **Rewetting/Lubricating Solutions** | |
| Boston Rewetting Drops | Hydroxyethyl cellulose; polyvinyl alcohol; cationic cellulose derivatives; poloxamer 407; chlorhexidine gluconate 0.006%; EDTA 0.05% |
| **Multipurpose Solutions** | |
| Boston Simplus | Poloxamine, hydroxyalkylphosphonate, boric acid, sodium borate, sodium chloride, hydroxypropylmethyl cellulose, Glucam, chlorhexidinegluconate (0.003%), polyaminopropyl biguanide (0.0005%) |
| Unique-pH Multipurpose | Hydroxypropyl guar; Tetronic 1304 |

Key: EDTA, ethylenediamine tetraacetic acid; NaCl, sodium chloride; PEG, polyethylene glycol.

* Preservative-free.

lenses should not be cleaned more than one time with MiraFlow. Cracking, changes in parameters, and brittleness have been noted when this type of lens is cleaned repeatedly with MiraFlow.

### Product Selection Guidelines

The appropriate lens care regimen for RGP lenses must be compatible with the particular lens. Lens wearers should be advised against substituting other products for those specifically recommended by their eye care practitioner. Patients wearing RGP lenses should be advised to purchase a surface-active cleaning product, an enzymatic product, and a conditioning or soaking solution, depending on the type of lens worn. A rewetting or reconditioning product should also be recommended. Table 29-8 lists examples of products for RGP lenses.

### *Insertion and Removal*

Wearers of RGP lenses should be counseled to follow the insertion and removal procedures for hard lenses (Tables 29-5 and 29-6).

## Soft Contact Lenses

The main chemical difference between the hydrophobic rigid lens and the hydrophilic soft lens is that the soft lens contains hydroxyl or hydroxyl and lactam groups, which allow it to absorb and hold water. Table 29-9 classifies the different types of soft contact lenses into four groups according to water content and ionic charge, based on 1986 FDA recommendations. Soft lenses are composed of hydrophilic groups, including hydroxyl, amide, lactam, and carboxyl, with small amounts of cross-linking agents that form a hydrophilic gel (hydrogel) network. The

**TABLE 29-9 Soft Contact Lens Classification***

| Classification | Water Content (%) |
|---|---|
| **Group I: Low Water, Nonionic** | |
| Hefilcon A and B | 45% |
| Polymacon | 38% |
| Tefilcon | 38% |
| Tetrafilcon A | 43% |
| **Group II: High Water, Nonionic** | |
| Lidofilicon A | 70% |
| Lidofilicon B | 79% |
| Nelfilcon A | 69% |
| **Group III: Low Water, Ionic** | |
| Bufilcon A | 45% |
| Deltafilcon A | 43% |
| Phemfilcon | 38% |
| **Group IV: High Water, Ionic** | |
| Bufilcon A | 55% |
| Etafilcon | 58% |
| Perfilcon A | 71% |
| Phemfilcon A | 55% |
| Vilfilcon A | 55% |

degree of cross-linking determines lens hydrophilicity and water content. Greater cross-linking means that fewer hydrophilic groups are available to interact with water, which in turn produces a less flexible, less hydrated lens than those originally available.

Ionic lenses have a negative surface charge, which tends to attract more protein deposits than nonionic lenses; soaking ionic lenses in sorbate-preserved saline yellows the lenses prematurely. Nonionic lenses are electrically neutral and tend to be less reactive with the tear film, resulting in a more deposit-resistant lens. High-water lenses (greater than 50%), which tend to attract tear film deposits into their matrix, usually cannot withstand daily heat disinfection. If soaked in enzymes for a prolonged period, these lenses may also cause sensitivity reactions.

The water content of soft lenses has gradually increased since they were introduced. Increasing the water content improves the oxygen permeability of a material. However, permeability also depends on lens thickness. Highly hydrated lenses are more comfortable but are also more fragile. Because these lenses must be thicker to offset their fragility, the two factors often cancel each other out regarding oxygen transmissibility. Lowering the water content produces a more durable and longer-lasting lens. The water content of a HEMA-type material can vary between 5% and 90%, but a theoretical ideal value might be 75% to 78%, matching the hydration of the corneal stroma. However, reducing the percentage of water in a soft HEMA lens also reduces the thickness of the hydrated lens, thereby improving the wearer's comfort. Thus, the optimal water content actually appears to be between 55% and 65%, given the thicknesses at which these materials can be reliably worn. Many lens wearers find they cannot tolerate lenses with a thickness above 0.4 mm because of lid discomfort. For those who cannot tolerate regular soft lenses, several ultrathin soft lenses are available with a thickness as low as 0.04 mm.

Soft lenses in the nonhydrated (dry) state are rigid and extremely brittle, and should not be handled by the wearer. When hydrated, the lenses expand as water is absorbed into the gel matrix. These lenses are most comfortable when they are larger than the diameter of the cornea, have thin edges, and undergo just enough movement on the eye to ensure lubrication of the ocular surface under the lens.

### *Types*

The increased oxygen permeability and reduced eyelid interaction of soft contact lenses enable certain lenses to be broken in more quickly and worn continuously. Table 29-10 lists examples of some of the soft contact lenses approved for wear in the United States.

#### Continuous-wear Lenses

In 1981, cosmetic, soft continuous-wear lenses were originally approved by FDA to be worn for 30 days. However, as with RGP continuous-wear lenses, problems with contamination, infection, and ulceration suggested that they should not be worn for more than 7 days and, in 1989, FDA rescinded its approval of 30-day continuous wear.[8] However, FDA recently approved certain contact lenses for up to 30 nights of continuous wear. Even though the lenses are approved for 30 days of continuous wear, some patients, depending on tear flow rate, sleep pattern, and ocular anatomy, may not be able to tolerate wearing them for this length of time.

#### Disposable and Planned Replacement Lenses

Disposable lenses represent the fastest-growing segment of the soft lens market. Depending on the lens, there are several approved wearing schedules. Some lenses are worn for 1 day and then discarded; others are worn daily for up to 2 weeks and then discarded; still others can be worn as continuous-wear lenses for up to 2 weeks, with the patient wearing them on various schedules (e.g., wearing them for 6 nights and then removing them for 1 night). Planned replacement lenses are discarded and replaced usually after 1 to 3 months of wear, depending on how quickly the lenses build up deposits and how well the patient complies with proper lens care. Planned replacement lenses and disposable lenses other than the daily disposables are cared for in a manner similar to other soft contact lenses. In most patients, an enzymatic cleaner is generally not necessary for disposable lenses that will be discarded after a few weeks of wear.

**TABLE 29-10 Examples of Soft Contact Lenses**

| Trade Name (Manufacturer) | Water/Saline Content (%) | Group Classification* |
|---|---|---|
| **Daily-wear Soft Lenses** | | |
| Cibasoft Visitint (CIBA Vision) | 37.5 | I |
| Hydrasoft Sphere (Coopervision) | 55.0 | IV |
| Satureyes (Metro) | 59.0 | II |
| Soflens (Bausch & Lomb Optics) | 38.0 | I |
| Soft Mate B (CIBA Vision) | 45.0 | III |
| **Continuous-wear Soft Lenses** | | |
| DuraSoft 3 (CIBA Vision) | 55.0 | IV |
| Focus Night and Day (CIBA Vision) | 24.0 | I |
| LL-70 (Unilens Corp.) | 70.0 | II |
| Permalens (Coopervision) | 71.0 | IV |
| **Disposable Soft Lenses** | | |
| Focus Dailies (CIBA Vision) | 69.0 | II |
| 1 Day Acuvue (Vistakon) | 58.0 | IV |
| Soflens one day (Bausch and Lomb) | 70.0 | II |
| **Soft Toric Lenses** | | |
| Frequency 55 Toric (Coopervision) | 55.0 | IV |
| Optima Toric (Bausch & Lomb Optics) | 45.0 | I |
| **Soft Bifocal Lenses** | | |
| Acuvue Bifocal (Vistakon) | 58.0 | IV |
| Hydrocurve II Bifocal (Ciba-Vision) | 45.0 | III |

* See Table 29-9 for group classifications.

Daily disposable lenses have the following advantages: (1) each lens is sterile prior to removal from its package for immediate insertion into the eye, (2) no cleaning regimen is necessary because the lens is discarded after wear, (3) deposit formation is minimal, and (4) lens-related problems, such as giant papillary conjunctivitis or allergic reactions to lens care solutions, occur less frequently. At a cost of $1 to $2 per day for daily disposable lenses to correct both eyes, they are sometimes considered to be too expensive by patients. However, if the cost of solutions is factored into the use of frequent replacement lenses, daily disposable lenses can actually be less expensive overall.

### Specialty Lenses

Some soft contacts are classified as specialty lenses. These include toric, bifocal, and tinted lenses. Toric soft lenses have been developed specifically to correct astigmatic (improper focusing attributed to an irregularly shaped cornea) visual conditions. Traditional soft lenses do not correct astigmatism because they conform to the corneal surface rather than retain their original shape, as do rigid lenses. Toric soft lenses are fabricated with both spherical and cylindrical optical corrections, and remain on axis because of design features such as weighting on the bottom edge of the lens. Spherical soft lenses can be fitted to eyes with an upper limit of astigmatism of about 1.00 diopters (a unit of refracting power used as a quantitative measure of the abnormal refraction of light at surfaces such as the cornea).

Bifocal lenses, which can be weighted in a fashion similar to that of toric lenses, are prescribed to correct presbyopia (ocular changes caused by age).

Tinted lenses are available to facilitate handling and for cosmetic purposes (i.e., to change eye color) as well as for corrective purposes. Three types of tinted lenses are available: translucent lenses, opaque lenses, and lenses that absorb ultraviolet radiation. Translucent lenses can be tinted in varying degrees, from light/number 1 intensity, to facilitate handling and increase the visibility of the lens, to medium/number 2 and dark/number 3 intensities to enhance eye color. Translucent lenses work best on light eye colors. Opaque lenses cover the iris and hide its natural color; they can completely change the apparent eye color, even in individuals with dark brown eyes. These lenses may also be used as a prosthetic to mask corneal scarring or to cover an amblyopic (lazy) eye. Some lenses incorporate designs such as cat eyes or football team logos and come in plano (no correction) and various corrections (e.g., WildEyes). Finally, some lenses have material incorporated into them that absorbs ultraviolet radiation; these lenses are used in patients with aphakia (patients in whom the crystalline lens of the eye is removed because of an opacified lens or cataract and an intraocular lens is not implanted).

### *Advantages*

Soft lenses are easier to remove and are considerably more comfortable than rigid lenses. This effect is most apparent during the initial break-in period. Photophobia is not likely to occur with soft lenses, and glare is significantly reduced. As with rigid lenses, however, flare around the periphery may be noticed at night, particularly in individuals who have large pupils. This flare is caused by refractive light entering the eye through the edge margin of the contact lens.

The typical soft lens wearer does not usually experience the spectacle blur common among hard lens wearers and even occasionally experienced by RGP wearers.

Soft lenses are less likely than rigid lenses to trap dust particles, eyelashes, or other foreign material under the lens. They are also less likely to become dislodged or fall out. Therefore, soft lenses are often better suited for occasional wear and for use during participation in sports, including contact sports.

### Disadvantages

Although many people prefer the comfort of soft lenses, not all soft lens wearers can achieve excellent visual acuity. The hydration of the lens may change either in or out of the eye, particularly with extreme temperatures and low relative humidity. This change can decrease the quality of the visual image. Because a soft lens conforms in large part to the corneal shape, it is difficult to project the degree of vision improvement before the lens is actually placed on the eye. Further, because soft lenses cannot be as precisely tailored to the specific requirements of an individual cornea, the fitting process is less exact than it is with rigid lenses. As a result, the overall quality of vision with soft contact lenses does not usually equal that of a properly fitted pair of rigid lenses. Fortunately, these differences are often small and should not concern many wearers.

Unlike rigid lenses, soft lenses can absorb chemical compounds from topically administered ophthalmic products.[9] As previously discussed, ocular irritation may result, and the lens may be damaged. With the exception of specially formulated rewetting solutions, no solution should be instilled into the eye with the soft lens in place. If a drug solution is instilled into the eye prior to lens insertion, the wearer must wait to insert a lens until the solution has cleared from the lower eyelid's precorneal (conjunctival) pocket (about 5 minutes). A nonprescription ophthalmic product not specifically designed for use with contact lenses should not be used when lenses are in the eye. When topical ophthalmic ointments, gels, or suspensions are being used, the lenses should not be worn at all.

Unlike rigid lenses, soft lenses cannot be easily marked to identify which is for the left and right eyes. A soft lens wearer who is uncertain of the identity of the lenses may have to see an eye care practitioner.

The care given to contact lenses varies considerably with each wearer. Soft lenses rapidly degenerate to useless pieces of plastic if they are neglected. However, when used with a fastidious care and cleaning program, daily-wear soft lenses can have an average life of 12 to 18 months, compared with 18 to 36 months for RGP lenses.

### Care of Soft Lenses

Conventional hard lens solutions should never be used with soft lenses because absorption of the ingredients can damage the lenses. Because soft lenses contain a high percentage of water, they are most prone to bacterial contamination. Lens disinfection is crucial to prevent ocular infection and damage to the lens by bacteria and fungi. Wearers of soft hydrophilic contact lenses should also be particularly cautious in exposing their lenses to chemicals. These chemicals, many of which penetrate and bind with the lens material, can come from cosmetics, environmental pollutants, and ophthalmic and systemic products.

The basic care regimen for soft lenses (Figure 29-3) is different from that for hard lenses. All steps must be completed to avoid ocular complications. The only exception is with daily-wear frequent replacement soft lenses. Because these lenses are disposed of within 2 weeks, enzymatic cleaners are usually not necessary. Frequent replacement lenses should, however, be cleaned and disinfected after each wearing until disposal.

#### Cleaning Products

A troublesome aspect of soft lens wear is the accumulation of deposits on the lens. The nature of these deposits varies, but generally they consist of proteins and lipids from the wearer's lacrimal secretions. Deposits are a greater problem with the more highly hydrated lenses, but the rate at which these deposits accumulate depends on the lens and the tears. Some wearers experience little difficulty and wear soft lenses for long periods without significant buildup; others may show deposits in as little as 2 or 3 days. Whatever the cause or accumulation rate, the result is an uncomfortable lens of poor optical quality.

Daily-wear soft contact lenses require two cleaning steps to rid them of debris (Tables 29-2 and 29-11). Cleaning with a surface-active cleaner must be done daily or, in the case of continuous-wear lenses, each time they are removed from the eyes. Cleaning with an enzymatic cleaner should be done daily (e.g., Supraclens) or weekly (e.g., Ultrazyme). Soft lens cleaning solutions generally contain a nonionic detergent, a wetting agent, a chelating agent, buffers, preservatives, and, in some cases, polymeric cleaning beads.

Although the surface-active cleaners are generally quite effective in removing lipid deposits, they remove tenacious protein debris less successfully. Enzymatic cleaners are an additional cleaning aid that can help solve this problem. These enzymes hydrolyze polypeptide bonds of protein and dissolve the protein deposits. For the enzyme solution to work properly, however, the lens must be cleaned with a surface-active cleaner first; enzymes are ineffective on debris that covers or is mixed with protein.

Enzymatic regimens were developed to be used simultaneously with chemical or hydrogen peroxide disinfection on either a daily or a weekly basis. Products that combine enzymatic cleaning and disinfecting steps tend to increase compliance by decreasing the number of lens care steps a patient must perform. Table 29-12 lists characteristics of various enzymatic products.

#### Disinfecting Methods

FDA recommends disinfecting soft contact lenses before each reinsertion. Disinfection is performed after the lens is cleaned. Two methods of cold disinfection are currently approved: chemical and hydrogen peroxide. A system that uses subsonic agitation and high-intensity ultraviolet light is also available (Purilens). Thermal disinfection has also

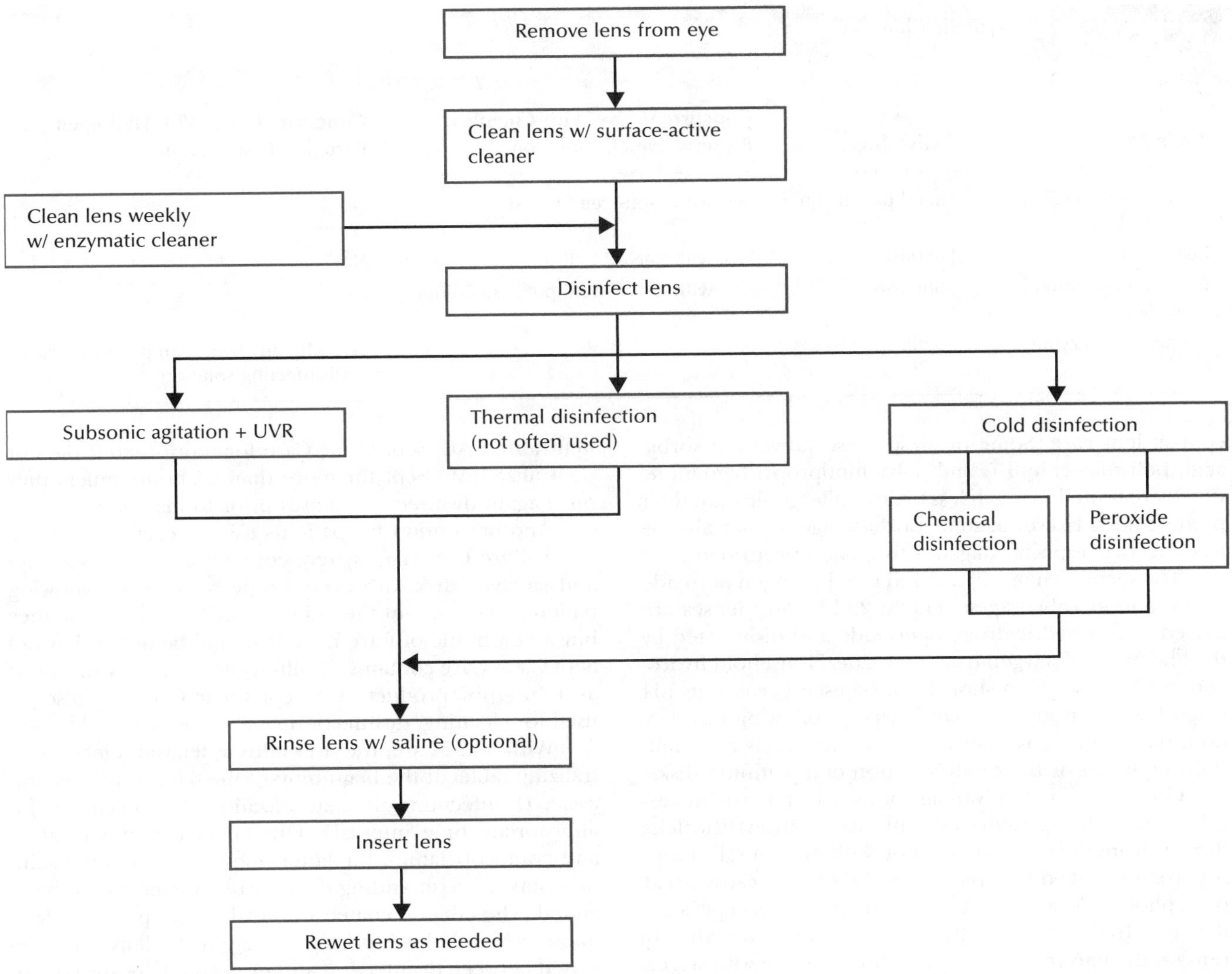


**FIGURE 29–3** Self-care of soft lenses. Key: UVR, ultraviolet radiation.

**TABLE 29-11 Specific Cleaning Procedures for Soft Lenses**

- Clean regular soft lenses daily with a surface-active cleaner. Clean continuous-wear and disposable soft lenses with a surface-active cleaner after each wearing.
- Place several drops of a cleaning product (if not using a no-rub product) on the lens; gently rub the lens between the thumb and forefinger or between the fingertip of the forefinger and the palm of the opposite hand for 20 to 30 seconds.
- Avoid cutting the lens with a fingernail or scratching the lens surface with grit or dirt on the hands.
- Rinse lenses with a sterile isotonic buffered solution. Never use tap water: it is not isotonic and contains harmful microorganisms.
- Clean lenses at least weekly (or every day if using a daily product) with enzymatic cleaners, either separately from disinfection or as part of the disinfecting process.
- When combining enzyme cleaning and disinfecting of the lenses as one step, see Table 29-12 for the appropriate combinations of products.
- Discard any enzyme cleaner that is discolored.

been used but has largely been replaced by cold disinfection systems. Studies have shown that microorganisms do not actually enter the matrix of soft lenses, but surface contamination can lead to ocular infection. Chemical disinfection with hydrogen peroxide has increased in popularity with certain types of lenses over earlier chemical disinfectants because of decreased ocular allergenicity and toxicity.

*Chemical Disinfection* In chemical disinfection, the lenses are stored for a prescribed period of time (usually 4-6 hours) in a solution containing bactericidal agents that are compatible with soft lens materials. Two basic chemical disinfection methods are available in the United States. The first is based on the original chemical disinfecting solutions, which consisted of antimicrobial preservatives of sufficient concentration in storage solutions primarily composed of saline. These initial disinfecting solutions contained chlorhexidine and thimerosal, either of which induce sensitivity reactions in many soft lens wearers. To avoid this problem, solutions with less sensitizing disinfecting preservatives are currently being marketed for soft

TABLE 29-12 **Enzymatic Cleaners**

| Trade Name | Active Ingredient | Concurrent Use With Chemical Preservative Disinfection | Concurrent Use With Hydrogen Peroxide Disinfection |
|---|---|---|---|
| Opti-Free SupraClens (used daily) | Liquid pancreatin | Yes, with Opti-Free Express | No |
| ReNu 1 Step | Subtilisin | Yes, with ReNu Multi-purpose Solution | No |
| ReNu 1-Step Liquid (daily use) | Subtilisin | Yes, with ReNu Multi-purpose Solution | No |
| Ultrazyme/Unizyme | Subtilisin | No | Yes, with any hydrogen peroxide 3% disinfecting solution |

contact lens care. Some of these preservatives are sorbic acid, polyquaternium-1, and polyaminopropyl biguanide, which are touted as much less toxic or allergenic than their predecessors. However, some of these agents may also be less effective, especially against fungi and protozoans.

The second chemical method uses hydrogen peroxide as the antimicrobial agent (Table 29-13). Soft lenses are placed in purified hydrogen peroxide and disinfected by the liberation of oxygen from peroxide. Household hydrogen peroxide solution should not be used because its pH is too low and it may discolor lenses.[10] Following disinfection, the peroxide is neutralized to trace levels by a neutralizing tablet or the catalytic action of a platinum disk.

One potential disadvantage of hydrogen peroxide disinfection is that patients may mistakenly insert the lens directly from the peroxide solution without neutralization. A peroxide-soaked lens placed on the eye will cause great pain, photophobia, redness, and, perhaps, corneal epithelial damage. If this occurs, the patient should immediately remove the lens from the eye and flush the eye with sterile saline solution. The pain should subside within a few hours. If it does not, the patient should consult an eye care practitioner. If the patient has any doubt as to whether the peroxide was neutralized, the entire disinfection cycle should be started over again to avoid the risk of inserting a peroxide-soaked lens without a neutralizing step.

Several hydrogen peroxide products help the patient avoid the possibility of forgetting to perform the neutralization step: AO Sept, AO Sept Clear Care, Pure Eyes, and Ultra-Care.

Patients who use the AO Sept platinum disk for neutralization should replace the disk after 100 uses or 3 months, whichever comes first. Failure to comply with these instructions may result in disk failure, and the patient may sustain a peroxide burn on the cornea. Although the catalytic disk systems require only one step, that step takes 6 hours for disinfection and neutralization, which decreases the system's flexibility and rules out morning use. Suboptimal disinfection is another concern with AO Sept. The catalytic disk will neutralize the surrounding peroxide quickly, and there may not be adequate time for disinfection. Once the catalytic disk neutralizes the peroxide, a nonpreserved solution remains. If the lenses are left in the case for long periods of time, bacterial contamination may occur. Patients should not store their lenses in neutralized AO Sept Clear Care for more than 7 days or neutralized AO Sept for more than 24 hours unless they once again disinfect the lenses prior to insertion.

Another option for patients using a catalytic disk system is Pure Eyes. This system contains a new storage case and catalytic disk with every bottle of solution, allowing patients to throw out the old case and disk each time they buy a new bottle of Pure Eyes. It should be noted that AO Sept Clear Care contains a built-in cleaner and is approved as a "no-rub" product. AO Sept Clear Care can also be used for cleaning, disinfection, and storage of RGP lenses.

With Ultra-Care, the user adds a delayed-release neutralizing tablet at the beginning of the 6-hour disinfecting cycle. Disinfection and neutralization then occur at the appropriate time intervals. This tablet contains catalase and cyanocobalamin; the latter ingredient turns the solution pink, thus reminding the user that the tablet has been added. The tablet is coated with hydroxypropyl methylcellulose, which helps lubricate the eye if the lens is not rerinsed between disinfection and insertion. Exposure of the lenses to the disinfecting effects of hydrogen peroxide before neutralization occurs allows optimal activity against *Acanthamoeba.* Patients using Ultra-Care should know the following:

- This product requires a minimum of 6 hours to complete disinfection and neutralization of the peroxide.
- The neutralizing tablet should not be crushed or used if there are cracks in the coating, or the tablet will start neutralizing the peroxide before adequate disinfection occurs.
- MiraFlow or Pliagel, which are used for surface-active cleaning, can leave a film on the lenses and lens cup if it is not carefully rinsed off the lens. This may result in foaming and overflow of the peroxide-neutralizer solution.[11] If this occurs, lenses should be rinsed more carefully or another surface-active cleaner should be used.
- Before lenses are removed from the eye, the lens container should be filled with fresh Ultra-Care disinfection solution and the neutralization tablet, the cap tightened, and the cup turned upside down, then right side up three times so the solution bathes the upper portion of the cup and the top.
- When lenses are to be inserted, the cup should be turned upside down to ensure full neutralization of all

**TABLE 29-13 Guidelines for Disinfecting RGP and Soft Lenses**

**Chemical Disinfection With Hydrogen Peroxide**

- Using the cup provided with the hydrogen peroxide product, soak lenses for the length of time specified by the manufacturer. Do not use lens cups or cases that came with other products.
- To disinfect and neutralize in one step, place platinum catalytic disk in lens case and leave the disk there until time to replace it. Add hydrogen peroxide, insert lenses, and leave for at least 6 hours.
- Never place neutralizing solution in lens case with a catalytic disk. An unwanted chemical reaction may occur, or a gummy residue may form on the disk.
- Make sure hydrogen peroxide is completely neutralized by carefully following product instructions before inserting lenses in the eyes.
- Rinse lenses thoroughly with saline before inserting them.

**Combination Enzyme Cleaning and Disinfection**

- When combining enzyme cleaning and disinfecting of the lenses as one step, select products compatible with your disinfecting system (see Table 29-12).
- Add appropriate solution (hydrogen peroxide or chemical disinfecting product) to storage case of disinfecting system.
- Add lenses, and then add appropriate enzymatic cleaner.
- Follow directions above for appropriate disinfecting system.
- Rinse lenses thoroughly with saline to remove residual enzymes.

**Thermal Disinfection**

- When heat disinfecting unit is not available, place tightly closed lens case containing lenses and saline solution in a pot of boiling water for at least 10 minutes (15 minutes if at an altitude above 7000 ft). Do not allow water to boil away.
- Remove pot from heat; allow to cool for 30 minutes.
- Rinse lenses with saline.
- Resume use of heat disinfecting unit as soon as possible.

**Chemical Preservative Disinfection**

- Store lenses for prescribed period of time (usually a minimum of 4 hours) in a preservative disinfecting solution appropriate for the lenses.
- If using Quick CARE, rub the hypertonic starting solution onto the lens to clean and disinfect. Then rinse lenses thoroughly with saline and soak in finishing solution for 5 minutes.
- Rinse lenses thoroughly with saline to remove disinfecting solution if you experience irritation.

---

residual disinfecting solution in the lens case, then the lenses are removed from the case and inserted.

- Ultra-Care should not be used with Illusions soft contact lenses. Lens damage may result.
- If the lenses are not going to be worn for a while, they can be stored unopened in the neutralized solution. However, they should be disinfected once weekly and just before wear.

## Multipurpose Products

Initially, manufacturers recommended three different products for the cleaning, protein removal, and disinfection of soft contact lenses. However, there has been a trend toward using multipurpose solutions for these functions; some single solutions claim to be effective for all three procedures.

The major problem with a multipurpose solution is that ingredients required in its formulation perform different and somewhat incompatible functions. For example, high concentrations of preservatives are necessary to kill bacteria; however, these same concentrations can cause ocular irritation when placed directly on the eye with a contact lens. If lenses are stored overnight in a cleaning solution containing an anionic surfactant, the detergent may eventually build up on the lens and cause irritation.

Some cold disinfection systems are considered multipurpose solutions, including ReNu MultiPlus MultiPurpose Solution, ReNu Multipurpose Disinfecting Solution, ReNu with MoistureLoc, OptiFree Express, SOLO-care 10 minute, and Complete Moisture Plus. All these solutions are indicated for surface-active cleaning of the lens as well as disinfection. Some of the products also perform protein removal. Some have also met FDA requirements to be labeled as "no rub required," meaning that no rubbing is needed during the cleaning step.[12] Examples include Opti-Free Express, ReNu Multi-Plus, Complete, and AO Sept Clear Care. It should be noted that all of the "no-rub" products require thoroughly rinsing the lenses with these solutions and not just soaking the lenses without first rinsing them.

These products are useful for patients with planned replacement lenses because these lenses are usually discarded before a significant amount of protein or lipid builds up on the lens. Patients who wear traditional soft contact lenses usually benefit from using separate solutions for cleaning, protein removal, and disinfection rather than multipurpose solutions.

## Saline Solutions

The hydrophilic soft contact lens must be maintained in a constant state of hydration. Furthermore, the hydrated lens must be isotonic with tears because changes in tonicity can alter the conformation and optical properties of the lens. Isotonic normal saline is the basic solution used for rinsing, thermally disinfecting, and storing soft contact lenses.

Prepared saline is available in either preserved or preservative-free forms. Because thimerosal and chlorhexidine can cause sensitivity reactions or irritation in many patients, sorbic acid–preserved products are commonly promoted for sensitive eyes and appear to be acceptable to most wearers.

Several preservative-free saline solutions are also available. Preservative-free buffered saline is available in multiuse bottles (which must be discarded 30 days after opening) and as aerosol sprays.

Patients using nonpreserved saline should be counseled that only aerosolized solutions can be used to rinse lenses just before insertion into the eye. Multipurpose nonpreserved saline (e.g., Unisol 4) should never be used to rinse lenses just before insertion, unless the bottle is new and has not been opened. Once these products have been opened, they should be used only if a disinfection step will be performed before insertion.

Patients should avoid using other forms of saline such as intravenous normal saline or saline squirts because these products are usually too acidic for use with soft contact lenses.

Some patients prepare their own preservative-free saline using salt tablets and USP purified water. Using salt tablets is inexpensive, but the clear superiority of commercial saline solutions argues strongly against use of homemade saline. This practice and the application of improper lens care are the greatest predisposing factors to *Acanthamoeba* keratitis and many anterior eye infections contracted by hydrophilic lens wearers.

When contact lens patients started using homemade salt tablet solutions, there was a resurgence of *Acanthamoeba* infections. *Acanthamoeba*, of which there are 15 species, is an opportunistic protozoan. Usually nonpathogenic, *Acanthamoeba* has been isolated from airborne dust, soils, surface water, tap water, and even distilled water. In unfavorable environments, it forms a very resistant cyst that can survive many antimicrobial agents, even though its vegetative form (trophozoite) may be susceptible. Viable cysts have been found in swimming pools and hot tubs that are adequately chlorinated to kill trophozoites. *Acanthamoeba* infection was very rare until contact lenses became popular. Most victims of *Acanthamoeba* keratitis have used improper lens hygiene, gone swimming without removing their contact lenses, used nonsterile saline solution made from salt tablets and distilled water, or used tap water in the maintenance of their soft contact lenses. Because they are very resistant, *Acanthamoeba* cysts often can survive attempts to eradicate them from the eye with antimicrobial agents. Multiple antibiotic regimens have been applied with variable or poor therapeutic response. Many cases of *Acanthamoeba* keratitis are severe enough to require keratoplasty (a partial or complete cornea transplant) in an attempt to save the eye. Unfortunately, the persistent presence of cysts gives this eye infection a poor prognosis, which, in many cases, ultimately leads to enucleation—the partial or total removal of the affected eye. For these reasons, FDA no longer condones the use of salt tablets, and neither should a concerned practitioner.

## Rewetting Solutions

Accessory solutions for use with soft lenses permit lubricating and rewetting (and, in some cases, cleaning) of the lens in the eye. These solutions typically contain a low concentration of a nonionic surfactant to promote cleaning and a polymer to lubricate the lens surface, along with buffering agents. Clerz Plus Lens Drops, contains Clens 100, a patented surfactant, that acts on protein, lipid, and calcium deposits. Besides rewetting activity, this product provides some on-the-eye cleaning, which can help improve lens comfort.[12] Other rewetting products, blink Contacts and AQuify, contain sodium hyaluronate, which strongly adheres to the mucin layer of the tear film. This allows for a water-retaining layer that resists evaporation.

Rewetting solutions are particularly useful to patients with highly hydrated lenses, such as the continuous-wear type. Exposing lenses to wind and high temperature causes some dehydration, even with the lens in the eye. The resulting discomfort is sometimes relieved by one or two drops of rewetting solution. To minimize contamination, the tip of the applicator bottle should not touch the eye, eyelid, or any other surface.

## Product Selection Guidelines

Many problems associated with soft lens wear arise from the way people handle their lenses; unsatisfactory results may stem from improper procedures rather than inadequate products. It should be noted, however, that patients who choose to buy generic (e.g. mass merchandiser labeled) multipurpose lens solutions may be purchasing older, potentially obsolete formulas. Mass merchandisers generally purchase older formulations of nationally known brands of multipurpose solutions and then label under their private label. In addition, the composition of a particular generic formulation can vary because the stores bid from manufacturers two to three times per year. Generally, it is preferable that patients not use generic brands unless they carefully read the label and compare all of the ingredients to the product that was recommended by their eye care professional or pharmacist. It is important to note that manufacturers are not required to use the same name for generic and brand-name ingredients, so it may be difficult to compare formulations.

Table 29-14 lists examples of products designed specifically for soft contact lenses. In one investigation, only 26% of contact lens wearers fully complied with care instructions, and the occurrence of signs and symptoms of potential wearing problems was directly correlated with noncompliance. Specific questions about the care and maintenance regimen a wearer uses can often bring these problems to light.

*Surface-active Cleaners* Some surface-active cleaners (e.g., Bausch & Lomb Sensitive Eyes Daily Cleaner) have a lower viscosity and may be easier to rinse off the lens. These products are good choices for patients who have difficulty completely rinsing the cleaner off their lens.

In addition to surfactants, some products (e.g., Opti-Clean II) contain mild abrasives that aid in the removal of lens deposits. Patients who have difficulty removing deposits from their lenses will benefit from this type of cleaner. These products should be shaken before use. Some patients may have difficulty rinsing these cleaners off their lenses. Care should be taken to be sure that no residue from the cleaning solution remains on the lens prior to insertion.

Finally, one surfactant cleaner (MiraFlow) contains isopropyl alcohol. This product is useful for patients who discover heavy lipid deposits on their lenses.

*Enzymatic Cleaners* Enzymatic cleaners can be recommended based on the disinfection system used by the patient. Ultrazyme and Unizyme are good choices for the patient using a hydrogen peroxide cleaning system. These

TABLE 29-14 Selected Products for Soft Lenses

| Trade Name | Primary Ingredients |
|---|---|
| **Surface-active Cleaning Solutions** | |
| Bausch & Lomb Sensitive Eyes Daily Cleaner | Hydroxypropyl methylcellulose; sorbic acid 0.25%; EDTA 0.5%; NaCl; borate buffer; poloxamine |
| MiraFlow Extra Strength | Isopropyl alcohol 20%; poloxamer 407; amphoteric 10 |
| Opti-Clean II Daily Cleaner | Nylon 11; polysorbate 21; hydroxyethyl cellulose; polyquaternium-1; EDTA; boric acid; sodium borate; NaCl |
| Opti-Free Daily Cleaner | Nylon 11; polysorbate 21; hydroxyethyl cellulose; polyquaternium-1, 0.001%; EDTA; boric acid; sodium borate; hydrochloric acid and/or sodium hydroxide |
| Pliagel | Sorbic acid 0.25%; EDTA 0.5%; poloxamer 407; KCl; NaCl |
| **Enzymatic Cleaning Products** | |
| AMO Complete Moisture Plus Weekly Enzymatic Cleaner Tablet | Subtilisin A |
| Opti-Free Enzymatic Cleaner for Sensitive Eyes Tablet | Pancreatin; povidone; citric acid; sodium bicarbonate; PEG; dehydrated alcohol |
| Opti-Free SupraClens Daily Protein Remover Solution* | Highly purified porcine pancreatin enzymes; PEG; sodium borate |
| Opti-Zyme Enzymatic Cleaner Tablet | Pancreatin |
| ReNu 1 Step Enzymatic Cleaner Tablet | Subtilisin; sodium carbonate; NaCl; boric acid |
| ReNu 1 Step Daily Protein Remover Liquid | Subtilisin; glycerin; borate buffers |
| Ultrazyme Enzymatic Cleaner Tablet | Subtilisin A; effervescing agents; buffers |
| Unizyme Tablet | Subtilisin |
| **Chemical Disinfecting Solutions** | |
| ReNu Multipurpose Solution | Poloxamine; polyaminopropyl biguanide; boric acid; edetate disodium |
| Opti-Free Rinsing, Disinfecting & Storage Solution | Polyquaternium-1, 0.001%; EDTA 0.05%; citrate buffer; NaCl |
| **Hydrogen Peroxide Disinfecting Solutions and Rinsing/Neutralizing Products** | |
| AO Sept | Disinfecting solution: hydrogen peroxide 3%; NaCl 0.85%; phosphate buffers; phosphoric acid<br>Neutralizer: platinum disk |
| AO Sept Clear Care | Hydrogen peroxide 3%; pluronic; platinum disk |
| Pure Eyes 2 | Hydrogen peroxide 3%; NaCl 0.85%; phosphate buffers; phosphoric acid; packaged with plastic lens case with built-in neutralizing disk |
| Ultra-Care | Disinfecting solution: hydrogen peroxide 3%; sodium stannate; sodium nitrate; phosphates<br>Neutralizer: catalase tablet; cyanocobalamin (color indicator) |
| **Preserved Saline Solutions** | |
| Bausch & Lomb Sensitive Eyes Saline | Sorbic acid 0.1%; NaCl; borate buffer; EDTA |
| **Preservative-free Saline Products** | |
| AMO Lens Plus | NaCl; boric acid |
| Unisol 4 Saline Solution | NaCl; sodium borate; boric acid |
| **Rewetting/Lubricating Solutions** | |
| Clerz Plus | Clens 100; Tetronic 1304 |
| Clerz 2 | Hydroxyethyl cellulose; sorbic acid 0.1%; EDTA 0.1%; NaCl; KCl; sodium borate |

TABLE 29-14 Selected Products for Soft Lenses (continued)

| Trade Name | Primary Ingredients |
|---|---|
| Opti-Free Rewetting Drops | Polyquaternium-1, 0.001%; citric acid; sodium citrate; NaCl |
| ReNu Rewetting Drops | Sorbic acid 0.15%; EDTA; borate buffer; poloxamine; NaCl |
| **Multipurpose Solutions** | |
| AQuify | Sorbitol, dexpanthenol, pluronic F127, tromethamine, polyhexanide, EDTA |
| Complete Moisture Plus Multi-Purpose Solution | Tyloxapol; hydroxypropyl methylcellulose; polyhexamethylene biguanide 0.0001%; EDTA; NaCl; tromethamine, Poloxamer 237 |
| Opti-Free Express Multipurpose Solution | Polyquaternium-1, 0.001%; EDTA; sodium citrate; NaCl; citric acid |
| Opti-One Multi-Purpose Solution | Polyquaternium-1, 0.0011%; EDTA 0.05%; sodium citrate; NaCl; citric acid; sodium hydroxide and/or hydrochloric acid |
| ReNu MultiPlus Solution | Polyaminopropyl biguanide; EDTA; NaCl; sodium borate; boric acid; poloxamine |
| ReNu Multi-Purpose Solution | Polyaminopropyl biguanide; EDTA; NaCl; sodium borate; boric acid; poloxamine |
| ReNu with MoistureLoc | Boric acid; sodium chloride; sodium phosphate; Hydranate (hydroxyalkylphosphonate); poloxamine; MoistureLoc (poloxamer, polyquaternium-10); alexidine 0.00045% |

Key: EDTA, ethylenediamine tetraacetic acid; KCl, potassium chloride; NaCl, sodium chloride; PEG, polyethylene glycol.
* Preservative-free.

products can be placed in the peroxide solution, thereby cleaning and disinfecting at the same time. If the patient uses Opti-Free disinfecting solution, Supra-Clens or Opti-Free Enzymatic Cleaner would be a good choice because they can be placed directly in the Opti-Free solution during the disinfection cycle. If the patient uses ReNu Multipurpose Disinfecting solution, then ReNu 1 Step tablets (weekly use) or ReNu 1 Step liquid (daily use) would be a good choice. If the patient uses another chemical disinfection system, product comparisons are very idiosyncratic unless the patient is allergic to one of the components.

*Disinfecting Methods* When counseling a patient about the best disinfecting method to use, compliance and convenience should be considered. Ultra-Care (2-hour exposure to hydrogen peroxide) is a good choice because it is the only method that eradicates *Acanthamoeba* besides heat disinfection, which is no longer commonly used. If a patient does not want to use a hydrogen peroxide system, a second-generation chemical system (i.e., Opti-Free Express or ReNu Multipurpose) can be recommended.

When choosing a chemical disinfection product, several factors should be considered. If the patient has a history of sensitivity reactions to lens solutions or is unsure if sensitivity exists, it is best to recommend a product containing one of the nonsensitizing preservatives. A recommendation can be made based on the brand and type of enzymatic cleaner the patient is using. For example, if the patient is using Supra-Clens Enzymatic cleaner, then Opti-Free or Opti-Free Express should be recommended as the disinfecting agent. If the patient is using ReNu 1 Step Enzymatic Cleaner, then the best recommendation is ReNu Multipurpose Disinfecting Solution. If a patient has no preference for a particular enzymatic product, then any of the chemical disinfection solutions that can be used concurrently with an enzymatic product are appropriate.

*Product Incompatibility* Several incompatibilities may occur when mixing soft lens products. Most manufacturers test for compatibility within their own product lines; however, compatibility with other manufacturers' products is usually not determined. Generally, chemical disinfecting solutions should not be interchanged or used concurrently. If a patient mixes a disinfecting solution containing chlorhexidine and thimerosal with a product containing a quaternary ammonium compound, a toxic keratopathy known as mixed solution syndrome may occur. Patients should be counseled not to switch from a chlorhexidine-containing chemical disinfection system to a hydrogen peroxide system, unless they procure new lenses. A fine black precipitate may form on the lenses if chlorhexidine is still present in the lens matrix. Other chemical disinfection system residue on soft lenses may cause the lens to turn pink, yellow, brown, black, or purple if the lens is exposed to a hydrogen peroxide system.[4]

### Insertion and Removal

See Table 29-15 for instructions on inserting and removing soft lenses.

### Lens Storage Case

Choice of a lens storage case is important. The case should have left and right clearly identified on the caps and in the lens wells. The lens wells should have ridges or flutes so the RGP lens does not adhere to the case, an occurrence that is common in smooth cases and can cause warpage of the lens or inversion on removal.

**TABLE 29-15 Insertion and Removal of Soft Lenses**

**Insertion**

- Wash the hands with noncosmetic soap and rinse thoroughly; dry the hands with a lint-free towel.
- Remove the lens for the right eye from its storage container.
- (Optional) Rinse the lens with saline solution to dilute any preservatives left from disinfection.
- Place the lens on the top of a finger and examine it to be sure it is not inside out. This can be done by using the "taco test." Gently fold the lens at the apex (not the edges) between the thumb and forefinger. The edges should look like a taco shell with the edges pointed inward. If the edges roll out, the lens is inverted and must be reversed.
- Examine the lens for cleanliness. If necessary, clean it and rinse again.
- Insert the lens on the right eye using the same procedure as for hard and RGP lenses (see Table 29-8).
- Repeat the process for the left eye.

**Removal**

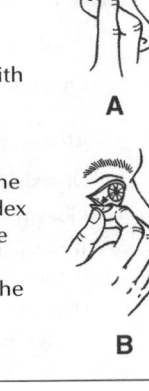

- Before removing the lenses, wash hands with a noncosmetic soap; rinse the hands thoroughly and dry them with a lint-free towel.
- Using the right middle finger, pull down the lower lid of the right eye. Touch the right index finger to the lens and slide the lens off the cornea as shown in drawing A.
- Using the index finger and thumb, grasp the lens and remove it (see drawing B).
- Repeat the procedure for the left eye.

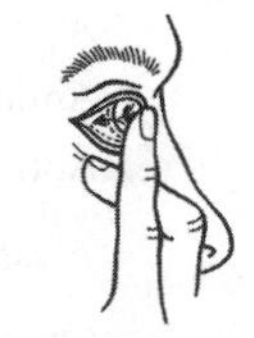

A

B

The proper care and cleaning of the contact lens storage case is as important as lens care itself. A storage case should be able to hold at least 2.5 mL of the storage solution.[13] This minimizes the chance that the soaking solution will be overwhelmed by an inoculum of bacteria. The lens case should be cleaned thoroughly on a routine basis and replaced at least every 3 months.[14] Routine cleaning entails air drying the case between periods of use and scrubbing it weekly. Air drying should be done daily as this discourages biofilm formation. Some manufacturers recommend cleaning the case twice weekly using a few drops of lens cleaner and hot water. If the case can withstand routine boiling (such as those cases made of polycarbonate or noryl plastic), it can be boiled in a pot of water for 10 minutes weekly. Examine the case for cracks and replace it periodically. Lens cases can be contaminated with a biofilm that will attract pathogens and increase the risk of infection.

## Assessment of Contact Lens–related Problems: A Case-based Approach

Although contact lenses are usually safe, lens wearers can experience a variety of problems. During the patient interview, the practitioner should first determine what type of eye problems exist and how long the patient has been experiencing them. Asking the patient whether a history of eye problems exists and what medications are currently being taken will give a general sense of the etiology and urgency of the current eye problem. The answers will also help the practitioner determine whether the problem is related to noncompliance with care regimens or to drug-lens interactions.

Determining which type of contact lenses a patient is wearing and for how long is crucial in assessing problems related to improper lens care or deteriorated lenses. Each type of lens has unique physical characteristics that in turn dictate which methods and products for cleaning and disinfecting lenses are appropriate. Patients should be asked to describe how they care for their lenses, which lens care products they use, and whether they have recently changed products. Many lens care–related problems are minor and can be easily solved by a knowledgeable practitioner.

The individual sections on types of contact lenses discuss problems related to lens care. The following sections discuss other types of lens-related problems and their symptoms, as well as problems that require medical referral.

### *Precautions for Contact Lenses*

Contact lenses generally can match or exceed the vision obtained with spectacles. However, depending on the type of lens, vision may become worse in certain situations. Some patients wearing lenses with high water content may experience hazy vision around the edges of objects. In some cases, patients wearing hard lenses experience nighttime ghosting, which occurs when the patient's pupil dilates enough to see the edges of the lens. This can sometimes be corrected with larger-diameter lenses. Other patients complain of spiderweb vision, usually at night; this can be due to crazing (i.e., the development of fine cracks) and is usually experienced with RGP lenses.

### *Potential Transmission of Viral Infections*

The human immunodeficiency virus (HIV) has been isolated from the tears of infected individuals as well as from the contact lenses worn by infected individuals. This seemingly becomes an issue in the case of trial contact lenses, which may be reused by different patients in the lens-fitter's office. Use of disposable contact lenses is advisable in this situation. Generally, trial lenses are not dispensed to a patient except as loaner lenses (i.e., to a patient waiting for new replacement lenses). Even in this scenario, after the lenses have been used in any patient, they are disinfected with heat or chemicals before being dispensed to another patient. Studies have shown that heat and the routinely available hydrogen peroxide products are effective in inactivating HIV.

### *Adverse Effects of Drugs*

Many undesired effects have been reported when a patient who wears contact lenses ingests, applies, or encounters certain drugs (Table 29-16). The practitioner must understand these drug-induced problems to counsel patients effectively.

**TABLE 29-16 Drug Contact Lens Interactions**

| | |
|---|---|
| **Changes in Tear Film and/or Production** | |
| ***Tear Volume Decreased*** | |
| Anticholinergic agents | Phenothiazines |
| Antihistamines | Serotonin reuptake inhibitors |
| β-Blockers | Sildenafil citrate |
| Benzodiazepines | Statins |
| Botulinum toxin type A (Botox) | Timolol (topical) |
| Conjugated estrogens | Tricyclic antidepressants |
| Diuretics | Vardenafil HCl |
| Oral contraceptives | |
| ***Tear Volume Increased*** | |
| Cholinergic agents | Reserpine |
| Garlic (dietary supplement) | |
| **Changes in Lens Color (Primarily Soft Lenses)** | |
| Diagnostic dyes (i.e., fluorescein) | Phenothiazines |
| Epinephrine (topical) | Phenylephrine |
| Fluorescein (topical) | Rifampin |
| Nicotine | Sulfasalazine |
| Nitrofurantoin | Tetracycline |
| Phenazopyridine | Tetrahydrozoline (topical) |
| Phenolphthalein | |
| **Changes in Tonicity** | |
| Pilocarpine (8%) | Sodium sulfacetamide (10%) |
| **Lid/Corneal Edema** | |
| Chlorthalidone | Oral contraceptives |
| Clomiphene | Primidone |
| Conjugated estrogens | |
| **Ocular Inflammation/Irritation** | |
| Diclofenac (topical ophthalmic) | Isotretinoin |
| Garlic (dietary supplement) | Salicylates |
| Gold salts | |
| **Changes in Refractivity (Induction of Myopia)** | |
| Acetazolamide | Sulfamethoxazole |
| Sulfadiazine | Sulfisoxazole |
| Sulfamethizole | |
| **Changes in Pupil Size** | |
| ***Pupillary Dilation*** | |
| Anticholinergic agents | CNS stimulants |
| Antidepressants | Kava |
| Antihistamines | Phenothiazines |
| ***Pupillary Miosis*** | |
| Opiates | |
| **Miscellaneous Agents (Effects)** | |
| Digoxin (increased glare) | |
| Ribavirin (cloudy lenses) | |
| Topical ciprofloxacin/prednisolone acetate (precipitate) | |
| Hypnotics/sedatives/muscle relaxants (decreased blink rate) | |

Key: CNS, central nervous system.

*Source:* Adapted with permission from Engle JP. Contact lens care. *Am Druggist*. 1990;201:5465.

## Topical Drugs

In general, patients should be counseled not to place any ophthalmic solution, suspension, gel, or ointment into the eye when contact lenses are in place. The only exceptions to this rule are products specifically formulated to be used with contact lenses, such as rewetting drops, or those products that an eye care practitioner has specifically recommended for use with contact lenses.

Topical administration of ophthalmic drugs may have physiologic consequences or may modify pharmacologic responses to drugs. The use of solutions that may be considered benign, such as artificial tears, may reduce tear breakup time and alter the distribution of the mucoid, aqueous, and lipid components of tears, perhaps causing initial discomfort on instillation of the drops.[4] The pharmacologic effect of a topically administered drug while soft lenses are in place may be exaggerated. The soft lens may absorb the drug and either release it over time, thus creating a sustained-release dosage form, or bind it tightly so that none of it is released into the eye. Furthermore, the presence of any kind of contact lens may increase the amount of time the medication is in contact with the eye. Finally, increased drug absorption may occur secondary to a compromised corneal epithelium during contact lens wear.[4]

In certain cases, patients will be treated with topical ophthalmic medications while wearing contact lenses. For example, such medications are used in conjunction with disposable soft contact lenses as an alternative to bandage contact lenses in the treatment of persistent epithelial corneal defects. Yet, an opaque precipitate has been noted in case reports of some patients using SeeQuence disposable contact lenses treated with topical ciprofloxacin and topical prednisolone acetate concurrently.[15] When studied in the laboratory, neither drug alone produced precipitates in the contact lens; white crystalline deposits were noted only when the two topical agents were used in combination. In another study, the combination of topical gentamicin and methylprednisolone produced precipitates.[16] Thus, if a patient who wears contact lenses is treated with a topical antibiotic and steroid combination, the eye care practitioner must carefully monitor for deposits in the lenses. If deposits are noted, the lenses should be removed and replaced with a new pair.

In addition, the preservatives, vehicles, tonicity, and pH of the solution instilled into the eye may alter the properties of the lenses. For instance, instillation of hypertonic solutions such as sodium sulfacetamide 10% or pilocarpine 8% may cause soft lens dehydration and lens disfigurement. Topical medications with an acidic pH promote lens dehydration and steepening; alkaline medications promote hydration and flattening.[17] Topical suspensions may lead to lens intolerance because particulate matter builds up and causes discomfort. Gel and oil formulations may alter the surface relationship between the contact lens and the cornea.[9] Finally, the active ingredient of certain topical products may discolor lenses. For example, exposure to light and air causes epinephrine to form adrenochrome deposits, which range in color from pink to brown.

#### Airborne Drugs and Particulate Matter

Some drugs present in indoor air may damage lenses. For example, nurses who care for patients receiving ribavirin have reportedly experienced cloudy lenses after repeated exposure to the drug.[18,19] Similarly, contact lens wearers who have been exposed to a large amount of cigarette smoke have discovered a brown discoloration and nicotine deposits on their lenses. This is especially true for those who smoke and have nicotine-stained fingers.[20]

#### Systemic Medications

Some systemic medications are secreted into tears and may interact with (primarily soft) contact lenses. For example, rifampin will stain both lenses and tears orange. Drugs and dietary supplements such as gold salts and garlic are secreted into the tears and may cause ocular irritation. Other drugs may affect tear production, the refractive properties of the eye, the shape of the cornea, or the actual lens (Table 29-16).[21] Some medications may influence the size of the pupil, causing complaints of glare or flare when lenses are in place. Visual performance may be diminished, especially in patients who wear multifocal lenses or gas-permeable lenses for which pupil size may determine placement of the reading segment or the optic zone of the lens, respectively.[22]

### *Use of Cosmetics*

Patients who wear contact lenses should choose—and use—cosmetics with care. Individuals should insert lenses before applying makeup and should avoid touching the lens with eyeliner or mascara. Cosmetics, moisturizers, and makeup removers with an aqueous base should be used because oil-based products may cause blurred vision and irritation if they are deposited on the lens. Cream eye shadows are preferable to powder shadows. Water-resistant (as opposed to waterproof) mascara (which requires an oil-based remover) should be applied only to the very tips of the lashes. Eyeliners should never be applied inside the eyelid margin as the liner can clog glands in the eyelid and contaminate the contact lens. Aerosol products, in particular, must be used with caution. Irritation may occur if some of the spray particles are trapped in the tear layer beneath the lens, and some sprays may actually damage the lens. One way to avoid this problem is to insert the lenses, go into another room, cover the eyes with a cloth, use the spray, and then leave the area with the eyes still closed.

Nail polish, hand creams, and perfumes should also be applied only after the lenses have been inserted. Nail polish and remover can destroy a lens. Men often contaminate their lenses with hair preparations and spray deodorants; they should take special care to clean their hands thoroughly before handling their lenses. Soaps that contain cold cream or deodorants should be avoided because they can leave a film on the fingers after rinsing. This residue readily transfers to a lens and can cause blurred vision. Moreover, if a lens comes in contact with residual petrolatum-based lotion on the patient's fingers, the lens's surface can be modified. This modification cannot be detected by inspection; it will be noted, however, once the lens is worn. The surface-wetting properties of the lens are disrupted approximately 20 to 30 minutes after insertion of the lens.

### *Corneal Hypoxia and Edema*

An adequate supply of oxygen exists only if the cornea is continuously bathed with oxygenated tears. During blinking, metabolic byproducts from the surface epithelium are flushed from under the contact lenses, and oxygen is brought in as the lenses move toward and away from the cornea. Even when properly fitted, however, both rigid and soft lenses can produce a progressive hypoxia of the cornea while the lenses are in place, especially in persons who have low blink frequency or incomplete blinks.

One major effect of this hypoxia is edema of the corneal tissues. It has been demonstrated that corneal thickness is increased by hard (PMMA) lenses. After approximately 16 hours of continuous wear, hard and, to a lesser extent, soft lenses cause the glycogen content of the cornea to fall to a level that is accompanied by significant edema. Symptoms associated with corneal edema include photophobia, rainbows around a light, sensations of hotness, grittiness and itchiness, fogging of vision, and blurred vision. Although it is not usually necessary, a patient experiencing corneal edema from overuse of contact lenses can be treated with one to two drops of a sodium chloride (2% or 5%) ophthalmic solution every 3 to 4 hours after the lenses have been removed (see Chapter 28) The patient should be counseled that transient stinging or burning may occur on instilling the drops. Furthermore, the patient should be counseled not to overuse the lenses.

Another effect of corneal hypoxia is neovascularization (the development of new vessels). This is potentially irreversible. Routine follow-up visits to the eye care practitioner are important to monitor this effect of contact lens wear.

### Corneal Abrasions

Corneal abrasions are surface defects in the epithelial layer of the cornea. The causes of these abrasions range from poorly fitted lenses or simple overwear to the entrapment of foreign bodies under the lens. The cornea is sensitive to abrasion, so blepharospasm (reflex lid closure), tearing, and rubbing the affected eye occur immediately. However, rubbing the eye must be avoided because it can cause more extensive damage while the lens remains in the eye.

Fortunately, the pain associated with corneal abrasion is usually of greater magnitude than the damage. The epithelium regenerates quickly; most minor epithelial defects (i.e., those 22 mm in diameter or less) generally heal within 12 to 24 hours. The lens should be left out for 2 to 7 days. The wearer may then proceed using a modified break-in schedule suggested by the eye care practitioner. More extensive abrasions require the attention of an eye care practitioner.

### Symptoms of Lens Problems

Patients may initially encounter various problems in adapting to contact lenses, particularly RGP lenses; even long-time wearers occasionally experience difficulty. Many of these problems arise from different causative factors, and identifying and solving a specific problem may require an eye care practitioner. The following list provides a perspective for counseling a lens wearer who seeks advice. Most of this information is particularly applicable to rigid lens wear.

- *Deep aching of eye:* This pain persists even after the lens is removed, and it may be caused by poorly fitted lenses. The eye care practitioner must be consulted.
- *Blurred vision:* This effect may be produced by improper refractive power, lenses switched right for left, lenses placed on the eye inside out, tear film buildup, cosmetic film buildup, corneal edema, or the use of oral contraceptives.
- *Excessive tearing:* Tearing is normal when lenses are first worn; however, poorly fitted lenses or chipped, rough edges on the lenses may also cause tearing.
- *Fogging:* Misty or smoky vision can be caused by corneal edema, overwearing of contact lenses, coatings or deposits on lens surfaces, or poor wetting of the lens while on the eye.
- *Flare:* Point sources of light having a sunburst or streaming quality can be caused by inadequate optic zone size or decentration of a poorly fitting lens.
- *Itching:* This symptom may be caused by allergic conjunctivitis and may be treated with short-term use of topical steroids (with the lenses out of the eyes).
- *Lens falling out of eye:* Poorly fitted lenses could be the cause. However, even properly fitted rigid lenses may occasionally slide off the cornea or be blinked out of the eye.
- *Inability to wear lenses in the morning:* This problem may be caused by corneal edema or mild conjunctivitis. The most likely cause is that the patient's eyes dry out overnight because of incomplete eyelid closure.
- *Pain after removal of lens:* This is usually caused by corneal abrasion. The presence of the lens anesthetizes the cornea because of hypoxia; sensation returns after 4 to 6 hours and pain develops.
- *Sudden pain in the eye:* A foreign body or chipped or a folded lens may be the problem.
- *Squinting:* This effect is caused by excessive movement of a lens or by a poorly fitted lens. The wearer will squint to center the optical portion of the lens over the pupil.

### Exclusions for Self-Care

When lens care is appropriate but the lenses are old or, in the case of hard lenses, chipped or scratched, the patient should see an eye care practitioner for replacement lenses. Other situations that require referral are suspected vision changes, deep aching of the eyes, last eye examination occurring longer than 1 year ago, and a suspected interaction between the lenses and oral contraceptives or other systemic medications. Patients experiencing lens problems related to the medical conditions or other factors discussed in Contraindications for Contact Lenses should also be referred for further evaluation. Cases 29-1 and 29-2 illustrate the assessment of patients with contact lens-related problems.

**CASE 29-1**

| Relevant Evaluation Criteria | Scenario/Model Outcome |
|---|---|
| **Information Gathering** | |
| 1. Gather essential information about the patient's symptoms, including: | |
| a. description of symptom(s) (i.e., nature, onset, duration, severity, associated symptoms) | Patient complains of eye discomfort associated with RGP contact lenses. Patient began wearing this particular pair of lenses 2 months ago. He is unsure of the exact brand name of the lenses but he knows they are Boston lenses. He did not experience discomfort when he first began wearing the lenses; however, during the past 2-3 weeks, he has noticed discomfort and some irritation that occurs only when he wears the lenses. He does not complain of other symptoms such as discharge from the eye. His last visit to the lens prescriber was 2 months ago when he received the RGP lenses. |

## CASE 29-1 (continued)

| Relevant Evaluation Criteria | Scenario/Model Outcome |
|---|---|
| b. description of any factors that seem to precipitate, exacerbate, and/or relieve the patient's symptom(s) | Patient is unable to associate the problem with specific factors and has taken no particular measures, except his usual lens care regimen, to relieve the symptoms |
| c. description of the patient's efforts to relieve the symptoms | Patient soaks his lenses in Boston Simplicity Solution every time he them takes out. Furthermore, he always uses fresh solutions and cleans his storage container once per week according to the manufacturer's recommendations. He also washes his hands with a noncosmetic soap before inserting the lenses. |
| 2. Gather essential patient history information: | |
| a. patient's identity | Mike Andrews |
| b. patient's age, sex, height, and weight | 25 y/o M |
| c. patient's occupation | Engineer |
| d. patient's dietary habits | N/A |
| e. patient's sleep habits | Stays up late on weekends; tries to get at least 8 hours of sleep each night |
| f. concurrent medical conditions, prescription and nonprescription medications, and dietary supplements | Ibuprofen as needed for occasional headaches |
| g. allergies | NKA |
| h. history of other adverse reactions to medications | None |
| i. other (describe)______ | Does not smoke; drinks 4-5 beers per week |
| **Assessment and Triage** | |
| 3. Differentiate the patient's signs/symptoms and correctly identify the patient's primary problem(s). | Lens discomfort secondary to lipid and protein build-up on the lens |
| 4. Identify exclusions for self-treatment. | None |
| 5. Formulate a comprehensive list of therapeutic alternatives for the primary problem to determine if triage to a medical practitioner is required, and share this information with the patient. | Options include:<br>(1) Refer Mike to his eye care practitioner.<br>(2) Recommend a change in his lens care routine.<br>(3) Take no action. |
| **Plan** | |
| 6. Select an optimal therapeutic alternative to address the patient's problem, taking into account patient preferences. | Start using the Boston Simplicity as directed on the label by including the digital rubbing step in his regimen. Consider adding an enzymatic product to his lens care regimen. |
| 7. Describe the recommended therapeutic approach to the patient. | Rather than just soaking the lenses, after removal of the lens from the eye place 2-4 drops of Boston Simplicity on each lens and rub the lens in his palm for 20 seconds. Rinse each lens for 5 seconds with a steady stream of Boston Simplicity solution. Once weekly, add 2 drops of Boston One Step Liquid Enzymatic Cleaner to the lens case completely filled with Boston Simplicity. Soak the lenses for at least 4 hours before wearing. Rinse and rub the lens with additional Simplicity solution for 5 seconds to ensure that the enzymatic cleaner is rinsed off the lens before insertion. |
| 8. Explain to the patient the rationale for selecting the recommended therapeutic approach from the considered therapeutic alternatives. | There are no symptoms of infection or of a poor-fitting lens. You should begin digital cleaning of your lenses with your solution before soaking them and add an enzymatic product to your lens care routine.<br>Boston One Step Liquid Enzymatic Cleaner is an appropriate choice because you use Boston Simplicity disinfection. The enzymatic product can be placed directly in the Simplicity solution to perform the enzymatic and disinfection step concurrently, which makes it easy to use. |

## CASE 29-1 (continued)

| Relevant Evaluation Criteria | Scenario/Model Outcome |
|---|---|
| **Patient Education** | |
| 9. When recommending self-care with nonprescription medications and/or nondrug therapy, convey accurate information to the patient, including: | |
| a. appropriate dose and frequency of administration | Use the Boston One Step Liquid Enzymatic Cleaner once weekly. If the lenses burn or sting when you insert them, you may need to rinse and rub them more thoroughly with Simplicity before insertion into the eye. |
| b. maximum number of days the therapy should be employed | N/A |
| c. product administration procedures | N/A |
| d. expected time to onset of relief | After one or two digital cleanings and one or two weekly uses of the enzymatic cleaner, the lenses should feel more comfortable. |
| e. degree of relief that can be reasonably expected | The lenses should feel as comfortable as when you first received them. |
| f. most common side effects | Stinging, burning, itching (uncommon for most people) |
| g. side effects that warrant medical intervention should they occur | Continued feelings of irritation and discomfort after two to three digital and enzymatic cleanings |
| h. patient options in the event that condition worsens or persists | The lens prescriber should be consulted if the discomfort or irritation persists or worsens, or if symptoms of infection appear, such as a thick discharge from either eye, or eyelids glued together when you awake. |
| i. product storage requirements | Store at room temperature in a dry place. Discard the Boston Simplicity Solution 90 days after opening. |
| j. specific nondrug measures | N/A |
| 10. Solicit patient's follow-up questions. | Could I use any other enzyme product to clean my lenses? |
| 11. Answer patient's questions. | You could use ProFree/GP Weekly Enzymatic Cleaner, but this product cannot be used in the Boston Simplicity Solution. You would need to perform an additional step by soaking the lenses in the ProFree/GP dissolved in a saline solution. This would add an extra step and more products to your lens care regimen so it is not the best choice in this situation. |

Key: N/A, not applicable; NKA, no known allergies; RGP, rigid gas permeable.

## CASE 29-2

| Relevant Evaluation Criteria | Scenario/Model Outcome |
|---|---|
| **Information Gathering** | |
| 1. Gather essential information about the patient's symptoms, including: | |
| a. description of symptom(s) (i.e., nature, onset, duration, severity, associated symptoms) | Patient began wearing frequent replacement soft contact lenses 1 week ago. She is looking for information about the proper care of her lenses. She is currently using the regimen she used with her old soft lenses. Her doctor told her she could eliminate some steps but she can't remember which ones. She is starting a new job that will involve travel, so she would like to simplify her care regimen. |

## CASE 29-2 (continued)

| Relevant Evaluation Criteria | Scenario/Model Outcome |
|---|---|
| b. description of any factors that seem to precipitate, exacerbate, and/or relieve the patient's symptom(s) | The patient had worn soft contact lenses for the prior 5 years. In the past she has used a surface active cleaner (Opti-Clean II), Ultracare hydrogen peroxide disinfection, and Ultrazyme for weekly enzymatic cleaning with good results, but she would like to eliminate some steps if possible. |
| c. description of the patient's efforts to relieve the symptoms | N/A |
| 2. Gather essential patient history information: | |
| a. patient's identity | Elizabeth Walsh |
| b. patient's age, sex, height, and weight | 43 y/o F |
| c. patient's occupation | Pediatrician |
| d. patient's dietary habits | N/A |
| e. patient's sleep habits | Has a regular sleep schedule except for the nights she is on call |
| f. concurrent medical conditions, prescription and nonprescription medications, and dietary supplements | Acetaminophen as needed for occasional headaches and pseudoephedrine for occasional nasal congestion |
| g. allergies | NKA |
| h. history of other adverse reactions to medications | History of sensitivity to topical thimerosal |
| i. other (describe)_______ | She does not smoke and is a social drinker (an occasional glass of wine or a cocktail). |
| **Assessment and Triage** | |
| 3. Differentiate the patient's signs/symptoms and correctly identify the patient's primary problem(s). | Elizabeth has switched to a frequent replacement lens and would like to simplify her lens care routine. |
| 4. Identify exclusions for self-treatment. | None |
| 5. Formulate a comprehensive list of therapeutic alternatives for the primary problem to determine if triage to a medical practitioner is required, and share this information with the patient. | Options include:<br>(1) Refer Elizabeth to her eye care practitioner.<br>(2) Recommend a change in her lens care routine.<br>(3) Take no action and have her continue with her current regimen. |
| **Plan** | |
| 6. Select an optimal therapeutic alternative to address the patient's problem, taking into account patient preferences. | Recommend a no-rub hydrogen peroxide product such as AO Sept Clear Care. |
| 7. Describe the recommended therapeutic approach to the patient. | Because you are wearing frequent replacement lenses, you can try a one-bottle simplified regimen such as Clear Care. Remove the lenses from your eye and place them in the lens holder. Thoroughly rinse each side of the lens for 5 seconds through the basket with the Clear Care solution.<br>Fill the lens case to the fill line with fresh solution. Place the lens basket into the solution and tighten the cap. Store lenses in the closed lens case overnight or at least 6 hours. After soaking, lenses are ready to wear. The lenses may be left in the unopened lens case for up to 7 days prior to wear. Never rinse your lenses with Clear Care prior to insertion. Fill your case with fresh solution every time you store your lenses. Never reuse solution. |
| 8. Explain to the patient the rationale for selecting the recommended therapeutic approach from the considered therapeutic alternatives. | Many options are appropriate to care for your lenses. Since you will be replacing them every 2 weeks, you can start out with a no-rub peroxide product such as AO-Sept Clear Care. Other options include multipurpose solutions such as ReNu with MoistureLoc, AMO Complete Moisture Plus, and Opti-Free Express. |

**CASE 29-2 (continued)**

| Relevant Evaluation Criteria | Scenario/Model Outcome |
|---|---|
| **Patient Education** | |
| 9. When recommending self-care with nonprescription medications and/or nondrug therapy, convey accurate information to the patient, including: | |
| a. appropriate dose and frequency of administration | Use this product every time you wear your contact lenses. |
| b. maximum number of days the therapy should be employed | N/A |
| c. product administration procedures | N/A |
| d. expected time to onset of relief | N/A |
| e. degree of relief that can be reasonably expected | N/A |
| f. most common side effects | Stinging, burning, itching (uncommon for most people) |
| g. side effects that warrant medical intervention should they occur | If the lenses stop feeling comfortable or visual acuity is lessened, a different lens care regimen may be necessary. Some patients are heavy depositors on their lenses and benefit from using cleaning products such as Mira Flow or Opti-Clean II and digital cleaning of their lenses. |
| h. patient options in the event that condition worsens or persists | The lens prescriber should be consulted if the patient does not get good results from the recommended lens care regimen. |
| i. product storage requirements | Store at room temperature. |
| j. specific nondrug measures | N/A |
| 10. Solicit patient's follow-up questions. | Are there other products that I could use? |
| 11. Answer patient's questions. | There are many other soft contact lens products that could be used. However, based on the fact that you have frequent replacement lenses, you can start out with one of the simpler regimens (no-rub, one bottle) to see if it is adequate for your needs. |

Key: N/A, not applicable; NKA, no known allergies.

## Key Points for Prevention of Contact Lens–related Disorders

- Following the prescribed lens care program is the best strategy for avoiding lens wear–related problems.
- The practitioner should explain the care regimen for the patient's particular lens type and stress that the patient should use only the products recommended for his or her lenses.
- Instructions on avoiding practices or situations that can cause eye irritation or lens damage are also important in educating the patient about successful wearing of contact lenses. The patient should also be advised of signs and symptoms that indicate medical care is needed.

## References


1. Weisbarth RE, McCartnery DL. In: Kastl PR, ed. *Contact Lenses, The CLAO Guide to Basic Science and Clinical Practice.* 3rd ed. Dubuque, Iowa: Kendall/Hunt Publishing; 1995;II:113-29.
2. Yamaguchi T, Hubbard A, Fukushima A, et al. Fungus growth on soft contact lenses with different water contents. *CLAO J.* 1984;10:166-71.
3. Contact Lens Council 2003. Available at: http://www.contactlenscouncil.org/stats.htm. Accessed February 16, 2005.
4. Rakow PL. Mixing contact lens solutions. *J Ophthalmic Nurs Technol.* 1989;8:67-8.
5. Diefenbach CB, Seibert CK, Davis LJ. Analysis of two home remedy contact lens cleaners. *J Am Optom Assoc.* 1988;59:518-21.
6. Bartlett JD. In: *Ophthalmic Drug Facts.* St. Louis: Facts and Comparisons; 2005:301-10.

## PATIENT EDUCATION FOR PREVENTING CONTACT LENS–RELATED DISORDERS

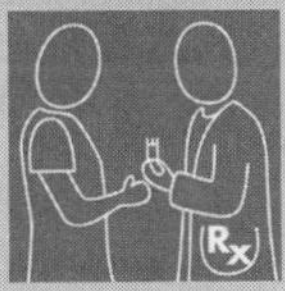

The objective of contact lens care is to prevent lens-related problems such as abrasions or infections of the cornea. For most patients, following the prescribed lens care regimen, product instructions, and self-care measures listed here will help ensure trouble-free use of contact lenses.

### General Instructions for All Contact Lens Types

- Wash hands with noncosmetic soap and rinse thoroughly before touching contact lenses.
- Avoid wearing oily cosmetics while wearing lenses. Bath oils or soaps with an oil or a cream base may leave an oil film on the hands that will be transferred to the lenses.
- To avoid mixing up the lenses, always work with the same lens first. Check hard lenses for a dot in the lens periphery to avoid confusing lenses.
- If the lenses are not comfortable after insertion or vision is blurred, check to see if they are on the wrong eyes or are inside out.
- To avoid damaging lenses, apply aerosol cosmetics and deodorants either before lens insertion or with eyes closed until the air is clear of spray particles.
- Except for prescription continuous-wear lenses, do not wear lenses while sleeping.
- To avoid excessive dryness of the eyes, do not wear lenses while sitting under a hair dryer, overhead fans, or air ducts.
- When lenses are worn outside on windy days, protect the eyes from soot and other particles that may become trapped under the lens and scratch the cornea.
- Use eye protection in industry, sports, or any other occupation or hobby that has the potential for eye damage.
- Store contact lenses in a proper lens case when not in use.
- Never reuse contact lens solutions.
- Replace soaking/disinfecting solutions in lens case after each use. Don't top off the storage solution in the case after it has been used.
- Never store lenses in tap water.
- Do not wear contact lenses in swimming pools, hot tubs, or natural bodies of water without external eye protection such as goggles.
- To prevent contamination, do not touch dropper tips or the tips of lens care product containers.
- While wearing lenses, apply to the eyes only ophthalmic solutions specifically formulated for contact lens use.
- Never use saliva to wet contact lenses. This practice can result in eye infections.

⚠ Do not insert lenses in red or irritated eyes. If the eyes become irritated while lenses are being worn, remove the lenses until the irritation subsides. If irritation or redness does not subside, consult an eye care practitioner.

⚠ If an eye infection is suspected, see an eye care practitioner immediately.

### Instructions for Hard Lenses

- Do not store lenses dry.
- Clean lenses every time they are removed from the eyes. See Tables 29-2 and 29-3 for cleaning procedures.
- Inspect lenses regularly for chips and scratches.
- Do not rub eyes while lenses are in place.
- Do not rinse contact lenses with very hot or very cold water because temperature extremes may warp the lenses.
- Do not get oils or lanolin on the lens.

### Instructions for RGP Lenses

- See Tables 29-2 and 29-7 for guidelines on cleaning RGP lenses.
- Do not use tap water to rinse off cleaner or to rewet lenses. If tap water is used, disinfect lenses before inserting them in the eyes.[23]
- Do not disinfect these lenses with thermal disinfecting systems.
- See Table 29-13 for guidelines on using other types of disinfecting systems.

### Instructions for Soft Lenses

- See Tables 29-2, 29-11, and 29-13 for guidelines on cleaning and disinfecting these lenses.
- Handle soft lenses carefully because they are very fragile and can easily be torn.
- Remove these lenses before instilling any ophthalmic preparation not specifically intended for concurrent use with soft contact lenses. Wait at least 20 to 30 minutes before reinserting the lenses unless directed otherwise by an eye care practitioner.
- Do not wear lenses when a topical ophthalmic ointment is being used.
- Do not wear soft contact lenses in the presence of irritating fumes or chemicals.

### Instructions for Continuous-wear Lenses (RGP or Soft)

- Remove mascara before sleeping because mascara can flake off during sleep and become trapped underneath the lens.[24]
- If lenses appear to be lost on awakening, check eyes to see if the lenses were displaced. Soft lenses can fold over on themselves and get lodged underneath the top or bottom eyelid.

⚠ Each morning, check eyes carefully for unusual, persistent redness, discharge, or pain. If redness does not abate within 45 minutes or discharge or pain is present, remove the lens and call the lens care practitioner.

⚠ Check vision after inserting lenses. (Some hazy vision is normal on awakening because of corneal hypoxia, which develops overnight.) Apply a few drops of rewetting solution to improve hydration of the lens and help resolve hypoxia. If the problem is not resolved, remove lenses, clean them, and reinsert. If vision is not improved within an hour, remove lenses and call your lens prescriber.

7. Key JE, Bennett ES. In: Kastl PR, ed. *Contact Lenses, The CLAO Guide to Basic Science and Clinical Practice.* 3rd ed. Dubuque, Iowa: Kendall/Hunt Publishing; 1995;II:51-74.
8. Nichols JJ. The controversy of contact lens convenience. *Contact Lens Spectrum.* January 2000;32-5.
9. Krezanoski JZ. Topical medications. *Int Ophthalmol Clin.* 1981;21: 173-6.
10. Harris MG. Practical considerations in the use of hydrogen peroxide disinfection systems. *CLAO J.* 1990;16(suppl 1):S53-60.
11. Wittman G. Personal communication of data on file at company. Irvine, Calif: Allergan, Inc; January 17, 1995.
12. Barr JT. Contact lens solutions and lens care update. *Contact Lens Spectrum.* June 2001;26-33.
13. Krezanoski JZ, Dabezies OH. In: Dabezies OH, ed. *Contact Lenses, The CLAO Guide to Basic Science and Clinical Practice.* 2nd ed. Boston: Little, Brown and Co; 1992:31.1-31.17.
14. Driebe WT. In: Kastl PR, ed. *Contact Lenses, The CLAO Guide to Basic Science and Clinical Practice.* 3rd ed. Dubuque, Iowa: Kendall/Hunt Publishing; 1995;II:237-62.
15. Macsai MS, Goel AK, Michael MM, et al. Deposition of ciprofloxacin, prednisolone phosphate, and prednisolone acetate in SeeQuence disposable contact lenses. *CLAO J.* 1993;19:166-8.
16. Lee BL, Matoba AY, Osato MS, et al. The solubility of antibiotic and corticosteroid combinations. *Am J Ophthalmol.* 1992;114:212-5.
17. Plotnik RD, Mannis MJ, Schwab IR. Therapeutic contact lenses. Int *Ophthalmol Clin.* 1991;31:35-52.
18. Diamond SA, Dupuis LL. Contact lens damage due to ribavirin exposure. *DICP Ann Pharmacother.* 1989;23:428-9.
19. Rodriguez WJ, Bui RH, Connon JD, et al. Environmental exposure of primary care personnel to ribavirin aerosol when supervising treatment of infants with respiratory syncytial virus infections. *Antimicrob Agents Chemother.* 1987;31:1143-6.
20. Broich J, Weiss L, Rapp J. Isolation and identification of biologically active contaminants from soft contact lenses. *Invest Ophthalmol Vis Sci.* 1980;19:1328-35.
21. Miller D. Systemic medications. *Int Ophthalmol Clin.* 1981;21:177-83.
22. Schornack JA. Drugs and pupillary interaction in contact lens practice. *Contact Lens Spectrum.* May 2003;46.
23. Campbell RC, Caroline PJ. RGPs and tap water. *Contact Lens Forum.* 1990;15:64.
24. Key JE, Bennett ES. In: Kastl PR, ed. *Contact Lenses, The CLAO Guide to Basic Science and Clinical Practice.* 3rd ed. Dubuque, Iowa: Kendall/Hunt Publishing; 1995;II:51-74.

CHAPTER 30

# Otic Disorders

*Linda Krypel*

Ear complaints are common and vary from simple complaints of excessive earwax (cerumen) or itching to painful ear infections. Ear disorders affect all ages, with younger patients and patients of advanced age being the most prone.

Self-treatment with nonprescription medications and complementary therapies should be restricted to external ear disorders, which include disorders of the auricle and the external auditory canal (EAC). Excessive cerumen and water-clogged ears are self-treatable EAC disorders for which the Food and Drug Administration (FDA) has approved nonprescription otic medications. Other self-treatable disorders of the auricle include allergic and contact dermatitis, seborrhea, psoriasis, and boils. Nonprescription medications used to treat the latter disorders when they appear on other parts of the body are also appropriate for treating the auricle. If improvement does not occur quickly, the patient should be referred to a physician.

Diseases in the head and neck can cause referred pain, which the patient often perceives as pain originating from the ear. The health care practitioner must determine the cause of pain prior to recommending self-treatment or referral to a primary care provider (PCP). Assessment of self-treatable disorders is covered in Patient Assessment of Otic Disorders. Collective discussions of patient counseling and evaluation of patient outcomes for the various self-treatable disorders are also presented at the end of the chapter.

## EPIDEMIOLOGY OF OTIC DISORDERS

Otic disorders account for 1.5% of ambulatory care visits per year.[1] Cerumen impaction can affect up to 6% of the general and almost 30% of the elderly population.[2,3] Hearing loss is the third most common chronic condition in older Americans after hypertension and arthritis.[4]

## ANATOMY AND PHYSIOLOGY OF THE EAR

The external ear consists of the auricle (also called the pinna) and the EAC (Figure 30-1), and is closed by the tympanic membrane (eardrum), which separates the external ear from the middle ear.[5] The auricle is composed of a thin layer of highly vascular skin that is tightly bound to cartilage. Adipose or subcutaneous tissue, which would insulate blood vessels, is absent except in the lobe. The lobe has fewer blood vessels and is composed primarily of fatty tissue. The triangular piece of cartilage in front of the ear canal adjacent to the cheek (not shown in Figure 30-1) is called the tragus.

The EAC consists of an outer cartilaginous portion, which comprises one third to one half of its length, plus an inner body or osseous portion.[5] The canal forms a blind cul-de-sac. Children have a shorter, straighter, and flatter EAC than adults, whose canals tend to lengthen and form an "S" shape.[5,6] At the same time, an adult's eustachian tube (part of the inner ear) lengthens downward as it enters the nasal cavity. This shape helps to promote drainage and inhibits aspiration of pharyngeal and nasal contents into the middle ear, which may help to explain why children suffer from more middle ear infections than do adults.[5,6]

The skin that covers the auricle is especially susceptible to bleeding when scratched because of the lack of flexibility usually afforded by a subcutaneous layer of fat and the large blood supply to the area.[5] The skin is highly innervated, causing a disproportionate otalgia (ear pain) when inflammation is present. Skin farther into the EAC is thicker and contains apocrine and exocrine glands as well as hair follicles.[7] The skin in the canal is continuous with the outer layer of the tympanic membrane.

Oily secretions from the exocrine glands mix with the milky, fatty fluid from the apocrine glands to form cerumen, which appears on the surface of the skin on the outer half of the EAC. Cerumen lubricates the canal, traps dust and foreign materials, and provides a waxy, waterproof barrier to the entry of pathogens.[7,8] It also contains various antimicrobial substances such as lysozymes, and it has an acidic pH, which aids in the inhibition of bacterial and fungal growth.[7,9]

The canal skin is shed continuously and mixes with cerumen. The debris-laden cerumen slowly migrates outward with jaw movements (such as chewing and talking). This serves as a process of self-cleaning.[8] Cerumen may appear dry and flaky or oily and pastelike. Color varies from light gray to orange or brown and may darken on exposure to air.[10]

The normal tympanic membrane or eardrum is smooth, translucent, and pearl gray. It is concave and oval with an average thickness of 0.074 mm and is composed of three layers. The continuous skin layer of the EAC forms the outer tympanic membrane layer. The middle layer is fibrous tissue, and the internal layer is a mucous membrane continuous with the lining of the middle ear.[5] The

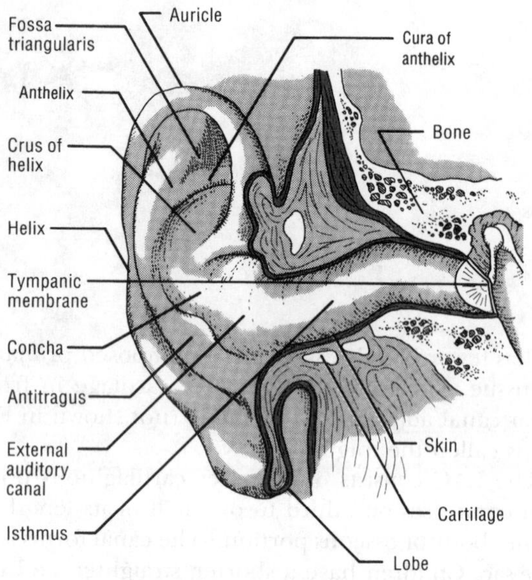


**FIGURE 30-1** Anatomy of the auricle and external ear.

tympanic membrane transmits sound waves and acts as a protective barrier to the middle ear.[8]

The natural defenses of the ear canal include the skin layer with its protective coating of cerumen, an acidic pH, and hairs that line the outer half of the canal. Together, they protect against injury from foreign material and infection. It is important for the clinician to explain the normal role and function of cerumen when educating patients.

## PATHOPHYSIOLOGY OF OTIC DISORDERS

Because the EAC forms a blind cul-de-sac, it is especially prone to collecting moisture. Its dark, warm, moist environment is ideal for fungal and bacterial growth. In the preinflammatory stage, moisture, local trauma, or both remove the lipid layer covering the skin. Local trauma from fingernails, cotton-tipped swabs, or other items inserted into the canal can abrade the skin and allow pathogens to enter. Because a normal, healthy ear canal is impervious to potentially pathogenic organisms, skin integrity generally must be interrupted before an organism can produce an infection. Trauma to the ear from thermal injuries, sports injuries, ear piercing, and poorly fitting or improperly cleaned ear molds or hearing aids can contribute to the breakdown of the EAC's natural defenses.[11] Dermatologic skin disorders, such as contact dermatitis, seborrhea, psoriasis, and malignancies, also compromise these defenses.[7]

Viral illnesses, such as colds and upper respiratory infections, can contribute to the breakdown of natural defenses of the middle and inner ear, especially in children, who are very susceptible to middle ear infections following such illnesses. Because a child's eustachian tube is shorter and angled flatter than an adult's, it is commonly believed that nasopharyngeal secretions can easily be aspirated and accumulate in the middle ear, leading to proliferation of bacteria. Holding back or trying to stifle a sneeze can force secretions into the middle ear and thus should be strongly discouraged, even in adults.

## EXCESSIVE/IMPACTED CERUMEN

Cerumen can be considered an undervalued defense system. Widespread misinformation has often led the public to believe that cerumen production is a pathologic condition and it must be continually removed. In fact, improper or excessive attempts to remove cerumen can actually damage the EAC.[9]

### Etiology/Pathophysiology of Excessive/Impacted Cerumen

Individuals with abnormally narrow or misshapen EACs and/or excessive hair growth in the canal are predisposed to impacted cerumen. These physiologic anomalies disrupt the normal migration of cerumen to the outer EAC. Individuals who have overactive ceruminous glands or who wear hearing aids, earplugs, and sound attenuators often suffer from impacted cerumen. Such devices worn in the ear can inhibit the migration of cerumen, causing wax buildup.[9,12]

Older adults often experience impacted cerumen resulting from atrophy of ceruminous glands.[8] This population secretes drier cerumen, which is more difficult to expel from the ear.

### Signs and Symptoms of Excessive/Impacted Cerumen

The most common symptoms of impacted cerumen are a sense of fullness or pressure in the ear and a gradual hearing loss. A dull pain is sometimes associated with this disorder.

### Complications of Excessive/Impacted Cerumen

Attempting to remove cerumen by means of cotton-tipped applicators, bobby pins, toothpicks, fingernails, or other such objects can force the cerumen into the inner half of the EAC, where it becomes hardened and compacted over time.[8,13] Hearing loss can occur as well as, rarely, vertigo (a sensation of spinning or whirling) or pain.[10] The delicate skin of the auditory canal can also be scratched or damaged, providing an entry point for water and pathogens.[8,9,12] Hardened cerumen generally does not cling to cotton-tipped applicators and using them may serve only to remove the protective waxy layer and force the cerumen plug further into the canal. Cerumen whose migration to the outer EAC is blocked by devices in the ear will also harden and become compacted. Frequent removal and proper cleaning of ear devices may help prevent wax buildup.

**Exclusions for Self-Treatment**

- Signs of infection
- Pain associated with ear discharge
- Bleeding or signs of trauma
- Presence of ruptured tympanic membrane
- Ear surgery within prior 6 weeks
- Tympanostomy tubes present
- Incapable of following proper instructions
- Hypersensitivity to recommended agents
- < 12 years of age

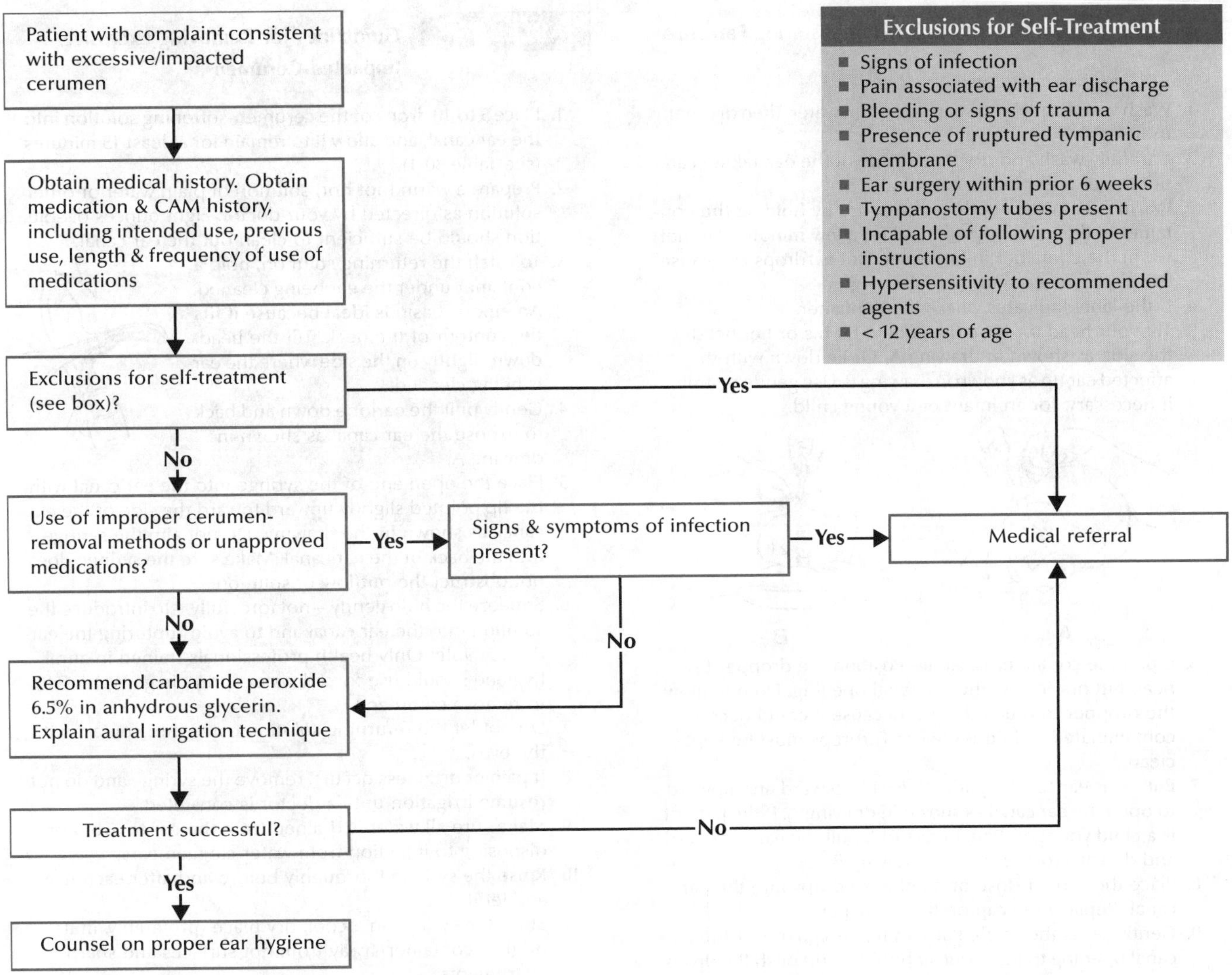


FIGURE 30-2 Self-care of excessive/impacted cerumen. Key: CAM, complementary and alternative medicine.

## Treatment of Excessive/Impacted Cerumen

### *Treatment Goals*

The goal of treatment of excessive/impacted cerumen is to soften it using proper methods and safe, effective agents. Proper treatment should eliminate temporary hearing loss and other symptoms.

### *General Treatment Approach*

The initial step in removing impacted cerumen is the use of a safe and effective agent to soften cerumen prior to gently irrigating the ear, using an otic bulb syringe filled with warm water. Caution must be used to ensure complete water removal, to avoid a possible infection because of water-clogged ears. Cotton-tipped swabs or other foreign objects should not be used to remove cerumen or water. The algorithm in Figure 30-2 outlines the appropriate self-treatment of excessive/impacted cerumen and lists exclusions for self-treatment.

### *Nonpharmacologic Therapy*

Earwax should be removed only when it has migrated to the outermost portion of the EAC. The only recommended nonpharmacologic method of removing cerumen is to use a wet, wrung-out washcloth draped over a finger. Making this procedure part of daily aural hygiene can prevent impacted cerumen if physiologic abnormalities or physical devices are not the cause of the impaction. This method is not effective once cerumen becomes impacted.

### *Pharmacologic Therapy*

Carbamide peroxide 6.5% in anhydrous glycerin is currently the only FDA-approved nonprescription cerumen-softening agent.[14] Other agents such as mineral oil, olive oil (sweet oil), glycerin, docusate sodium, and dilute hydrogen peroxide have been used by primary care providers and patients as inexpensive home remedies to soften cerumen. There are no data, however, to support these remedies as being more effective than carbamide peroxide in anhydrous glycerin.

**TABLE 30-1 Guidelines for Administering Eardrops**

1. Wash your hands with soap and warm water; then dry them thoroughly.
2. Carefully wash and dry the outside of the ear, taking care not to get water in the ear canal.
3. Warm eardrops to body temperature by holding the container in the palm of your hand for a few minutes. Do not warm the container in hot water. Hot eardrops can cause ear pain, nausea, and dizziness.
4. If the label indicates, shake the container.
5. Tilt your head (or have the patient tilt his or her head) to the side as shown in drawing A. Or lie down with the affected ear up as shown in drawing B. Use gentle restraint, if necessary, for an infant or a young child.

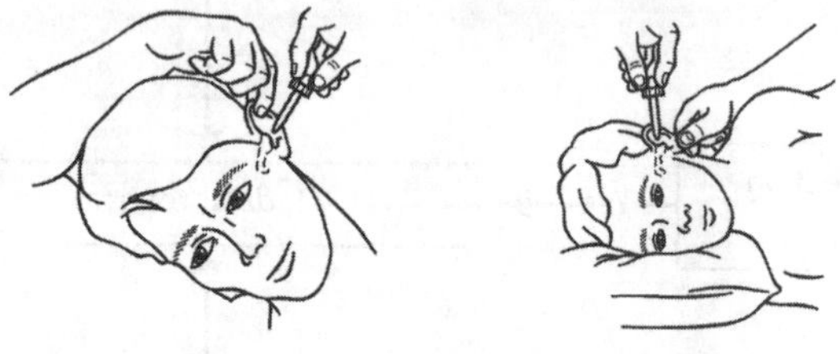

A B

6. Open the container carefully. Position the dropper tip near, but not inside, the ear canal opening. Do not allow the dropper to touch the ear, because it could become contaminated or injure the ear. Eardrops must be kept clean.
7. Pull your ear (or the patient's ear) backward and upward to open the ear canal as shown in drawing A. If the patient is a child younger than 3 years old, pull the ear backward and downward as shown in drawing B.
8. Place the proper dose or number of drops into the ear canal. Replace the cap on the container.
9. Gently press the small, flat skin flap (tragus) over the ear canal opening to force out air bubbles and push the drops down the ear canal.
10. Stay (or keep the patient) in the same position for the length of time indicated in the product instructions. If the patient is a child who cannot stay still, the doctor may tell you to place a clean piece of cotton gently into the child's ear to prevent the medication from draining out. Use a piece large enough to remove easily, and do not leave it in the ear longer than an hour.
11. Repeat the procedure for the other ear, if needed.
12. Gently wipe excess medication off the outside of the ear, using caution to avoid getting moisture in the ear canal.
13. Wash your hands.

*Source: APhA Special Report: Medication Administration Problem Solving in Ambulatory Care.* Washington, DC: American Pharmaceutical Association; 1994:9.

## Carbamide Peroxide

Carbamide peroxide 6.5% in anhydrous glycerin is approved as safe and effective in softening, loosening, and removing excessive earwax in adults and in children 12 years and older.[14] (See Table 30-1 for the proper instillation of eardrops.) Carbamide peroxide is prepared from hydrogen peroxide and urea. When carbamide peroxide is exposed to moisture, nascent oxygen is released slowly and acts as a weak antibacterial. The effervescence that occurs during this process, along with urea's effect on tissue debridement, helps to mechanically break down and loosen cerumen that has been softened by anhydrous glycerin.

Any cerumen remaining after treatment may be removed with gentle, warm-water irrigation using a rubber otic bulb syringe (Table 30-2). Improper use of an otic syringe or using an oral jet irrigator to remove cerumen can leave excess moisture in the canal or further compress cerumen. These actions can also cause otitis externa, perforated tympanic membrane, pain, vertigo, otitis media, tinnitus (ringing, hissing, or buzzing noises in the ear), and cough.[12,15,16]

Carbamide peroxide solution is nonirritating and may be used twice daily for up to 4 days. If symptoms persist after 4 days, the patient should see a primary care provider for evaluation.[17]

**TABLE 30-2 Guidelines for Removing Excessive/Impacted Cerumen**

1. Place 5 to 10 drops of the cerumen-softening solution into the ear canal, and allow it to remain for at least 15 minutes (see Table 30-1).
2. Prepare a warm (not hot) solution of plain water or other solution as directed by your doctor. Eight ounces of solution should be sufficient to clean out the ear canal.
3. To catch the returning solution, hold a container under the ear being cleaned. An emesis basin is ideal because it fits the contour of the neck. Tilt the head down slightly on the side where the ear is being cleaned.

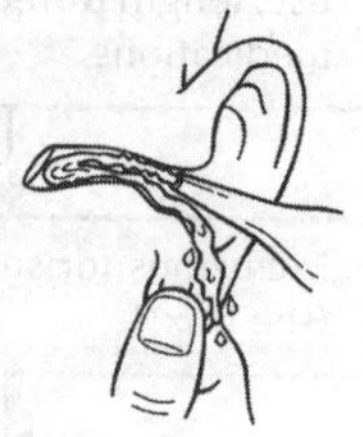

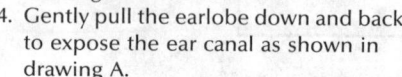

4. Gently pull the earlobe down and back to expose the ear canal as shown in drawing A.
5. Place the open end of the syringe into the ear canal with the tip pointed slightly upward toward the side of the ear canal, as shown in the drawing. Do not aim the syringe into the back of the ear canal. Make sure the syringe does not obstruct the outflow of solution.
6. Squeeze the bulb gently—not forcefully—to introduce the solution into the ear canal and to avoid rupturing the eardrum. (Note: Only health professionals trained in aural hygiene should use forced water sprays [e.g., Water Pik] to remove cerumen.)
7. Do not let the returning solution come into contact with the eyes.
8. If pain or dizziness occurs, remove the syringe and do not resume irrigation until a doctor is consulted.
9. Make sure all water is drained from the ear to avoid predisposing to infection from water-clogged ears.
10. Rinse the syringe thoroughly before and after each use, and let it dry.
11. Store the syringe in a cool, dry place (preferably, in its original container) away from hot surfaces and sharp instruments.
12. Do this procedure twice daily for no longer than 4 consecutive days.

*Source:* Adapted with permission from *Ohio Clinician*. 1996; 14(5):10.

**TABLE 30-3 Selected Products for Otic Disorders**

| Trade Name | Primary Ingredients |
|---|---|
| **Cerumen-softening Products** | |
| Auro Ear Drops | Carbamide peroxide 6.5%; anhydrous glycerin |
| Debrox | Carbamide peroxide 6.5%; glycerin; propylene glycol; sodium stannate |
| E.R.O. Ear | Carbamide peroxide 6.5%; anhydrous glycerin |
| Mollifene Ear Wax Removal Formula | Carbamide peroxide 6.5%; anhydrous glycerin; propylene glycol; sodium stannate |
| Murine Earwax Removal System | Carbamide peroxide 6.5%; glycerin; alcohol 6.3%; polysorbate 20; packaged with syringe |
| **Ear-drying Products** | |
| Auro-Dri Drops | Isopropyl alcohol 95%; boric acid 2.75% |
| Dri Ear | Isopropyl alcohol 95%; boric acid 2.75% |
| Ear Dry Drops | Isopropyl alcohol 95%; boric acid 2.75% |
| Swim Ear Drops | Isopropyl alcohol 95%; anhydrous glycerin |
| **Botanical and Homeopathic Products** | |
| Earsol Drops | Alcohol 44%; propylene glycol; yerba santa; benzyl benzoate |
| Earsol-HC Drops | Alcohol 44%; hydrocortisone 1%; propylene glycol; yerba santa; benzyl benzoate |
| Similasan Healthy Relief Homeopathic Ear Drops | Chamomilla HPUS 10X; Mercurius solubus HPUS 15X; sulfur HPUS 12X |
| **Acidifying Products** | |
| Star Otic Solution | Nonaqueous acetic acid; Burow's solution; boric acid; propylene glycol |

Key: *HPUS, Homeopathic Pharmacopoeia of the United States.*

### Docusate Sodium

Docusate sodium is classified as an emollient and has been used by some physicians to soften earwax. Evidence for its effectiveness over approved agents is lacking.

### Glycerin

Glycerin has emollient and humectant properties and is widely used as a solvent and vehicle.[18] It is safe and nonsensitizing when applied to abraded skin. It has been used to soften earwax.

### Hydrogen Peroxide

Hydrogen peroxide releases nascent oxygen when exposed to moisture and acts as a weak antibacterial.[18] A 1:1 solution of warm water and hydrogen peroxide 3% can be used to flush the ear canal when softening or removing earwax.[19] This solution, however, is not an effective ear-drying agent. Overuse of 1:1 aqueous hydrogen peroxide solutions may predispose the ear to infection from tissue maceration because of excessive water left in the canal.

### Olive Oil (Sweet Oil)

Olive oil is used as an emollient and has been used to soften earwax.[18] It has also been used in the ear canal to alleviate itching.[20]

### Product Selection Guidelines

Although overall costs of FDA-approved and nonapproved agents are low, docusate sodium is more expensive, has poor results, and causes superficial erythema in some cases and thus should not be recommended.[21,22] Table 30-3 lists examples of cerumen-softening and other otic products.

## *Complementary Therapies*

Although major herbal references do not list herbal remedies for otic disorders,[23-25] some folk remedies remain popular in many regions. One of the more interesting—and dangerous—is the use of ear candles to remove cerumen. A hollow candle is burned with one end inserted in the ear canal. The intent is to create negative pressure and draw cerumen from the ear. Studies have shown this method does not aid in removing cerumen but has caused serious ear injuries.[26] Candle wax was deposited in the ear canal in some patients, and severe blockages and burns have occurred. One survey of 122 otolaryngologists identified 21 ear injuries resulting from the use of ear candles.[26]

The herb yerba santa is listed as an ingredient in two available products. It contains flavonoids such as eriodictyol and tannins. Eriodictyol is reported to exert an expectorant effect when taken orally. Although the manufacturer lists yerba santa as a dermprotective factor, there is no evidence for safety and effectiveness of yerba santa used topically.[23-25] A homeopathic product is available, but no published studies document safety and effectiveness (Table 30-3).

## WATER-CLOGGED EARS

Water-clogged ears is a separate disorder from swimmer's ear (external otitis). FDA has not approved any nonprescription products for preventing or treating external otitis. Manufacturers have argued that removing moisture from a water-clogged ears with an approved agent may prevent tissue maceration, a process that can lead to inflammation and infection of the EAC (commonly referred to as swimmer's ear). FDA, however, prohibits this extrapolation and manufacturers may no longer label their products as preventing swimmer's ear.[27,28] Most available nonprescription products for water-clogged ears have been reformulated to contain only FDA-approved ingredients.

### Etiology of Water-clogged Ears

Some patients are more prone to retaining water because of the shape of their ear canals or the presence of excessive cerumen,[7] which can swell, thereby trapping water. Excessive moisture in the ears can result from hot, humid climates, sweating, swimming, bathing, or improper use of aqueous solutions to cleanse the ear. Thus, simple attempts to remove water by mechanical manipulation may be insufficient.

### Signs and Symptoms of Water-clogged Ears

A feeling of wetness or fullness in the ear, accompanied by gradual hearing loss, can occur after exposure to any of the etiologic factors. The trapped moisture can compromise the natural defenses of the EAC, causing tissue maceration that, in turn, can lead to itching, pain, inflammation, or infection.[9]

### Treatment of Water-clogged Ears

#### *Treatment Goals*

The goals of treating a water-clogged ears are to dry it using a safe and effective agent, and to prevent recurrences in persons who are prone to retaining moisture in the ears.

#### *General Treatment Approach*

Before recommending an agent to treat water-clogged ears, the clinician should determine whether a patient has a ruptured tympanic membrane or has a tympanostomy tube in place. Ear-drying agents are very painful if instilled in either of these situations. Figure 30-2 lists additional exclusions to self-treatment.

The algorithm in Figure 30-3 outlines the appropriate treatment of water-clogged ears. The clinician should recommend either a product containing isopropyl alcohol 95% in anhydrous glycerin 5% or an extemporaneously compounded 50:50 mixture of isopropyl alcohol 95% and acetic acid 5%.

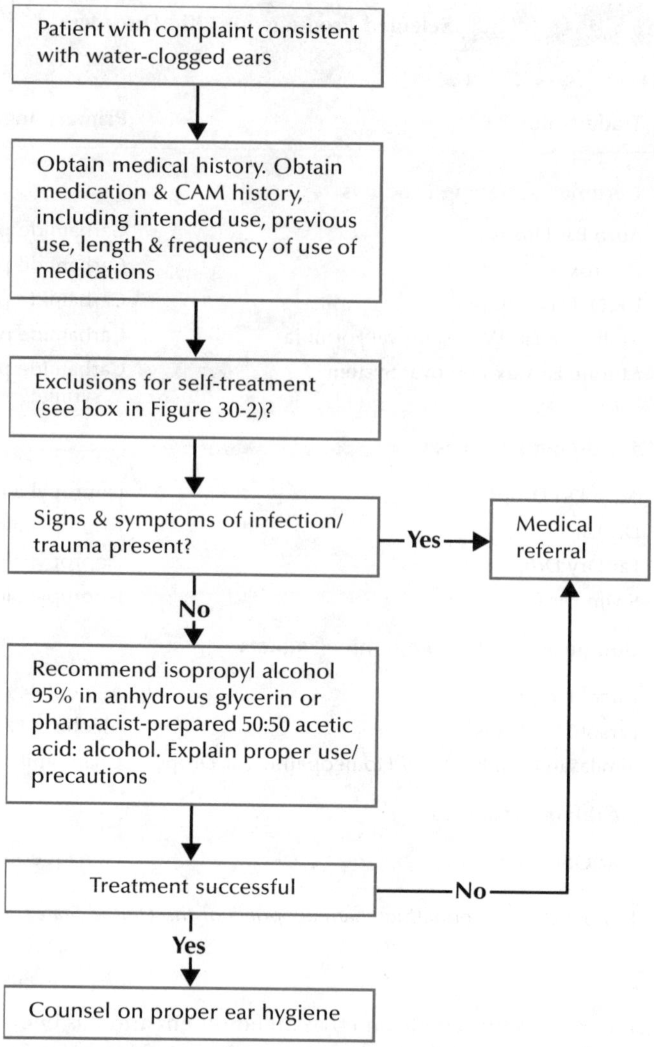


FIGURE 30-3 Self-care of water-clogged ears. Key: CAM, complementary and alternative medicine.

#### *Nonpharmacologic Therapy*

Tilting the affected ear downward and gently manipulating the auricle can expel excessive water from the ear. This procedure should be performed after swimming or bathing, or during periods of excessive sweating, especially by persons who are prone to developing this disorder. Using a blow-dryer on a low setting around (not directly into) the ear immediately after swimming or bathing may help dry the ear canal.

#### *Pharmacologic Therapy*

FDA has approved only isopropyl alcohol 95% in anhydrous glycerin 5% as a safe and effective "ear-drying aid."[29] (See Table 30-3 for examples of products containing these agents.) In addition, a 50:50 mixture of acetic acid 5% (white household vinegar) and isopropyl alcohol 95% has also commonly been recommended to help dry a water-clogged ears.[7,13,30]

### Isopropyl Alcohol in Anhydrous Glycerin

Alcohol is highly miscible with water and acts as a drying agent. In concentrations greater than 70%, it is also an effective skin disinfectant. Glycerin has been used in pharmaceutical preparations for its solvent, emollient, or hygroscopic properties. It is safe and nonsensitizing when applied to open wounds or abraded skin. Combined with alcohol, glycerin provides a product that reduces moisture in the ear without overdrying.

Ear-drying agents, which are recommended for use in adults and children ages 12 years and older, may be used whenever ears are exposed to water. Table 30-1 presents guidelines for administering these agents. Medical referral is necessary if symptoms persist after several days of simultaneous use of ear-drying agents and prevention of exposure of ears to water. Symptoms of infection also require medical referral.

### Acetic Acid

The acetic acid in a 50:50 mixture of acetic acid 5% and isopropyl alcohol 95% has bactericidal and antifungal properties.[30] Species of *Pseudomonas, Candida,* and *Aspergillus* are particularly sensitive to this agent. As discussed previously, alcohol has anti-infective properties as well, is highly miscible with water, and helps remove water from the ear. Care must be taken to advise patients against using cider vinegar instead of white vinegar. Cider vinegar is produced from fruit and contains impurities that could hinder antibacterial activity.

A 50:50 mixture of these two agents provides an acetic acid 2.5% solution. Concentrations of acetic acid between 2% and 3% may lower the pH of the ear canal below the optimal pH of 6.5 to 7.5 needed for bacterial growth.[31] This solution is well tolerated and nonsensitizing, and does not induce resistant organisms. It may sting or burn slightly, especially if the skin is abraded. The clinician should provide an accurately compounded solution in a proper dropper bottle.

### Boric Acid

Boric acid is added to some commercially prepared ear products to increase product acidity. It is also a very weak germicide. Solutions containing boric acid should be applied only to unbroken skin because it may be toxic if absorbed through broken skin or accidentally swallowed. As little as 5 g of boric acid powder ingested orally can cause serious poisonings.[18] Children are particularly vulnerable to the risk of accidental ingestion. Home preparation and use of extemporaneous solutions of boric acid should not be recommended.

## DERMATOLOGIC DISORDERS OF THE EAR

Self-treatable dermatologic disorders of the external ear include contact dermatitis, seborrhea, psoriasis, and boils.

### Contact Dermatitis

Contact dermatitis is categorized as either allergic contact dermatitis or irritant contact dermatitis. The external ear is susceptible to both types of this dermatitis.

#### *Etiology of Contact Dermatitis*

Topical neomycin, nickel in earrings, poison ivy, and the chemicals used to process the rubber or plastic of hearing aid molds or earphones typically cause allergic reactions of the external ear.[8,9] Soaps and detergents are mild irritants, which generally require repeated or extended contact to cause a significant inflammatory response. However, such substances have been shown to cause reactions similar to allergic contact dermatitis.[8,9] See Chapter 35 for a detailed discussion of the etiology of these disorders.

#### *Signs and Symptoms of Contact Dermatitis*

Allergic dermatitis is associated with various skin manifestations, including maculopapular rash and formation of vesicles. The rash, in turn, causes pruritus, erythema, and edema.

#### *Treatment of Contact Dermatitis*

Dermatitis of the ear frequently is treated with an astringent such as 1:40 aluminum acetate (Burow's solution). Solutions of aluminum acetate have antipruritic, anti-inflammatory, and limited antibacterial properties. They are useful for treating itchy, weeping, swollen conditions of the external ear when diluted to concentrations of 1:10 to 1:40.[18] Astringents precipitate proteins and dry the affected area by reducing the secretory function of skin glands.[18] The dilute solution has an acidic pH that inhibits bacterial and fungal growth. A wet compress of diluted aluminum acetate solution applied several times per day is useful for acute contact dermatitis (see Chapter 35).

### Seborrhea and Psoriasis

Seborrhea and psoriasis are chronic dermatologic disorders usually associated with the scalp, face, and trunk. Seborrhea can usually be managed with nonprescription medications. Psoriasis that involves mild inflammation is sometimes responsive to nonprescription medications. However, a primary care provider or dermatologist should make the initial diagnosis of psoriasis.

#### *Etiology/Signs and Symptoms of Seborrhea and Psoriasis*

Pruritus with visible drying and flaking of the skin is the most common manifestation of seborrhea. Skin fissures may develop, compromising the skin's protective barrier and possibly leading to acute bacterial external otitis.[9,11] Psoriasis of the scalp can extend to the external ear. Psoriasis appears as thickened, erythematous, silvery scaling lesions that occur most frequently on the knees, elbows, torso, and scalp. Cold weather and stress appear to aggravate psoriasis.[32] See Chapter 34 for a detailed discussion of the etiology of these disorders.

**TABLE 30-4 Differentiation of Common Otic Disorders**

| Disorder | Etiology | Pain |
|---|---|---|
| Ruptured tympanic membrane | Otitis media or trauma to ear such as sharp blows, diving into water, forceful irrigation of ear | Brief, severe |
| External otitis (swimmer's ear) | Local trauma to EAC caused by excessive moisture or abrasions; subsequent fungal/bacterial infections | Acute onset, varies from mild to severe, increases with movement of tragus or auricle |
| Otitis media | Bacterial infection of middle ear, usually following upper respiratory tract infections | Sharp, steady, frequently unilateral; does not increase with movement of tragus or auricle |
| Foreign object in ear | Insects, insertion of objects by children, hearing aids, sound attenuators | Dull to severe pain with sense of fullness or pressure while chewing |
| Trauma to ear | Burns from curling iron, frostbite, hematomas/injuries from contact sports or ill-fitting helmets, ear piercing, improper cerumen removal techniques, abrasions of EAC, rapid changes in air pressure | Varies from sharp and steady to brief and severe |
| Tinnitus | Hearing disorders, blockage of EAC, exposure to high noise levels, acoustic trauma, systemic diseases, drug toxicities (salicylate, quinidine, aminoglycosides, and other antibiotics) | Possible |
| Excessive/impacted cerumen | Overactive ceruminous glands, obstructed migration of cerumen | Rare, dull pain if present |
| Water-clogged ears | Excessive moisture in EAC | None |
| Boils | Localized staphylococcal infections of hair follicles | Often |

Key: EAC, external auditory canal.

### *Treatment of Seborrhea and Psoriasis*

Treating the scalp with antiseborrheic shampoos often relieves the symptoms of this disorder. Medicated shampoos can be used to treat mild cases of psoriasis of the scalp. Topical hydrocortisone is also useful in treating these disorders (see Chapter 34).

## Boils

Boils (furuncles) are usually localized infections of the hair follicles. Boils on the auricle are self-treatable; those that appear in the EAC require medical referral.

### *Etiology of Boils*

In a high percentage of cases in young adults, no specific causative or predisposing factor for boils can be established. Poor body hygiene may contribute to their development. The etiologic organism is usually a *Staphylococcus* species.[8]

### *Signs and Symptoms of Boils*

A boil often involves the anterior portion of the EAC. It usually begins as a red papule and develops into a round or conical superficial pustule with a core of pus and erythema around the base. The lesion gradually enlarges, becomes firm, and then generally softens and opens within 2 weeks, discharging its purulent contents. Because the skin is very taut, even minimal swelling may cause severe pain.

### *Treatment of Boils*

Boils are usually self-limiting; however, they may be severe, autoinoculable, and multiple. Warm compresses followed by a topical antibiotic, such as bacitracin, are often recommended. Antibiotics do not readily penetrate boils; therefore, incision and drainage by a primary care provider may be required. Multiple boils, boils that do not respond rapidly to topical treatment, or boils in the EAC should be referred to a primary care provider.[8]

## ASSESSMENT OF OTIC DISORDERS: A CASE-BASED APPROACH

The most common complaints of ear disorders are otalgia, pruritus (itching), and hearing loss. Evaluating the characteristics of particular symptoms, such as pain and hearing loss, and the specific combination of symptoms is the key to assessing otic disorders. To that end, the following discussion of common otic symptoms describes their possible causes. Further, Table 30-4 compares the signs and symptoms and other features of common otic disorders, and Table 30-5 describes the common etiologies and treatments for otalgia, otic pruritus, hearing loss, dizziness, and tinnitus. A verbal 5-minute hearing loss test is available at the American Academy of Otolaryngology Head and Neck Surgery, Inc. Web site: http://www.entnet.org/healthinfo/hearing/hearing_test.cfm. Finally, Cases 30-1 and 30-2 give examples of the assessment of patients with otic disorders.

| Itching | Loss of Hearing | Discharge | Other Features |
|---|---|---|---|
| No | Abrupt | If associated with otitis media | May be associated with otitis media (see below) |
| Yes | Occasional | Occasionally, clear discharge changing to seropurulent | Swollen ear canal, stuffiness, discharge, swollen lymph nodes, fever, usually occurring in summer or in warm, humid climates |
| No | Is sometimes decreased | Possible exudate through perforated eardrum | Perforated or bulging eardrum, lymph nodes sometimes swollen, fever, dizziness, usually occurring in winter |
| Yes | Yes | Possible exudate from secondary bacterial infection | If obstruction not removed promptly, acute otitis externa and tinnitus may develop |
| Rare | Varies, can be abrupt to seldom | Seldom | Untreated hematomas may cause swelling/ scarring; ear piercing may cause metal sensitivities, keloids, perichondritis, toxic shock syndrome, hepatitis B |
| No | Sometimes | No | Continuous or intermittent alien noises in ear such as ringing, roaring, or humming |
| No | Often | None | Sense of fullness or pressure in the ears |
| No | Often | None | Sense of fullness or wetness |
| No | Rare | Rare, except on rupture | Round or conical, superficial pustules with cores of pus |

**TABLE 30-5 Treatment of Common Otic Disorders[33-37]**

| Disorder | Etiology | Treatment |
|---|---|---|
| Otalgia | Intrinsic: infection, trauma, foreign objects, perichondritis<br>Extrinsic: dental or jaw problems, nasopharyngeal infections, tumors, cysts, migraine headaches, neuralgias, cervical arthritis | Medical referral unless cause is clearly obvious, self-limiting, and self-treatable; always refer infections; do not use olive oil |
| Otic pruritus | Contact dermatitis, seborrhea, psoriasis, infection (external otitis), excessive dryness related to decreased sebum production | Excessive dryness: 1-2 drops of mineral oil; avoid application of alcohol, insertion of foreign objects; medial referral if severe |
| Hearing loss | Foreign objects, water trapped in canal, infection, upper respiratory tract congestion, neoplasms, tympanic membrane perforation (abrupt), excessive pressure in ear canal, excessive cerumen, excessive noise, medications | Medical referral unless hearing loss is related to excessive water or impacted cerumen |
| Dizziness | Inner ear lesions, otitis media, rapid change in pressure on the tympanic membrane, migraine headache, ototoxic drugs, postural hypotension, cardiac disease, neoplasms. Irrigation of ear canal with very hot or cold water, motion sickness. | Medical referral unless related to motion sickness |
| Tinnitus | Hearing disorders, blockage of EAC, exposure to high noise levels, acoustic trauma, systemic diseases, drug toxicities (salicylate, quinidine, aminoglycosides, and other antibiotics) | Discontinuation of offending drug; medical referral for all other causes (OTC medications are ineffective) |

## PATIENT COUNSELING FOR OTIC DISORDERS

Patients who self-treat otic disorders must understand how easily the EAC can be injured. The clinician should discourage common harmful practices of relieving itching of the ear and instruct patients on the proper methods of removing excessive cerumen and moisture from the ears. Patients who are susceptible to these disorders should be advised to incorporate the removal methods as part of their aural hygiene. The clinician should explain the proper use and possible adverse effects of all recommended medications. The box Patient Education for Self-treatable Otic Disorders lists specific information to provide patients.

## CASE 30-1

| Relevant Evaluation Criteria | Scenario/Model Outcome |
|---|---|
| **Information Gathering** | |
| 1. Gather essential information about the patient's symptoms, including: | |
| a. description of symptom(s) (i.e., nature, onset, duration, severity, associated symptoms) | Patient reports a gradual hearing loss over the past month in the left ear that has recently turned painful with a discharge. |
| b. description of any factors that seem to precipitate, exacerbate, and/or relieve the patient's symptom(s) | Pain started 2 days ago after the patient attempted to remove the wax in his ear with a toothpick. Removal was not successful. The pain is preventing his using a sound attenuator in the affected ear. The pain is worse when he bends over. |
| c. description of the patient's efforts to relieve the symptoms | Patient used sweet oil in affected ear with poor results. |
| 2. Gather essential patient history information: | |
| a. patient's identity | Max Johnson |
| b. patient's age, sex, height, and weight | 55 y/o M, 5'9", 220 lb |
| c. patient's occupation | Night-shift supervisor |
| d. patient's dietary habits | Balanced diet with occasional alcohol |
| e. patient's sleep habits | Sleeps 6-7 hours between 7 AM-2 PM |
| f. concurrent medical conditions, prescription and nonprescription medications, and dietary supplements | Hypertension, hypercholesterolemia; losartan 50 mg daily; simvastatin 40 mg daily; aspirin 81 mg daily |
| g. allergies | NKA |
| h. history of other adverse reactions to medications | None |
| i. other (describe)______ | Started using sleep attenuators to aid sleep during the day 6 months ago after switching to overnight shift. |
| **Assessment and Triage** | |
| 3. Differentiate the patient's signs/symptoms and correctly identify the patient's primary problem(s) (see Table 30-4). | Improper removal of excessive cerumen has resulted in a probable infection. |
| 4. Identify exclusions for self-treatment (see Figure 30-2). | Signs of infection; pain associated with ear discharge |
| 5. Formulate a comprehensive list of therapeutic alternatives for the primary problem to determine if triage to a medical practitioner is required, and share this information with the patient. | Options include:<br>(1) Refer patient to a PCP for a differential diagnosis.<br>(2) Recommend OTC cerumen-softening agent with proper ear hygiene.<br>(3) Take no action. |
| **Plan** | |
| 6. Select an optimal therapeutic alternative to address the patient's problem, taking into account patient preferences. | Refer the patient to a PCP for a differential diagnosis. |
| 7. Describe the recommended therapeutic approach to the patient. | N/A |
| 8. Explain to the patient the rationale for selecting the recommended therapeutic approach from the considered therapeutic alternatives. | Seeing a primary care provider is necessary because of the signs and symptoms of a possible infection. OTC therapy is not appropriate. |

## CASE 30-1 (continued)

| Relevant Evaluation Criteria | Scenario/Model Outcome |
|---|---|
| **Patient Education** | |
| 9. When recommending self-care with nonprescription medications and/or nondrug therapy, convey accurate information to the patient. | For future prevention of complaint, use proper ear hygiene along with regular cleaning of sound attenuators. See the box Patient Education for Self-treatable Otic Disorders. |
| 10. Solicit patient's follow-up questions. | Is there any OTC product I can use in the future to help remove excessive cerumen? |
| 11. Answer patient's questions. | Yes. Refer to Tables 30-2 and 30-3. |

Key: N/A, not applicable; NKA, no known allergies; OTC, over-the-counter; PCP, primary care provider.

## CASE 30-2

| Relevant Evaluation Criteria | Scenario/Model Outcome |
|---|---|
| **Information Gathering** | |
| 1. Gather essential information about the patient's symptoms, including: | |
| a. description of symptom(s) (i.e., nature, onset, duration, severity, associated symptoms) | Patient describes right ear as being plugged-up for 2 days. Hearing is diminished in that ear but no pain, discharge, or fever exists. |
| b. description of any factors that seem to precipitate, exacerbate, and/or relieve the patient's symptom(s) | Symptoms appeared after the patient went snorkeling on spring break vacation. Swimming makes it worse. No relief has been observed. |
| c. description of the patient's efforts to relieve the symptoms | Patient applied several drops of hydrogen peroxide 3% to affected ear and has attempted to remove the excess water by using a cotton-tipped applicator with poor results. |
| 2. Gather essential patient history information: | |
| a. patient's identity | Amanda Brownsfield |
| b. patient's age, sex, height, and weight | 19 y/o F, 5'8", 130 lb |
| c. patient's occupation | College student |
| d. patient's dietary habits | Balanced diet |
| e. patient's sleep habits | Normal for college student |
| f. concurrent medical conditions, prescription and nonprescription medications, and dietary supplements | Ortho-Tri-Cyclen 1 tablet daily; multiple vitamin/minerals, and extra calcium 1 tablet daily |
| g. allergies | Penicillin |
| h. history of other adverse reactions to medications | None |
| i. other (describe)_______ | Patient wants to continue to swim during remainder of vacation. |
| **Assessment and Triage** | |
| 3. Differentiate the patient's signs/symptoms and correctly identify the patient's primary problem(s) (see Table30-4). | Excessive water in the ear caused by snorkeling/swimming and improper methods of removal |

## CASE 30-2 (continued)

| Relevant Evaluation Criteria | Scenario/Model Outcome |
|---|---|
| 4. Identify exclusions for self-treatment (see Figure 30-2). | None |
| 5. Formulate a comprehensive list of therapeutic alternatives for the primary problem to determine if triage to a medical practitioner is required, and share this information with the patient. | Options include:<br>(1) Refer patient to her PCP for further evaluation.<br>(2) Recommend isopropyl alcohol 95% in anhydrous glycerin.<br>(3) Recommend a pharmacist-compounded solution of 50:50 acetic acid/alcohol.<br>(4) Take no action. |
| **Plan** | |
| 6. Select an optimal therapeutic alternative to address the patient's problem, taking into account patient preferences. | The patient prefers an FDA-approved product containing isopropyl alcohol 95% in anhydrous glycerin. |
| 7. Describe the recommended therapeutic approach to the patient. | You should use proper ear hygiene and avoid placing foreign objects, including cotton-tipped swabs, in your ear. Don't use any solutions that contain water. See the box Patient Education for Self-treatable Otic Disorders and Table 30-1. |
| 8. Explain to the patient the rationale for selecting the recommended therapeutic approach from the considered therapeutic alternatives. | Seeking care with a primary care provider may not be necessary if you follow administration guidelines and proper ear hygiene. Solutions of 50:50 acetic acid/alcohol may overdry the ears. |
| **Patient Education** | |
| 9. When recommending self-care with nonprescription medications and/or nondrug therapy, convey accurate information to the patient. | |
| a. appropriate dose and frequency of administration | See Table 30-1 and the box Patient Education for Self-treatable Otic Disorders. |
| b. maximum number of days the therapy should be employed | You may use ear-drying agents whenever your ears have been exposed to water. |
| c. product administration procedures | See Table 30-1 and the box Patient Education for Self-treatable Otic Disorders. |
| d. expected time to onset of relief | With use of medication and proper ear hygiene, there should be noticeable improvement within one to two applications. |
| e. degree of relief that can be reasonably expected | Complete relief of symptoms should be seen. |
| f. most common side effects | Slight stinging may occur if ear canal is abraded. |
| g. side effects that warrant medical intervention should they occur | Pain, discharge (other than OTC product), fever |
| h. patient options in the event that condition worsens or persists | Consult a primary care provider if symptoms do not improve. |
| i. product storage requirements | Keep product tightly closed in a cool, dry area. |
| j. specific nondrug measures | See the box Patient Education for Self-treatable Otic Disorders. |
| 10. Solicit patient's follow-up questions. | Is there anything I can do to prevent water from entering my ears during swimming? |
| 11. Answer patient's questions. | Yes. Specific products are available that can be inserted into the ears prior to swimming that, if used correctly, will prevent water from entering. |

Key: OTC, over-the-counter; PCP, primary care provider.

## PATIENT EDUCATION FOR SELF-TREATABLE OTIC DISORDERS

### Excessive/Impacted Cerumen

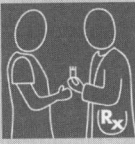

The objective of self-treatment is to soften and remove excessive or impacted cerumen (earwax) that is already present or to prevent the disorder from recurring in susceptible patients. For most patients, carefully following product instructions and the self-care measures listed here will help ensure optimal therapeutic outcomes.

#### *Nondrug Measures for Excessive/Impacted Cerumen*

- Use a washcloth draped over a finger to remove earwax from the outer canal.
- Do not insert objects in the ear to remove earwax. Such attempts may injure the ear canal or push the wax further into the canal.
- Never use the hollow candle method to remove earwax; it can cause serious ear injury.

#### *Nonprescription Medications for Excessive/Impacted Cerumen*

- See Tables 30-1 and 30-2 for guidelines on using carbamide peroxide to remove excessive or impacted earwax.
- Do not let the medication come into contact with the eyes.
- Do not use this medication if you have a fever, ear drainage, pain more severe than a dull pain, dizziness, or a ruptured eardrum, or if you had ear surgery within the past 6 weeks.
- Do not use this medication to treat inflamed ear tissue, swimmer's ear, or itching of the ear canal.
- Prolonged contact between carbamide peroxide solution and skin of the ear canal can cause dermatitis. Discontinue treatment if irritation or a rash appears.

Monitor your hearing and symptoms of infection such as pain and itching. If severe pain occurs or your hearing worsens, see a primary care provider immediately. Severe pain may indicate a ruptured eardrum.

### Water-clogged Ears

The objective of self-treatment is to remove water from ears already clogged with water or to prevent the disorder in persons who are susceptible to excessive moisture in the ears. For most patients, carefully following product instructions and the self-care measures listed here will help ensure optimal therapeutic outcomes.

#### *Nondrug Measures for Water-clogged Ears*

- Tilt the affected ear down, and gently manipulate it to help drain water from the ear.
- Immediately after swimming or bathing, use a blow-dryer on a low setting to help dry the ear canal. Do not blow directly into the ear canal.

#### *Nonprescription Medications for Water-clogged Ears*

- Use a product that reduces moisture content in the ear without overdrying. Isopropyl alcohol 95% in anhydrous glycerin 5% or a solution of one part isopropyl alcohol to one part white (not cider) vinegar is acceptable.
- Do not use the medications if you have a ruptured eardrum or have tympanostomy tubes in place.
- Place 5 to 10 drops of the solution in the ear canal, and allow the solution to remain for 1 to 2 minutes.
- See Table 30-1 for instructions on instilling the medication.
- Do not let the medication come into contact with the eyes.
- Discontinue the medication if stinging or burning occurs.

If pain, fever, or discharge develops, see a primary care provider immediately.

### Dermatologic Disorders of the Ear

The objective of self-treatment is to relieve the symptoms. For most patients, carefully following product instructions and the self-care measures listed here will help ensure optimal therapeutic outcomes.

#### *Contact Dermatitis*

- Avoid substances known to cause allergic or irritant reactions.
- Apply a wet compress of diluted (1:10 to 1:40) aluminum acetate solution several times per day to relieve itching and weeping of affected areas.

#### *Seborrhea and Psoriasis*

- Treat the scalp and the external ear with the appropriate medicated shampoo.
- If needed, apply nonprescription hydrocortisone cream to relieve inflammation.

#### *Boils*

- Do not self-treat multiple boils or a boil in the ear canal.
- Apply warm compresses to a boil located on the outside of the ear; then apply topical antibiotics.

If the boil does not respond to the topical treatment within 4 days, see a primary care provider.

## EVALUATION OF PATIENT OUTCOMES FOR OTIC DISORDERS

If the symptoms of excessive/impacted cerumen, water-clogged ears, or self-treatable dermatologic disorders of the ear persist or worsen after 4 days of proper treatment, the patient should consult a primary care provider. The patient should also consult a primary care provider if ear pain or discharge develops during treatment. The clinician can follow up by phone in 4 days to determine if therapy is successful.

## A WORD ABOUT
## Fluid Monitors

In 1997, a medical device that detects the presence of fluid in the middle ear was approved for marketing and for use by patients ages 6 months to adult.[38] It is marketed as an aid to monitoring fluid resolution in the middle ear following middle ear infections. The device uses sonarlike technology to detect the presence of fluid by measuring reflected sound. An acoustic transducer emits a soft, complex series of sound waves into the ear canal. In a normal ear, the tympanic membrane is flexible and vibrates when sound waves reach it. When fluid is in the middle ear, the tympanic membrane is not as mobile and reflects sound waves differently from that of the normal ear. The intensity of the reflected sound is measured by the device, using a microphone and microprocessor.[39] While used primarily by clinicians, this device is available to the public, although expense limits public use. Three color levels are coded according to the probability of fluid being present. Users of the device should be reminded that the presence of fluid in the middle ear does not always indicate an infection. The device will not work if a tympanostomy tube, a ruptured eardrum, or impacted cerumen is present. Normal amounts of cerumen in the canal do not appear to affect the results. Precautions for use of the device include not reusing the disposable tips and not forcing the tip far into the ear.

## KEY POINTS FOR OTIC DISORDERS

- Limit the self-treatment of otic disorders to minor symptoms such as a sense of fullness, pressure, or wetness in the ears.
- Refer patients with acute onset of hearing loss, dizziness, pain, discharge, or other symptoms associated with infection, tympanostomy tubes, or ear surgery within the last 6 weeks for further evaluation.
- Instruct patients on how to use specific otic products that have been proven safe and effective (Tables 30-1 and 30-2).
- Advise patients with self-treatable symptoms to contact a primary care provider if symptoms worsen or do not improve after 4 days.
- Advise patients about proper ear hygiene and the importance of cerumen to prevent further problems or complaints.

## References


1. CDC Advance Data from Vital and Health Statistics; No. 346, Table 9. Aug 2004. Available at: http://wwwcdc.gov.nchs/fastats/docvisit.htm. Accessed February 19, 2005.
2. Jabor MA. Cerumen impaction. *J La State Med Soc.* 1997;149:358-62.
3. Aung T, Mulley GP. Removal of earwax. *BMJ.* 2002;325:27.
4. Cruickshanks KJ, Wiley TL, Tweed TS, et al. Prevalence of hearing loss in older adults in Beaver Dam, Wisconsin: the Epidemiology of Hearing Loss Study. *Am J Epidemiol.* 1998;148:879-86.
5. Bluestone CD. Anatomy and physiology of the eustachian tube system. In: Bailey BJ, Calhoun KH, Healy GB, et al., eds. *Head and Neck Surgery—Otolaryngology.* 3rd ed. Philadelphia: Lippincott Williams & Wilkins; 2001:1059-69.
6. Hoppe MW, Kolling WM. Ear infections and their treatment in pediatrics. *Drug Topics.* August 17, 1998:93-7.
7. Kryzer TC, Lambert PR. Diseases of the external auditory canal. In: Canalis RF, Lambert PR, eds. *The Ear: Comprehensive Otology.* Philadelphia: Lippincott Williams & Wilkins; 2000:341-57.
8. Linstrom CJ, Lucente FE, Joseph EM. Infections of the external ear. In: Bailey BJ, Calhoun KH, Healy GB, et al., eds. *Head and Neck Surgery—Otolaryngology.* 3rd ed. Philadelphia: Lippincott Williams & Wilkins; 2001:1711-24.
9. Hughes E, Lee JH. Otitis externa. *Pediatr Rev.* 2001;22:191-7.
10. Roeser RJ, Ballachanda BB. Physiology, pathophysiology, and anthropology/epidemiology of human ear canal secretions. *J Am Acad Audiol.* 1997;8:391-8.
11. Holten KB, Gick J. Management of the patient with otitis externa. *J Fam Prac.* 2001;50:353.
12. Nichols A. Nonorthopaedic problems in the aquatic athlete. *Clin Sports Med.* 1999;18:405-9.
13. Beers MH, Berkow R, eds. External ear. In: *The Merck Manual of Diagnosis and Therapy.* 17th ed. Available at: http://www.merck.com/mrkshared/mmanual/section7/sec7.jsp. Accessed February 25, 2005.
14. *Federal Register.* 1986;51:28656-61.
15. Grossan M. Cerumen removal—current challenges. *Ear Nose Throat J.* 1998;77:541-6.
16. Wilson PL, Roeser RJ. Cerumen management: professional issues and techniques. *J Am Acad Audiol.* 1997;8:428.
17. Cada DJ, Covington TR, Generali JA, et al., eds. *Drug Facts and Comparison.* St. Louis: Facts and Comparisons; 2001:1802-5.
18. Gennaro AR, DerMarderosian AH, Hanson GR, eds. *Remington: The Science and Practice of Pharmacy.* 20th ed. Baltimore: Lippincott Williams & Wilkins; 2000:417, 1040, 1045, 1205-6, 1509.
19. Otic preparations: hydrogen peroxide 3%. In: *eFacts Nonprescription Drug Therapy.* Available at: http://www.efactsonline.com. Accessed February 25, 2005.
20. Otic preparations: Olive oil (sweet oil). In: *eFacts Nonprescription Drug Therapy.* Available at: http://www.efactsonline.com. Accessed February 25, 2005.
21. Spiro SR. A cost-effectiveness analysis of earwax softeners. *Nurse Pract.* 1997;22(8):28-31, 166.
22. Whatley VN, Dodds CL, Paul RI. Randomized clinical trial of docusate, triethanolamine polypeptide, and irrigation in cerumen removal in children. *Arch Pediatr Adolesc Med.* 2003;157;1181-3.
23. Blumenthal M, Busse WR, Goldberg A, et al. *The Complete German Commission E Monographs: Therapeutic Guide to Herbal Medicines.* Boston: Integrative Medicine Communications; 1998.
24. National Center for Complementary and Alternative Medicine Web site. Available at: http/www.nccam.nih.gov. Accessed February 25, 2005.
25. Robbers JE, Tyler VE. *Tyler's Herbs of Choice: The Therapeutic Use of Phytomedicinals.* 2nd ed. Barrington, NY: Haworth Press; 1999.
26. Seely DR, Quigley SM, Langman AW. Ear candles: efficacy and safety. *Laryngoscope.* 1996;106:1226-9.
27. *Federal Register.* 1995;60:8915.
28. *Federal Register.* 1995;60:42435.
29. "Ear drying aids" monograph status proposed by FDA. *FDC Reports—The Tan Sheet.* 1999;7(34):4.

30. Otic preparations: acetic acid 2.5% in 70% alcohol. In: *eFacts Nonprescription Drug Therapy.* Available at: http://www.efactsonline.com. Accessed February 25, 2005.
31. Aminifarshidmehr N. The management of chronic suppurative otitis media with acid media solution. *Am J Otol.* 1996;17:24-5.
32. Patel NM, Elias SS, Cheigh NH. Acne and psoriasis. In: DiPiro JT, Talbert RL, Yee GC, et al., eds. *Pharmacotherapy: A Pathophysiologic Approach.* 5th ed. New York: McGraw-Hill Inc; 2002:1689-705.
33. Lau D, Watson D. Referred otalgia: an unusual presentation of a laryngeal foreign body. *Hosp Med.* 1998;59:161.
34. Oliveira RJ. The active ear canal. *J Am Acad Audiol.* 1997;8:409-10.
35. Snow JB, Martin JB. Disturbances of smell, taste, and hearing. In: Fauci AS, Braunwald E, Isselbacher KJ, et al., eds. *Harrison's Principles of Internal Medicine.* 14th ed. New York: McGraw-Hill Inc; 1998:173-8.
36. Cada DJ, Covington TR, Generali JA, et al., eds. *Drug Facts and Comparison.* St. Louis: Facts and Comparisons; 2003:703, 899, 920, 1437, 1461, 2182.
37. Baloh RW. Vertigo of peripheral origin. In: Canalis RF, Lambert PR, eds. *The Ear, Comprehensive Otology.* Philadelphia: Lippincott Williams & Wilkins; 2000: 647-63.
38. *FDA Consumer.* 1997;31(4):37.
39. *How EarCheck* Works. Woburn, Mass: MDI Instruments, Inc; 1999.

CHAPTER 31

# Prevention of Hygiene-related Oral Disorders

*Gary D. Klasser and Michael Colvard*

Dental diseases are the most prevalent chronic diseases in American society. Each year, dental conditions cause 7.05 million days of work loss. Among all Americans, 50% need dental treatment, and nearly 80% have some form of periodontal disease. Of all 12- to 17-year-olds, 68% have experienced tooth decay; the average adult has 21.5 decayed or filled tooth surfaces. Only 42% of adults 65 years and older visit a dentist during a given year. Furthermore, nearly 44% of Americans 75 years and older have lost all their natural teeth, but that percentage is declining. The increasing number of persons of advanced age with natural teeth has many dental implications.[1]

Improper oral hygiene is a direct cause of dental caries (decay), periodontal disease (gingivitis and periodontitis), halitosis, and some cases of denture-related discomfort. Nonprescription products for prevention of oral disease are widely available in pharmacies, food stores, and other retail stores; therefore, educating the public about proper use of these products is the key to preventing dental diseases.

## ANATOMY AND PHYSIOLOGY OF THE ORAL CAVITY

The teeth and supporting structures are necessary for normal mastication and articulation as well as for appearance. The primary (deciduous) dentition first appears at approximately age 6 months, when the mandibular (lower jaw) central incisors erupt; it is usually complete with the eruption of the upper second molars at approximately age 24 months. There are 20 deciduous (baby) teeth, 10 in each arch. Generally, the permanent dentition first appears when the mandibular first molar erupts behind the deciduous second molar at approximately age 6 years, and it continues in a regular pattern, usually replacing shedding deciduous teeth. All permanent teeth are present by age 14, except third molars (wisdom teeth), which may appear between the ages of 17 and 21 years.

Anatomically, the teeth are grossly viewed as having two parts, the roots and the crown (Figure 31-1). The roots are normally below the gingival (gum) line or margin and are essential in supporting and attaching the tooth to the surrounding tissues. The crown is above the gingival margin and is responsible for mastication. Each tooth has four basic components: enamel, dentin, pulp, and periodontium.

Enamel is composed of very hard, crystalline calcium phosphate salts (hydroxyapatite). It is 1.5 to 2 mm thick at its thickest part and protects the underlying tooth structure. It covers the crown of the tooth, ending around the gum line at the cementoenamel junction. Its hardness enables the crown to withstand the wear of mastication. Dentin, which is softer, lies beneath the enamel and makes up the largest part of the tooth structure. It is transected by microscopic tubules that transport nutrients from the dental pulp. Dentin protects the dental pulp from mechanical, thermal, and chemical irritation.

The pulp occupies the pulp chamber and is continuous with the tissues surrounding the tooth by an opening at the apex of the root (apical foramen). The pulp consists primarily of vascular and neural tissues. The only nerve endings in the pulp are free nerve endings; thus, any type of stimulus to the pulp is interpreted as pain.

The periodontium comprises the tissúes that support the teeth, including the cementum, the periodontal ligament, the encompassing alveolar bone, and the gingiva. The bonelike cementum is softer than dentin and covers the root of the tooth, extending apically from the cementoenamel junction. Thus, the tooth is suspended in bone, but is not continuous with it. Its major function is to attach the tooth to the periodontal ligament by periodontal fibers. The periodontal ligament is connective tissue that attaches the tooth to the surrounding alveolar bone and gingival tissue. The four functions of the periodontal ligament are supportive, formative, sensory, and nutritive. The alveolar bone forms the sockets of the teeth. Alveolar bone is thin and spongy, and it attaches to the principal fibers of the periodontal ligament, as well as to the gingiva. The gingiva is the soft tissue surrounding the teeth. It is normally pink, stippled (looking like an orange peel) and keratinized, and it is attached to the cementum by the gingival group of periodontal ligament fibers.

The mucosa covering the pharyngeal region, soft palate, floor of the mouth, vestibule (between the alveolar ridge and cheek), and cheeks is normally more pinkish red than the gingiva. This coloration occurs because the tissue is more vascularized and the outer surface of the mucosa, which is stratified squamous epithelium, lacks the keratinized stratum corneum outer layer found in the gingiva and hard palate.

---

**Editor's Note:** This chapter is based, in part, on the 14th edition chapter with the same title, which was written by Robert G. Smith.

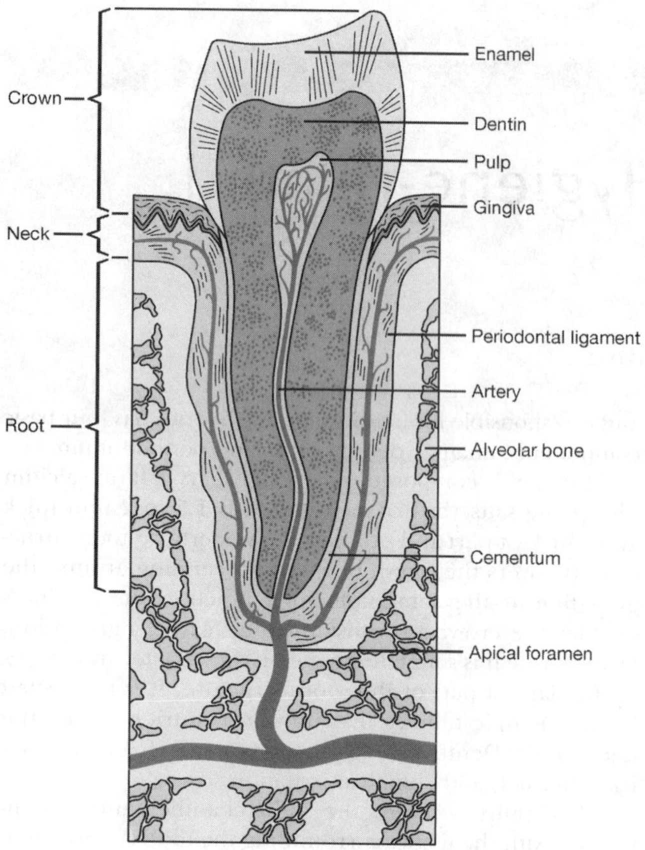


FIGURE 31-1 Anatomy of the tooth.

The tongue functions in mastication, swallowing, taste, and speech. Its dorsal or upper surface is usually irregular and rough in appearance. Taste buds located on the dorsum and lateral borders of the tongue usually are small, oval organs of flat epithelial cells surrounding a small opening (taste pore).

The major salivary glands (parotid, submandibular, and sublingual) are responsible for secreting saliva, an alkaline, slightly viscous, clear secretion that contains enzymes (lysozymes and ptyalin), albumin, epithelial mucin (a mucopolysaccharide), immunoglobulin, leukocytes, and minerals. Normal salivary gland function promotes good oral health in several ways. Saliva lubricates and facilitates the removal of carbohydrates and microorganisms from the oral cavity. Saliva also buffers the decline in pH caused by the acid formed by carbohydrate fermentation. Its mineral components have a protective role in the demineralization and remineralization of tooth enamel.

## CARIES

Since the 1970s, the incidence of dental caries has declined significantly in school-age children in the United States, and the proportion of children who are caries-free has increased. The percentage of 12- to 17-year-old children in the United States who are free of caries has increased threefold, from 10.4% in the early 1970s to 32.7% in the late 1980s. Similar declines are reported in younger children. The 1988 to 1991 survey of the National Health and Nutrition Examination III reported that 50% of 5- to 9-year-olds and 83% of 2- to 4-year-old children were free of caries in the primary dentition.[2] This reduction in caries most likely results from the presence of fluoride in public water supplies and toothpastes, even though many people still believe that fluoride in the water might be a health hazard. In fact, Los Angeles began to add fluoride to its water only in August 1999.[3] Nevertheless, dental caries remains a public health problem, and the importance of prevention should not be ignored.

Edentulism (toothlessness) is decreasing; more than one half of older Americans have retained their natural dentition. This has many dental implications. Root caries, an age-related problem that affects the root surfaces of adult teeth exposed by gingival recession, is becoming more prevalent as adults retain greater numbers of teeth later in life.[2]

### Epidemiology of Caries

Patients with poor oral hygiene are at greatest risk for developing caries. Patients at increased risk for caries include those with orthodontic appliances, xerostomia (dry mouth), and gum tissue recession that exposes root surfaces. Certain prescription medications may cause xerostomia (see Chapter 32). Patients who received head and neck radiation therapy, may also be more likely to manifest xerostomia.

Evidence also supports the association of smokeless tobacco with increased dental caries (because these products contain sugar that is kept in contact with the teeth) and with cervical erosion of the teeth.[4] The use of tobacco (both smoked and smokeless) has been linked to the formation of dental caries, gum and bone disease, and discoloration of teeth. Because alcohol consumption can cause xerostomia, individuals who consume alcohol may also have a higher risk of caries.

### Etiology of Caries

Dental caries is now considered to be an infectious disease that affects the calcified tissues of the teeth. Certain plaque bacteria generate acid from dietary carbohydrates; the acid demineralizes tooth enamel, leading to the formation of carious lesions (pits or perforations) which, if left untreated, will eventually destroy the tooth. Dental caries formation requires growth and attachment of many cariogenic microorganisms (e.g., *Streptococcus mutans, Lactobacillus casei, Actinomyces viscosus*) to exposed surfaces. *S. mutans* is the primary organism to initiate the carious process. Lactobacilli continue the process after entering established pits and fissures in biting surfaces of teeth, whereas *A. viscosus* is associated with root caries. These organisms are spread by saliva: from mother to infant by sharing a spoon, kissing, blowing on food, and other shared activities. Most children are infected by age 2 years, and 83% are infected by age 4 years.[5] If oral hygiene is neglected, dental plaque containing these organisms remains on the tooth surfaces and, in time, attracts more bacteria, thereby promoting decay.

## Pathophysiology of Caries

The carious process is characterized by alternating periods of destruction (demineralization) and repair (remineralization). Demineralization is caused by organic acids, such as lactic and formic acids, which are produced (usually anaerobically) by microbial metabolism of low-molecular-weight carbohydrates (sugars) that readily diffuse into plaque. The resulting reduction in pH on the tooth surface causes demineralization of dental enamel. Saliva, rich in calcium and phosphate ions, is crucial in remineralizing early carious lesions. The presence of fluoride ions in the mouth also promotes remineralization and slows demineralization, thus retarding enamel dissolution.

Repeated and frequent sugar intake keeps plaque pH low and prolongs demineralization. A carious lesion starts slowly on the enamel surface and initially produces no clinical symptoms. Once demineralization progresses through the enamel to the softer dentin, the destruction proceeds much more rapidly, becoming clinically or radiographically evident as a carious lesion. At this point, the patient can become aware of the process by either observing it or experiencing symptoms of sensitivity to stimuli (such as heat, cold, or sweet foods) or chewing. If untreated, the carious lesion can result in damage to the dental pulp itself (with continuous pain as a common symptom) and, eventually, in necrosis of vital pulp tissue. Because an opening exists between the pulp and surrounding supporting tissues through the apical foramen, the infectious process can progress apically, resulting in bone loss, abscesses, cellulitis, or osteomyelitis.

Plaque is commonly recognized as the source of microbes that cause caries and periodontal disease; thus, plaque buildup is directly related to the incidence of oral disease. Plaque begins with the formation of acquired pellicle on a clean tooth surface. Pellicle appears to be a thin, acellular, glycoprotein/mucoprotein coating that adheres to the enamel within minutes after a tooth is cleaned. Its source is believed to be saliva. The pellicle seems to serve as an attachment for cariogenic bacteria that, along with acids, produces long-chain polymers such as dextrans and levans that adhere to the pellicle and tooth surface. The resulting sticky, adherent mass is soft and readily disrupted by toothbrushing or flossing.

After meals, food residue may be incorporated into plaque by bacterial degradation. Left undisturbed, plaque thickens and bacteria proliferate. Plaque growth begins in protected cracks and fissures, and along the gingival margin. If not removed within 24 hours, dental plaque (especially in areas opposite the salivary glands) begins to calcify by calcium salt precipitation from the saliva, forming calculus, or tartar. This hardened, adherent deposit is removable only by professional dental cleaning.

Calculus is generally considered to be a substrate on which additional plaque can develop, and it is not regarded as the primary cause in periodontal disease. However, most periodontists agree that supragingival (above) and subgingival (below the gingival margin) calculus can promote the progression of periodontal disease by accumulating new bacterial plaque in contact with sensitive tissue sites and by interfering with local self-cleaning efforts to remove plaque. Subgingival calculus may also intensify the inflammatory process. Thorough removal of subgingival calculus in periodontal therapy is an important step in delaying the reestablishment of periodontal pathogens and resolution of inflammation.

## Prevention of Caries

The key to preventing caries is controlling dental plaque. Because a combination of diet (carbohydrate substrate), oral bacteria, and host resistance is involved in developing caries, prevention should be aimed at modifying these factors. The frequency of refined carbohydrate intake should be reduced; plaque, which supports cariogenic bacterial growth, should be removed, usually by mechanical means (brushing and flossing); and host resistance should be increased through appropriate exposure to fluoride ion. Antiplaque products aid in mechanical removal of plaque or retard its buildup. The declining prevalence of dental caries in children may be attributed to a combination of these interventions (e.g., increased exposure to fluoride in drinking water, dentifrices, and mouth rinses; changed patterns of diet; and overall improved oral hygiene).

### *Dietary Measures*

Cariogenic foods should be avoided in favor of less cariogenic foods. A food is considered highly cariogenic if it contains more than 15% sugar, clings to the teeth, and remains in the mouth after it is eaten. Conversely, foods are less cariogenic if they have a high water content (e.g., fresh fruit), stimulate the flow of saliva (i.e., fibrous foods that require lots of chewing), or are high in protein (e.g., dairy products). Both the water content of fresh fruit and the flow of saliva tend to wash the sugar away and neutralize the acid it creates. Milk protein also raises pH and tends to inhibit binding of bacteria.

Although sucrose is the most cariogenic sugar, other types of fermentable carbohydrates, such as fructose and lactose, also are cariogenic. Oral hygiene products such as mouth rinses and dentifrices may contain a low concentration of saccharin, which is a potent noncariogenic sugar substitute that appears to present no caries hazard. The Food and Drug Administration's (FDA) limit on saccharin is 1.0 g/day for adults; ingestion from normal use of both mouth rinse and dentifrice would result in a total saccharin exposure of only about 20 to 40 mg/day. Other noncariogenic sugar substitutes such as sugar alcohols (sorbitol, xylitol) and aspartame (amino acid methyl ester) are currently used as sweetening agents.

In 1996, FDA approved health-claim labeling of foods that contain sugar alcohol. The approved sugar alcohols are xylitol, sorbitol, mannitol, maltitol, isomalt, lactisol, hydrogenated starch hydrolysates, hydrogenated glucose syrups, erythritol, and combinations of these. Products that contain these syrups may claim that they reduce the risk of dental caries, that the sugar alcohol in the food does not promote tooth decay, or both. Claims for the noncariogenicity of sorbitol, however, need substantiation through further clinical trials.[1] Xylitol has been shown to be noncariogenic. Some clinical trials have reported that xylitol-containing chewing gum is cariostatic and others have shown that xylitol activity may aid in remineralization.[1]

### Chemical Management of Plaque

Mechanical methods of plaque removal (i.e., brushing with a dentifrice and flossing) are most frequently used. However, chemical management of plaque (i.e., using specific products to prevent plaque accumulation or aid in its removal) is a more recent innovation in oral hygiene. The best way to ensure healthy teeth and gingival tissues is to mechanically remove plaque buildup by brushing at least twice daily and flossing at least once a day. Toothbrushing removes plaque from the lingual (tongue) side, buccal (cheek) side, and occlusal (biting) surfaces of the teeth. Plaque found on interproximal (between the teeth) surfaces can be removed efficiently only with dental floss and other interdental cleaning aids (e.g., interproximal brush, dental tape, or tapered picks).

Chemical management of plaque and calculus can enhance mechanical removal either by acting directly on the plaque bacteria or by disrupting components of plaque to aid in its removal during routine oral hygiene. The use of chemical agents in plaque control may be particularly appropriate for selected patients who may be unable to brush and floss effectively. Physically or mentally disabled individuals (who may not be able to master the necessary manual techniques) and orthodontia patients (i.e., those with fixed prostheses) may benefit from adding antiplaque agents to their oral hygiene regimen.

Desirable characteristics for antiplaque agents include the following:

- Selective antibacterial activity, interference with the rate of accumulation, or metabolism of supragingival plaque
- Substantivity (sustained retention of the agent in the mouth)
- Compatibility with dentifrice ingredients
- Lack of undesirable side effects for the user
- Noninterference with the natural ecology of the normal oral microflora

### Dentifrices

Dentifrices are used with a toothbrush for cleaning accessible tooth surfaces. Use of a dentifrice enhances removal of dental plaque and stain, resulting in a decreased incidence of dental caries and gum disease, reduced mouth odors, and enhanced personal appearance.

Dentifrices are available as powders, pastes, or gels (Table 31-1). The powder forms commonly contain abrasive and flavoring agents and sometimes a surfactant (foaming agent). Dentifrice powders are either moistened to form a slurry and applied with a dry brush, or used dry with a brush moistened with water. The powder is more abrasive when it is used dry. In the final rule for anticaries drug products, monograph status is approved for powdered dentifrice containing sodium fluoride with a sodium bicarbonate abrasive. The gels and pastes commonly contain an abrasive, a surfactant, a humectant (moistening agent), a binder/thickener, a sweetener, flavoring agents, and a therapeutic agent such as fluoride for anticaries activity.

#### Abrasive Ingredients

Dentifrice abrasives are pharmacologically inactive and insoluble compounds. Common abrasives include silicates, dicalcium phosphate, alumina trihydrate, calcium pyrophosphate, calcium carbonate, and sodium metaphosphate. Although dentifrices vary in their degree of abrasiveness, abrasion is an essential property for removing stained pellicle from teeth.[1] The ideal abrasive would maximally aid in cleaning and cause minimal damage to tooth surfaces. Unfortunately, because of the variability in patient brushing techniques and oral conditions, the ideal dentifrice abrasive does not exist. Low-abrasive dentifrices, which include most dentifrice formulations currently marketed in the United States, usually have a low concentration (10%-25%) of silica abrasives, whereas high-abrasive dentifrices typically have higher concentrations (40%-50%) of the inorganic calcium or aluminum salts mentioned previously. Baking soda, a mild abrasive, is found in a number of dentifrices. Although they are safe to use, toothpastes with baking soda have not been shown to clean teeth better than toothpastes without this substance.

#### Whitening/Antistain Ingredients

Cosmetic dentifrices make no therapeutic claims and are usually chosen by patients because of taste, whitening ability, or antistain properties. Some dentifrices claiming to

**TABLE 31-1 Selected Dentifrices**

| Trade Name | Primary Ingredients |
|---|---|
| **Fluoride Toothpastes** | |
| Aim Regular Strength Gel | Hydrated silica; sodium monofluorophosphate (fluoride 0.14%) |
| Aquafresh Extra Fresh Toothpaste | Calcium carbonate; hydrated silica; sodium monofluorophosphate (fluoride 0.15%) |
| Colgate Toothpaste | Dicalcium phosphate dihydrate; sodium monofluorophosphate (fluoride 0.15%) |

**TABLE 31-1 Selected Dentifrices (continued)**

| Trade Name | Primary Ingredients |
|---|---|
| Crest Cavity Protection Gel | Hydrated silica; sodium fluoride (fluoride 0.15%) |
| Pepsodent Original Toothpaste | Hydrated silica; sodium monofluorophosphate (fluoride 0.14%) |
| **Tartar-control Toothpastes** | |
| Aquafresh Tartar Control Toothpaste | Hydrated silica; sodium fluoride; tetrapotassium pyrophosphate; tetrasodium pyrophosphate |
| Colgate Baking Soda and Peroxide Tartar Control Toothpaste | Hydrated silica; sodium monofluorophosphate (fluoride 0.15%); pentasodium triphosphate; tetrasodium pyrophosphate |
| Crest Tartar Protection Gel/Toothpaste | Silica; sodium fluoride (fluoride 0.15%); tetrapotassium pyrophosphate; disodium pyrophosphate; tetrasodium pyrophosphate |
| Viadent Advanced Care | Hydrated silica; sodium monofluorophosphate (fluoride 0.13%); zinc citrate trihydrate |
| **Antiplaque/Antigingivitis Toothpastes** | |
| Colgate Total Toothpaste | Hydrated silica; sodium bicarbonate; sodium fluoride (fluoride 0.14%); triclosan 0.3% |
| Crest Multicare Toothpaste | Hydrated silica; sodium fluoride (fluoride 0.15%); sodium bicarbonate; tetrasodium pyrophosphate |
| **Whitening Toothpastes** | |
| Aquafresh Whitening Gel/Toothpaste | Hydrated silica; sodium fluoride; titanium dioxide |
| Colgate Baking Soda Peroxide Whitening Toothpaste | Hydrated silica; sodium bicarbonate; aluminum oxide; sodium monofluorophosphate (fluoride 0.14%); titanium dioxide |
| Mentadent Advanced Whitening Gel/Toothpaste | Hydrated silica; sodium bicarbonate; sodium fluoride (fluoride 0.24%); titanium dioxide |
| Ultrabrite Toothpaste | Hydrated silica; alumina; sodium monofluorophosphate (fluoride 0.14%); titanium dioxide |
| **Sodium Lauryl Sulfate-free Toothpastes** | |
| Biotène Dry Mouth Toothpaste | Lactoperoxidase, glucose oxidase, lysozyme; sodium monofluorophosphate 0.15% |
| Oral B Rembrandt Whitening Natural Toothpaste | Dicalcium phosphate; silica; sodium monofluorophosphate; papain |
| Sensodyne Original Flavor Toothpaste | Potassium nitrate 5%; sodium fluoride (fluoride 0.13%) |
| **Botanical-based Toothpastes** | |
| Biocalor | Licorice extract; ginseng extract; aloe; augustifolia; eucalyptol; chile; saragundi |
| Calendula | Calendula |
| Colgate Herbal | Lemon; salvia; myrrh; chamomile; eucalyptus; manzanilla |
| Dabur Ayurvedic | Bulletwood; acacia; lotur bark; blackberry; pellitory root; basil; peppermint; spearmint; coriander; ginger; eucalyptus |
| Dr. Burt's | Peppermint; coconut oil; lavender oil; rosemary; eucalyptus; comfrey |
| Dr. Tichenor's | Peppermint |
| Herbal Toothpaste and Gum Therapy | Aloe vera; goldenseal; echinacea; carrageenan |
| Listerine | Thymol; eucalyptol; methyl salicylate and menthol |
| Natural Toothpaste | Goldenseal; mint; carrot root; annatto; azulene |
| Optifresh | Sorbitol; spearmint and peppermint oils; echinacea; olive leaf; neem; citric acid |
| Shane | Aloe vera |
| Tea Tree | Tea tree oil; aloe; witch hazel; spearmint oil; alcohol |
| Tom's of Maine | Peppermint; spearmint; orange; mango; fennel; carrageenan; propolis; cassia; myrrh; cinnamon |
| Tru-Dent | Carrageenan; peppermint; cinnamon; papain |
| Viadent Original | Sanguinaria |

## A WORD ABOUT Tooth-bleaching Products

During the past 5 to 10 years, the popularity of tooth bleaching has increased in the United States. Three methods are currently in use: (1) in-office dental bleaching, (2) dental office–supported home bleaching, and (3) nonprescription home bleaching. All three use basically the same chemical agents: carbamide peroxide or hydrogen peroxide in various strengths. The in-office method has the advantage of a one-time treatment, but the stronger bleach and the accelerator light are not necessary to obtain the same result as with the dental office–supported home-bleaching process, which involves the use of custom trays. With this process, patients can fine tune the extent of lightening to their own preferences. The following two nonprescription products (among the many) may aid in lightening:

- Rembrandt Plus Superior Bleaching System includes a lower concentration of the company's professional product, which contains carbamide peroxide gel and fluoride. The kit contains a mouth guard that is boiled to form a one-size-fits-all tray similar to nonprescription athletic mouth guards. Because the tray cannot be trimmed exactly to the gumline, there is no way to keep the bleaching gel away from the gingival tissue (gums), and a large quantity of product is required to fill the tray. A kit contains enough for 30 doses.
- Crest WhiteStrips are translucent film strips impregnated with hydrogen peroxide and other ingredients. The strips are peeled away from a protective backing and folded over the six upper or lower front teeth (different strips are provided for upper and lower teeth). The teeth will look as though they are covered with small pieces of transparent food wrap. The strips are applied twice a day and left in place for 30 minutes. A kit contains enough strips for 14 days. A stronger version of the same system is available only through a dentist.

remove stubborn coffee or tobacco stains may contain higher concentrations of abrasives. High-abrasive formulations are not advised for long-term use or for use by patients with exposed root surfaces. Plain baking soda, which is a water-soluble mild abrasive, or toothpastes containing baking soda have limited polishing and stain-removal capacity. Other products may contain a pigment (e.g., titanium dioxide) that produces a temporary brightening effect. Rembrandt Whitening Toothpaste contains a chemical complex of aluminum oxide, a citrate salt, and papain. Whitening dentifrices containing oxygenating agents rely on a debriding action to remove stained pellicle. Numerous products offer a combination of baking soda and peroxide with fluoride. Whitening dentifrices should not be confused with tooth-bleaching products (see box A Word About Tooth-bleaching Products).

### Chemotherapeutic Ingredients

Fluoride, the most common therapeutic agent added to dentifrices, is used for its anticaries activity. Other therapeutic ingredients include potassium nitrate to treat hypersensitive dentin; triclosan, an antibacterial ingredient, for its antigingivitis properties; and stabilized stannous fluoride for its antigingivitis/antiplaque and anticaries properties. An FDA advanced notice of proposed rulemaking (ANPR) reaffirms stannous fluoride 0.454% as the only Category I antigingivitis/antiplaque agent for use in dentifrices. Category III combination active ingredients often added to dentifrices include zinc citrate and stannous pyrophosphate and hydrogen peroxide and sodium bicarbonate. The essential oils thymol and eucalyptol have also been added to dentifrices, but the ANPR designates cetylpyridinium chloride 0.045% to 0.1%, and the combination of eucalyptol 0.092%, menthol 0.042%, methyl salicylate 0.060%, and thymol 0.064% as Category I antigingivitis/antiplaque agents for use in mouth rinses.[6] FDA had not issued a final rule at the time this book went to print. More information may be found by searching for "plaque committee" on the FDA Web site (www.fda.gov).

**TABLE 31-2 FDA-approved Active Ingredients for Anticaries Dentifrices**

| Ingredient | Concentration (ppm) (Dosage Form) |
|---|---|
| Sodium fluoride | 850-1150 (paste)<br>850-1150 (powder) |
| Sodium monofluorophosphate | 850-1150 (paste)<br>1500 (paste) |
| Stannous fluoride | 850-1150 (paste) |

### Fluoride

Fluoride dentifrices are indicated for both preventing and treating carious lesions. Use of fluoride-containing dentifrices is the one method of caries prevention that is common to all countries that show a reduction in caries. The American Dental Association (ADA) accepts as safe and effective fluoride-containing toothpaste and fluoride-containing gel dentifrice formulations with compatible abrasives. FDA promulgated a final rule for nonprescription anticaries drug products in 1995 and determined that sodium fluoride 0.22%, sodium monofluorophosphate 0.76%, and stannous fluoride 0.4% dentifrices containing 850 to 1150 ppm of theoretical total fluorine in a compatible base will meet monograph conditions (Table 31-2). Although it was previously recognized as safe, clinical data submitted in the final rulemaking process established efficacy for enhanced anticaries benefit from a theoretical total fluorine concentration of sodium monofluorophosphate 1500 ppm.

The possibility of staining exists with the use of stannous fluoride. About 10% to 20% of patients experience slight, but noticeable, tooth discoloration after 2 to 3 months of continuous use. The discoloration is not permanent and is readily removed at the next professional

## THE AMERICAN DENTAL ASSOCIATION SEAL OF ACCEPTANCE

ADA evaluates the safety and efficacy of dental products used by dental professionals and the public through the Seal of Acceptance's evaluation program of its Council on Scientific Affairs. Manufacturers of dentifrices or mouth rinses with therapeutic potential for gingivitis and supragingival dental plaque control may voluntarily submit data to ADA for evaluation. Product labels and promotional material must also comply with ADA standards.[7]

The ADA Council on Scientific Affairs awards allows only products that demonstrate a significant effect against gingivitis to make plaque control or plaque modification claims. A product that can demonstrate significant plaque reduction but no concomitant significant reduction in gingivitis will not be eligible for Acceptance.[8] ADA has approved two statements to be used for products classified under these guidelines—one for both gingivitis and plaque reduction and one for gingivitis reduction only:

- [Product name] has been shown to help to prevent and reduce [whichever is appropriate] gingivitis [and supragingival plaque accumulation] when used as directed in a conscientiously applied program of oral hygiene and regular professional care. Its effect on periodontitis has not been determined.[8]
- Once a product has earned the ADA seal, it may display that seal for 3 years, provided it continues to meet all the requirements.[7] The ADA's online home page www.ada.org provides searchable access to a current listing of dental consumer products that have been awarded the ADA Seal of Acceptance.

dental cleaning. This product is for use by adults and children ages 12 years and older.

### Triclosan

Colgate Total contains triclosan, an antibacterial agent and promoter of substantivity that has antigingivitis and antiplaque activity. The product also contains fluoride for caries protection and a copolymer delivery system for the triclosan. It is also the only toothpaste currently accepted by ADA for this indication (see the box American Dental Association Seal of Acceptance).[7,8] Approval was based on clinical data for safety and efficacy. The product is not intended for use in children younger than 6 years of age.

The FDA Dental Plaque Subcommittee evaluated data on the safety and effectiveness of triclosan but did not include it in the ANPR, published in the May 29, 2003, *Federal Register,* because triclosan has not been marketed as an antigivitis/antiplaque agent in the United States for a "material time and to a material extent."[6] However, the company that produces triclosan submitted a time and extent application on November 25, 2003, asking FDA to consider the fact that 3.5 billion units of toothpaste containing triclosan have been used in 13 selected countries over the past 6 years.[9]

### Zinc Chloride, Zinc Citrate, and Soluble Pyrophosphates

A number of fluoride dentifrices contain anticalculus, or tartar-control, compounds. Although plaque—not supragingival calculus—is the primary etiologic factor in marginal periodontal disease, reducing calculus formation is still a goal of good oral hygiene. The ingredients that prevent or retard new calculus formation are zinc chloride, zinc citrate, and soluble pyrophosphates (which act to inhibit crystal growth). Placebo-controlled clinical studies have reported a significant reduction in calculus occurrence and severity.[10]

ADA regards the inhibition of supragingival calculus as a nontherapeutic use and, therefore, does not evaluate anticalculus claims. However, all advertising claims made for accepted products are reviewed for accuracy. ADA has directed that the following additional statement appear on all package and container labeling for accepted fluoride dentifrice products with calculus-control activity: "[Product name] has been shown to reduce the formation of tartar above the gumline, but has not been shown to have a therapeutic effect on periodontal diseases."[8]

The use of tartar-control toothpastes has been associated with a type of contact dermatitis in the perioral region. Adding pyrophosphate compounds to these products increases alkalinity and requires increased concentrations of other components, such as flavorings and surfactants, for solubilizing. It is hypothesized that the pyrophosphates, either alone or combined with the higher concentrations of inactive ingredients, are implicated as the cause of irritant contact dermatitis. Patients experiencing such a reaction should be advised to discontinue the tartar-control dentifrice and should switch to a non–tartar-control fluoride product. The skin eruption resolves by decreasing or eliminating exposure.[11]

### Administration Guidelines

Table 31-3 describes the proper method for brushing teeth using a fluoride dentifrice. Children are usually unable to brush by themselves until they are 4 or 5 years of age, and they may require supervision until age 8 or 9 years to clean effectively. FDA recommends that parents instruct children ages 6 to 12 years about good brushing and rinsing habits to minimize swallowing of fluoride. Parents should apply the toothpaste (only a pea-sized amount) to a child-sized toothbrush and should brush the teeth of preschoolers until the children can manage it properly by themselves. Children should be taught to rinse thoroughly and expectorate after brushing. Only regular-strength fluoride toothpaste is recommended for use in children from 2 to 6 years of age. Use in children younger than 2 years should be under the direction of a dentist or primary care provider.

All fluoride dentifrice products must contain the following warning on the labeling: "Warning: Keep out of the reach of children under 6 years of age. If you accidentally swallow more than used for brushing, seek professional assistance or contact a Poison Control Center immediately."

**TABLE 31-3 Guidelines for Brushing Teeth**

- Brush teeth after each meal, or at least twice a day.
- If using a toothpaste, apply a small amount of paste to the toothbrush.
- If using a powder, apply the powder to a wet toothbrush, completely covering all bristles.
- Use a gentle scrubbing motion with the bristle tips at a 45° angle against the gumline so that the tips of the brush do the cleaning.
- Do not use excessive force because such force may result in bristle damage, cervical abrasion, irritation of delicate gingival tissue, and gingival recession with associated hypersensitivity.
- Brush for at least 30 seconds, cleaning all tooth surfaces systematically.
- Gently brush the upper surface of the tongue to reduce debris, plaque, and bacteria that can cause oral hygiene problems.
- If using a powder, reapply powder as before and brush again. (Two applications of powder are needed to deliver an amount of sodium fluoride comparable to one application of a paste formulation.)
- Rinse the mouth, and spit out all the water.

### Product Selection Guidelines

Unless advised otherwise by their dentists, patients—especially those with periodontal disease, significant gum recession, and/or exposed root surfaces—should choose the least abrasive dentifrice that effectively removes stained pellicle. Although dentifrice abrasives do not pose a risk to dental enamel, toothbrushing action and excessive abrasiveness, which may lead to tooth hypersensitivity, can damage the softer material of exposed root surfaces (cementum) and dentin.

Children younger than 6 years should not use a fluoride dentifrice. Extra-strength fluoride dentifrices, however, may be beneficial to patients who have a greater tendency to develop cavities or who reside in an area with nonfluoridated water.

Popular gel dentifrices are flavored and disperse rapidly in the mouth. Manufacturers of gel dentifrices have advertised that children brush longer and more thoroughly because of the gel's consistency, translucence, dispersibility, and flavor. This claim has not been substantiated, but many dentifrices marketed for children are of the gel type. The children's products usually have fruit flavors rather than the breath-freshening minty or cinnamon flavors that adults prefer.

## *Plaque Removal Devices*

Toothbrushes, dental floss, specialty aids (e.g., interproximal dental brushes), and oral irrigating devices are the primary devices used in facilitating plaque removal.

### Toothbrushes

The toothbrush is the most universally accepted device available for removing dental plaque and maintaining good oral hygiene. Estimated yearly retail sales of toothbrushes is $500 million.

The proper frequency and method of brushing will vary from patient to patient. Thoroughness of plaque removal without gingival trauma is more important than the method used. Table 31-3 describes the proper method of brushing teeth

*Types of Toothbrushes* Manual toothbrushes vary in size, shape, texture, and design, with new product designs proliferating rapidly. These toothbrushes have either nylon or natural bristles. The firmness of the bristles is usually rated as soft, medium, or firm.

Electric toothbrushes, of which there are many on the market, are either battery operated or have a rechargeable battery system. The battery-operated variety, such as the Crest Spinbrush or Colgate Powered Toothbrush, use a rotary and/or vibratory motion, and are less expensive, but the efficiency of their actions deteriorates as a result of the inherent properties of the disposable battery. Rechargeable battery toothbrushes, such as the Oral B Braun and Sonicare, use a rotary and/or vibrating motion (Oral B Braun) or high-frequency sound (Sonicare) to remove plaque. These power brushes tend to be more expensive, but they maintain constant efficiency because of their rechargeability. Dental professionals consider the power toothbrush to have a positive effect on the oral health of 80.5% of their patients.[12] Electric toothbrushes may also benefit certain patients, such as those who are disabled or of advanced age, patients with orthodontic devices, and those who may have difficulty mastering manual brushing techniques.

Best results can be expected if a patient uses a brush carrying the ADA seal of acceptance and follows a dental professional's specific directions for use. ADA's criteria for acceptance are based on safety and efficacy concerns. Advertisements may mention plaque reduction but may not claim to improve any existing oral disease.[1] Comparative studies to date have yielded mixed results and modest differences. Variations in study design and specific patient factors or situations have influenced interpretation of the results. Positive results (i.e., significant reductions in dental plaque accumulation) depend, to some extent, on the proper use of the device, implying a need for patient education.

*Replacement of Toothbrushes* There is no definite guideline as to how often a patient should buy a new toothbrush, although 3 months has been suggested as the average toothbrush life expectancy. Marketing data suggest that consumers, on average, replace their toothbrushes only 1.7 times per year. Two major reasons exist for replacing toothbrushes frequently: wear and bacterial accumulation. Different methods of brushing cause bristles to wear differently. Worn, bent, or matted bristles do not remove plaque effectively. Thus, patients should replace toothbrushes at the first sign of bristle wear rather than after a defined period of use. Ideally, they should rotate two or three toothbrushes to allow each to dry completely between uses, thereby decreasing bristle wear and matting. Some brands of toothbrushes have color-impregnated bristles that indicate the need for replacement when the color disappears halfway down the brush.

*Product Selection Guidelines* Dental professionals recommend toothbrushes based on the individual patient's manual dexterity, oral anatomy, and periodontal health. The toothbrush should be of a size and shape to allow the patient to reach every tooth in the mouth. Many dentists and dental hygienists prefer soft, rounded, multitufted, nylon bristle brushes because nylon bristles are more durable and easier to clean than natural bristles and soft, rounded bristle tips are also more effective in removing plaque below the gingival margin and on proximal tooth surfaces. Unfortunately, toothbrush firmness is not standardized; toothbrushes designated as soft, medium, or hard may not be comparable across manufacturers. Most dental professionals recommend a soft brush, even though many individuals may believe that a firm brush will do a better job of cleaning. The softer bristles are more effective at working themselves into crevices and spaces between the teeth and are less abrasive on teeth with exposed recession. Innovations in head shapes and bristle configurations continue to be introduced in an attempt to improve cleaning contact with tooth and gumline surfaces.

The handle size and shape of a toothbrush should allow the individual to maneuver the brush easily while maintaining a firm grasp. Many modifications (e.g., angle bends or flexible areas in the handle) have been introduced that may improve contact between the bristles and some less-accessible tooth surfaces. The dentist can fabricate customized handles for physically impaired individuals by adding moldable acrylic to the handles.

Soft bristles are recommended for children's toothbrushes. Children's toothbrushes are smaller than an adult's and are available in baby (for children up to age 6 or 7 years) and junior (ages 7 years to teens) sizes. Toothbrush size and shape should be individualized according to the size of the child's mouth. Children can usually remove plaque more easily with a brush that has short and narrow bristles.

## Dental Floss

Plaque accumulation in the interdental spaces contributes to proximal caries and periodontal pocketing. Interdental plaque removal has been reported to reduce gingival inflammation and prevent periodontal disease and dental caries. Dental flossing is the most widely recommended method of removing dental plaque from proximal tooth surfaces that are not adequately cleaned by toothbrushing alone. Besides removing plaque and debris interproximally, proper flossing also polishes the tooth surfaces, massages interdental papillae, and reduces gingival inflammation. Proper flossing technique requires some finger dexterity and practice. If performed improperly, flossing can injure gingival tissue and cause cervical wear on proximal root surfaces.[1] Table 31-4 describes the proper use of dental floss.

**TABLE 31-4 Guidelines for Using Dental Floss**

- Pull out approximately 18 in. of floss, and wrap most of it around the middle finger.
- Wrap the remaining floss around the same finger of the opposite hand. About an inch of floss should be held between the thumbs and forefingers.
- Do not snap the floss between the teeth; instead, use a gentle, sawing motion to guide the floss to the gumline.
- When the gumline is reached, curve the floss into a C-shape against one tooth, and gently slide the floss into the space between the gum and tooth until you feel resistance
- Hold the floss tightly against the tooth, and gently scrape the side of the tooth while moving the floss away from the gums.
- Curve the floss around the adjoining tooth, and repeat the procedure.

*Types of Dental Floss* Most floss is a multifilament nylon yarn that is available in waxed or unwaxed form and in varying widths, from thin thread to thick tape. Many brands feature product lines of flosses that are impregnated or coated with additives, such as flavoring, baking soda, and fluoride. Also, several manufacturers are marketing floss made of materials with superior antishredding properties (e.g., Colgate Total, Glide, Reach Floss Easy Slide). ADA has recognized nearly 100 brands of dental floss and tape as safe and effective.[7]

*Product Selection Guidelines* Because no particular product has been proven to be superior, patient factors (e.g., tightness of tooth contacts, tooth roughness, manual dexterity, personal preference) should be considered in product selection. Similarly, clinical studies show no difference between waxed and unwaxed floss in terms of removing plaque and preventing gingivitis.[13] Evidence does not support concern about waxed floss leaving a residual wax film deposited on tooth surfaces.

Waxed floss may pass interproximally between tight-fitting teeth without shredding more easily than unwaxed floss can. Teflon floss, such as Glide, also resists shredding and slips easily between tight teeth. If contacts at the crowns of teeth are too tight to force floss interdentally, floss threaders can be used to pass floss between the teeth and under the replacement teeth (pontics) of fixed bridges. Floss threaders, which are available in reusable and disposable forms, are usually thin plastic loops or soft plastic, needle-like appliances. Electrically powered (flossing) interdental cleaning devices may be used to remove interproximal debris. However, electrically powered interdental devices or floss threaders should be used cautiously to avoid physical trauma of the gingiva.[14] Floss holders have one or two forks rigid enough to keep floss taut and a mounting mechanism that allows quick rethreading of floss. Both floss and electrically powered interdental cleaning devices may improve compliance among some people, and are recommended for patients who lack manual dexterity and for caregivers who assist disabled or hospitalized patients. Yet, studies comparing these devices with conventional dental floss have not documented any improvement in gingival health or plaque removal.[15]

### Specialty Aids

Cleaning devices that adapt to irregular tooth surfaces better than dental floss are recommended for interproximal cleaning of teeth with large interdental spaces, such as is found in patients with periodontal disease. The Flossbrush is such a device; it features woven dental floss with a time-release fluoride system that is molded into a plastic handle for interdental cleaning. The most common aids are tapered triangular wooden toothpicks (Stim-U-Dent), holders for round toothpicks (Perio-aid), miniature bottle brushes (Py-Co-Prox or Proxabrush), rubber stimulator tips, denture brushes, and denture clasp brushes.

The evidence for plaque-removal efficacy among these interproximal cleaning devices is conflicting. Differences in methodology and patient populations prevent generalizations from being made, whereas individual patient motivation and dexterity may also influence results. The dental professional considers the patient's oral anatomy, the presence of periodontal disease, the size of the interproximal spaces, and the patient's dexterity when recommending an interdental cleaning aid.

### Oral Irrigating Devices

Oral irrigators work by directing a high-pressure stream of water through a nozzle to the tooth surfaces. These devices can remove only a minimal amount of plaque from tooth surfaces. Thus, oral irrigators cannot be viewed as substitutes for a toothbrush, dental floss, or other plaque-removal devices but should be considered as adjuncts in maintaining good oral hygiene. These devices are useful for removing loose debris from those areas that cannot be cleaned with the toothbrush (e.g., around orthodontic bands and fixed bridges). Several brands on the market carry the ADA seal of acceptance.[7]

A multicenter study of periodontitis patients receiving supportive periodontal treatment (maintenance phase) determined that adjunctive daily water irrigation resulted in meaningful clinical outcomes.[16] Oral irrigators have also been valuable as vehicles for administering chemotherapeutic agents that inhibit microbial growth in inaccessible regions of the mouth. Patients with advanced periodontal disease should use these devices only under professional supervision because it is possible for transient bacteremia to occur after manipulative procedures with the oral irrigator. Oral irrigation devices are also contraindicated in patients who are predisposed to bacterial endocarditis.

## *Other Antiplaque Products*

Two classes of oral health care products have made antiplaque claims: (1) products that rely on the mechanical action of abrasives to remove plaque, and (2) those that claim to reduce or remove plaque by chemical or antimicrobial activity. These products are available in multiple forms (e.g., dentifrices and mouth rinses). The FDA Dental Plaque Subcommittee has proposed only the quaternary ammonium compound cetylpyridinium chloride 0.045% to 0.1%, and the aromatic oils combination of eucalyptol 0.092%, menthol 0.042%, methyl salicylate 0.060%, and thymol 0.064% as Category I antigingivitis/antiplaque agents for mouth rinses.[6]

ADA has adopted Acceptance Program Guidelines for Adjunctive Dental Therapies for the Reduction of Plaque and Gingivitis. The guidelines apply to the design of clinical trials that will evaluate the safety and effectiveness of products intended to mechanically remove dental plaque and reduce gingivitis. Separate guidelines evaluate products that contain chemotherapeutic agents for control of gingivitis.

### Mouth Rinses and Gels

A mouth rinse with plaque or calculus control properties is indicated as an adjunct to proper flossing and toothbrushing with a fluoride toothpaste. Further research is necessary to determine the efficacy of the antiplaque activity of these products.

Mouth rinse and dentifrice formulations are very similar. Like dentifrices, mouth rinses may be cosmetic or therapeutic (Table 31-5). Both may contain surfactants, humectants, flavor, coloring, water, and therapeutic ingredients.

*Cosmetic Mouth Rinses* A mouth rinse approximates a diluted liquid dentifrice that contains alcohol but no abrasive. Alcohol adds bite and freshness, enhances flavor, solubilizes other ingredients, and contributes to the mouth rinse's cleansing action and antibacterial activity. Flavor contributes to pleasant taste and breath freshening. Surfactants are foaming agents that aid in the removal of debris. Other active ingredients may include astringents, demulcents (soothing agents), antibacterial agents, and fluoride.

Cosmetic mouth rinses freshen the breath and clean some debris from the mouth. Mouth rinses can be classified by appearance, alcohol content, and active ingredients. In general, mouth rinses are minty (green or blue) or spicy (red), medicinal (phenolic) or alcoholic, and contain various miscellaneous ingredients such as (1) glycerin, a topical protectant that tastes sweet and is soothing to oral mucosa; (2) benzoic acid, an antimicrobial agent; or (3) zinc chloride/citrate, an astringent that neutralizes odoriferous sulfur compounds produced in the oral cavity. The most popular cosmetic mouth rinses are medicinal and mint flavored. It is normal for healthy individuals to have some degree of oral malodor (e.g., morning breath). This malodor results from reduced activity of tongue, cheeks, and salivary flow, which enhances bacterial activity and production of odoriferous sulfur compounds. Thus, products that are intended to eliminate or suppress mouth odor of local origin in healthy people with healthy mouths are considered by the FDA Advisory Review Panel on Over-the-Counter Oral Health Care Products to be cosmetics, unless they contain antimicrobial or other therapeutic agents. ADA's acceptance program does not evaluate mouth rinses labeled and advertised only as cosmetic agents.

An important consideration is the potential for breath-freshening mouth rinses to disguise or delay treatment of pathologic conditions that may contribute to lingering oral malodor (e.g., periodontal disease, purulent oral infections, and respiratory infections). If marked breath odor

**TABLE 31-5 Selected Mouth Rinses**

| Trade Name | Primary Ingredients |
|---|---|
| **Cosmetic Mouth Rinses** | |
| Biotène*† | Lysosyme; lactoferrin; glucose oxidase; lactoperoxidase |
| Lavoris† | Zantate; clove oil; zinc chloride |
| Oral B Rembrandt Dazzling Fresh*† | Methylparaben |
| Targon† | Polyethylene glycol 40; hydrogenated castor oil |
| **Therapeutic Mouth Rinses** | |
| Cepacol† | Cetylpyridinium chloride 0.05% |
| Crest Pro-Health Rinse* | Cetylpyridinium chloride 0.07% |
| Listerine Tartar Control Antiseptic | Sodium lauryl sulfate; tetrasodium pyrophosphate |
| Scope† | Cetylpyridinium chloride; domiphen |
| **Botanical-based Mouthwashes** | |
| Dr Tichenor's | Alcohol; peppermint oil; arnica |
| Gyloxide* | Carbamide peroxide |
| Herbal Mouth and Gum* | Echinacea; goldenseal; calendula; aloe; bloodroot; grapefruit seed |
| Ipsab* | Prickly ash; iodine tetrachloride; peppermint oils |
| Ipsadent | Iodine; prickly ash; stevia; cinnamon; clove; alcohol |
| Listerine* | Thymol; eucalyptol; methyl salicylate and menthol |
| Optifresh* | Sorbitol; spearmint and peppermint oils; echinacea; olive leaf; neem; citric acid |
| Tea Tree | Tea tree oil; aloe; witch hazel; spearmint oil; alcohol |
| Tom's of Maine* | Peppermint; spearmint; cinnamon; fennel; aloe vera; witch hazel |
| Viadent Original* | Sanguinaria |

*Alcohol-free; †sodium lauryl sulfate–free.

persists after proper toothbrushing, the cause should be investigated and not masked with mouth rinse.

*Therapeutic Mouth Rinses* Since the 1990s, nonprescription mouth rinses promoted for antiplaque or tartar control activity have proliferated. Ingredients added to mouth rinses for plaque control include (1) aromatic oils (thymol, eucalyptol, menthol, and methyl salicylate), which are antibacterial and have some local anesthetic activity; and (2) agents with antimicrobial activity (e.g., quaternary ammonium compounds). Of the latter, cetylpyridinium chloride is a cationic surfactant capable of bactericidal activity, although it does not penetrate plaque well. Domiphen bromide is a bactericidal agent similar to cetylpyridinium. Another ingredient, phenol, is a local anesthetic, antiseptic, and bactericidal agent that penetrates plaque better than either cetylpyridinium or domiphen.

Listerine, containing the active ingredients thymol, eucalyptol, methyl salicylate, and menthol, was the first mouth rinse to be accepted by ADA as a nonprescription antiplaque/antigingivitis mouth rinse. The phenol oils (active ingredients) control plaque by destroying bacterial cell walls, inhibiting bacterial enzymes, and extracting bacterial lipopolysaccharides. ADA has since added Cool Mint and FreshBurst Listerine and more than 100 similarly formulated private-label antiseptic mouth rinses to the antiplaque/antigingivitis category of accepted therapeutic products.[7]

Many practitioners have found anecdotally that use of rinses containing phenol oils, methyl salicylate, and alcohol often brings about a sloughing of the oral epithelium, which subsides when the rinse is discontinued. A similar event seems to occur with the use of lozenges or candies containing cinnamon or other common flavoring substances.

Clinical trials with mouth rinses containing cetylpyridinium chloride alone or in combination with domiphen bromide have reported reductions in plaque accumulation.[17] On the basis of available data, the potential for oral toxicity with these agents is low, and the potential for a gingival health benefit exists. However, studies consistent with ADA guidelines have not been evaluated, and further study is needed to substantiate their antigingivitis efficacy. At least one study has reported no difference in plaque control and gingival health between a cetylpyridinium rinse and a placebo when the former was used as a prebrushing rinse.[18] It was suggested that the order of rinsing and brushing may be relevant; reduced activity may have been influenced by the interaction of the cationic surfactant with anionic detergents in the toothpaste. Rinsing after brushing or at a time separate from brushing may be more appropriate. Cepacol, Scope, Clear Choice, and Oral-B Anti-Plaque Rinse are examples of products in this category. Because cetylpyridinium is chemically related to chlorhexidine, it may also stain teeth but to a much lesser degree. Staining is usually associated with overuse.

Another approach to plaque control does not rely on antimicrobial activity but is based on principles of surfactant action to loosen plaque. Plax, intended for use as a prebrushing rinse, has been reformulated. The new product, Advanced Formula Plax, contains an enhanced level of detergent (sodium lauryl sulfate) and the addition of detergent builders, tetrasodium pyrophosphate, and sodium benzoate. Approximately 1 to 2 tbsp of the product is vigorously swished between the teeth and then expectorated. Patients should refrain from eating, drinking, or smoking for 30 minutes after use. The FDA Dental Plaque Subcommittee concluded in the recent ANPR that insufficient data are available to classify sodium lauryl sulfate as an effective antigingivitis/antiplaque agent.[6]

Anticavity fluoride treatment mouth rinses and gels are therapeutic topical applications of fluoride for prevention of dental caries (see Use of Fluoride).

*Usage Guidelines* With the exception of Advanced Formula Plax, plaque- or calculus-control mouth rinses are intended for use twice daily after brushing. In general, an amount equal to 1 to 2 tbsp of rinse should be swished vigorously in the mouth and between the teeth for about 30 seconds and then expectorated; the rinse should not be swallowed. Patients should be advised to refrain from smoking, eating, or drinking for 30 minutes following use. Children younger than 12 years should be instructed to develop good rinsing habits (to minimize swallowing) until they are capable of using mouth rinses without supervision.

*Safety Considerations* Mouth rinses and gels are generally safe when used as directed, but occasional adverse reactions (e.g., burning sensation or irritation) have been reported. Overuse should be discouraged. Consultation with a health professional is indicated if irritation occurs and persists after the patient discontinues use of the product. The detergent sodium lauryl sulfate is also present in nearly all toothpastes and has been implicated as a cause of aphthous ulcers (canker sores).[19] Some dentifrices that do not contain sodium lauryl sulfate are listed in Table 31-1. Aphthous ulcers are discussed in Chapter 32.

Unsupervised use is contraindicated in patients with mouth irritation or ulceration. These products should be kept out of the reach of children. In case of accidental ingestion, the caregiver should seek professional assistance or contact a poison control center.

The alcohol content in mouth rinses ranges from 0% to 27%; the most popular adult mouth rinses contain between 14% and 27%. This issue has drawn attention for two reasons. Ingestion of alcohol-containing products poses a danger for children, who may be attracted by bright colors and pleasant flavors, and concern exists about a potential association between the use of mouth rinses containing alcohol and an increased risk of oral cancer.

Toxicity data concerning a child's ingestion of an alcohol-containing mouth rinse demonstrate that the amount of alcohol in available mouth rinse preparations is sufficient to cause serious illness and injury. Acute alcoholic intoxication and death resulting from high-dose ingestion is possible. For a child weighing 26 lb, 5 to 10 oz of a mouth rinse containing alcohol can be lethal.[1] Responding to concern over the potential danger to children, the Consumer Products Safety Commission issued a final rule in January 1995 that required child-resistant packaging for mouth rinses with 3 g or more of absolute alcohol per package—the amount that is present in a small quantity (approximately 2.6 oz) of a mouth rinse with alcohol 5%: "For the purposes of this final rule, the term *mouthwash* includes liquid products that are variously called mouthwashes, mouth rinses, oral antiseptics, gargles, fluoride rinses, antiplaque rinses, and breath fresheners. It does not include throat sprays or aerosol breath fresheners." These products should be kept out of the reach of children and should not be administered to children younger than 12 years. Labeling includes a warning not to swallow but to seek professional assistance or contact a poison control center immediately in case of accidental ingestion.

The Dental Products Panel considered the use of alcohol in oral health care products in 1994 and again in 1996.[20] A 2003 ANPR would permit the proposed Category I antigingivitis/antiplaque single active ingredient cetylpyridinium chloride, and the combination active ingredients eucalyptol, menthol, methyl salicylate, and thymol to be combined in a hydroalcoholic vehicle containing 21.6% to 26.9% alcohol in a mouth rinse provided the alcohol content is clearly stated on the principal display panel.[6] Alcohol-free formulations in the various mouth rinse categories also are available (Table 31-5).

## Plaque-control Chewing Gum and Lozenges

Additions to the plaque-control market include baking soda chewing gum (e.g., Arm & Hammer Dental Care Chewing Gum, Trident Advantage) for plaque reduction. Gum chewing contributes to increased saliva flow that apparently produces a beneficial buffering effect against acids in the oral cavity. Thus, especially for patients with xerostomia, these products may have some value as an adjunct to their oral hygiene. In addition, the chewing gums are sugar-free and sweetened with sugar alcohols (e.g., xylitol and sorbitol) that do not promote caries and may reduce the risk of caries formation. Furthermore, Aquafresh now makes a lozenge that may aid in plaque control by increasing saliva flow.

The patient is directed to chew two pieces of gum daily after eating. These products are not regulated for their antiplaque claims by FDA and should not substitute for a regular program of brushing, flossing, and rinsing to remove plaque.

## Special Population Considerations for Plaque Removal

At birth, the 20 primary teeth that will erupt are present but not visible. It is important to start oral hygiene early in life. Thus, the practitioner should recommend removal of plaque and milk residue by wiping the baby's gums with a wet gauze pad after each feeding. The deciduous teeth will usually start to erupt at about age 6 months and can decay at any time. "Baby bottle caries" results when an infant is allowed to nurse continuously from a bottle of juice, milk, or sugar water. The prolonged contact of teeth with the cariogenic liquid promotes caries. When the teeth have erupted, a soft, child-sized toothbrush can be used for cleaning. Parents must do the brushing and should take care to use only a very small amount of fluoride toothpaste or none at all. Children at this age will swallow the toothpaste, which will contribute to overall systemic fluoride ingestion. Therefore, younger children need to be taught the proper brushing technique or be supervised while brushing.

In patients with fixed orthodontia, very careful attention to oral hygiene to prevent gingivitis and caries is required because of the ease with which plaque accumulates along the orthodontic brackets. Patients with these appliances require a combination of toothbrush types to clean all surfaces effectively. Use of power toothbrushes or oral irrigating devices may help remove plaque and debris around orthodontic bands. It may be advisable for orthodontic patients to use a nonprescription fluoride mouth rinse while undergoing treatment.

Patients with removable orthodontic appliances should consult their orthodontist about using a denture cleanser. Some dental practitioners have recommended, in addition to brushing, a denture cleanser to remove plaque, tartar, odor-causing bacteria, and stain that accumulates on orthodontic appliances.

In patients of advanced age who have natural dentition, topical fluoride application in the form of a dentifrice, rinse, or gel is indicated to prevent coronal and root caries. Practitioners should continue to recommend fluoride anticaries products to their older adult patients. When a practitioner counsels these patients on oral health care, it becomes very important to consider the patients' medication use. Because this population is more likely to be taking multiple medications, incidence of drug-induced or disease-related changes in oral physiology is increased.

### *Botanical Nonprescription Preparations*

Ethnomedical survey research continues to identify, catalog, and tabulate the most common natural products, derivatives, and nonprescription remedies advocated for oral medicine conditions within North, Central, and South America. Numerous commercial products, such as dentrifices (Table 31-1) and mouthwashes (Table 31-5), that contain a variety of natural agents are available. Many popular, commonly used products, such as Listerine, are botanically based, but often are not recognized as such by patients and health care professionals.

Evidence-based research is lacking to verify the identification, use, and standardized dosage of most naturally occurring nonprescription compounds for oral medicine applications.[21,22] Evidence-based research is needed to verify the indications, safety, dosage, efficacy,[21,23-25] and potential herb–drug interactions[26-28] of these products and compounds to justify their role in contemporary oral medicine.

### *Use of Fluoride*

Fluoride is believed to help prevent dental caries through a combination of effects. When it is incorporated into developing teeth, fluoride systemically reduces the solubility of dental enamel by enhancing the development of a fluoridated hydroxyapatite (which is more resistant to demineralizing acids) at the enamel surface. The topical effect facilitates remineralization of early carious lesions during repeated cycles of demineralization and remineralization. Some evidence exists that fluoride interferes with the bacterial cariogenic process. Fluoride that is chemically bound to organic constituents of plaque may interfere with plaque adherence and inhibit glycolysis, the process by which sugar is metabolized to produce acid.[1]

#### Fluoridated Water Supplies

Fluoridation of the public water supply is an effective and economically sound public health measure that has played a major role in decreasing the incidence of caries.[29] More than one half of the U.S. population resides in communities in which the public water supply contains either naturally occurring or added fluoride at optimal levels for decay prevention (e.g., 1 ppm or 1 mg/L). Besides reducing dental caries in children, fluoridation has benefits that extend through adulthood, resulting in (1) fewer decayed, missing, or filled teeth; (2) greater tooth retention; and (3) a lower incidence of root caries. Systemic fluoride supplementation in children is based on the preventive mechanism of fluoride when incorporated into developing enamel. Current concepts of the action of fluoride relative to its presence in saliva and plaque provide a rationale for its topical application to prevent caries in all age groups. It must be noted, however, that any decision to supplement fluoride intake must take into account the concentration of fluoride present in the drinking water.[1] Bottled water does not contain fluoride.

#### Fluoride Rinses and Gels

Mouth rinses and gels that contain sodium fluoride are therapeutic topical applications of fluoride for prevention of dental caries (Table 31-6). Fluoride mouth rinsing enables patients to apply fluoride interproximally. Studies of fluoride mouth rinsing have shown consistently positive

**TABLE 31-6 Selected Topical Fluoride Products**

| Trade Name | Primary Ingredients |
|---|---|
| Act for Kids* | Sodium fluoride 0.05%; cetylpyridinium chloride |
| Fluorigard Anti-Cavity Rinse† | Sodium fluoride 0.05% |
| GelKam Gel | Stannous fluoride 0.4% |
| Oral-B Anti-Cavity Rinse* | Sodium fluoride 0.05% |
| Reach Act Adult Anti-Cavity Rinse* | Sodium fluoride 0.05%; cetylpyridinium chloride |

*Alcohol-free; †dye-free.

**TABLE 31-7 Guidelines for Using Topical Fluoride Treatments[2]**

- Use topical fluoride treatments no more than once a day.
- Brush teeth with a fluoride dentifrice before using a fluoride treatment.
- If using a fluoride rinse, measure the recommended dose (most commonly 10 mL), and vigorously swish it between the teeth for 1 minute.
- If using a fluoride gel, brush the gel on the teeth. Allow the gel to remain for 1 minute.
- After 1 minute, spit out the fluoride product. Do not swallow it.
- Do not eat or drink for 30 minutes after the treatment.
- Supervise children as necessary until they can use the product without supervision.
- Instruct children younger than 12 years in good rinsing habits to minimize swallowing of the product.
- Consult a dentist or primary care provider before using fluoride products in children younger than 6 years.

results.[30] Studies in which subjects used sodium fluoride 0.05% rinse once daily have demonstrated a significant reduction in the incidence of caries, especially among children living in areas with nonfluoridated water.[31]

Examples of patients who may benefit from fluoride rinsing are those with orthodontic appliances, those with decreased salivary flow, those at risk for developing root caries, and anyone with difficulty maintaining good oral hygiene. Orthodontic patients are at risk of developing decalcified areas while under treatment, and their ability to thoroughly clean interdental spaces may be inhibited.

Because fluoride rinses and gels provide a therapeutic fluoride treatment, package directions should be followed closely. To maximize the safe and effective use of these products, FDA requires labeling to instruct consumers to read the directions. Table 31-7 describes the proper method of applying fluoride rinses and gels. When recommending a nonprescription fluoride mouth rinse, the practitioner should stress that children younger than 12 years of age should be supervised as necessary until they are capable of using the product correctly. Further, children younger than 6 years of age should use these products only as directed by a dentist or primary care provider. Concern has been raised about whether unsupervised home use of fluoride gels is justified.

### Fluoride Dentifrices

Fluoride dentifrices provide a means of increasing the contact of fluoride with the tooth surfaces, where it exerts its greatest protection. Brushing with a fluoride dentifrice provides anticaries protection; however, the fluoride does not adequately reach the surfaces between teeth. Thus, the high-risk patients mentioned previously may especially benefit from multiple sources of fluoride application. Fluoride-containing dental products are believed to be of greatest benefit when used in areas with a nonfluoridated public water supply. However, they can help reduce the incidence of caries, even in patients residing in communities with a fluoridated water supply.

Patients who form heavy calculus between dental visits may consider using a fluoride dentifrice with added tartar control ingredients instead of a plain fluoride dentifrice. A patient's appearance may benefit from a lessening of visible supragingival calculus buildup, and reports indicate that professional dental cleaning may be easier because the calculus that does form is less adherent.

### Dental Fluorosis

Fluoride dentifrices contribute to the total amount of fluoride ingested by children. Other sources are dietary products, recommended systemic supplements, and any other topical fluoride preparations. When chronic fluoride ingestion from all sources is considered, children who live in a community with an optimally fluoridated water supply may exceed optimal daily amounts. This places them at risk for mild forms of dental fluorosis, a mottled appearance of surface enamel. Although a mild degree of fluorosis is an esthetic concern, more severe cases can result in pitting and surface defects (see Color Plates, photograph 7).

Related to this concern, FDA considered comments regarding formulation of a reduced-strength fluoride dentifrice during the anticaries final rule process. It was determined that mild dental fluorosis does not compromise oral health or tooth function as do dental caries. Therefore, the risk of dental caries from inadequate fluoride protection is a greater health hazard than the cosmetic effect of fluorosis.

Because of the concerns about dental fluorosis in children, FDA required that dentifrice products with sodium monofluorophosphate containing 1500 ppm of theoretical total fluorine carry the following label: "Keep out of the reach of children under 6 years of age." Aim Extra Strength toothpaste is an extra-strength monofluorophosphate fluoride product that is accepted by ADA; data support its clinical and statistical superiority over its regular-strength counterpart.

In 1994, ADA revised its recommendations for fluoride supplement dosing in children. The new schedule slightly lowers the dose amounts, recommends beginning treatment not earlier than age 6 months, and extends the age limit from 13 to 16 years. Evaluation of studies reporting on the intake of fluoride among children prompted the revision.

Studies of dentifrice ingestion by children show great variation in the amount of dentifrice retained and consistently show that younger children are more likely than older ones to swallow some dentifrice. Limiting ingestion of fluoride dentifrice is advised (see Administration Guidelines under Dentifrices).

Fluoride rinsing presents a similar problem for children (ages 3 to 5 years) who may swallow significant amounts of rinse each time they swish. A usual dose of fluoride 0.05% rinse contains 2 mg of fluoride ion and may contribute to mild fluorosis in the presence of a fluoridated public water supply. Fluoride rinses should be used only by children 6 years and older who have mastered the swallowing reflex. These products should be kept out of the reach of children, and children younger than

12 years should be supervised when rinsing. High-dose ingestion requires prompt medical care. Toxicity is related to both the fluoride and the alcohol content. Parents should be able to identify the product and to estimate the amount ingested.

## Assessment of Caries: A Case-based Approach

When asked to recommend plaque control products, the practitioner should determine what dental care measures the patient is taking, whether these measures meet recommended oral hygiene standards, and how often the patient sees a dentist. The patient's concern about caries should alert the practitioner to ask whether the patient has a history of caries or suspects a new carious lesion has developed. Case 31-1 illustrates the assessment of patients with caries.

## Patient Counseling for Caries

The practitioner should tailor all explanations of the purpose of various oral hygiene products and the methods for using them to the patient's level of knowledge. Patients with a history of caries should be encouraged to brush after meals and to consult with a dentist regarding the use of topical fluoride products. If caries recur or are widespread, the patient should be encouraged to visit a dentist for treatment. The practitioner may recommend products with anticaries agents (e.g., chlorhexidine, povidone iodine, or xylitol). The practitioner should explain the precautions for these products as well as the possible adverse effects of some therapeutic ingredients in other products. Patients should be advised of signs and symptoms that indicate a dental evaluation is necessary. The box Patient Education for Prevention of Caries, Gingivitis, and Halitosis lists specific information to provide patients about plaque-induced oral disorders.

Because dental disease is the most frequently encountered health problem in the United States, and practitioners see many people with dental problems, the practitioner needs a well-developed knowledge of oral health care products and their use. Useful resources, references, and information related to ongoing FDA and ADA evaluations of nonprescription dental products are easily available on the Internet. Sites maintained by government agencies, industry, and professional associations provide valuable professional and patient education material. Table 31-8 lists some of these organizations.

### CASE 31-1

| Relevant Evaluation Criteria | Scenario/Model Outcome |
|---|---|
| **Information Gathering** | |
| 1. Gather essential information about the patient's symptoms, including: | |
| a. description of symptom(s) (i.e., nature, onset, duration, severity, associated symptoms) | Patient has suffered from a toothache for several days. The pain is in the lower right jaw, intermittent with varying intensities. |
| b. description of any factors that seem to precipitate, exacerbate, and/or relieve the patient's symptom(s) | Symptoms began when the patient bit down on a popcorn kernel and seemed to subside after he rinsed with water. |
| c. description of the patient's efforts to relieve the symptoms | Patient has tried Anbesol, to no avail. |
| 2. Gather essential patient history information: | |
| a. patient's identity | Jim Williams |
| b. patient's age, sex, height, and weight | 35 y/o M, 6'0", 205 lb |
| c. patient's occupation | Attorney |
| d. patient's dietary habits | Well-balanced diet, but likes chewing gum |
| e. patient's sleep habits | Good |
| f. concurrent medical conditions, prescription and nonprescription medications, and dietary supplements | Allegra 180 mg once daily |
| g. allergies | Pollen, sulfa-containing medications |
| h. history of other adverse reactions to medications | Codeine upsets his stomach. |
| i. other (describe)_______ | Jim likes sucking on mint candies as breath fresheners and chewing gum, but now chews only sugar-free gum. |

## CASE 31-1 (continued)

| Relevant Evaluation Criteria | Scenario/Model Outcome |
|---|---|
| **Assessment and Triage** | |
| 3. Differentiate the patient's signs/symptoms and correctly identify the patient's primary problem(s). | Patient appears to have dental caries or cracked tooth caused by poor hygiene and heavy sugar consumption related to mint candies and regular gum chewing. |
| 4. Identify exclusions for self-treatment. | None |
| 5. Formulate a comprehensive list of therapeutic alternatives for the primary problem to determine if triage to a medical practitioner is required, and share this information with the patient. | Options include:<br>(1) Refer Jim to a dentist.<br>(2) Recommend appropriate OTC products with lifestyle modifications and refer to a dentist.<br>(3) Take no action. |
| **Plan** | |
| 6. Select an optimal therapeutic alternative to address the patient's problem, taking into account patient preferences. | Take OTC NSAIDs for pain and inflammation; I suggest a thorough cleaning with a fluoride-containing toothpaste. Modify your diet by using sugar-free mint candies to freshen breath. |
| 7. Describe the recommended therapeutic approach to the patient. | NSAIDs, pain relievers such as ibuprofen, aspirin, or naproxen, will reduce pain and particularly tooth nerve inflammation. Also, discontinue use of sugar-containing breath mint fresheners, which contribute to the pain, and discontinue chewing gum, which applies pressure to your tooth. |
| 8. Explain to the patient the rationale for selecting the recommended therapeutic approach from the considered therapeutic alternatives. | You need to see a dentist to completely solve the problems of caries and/or a possible cracked tooth. The suggested actions are palliative and will aid in preventing future disease. |
| **Patient Education** | |
| 9. When recommending self-care with nonprescription medications and/or nondrug therapy, convey accurate information to the patient, including: | |
| a. appropriate dose and frequency of administration | Take one of the following for pain relief: 400 mg of ibuprofen 4 to 6 times a day; 650 mg of aspirin every 4 hours as needed; or 220 mg of naproxen every 8 to 12 hours. |
| b. maximum number of days the therapy should be employed | Use palliative treatment for the shortest time possible before seeing dentist. |
| c. product administration procedures | Remember to take NSAIDs with food and plenty of fluids. |
| d. expected time to onset of relief | Relief should come within an hour. |
| e. degree of relief that can be reasonably expected | Total relief will not occur until caries is removed and tooth is restored. |
| f. most common side effects | Dyspepsia, heartburn, and nausea |
| g. side effects that warrant medical intervention should they occur | Gastrointestinal bleeding; severe dyspepsia, heartburn, or nausea |
| h. patient options in the event that condition worsens or persists | If no pain relief occurs after 1 hour of taking the medication, seek emergency dental treatment. |
| i. product storage requirements | Keep NSAIDs in a tightly closed container at room temperature or below. |
| j. specific nondrug measures | Avoid hard and/or sweet foods. |

CASE 31-1 (continued)

| Relevant Evaluation Criteria | Scenario/Model Outcome |
|---|---|
| 10. Solicit patient's follow-up questions. | May I double my dose of any of these products if needed? |
| 11. Answer patient's questions. | No. You should seek emergency dental treatment if the pain isn't relieved within an hour of taking the medication. |

Key: NSAID, nonsteroidal anti-inflammatory drug; OTC, over-the-counter.

**TABLE 31-8 Internet Oral Health Care Resources for the Pharmacist**

| Agency/Organization | Web Site | Available Resources/Services |
|---|---|---|
| American Dental Association | www.ada.org | Patient education, product news, research, publications, references, accepted products |
| Federal Register | www.access.gpo.gov | OTC advisory committee actions and recommendations; proposed and final rules, etc. |
| National Institute of Dental and Craniofacial Research | www.nidr.nih.gov (site maintained by National Institutes of Health) | Health care and patient information, *NIDCR Research Digest*, and links to oral health resources |
| Academy of General Dentistry | www.agd.org | Reliable source for consumer dental health information |
| American Dental Hygienists' Association | www.adha.org | Consumer oral health information and related links |
| American Association of Public Health Dentistry | www.pitt.edu/~aaphd | Databases and links to Internet resources on oral health |
| National Oral Health Information Clearinghouse | www.aerie.com/nohicweb | Information for special care populations; Oral Health Database; resource links |
| Combined Health Information Database | www.chid.nih.gov | Database produced by health-related agencies of the federal government; health information and health education resources |
| Various manufacturers of oral health care products | Search for home pages on the Internet | Product information and links to related dental sites |

## GINGIVITIS

Periodontal disease, the prevalence and severity of which is related primarily to the degree and quality of oral health care, remains the principal cause of tooth loss in adults older than 45 years.[2] Controlling buildup of plaque and calculus can prevent or control this common and significant public health problem. All forms of periodontal disease are associated with oral hygiene status, not with age. However, as lifespans increase and people retain more teeth later in life, both the number of teeth at risk and the time for risk of periodontal disease increases.[1]

Gingivitis, the mildest form of periodontal disease, is reversible and affects nearly everyone. Gingivitis may progress to more severe periodontal diseases, such as acute necrotizing ulcerative gingivitis and periodontitis. The latter can cause significant, irreversible alveolar bone loss.

Acute necrotizing ulcerative gingivitis, also referred to as Vincent's stomatitis and trench mouth, is an acute bacterial infection characterized by necrosis and ulceration of the gingival surface with underlying inflammation. The disease may involve a single tooth, a group of teeth, or the entire oral cavity. Localized symptoms often include severe pain, bleeding gingival tissue, halitosis, foul taste, and increased salivation. Lymphadenopathy, fever, and malaise may accompany the localized symptoms.

Trench mouth is seen most frequently in the United States in teenagers and young adults. Predisposing factors include anxiety, emotional stress, smoking, malnutrition, and poor oral hygiene.[32] Factors resulting in decreased host resistance and an altered host-bacteria relationship have been implicated.[33] Professional dental treatment is indicated and consists of local debridement and systemic drug therapy, coupled with elimination of the predisposing factors.

Periodontitis and gingivitis can be distinguished in the following way. Whereas gingivitis is the inflammation of the gingiva without loss or migration of epithelial attachment to the tooth, periodontitis occurs when the periodontal ligament attachment and alveolar bone support of the tooth have been compromised or lost. This process involves apical migration of the epithelial attachment from the enamel to the root surface (see Color Plates, photographs 8 and 9).

Most adults with periodontitis have moderately progressing disease, and perhaps 10% have rapidly progressing disease. Prognosis is good if an initial comprehensive course of therapy is successful. In some cases, unfortunately, alveolar bone loss is irreversible. Prospects for disease control are not good if plaque and calculus control is poor or resolution of inflammation is inadequate despite comprehensive treatment.

Practitioners can assist patients in preventing gingivitis and the more advanced periodontal diseases by counseling them on the selection of oral hygiene products and encouraging good oral hygiene.

## Epidemiology of Gingivitis

Because caries and gingivitis can result from buildup of plaque, the epidemiology of caries can be extended to that of gingivitis (see Epidemiology of Caries). In addition, hormonal changes influence gingivitis, accounting for its increased frequency during puberty and pregnancy.

Pregnant patients are more susceptible to both dental caries and gingivitis. An inflammatory condition so common that it is called pregnancy gingivitis is characterized by red, swollen gingival tissue that bleeds easily. Local factors cause this gingivitis, as in any patient. Pregnancy modifies the host's response, however, making gingival tissue more sensitive to bacterial dental plaque. Hormone level and increased production of prostaglandins have been implicated in the heightened inflammatory response.[1] Pregnancy gingivitis can be prevented or resolved with thorough plaque control. The severity of the inflammatory response and the resulting gingivitis decrease postpartum and return to prepregnancy levels after approximately 1 year.

## Etiology of Gingivitis

Gingivitis results from the accumulation of supragingival bacterial plaque. If this accumulation is not controlled, the plaque proliferates and invades subgingival spaces. At the same time, as specific types of bacteria are associated with plaque at different stages of accumulation, the composition of the bacterial flora changes to a more complex mix of organisms. The transition from supragingival to subgingival plaque accumulation is significant because the patient cannot adequately remove the subgingival plaque mechanically. Thus, the accumulation of supragingival plaque over time can eventually result in gingivitis. Although not all gingivitis progresses to periodontitis, the progression from supragingival plaque to gingivitis to periodontitis is relatively common, so that controlling gingivitis is a reasonable approach to limiting periodontitis.[1]

Gingivitis also may manifest as a result of (1) blood dyscrasias such as leukemia, (2) mucocutaneous diseases such as lichen planus, and (3) viral infections such as acute herpetic gingivostomatitis. Most important, disturbances of the immune system (e.g., AIDS) can lead to a severe form of this disease.[34]

Other possible etiologies include medications such as calcium channel blockers, cyclosporine, and phenytoin. Anticholinergics and antidepressants may cause gingivitis by reducing the flow of saliva. The use of tobacco (both smokeless and smoked) has also been linked to periodontal disease.

## Pathophysiology/Signs and Symptoms of Gingivitis

The basic pathologic process of gingivitis is an inflammatory reaction caused by bacterial plaque. If dental plaque is not controlled, specific bacteria (initially, gram-positive cocci such as *Streptococcus sanguis* and *S. mitis* and, later, *Actinomyces* spp. and gram-negative organisms) colonize the gum tissue to cause swelling, redness, changes in gum form and position, and bleeding (when gums are brushed or probed). Pink-tinted toothbrush bristles should be a sign to patients of possible gingivitis.

The marginal gingiva (the border of the gingiva surrounding the neck of the tooth) is held firmly to the tooth by a network of collagen fibers. Microorganisms present in the plaque in the gingival sulcus (the space between the gingiva and the tooth) are capable of producing harmful products, such as acids, toxins, and enzymes that damage cellular and intercellular tissue. Dilation and proliferation of gingival capillaries, increased flow of gingival fluid, and increased blood flow with resultant erythema of the gingiva are found in early stages. The gingiva may also enlarge, change contour, and appear puffy or swollen as a result of the inflammation (see Color Plates, photograph 8). In the early stage of gingivitis, the inflammatory process is reversible with effective oral hygiene.

In time and with neglect, the condition becomes chronic as capillaries become engorged, venous return is slowed, and localized anoxemia results in a bluish hue to areas of the reddened gingiva. Chronic gingivitis may be localized to the area around one or several teeth, or it may be generalized, involving the gingiva around all the teeth. The inflammation may involve just the marginal gingiva or it may be more diffuse, involving all the gingival tissue surrounding the tooth. Changes in gingival color, size, and shape, as well as the ease with which gingival bleeding occurs, are common indications of chronic gingivitis that both the patient and the practitioner can recognize. The flat knife-edge appearance of healthy gingiva is replaced by a ragged or rounded edge. The presence of red cells in extravascular tissue and the breakdown of hemoglobin also deepen the color of gingival tissue. Progression of these conditions is usually slow and insidious—and often painless.

Left untreated, chronic gingivitis may advance to the inflammatory condition of chronic destructive periodontal disease, or periodontitis (see Color Plates, photograph 9). Bacterial species that predominate in periodontitis, but are not present in healthy periodontium, have been found in low proportions in gingivitis. Progression of gingivitis may parallel the increasing proportions of bacterial species implicated in the genesis of periodontitis.

## Prevention of Gingivitis

Because prevention of gingivitis and caries depends on calculus prevention and plaque control, the same measures described in Prevention of Caries pertain to gingivitis. The active antigingivitis ingredients in dentifrices, mouth rinses, and other plaque removal and antiplaque products are triclosan (an antibacterial ingredient introduced for its antigingivitis properties) and a stabilized stannous fluoride added for its antigingivitis and anticaries properties. Stannous fluoride inhibits the types of bacteria that infect supragingival spaces.[35] Triclosan is both an antiplaque and an anti-inflammatory agent; it inhibits production of prostaglandins by several means.[36]

Brushing and flossing can cure early gingivitis that arises from irritating food debris and plaque. Adequate removal and control of supragingival plaque is the single most important factor in reversing gingivitis, and in preventing and controlling periodontal disease. Gum massage is also recommended, with such devices as soft brushes, special rubber cup massagers, a Stim-U-Dent, or toothpicks. Practitioners should immediately refer for dental care any patient who describes bleeding during brushing or shows signs of early gingivitis.

## Assessment of Gingivitis: A Case-based Approach

Before recommending oral hygiene products, the practitioner should evaluate the patient's oral hygiene regimen. At a minimum, the practitioner should find out whether the patient has a history of gingivitis, whether signs and symptoms of gingivitis are currently present, and what preventive measures the patient has tried or is using. Checking the patient's medical and medication history will identify asymptomatic patients who are at risk for gingivitis.

The practitioner is quite often alerted to pregnancy gingivitis during counseling on prescription prenatal vitamins. Besides monitoring the pregnant patient's medications for safety, the practitioner has an opportunity to encourage the patient to have a dental checkup and to stress the importance of careful attention to brushing and flossing to avoid oral health complications. Case 31-2 gives an example of the assessment of patients with gingivitis.

### CASE 31-2

| Relevant Evaluation Criteria | Scenario/Model Outcome |
|---|---|
| **Information Gathering** | |
| 1. Gather essential information about the patient's symptoms, including: | |
| a. description of symptom(s) (i.e., nature, onset, duration, severity, associated symptoms) | Patient has suffered from red, bleeding, sore and enlarged gums for a number of weeks. |
| b. description of any factors that seem to precipitate, exacerbate, and/or relieve the patient's symptom(s) | Gingival tissues bleed easily during brushing. |
| c. description of the patient's efforts to relieve the symptoms | Patient has tried a mouth rinse that contains natural oils, but the bleeding continues. |
| 2. Gather essential patient history information: | |
| a. patient's identity | Kim Johnson |
| b. patient's age, sex, height, and weight | 40 y/o F, 5'2",124 lb |
| c. patient's occupation | Registered nurse |
| d. patient's dietary habits | Lots of fast food and cigarettes |
| e. patient's sleep habits | Off and on night shift |
| f. concurrent medical conditions, prescription and nonprescription medications, and dietary supplements | Fluoxetine 20 mg once daily |
| g. allergies | Penicillin |
| h. history of other adverse reactions to medications | Erythromycin upsets her stomach. |
| i. other (describe)______ | Kim has tried hypnosis to stop smoking, with some success. |

## CASE 31-2 (continued)

| Relevant Evaluation Criteria | Scenario/Model Outcome |
|---|---|
| **Assessment and Triage** | |
| 3. Differentiate the patient's signs/symptoms and correctly identify the patient's primary problem(s). | Kim appears to have gingivitis and possibly severe periodontal disease. |
| 4. Identify exclusions for self-treatment. | None |
| 5. Formulate a comprehensive list of therapeutic alternatives for the primary problem to determine if triage to a medical practitioner is required, and share this information with the patient. | Options include: (1) Refer Kim to a dentist. (2) Recommend proper OTC products with lifestyle modifications and refer Kim to a dentist. (3) Take no action. |
| **Plan** | |
| 6. Select an optimal therapeutic alternative to address the patient's problem, taking into account patient preferences. | NSAIDs for pain and inflammation and thorough cleaning with a fluoride-containing toothpaste will help. Suggest use of dental floss and smoking cessation aids. A visit to the dentist for a thorough assessment is absolutely necessary. |
| 7. Describe the recommended therapeutic approach to the patient. | You should take NSAIDs for pain, and use a fluoride-containing toothpaste and dental floss regularly. You should continue efforts to stop smoking. You need to see a dentist for evaluation and a professional cleaning. |
| 8. Explain to the patient the rationale for selecting the recommended therapeutic approach from the considered therapeutic alternatives. | The services of a dentist are ultimately needed to completely solve the problems of periodontal disease. The suggested actions are palliative and will aid future disease prevention. |
| **Patient Education** | |
| 9. When recommending self-care with nonprescription medications and/or nondrug therapy, convey accurate information to the patient, including: | |
| a. appropriate dose and frequency of administration | Brush at least 2 times/day for at least 2 minutes and floss at least once a day. Use OTC NSAIDs at recommended dosages. |
| b. maximum number of days the therapy should be employed | Lifetime |
| c. product administration procedures | Use a pea-sized quantity of toothpaste. |
| d. expected time to onset of relief | Relief should come within a few days. |
| e. degree of relief that can be reasonably expected | Total relief will not occur until calculus is removed by a dentist or dental hygienist. |
| f. most common side effects | Tissue edema and sloughing |
| g. side effects that warrant medical intervention should they occur | Sensitivity to flavoring oils in dentifrice |
| h. patient options in the event that condition worsens or persists | See a dentist for evaluation. |
| i. product storage requirements | Keep fluoride dentifrices out of reach of small children. |
| j. specific nondrug measures | Electric rotary toothbrushes are quite helpful. |
| 10. Solicit patient's follow-up questions. | Isn't there a good essential oils dental rinse that will kill the plaque bacteria in my mouth? |
| 11. Answer patient's questions. | No. You must remove the plaque mechanically by brushing and flossing. However, your dentist may recommend the use of a certain mouth rinse as an adjunct to your oral hygiene procedures. |

Key: NSAID, nonsteroidal anti-inflammatory drug; OTC, over-the-counter.

### Patient Counseling for Gingivitis

Because gingivitis is usually not associated with pain, patients are unlikely to seek a practitioner's advice for this problem alone. More likely, patients will ask for oral hygiene information and product recommendations. The practitioner may have to suggest oral hygiene methods and alert the patient to the possible adverse effects of certain products. The box Patient Education for Prevention of Caries, Gingivitis, and Halitosis lists specific information to provide patients.

The practitioner should also use this opportunity to warn patients with suspected gingivitis (bleeding, swollen gums) that this disease is a serious problem warranting professional attention. The practitioner should stress, especially to pregnant patients and teenagers, that adherence to an oral hygiene program is vital to preventing gingivitis.

## HALITOSIS

Halitosis, oral malodor usually known as bad breath, may be a symptom of oral pathology. However, in 90% of cases, poor oral hygiene is the cause.

### Etiology of Halitosis

Common oral causes related to poor oral hygiene include malodorous decaying food particles, tonsillar crypt debris, plaque on the dorsum of the tongue (particularly the posterior third), caries, and periodontal disease.[37] Xerostomia can also cause mouth odor. Medications that have anticholinergic properties often cause xerostomia. Garlic, tobacco, onions, alcohol, and other substances commonly placed into the mouth have their own odors that are not always appreciated by others.

Pulmonary diseases such as purulent lung infections, tuberculosis, bronchiectasis, sinusitis, tonsillitis, and rhinitis are responsible for a small percentage of mouth odors. Renal failure, carcinoma, hepatic failure, and hyperglycemic acetone breath (ketosis) are also examples of nonoral causes.[38]

### Pathophysiology of Halitosis

Most foul breath odors occur because of a breakdown of sulfur-containing proteins into volatile sulfur compounds (VSCs) including hydrogen sulfide, methylmercaptan, and dimethyl sulfide.[39]

### Prevention of Halitosis

Prevention of halitosis relies on the removal of plaque and the prevention of calculus formation as described in Prevention of Caries. One of the primary sites for the formation of VSCs is the back of the tongue. Plaque and VSCs in this area of the mouth can seed the tonsillar crypts with malodorous debris. Brushing the teeth and tongue are helpful, but some dentists have found that the use of a tongue cleaning device such as the Orafresh tongue blade (Alwin Enterprises) may be the best way to clean the circumvallate papillae area of the tongue. Cleaning this posterior dorsal area will not only remove the fetid VSCs but also prevent them from spreading to the tonsils.

Zinc salts and chlorine dioxide are most effective in the chemical prevention of oral malodor. The two are combined in two-part rinses such as Tri-Oral (Triumph Pharmaceuticals). Zinc chloride, citrate, and acetate reduce the receptor binding necessary for VSC production. Chlorine dioxide breaks disulfide bonds and oxidizes the precursors of VSCs. The zinc salts also kill gram-negative bacteria.

Any patient who complains of severe or lingering halitosis without a readily identifiable cause (e.g., smoking) should be advised to see a dentist for a thorough evaluation. Masking foul taste and odor with cosmetic mouth rinses may delay necessary dental or medical assessment and any needed treatment.

### Assessment of Halitosis: A Case-based Approach

When assessing a patient for halitosis, the practitioner should evaluate the patient's dental hygiene. Ideally, the practitioner should obtain a medication and medical history to determine whether the halitosis might arise from one of the illnesses discussed in Etiology of Halitosis (see also Xerostomia in Chapter 32.)

### Patient Counseling for Halitosis

For patients with mouth odor related to poor dental hygiene, the practitioner should recommend the appropriate products and explain their use. Nonpharmacologic measures should also be explained. The practitioner should stress to patients whose mouth odor is related to medical conditions that proper oral hygiene is still necessary to prevent tooth and gum problems. The box Patient Education for Prevention of Caries, Gingivitis, and Halitosis lists specific information to provide patients. Case 31-3 illustrates the assessment of patients with halitosis.

## HYGIENE-RELATED DENTURE PROBLEMS

Pain along the gingival ridge under a denture prosthesis suggests conditions such as denture stomatitis (an inflammation of the oral tissue in contact with a removable denture), inflammatory papillary hyperplasia, and chronic candidiasis. Denture stomatitis, which results from poor cleaning of dentures, can lead to chronic candidiasis (fungal infection).

### Etiology/Pathophysiology of Hygiene-related Denture Problems

Dentures accumulate plaque, stain, and calculus by a process very similar to that occurring on natural teeth. The denture plaque mass that is in contact with oral tissues produces predictable toxic results. Poor denture hygiene contributes to fungal and bacterial growth, not only affecting the patient esthetically (unpleasant odors and staining), but

## CASE 31-3

| Relevant Evaluation Criteria | Scenario/Model Outcome |
|---|---|
| **Information Gathering** | |
| 1. Gather essential information about the patient's symptoms, including: | |
| a. description of symptom(s) (i.e., nature, onset, duration, severity, associated symptoms) | Patient has noticed a bad odor coming from his mouth and has been directed by his wife to do something about it. |
| b. description of any factors that seem to precipitate, exacerbate, and/or relieve the patient's symptom(s) | The mouth odor seems to be present even when the patient has avoided eating garlic, onions, or other suspicious food items. He also notices the odor is more offensive when he awakes in the morning. |
| c. description of the patient's efforts to relieve the symptoms | Patient has tried brushing, flossing, and using several mouth rinses with only minimal improvement. |
| 2. Gather essential patient history information: | |
| a. patient's identity | George Smith |
| b. patient's age, sex, height, and weight | 45 y/o M, 5'11", 155 lb |
| c. patient's occupation | Pediatrician |
| d. patient's dietary habits | Excellent |
| e. patient's sleep habits | Good |
| f. concurrent medical conditions, prescription and nonprescription medications, and dietary supplements | Celebrex 200 mg once daily for joint pain |
| g. allergies | None |
| h. history of other adverse reactions to medications | GI distress with some NSAIDs |
| i. other (describe)_______ | N/A |
| **Assessment and Triage** | |
| 3. Differentiate the patient's signs/symptoms and correctly identify the patient's primary problem(s). | George has the fetid odor of volatile sulfur compounds in his mouth. |
| 4. Identify exclusions for self-treatment. | The halitosis may be an indication of systemic disorder. |
| 5. Formulate a comprehensive list of therapeutic alternatives for the primary problem to determine if triage to a medical practitioner is required, and share this information with the patient. | Options include:<br>(1) Refer George to a dentist.<br>(2) Recommend proper OTC products with lifestyle modifications and refer George to a dentist.<br>(3) Take no action. |
| **Plan** | |
| 6. Select an optimal therapeutic alternative to address the patient's problem, taking into account patient preferences. | Patient would like to try appropriate OTC products. |
| 7. Describe the recommended therapeutic approach to the patient. | Use a tongue cleaner to clean plaque from the posterior area of tongue, a zinc salt and/or chlorine dioxide rinse to deactivate the volatile sulfur compounds, and standard brushing and flossing. |
| 8. Explain to the patient the rationale for selecting the recommended therapeutic approach from the considered therapeutic alternatives. | Removing the volatile sulfur compounds instead of just masking the odor is the appropriate approach. If these measures are ineffective, you should see a dentist or your primary care provider. |

## CASE 31-3 (continued)

| Relevant Evaluation Criteria | Scenario/Model Outcome |
|---|---|
| **Patient Education** | |
| 9. When recommending self-care with nonprescription medications and/or nondrug therapy, convey accurate information to the patient, including: | |
| a. appropriate dose and frequency of administration | Two-part rinse with zinc salt and chlorine dioxide will be effective for 6-8 hours. |
| b. maximum number of days the therapy should be employed | No limit |
| c. product administration procedures | After cleaning tongue, rinse for at least 30 seconds. |
| d. expected time to onset of relief | Relief should be immediate. |
| e. degree of relief that can be reasonably expected | Complete relief in the absence of systemic disease |
| f. most common side effects | Gagging |
| g. side effects that warrant medical intervention should they occur | Sensitivity to flavoring |
| h. patient options in the event that condition worsens or persists | Seek aid from a dentist or primary care provider. |
| i. product storage requirements | Keep two components unmixed and watch expiration date. |
| j. specific nondrug measures | Tongue cleaning device |
| 10. Solicit patient's follow-up questions. | May I double my dose of any of these products if needed? |
| 11. Answer patient's questions. | Yes. |

Key: GI, gastrointestinal; N/A, not applicable; NSAID, nonsteroidal anti-inflammatory drug; OTC, over-the-counter.

also seriously affecting the patient's oral health (inflammation and mucosal disease) and ability to successfully wear the dentures.

Chronic atrophic candidiasis, sometimes referred to as denture stomatitis or denture sore mouth, is common in patients with full or partial dentures. This condition may be attributed to infection with *Candida albicans*, which can be found resident on the denture base.[40] Symptomatically, the inflamed denture-bearing area may appear granular or erythematous and edematous with soreness or a burning sensation (see Color Plates, photograph 10). Inflammation secondary to *Candida* organisms is generalized to the entire denture-bearing tissue area, whereas inflammation secondary to the trauma of ill-fitting dentures is usually localized to the specific area of the trauma. It appears that the candida organisms either adhere to the denture material or reside in pores of the denture material and can reinfect the mouth. Failure to remove the denture at bedtime and clean it regularly worsens this condition. Angular cheilitis (soreness and cracking at corners of the mouth) is commonly associated with chronic atrophic candidiasis and other forms of oral candidiasis. The corners of the mouth can often be effectively treated with terbinafine cream, or if a staphylococcal organism is also involved, a prescription will be needed.

## Prevention of Hygiene-related Denture Problems

Removing plaque from dentures helps prevent gum infections, staining of dentures, and mouth odor. Specialty brushes and aids are available to remove plaque from hard-to-clean areas (e.g., spaces around a fixed bridge, implants, or orthodontic bands) and dentures. Dentures should be cleaned thoroughly at least once daily to remove unsightly stain, debris, and plaque. Abrasive and chemical cleansers formulated specifically for dentures are available (Table 31-9). A combination regimen of brushing dentures with an abrasive cleaner and soaking them in a chemical cleanser is recommended.

### *Abrasive Denture Cleansers*

Denture (paste or powder) cleansers containing mild abrasives (e.g., calcium carbonate) must be applied properly with specialty brushes adapted to the denture's contour to remove stains, plaque, and calculus. Overly vigorous scrubbing can abrade the acrylic materials of dentures and bend the metal clasps. To prevent irritation of oral tissues, the patient should thoroughly rinse the abrasive cleaner from the denture.

The brushing routine can be followed by soaking the denture in an alkaline peroxide cleansing solution to help

## PATIENT EDUCATION FOR PREVENTION OF CARIES, GINGIVITIS, AND HALITOSIS

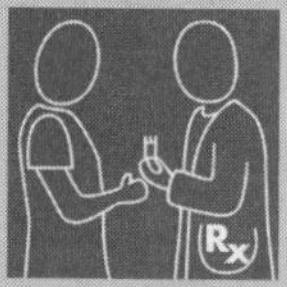

The primary objective of self-care is the removal of plaque to prevent caries, gingivitis, and halitosis. For most patients, carefully following product instructions and the self-care measures listed here will help ensure good oral hygiene.

### Nondrug Measures and Other Considerations

- Avoid cariogenic foods, such as foods that contain more than 15% sugar, that cling to the teeth, and that remain in the mouth after they are eaten.
- Eat low-cariogenic foods, such as foods that have a high water content (e.g., fresh fruit), that stimulate the flow of saliva (e.g., fibrous foods that require lots of chewing), or that are high in protein (e.g., dairy products).
- To help prevent mouth odor, drink at least eight 8-oz glasses of water a day, if possible. Also, if you wear dentures, do not wear them while sleeping.
- Note that use of alcohol and tobacco can cause caries, gingivitis, and halitosis.
- Note that hormonal changes during pregnancy increase the risk of gingivitis.
- Consider incorporating gum massage as an antigingivitis measure, using such devices as soft brushes, special rubber cup massagers, a Stim-U-Dent, or toothpicks.

### Plaque Removal

#### *Brushing Teeth*

- Mechanically remove plaque buildup by brushing teeth at least twice daily with a fluoride dentifrice. (See Table 31-3 for proper brushing technique.)
- Use a brush with soft nylon bristles.
- Replace the brush when the bristles show signs of wear.
- For children younger than 2 years, clean the teeth with a soft cloth, and massage the gums.
- For preschool children, apply a pea-sized amount of toothpaste to a child-sized toothbrush, and brush the child's teeth until the child can brush properly.
- Use only regular-strength fluoride toothpaste for children from ages 2 to 6 years. Consult a dentist before using fluoride toothpastes in children younger than 2 years.
- Teach children how to rinse the mouth and spit out the toothpaste to avoid swallowing fluoride.
- Note that tartar control toothpastes have been related to a type of contact dermatitis in the perioral region. Discontinue the tartar control dentifrice, and switch to a non–tartar control fluoride toothpaste if you experience itching or irritation of the mouth after brushing.
- If you are prone to developing caries or gingivitis, consider using a toothpaste classified as having antiplaque/antigingivitis activity. Such toothpastes contain stannous fluoride.

#### *Flossing Teeth*

- Floss your teeth at least once a day. (See Table 31-4 for proper flossing technique.)
- Use a waxed or Teflon-coated floss for teeth with tight contacts.

#### *Using Plaque-disclosing Products*

- For maximum plaque removal, use a plaque-disclosing product to see whether toothbrushing and flossing have removed all the plaque.
- Rinse the mouth with water.
- Chew a disclosing tablet, or apply a solution to the teeth with a cotton-tipped applicator.
- Swish the product around the mouth for 30 seconds, and then spit out the product.
- Rinse the mouth with water, and spit out the solution. Look for red areas on the teeth that indicate areas of plaque accumulation. If teeth are red, brush and floss again.

#### *Using Mouth Rinses and Gels*

- To freshen breath, use a mouth rinse that contains zinc chloride (Viadent) and zinc citrate. Zinc chloride and chlorine dioxide are found in Tri-Oral two-part rinse. These ingredients eliminate odoriferous volatile sulfur compounds.
- If you are prone to developing caries or gingivitis, consider using a mouth rinse classified as having antiplaque/antigingivitis activity. Such mouthwashes contain cetylpyridinium chloride or a combination of thymol, eucalyptol, methyl salicylate, and menthol.
- To use plaque-softening mouth rinses (Advanced Formula Plax) effectively, use them before brushing. Vigorously swish 1 to 2 tbsp of rinse in the mouth and between the teeth for about 30 seconds, and spit out the rinse. Do not smoke, eat, or drink for 30 minutes following use.
- Note that overuse of mouth rinses containing cetylpyridinium can stain teeth.

### Using Topical Fluoride Treatments

- If your drinking water is not fluoridated (including bottled water) or if you are prone to developing caries, consider using topical fluoride treatments. (See Table 31-7 for proper use of these products.)
- Supervise children younger than 12 years until they are capable of using the product correctly.
- Consult a dentist or primary care provider before using these products in children younger than 6 years.

See a dentist if any of the following occur:

- You develop symptoms of a toothache.
- Your teeth develop a mottled appearance.
- Your gums bleed, swell, or become red.
- Mouth odor persists despite regular use of a fluoride toothpaste, or the cause of the odor cannot be identified.

**TABLE 31-9 Selected Denture Cleansers**

| Trade Name | Primary Ingredients |
|---|---|
| Ban-A-Stain Liquid | Phosphoric acid 25% |
| Dentu-Cream Paste | Dicalcium phosphate dihydrate; calcium carbonate; aluminum silicate |
| Efferdent Antibacterial Tablets | Sodium carbonate; sodium bicarbonate; potassium monopersulfate; sodium perborate |
| Efferdent Plus Tablets | Sodium bicarbonate; sodium perborate; potassium monopersulfate; detergents |
| Polident Tablets | Potassium monopersulfate; sodium perborate monohydrate; sodium carbonate; sodium bicarbonate; citric acid; surfactant; chelating agents |

remove remaining plaque and bacteria. Plaque removal is then enhanced by brushing the denture after it has soaked; instructions for this procedure are included on some products.

### *Chemical Denture Cleansers*

The other method of cleaning is to use a soaking solution containing one of the three chemical cleansers: hypochlorite, alkaline peroxide, or dilute acids.

Alkaline peroxide cleaners are the most commonly used chemical denture cleansers. These powders or tablets become alkaline solutions of hydrogen peroxide when dissolved. The ingredients are alkaline detergents and perborates, the latter of which cause oxygen release for a mechanical cleaning effect. These products are most effective on new plaque and stains that are soaked for 4 to 8 hours. The alkaline peroxides have few serious disadvantages and do not damage the surface of acrylic resins.

Hypochlorites (bleach) remove stains, dissolve mucin, and are both bactericidal and fungicidal. Denture plaque consists of cells embedded in a matrix that serves as a surface on which calculus may develop. Hypochlorite cleansers act directly on the organic plaque matrix to dissolve its structure, but they cannot dissolve calculus once it has formed. The most serious disadvantage of hypochlorite is that it corrodes metal denture components such as the framework and clasps of removable partial dentures, solder joints, and possibly the pins holding the teeth. The addition of anticorrosive phosphate compounds has greatly reduced this problem, but these products should be used only for 15-minute soaks to limit exposure and not more often than once a week.

Acid-containing soaking solutions can also be corrosive to metals, and short soaking times in these solutions are recommended. A sonic or ultrasonic cleaning device, when used with a commercially prepared solution, is easier to use and cleans more effectively than soaking alone. However, some hand brushing may still be required.

#### Safety Considerations

All denture-cleansing products should be completely rinsed off the denture before it is inserted into the mouth. Abrasive cleansers coming in contact with oral or other mucous membranes may cause tissue irritation. Chemical cleansers may cause tissue irritation or possibly severe chemical burns. All denture cleansers should be kept out of the reach of children because of the potential for eye or skin irritation or for toxicity from accidental ingestion. A dentist should evaluate stains that are resistant to proper denture brushing and soaking in available solutions.

#### Unapproved Denture Cleansers

Only products that are specifically formulated for denture cleansing should be used. Household cleansers (used for soaking) are not appropriate and may either be ineffective or damage the denture material. The use of whitening toothpastes intended to be used with natural dentition should be discouraged because they are too abrasive to be used safely on denture material.

Patients should not soak or clean dentures in hot water or hot soaking solutions because distortion or warping may occur.

#### Product Selection Guidelines

Patients of advanced age or disabled patients may prefer an alkaline peroxide soak solution for daily, overnight cleaning. Alkaline peroxide cleansers do not corrode metal components of dentures as do alkaline hypochlorite and acid cleansers.

## Assessment of Hygiene-related Denture Problems: A Case-based Approach

Before recommending any type of oral hygiene product, the practitioner should determine what denture care measures the patient is taking and whether those measures are adequate. At a minimum, the practitioner should determine whether the patient suffers from denture stomatitis or inflammation secondary to ill-fitting dentures. Case 31-4 provides an example of the assessment of patients with hygiene-related denture problems.

## Patient Counseling for Hygiene-related Denture Problems

Denture wearers may tend to blame any oral discomfort on the appliances rather than their hygiene regimen. The practitioner should stress that diligent plaque removal from dentures is the key to preventing denture stomatitis. The methods of cleaning dentures, including their advantages and

## CASE 31-4

| Relevant Evaluation Criteria | Scenario/Model Outcome |
|---|---|
| **Information Gathering** | |
| 1. Gather essential information about the patient's symptoms, including: | |
| a. description of symptom(s) (i.e., nature, onset, duration, severity, associated symptoms) | Patient has had upper and lower dentures for a long time. She has not visited a dentist since she received these dentures. She complains of a sore mouth accompanied by red and cracked regions along the corners of her mouth. |
| b. description of any factors that seem to precipitate, exacerbate, and/or relieve the patient's symptom(s) | Soreness subsides slightly when both dentures are left out for a few hours. |
| 2. Gather essential patient history information: | |
| a. patient's identity | Francis Thompson |
| b. patient's age, sex, weight, and height | 75 y/o F, 5'4", 115 lb |
| c. patient's occupation | Retired librarian |
| d. patient's dietary habits | Good |
| e. patient's sleep habits | Patient has trouble falling asleep and awakes early in the morning. |
| f. concurrent medical conditions, prescription and nonprescription medications, and dietary supplements | ASA 81 mg for cardioprotection; atenolol 50 mg for hypertension; calcium supplements for osteoporosis |
| g. allergies | Dairy products, fresh-cut grass, shellfish, penicillin |
| h. history of other adverse reactions to medications | GI upset with some NSAIDs |
| i. other (describe)_______ | N/A |
| **Assessment and Triage** | |
| 3. Differentiate the patient's signs/symptoms and correctly identify the patient's primary problem(s). | Francis seems to have an oral yeast infection extending to the corners of her mouth. |
| 4. Identify exclusions for self-treatment. | None |
| 5. Formulate a comprehensive list of therapeutic alternatives for the primary problem to determine if triage to a medical practitioner is required, and share this information with the patient. | Options include:<br>(1) Refer Francis to a dentist and recommend lifestyle modifications.<br>(2) Recommend proper OTC products with lifestyle modifications.<br>(3) Take no action. |
| **Plan** | |
| 6. Select an optimal therapeutic alternative to address the patient's problem, taking into account patient preferences. | Refer to dentist for assessment of oral cavity and existing dentures and antifungal prescription. Recommend appropriate lifestyle modifications. |
| 7. Describe the recommended therapeutic approach to the patient. | Your dentist will assess your oral cavity and make recommendations regarding your current dentures in addition to prescribing an antifungal for the yeast infection. To prevent future yeast infections, clean your dentures and tongue thoroughly, leave dentures out at night, and do not use antibacterial mouthwashes. |
| 8. Explain to the patient the rationale for selecting the recommended therapeutic approach from the considered therapeutic alternatives. | Removing the cause of the problem is usually the most effective choice of treatment. Your mouth and dentures need to be assessed because you have not had this done for a long time and changes in the mouth may have occurred. Avoiding use of an antibacterial mouthwash and using an antifungal will help the "good" bacteria to repopulate the mouth. |

## CASE 31-4 (continued)

| Relevant Evaluation Criteria | Scenario/Model Outcome |
|---|---|
| **Patient Education** | |
| 9. When recommending self-care with nonprescription medications and/or nondrug therapy, convey accurate information to the patient. | Criterion does no apply in this case. |
| 10. Solicit patient's follow-up questions. | Why does my breath smell? |
| 11. Answer patient's questions. | The bad breath is caused by not cleaning your dentures and tongue properly as well as the possibility that you have poor-fitting dentures. The combination of these factors has resulted in a yeast infection, which contributes to the malodor. |

Key: ASA, aspirin; GI, gastrointestinal; NSAID, nonsteroidal anti-inflammatory drug; OTC, over-the-counter.

## PATIENT EDUCATION FOR HYGIENE-RELATED DENTURE PROBLEMS

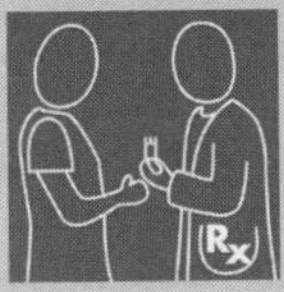

The objective of self-care is to prevent bacterial or fungal infections of the mouth by removing plaque from the dentures. For most patients, carefully following product instructions and the self-care measures listed here will help ensure good denture hygiene.

- Clean dentures thoroughly at least once daily to remove unsightly stain, debris, and potentially harmful plaque.
- Preferably, brush dentures with an abrasive cleaner, and then soak them in a chemical cleanser. This combination regimen is more effective in removing plaque and bacteria.
- Apply the abrasive cleaner to the denture, using a brush designed to adapt to the denture's contour.
- Do not scrub the denture surface vigorously; such action can abrade the acrylic materials and bend the metal clasps.
- To prevent irritation of oral tissues, rinse the abrasive cleaner thoroughly from the denture.
- After brushing the dentures, soak them in an alkaline peroxide cleansing solution for 4 to 8 hours. Rinse the dentures thoroughly to avoid chemical burns of the mouth.
- If possible, brush the dentures again, and rinse them thoroughly.
- Note that alkaline peroxide cleansers cannot damage the denture as can hypochlorite or dilute acid (phosphoric acid) cleansers.
- If using an alkaline peroxide or acid cleanser, soak the dentures for only 15 minutes to avoid corrosion of metal denture components.
- Keep all denture cleansers out of the reach of children. These agents can cause eye or skin irritation or toxicity if accidentally ingested.
- Do not use household cleansers or whitening toothpastes to clean dentures. These agents may damage denture material.
- Do not soak or clean dentures in hot water or hot soaking solutions. Distortion or warping of the denture may occur.
- Do not sleep while wearing your dentures. Decreased levels of saliva during sleep may contribute to plaque buildup on the denture.

⚠ If your mouth becomes sore or shows sign of infection, see a dentist.

disadvantages, should be explained. Using the patient's preferences, the practitioner should recommend a denture cleanser and reinforce the methods of use. The box Patient Education for Hygiene-related Denture Problems lists specific information to provide patients.

## KEY POINTS FOR PREVENTION OF HYGIENE-RELATED ORAL DISORDERS

- Removing plaque and modifying diet are the main goals of self-care to prevent caries, gingivitis, and halitosis.
- Mechanical removal of plaque by brushing and flossing is essential for good oral health.
- Mouth rinses may augment brushing and flossing procedures and be used to freshen breath and/or as antiplaque/antigingivitis adjuncts.
- Topical fluorides may be used in individuals with high caries activity.
- Supervision of children younger than 12 years of age or until they are capable of using the products correctly must be enforced.
- Denture cleaners may be used, in addition to physically removing debris, to prevent bacterial and/or fungal infections.
- If individuals have specific problems relating to the purpose or use of these products, a consultation with a dentist should be recommended.

## References


1. Harris NO, Garcia-Godoy F. *Primary Preventive Dentistry.* 6th ed. Stamford, Conn: Appleton & Lange; 2004:76-85, 96-102, 124-5, 128-30, 165-6, 242-7, 249-53, 419, 440, 471, 489-90, 655-9.
2. Gluck GM, Morganstein WM, eds. *Jong's Community Dental Health.* 4th ed. St. Louis: Mosby–Year Book, Inc; 1998:127-33.
3. Los Angeles Department of Water and Power. Water Quality—Frequently Asked Questions—Q8: Fluoride. Available at: http://www.ladwp.com/ladwp/cms/ladwp000499.jsp. Accessed December 1, 2003.
4. Federal Trade Commission. *1997 Smokeless Tobacco Report.* Washington, DC: Federal Trade Commission; 1997.
5. Mandel ID. The new toothpastes. *Texas Dent J.* December 1998: 8-13.
6. *Federal Register.* May 29, 2003;68:32235,32263,32285-6. Available at: http://a257.g.akamaitech.net/7/257/2422/14mar20010800/edocket.access.gpo.gov/2003/pdf/ 03-12783.pdf. Accessed December 7, 2003.
7. Council on Scientific Affairs. *Products of Excellence ADA Seal Program.* Chicago: American Dental Association; 1998.
8. Council on Scientific Affairs. *Guidelines for Acceptance of Chemotherapeutic Products for the Control of Gingivitis.* Chicago: American Dental Association; 1997.
9. Triclosan antigingivitis/antiplaque monograph status sought by Ciba. *F-D-C Reports—The Tan Sheet.* December 8, 2003;11(49):8.
10. Fairbrother KJ, Heasman PA. Anticalculus agents. *J Clin Periodontol.* 2000;27:285-301.
11. DeLattre VF. Factors contributing to adverse soft tissue reactions due to the use of tartar control toothpastes: report of a case and literature review. *J Periodontol.* 1999;70:803-7.
12. Warren PR, Ray TS, Cugini M, et al. A practice-based study of a power toothbrush: assessment of effectiveness and acceptance. *J Am Dent Assoc.* 2000;131:389.
13. Carr MP, Rice GL, Horton JE. Evaluation of floss types for interproximal plaque removal. *Am J Dent.* 2000;13:212-4.
14. Rawal SY, Claman LJ, Kalmar JR, et al Traumatic lesions of the gingiva: a case series. *J Periodontol.* 2004;75:762-9.
15. Isaacs RL, Beiswanger BB, Crawford JL, et al. Assessing the efficacy and safety of an electric interdental cleaning device. *J Am Dent Assoc.* 1999;130:104-8.
16. Newman MG, Cattabriga M, Etienne D, et al. Effectiveness of adjunctive irrigation in early periodontitis: multi-center evaluation. *J Periodontol.* 1994;65:224-9.
17. Renton-Harper P, Addy M, Moran J, et al. A comparison of chlorhexidine, cetylpyridinium chloride, triclosan, and C31G mouthrinse products for plaque inhibition. *J Periodontol.* 1996; 67:486-9.
18. Moran J, Addy M. The effects of a cetylpyridinium chloride prebrushing rinse as an adjunct to oral hygiene and gingival health. *J Periodontol.* 1991;62:562-4.
19. Herlofson BB, Barkvoll P. The effect of two toothpaste detergents on the frequency of recurrent aphthous ulcers. *Acta Odontol Scand.* 1996;54:150-3.
20. *NDMA Executive Newsletter.* 1996;12:1.
21. Blumenthal M, Goldberg A, Brinckmann J. eds. *Herbal Medicine: Expanded Commission E Monographs.* Boston: Integrative Medicine Communications; 2000.
22. Roth I, Lindorf H. *South American Medicinal Plants: Botany, Remedial Properties and General Uses.* Berlin: Springer-Verlag; 2002.
23. Cordell GA. ed. *The Alkaloids, Chemistry and Biology.* Vol 53. San Diego, Calif: Academic Press; 1999.
24. Dewick P. *Medicinal Natural Products: A Biosynthetic Approach.* 2nd ed. Chester, England: John Wiley and Sons; 2002.
25. Gage T, Pickett F. *Mosby's Dental Drug Reference.* 7th ed. St Louis: Mosby; 2005.
26. Abebe W. An overview of herbal supplement utilization with particular emphasis on possible interactions with dental drugs and oral manifestations. *J Dent Hyg.* 2003;77:37-46.
27. Fugh-Berman A. Herb-drug interactions. *Lancet.* 2000;355:134-8.
28. Iraskin I, Ribnicky D, Komarnytsky S, et al. Plants and human health in the twenty-first century. *Trends Biotechnol.* 2002;20:522-31.
29. Petersen PE, Lennon MA. Effective use of fluorides for the prevention of dental caries in the 21st century: the WHO approach. *Community Dent Oral Epidemiol.* 2004;32:319-21.
30. Marinho VC, Higgins JP, Logan S, et al. Fluoride mouthrinses for preventing dental caries in children and adolescents. *Cochrane Database Syst Rev.* 2003(3):CD002284.
31. Kobayashi S, Kishi H, Yoshihara A, et al. Treatment and post-treatment effects of fluoride mouthrinsing after 17 years. *J Public Health Dent.* 1995;55:229-33.
32. Wade DN, Kerns DG. Acute necrotizing ulcerative gingivitis-periodontitis: a literature review. *Mil Med.* 1998;163:337-42.
33. Murayama YKH, Nagai A, Dompkowski D, et al. Acute necrotizing ulcerative gingivitis: risk factors involving host defense mechanisms. *Periodontology.* October 2000;(6):116-24.
34. Eisen DE, Lynch DP. *The Mouth: Diagnosis and Treatment.* St. Louis: Mosby; 1998.
35. Mengel R, Wissing E, Smitz-Habben A, et al. Comparative study of plaque and gingivitis prevention by AmF/SnF2 and NaF: a clinical and microbiological 9-month study. *J Clin Periodont.* 1996; 23:372-8.
36. Modeer T, Bengtsson A, Rolla G. Triclosan reduces prostaglandin biosynthesis in human gingival fibroblasts challenged with interleukin-1 in vitro. *J Clin Periodont.* 1996;10:927-33.
37. Sanz M, Roldan S, Herrera D. Fundamentals of breath malodor. *J Contemp Dent Pract.* 2001;2:1-17.
38. Tangerman A. Halitosis in medicine: a review. *Int Dent J.* 2002; 52(suppl 3):201-6.
39. ADA Council on Scientific Affairs. Oral malodor. *J Am Dent Assoc.* 2003;134:209.
40. Kulak-Ozkan Y, Kazazoglu E, Arikan A. Oral hygiene habits, denture cleanliness, presence of yeasts and stomatitis in elderly people. *J Oral Rehabil.* 2002;29:300.

CHAPTER 32

# Oral Pain and Discomfort

*Gary D. Klasser and Charles S. Greene*

Everyone has experienced oral pain and discomfort. Pain can accompany many common oral problems. Different features of pain indicate different underlying problems. For example, tooth pain that is triggered or worsened by stimuli such as heat, cold, or pressure on biting will often indicate a pulpal response to deep carious lesions or a cracked or broken tooth. Continuous tooth pain may indicate a pulpal infection and necrosis, an abscess, or serious periodontal disease. Fever, malaise, and swelling may indicate an oral abscess; a patient who exhibits such symptoms should be referred to a dentist for immediate professional care.

Similarly, pain in the mucosa of the oral cavity and lips can be generated by many types of problems, ranging from injury to the mouth to recurrent aphthous stomatitis (canker sores) and herpes simplex labialis (cold sores). Some of these problems are self-limiting and may be treated with nonprescription products. By distinguishing the patient's self-treatable problems from those potentially requiring professional dental or medical care, the health care practitioner plays an important advisory role in oral health care.

## OROFACIAL PAIN

Orofacial pain attributable to tooth hypersensitivity or teething pain is not serious and is self-treatable. Resolution of pain associated with toothache or ill-fitting dentures requires professional dental care. Although denture adhesives and so-called reliners are available as nonprescription products, their use can delay treatment and worsen the condition. Loose, poorly fitting, or broken removable dental prostheses (partial or full dentures) can also contribute to accelerated bone loss, ulceration, irritation, tumorous growths, and compromised oral function. Refitting, relining, or repairing dentures to ensure proper functioning requires professional dental treatment.

### Tooth Hypersensitivity

Varying degrees of pulp injury can cause toothache. The mildest form is called hypersensitivity, and this is the only form that can be treated with nonprescription products. Tooth hypersensitivity (as opposed to toothache) affects approximately 40 million adults at some time, and about one fourth of this population has chronic hypersensitivity.[1]

#### *Etiology of Toothache and Tooth Hypersensitivity*

Hypersensitivity of teeth is a pathologic condition in which the teeth are sensitive to thermal, chemical, or physical stimuli. The patient with hypersensitivity experiences pain from hot/cold and sweet/sour solutions as well as when hot/cold air touches the teeth. It varies in degree from mild to sharp and excruciating pain. Dentin hypersensitivity occurs when dentinal tubules are exposed as a result of attrition, abrasion (excessive brushing with an abrasive dentifrice or hard-bristle toothbrush), erosion, fracture of a tooth, chipping of a tooth, or a faulty restoration. It can also occur after periodontal scaling and root planing, orthodontic tooth movement,[2] occlusal imbalance,[3] gingival recession, or periodontal surgery (shrinkage of the swollen gingiva after curettage or elimination of tissue by gingivectomy).

#### *Pathophysiology of Toothache and Tooth Hypersensitivity*

Exposed dentin allows stimuli (heat, cold, pressure, and acid) to reach the nerve fibers within the pulp. These irritations do not damage the pulp and, over time, secondary dentin (reparative dentin) will be created. The generation of new dentin will eventually eliminate pain impulses; however, while the nerve fibers are frequently stimulated, the pain may be intense and condition patients to limit oral hygiene which, in turn, contributes to plaque accumulation and the progression of oral plaque diseases.[4] (See Anatomy and Physiology of the Oral Cavity in Chapter 31.)

Two processes are essential for the development of dentin hypersensitivity: dentin must become exposed (lesion localization), through either loss of enamel or gingival recession, and the dentin tubules must be open to both the oral cavity and the pulp (lesion initiation).[5]

The roots of teeth are usually covered by gum tissues, but with time the processes of attrition, abrasion, and erosion reduce the outer layer of cementum, eventually exposing the underlying porous dentine. Root surface exposure allowing contact with stimuli may also be caused by gingival recession or some types of periodontal treatment. These stimuli may elicit pain because dentine tubules contain fluid, which hot or cold stimuli cause to expand or shrink, stimulating the underlying pulpal nerves and resulting in

**Editor's Note:** This chapter is based, in part, on the 14th edition chapter with the same title, which was written by Pamela J. Sims and Kevin M. Sims.

**TABLE 32-1 Differentiation of Tooth Hypersensitivity and Toothache**

| | Tooth Hypersensitivity | Toothache |
|---|---|---|
| Etiology | Exposed and open dentin tubules | Bacterial invasion to the pulp |
| Pathophysiology | Stimuli (heat, cold, pressure, and acid) cause fluid in the dentinal tubules to expand and shrink stimulating pulp nerve fibers; resulting in pain | Inflammatory response to invading bacteria stimulates free nerve endings in the pulp |
| Signs | Attrition, abrasion, erosion, tooth/restoration fracture, faulty restoration, or gingival recession | Cavitation/decay present in tooth/teeth under existing restoration, tooth/restoration fracture, or trauma to the dentition |
| Symptoms | A quick, fleeting, sharp, or stabbing pain on stimulation by thermal, chemical, or physical stimuli, which stops after stimuli are no longer present | Intermittent, short, and sharp pain on stimulation may indicate reversible damage; continuous, dull, and throbbing pain without stimulation usually indicates irreversible damage |
| Assessment | Nonserious and self-treatable | Requires professional care for resolution |

pain.[5] Both clinical and laboratory evidence suggest that enamel at the buccal (cheek side) cervical region is lost through a combination of erosion and abrasion.[5] Enamel is resistant to abrasion by normal tooth brushing, with or without a nonabrasive toothpaste, but is particularly sensitive to the effects of acid; thus, brushing of acid-softened (eroded) enamel has a marked abrasive effect.[5]

Cervical dentin wear (at the junction of the crown and root of a tooth) is commonly observed, and may be associated with dentin hypersensitivity. Erosion is thought to play a part in both conditions.[6] The etiology of dental erosion is primarily attributed to the presence of extrinsic or intrinsic acid.[7,8] Extrinsic sources of acid include frequent consumption of acidic foods and drinks, and acidic medications.[7,8] Older cements used to secure crowns were acidic and had the potential to cause hypersensitivity. Tooth sensitivity related to crowns rarely occurs now that hybrid ionomer/resin cements are used. Regurgitation of gastric contents into the mouth, which occurs with gastroesophageal reflux, is the most common source of intrinsic acid in children and adults.[7] In addition, erosion of tooth enamel and dentin by acidic vomitus is the most notable and least controversial oral consequence of frequent purging in patients suffering from bulimia nervosa.[8] According to one report, one third of patients with bulimia will exhibit erosion of their anterior teeth.[8] Brushing immediately after purging traditionally has not been recommended, as it is thought to remove acid-weakened enamel.[8] Patients should rinse with water instead.

The next level of injury involves further exposure or loss of dentin. If left untreated, dental caries will progress to destroy the enamel and dentin layers of the tooth, allowing bacteria to reach the pulp. The inflammatory response to bacteria in the pulp (pulpitis) stimulates free nerve endings, resulting in pulpalgia, or common toothache.

Over the past several years, patients have become increasingly interested in the esthetic benefits of whitening systems that can be used at home.[9] Tooth-whitening procedures may adversely affect both hard and soft tissues in the oral cavity, as well as the dental pulp.[9] A recent study showed that mild tooth sensitivity can be expected in approximately half of patients who undergo home whitening treatment; approximately 10% experience moderate sensitivity and 4% experience severe sensitivity.[9]

Patients with poor oral hygiene practices or systemic illness are prone to dental decay and toothaches. Although toothache usually indicates dental pathology involving the tooth substance, dental pulp, or supporting periodontium, pain may also be referred to the teeth from nondental sources.[10,11] Possible sources of such referred pain may be muscular (masticatory and cervical), neurovascular (migraine headache), cardiac, neuropathic (episodic and continuous), sinus/nasal mucosa, cancer-related, or psychogenic. Often, the resulting toothache is resolved after proper management of the true source of pain.

### *Signs and Symptoms of Toothache and Tooth Hypersensitivity*

Whereas the pain of tooth hypersensitivity tends to be short and stabbing, the pain of pulpitis is prolonged and throbbing (Table 32-1). Pulpitis from dental caries or hypersensitivity can be either reversible (after removing decay and repairing the tooth) or irreversible (requiring root canal therapy or extraction). Intermittent, short, sharp pain often indicates a viable pulp with reversible damage, whereas continuous, dull, throbbing pain usually indicates irreversible pulp damage.

Sensitivity to hot and cold for several weeks following dental therapy is normal. It also occurs as a result of clenching or grinding teeth (bruxism) and from gumline grooves (abfraction lesions or toothbrush abrasions) formed by abrasive or inappropriate toothbrushing technique.

This problem can be reversed after cessation of these activities or with dental treatment.

### *Treatment of Toothache and Tooth Hypersensitivity*

Effective nonprescription oral products are available for treating tooth hypersensitivity. Self-treatment of toothache, however, is limited to the use of oral and topical analgesics for temporary pain relief until the cause of the problem is found and corrected.

### Treatment Goals

The goals of self-treating tooth hypersensitivity are to (1) alter the damaged tooth surface using the appropriate toothpaste and (2) stop abrasive toothbrushing practices. When these goals have been achieved, tooth hypersensitivity may be eliminated.

### General Treatment Approach

Most patients seek care early in the course of their symptoms.[12] Patients frequently report an inability to cope with toothache and often consult nondental health care professionals, such as physicians or pharmacists.[13] The patient with a toothache should be advised to seek professional dental assistance as soon as possible. The presence of swelling or fever usually indicates the need for antibiotic therapy as well as dental treatment. If the patient wears a removable prosthesis that attaches to the painful tooth, removing the appliance may help temporarily. Nonprescription systemic analgesics such as ibuprofen, aspirin, or acetaminophen may be taken for short-term pain relief until a dentist corrects the problem. (See Chapter 5 for a discussion of these agents.) None of these products—particularly aspirin—should ever be placed locally on gingival tissue or in a cavity; doing so can result in chemical burns of sensitive tissue (see Color Plates, photograph 11). For temporary relief, nonprescription topical anesthetic products containing lidocaine or benzocaine may also be used (see Treatment of Recurrent Aphthous Stomatitis). Patients with allergy to common local anesthetics should not use these products. These topical anesthetics are also indicated for posttreatment pain associated with tooth extractions or root canals.

The American Dental Association (ADA) has not accepted eugenol or clove oil as being safe and effective nonprescription drugs for toothache. These types of medicaments are generally ineffective and can damage viable pulp and soft tissue.

Once a dentist has diagnosed tooth hypersensitivity, the patient should brush with a desensitizing toothpaste. A single application of these toothpastes has no effect; for some patients, long-term use (2 to 4 weeks or more) may be necessary to relieve the symptoms. Figure 32-1 outlines the self-treatment of tooth hypersensitivity and lists exclusions for self-care.

### Nonpharmacologic Therapy

Ice applied in 10-minute increments may provide temporary relief for toothaches, but not all toothaches respond to it. Heat from hot packs may cause a bacterial infection to spread by increasing local blood flow, and therefore is contraindicated. If the tooth is infected, hot or sweet foods may exacerbate the problem. Patients should be advised not to delay treatment of a toothache, even if palliative self-care measures provide relief.

### Pharmacologic Therapy (Desensitizing Dentifrices)

Patients with hypersensitive teeth may get pain relief from brushing less vigorously with standard fluoride toothpaste and a soft-bristle toothbrush. Dentists typically recommend toothpastes that contain sodium fluoride, potassium nitrate, strontium chloride, or potassium chloride (Table 32-2).[4,14] Two well-controlled clinical studies and three supportive studies provided sufficient data to the Food and Drug Administration (FDA) to establish the effectiveness of potassium nitrate 5% for protection against painful sensitivity of the teeth caused by cold, heat, acids, sweets, or contact. As a tooth desensitizer, potassium nitrate 5% currently remains the only Category I agent.[15] Two recent studies demonstrated that the dentifrice containing potassium nitrate 5% and stannous fluoride 0.454% (Colgate Sensitive Maximum Strength) is superior to products containing potassium nitrate 5.0% and sodium monofluorophosphate 0.76% (Fresh Mint Sensodyne).[16,17] Dibasic sodium citrate (used in Pluronic gel) and strontium chloride 10% were classified as Category III, pending further evidence of effectiveness. FDA has proposed a Category I classification for the combination of a Category I fluoride ingredient with potassium nitrate 5% to be used to relieve dentinal hypersensitivity and prevent dental caries.[18] Such a combination product would be a good recommendation. New combination dentifrices in development that contain potassium nitrate, stannous fluoride, and sodium fluoride have demonstrated significantly better reduction in dentin hypersensitivity compared with dentifrices containing sodium fluoride or potassium chloride, triclosan, and sodium fluoride (Sensodyne F).[19] Other studies have demonstrated benefit in combining potassium nitrate with dimethyl isosorbide.[20]

If these measures do not relieve the sensitivity after 7 to 10 days, the dentist may prescribe the use of topical fluoride for patients with a high degree of dentinal sensitivity. Other agents under investigation for the treatment of dentin sensitivity include a Bioglass dentifrice and an intraoral fluoride-releasing device.[21,22]

*Mechanism of Action/Indication* A tooth desensitizer acts on the dentin to block the perception of stimuli that patients with normal teeth usually do not perceive. Because the most common cause of tooth sensitivity is exposed dentin, a desensitizing dentifrice must inhibit sensitization while also being nonabrasive.

*Dosage and Administration Guidelines* For optimum effectiveness, patients should apply at least a 1-inch strip of the desensitizing dentifrice to a soft-bristle toothbrush and use the product twice daily. Brushing thoroughly for at least 1 minute will apply the desensitizing agent to all sensitive surfaces. Onset of effect is not immediate and may take from several days to 5 weeks. The desensitizing dentifrice should be used until the sensitivity subsides or as long as a dentist recommends its use. The patient should then switch to a low-abrasion dentifrice. If there are isolated teeth with areas of hypersensitivity, the patient may burnish the desensitizing dentifrice into the appropriate area using a finger as an applicator. In about 25% of adults,

**Exclusions for Self-Treatment**

- Toothache (see Table 32-1)
- Mouth soreness associated with poor-fitting dentures
- Presence of fever or swelling
- Loose teeth
- Bleeding gums in the absence of trauma
- Broken or knocked-out teeth
- Severe tooth pain triggered or worsened by hot, cold, or chewing
- Trauma to the mouth with bleeding, swelling, and soreness

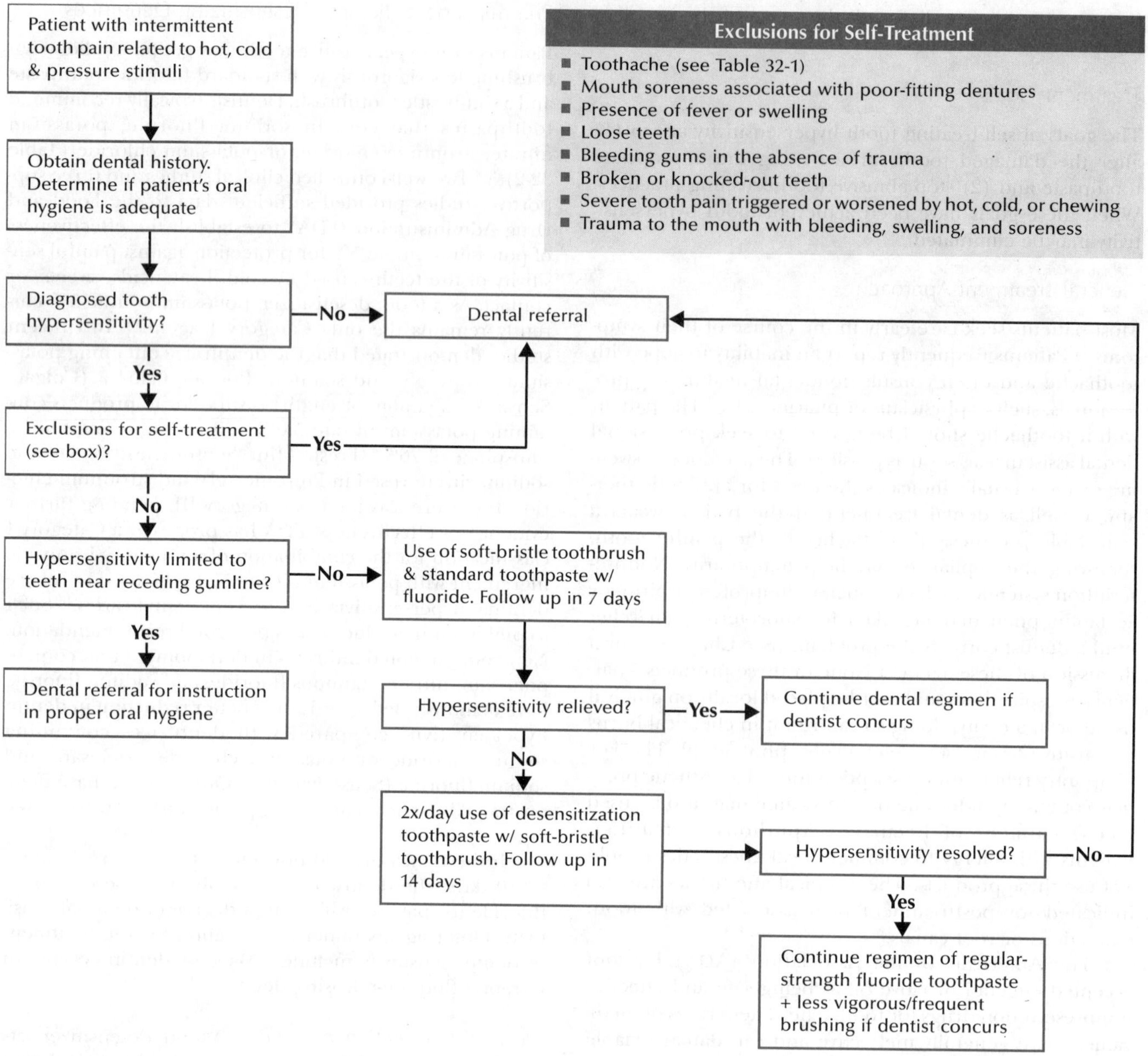

Patient with intermittent tooth pain related to hot, cold & pressure stimuli
Obtain dental history. Determine if patient's oral hygiene is adequate
Diagnosed tooth hypersensitivity?
No
Dental referral
Yes
Exclusions for self-treatment (see box)?
Yes
No
Hypersensitivity limited to teeth near receding gumline?
No
Use of soft-bristle toothbrush & standard toothpaste w/ fluoride. Follow up in 7 days
Yes
Dental referral for instruction in proper oral hygiene
Hypersensitivity relieved?
Yes
Continue dental regimen if dentist concurs
No
2x/day use of desensitization toothpaste w/ soft-bristle toothbrush. Follow up in 14 days
Hypersensitivity resolved?
No
Yes
Continue regimen of regular-strength fluoride toothpaste + less vigorous/frequent brushing if dentist concurs

**FIGURE 32-1** Self-care of tooth hypersensitivity.

**TABLE 32-2 Selected Desensitizing Toothpastes**

| Trade Name | Primary Ingredients |
|---|---|
| Colgate Sensitive Maximum Strength | Potassium nitrate 5%; stannous fluoride 0.454% |
| Crest Sensitivity Protection Toothpaste* | Potassium nitrate 5%; sodium fluoride 0.15% |
| Orajel Sensitive Pain-Relieving Toothpaste for Adults | Potassium nitrate 5%; sodium monofluorophosphate 1.15% |
| Oral B Extra Rembrandt Whitening Toothpaste for Sensitive Teeth | Potassium nitrate 5%; sodium monofluorophosphate 0.76% |
| Sensodyne Extra Whitening† | Potassium nitrate 5%; sodium monofluorophosphate 0.15% |

*Dye-free; †sucrose-free.

# Color Plates

# Color Illustration Contributors

Allergan, Inc.

Lawrence R. Ash

Umberto Benelli (eyeatlas.com)

Jean A. Borger

Richard C. Childers

Stanley Cullen

eMedicine.com, Inc.

Jeffrey A. Goad

Alfred C. Griffin (deceased)

Harold L. Hammond

Hollister Incorporated

Christopher Huerter

Thomas C. Orihel

Joan Lerner Selekof

R. Gary Sibbald

George Yatskievych

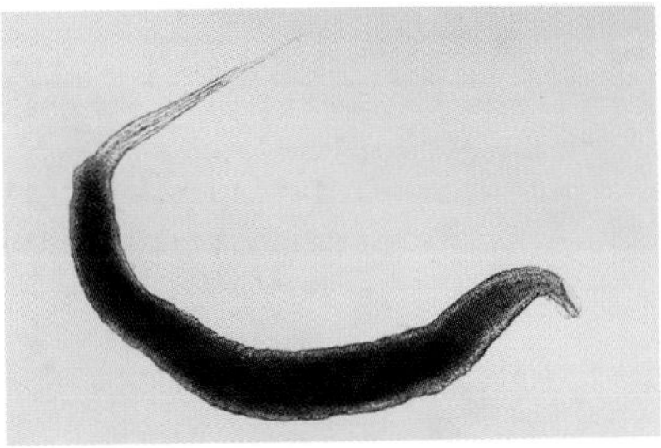

1A

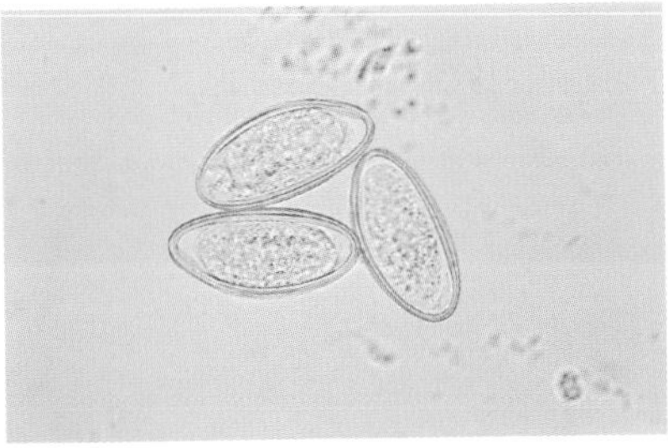

1B

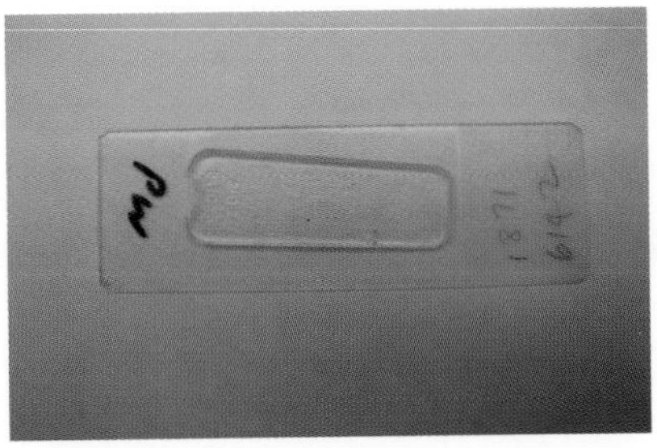

1C

**1A, B, and C** **Pinworm infection,** the most common worm infestation in the United States, is caused by ingestion of pinworm eggs from fecally contaminated hands, food, clothing, or bedding. **A,** The adult pinworm is a small (1-cm long), white, threadlike worm with a pin-shaped, pointed tail. **B,** The mature female stores approximately 11,000 eggs in her body, which she deposits in the perianal region of the host, usually at night. Reinfection occurs when the hatched larvae return to the large intestine or when eggs are transferred from the anus to the mouth and swallowed. **C,** Commercial pinworm detection kits use a sticky paddle, instead of tape, to affix the adult pinworm to a slide, which is then examined microscopically (see Chapter 19). (Photographs 1A and B courtesy of Lawrence R. Ash, PhD, and Thomas C. Orihel, PhD, © 1997, *Atlas of Human Parasitology.* 4th ed. Chicago: ASCP Press; 1997. Photograph 1C courtesy of Jeffrey A. Goad, PharmD, University of Southern California, School of Pharmacy, Los Angeles, © 2003.)

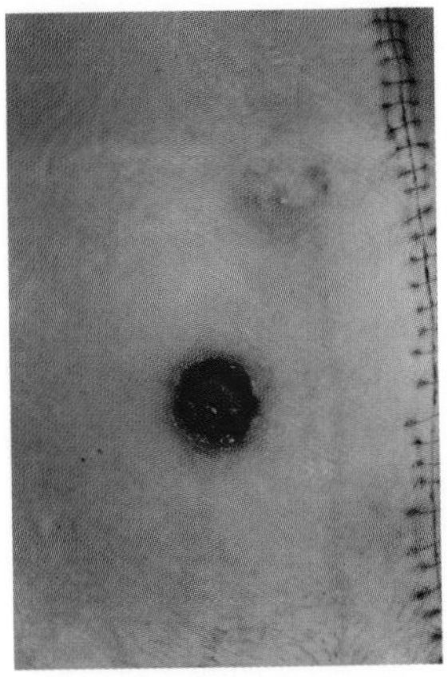

2A

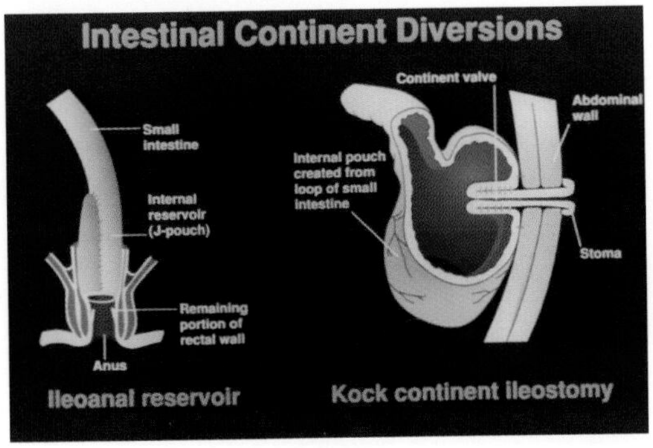


2B

**2A-B** There are three major types of ostomies: ileostomy, colostomy, or urinary diversion. **A,** In an ileostomy, a portion of the ileum is brought through the abdominal wall. **B,** The two most common types of continent ileostomies are the ileoanal reservoir and the Kock continent ileostomy. The ileoanal reservoir is created by stripping diseased mucosa from the rectum, creating an internal pouch from the ileum, and pulling the distal end of the pouch through the rectum and attaching it. In the Kock continent ileostomy, an internal pouch is created from the ileum and an intussusception of the bowel is used to create a "nipple."

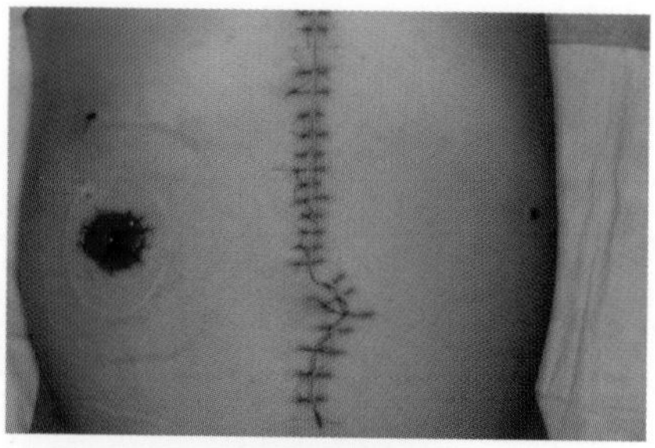

2C

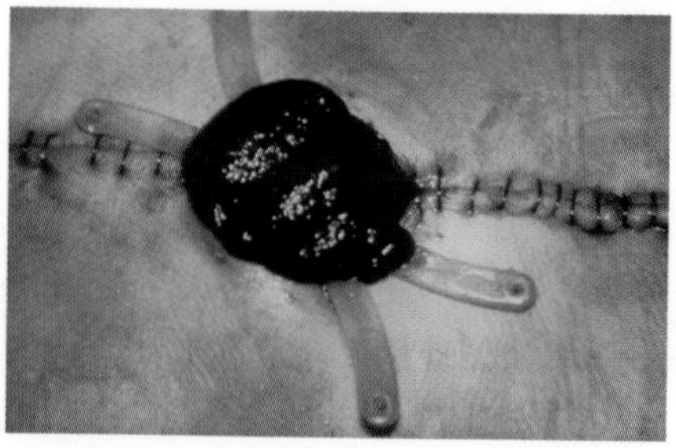

2D

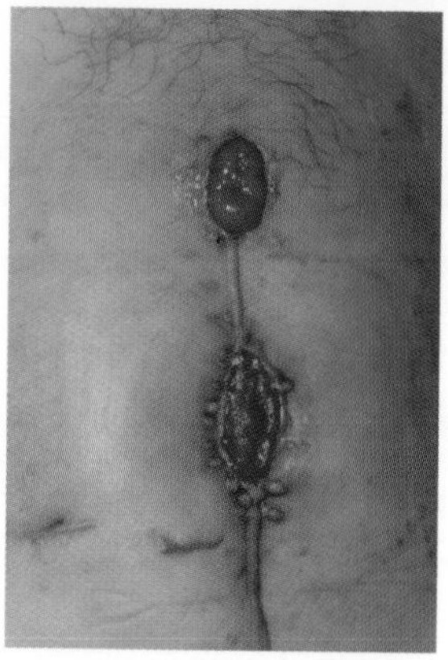

2E

2C-F Colostomies are located on the ascending, transverse, or descending/sigmoid colon. **C,** Ascending colostomies are uncommon. The ascending colon is retained, but the rest of the large bowel is removed or bypassed. The stoma is usually on the right side of the abdomen. The transverse colon is the site of most temporary colostomies. A loop of the transverse colon is lifted through the abdominal incision, and a rod or bridge is placed under the loop to give it support. **D,** Loop colostomies have one large opening, but two tracts. The proximal tract discharges fecal material; the distal tract secretes small amounts of mucus. **E,** In a double-barrel transverse colostomy, the bowel is completely divided by bringing both the proximal end and the distal end through the abdominal wall and suturing it to the skin. **F,** Descending and sigmoid colostomies are fairly common and generally are on the left side of the abdomen.

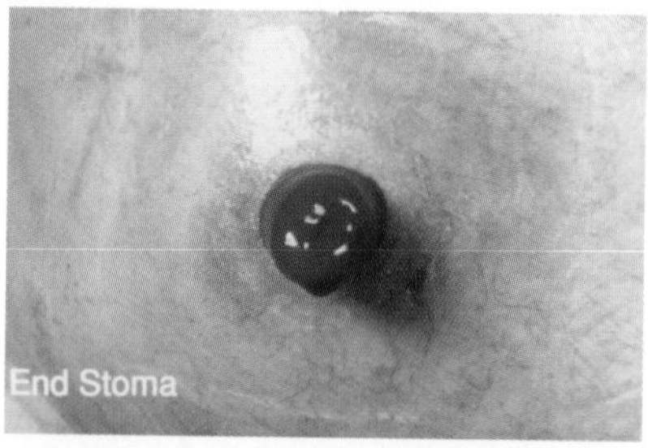


2F

2G-I Urinary diversion surgery diverts the urinary stream through an opening in the abdominal wall. **G,** In the ileal conduit, the most common type of urinary diversion, ileal and colon conduits are created after removal of the bladder by implanting the ureters into an isolated loop of bowel, the distal end of which is brought to the surface of the abdomen. **H,** Mucous shreds will be present if the bowel is used to create the diversion. **I,** In an ureterostomy, one or both ureters are detached from the bladder and brought to the outside of the abdominal wall, where a stoma is created. This procedure is used less frequently because the ureters tend to narrow unless they have been dilated permanently by previous disease (see Chapter 22). (Copyrighted photographs 2B, D, and G courtesy of Hollister Incorporated, Libertyville, Illinois. Copyrighted photographs 2A, C, E, F, H, and I courtesy of Joan Lerner Selekof, BSN, CWOCN, University of Maryland Medical Center, Baltimore, Maryland.)

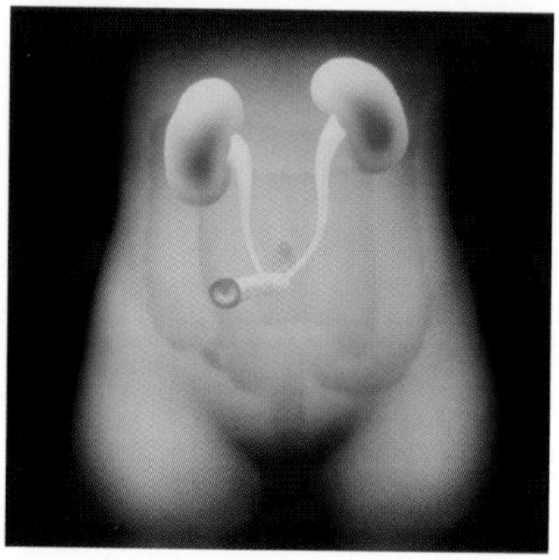

2G

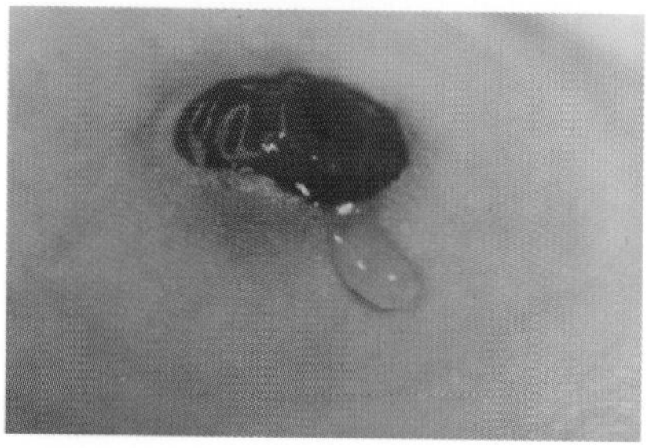

2H

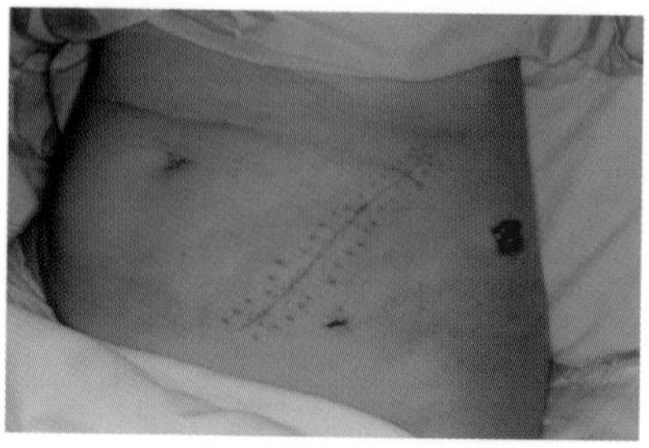

2I

3
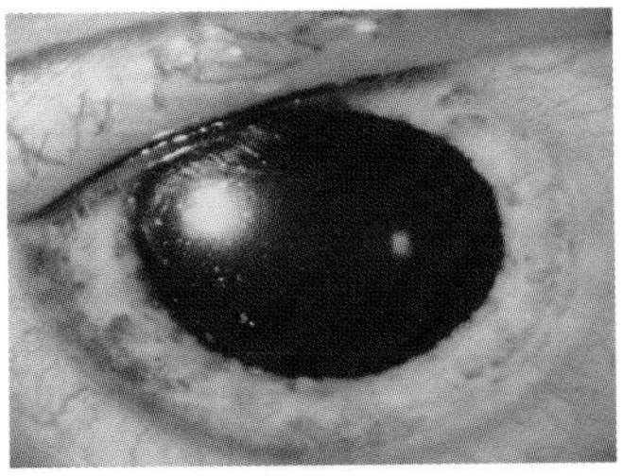

3 **Severe dry eye** can result from failure to properly diagnose and treat dry eye syndromes. Severe damage to eye tissue, particularly the corneal surface, can occur (see Chapter 28). (Photograph courtesy of Allergan, Inc., Irvine, California.)

4
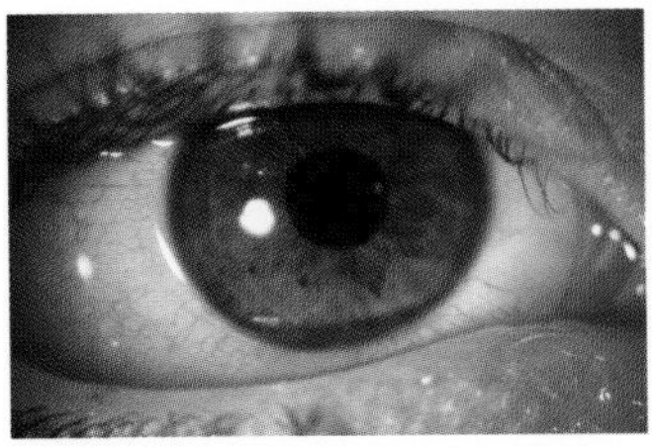

4 **Allergic conjunctivitis** is characterized by itchy, red eyes with a watery discharge. Vision is usually not impaired, but it may be blurred because of excessive tearing (see Chapter 28).

5
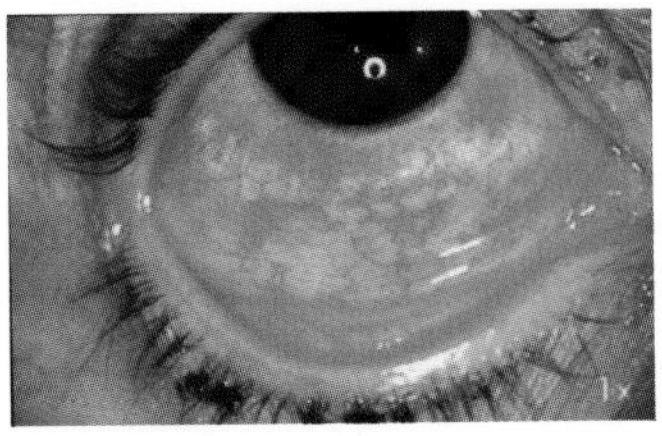

5 **Viral conjunctivitis,** the most common form of conjunctivitis, is usually characterized by a "pink eye" with a copious amount of watery discharge. A recent cold, sore throat, or exposure to someone with viral conjunctivitis is a common precursor of this condition (see Chapter 28). (Copyrighted photograph courtesy of Umberto Benelli, MD, eyeatlas.com.)

6
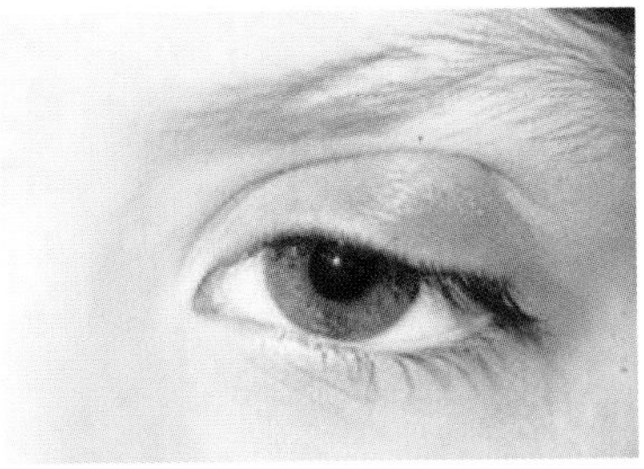

6 **Chalazion** is a sterile granuloma that may involve one of the lid glands or be located near (but not on) the eyelid. Unlike a hordeolum, a chalazion is neither infectious nor tender to gentle touching (see Chapter 28). (Copyrighted photograph courtesy of Umberto Benelli, MD, eyeatlas.com.)

7
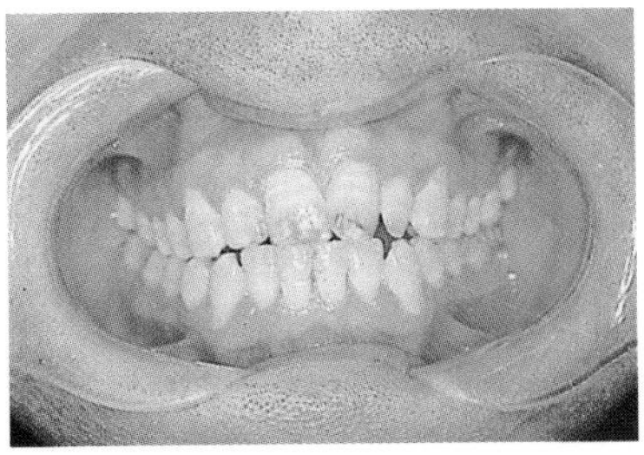

7 **Dental fluorosis (mottled enamel)** occurs during the time of tooth formation and is caused by the long-term ingestion of drinking water containing fluoride at concentrations greater than 1 ppm. Discoloration of the teeth varies, depending on the level of fluoride in the water, and ranges from white flecks or spots to brownish stains, small pits, or deep irregular pits that are dark brown in color (see Chapter 31).

8
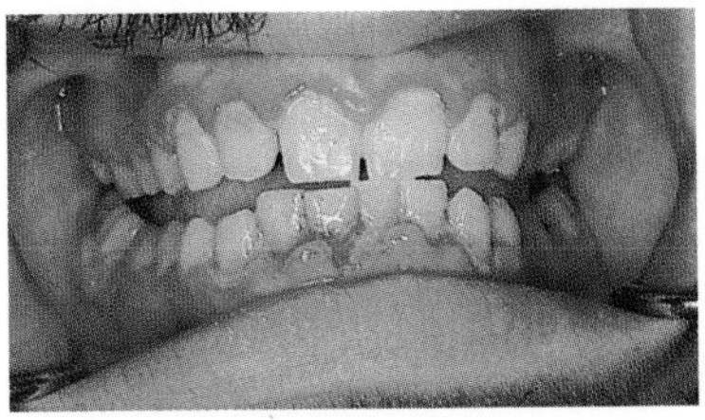

8 **Chronic gingivitis,** an asymptomatic inflammation of the gingivae (gums) at the necks of the teeth, is an early stage of periodontitis and is usually caused by poor oral hygiene. The gingivae are erythematous (red) and may have areas that appear swollen and glossy. In addition, mild hemorrhage may occur during teeth brushing (see Chapter 31).

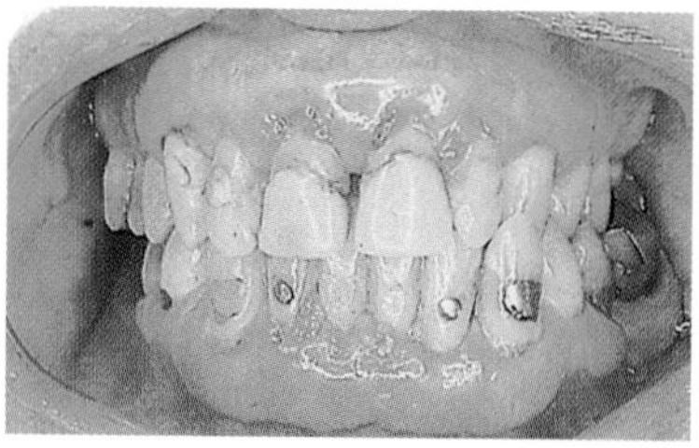

9

**9 Chronic periodontitis (pyorrhea),** an inflammation of the tissues surrounding the teeth, including the gingivae, periodontal ligaments, alveolar bone, and the cementum (bony material covering the root of a tooth), is caused by plaque accumulation resulting from poor oral hygiene. The gingivae may be erythematous and swollen, and may recede from the necks of the teeth. The condition is not painful and usually is accompanied by halitosis, loosening of the teeth, and mild hemorrhage during teeth brushing (see Chapter 31).

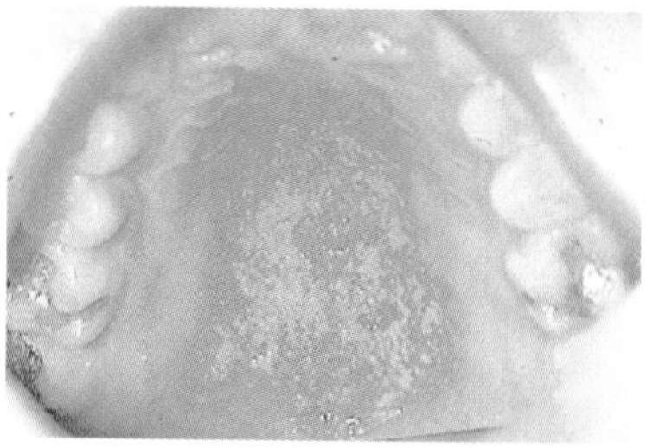

10

**10 Candidiasis (candidosis, moniliasis, thrush),** an infection caused by overgrowth of *Candida albicans*, tends to occur in people with debilitating or chronic systemic disease or those on long-term antibiotic therapy. Candidiasis commonly presents as a whitish-gray to yellowish, soft, slightly elevated pseudomembrane-like plaque on the oral mucosa; the plaque is often described as having a milk curd appearance. If the membrane is stripped away, a raw bleeding surface remains. A dull, burning pain is often present (see Chapters 31 and 32).

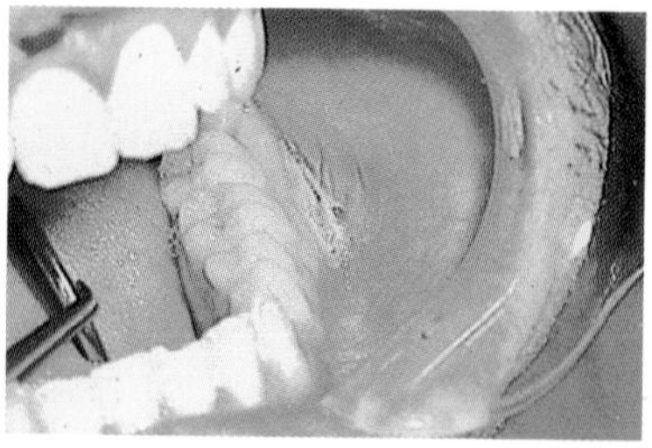

11

**11 Aspirin burn** results from the topical use of aspirin to relieve toothache. An aspirin tablet is placed against the tooth, where it is held in place by pressure from the buccal (cheek) mucosa. The mucosa becomes necrotic and is characterized by a white slough that rubs away, revealing a painful ulceration (see Chapter 32).

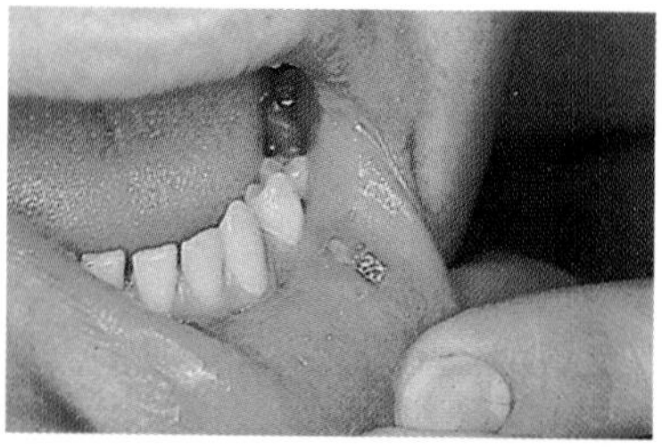

12

**12 Recurrent aphthous ulcers (canker sores)** are recurrent, painful, single or multiple ulcerations of bacterial origin. The central ulceration is sharply demarcated, often has a yellow to white surface of necrotic debris, and is surrounded by an erythematous margin (see Chapter 32).

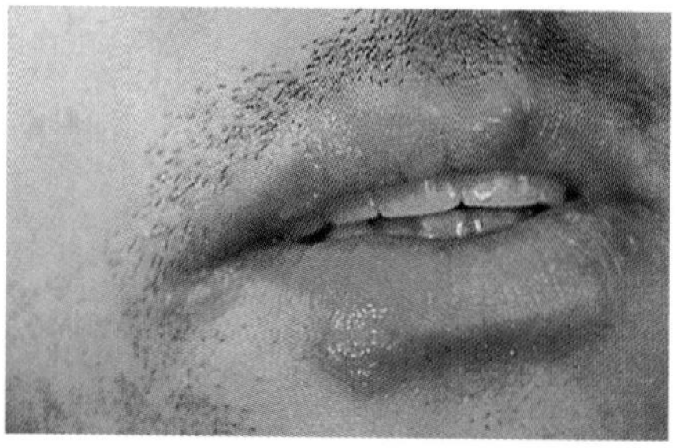

13

**13 Herpes simplex** lesions of the mouth and the eye usually start as a small cluster of vesicles (tiny blisters) that subsequently heal over with a serosanguinous (blood-tinged) crust. Local stinging, burning, and pain often herald the onset of lesions. Eye involvement should always be referred to an ophthalmologist (see Chapter 32).

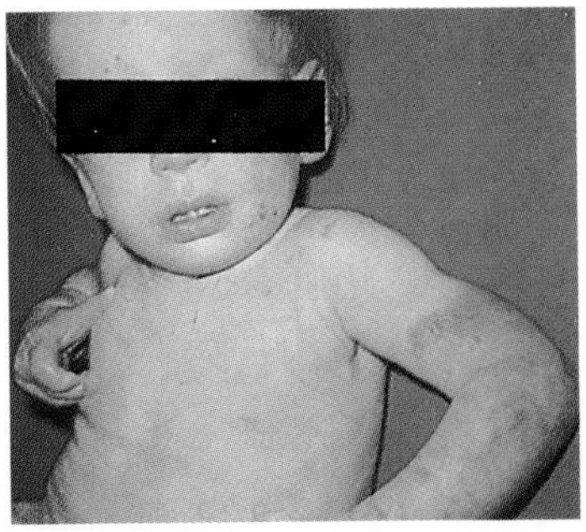

14A

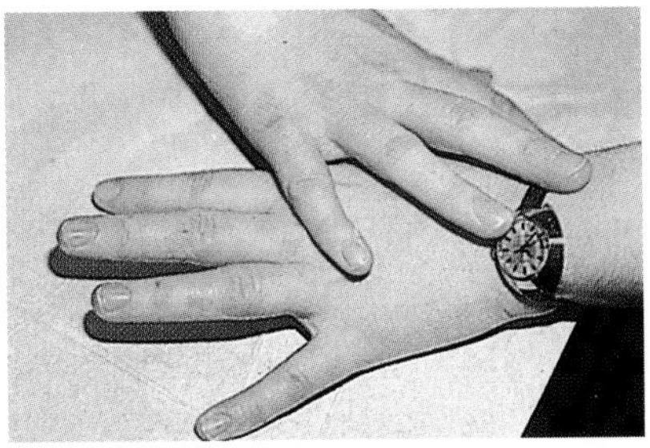

14B

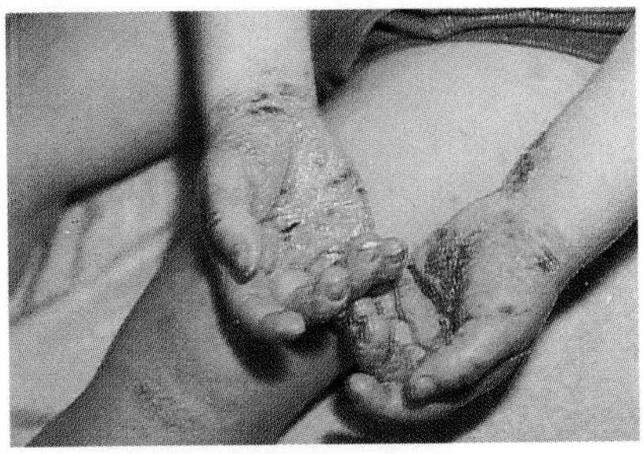

14C

**14A, B, and C** **Atopic dermatitis (eczema)** is an inflammatory condition that occurs **(A)** on the extensor surface of the elbows and knees during the first year of life and then **(B)** involves predominantly the flexors. **C,** The hands, feet, and face are often involved as well. The dermatitis is characterized by erythema, scale, increased skin surface markings, and crusting; secondary infection is common (see Chapter 33).

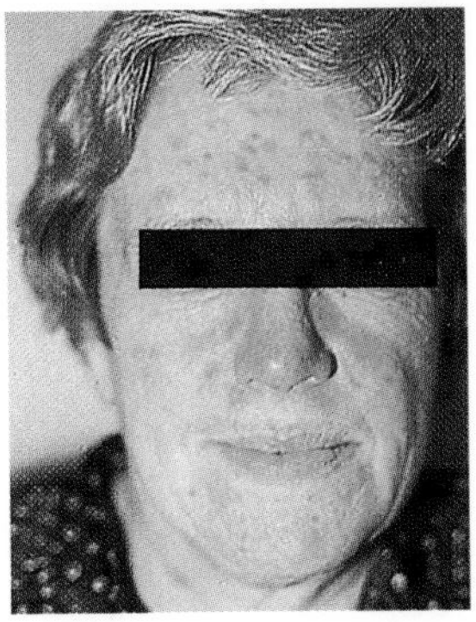

15

**15** **Seborrheic dermatitis** is a red scaling condition of the scalp, midface, and upper midchest of adults. This dermatitis is marked by characteristic greasy, yellowish scaling and is associated with erythema (see Chapter 34).

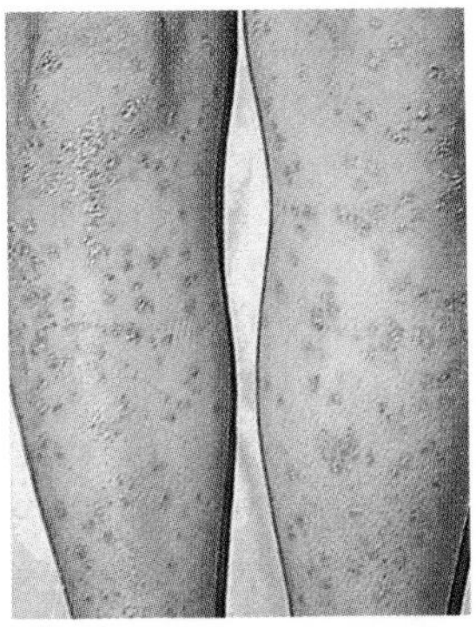

16A

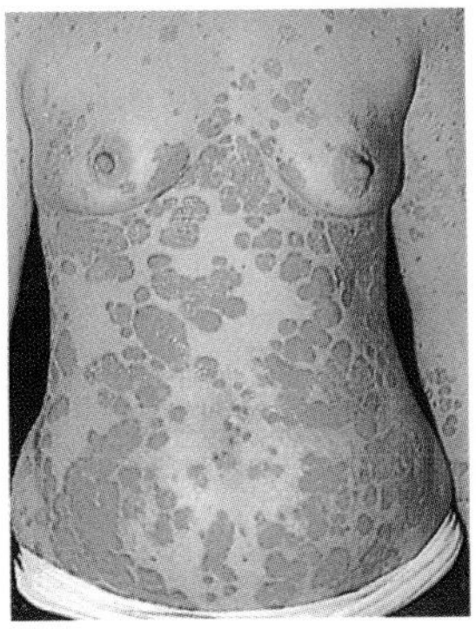

16B

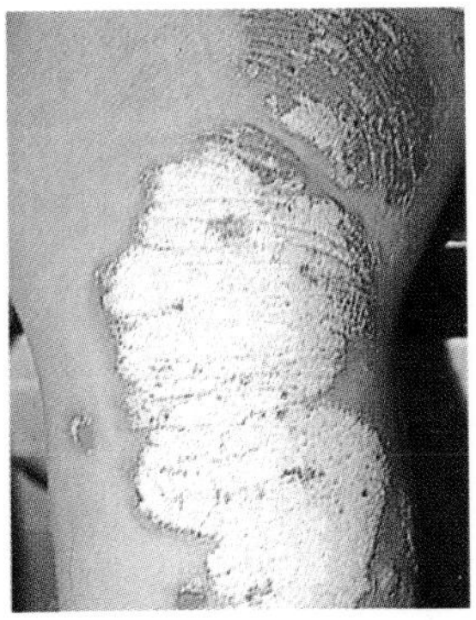

16C

**16A, B, and C** **Psoriasis** is a scaling condition in which erythematous plaques (red raised areas) are covered by a thick adherent scale. The borders of the lesions are well developed and vary from guttate (very small drop-shaped plaques) to much larger plaques: (**A**) guttate, (**B**) medium-size plaques, (**C**) large plaques (see Chapter 34).

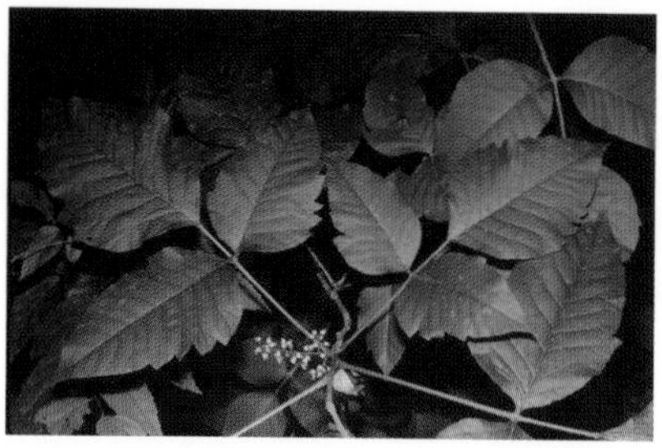

17A

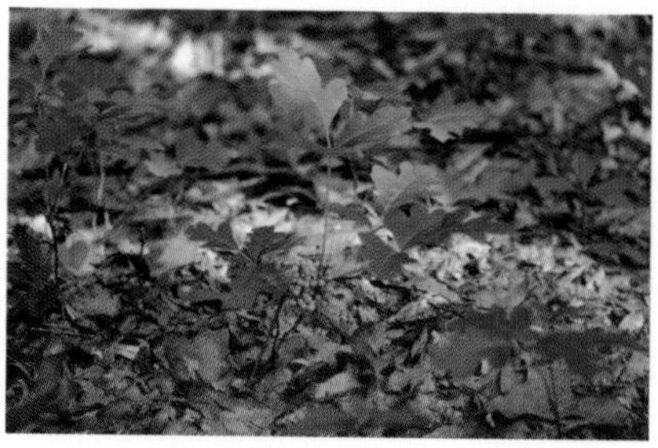

17B

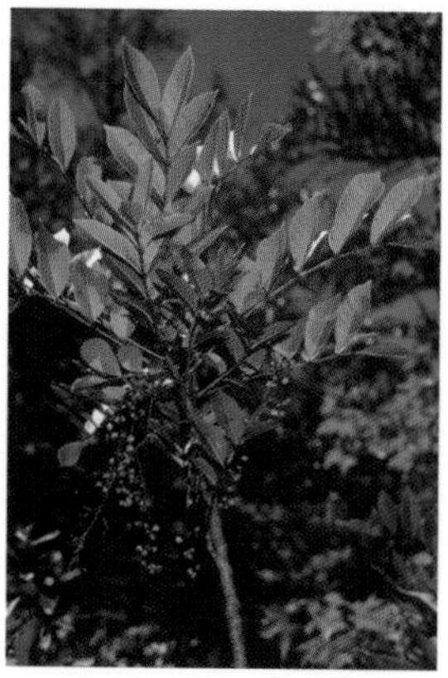

17C

**17A, B, and C** **Poison ivy, oak, and sumac** account for the majority of plant-induced allergic contact dermatitis. **A,** In the United States, poison ivy is the most common of the three plants. It usually grows as a scrambling shrub or a climbing hairy vine that often grows up poles, trees, and building walls. Its leaves are usually large, broad, and spoon-shaped. **B,** Two species of poison oak are indigenous to the United States; both possess leaves with unlobed edges that look similar to those of oak trees. Eastern poison oak (*T. toxicarium*) commonly displays three leaflets, whereas Western poison oak (*T. diversilobum*) has between 3 and 11 leaflets per stem. Poison oak usually grows as a shrub capable of reaching heights of 131 feet (40 m). **C,** Poison sumac (*T. vernix*) grows in remote areas of the eastern one third of the United States in peat bogs and swampy areas. It grows as a shrub or small tree and attains a height of about 9.8 feet (3 m). Its pinnate leaves have smooth edges that come to a tip and may be almost 16 inches (40 cm) in length. The leaves are odd numbered, ranging between 7 and 13 leaflets (see Chapter 35). (Photographs courtesy of George Yatskievych, PhD, Missouri Botanical Garden, St. Louis, © 2000.)

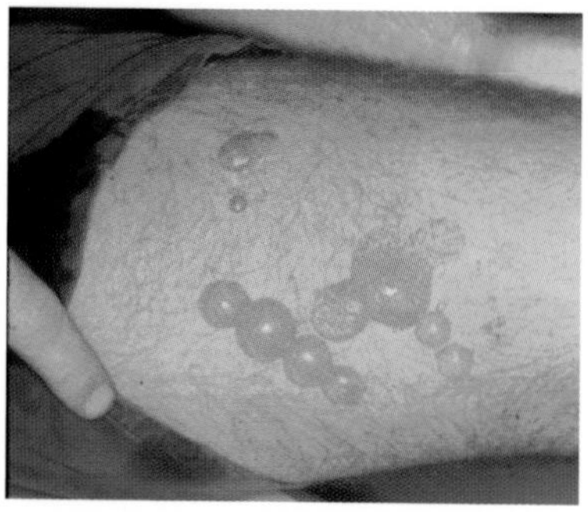

18A

**18A, B, and C** **Poison ivy** dermatitis is often associated with **(A)** fluid-filled vesicles (blisters) or bullae, depending on a person's sensitivity. **B,** Oozing and weeping of the vesicular fluid occurs for several days, until the affected area develops crusts and begins to dry. **C,** Streaks of vesicles that correspond to the points of urushiol contact from the damaged plant are highly suggestive of poison ivy exposure. Similar reactions can also be caused by poison oak and poison sumac (see Chapter 35). (Photographs courtesy of Christopher Huerter, MD, Creighton University Medical Center, Omaha, Nebraska, © 2002.)

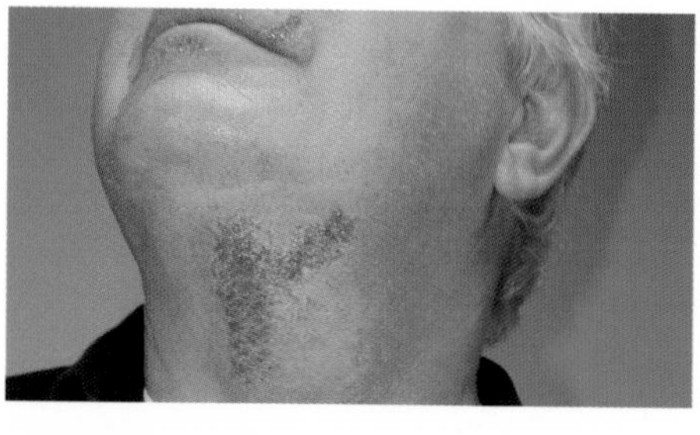

18B

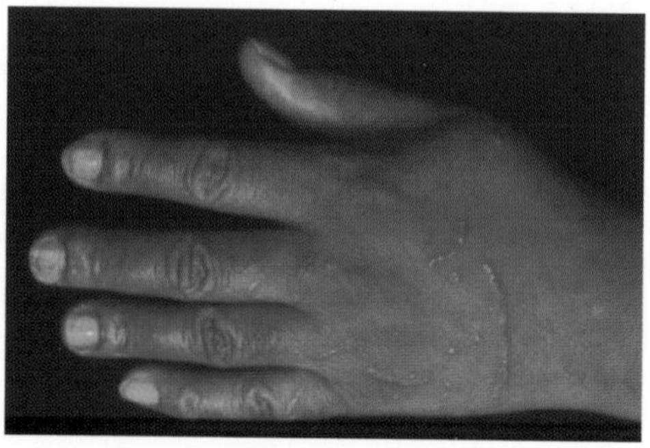

18C

19 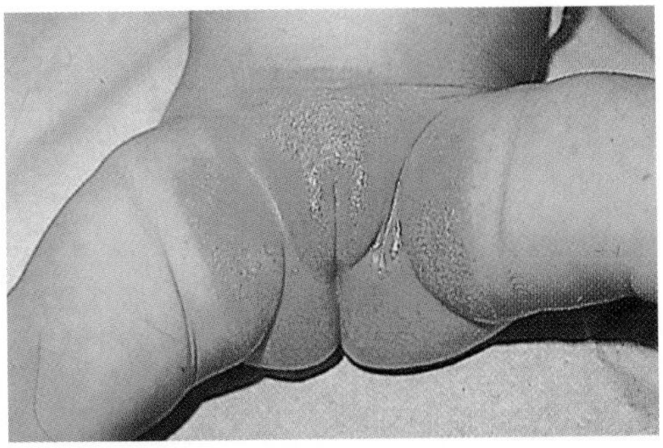

**19 Diaper dermatitis** presents as erythema of the groin (crease area around the genitals) and is common in infants. The case shown here was caused by a contact allergen. Contact irritants, such as urine and feces, and secondary bacterial and yeast infections may also cause problems in this area (see Chapter 36).

20 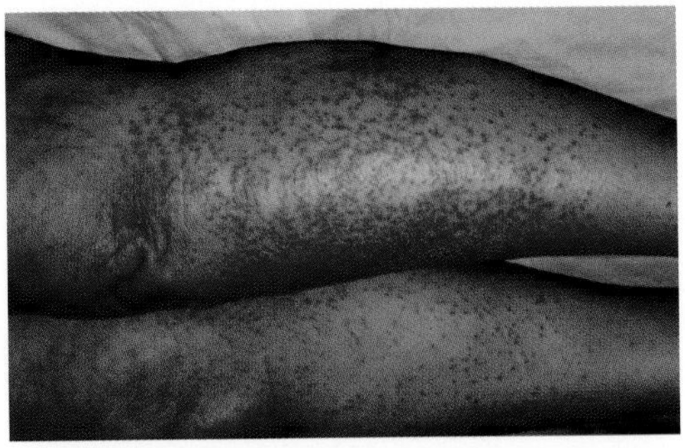

**20 Miliaria rubra (heat rash)** is an obstruction of sweat glands. Superficial involvement results in only tiny vesicles (blisters) appearing on the skin surface (miliaria crystallina). When deeper inflammation is present, the surrounding erythema is characteristic of miliaria rubra (see Chapter 36). (Photograph reprinted with permission from eMedicine.com, Inc., © 2003.)

21 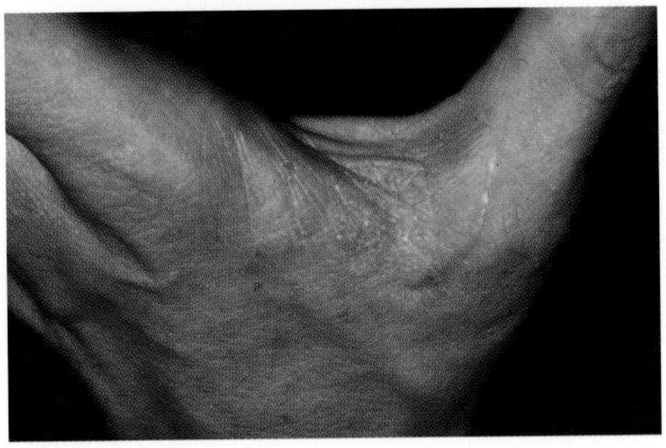

**21 Scabies** is caused by a small mite that burrows under the superficial skin layers. Small linear blisters that cause intense itching can be seen between the finger webs, on the inner wrists, in the axilla, around the areola (nipple) of the breast, and on the genitalia (see Chapter 37). (Photograph reprinted with permission from eMedicine.com, Inc., © 2003.)

22 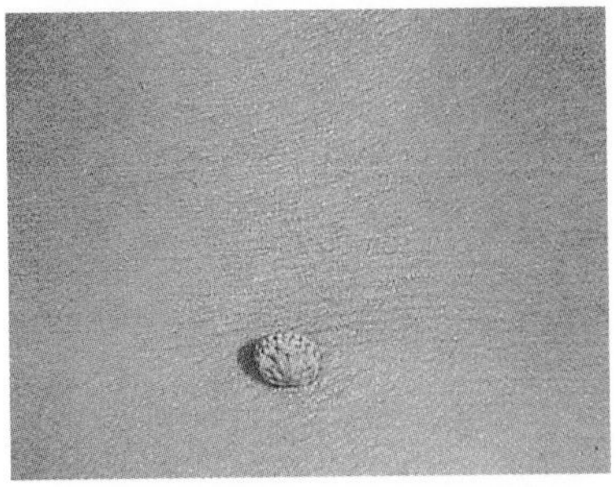

**22 Ticks** can attach to human skin and burrow into superficial skin layers. With careful examination, the back of the organism is usually visible on the skin surface. Ticks are vectors of several systemic diseases (see Chapter 37).

23A 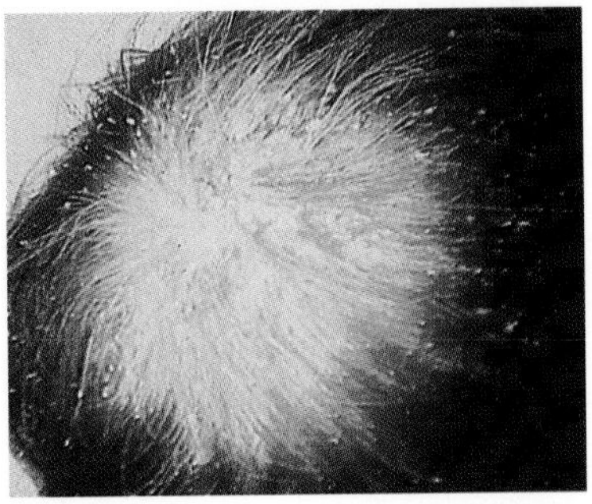

23B 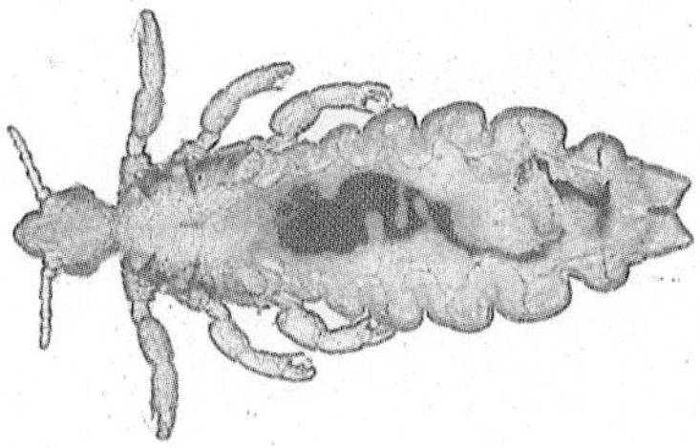

**23A and B Pediculosis humanus capitis** is a louse infestation of the scalp. **A,** Examination of the scalp hair in this infestation shows tiny nits (eggs) attached to the hair shaft. **B,** The organism shown is only occasionally seen (see Chapter 37).

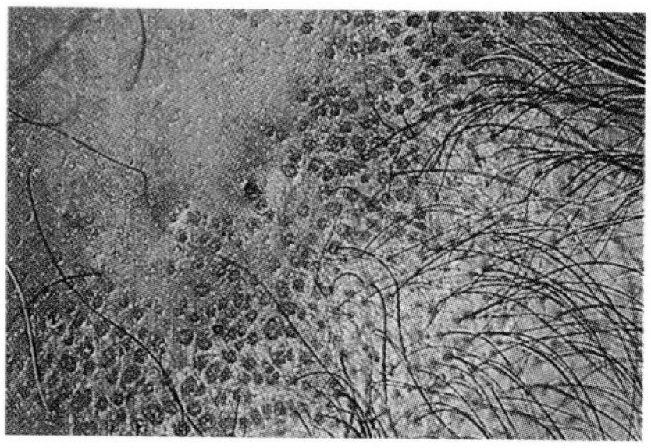

24

24 **Comedonic acne (noninflammatory)** occurs when follicles become plugged with sebum, forming a comedone on the surface. The black color is caused by oxidation of lipid and melanin, not dirt as is commonly believed (see Chapter 38).

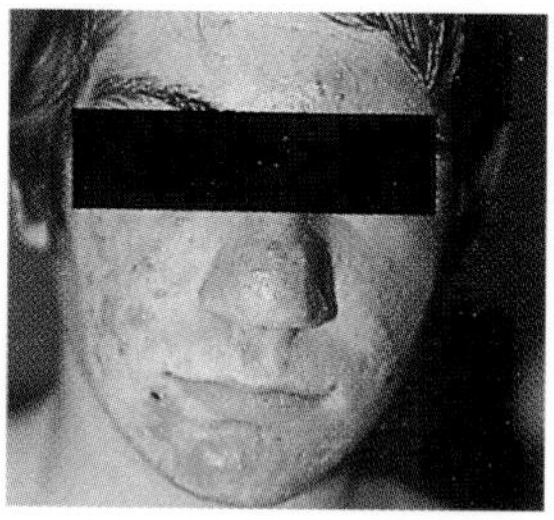

25

25 **Pustular acne (inflammatory)** presents as inflamed papules that are formed when superficial hair follicles become plugged and rupture at a deeper level. Superficial inflammation results in pustules; deep lesions cause large cysts to form with possible resultant scarring (see Chapter 38).

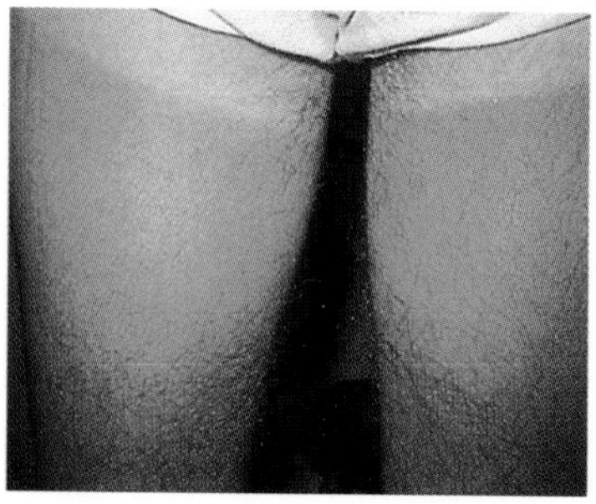

26

26 **Sunburn** presents as an erythema that occurs after excessive sun exposure; severe burns can result in large blister formation. Proper sunscreen application can provide photoprotection for susceptible patients (see Chapters 39 and 41).

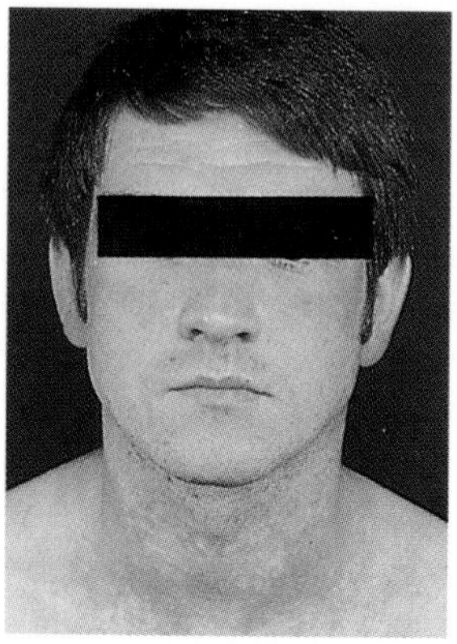

27

27 **Drug-induced photosensitivity** is a reaction that occurs on sun-exposed surfaces of the head, neck, and dorsum (back) of the hands. The erythema does not occur on photoprotected areas, such as under the nose and chin, behind the ears, and between the fingers (see Chapters 39 and 41).

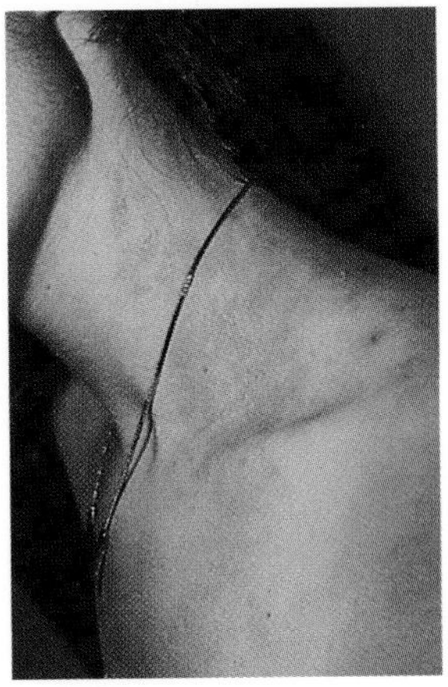

28

**28 Cosmetic-induced photosensitivity** can be caused by ingredients in certain topical colognes and perfumes. This immunologic reaction produces a local erythema that leaves characteristic postinflammatory pigmentation (see Chapters 39 and 41).

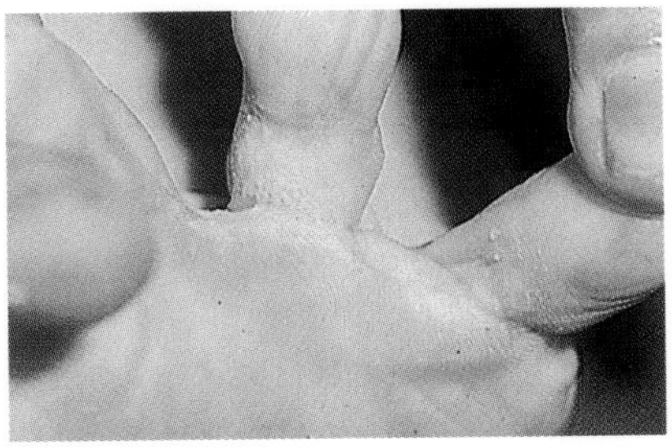

29

**29 Tinea pedis** infection of the toes characteristically starts between the fourth and fifth web space and spreads proximally. Scaling can progress to maceration with resultant small fissures (see Chapter 43).

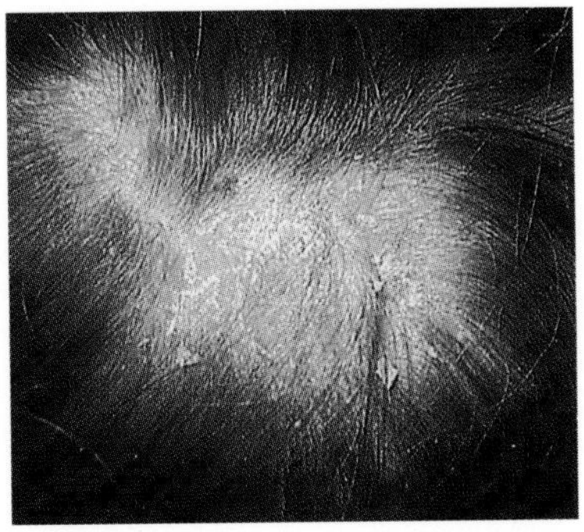

30

**30 Tinea capitis,** a fungal infection of the scalp, is marked by scale on the scalp with local breaking or loss of hair; erythema (redness) is usually not observed (see Chapter 43).

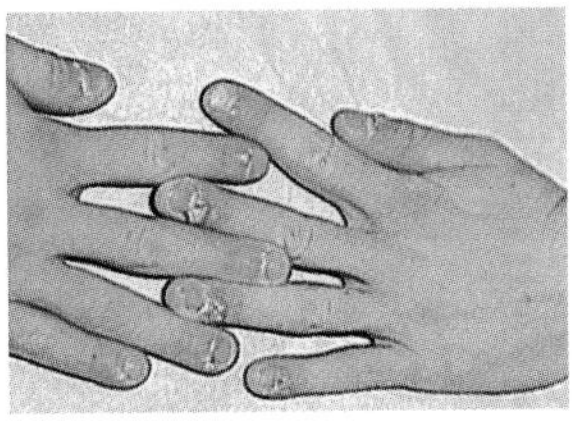

31

**31 Common warts** are viral-induced lesions that present as localized rough accumulations of keratin (hyperkeratosis) containing many tiny furrows. If the wart's surface is pared, small bleeding points can be seen (see Chapter 44).

32 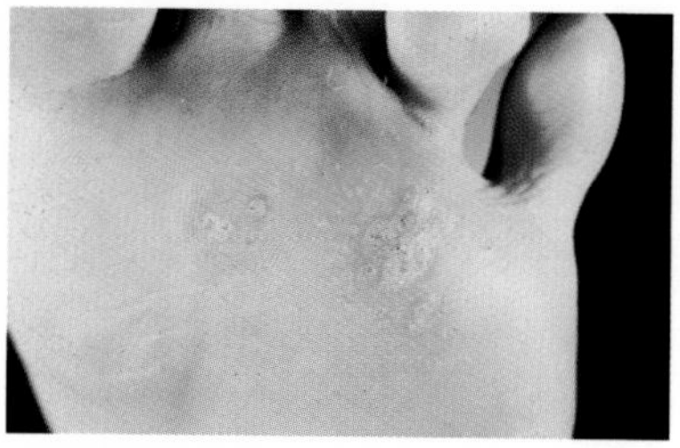

32 **Plantar warts,** caused by a viral infection, are often found on the plantar surface of the foot and present with hard localized accumulations of keratin. The punctate bleeding points seen when the lesions are pared distinguish plantar warts from calluses (see Chapter 44). (Photograph reprinted with permission from eMedicine.com, Inc., © 2003.)

33 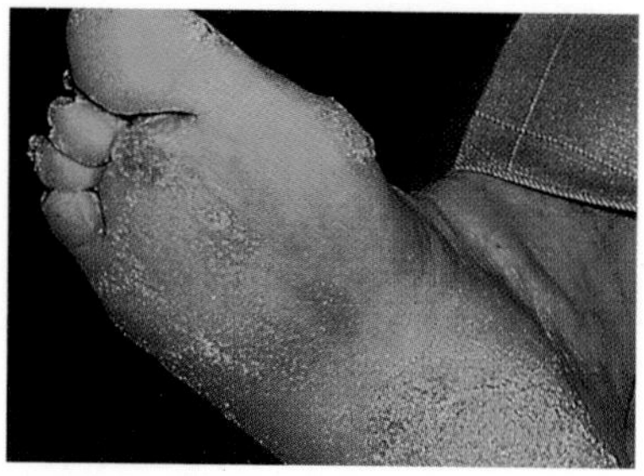

33 **Calluses** are thickened scales that often form on joints and weight-bearing areas. A callus on the plantar surface of the foot is shown here (see Chapter 45).

hypersensitive teeth are a chronic problem and require long-term treatment provided by a dentist.

*Safety Considerations* Dentifrices containing potassium nitrate 5% are not recommended for children younger than 12 years. Patients with hypersensitive teeth should be cautioned against using high-abrasion toothpastes such as cosmetic pastes that whiten teeth or remove stains.

*Product Selection Guidelines* Presently, the best choice of products is limited to either a desensitizing toothpaste containing the only Category I agent, potassium nitrate 5%, or a combination product containing this desensitizing agent and fluoride. FDA has proposed a Category I classification for this combination product. Such a product, when used as directed, can relieve dentinal hypersensitivity and prevent dental caries, making it a good recommendation.

### *Assessment of Toothache and Tooth Hypersensitivity: A Case-based Approach*

Before recommending self-treatment of tooth pain, the practitioner should determine whether a dentist has already diagnosed the cause. The practitioner should also determine whether the patient has a history of dental problems (caries, periodontal, or endodontic problems) and how the patient removes plaque from the teeth. This information will help determine whether the patient's oral hygiene is adequate. Use of plaque removal products should be evaluated for possible misuse, abuse, or inappropriate response. Case 32-1 illustrates the assessment of patients with toothache.

**CASE 32-1**

| Relevant Evaluation Criteria | Scenario/Model Outcome |
|---|---|
| **Information Gathering** | |
| 1. Gather essential information about the patient's symptoms, including: | |
| a. description of symptom(s) (i.e., nature, onset, duration, severity, associated symptoms) | Patient is having persistent tooth pain in the left side of her mouth. |
| b. description of any factors that seem to precipitate, exacerbate, and/or relieve the patient's symptom(s) | Drinking hot coffee, breathing in cold air, and brushing teeth increase pain. |
| c. description of the patient's efforts to relieve the symptoms | Patient went to her dentist and has used a desensitizing dentifrice. |
| 2. Gather essential patient history information: | |
| a. patient's identity | Mary Harper |
| b. patient's age, sex, height, and weight | 24 y/o F |
| c. patient's occupation | Graduate student |
| d. patient's dietary habits | Eats a lot of fast food |
| e. patient's sleep habits | Good, except around exam time |
| f. concurrent medical conditions, prescription and nonprescription medications, and dietary supplements | None |
| g. allergies | None |
| h. history of other adverse reactions to medications | None |
| i. other (describe)______ | N/A |
| **Assessment and Triage** | |
| 3. Differentiate the patient's signs/symptoms and correctly identify the patient's primary problem(s) (see Table 32-1). | Patient appears to have tooth hypersensitivity. Mary's tooth pain was not resolved with the desensitizing dentifrice recommended by dentist. Dentist also recommended a nonprescription fluoride rinse. |

## CASE 32-1 (continued)

| Relevant Evaluation Criteria | Scenario/Model Outcome |
|---|---|
| 4. Identify exclusions for self-treatment (see Figure 32-1). | None |
| 5. Formulate a comprehensive list of therapeutic alternatives for the primary problem to determine if triage to a medical practitioner is required, and share this information with the patient. | Options include:<br>(1) Recommend a different desensitizing dentifrice.<br>(2) Recommend appropriate use of a fluoride rinse.<br>(3) Suggest that Mary return to her dentist.<br>(4) Take no action. |
| **Plan** | |
| 6. Select an optimal therapeutic alternative to address the patient's problem, taking into account patient preferences. | Recommend patient continue twice-daily use of a desensitization toothpaste with a soft-bristle toothbrush, as it may take several weeks for sensitivity to resolve. |
| 7. Describe the recommended therapeutic approach to the patient. | Use a soft-bristle brush and light pressure to apply the desensitizing toothpaste; brush your teeth twice a day.<br>You may purchase toothpaste that also contains fluoride or a fluoride rinse for adults. |
| 8. Explain to the patient the rationale for selecting the recommended therapeutic approach from the considered therapeutic alternatives. | Another brand of desensitizing toothpaste may work better for you if you follow the usage instructions carefully. A toothpaste with fluoride or an adult fluoride rinse will help prevent tooth decay. |
| **Patient Education** | |
| 9. When recommending self-care with nonprescription medications and/or nondrug therapy, convey accurate information to the patient, including: | |
| a. appropriate dose and frequency of administration | See the box Patient Education for Tooth Hypersensitivity. |
| b. maximum number of days the therapy should be employed | See the box Patient Education for Tooth Hypersensitivity. |
| c. product administration procedures | See the box Patient Education for Tooth Hypersensitivity. |
| d. expected time to onset of relief | See the box Patient Education for Tooth Hypersensitivity. |
| e. degree of relief that can be reasonably expected | See the box Patient Education for Tooth Hypersensitivity. |
| f. most common side effects | See the box Patient Education for Tooth Hypersensitivity. |
| g. side effects that warrant medical intervention should they occur | See the box Patient Education for Tooth Hypersensitivity. |
| h. patient options in the event that condition worsens or persists | See the box Patient Education for Tooth Hypersensitivity. |
| i. product storage requirements | See the box Patient Education for Tooth Hypersensitivity. |
| j. specific nondrug measures | See the box Patient Education for Tooth Hypersensitivity. |
| 10. Solicit patient's follow-up questions. | May I use the desensitizing toothpaste more often? |
| 11. Answer patient's questions. | Yes. Instead of using a toothbrush to apply the desensitizing toothpaste on your teeth you may want to place a small amount on your finger and rub into the area(s) that you have sensitivity. |

Key: N/A, not applicable.

## PATIENT EDUCATION FOR TOOTH HYPERSENSITIVITY

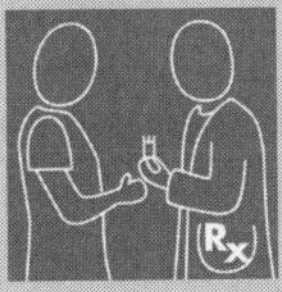

The objectives for self-care of diagnosed tooth hypersensitivity are to (1) repair the damaged tooth surface using the appropriate toothpaste and (2) stop abrasive toothbrushing practices. For most patients, carefully following product instructions, the dentist's recommendations, and the self-care measures listed here will help ensure optimal therapeutic outcomes.

- Use a soft-bristle toothbrush, and brush with light pressure with a fluoride toothpaste for sensitive teeth at or near a receding gumline.
- If correct brushing techniques with a fluoride toothpaste are ineffective, a desensitizing toothpaste should be used.
- If a desensitizing toothpaste is needed, apply a 1-inch strip of toothpaste to a soft-bristle toothbrush. Brush for at least 1 minute twice daily.
- Note that relief of the sensitivity may take several days to several weeks. The better the patient is at removing bacterial plaque, the quicker the sensitivity will resolve.
- Use the toothpaste as long as the dentist recommends, and then switch to a low-abrasion (nonwhitening) fluoride dentifrice.
- Note that some cases of hypersensitive teeth require long-term treatment or several repeated treatments.
- Do not use desensitizing toothpastes in children younger than 12 years of age.
- Do not use high-abrasion toothpastes such as cosmetic pastes that whiten or remove stains.

⚠ See a dentist if the pain worsens during treatment or if new symptoms develop.

### *Patient Counseling for Toothache and Tooth Hypersensitivity*

Patients should be counseled that, because a differential diagnosis of toothache is needed to rule out other conditions that produce this pain, the problem can be serious and warrants the attention of a dentist. A nonprescription analgesic can be recommended to relieve toothache pain prior to the patient's dental appointment.

Subsequent to a definite diagnosis of tooth hypersensitivity, the practitioner should explain the proper use of desensitizing toothpastes and safe methods of toothbrushing. The practitioner should also explain precautions for using the toothpastes.

### *Evaluation of Patient Outcomes for Toothache and Tooth Hypersensitivity*

The patient with hypersensitive teeth should return for evaluation after 14 days of treatment with desensitizing toothpaste. If the pain is resolved, the patient should continue treatment as recommended by a dentist. The patient should be advised to continue the recommended dental hygiene measures. If the pain persists or worsens or if new symptoms develop, the patient should see a dentist for further evaluation.

## Teething Discomfort

Not all babies suffer discomfort during teething. For those who do, nonprescription products can provide symptomatic relief.

### *Etiology of Teething Discomfort*

Teething is the eruption of the deciduous (primary or baby) teeth through the gingival tissues. Usually, this normal physiologic process is uneventful. However, it can cause sleep disturbances or irritability in some infants.

### *Signs and Symptoms of Teething Discomfort*

Teething is not associated with vomiting, diarrhea, nasal congestion, malaise, fever, or rashes, but these symptoms may be a sign of ear or stomach infection. Mild pain, irritation, reddening, excessive drooling or slight swelling of the gums may precede or accompany the other symptoms (sleep disturbances or irritability).

Bluish, soft, and round swellings (called eruption cysts) sometimes form over emerging incisors and molars. Eruption cysts are not the result of infection and will disappear if left alone. In addition, three bumps (called mamelons) may be present on the biting surfaces (incisal edges) of emerging incisors. The mamelons will wear away as the teeth begin to occlude against the opposing dentition. If the underside of the tongue becomes irritated, a dentist may try to smooth the edges of the mamelons to prevent further irritation.

### *Treatment of Teething Discomfort*

#### Treatment Goals

The goal of self-care of teething discomfort is to relieve gum pain and irritation, thereby reducing the child's irritability and sleep disturbances.

#### General Treatment Approach

Parents should be cautioned to exercise restraint in treating a child's teething discomfort. Eruption cysts are a part of the normal physiologic process and should be left alone to resolve spontaneously. If cut or punctured, the cysts will leave scars that may delay the tooth's eruption. Parents should also exercise restraint in the use of nonprescription teething products.

Various nonpharmacologic measures are recommended for alleviating teething discomfort. Parents should try all measures to determine which are helpful. If additional treatment is needed, topical analgesics that are approved specifically for teething discomfort can be used.

**TABLE 32-3 Selected Teething Products***

| |
|---|
| **Benzocaine 7.5% Products** |
| Anbesol Grape Baby Gel |
| Anbesol Original Baby Gel |
| Num-Zit Teething Gel |
| Orajel Baby Gel/Liquid |
| **Benzocaine 10% Products** |
| Orajel Baby Nighttime Gel |

* All products are alcohol-free.

## Nonpharmacologic Therapy

If the baby cooperates, massaging the gum around the erupting tooth may provide relief. Babies may be made more comfortable by giving them a frozen pacifier (teething ring), a cold wet cloth, or if they are at an age to tolerate food (such as dry toast), they may given such food to chew.

## Pharmacologic Therapy

Pharmacologic management of teething discomfort is limited to topical analgesics that are approved for use in infants and pediatric doses of systemic analgesics.

*Topical Oral Analgesics* The FDA review of nonprescription drug products for relief of oral discomfort has classified benzocaine 5% to 20% and phenol 0.5% preparations as Category I topical anesthetic/analgesics for teething pain. Currently, no phenol 0.5% products are marketed for teething pain, although phenol products are marketed for other mouth pain. Table 32-3 lists selected trade-name products.

Indications Teething products are labeled, "For the temporary relief of sore gums due to teething in infants and children 4 months of age and older."[15]

Dosage and Administration Guidelines Products containing benzocaine in solution or suspension should be rubbed onto the gums not more than four times daily. Concentrations of benzocaine in commercial teething products range from 7.5% to 10%. Many of them are alcohol-free. Teething preparations containing phenol or phenolate sodium equivalent to phenol 0.5% in aqueous solution or suspension may be applied to the affected area up to six times daily.

Safety Considerations In the highest (20%) concentration that is approved for nonprescription use, benzocaine is too potent for infants and can even cause death from drug overdose. This is why most pediatric products contain only benzocaine 7.5%. Purchasers of these products should be careful to select only those that are labeled for teething. The risk of hypersensitivity to common local anesthetics also exists.

Teething products must carry a warning that fever and nasal congestion are not symptoms of teething and may indicate the presence of an infection.

*Systemic Analgesics* Pediatric doses of systemic nonprescription analgesics (e.g., acetaminophen) may be used to relieve teething discomfort (see Chapter 5 for appropriate doses).

*Product Selection Guidelines* Most commercially available teething products contain benzocaine 7.5% (Table 32-3). As the trade name indicates, a product containing benzocaine 10% (Oragel Baby Nighttime) might be preferable for nighttime use to help babies sleep.

For ease of application, gels are the best choice; unlike liquids, they do not drip when applied. ADA recommends using an alcohol-free product. Parents should be advised to check the ingredients of teething products for the presence of alcohol.

### *Assessment of Teething Discomfort: A Case-based Approach*

In most cases, the practitioner must assess teething discomfort based on the parent's description of the child's symptoms. If the child cooperates, visual inspection of the gums may confirm that the child is teething. Nonetheless, the practitioner must distinguish the signs and symptoms of teething from those of an infection. Case 32-2 illustrates this approach to assessing patients with teething discomfort.

**CASE 32-2**

| Relevant Evaluation Criteria | Scenario/Model Outcome |
|---|---|
| **Information Gathering** | |
| 1. Gather essential information about the patient's symptoms, including: | |
| a. description of symptom(s) (i.e., nature, onset, duration, severity, associated symptoms) | Mother says that baby is crying, fussy, and chewing on everything. She has noticed increased drooling, red cheeks, and loose stools for 36 hours. |

## CASE 32-2 (continued)

| Relevant Evaluation Criteria | Scenario/Model Outcome |
|---|---|
| b. description of any factors that seem to precipitate, exacerbate, and/or relieve the patient's symptom(s) | Chewing on frozen teething ring seems to help. |
| c. description of the patient's efforts to relieve the symptoms | Sucking on fingers |
| 2. Gather essential patient history information: | |
| a. patient's identity | Timmy Taylor |
| b. patient's age, sex, height, and weight | 7-month-old M, 15 lb |
| c. patient's occupation | N/A |
| d. patient's dietary habits | Breast-feeding, cereal |
| e. patient's sleep habits | Usually sleeps from 9 PM until 7 AM |
| f. concurrent medical conditions, prescription and nonprescription medications, and dietary supplements | Tri-Vi-Flor 0.25 mg 1 mL by mouth once daily as nutritional supplement |
| g. allergies | NKA |
| h. history of other adverse reactions to medications | None |
| i. other (describe)_______ | Not feeding well |
| **Assessment and Triage** | |
| 3. Differentiate the patient's signs/symptoms and correctly identify the patient's primary problem(s). | Infant teething |
| 4. Identify exclusions for self-treatment. | None |
| 5. Formulate a comprehensive list of therapeutic alternatives for the primary problem to determine if triage to a medical practitioner is required, and share this information with the caregiver. | Options include:<br>(1) Recommend proper OTC products and nondrug therapies.<br>(2) Suggest that Timmy's mother take him to a dentist or PCP.<br>(3) Take no action. |
| **Plan** | |
| 6. Select an optimal therapeutic alternative to address the patient's problem, taking into account patient/caregiver preferences. | Topical application of teething gel and orally administered analgesics |
| 7. Describe the recommended therapeutic approach to the caregiver. | Rub teething gel onto Timmy's gums and give him acetaminophen drops orally for discomfort. |
| 8. Explain to the caregiver the rationale for selecting the recommended therapeutic approach from the considered therapeutic alternatives. | Timmy's discomfort is normal, and can be treated without need for dentist or PCP visit. |
| **Patient Education** | |
| 9. When recommending self-care with nonprescription medications and/or nondrug therapy, convey accurate information to the caregiver, including: | |
| a. appropriate dose and frequency of administration | Apply small amount of gel directly to gum where teeth are erupting. Apply 3-4 times/day. Give acetaminophen drops or liquid per package directions. |

| CASE 32-2 (continued) | |
|---|---|
| **Relevant Evaluation Criteria** | **Scenario/Model Outcome** |
| b. maximum number of days the therapy should be employed | Use until teeth have erupted. |
| c. product administration procedures | Avoid excessive gel application to prevent Timmy from swallowing it. |
| d. expected time to onset of relief | Some immediate relief should be expected. |
| e. degree of relief that can be reasonably expected | There may not be complete relief. |
| f. most common side effects | Redness or irritation of gum that increases after use of the teething gel |
| g. side effects that warrant medical intervention should they occur | Increased discomfort or GI complaints, decreased feeding |
| h. patient options in the event that condition worsens or persists | See PCP. |
| i. product storage requirements | Store gel and acetaminophen out of reach of children. |
| j. specific nondrug measures | Gel-filled teething rings that can be chilled/frozen may also give some relief. |
| 10. Solicit caregiver's follow-up questions. | What type of teething product should I buy? |
| 11. Answer caregiver's questions. | A gel will be easier to apply to the gums than a liquid. Also, check the label to make sure the product does not contain alcohol. |

Key: N/A, not applicable; NKA, no known allergies; OTC, over-the-counter; PCP, primary care provider.

### *Patient Counseling for Teething Discomfort*

The practitioner should be prepared to suggest both pharmacologic and nonpharmacologic remedies for teething discomfort. Parents should be urged to contact a primary care provider when symptoms uncharacteristic of teething discomfort are present.

### *Evaluation of Patient Outcomes for Teething Discomfort*

The practitioner should ask the parent to call back after 3 to 5 days of treatment. If neither nonpharmacologic therapy nor nonprescription medications are relieving the symptoms, the parent should be advised to take the baby to a primary care provider, pediatrician, or pediatric dentist. Furthermore, if symptoms uncharacteristic of teething discomfort have developed, the baby should be evaluated by a primary care provider or pediatrician.

## Fractured Dentition and Restorations

Teeth, fillings, or crowns (caps) may crack, break, or be knocked out. These problems may occur as a result of trauma (an accident or fight), chewing on a hard object, decay, or the abrasive action of a filling. They may also appear for no apparent reason.

Pain may be associated with sudden exposure of or damage to nerves in a fractured tooth. Irritation of or injury to gums, mucosa, lips or tongue can also cause pain. Complications include malocclusion, rapid carious breakdown, compromised mastication, and infection. Loose, displaced, or broken fillings, crowns, or bridges may cause loss of normal tooth function, tooth breakdown, malocclusion, or accidental aspiration of the object. Only a dentist can adequately evaluate and treat these conditions. As with other disorders involving tooth pain, the practitioner should advise the patient to see a dentist without delay.

# ORAL MUCOSAL DISORDERS

Two of the most common oral problems for which patients seek treatment advice are recurrent aphthous stomatitis (RAS, canker sores) and herpes simplex labialis (HSL, cold sores/fever blisters). Both disorders respond to symptomatic self-treatment and should be self-limiting, unless a secondary infection occurs. Patients frequently seek a practitioner's recommendations for nonprescription products to relieve symptoms of these disorders. Although many nonprescription products are available for symptomatic treatment of cold sores and canker sores, none has been shown conclusively to decrease the recurrence rate of lesions or to be curative.

## Recurrent Aphthous Stomatitis

RAS, also known as a canker sore or aphthous ulcer, occurs in three clinical forms: minor, major, and herpetiform. Table 32-4 compares the features of these three forms.

### *Epidemiology of RAS*

RAS affects approximately 25% of Americans and has a recurrence rate of 50% within 3 months.[23,24] RAS occurs more commonly during the second and third decades of life. There may be a female predominance in some adult and child patient groups, and children of higher socioeconomic status may be more commonly affected than those from lower socioeconomic groups.[25] Also, the incidence is slightly

## PATIENT EDUCATION FOR TEETHING DISCOMFORT

The objective of self-care for teething discomfort is to relieve gum pain and irritation, thereby reducing the child's irritability and sleep disturbances. For most patients, the parent's careful following of product instructions and the self-care measures listed here will help ensure optimal therapeutic outcomes.

### Nondrug Measures

- To reduce irritation of the underside of the tongue, have a dentist smooth the edges of the erupting teeth.
- Do not cut or puncture gum cysts. Doing so will leave scars that may delay the tooth's eruption.
- If possible, massage the gum around the erupting tooth to provide relief.
- Give the baby a frozen pacifier (teething ring), a cold wet cloth, or food (such as dry toast) to chew.

### Nonprescription Medications

#### *Topical Analgesics*

- Rub commercial teething products containing benzocaine onto the gums not more than four times daily.
- Note that although benzocaine in concentrations of 5% to 20% was approved for teething preparations, the 20% concentration is too potent for infants and can even cause death from drug overdose. Use only products that are labeled for teething.
- Rub teething products containing phenol 0.5% onto the gums not more than six times daily.
- Use alcohol- and sucrose-free products that carry the ADA acceptance seal.
- Note that benzocaine can cause hypersensitivity. If redness or irritation of the gum increases after use of this medication, stop using it.

#### *Systemic Analgesics*

- If desired, use pediatric formulations of oral nonprescription analgesics such as acetaminophen to relieve teething discomfort.
- Read the label carefully, and do not exceed recommended doses or frequency of use.

⚠ If the baby is vomiting or has diarrhea, fever, nasal congestion, malaise, pain, or other symptoms not typical of teething discomfort, take the baby to a primary care provider or pediatrician.

**TABLE 32-4 Differentiation of RAS and HSL**

| | RAS (Canker Sores) | | | |
|---|---|---|---|---|
| | Minor Aphthae | Major Aphthae | Herpetiform Aphthae | HSL (Cold Sores) |
| Manifestations | Oval, flat ulcer; erythematous tissue around ulcer | Oval, ragged, gray/yellow ulcers; crater form | Small ulcers in crops, similar to minor aphthae | Red, fluid-filled vesicles; lesions may coalesce; crusted when mature |
| Incidence | 85% | 5% | 10% | |
| Number of lesions | Usually one | Several (1-10) | Multiple (crops) | Several |
| Pain | None-moderate | None-moderate | Moderate-severe | None-moderate |
| Size of ulcers | <1 cm | 0.5-2 cm | 1-4 cm | 1-4 mm |
| Duration (days) | 5-7 | 7-14 | 60 | 10-14 |
| Scarring | None | Rare | Common | Rare |
| Location | All areas except gingiva, hard palate, vermilion (border of the oral mucosa and external skin) | All areas except gingiva, hard palate, vermilion (border of the oral mucosa and external skin) | Any intraoral area | Junction of oral mucosa and skin of lip and nose |
| Comments | Immunologic defect | Immunologic defect | Immunologic defect | Induced by HSV-1 |

Key: HSV-1, herpex simplex virus-1; HSL, herpes simplex labialis; RAS, recurrent aphthous stomatitis.

higher in stressed than in nonstressed populations. Minor RAS is the most common form of RAS, representing 80% to 90% of all cases,[26] and is the most likely form for which patients will consult a practitioner. The disease usually begins in childhood or early adolescence. In patients over 50 years of age, RAS declines in both frequency and severity.

### *Etiology of RAS*

The cause of RAS is unknown in most patients. The most likely precipitating factors are stress and local trauma. Trauma (e.g., chemical irritation, biting the inside of cheeks or lips, or injury caused by toothbrushing or braces) has been implicated as a leading cause of lesions.[27] Systemic conditions associated with RAS include Behçet's disease, systemic lupus erythematosus,[2] neutrophil dysfunction, allergy, nutritional deficiencies, inflammatory bowel disease, and HIV/AIDS.[28-31] Associated precipitating or contributing factors may include food allergy, genetic predisposition, and hormonal changes. RAS may also occur following smoking cessation. This may be a result of the stress of cessation or the changes that occur to the oral mucosa after cessation. Smoking is an irritant to the oral mucosa that results in a thickening process that may protect the oral mucosa from traumatic injury. Ex-smokers need reassurance during this time period to be successful in giving up this habit.

Infectious agents, immune dysfunction, and humoral and cellular factors are being evaluated as causes of RAS.[31] In a recent study, *Helicobacter pylori* was found in RAS lesions.[32] RAS are not viral in origin nor does it appear to be contagious.

### *Signs and Symptoms of RAS*

RAS appears as an epithelial ulceration on nonkeratinized mucosal surfaces of movable mouth parts, such as the tongue, floor of the mouth, soft palate, or the inside lining of the lips and cheeks. Rarely, ulcerations affect keratinized tissue such as gingiva. Most recurrent aphthous ulcerations persist for 5 to 14 days and heal spontaneously without scarring.[24] The ulcers usually range from 0.5 to 2.0 cm in diameter; however, larger lesions can develop in clusters. Individual ulcers are usually (1) round or oval, (2) flat or craterlike in appearance, and (3) gray to grayish yellow with an erythematous halo of inflamed tissue surrounding the ulcer (see Color Plates, photoraph 12).

Some patients may experience a painful sensation before the lesion actually appears. Patients may develop single or multiple lesions. The lesions can be very painful—with the pain increasing on eating and drinking—and may inhibit normal eating, drinking, swallowing, and talking, as well as routine oral hygiene. Although many patients have recurrent episodes of oral lesions with periods of remission, some patients chronically experience one or more lesions in the mouth for very long periods without the knowledge of their presence. Usually, fever or lymphadenopathy does not accompany RAS; however, such symptoms may arise if a secondary bacterial infection is present.

### *Treatment of RAS*

RAS cannot be cured; however, nonprescription medications can provide symptomatic relief.

#### Treatment Goals

The goals in treating RAS are to (1) control pain of the ulcer, (2) promote ulcer healing, (3) prevent recurrence, and (4) prevent complications such as secondary infection.[26]

#### General Treatment Approach

Treatment should focus on protecting the ulcerations from irritating stimuli and reducing the duration and severity of pain and irritation. Figure 32-2 outlines the self-treatment of RAS and exclusions for self-care.

#### Nonpharmacologic Therapy

If a nutritional deficiency (e.g., iron, folate, or vitamin $B_{12}$) is suspected as a contributing factor, the patient should increase consumption of foods high in these nutrients or take nutritional supplements. Spicy foods and foods that have the potential to cause local injury should be avoided until ulcerations improve.

Ice applied in 10-minute increments directly to the lesions can give temporary relief. However, heat may cause the spread of infection (if present) and should not be used.

#### Pharmacologic Therapy

Several types of nonprescription medications (oral debriding and wound cleansing agents, topical oral anesthetics, topical oral protectants, oral rinses, and systemic analgesics) provide symptomatic relief of RAS, but they do not prevent its recurrence. Table 32-5 lists a variety of commercial products containing these agents. Cauterizing lesions with silver nitrate is not effective. Furthermore, this agent may stain teeth and damage healthy tissue.

*Oral Debriding and Wound Cleansing Agents* Products that release nascent oxygen can be used as debriding and cleansing agents to provide temporary relief of RAS discomfort. After a thorough review process, FDA has determined that carbamide peroxide 10% to 15% in anhydrous glycerin, hydrogen peroxide 3%, sodium perborate monohydrate (1.2 g), and sodium bicarbonate are Category I (safe and effective) for use as nonprescription debriding agents or oral wound cleansers for oral health care.[33] FDA has determined that no ingredient is generally recognized as safe and effective for use as a nonprescription healing agent for oral wounds.

Mechanism of Action Peroxides and perborates release molecular oxygen. Hydrogen peroxide and carbamide peroxide do so immediately on contact with tissue enzymes (catalase and peroxidase), but tissue and bacterial exposure to the oxygen is very brief.[34] The foaming of the liberated oxygen has a mechanical effect, which loosens particulate matter and cleanses debris from wounds. The efficacy of oxidizing products in killing anaerobic bacteria when treating infections and periodontitis has not been established.

Dosage and Administration Guidelines For direct application, a few drops of carbamide peroxide or hydrogen peroxide are applied to the affected area and allowed

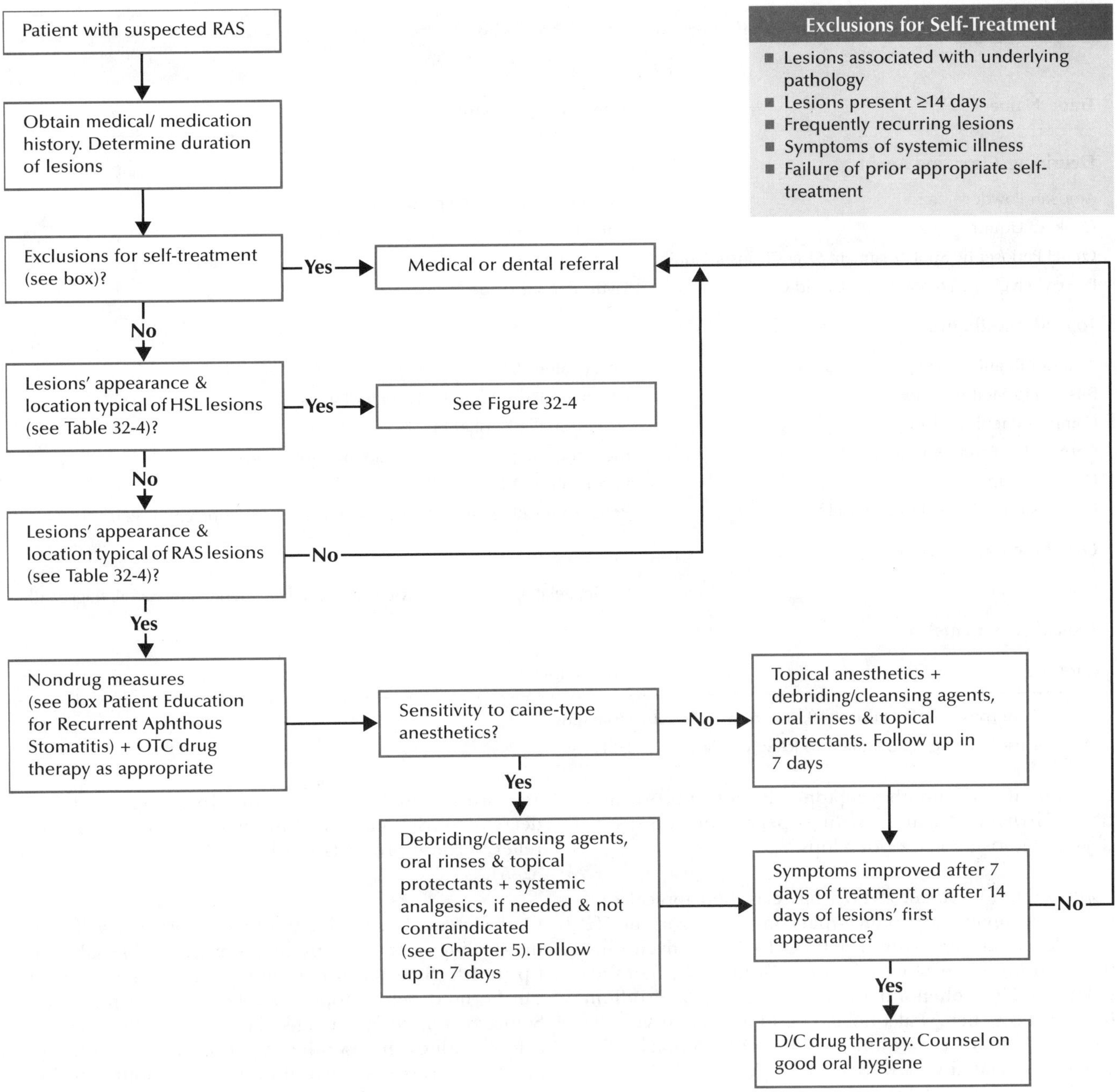


**FIGURE 32-2** Self-care of recurrent aphthous stomatitis; Key: D/C, discontinue; HSL, herpes simplex labialis; OTC, over-the-counter; RAS, recurrent aphthous stomatitis.

to remain in place for 1 minute. As a rinse, carbamide peroxide drops are placed on the tongue, mixed with saliva, and swished in the mouth for 1 minute. An aqueous solution of hydrogen peroxide 3% should be mixed with an equal amount of water before rinsing the mouth. Some products (e.g., Peroxyl Rinse, Perimed) are a solution of hydrogen peroxide 1.5% and should be used without dilution. Sodium perborate monohydrate powder (1.2 g) should be dissolved in 1 oz of water and used immediately.

Such products can be used up to four times daily (after meals) for no longer than 7 days. In all cases, it is important to follow package directions carefully. The solution should be expectorated, not swallowed.

Safety Considerations Prolonged rinsing with oxidizing products can lead to soft-tissue irritation, transient tooth sensitivity from decalcification of enamel, cellular changes, and overgrowth of undesirable organisms that will possibly lead to a black hairy tongue.[35,36]

Labeling of these products includes the following warning: "Do not use this product more than 7 days unless directed by a dentist or doctor. See your doctor or dentist

**TABLE 32-5 Selected Nonprescription Products for RAS and HSL**

| Trade Name | Primary Ingredients |
|---|---|
| **Debriding/Cleansing Agents*** | |
| Amosan Powder | Sodium peroxyborate monohydrate |
| Cankaid Liquid | Carbamide peroxide 10% |
| Orajel Perioseptic Spot Treatment Oral Cleanser Liquid | Carbamide peroxide 15% |
| Peroxyl Hygienic Dental Rinse Liquid/Gel | Hydrogen peroxide 1.5% |
| **Topical Anesthetics** | |
| Anbesol Regular Strength Gel/Liquid | Benzocaine 10% |
| Blistex Lip Medex Ointment | Camphor 1%; menthol 1%; phenol 0.5% |
| Campho-Phenique Gel | Camphor 10.8%; phenol 4.7% |
| Carmex Lip Balm Ointment | Menthol; camphor; salicylic acid; phenol |
| Colgate Orabase Gel | Benzocaine 20% |
| Orajel Mouth Sore Medicine Gel | Benzocaine 20%; benzalkonium chloride 0.02%; zinc chloride 0.1% |
| **Oral Mucosal Protectants†** | |
| Orabase Plain | Pectin; gelatin; carboxymethylcellulose; polyethylene; mineral oil; tragacanth |
| **Topical Treatments‡** | |
| Abreva | Docosanol 10% |

Key: HSL, herpes simplex virus; RAS, recurrent aphthous stomatitis.
*Not for use on HSL; †use limited to RAS; ‡use limited to HSL.

promptly if sore mouth symptoms do not improve in 7 days; if irritation, pain, or redness persists or worsens; or if swelling, rash, or fever develops."[3]

*Topical Oral Anesthetics* FDA has classified topical oral anesthetic/analgesic products that contain benzocaine 5% to 20%, butacaine sulfate 0.05% to 0.1%, dyclonine 0.05% to 0.1%, hexylresorcinol 0.05% to 0.1%, menthol 0.04% to 2.0%, phenol 0.5% to 1.5%, phenolate sodium 0.5% to 1.5%, benzyl alcohol 0.05% to 0.1%, and salicylic alcohol 1% to 6% as safe and effective for temporary relief of pain associated with RAS.[3]

Benzocaine and butacaine are the most commonly used local anesthetics in nonprescription products. However, benzocaine is a known sensitizer (allergen) and should not be used by patients with a history of hypersensitivity to other common local anesthetic products.

The patient should avoid using potentially inflammatory products containing ketone or alcohol counterirritants (e.g., menthol, phenol, camphor, and eugenol) as anesthetic, counterirritant, or antiseptic treatments for RAS. These agents may cause tissue irritation and damage, which may prevent spontaneous healing or cause systemic toxicity, especially if overused. To reduce the incidence irritation of RAS, patients should also be advised to avoid the use of dentifrices containing sodium lauryl sulfate.[34]

*Topical Oral Protectants* Coating the ulcers with topical oral protectants (e.g., Orabase, Zilactin,[26] or denture adhesives) can be effective in protecting ulcerations, decreasing friction, and affording temporary symptomatic relief.[34] These products can be applied as needed (Table 32–5).

*Oral Rinses* Rinsing the mouth with Listerine will hasten the healing of the lesions. Saline rinses (table salt 1 to 3 tsp in 4 to 8 oz warm tap water) may soothe ulcers and can be used before topical application of a medication. Similarly, a paste of baking soda applied to the lesions for a few minutes may soothe irritation. Zinc in astringent mouth rinses is of equivocal value in promoting healing.

*Systemic Analgesics* Systemic nonprescription analgesics (e.g., aspirin, nonsteroidal anti-inflammatory drugs, and acetaminophen) afford additional relief of mouth discomfort. (See Chapter 5 for discussion of these agents and their recommended dosages.)

As with toothache, aspirin should not be retained in the mouth before swallowing or placed in the area of the oral lesions. The acid can cause a chemical burn with subsequent tissue damage (see Color Plates, photograph 11).

*Product Selection Guidelines* Of the four oral debriding and wound cleansing agents, sodium bicarbonate is the least expensive because rinses or pastes of the agent can be made at home. This agent also temporarily soothes discomfort.

Patients with known hypersensitivity to common local anesthetics should use a product containing one or more of the other Category I agents. Patients with known sensitivity to aspirin should avoid salicylic acid. Only products containing menthol, phenol, and/or camphor in the concentrations approved as Category I should be used for RAS. Higher concentrations are potentially inflammatory.

### *Assessment of RAS: A Case-based Approach*

The practitioner should determine whether the patient has a history of RAS. If possible, the lesions should be inspected to determine whether their appearance and location are characteristic of RAS. The patient's medical history will help rule out underlying pathology that can cause lesions resembling RAS. Finally, the practitioner should ask about previous self-treatments and their effectiveness. Case 32-3 illustrates the assessment of patients with RAS.

### *Patient Counseling for RAS*

The practitioner should explain all pharmacologic and nonpharmacologic measures for treating RAS. The patient

## CASE 32-3

| Relevant Evaluation Criteria | Scenario/Model Outcome |
|---|---|
| **Information Gathering** | |
| 1. Gather essential information about the patient's symptoms, including: | |
| a. description of symptom(s) (i.e., nature, onset, duration, severity, associated symptoms) | Patient complaining of painful white sores in mouth. Pain is worse when he eats pizza and has a soft drink. |
| b. description of any factors that seem to precipitate, exacerbate, and/or relieve the patient's symptom(s) | Anything that touches the sores causes extreme pain. |
| c. description of the patient's efforts to relieve the symptoms | Patient has tried taking OTC analgesics. |
| 2. Gather essential patient history information: | |
| a. patient's identity | David Thompson |
| b. patient's age, sex, height, and weight | 25 y/o M, 6', 175 lb |
| c. patient's occupation | Plumber |
| d. patient's dietary habits | Lots of fast food and cigarettes |
| e. patient's sleep habits | Good |
| f. concurrent medical conditions, prescription and nonprescription medications, and dietary supplements | Pepcid AC 10 mg 1-2 tablets once daily as needed for gastritis |
| g. allergies | None |
| h. history of other adverse reactions to medications | Erythromycin upsets stomach. |
| i. other (describe)_______ | Patient has tried nicotine patches and gum to stop smoking without success. |
| **Assessment and Triage** | |
| 3. Differentiate the patient's signs/symptoms and correctly identify the patient's primary problem(s). | David appears to have recurrent aphthous stomatitis. |
| 4. Identify exclusions for self-treatment (see Figure 32-2). | None |
| 5. Formulate a comprehensive list of therapeutic alternatives for the primary problem to determine if triage to a medical practitioner is required, and share this information with the patient. | Options include:<br>(1) Recommend appropriate OTC products with lifestyle modifications.<br>(2) Refer David to a dentist.<br>(3) Take no action. |

| CASE 32-3 (continued) | |
|---|---|
| **Relevant Evaluation Criteria** | **Scenario/Model Outcome** |
| **Plan** | |
| 6. Select an optimal therapeutic alternative to address the patient's problem, taking into account patient preferences. | Recommend appropriate OTC products with lifestyle modifications. |
| 7. Describe the recommended therapeutic approach to the patient. | You should take NSAIDs for pain and inflammation, use a mouth rinse, then apply a topical oral anesthetic. Identify triggers (stress, smoking, and poor diet). Improve nutrition, and consider taking a multivitamin. Stop smoking. |
| 8. Explain to the patient the rationale for selecting the recommended therapeutic approach from the considered therapeutic alternatives. | Identification and avoidance of triggers can reduce frequency of recurrence. Improving health will increase immune response. |
| **Patient Education** | |
| 9. When recommending self-care with nonprescription medications and/or nondrug therapy, convey accurate information to the patient, including: | |
| a. appropriate dose and frequency of administration | For pain relief, apply a baking soda paste to the lesions for a few minutes, apply a topical anesthetic, or take an oral analgesic as directed. Rinse with a mouth rinse several times a day. |
| b. maximum number of days the therapy should be employed | 7 days |
| c. product administration procedures | Apply products directly to affected area. |
| d. expected time to onset of relief | Relief should come within a few days. |
| e. degree of relief that can be reasonably expected | Total relief will not occur until lesion is healed. |
| f. most common side effects | See the box Patient Education for Recurrent Aphthous Stomatitis. |
| g. side effects that warrant medical intervention should they occur | See the box Patient Education for Recurrent Aphthous Stomatitis. |
| h. patient options in the event that condition worsens or persists | If lesions are not healed within 7 days, see a dentist or primary care provider. |
| i. product storage requirements | Keep medications out of young children's reach. |
| j. specific nondrug measures | Improve nutrition by changing diet. Stop smoking. |
| 10. Solicit patient's follow-up questions. | Is there any specific mouth rinse that I should be using? |
| 11. Answer patient's questions. | Yes. You should avoid alcohol-containing mouth rinses as these may be more irritating to your mouth sores. |

Key: NSAID, nonsteroidal anti-inflammatory drug; OTC, over-the-counter.

should be cautioned about using ineffective or harmful therapies. Possible adverse effects, contraindications, and precautions should be explained for all nonprescription agents. In addition, the practitioner must alert patients to the conditions that warrant dental or medical evaluation.

### *Evaluation of Patient Outcomes for RAS*

The patient should return for reevaluation after 7 days of treatment with debriding and cleansing agents. If the symptoms have improved, the patient should discontinue treatment but continue other dental hygienic measures. Symptoms that are unimproved or that have worsened during treatment require dental/medical evaluation.

The patient should return for reevaluation after 14 days of treatment. If the ulcerations have healed, the patient should continue other dental hygienic measures. Lesions that do not heal in 14 days should be evaluated by a dentist or primary care provider.

## PATIENT EDUCATION FOR RECURRENT APHTHOUS STOMATITIS

The primary objective of self-treatment for RAS is to relieve pain and irritation so the lesions can heal and the patient can eat, drink, and perform routine oral hygiene. The secondary objective is to prevent complications, such as secondary infection. For most patients, carefully following product instructions and the self-care measures listed here will help ensure optimal therapeutic outcomes.

### Nondrug Measures

- If a deficiency of iron, folate, or vitamin B12 is suspected as a contributing factor, increase consumption of foods high in these nutrients, or take nutritional supplements.
- Avoid spicy foods until the lesions heal.
- Avoid sharp foods that may cause increased trauma to the lesion.
- If desired, apply ice in 10-minute increments directly to the lesions.
- Do not use heat. If infection is present, heat may spread the infection.
- Apply a paste of baking soda directly to the lesions to soothe discomfort.

### Nonprescription Medications

- If longer-lasting relief is desired, ask your pharmacist to recommend one or more of the following types of nonprescription medications: debriding and cleansing agents, topical oral anesthetics, topical oral protectants, oral rinses, and systemic analgesics.
- Do not cauterize lesions with silver nitrate. This treatment is not effective and may stain teeth and damage healthy tissue.

#### *Debriding and Cleansing Agents*

- Use a product containing one of the following ingredients: carbamide peroxide 10% to 15%, hydrogen peroxide 1.5%, or perborates. Apply after meals up to four times daily.
- Do not use these medications longer than 7 days. Chronic use can cause tissue irritation, decalcification of enamel, and black hairy tongue.
- Do not swallow these medications.

#### *Topical Oral Anesthetics*

- Ask your pharmacist to recommend a product containing one of the following medications: benzocaine 5% to 20%, benzyl alcohol 0.05% to 0.1%, butacaine sulfate 0.05% to 0.1%, dyclonine 0.05% to 0.1%, hexylresorcinol 0.05% to 0.1%, or salicylic alcohol 1% to 6%.
- Do not use benzocaine if you have a history of hypersensitivity to other benzocaine-containing products.
- Avoid potentially inflammatory products containing substantial amounts of menthol, phenol, camphor, or eugenol. These agents may cause tissue irritation and damage or systemic toxicity.

#### *Topical Oral Protectants*

- Use topical oral protectants (e.g., Orabase Plain) or denture adhesives to coat and protect the lesions. These agents will also provide temporary relief of discomfort.
- Apply these products as needed.

#### *Oral Rinses*

- Rinse the mouth with Listerine to hasten healing of the lesions.
- Rinse the mouth with a saline solution to soothe discomfort or to prepare the lesion for application of a topical medication. For saline solution, add 1 to 3 tsp of table salt to 4 to 8 oz of warm tap water.

#### *Systemic Analgesics*

- If desired, take an oral analgesic (e.g., aspirin, ibuprofen, or acetaminophen) for additional relief of mouth discomfort.
- Do not hold aspirin in the mouth or place it on oral lesions. The acid can cause a chemical burn with tissue damage.

See a primary care provider if any of the following occur:

- Symptoms do not improve after 7 days of treatment with debriding/wound cleansing agents.
- The lesions do not heal in 14 days.
- Symptoms worsen during self-treatment.
- Symptoms of systemic infection such as fever, rash, or swelling develop.

## Minor Oral Mucosal Injury or Irritation

### *Etiology of Minor Oral Mucosal Injury or Irritation*

Minor wounds or inflammation resulting from minor dental procedures, accidental injury (e.g., biting the cheek or abrasion from sharp, crisp foods), or other irritations of the mouth, gums, or palate may be treated with various nonprescription medications.

### *Treatment of Minor Oral Mucosal Injury or Irritation*

Treatment of mouth injury and irritation is similar to that of RAS. It differs from RAS, however, in its etiology and certain treatment considerations.

#### Treatment Goals

The goals of treating minor mucosal injury and irritation are to (1) control discomfort and pain, (2) aid healing with the appropriate use of pharmacologic and nonpharmacologic measures, and (3) prevent secondary bacterial infection.

#### General Treatment Approach

Treatment should focus first on relieving discomfort. Local anesthetics, oral analgesics, and saline rinses are safe and effective choices. Application of ice can also relieve discomfort. Once the discomfort has resolved, patients should focus on healing the affected area. Homemade

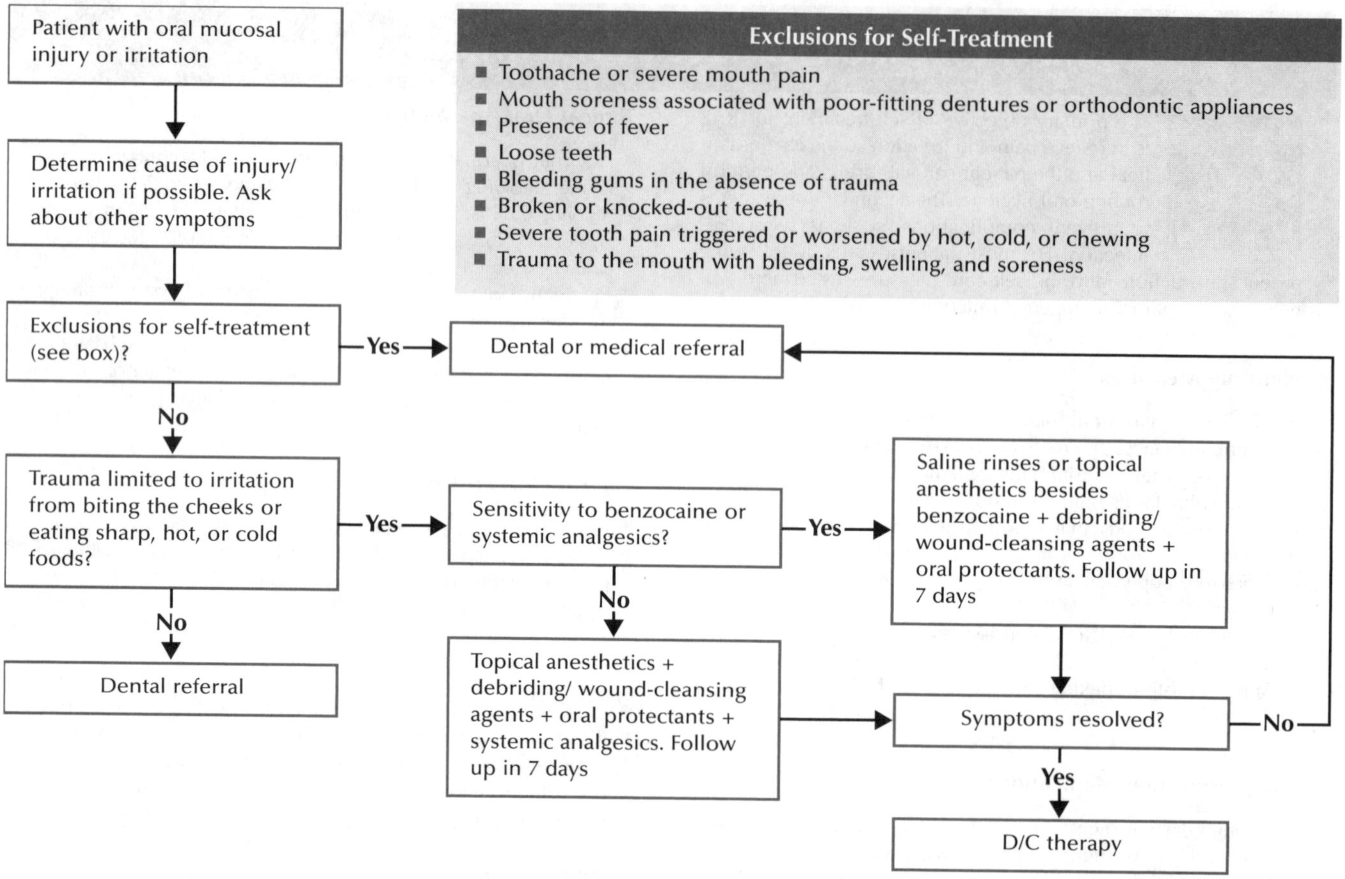


**FIGURE 32-3** Self-care of minor oral mucosal injury or irritation. Key: D/C, discontinue.

sodium bicarbonate rinses and oral debriding/cleansing agents can help achieve this objective. Finally, concomitant use of oral protectants can relieve discomfort and aid healing by protecting the area from further irritation. Figure 32-3 outlines this approach and lists exclusions for self-care.

## Nonpharmacologic Therapy

Sodium bicarbonate (household baking soda 1/2 to 1 tsp in 4 oz of water) solutions can act as an oral debriding agent/wound cleanser. The solution is swished in the mouth over the affected area for at least 1 minute and then expectorated. Sodium bicarbonate's mucolytic action is related to its alkalinity. Saline rinses can cleanse and soothe the affected area. The patient should add 1 to 3 tsp of salt to 4 to 8 oz of warm tap water.

When tissues of the lips, cheeks or palate are bruised, direct application of ice may reduce the swelling. Ice should be applied in 10-minute increments. Longer application times may cause local tissue damage.

## Pharmacologic Therapy

As with RAS, topical analgesics/anesthetics, oral protectants, and oral debriding/wound cleansing agents are the mainstay of pharmacologic therapy. In addition, astringents may be used.

Topical analgesics/anesthetics are applied for pain relief. Astringents cause tissues to contract or arrest secretions by causing proteins to coagulate on a cell surface.[3] Oral mucosal protectants are pharmacologically inert substances that coat and protect the area. Debriding agents/oral wound cleansers may be used to (1) aid in the removal of debris or phlegm, mucus, or other secretions associated with sore mouth; (2) cleanse minor wounds or minor gum inflammation; and (3) cleanse recurrent aphthous ulcers (see Treatment of Recurrent Aphthous Stomatitis).

Dentists may suggest that their patients use oxidizing mouth rinses or topically applied steroids (which are available only by prescription) as an adjunctive treatment of specific conditions or a postoperative aid to cleaning and relieving discomfort and assisting the healing process.

The FDA review of oral antiseptic products found insufficient data to support efficacy for oral antiseptic use (i.e., to decrease the chance of infection in minor oral irritation).[33]

Patients who dislike complicated regimens may want to use a combination preparation (Table 32-5). These preparations may contain (1) a single anesthetic/analgesic with a single astringent, an oral mucosal protectant, or a denture adhesive; or (2) benzocaine combined with menthol or phenol.

### *Assessment of Minor Oral Mucosal Injury or Irritation: A Case-based Approach*

The cause and nature of the injury or irritation are the primary considerations in patient assessment. If the disorder is self-treatable, the practitioner should determine whether the patient has had previous episodes, how they were treated, and whether the patient has known contraindications to the nonprescription medications used to treat these disorders (Case 32-4).

### *Patient Counseling for Minor Oral Mucosal Injury or Irritation*

Once the problem is determined to be minor irritation or injury of the mouth, the practitioner should explain (1) the steps in the treatment regimen, (2) the purpose of each agent, and (3) the length of time the products can be used safely. Signs and symptoms that indicate infection should also be explained.

### *Evaluation of Patient Outcomes for Minor Oral Mucosal Injury or Irritation*

The patient should return for reevaluation after 7 days of treatment with oral mucosal healing agents. If the symptoms are resolved, no further treatment is necessary. If symptoms persist or worsen or swelling, rash, or fever develops, the patient should see a dentist or primary care provider for evaluation.

**CASE 32-4**

| Relevant Evaluation Criteria | Scenario/Model Outcome |
|---|---|
| **Information Gathering** | |
| 1. Gather essential information about the patient's symptoms, including: | |
| a. description of symptom(s) (i.e., nature, onset, duration, severity, associated symptoms) | Patient has complained of sore, red, and bleeding tissue on the inner aspect of her lips for several days. |
| b. description of any factors that seem to precipitate, exacerbate, and/or relieve the patient's symptom(s) | It hurts to smile, talk, chew, and play the flute. |
| c. description of the patient's efforts to relieve the symptoms | Patient has tried rinsing with Listerine. |
| 2. Gather essential patient history information: | |
| a. patient's identity | Jessica Wallace |
| b. patient's age, sex, height, and weight | 14 y/o F, 5'2",114 lb |
| c. patient's occupation | 9th-grade student |
| d. patient's dietary habits | Soft foods after orthodontic visit |
| e. patient's sleep habits | Good |
| f. concurrent medical conditions, prescription and nonprescription medications, and dietary supplements | None |
| g. allergies | None |
| h. history of other adverse reactions to medications | None |
| i. other (describe)_______ | Jessica has braces. |
| **Assessment and Triage** | |
| 3. Differentiate the patient's signs/symptoms and correctly identify the patient's primary problem(s). | Soft tissue irritation from braces |
| 4. Identify exclusions for self-treatment (see Figure 32-3). | Do not try to self-remove the braces. |
| 5. Formulate a comprehensive list of therapeutic alternatives for the primary problem to determine if triage to a medical practitioner is required, and share this information with the patient. | Options include:<br>(1) Recommend appropriate OTC products.<br>(2) Refer Jessica to her orthodontist.<br>(3) Take no action. |

## CASE 32-4 (continued)

| Relevant Evaluation Criteria | Scenario/Model Outcome |
|---|---|
| **Plan** | |
| 6. Select an optimal therapeutic alternative to address the patient's problem, taking into account patient preferences. | Use appropriate OTC products for pain and inflammation. |
| 7. Describe the recommended therapeutic approach to the patient. | Coat the rough edges of your braces with wax. Keep mouth and lips lubricated. Apply local anesthetic gel as needed. Keep mouth, teeth, and braces clean. You may take NSAIDs as needed for pain. |
| 8. Explain to the patient the rationale for selecting the recommended therapeutic approach from the considered therapeutic alternatives. | Topical treatments alone usually relieve this problem. |
| **Patient Education** | |
| 9. When recommending self-care with nonprescription medications and/or nondrug therapy, convey accurate information to the patient, including: | |
| a. appropriate dose and frequency of administration | Apply local anesthetic gel as needed. Follow good oral hygiene practice after meals. |
| b. maximum number of days the therapy should be employed | Continue to use as long as braces are in place. |
| c. product administration procedures | Use a small amount of gel. |
| d. expected time to onset of relief | Relief should come within a few days. |
| e. degree of relief that can be reasonably expected | Total relief will occur when tissues heal. |
| f. most common side effects | Bad taste, excessive numbness of the mouth (if excessively applied), allergic reactions |
| g. side effects that warrant medical intervention should they occur | Significant symptoms of allergy (hives, shortness of breath, wheezing, swelling of throat or tongue, hypotension) |
| h. patient options in the event that condition worsens or persists | If swelling, bleeding, or infection occurs, see orthodontist. |
| i. product storage requirements | Keep products out of young children's reach. |
| j. specific nondrug measures | Apply wax coating on rough surfaces of braces. Keep mouth and lips lubricated with emollient cream. |
| 10. Solicit patient's follow-up questions. | What kind of wax should I use? |
| 11. Answer patient's questions. | Use a soft wax that will not cause damage to your braces and that will not stick to them permanently. |

Key: NSAID, nonsteroidal anti-inflammatory drug; OTC, over-the-counter.

## Herpes Simplex Labialis

HSL (cold sores) is a disorder caused by a virus of the family Herpesviridae. Anyone who comes in contact with the virus can potentially become infected. Once the virus has infected a host, it can go through periods of dormancy and reactivation, but that person is infected for life.

### *Epidemiology of HSL*

Cold sores or fever blisters are lesions generally caused by herpes simplex virus 1 (HSV-1). Each year 500,000 individuals experience primary eruptions, often during childhood. These primary eruptions represent only 1% of the exposed population; 99% of exposed individuals have subclinical

## PATIENT EDUCATION FOR MINOR ORAL MUCOSAL INJURY OR IRRITATION

The objectives of self-treatment for minor oral mucosal injury or irritation are to (1) control discomfort and pain, (2) aid healing with the appropriate use of drug and nondrug measures, and (3) prevent secondary bacterial infection. For most patients, carefully following product instructions and the self-care measures listed here will help ensure optimal therapeutic outcomes.

### Nondrug Measures

- Rinse with a sodium bicarbonate solution to remove injured tissue and cleanse the affected area. Add 1/2 to 1 tsp of sodium bicarbonate to 4 oz of water. Swish the solution in the mouth over the affected area for 1 minute; then spit out the solution.
- Use saline rinses to cleanse and soothe the affected area. Add 1 to 3 tsp of salt to 4 to 8 oz of warm tap water.
- For bruised lips or cheeks, apply ice in 10-minute increments to reduce swelling. Do not apply ice longer than 20 minutes in a given hour.

### Nonprescription Medications

- If longer-lasting relief is desired, ask your pharmacist to recommend one or more of the following types of nonprescription medications: debriding and cleansing agents, topical oral anesthetics, topical oral protectants, and systemic analgesics.

#### *Debriding and Cleansing Agents*

- Use a product containing one of the following ingredients: carbamide peroxide 10% to 15%, hydrogen peroxide 1.5%, or perborates. Apply after meals up to four times daily.
- Do not use these medications longer than 7 days. Chronic use can cause tissue irritation, decalcification of enamel, and black hairy tongue.
- Do not swallow these medications.

#### *Topical Oral Anesthetics*

- Ask your pharmacist to recommend a product containing one of the following medications: benzocaine 5% to 20%, benzyl alcohol 0.05% to 0.1%, butacaine sulfate 0.05% to 0.1%, dyclonine 0.05% to 0.1%, hexylresorcinol 0.05% to 0.1%, or salicylic alcohol 1% to 6%.
- Do not use benzocaine if you have a history of hypersensitivity to other benzocaine-containing products.
- Avoid potentially inflammatory products containing substantial amounts of menthol, phenol, camphor, or eugenol. These agents may cause tissue irritation and damage or systemic toxicity.

#### *Topical Oral Protectants*

- Use topical oral protectants (e.g., Orabase Plain) or denture adhesives to coat and protect the lesions.
- Apply these products as needed.

#### *Systemic Analgesics*

- If desired, take an oral analgesic (e.g., aspirin, ibuprofen, acetaminophen) for additional relief of mouth discomfort.
- Do not hold aspirin in the mouth or place it on oral lesions. The acid can cause a chemical burn and tissue damage.

⚠ See a primary care provider if any of the following occur:

- Symptoms persist after 7 days of treatment.
- Symptoms worsen during self-treatment.
- Symptoms of systemic infection such as fever, redness, or swelling develop.

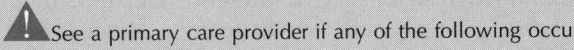

cases on primary exposure. However, after first exposure, when the virus resides in the trigeminal ganglia, reactivation occurs, often following trigger factors, with 98 million recurrent eruptions reported each year. By the age of 40 years, 84% of the population has positive antibodies for HSV-1.[37] Triggers of viral reactivation include ultraviolet radiation, stress, fatigue, cold, and windburn. Other possible triggers include fever, injury, menstruation, dental work, infectious diseases, and factors that depress the immune system (e.g., chemotherapy or radiation therapy).

### *Etiology of HSL*

Cold sores and fever blisters are referred to as herpes simplex labialis because they commonly occur on the lip or on areas bordering the lips; the usual site is at the junction of mucous membrane and skin of the lips or nose. However, these lesions may also occur intraorally. The lesions are recurrent, painful, and cosmetically objectionable. About one half of all patients who have sustained a primary (initial) HSV-1 infection will experience recurrent local lesions after some unpredictable latent interval; the lesions often arise repeatedly in the same location. After the primary infection, the virus apparently remains in host cells. The primary infection is reported most frequently in childhood. Patients may relate a history of primary herpetic stomatitis (viral-induced inflammation of the mouth), which usually manifests itself as vesicles (blisters) in the mouth. However, most primary oral infections of herpes virus seem to be subclinical, and most patients are unaware of their previous primary exposure.

Any of the human herpesviruses (cytomegalovirus, Epstein-Barr virus, and others), not just HSV-1 and 2, can cause oral lesions. Most people are sufficiently protected by their immune systems from manifesting symptoms. But when immunosuppression is present, repeated reactivation of the latent infection becomes possible.

### *Pathophysiology of HSL*

HSV-1 is contagious and is believed to be transmitted by direct contact. Fluid from herpes vesicles contains live virus and may serve to transmit the virus from patient to patient. Herpes simplex virus 2 (HSV-2), which causes genital lesions, can be transmitted through either sexual or oral contact with an infected individual. In addition, it has been demonstrated that herpes lesions of the lip can be caused by oral-genital contact or hand-to-mouth transfer.[37]

HSL enters the host through a break in the skin or intact mucous membranes. Invasion of sensory neurons follows, and then the virus migrates to sensory ganglia where it may remain dormant. Because the virus remains viable on surfaces for several hours, contaminated objects may also be a source of infection. Once infected, an individual may have recurrent lesions throughout life. HSL is self-limiting and heals without scarring, usually within 10 to 14 days. The recurrence rate and extent of lesions vary greatly among patients. Some patients may experience several large lesions every few weeks; other patients may have only a single small lesion at infrequent intervals.

### *Signs and Symptoms of HSL*

HSL lesions are often preceded by a prodrome in which the patient notices burning, itching, tingling, or numbness in the area of the forthcoming lesion. Other symptoms include pain, fever, bleeding, swollen lymph nodes, and malaise. The lesion first becomes visible as small, red papules of fluid-containing vesicles 1 to 3 mm in diameter. Often, many lesions coalesce to form a larger area of involvement. An erythematous, inflamed border around the fluid-filled vesicles may be present. A mature lesion often has a crust over the top of many coalesced, burst vesicles; its base is erythematous. Pustules or pus present under the crust of a herpes virus lesion may indicate a secondary bacterial infection and should be evaluated promptly and treated with an appropriate antibiotic, if indicated (see Color Plates, photograph 13).

A related disease, acute herpetic gingivostomatitis, is seen mainly in children but can occur in adults, especially those who are immunocompromised. Although the oral lesions of this disease can develop anywhere on the oral mucosal surface, they commonly occur on the lips or bordering areas or the gums. Herpetic gingivostomatitis is distinguished from RAS gingivostomatitis by infected gums that are very red and covered by a pseudomembrane or are studded with ulcerations.

The appearance of HSL and RAS should easily be distinguished from candidal plaque, which develops as part of yeast infections. In the mouth, candidiasis is often referred to as thrush, and is characterized by white plaques with a milk curd appearance. Such plaques, which are attached to the oral mucosa, can usually be detached easily, displaying erythematous, bleeding, sore areas beneath (see Color Plates, photograph 10).

### *Treatment of HSL*

Although the etiologies of HSL and RAS differ, global treatment of these disorders is similar. The patient should be instructed to avoid circumstances that induce more lesions (e.g., stress), keep the lesions free of counterirritants, and keep existing lesions as clean as possible, thus avoiding secondary infections. Of the products listed in Table 32-5, debriding and cleansing agents are not used to treat HSL.

#### Treatment Goals

The goals of treating HSL are to (1) relieve the discomfort of the lesions, (2) prevent secondary bacterial infection, and (3) prevent autoinoculation or spread of the virus to others.

#### General Treatment Approach

Cleansing the affected area and using topical skin protectants can protect the lesions from infection. These agents can also relieve dryness and keep the lesions soft. Topical local anesthetics in bland, emollient vehicles help relieve the discomfort of burning, itching, and pain. If evidence of secondary bacterial infection is seen, topical application of a thin layer of triple-antibiotic ointment (e.g., Mycitracin or Neosporin) three to four times daily is recommended, along with systemic antibiotics, if indicated. Figure 32-4 outlines the self-treatment of HSL and lists exclusions for self-care. Systemic nonprescription analgesics may provide additional pain relief.

#### Nonpharmacologic Therapy

Lesions should be kept clean by gently washing with mild soap solutions. Handwashing is important in preventing lesion contamination and minimizing autoinoculation of herpes virus. The lesion should be kept moist to prevent drying and fissuring. Cracking of the lesions may render them more susceptible to secondary bacterial infection, may delay healing, and usually increases discomfort.

Factors that delay healing (e.g., stress, local trauma, wind, excessive sun exposure, and fatigue) should be avoided. Patients who identify sun exposure as a precipitating event should be advised to use a lip and face sunscreen product routinely.

#### Pharmacologic Therapy

FDA approved docosanol 10% (Abreva) as the only nonprescription product proven to reduce the severity and duration of symptoms. The agent inhibits direct fusion between the herpes virus and the human cell plasma membrane, thereby preventing viral replication.[38]

Studies suggest that patients suffering from sideropenia, a condition resulting from a deficiency of iron in the body, who have recurrent HSL may experience fewer episodes following treatment with iron replacement therapy.[39]

FDA has proposed the use of topically applied nonprescription skin protectants or externally applied analgesic/anesthetic drug products as effective nonprescription treatment for relieving the discomfort of HSL, but not for reducing the duration of symptoms.[40]

The FDA review of OTC products for HSL classified external analgesics, alcohols, ketones, and amine- and caine-type local anesthetics as Category I.[41] A partial listing of Category I ingredients includes benzocaine 5% to 20%, dibucaine 0.25% to 1%, dyclonine hydrochloride 0.5% to 1%, benzyl alcohol 10% to 33%, camphor 0.1% to 3%, and menthol 0.1% to 1%. These ingredients offer analgesic,

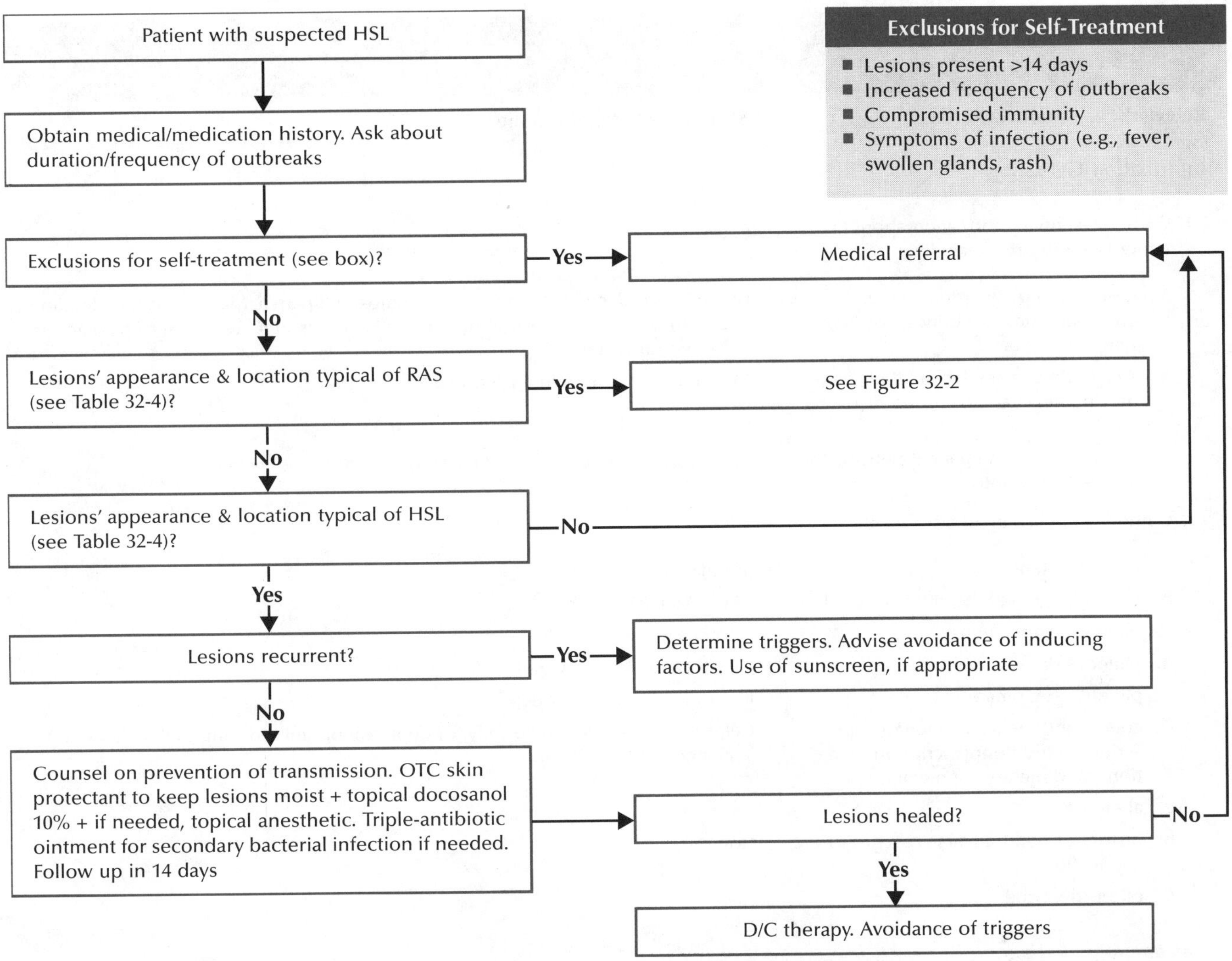


**FIGURE 32-4** Self-care of herpes simplex labialis. Key: D/C, discontinue; HSL, herpes simplex labialis; OTC, over-the-counter; RAS, recurrent aphthous stomatitis.

anesthetic, and antipruritic effects in relieving the pain and itching of HSL. Higher concentrations of certain ingredients (i.e., camphor >3% and menthol >1%) that stimulate cutaneous sensory receptors and produce a counterirritant effect are contraindicated.[42]

HSL is not considered to be a steroid-responsive dermatosis; therefore, the use of topical steroids is contraindicated.

Products that are highly astringent should be avoided. Tannic acid and zinc sulfate are Category II agents for topical management of HSL42 because their frequent application to the lip and oral cavity could cause oral mucosal absorption and toxicity.

Lesions that are secondarily infected with bacteria can also be coated three times a day with a triple-antibiotic ointment (see Chapter 42 for more information about these agents).

### Complementary Therapies

The essential oil of *Melaleuca alternifolia*, or tea tree oil, has activity against HSV in vitro. Studies have shown healing time with tea tree oil is reduced versus placebo and similar to topical acyclovir 5%.[43,44] Lysine has preventive effects and has been shown to decrease the frequency of outbreaks when taken daily.[45] LongoVital, a vitamin tablet supplemented with dried and ground herbs, has been shown to decrease the frequency of episodes after 2 months of therapy.[46]

### *Assessment of HSL: A Case-based Approach*

Although many of the same nonprescription medications are indicated for RAS and HSL, the practitioner still needs to differentiate the disorders as illustrated in Case 32-5. Because herpes simplex lesions are contagious, additional measures are necessary to prevent transmission of the virus. The practitioner should obtain the patient's medical and medication history to determine whether an underlying pathology predisposes the patient to recurrent HSL or could complicate treatment.

## CASE 32-5

| Relevant Evaluation Criteria | Scenario/Model Outcome |
|---|---|
| **Information Gathering** | |
| 1. Gather essential information about the patient's symptoms, including: | |
| a. description of symptom(s) (i.e., nature, onset, duration, severity, associated symptoms) | Patient has red, crusty lesions covering most of lip area. Many areas are bleeding. Lesions have been present for 4 days. Patient is in a great deal of pain and is having difficulty eating. |
| b. description of any factors that seem to precipitate, exacerbate, and/or relieve the patient's symptom(s) | Movement of mouth in any way causes pain. |
| c. description of the patient's efforts to relieve the symptoms | Patient has been applying antibiotic ointment to the lesions. |
| 2. Gather essential patient history information: | |
| a. patient's identity | Joe Blanchard |
| b. patient's age, sex, height, and weight | 24 y/o M, 6'0", 130 lb |
| c. patient's occupation | Painter |
| d. patient's dietary habits | Usually eats a healthy diet |
| e. patient's sleep habits | Has difficulty falling asleep |
| f. concurrent medical conditions, prescription and nonprescription medications, and dietary supplements | Celexa 20 mg 1 tablet once daily for depression; Ambien 5 mg 1 tablet at bedtime as needed for insomnia |
| g. allergies | NKA |
| h. history of other adverse reactions to medications | None |
| i. other (describe)_______ | N/A |
| **Assessment and Triage** | |
| 3. Differentiate the patient's signs/symptoms and correctly identify the patient's primary problem(s). | Joe has an extensive case of herpes simplex labialis. |
| 4. Identify exclusions for self-treatment (see Figure 32-4). | None |
| 5. Formulate a comprehensive list of therapeutic alternatives for the primary problem to determine if triage to a medical practitioner is required, and share this information with the patient. | Options include:<br>(1) Refer Joe to a dentist or PCP.<br>(2) Recommend appropriate OTC products. If symptoms do not resolve in several days, refer Joe to a dentist or PCP.<br>(3) Take no action. |
| **Plan** | |
| 6. Select an optimal therapeutic alternative to address the patient's problem, taking into account patient preferences. | Appropriate OTC products, with medical/dental referral if symptoms do not resolve in several days |
| 7. Describe the recommended therapeutic approach to the patient. | Try a local anesthetic and application of Abreva (see the box Patient Education for Herpes Simplex Labialis). You also may use NSAIDs or acetaminophen to help with the pain. Extensive outbreaks generally require prescription drug therapy. You should see a dentist or PCP, that is, primary care provider, if the symptoms continue for more than a few more days. Avoid touching these areas with your fingers to prevent spread to other areas. |

**CASE 32-5 (continued)**

| Relevant Evaluation Criteria | Scenario/Model Outcome |
|---|---|
| 8. Explain to the patient the rationale for selecting the recommended therapeutic approach from the considered therapeutic alternatives. | Topical and oral prescription drug therapy is warranted in extensive outbreaks. |
| **Patient Education** | |
| 9. When recommending self-care with nonprescription medications and/or nondrug therapy, convey accurate information to the patient, including: | |
| a. appropriate dose and frequency of administration | Apply as directed on package. |
| b. maximum number of days the therapy should be employed | 7 days |
| c. product administration procedures | See the box Patient Education for Herpes Simplex Labialis. |
| d. expected time to onset of relief | 7 days |
| e. degree of relief that can be reasonably expected | Should resolve completely |
| f. most common side effects | See the box Patient Education for Herpes Simplex Labialis. |
| g. side effects that warrant medical intervention should they occur | See the box Patient Education for Herpes Simplex Labialis. |
| h. patient options in the event that condition worsens or persists | See dentist or PCP if lesions have not healed in 7 days or if infection develops. |
| i. product storage requirements | Keep all products out of young children's reach. |
| j. specific nondrug measures | Identify triggers for future prevention of outbreaks. Keep lips moist. |
| 10. Solicit patient's follow-up questions. | Are my sores contagious? |
| 11. Answer patient's questions. | Yes. You should avoid any intimate contact with other individuals. |

Key: N/A, not applicable; NKA, no known allergies; NSAID, nonsteroidal anti-inflammatory drug; OTC, over-the-counter; PCP, primary care provider.

### *Patient Counseling for HSL*

The practitioner should stress that herpes simplex lesions are contagious and should explain to the patient appropriate measures to prevent transmission of the virus. Patients should be advised that the disorder is self-limiting and pharmacologic therapy can keep the lesions moist and supple, decrease the itch and pain, protect the lesions from secondary bacterial infection, and help reduce the duration of active infection. The practitioner should explain the action of each recommended product, its proper use, and possible adverse effects.

### *Evaluation of Patient Outcomes for HSL*

The patient should return for reevaluation after 14 days. If the symptoms have resolved, no further treatment is necessary. However, if the condition worsens (pain and itching persist, redness increases, or signs of secondary infection are apparent), the patient should see a primary care provider or dentist for evaluation.

## XEROSTOMIA

Xerostomia, commonly referred to as dry mouth, is a disorder in which salivary flow is limited or completely arrested. A person with normal salivary flow reportedly produces up to 1.5 L of saliva every 24 hours.[47]

### *Epidemiology/Etiology of Xerostomia*

Epidemiologic factors for dry mouth correlate with its causes. Patients with certain disease states (e.g., Sjögren's syndrome, diabetes mellitus, depression, and Crohn's disease) or who are undergoing head and neck radiation therapy and/or chemotherapy, taking certain medications, or exhibiting certain lifestyle behaviors (e.g., excessive alcohol intake) are most prone to this disorder. About 20% of older adult patients are affected with dry mouth. Estimates of the total number of U.S. cases of Sjögren's syndrome (an autoimmune disease in which the salivary glands become partly or completely dysfunctional) range

## PATIENT EDUCATION FOR HERPES SIMPLEX LABIALIS

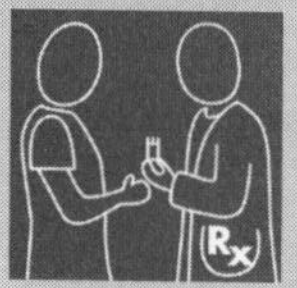


The objectives of self-treatment for herpes simplex labialis (cold sores) are to (1) relieve pain and irritation while the sores are healing, (2) prevent secondary infection, and (3) prevent spread of the lesions. For most patients, carefully following product instructions and the self-care measures listed here will help ensure optimal therapeutic outcomes.

### Nondrug Measures

- Keep lesions clean by gently washing them with mild soap solutions.
- Wash hands frequently to prevent contaminating the lesions and to avoid spreading the virus.
- Avoid factors believed to delay healing such as stress, injury to the lesions, wind, excessive sun exposure, and fatigue.
- If outbreaks are related to sun exposure, use a lip and face sunscreen routinely.

### Nonprescription Medications

- Use skin protectants such as allantoin, petrolatum, and cocoa butter to keep lesions moist and prevent cracking of the lesions. (See Chapter 41 for discussion of these agents.) These measures help prevent secondary bacterial infection.
- Use topical anesthetics such as benzocaine or dibucaine to relieve burning, itching, and pain. Do not use benzocaine if you have a history of hypersensitivity to other benzocaine-containing products.
- If using products containing camphor and menthol, make sure the concentration of camphor does not exceed 3% and the concentration of menthol does not exceed 1%.
- Do not apply hydrocortisone to the lesions.
- If evidence of secondary bacterial infection is seen, apply a thin layer of triple-antibiotic ointment (e.g., Mycitracin or Neosporin) three to four times daily.
- Apply topical agent docosanol 10% (Abreva) to limit the burning, tingling, and itching sensations. Docosanol 10% can also speed up the healing process, thus reducing the duration of the symptoms.
- If desired, take oral nonprescription analgesics (e.g., aspirin, ibuprofen, acetaminophen) for additional pain relief.
- Do not hold aspirin in the mouth or place it on oral lesions. The acid can cause a chemical burn and tissue damage.

⚠ See a primary care provider if any of the following occurs:

- The lesions do not heal in 14 days.
- The self-treatment measures do not relieve discomfort.
- Symptoms of systemic illness such as fever, malaise, rash, or swollen lymph glands occur.

from 1 to 4 million.[48] Radiation therapy of the head and neck can cause atrophy of the salivary glands. Following treatment, the vast majority of patients have compromised salivary function for the rest of their lives. Drugs with anticholinergic activity and drugs that cause depletion of salivary flow volume (e.g., antihypertensives, antihistamines, antipsychotics, stimulants, tricyclic antidepressants, tranquilizers, diuretics)[49] can cause xerostomia. Older patients who are more likely to be taking multiple medications for chronic diseases may be more greatly affected. However, if xerostomia is drug-induced and the medication can be discontinued, the condition may be reversed in some cases.[50] Nonpharmacologic causes include use of alcohol, tobacco, caffeine, and breathing through the mouth.

### *Signs and Symptoms of Xerostomia*

Xerostomia can result in difficulty talking and swallowing, stomatitis, burning tongue, and halitosis. Unmoistened food cannot be tasted; thus, xerostomia can cause loss of appetite and eventual decline in nutritional status. Patients' teeth can become hypersensitive, which can be related to a decrease in salivary flow and the lack of buffering capacity saliva provides.[51] Xerostomia can also result in a higher than normal incidence of cervical caries (decay around the root surfaces of teeth) despite excellent oral hygiene.[52]

### *Complications of Xerostomia*

Depending on the status of a patient's dentition, this disorder also can increase the incidence of caries, gingivitis, and more severe periodontal disease or reduce denture-wearing time. Furthermore, reduced flow of saliva can disturb the balance of microflora in the oral cavity and predispose it to candidiasis. The absence of lubrication and buffering can lead to tooth erosion, decalcification, and decay.[53]

### *Treatment of Xerostomia*

Dry mouth should never be discounted as inconsequential. Failure to treat it can result in serious complications for some patients.

#### Treatment Goals

The goals in treating dry mouth are to (1) relieve discomfort, (2) prevent and treat oral infections and periodontal disease, and (3) reduce the risk of dental caries by either replacing lost saliva with exogenous sources, or stimulating the remaining functional gland tissue to produce saliva.[54]

#### General Treatment Approach

The patient should discontinue using substances that dry the mouth or erode tooth enamel. Commercial artificial saliva products can be used as needed to relieve soft-tissue discomfort as outlined in Figure 32-5. The figure also lists exclusions for self-treatment. These products are more effective and longer lasting than simple rinses and lozenges. To reduce the risk of caries, it is necessary for the patient to maintain good oral hygiene and use sugarless sweets and chewing gums to stimulate residual salivary flow.[54]

**Exclusions for Self-Treatment**

- Tooth erosion, decalcification, and decay
- Candidiasis, gingivitis, and periodontitis
- Reduced denture-wearing time
- Mouth soreness associated with poor-fitting dentures
- Presence of fever or swelling
- Loose teeth
- Bleeding gums in the absence of trauma
- Broken or knocked-out teeth
- Severe tooth pain triggered or worsened by hot, cold, or chewing
- Trauma to the mouth with bleeding, swelling, and soreness

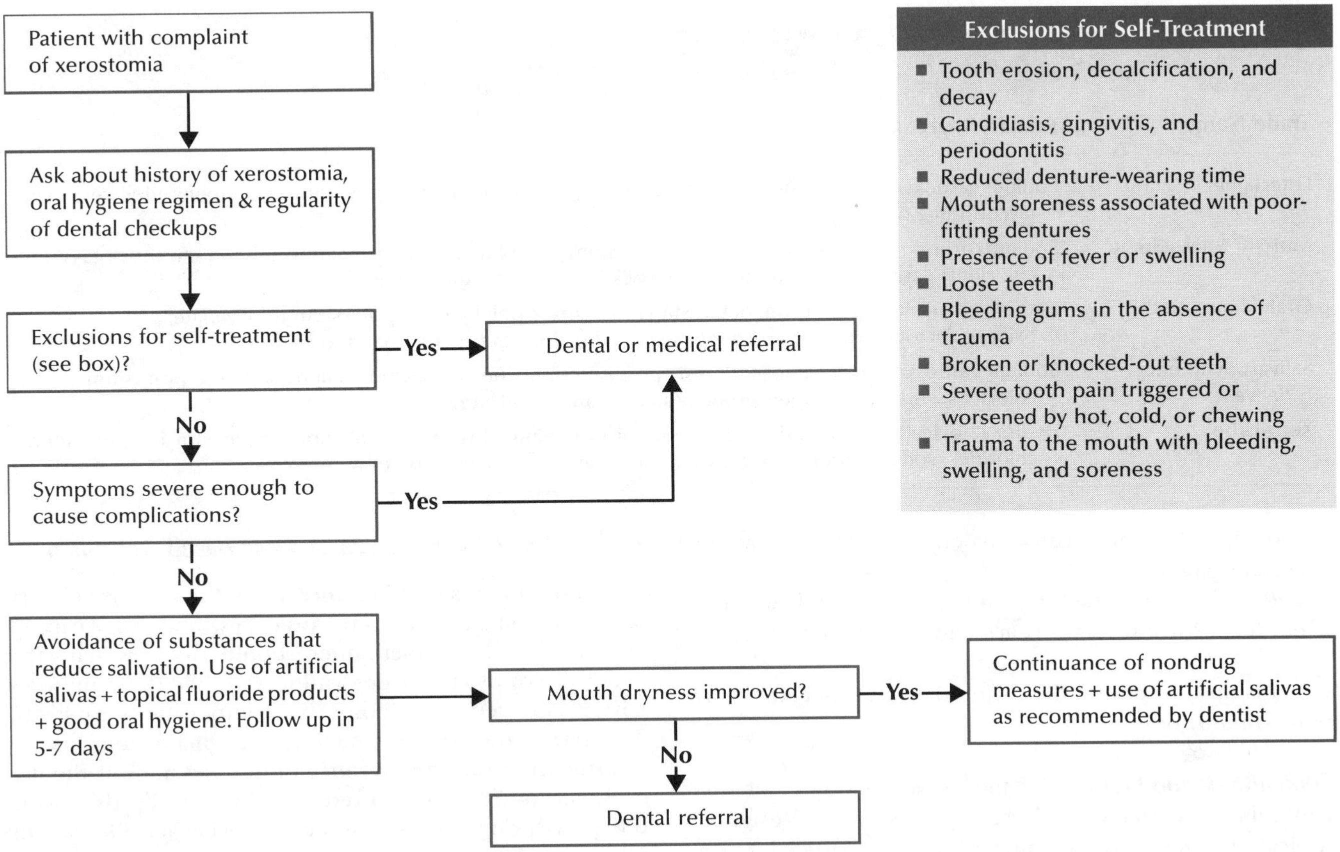


**FIGURE 32-5** Self-care of xerostomia.

## Nonpharmacologic Therapy

The patient should avoid substances that reduce salivation. Tobacco (smoked and smokeless) and products that contain alcohol (including mouth rinses), antihistamines, or central nervous system stimulants (pseudoephedrine) are common causes of impaired salivation. Modification of medication schedules, in consultation with the treating physician, to coincide with periods of natural stimulation should be considered. For example, patients could take medications that cause dry mouth 1 hour prior to meals because eating naturally stimulates an increase in salivary flow. Consequently, the duration of dry mouth would be reduced.

To prevent tooth decay, the xerostomic patient should limit intake of sugary and acidic foods that may have been tolerated before, but now pose significant danger to the patient's oral health. The sugar promotes bacterial growth, and the acid creates caries and increases tooth erosion. Similarly, the patient should avoid sucking on hard candy or lozenges sweetened with sugar because of their cariogenic potential. Chewing gum sweetened with sugar alcohols (e.g., xylitol), however, may be beneficial. Chewing gum increases salivary flow, and xylitol has not been shown to be cariogenic.[35] Increasing water intake, especially if it is fluoridated, would also be of benefit. Finally, the use of very soft toothbrushes will help prevent decay by minimizing tissue abrasion.

## Pharmacologic Therapy

Artificial saliva products are the primary agents for relieving the discomfort of dry mouth. Topical fluoride products help reduce the risk of caries.

*Artificial Saliva Products* Artificial salivas are of value and can be used on an as-needed basis in patients with little or no saliva flow. An ADA-accepted artificial saliva is Salivart Synthetic Saliva. (Table 32-6 lists other examples.)

Artificial saliva products are designed to mimic natural saliva both chemically and physically. However, they do not contain the many naturally occurring protective components that are present in innate saliva. Because they do not stimulate natural salivary gland production, however, they must be considered replacement therapy, not a cure for xerostomia. Closely resembling natural saliva, artificial saliva is formulated with the following properties:

- *Viscosity:* Carboxymethylcellulose and glycerin are used to mimic natural saliva viscosity.
- *Mineral content:* All products contain calcium and phosphate ions, and some also contain fluoride. With normal use, no product has demonstrated the ability to remineralize enamel. Therefore, ADA does not recognize any such claims made by the manufacturers.
- *Preservatives:* Salivart does not contain preservatives because it is packaged as a sterile aerosol. Other products containing preservatives, such as methyl- or

**TABLE 32-6 Selected Nonprescription Saliva Substitutes**

| Trade Name | Primary Ingredients |
|---|---|
| Entertainer's Secret | Sodium carboxymethylcellulose; dibasic sodium phosphate; potassium chloride; parabens; aloe vera gel; glycerin in 2-oz spray |
| Moi-Stir Sticks/Spray | Sodium carboxymethylcellulose; dibasic potassium phosphate; calcium; magnesium; sodium and potassium chlorides; parabens; sorbitol in 3-stick pack and 120 mL pump spray |
| Oralbalance Gel | Hydroxyethylcellulose; hydrogenated starch; glycerate polyhydrate; potassium thiocyanate; glucose oxidase; lactoperoxidase; lysozyme; lactoferrin; aloe vera; xylitol in gel form |
| Salivart Synthetic Saliva | Sodium carboxymethylcellulose; dibasic potassium phosphate; calcium; magnesium and potassium chlorides; sorbitol; nitrogen propellant in 25 and 75 mL spray |
| Xero-Lube | Hydroxyethylcellulose; dibasic and monobasic potassium phosphates; calcium; magnesium and potassium chlorides; sodium fluoride; methylparaben; flavor; xylitol in 6-oz spray |

propylparaben, may cause hypersensitivity reactions in certain patients.

- *Palatability:* Flavorings (e.g., mint, lemon) and sweeteners (e.g., sorbitol, xylitol) are commonly used.

Patients on low-sodium diets should avoid artificial salivas that contain sodium.

*Topical Fluoride Products* Patients with a history of susceptibility to caries should use a professionally designed topical fluoride program in addition to artificial saliva products. (Chapter 31 discusses the use of topical fluoride products and other oral hygiene measures.)

### *Assessment of Xerostomia: A Case-based Approach*

The practitioner should inquire about the patient's history of xerostomia, oral hygiene practices, and regularity of dental visits. The practitioner should then evaluate the patient's symptoms to determine whether the symptoms have progressed to the point that complications are likely. A review of the patient's medical and medication history will rule in or out the presence of diseases and/or the use of medications known to reduce salivation. Furthermore, the practitioner should determine whether lifestyle or other practices could be contributing to dry mouth. Case 32-6 illustrates this approach to assessing patients with xerostomia.

**CASE 32-6**

| Relevant Evaluation Criteria | Scenario/Model Outcome |
|---|---|
| **Information Gathering** | |
| 1. Gather essential information about the patient's symptoms, including: | |
| a. description of symptom(s) (i.e., nature, onset, duration, severity, associated symptoms) | Patient has difficulty talking and chewing because of dryness in mouth. She has lost several pounds over the past few weeks. She sometimes has a metallic taste in her mouth and a burning sensation in the back of her throat. |
| b. description of any factors that seem to precipitate, exacerbate, and/or relieve the patient's symptom(s) | None |
| c. description of the patient's efforts to relieve the symptoms | She has seen a PCP and a periodontist. The periodontist recommended a saliva substitute and prescribed an antifungal for an oral "yeast infection." Patient is confused about which saliva substitute to use. |
| 2. Gather essential patient history information: | |
| a. patient's identity | Bobbi Winston |
| b. patient's age, sex, height, and weight | 76 y/o F; 5'2", 103 lb |
| c. patient's occupation | Retired teacher |
| d. patient's dietary habits | Difficulty eating because of dry mouth; weight loss |
| e. patient's sleep habits | N/A |

## CASE 32-6 (continued)

| Relevant Evaluation Criteria | Scenario/Model Outcome |
|---|---|
| f. concurrent medical conditions, prescription and nonprescription medications, and dietary supplements | Diagnosed Sjögren's syndrome; extensive dental work over past few years; Salagen 5 mg 1 tablet 4 times/day for dry mouth; Cardizem CD 240 mg 1 capsule once daily for hypertension; Premarin 0.625 mg 1 tablet once daily for osteoporosis; Atrovent inhaler 2 puffs 4 times/day for emphysema; albuterol inhaler 2 puffs 4 times/day for emphysema; meclizine 12.5 mg 1 tablet 3 times/day as needed for dizziness; quinine sulfate 325 mg 1 tablet at bedtime as needed for leg cramps; Mycelex 10 mg 1 troche dissolved in mouth 5 times/day for 14 days for thrush |
| g. allergies | None |
| h. history of other adverse reactions to medications | None |
| i. other (describe)_______ | Bobbi's teeth are capped and she has an upper partial denture. She lives by herself and never removes her partial denture. |
| **Assessment and Triage** | |
| 3. Differentiate the patient's signs/symptoms and correctly identify the patient's primary problem(s). | Bobbi has disease- and drug-induced xerostomia, and a secondary oral yeast/fungal infection. |
| 4. Identify exclusions for self-treatment (see Figure 32-5). | None |
| 5. Formulate a comprehensive list of therapeutic alternatives for the primary problem to determine if triage to a medical practitioner is required, and share this information with the patient. | Options include:<br>(1) Recommend saliva substitute.<br>(2) Provide information on oral hygiene including care of removable partial denture.<br>(3) Evaluate drug therapy for contribution to xerostomia.<br>(4) Take no action. |
| **Plan** | |
| 6. Select an optimal therapeutic alternative to address the patient's problem, taking into account patient preferences. | Use of saliva substitute, good oral hygiene, and return visit to periodontist and PCP if symptoms are not resolved. |
| 7. Describe the recommended therapeutic approach to the patient. | Saliva is important to your oral health, including the ability to chew food effectively and talk clearly, so you need to use a saliva substitute on a regular basis. The prescription antifungal lozenge will help get rid of the yeast infection. You need to use a fluoride toothpaste and rinse, and take out your partial denture and clean it daily. We can consult with your PCP, that is, primary care provider, and make some changes to your medication administration techniques and schedules to help reduce your dry mouth. |
| 8. Explain to the patient the rationale for selecting the recommended therapeutic approach from the considered therapeutic alternatives. | This combination of steps is needed to treat all your symptoms. |
| **Patient Education** | |
| 9. When recommending self-care with nonprescription medications and/or nondrug therapy, convey accurate information to the patient, including: | |
| a. appropriate dose and frequency of administration | Use saliva substitute several times daily. Brush teeth with fluoride toothpaste and soft brush twice daily. Remove partial denture at night and mechanically clean it and place in a denture cleanser |

## CASE 32-6 (continued)

| Relevant Evaluation Criteria | Scenario/Model Outcome |
|---|---|
| b. maximum number of days the therapy should be employed | If burning in back of throat does not resolve in 7 days, see your periodontist and/or PCP again. |
| c. product administration procedures | Make sure you are using your inhalers properly. Your medications also contribute to dry mouth. |
| d. expected time to onset of relief | Dry mouth should improve with regular saliva substitute. Burning in throat should improve in 7 days. |
| e. degree of relief that can be reasonably expected | Dry mouth will probably be a continual problem, as a result of your medications. |
| f. most common side effects | N/A |
| g. side effects that warrant medical intervention should they occur | N/A |
| h. patient options in the event that condition worsens or persists | See periodontist or PCP. |
| i. product storage requirements | See package. |
| j. specific nondrug measures | Drink water and rinse mouth with water. See the box Patient Education for Xerostomia. |
| 10. Solicit patient's follow-up questions. | May I soak my partial denture in household bleach? |
| 11. Answer patient's questions. | No. This will damage the partial denture. |

Key: N/A, not available; PCP, primary care provider.

## PATIENT EDUCATION FOR XEROSTOMIA

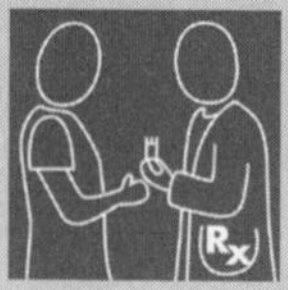

The objectives of self-treatment for xerostomia (dry mouth) are to (1) relieve the discomfort of dry mouth, (2) reduce the risk of dental decay, and (3) prevent and treat infections and periodontal disease. For most patients, carefully following product instructions and the self-care measures listed here will help ensure optimal therapeutic outcomes.

### Nondrug Measures

- To prevent reduced levels of saliva, avoid use of cigarettes and smokeless tobacco.
- Do not use products that contain alcohol (including mouth rinses), antihistamines, or the drug pseudoephedrine. These substances reduce saliva levels.
- Avoid food or drinks that contain caffeine.
- To prevent tooth decay, limit consumption of sugary and acidic foods. Do not suck on hard candy or lozenges sweetened with sugar.
- If desired, chew gum sweetened with sugar alcohols such as xylitol to help increase flow of saliva.
- If possible, take medications 1 hour before meals so that the natural saliva flow caused by food can counteract any mouth dryness.
- To help prevent tooth decay, use a very soft toothbrush to reduce abrasion of the teeth.

### Nonprescription Medications

- Use artificial saliva products that contain fluoride to relieve the discomfort of dry mouth and prevent tooth decay.
- If you are on a low-sodium diet, avoid artificial salivas that contain sodium.
- Use an additional topical fluoride product to help reduce the risk of tooth decay. Also, brush and floss your teeth at least twice daily using a regular toothpaste with fluoride, and see your dentist regularly.

If your symptoms do not improve or if they worsen, see a dentist.

### *Patient Counseling for Xerostomia*

It is generally necessary for xerostomic patients to have professional dental management of their condition as well as the self-care methods discussed above. Patients should be encouraged to practice good oral hygiene measures and to see their dentist regularly. In addition, the practitioner also should be advising patients about what they need to know regarding which pharmacologic and nonpharmacologic measures will keep the oral cavity moist and can be used to treat dry mouth to minimize the increased risk for tooth decay associated with xerostomia. Finally, the practitioner must alert patients to signs and symptoms that indicate complications from dry mouth.

### *Evaluation of Patient Outcomes for Xerostomia*

The patient with xerostomia should return for evaluation after 5 to 7 days of self-treatment. If the mouth dryness is improved, the patient should continue using artificial saliva and fluoride products as recommended by a dentist. The patient should also be advised to continue the nonpharmacologic measures. If the dryness becomes worse or symptoms of complications develop, the patient should return to the dentist for further evaluation.

## KEY POINTS FOR ORAL PAIN AND DISCOMFORT

- Tooth hypersensitivity and teething are nonserious and self-treatable problems.
- Self-treatment of toothache should be limited to the temporary relief of pain as professional treatment is required for complete resolution of pain.
- RAS is amenable to self-treatment for the relief of pain and irritation so the lesions can heal, thus allowing the patient the ability to eat, drink, and perform routine oral hygiene while preventing further complications.
- Minor oral mucosal injury or irritation may be self-treated by controlling discomfort and pain, aiding healing with the appropriate use of drug and nondrug measures, and preventing secondary bacterial infection.
- The goals of self-treatment for herpes simplex labialis (cold sores) are to relieve pain and irritation while the sores are healing, prevent secondary infection, and prevent spread of the lesions to other areas of the body and other individuals.
- Xerostomia (dry mouth) can be aided by self-treatment for the relief of discomfort from dry mouth, reducing the risk of dental decay and preventing and at times, treating infections.
- It is critical for practitioners to recognize and understand that, in the event conditions worsen or persist after self-treatment and nonprescription measures, it is imperative to strongly advise the individual to seek professional assistance form their dentist or PCP.

## References

1. Kanapka JA. Over-the-counter dentifrices in the treatment of tooth hypersensitivity. *Dent Clin North Am.* 1990;34:545-60.
2. Leavitt AH, King GJ, Ramsay DS, et al. A longitudinal evaluation of pulpal pain during orthodontic tooth movement. *Orthod Craniofacial Res.* 2002;5:29-37.
3. Simon J. Biomechanically-induced dental disease. *Gen Dent.* 2000;48:598-605.
4. Paine ML, Slots J, Rich SK. Fluoride use in periodontal therapy: a review of the literature. *J Am Dent Assoc.* 1998;129:69-77.
5. Canadian Advisory Board on Dentin Hypersensitivity. Consensus-based recommendations for the diagnosis and management of dentin hypersensitivity. *J Can Dent Assoc.* 2003;69:221-6.
6. Vanuspong W, Eisenburger M, Addy M. Cervical tooth wear and sensitivity: erosion, softening and rehardening of dentine; effects of pH, time and ultrasonication. *J Clin Periodontol.* 2002;29:351-7.
7. Linnett V, Seow WK. Dental erosion in children: a literature review. *Pediatr Dent.* 2001;23:37-43.
8. Woodmansey KF. Recognition of bulimia nervosa in dental patients: implications for dental care providers. *Gen Dent.* 2000; 48:48-52.
9. Jorgensen MG, Carroll WB. Incidence of tooth sensitivity after home whitening treatment. *J Am Dent Assoc.* 2002;133:1076-82.
10. DuPont JS Jr. Neuritic toothache. *Gen Dent.* 2001;49:178-81.
11. Okeson JP. Non-odontogenic toothache. *Northwest Dent.* 2000; 79(5):37-44.
12. Riley JL III, Gilbert GH, Heft MW. Race/ethnic differences in health care use for orofacial pain among older adults. *Pain.* 2002; 100:119-30.
13. Pau AKH, Croucher R, Marcenes W. Perceived inability to cope and care seeking in patients with toothache: a qualitative study. *Br Dent J.* 2000:189:500-2.
14. Gilliam DG, Bulman JS, Jackson RJ, et al. Comparison of two desensitizing dentifrices with a commercially available fluoride dentifrice in alleviating cervical dentine sensitivity. *J Periodontol.* 1996;67:737-42.
15. *Federal Register.* 1991;56:48308-10,48315-6,48325, 48335-46.
16. Sowinski JA, Bonta Y, Battista GW, et al. Desensitizing efficacy of Colgate Sensitive Maximum Strength and Fresh Mint Sensodyne denitrifies. *Am J Dent.* 2000;13:116-20.
17. Schiff T, Bonta Y, Proskin HM, et al. Desensitizing efficacy of a new dentifrice containing 5.0% potassium nitrate and 0.454% stannous fluoride. *Am J Dent.* 2000;13:111-5.
18. *Federal Register.* 1992;57:20115.
19. Sowinski J, Ayad F, Petrone M, et al. Comparative investigations of the desensitizing efficacy of a new dentifrice. *J Clin Periodontol.* 2001;28:1032-6.
20. Hodosh M. Potentiating potassium nitrate's desensitization with dimethyl isosorbide. *Gen Dent.* 2001;49:531-6.
21. Gillam DG, Tang JY, Mordan NJ, et al. The effects of a novel Bioglass dentifrice on dentine sensitivity: a scanning electron microscopy investigation. *J Oral Rehabil.* 2002;29:305-13.
22. Marini I, Checchi L, Vecchiet F, et al. Intraoral fluoride releasing device: a new clinical therapy for dentine sensitivity. *J Periodontol.* 2000;71:90-5.
23. Eisen DE, Lynch DP. *The Mouth: Diagnosis and Treatment.* St. Louis: Mosby; 1998.
24. Barrons RW. Treatment strategies for recurrent aphthous ulcers. *Am J Health-Syst Pharm.* 2001;58:41-53.
25. Porter SR, Hegarty A, Kaliakatsou F, et al. Recurrent aphthous stomatitis. *Clin Dermatol.* 2000;18:569-78.
26. Shashy RG, Ridley MB. Aphthous ulcers: a difficult clinical entity. *Am J Otolaryngol.* 2000;21:389-93.
27. Woo SB, Sonis ST. Recurrent aphthous ulcers: a review of diagnosis and treatment. *J Am Dent Assoc.* 1996;127:1202-13.
28. Rehberger A, Puspok A, Stallmeister T, et al. Crohn's disease masquerading as aphthous ulcers. *Eur J Dermatol.* 1998;8:274-6.
29. Bonaccorso A, Tripi TR. Oral lesions in systemic lupus erythematosus, I: the etiopathogenic aspects of lupus erythematosus. *Minerva Stomatol.* 1998;47:27-31.
30. Krause I, Rosen Y, Kaplan I, et al. Recurrent aphthous stomatitis in Behçet's disease: clinical features and correlation with systemic disease expression and severity. *J Oral Pathol Med.* 1999;28:193-6.
31. Casiglia JM, Recurrent aphthous stomatitis: etiology, diagnosis, and treatment. *Gen Dent.* 2002;50:157-66.
32. Riggio MP, Lennon A, Wray D. Detection of Helicobacter pylori DNA in recurrent aphthous stomatitis by PCR. *J Oral Pathol Med.* 2000;29:507-13.
33. *Federal Register.* 1994;59:6084.

34. Greenberg MS. Drug use for connective tissue disorders and oral mucosal diseases. In: Ciancio SG, ed. *ADA Guide to Dental Therapeutics.* 2nd ed. Chicago: ADA Business Enterprises, Inc; 2000: 450-1.
35. Harris NO, Garcia-Godoy F. *Primary Preventive Dentistry.* 6th ed. Stamford, Conn: Appleton & Lange; 2004:76-85, 96-102, 124-5, 128-30, 165-6, 242-7, 249-53, 419, 440, 471, 489-90, 655-9.
36. American Dental Association. *ADA Statement on the Safety of Hydrogen-Peroxide-Containing Dental Products Intended for Home Use.* Chicago: American Dental Association; 1997.
37. Slavkin HC. Infection and immunity. *J Am Dent Assoc.* 1996;127: 1792-6.
38. ADA news. *J Am Dent Assoc.* 2000;131:1256-60.
39. Wilis A, Hyland P, Lamey P-J. Response to replacement iron therapy in sideropenic individuals with recrudescent herpes labialis. *Eur J Clin Microbiol Infect Dis.* 2000;19:355-7.
40. *Federal Register.* 1992;57:29173.
41. *Federal Register.* 1990;55:3372,3379.
42. *Federal Register.* 1993;58:27638.
43. Carson CF, Ashton L, Dry L., et al. Melaleuca alternifolia (tea tree) oil gel (6%) for the treatment of recurrent herpes labialis. *J Antimicrob Chemother.* 2001;48:450-1.
44. Allen P. Tea tree oil: the science behind the antimicrobial hype. *Lancet.* 2001;13:1245.
45. Tomblin FA, Lucas KH. Lysine for management of herpes labialis. *Am J Health-Syst Pharm.* 2001;58:298-304.
46. Pederson A. LongoVital and herpes labialis: a randomised, double-blind, placebo-controlled study. *Oral Dis.* 2001;7:221-5.
47. Guyton AC. *Textbook of Medical Physiology.* 8th ed. Philadelphia: WB Saunders; 1991:711-2.
48. Fox PC. Management of dry mouth. *Dent Clin North Am.* 1997; 41:863-75.
49. Smith RG, Burtner PA. Oral side-effects of the most frequently prescribed drugs. *Spec Care Dent.* 1994;14:96-108.
50. Wynn RL, Meiller TF, Crossly HL. *Drug Information Handbook for Dentistry.* 9th ed. Hudson, Ohio: Lexi-Comp; 2003:1553-61.
51. Garg AK, Malo M. Manifestations and treatment of xerostomia and associated oral effect secondary to head and neck radiation therapy. *J Am Dent Assoc.* 1997;128:1128-33.
52. Atkinson JC, Wu AJ. Salivary gland dysfunction: causes, symptoms, treatment. *J Am Dent Assoc.* 1994;125:409-16.
53. Yagiela JA. Agents affecting salivation. In: Ciancio SG, ed. *ADA Guide to Dental Therapeutics.* 2nd ed. Chicago: ADA Business Enterprises, Inc; 2000:198-210.
54. Jonsson R, Moen K, Vestrheim D, et al. Current issues in Sjögren's syndrome. *Oral Dis.* 2002;8:130-40.

SECTION VIII

# Dermatologic Disorders

CHAPTER 33

# Atopic Dermatitis and Dry Skin

*Steven A. Scott and Robert W. Martin III*

An estimated 5% of the population suffer from a chronic skin, hair, or nail condition, and many others experience acute or seasonal disorders. Numerous skin disorders present as early as infancy and continue to appear throughout childhood and adulthood. A majority of people 65 years of age and older have two or more skin conditions such as contact dermatitis, seborrheic dermatitis, fungal infections, and neoplastic growths.[1]

Patients with skin disorders typically present with some type of rash and/or itching (pruritus), which may indicate dermatitis. It is essential for clinicians to be able to recognize, differentiate, and suggest appropriate treatment for common skin conditions and to know when to refer patients to a primary care provider or dermatologist for severe skin disorders.

Dermatitis is a nonspecific term describing numerous dermatologic conditions that are generally characterized by erythema (redness). The terms eczema and dermatitis are used interchangeably to describe a group of inflammatory skin disorders of unknown etiology. When the cause of a particular skin condition is elucidated, the disorder is given a specific name. Known causes of dermatitis include allergens, irritants, and infections; however, several distinct forms of dermatitis exist for which the causes remain unclear.

This chapter discusses atopic dermatitis, a common form of dermatitis, and dry skin, another frequent dermatologic complaint. Almost everyone will experience dry or chapped skin (xerosis) at some point, and the incidence increases with age. It is a seasonal occurrence in some and a chronic condition in others. Although dry skin is often not severe, it may be annoying and uncomfortable for patients with mild to moderate dryness because of the attendant pruritus, and, in some cases, infection, pain, and inflammation occur.

## ANATOMY AND PHYSIOLOGY OF SKIN

The skin is involved in numerous physical and biochemical processes.[2] Skin thickness is variable but averages about 1 to 2 mm, with the thickest skin on the palms and soles, and the thinnest skin on the scrotum. Thinner areas are more permeable, allowing substances to be absorbed more easily than through thicker skin. Although skin is exposed to a variety of chemical and environmental insults, it demonstrates remarkable resiliency and recuperative ability.

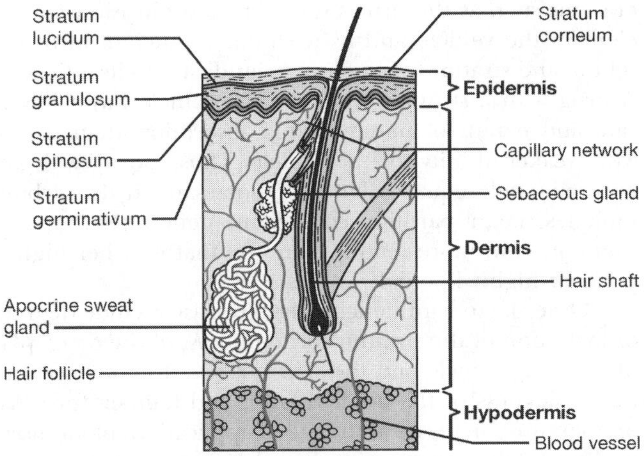


**FIGURE 33-1** Cross-section of human skin.

### Skin Regions and Functions

Human skin has three functionally distinct regions: epidermis, dermis, and hypodermis (Figure 33-1). The epidermis, the outermost thin layer of the skin, regulates the water content of the skin and controls drug transport into the lower layers and systemic circulation. The dermis is 40 times thicker than the epidermis and contains nerve endings, vasculature, and hair follicles. The hypodermis primarily provides nourishment and cushioning for the upper two layers.

The most important function of skin and its appendages (hair and nails) is to protect the body from external harmful agents, such as pathogenic organisms and chemicals. The skin's ability to do this depends on age, immunologic status, underlying disease states of the individual, concurrent medications, and preservation of an intact stratum corneum.[3]

The acid mantle (pH approximately 4.5-5.5) serves as a protective mechanism, inhibiting the growth of pathogens. Normal skin flora also acts as a defense mechanism by controlling the growth of potential pathogenic organisms and preventing their possible invasion of the skin and body. The skin also contributes to sensory experiences, and is involved in temperature control, pigment development, and synthesis of some vitamins. It is important in hydroregulation as well, controlling moisture loss from the body and moisture penetration into the body. If the stratum corneum becomes dehydrated, it loses elasticity and its permeation characteristics are altered. Aging skin becomes more fragile, requiring a longer recovery time after injury.

Excessive or aggressive bathing insults aging skin more than younger skin.

## Percutaneous Absorption of Drugs

A drug must be released from its vehicle if it is to exert an effect at the desired site of activity (skin surface, epidermis, or dermis). Release occurs at the interface between the skin surface and the applied layer of product. The physical-chemical relationship between the drug and the vehicle determines the rate and amount of drug released. Considerations such as the drug's solubility and diffusion coefficient in the vehicle and its partition coefficient into the sebum and stratum corneum are significant to its efficacy.[3] A drug with a strong affinity for the vehicle has a lower rate and extent of percutaneous absorption than drugs with weaker affinity for the vehicle. Thus, a drug with an approximately equal balance of polar and hydrocarbon moieties (i.e., a partition coefficient) penetrates the stratum corneum more readily than one that is either highly polar or highly lipoidal.

Other factors influencing drug release include degree of hydration of the stratum corneum, $pK_a$ of the drug, pH of the drug vehicle and the skin surface, drug concentration, thickness of the applied layer, and temperature. As temperature increases at the site of application, blood flow in the area also increases, as does the rate of percutaneous absorption. These factors apply to drug flux from all topical forms (e.g., powders, ointments, pastes, emulsified creams or lotions, gels, suspensions, and solutions).

Oily hydrocarbon bases such as petrolatum are transiently occlusive, promote hydration, and generally enhance the transport of agents through the skin layers. Hydrous emulsion bases are less occlusive. Water-soluble bases (polyethylene glycols) are minimally occlusive, may attract water from the stratum corneum, and may decrease drug transport. Powders with hydrophilic ingredients presumably decrease hydration because they promote evaporation from the skin by absorbing available water.

Substances are transported from the skin surface to the general circulation through percutaneous absorption. The routes of such transport are presumed to involve passages through skin between the keratinized units of the stratum corneum and through skin appendages (e.g., hair follicles, sweat glands, and sebaceous glands). The major mechanism of drug absorption is passive diffusion through the stratum corneum, followed by transport through the deeper epidermal regions and then the dermis.

Drug movement into and through the skin is enhanced or inhibited to varying degrees, depending on the physical-chemical properties of a drug, the sebum, and area of skin. The stratum corneum provides the greatest resistance and is often a rate-limiting barrier to percutaneous absorption. Because it is nonliving tissue, the stratum corneum may be viewed as having the general characteristics of an artificial and semipermeable membrane. Molecular passage through the stratum corneum occurs mostly by passive diffusion. Once a molecule has crossed this layer, there is much less resistance to its transport through the rest of the epidermis and into the dermis.

When the stratum corneum is hydrated, drug diffusion is sometimes accelerated. Hydration swells the stratum corneum, loosening its normally tight, densely packed arrangement, thus making diffusion easier. Occlusion also increases hydration of the stratum corneum, which enhances the transfer of most drugs. The increased amount of water present in the skin under such conditions probably further enhances the transfer of polar molecules.

Wounds, burns, chafed areas, and dermatitis can alter the integrity of the stratum corneum, and can result in artificial shunts of the percutaneous absorption process. Inflammation can also enhance percutaneous absorption of topically applied medications, which may result in dangerous systemic drug levels. Therefore, caution should be used in applying topical medication to compromised skin, particularly if large surface areas are involved.

Topical medications should not be used on children ages 2 years or younger, except under the advice and supervision of a primary care provider. Infants have a reduced capability to biotransform drugs absorbed by the cutaneous route and immature hepatic enzyme systems. Also, because the ratio of surface area to body weight in a newborn is approximately two to three times that of an adult, the proportion of drug absorbed per kilogram of body weight is greater in a newborn.[4] Infants are, therefore, at increased risk for systemic effects from topically applied drugs.

# ATOPIC DERMATITIS

## Epidemiology of Atopic Dermatitis

Atopy is a genetically predisposed tendency to exaggerated skin and mucosal reactivity in response to environmental stimuli. The atopic triad is asthma, allergic rhinitis (hay fever), and atopic dermatitis (AD). AD is a chronic, relapsing, skin disorder that typically begins during infancy or early childhood and often lasts into adulthood. Over time it moves through three age-related phases (infancy, childhood, and adult phases).[5] The incidence of AD may be increasing (from 3% of children after World War II to 10%-15% today) possibly in part because of increased exposure to pollutants, irritants, indoor allergens (particularly house-dust mites), and a decline in breast-feeding.[6]

The estimated worldwide incidence of AD is 5% to 10% of the children under the age of 14 years, and occurs in 2% to 5% of adults.[6] It is considered the most common dermatologic condition of children, with more than 5% of children affected by age 6 months. AD persists or recurs in about 60% of affected individuals and is more common in boys, whites, higher socioeconomic classes, and urban areas.[6] Allergic rhinitis (hay fever) and asthma occur in 30% to 80% of cases of AD. Areas commonly affected (e.g., face, flexural areas on the inside of the knees and elbows, collar area of the neck) depend on the patient's age.

AD accounts for many of the skin consultations in general medical practice and constitutes a significant number of all referrals to dermatologists. Two thirds to three quarters of patients with AD do not seek medical care and thus are likely to look for advice regarding self-care of this condition.[6]

**TABLE 33-1 Diagnostic Criteria for Atopic Dermatitis**

An itchy skin condition, plus three or more of the following criteria:

- Onset at <2 years of age
- History of skin crease involvement (including cheeks in children <10 years of age)
- History of generally dry skin
- Personal history of other atopic disease (or history of any atopic disease in first-degree relative in children <4 years of age)
- Visible flexural dermatitis (or dermatitis of cheeks/forehead and other outer limbs in children <4 years of age)

## Etiology/Pathophysiology of Atopic Dermatitis

AD has a genetic basis, but its expression is modified by a broad spectrum of exogenous manifestations.[7] Seventy percent of cases have an atopic family history. For example, if one parent (especially the father) has an atopic disorder, there is a 60% chance of the child being atopic. If both parents are affected, the likelihood is 80%. In nonatopic families, the likelihood of having an atopic child is roughly 20%. Twin studies have shown a much higher occurrence of atopy in monozygotic rather than dizygotic twins (85% versus 21%).

AD is diagnosed according to clinical criteria (Table 33-1). No established laboratory tests exist, although many patients have shown an elevated immunoglobulin E level and peripheral blood eosinophilia. Atopic dermatitis may be accompanied by allergic respiratory disease, but often is the initial clinical manifestation of an allergic disease.

Common exacerbating factors include foods, soaps, detergents, fragrances, chemicals, temperature changes, dust, pollens, certain bacteria, and emotional changes. Clinically relevant food allergy in AD is estimated to range up to 33% to the age of 24 months. Patients with AD may be more sensitive to irritants than the general population; thus, it is important for affected patients to minimize exposure to known irritants and allergens.[8]

AD may be exacerbated by factors such as irritants, allergens, extremes of temperature and humidity, dry skin, emotional stress, and local infection. The patient should be encouraged to identify the role of these factors (if any) so they may be minimized or avoided.

Irritants (e.g., solvents, industrial chemicals, fragrances, soaps, fumes, paints, bleach, wool, and astringents) may cause burning, itching, or redness. Patients with AD may be especially sensitive to low concentrations of irritants that would not generally cause a reaction on normal skin.[9]

Allergens—typically, plant or animal proteins from food, pollens, or pets—may aggravate AD. However, the role of food allergies in exacerbating AD is unclear. It is claimed that up to 20% of children under 2 years with AD are affected by allergic reactions to foods through either ingestion or skin contact, and specific hypersensitivities to milk products and eggs have been identified. Restricting offending foods, especially in children, creates overwhelming compliance problems. Moreover, although dietary restriction may produce some improvement in the condition initially, complete resolution is unlikely to occur. Thus, it is probably best to reserve dietary management for patients who have severe symptoms and are unresponsive to other treatments.[10]

Patients with AD are often intolerant of sudden and extreme changes in temperature and humidity. High temperature may enhance perspiration, leading to increased itching. Low humidity, often found in heated buildings during the winter, dries the skin and increases itching. Use of humidifiers in dry environments will provide some benefit. As with asthma, emotional stress is an exacerbating factor in some patients.

## Signs and Symptoms of Atopic Dermatitis

Although AD is often first manifested in infancy, it is rarely present at birth. If it does develop early in life, it typically occurs within the first year (often beginning at age 2-3 months) in approximately 80% of the cases. It initially appears as redness and chapping of the infant's cheeks, which may continue to affect the face, neck, and trunk (Table 33-2). At times, this dermatitis may progress to become more generalized, with crusting developing on the forehead and cheeks.[10] Crusts consist of dried exudate containing proteinaceous and cellular debris from erosion or ulceration of primary skin lesions. Remission usually occurs between the ages of 2 and 4 years, with recurrences often diminishing in intensity or even disappearing as the child approaches adulthood.

A classic case of infantile or childhood AD involves the cheeks and extensor surfaces of the forearms and legs (see Color Plates, photographs 14A, B, and C). Later manifestations of atopic dermatitis typically present on flexor surfaces. Lesions are typically symmetric in patients with AD.

**TABLE 33-2 Characteristics of Atopic Dermatitis by Age**

| Age | Location | Signs |
|---|---|---|
| 2 months | Chest, face | Red, raised vesicles; dry skin; oozing |
| 2 years | Scalp, neck, and extensor surface of extremities | Less acute lesions; edema; erythema |
| 2-4 years | Neck, wrist, elbow, knee | Dry, thickened plaques; hyperpigmentation |
| 12-20 years | Flexors, hands | Dry, thickened plaques; hyperpigmentation |

The primary sign of AD is intense pruritic papules (solid, circumscribed, elevated lesions less than 1 cm in diameter) and vesicles (sharply circumscribed, elevated lesions containing fluid). Pruritus is common and causes significant morbidity in AD. Patients with AD react more readily and more persistently to pruritic-inducing stimuli. Scratching and lichenification (increased epidermal markings) can produce a vicious cycle and lead to excoriation (abrasion of the epidermis by trauma).[11]

AD has three clinical forms. Acute AD is characterized by intensely pruritic, erythematous papules or vesicles over erythematous skin, and is often associated with excoriation and serous exudate. Subacute AD is characterized by erythematous, excoriated, scaling papules. Chronic AD is characterized by thickened plaques of skin and accentuated skin markings (lichenification). In chronic AD, all three stages of skin reactions frequently coexist in the same individual.

## Complications of Atopic Dermatitis

Secondary or associated cutaneous infections, especially bacterial, can be common, difficult to prevent, and typically aggravate AD. Over 90% of the skin lesions in patients with AD (in contrast to 5% of unaffected individuals) harbor *Staphylococcus aureus*.[6] Although *S. aureus* is the most common cause, streptococci may also be found alone or in association with *S. aureus*. Infections present as yellowish crusting of the eczematous lesions. Patients should be counseled to seek medical attention promptly when signs of bacterial or viral skin infection such as pustules (circumscribed, elevated lesions less than 1 cm in diameter containing pus), vesicles (especially exudate or pus filled), and crusting (dried exudate) are noticed.

## Treatment Overview of Atopic Dermatitis

### Treatment Goals

The goals of self-treatment of AD are to (1) stop the itch-scratch cycle, (2) maintain skin hydration, and (3) avoid or minimize factors that trigger or aggravate the disorder.

### General Treatment Approach

To prevent unrealistic expectations, clinicians should stress to patients that AD cannot be cured but most patients' symptoms can be managed satisfactorily. The condition should be explained as a multifactorial disorder, and it must be appreciated that just as there is no "cure" there is no single "cause." Often no explanation can be found for a particular flare-up of the condition, and many factors are probably working in combination at all times.

Regardless of a patient's age, the stratum corneum in patients with AD contains less moisture than that of normal skin. Enhancing skin hydration can be achieved through nonpharmacologic measures, as well as through the use of emollients and moisturizers. Hydrocortisone relieves itching and inflammation, and cool water compresses relieve weeping vesicles. An effective preventive measure is to minimize exposure to factors known to trigger AD. The algorithm in Figure 33-2 outlines the self-treatment of this disorder and lists exclusions for self-treatment.

### Nonpharmacologic Therapy

The variability in severity and age of onset requires tailoring treatment to an individual's needs, bearing in mind their age, gender, and social conditions, and the site(s) and severity of the lesions.[11] Extensive patient education about the skin disorder is paramount at the onset. Successful treatment of AD requires a systematic, multipronged approach that incorporates (1) skin hydration, (2) the identification and elimination of flare factors such as irritants, allergens, infectious agents, and emotional stressors, and (3) topical and systemic therapy.

Patients with AD may be more susceptible to irritants than normal individuals. Reducing or eliminating exposure to or contact with trigger factors (soaps, cigarette smoke, animal dander, molds, pollens, etc.) is crucial. Laundering all new clothing with liquid detergent and a second rinse cycle prior to wearing them decreases potential exposure to allergens and other irritating substances. Placing a humidifier in the patient's room and having the patient wear cotton clothing reduces itching. Normal activities are encouraged. Swimming is better tolerated than sports that cause intense perspiration. After swimming, the patient should immediately rinse the chlorine off and lubricate the skin. Ultraviolet light may be beneficial to some patients with AD, but nonirritating sunscreens should be used to avoid sunburn.

Errors in bathing and moisturizing are by far the most common factors in persistent AD. Some dermatologists oppose daily bathing because it dries the skin, causing microfissures and cracks that serve as portals of entry for skin pathogens, irritants, and allergens. In contrast, other dermatologists claim that "appropriate" bathing in AD sufferers hydrates the stratum corneum, removes allergens and irritants, cleanses and debrides crusts, and enhances the effects of moisturizers and topical steroids.[12] The answer to the apparent paradox is that bathing hydrates the skin as long as an effective moisturizer is applied within 3 minutes to prevent evaporation from the stratum corneum. When evaporation occurs, this barrier dries and cracks. Patients should bathe for only 3 to 5 minutes using nonperfumed bath oils to soothe the skin, or else dehydration of the skin occurs. Common bar soaps are often too drying and irritating for some AD patients.[13] Preferred frequency of bathing is every other day (to minimize removal of natural oils), with tepid rather than hot water. Because of the significant drying effect of most soaps, mild nonsoap cleansers (e.g., Cetaphil) are recommended.

After bathing, moisturizers can be applied and excessively dry areas of skin covered with a lubricating ointment. Topical corticosteroids can be applied to any inflamed areas.

Treatment of acute weeping or oozing lesions is directed toward drying the lesions. Wet compresses using tap water should be applied for 20 minutes, four to six times daily. Bathing with tepid water containing colloidal oatmeal may also be soothing.

**Exclusions for Self-Treatment**

- Severe condition with intense pruritis
- Involvement of large area of body
- <2 years of age
- Skin appears to be infected

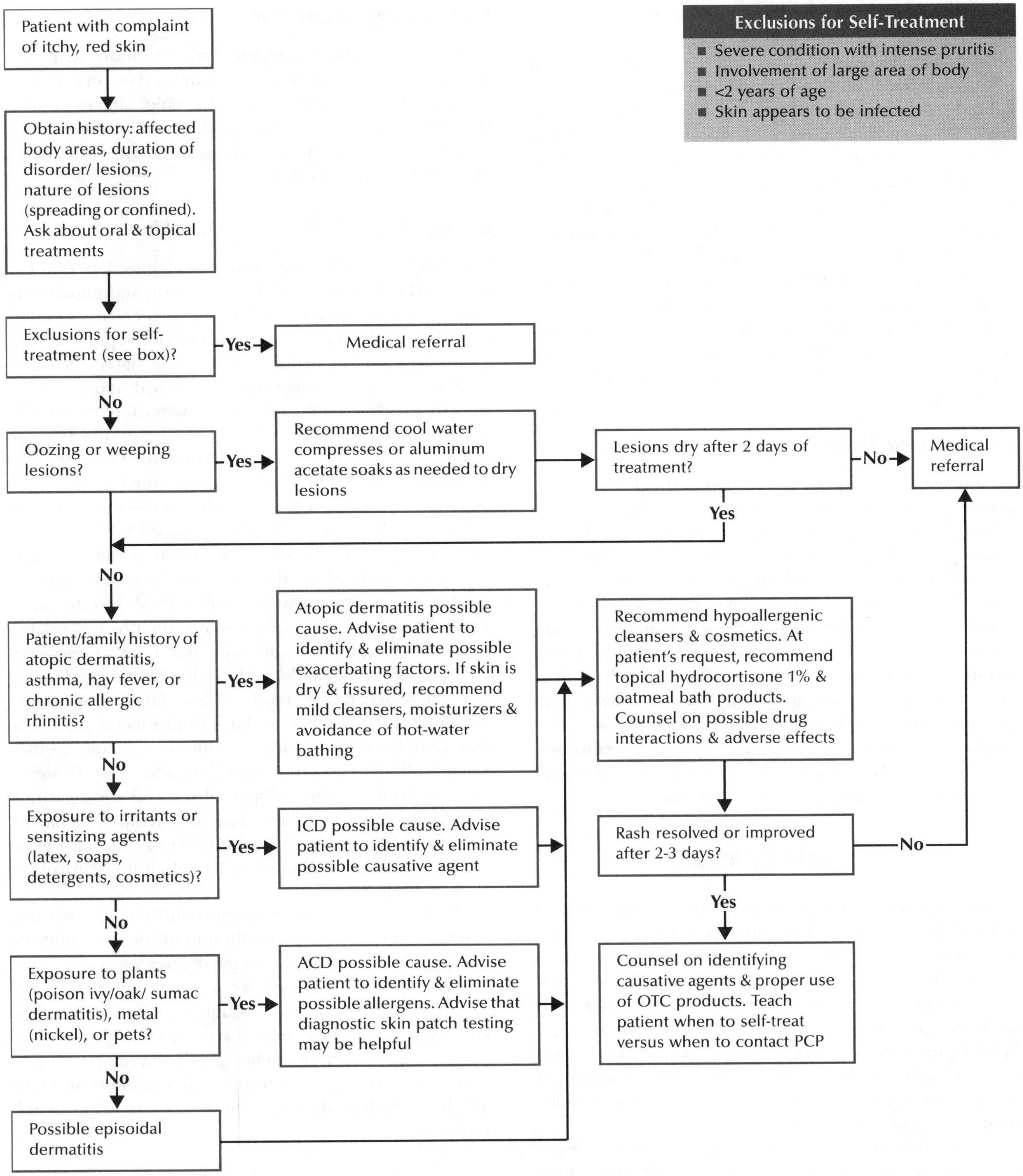


**FIGURE 33-2** Self-care of dermatitis. Key: ACD, allergic contact dermatitis; ICD, irritant contact dermatitis; OTC, over-the-counter; PCP, primary care provider.

For itching, simply telling a patient not to scratch is generally ineffective. Therefore, adjunctive measures may be used to minimize scratching and the damage it produces. Fingernails should be kept short, smooth, and clean. Because scratching may increase at night, even while the patient is sleeping, wearing cotton gloves or socks on the hands at night may lessen scratching. Patients should avoid occlusive, tight clothing. If possible, patients should remain in moderate temperature settings and moderate relative humidity conditions.

Treatment of chronic lesions focuses on measures to maintain skin hydration and decrease itching. A water-miscible bath oil may be added to the water near the end of the bath. The skin should be patted dry gently; vigorous rubbing produces irritation. An emollient should be applied within 3 minutes while the skin is still damp. Although ointments with a petrolatum or water-in-oil base maintain hydration best, sweating after the application of heavy ointments may add to the propensity for itching. Patients should be instructed to rub a very small amount of ointment into the affected area very well. Oil-in-water preparations (creams and lotions) are often more cosmetically acceptable, but they may need to be applied more frequently than ointments as their ability to maintain moisture in the skin is often more short-lived. If applied correctly, they should have a good emollient effect and not produce dryness.

#### *Pharmacologic Therapy*

Hydrocortisone in an oil-in-water base is the primary pharmacologic nonprescription agent used to treat AD. Although these preparations may be used to dry weeping lesions, they are primarily indicated to relieve itching.

Magnesium ions inhibit the antigen-presenting function of skin cells and thereby may decrease cutaneous irritation and inflammation.[14] Topical magnesium salts (chloride and sulfate) are, therefore, used as nonprescription products to provide anti-inflammatory benefit in dermatoses that include psoriasis and AD. Several products (shampoo and topical cream as well as bathing salts) that contain salt from the Dead Sea (46% magnesium chloride) have been used to manage these dermatoses, although there is little evidence to support their use.

## DRY SKIN (XEROSIS)

Xerosis, or dry skin, is the result of decreased water content of the skin with resulting abnormal loss of cells from the stratum corneum. Normal stratum corneum requires a 10% or higher water content. In low humidity, water lost through evaporation must be replenished by water from the lower epidermal and dermal layers. Three intercellular lipids (sphingolipids, free sterols, and free fatty acids) play a key role in barrier function and are essential to trap water and prevent excessive water loss. Most xerosis is either undertreated or ignored as a cause of the patient's problem.

Environmental dry skin is usually associated with the patient's taking long, hot showers or not consuming enough water. The prevention and care of dry skin may become a major focus for practitioners as the population of persons of advanced age continues to increase. There is a heightened awareness among those caring for persons of advanced age that prophylactic dry skin care can reduce morbidity by minimizing the risk of skin breakdown, and thus can ultimately reduce the cost of dermatologic health care.[15]

### Epidemiology of Dry Skin

Xerosis is a common problem, affecting more than 50% of older adults, and is the most common cause of pruritus.[6] It is a frequent cause of pruritus in cooler climates during the winter season (i.e., "winter itch"). Individuals who live or work in arid, windy, or cold environments also have an increased risk for dry skin.

### Etiology/Pathophysiology of Dry Skin

Dry skin can result from various etiologies. Dry skin can be caused by disruption of keratinization and impairment of water-binding properties.[16] It may also occur secondary to prolonged detergent use, malnutrition, or physical damage to the stratum corneum. It may also signal a systemic disorder such as hypothyroidism or dehydration.

Dry skin is related to decreased water retention in the stratum corneum, not a lack of natural skin oils. Dry skin pathophysiology, therefore, can be described by examining the factors involved in skin hydration. One major factor is frequent or prolonged bathing or showering with hot water, as well as excessive use of soap, both of which increase dryness of the skin. Soap removes the skin's natural oils, and the short duration of contact with water is usually insufficient to hydrate dry skin. A second factor relates to environmental conditions, such as low relative humidity. Dry air allows the outer skin layer to lose moisture, become less flexible, and crack when flexed, leading to an increased rate of moisture loss. High wind velocity also causes moisture loss in skin. A third factor is physical damage to the stratum corneum, such as a leg ulcer, which dramatically increases transepidermal water loss. However, after the insult is removed, partial recovery occurs within 1 or 2 days with the formation of a temporary barrier consisting of incompletely keratinized cells. The maximum barrier effect is restored in 2 to 3 weeks if the skin barrier is not severely disrupted.

With advancing age, the epidermis changes because of abnormal maturation or adhesion of the keratinocytes, resulting in a superficial, irregular layer of corneocytes. This condition may be described as a thinning of the entire epidermis, which produces a roughened skin surface. The skin's hygroscopic substances also decrease in quantity with advancing age. Hormonal changes that accompany aging result in lowered sebum output. Older patients also typically have inadequate water intake, contributing to this condition.

### Signs and Symptoms of Dry Skin

Xerosis is characterized by one or more of the following signs and symptoms: roughness, scaling, loss of flexibility, fissures, inflammation, and pruritus. Clinically fine plate-like scaling particularly on the arms and legs that may be associated with a "cracked" appearance (eczema craquelé) or fish scaling (ichthyosis) appearance of the skin is common.

**TABLE 33-3 Dry Skin Therapy**

- Tub baths 2-3 times per week, with bath oil for brief periods (3-5 minutes). Sponge bath on other days.
- The water should be tepid, not more than 3°F above body temperature.
- Stay in water only 3-5 minutes.
- Within 3 minutes of getting out of the tub, pat the body dry, leaving beads of moisture, and generously apply body lotion to trap in the moisture.
- Apply the body lotion at least three more times during the day to (preferably) the whole body or at least the most affected areas.
- In addition:
  - Use only corticosteroid ointments rather than creams.
  - Keep room humidity higher.

## Treatment Overview of Dry Skin

### *Treatment Goals*

The goals of self-treatment of dry skin are to (1) restore skin hydration, (2) restore the skin's barrier function, and (3) educate the patient about this chronic condition

### *General Treatment Approach*

Treatment involves recognizing the problem as well as modifying the environment (humidity) and bathing habits to maintain skin hydration. Nonprescription products such as bath oils, emollients/moisturizers, humectants, and keratolytic agents also aid in restoring and maintaining barrier function. If needed, topical hydrocortisone can be used to reduce pruritus and erythema. Dry skin responds minimally to topical corticosteroid therapy, although short-term use of topical corticosteroids may reduce symptoms of erythema and pruritus.[17,18]

### *Nonpharmacologic Therapy*

The most important aspects of care are the proper use of emollients and modifications to bathing practices. Products such as oilated oatmeal or bath oil added near the end of the bath may be used to enhance skin hydration. The patient should apply oil-based emollients immediately after bathing while the skin is damp and should reapply them frequently. The room humidity should be increased with a humidifier or even a vaporizer. The patient, if medical conditions allow, should be encouraged to drink at least six 8-oz glasses of water daily. Table 33-3 reviews nonpharmacologic therapy of dry skin.

### *Pharmacologic Therapy*

More severe cases of dry skin may require a urea-containing or lactic acid–containing product to enhance hydration. The patient may apply topical hydrocortisone ointment on a short-term basis (no longer than 7 days) to reduce inflammation and itching. If resolution does not occur within 1 or 2 weeks, a primary care provider should be consulted as higher potency corticosteroid products (such as betamethasone or halobetasol) or one of the new immunomodulatory agents (such as pimecrolimus or tacrolimus), may be required to control the skin disorder.[5] Dry skin is more prone to itching, inflammation, and development of secondary infections. Most moisturizers are mixtures of oils and water. Moisturizers containing ammonium lactate 12% have improved the appearance of skin covered with cracks and fissures.[19] $\alpha$-Hydroxy acids (AHAs) and related compounds have been shown to normalize keratinization and to result in more normal stratum corneum.[16] Indications for using AHA products include treatment of xerosis (dry skin), melasma, acne, and photoaging. The emergence of such products allows the practitioner to choose from a vast array of nonprescription products.

# TREATMENT OF ATOPIC DERMATITIS AND DRY SKIN

Nonprescription products for dermatitis and dry skin that restore skin hydration include bath products, emollients, hydrating agents, and keratin-softening agents (Table 33-4). Astringents, antipruritics, protectants, and hydrocortisone are used to relieve weeping and/or itching of lesions and to protect the affected area.

## Bath Products

### *Bath Oils*

Bath oils generally consist of a mineral or vegetable oil, plus a surfactant. Mineral oil products are adsorbed better than vegetable oil products. Adsorption onto and absorption into the skin increase as temperature and oil concentration increase. Bath oils are minimally effective in improving a dry skin condition because they are greatly diluted in water. Their major effect is the slip or lubricity they impart to the skin, which may be important to the patient. When applied as wet compresses, however, bath oils (1 tsp in 1/4 cup of warm water) help lubricate dry skin and may allow a decrease in the frequency of full-body bathing.[5,18] Bath oils make the tub and floor slippery, creating a safety hazard, especially for patients of advanced age or children. They also make cleansing the skin with soaps more difficult.

### *Oatmeal Products*

Colloidal oatmeal bath products contain starch, protein, and a small amount of oil. They are less effective than bath oils; however, oilated oatmeal products combine the effect of oatmeal and a bath oil. Although evidence-based efficacy is minimal, colloidal oatmeal is claimed to be soothing and antipruritic, and it does have a lubricating effect.

### *Cleansers*

Typical bath soaps generally contain salts of long-chain fatty acids (commonly oleic, palmitic, or stearic acid) and alkali metals (e.g., sodium or potassium). Combined with

**TABLE 33-4 Selected Dry Skin Products**

| Trade Name | Primary Ingredients |
|---|---|
| Absorbase Ointment* | Petrolatum; mineral oil; ceresin wax; wool wax alcohol; potassium sorbate |
| Alpha Keri Moisture Rich Cleansing Bar | Mineral oil; lanolin oil; glycerin |
| AmLactin Cream/Lotion | Ammonium lactate 12% |
| Aquaphor Ointment | Petrolatum 41%; water |
| Aveeno Cleansing Bar* | Disodium lauryl sulfosuccinate; cetyl alcohol; wheat starch; paraffin |
| Aveeno Daily Moisturizing Lotion* | Dimethicone 1.25%; cetyl alcohol; oat kernel flour; glycerin |
| Aveeno Moisturizing Bath Treatment Formula* | Mineral oil; colloidal oatmeal 43% |
| Aveeno Moisturizing Cream/Lotion* | Petrolatum; dimethicone; isopropyl palmitate; cetyl alcohol; colloidal oatmeal 1%; glycerin |
| Aveeno Skin Relief Moisturizing Lotion* | Dimethicone 1.25%; menthol 0.1%; oat kernel flour |
| Aveeno Soothing Bath Treatment Formula* | Colloidal oatmeal 100% |
| Carmol 10 Lotion | Urea 10% |
| Carmol 20 Cream | Urea 20% |
| Cetaphil Gentle Cleansing Bar* | Sodium cocoyl isethionate; stearic acid; sodium tallousate; PEG-20; petrolatum |
| Cetaphil Gentle Skin Cleanser Liquid* | Cetyl alcohol; stearyl alcohol; PEG |
| Corn Huskers Lotion | Glycerin 6.7%; SD alcohol 40, 5.7%; algin; guar gum |
| Curél Ultra Healing Lotion | Petrolatum; dimethicone; isopropyl palmitate; glycerin |
| Dermabase Cream | Mineral oil; petrolatum; cetostearyl alcohol; propylene glycol; sodium lauryl sulfate; isopropyl palmitate; imidazolidinyl urea |
| Eucerin Cream* | Petrolatum; mineral oil; mineral wax; wool wax alcohol |
| Jergens Advanced Therapy Ultra Healing Lotion | Petrolatum; mineral oil; dimethicone; cetearyl alcohol; cetyl alcohol; glycerin; allantoin |
| Keri Original Formula Therapeutic Dry Skin Lotion | Mineral oil; lanolin oil; glyceryl stearate; propylene glycol |
| Lac-Hydrin Five Lotion | Urea 5% |
| Lubriderm Advanced Therapy Lotion | Cetyl alcohol; glycerin; mineral oil; PEG-40; emulsifying wax; vitamin E |
| Lubriderm Bath and Shower Oil | Mineral oil |
| Lubriderm Daily Moisturizing Lotion | Mineral oil; petrolatum; sorbitol; lanolin; lanolin alcohol; triethanolamine |
| Moisturel Cream/Lotion* | Petrolatum; dimethicone; cetyl alcohol; glycerin |
| Neutrogena Body Oil | Isopropyl myristate; sesame oil |
| Neutrogena Norwegian Formula Body Moisturizing Lotion* | Glycerin; distearyldimonium chloride; petrolatum; cetyl alcohol; dimethicone; colloidal oatmeal |
| Neutrogena Norwegian Formula Hand Cream | Glycerin 41% |
| Neutrogena Soap | TEA-stearate; triethanolamine; glycerin |
| Nivea Body Lotion | Mineral oil; glycerin isopropyl palmitate; vitamin E; lanolin alcohol |
| Purpose Gentle Cleansing Bar | Sodium tallowate; sodium cocoate; glycerin; BHT |
| Sardo Bath Oil | Mineral oil; isopropyl palmitate |
| Sarna Anti-Itch Lotion | Camphor 0.5%; menthol 0.5%; carbomer 940; cetyl alcohol; DMDM hydantoin, glyceryl stearate; petrolatum |
| Vaseline Dermatology Formula Lotion | White petrolatum 5%; mineral oil 4%; dimethicone 1%; glyceryl stearate; cetyl alcohol; glycerin |

* Fragrance-free.

water, such products act as surfactants that will remove many substances from the skin, including the lipids that normally keep the skin soft and pliable. Some authorities recommend special soaps that contain extra oils to minimize the drying effect of washing. However, these soaps usually lather and clean poorly.

Glycerin soaps, which are transparent and more water soluble, have a higher oil content than standard toilet soaps because of the addition of castor oil. They are closer to a neutral pH and are, therefore, regarded as less drying than soaps, which are alkaline. Although little objective proof exists to prove their superiority, glycerin soaps are advertised for, and well accepted by, people with skin conditions.

Practitioners may choose to recommend mild cleansers such as Cetaphil or pHisoDerm, if soap is to be avoided. Most of these products consist primarily of surfactants and may contain oil. Although these products claim to have a low potential for irritation, clear evidence of their superiority over soaps is lacking. On application, they foam mildly, and on gentle wiping, they leave a thin layer of lipid material on the skin, which helps retain water in the stratum corneum. Leave-on, no-rinse skin cleansers are a useful tool to minimize the skin barrier disruption seen with traditional soaps and body bathing.

### *Emollients/Moisturizers*

Emollients function by filling the spaces between the desquamating skin scales with oil droplets, but their effect is only temporary. Many terms are used to describe the effects of creams and lotions such as lubricants (i.e., products that increase skin slip in dry skin), moisturizers (i.e., products imparting moisture to the skin, increasing skin flexibility), repair or replenishing products (i.e., intended to reverse the appearance of aging skin), emollients, and so forth.

Most moisturizers consist of the following:

- Water (60% to 80%), which functions as a diluent and evaporates, leaving behind the active agents
- Lipids (essential fatty acids)
- Emulsifiers, which keep water and lipids in one continuous phase
- Humectants, which help skin retain water
- Preservatives
- Fragrance (or may be fragrance-free)
- Color
- Specialty additives, such as (1) vitamins (vitamin A, C, D, and B complex), which have no effect, and (2) natural moisturizing factors (NMF), a group of substances (e.g., lactate, urea, ammonia, uric acid, glucosamine) reported to regulate the moisture content of the stratum corneum.

Facial moisturizers are either oil-in-water emulsions or water-in-oil emulsions. The differences between moisturizer products are caused by the addition of fragrances, exotic oils, vitamins, protein or amino acid products, and other minor moisturizing aids. The selection of an appropriate facial moisturizer depends on skin type. Oily complexion products are oil-free or contain small amounts of light oils (mineral oil) with silicone derivatives and talc, clay, starch, or synthetic polymers (oil control). Normal skin products contain predominantly water, mineral oil, and propylene glycol with very small amounts of petrolatum or lanolin. These leave an oilier residue on the face than oil-free formulations. Dry skin products contain water, mineral oil, propylene glycol, and larger amounts of petrolatum or lanolin.[20]

Body moisturizers come in lotion, cream, and ointment. Lotions are the most popular. Creams and ointments are more difficult to spread, especially in hair-bearing areas. Body lotions are generally oil-in-water emulsions containing 10% to 15% oil phase, 5% to 10% humectant, and 75% to 85% water phase.

Hand moisturizers are much heavier than body or facial emollients. The simplest and most economical hand ointment is petroleum jelly. Although it is greasy, which leads to poor compliance, it is effective when applied correctly. Hand creams are nongreasy oil-in-water emulsions with 15% to 40% oil phase, 5% to 15% humectant, and 45% to 80% water phase. Adding silicone derivatives renders hand cream water-resistant through four to six washings.

Because sebum and skin surface lipids contain a relatively high concentration of fatty acid glycerides, vegetable and animal oils derived from avocado, cucumber, mink, peanut, safflower, sesame, turtle, and shark liver are included in dry skin products, presumably because of their unsaturated fatty acid content. However, although use of such oils contributes to skin flexibility and lubricity, their occlusive effect is less than that of white petrolatum.

#### Mechanism of Action

Emollients are occlusive agents and moisturizers that are used to prevent or relieve the signs and symptoms of dry skin. Such products act primarily by leaving an oily film on the skin surface through which moisture cannot readily escape.

Cosmetically, emollients make the skin feel soft and smooth by helping to reestablish the integrity of the stratum corneum. Lipid components make the scales on the skin translucent and flatten them against the underlying skin. This flattening eliminates air between the scales and the skin surface, which is partly responsible for a white, scaly appearance.[15]

#### Dosage and Administration Guidelines

Some clinicians believe that minimizing transepidermal water loss is not enough to maintain adequate hydration. Therefore, a patient may be advised to hydrate the skin by soaking the affected area in water for 5 to 10 minutes, patting it dry, and applying an occlusive agent (within 3 minutes) while the skin is still damp. In this way, moisture is retained more adequately in the skin.

Frequency of application depends on the severity of the dry skin condition, as well as on the hydration efficiency of the occlusive agent. Generally, moisturizers must be applied three to four times daily to achieve maximum benefit. For dry hands, the patient may need to apply the occlusive agent after each hand washing, as well as at numerous other times during the day.

#### Dosage Forms

Emollient products are available as ointments containing petrolatum that are typically very greasy and generally lack consumer appeal because of their texture, difficulty of spreading and removing, and staining properties. To avoid a greasy feel, patients should be advised to gently warm the product in the hands, apply a very thin layer, and massage it into the skin gently, but well. Ointments are inappropriate for an oozing AD, as they do not allow the lesions to dry and ultimately heal.

Lotions and creams are either water-in-oil or oil-in-water emulsions. For non-oozing AD/dry skin, the higher the lipid content, the greater the occlusive effect. In most cases, patients prefer the less effective but more esthetic oil-in-water emulsions for their cosmetic acceptability. Such agents help alleviate the pruritus associated with dry skin by virtue of their cooling effect as water evaporates from the skin surface. Moreover, enough oil exists in most oil-in-water emulsions to form a continuous occlusive film.[5,15]

### Safety Considerations

Lanolin, a natural product derived from sheep wool, is found in many nonprescription moisturizing products. Rarely, patients develop an allergic reaction to this substance presumably because its wool wax fraction is recognized as antigenic. Patients with a previous history of allergic reactions to lanolin should generally avoid lanolin-containing products. However, products containing refined lanolin are generally less likely to be sensitizing and may even be tolerated by those with a history of allergic contact reactions to unrefined lanolin.

Although most commercial formulations generally are bland, contact with the eye or with broken or abraded skin should be avoided because formulation ingredients may cause irritation. This irritation is especially true with emulsion systems because the surfactants in them denature protein and may thus produce further irritation.

Petrolatum should not be applied over puncture wounds, infections, or lacerations because its high occlusive ability may lead to maceration and further inflammation. Application of petrolatum to intertriginous areas, mucous membranes, and acne-prone areas should be minimized as it is tolerated only when the concentration of petrolatum in the preparation is low.

#### *Humectants*

Humectants or hydrating agents are hygroscopic materials that may be added to an emollient base. Commonly used hydrating agents are glycerin, propylene glycol, and phospholipids.

Humectants draw water into the stratum corneum to hydrate the skin. Water may come from the dermis or from the atmosphere. However, high relative humidity (80% or greater) is necessary for the latter to occur. Humectants are distinct from emollients, which serve to retain water already present.

Because of glycerin's hygroscopic properties, high concentrations may actually increase water loss by drawing water from the skin rather than from the atmosphere. At lower concentrations (i.e., 5%), however, humectants such as glycerin help decrease water loss by keeping water in close contact with skin and accelerating moisture diffusion from the dermis to the epidermis. In addition, glycerin lubricates the skin surface.

Propylene glycol is a viscous, colorless, odorless solvent with hygroscopic properties. It is less viscous than glycerin and is included in many skin care formulations for its humectant action. However, it can cause skin irritation, usually on a concentration-dependent basis. Phospholipid products contain lecithin, a water-binding compound normally present in the skin. Each phospholipid molecule can complex with up to 15 molecules of water.

#### *Urea*

Urea in concentrations of 10% to 30% is mildly keratolytic and increases water uptake in the stratum corneum, giving it a high water-binding capacity. Urea has a direct effect on stratum corneum elasticity because of its ability to bind to skin protein. It is considered safe and has been recommended for use on crusted, necrotic tissue. Concentrations of 10% have been used on simple dry skin; 20% to 30% formulations have been used for treating more resistant dry skin conditions. Lotion and cream formulations containing urea may better help remove scales and crusts, whereas urea in emollient ointments (e.g., urea in a hydrophilic ointment base) may be better at rehydrating the skin. However, urea preparations can cause stinging, burning, and irritation, particularly on broken skin.[19]

#### *Lactic Acid/α-Hydroxy Acids*

Lactic acid is an α-hydroxy acid that has been useful in concentrations of 2% to 5% for treating dry skin conditions. Lactic acid increases the hydration of human skin and may act as a modulator of epidermal keratinization rather than a keratolytic agent at low concentrations. Lactic acid may be added to urea preparations for both its stabilizing and its hydrating effects.

Other α-hydroxy acids, derived from fruits, are used for a number of common skin conditions such as dry skin, acne, melasma, and photoaging (see Chapter 40). Such acids include malic acid (in apples), citric acid (in oranges and lemons), tartaric acid (in grapes), and glycolic and gluconic acids (in sugar cane).[21]

#### *Allantoin*

Allantoin and allantoin complexes soften keratin by disrupting its structure. A product of purine metabolism, allantoin is considered to be a relatively safe compound. However, it is less effective than urea. The Food and Drug Administration (FDA) classifies allantoin as a Category I (safe and effective for nonprescription use) skin protectant for adults, children, and infants when applied in concentrations of 0.5% to 2.0%.[19]

#### *Astringents*

Astringents retard oozing, discharge, or bleeding of dermatitis when applied to unhealthy serous skin or mucous membranes. When applied as a wet dressing or compress, they cool and dry the skin through evaporation. They cause vasoconstriction and reduce blood flow in inflamed tissue. They also cleanse the skin of exudates, crust, and debris. Because they generally have a low cell penetrability, their activity is limited to the cell surface and interstitial spaces. The protein precipitate that forms may serve as a protective coat, allowing new tissues to grow underneath.[19]

FDA has identified two astringent solutions as Category 1: aluminum acetate (Burow's solution) and witch hazel (hamamelis water). Aluminum acetate solution USP contains approximately 5% aluminum acetate. The solution must be diluted 1:10 to 1:40 with water before use. It is commercially available in tablet or powder form. Witch hazel has been used for centuries as an astringent. A natural product prepared from the twigs of *Hamamelis virginiana*, it contains tannins, trace amounts of volatile oils (which give it a characteristic pleasant odor), and alcohol 14% to 15%, all of which contribute to its astringent activity. The product may be applied as often as necessary in the treatment of minor skin irritations. Numerous other ingredients, including alum and zinc oxide, have been promoted as astringents, but data demonstrating their safety and effectiveness are lacking.

The patient may soak the affected area two to four times daily for 15 to 30 minutes. Alternatively, the patient may loosely apply a compress of washcloths, cheesecloth, or small towels soaked in the solution and then wrung gently so they are wet but not dripping. The dressings should be rewetted and applied every few minutes for 20 to 30 minutes, four to six times daily. Less expensive alternatives to aluminum acetate include isotonic saline solution (1 tsp salt in 2 cups of water), tap water, diluted white vinegar (1/4 cup per pint of water), plain water.

### Topical Hydrocortisone

Hydrocortisone is currently the only corticosteroid available without a prescription for the topical treatment of dermatitis. Although its exact mechanism is unknown, it most likely suppresses cytokines associated with the development of inflammation and itching associated with various dermatoses. FDA monograph indications for its use include temporary relief of itching associated with minor skin irritations, inflammation, and rashes caused by dermatitis, seborrheic dermatitis, insect bites, poison ivy, poison oak, poison sumac, soaps, detergents, cosmetics, and jewelry. Concentrations of 0.5% to 1% are regarded as appropriate for treating localized dermatitis (Table 33-5).

**TABLE 33-5 Selected Dermatitis Products**

| Trade Name | Primary Ingredients |
|---|---|
| Cortaid Maximum Strength Ointment/Cream<br>Cortizone-10 Ointment | Hydrocortisone 1% |
| Cortaid Sensitive Skin Cream<br>Cortizone-5 Ointment | Hydrocortisone 0.5% |
| Cortizone-5 Cream | Hydrocortisone 0.5%; aluminum sulfate; calcium acetate |
| Cortizone-10 Cream | Hydrocortisone 1%; aluminum sulfate; calcium acetate |
| Lanacort-5 Cream/Ointment | Hydrocortisone 0.5%; aloe |

Hydrocortisone should be applied sparingly to the affected area three or four times a day. An ointment formulation generally provides the best results for chronic, non-oozing dermatoses. The drug should not be applied to infected skin as it may mask the symptoms of dermatologic infections and allow the infection to progress.

Topical hydrocortisone rarely produces systemic complications because systemic absorption is relatively minimal. Approximately 1% of hydrocortisone solution applied to normal skin on the forearm is absorbed systemically. Absorption increases in the presence of skin inflammation, with the use of occlusive dressings, or when the temperature of the skin is elevated. Certain local adverse effects such as skin atrophy may arise with prolonged use because collagen production is inhibited, which thereby weakens the skin's "infrastructure." In practice, however, clinically detectable atrophy rarely occurs with nonprescription concentrations; it is more common with the more potent prescription products. Because response to topical corticosteroids may decrease with continued use, intermittent courses of therapy are advised when possible.[5]

### Antipruritics

The itching associated with dermatitis may be mediated through several mechanisms, which may explain how three major classes of pharmacologic agents—local anesthetics, antihistamines, and corticosteroids (discussed previously)—are useful as antipruritics. Cooling the area through application of a soothing, bland lotion may reduce the extent of the pruritus, but this effect is only transitory.

The itching sensation is mediated by the same nerve fibers that carry pain impulses. Local anesthetics block conduction along axonal membranes, thereby relieving itching as well as pain. However, because local anesthetics may cause systemic side effects, they should not be used in large quantities or over long periods of time, particularly if the skin is raw or blistered. Nonprescription topical anesthetics that appear to be safe and effective are pramoxine, lidocaine, and benzocaine. Topical anesthetics may be applied to affected areas three or four times daily, but caution should be used as these agents may have a sensitizing effect in a small number of people. Counterirritants such as camphor and menthol, in concentrations of 0.5% to 1%, are available in or can also be added to lotions and creams to serve as an inexpensive antipruritic.[19]

Itching may also be mediated by various endogenous substances, including histamine. Accordingly, topical antihistamines such as diphenhydramine are effective in alleviating this symptom. Their activity stems from an ability to compete with histamine at $H_1$-receptor sites and to exert a topical anesthetic effect. Local anesthesia may be the more important mechanism of action because the cause of itching in many conditions (e.g., atopic dermatitis) is most likely cytokine release and may not be related to histamine release at all. Antihistamines are considered safe and effective for use as nonprescription external analgesics. However, because of their significant sensitizing potential, FDA does not recommend the topical use of such agents for more than 7 consecutive days except under the advice and supervision of a primary care provider.[22]

Oral antihistamines have been used to treat the itching of dermatologic disorders with variable results. Some researchers claim that the antipruritic effect is a result of the sedative side effect; others claim the efficacy is caused by antihistaminic activity, although with a delayed onset of several days. If histamine is involved, it has already reached and stimulated the receptor sites to produce itching, and the antihistamine requires a finite amount of time to displace it. In either case, central nervous system depression may be a problem, as may the anticholinergic side effects in patients with conditions such as prostatic hypertrophy or closed-angle glaucoma.[10]

### Product Selection Guidelines

When deciding which product to recommend for dermatitis or dry skin, the practitioner must evaluate the active ingredients and the vehicle. Primary active ingredients contained in nonprescription skin products are water and oil. However, a variety of secondary ingredients are added to enhance product elegance and stability, and many of them have the potential for producing contact dermatitis through either an irritant or a sensitizing effect. The agents may include the following:

- *Emulsifiers:* cholesterol, magnesium aluminum silicate, polyoxyethylene lauryl ether, polyoxyethylene monostearate, polyoxyethylene sorbitan monolaurate (Tween), propylene glycol monostearate, sodium borate plus fatty acid, sodium lauryl sulfate, sorbitan monopalmitate (Span), or triethanolamine plus fatty acid
- *Emulsion stabilizers (thickening agents):* carbomer, cetyl alcohol, glyceryl monostearate, methylcellulose, spermaceti, or stearyl alcohol
- *Preservatives*

The type of vehicle (e.g., ointment, cream, lotion, gel, solution, or aerosol) may have a significant effect on dermatitis. The following guidelines may be used to choose an appropriate vehicle:

1. *"If it's wet, dry it."* If a drying effect is desired, the practitioner may recommend solutions, gels, and occasionally creams. However, components of these systems may quickly diffuse into the underlying tissue and possibly cause irritation.
2. *"If it's dry, wet it."* If slight lubrication is needed, creams and lotions are be preferred. If the lesion is very dry and fissured, an ointment is the vehicle of choice. However, avoid use in intertriginous areas because of the potential for maceration. Also, in an acute process, the occlusive effects of an ointment may cause further irritation.

In recommending aerosols, gels, or lotions for dermatitis affecting a hair-covered area of the body, the practitioner must keep in mind that gels can be very drying when used for prolonged periods of time.

Numerous cosmetic dry skin formulations are available and may contain natural oils, vitamins, or fragrances that have psychologic appeal. However, the fragrances found in many formulations may be allergenic to sensitive, dry skin and should be avoided. Efficacy of any skin care product may need to be sacrificed or compromised somewhat to achieve patient acceptance. The practitioner should recommend the most efficacious product that the patient will accept.

**TABLE 33-6 Amount of Topical Medication Needed for Three Times Daily Application for 1 Week**

| Part of Body | Cream/ Ointment (g) | Lotion/Solution/ Gel (mL) |
|---|---|---|
| Face | 5-10 | 100-120 |
| Both hands | 25-50 | 200-240 |
| Scalp | 50-100 | 200-240 |
| Both arms or both legs | 100-200 | 240-360 |
| Trunk | 200 | 360-480 |
| Groin and genitalia | 15-25 | 120-180 |

*Source:* Adapted from Bingham EA. Topical dermatologic therapy. In: Rook A, Parish LC, Beare JM, eds. *Practical Management of the Dermatologic Patient*. Philadelphia: JB Lippincott; 1986: 2278.

Topical nonprescription products come in varying package sizes and strengths. Table 33-6 lists the amount of drug needed to cover a given area of the body three times daily over a 1-week period. By being aware of such details, the practitioner can serve the patient economically as well as therapeutically.

## ASSESSMENT OF ATOPIC DERMATITIS AND DRY SKIN: A CASE-BASED APPROACH

Initially, the signs and symptoms are similar for most forms of dermatitis. A diagnosis of atopic dermatitis is often made after excluding other dermatologic conditions such as contact dermatitis or scaly dermatoses. Because AD is primarily a disease of the young, patient age is important in assessment. The practitioner should determine whether the patient (or patient's family) has a history of atopic disorders. Inquiries should be made regarding onset and duration of the eruption, anatomic location, and distribution of the lesions (Table 33-1).

When recommending the use of an appropriate nonprescription product or referring the patient to a primary care provider, the practitioner must consider the cosmetic, psychologic, and work- or recreation-related aspects of a dermatologic disorder, in addition to the underlying pathology

Dry skin is typically visible, with roughness and scaling. Practitioners can question patients about their bathing habits, the soaps and detergents used, and any other medical condition that may predispose them to excessive dryness. Patients should note that changes in climate can also affect their skin, such as winter air drying the skin, even though it may be raining. Cases 33-1 and 33-2 give examples of the assessment of patients with atopic dermatitis and dry skin.

## CASE 33-1

| Relevant Evaluation Criteria | Scenario/Model Outcome |
|---|---|
| **Information Gathering** | |
| 1. Gather essential information about the patient's symptoms, including: | |
| a. description of symptom(s) (i.e., nature, onset, duration, severity, associated symptoms) | Patient has persistent itching in the flexural areas of the knees and elbows. The affected areas appear erythematous, excoriated, and lichenified, with fine scaling. |
| b. description of any factors that seem to precipitate, exacerbate, and/or relieve the patient's symptom(s) | Symptoms seem to worsen during the winter and summer months. Sweating seems to make condition worse. |
| c. description of the patient's efforts to relieve the symptoms | Washing with soap and water regularly after workouts and use of Jergens Lotion has not helped to date. |
| 2. Gather essential patient history information: | |
| a. patient's identity | Fred Meyers |
| b. patient's age, sex, height, and weight | 21 y/o M, 6'1", 200 lb |
| c. patient's occupation | College student |
| d. patient's dietary habits | Normal diet with occasional junk food |
| e. patient's sleep habits | Stays up late and sleeps in as allowed by his schedule |
| f. concurrent medical conditions, prescription and nonprescription medications, and dietary supplements | Claritin 10 mg once daily for relief of allergic rhinitis |
| g. allergies | House dust, cats, and grass pollen |
| h. history of other adverse reactions to medications | Experienced severe drowsiness when Benadryl was used in the past |
| i. other (describe)_______ | The patient had atopic dermatitis rashes as a child. |
| **Assessment and Triage** | |
| 3. Differentiate the patient's signs/symptoms and correctly identify the patient's primary problem(s). | The patient has atopic dermatitis that may be exacerbated by sweating and allergens. |
| 4. Identify exclusions for self-treatment (see Figure 33-2). | None |
| 5. Formulate a comprehensive list of therapeutic alternatives for the primary problem to determine if triage to a medical practitioner is required, and share this information with the patient. | Options include:<br>(1) Refer Fred to a PCP or dermatologist.<br>(2) Recommend an appropriate OTC product with nondrug measures.<br>(3) Recommend an appropriate OTC product until Fred can be seen by a PCP or dermatologist.<br>(4) Take no action. |
| **Plan** | |
| 6. Select an optimal therapeutic alternative to address the patient's problem, taking into account patient preferences. | See Figure 33-2. A hydrocortisone 1% cream will be appropriate for Fred to use in an effort to stop the itch-scratch cycle. An ointment base should be used if the skin is especially dry, but the patient may prefer the cream base. The number and length of hot showers should be minimized and moisturizer should be applied frequently. |
| 7. Describe the recommended therapeutic approach to the patient. | See the box Patient Education for Atopic Dermatitis and Dry Skin. Apply the hydrocortisone cream three to four times daily for 7 days. You should avoid scratching the affected areas and avoid practices that promote drying of the skin. |

## CASE 33-1 (continued)

| Relevant Evaluation Criteria | Scenario/Model Outcome |
|---|---|
| 8. Explain to the patient the rationale for selecting the recommended therapeutic approach from the considered therapeutic alternatives. | It is not necessary that you see your PCP, that is, primary care provider, because the rash is relatively minor. The rash and itching should respond to the suggested drug and nondrug therapy. A medical referral may be necessary if the rash does not respond, if any signs of a skin infection develop, or if exacerbations of the condition become more frequent. |
| **Patient Education** | |
| 9. When recommending self-care with nonprescription medications and/or nondrug therapy, convey accurate information to the patient, including: | |
| a. appropriate dose and frequency of administration | See the box Patient Education for Atopic Dermatitis and Dry Skin. |
| b. maximum number of days the therapy should be employed | See the box Patient Education for Atopic Dermatitis and Dry Skin. |
| c. product administration procedures | See the box Patient Education for Atopic Dermatitis and Dry Skin. |
| d. expected time to onset of relief | See the box Patient Education for Atopic Dermatitis and Dry Skin. |
| e. degree of relief that can be reasonably expected | See the box Patient Education for Atopic Dermatitis and Dry Skin. |
| f. most common side effects | See the box Patient Education for Atopic Dermatitis and Dry Skin. |
| g. side effects that warrant medical intervention should they occur | See the box Patient Education for Atopic Dermatitis and Dry Skin. |
| h. patient options in the event that condition worsens or persists | A PCP or dermatologist should be consulted if the rash does not improve or if irritation is intolerable after 7-10 days. |
| i. product storage requirements | See the box Patient Education for Atopic Dermatitis and Dry Skin. |
| j. specific nondrug measures | See the box Patient Education for Atopic Dermatitis and Dry Skin. |
| 10. Solicit patient's follow-up questions. | Will Claritin help with the itching? |
| 11. Answer patient's questions. | No. It is unlikely Claritin will help with your skin symptoms as the itching is not related to histamine release. You should, however, continue to take Claritin if you have been experiencing symptoms of allergic rhinitis. |

Key: OTC, over-the-counter; PCP, primary care provider.

## CASE 33-2

| Relevant Evaluation Criteria | Scenario/Model Outcome |
|---|---|
| **Information Gathering** | |
| 1. Gather essential information about the patient's symptoms, including: | |
| a. description of symptom(s) (i.e., nature, onset, duration, severity, associated symptoms) | Patient has pruritic, fine, scaly skin on the exterior surfaces of her arms and lower legs. Physical observation reveals no evidence of weeping, vesicles, or crusting. |

## CASE 33-2 (continued)

| Relevant Evaluation Criteria | Scenario/Model Outcome |
|---|---|
| b. description of any factors that seem to precipitate, exacerbate, and/or relieve the patient's symptom(s) | Symptoms are more bothersome in the winter months. |
| c. description of the patient's efforts to relieve the symptoms | Use of a generic dry skin lotion product on a daily basis only alleviates symptoms briefly. |
| 2. Gather essential patient history information: | |
| a. patient's identity | Sara Lacy |
| b. patient's age, sex, height, and weight | 75 y/o F, 5'1", 115 lb |
| c. patient's occupation | Retired school teacher |
| d. patient's dietary habits | Normal healthy diet |
| e. patient's sleep habits | 7-8 hours of sleep per night |
| f. concurrent medical conditions, prescription and nonprescription medications, and dietary supplements | HCTZ 25 mg once daily and lisinopril 20 mg once daily for HTN; Zantac 75 mg once daily for dyspepsia; Os-Cal D 500 mg 3 times/day and risedronate 35 mg once a week for osteoporosis |
| g. allergies | Penicillin (rash) |
| h. history of other adverse reactions to medications | GI upset with use of NSAIDs resulted in use of Zantac on a daily basis. |
| i. other (describe)_______ | Sara takes long hot showers in the winter to warm her. She lives in Madison, Wisconsin, and says she does not have a humidifier in her apartment. |
| **Assessment and Triage** | |
| 3. Differentiate the patient's signs/symptoms and correctly identify the patient's primary problem(s). | Sara has dry skin most likely caused by environmental factors combined with her advancing age. |
| 4. Identify exclusions for self-treatment (see Figure 33-2). | None |
| 5. Formulate a comprehensive list of therapeutic alternatives for the primary problem to determine if triage to a medical practitioner is required, and share this information with the patient. | Options include:<br>(1) Refer Sara to a PCP or dermatologist.<br>(2) Recommend an appropriate OTC product with nondrug measures.<br>(3) Recommend an appropriate OTC product for use until Sara can be seen by a PCP.<br>(4) Take no action. |
| **Plan** | |
| 6. Select an optimal therapeutic alternative to address the patient's problem, taking into account patient preferences. | OTC treatment with moisturizing cream will be appropriate for this patient. Use of a store brand or generic formulation is preferred by the patient because of limited resources. See Table 33-3. |
| 7. Describe the recommended therapeutic approach to the patient. | See Table 33-3 and the box Patient Education for Atopic Dermatitis and Dry Skin. |
| 8. Explain to the patient the rationale for selecting the recommended therapeutic approach from the considered therapeutic alternatives. | Your condition should be easily managed with nonprescription topical therapy plus modification of your bathing habits. |
| **Patient Education** | |
| 9. When recommending self-care with nonprescription medications and/or nondrug therapy, convey accurate information to the patient, including: | |

## CASE 33-2 (continued)

| Relevant Evaluation Criteria | Scenario/Model Outcome |
|---|---|
| a. appropriate dose and frequency of administration | See the box Patient Education for Atopic Dermatitis and Dry Skin. |
| b. maximum number of days the therapy should be employed | See the box Patient Education for Atopic Dermatitis and Dry Skin. |
| c. product administration procedures | See the box Patient Education for Atopic Dermatitis and Dry Skin. |
| d. expected time to onset of relief | See the box Patient Education for Atopic Dermatitis and Dry Skin. |
| e. degree of relief that can be reasonably expected | See the box Patient Education for Atopic Dermatitis and Dry Skin. |
| f. most common side effects | See the box Patient Education for Atopic Dermatitis and Dry Skin. |
| g. side effects that warrant medical intervention should they occur | See the box Patient Education for Atopic Dermatitis and Dry Skin. |
| h. patient options in the event that condition worsens or persists | See the box Patient Education for Atopic Dermatitis and Dry Skin. |
| i. product storage requirements | See the box Patient Education for Atopic Dermatitis and Dry Skin. |
| j. specific nondrug measures | See the box Patient Education for Atopic Dermatitis and Dry Skin. |
| 10. Solicit patient's follow-up questions. | Will putting Vaseline on my arms and legs at bedtime produce better results than using a cream? |
| 11. Answer patient's questions. | Yes, most likely. Ointments, such as Vaseline, do a better job of holding moisture in the skin than do creams or lotions. You will need to wear cotton pajamas to prevent staining your bed linens. |

Key: GI, gastrointestinal; HCTZ, hydrochlorothiazide; HTN, hypertension; NSAID, nonsteroidal anti-inflammatory drug; OTC, over-the-counter; PCP, primary care provider.

## PATIENT COUNSELING FOR ATOPIC DERMATITIS AND DRY SKIN

Patients with atopic dermatitis should be educated on achieving control of their disease with proper information on the chronic nature of the disease, exacerbating factors, and appropriate treatment options.

Patients with dry skin should be informed that they have more control over mild to moderate forms of this disorder than most other types of dermatologic disorders. The practitioner should also explain factors that cause dry skin and the appropriate measures for restoring barrier function. The box Patient Education for Atopic Dermatitis and Dry Skin lists specific information to provide patients.

## EVALUATION OF PATIENT OUTCOMES FOR ATOPIC DERMATITIS AND DRY SKIN

The practitioner should reevaluate a patient with atopic dermatitis within 2 to 3 days of the patient's initial visit. A patient with dry skin should be reevaluated in 7 days.

Visual assessment is the best method of determining treatment response. Therefore, a scheduled visit is the preferred follow-up method. If the symptoms have not improved or have worsened (continued or additional itching, redness, scaling, lesions, or tissue breakdown), the patient should see a primary care provider.

## KEY POINTS FOR ATOPIC DERMATITIS AND DRY SKIN

- Note that most patients with mild to moderate atopic dermatitis or dry skin are candidates for self-treatment with a combination of nonprescription and nonpharmacologic therapies.
- Refer patients with yellow, crusting, eczematous atopic dermatitis lesions and all children younger than 2 years with atopic dermatitis to a primary care provider or dermatologist for evaluation and treatment.
- Question patients presenting with dry or eczematous skin lesions about exposure to soaps, detergents, fragrances, chemicals, irritants, changes in temperature, allergens, and bathing.
- Counsel patients with dry skin conditions to take brief baths, using tepid water, and apply moisturizers within 3 minutes of completing the bath or shower.
- Advise patients to use mild skin cleansers, to avoid products with fragrances or other potential irritants, and to apply copious quantities of moisturizers three to four times daily.
- Educate the patient with chronic dry skin conditions about the importance of stopping the itch-scratch cycle, maintaining adequate hydration, and avoiding triggers of the condition.

## PATIENT EDUCATION FOR ATOPIC DERMATITIS AND DRY SKIN

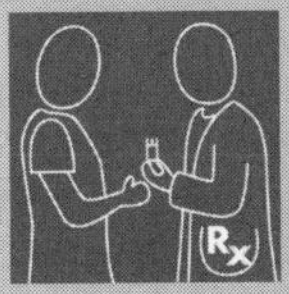

The primary objectives of self-treating atopic dermatitis are to (1) relieve symptoms of itching and weeping and (2) avoid or minimize exposure to factors that trigger or aggravate the disorders. The primary objectives in self-treating dry skin—restoring skin moisture and the skin's barrier function—can also help relieve the discomfort of atopic dermatitis. For most patients, carefully following product instructions and the self-care measures listed here will help ensure optimal therapeutic outcomes.

### Atopic Dermatitis

#### *Nondrug Measures*

- Avoid factors that trigger allergic reactions. Do not wear occlusive, tight clothing. Remain in areas with a moderate temperature and low humidity.
- Bathe or shower every other day, if possible. Take short showers or baths, using warm (tepid) water and a nonsoap cleanser.
- If possible, substitute sponge baths with tepid water for full-body bathing.
- To dry weeping lesions, apply cool tap water compresses for 5 to 20 minutes, four to six times daily.
- To prevent injury to the affected area caused by scratching, keep your fingernails short, smooth, and clean. At night, wear cotton gloves or socks on your hands to lessen scratching.
- Nonprescription Medications
- To decrease itching, bathe in tepid water that contains colloidal oatmeal or add a water-miscible bath oil to the water near the end of the bath.
- Gently wash the affected areas with a nonsoap cleanser prior to applying any emollient or medication. Gently pat your skin dry, and apply an emollient within 3 minutes after washing, while your skin is still damp.
- Wash hands before and after applying any medication.
- Apply a thin layer of medication over the affected areas.
- Apply hydrocortisone three to four times daily to dry weeping lesions and to relieve itching. Do not use this medication for longer than 7 days.
- With proper use of medication and nondrug measures, noticeable improvement can be observed in 24 to 48 hours.
- Although complete eradication of the rash and itching is possible, it is likely that exacerbation may occasionally appear, especially during the winter and summer months.
- Atrophy of the skin while using hydrocortisone should be reported to a primary care provider.
- If the atopic dermatitis does not improve or worsens after 2 to 3 days of treatment, consult a primary care provider.

### Dry Skin

#### *Nondrug Measures*

- Avoid excessive bathing; take brief (3- to 5-minute) full-body baths two to three times per week, using bath oil.
- Do not take hot baths; use tepid water.
- If possible, take sponge baths on other nights, using warm water to maintain skin hydration.
- Drink plenty of water daily. Do not substitute sodas, coffee, or tea for water.
- Copious quantities of moisturizer should be applied three to four times daily and continued as long as dry skin persists.
- Moisturizers should be applied within 3 minutes after bathing plus an additional three times per day.
- Complete eradication of dry skin is unlikely, but significant symptomatic improvement should start to be observed within 24 hours.
- Avoid caffeine, spices, and alcohol as these can contribute to dehydration.
- Keep the room humidity higher than normal to minimize evaporation from the skin.

#### *Nonprescription Medications*

- Add products such as oilated oatmeal or bath oil near the end of your bath to enhance skin hydration. Colloidal oatmeal products, if used on a regular basis, may clog plumbing pipes and can leave the tub slick.
- Apply an oil-based emollient immediately after bathing while your skin is damp. Reapply the emollient frequently.
- For more severe cases of dry skin, use a product that contains urea or lactic acid.
- Apply topical hydrocortisone ointment to reduce inflammation and itching. Do not use this medication for longer than 7 days.
- If skin dryness worsens after 7 days of treatment, consult a primary care provider.

---

- Advise patients to use cream base products, whenever possible, to maximize the hydrating properties of the product and compliance. Ointment base products should be recommended for patients not responding adequately to creams.
- Instruct patients on how to properly apply topical emollients, anti-inflammatory, and antipruritic agents.
- Advise patients with self-treatable symptoms to contact their primary care provider if symptoms worsen or do not improve within 7 days.

## References


1. Kligman AM, Koblenzer C. Demographics and psychological implications for the aging population. *Dermatol Clin.* 1997;15:549-53.
2. MacKie RM. *Clinical Dermatology.* 4th ed. Oxford: Oxford University Press; 1997:3-4.
3. Micali G, Lacarrubba F, Bongu A, et al. The skin barrier. In: Freinkel R, Woodely D, eds. *The Biology of the Skin.* New York: Parthenon; 2001:227.
4. Micali G, West D. Poisoning and paediatric skin. In: Harper J, Oranje A, Prose N, eds. *Textbook of Pediatric Dermatology.* Oxford: Blackwell Scientific; 2000:1753-4.

5. Leung DY, Tharp M, Boguniewicz M. Atopic dermatitis. In: Freedberg IM, Eisen AZ, Wolff K, eds. *Fitzpatrick's Dermatology in General Medicine.* 5th ed. New York: McGraw-Hill, Inc; 1999:1464-80.
6. Williams H, Burr M, Clayton T, et al. Worldwide variations in the prevalence of symptoms of atopic eczema in the international study of asthma and allergies in childhood. *J Allergy Clin Immunol.* 1999;103:125-38.
7. Ruzicka T. Atopic eczema between rationality and irrationality. *Arch Dermatol.* 1998;134:1462-9.
8. Leung DY, Hanifin JM, Charlesworth EN, et al. Disease management of atopic dermatitis: a practice parameter. Joint Task Force on Practice Parameters, representing the American Academy of Allergy, Asthma and Immunology, the American College of Allergy, Asthma and Immunology, and the Joint Council of Allergy, Asthma and Immunology, Work Group on Atopic Dermatitis. *Ann Allergy Asthma Immunol.* 1997;79:197-209.
9. Zhai H, Maibach HI. *Dermatoxicology.* 6th ed. Boca Raton, Fla: CRC Press; 2004:795-800.
10. Greaves MW. Antihistamines. In: Wolverton SE, ed. *Comprehensive Dermatologic Drug Therapy.* Philadelphia: WB Saunders; 2001:360-72.
11. Holden CA, Parish WE. In: Champion RH, Burton JL, Burns DA, et al., eds. *Textbook of Dermatology.* 6th ed. Oxford: Blackwell Scientific; 1998:681-708.
12. Hanifin JM, Cooper KC, Ho CV, et al. Guidelines of care for atopic dermatitis. *J Am Acad Dermatol.* 2004;50:391-404.
13. White MI, McElwan-Jenkinson D, Lloyd DH. The effect of washing on the thickness of the stratum corneum in normal and atopic individuals. *Br J Dermatol.* 1987;116:525-30.
14. Schempp CM, Dittmar HC, Hummler D, et al. Magnesium ions inhibit the antigen-presenting function of human epidermal Langerhans cells in vivo and in vitro: involvement of ATPase, HLA-DR, B7 molecules, and cytokines. *J Invest Dermatol.* 2000; 115:680-6.
15. Lazar AP, Lazar P. Dry skin, water, and lubrication. *Dermatol Clin.* 1991;9:45-51.
16. Kempers S, Katz HI, Wildnauer R, et al. An evaluation of the effect of an alpha-hydroxy acid-blend skin cream in the cosmetic improvement of symptoms of moderate to severe xerosis, epidermolytic hyperkeratosis, and ichthyosis. *Cutis.* 1998;61:347-50.
17. Shwayder T, Ott F. All about ichthyosis. *Pediatr Clin North Am.* 1991;38:835-57.
18. Draelos ZK. Cosmetics *in Dermatology.* 2nd ed. New York: Churchill-Livingstone; 1995.
19. Knutson K, Pershing LK. Topical Drugs. In: Hendrickson, R, Beringer, P, Der Marderosian AH, et al., eds. *Remington: The Science and Practice of Pharmacy.* 21st ed. Philadelphia: Lippincott Williams & Wilkins; 2005:1277-93.
20. Loden M, Maiback HI. *Dry Skin and Moisterizers: Chemistry and Function.* Boca Raton, Fla: CRC Press; 1999:323-8.
21. Jackson EM. AHA-type products proliferate in 1993. *Cosmet Dermatol.* 1993;6:22-4.
22. Gebhardt M, Elsner P, Marks JG. *Handbook of Contact Dermatitis.* Boca Raton, Fla: CRC Press; 2004:125-30.

CHAPTER 34

# Scaly Dermatoses

*Robert W. Martin III and Steven A. Scott*

Dandruff, seborrheic dermatitis (seborrhea), and psoriasis are chronic, scaly dermatoses. They may be placed on a spectrum ranging from dandruff (a less inflammatory form of seborrheic dermatosis with relatively fine scaling confined to the scalp) to seborrhea (inflammatory seborrheic dermatitis involving scalp, face, and trunk) to psoriasis (an inflammatory clinical condition with plaques and relatively adherent thick scales that can have profound physical, psychologic, and economic consequences). These conditions involve the uppermost layer of skin, the epidermis. The lowest layer of the epidermis is the stratum germinativum, where germinative "basal cells" divide and then migrate upwards to the uppermost layer, the stratum corneum. This outer layer of dead keratinized cells prevents substances from entering the body and body fluids from escaping the underlying living cells of the epidermis.[1]

Nonprescription products are appropriate treatment for most cases of seborrheic dermatitis. Mild psoriasis may be responsive to nonprescription treatment, but the initial diagnosis of psoriasis and the management of acute flare-ups require the attention of a primary care provider.[1]

## DANDRUFF

Dandruff is a chronic, noninflammatory scalp condition that results in excessive scaling of the scalp. It is a substantial cosmetic concern and is associated with social stigma. This disorder represents the less inflammatory end of the seborrheic dermatitis spectrum. Authorities disagree over whether inadequate shampooing exacerbates dandruff; however, they agree that a consistent washing routine is important in managing the condition.[1,2]

### Epidemiology of Dandruff

Dandruff occurs in approximately 1% to 3% of the population.[3] Dandruff is uncommon in children and generally appears at puberty, reaches a peak in early adulthood, levels off in middle age, and is less prominent after 75 years of age.[1] There is no gender preference, and bald spots on males are typically dandruff free. Dandruff is less severe during the summer.[1,2]

### Etiology of Dandruff

The specific cause of accelerated cell growth seen in dandruff is unknown. Debate continues as to whether dandruff is a result of accelerated cell turnover or of elevated microorganism levels—particularly of *Pityrosporum* (a yeast-like fungus that is normal flora of the scalp).[4]

### Pathophysiology of Dandruff

Dandruff is a hyperproliferative epidermal condition, characterized by accelerated epidermal cell turnover (twice that of normal scalp[5]) and irregular keratin breakup pattern resulting in the shedding of large, nonadherent white scales. The horny layer of the scalp normally consists of 25 to 35 fully keratinized, closely coherent cells per square millimeter arranged in an orderly fashion. However, in dandruff, the intact horny layer has fewer than 10 normal cells per square millimeter, and nonkeratinized cells are common. With dandruff, crevices occur deep in the stratum corneum, resulting in cracking, which generates relatively large scales.[1] If the large scales are broken down to smaller units, the dandruff becomes less visible.

### Signs and Symptoms of Dandruff

Dandruff is diffuse rather than patchy and is minimally inflammatory. Scaling, the only visible manifestation of dandruff, is the result of an increased rate of horny substance production on the scalp and the sloughing of large white or gray scales. Pruritus, although not universal in all patients, is common. The condition affects the pate diffusely, but the crown is often a prime location for dandruff flake formation.

### Treatment Overview of Dandruff

#### *Treatment Goals*

The goals of self-treating dandruff are to (1) reduce the epidermal turnover rate of the scalp skin, (2) minimize the cosmetic embarrassment of visible scaling, and (3) minimize itch.

#### *General Treatment Approach*

Washing the hair and scalp with a general-purpose nonmedicated shampoo every other day or daily is often sufficient to control mild to moderate dandruff. If it is not, the practitioner may recommend medicated nonprescription antidandruff products.

With medicated shampoos, contact time is the key to effectiveness. The patient should massage the shampoo into the scalp with a scalp scrubber and leave the medicated shampoo on the hair for 5 minutes before rinsing and repeating. Medicated shampoos need only be used two to three times weekly for 2 to 3 weeks and then once weekly or every other week to control the condition. Thorough rinsing is important in the use of all shampoo products. It is the scalp, not the hair, that is being treated, and thus use of a "scalp scrubber" will help ensure adequate contact of the medicated shampoo with the scalp.

A cytostatic agent (e.g., pyrithione zinc, selenium sulfide, or coal tar) is generally initially recommended. Such agents reduce scaling by decreasing the epidermal turnover rate. However, shampoos containing coal tar may tend to discolor light hair as well as clothing and jewelry and thus may not appeal to some patients. A keratolytic shampoo, containing salicylic acid or sulfur, or ketoconazole shampoo may also be used (see Treatment of Scaly Dermatoses). If dandruff proves resistant to these agents after 4 to 8 weeks of use, the patient should be referred to a primary care provider for treatment with products containing a higher concentration of selenium sulfide, ketoconazole, or coal tar.[1]

## SEBORRHEIC DERMATITIS

Seborrheic dermatitis is a subacute or chronic inflammatory disorder that occurs predominantly in the areas of greatest sebaceous gland activity (e.g., scalp, face, trunk).[6]

### Epidemiology of Seborrheic Dermatitis

Seborrheic dermatitis is a common chronic red, scaly, itchy rash with two age peaks of occurrence, one within the first 3 months of life and the second around the fourth to the seventh decade of life. Seborrheic dermatitis is common in infants and affects 2% to 5% of adults, more commonly men. There is no ethnic predilection. Seborrheic dermatitis is more severe in winter and is commonly found in people with parkinsonism, zinc deficiency, endocrine states associated with obesity, and human immunodeficiency virus (HIV) infection.

### Etiology of Seborrheic Dermatitis

The cause of seborrheic dermatitis is unknown, although the lipophilic, pleomorphic fungus *Pityrosporon* has been proposed as contributing to seborrheic dermatitis. Emotional stress may serve as an aggravating factor.

### Pathophysiology of Seborrheic Dermatitis

Seborrheic dermatitis is more inflammatory than dandruff and is marked by accelerated epidermal proliferation in areas with dense distribution of sebaceous glands.[7] Cell turnover rate for seborrheic dermatitis is 9 to 10 days, compared with 13 to 15 days for dandruff.[1] The characteristic accelerated cell turnover and enhanced sebaceous gland activity give rise to the prominent scale displayed in the condition.

### Signs and Symptoms of Seborrheic Dermatitis

Seborrheic dermatitis occurs in the scalp, eyebrows, glabella, eyelid margins (often with conjunctivitis), cheeks, paranasal areas, nasolabial folds, beard area, presternal area, central back, retroauricular (behind the ear) creases, and in and about the external ear canal. The disorder typically presents as dull, yellowish, oily, scaly areas on red skin that are fairly well-demarcated. Pruritus is common.[8] In the axillae, inframammary, umbilicus, groin, and intergluteal cleft (i.e., intertriginous) areas, the lesions consist of bright erythema with or without fissures but are usually devoid of scale.

The infantile form occurs in the first months of life, affecting the scalp (cradle cap), retroauricular creases, lateral neck, and intertriginous folds with greasy scales and scale crusts on a bright erythematous base. Cradle cap usually clears without treatment by age 8 to 12 months (because of the gradual disappearance of hormones passed from the mother to the child before birth), after which the disease is rare until puberty. The center of the face, chest, and neck may also be affected.

The most common form in adults is seborrhea of the scalp, characterized by greasy scales on the scalp that often extend to the middle third of the face with subsequent eye involvement (see Color Plates, photograph 15).

Asymptomatic, fluffy white dandruff of the scalp represents the mild end of the spectrum of seborrheic dermatitis and has been referred to as pityriasis sicca. An oily type, pityriasis steatoides, at times accompanied by erythema and an accumulation of thick crusts, is also encountered. Other types of seborrheic dermatitis on the scalp are more severe and are manifested by greasy, scaling, patches or plaques, exudation, and thick crusting.

On the face, flaky scales or yellowish scaling patches on red, itchy skin are seen in the eyebrows and glabella. The eyelid edges may be erythematous and granular (marginal blepharitis) with injected conjunctivae. There may be yellowish or reddish-yellow scaling macules, sometimes with fissures in the nasolabial creases. In men, folliculitis of the upper lip may occur. Red scaling, fissures, and swelling may be present in the ear canals, around the auditory meatus, in the postauricular region, or under the earlobe.

V-shaped areas of the chest and back and less frequently, intertriginous areas such as the side of the neck, axillae, submammary region, umbilicus, and genitocrural folds may also be involved. The involvement may vary from simple yellowish erythema and scaling to more pronounced thick patches with fissures. Seborrheic dermatitis in the groin and gluteal crease is scaly with less definite borders, and is bilateral and symmetrical with fissures or psoriasiform thick scales.

In adults the disease lasts for years to decades with periods of improvement in warmer seasons and periods of exacerbation in the colder months.

## Treatment Overview of Seborrheic Dermatitis

### Treatment Goals

The goals of self-treatment of seborrheic dermatitis are to (1) reduce inflammation and the epidermal turnover rate of the scalp skin and (2) minimize or eliminate visible erythema and scaling.

### General Treatment Approach

The treatment of seborrheic dermatitis is similar to that of dandruff. There is no way to cure seborrheic dermatitis. Patients should be informed about the chronic nature of the disease and understand that therapy works by controlling the disease rather than curing it. Therapy is directed toward loosening and removal of scales and crusts, inhibiting yeast colonization, controlling secondary infection, and reducing erythema and itching. When a medicated shampoo is used for treatment, patients should be instructed to work the shampoo into the scalp and then leave the lather on the hair and affected areas for 3 to 5 minutes three times per week, initially. A double application of medicated shampoos and use of a scalp scrubber ensures penetration to the scalp.

In infants, seborrheic dermatitis is usually self-limited and treated primarily by gently massaging the scalp with baby oil, followed by the use of a nonmedicated shampoo to remove scales.[1,6,8] For more severe cases, crusts can be removed with salicylic acid 3% to 5% in olive oil or a water-soluble base and warm olive oil compresses followed by gentle shampooing with a mild shampoo or a shampoo containing salicylic acid. Following shampooing, a low-potency OTC glucocorticoid (e.g., hydrocortisone 1%) in a cream or lotion may be tried for a few days in children 2 years of age and older. When the face is involved in infants, gentle washing with mild soap and application of a facial emollient are all that is necessary. The application of corticosteroids to an infant's face is to be avoided unless its use is directed by a dermatologist to avoid adverse reactions.

In adults, shampooing is the foundation of treatment. The scalp should be shampooed several times per week with shampoos containing pyrithione zinc, selenium sulfide, sulfur, ketoconazole, salicylic acid, or coal tar. If the odor of a medicated shampoo is objectionable, it can be followed by a more cosmetically acceptable shampoo/conditioner. A regular nonmedicated shampoo or liquid dishwashing soap (e.g., Dawn) can be used to soften and remove crusts or scales.[9]

Seborrheic dermatitis involving the ears can be treated with a medicated shampoo during a bath or shower followed by application of an emollient and hydrocortisone 0.5% to 1.0% cream. Adult patients should avoid greasy ointments and pre- or aftershave lotions containing alcohol, and reduce the use of soaps. It is the primary author's personal observation that washing the face with an over-the-counter (OTC) pyrithione zinc bar (e.g., ZNP bar) or shampoo or another OTC medicated shampoo (e.g., selenium sulfide, ketoconazole) may be sufficient in mild cases.

The primary difference between the treatment of dandruff and that of seborrheic dermatitis is the frequency of topical corticosteroid use. Such products may be used to manage seborrheic dermatitis whenever erythema is persistent after therapy with medicated shampoos or creams. Hydrocortisone should be applied two to three times a day until symptoms subside, and then intermittently to control acute exacerbations. Lotions are preferred for hairy areas, and care should be taken to prevent any corticosteroid from being used on eyelids or entering the eyes. The hair should be parted, and the product applied directly to the scalp and massaged in thoroughly. The patient should repeat this process until desired coverage of the affected area is achieved. The absorption of medication into the scalp is enhanced by applying the lotion after shampooing; skin hydration promotes drug absorption. Shampooing removes natural body oils, which also allows for better medication penetration.

Use of nonprescription hydrocortisone should not exceed 7 days. If the condition worsens or symptoms persist longer than 7 days, a primary care provider should be consulted. A more potent topical corticosteroid may be indicated.[5]

# PSORIASIS

Psoriasis is a noncontagious, chronic inflammatory disease estimated to afflict 1% to 3% of Americans.[10] Lesions are often localized but may become generalized over much of the body surface and result in disability caused by deformities that impair use of the hands and feet.[11] Remissions and exacerbations are unpredictable. Approximately 30% of people with psoriasis find that lesion involvement clears spontaneously.[10] Unrelenting generalized psoriasis may cause enough psychologic distress to adversely affect the patient's quality of life. Psoriatic arthritis may result in joint deformity and, in some cases, disability.[12] Treatment of severe psoriasis can also produce a significant physical and economic burden.[13]

## Epidemiology of Psoriasis

The incidence of psoriasis is distributed almost equally among men and women. Psoriasis is seen in all races and geographic regions, but the incidence is lower among people living in countries close to the equator and among blacks, Native Americans, and Asians.[10,13,14]

Psoriasis may be categorized into two types. Patients with Type I disease typically present at an early age, have a strong family history of the disorder (36% of patients have relatives with psoriasis, but the mode of inheritance is not clear), and have a higher frequency of human lymphocyte antigen. On the other hand, Type II psoriasis develops in the later decades of life and does not show a high incidence of family history.

## Etiology of Psoriasis

The cause of psoriasis is unknown. However, environmental factors such as physical, ultraviolet (UV), and chemical injury; various infections (streptococcal infections, but also acute viral infections and HIV infection); prescription drug use (β-blockers, lithium, antimalarials, indomethacin, quinidine, withdrawal of systemic corticosteroids); psychologic stress; endocrine/hormonal changes; obesity; and the use of alcohol and tobacco can trigger the onset of psoriasis. There is a distinct tendency for improvement or even temporary disappearance during pregnancy. After childbirth, there is a tendency for exacerbation of lesions. During menopause, lesions may change for better or worse, with no set pattern of behavior. Hot weather and sunlight exposure improves the lesions in many patients.[13]

## Pathophysiology of Psoriasis

Accelerated epidermal proliferation leading to excessive scaling is one hallmark symptom of psoriasis. Normal epidermal cell turnover is 25 to 30 days, whereas it is approximately 4 days in a psoriatic plaque. The duration of psoriasis is variable, and lesions may last a lifetime or disappear quickly. When lesions disappear, they may leave the skin either hypopigmented or hyperpigmented. The disease course is marked by spontaneous exacerbations and remissions, and it tends to be chronic and relapsing. Classic psoriasis is characterized by defects in the normal cycle of epidermal development that lead to epidermal hyperproliferation, altered maturation of the skin, inflammation, and vascular alterations.[13]

## Signs and Symptoms of Psoriasis

There are several clinical forms of psoriasis including plaque, inverse, guttate, pustular, and erythrodermic. Regardless of the type, psoriasis is usually symmetrical, with minimal itching. The isomorphic response, commonly known as the Koebner reaction, is the appearance of psoriatic lesions at sites of injuries.

Plaque psoriasis is by far the most common form, occurring in about 90% of patients. Lesions start as small papules that grow and unite to form plaques. These lesions are well circumscribed, sharply demarcated, light pink to bright red or maroon plaques with overlying opaque, thick, adherent, white scale that can be pulled off in layers (see Color Plates, photographs 16A, B, and C.) This typical feature has been likened to the mineral mica and descriptively termed *micaceous scale.* When scale is lifted from the base of the plaque, punctate bleeding points sometimes occur at the sites of scale removal (Auspitz sign). The most common locations are the extensor surfaces of the elbow and knees, the lumbar region of the back, the scalp, the posterior auricular area, the external auditory canal, and the glans penis.

Inverse or flexural psoriasis involves folds, recesses, and flexor surfaces: ears, axillae, groin, inframammary folds, navel, intergluteal crease, glans penis, lips, and above all, the palms, soles, and nails.

Guttate (droplike) psoriasis is characterized by the rapid onset of "crops" of uniformly sized, scattered papules with light pink, flaking scale on the trunk and proximal extremities. This form of psoriasis is often seen in adolescents. When it occurs in children, it is often preceded by streptococcal throat infections. In patients with chronic, persistent plaque-type psoriasis, guttate psoriasis is a sign of an acute exacerbation. Guttate psoriasis arises very rapidly but responds to antibiotic treatment and ultraviolet light therapies better than psoriatic lesions that have a longer onset.[13,15]

Pustular psoriasis is either localized to hands or widespread over the entire body. Erythrodermic psoriasis may present as widespread chronic redness and scaling of the skin in a medically stable patient or an exfoliative phase involving almost all of the skin. The second form of erythrodermic psoriasis is a medical emergency with pustular psoriasis patients becoming febrile and medically unstable with widespread sloughing of skin.

Psoriasis may also involve the nails and synovium. Nail involvement may include onycholysis (separation of the nail from the nail bed), pitting, and yellow discoloration. In many patients with coexisting joint disease and psoriasis, the arthritic component is not easily distinguishable from rheumatoid arthritis. An estimated 7% of psoriatic patients have psoriatic arthritis. Unlike rheumatoid arthritis, psoriatic arthritis often has asymmetric joint involvement. Usually, rheumatoid factor is absent, and prognosis is better than it is with rheumatoid arthritis.

## Treatment Overview of Psoriasis

### Treatment Goals

The goals of self-treatment of psoriasis are to (1) control or eliminate the signs and symptoms (inflammation, scaling, and itching) and (2) prevent or minimize the likelihood of flares.

### General Treatment Approach

The Food and Drug Administration (FDA) recommends that only mild cases of psoriasis be self-treated. Individuals with moderate to severe cases, involving more than 10% of body surface area, should be treated by a primary care provider.[2] Severe, generalized psoriasis sometimes necessitates day care or hospitalization. Furthermore, recalcitrant cases (cases not responding to emollients and nonprescription strengths of hydrocortisone) or cases in children younger than 2 years should be referred to a primary care provider for evaluation.

Numerous nondrug measures can be used by patients in the treatment of psoriasis. However, it is unlikely that these measures alone will control the signs and symptoms of the disorder. Patients should avoid psychologic stress, as well as, physical, UV, and chemical injury of the skin. Overweight patients should be encouraged to lose weight, smoking should be stopped, and alcohol consumption should be discouraged. Patients with psoriasis should be encouraged to bathe with lubricating bath products two to three times per week using tepid water. Scales can be removed by gently rubbing with a soft cloth. Emollients should be applied to the lesions within 3 minutes of bathing.

The selection of the most effective but appropriate therapy depends on the site, severity, duration, previous treatment, and age of the patient. Treatment may be topical, systemic, or a combination of both. The treatment selected will be more accepted if the patient and/or the parent/guardian are educated about the nature of psoriasis and the alternatives available for treatment.

Factors in determining appropriate therapy include the morphologic type of psoriasis, extent, age, cost, and ability of the patient to comply with the regimen.

Topical treatment of psoriasis is usually the first line of therapy. Pruritic dry skin is common in psoriasis, and emollients and lubricating bath products often provide relief for these symptoms (see Chapter 33). Daily lubrication of the skin after a bath or shower is an essential part of therapy. Emollients moisturize, lubricate, and soothe dry and flaky skin, as well as reduce fissure formation within plaques and help maintain flexibility of the surrounding skin. To be effective, they need to be applied liberally, four to six times daily. Gentle rubbing of affected areas with a soft cloth following the bath helps to mechanically remove scales. Depending on the anatomic site, self-treatment may progress to the use of topical hydrocortisone, coal tar products, and/or keratolytic agents such as salicylic acid.[2] The patient should avoid vigorous rubbing, which can aggravate the lesions.

Acute localized flares, characterized by bright red lesions, call for soothing local therapy with emollients and hydrocortisone. Tars, salicylic acid, and aggressive UV radiation therapy at this stage may exacerbate the disease. After the flare has subsided and the usual thick-scaled plaques appear, the patient may use agents such as keratolytics. Many patients respond well to simple measures, whereas others have disease that is refractory even to aggressive treatments.[5]

Psoriatic arthritis is treated with nonsteroidal anti-inflammatory drugs (NSAIDs; see Chapter 5) or with prescription agents such as methotrexate and entanercept.[13] No reliably effective nonprescription treatment is available for nail psoriasis.

In many cases, psoriasis will not be controlled by nonprescription treatment, and a dermatologic referral from the practitioner will be necessary. Prescription topical agents such as calcipotriol, topical retinoids (tazarotene), and anthralin are effective. For severe or recalcitrant psoriasis, systemic agents may be necessary. These include oral retinoids (acitretin), methotrexate, cyclosporine, and the newer biologicals (alefacept, efalizumab, etanercept, and infliximab). Phototherapy with narrow-band UVB or PUVA (ultraviolet light-A [UVA]) in combination with methoxsalen (a chemical photosensitizing psoralen [P]) is also a treatment option available in many dermatologists' offices.

Scalp psoriasis can be treated with tar-based and salicylic acid–based nonprescription shampoos. Again, sufficient contact time is the key to successful therapy, the goal of which is scale removal. In addition, although hydrocortisone 1% products may be used for scalp itching and mild lesional skin involvement, widespread involvement and involvement of the face dictates that the patient be treated by a dermatologist for more effective prescription medications. If a nonprescription product is used, the practitioner should counsel the patient to consult a primary care provider if the condition does not improve in 7 days, or if it worsens.

Agents such as coal tar and salicylic acid should be used with extreme caution, if at all, to treat psoriasis in intertriginous areas (e.g., armpits and genital/anal region). Instead, hydrocortisone cream may be applied sparingly two or three times a day for up to 2 weeks and should be used less often as improvement occurs.

Salicylic acid products, which are most useful if thick scales are present, may be more cosmetically acceptable than coal tar products to some patients and encourage compliance. Soaking the affected area in warm (not hot) water for 10 to 20 minutes before applying a salicylic acid product enhances keratolytic activity.

Coal tar products may be applied to the body, arms, and legs preferably at bedtime. Because coal tar stains most materials, the patient should be advised to use bed linen and clothing for which staining would not present a problem. Overnight application is followed by a bath in the morning to remove residual coal tar and loosen psoriatic scales. Patients using coal tar preparations should avoid sun exposure for 24 hours after application. Topical hydrocortisone 1% ointment for the body may be applied sparingly to lesions and massaged into the skin thoroughly but gently (see Treatment of Scaly Dermatoses).

Psoriasis cannot be cured, but signs and symptoms can usually be controlled adequately with appropriate patient education and treatment, and remissions do occur. The patient should be reassured that, in most cases, control is possible. Such reassurance increases compliance with burdensome and prolonged treatment regimens. Also, if the practitioner can help the patient gain some understanding and acceptance of the condition, that knowledge may reduce the patient's emotional stress and psychogenic exacerbations. Prevention of flares, which can be achieved by minimizing identified precipitating factors such as emotional stress, skin irritation, and physical trauma, should be emphasized.

## TREATMENT OF SCALY DERMATOSES

Cytostatic agents and keratolytic agents, usually in the form of medicated shampoos, are used to reduce epidermal turnover rate. Ketoconazole, an antifungal agent, is used in self-treatment of seborrheic dermatitis and dandruff. Hydrocortisone controls the inflammation associated with seborrheic dermatitis and psoriasis. Table 34-1 summarizes the concentrations and indications of currently approved agents, and the algorithm in Figure 34-1 outlines self-treatment with these agents. FDA also has published two announcements seeking safety and efficacy data on two potential nonprescription antidandruff agents. The December 9, 2005, *Federal Register* proposes to amend the final monograph for nonprescription dandruff, seborrheic dermatitis, and psoriasis drug products to include the combination of 1.8% coal tar solution and 1.5% menthol in a dandruff shampoo drug product.[16] This action was prompted by information submitted in a citizen petition. The deadline for comments is March 8, 2006. The December 5 issue of the *Federal Register* requests data for 0.1% to 0.5% and 0.5% to 2.0% climbazole for use as an active dandruff control ingredient in leave-on and rinse-off dosage forms, respectively.[17] The deadline for comments is March 6, 2006.

**TABLE 34-1 Concentrations of Approved Nonprescription Ingredients for Products Used to Treat Scaly Dermatoses[11]**

| Ingredient | Concentration (%) Dandruff | Seborrheic Dermatitis | Psoriasis |
|---|---|---|---|
| Coal tar | 0.5-5.0 | 0.5-5.0 | 0.5-5.0 |
| Ketoconazole | 1 | 1 | 1 |
| Pyrithione zinc (brief exposure) | 0.3-2.0 | 0.95-2.0 | 2.0 |
| Pyrithione zinc (residual) | 0.1-0.25 | 0.1-0.25 | .25 |
| Salicylic acid | 1.8-3 | 1.8-3.0 | 1.8-3.0 |
| Selenium sulfide | 1 | 1 | 1 |
| Sulfur | 2-5 | 2-5 | |
| Hydrocortisone | | 0.5-1.0 | 0.5-1.0 |

Patients should shampoo with a nonmedicated, nonresidue shampoo to remove scalp and hair dirt, oil, and scale before using a medicated shampoo. Many shampoos leave a residue on the hair shaft and scalp that may aggravate scaly dermatoses of the scalp. Nonresidue shampoos (e.g., Prell, Breck, Johnson's Baby Shampoo) do not interfere with these scalp conditions, but rather leave the scalp clean and receptive to optimal effects from medicated shampoos. A nonresidue shampoo application and rinse may be followed by a medicated shampoo left on the scalp for the labeled length of time. The patient can use this treatment as often as daily until symptoms are relieved, then two to three times weekly or as needed.[5]

### *Cytostatic Agents*

Although their mechanism of action is not completely understood, topical cytostatic agents are known to decrease the rate of epidermal cell replication. This action increases the time required for epidermal cell turnover, which, in turn, allows the possibility of normalizing epidermal differentiation, resulting in a dramatic decline in visible scales. Thus, use of products containing cytostatic agents (Table 34-2) represents a direct approach to controlling dandruff and seborrheic dermatitis.

#### Pyrithione Zinc

Pyrithione zinc's action is likely caused by a nonspecific toxicity for epidermal cells. The pyrithione moiety is apparently the active part of the molecule. Product effectiveness is influenced by several factors. Pyrithione zinc is strongly bound to both hair and the external skin layers, and the extent of binding correlates with clinical performance. The drug's absorption increases with contact time, temperature, concentration, and frequency of application. Some researchers consider pyrithione zinc to be slower acting than selenium sulfide.[2]

For pyrithione zinc products intended to be applied and washed off within minutes, FDA allows concentrations of 0.3% to 2.0% for treating dandruff and 0.95% to 2.0% for treating seborrheic dermatitis. Concentrations for products intended to be applied and then left on the skin or scalp are 0.1% to 0.25% for treating both dandruff and seborrheic dermatitis.[7] Shampoos and soaps are currently available in 1% and 2% concentrations.

Long-term use of pyrithione zinc 1% to 2% rinse-away products has rarely been associated with toxicity. Rare cases of contact dermatitis have been reported with use of this agent on broken or abraded skin.[4]

#### Selenium Sulfide

Selenium sulfide is believed to have a direct antimitotic effect on epidermal cells.[4] Like pyrithione zinc, it is more effective with longer contact time and thus should be applied in a similar manner.[4] The product must be rinsed from the hair thoroughly or discoloration may result, especially in blond, gray, or dyed hair. Frequent use of selenium sulfide tends to leave a residual odor and an oily scalp.

Selenium sulfide has been approved in a 1% concentration as an active ingredient in nonprescription products to treat dandruff and seborrhea.[18] A higher concentration is available by prescription for use in resistant cases.

Irritation from selenium sulfide is minimal. Contact with the eyelids should be avoided because of the potential for eye irritation. If such contact does occur, the patient should flush the eyes with copious amounts of water. Selenium sulfide is toxic if ingested. Because of the risk of systemic toxicity, it should be applied only to intact skin.

#### Coal Tar

Coal tar products have long been popular for treating dandruff, seborrheic dermatitis, and psoriasis. Many nonprescription products are available. Crude coal tar, which consists of a heterogeneous mixture of thousands of hydrocarbon compounds, is produced by the destructive distillation of bituminous coal. Its composition varies, depending on the source of the coal and the process used.

Crude coal tar 1% to 5% and UV radiation therapy have been used to treat psoriasis since 1925 in a method known as the Goeckerman treatment. A therapeutic benefit has been demonstrated for both the tar alone and the irradiation alone, but the combination is more effective than either agent by itself. Rare remissions lasting up to 12 months have been reported after 2 to 4 weeks of therapy. The coal tar is removed from the skin before irradiation takes place; otherwise, the UV radiation will not reach the skin.

For many years, the therapeutic response to this form of therapy was believed to be caused solely by its phototoxicity. Now it is believed that the beneficial effect of coal tar lies primarily in its ability to cross-link with DNA.[4] Coal tar in combination with UV radiation may also increase prostaglandin synthesis in the skin, which may contribute to its beneficial effect. Comparison of 1% versus 6% crude coal tar with UVB radiation showed each concentration to be equally effective. Hence, only modest levels of coal tar are needed.[5]

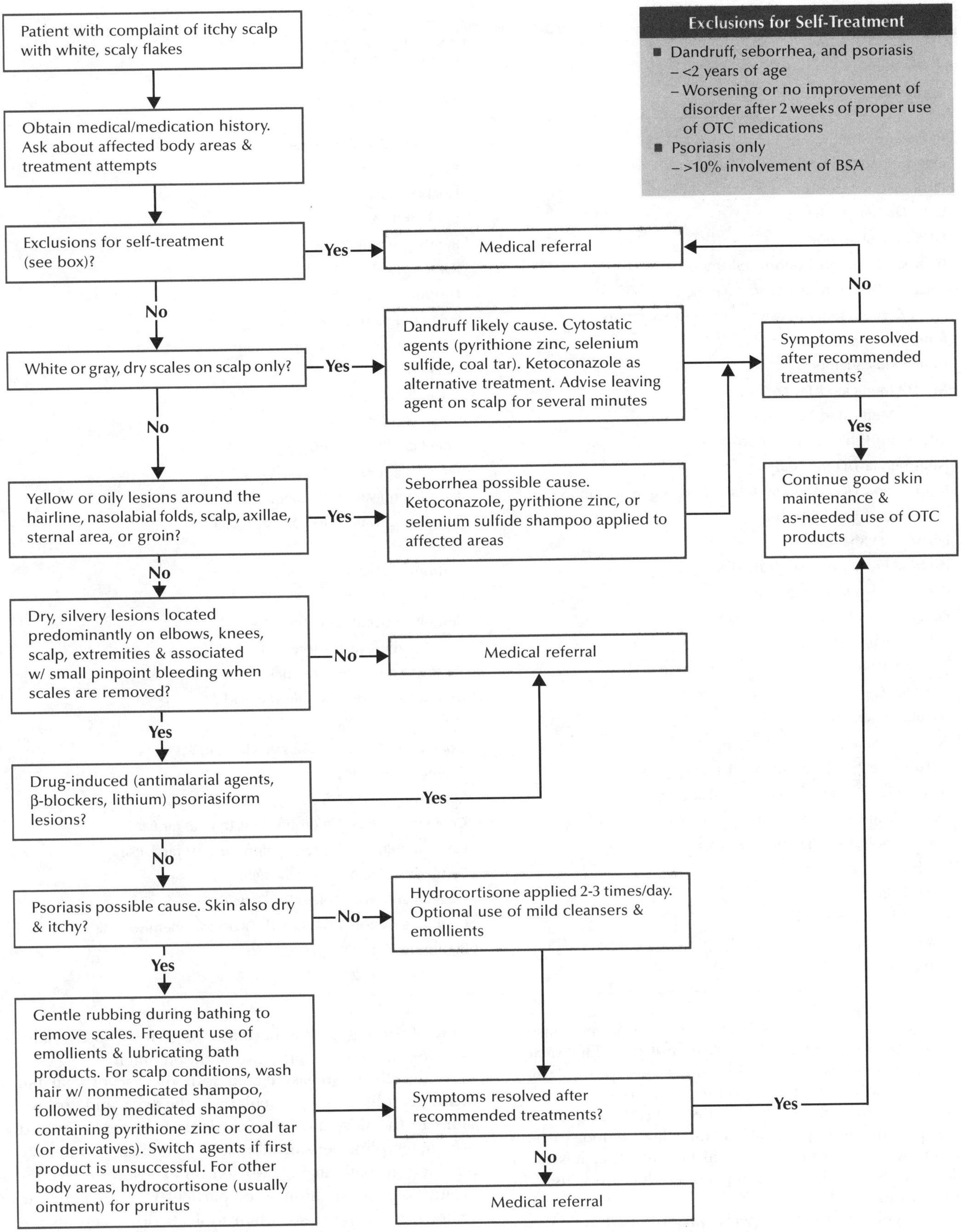


**FIGURE 34-1** Self-care of scaly dermatoses. BSA, body surface area; OTC, over-the-counter.

**TABLE 34-2 Cytostatic Products for Scaly Dermatoses**

| Trade Name | Primary Ingredients |
|---|---|
| Balnetar Bath Oil | Coal tar 2.5% in mineral oil |
| Denorex Advanced Formula Shampoo | Pyrithione zinc 2% |
| DHS Tar Shampoo | Coal tar 0.5% |
| DHS Tar Gel Shampoo | Coal tar 0.5% |
| DHS Zinc Shampoo | Pyrithione zinc 2% |
| Head & Shoulders Dandruff Shampoo | Pyrithione zinc 1% |
| Head & Shoulders Dry Scalp Shampoo | Pyrithione zinc 1% |
| Head & Shoulders Intensive Treatment Shampoo | Selenium sulfide 1% |
| Ionil T Shampoo | Coal tar solution 5% (equivalent to coal tar 1%) |
| Ionil T Plus Shampoo | Coal tar 2% |
| MG217 Medicated Tar Lotion | Coal tar solution 5% |
| MG217 Medicated Tar Ointment | Coal tar solution 10% |
| MG217 for Psoriasis Shampoo | Coal tar solution 15% |
| Neutrogena T/Derm Body Oil | Tar 5% (equivalent to coal tar 1.2%) |
| Neutrogena T/Gel Extra Strength Therapeutic Shampoo | Tar 4% (equivalent to coal tar 1%) |
| Neutrogena T/Gel Shampoo | Tar 2% (equivalent to coal tar 0.5%) |
| Nizoral AD Shampoo | Ketoconazole 1% |
| Pantene Pro-V Anti-Dandruff Shampoo | Pyrithione zinc 1% |
| Pert Plus Dandruff Shampoo | Pyrithione zinc 1% |
| Pentrax Gold Shampoo | Solubilized coal tar extract 4% |
| Polytar Shampoo | Tar 4.5% (equivalent to coal tar 0.5%) |
| Polytar Cleansing Bar | Tar 2.5% (equivalent to coal tar 0.5%) |
| P&S Plus Gel | Coal tar solution 8%; salicylic acid 2% |
| Sebulon Shampoo | Pyrithione zinc 2% |
| Sebutone Shampoo | Coal tar 0.5%; sulfur 2%; salicylic acid 2% |
| Selsun Blue 2-in-1 Treatment Shampoo | Selenium sulfide 1% |
| Selsun Blue Balanced Treatment Shampoo | Selenium sulfide 1% |
| Tegrin Cleansing Bar/Cream | Coal tar solution 5% (equivalent to coal tar 0.8%) |
| Tegrin Medicated Shampoo | Coal tar solution 7% (equivalent to coal tar 1.1%) |
| X-Seb Plus Shampoo | Pyrithione zinc 1%; salicylic acid 2% |
| X-Seb T Shampoo | Coal tar solution 10%; salicylic acid 4% |
| X-Seb T Plus Shampoo | Coal tar solution 10%; salicylic acid 3%; menthol 1% |
| Zincon Shampoo | Pyrithione zinc 1% |
| ZNP Cleansing Bar | Pyrithione zinc 2% |

Coal tar is available in creams, ointments, pastes, lotions, bath oils, shampoos, soaps, and gels. This variety of dosage forms is partly a result of an attempt to develop a cosmetically acceptable product, one that masks the odor, color, and staining properties of crude coal tar that most patients find esthetically unappealing. Liquor carbonis detergens is a tincture of coal tar 20% that has been useful in developing acceptable tar products. It is used in concentrations of 3% to 15%.

Tar gels represent a special product that appears to deliver the beneficial elements of crude coal tar in a form both convenient to apply and cosmetically acceptable. These gels are nongreasy, nonstaining, and nearly colorless. Many of these gels may have a drying effect on the skin, however, necessitating the use of an emollient.

Side effects are associated with the use of coal tar, including folliculitis (particularly of the axilla and groins), stains to the skin and hair (particularly blond, gray, and dyed hair), photosensitization, and irritant contact dermatitis.[2] Rarely, patients may worsen on exposure to coal tar products. This situation is of particular concern in the acute phase of psoriasis, when topical corticosteroids are recommended to reduce inflammation before coal tar preparations are used. Allergic contact dermatitis, however, is rare with coal tar in topical medications.

TABLE 34-3 Selected Keratolytic Products for Scaly Dermatoses

| Trade Name | Primary Ingredients |
|---|---|
| MG217 Medicated Tar-Free Shampoo | Salicylic acid 3%; sulfur 5% |
| Neutrogena Healthy Scalp Anti-Dandruff Shampoo | Salicylic acid 1.8% |
| Neutrogena T/Sal Maximum Strength Therapeutic Shampoo | Salicylic acid 3%, coal tar extract 2% |
| Scalpicin Maximum Strength Foam/Solution | Salicylic acid 3%; menthol |
| Sebucare Lotion | Salicylic acid 1.8% |
| Sebulex Conditioning Shampoo with Protein | Salicylic acid 2%; sulfur 2% |
| Sulfoam Medicated Antidandruff Shampoo | Sulfur 2% |
| Sulray Cleansing Bar | Sulfur 5% |
| Sulray Dandruff Shampoo | Sulfur 2% |
| X-Seb Shampoo | Salicylic acid 4% |

Coal tar contains known human carcinogens. However, because of the relatively short contact time and thus the low lifetime exposure, FDA considers the benefits of coal tar to outweigh the risks for use in topical formulations. Thus, coal tar is available in concentrations of 0.5% to 5% for the self-treatment of scalp conditions such as dandruff, seborrheic dermatitis, and psoriasis.[18]

## Keratolytic Agents

The keratolytic agents salicylic acid and sulfur are used in dandruff and seborrheic dermatitis products to loosen and lyse keratin aggregates, thereby facilitating their removal from the scalp in smaller particles. These agents act by dissolving the "cement" that holds epidermal cells together. Vehicle composition, contact time, and concentration are important factors in the success of a keratolytic agent. The keratolytic concentrations in nonprescription scalp products (Table 34-3) are not sufficient to impair the normal skin barrier, but do affect the abnormal, incompletely keratinized stratum corneum.

Keratolytic agents may produce several adverse effects, and patients should be counseled accordingly. These agents have a primary, concentration-dependent irritant effect, particularly on mucous membranes and the conjunctiva of the eye. They also have the potential of acting on hair and skin keratin. Thus, extended use may alter hair appearance. The directions and precautions for the use of keratolytic shampoos are similar to those for shampoos containing cytostatic agents.

### Salicylic Acid

Salicylic acid decreases skin pH, which causes increased hydration of keratin and thus facilitates its loosening and removal. Because contact time is minimal for a shampoo, percutaneous absorption of the agent is minimal.[4]

Topical salicylic acid is useful for psoriasis when thick scales are present. However, application over extensive areas should be avoided because of the potential for percutaneous absorption and systemic toxicity, as evidenced by symptoms of salicylism such as tinnitus. Initially, the patient should use lower concentrations to minimize the possibility of causing irritation and worsening the condition.[5]

Salicylic acid has been approved in concentrations of 1.8% to 3% for the self-treatment of dandruff, seborrheic dermatitis, and psoriasis.[18] At these concentrations, the keratolytic effect typically takes 7 to 10 days. In higher concentrations for other uses, the keratolytic effect may be evident in 2 to 3 days.

### Sulfur

Sulfur is believed to cause increased sloughing of cells and to reduce corneocyte counts. Sulfur has been approved in concentrations of 2% to 5% for the self-treatment of dandruff only. Although it is approved as a single-entity active ingredient, sulfur is often combined with salicylic acid.[18] Although not FDA-approved indication, this combination has been commonly used for the self-treatment of seborrheic dermatitis.[6]

## Topical Hydrocortisone

Topical hydrocortisone 0.5% and 1% is available without a prescription and is FDA approved for the temporary relief of itching associated with minor skin irritations, inflammation, and rashes caused by eczema, psoriasis, seborrheic dermatitis, poison ivy, poison oak, poison sumac, insect bites, soaps, detergents, cosmetics, and jewelry and for external feminine and anal itching. It is not indicated, nor is evidence available that it is effective, in treating dandruff. However, it may be useful for seborrhea accompanied by inflammation that is unresponsive to medicated shampoos.[6]

Nonprescription hydrocortisone products (Table 34-4) can play a role in managing mild psoriasis. Relapse occurs more quickly after use of topical corticosteroids than after use of tar therapy. Nevertheless, corticosteroids are more appealing to patients on cosmetic grounds, which is a consideration in long-term therapy.[13]

Topical corticosteroids have several effects (e.g., anti-inflammatory, antimitotic/antisynthetic, antipruritic, vasoconstrictive, immunosuppressive) on cellular activity. Efficacy may be enhanced by using the ointment dosage form

**TABLE 34-4 Distinguishing Features of Scaly Dermatoses**

| | Dandruff | Seborrheic Dermatitis | Psoriasis |
|---|---|---|---|
| Location | Scalp | Adults and children: head and trunk; children only: back, intertriginous areas | Scalp, elbows, knees, trunk, lower extremities |
| Exacerbating factors | Generally a stable condition, exacerbated by dry climate | Exacerbated by many external factors, notably stress | Exacerbated by irritation, stress, climate, medications, infection, endocrine factors |
| Appearance | Thin, white, or grayish flakes; even distribution on scalp | Macules, patches, and thin plaques of discrete yellow, oily scales on red skin | Discreet symmetrical, red plaques with sharp border; silvery white scale; small bleeding points when removed; difficult to distinguish from seborrhea in early stages or in intertriginous zones |
| Inflammation | Absent | Present | Present |
| Epidermal hyperplasia | Absent | Present | Present |
| Epidermal kinetics | Turnover rate 2 times faster than normal | Turnover rate about 3 times faster than normal | Turnover rate about 5-6 times faster than normal |
| Percentage of incompletely keratinized cells | Rarely exceeds 5% of total corneocyte count | Commonly makes up 15%-25% of corneocyte count | Commonly makes up 40%-60% of corneocyte count |

*Source:* Adapted from reference 3 and McGinley KJ, Marples RR, Plewig G, et al. A method for visualizing and quantitating the desquamating portion of the human stratum corneum. *J Invest Dermatol.* 1969;53:107.

and an occlusive dressing (cover with Saran Wrap for 12 to 24 hours). If the patient does not respond adequately to hydrocortisone, referral to a primary care provider is appropriate because the use of more potent corticosteroids may be in order.

Adverse effects associated with the use of topical corticosteroids include local atrophy after prolonged use as well as the aggravation of certain cutaneous infections. The possibility of systemic sequelae exists and is enhanced by the use of the more potent compounds, by occlusive dressings, or by application to large areas of the body. Because children have a greater surface area-to-body mass ratio, they are at greater risk for developing systemic complications. In general, however, the concentrations of hydrocortisone available in nonprescription preparations are highly unlikely to cause systemic sequelae.

### Other Agents

*Ketoconazole* Ketoconazole, a synthetic azole antifungal agent, is available as a nonprescription shampoo formulation. Nizoral AD (ketoconazole 1%) is active against most pathogenic fungi but is indicated specifically for *Pityrosporon yeast.* Thus, it is used to treat dandruff and seborrheic dermatitis of the scalp. Although the fungal etiology of dandruff and seborrhea has been debated in the past, the efficacy of newer antifungal agents against these conditions has resulted in FDA OTC review panel endorsement of these agents for treatment of these two common skin disorders. In addition to ketoconazole shampoo, other antifungals such as clotrimazole and miconazole (cream or solution) have been used to treat seborrheic dermatitis of areas other than the scalp.

As with other medicated shampoos, contact time is crucial. The scalp and hair should be wet; then the shampoo should be massaged well into the scalp and left on for 3 to 5 minutes. The scalp and hair should be thoroughly rinsed and the process repeated. The patient should use ketoconazole shampoo twice a week for 4 weeks, with at least 3 days between each treatment. Once the condition is controlled, the shampoo can be applied once weekly or once every other week.

Adverse effects are minimal, but hair loss, skin irritation, abnormal hair texture, and dry skin have been reported.

*Detergents* Detergents are not generally considered to be active ingredients in antidandruff products. However, for mild forms of dandruff, frequent and vigorous washing with a nonmedicated shampoo may help control excess scaling. Massaging the scalp produces a dispersion of scales into smaller, less-visible subunits. Detergents may contribute to this effect by virtue of their surfactant activity. Detergents found in shampoos include sodium lauryl sulfate, polyoxyethylene ethers, triethanolamine, and quaternary ammonium compounds such as benzalkonium chloride, benzethonium chloride, and isoquinolinium bromide.[5]

## ASSESSMENT OF SCALY DERMATOSES: A CASE-BASED APPROACH

Differentiation of the scaly dermatoses involves several factors. The appearance of the scales in the early stages of a disorder is not always definitive. In these cases, the presence and nature of other symptoms or the location of the dermatitis provide additional important clues to its assessment. Factors that precipitate or exacerbate the disorder are also helpful in defining the disorder. Table 34-4 describes the distinguishing features of these three dermatoses. Cases 34-1 and 34-2 illustrate the assessment of patients with scaly dermatoses.

## CASE 34-1

| Relevant Evaluation Criteria | Scenario/Model Outcome |
|---|---|
| **Information Gathering** | |
| 1. Gather essential information about the patient's symptoms, including: | |
| a. description of symptom(s) (i.e., nature, onset, duration, severity, associated symptoms) | Patient has had excessive dandruff with itchy, flaky scalp during the past several months. He also has some yellow, oily scales around his nose and mouth. |
| b. description of any factors that seem to precipitate, exacerbate, and/or relieve the patient's symptom(s) | The condition has grown worse with the onset of winter. |
| c. description of the patient's efforts to relieve the symptoms | Daily shampooing with Head and Shoulders Shampoo for the past 2 weeks has not improved the condition. |
| 2. Gather essential patient history information: | |
| a. patient's identity | Joel Barker |
| b. patient's age, sex, height, and weight | 24 y/o M, 5'8", 175 lb |
| c. patient's occupation | Computer programmer |
| d. patient's dietary habits | Normal diet |
| e. patient's sleep habits | 6-7 hours of sleep per night |
| f. concurrent medications and medical conditions | Takes a daily vitamin supplement; no known medical conditions |
| g. allergies | None |
| h. history of other adverse reactions to medications | None |
| i. other (describe)_______ | Joel has experienced some mild dandruff symptoms in the past but nothing this severe until recently. Previous episodes of dandruff have responded to Head & Shoulders Shampoo or Pert Plus Dandruff Shampoo. |
| **Assessment and Triage** | |
| 3. Differentiate the patient's signs/symptoms and correctly identify the patient's primary problem(s) (see Table 34-4). | Joel appears to have seborrheic dermatitis on his face and possibly his scalp. The scales on his scalp should be examined to determine if they are dry or oily. If dry, his scalp condition may be classic dandruff. |
| 4. Identify exclusions for self-treatment (see Figure 34-1). | None |
| 5. Formulate a comprehensive list of therapeutic alternatives to address the primary problem and share this information with the patient. | Options include:<br>(1) Recommend self-care with an appropriate OTC product (pyrithione zinc, selenium sulfide, coal tar, or ketoconazole shampoo) with nondrug measures.<br>(2) Refer Joel to a PCP or dermatologist.<br>(3) Recommend self-care until a PCP or dermatologist can be consulted.<br>(4) Take no action. |
| **Plan** | |
| 6. Select an optimal therapeutic alternative to address the patient's problem, taking into account patient preferences. | OTC treatment with Nizoral AD (ketoconazole). Shampoo may be the best option for Joel initially. A mild soap may also be recommended for his face. Hydrocortisone 1% cream can be applied to the face if redness persists after using the medicated shampoo. See Figure 34-1 and Table 34-2 for product options. |

## CASE 34-1 (continued)

| Relevant Evaluation Criteria | Scenario/Model Outcome |
|---|---|
| 7. Describe the recommended therapeutic approach to the patient. | Apply the ketoconazole shampoo to your scalp and affected areas of your face two times a week (with at least 3 days between applications) for 4 weeks. Once the condition is controlled, it can be applied once weekly or once every other week. If hydrocortisone cream is used, it should be applied two to three times daily for 7 days. |
| 8. Explain to the patient the rationale for selecting the recommended therapeutic alternatives that were considered. | Ketoconazole shampoo was selected since you have had limited success with pyrithione zinc and the use of selenium products may increase oiliness in patients with seborrheic dermatitis. Coal tar shampoo is an option, but many patients find the odor unacceptable. |
| **Patient Education** | |
| 9. When recommending self-care with nonprescription medications and/or nondrug therapy, convey accurate information to the patient, including: | |
| a. appropriate dose and frequency of administration | See the box Patient Education for Scaly Dermatoses. |
| b. maximum number of days the therapy should be employed | See the box Patient Education for Scaly Dermatoses. |
| c. product administration procedures | See the box Patient Education for Scaly Dermatoses. |
| d. expected time to onset of relief | See the box Patient Education for Scaly Dermatoses. |
| e. degree of relief that can be reasonably expected | See the box Patient Education for Scaly Dermatoses. |
| f. most common side effects | See the box Patient Education for Scaly Dermatoses. |
| g. side effects that warrant medical intervention should they occur | See the box Patient Education for Scaly Dermatoses. |
| h. patient options in the event that condition worsens or persists | See the box Patient Education for Scaly Dermatoses. |
| i. product storage requirements | See the box Patient Education for Scaly Dermatoses. |
| j. specific nondrug measures | See the box Patient Education for Scaly Dermatoses. |
| 10. Solicit follow-up questions from patient. | I have never left a shampoo on my hair for more than about 30 seconds. Is it really necessary to leave it on for 3-5 minutes? |
| 11. Answer patient's questions. | Yes. The effectiveness of the medicated shampoo is directly associated with scalp contact time. The Head and Shoulders shampoo may not have been left on long enough to be effective. |

Key: OTC, over-the-counter; PCP, primary care provider.

## CASE 34-2

| Relevant Evaluation Criteria | Scenario/Model Outcome |
|---|---|
| **Information Gathering** | |
| 1. Gather essential information about the patient's symptoms, including: | |
| a. description of symptom(s) (i.e., nature, onset, duration, severity, associated symptoms) | Patient has new "scales" around her knees and legs. She admits to "picking" at her lesions and noticing some little bleeding marks. |

## CASE 34-2 (continued)

| Relevant Evaluation Criteria | Scenario/Model Outcome |
|---|---|
| b. description of any factors that seem to precipitate, exacerbate, and/or relieve the patient's symptom(s) | Being out in the sun appears to be beneficial. The scaling is worse when patient feels stressed. |
| c. description of the patient's efforts to relieve the symptoms | Use of Vaseline Intensive Care Lotion on a daily basis has produced minimal benefit. |
| 2. Gather essential patient history information: | |
| a. patient's identity | Ileana Bradenburg |
| b. patient's age, sex, height, and weight | 50 y/o F, 5'3", 165 lb |
| c. patient's occupation | Factory worker |
| d. patient's dietary habits | Normal diet |
| e. patient's sleep habits | 6-7 hours of sleep per night |
| f. concurrent medications and medical conditions | Hypertension diagnosed 6 months ago; started therapy with atenolol 50 mg by mouth once daily approximately 4 months ago |
| g. allergies | Sulfa (rash) |
| h. history of other adverse reactions to medications | None |
| i. other (describe)_______ | Ileana takes long hot showers, especially in the winter. |
| **Assessment and Triage** | |
| 3. Differentiate the patient's signs/symptoms and correctly identify the patient's primary problem(s) (see Table 34-4). | Ileana has dry scaly skin most likely caused by psoriasis. The condition may have been triggered by atenolol, a β-blocker. |
| 4. Identify exclusions for self-treatment (see Figure 34-1). | None |
| 5. Formulate a comprehensive list of therapeutic alternatives to address the primary problem, and share this information with the patient. | Options include:<br>(1) Recommend self-care with a proper OTC product (hydrocortisone) with modification of her bathing habits.<br>(2) Refer Ileana to a PCP or dermatologist.<br>(3) Recommend self-care until an appropriate health care provider can be consulted.<br>(4) Take no action. |
| **Plan** | |
| 6. Select an optimal therapeutic alternative to address the patient's problem, taking into account patient preferences. | Treatment with a moisturizing cream after bathing. Scales can be removed by gentle rubbing during bathing. Hydrocortisone 1% ointment can be applied to relieve itching. |
| 7. Describe the recommended therapeutic approach to the patient. | Apply emollients to the affected areas three to four times daily. Hydrocortisone 1% ointment should also be applied three to four times per day. You should attempt to minimize stressful situations. |
| 8. Explain to the patient the rationale for selecting the recommended therapeutic approach from the considered therapeutic alternatives. | Mild psoriasis may be managed with nonprescription topical therapy plus modification of your bathing habits. Hydrocortisone was chosen over coal tar or salicylic acid preparations because of better patient acceptance and faster relief of itching. |
| **Patient Education** | |
| 9. When recommending self-care with nonprescription medications and/or nondrug therapy, convey accurate information to the patient, including: | See the box Patient Education for Scaly Dermatoses. |

**CASE 34-2 (continued)**

| Relevant Evaluation Criteria | Scenario/Model Outcome |
|---|---|
| a. appropriate dose and frequency of administration | See the box Patient Education for Scaly Dermatoses. |
| b. maximum number of days the therapy should be employed | See the box Patient Education for Scaly Dermatoses. |
| c. product administration procedures | See the box Patient Education for Scaly Dermatoses. |
| d. expected time to onset of relief | See the box Patient Education for Scaly Dermatoses. |
| e. degree of relief that can be reasonably expected | See the box Patient Education for Scaly Dermatoses. |
| f. most common side effects | See the box Patient Education for Scaly Dermatoses. |
| g. side effects that warrant medical intervention should they occur | See the box Patient Education for Scaly Dermatoses. |
| h. patient options in the event that condition worsens or persists | Your primary care provider or a dermatologist should be consulted if the condition does not improve. Topical coal tar, salicylic acid, or a higher-potency corticosteroid ointment may be required. In addition, your skin condition may be related to the use of atenolol. Your primary care provider may decide to prescribe an alternative hypertensive agent. |
| i. product storage requirements | See the box Patient Education for Scaly Dermatoses. |
| j. specific nondrug measures | See the box Patient Education for Scaly Dermatoses. |
| 10. Solicit follow-up questions from patient. | What types of moisturizers work best? |
| 11. Answer patient's questions. | Moisturizers with an ointment base do a better job of holding moisture in the skin. Try to use them at night. You will need to wear cotton pajamas to prevent your bed linens from becoming greasy. Creams and lotions can be used during the daytime hours. |

Key: OTC, over-the-counter; PCP, primary care provider.

## PATIENT COUNSELING FOR SCALY DERMATOSES

Patients need to know that scaly dermatoses are rarely cured by pharmacotherapy; rather, nonprescription agents help control the signs and symptoms of the disorders. The practitioner should also explain that fluctuation in severity of seborrhea and psoriasis may be related to emotional, physical, or environmental factors.

Explanations of the proper use of cytostatic and keratolytic agents should include information about the length of time to leave the agent on the affected area. The practitioner should also explain possible adverse effects and drug interactions with recommended agents. Finally, the practitioner should advise the patient what signs and symptoms indicate medical attention is needed. The box Patient Education for Scaly Dermatoses lists specific information to provide to patients.

## EVALUATION OF PATIENT OUTCOMES FOR SCALY DERMATOSES

Follow-up on the patient's progress should occur after 1 week of self-treatment. A scheduled visit to the practitioner is preferable if the lesions are on a part of the body that can be inspected. If the symptoms persist or have worsened after 1 week of treatment, the patient should consult a primary care provider. If the disorder has not worsened, the practitioner should ask the patient to return after a second week of treatment. If the symptoms persist or have worsened after this period, the patient should consult a primary care provider.

## KEY POINTS FOR SCALY DERMATOSES

- Mild to moderate scaly dermatoses can often be effectively managed with topical nonprescription products.
- Products should be selected on the basis of the patient's history and prior response to treatment, as well as on the basis of a careful evaluation of the risks and benefits of using the nonprescription products.
- The practitioner should be sure to educate patients about the proper application of topical therapy as it greatly impacts the efficacy of therapy.

### References

1. Odom RB, James WD, Berger T. *Andrews Diseases of the Skin: Clinical Dermatology.* 9th ed. Philadelphia: WB Saunders; 2000.
2. Hay RJ, Graham-Brown RAC. Dandruff and seborrheic dermatitis: causes and management. *Clin Exp Dermatol.* 1997;22:3-6.

## PATIENT EDUCATION FOR SCALY DERMATOSES

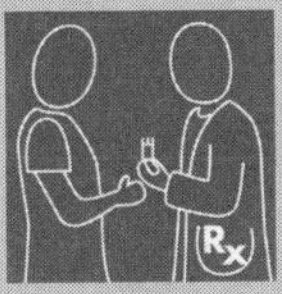

The primary objective for self-treating dandruff, seborrhea, and psoriasis is to reduce the turnover rate of skin cells, which is responsible for the scaly lesions. Controlling inflammation and itching of the affected areas is another treatment objective for seborrhea and psoriasis. Although the chronicity and incurability of these disorders carefully following product instructions and the self-care measures can help ensure optimal therapeutic outcomes for many patients.

### General Measures

- Shampoo the hair with the medicated shampoo three times per week initially, leaving the shampoo on the hair for 3 to 5 minutes. Work the shampoo into the scalp and affected area of the face. Use a scalp scrubber to ensure penetration to the scalp. Repeat application.
- If used, apply a thin layer of the hydrocortisone cream two to three times daily. Wash the affected areas before use.
- Use the shampoo for a minimum of 2 weeks to determine effectiveness and then on a weekly or biweekly basis to control the condition.
- With usage of medication and proper nondrug therapy, noticeable improvement could be observed within 7 to 14 days. Complete control of the condition is possible with periodic use of the medicated shampoo. It is likely that exacerbations may occasionally appear, especially during the winter months.
- Stinging or burning may occur if medicated shampoo enters the eyes.
- Use of coal tar products can stain light-colored hair and sensitize patients to the sun.

### Dandruff

- Use a medicated shampoo containing ketoconazole, pyrithione zinc, selenium sulfide, or coal tar. If these agents are ineffective, use a medicated shampoo containing sulfur or salicylic acid.
- Coal tar can stain light hair, and cause folliculitis (inflammation of hair follicles), dermatitis, and photosensitization (sensitivity of the skin to sunlight).
- Shampoo the hair with the medicated shampoo, and leave it on the hair for several minutes. Rinse the hair thoroughly and repeat.

### Seborrhea

- Use a medicated shampoo containing ketoconazole, pyrithione zinc, or selenium sulfide. Note that selenium sulfide may increase scalp oiliness or worsen seborrhea in some individuals.
- If redness persists after therapy with medicated shampoos, apply hydrocortisone two to three times a day until symptoms subside and then intermittently to control acute exacerbations. Do not use this agent longer than 7 days. Prolonged use can cause rebound flare-ups when the hydrocortisone is discontinued.
- After shampooing, part the hair, apply the product directly to the scalp, and massage it in thoroughly. Repeat this process until the affected area is covered.

### Psoriasis

- For itchy, dry skin, use emollients and lubricating bath products (see Chapter 33, Table 33-4). Remove scales by gently rubbing them with a soft cloth following the bath. Do not rub vigorously. Avoid alcohol and smoking. Obese patients should lose weight.
- For scalp psoriasis, use medicated shampoos containing coal tar or salicylic acid.
- For daytime treatment of itchiness, apply hydrocortisone 1% cream three to four times daily. Reduce frequency of application as the condition improves. Do not use this agent longer than 7 days.
- To help loosen and remove scales during the day, soak the affected body area in warm (not hot) water for 10 to 20 minutes. Then apply a salicylic acid product. Do not apply salicylic acid to extensive areas of the body. The agent may be absorbed into the bloodstream.
- For more effective removal of scales, apply coal tar products to lesions on the body, arms, and legs at bedtime. Note that this agent stains bed linen and clothing. Bathe in the morning to remove residual coal tar and also to loosen psoriatic scales. If preferred, apply salicylic acid at bedtime.
- For psoriasis of the armpits, genital areas, and anus, use hydrocortisone instead of coal tar or salicylic acid.
- When bright red lesions are present, use only emollients and hydrocortisone until the flare-up has subsided. Resume therapy with coal tar and salicylic acid when the thick-scaled plaques appear.
- Prevent flare-ups by minimizing factors such as emotional stress, skin irritation, and physical trauma that you know will exacerbate the disorder.
- Consult a primary care provider before treating psoriasis with sun exposure.
- Take an NSAID (e.g., aspirin, ibuprofen, naproxen, or ketoprofen) for swelling of joints associated with psoriatic arthritis (see Chapter 7).

⚠ Consult a primary care provider if the condition does not improve or if it worsens after 1 to 2 weeks of treatment with nonprescription medications.


3. Johnson M-Lt, Roberts J. *Prevelance of Dermatological Diseases Among Persons 1-74 Years of Age.* Washington, DC: US Department of Health and Education, National Center of Health Statistics; 1978.
4. Brodell RT, Cooper KD. Therapeutic shampoo. In: Wolverton SE, ed. *Comprehensive Dermatologic Drug Therapy.* Philadelphia: WB Saunders; 2001:647-58.
5. Han NH, West DP. Scaly dermatoses. In: Berardi RR, DeSimone EM, Newton GD, et al., eds. *Handbook of Nonprescription Drugs.* 12th ed. Washington, DC: American Pharmaceutical Association; 2000:633-45.
6. Cropley TG, Wintroub BU. Seborrheic dermatitis. In: Arndt KA, Wintroub BU, Robinson JK, et al., eds. *Primary Care Dermatology.* Philadelphia: WB Saunders; 1997:193-5.
7. Burton JL, Holden CA. Atopic dermatitis. In: Champion RH, Burton JL, Ebling FJG, eds. *Textbook of Dermatology.* 6th ed. Oxford, England: Blackwell Science; 1998:638-43.
8. Plewig G, Jansen T. Seborrheic dermatitis. In: Freedberg IM, Eisen AZ, Wolff K, et al., eds. *Fitzpatrick's Dermatology in General Medicine.* 5th ed. New York: McGraw-Hill, Inc; 1999:1482-3.
9. Holden CA, Berth-Jones J. Eczema, lichenfication, prurigo and erythroderma. In: Burns T, Breathnach S, Cox N, Griffiths C,

eds. *Rook's Textbook of Dermtology.* 7th ed. Malden, Mass: Blackwell Publishing; 2004:17:10-17:15.
10. Griffiths CEM, Camp RDR, Barker JNWN. Psoriasis. In: Burns T, Breathnach S, Cox N, Griffiths C, eds. *Rook's Textbook of Dermtology.* 7th ed. Malden, Mass: Blackwell Publishing; 2004:35.1-35.51.
11. Christophers E, Mrowietz U. Psoriasis. In: Freedberg IM, Eisen AZ, Wolff K, et al., eds. *Fitzpatrick's Dermatology in General Medicine.* 5th ed. New York: McGraw-Hill, Inc; 1999:495-521.
12. Sege-Peterson K, Winchester RJ. Psoriatic arthritis. In: Freedberg IM, Eisen AZ, Wolff K, et al., eds. *Fitzpatrick's Dermatology in General Medicine.* 5th ed. New York: McGraw-Hill, Inc; 1999:522-33.
13. Stern RS. Psoriasis. In: Arndt KA, Wintroub BU, Robinson JK, et al., eds. *Primary Care Dermatology.* Philadelphia: WB Saunders; 1997:177-81.
14. MacKie RM. Psoriasis, papulosquamous diseases, and disorders of keratinization. In: *Clinical Dermatology.* 4th ed. Oxford, England: Oxford University Press; 1997:44-62.
15. Camp RD. Psoriasis. In: Champion RH, Burton JL, Burns DA, et al., eds. *Textbook of Dermatology.* 6th ed. Oxford, England: Blackwell Science; 1998:1595-6.
16. *Federal Register.* 2005;70:73178-81.
17. *Federal Register.* 2005;70:72448-9.
18. *Federal Register.* 1991;56:63554-69.

CHAPTER 35

# Contact Dermatitis

*Kenneth R. Keefner*

Contact dermatitis accounts for 5.7 million primary care provider (PCP) visits per year, not to mention the number of requests for the clinician to evaluate and help relieve this condition. Contact dermatitis is defined as an inflammatory skin condition characterized by inflammation, redness, itching, burning, stinging, and vesicle and pustule formation on dermal areas exposed to irritant or allergenic agents.[1-3] Irritant contact dermatitis (ICD) is an inflammatory reaction of the skin caused by exposure to an irritant. Allergic contact dermatitis (ACD) is an inflammatory reaction of the skin caused by exposure to an allergen.[3] In industrial societies, ICD and ACD commonly occur in 1% to 10% of the population.

## IRRITANT CONTACT DERMATITIS

### Epidemiology of ICD

The majority of ICD cases are related to occupation, especially jobs that involve exposure to irritant chemicals. Although contact dermatitis may be caused by chemical exposure in the home, available statistics cover only contact dermatitis associated with occupations and job tasks. According to a recent report, work-related dermatoses comprise 15% of the total workplace injuries.[4] Overall, persons employed in forestry, agriculture, and fishing industries have the greatest incidence at 155 per 100,000 workers. Workers in the manufacturing and service sectors follow with 110 and 50 incidents per 100,000 workers, respectively.[5,6]

An analysis of several occupational disorders, dermatitis among them, showed the highest incidence of contact dermatitis in health care professionals (physicians, nurses, pharmacists, dietitians, and others in related professions); second highest were individuals in personal service occupations; and third highest were health care therapists, technologists, technicians, and assistants.[7] The Bureau of Labor Statistics (BLS) annual survey of occupational illnesses reveals that occupational contact dermatitis accounts for 90% to 95% of all occupational skin diseases. Of this, 80% is related to ICD. In 1999, the BLS identified that 12% of all occupational illnesses reported are skin diseases/disorders and make up the highest percentage of nontraumatic work-related illness. The number of cases is estimated to be 10 to 50 times greater than actually reported because of changes in industry procedure, underreporting of incidents, and limitations in data collection for the BLS survey. A 1984 report estimated that the national medical costs for treating occupational skin diseases at that time was $4.7 million annually.[5]

### Etiology of ICD

Approximately 80% to 90% of the cases of contact dermatitis are caused by exposure to irritants such as harsh chemicals and solvents (Table 35-1).[8-10]

### Pathophysiology of ICD

Contact dermatitis may appear after a single exposure or following multiple exposures to the same agent. Several mechanisms may be responsible for inciting ICD. First, the chemical may directly damage the dermal cells by direct absorption through the cell membrane, destroying cell systems. A second mechanism may be through mediators released by nonspecifically activated T cells.[3,11] The reaction has no immune basis and does not require previous exposure to an irritant for a reaction to appear.

Several factors may affect the magnitude of the skin response. The presence of existing skin diseases or conditions can result in a more profound dermatitis by allowing the irritant to easily enter the dermis. The quantity and concentration of chemical exposure are also important. The greater the concentration and length of exposure, the more likely a severe dermatitis will occur. Strong chemical irritants, acids, and alkalis are more likely to produce immediate and severe inflammatory reactions. Mild irritants, such as detergents, soaps, and solvents, may require successive exposures before the dermatitis appears. Occlusion of skin areas by shoes, gloves, and other protective clothing may lead to more severe reactions when exposure to irritants occurs because the protective clothing harbors the irritants. This reaction develops simply through normal skin respiration and humidification; the occluded skin allows greater skin penetrability of the irritant. In addition, environmental factors, such as warmer ambient temperature and higher humidity, or wet work, may contribute to more severe dermatologic conditions.[1,9]

### Signs and Symptoms of ICD

On exposure to an irritant, the skin becomes inflamed and swollen, turns red, and may develop small vesicles or papules that ooze fluid when opened. Itching, stinging, and burning commonly accompany the rash. The inflammatory reaction is variable, and may range from these initial symptoms to ulcer formation and localized necrotic areas

**TABLE 35-1 Selected Common Irritants Associated with Contact Dermatitis**

| |
|---|
| Strong acids (hydrochloric, nitric, sulfuric, hydrofluoric) |
| Strong alkalis (sodium, potassium, calcium hydroxides) |
| Detergents |
| Epoxy resins |
| Ethylene oxide |
| Fiberglass |
| Leather tanning agents |
| Oils (cutting, lubricating, etc.) |
| Solvents |
| Oxidizing agents |
| Reducing agents |
| Oxidants, plasticizers, and activators in athletic shoes |
| Wood dust and products |

*Source:* Adapted from references 8-10.

of skin. Within several days, the dermatitis may crust, especially if the irritant is avoided. If the patient remains free of the irritant, the dermatitis will resolve in several days. In patients chronically exposed to an irritant, the affected areas of skin will remain inflamed, begin to furrow and scale, and may become hyper- or hypopigmented.[1,9,11,12] A portion of patients chronically exposed to irritants recover completely, whereas a majority improve but continue to have recurrences. The remainder continue to have an inflammatory process comparable to or worse than the original insult. This latter condition has come to be known as "persistent postoccupational dermatitis," in that the dermatitis persists though there is no identifiable irritant source.[13]

Most instances of ICD occur on exposed or unprotected skin surfaces, especially the face and dorsal surfaces of the hands and arms, because of heightened exposure. Approximately 80% of the cases of ICD involve the hands and 10% involve facial dermatitis.[6]

## Treatment of ICD

### *Treatment Goals*

The goals in self-treating ICD are to (1) relieve the inflammation, dermal tenderness, and irritation; (2) prevent continued exposure to the irritant substance; and (3) educate the patient on methods to prevent recurrence.

### *General Treatment Approach*

The approach to treating ICD will depend primarily on the severity of the reaction. Regardless of the severity, the area of initial exposure to the irritant substance should be washed with copious amounts of water and cleansed with a mild or hypoallergenic soap. Avoidance of the irritant is a hallmark of treatment and patient education. Application of wet compresses of the astringent aluminum acetate soothes and dries weeping lesions. Hydrocortisone, calamine lotion, and colloidal oatmeal baths are helpful in relieving associated itching. The use of topical local caine-type anesthetics should be avoided because of their ability to generate a contact dermatitis. Figure 35-1 outlines self-treatment of ICD and lists exclusions for self-treatment.

### *Nonpharmacologic Therapy*

Immediately washing exposed areas will reduce the contact time of the offending substance and, if a dermal response occurs, help prevent the spread of the dermatitis. (See Hygienic Measures for specific bathing/showering information.) Any substance that has created a dermal response should be avoided. Educating the patient in techniques to reduce risk of exposure is fundamental. Using protective clothing, gloves, and other protective equipment and limiting the time skin areas are occluded through frequent changes in coverings will aid in reducing irritant exposure. Hydropel and Hollister Moisture Barrier Cream claim to prevent ICD if applied before contact with an irritant.[14]

### *Pharmacologic Therapy*

The same pharmacologic treatment is used for ICD, ACD, and poison ivy/oak/sumac dermatitis. (See Treatment of ACD for a detailed discussion of the appropriate pharmacologic agents.)

# ALLERGIC CONTACT DERMATITIS

Although ACD accounts for a small percentage of contact dermatitis cases, poison ivy/oak/sumac dermatitis is responsible for a large number of field occupational injuries and is the primary cause of ACD. For these reasons, poison ivy/oak/sumac dermatitis is discussed in more detail than other ACDs.

## Epidemiology of ACD

Allergen exposure is the cause of 10% to 20% of contact dermatitis cases. Poison ivy/oak/sumac dermatitis, also referred to as *Rhus* dermatitis, is the principal cause of ACD in the United States and exceeds the incidence of all other causes of ACD combined. Several million cases of poison ivy are reported each year in the United States, and they account for the largest number of worker's compensation claims. These plants are the primary cause of injuries in the field for U.S. Forestry Service personnel.[15] After poison ivy/oak/sumac, metal allergy, most often caused by nickel, is the most common form of ACD. In fact, approximately 14.2% of all patients patch tested for allergies are allergic to nickel.[16] Cosmetics and skin care products can also cause ACD. Although they are not common, dermatologists estimate that 1 in 5000 (0.21%) people may suffer from such dermatoses.[17]

No other plant in the United States can compare with the *Toxicodendron* genus in the magnitude of disease caused.[18] Dermatitis caused by this family of plants provides an excellent opportunity for practitioners to apply the tenets of good pharmaceutical care, while directing the care and treatment of patients afflicted with this uncomfortable rash.

**Exclusions for Self-Treatment**

- <2 years of age
- Dermatitis present >2 weeks
- Involvement of >25% of body surface area
- Presence of numerous bullae
- Extreme itching, irritation, or severe vesicle and bullae formation
- Swelling of the body or extremities
- Swollen eyes or eyelids swollen shut
- Discomfort in genitalia from itching, redness, swelling, or irritation
- Involvement and/or itching of mucous membranes of the mouth, eyes, nose, or anus
- Low tolerance for pain, itching, or symptom discomfort
- Impairment of daily activities

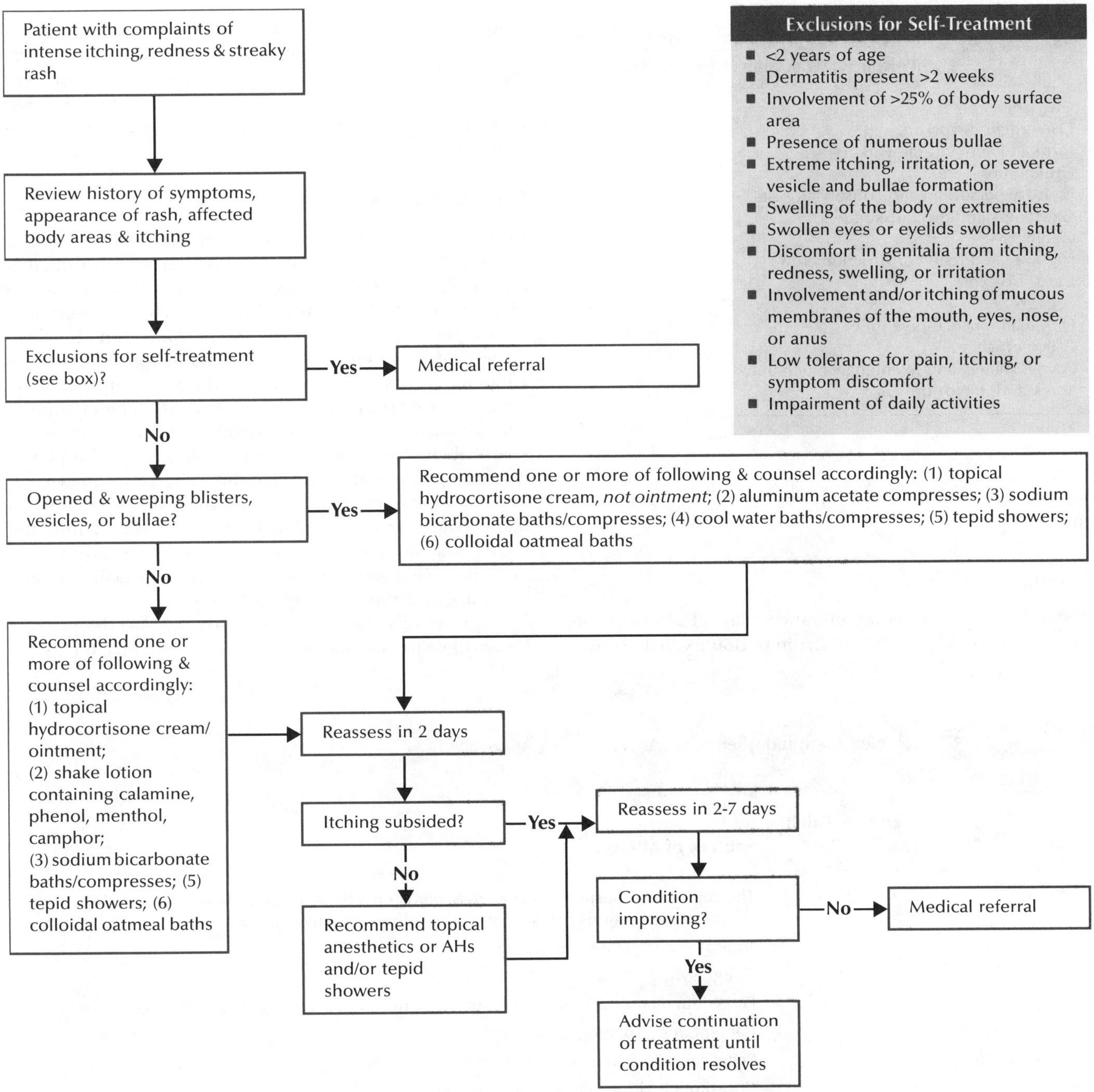


**FIGURE 35-1** Self-care of contact dermatitis. Key: AH, antihistamine.

The incidence of poison ivy/oak/sumac dermatitis begins in patients as young as 3 years old. It continues to rise through early adulthood and begins to decline only during the mid-30s. After this period, its incidence peaks once again and continues to climb throughout the fifth decade of life. Primarily because of diminished exposure after age 65 years, the incidence of this dermatitis again declines and remains low throughout the remainder of the human life cycle.

As much as 80% of the U.S. population is estimated to be sensitive to poison ivy's urushiol, the oleoresin that causes the dermatitis, whereas only 50% of the population will show a dermatologic reaction to urushiol. (Ordinary patch testing is not used to confirm poison ivy sensitivity. Many researchers believe that patch testing will sensitize the patient who is not already sensitive to urushiol.)

The peak ages at which adults show their greatest reactivity and sensitivity to urushiol are between 25 and 50 years. Several reports exist of dark-skinned people being less susceptible to urushiol than other individuals.[19]

The primary incidences of poison ivy rash occur through outdoor recreation and exercise. Of equal importance are various occupations linked with Toxicodendron exposure in the daily work environment, as shown in Table 35-2.

In the past, poison ivy/oak/sumac dermatitis has been the major cause of occupational skin diseases. It accounts

**TABLE 35-2 Occupations at Risk for Developing Poison Ivy/Oak/Sumac Dermatitis**

Civil engineers
Construction workers
Farm and agricultural workers
Firefighters
Forestry personnel and conservationists
Gardeners and groundskeepers
Geologists
Highway and road construction crews
Land surveyors
Loggers
Park maintenance personnel
Police officers
Power utilities and maintenance personnel
Truck and tractor drivers

for 9.94% of occupational injuries caused by a plant dermatitis.[20,21]

## Etiology of ACD

Numerous environmental substances may act as an antigen in the right patient. Urushiol (from poison ivy/oak/sumac plants), nickel salts (in jewelry, clothing), and fragrances (in cosmetics) are examples of allergens capable of producing ACD. Table 35-3 lists *selected* allergenic substances and is not comprehensive. The reader is directed to review the references used to generate this table for more comprehensive information.

### *Urushiol-induced ACD*

In the United States, five species of *Toxicodendron* plants, which belong to the family Anacardiaceae, are primarily responsible for dermatoses associated with exposure to plants (Table 35-4).[22] Many of these plants were previously considered to belong to the genus *Rhus*, but the term *Toxicodendron* is now the accepted genus for this group of antigenic plants. This genus is used throughout the chapter to appropriately refer to these plants. The change in genus and the difficulty in classifying these plants is the result of the variability in the morphology of the plants. Botanists claim that such variability is based on the effects associated with geographic location, soil, water, and climatic conditions. The plants were reclassified into the genus *Toxicodendron*, but terms such as *Rhus radicans*, *Rhus rash*, and *Rhus dermatitis* are still used, especially in early literature and reference works.

Species of poison ivy and poison oak are the primary causes of rashes induced by *Toxicodendron* plants. If patients

**TABLE 35-3 Selected Common Allergens Associated with ACD**

| Allergen | Positive Patch Test (%)* | Sources of Allergen |
|---|---|---|
| Benzocaine | 2 | The caine-type anesthetics have crossover allergy to other caine-type local anesthetics, topical medications (for skin, eye, ear), other oral medications |
| Bacitracin | 8.7 | Topical and injectable medications |
| Balsam of Peru | 11.9 | Cough syrups, flavors |
| Chromium salts | 2.8 | Potassium dichromate-electroplating, cement, leather tanning agents, detergents, dyes |
| Cobalt chloride | 9 | Cement, metal plating, pigments in paints |
| Colophony (rosin) | 2 | Rosin cake for string instrument bows, sport rosin bags, cosmetics, adhesives |
| Epoxy resins | 1.9 | Constituents prior to mixing and hardening |
| Formaldehyde | 9.3 | Germicides, plastics, clothing, glue, adhesives |
| Fragrances | 11.7 | Cosmetics, household products, eugenol, cinnamic acid, geraniol, oak moss absolute |
| Lanolin | 3.3 | Lotions, moisturizers, cosmetics, soaps |
| Latex | 7.3 | Gloves, syringes, vial closures |
| Nickel sulfate | 14.2 | In jewelry, blue jean studs, utensils, pigments, coins, tools, many metal alloys encountered daily |
| Neomycin sulfate | 13.1 | Medications, antibiotic ointments, other aminoglycosides |
| Plants | Not tested | *Toxicodendron* species (poison ivy, oak, sumac), primrose (*Primula obonica*), tulips, others |
| Rubber (Carba Mix) | 7.3 | Added ingredients, accelerators, activators, other processing chemicals |
| Thiomersal | 10.9 | Preservative in many medications, injectables, cosmetics |

* Percentages are based on the number of participants in a large, national patient population study who reacted to patch testing with these common allergens. Note that the *Toxicodendron* family of plants was not tested.

**TABLE 35-4 Toxicodendron Plants Indigenous to North America**

| Plant (Genus, Species) | Other Common Names | Common Geographic Location |
|---|---|---|
| **Poison Ivy** | | |
| *T. radicans* | Poison vine, mark weed, three-leaved ivy, poor man's liquid amber | Several subspecies exist throughout North America, ranging throughout the United States (central, midwest, south central, southeastern, lower Mississippi Valley regions; specifically, SE Arizona, SW and E Texas, Great Lakes states, and Oklahoma); Canada (Ontario, Nova Scotia); and Mexico. |
| *T. rydbergii* | | The most northerly species exists in southern Canada, United States (Texas and Arizona). |
| **Poison Sumac** | | |
| *T. vernix* | Poison elder, poison ash | Species commonly exists from Quebec to Florida in primarily the eastern third of the U.S. coast. |
| **Western Poison Oak** | | |
| *T. diversilobum* | | Species exists from Baja, California, to British Columbia, Canada, but less so in the northern ranges. |
| **Eastern Poison Oak** | | |
| *T. toxicarium* | | Species exists widely in the southeastern United States. |

*Source:* Adapted with permission from reference 22.

have sensitivity to any one species, they are usually allergic to all members of the genus. Although all five species are common to the United States, they are somewhat indigenous to specific regions of the country. These species are most easily identified as having three leaves emanating from a central stem, with the middle leaflet appearing at the terminal end of the stem. The plants flower in the spring and produce small, waxy, white five-petaled flowers. In the late fall, the plants develop berries that are greenish white, pale yellow, or tan. In the fall, the leaves turn brilliant red or orange. A saying taught to youngsters to help identify the plant and to avoid exposure to urushiol is "Leaves of three; let it be!" In general, this statement is true, but other members of the genus differ in the number of leaflets attached to the central stalk, and in the berry and leaf morphology.

## Poison Ivy

The most common *Toxicodendron* plant found throughout the United States is poison ivy (*T. radicans* and *T. rydbergii*). It is quite common throughout central and northeastern United States and Canada. Poison ivy has been described as a scrambling shrub or a climbing hairy vine that commonly grows up poles, trees, and building walls (see Color Plates, photograph 17A). It also grows along roads, hiking trails, streams, dry rocky canyons, and embankment slopes. *T. radicans* is composed of nine subspecies that can exist as a shrub or a climbing vine, whereas *T. rydbergii* is a dwarf shrub that has large, broad, spoon-shaped leaves with a hairy underside. *T. rydbergii* is the principal variety of poison ivy that grows in the northern United States and southern Canada. *T. radicans* grows over much of the United States as a climbing vine with aerial rootlets.

## Poison Oak

Poison oak has two species indigenous to the United States: *T. diversilobum*, which inhabits the West Coast, and *T. toxicarium*, which inhabits the East Coast. Both species possess leaves similar to those of oak trees; most have an unlobed leaf edge and commonly display three leaflets per stem (see Color Plates, photograph 17B). The leaves and berries of eastern poison oak (*T. toxicarium*) are covered with fine hairs. The plant ordinarily exists as a nonclimbing shrub. Western poison oak (*T. diversilobum*) differs by usually possessing between three and 11 leaflets per stem; its leaves are quite similar to California live oak. Poison oak bears fruit covered with numerous fine hairs. It exists as a shrub capable of climbing to distances as high as 131 ft (40 m). Poison oak grows along streams, in thickets, on wooded slopes, and in dry woodlands. As a rule, poison oak grows well at altitudes below 4000 to 5000 feet.

## Poison Sumac

Poison sumac (*T. vernix*) grows in remote areas of the eastern third of the United States in peat bogs and swampy areas. Although highly antigenic, its remoteness from human contact limits the incidence of human dermatoses. It appears as a shrub or small tree, attains a height of roughly 9.8 ft (3 m), and may resemble, to some extent, either elder or ash trees. Hence, it has been given the names "poison elder" or "poison ash." Its leaves are pinnate and may be almost 16 in. (40 cm) in length; they are odd numbered, ranging between 7 and 13 leaflets. The edges of the leaves are smooth and come to a tip (see Color Plates, photograph 17C).

### Other Causative Plants

In addition to the genus *Toxicodendron*, several other plants are known to have cross-sensitivity with urushiol, causing a poison ivy–like dermatitis in individuals who have been previously sensitized to urushiol. Although this discussion is not all-inclusive, several plants deserve specific mention. The cashew nut tree (*Anacardium occidentale* L.) bears an edible nut, the shells of which contain oils that share a cross-sensitivity to urushiol and produce a similar rash. The peel of the mango fruit (*Magnifera indica* L., Indian mango, king of the fruits, apples of the tropics)[23] contains an antigenic substance that has been responsible for facial, oral, and lip dermatitis and cheilosis. The mango allergen is found in the stems, leaves, and peel, but not in the edible fruit of the mango itself. Even poison ivy–sensitive patients can freely eat the fruit after it has been peeled. Such rashes are commonly encountered in Malaysia and Hawaii when urushiol-sensitive visitors to these locations are exposed to the peels of fresh mangoes.

Lacquer from the Japanese lacquer tree (*T. vernicifluum*) is used as an ingredient in the finish of varnished boxes, rifle stocks, floors, bar rails, teapots, canes, and toilet seats. Urushiol-sensitive individuals who are exposed and reexposed to these lacquered products may have recurrent episodes of ACD. In Korea, the sap of the Japanese lacquer tree is used as an herbal medicament and in basting and boiling chicken. Currently, there are two Korean reports of patients developing generalized dermal reactions to ingestion of the lacquer.[24,25] The fruit of the ginkgo tree (*Ginkgo biloba* L.) contains a cross-sensitive resin that leads to rashes on the lower extremities (caused by walking through an area with fallen fruit) and to dermatitis of the mucous membranes, cheilitis, stomatitis, proctitis, or rectal itching associated with consumption of the fruit.

## Pathophysiology of ACD

Allergic contact dermatitis is an inflammatory dermal reaction related to exposure to an allergen that activates sensitized T cells, which migrate to the site of contact and release their inflammatory mediators. The most well-known and highly publicized ACD is exposure to the poison ivy plant, which is discussed in detail below. ACD ordinarily does not appear on first contact because poison ivy allergens, as well as other allergens responsible for ACD, are immunologically connected, and several steps must occur before the dermatitis is manifested. The immunologic reaction is briefly explained here. First, an initial exposure to the antigen must take place to sensitize the immune system. This is known as the induction phase. With the immune system now sensitized, the next contact with the allergen induces a type IV delayed hypersensitivity reaction, which is a cell-mediated (allergen-sensitized T cells) allergic reaction that can take 24 to 48 hours or longer to develop. This reaction results in the symptoms and dermatitis associated with ACD.[26-28]

The allergenic substance responsible for the dermatologic conditions caused by this genus of plant is known as urushiol. Urushiol has been identified as several chemically similar catechols (3-*n*-alk-[en]-*Y* chols) that vary in concentration according to the species of plant. Urushiol is quite sensitive to oxidation by ambient air. It changes in appearance from clear fluid to a black inky lacquer that becomes tarry and may harden on the damaged portion of the plant in a matter of minutes. This oddity has been used as a visual identifier to confirm the existence of poison ivy, oak, or sumac in the surrounding foliage.[29]

The release of urushiol from the plant can occur only through damage to some portion of the plant itself, either through direct damage by an individual who bruises the plant by lying, sitting, kneeling, or stepping on it, or by contact after damage by natural causes (e.g., wind, rain, insects, or animals eating or damaging the plant). The antigenic urushiol is contained and carried only within resin canals of the plant that do not communicate to the surface of the plant.

Urushiol is not a volatile substance, but it has been implicated in dermatitis when the plant is burned because smoke emanating from burned plants contained the antigen. Urushiol carried by smoke particulates is capable of affecting body surface areas ordinarily viewed as protected (e.g., genitals, buttocks, anus, lungs). This source of exposure is a primary occupational cause of poison ivy and poison oak in personnel who fight forest fires, especially in California and other states along the West Coast.

Patients presenting with poison ivy dermatitis in midwinter or off-season periods may have recently used urushiol-contaminated fomites (inanimate objects). It is well known that urushiol can remain active for long periods of time on inanimate objects, and that it continues to be active within dead and dried parts of plants, especially if they are kept in a dry location. For example, the urushiol contained in dried plants stored at a herbarium—for more than 100 years—has been reported to still retain its ability to incite a dermal rash. The oleoresin is inactivated by exposure to wet environmental conditions. A fomite is easily contaminated with the oleoresin, and is a common source of oddly timed dermatitis. It is not unusual for fomites to become contaminated in one growing season; the contaminating urushiol retains its antigenicity throughout the winter and causes rashes with each use of the fomite in succeeding seasons. Urushiol-contaminated shoes, boots, clothing, garden and work tools, golf clubs, baseball bats, fishing rods, and other recreational equipment, or the fur of domestic pets, have all been implicated as sources of nonseasonal poison ivy rash, as well as of recurrent seasonal rashes.

The reaction to poison ivy is described as a type IV delayed hypersensitivity reaction, or ACD, which requires an initial exposure to the antigenic substance (urushiol). This initial exposure causes a dermal sensitization to the offending allergen to develop. Most clinicians think that the initial exposure is not ordinarily associated with dermal symptoms, although some reports suggest that the initial exposure in very sensitive patients may not only sensitize the patient to urushiol, but also lead to dermatitis as much as 2 to 10 days later.[30] The first sensitizing dose may not produce a rash until as long as 3 weeks after the initial exposure. Other reports suggest that numerous, recurrent exposures may be needed to develop the clinical dermatitis in highly resistant or tolerant patients. In people previously sensitized, the rash and related symptoms may appear at any time between 2 and 48 hours after the second exposure.

The allergic response appears to be a two-step process: initial sensitization (step one), followed by a delayed hypersensitivity reaction (step two) in the dermal layers of the skin. Some clinicians think the urushiol rapidly (10 minutes) enters the skin and attaches to protein molecules found on the surface of Langerhans cells (specialized white blood cells) in the epidermis and to macrophages in the dermis. The Langerhans cells communicate the antigen information to lymphocytes (inducer cells); these cells, in turn, proliferate into circulating T-effector and T-memory lymphocytes. This process allows the immune lymphocytes to become sensitized to future entry of urushiol into the skin layers. With succeeding urushiol exposure, the patient has a delayed hypersensitive reaction that allows T cells to invade the skin area containing the newly deposited urushiol. It has been reported that as little as 2 to 2.5 mg or less of urushiol is enough to stimulate the typical dermal rash in sensitive patients.[31] In patients who are tolerant or show subclinical reactions to the same level of urushiol, as much as 5, 10, or 50 mg may be necessary to elicit an allergic response. Symptoms of pruritus, erythema, vesiculation, and local edema are the result of this cytotoxic immune response.[32,33]

Newborn infants are not sensitive to poison ivy, although experimental results show that 70% to 85% of infants and children may be easily sensitized to poison ivy or urushiol through a single exposure to the plant or its constituents. Although not born sensitive to urushiol, newborns may be sensitized with as little as one application in a localized area, and by 3 years of age they demonstrate peak reactivity to urushiol exposure. Patients of advanced age, in contrast, appear to have a declining sensitivity because of reduced response but have a prolonged duration of symptoms. Itching in patients of advanced age has been observed to be greater than in younger adults. Presentation of symptoms in the older patient may be explained in part by a general decline in immune competence that occurs with age and a reduced ability to be sensitized to a new antigen.

## Signs and Symptoms of ACD

### *General Presentation*

Signs and symptoms of ACD vary depending on the allergen, site and duration of exposure and host factors. Typically, the skin appears red and swollen. Blisters may also appear and form crusts or scales when they break open. Itching, burning, and pain are common symptoms of ACD. A more detailed discussion of the signs and symptoms of the primary plant-induced dermatitis follows.

### *Presentation of Urushiol-induced Dermatitis*

After exposure to urushiol, erythematous itchy patches begin to develop on the affected, exposed areas of the body. The intensity and magnitude of the rash may continue to increase for several days and will depend on the sensitivity of the specific body area exposed, the amount of urushiol on the skin surface, the amount of urushiol that entered the dermis, the duration of the exposure, the rapidity with which the area was cleaned after exposure, and the individual's sensitivity and genetic makeup.

The initial dermal reaction to urushiol is an intense itching of the skin's surface areas exposed to the antigen, followed by erythema. Scratching the area may spread the urushiol to other unexposed skin surfaces if it has not been previously washed from the skin. As the dermatitis progresses, vesicles (blisters) or bullae form, depending on an individual's sensitivity. The vesicles/bullae may break open, releasing their fluid (see Color Plates, photograph 18A). Vesicular fluid does not contain any antigenic material to further spread the dermatitis. Patients may continue to scratch for several days after exposure and excoriate the surface dermal layer, leading to open lesions and the potential for secondary wound infections. Common microbes found in infected poison ivy dermatitis consist of *Staphylococcus aureus*, group A *Streptococcus*, and *Escherichia coli*.[34] In addition to these microbes, other organisms identified depended on where the infection arose on the skin. Oozing and weeping of the vesicular fluid continues to occur for several days, until the affected area develops crusts and begins to dry (see Color Plates, photograph 18B).

Poison ivy rash usually occurs on skin unprotected by clothing. Poison ivy rashes on the East Coast generally occur in the spring and summer, whereas in the southwestern United States poison oak rashes may appear any time, because outdoor living is common throughout the year.[23] Rashes commonly occur on exposed or unprotected skin surfaces, such as the hands and fingers, forearms, ankles, calves of the legs, and areas with thin skin, especially around the eyes, face, and neck. A common patient description that highly suggests poison ivy or oak exposure is streaks of vesicles that correspond to the points of urushiol contact from the damaged plant (see Color Plates, photograph 18C). In fact, specks of black oxidized urushiol may form on the skin and clothing after contamination.

Lesions may develop on skin that is ordinarily considered protected (e.g., the genitals, anus, buttocks, or other covered body surfaces), and occurs primarily through contact with urushiol-contaminated fingers and hands. Unwashed, contaminated hands and fingernails are the principal sources of rash on protected areas of the body. Numerous reports describe the dermatitis on the face and around the eyes, lips, underarms, buttocks, and anus, as well as on the genitalia of the affected patient and his or her sexual partner.

#### Mild Poison Ivy/Oak/Sumac Dermatitis

Mild dermatitis characteristically consists of localized patches of pruritus and erythema, followed by the appearance of vesicles and papules, often in a linear streaking arrangement. Marked swelling of the eyelids without associated swelling of other parts of the face may occur[23] and is caused by rubbing the eyelids with urushiol-contaminated fingers and hands. Clinically, the dermatitis is localized in distinct patches on the unprotected lower and upper extremities.

#### Moderate Poison Ivy/Oak/Sumac Dermatitis

Signs and symptoms of moderate dermatitis include the appearance of bullae and edematous swellings of various body parts, in addition to the pruritus, erythema, papules, and vesicles of mild dermatitis.

#### Severe Poison Ivy/Oak/Sumac Dermatitis

Severe dermatitis is distinguished by extensive involvement and edema of the extremities and the face. Often the eyelids are swollen closed. Extreme itching, irritation, and formation of severe vesicles, blisters, and bullae may also be present. Furthermore, daily activities may be hampered in some patients. Dermatitis or edema affecting large areas of the face, eyes, or genitalia requires immediate medical referral for systemic or parenteral therapy.

Dark-skinned patients may experience a permanent discoloration in areas of dermatitis where severe inflammatory changes and blistering have occurred.

#### Complications

On rare occasions, various other diseases have been associated with exposure to Toxicodendron plants and the development of ACD. Such diseases have included eosinophilia (ordinarily seen with exposure to poison ivy), secondary mania,[35] erythema multiforme,[36] acute respiratory distress syndrome (caused by inhaling urushiol particles carried in smoke),[37] renal failure, dyshydrosis of the hands and feet,[30] and urethritis.

## Treatment of ACD

### *Treatment Goals*

The goals of self-treating ACD are to (1) protect the area affected during the acute phase of the rash, (2) prevent itching and excessive scratching that may lead to open lesions and potential secondary skin infections, and (3) prevent the accumulation of debris that arises from the vesicle fluids oozing, crusting, and scaling, thereby preventing spread of the dermatitis to the surrounding area of inflammation.

Customarily, the first several days following the initial appearance of ACD are usually the most uncomfortable for the patient. Treated or untreated dermatitis will naturally resolve in approximately 10 to 21 days as a result of the patient's own immune system. Topical nonprescription products may be used for symptomatic relief. Patients will seek the practitioner's counsel principally because of the intensity of itching, burning, and pain associated with a mild localized rash, or because of the widespread nature of the dermatitis and the magnitude of symptoms.

The following discussion deals primarily with treatment of poison ivy dermatitis, but the same therapeutic approaches apply to ICDs as well as other ACDs. Therapy is indicated primarily to relieve symptoms associated with the dermatitis and to avoid secondary infection of excoriated portions of the skin caused by excessive scratching.

### *General Treatment Approach*

Cleansing the affected area within the first 10 minutes of exposure reduces the immune response in poison ivy/oak/sumac dermatitis. Removing known allergen from the skin as soon as possible may reduce the chance and/or severity of the immune response.

#### Measures for All ACDs

The aggressiveness and type of treatment for the allergic reaction depends on the severity of the allergic reaction: mild, moderate to severe, or severe. (See the algorithm in Figure 35-1 for a summary of appropriate treatments and exclusions for self-treatment.) If, at the time of presentation, the patient exhibits mild dermatitis (only localized patches of rash with intense pruritus and erythema), the practitioner may initially recommend treatment that includes the topical application of an antipruritic (shake) lotion containing calamine, menthol, phenol, camphor, and antipruritic agents, or the application of a hydrocortisone cream or ointment. As long as the rash does not begin to weep and remains dry, the patient may use shake lotions and ointments. When a rash is present, the patient should avoid further exposure to allergens, *Toxicodendron* plants, or plants with cross-sensitivity to prevent exacerbating the dermatitis. If the rash spreads to larger areas but does not affect the eyes or genitals and does not cover the body (moderate to severe reaction), the patient may use astringent compresses and baths to treat the rash.

#### Measures for Urushiol-induced Dermatitis

*Mild Poison Ivy/Oak/Sumac Dermatitis* Initial treatment recommendations may consist of several options to relieve pruritic symptoms. One option is the use of a shake lotion consisting of calamine lotion with the addition of phenol (1%) and/or menthol (0.25%). The lotion should be shaken well then applied topically to the itchy or erythematous areas every 4 hours as needed for relief of pruritus. The lotion should not be applied if open lesions are present. Calamine leaves a light pink film in the application area, and the patient may find it cosmetically distasteful, especially when applied to the face. Instead, the patient may find a hydrocortisone cream or ointment more esthetically acceptable. These dosage forms, especially the cream, do not bring attention to the affected areas.

Alternatively, patients may use sodium bicarbonate (baking soda) as either a paste or a cool compress to relieve itching and irritation. For paste application, cool tap water is added to sodium bicarbonate powder in sufficient quantity to prepare a paste for direct application to the vesicles. In addition, 1 or 2 cups of sodium bicarbonate powder may be added to a warm bath. The affected areas should be soaked for 15 to 30 minutes and then the paste applied.

The skin should be dried by patting rather than wiping so a film of baking soda will remain on the skin. For very localized dermatitis, baking soda compresses may be applied for 15 to 30 minutes and repeated as needed. Patients should be warned not to use baking soda near the eyes and to consult a PCP if relief is not obtained within 7 days of treatment. Baking soda should not be applied to patients younger than 2 years.

Topical ointments and creams containing anesthetics (benzocaine) or antihistamines (diphenhydramine), which are used for their antipruritic qualities, or antibiotics (neomycin), which are used for secondary infections of the blisters, should not be used. These agents are known sensitizers and can cause a drug-induced dermatitis along with the existing dermatitis. However, when traditional treatments have failed, pramoxine or benzocaine may be used on a trial basis if the patient is monitored closely for untoward dermatologic reactions.

*Moderate to Severe Poison Ivy/Oak/Sumac Dermatitis* Treatment of numerous large, coalesced bullae should be referred to a PCP, who may open and drain them under sterile conditions. A safe initial recommendation is the application of a cool water compress to the affected area for as long and as often as needed. Mild edema or swelling of the eyelids should be treated with only cold water dressings. Cool compresses of aluminum acetate solution (Burow's) may be applied to other affected areas.

A 1:40 dilution of Burow's solution may be prepared from prepackaged tablets or powder by adding 1 tablet or package to 1 pint of cool tap water. Clean white compresses are soaked in the solution and then applied to the affected areas for 30 minutes, four times a day or as often as needed. Any remaining solution should be discarded and a fresh solution prepared for each application. Burow's solution provides an astringent action on the papulovesicular lesions of the dermatitis that dries the weeping vesicles.[38] In addition, Burow's solution is useful in softening and removing crusting, and in preparing the skin for the application of a hydrocortisone cream or ointment.

Shake lotions are not recommended for treating large areas of weeping dermatitis on the face because the lotions have a tendency to cake and generate debris that can make the skin uncomfortable and stiff. An application of Burow's compresses may help the patient, and should be followed with a cream or lotion application that will provide an emollient effect and may be better tolerated.

Colloidal oatmeal baths can cleanse and soothe the lesions, and reduce the itch. One packet (30 g) of colloidal oatmeal per tub of water is sprinkled into warm, running water to allow for good mixing of the milled oatmeal. Stirring the bath water occasionally will help prevent lumps from developing. Colloidal oatmeal makes bath water extremely slippery. Placing a rubber mat in the tub and a dry rug or towel on the floor will help prevent falling. Holding a grab rail/bar or other such convenience securely will provide additional safety for entering and exiting the tub. Soaking for 15 or 20 minutes at least twice each day is recommended; the oatmeal bath water should be drizzled over areas that cannot be soaked. The skin should be patted dry (not wiped) to leave a film of colloidal oatmeal on the skin.

*Severe Poison Ivy/Oak/Sumac Dermatitis* Symptomatic topical treatment of severe dermatitis remains quite similar to that used in moderately severe cases, except that the PCP will likely prescribe a potent anti-inflammatory glucocorticoid systemically as well as topically. The prescriber should ensure a good treatment outcome by recommending a systemic glucocorticoid that consists of a tapering dosage of not fewer than 12 days to as long as 21 days of therapy. On average, about 1 mg/kg body weight per day (approximately 40-100 mg) of prednisone is used when initiating therapy and is tapered over the next 2 to 3 weeks. The use of prepackaged dosage packs of glucocorticoid (tapered over 6 days) in numerous instances has led to the use of a second or third dose pack, or may even lead to rebound dermatologic symptoms if this shorter therapy period is selected.[39]

### *Nonpharmacologic Therapy*

Nonpharmacologic treatment of the allergic reaction is limited primarily to showers. However, hypersensitive patients who suspect poison ivy exposure can take measures to prevent or lessen the severity of the dermatitis. All individuals should avoid contact with *Toxicodendron* plants or other allergens, and, if exposed, should take the following steps to remove the offending substance from the skin.

#### Hygienic Measures

The primary nondrug measure to relieve symptoms of contact dermatitis is to take cold or tepid soapless showers to temporarily relieve the pruritus. A tepid shower is approximately 90°F (32.2°C) or cooler. The clinician should recommend that a patient be cautious about taking a hot shower (temperatures greater than 105°F [40.5°C]), because it may cause scalding or thermal skin injuries (second-degree burns). The clinician may recommend that patients bathe or shower using hypoallergenic face soap to maintain cleanliness; they should never use harsh soaps. Furthermore, when a rash is present, affected areas should not be vigorously scrubbed. Men should be encouraged to shave because shaving cleanses the facial area of caked and crusted fluid from pustules or bullae. If the dermatitis is allowed to become crusted and hardened in the hairs and stubble of the beard, shaving will become very uncomfortable. Along with applying topical treatment, all patients, both adults and children, should trim their fingernails to help reduce the degree of scratching injury.

#### Preventive/Protective Measures

For any individual who is sensitive to urushiol from *Toxicodendron* plants or other allergens, the best preventive measure against exposure is total avoidance of the substances or plants (Table 35-5). In the case of *Toxicodendron* plants, any recreational or work-related outdoor activity should include a brief survey of the surrounding vegetation to determine the potential risk of exposure. The individual

**TABLE 35-5 Preventive and Protective Measures for Poison Ivy/Oak/Sumac Dermatitis**

**Preventive Measures**

- Learn the physical characteristics and usual habitat of *Toxicodendron* plants.
- Eradicate *Toxicodendron* plants near your residence either by mechanically removing the plant and its roots or by applying a herbicide recommended by the state Farm Bureau or the USDA Extension Services.
- Apply bentoquatam on exposed areas of body to reduce the risk of contamination before visiting an outdoor site. Repeat application every 4 hours until your potential exposure has ended. This application should be followed by flushing the area with water to remove bentoquatam and any urushiol deposited on the skin surface.
- Survey the area of an outdoor visit, identify surrounding plants, and assess potential risk for exposure to *Toxicodendron* plants.
- Take the protective measures listed here for suspected exposure.

**Protective Measures**

- Remove all clothing worn during exposure.
- Wash the suspected area with soap and water as soon as possible.
- If thorough washing is not possible, rinse with water as soon as possible.
- At earliest convenience, take a complete shower instead of a bath, using soap and water. Avoid tub baths right after exposure, because oleoresin may remain in the tub and potentially affect other unaffected areas.
- Meticulously clean under the fingernails to avoid transferring trapped urushiol to clean skin surfaces.
- Wash all clothing exposed to urushiol separate from other clothes in a washing machine using ordinary detergent. If clothes are dry cleaned to remove urushiol, warn cleaning personnel of the possible contamination. Put contaminated clothing in a plastic bag for transport.
- Thoroughly wash with soap and water, or with water alone, any shoes, gloves, jackets, or other protective garments; sports equipment; garden and work tools; and any equipment that is capable of carrying urushiol, as soon after use as possible. Wear vinyl gloves for washing contaminated objects. Allow this clothing and equipment to dry and then store them for the next use.
- Cleanse the fur of pets after known or suspected exposures to poison ivy plants

should avoid frequenting areas that have indigenous poison ivy or poison oak plants. In addition, a proactive educational process that includes descriptive and photographic representations of the plants should help patients identify the plants that naturally occur in the areas in which they live. From the description of the *Toxicodendron* genus and from observations of other experts in this field,[31,40] readers will know that the plants vary in morphology according to geographic location, soil, and climate.

*Use of Protective Clothing* Individuals should wear additional protective clothing that can be removed and immediately washed after exposure. They should use ordinary laundry detergent to wash clothes contaminated with urushiol separate from noncontaminated clothing.

*Removal of Urushiol or Other Allergens from Skin* To reduce the contact and spread of the dermatitis, the individual should immediately wash the area that was exposed to poison ivy plants or other allergens. Even though urushiol is a water-insoluble compound, clinicians have shown that immediate and early washing of urushiol-exposed areas with soap and water may avoid or reduce the severity of the rash. Researchers have shown[19] that washing the contaminated area must take place within 10 minutes of exposure to significantly reduce the risk of dermatitis. Studies have also revealed that, for up to 30 minutes after exposure, washing will remove unreacted oleoresin. Therefore, washing after the initial 10-minute period is still useful in removing any oleoresin that remains on the skin's surface and has not entered the dermal layers. Once urushiol has entered the skin and attached to tissue proteins, it can no longer be removed.

"In the field" washing is difficult, but simply using large volumes of water will rinse away much of the surface irritant and oleoresin. Historically, PCPs and many home remedies recommended vigorous scrubbing of contaminated skin surfaces with a harsh soap (e.g., Fels Naphtha or homemade lye soap). Instead, the current recommendation is to use a mild face soap and water to wash all body areas believed to have been exposed to urushiol. In lieu of this approach, copious amounts of plain water may be sufficient to reduce the chance of dermatitis. In addition, it is crucial that at-risk patients practice good handwashing, including meticulous cleansing under the fingernails, to avoid contaminating other clean skin surfaces with allergen trapped under the fingernails.

Other cleansers and organic solvents have been used to rinse off skin surface urushiol, including isopropyl alcohol. However, general thought holds that although urushiol is soluble in alcohol, its use should be followed immediately by a mild soap and water wash to remove any remaining surface oleoresin. Alcohol may dissolve and transport the surface oleoresin to clean skin surfaces and thus generate additional areas of dermatitis. Alcohol may also remove natural protective oils from the skin and can be a source of irritation.

One product used as a cleanser for urushiol is Technu Outdoor Skin Cleanser, whose constituents include mineral spirits, water, a soap, and a surface-active agent. The cleanser was originally developed as an agent to wash away radioactive matter from the skin surface of exposed individuals. This product is recommended for use after exposure and should be rubbed into the affected area as soon after exposure as possible. The patient should use the liquid to cleanse the contaminated area for a minimum of 2 minutes. No water is required for the initial cleansing application, but the cleanser may be wiped away with a cloth or rinsed with cool water. The manufacturer recommends using the product before eating, smoking, or using the bathroom in an effort to minimize spreading urushiol to uncontaminated skin. In a study comparing untreated urushiol exposures with those cleansed with Technu, Dial Ultra dishwashing soap, and Goop grease remover, it was found that any of the three provided good protection against poison ivy rash when used to cleanse skin exposed to urushiol.[41] The difference in protective ability among the products is insignificant.

*Use of Barrier Products for Poison Ivy/Oak/Sumac* Several studies have evaluated the use of barrier creams and lotions as agents to prevent urushiol from entering the skin. A comprehensive study[14] identified three products that had notable protective qualities when used in subjects who were experimentally challenged with *Toxicodendron* extract. The three products (Hydropel, Hollister Moisture Barrier, and Stokogard Outdoor Cream) reduced dermatitis severity by 48%, 52%, and 59%, respectively. At the present time, Stokogard is in extremely short supply and is available from only one midwestern supplier. The manufacture of additional product is not planned. The active ingredient was a dimer of linoleic acid, whose presumed mechanism of action was probably the obstruction of urushiol penetration into the skin. Disadvantages of this product included its tacky, greasy nature and an unpleasant fishy odor.[40] The remaining two products (Hydropel and Hollister Moisture Barrier Cream) do not claim protection from poison ivy dermatitis, but instead prevention of ICD or diaper rash.

IvyBlock Lotion is the first barrier product approved by the Food and Drug Administration (FDA) via a New Drug Application to provide protection against exposure to poison ivy, oak, and sumac. This product's active ingredient is an organoclay known as quaternium-18 bentonite (bentoquatam),[42,43] which is manufactured by reacting bentonite clay with quaternium-18 (a dimethyl dihydrogenated tallow quaternary ammonium compound). The product contains 5% bentoquatam in a lotion containing alcohol. Bentoquatam is a nonsensitizing and nonirritating organoclay that appears to possess little antigenicity or toxicities when it is applied topically. The mechanism by which this ingredient works is not presently known, but it is believed to physically block urushiol from being absorbed into the skin. It is effective in protecting patients from exposure to the urushiol common to all *Toxicodendron* plants, as well as urushiol that adheres to smoke particles from burned plants.

This barrier lotion claims protection when it is topically applied at least 15 minutes before exposure to *Toxicodendron*. It should be reapplied once every 4 hours or as needed after the initial application to maintain effective protection. The lotion should be shaken vigorously before applying to skin that is likely to be exposed to poison ivy, oak, or sumac. The individual must apply the lotion generously to clean dry skin, leaving a smooth wet film of lotion where it is applied. One may determine skin coverage by looking for the faint white coating that appears when the lotion has dried. After the period of exposure has ended, the patient may remove the lotion by washing with soap and water.[44] This product is flammable and should be not be used around the eyes or applied to an existing poison ivy rash. In addition, its use is not recommended in children younger than 6 years.

*Eradication of Toxicodendron Plants* The eradication of Toxicodendron plants has been suggested in situations in which extremely sensitive individuals are affected by close proximity to the plant and its oleoresin. Two methods of eradication have been recommended: either mechanically removing (hand grubbing of plants and the root system) or applying an appropriate herbicide. When considering the use of herbicides, patients should contact the U.S. Department of Agriculture (USDA, http://www.csrees.usda.gov/Extension/index.html) Extension Service or the appropriate state or county agency to determine the recommended herbicide and prescribed methods of application for *Toxicodendron* species indigenous to the area.

*Hyposensitization to Toxicodendron Plants* History and scientific literature are replete with folklore and stories of Native Americans who ate poison ivy to desensitize themselves. Beginning in the early 1940s, numerous oral and injectable forms of poison ivy extract products were available for use. Their purpose was to desensitize patients to urushiol. From the numerous studies published since these products were introduced, clinicians have learned that such desensitization methods are incapable of adequately desensitizing the patient to poison ivy. Although hyposensitization was possible, it could be maintained only with consistent maintenance doses of injectable extracts. Any protection provided through hyposensitization was lost within 3 months of discontinuing maintenance doses. Several hundred milligrams of urushiol were required to provide clinical hyposensitization. Injectable products could be given only in small doses because of the development of poison ivy symptoms and the side effects associated with administering higher doses. PCPs have long doubted the potency of such commercial products. However, some clinicians prepared their own injectables, which then led to overall claims that were confusing and did not convincingly support the hyposensitization process.

FDA took actions in 1994 and 1995 to remove injectable *Toxicodendron* oleoresin extracts (poison ivy or poison oak) from the marketplace.[45,46] No products can currently be recommended as hyposensitization programs for human use.[47]

### Pharmacologic Therapy

The agents used for topical relief of symptoms come from several therapeutic classes. Because treatment is primarily aimed at relieving itching, patients should use topical hydrocortisone, topical antihistamines, and other antipruritic agents. Patients can use astringents to promote drying of the moist, wet, oozing lesions and provide a protective covering for the inflamed, tender skin beneath the lesional areas. Combination products that contain one or more of these ingredients are available for use. Many dosage forms are available for use on the dermatitis, according to the skin condition and patient-specific preferences. In addition, antiseptics can be included in the formulation theoretically to provide antimicrobial protection. The FDA recently provided final monograph approval for the antipruritic and astringent ingredients discussed in this section.[48,49]

## Topical Anesthetics

Two topical anesthetic agents appear in most nonprescription drug products that relieve itching: benzocaine and pramoxine (see Chapter 41). Benzocaine is available in concentrations as high as 20%. Pramoxine is ordinarily used in a concentration of 1%. Anesthetic agents affect the impulses carried by the sensory neurons emanating in the areas affected by the dermatitis. By relieving the itch, anesthetic agents indirectly protect the inflamed tissues from further scratching injury and may reduce the risk of a secondary infection. Available dosage forms include creams, ointments, sprays, and gels. In many instances, these agents are formulated in combination with other antipruritic agents such as camphor and menthol. The practitioner should reserve these topical anesthetic ingredients for treatment only after other forms of antipruritic therapy have failed to relieve the itching. These agents should be applied no more than three to four times daily. As previously mentioned, benzocaine may be the source of a secondary dermatitis and increased itching because it has known sensitizing capabilities. If the patient experiences additional itching, redness, or worsening of the dermatitis or urticaria after applying the anesthetic, the product should be washed off with mild soap and water and not applied again.

## Hydrocortisone

Hydrocortisone is the most effective form of topical therapy for treating symptoms of mild to moderately severe ICD or ACD that does not involve extensive areas of the skin and edema. Hydrocortisone is a low-potency, naturally occurring corticosteroid capable of relieving pruritus and reducing inflammation associated with dermatitis (see Chapter 34). FDA's advisory panel and dermatologists believe that hydrocortisone is safe to apply to all parts of the body except the eyes and eyelids. It may be applied to large areas of dermatitis, including areas that contain open lesions. It is free of systemic side effects such as adrenal suppression that may result from the absorption of more potent topically or systemically administered anti-inflammatory steroids. Hydrocortisone may be applied up to three or four times a day and is available without a prescription in concentrations from 0.25% to 1%. Topical hydrocortisone should not be used for children younger than 2 years, except on a PCP's advice. Practitioners should advise patients that hydrocortisone dosage forms should not be used if the dermatitis persists for longer than 7 days, or if symptoms clear and then reappear in a few days, unless patients have consulted with a PCP.

## Other Topical Antipruritics

Several longstanding external analgesics have been used for their local antipruritic and anesthetic properties, and are incorporated into nonprescription products to relieve the pruritus of ICD or ACD (see Chapter 7). Phenol, camphor, and menthol appear in numerous products at various low concentrations. All three are capable of depressing the skin's sensory receptors, which contributes to their topical analgesic effectiveness. Using such products on open lesions and tender, inflamed tissues may cause local burning and irritation at the application site.

## Astringents

Astringents are pharmacologic entities that are known protein precipitants used to stop or reduce the oozing of capillaries or the fluid release from blisters or inflamed tissues. These substances promote drying of wet dermatitis and in turn promote reduced inflammation and healing. FDA-approved astringents include aluminum acetate (Burow's solution), zinc oxide, zinc acetate, sodium bicarbonate, calamine, and witch hazel (hamamelis water).[48] They are often used as soaks or in wet compresses applied to the affected area several times a day. This type of application aids in cleansing and removing crusting or surface debris that arises from the natural progression of poison ivy or poison oak dermatitis. Therapy may be continued for approximately 5 to 7 days, when the dermatitis is moist and oozing.

After the use of astringents, patients may notice drying, tightening, and contracting of the skin. As a note of caution, prolonged use of calamine lotion or zinc oxide lotion or paste may lead to a buildup of debris and caked material on the skin, which will lead to further irritation and discomfort. Regular cleansing of the affected area to avoid buildup is recommended. The clinician may recommend the use of colloidal oatmeal baths to help provide skin hydration, to aid in cleansing or removing skin debris, and to allay the drying and tightening symptoms noted after frequent use. Also available is an oileated form of colloidal oatmeal, which contains mineral oil to provide an emollient action on the skin.

## Antihistamines

Antihistamines are used for their topical anesthetic activity (see Chapter 37) to treat poison ivy. Although antihistamines block the histamine$_1$ ($H_1$) receptor, such receptors do not play a significant role in type IV cell-mediated responses. Other antihistamines have been included in topical formulations for a similar anesthetic action. Topical antihistamines can act as dermatologic sensitizers, which are responsible for causing secondary inflammatory dermatologic conditions. Just as with topical anesthetics, if additional itching or redness occurs or the dermatitis or urticaria worsens after a topical antihistamine is applied, the product should be washed off with mild soap and water and not applied again.

## Nonmonograph Agents

Formerly, some nonprescription products used zirconium for its drying and astringent action on poison ivy/oak rashes and other forms of weeping dermatitis. Reports have appeared in the literature showing that zirconium caused lesions known as zirconium granulomas on the skin where it was applied. Superimposed on the existing dermatitis, the granulomas complicated the existing condition. Products that contain zirconium are no longer available on the market, although some brand names once connoted zirconium content remain in use today. Such products do not contain zirconium, but they may contain other approved nonprescription ingredients.

### Product Selection Guidelines

Numerous dosage forms are available for nonprescription recommendation by the clinician. The choice of dosage form depends on several factors, especially the severity of the dermatitis and the presence of vesicles (dry or weeping). Ointments hold moisture within the skin and act as a reservoir for the active ingredient, keeping it on the affected site. Ointments are effective agents when they are applied before the lesions open and begin oozing fluid. Ointments should not be applied to open lesions for several reasons: removal of ointments from the skin is more difficult, and they may trap bacteria beneath the oleaginous film, leading to secondary infections.

Applying a cream base allows vesicle fluid to flow freely from the blisters and does not trap bacteria because it is quickly absorbed into the skin. Gels offer ease of application and a rapid absorption of active ingredients into the skin. Some gels may contain alcohol or similar organic solvents that may cause irritation or burning when applied to open lesions.

Spray products provide the easiest form of drug application. They allow even distribution to relatively larger areas and are convenient to use, but they are somewhat more expensive. One advantage of a spray product is that touching the area of dermatitis is not necessary, which may curtail additional scratching. Aerosol sprays may contain propellants that cause additional inflammation. Table 35-6 lists selected products containing primarily colloidal oatmeal, astringents, or bentoquatam. (See Chapter 37 for products that contain local anesthetics, hydrocortisone, or topical antihistamines.)

### *Complementary Therapies*

Jewel weed (*Impatiens biflora, Impatiens pallida*) is a well-known natural product and folk remedy used by Native Americans to treat a vast array of dermal conditions, including the prevention of poison ivy/oak/sumac dermatitis. The juice of the stems is applied to the area where urushiol contact occurred to prevent the ensuing rash. In a double-blind study,[50] fresh juice from the stems of *Impatiens pallida* was applied to the skin where freshly crushed poison ivy (*T. radicans*) had been applied for 15 minutes. Three treatment approaches were tried: (1) application of jewel weed juice, (2) application of saline solution, and (3) no treatment. The study's conclusions revealed that jewel weed juice applied directly after fresh poison ivy exposure did not reduce or prevent poison ivy dermatitis in humans. A second study[51] concluded that boiled jewel weed extract was not an effective treatment for preventing poison ivy/oak dermatitis.

**TABLE 35-6 Selected Products for Poison Ivy/Oak/Sumac Dermatitis**

| Trade Name | Primary Ingredients |
|---|---|
| Aveeno Bath Treatment Moisturizing Formula Powder | Colloidal oatmeal 43% |
| Aveeno Bath Treatment Soothing Formula Powder | Colloidal oatmeal 100% |
| Bluboro Powder | Aluminum sulfate 53.9% |
| Domeboro Powder | Aluminum sulfate 1191 mg |
| Ivarest 8-Hour Medicated Cream | Diphenhydramine hydrochloride 2%; calamine 14% |
| Ivy Dry Cream | Benzyl alcohol 10 mg/g; camphor 6 mg/g; menthol 4 mg/g; zinc acetate 20 mg/g |
| Ivy Dry Liquid | Isopropyl alcohol 12.5%; zinc acetate 20 mg/mL |
| Ivy Super Dry Liquid | Benzyl alcohol 0.1 mg/g; camphor 4 mg/g; menthol 2 mg/g; isopropyl alcohol 35%; zinc acetate 20 mg/mL |
| IvyBlock Lotion | Benzyl alcohol; SDA alcohol 40 25%; bentoquatam (quaternium-18 bentonite) 5% |

## ASSESSMENT OF CONTACT DERMATITIS: A CASE-BASED APPROACH

Diagnostically, ICD and ACD are difficult to differentiate from each other (Table 35-7). Circumstances surrounding the occurrence of the dermatitis, including the time relationship to irritant or allergen exposure (at home, work, or recreation), the distribution of the dermatitis on exposed skin areas, symptomatology, and whether dermatitis improves with avoidance, help the clinician determine the type of dermatitis.[3]

Assessment of a suspected irritant, allergic, or plant-induced dermatitis is based on characteristic symptoms, history of sensitivity, and activities that indicate exposure to causative substances. Determining the type and success of previous treatments of such rashes will aid in recommending the appropriate nonprescription medications. Cases 35-1 and 35-2 illustrate the assessment of patients with contact dermatitis.

## PATIENT COUNSELING FOR CONTACT DERMATITIS

When approached by a patient with ICD or ACD, the practitioner should take the opportunity to explain preventive and protective measures, as well as treatment measures. If the patient cannot identify contact with irritant chemicals, allergens, or *Toxicodendron* plants, the practitioner should review chemicals or allergens likely to cause

**TABLE 35-7 Differentiation of ICD and ACD**

| Symptom or Characteristic | ICD | ACD |
|---|---|---|
| Itching | Yes, later | Yes, early |
| Stinging, burning | Early | Late or not at all |
| Erythema | Yes | Yes |
| Vesicles | Yes, minimal | Yes, early |
| Pustules | Yes | Yes, minimal |
| Dermal edema | Yes | Yes |
| Delayed reaction to exposure | Minutes to hours | Days, slower reaction |
| Appearance of symptoms in relation to exposures | Single or multiple exposures | Delayed |
| Causative chemical substances | Alkalis, acids, solvents, salts, surfactants, oxidizers | Low-molecular-weight and lipid-soluble substances, fragrances, metals |
| Substance concentration at exposure | Very important | Less important |
| Mechanism of reaction | Direct tissue damage | Immunologic reaction |

Key: ACD, allergic contact dermatitis; ICD, irritant contact dermatitis.
*Source:* Adapted from references 1, 11, and 12.

## CASE 35-1

| Relevant Evaluation Criteria | Scenario/Model Outcome |
|---|---|
| **Information Gathering** | |
| 1. Gather essential information about the patient's symptoms, including: | |
| a. description of symptom(s) (i.e., nature, onset, duration, severity, associated symptoms) | Patient has irritated hands and wishes to treat the condition. He is working during the summer as a restaurant clean-up person and dishwasher. His job consists of cleaning kitchen equipment and washing dishes many hours a day. He does not use gloves while working and noticed that his hands have become more irritated since he began this job approximately 4 weeks ago.<br>Patient's hands appear dry, red, with little fissure formation at the knuckles and joints; no vesicles, weeping, or infection is noted. Irritation is confined to the hands. The patient complains of periodic itching and a feeling of "tightness" across the skin of the hands. |
| b. description of any factors that seem to precipitate, exacerbate, and/or relieve the patient's symptom(s) | Skin dryness, rash, and tightness began to occur shortly after patient began work as a dishwasher for the restaurant. |
| c. description of the patient's efforts to relieve the symptoms | Patient has not tried anything yet. |
| 2. Gather essential patient history information: | |
| a. patient's identity | Pat Bannon |
| b. patient's age, sex, height, and weight | 19 y/o M |
| c. patient's occupation | Full-time college student; clean-up and dishwashing attendant during the summer |
| d. patient's dietary habits | Generally healthy |
| e. patient's sleep habits | 8 hours per night |
| f. concurrent medical conditions, prescription and nonprescription medications, and dietary supplements | None |
| g. allergies | NKA |

## CASE 35-1 (continued)

| Relevant Evaluation Criteria | Scenario/Model Outcome |
|---|---|
| h. history of other adverse reactions to medications | None |
| i. other (describe)_______ | No history of similar reactions |
| **Assessment and Triage** | |
| 3. Differentiate the patient's signs/symptoms and correctly identify the patient's primary problem(s) (see Tables 35-1, 35-3, and 35-7). | Pat is suffering from irritant contact dermatitis, and the likely source of irritation is the detergents used in washing dishes and general kitchen clean-up. |
| 4. Identify exclusions for self-treatment (see Figure 35-1). | None |
| 5. Formulate a comprehensive list of therapeutic alternatives for the primary problem to determine if triage to a medical practitioner is required, and share this information with the patient. | Options include:<br>(1) Refer Pat to an appropriate health care professional.<br>(2) Recommend self-care with a nonprescription product and/or nondrug measures.<br>(3) Recommend self-care until Pat can see an appropriate health care professional.<br>(4) Take no action. |
| **Plan** | |
| 6. Select an optimal therapeutic alternative to address the patient's problem, taking into account patient preferences. | Pat should use protective measures while performing his cleaning chores. In addition, the use of a nonprescription antipruritic product and a hypoallergenic hand lotion should relieve the irritation and dryness. |
| 7. Describe the recommended therapeutic approach to the patient. | Use protective gloves (water and soap impermeable with high sleeves) while cleaning. Every effort should be taken to regularly and thoroughly wash and completely dry your hands throughout the day, and then use a hypoallergenic hand lotion. Apply hydrocortisone cream (1%) 3-4 times daily to the affected area. |
| 8. Explain to the patient the rationale for selecting the recommended therapeutic approach from the considered therapeutic alternatives. | Using protective gloves while cleaning is the most effective way of reducing the irritation to your hands. Washing and thoroughly drying your hands will cleanse them of detergent irritants and also help reduce symptoms. The hydrocortisone cream will relieve the itching, and the hand lotion will help relieve skin tightness. |
| **Patient Education** | |
| 9. When recommending self-care with nonprescription medications and/or nondrug therapy, convey accurate information to the patient, including: | |
| a. appropriate dose and frequency of administration | See the box Patient Education for Irritant Contact Dermatitis. |
| b. maximum number of days the therapy should be employed | See the box Patient Education for Irritant Contact Dermatitis. |
| c. product administration procedures | See the box Patient Education for Irritant Contact Dermatitis. |
| d. expected time to onset of relief | See the box Patient Education for Irritant Contact Dermatitis. |
| e. degree of relief that can be reasonably expected | Complete symptomatic relief is likely. |
| f. most common side effects | See the box Patient Education for Irritant Contact Dermatitis. |
| g. side effects that warrant medical intervention should they occur | See the box Patient Education for Irritant Contact Dermatitis. |
| h. patient options in the event that condition worsens or persists | See the box Patient Education for Irritant Contact Dermatitis. |

## CASE 35-1 (continued)

| Relevant Evaluation Criteria | Scenario/Model Outcome |
|---|---|
| i. product storage requirements | See the box Patient Education for Irritant Contact Dermatitis. |
| j. specific nondrug measures | See the box Patient Education for Irritant Contact Dermatitis. |
| 10. Solicit patient's follow-up questions. | How long may I continue to use the hydrocortisone cream on my hands? |
| 11. Answer patient's questions. | You may continue to use the cream for a maximum of 7 days. |

Key: NKA, no known allergies.

## CASE 35-2

| Relevant Evaluation Criteria | Scenario/Model Outcome |
|---|---|
| **Information Gathering** | |
| 1. Gather essential information about the patient's symptoms, including: | |
| a. description of symptom(s) (i.e., nature, onset, duration, severity, associated symptoms) | Patient complains of intense itching, redness, and streaking around the ankles and wrists. Symptoms have developed within the last 24-36 hours. Patient says the itching is intense, especially at night, and blisters have begun forming on his ankles. |
| b. description of any factors that seem to precipitate, exacerbate, and/or relieve the patient's symptom(s) | A warm shower this morning seemed to provide only temporary relief from the itching in both areas. |
| c. description of the patient's efforts to relieve the symptoms | The patient has only applied calamine lotion during the night and this morning. This has not provided good relief from the itching. |
| 2. Gather essential patient history information: | |
| a. patient's identity | Peter Charles |
| b. patient's age, sex, height, and weight | 26 y/o M, 5'11", 145 lb |
| c. patient's occupation | Patient is employed as an editor for a publishing company; on weekends he is outside maintaining a lake property and enjoying time with his family. |
| d. patient's dietary habits | Generally a healthy diet |
| e. patient's sleep habits | 7 to 8 hours per night |
| f. concurrent medical conditions, prescription and nonprescription medications, and dietary supplements | No current medications other than a daily multivitamin |
| g. allergies | NKA |
| h. history of other adverse reactions to medications | None |
| i. other (describe)______ | Patient's symptoms occurred within 24 to 48 hours of trying to remove a fallen tree covered with vines. He pulled the vines from the tree bark to remove it from the road, then drove 90 minutes home before washing or showering affected areas. |
| **Assessment and Triage** | |
| 3. Differentiate the patient's signs/symptoms and correctly identify the patient's primary problem(s) (see Tables 35-1, 35-2, 35-3, and 35-7). | Peter is suffering from poison ivy rash caused by exposure to urushiol from the damaged vines and leaves covering the tree. He had mistakenly thought the poison ivy vine was Virginia Creeper. He did not realize he was exposed to poison ivy and therefore did not wash his ankles, wrists, or other exposed body areas until he returned home 90 minutes later. He does realize he is sensitive to poison ivy. |

## CASE 35-2 (continued)

| Relevant Evaluation Criteria | Scenario/Model Outcome |
|---|---|
| 4. Identify exclusions for self-treatment (see Figure 35-1). | None |
| 5. Formulate a comprehensive list of therapeutic alternatives for the primary problem to determine if triage to a medical practitioner is required, and share this information with the patient. | Options include:<br>(1) Refer Peter to an appropriate health care professional.<br>(2) Recommend hydrocortisone and the use of sodium bicarbonate soaks until the rash begins to weep, and then recommend Burow's solution to minimized crusting.<br>(3) Recommend self-care until Peter can see an appropriate health care professional.<br>(4) Take no action. |
| **Plan** | |
| 6. Select an optimal therapeutic alternative to address the patient's problem, taking into account patient preferences. | Peter should use a topical anti-inflammatory agent (cream or ointment) as long as the areas of rash are relatively small and do not enlarge. Astringent or antipruritic soaks may be applied as needed to relieve the itch. Oatmeal baths may also be recommended several times a day and just before bedtime. |
| 7. Describe the recommended therapeutic approach to the patient. | Apply hydrocortisone cream/ointment (1%) 3-4 times daily to affected areas. In addition, astringent and antipruritic soaks may be used to help reduce itching and inflammation. Continue to use this treatment as long as the areas of rash and vesicles do not increase in size. If the area of rash worsens or blisters become large (bullae), you should see your primary care provider. |
| 8. Explain to the patient the rationale for selecting the recommended therapeutic approach from the considered therapeutic alternatives. | It is important to use these measures to reduce itching and avoid opening the blisters and the chance for a skin infection. Use the soaks and oatmeal baths as often as needed to reduce itching and cleanse the area when it begins to weep. If the area of rash or blisters get larger (bullae), you should see your primary care provider. In the future if you are exposed to vines or poison ivy, you should immediately wash or shower the exposed areas. Clean you hands and fingernails thoroughly after exposure. |
| **Patient Education** | |
| 9. When recommending self-care with nonprescription medications and/or nondrug therapy, convey accurate information to the patient, including: | |
| a. appropriate dose and frequency of administration | See the box Patient Education for Irritant Contact Dermatitis. |
| b. maximum number of days the therapy should be employed | See the box Patient Education for Irritant Contact Dermatitis. |
| c. product administration procedures | See the box Patient Education for Irritant Contact Dermatitis. |
| d. expected time to onset of relief | See the box Patient Education for Irritant Contact Dermatitis. |
| e. degree of relief that can be reasonably expected | Complete symptomatic relief is likely within 14 to 21 days. |
| f. most common side effects | See the box Patient Education for Irritant Contact Dermatitis. |
| g. side effects that warrant medical intervention should they occur | See the box Patient Education for Irritant Contact Dermatitis. |
| h. patient options in the event that condition worsens or persists | See the box Patient Education for Irritant Contact Dermatitis. |
| i. product storage requirements | See the box Patient Education for Irritant Contact Dermatitis. |
| j. specific nondrug measures | See the box Patient Education for Irritant Contact Dermatitis. |
| 10. Solicit patient's follow-up questions. | Why can't I just use hydrocortisone cream on the rash instead of all the other agents? |

## CASE 35-2 (continued)

| Relevant Evaluation Criteria | Scenario/Model Outcome |
|---|---|
| 11. Answer patient's questions. | Hydrocortisone can affect skin integrity causing skin disintegration. The other agents will relieve itch and cleanse the area of crusting, keeping the skin supple. |

Key: NKA, no known allergies.

## PATIENT EDUCATION FOR IRRITANT CONTACT DERMATITIS

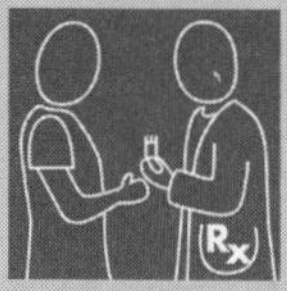

The primary objectives of self-treating irritant contact dermatitis are to (1) relieve symptoms of itching and weeping, and (2) avoid or minimize exposure to factors that trigger or aggravate the disorders. For most patients, carefully following product instructions and the self-care measures listed here will help ensure optimal therapeutic outcomes.

### Nondrug Measures

- Decrease exposure to common skin irritants such as detergents, soaps, and solvents.
- Avoid occlusion of the skin, which can make it more permeable to chemicals, by changing gloves (especially latex gloves used for cleaning chores), diapers, and clothing more frequently.
- Wash the affected area gently to remove traces of the offending agent.

### Nonprescription Medications

- To help the lesions dry, apply compresses of cool tap water or aluminum acetate for 20 minutes, four to six times daily.
- Apply calamine lotion between compress applications, and take colloidal oatmeal baths to soothe and help relieve itching.
- Apply a thin layer of hydrocortisone cream/ointment to the affected area three or four times daily for up to 7 days to relieve itching and/or inflammation.
- If itching keeps you awake at night, take an antihistamine that has a sedative effect, such as diphenhydramine or doxylamine, which have labeled instructions to help you sleep. Be aware that such medications can cause drowsiness the next morning.
- Store nonprescription medications in a cool, dry place and out of the reach of children.

If the contact dermatitis does not begin to improve in 2 to 3 days or if it worsens, consult a primary care provider.

dermatitis, show illustrations of *Toxicodendron* plants, if possible, or refer the patient to an appropriate reference. The practitioner should also explain the purpose and appropriate use of nonprescription agents, their possible adverse effects, and signs and symptoms that indicate one should see a clinician. The boxes Patient Education for Irritant Contact Dermatitis and Patient Education for Allergic Contact Dermatitis list specific information to provide patients.

## EVALUATION OF PATIENT OUTCOMES FOR CONTACT DERMATITIS

After recommending treatment for a contact dermatitis, the practitioner may choose to follow up with the patient after several days of treatment, or may instead encourage the patient to call for additional advice if the itching has not subsided significantly within 5 to 7 days. If, at follow-up, the rash has significantly increased in size, affects the eyes or genitals, or covers extensive areas of the face, the practitioner must reassess the patient for further therapy or referral to a PCP. Overall, complete remission of the dermatitis may take up to 3 weeks. However, the patient should see slow but steady reduction in itching, weeping, and dermatitis after 5 to 7 days of therapy.

## KEY POINTS FOR CONTACT DERMATITIS

- The leading cause of irritant contact dermatitis is exposure to a chemical irritant, primarily related to occupation. Irritants include such agents as acids, alkalis, solvents, and numerous other harsh chemicals.
- Allergic contact dermatitis, the next largest segment of contact dermatitis, is produced through sensitization to an antigenic substance.
- Many substances are antigenic, such as fragrances, metals, medications, plants, and chemicals. Urushiol from poison ivy/oak/sumac is the best-known allergen.
- Patients who are sensitive to irritants, allergens, or urushiol may take precautions to eliminate unnecessary exposure by avoiding these agents, limiting exposure time, and wearing protective clothing and equipment.
- In the case of poison ivy, avoiding geographic areas endemic with *Toxicodendron* plants is helpful. In addition, patients sensitive to urushiol should make liberal and timely applications of bentoquatam barrier lotion every 4 hours until the exposure period is over to reduce risk of dermatitis.
- Once exposed to an irritant or allergen, the patient can take protective measures that include bathing with mild soap and water or using large volumes of cool water immediately after exposure to reduce the risk of dermatitis.

## PATIENT EDUCATION FOR ALLERGIC CONTACT DERMATITIS

The objectives of self-treatment of allergic contact dermatitis are to (1) reduce or prevent itching and excessive scratching that may lead to secondary skin infections, (2) protect the affected area, and (3) prevent the accumulation of skin debris and oozing, crusting, and scaling of vesicle fluids, which could spread the infection to the area surrounding the inflammation. For most patients, carefully following product instructions and the self-care measures listed here will help ensure optimal therapeutic outcomes.

### Nondrug Measures

- Take the preventive measures outlined in Table 35-5 to prevent poison ivy/oak/sumac dermatitis.
- If exposure is suspected and if preventive measures were not taken, implement the protective measures outlined in Table 35-5.
- Take tepid, soapless showers to relieve itching.
- When cleansing the affected areas, do not use harsh cleansers or scrub vigorously.
- If you have experienced topical allergic reactions, avoid contact with known allergens.
- To avoid potential allergic reactions, use hypoallergenic cosmetics and soapless cleansers.

### Nonprescription Medications

- Note that the dermatitis will subside with or without treatment in 14 to 21 days.
- If treatment is desired, consult a clinician about the use of one or more of the following nonprescription medications to relieve the intense itching, inflammation, weeping, and crusting that may accompany this dermatitis.
- If desired, use sodium bicarbonate paste or compresses as follows to relieve itching:
  - Apply paste directly to the rash to reduce itching.
  - Use clean white cloths to apply cool water compresses and apply for 20 to 30 minutes as often as needed or desired. Use a fresh solution with each new application.
- If desired, apply topical hydrocortisone cream or ointment as follows to reduce the itching and dissipate the dermal inflammation and erythema:
  - Apply sparingly to affected areas four times a day.
  - Avoid direct application around the eyes or eyelids.
  - Note that ointment dosage forms appear to maintain hydrocortisone application for longer periods of time than cream forms.
- To avoid potential dermal infections, do not apply ointments to open or excoriated pustules or lesions.
- Use aluminum acetate (Burow's solution) compresses as follows to dry open and weeping pustules or lesions:
  - Mix a prepackaged tablet or packet of aluminum acetate with a pint of cool tap water and use it to wet cloth compresses for application to rash areas.
  - Apply compresses for 30 minutes at least four times a day or as needed.
  - Prepare fresh Burow's solution for each application period.
- Use colloidal oatmeal baths or soaks as follows to soothe and cleanse areas of rash, as well as reduce pruritus:
  - Sprinkle a 30-g packet or a cup full of milled oatmeal into fast-running bath water and mix water periodically to avoid lumping of the oatmeal.
  - Soak for 15 to 20 minutes in the oatmeal bath at least twice a day. Pat skin dry rather than wiping it.
  - Be cautious on entry and exit from the bathtub because oatmeal baths are quite slippery.
- If the measures listed above have not been successful and you are not sensitive to local anesthetics (e.g., benzocaine) or topical antihistamines (e.g., diphenhydramine), use these agents as follows to provide relief of itching:
  - Apply agents sparingly to the affected area three or four times a day.
  - Avoid prolonged use beyond 7 days unless directed by your primary care provider.
  - Note that antihistamines and anesthetic agents are sensitizing agents, and may cause additional dermatitis and inflammation in areas where they are applied.
- Store nonprescription medications in a cool, dry place and out of the reach of children.

Contact a primary care provider for systemic and topical treatment in the following situations:

- Symptoms become worse.
- The rash becomes more widespread on the body.
- The rash covers large areas of the face or causes swelling of the eyelids.
- The rash involves the genitalia.

---

- Dermatitis may begin as localized streaks or patches of highly pruritic rash proceeding to larger areas on exposed dermal areas. The rash may affect the eyelids or face and, in some cases, areas ordinarily considered to be protected.
- The practitioner should refer patients to a PCP if the rash causes edema of the eyelids, closes the eyelids, affects the external genitalia or anus, or produces massive areas of body rash or edema.
- Treatment of localized, pruritic rash consists of a topical application of hydrocortisone cream or ointment, sodium bicarbonate paste, compresses, or baths. Weeping of vesicles or bullae, which is caused by the patient's scratching, may be treated with aluminum acetate compresses as an astringent to soothe and dry the weeping. Colloidal oatmeal baths may be used to treat the pruritic rash, to soothe, and to provide an emollient action on dry skin.
- For pruritus that has not resolved with the use of hydrocortisone products, the patient may topically apply a local anesthetic or antihistamine agents for additional anesthetic activity. The clinician should advise caution when recommending these agents because they are sensitizing substances and capable of producing additional dermatitis and itching.
- Irritant, allergic, and poison ivy/oak/ sumac dermatitis will resolve in approximately 7 to 21 days with or without topical therapy. Nonprescription medication recommendations serve in part to relieve the intense itching, inflammation, weeping, and crusting that may accompany these dermatoses.

## References


1. Wigger-Alberti W, Iliev D, Elsner P. Contact dermatitis due to irritation. In: RM Adams, ed. *Occupational Skin Disease.* 3rd ed. Philadelphia: WB Saunders; 1999:1-22.
2. Drake LA, Dorner W, Gottz RW, et al. Guidelines of care for contact dermatitis. Available at: http://www.aad.org/Guidelines/contderm.html. Accessed February 26, 2005.
3. Beltrani VS, Beltrani VP. Contact dermatitis. *Ann Allergy Asthma Immunol.* 1997;78:160-75.
4. McCall BP, Horwitz IB, Feldman SR, et al. Incidence rates, costs, severity, and work-related factors of occupational dermatitis. *Arch Dermatol.* June 2005;141:713-8.
5. Occupational dermatoses: a program for physicians. Available at: http://www.cdc.gov/niosh/ocderm1.html. Accessed February 26, 2005.
6. Lushniak BD. Occupational skin diseases. Occupational and environmental medicine. *Prim Care.* December 2000;27:895-915.
7. Behrens V, Seligman P, Cameron L, et al. The prevalence of back pain, hand discomfort, and dermatitis in the US working population. *Am J Public Health.* 1994;84:1780-5.
8. Koch, P Occupational contact dermatitis, recognition and management. *Am J Dermatol.* 2001;2:353-65.
9. Belisto DV. Allergic contact dermatitis. In: Freedberg IM, Eisen AZ, Wolff K, et al., eds. *Fitzpatrick's Dermatology in General Medicine.* 5th ed. New York: McGraw-Hill Inc;1999:1447-61.
10. Belisto DV. The diagnostic evaluation, treatment, and prevention of allergic contact dermatitis in the new millennium. *J Allergy Clin Immunol.* 2000;105:409-20.
11. Marks JG, DeLeo VA. Allergic and irritant contact dermatitis. In: *Contact & Occupational Dermatology.* 2nd ed. St. Louis: Mosby; 1997:1-14.
12. Adams RM. Occupational skin disease. In: Freedberg IM, Eisen AZ, Wolff K, et al., eds. *Fitzpatrick's Dermatology in General Medicine.* 5th ed. New York: McGraw-Hill Inc; 1999:1609-31.
13. Aajjachareonpong P, Cahill J, Keegel T, et al. Persistent post-occupational dermatitis. *Contact Dermatitis.* 2004;51:278-81.
14. Grevelink SA, Murrell DF, Olsen EA. Effectiveness of various barrier preparations in preventing and/or ameliorating experimentally produced *Toxicodendron* dermatitis. *J Am Acad Dermatol.* 1992;27(2 pt 1):182-8.
15. Klingman DL, Davis DE, Knake ED, et al. *Poison Ivy, Poison Oak, Poison Sumac.* Washington, DC: Extension Service, U.S. Department of Agriculture; 1983.
16. The itch that won't quit. Available at: http://www.aad.org/PressReleases/Fowler-MetalItch.html. Accessed February 26, 2005.
17. Solving problems related to the use of cosmetics and skin care products. Available at: http://www.aad.org/pamphlets/cosmetic.html. Accessed August 12, 2003.
18. Dannaker C, Maibach HI. Allergic contact dermatitis due to plants. In: Lovell CR, ed. *Plants and the Skin.* London: Blackwell Scientific Publications; 1993:105-20.
19. Fisher AA. Poison ivy/oak dermatitis, part 1: prevention soap and water, topical barriers, hyposensitization. *Cutis.* 1996;57:384-6.
20. Bureau of Labor Statistics, Department of Labor. Table R 25 Number of nonfatal occupational injuries and illnesses involving days away from work by source of injury or illness and selected natures of injury or illness, 2001. Available at: http://www.bls.gov/iif/oshwc/osh/case/ostb1180.txt. Accessed September 1, 2005.
21. Bureau of Labor Statistics, U.S. Department of Labor. Table R 28 Incidence rates for nonfatal occupational injuries and illnesses involving days away from work per 10,000 full-time workers by source of injury or illness and selected natures of injury or illness, 2001. Available at: http://www.bls.gov/iif/oshwc/osh/case/ostb1183.txt. Accessed September 1, 2005.
22. Botanical Dermatology Database. Anacardiaceae. Available at: http://www.uwcm.ac.uk/uwcm/dm/BoDD/BotDermFolder/BotDermA/ANAC.html. Accessed February 26, 2005.
23. Reitschel RL, Fowler JF, eds. *Fisher's Contact Dermatitis: Toxicodendron Plants and Spices.* 4th ed. Baltimore: Williams & Wilkins; 1995:461-74.
24. Park YM, Park JG, Kang H, et al. Acute generalized exanthematous pustulosis induced by ingestion of lacquer chicken. *Br J Derm.* 2000;143:230-3.
25. Park SD, Lee S-W, Chun JH, et al. Clinical features of 31 patients with systemic contact dermatitis due to the ingestion of Rhus (lacquer). *Br J Derm.* 2000;142:937-42.
26. Funk JO, Maibach HI. Horizons in pharmacologic intervention in allergic contact dermatitis. *J Am Acad Derm.* 1994;31:999-1014.
27. Gayer KD, Burnett JW. Toxicodendron dermatitis. *Cutis.* 1988; 42:99-100.
28. Epstein WL. Plant-induced dermatitis. *Ann Emerg Med.* 1987;16: 950-5.
29. Guin JD. The black spot test for recognizing poison ivy and related species. *J Am Acad Dermatol.* 1980;2:332-3.
30. Klingman AM. Poison ivy (Rhus) dermatitis: an experimental study. *Arch Dermatol.* 1958;77:149-80.
31. Epstein WL, Epstein JH. Plant induced dermatitis. In: Auerbach PL, ed. *Wilderness Medicine Management of Wilderness and Environmental Emergencies.* 3rd ed. St. Louis: Mosby-Yearbook; 1995:843-61.
32. Gayer KD, Burnett JW. Toxicodendron dermatitis. *Cutis.* 1988; 42:99-100.
33. Epstein WL. Plant-induced dermatitis. *Ann Emerg Med.* 1987;16: 950-5.
34. Brook I. Secondary bacterial infections complicating skin lesions. *J Med Microbiol.* 2002;51:808-12.
35. D'Mello DA, MacAuley L. Poison ivy dermatitis and secondary mania. *J Nerv Ment Dis.* 1994;182:116-7.
36. Werchniak AE, Schwarzenberger K. Poison ivy: an underreported cause of erythema multiforme. *J Am Acad Dermatol.* 2004: 51:S87-8.
37. Gealt L, Osterhoudt KC. Adult respiratory distress syndrome after smoke inhalation from burning poison ivy. *JAMA.* 1995;274: 358-9.
38. Williford PM, Sheretz EF. Poison ivy dermatitis: nuances in treatment. *Arch Fam Med.* 1994;3:184-8.
39. Ives TJ, Tepper RS. Failure of a tapering dose of oral methylprednisolone to treat reactions to poison ivy. *JAMA.* 1991;266:1362.
40. Epstein WL. Occupational poison ivy and oak dermatitis. *Dermatol Clin.* 1994;12:511-6.
41. Stibach AS, Yagan M, Sharma V, et al. Cost-effective post-exposure prevention of poison ivy dermatitis. *Intl J Derm.* 2000;39:515-8.
42. Epstein WL. Topical prevention of poison ivy/oak dermatitis. *Arch Dermatol.* 1989;125:499-501.
43. Marks JG Jr, Fowler JG Jr, Sheretz EF, et al. Prevention of poison ivy and poison oak allergic contact dermatitis by quaternium-18 bentonite. *J Am Acad Dermatol.* 1995;33(2 pt 1):212-6.
44. EnviroDerm Pharmaceuticals, Inc. IvyBlock Lotion product information. Plymouth, Mass; 1998.
45. Biological products; allergenic extracts; implementation of efficacy review. *Federal Register.* 1985;50:3082-288.
46. Biological products; allergenic extracts classified in category IIIB; final order; revocation of licenses. *Federal Register.* 1994;59:59228-37.
47. Scott PM. Personal communication. Bayer Allergy Products, Miles, Inc., Spokane, WA, confirmed the fact that Bayer Allergy Products will no longer manufacture the oral poison/oak extract capsule for hyposensitization use; March 1999.
48. Skin protectant drug products for over-the-counter human use; final monograph. *Federal Register.* 2003;68:33362-81.
49. Skin protectant drug products for over-the-counter human use; final monograph; Technical Amendment. *Federal Register.* 2004; 69:51362.
50. Zink BJ, Otten EJ, Rosenthal M, et al. The effect of jewel weed in preventing poison ivy dermatitis. *J Wilderness Med.* 1991;2:178-82.
51. Long D, Ballentine NH, Marks JG Jr. Treatment of poison ivy/oak allergenic contact dermatitis with an extract of jewelweed. *Am J Contact Dermat.* 1997;8:150-3.

CHAPTER 36

# Diaper Dermatitis and Prickly Heat

*Victor A. Padrón*

"Diaper rash" is the common name for diaper dermatitis, which is an acute dermatitis of the skin. It is an inflammatory condition in the region of the perineum, buttocks, lower abdomen, and inner thighs. In some countries the diaper is called a napkin or nappy (nappie), and diaper rash may be referred to as nappy rash. Diaper rash can appear in adults or children on any skin surface area enclosed by a diaper.

Prickly heat (miliaria or miliaria rubra) is a transient inflammation of the skin that appears as a very fine, usually red, rash. It can appear on any part of the body that has sweat glands (e.g., groin, chest, axilla regions).

In most circumstances neither diaper rash nor prickly heat causes serious illness. These conditions typically produce discomfort, irritation, or itching. They may lead to fussiness, agitation, and easy irritability in infants. These dermatoses can also be devoid of any discomfort or may be only a minor annoyance in either adults or infants.

## DIAPER DERMATITIS

### Epidemiology of Diaper Dermatitis

The majority of diaper dermatitis cases appear in diapered infants younger than 20 months. Approximately 70% of infants exhibit some features of diaper-induced skin compromise as early as 7 days after birth.[1] Two thirds of all infants have overt symptoms of diaper rash at some time in their infancy. The steady decline in the number of cases of diaper rash in infants since the 1970s is attributed to the rise in affordability, widespread acceptability, use of, and advertising of disposable diapers. The decline was accelerated in the 1980s and 1990s with improvements in diaper technology and the rise of superabsorbent core materials and breathable coverings.[2] Breast-fed infants have less diaper rash than bottle-fed infants. The feces of breast-fed infants are less copious, less alkaline, and less caustic to the skin. Studies have shown that starting a child on solid food early, of itself, has no effect on the incidence of diaper rash in infants, but foods that increase the urinary and fecal pH, such as high-protein diets, may contribute to diaper rash.

Diaper rash can also be a manifestation of other diseases such as Kawasaki's syndrome, granuloma gluteale infantum, and cytomegalovirus infection. Infants born to compromised mothers (e.g., HIV-positive; genital herpes; other chronic, congenital, or sexually transmitted infections) should be considered at increased risk for unusual manifestations of diaper rash or diaper rash–like presentations. Infections of the skin by yeasts (candidiasis), staphylococci (erysipelas), streptococci (impetigo), clostridia, and other bacteria may initially resemble diaper rash and be misdiagnosed. Inguinal swelling, fever, chills, tachycardia, blisters, vesicles, irregular borders bounded by bumps or vesicles are a few of the indicators of secondary infections that require medical referral.

The rapid rise in the number of patients of advanced age in the population has been accompanied by an increase in the cases of adult incontinence. Improved public awareness and advertising of adult incontinence products (see Chapter 52) have led to increased use of adult diapers and increased reporting of diaper dermatitis (incontinence dermatitis) in persons of advanced age. There are no known racial or gender differences in the incidence of diaper rash. Infant caregivers may need to be reassured that, at one time or another, most infants have an episode of diaper rash and that this pathology is not a social stigma.

### Etiology of Diaper Dermatitis

Diaper dermatitis is most likely caused by a combination of factors. Occlusion, moisture, bacteria, a shift away from the normal acidic skin pH (pH 4.0-5.5) to a more alkaline pH, mechanical chafing and friction (as the infant becomes more active and more mobile), and proteolytic enzymes and bile salts from the gastrointestinal (GI) tract all combine in additive or synergistic ways to cause diaper rash.

Urine and fecal bacteria can contribute to skin breakdown; urea-splitting bacteria from the colon are believed to convert urine contents into ammonia. Ammonia can raise the pH of the skin, making it more susceptible to damage or infection; ammonia from urine can also rapidly produce a serious chemical burn. Mechanical irritation of the skin can also be the initial insult that breaks down the epidermis, allowing other irritants to assault the skin.

Tight-fitting, stiff, or rough diapers and the use of occlusive plastic or rubberized covers or pants over the diaper can contribute to occlusion and mechanical friction of the skin. Infrequent changing of the diaper contributes to increased skin moisture. Skin left in contact with wetness for long periods becomes waterlogged or hyperhydrated, which plugs sweat glands and makes skin more susceptible to irritation and absorption of chemicals. The typical infant begins to urinate within 24 hours after birth. Urination occurs in infants up to 20 times a day until they are approximately 2 months old; the frequency falls to about 8 times a day until age 8 months. Defecation occurs from 3 to 6 times a day up to about age 8 months. As the infant's autonomic and muscular control develops, defecation gradually declines to 1 to 3 times a day. In the first months of life, it is common for infants to need an average of six diaper changes per day.

Reusable cloth diapers can contribute to diaper rash and skin irritation if not adequately washed and rinsed. Harsh chemicals to clean and sanitize the diapers may leave chemical residues on the diaper that then come into contact with the skin.

Medications that affect the motility and microbial flora of the GI tract, and that hinder autonomic control of urination and defecation may contribute to diaper rash. Intolerance to certain foods, excessive dietary sugar, and dairy products are known to induce diarrhea. Apple juice, mints, candies, chocolates, honey, fruit-flavored soft drinks, grapes, and other foods high in hexitols, sorbitol, sucrose, and fructose may induce diarrhea and predispose to diaper rash. Diary products, such as ice cream, frozen yogurt, and cheeses, may induce diarrhea, especially in the presence of lactose intolerance. Antibiotics can alter microbial flora and induce diarrhea. Caffeine- or magnesium-containing products, such as teas or antacids, may cause diarrhea. Some products, such as antioxidants, detergent or soap residues, household cleaning products, lotions, sunscreens, insect repellents, and plant materials such as ragweed and thistle, can produce a contact dermatitis that resembles diaper rash or predisposes the infant to diaper rash, While many of these agents commonly are not used in the diaper region, they may have an unexpected effect on skin under a diaper should they be placed in the diaper region through accident or ignorance.

## Pathophysiology of Diaper Dermatitis

The skin of the infant perineal region is about one half to one third of the thickness of adult skin. Because the area is typically enclosed by a diaper and has little exposure to the outside environment, it tends to hold moisture and wetness, predisposing it to irritation and infection. It is also a less effective barrier to the absorption of drugs and toxins. Adult skin, being thicker, is less susceptible to this irritation and to the penetration of drugs and chemicals.[1]

## Signs and Symptoms of Diaper Dermatitis

Diaper rash usually presents as red to bright red (erythematous), sometimes shiny, wet-looking patches and lesions on the skin (see Color Plates, photograph 19). They may appear dusky maroon or purplish on darker skin. Severe diaper rash can progress to maceration, papule formation, the presence of vesicles or bullae, oozing, erosion of the skin, or ulceration. Such developments require intervention by a primary care provider (PCP).

Generally, diaper rash occurs on the skin spaces covered by the diaper, but severe cases can spread outside the diaper area, moving up the abdomen or onto the upper buttocks and lower back. If the infant lies primarily on his or her abdomen, the rash may appear more forward of the perineum. If the infant lies primarily on his or her back, the rash may appear more posterior to the perineum.

A very disconcerting feature of diaper rash is that it can occur in a matter of hours and take days or weeks to completely resolve. The onset of clearly observable diaper rash can occur in the time between two diaper changes. Most likely, the process of skin breakdown is not pronounced or observable initially, and the breakdown goes from unobservable to observable in a matter of hours. The entire process from normal to noticeably inflamed skin takes longer than the time between normal diaper changes. It is noteworthy that no diaper rash is found in cultures in which infants are kept essentially naked, wear loincloths that leave the genitals uncovered, or wear clothing with slits.

## Complications of Diaper Dermatitis

Diaper rash can predispose to secondary infection and genital damage. As skin pH changes, it can foster the growth of opportunistic infections that can be bacterial (e.g., streptococci or staphylococci), fungal (e.g., yeasts), and even viral (e.g., herpes simplex). Untreated or infected diaper rash can progress to skin maceration and ulceration, infection of the penis or vulva itself, and urinary tract infection. If left untreated, adhesions and scarring of the genitals can occur, necessitating cosmetic or reconstructive surgery.

In addition to secondary infection, diaper rash can exist concurrent with other skin conditions such as psoriasis and seborrhea. Skin conditions that can occur on other parts of the body can exist in the diaper region and may be misdiagnosed as diaper rash.

## Treatment of Diaper Dermatitis

### Treatment Goals

The overall goals of diaper rash treatment are to (1) relieve the symptoms, (2) rid the patient of the rash, and (3) prevent recurrences.

### General Treatment Approach

The general approach to diaper rash is the use of nondrug therapy or a combination of drug and nondrug therapy as outlined in Figure 36-1.

The best treatment for diaper rash is prevention. The ideal preventive therapy would be to change the diaper each time the child defecates or urinates. This treatment is impractical because it would require a 24-hour vigil and a way to know immediately when the infant has defecated or urinated. It is difficult enough for modern parents and caregivers to make six or more diaper changes in a typical day. Electronic devices (moisture alarms) for constant monitoring of when infants urinate are available. These devices are not without problems as they may not be loud enough or lose battery power without warning, children may tamper with them or deactivate them by accident, drink spills can give false alarms, and the parent may need some training in their use. These devices are better used

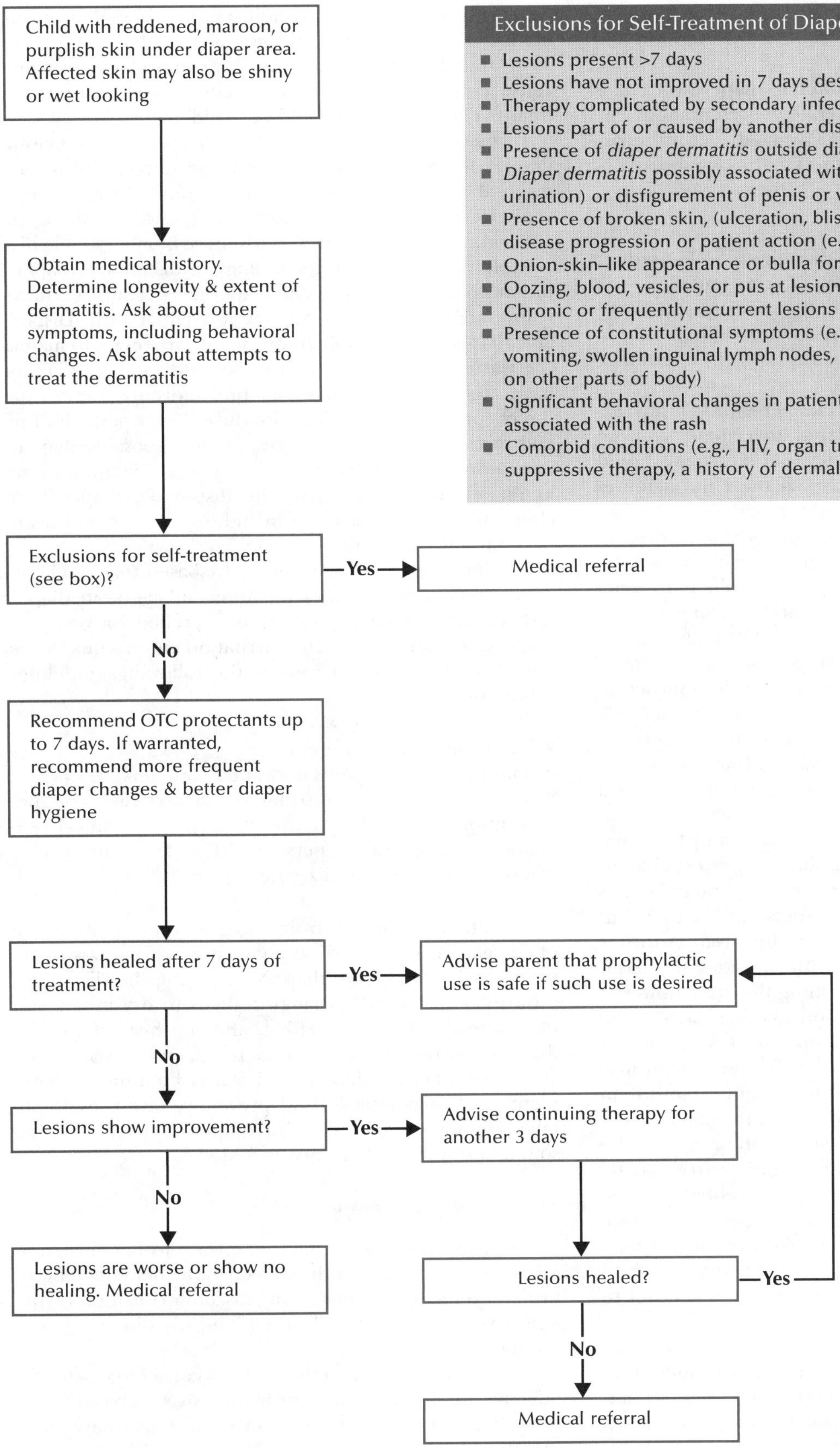
Child with reddened, maroon, or purplish skin under diaper area. Affected skin may also be shiny or wet looking
Obtain medical history. Determine longevity & extent of dermatitis. Ask about other symptoms, including behavioral changes. Ask about attempts to treat the dermatitis
Exclusions for self-treatment (see box)?
Yes
Medical referral
No
Recommend OTC protectants up to 7 days. If warranted, recommend more frequent diaper changes & better diaper hygiene
Lesions healed after 7 days of treatment?
Yes
Advise parent that prophylactic use is safe if such use is desired
No
Lesions show improvement?
Yes
Advise continuing therapy for another 3 days
No
Lesions are worse or show no healing. Medical referral
Lesions healed?
Yes
No
Medical referral

**Exclusions for Self-Treatment of Diaper Dermatitis and Prickly Heat**

- Lesions present >7 days
- Lesions have not improved in 7 days despite appropriate care
- Therapy complicated by secondary infection (viral, bacterial, or fungal)
- Lesions part of or caused by another disease state
- Presence of *diaper dermatitis* outside diaper region
- *Diaper dermatitis* possibly associated with urinary tract infection (painful urination) or disfigurement of penis or vulva
- Presence of broken skin, (ulceration, blistering, or peeling of skin) due to disease progression or patient action (e.g., scratching)
- Onion-skin–like appearance or bulla formation in affected area
- Oozing, blood, vesicles, or pus at lesion sites
- Chronic or frequently recurrent lesions
- Presence of constitutional symptoms (e.g., fever, diarrhea, nausea, vomiting, swollen inguinal lymph nodes, rapid pulse or rash or skin lesions on other parts of body)
- Significant behavioral changes in patient (e.g., lethargy, incessant crying) associated with the rash
- Comorbid conditions (e.g., HIV, organ transplantation, immune suppressive therapy, a history of dermal hepatic infections)

**FIGURE 36-1** Self-care of diaper dermatitis. Key: HIV, human immunodeficiency virus; OTC, over-the-counter.

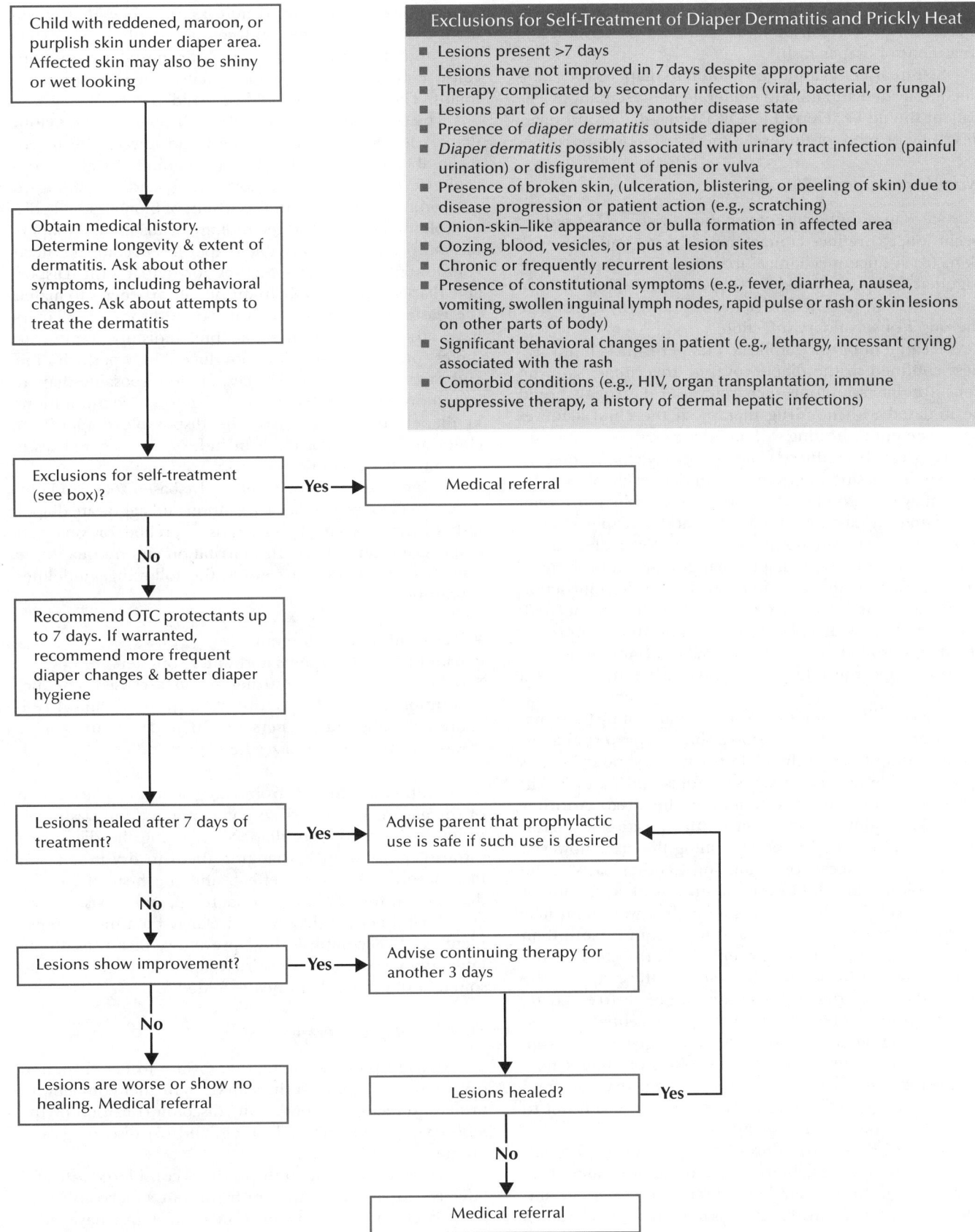

for bedwetting and potty training in the older child. In infants it is more realistic to use standard prevention and treatment of diaper rash.

Self-treatment should be limited to diaper rash that is uncomplicated and mild to moderate in presentation. The patient should be referred to a PCP when diaper rash manifests one or more of the exclusions listed in Figure 36-1.

### Nonpharmacologic Therapy

The steps in nonpharmacologic therapy are to (1) reduce occlusion, (2) reduce contact time of urine and feces with skin, (3) reduce mechanical irritation and trauma to the inguinal and perineal skin, (4) protect the skin from further irritation, (5) encourage healing, and (6) discourage the onset of secondary infection.

Treatment of uncomplicated diaper rash (simple redness confined to the diaper-covered area, intact skin, no constitutional symptoms such as fever or diarrhea) should be initiated with nondrug therapy. If the child achieves improvement or healing with nondrug methods, exposure to drugs can be reduced, and the drugs can be held in reserve. Increasing the frequency of diaper changes to six a day may be a good starting place. If feasible, more than six changes a day combined with careful diaper change procedures may ameliorate mild symptoms of redness. During each and every diaper change, careful flushing of the skin with plain water followed by gentle nonfriction drying is to be encouraged. Should wiping be needed, gentle rubbing with a bland soft cloth or wipe is appropriate. The unsoiled part of a diaper should not be used to clean or wipe the infant as it may harbor unseen fecal bacteria.

Anecdotally, both professional and nonprofessional caregivers have suggested using a shower sprayer on a low power setting to rinse the child because a sprayer head is maneuverable and can flush skin folds and natural skin creases without directly touching the area. Another method is holding the infant in a sitting position in a basin of lukewarm water and gently washing the area; however, this may spread fecal contamination to other parts of the body. Holding the child over a basin or sink as the infant is washed is better, but holding a wiggling wet infant may not be as simple as it sounds and may require more than one set of hands. Some caregivers will let the child air dry and run naked for a spell, but there is the risk that the infant has more urine or bowel contents ready to evacuate. Thorough drying before rediapering is essential to good diaper-changing procedures. Other caregivers have ventured to use a hair dryer set to its lowest or coolest temperature setting and lowest speed to help dry the child more thoroughly and quickly. Care must be taken not to burn, shock, or scald the infant.

None of these procedures has been subjected to scientific analysis for reliability, safety, or clinical value. Caregivers are, unfortunately, left to their own devices to find safe, effective, and convenient ways to clean and dry infants during diaper changes.

The use of commercial baby wipes is no longer controversial. Most are now low in abrasives and chemically bland for use on diaper rash. Used with finesse and gentle wiping, infant wipes are as mild as or milder than washcloths.[3] Few baby wipes still contain alcohol, perfumes, soap, and other unnecessary or exotic ingredients that can cause contact dermatitis or actually burn or sting the infant. Those that do should be avoided.

The controversy over the use of disposable versus cloth diapers is becoming moot. The trend toward the use of disposable diapers has been overwhelming, driven by convenience to the caregiver, advertising, and a quelling of environmental issues with the advent of biodegradable disposable diapers. As the technology of disposable diapers has improved, the disposable diaper has become a critical component of nondrug therapy for diaper rash. Disposable diapers are available in various absorbencies to match the waste output of the infant. Some disposable diapers have absorptive materials that pull moisture away from direct contact with the skin to reduce skin hyperhydration and mixing of urine with feces. Some disposable diapers have a protectant already in the diaper. These innovations in diaper technology favor the disposable diaper over cloth, and the use of cloth in industrialized countries is becoming the exception.[4]

Using detergents or ordinary lye-based soaps to launder cloth diapers may cause irritation and aggravate diaper rash or cause contact dermatitis. Starched or very stiff diapers can cause mechanical irritation and trauma to the skin. If cloth diapers are used, the following guidelines should be observed:

- Wash with mild detergent.
- Avoid harsh detergents and water softeners.
- If bleach or other sanitizing agents are used, conduct additional rinses to remove chlorine or chemical residues; boiling the diapers for 10 to 15 minutes after washing will also sterilize the diapers.

Another suggestion from caregivers is to place a cup of vinegar in the final rinse water of a half-full wash load to lower the pH of the diapers. Exposing the diapers to ultraviolet radiation by hanging them to dry in the sun may have a bactericidal effect, and the heat of ironing diapers may further kill bacteria, fungi, and yeasts.[5,6] However, a commercial diaper service may be a more convenient way to accomplish these preventive measures. Reputable diaper services sterilize diapers and then press, soften, and return them neatly folded.

### Pharmacologic Therapy

The steps in pharmacologic therapy are to (1) clean and dry the skin, (2) protect the skin from further contact with urine and feces, (3) soothe any discomfort caused by the lesion(s), (4) encourage healing, and (5) discourage the onset of secondary infection.

Protectants are the only products considered safe and effective for use in diaper rash without supervision by a PCP. Twelve ingredients, all skin protectants, have been proposed for treating diaper rash (Table 36-1). It is common for two or more of the proposed ingredients to be combined in commercial products for treating diaper rash. Some products that contain a proposed ingredient have

**TABLE 36-1 Skin Protectants Approved to Treat Diaper Rash[7]**

| Agent | Concentration (%) |
|---|---|
| Allantoin | 0.5-2.0 |
| Calamine | 1-25 |
| Cod liver oil (in combination) | 5.0-13.5 |
| Dimethicone | 1-3 |
| Kaolin | 4-20 |
| Lanolin (in combination) | 15.5 |
| Mineral oil | 50-100 |
| Petrolatum | 30-100 |
| Talc | 45-100 |
| Topical cornstarch | 10-98 |
| White petrolatum | 30-100 |
| Zinc oxide | 1-25 |
| Zinc oxide ointment | 25-40 |

been combined with other ingredients that are unsafe or of dubious value for treating diaper rash. The other ingredient(s) may be unsuitable or even toxic when applied to skin compromised by diaper rash.

Hence, practitioners should recommend only those products that are labeled for diaper rash or contain only 1 or more of the 12 proposed ingredients. Products that contain antimicrobials, external analgesics, and antifungals legally cannot claim they are for treatment of diaper rash.

Because skin protectants are remarkably safe, their use either as treatment or prophylaxis is acceptable. An infant with no diaper rash symptoms should not be exposed needlessly to diaper rash products unless a diaper rash is anticipated on the basis of previous history (e.g., diaper rash occurred during a previous episode of diarrhea or while infant was on antibiotic therapy). In such cases preventive therapy is reasonable.

## Skin Protectants

Skin protectants serve as a physical barrier between the skin and external irritants. They are removed and reapplied with each diaper change. By preventing further insult or aggravation, they protect surfaces that are healing. Protectants serve as lubricants in areas in which skin-to-skin or skin-to-diaper friction could aggravate diaper rash or could predispose the area to diaper rash. Protectants absorb moisture or prevent moisture from coming into direct contact with skin. Protective effects of these products allow the body's normal healing processes to work.

Zinc oxide, a mild astringent with minor antiseptic properties, is an excellent protectant. Zinc oxide typically is formulated as a powder or ointment. The ointment is acceptable in concentrations of 1% to 40%. The concentration in other dosage forms is acceptable only up to 25%. Zinc oxide paste USP is a classic example of the protectant group of products; it contains zinc oxide 25%, cornstarch

**TABLE 36-2 Selected Nonmonograph Ingredients Found in Diaper Rash Products**

| | |
|---|---|
| *Aloe vera* sp., aloe | Plantain |
| Aluminum acetate or hydroxide | Poplar bud |
| Arnica (flower) | Shepherd's purse |
| Bovine collagen | Silicone |
| Castor oil | Sodium bicarbonate |
| Comfrey (herb) | Sweet clover |
| Emu oil | St. John's wort |
| Goldenseal | Tea tree oil |
| Jambolan bark | Vitamins A and D |
| Melissa (lemon balm) | Vitamin E |
| Peruvian balsam | Walnut leaf |
| | Witch hazel |

25%, and white petrolatum 60%. The paste's major drawback is that it is thick and tacky to the touch. Removal from the skin requires wiping with mineral oil. There are zinc oxide preparations formulated to be less difficult to use, more washable, more creamlike, and easier to apply and remove. Zinc oxide is often combined with other ingredients that may or may not have Food and Drug Administration (FDA) approval (Table 36-2). Use of plain approved ingredients avoids irritation and possible allergic response from additive ingredients. Few useful comparative studies of the protectants are available.

Calamine is a mixture of zinc and ferrous oxides, has absorption properties, and is available in numerous dosage forms. Allantoin rarely is seen as a single-entity product. It is a purine that complexes with and renders harmless many sensitizing agents on the skin. Mineral oil coats the skin with a water-impenetrable film that must be washed off with each diaper change to avoid buildup in pores and subsequent folliculitis. Lanolin is proposed for use only in combination with other ingredients. By itself, lanolin is very tacky and difficult to wash off, and some people are allerigc to it. It should not appear in products at more than 20% concentration.

Petrolatum is a yellow oleaginous hydrocarbon that, when decolorized, becomes white petrolatum. In either form, it is an excellent protectant and a ubiquitous ointment base. Plain white petrolatum or white petrolatum combined with mineral oil and wax is superior to all other product choices for newborns with uncomplicated diaper dermatitis.[8] Kaolin is a claylike material of hydrated aluminum silicate. It is mined from the earth and then highly purified. This protectant absorbs moisture and perspiration. Cod liver oil is a protectant rich in vitamin A. Dimethicone is a silicone-based oil that repels water and soothes and counteracts inflammation.

Talc and topical cornstarch are used almost exclusively as loose powders, and have a long history of use in diaper rash and prickly heat. Talc is a finely milled form of hydrous magnesium silicate and is more a lubricant than an absorbent. It reduces friction between body parts, such as the thighs, buttocks, and inguinal area skin folds. It adheres well to the skin but should never be applied to broken or oozing skin; it can cake on the edges of wounds and precipitate infection or retard healing.

Talc and cornstarch carry a warning against inhalation of the powders because of a history of injury and fatality from improper use of the powder around infants. The warning states: "Do not use on broken skin. Keep powder away from child's face to avoid inhalation, which can cause breathing problems." Powders should be carefully applied with as little aerosolization as possible. Concerns about inhalation of powders has caused some practitioners to suggest pouring the powder into the hands away from the infant and gently rubbing it onto the perineal area, while others recommend avoiding any use of powders around infants.

Cornstarch, which is literally derived from the grain heads of corn plants, is an effective absorbent. Controlled studies have failed to substantiate fears that cornstarch encourages yeast infection and fermentation to alcohol. Cornstarch and talc are sometimes combined with other ingredients (e.g., magnesium stearate, calcium carbonate, zinc stearate, microporous cellulose, skin-soothing agents, fragrance), which may increase the product's adhesion to skin, increase moisture absorption, soothe skin, avoid caking of the powder, and improve product acceptability and marketability.

### Contraindicated Agents

Topical nonprescription antibiotic and antifungal agents are not appropriate to use in diaper rash. The general public is not considered adequately educated to diagnose and treat infectious diseases in infants' inguinal area. External analgesics are not recommended as they can alter sensory perception in a population that cannot communicate perceptual changes. They may also excoriate macerated skin, be painful, retard healing, and further complicate diaper rash. Products containing boric acid or baking soda (sodium bicarbonate) should be avoided because of case reports of toxicity.[9]

Hydrocortisone is indicated for minor skin irritation, but should not be used in diaper rash without supervision by a PCP. This contraindication is especially true in infants. First, hydrocortisone may suppress local immune response, an action that may be undesirable when secondary infection is possible. Second, the diaper area is a significant portion of the infant's body surface area. Hydrocortisone absorption into the skin is enhanced under occlusive conditions. When applied to macerated skin or a large surface area, absorption of hydrocortisone may lead to blood levels that interfere with the infant's pituitary-adrenal axis. Nonprescription hydrocortisone is labeled not to be used in patients younger than 2 years[2] (see Chapter 33).

### Product Selection Guidelines

Drug therapy is only an adjunct to good diaper hygiene and diaper-changing practices. When diaper rash is present and pharmacologic therapy is indicated, the practitioner should inform caregivers about their choices between semisolid and powdered protectants. Caregivers may be more comfortable with a semisolid product if they are anxious about the inhalation warning on powders or when hands-on application is not painful or uncomfortable to the patient. Fortunately, the products in this category are relatively inexpensive, and socioeconomic status tends not to be a major issue in treating diaper rash. Table 36-3 lists selected trade-name products and their ingredients.

Despite their popularity, some commonly used products contain nonapproved (nonmonograph) ingredients, which possibly are used for formulation purposes, present in nonpharmacologic concentrations, unregulated nutraceuticals, listed as inactive ingredients, or listed to support marketing claims. For example; camphor may be present to provide a "medicated' fragrance; aloe may be present to appeal to the public perception that aloe is a wound healer; or vitamins may be present to sound "natural." To make the claim to treat diaper rash, the product must, however, meet the FDA-published guidelines for active ingredients. Although the products used in diaper dermatitis generally have a wide margin of safety, the practitioner should not recommend them indiscriminately.

### *Complementary Therapies*

Products containing complementary therapies (Table 36-2) are not recommended for use on newborn and infant skin for several reasons. Not enough is known about their effects on infant skin. The amount and effect of systemic absorption are unknown. What product strength to use is unknown. While some of these agents have been used without incidence in adults, there is no credible data on their safety or efficacy in infants. Infants and children should be treated with the mildest and most bland effective products available.

## Assessment of Diaper Dermatitis: A Case-based Approach

When a caregiver consults a practitioner about a suspected diaper rash, the practitioner should find out whether factors conducive to diaper dermatitis are present. Specifically, the caregiver should be asked what type of diaper is being used and how frequently diapers are changed. Drawing on that response, the practitioner must consider whether increasing the frequency of diaper changes would reduce the diaper rash problem or whether medication is warranted.

If cloth diapers are used, the practitioner should find out how they are laundered and should determine whether the laundering method is adequate to remove chemical residues or fecal bacteria. The practitioner should also ask how the infant is cleaned during diaper changes. The parent's response may indicate a cleaning method that does not remove all fecal bacteria or the use of a disposable wipe that may cause skin irritation. To find out whether occlusion of the diaper area is a problem, the practitioner should find out whether plastic pants are being used over the diaper or whether high-absorbency diapers are being used. The practitioner should ask questions to determine whether self-care is appropriate. Case 36-1 illustrates assessment of patients with diaper dermatitis.

**TABLE 36-3 Selected Products for Diaper Dermatitis**

| Trade Name | Primary Ingredients |
|---|---|
| A + D Ointment with Zinc Oxide | Zinc oxide 10%; dimethicone 1% |
| Amerigel Lotion | Glycerin; lemon oil; parabens; oak extract |
| Aquaphor Original Ointment* | Petrolatum; mineral oil; ceresin; lanolin alcohol |
| Aveeno Bath Treatment Soothing Formula Powder | Colloidal oatmeal 100% |
| Aveeno Lotion | Colloidal oatmeal 1%; glycerin; phenylcarbinol; petrolatum; dimethicone; benzyl alcohol |
| Aveeno Moisturizing Cream | 1% colloidal oatmeal; glycerin; petrolatum; dimethicone; phenylcarbinol |
| Balmex Diaper Rash Ointment | Zinc oxide; aloe vera; vitamin E† |
| Boudreaux's Butt Paste | Zinc Oxide 16% ; Peruvian balsam,† boric acid,‡ castor oil, mineral oil, white wax, petrolatum |
| Caldesene Powder | Talc 81%; zinc oxide 15% |
| Desitin Diaper Rash Ointment | Zinc oxide 40%; cod liver oil; petrolatum; lanolin; talc |
| Desitin with Zinc Oxide Powder | Cornstarch 88.2%; zinc oxide 10% |
| Desitin Creamy Ointment | Zinc oxide 10%; parabens; petrolatum; mineral oil |
| Diaper Guard Ointment | Dimethicone 1%; white petrolatum 66%; cocoa butter; parabens; vitamins A, D, and E;† zinc oxide |
| Diaparene Cornstarch Baby Powder | Corn starch; aloe† |
| Dyprotex pads | Micronized zinc oxide 4%; petrolatum 37.6%; dimethicone 2.5%; cod liver oil; aloe† |
| Eucerin Cream | Petrolatum; mineral oil; mineral wax |
| Gold Bond Triple Action Medicated Baby Powder | Zinc oxide 10%; talc 89% |
| Johnson & Johnson No More Rash Cream with Zinc Oxide | Zinc oxide 13%; water; mineral oil; dimethicone; glycerin; lanolin; petrolatum |
| Mexsana Medicated Powder | Kaolin; eucalyptus oil; camphor; corn starch; lemon oil; zinc oxide |
| Vaseline Pure Petroleum Jelly | White petrolatum 100% |

*Not to be confused with Aquaphor Healing Ointment; †nonmonograph ingredients; ‡potentially hazardous ingredient.

## CASE 36-1

| Relevant Evaluation Criteria | Scenario/Model Outcome |
|---|---|
| **Information Gathering** | |
| 1. Gather essential information about the patient's symptoms, including: | |
| a. description of symptom(s) (i.e., nature, onset, duration, severity, associated symptoms) | A frustrated mother calls you and says that her 8- month-old child has had diaper rash intermittently over a 6-week period. |
| b. description of any factors that seem to precipitate, exacerbate, and/or relieve the patient's symptom(s) | She started out using the standard therapy of a zinc oxide ointment; for several days, the diaper rash got better. She increased the frequency of diaper changes, even resorting to changing the diaper during the night. After 3 days of improvement, she opened the diaper one morning and found that full-blown diaper rash had returned. |

## CASE 36-1 (continued)

| Relevant Evaluation Criteria | Scenario/Model Outcome |
|---|---|
| c. description of the patient's efforts to relieve the symptoms | The mother informed her child's PCP by telephone of the status of the rash. The PCP recommended bathing the child twice daily in colloidal oatmeal, use of Mycolog II Ointment, and use of Tucks disposable wipes to clean the child during diaper changes. The PCP also recommended that the child be seated for 15 minutes in a solution of aluminum acetate each evening before bedtime. The mother also changed to a so-called rash prevention diaper. She followed this regimen over a 2-week period, and the skin seemed to return to normal.<br>An additional 5 days went by, and the child once again developed a bright red, wet-looking bottom. The mother called the PCP, who told her the child had the "most stubborn case of diaper rash I have ever seen." The mother scheduled another appointment for the following week with the PCP, but in frustration she called her pharmacist because she and the PCP "seemed to have tried everything" to give the child relief. |
| 2. Gather essential patient history information: | |
| a. patient's identity | Mona Vana |
| b. age, sex, height, and weight | 8-month-old F, 30", 26 lb |
| c. patient's occupation | N/A |
| d. patient's dietary habits | Normal healthy diet for age |
| e. patient's sleep habits | Normal for age |
| f. concurrent medical conditions, prescription and nonprescription medications, and dietary supplements | Only those topical products stated above |
| g. allergies | NKA |
| h. history of other adverse reactions to medications | None |
| i. other (describe)_______ | The child has not displayed any fussiness, distress or behavioral changes during the acute flare-ups. |
| **Assessment and Triage** | |
| 3. Differentiate the patient's signs/symptoms and correctly identify the patient's primary problem(s). | Recurrent diaper rash–like symptoms in the inguinal area |
| 4. Identify exclusions for self-treatment (see Figure 36-1). | Frequently recurring lesions |
| 5. Formulate a comprehensive list of therapeutic alternatives for the primary problem to determine if triage to a medical practitioner is required, and share this information with the caregiver. | Options include:<br>(1) Recommend self-care with OTC products.<br>(2) Recommend self-care with nonpharmacologic methods.<br>(3) Refer Mona's mother immediately to an appropriate PCP.<br>(4) Recommend self-care until an appropriate PCP can be consulted.<br>(5) Take no action. |
| **Plan** | |
| 6. Select an optimal therapeutic alternative to address the patient's problem, taking into account patient preferences. | Recommend the mother take Mona to a pediatric or dermatology specialist to obtain a second medical opinion. |
| 7. Describe the recommended therapeutic approach to the caregiver. | When standard therapy fails, we should suspect the presence of underlying disease that is not being addressed or possible misdiagnosis of the condition. |
| 8. Explain to the caregiver the rationale for selecting the recommended therapeutic approach from the considered therapeutic alternatives. | This patient meets one of the exclusion criteria for self-care (see Figure 36-1). A second medical opinion by a specialist may be warranted. |

## CASE 36-1 (continued)

| Relevant Evaluation Criteria | Scenario/Model Outcome |
|---|---|
| **Patient Education** | |
| 9. When recommending self-care with nonprescription medications and/or nondrug therapy, convey accurate information to the caregiver, including: | Criterion does not apply in this case. |
| 10. Solicit follow-up questions from caregiver. | Is it something really serious? |
| 11. Answer caregiver's questions. | We cannot know until a cause of the recurrence is known or the actual diagnosis is identified. Since the child is otherwise normal and exhibiting no signs or symptoms of distress, it is not likely to be life threatening. |

Key: N/A, not applicable; NKA, no known allergies; OTC, over-the-counter; PCP, primary care provider.

## PATIENT EDUCATION FOR DIAPER DERMATITIS

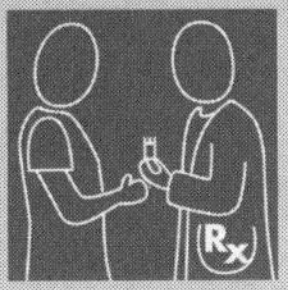

The objectives of self-treatment are to (1) eliminate the rash, (2) relieve the symptoms, and (3) prevent recurrent rashes. For most patients, carefully following product instructions and the self-care measures listed here will help ensure optimal therapeutic outcomes.

### Nondrug Measures

- Change diapers frequently, at least six times a day, to prevent prolonged exposure of the infant's skin to moisture and feces.
- To prevent occlusion of skin in the diaper area, avoid putting rubber pants over cloth diapers. Tightly covering the skin causes it to break down.
- During every diaper change, flush the infant's skin with plain water and gently pat it dry or allow it to air dry.
- Do not wipe the infant with any part of the diaper. Even areas that appear unsoiled may be contaminated with fecal bacteria.
- To prevent irritating the infant's skin, do not use detergent or ordinary lye-based soaps to launder cloth diapers; avoid starched or very stiff diapers; and avoid commercial baby wipes that contain alcohol, perfumes, and soap, which may burn or sting the skin.

### Nonprescription Medications

- To treat diaper rash, use a product containing one or more of the skin protectants listed in Table 36-1. The product can be used even after the rash clears to prevent recurrences, but use should be stopped for short periods to see whether the rash returns and the product is still needed.
- Do not use products that contain ingredients listed in Table 36-1 if they are combined with benzocaine or an antibacterial such as benzethonium chloride. Benzocaine can cause an allergic reaction; antibacterials are not suitable for use on diaper rash.
- Do not use hydrocortisone.
- Do not use external analgesics such as phenol, menthol, methyl salicylate, or capsaicin to treat diaper rash. These medications are inappropriate for use on infant skin and may cause harm.
- Powders for children or infants should be gently poured into the hands then rubbed onto the skin, using a sufficient amount to cover the affected area. Do not vigorously shake powders near infants and keep powders away from the child's face to avoid their inhalation.
- Semisolid products can be applied by hand, or with disposable tongue depressors or washable rubber spatulas.
- Apply sufficient cream or ointment, by hand or with a disposable or washable spatula, to cover the affected area.
- If using mineral oil, wash it off at every diaper change to avoid clogging skin pores, which may lead to prickly heat and folliculitis.
- Do not apply products containing talc to broken or oozing skin because it can cake on the edges of wounds and lead to infection or retard healing.
- Discard products that are discolored or whose expiration date has passed. (The practitioner should point out expiration dates on the products.)

⚠ Consult a primary care provider if any of the exclusions in Figure 36-1 apply.

## Patient Counseling for Diaper Dermatitis

The practitioner should review with the caregiver proper cleaning of the diaper area, and caution the caregiver to avoid occlusion of the area and prevent prolonged contact of urine or feces with the infant's skin. The practitioner should explain the proper methods of applying nonprescription skin protectants and should warn the caregiver of signs and symptoms that indicate the dermatitis has worsened and needs medical attention. The box Patient Education for Diaper Dermatitis lists specific information to provide to patients.

### Evaluation of Patient Outcomes for Diaper Dermatitis

Treatment of diaper dermatitis should be relatively short, approximately 1 week. If 7 days have elapsed and the condition is improved but not healed, therapy should be continued for another 3 days or until complete healing has occurred. If the condition has not improved or has worsened at the seventh day, a PCP should be consulted. At each diaper change, the parent should inspect the lesions for signs of improvement. At the end of therapy, the skin should have returned to normal.

## PRICKLY HEAT

### Epidemiology of Prickly Heat

Prickly heat (also called heat rash or miliaria) can occur at any age in anyone who has active sweat glands. It probably is significantly underreported because it is less troublesome than diaper rash and clears up very rapidly if left alone and/or if its cause is removed. Because persons of advanced age are less tolerant to heat, sweat less, are less physically active, and spend more time indoors and in controlled environments than younger people, they may have less opportunity to develop prickly heat.

### Etiology of Prickly Heat

Prickly heat results from blocked or plugged sweat glands. Prickly heat can arise from normal skin with little or no anatomic prodrome. The condition is most often associated with very hot, humid weather or can occur during illnesses that cause significant or profuse sweating. It also results from inability of the skin to "breathe" (interact with air) because of excessive clothing, very tight clothing, or clothing that is occlusive, such as leather and polyester, or athletic protective or safety garments and devices.

### Pathophysiology of Prickly Heat

The pores that house the sweat glands are obstructed in prickly heat. The inability of sweat to be secreted and escape the pore causes dilation and rupture of epidermal sweat pores. This situation causes an acute inflammation of the dermis that may manifest as stinging, burning, or itching.

### Signs and Symptoms of Prickly Heat

The pinpoint-size lesions are raised and red or maroon, forming erythematous papules (see Color Plates, photograph 20). The pinhead-size lesions may appear in small numbers clustered together or spread out over the occluded area on a pink to red field ("miliaria rubra"). Common sites for prickly heat dermatitis include the axilla (armpits), chest, upper back, back of the neck, abdomen, and inguinal area (groin). The lesions usually trace the pattern of the occlusion and, in uncomplicated cases, do not extend beyond the occluded area. Lesions can occur on the body wherever occlusion occurs and active sweat glands are present. If lesions are not resolved in a reasonable length of time (approximately 3-10 days), they can evolve into the same kinds of complications seen in diaper rash (e.g., infection, pustule formation, generalized dermatitis). Complications are extremely rare.

### Treatment of Prickly Heat

#### *Treatment Goals*

The lesions of prickly heat will resolve without pharmacologic treatment if the cause is removed; therefore, eliminating the cause is the primary goal.

#### *General Treatment Approach*

The steps in nonpharmacologic therapy of prickly heat include (1) eliminating occlusion of skin, (2) protecting skin from further irritation, (3) promoting healing of skin, and (4) discouraging onset of secondary infection.

Pharmacologic therapy and nondrug therapy have the same goals. The pharmacologic products help to (1) keep skin dry, (2) promote healing, (3) soothe any discomfort caused by lesion(s), and (4) discourage onset of secondary infection. The algorithm in Figure 36-2 outlines the self-treatment of prickly heat.

#### *Nonpharmacologic Therapy*

Nondrug therapy for prickly heat consists of decreasing sweating. Letting the patient rest, cool off, or enter a cool environment is a start. If the sweating is caused by a fever, the use of internal antipyretics, if not contraindicated, is appropriate. Wearing loose, light-colored, and lightweight clothing is palliative in prickly heat and is also good prevention because it allows air flow to the skin. In infants, frequent diaper changes and sparing use of soap or chemical irritants can reduce discomfort of existing prickly heat. Practitioners should warn patients not to apply oleaginous or oily substances to prickly heat lesions because these substances plug pores that need to be patent.

#### *Pharmacologic Therapy*

Nonprescription treatment of prickly heat should be limited to mild to moderate, uncomplicated cases. Prickly heat should not be occluded during therapy. This disorder can be ameliorated in less time and with less total drug exposure than diaper rash.

##### Emollients, Skin Protectants, and Antipruritics

For prickly heat, washing the skin with bland soap and soaking in colloidal oatmeal may be all that is needed. The choice of a drug product should be limited to one product that relieves burning and itching and does not block skin exposure to the air. Water-washable antipruritic products and bland emollients and protectants that soothe the skin

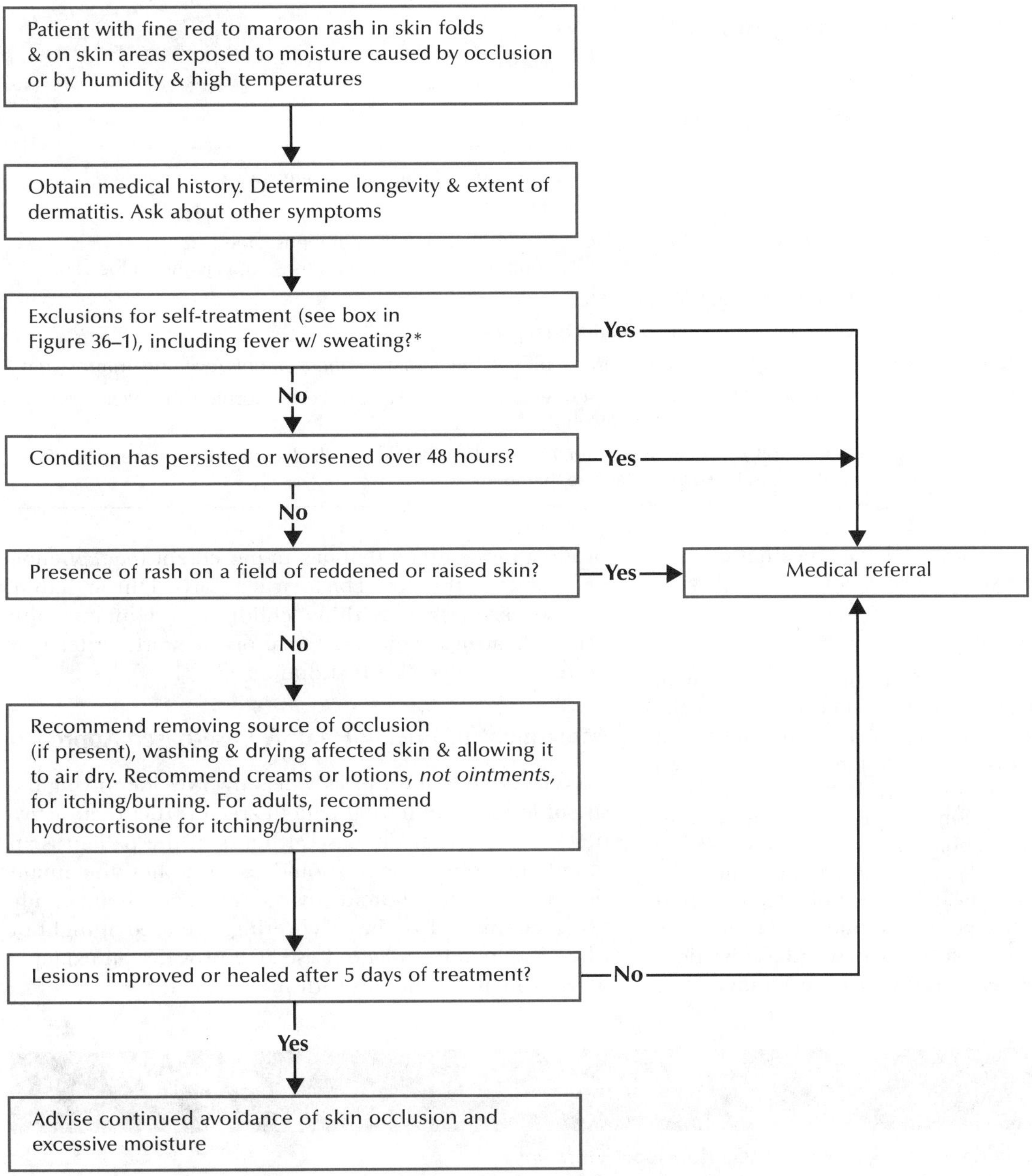


* High fever without sweating, high pulse rate, possible increased respiration, or hot, flushed dry skin (patient seems to be "burning up") may indicate hyperpyrexia ("heatstroke" or "sunstroke"). Refer the patient immediately to a PCP and/or transport patient to an emergency facility. Slow or weak pulse, lethargy, cold, pale clammy skin, absence of fever, or disorientation may indicate heat exhaustion. Move patient to a cool environment, and have the patient recline and take regular sips of water or slightly salty liquids or electrolyte solutions every few minutes.

**FIGURE 36-2** Self-care of prickly heat. Key: PCP, primary care provider.

and maintain skin moisture and texture may be all that is needed to treat the symptoms of prickly heat while they resolve. Powders should be used only prophylactically to absorb moisture and keep skin dry rather than as treatment of active prickly heat. They can actually clog pores and complicate therapy. (See Table 36-4 for selected trade-name products and Chapter 33 for a discussion of skin emollients.)

## Other Pharmacologic Agents

As in diaper rash, hydrocortisone is contraindicated in infants. In adults, hydrocortisone may be useful if the surface area involved is equal to or less than approximately 10% of body surface area. (See Figure 41-3 for information on calculating body surface area.) Because prickly heat rapidly clears without drug therapy, the only real use for hydrocortisone is to relieve itching.

**TABLE 36-4 Selected Products for Prickly Heat**

| Trade Name | Primary Ingredients |
|---|---|
| Aveeno Moisturizing Cream | Colloidal oatmeal 1%; glycerin; petrolatum; dimethicone; phenylcarbinol |
| Band-Aid Itch Relief Gel Spritz | Camphor 0.5% |
| Benadryl Maximum Strength Itch Relief | Cream: diphenhydramine HCl 2%; zinc acetate 0.1%; parabens; aloe vera<br>Stick: diphenhydramine HCl 2%; zinc acetate 0.1%; parabens; 73.5% alcohol ; aloe vera |
| Cortizone-5, Cortizone-10 Cream | Hydrocortisone 0.5% or 1.0% |
| Curel Moisturizing Cream | Glycerin; petrolatum; dimethicone; parabens |
| Eucerin Itch-Relief Moisturizing Spray | Menthol 0.15%; glycerin; mineral oil; cetyl alcohol; *Oenohera biennis* (evening primrose oil) |
| Eucerin Moisturizing Lotion | Mineral oil; PEG-40 sorbitan peroleate; lanolin acid glycerin ester; sorbitol; propylene glycol; cetyl palmitate; lanolin alcohol |
| Lubriderm Cream | Mineral oil; petrolatum; lanolin; lanolin alcohol; lanolin oil; glycerin; glyceryl stearate; PEG-100 stearate; sorbitan laurate; parabens |

Topical antihistamines and local anesthetics (see Chapter 37) carry the risk of sensitization.

### Product Selection Guidelines

Petrolatum and oils are not desirable in prickly heat because they trap moisture beneath them and keep the area hydrated. In prickly heat, the skin needs to dry and dissipate moisture. Only water-washable, cream-based products should be applied to prickly heat to relieve symptoms. For moisture absorption and prevention of wetness, powders are a reasonable choice. However, prolonged use or overuse of powders can lead to clogged pores and actually can precipitate prickly heat. When applied to the chest or neck, cornstarch or talc powder should be placed in the hand and applied manually to the skin with light friction. Practitioners should be very careful not to recommend any product for an infant that has an ingredient (e.g., phenols or boric acid) that could be toxic if absorbed through thin, compromised skin. Bathing children and infants with prickly heat in colloidal oatmeal or lukewarm water may be recommended as a first option.

## Assessment of Prickly Heat: A Case-based Approach

Patient assessment for prickly heat involves identifying the site of lesions and having patients reconstruct their activities and attire over the past 24 hours. If the patient is an infant, the practitioner should ask whether the infant sleeps in a warm or humid environment and whether additional clothing or occlusive coverings are used at night or when the infant is asleep. Case 36-2 provides an example of assessment of patients with prickly heat.

**CASE 36-2**

| Relevant Evaluation Criteria | Scenario/Model Outcome |
|---|---|
| **Information Gathering** | |
| 1. Gather essential information about the patient's symptoms, including: | |
| a. description of symptom(s) (i.e., nature, onset, duration, severity, associated symptoms) | Patient has a fine rash on the upper chest, upper back, and inner surface of his upper arms, which he discovered upon awakening about 2 hours ago. He had itching at the site of the lesions and only one other symptom: sour stomach. Patient suspected insect bites, but the lesions don't have any sign of skin penetration. |
| b. description of any factors that seem to precipitate, exacerbate, and/or relieve the patient's symptom(s) | Patient experienced much reduced itching following a hot shower. However, there was no change in the lesions. The sour stomach resolved after having breakfast. |
| c. description of the patient's efforts to relieve the symptoms | Showering provided some relief from itching, but skin feels uncomfortable. |
| 2. Gather essential patient history information: | |
| a. patient's identity | Dewey Edwards |

## CASE 36-2 (continued)

| Relevant Evaluation Criteria | Scenario/Model Outcome |
|---|---|
| b. age, sex, and height, and weight | 26 y/o M, 5'11", 160 lb |
| c. patient's occupation | Mechanic and student |
| d. patient's dietary habits | Normal healthy diet, occasional junk food |
| e. patient's sleep habits | Stays up late, and sleeps in late as allotted by his schedule |
| f. concurrent medical conditions, prescription and nonprescription medications, and dietary supplements | N/A |
| g. allergies | NKA |
| h. history of other adverse reactions to medications | None |
| i. other (describe)_______ | The patient reports that he country danced for about 4 hours at a party the previous night then went to bed in his clothes around 2 AM: He wore a Western style shirt of luminescent polyester material with faux leather yoke, blue jeans, boots, and a leather rodeo belt. The patient reports that the shirt was still "pretty yucky" when he awoke this morning. He denies having symptoms such as headache, fever, nausea, and vomiting. |
| **Assessment and Triage** | |
| 3. Differentiate the patient's signs/symptoms and correctly identify the patient's primary problem(s) | Prickly heat secondary to heavy sweating and occlusive clothing |
| 4. Identify exclusions for self-treatment (see Figure 36-1). | None |
| 5. Formulate a comprehensive list of therapeutic alternatives for the primary problem to determine if triage to a medical practitioner is required, and share this information with the patient. | Options include:<br>(1) Recommend self-care with OTC products.<br>(2) Recommend self-care with nonpharmocologic methods.<br>(3) Refer Dewey to an appropriate PCP.<br>(4) Recommend self-care until an appropriate PCP can be consulted.<br>(5) Take no action. |
| **Plan** | |
| 6. Select an optimal therapeutic alternative to address the patient's problem, taking into account patient preferences. | A topical emollient may be palliative (physically and psychologically) until the skin heals and may relieve the discomfort. Patient education about the cause of prickly heat is a must to prevent future occurrences. |
| 7. Describe the recommended therapeutic approach to the patient. | Because your itching is mild and was apparently reduced by the shower, you can apply an emollient skin lotion twice a day. Shower tomorrow morning and apply the product again if the lesions are still present. |
| 8. Explain to the patient the rationale for selecting the recommended therapeutic approach from the considered therapeutic alternatives. | Since your symptoms are mild, a skin lotion should help clear up the lesions. To avoid this condition in the future, you should change clothes and shower as soon as possible after sweating heavily. |
| **Patient Education** | |
| 9. When recommending self-care with nonprescription medications and/or nondrug therapy, convey accurate information to the patient, including: | |
| a. appropriate dose and frequency of administration | See the box Patient Education for Prickly Heat. |

**CASE 36-2 (continued)**

| Relevant Evaluation Criteria | Scenario/Model Outcome |
|---|---|
| b. maximum number of days the therapy should be employed | See the box Patient Education for Prickly Heat. |
| c. product administration procedures | See the box Patient Education for Prickly Heat. |
| d. expected time to onset of relief | See the box Patient Education for Prickly Heat. |
| e. degree of relief that can be reasonably expected | See the box Patient Education for Prickly Heat. |
| f. most common side effects | See the box Patient Education for Prickly Heat. |
| g. side effects that warrant medical intervention should they occur | See the box Patient Education for Prickly Heat. |
| h. patient options in the event that condition worsens or persists | See the box Patient Education for Prickly Heat. |
| i. product storage requirements | Keep in a tightly closed container in close proximity to shower or grooming area. |
| j. specific nondrug measures | See the box Patient Education for Prickly Heat. |
| 10. Solicit follow-up questions from patient. | Is this condition contagious? |
| 11. Answer patient's questions. | No. |

Key: N/A, not applicable; NKA, no known allergies; OTC, over-the-counter; PCP, primary care provider.

## Patient Counseling for Prickly Heat

The practitioner should stress to the patient that prickly heat is easily prevented by removing factors that clog skin pores, and explain appropriate nondrug and drug measures for healing prickly heat rash. The practitioner should explain that excessive use of skin protectants can exacerbate the disorder. The box Patient Education for Prickly Heat lists specific information to provide patients.

## Evaluation of Patient Outcomes for Prickly Heat

Treatment of prickly heat should be relatively short, approximately a week; it may take even less time. If the condition is improved but not completely resolved after 7 to 10 days of treatment, therapy can be continued another 3 to 4 days until complete healing has occurred. If the condition has not improved or has worsened by the seventh day, the patient should be referred for further evaluation. If extending treatment after improvement has been seen still does not result in healing, a PCP should be consulted. Monitoring of treatment success involves simple observation of lesions. At the end of therapy, skin should have returned to normal.

## Key Points for Diaper Dermatitis and Prickly Heat

- Diaper rash is caused by moisture and occlusion.
- The frequency of diaper changes (at least 6 per day) is a major factor in the prevalence of diaper rash.
- Pharmacologic treatment should be limed to the mildest most bland products with the fewest ingredients and avoiding exotic additives.
- Products containing petrolatum and zinc oxide are the favored semi-solid dosage forms; talc, cornstarch and zinc oxide are the favored powders.
- Do not use hydrocortisone on diaper rash.
- Caution should be used with powders to prevent infant inhalation of powders.
- The majority of diaper rash will resolve itself when occlusion and wetness are adequately suppressed.
- Help the patient to distinguish between ordinary diaper rash and complicated cases that warrant referral to a PCP.
- Cases that do not resolve in 10 days should be referred for further evaluation.
- Prickly heat is caused by occluded sweat glands.
- By removing the occlusion, prickly heat will generally heal itself.
- Pharmacologic treatment is directed to providing relief from itching or burning.
- Products containing emollients and/or anti-itch ingredients in water-washable dosage forms are favored; powders may be used to help dry the skin, but must be used judiciously to prevent clogging pores.
- Caution should be used with powders to prevent inhalation of powders by children infants and elderly patients.
- Help the patient to distinguish between ordinary prickly heat and complicated cases that warrant referral to a PCP.

## PATIENT EDUCATION FOR PRICKLY HEAT

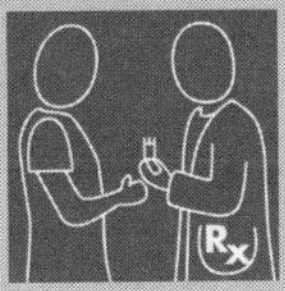


The objectives of self-treatment are to (1) relieve the discomfort of prickly heat and (2) eliminate its cause. For most patients, following product instructions and the self-care measures listed here will help ensure optimal therapeutic outcomes.

### Nondrug Measures

- To prevent clogging skin pores, avoid excessive sweating by resting, cooling off, or going to a cool environment.
- Wear loose, light-colored, porous, and/or lightweight clothing to allow air flow to the skin.
- Decrease the discomfort of prickly heat in infants by changing diapers frequently and by using soaps or possible chemical irritants (e.g., baby wipes) sparingly.
- Shower, bathe, or at least change clothes immediately after heavy sweating and wear loose fitting clothes when such activity is anticipated. Remember to drink plenty of fluids and allow the body to cool down after any strenuous activity.

### Nonprescription Medications

- Unless a primary care provider advises otherwise, use internal analgesics (e.g., aspirin, acetaminophen, ibuprofen, ketoprofen, or naproxen) to reduce a fever and the sweating it can cause.
- Do not apply oleaginous or oily substances to prickly heat lesions because they clog skin pores.
- Use powdered skin protectants to absorb moisture and help prevent wetness (see Table 36-3). Place cornstarch or talc powder in the hand, and apply to the skin with light friction. Note that prolonged use or overuse of powders can lead to clogged pores and can precipitate prickly heat.
- Do not use hydrocortisone on infants. However, it may be used to relieve itching in adult cases of prickly heat if no more than 10% of the body surface area is involved.
- Water washable emollients applied in a thin film twice a day can help the skin return to normal.
- If redness, burning, itching, peeling, or swelling develop after a product is applied, rinse any remaining product off the skin and avoid further use.
- For older children and adults, consider using oral antihistamines for relief of itching. Note that topical antihistamines can cause allergic reactions (see Chapter 11).
- To soothe discomfort in adults or infants, wash the affected skin with bland soap or soak the skin in a colloidal oatmeal solution.
- The condition should show observable improvement in 24 hours.
- The skin should return to normal without scarring.
- If the condition has not improved or has worsened after 7 days of treatment, consult a primary care provider.

## References


1. Visscher MO, Chatterjee R, Munson KA, et al. Development of diaper rash in the newborn. *Pediatr Dermatol.* 2000;17:52-7.
2. Spraker M, Krafchik B, Leyden J, et al. Clinical impact of disposable diapers. *Supplement to Contemporary Pediatrics.* Montvale, NJ: Medical Economics Company; 2001:1-18. Available at: http://cp.pdr.net/cp/docs/papc_diapers_site/clinical.htm#. Accessed August 23, 2001.
3. Odio M, Streicher-Scott J, Hansen RC. Disposable baby wipes: efficacy and skin mildness. *Dermatol Nurs.* 2001; 13:107-13.
4. Odio M, Friedlander SF. Diaper dermatitis and advances in diaper technology. *Curr Opin Pediatr.* 2000;12:342-6.
5. Lazarova V, Savoye P, Janex ML, et al. Advanced wastewater disinfection technologies: state of the art and perspectives. *Water Sci Tech.* 1999;40:203-13.
6. Wojtenko I, Stinson MK, Field R. Challenges of combined sewer overflow disinfection by ultraviolet light irradiation. *Crit Rev Environ Sci Tech.* 2001;31:223-39.
7. *Federal Register.* 1990;55:25204-46.
8. Ruchir A, Sammeta V, Thomas I, et al. Diaper dermatitis. Available at: http://www.emedicine.com/ped/topic2755.htm. Accessed Auguest 19, 2005.
9. Mancini, AJ. Skin. *Pediatrics.* 2004;113:1114-9.

CHAPTER 37

# Insect Bites and Stings and Pediculosis

*Wayne Buff and Cliff Fuhrman*

Insect bites and stings are common. The reaction to these injuries is usually confined to the injury site; however, for a group of sensitive individuals, stings from some insects can produce allergic reactions that range from a mild response to life-threatening anaphylaxis. Thousands of people are hospitalized annually because of allergic reactions precipitated by insect stings. Initiation of adequate precautions and treatment could prevent many deaths resulting from anaphylaxis.

Most encounters with biting and stinging insects are brief. Pediculosis (lice infestation) and scabies, however, are parasitic infections; these arachnids remain on the host until eradicated. Pediculosis occurs frequently among children.

Although the public usually refers to all biting and stinging invertebrate animals as "insects," such animals are members of the phylum Arthropoda, which includes insects, arachnids, and crustaceans. This chapter covers the stings of insects only, but discusses the bites of both insects and arachnids (e.g., ticks, mites, spiders, lice). The term *insect* is used to cover general statements about these invertebrates.

## INSECT BITES

### Epidemiology of Insect Bites

Individuals who enjoy outdoor activities or spend time in their yard, as well as those whose occupation requires them to remain outdoors, are at risk for insect bites and stings. Almost all victims of insect bites experience local reactions at the injury site. The exact number of people who experience systemic allergic reactions to salivary secretions of biting insects is unknown.

### Etiology of Insect Bites

Bites from insects, such as mosquitoes, fleas, and bedbugs, and from arachnids, such as ticks and chiggers, are nonvenomous. These insects usually attack by insert their biting organs into the skin to pierce it and then feed by sucking blood from their hosts. An anticoagulant saliva, consisting of antigenic substances, is introduced into the pierced skin to keep the victim's blood flowing.

#### *Mosquitoes*

Mosquitoes are found in abundance worldwide, particularly in humid, warm climates. These insects always live and breed near wet areas because their larvae can live only in water. The adult mosquitoes become most active in the evening. Some transmit diseases such as malaria and West Nile virus.

#### *Fleas*

Fleas are tiny (1.5 to 4 mm long), bloodsucking, wingless, laterally compressed insects with strongly developed posterior legs used for leaping. These insects are found worldwide, including arctic regions, but they breed best in warm areas with relatively high humidity. Fleas act as parasites on birds and mammals. Body warmth and exhaled carbon dioxide are believed to attract fleas to the host. They may survive and multiply without food for several weeks, but females need a blood meal to deposit eggs. Places that have been vacant for weeks may be heavily infested, partly because of hatching of eggs usually deposited in floor crevices or on rugs, particularly those on which pets have been sleeping. Humans are often bitten after moving into a vacant, flea-infested habitat or when living with infested pets. Fleas are not only annoying; they transmit diseases, such as bubonic plague and endemic typhus.

#### *Sarcoptes scabiei*

Scabies, commonly called "the itch," is a contagious parasitic skin infection caused by *Sarcoptes scabiei*, a very small and rarely seen arachnid mite. The mites burrow into the stratum corneum, and the females deposit eggs in their "tunnels." Mites are transmitted from an infected individual to others through physical contact.

#### *Bedbugs*

Bedbugs have a short head and a broad, flat body (4 to 5 mm long and 3 mm wide). Bedbugs usually hide and deposit their eggs in crevices of walls, floors, picture frames, bedding, and furniture, and may survive for up to 6 months in the absence of blood feedings.[1] They normally hide during the day, become active at night, and bite their sleeping victims. People may also be bitten in subdued light while sitting in theaters or other public places. The increased mobility of society worldwide has heightened concern for an increased incidence of bedbug infestations in the United States in places frequented by travelers, such as hotels.[1]

### Ticks

Ticks feed on the blood of humans and both wild and domesticated animals. Certain species of ticks can transmit systemic diseases, such as Rocky Mountain spotted fever and Lyme disease.

### Chiggers

Chiggers, or redbugs, are annoying pests that live in shrubbery, trees, and grass. Only the chigger larvae bite. The larvae insert their mouthpart into the skin and secrete a digestive fluid that causes cellular disintegration of the affected area and intense itching.

### Spiders

An estimated 60 species of spiders that can bite humans exist in the United States; most cause only local reactions.[2] The black widow and brown recluse are two varieties whose bites are serious. The black widow's bite may not be noticed initially, but the victim may develop symptoms from the bite within a short period. Bites from the brown recluse spider also are painless initially, but later may cause local and/or systemic reactions.[2]

## Pathophysiology/Signs and Symptoms of Insect Bites

Each biting arthropod has distinctive biting organs and salivary secretions. These factors produce characteristic signs and symptoms for each type of bite.

### Mosquitoes

When a mosquito lands on the skin, it cuts through the skin with its mandibles and maxillae. The proboscis, a fine, hollow, flexible structure, is introduced into the cut and probes the tissue for a blood vessel. The insect sucks blood directly from a capillary lumen or sucks extravasated blood from previously lacerated capillaries. During feeding, the mosquito injects a salivary secretion containing an anticoagulant and antigenic components that cause the characteristic sign of a welt and itching. The bites usually occur on exposed parts (face, neck, forearms, legs), but mosquitoes can also bite through thin clothing.

West Nile virus is transmitted by mosquitoes, with several types of birds serving as hosts for the virus as it multiplies. The disease was first diagnosed in the United States in 1999 in New York and has been detected in forty-seven states.[3] The most common symptoms are flulike with fever and fatigue; however, symptoms can progress to muscle weakness, encephalitis, or meningitis. Patients 50 years of age or older are at greatest risk for more serious illness:[4] Statistics from CDC for 2004 reflect a 3.6% death rate in reported human cases.[3] Health officials continue to monitor for trends toward increased incidence of West Nile virus in the United States. Research is underway to develop a vaccine; [5] however, currently available treatments are supportive only, with primary emphasis on control of mosquito populations to prevent spread of the disease.[6,7]

### Fleas

Flea bites are usually multiple and grouped, and, in humans, occur primarily on legs and ankles. Each lesion is characterized by an erythematous region around the puncture and causes intense itching.

### *Sarcoptes scabiei*

The impregnated female *S. scabiei* is responsible for scabies. She uses her jaws and first two pairs of legs to burrow into the stratum corneum, forming tunnels up to 1 cm long in which she lays eggs and excretes fecal matter. In a few days, the hatched larvae form their own burrows and develop into adults. The adult mites copulate, and the impregnated females burrow into the stratum corneum to start a new life cycle. Common infestation sites are interdigital spaces of fingers, flexor surface of the wrists, external male genitalia, buttocks, and anterior axillary fold (see Color Plates, photograph 21). Scabies infection is characterized by inflammation and intense itching secondary to an immunologic response.

### Bedbugs

A bedbug uses its mouth parts consisting of two pairs of stylets to pierce skin. The outer part has barbs that saw the skin; the inner part is used to suck blood and allow salivary secretions to flow into the wound. A bedbug can engorge itself with blood within 3 to 5 minutes and then typically seeks its hiding place. The reaction may range from irritation at the site of the bite to a small dermal hemorrhage, depending on the sensitivity of the bitten individual. Hepatitis B possibly is transferred through bedbug bites, but potential for this type of transmission has not been determined yet.[8]

### Ticks

During feeding, the tick's mouth parts are introduced into the skin, enabling it to hold firmly. If the tick is removed, the mouth parts are torn from the tick and remain embedded, causing intense itching and nodules, which may require surgical excision (see Color Plates, photograph 22). If the tick is left attached, it becomes fully engorged with blood and remains for as long as 10 days before dropping off. Ticks should be removed intact from the skin by using fine tweezers. If fingers are used, they should be protected by using gloves and washed afterward. The tick should be grasped as close to the head as possible, roughly parallel to the skin, and then pulled gently to facilitate its complete release from skin. Complete removal, including the head, is the goal. It is generally recommended that mineral oil, petrolatum, or other irritants not be applied to the tick in an effort to aid removal.[2] These treatments may induce salivation by the tick and possibly contribute to infection in the bite area.[9] The local reaction to tick bites consists of itching papules that disappear within 1 week.

Lyme disease, first identified in 1977, is an inflammatory systemic infection affecting the joints, heart, and nervous system. It is caused by a spirochete found in deer ticks that is transmitted into the victim after tick bites.[10] The deer tick is about one-eighth inch in diameter and thus is difficult to find as a parasite on animals. As the tick inserts its mouthpiece into its prey to suck blood, the spirochetes are released at the bite site and spread throughout the body by the circulatory system. Most acute stages of Lyme disease are heralded by skin rash and flulike symptoms. The rash appears first as a papule at the bite site and may become an enlarged circle with a clear center referred to as a "bull's-eye." The infection then spreads gradually to various parts of the body. Lesions, usually tender and urticarial in nature, appear 3 to 30 days after the bite and disappear spontaneously within 3 to 4 weeks. When antibiotic treatment is initiated, remission occurs within several days. The flulike symptoms include fever and muscle and joint pain. If left untreated, neurologic symptoms ranging from headache and stiff neck to partial paralysis or aseptic meningitis may occur. Cardiac disturbances and musculoskeletal symptoms may develop and last up to several months. Finally, the patient may experience arthritis and a red discoloration of the skin on hands, wrists, feet, or ankles.[2] Early diagnosis and prompt treatment of Lyme disease can prevent development of serious neurologic, cardiac, and rheumatologic manifestations.

### *Chiggers*

The nearly microscopic chigger larvae attack the host by attaching to skin and sucking blood. Upon attachment, larvae insert their mouth parts into skin and secrete a digestive fluid that causes cellular disintegration of the affected area, a red papule, and intense itching. Chiggers do not burrow in the skin; however, the injected fluid causes the skin to harden and a tiny tube is formed. The chigger lies in this tube and continues to feed until engorged, after which it drops off and changes into an adult.

### *Spiders*

Even though spider bites are seldom fatal, infants, older persons, and individuals with allergies are at risk. Reaction to black widow bites includes delayed intense pain, stiffness and joint pain, abdominal disturbances, fever, chills, and dyspnea. In addition to these symptoms, brown recluse spiders may cause a spreading, ulcerated wound at the bite site. If a spider bite is suspected but cannot be identified clearly, the wound area should be monitored for these symptoms.[2]

## Complications of Insect Bites

Secondary bacterial infection of insect bites can occur if, during scratching, skin of the affected area is abraded. Skin infections such as impetigo may be a complication of insect bites; these infections may appear as yellow crusting, purulent drainage, and/or significant redness and swelling of the skin around the bite.

## Treatment of Insect Bites

Specific nonprescription external analgesics are labeled for use in treating minor insect bites. These agents are not, however, effective for treating scabies.

### *Treatment Goals*

The goals of self-treating insect bites are to relieve symptoms and prevent secondary bacterial infections.

### *General Treatment Approach*

Application of an ice pack may provide sufficient relief of pain and irritation of bites from mosquitoes, chiggers, bedbugs, or fleas. If this does not work, applying an external analgesic to the site should relieve symptoms. Patients should be advised to avoid scratching the bite. For children, trimming their fingernails may prevent further injury from scratching. Prevention of future insect bites is also important.

Self-treatment of insect bites with a nonprescription product is appropriate if the reaction is confined to the site and the patient is older than 2 years; parents should seek a primary care provider's advice for treatment of children younger than 2 years. No effective nonprescription product is available to treat scabies. Because of possible systemic effects, a primary care provider should evaluate and treat bites from ticks and spiders. There are no nonprescription drug treatments for Lyme disease; the disease is treated with prescription antibiotics such as tetracycline, doxycycline, amoxicillin, and cephalosporins.[2] If a black widow or brown recluse spider bite is suspected, immediate medical attention should be sought. Figure 37-1 outlines treatment of insect bites and lists exclusions for self-treatment.

### *Nonpharmacologic Therapy*

Nondrug measures include the two methods of preventing insect bites: avoiding insects and using repellents. Other measures are discussed in the box Patient Education for Insect Bites.

#### Avoidance of Insects

Measures to avoid insect bites include covering skin as much as possible with clothing, hats, and shoes; cuffing clothing around ankles, wrists, and neck; avoiding swamps, dense woods, and brush that harbors ticks, mosquitoes, and chiggers; keeping pets free of pests; and removing standing water, when possible, to reduce breeding areas for mosquitoes. It should be noted that scabies is transmitted by close, prolonged personal contact with an infected individual.[2]

#### Use of Insect Repellents

Insect repellents are useful in preventing bites from insects such as mosquitoes, fleas, and ticks, but these products are not effective in repelling stinging insects, such as wasps, hornets, bees, or yellow jackets. An insect repellent should have an inoffensive odor, protect for several hours, be

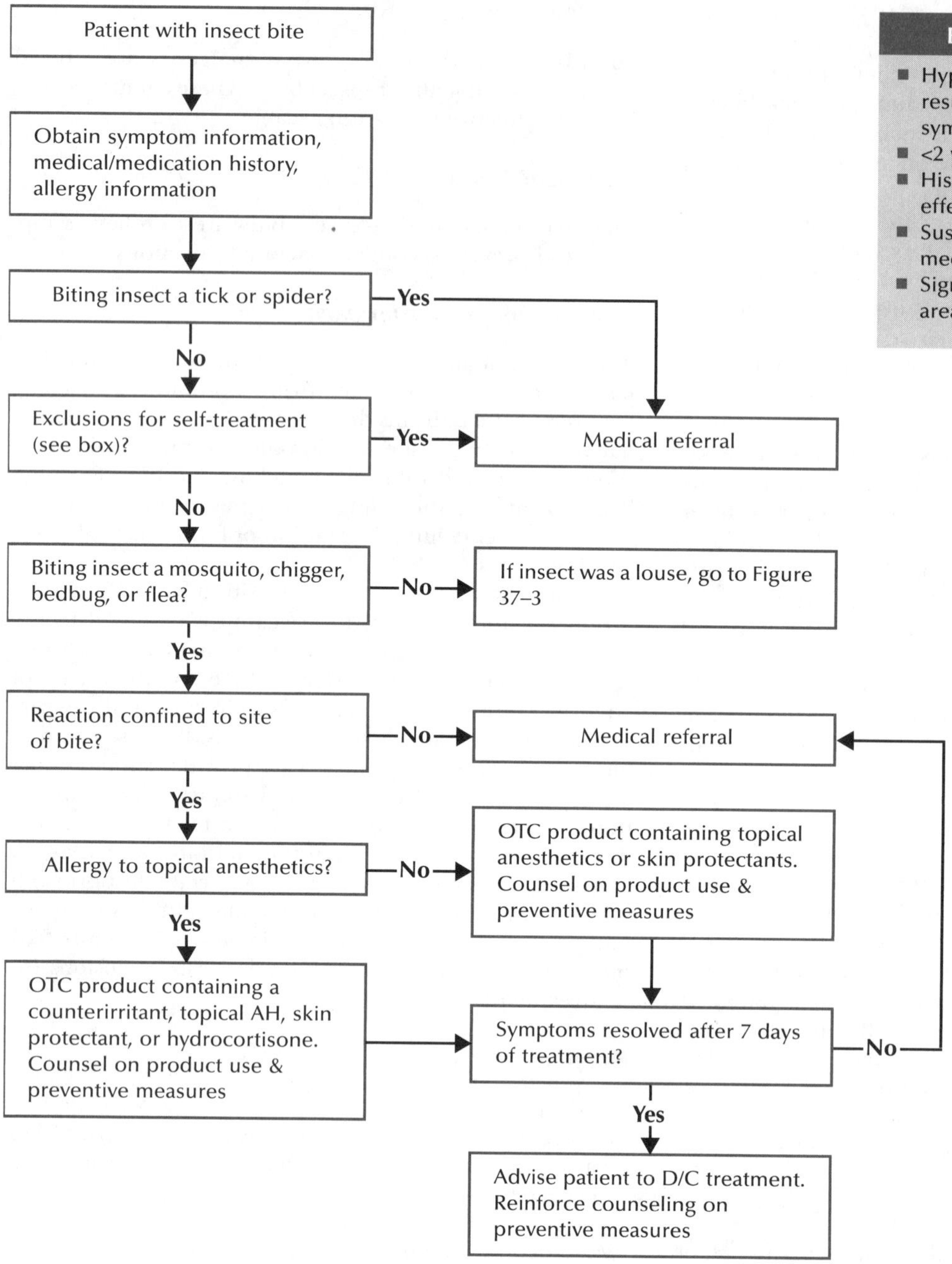


**Exclusions for Self-Treatment**

- Hypersensitivity to insect bites, resulting in systemic symptoms or symptoms away from bite area
- <2 years of age
- History of tick bite and systemic effects indicating possible infection
- Suspected spider bite requiring medical attention
- Signs of secondary infection of bite area

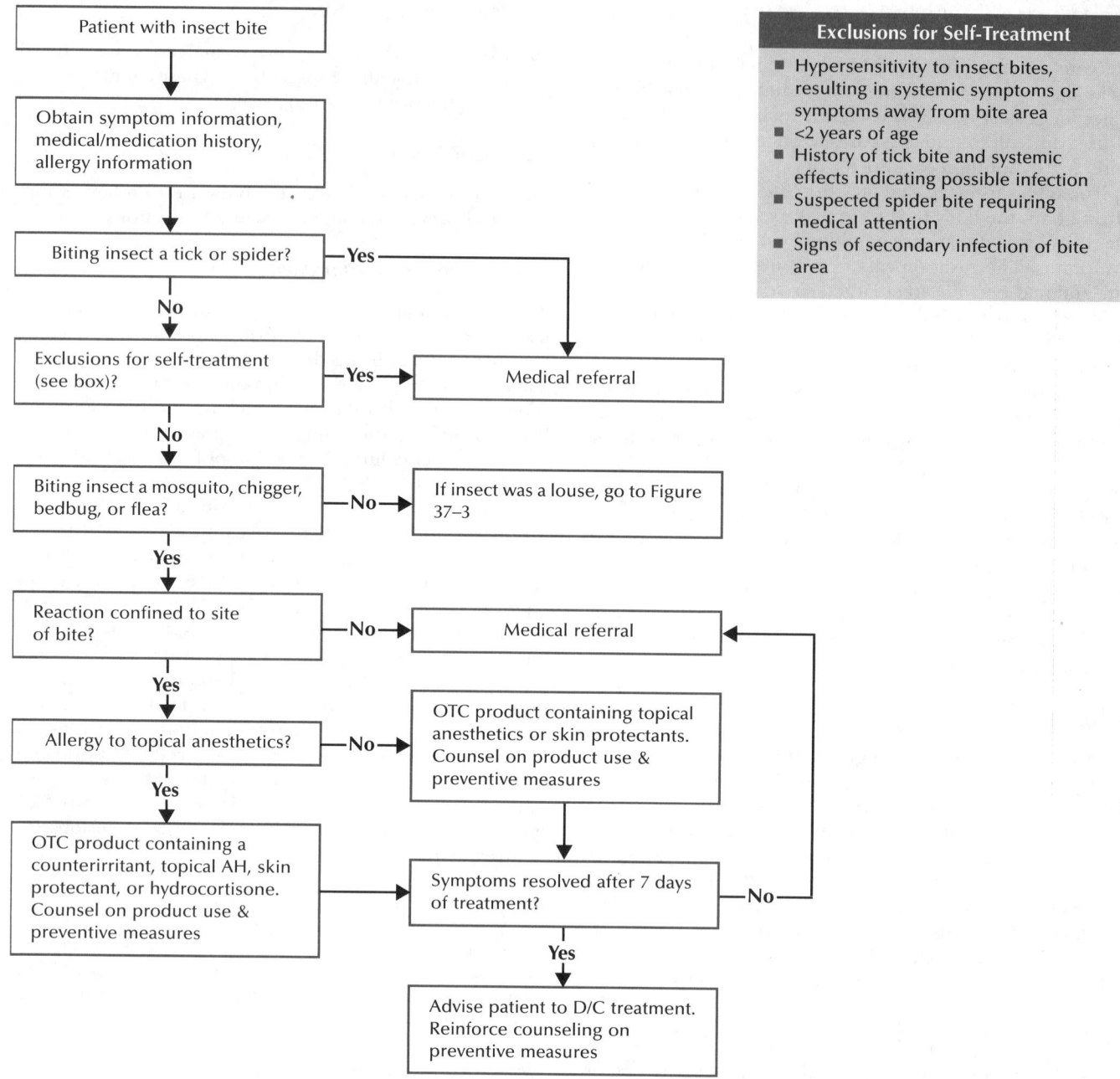

**FIGURE 37-1** Self-care of insect bites. Key: AH, antihistamine; D/C, discontinue; OTC, over-the-counter.

effective against as many insects as possible, be relatively safe, withstand all weather conditions, and have an esthetic feel and appearance. Most commercial products contain n,n-diethyl-m-toluamide, commonly called DEET, in concentrations ranging from 7% to 40%, which are effective concentrations for routine insect exposure situations. Products containing up to 100% DEET are also available. Other ingredients that may be combined with DEET include ethylbutylacetylaminopropionate and dimethylpthalate (Table 37-1).

*n,n-Diethyl-m-toluamide* The best all-purpose repellent is n,n-diethyl-m-toluamide, or DEET.

Mechanism of Action/Indication Repellents protect the skin against insect bites. The exact mechanism of action is not known fully, but DEET, like other repellents, does not kill insects. The volatile repellent, when applied to skin or clothing, releases vapors that tend to discourage the approach of insects and prevents them from alighting.

Dosage and Administration Guidelines Repellents, available in sprays, solutions, creams, wipes, and other forms, are applied to skin or clothing according to package directions as needed, which usually is no more frequent than every 4 to 8 hours. Concentrations below 30% are preferable for children, but use of DEET insect repellents

**TABLE 37-1 Selected Insect Repellents**

| Trade Name | Primary Ingredients |
|---|---|
| Cutter Skinsations Pump | DEET 7%; aloe vera; vitamin E |
| Cutter Advanced Pump | Picaridin 7% |
| Deep Woods Off! For Sportsmen Insect Repellent I Pump Spray | DEET 100% |
| Off Insect Repellent II Aerosol | DEET 15% |
| Off Skintastic Family Formula Pump or Aerosol | DEET 7% |
| Off Botanicals Insect Repellent Lotion | Eucalyptus oil |
| Repel Lemon Eucalyptus Lotion | Lemon eucalyptus oil |
| Repel Sportsman Formula Aerosol | DEET 29% |
| Repel Sun and Bug Lotion | DEET 20%; ethyl hexyl-p-methoxy-cinnamate 7.5%; oxybenzone 5% |

Key: DEET, n,n-diethyl-m-toluamide.

**TABLE 37-2 EPA Guidelines for Safe Use of DEET[14]**

- Follow label directions; avoid overuse of product.
- Do not apply to broken or irritated skin.
- Avoid application to hands or near mouth, eyes of young children.
- Adults should apply the product to children; children should not apply it.
- Use only sufficient amount to cover exposed skin and/or clothing.
- Spray on hands and then apply to areas around face.
- Wash skin thoroughly when back indoors.
- Product can be applied to clothing, but should not be applied under clothing.
- Any clothing that was sprayed should be washed before wearing again.
- Watch for possible skin irritation from the product.
- Apply only in open areas with good ventilation.
- Use caution during application; product may damage some synthetic fabrics, painted surfaces, leather, and plastics.

on children younger than 2 months should be discouraged;[11] appropriate clothing may offer some protection against insect bites in these younger children. Products with DEET concentrations ranging from 10% to 40% provide adequate effect and sufficient protection for adults in routine situations. Products containing 50% to 100% DEET generally are promoted for adults with high exposure to insects for long periods and when high heat and humidity may decrease adherence of the product; higher concentrations of DEET may be associated with higher incidence of skin reactions.[12] A unique polymer formulation of 25% or 33% DEET is also available; it is promoted as an extended duration product offering 8 to 12 hours of protection.[13] Table 37-2 provides a summary from the Environmental Protection Agency regarding the application and safe use of DEET products.[14]

Safety Considerations Skin irritation is the most frequent DEET-related problem, with occlusion of application area possibly contributing to skin rashes or eruptions.[13,14] Central nervous system reactions, including seizures, ataxia, hypotension, and angioedema, have been reported, primarily associated with improper use or ingestion.[13,15] These products are considered safe if used appropriately, even in women who are pregnant or breast feeding.[13,15] Table 37-2 lists warnings and precautions for use of DEET.

*Other Insect Repellents* Alternative products include citronella, lemon eucalyptus oil, soybean oil, cedar oil, lavender oil, tea tree oil, garlic, thiamin, and fragranced moisturizers in mineral oil, such as Skin So Soft. They generally have been found to be less effective than DEET as repellents against mosquitoes, particularly with regard to length of action; soybean oil products have shown promise as potential repellents, providing 90 minutes of protection against mosquito bites in one test.[12] A new insect repellent, picaridin, has been marketed as an alternative to DEET; it is being promoted as having less odor and being less irritating to skin.[13]

## *Pharmacologic Therapy*

External analgesics such as local anesthetics, topical antihistamines, hydrocortisone, and some counterirritants are approved for treating pain and itching from insect bites. These agents are not approved for use in children younger than 2 years; a physician should be consulted about treatment of these children.

Topical skin protectant agents may be used to reduce inflammation and promote healing. First-aid antiseptics and antibiotics can help prevent secondary infections (see Chapter 42).

Systemic antihistamines often are used in treating itching related to insect bites, but this is not a label indication. Chapter 11 discusses systemic antihistamines in detail.

### Local Anesthetics

Local anesthetics such as benzocaine, pramoxine, benzyl alcohol, lidocaine, dibucaine, and phenol are used in topical preparations for relief of itching and irritation caused by insect bites.

*Mechanism of Action* Local anesthetics cause a reversible blockade of conduction of nerve impulses at the site of application, thereby producing loss of sensation. Phenol exerts topical anesthetic action by depressing cutaneous sensory receptors.

*Indications* Local anesthetics are approved for use on burns, sunburns, minor cuts, insect bites, and minor skin irritation to relieve pain and itching.[16]

*Dosage and Administration Guidelines* Topical preparations containing local anesthetics are applied in the form of creams, ointments, aerosols, or lotions. These products are generally applied to the bite area up to three to four times daily for no longer than 7 days.

*Safety Considerations* Even though local anesthetics, including benzocaine, are relatively nontoxic when applied topically, allergic contact dermatitis may occur. Pramoxine and benzyl alcohol do not commonly cause adverse effects and exhibit less cross-sensitivity than other local anesthetics. Dibucaine, a common allergen, may cause systemic toxicity if there is excessive absorption. Phenol solutions of greater than 2% are irritating and may cause sloughing and necrosis of skin, but the concentration of phenol in nonprescription products ranges from 0.5% to 1.5%.

Local anesthetics should not be used longer than 7 days. Some individual agents have specific precautions or warnings.

Preparations containing benzocaine should not be applied to skin of individuals with confirmed or suspected hypersensitivity (typically allergic contact dermatitis) to benzocaine or other ester-type local anesthetics.

Although in the same class as benzocaine, dibucaine products carry additional labeling warning against use of large quantities, especially over raw surfaces or blistered areas.[17] Convulsions, myocardial depression, and death have been reported from systemic absorption.

Nonprescription products containing phenol should not be applied to extensive areas of the body, especially under compresses or bandages, because of risk of skin damage and systemic absorption;[17] systemic toxicities of phenol include convulsions and cardiac failure. Products containing phenol should be avoided in pregnant patients and children.

### Topical Antihistamines

Diphenhydramine hydrochloride in concentrations of 0.5% to 2% is the agent used in most products that contain a topical antihistamine.

*Mechanism of Action* Topical antihistamines exert an anesthetic effect by depressing cutaneous receptors, thereby relieving pain and itching.

*Indications* Topical antihistamines are approved for temporary relief of pain and itching related to minor burns; sunburns; insect bites; poison oak, ivy, and sumac; and minor skin irritation.[18]

*Dosage and Administration Guidelines* Products are available in several topical dosage forms; they are generally applied to the bite area up to three to four times daily for no longer than 7 days.

*Safety Considerations* Although absorption occurs through skin, topical antihistamines generally are not absorbed in sufficient quantities to cause systemic side effects, even when applied to damaged skin. Systemic absorption is of more concern when these products are used over large body areas, especially in young children. Topical antihistamines are capable of producing hypersensitivity reactions, specifically allergic and photoallergic contact dermatitis; continued use of these agents for 3 to 4 weeks increases the possibility of contact dermatitis

Topical antihistamines should not be used longer than 7 days, except as advised by a primary care provider.

### Counterirritants

Low concentrations of the counterirritants camphor and menthol are used in some external analgesic products. Chapter 7 discusses these agents in more detail. These products generally are applied to the bite area three or four times daily for up to 7 days.

*Camphor* At concentrations of 0.1% to 3%, camphor depresses cutaneous receptors, thereby relieving itching and irritation by exerting an anesthetic effect. However, camphor-containing products can be very dangerous if ingested. Patients should be warned to keep these products out of children's reach.

*Menthol* In concentrations of less than 1%, menthol depresses cutaneous receptors and exerts an analgesic effect. Menthol is considered a safe and effective antipruritic when applied to affected area in concentrations of 0.1% to 1%.

### Hydrocortisone

The Food and Drug Administration (FDA) has approved topical preparations containing hydrocortisone in concentrations up to 1% for nonprescription use.

*Mechanism of Action* Topically applied, hydrocortisone is an antipruritic and anti-inflammatory agent capable of preventing or suppressing development of edema, capillary dilation, swelling, and tenderness that accompanies inflammation. Reduction in inflammation results in relief of pain and itching.

*Pharmacokinetics* Topical absorption of hydrocortisone is increased after prolonged use of occlusive dressings. After application, a minimal amount of hydrocortisone may enter circulation; however, this penetration increases if skin is broken or inflamed.

*Indications* Hydrocortisone topical preparations are indicated for temporary relief of minor skin irritations, itching, and rashes caused by dermatitis, insect bites, poison ivy/oak/sumac, soaps, cosmetics, and jewelry.

*Dosage and Administration Guidelines* A wide variety of topical hydrocortisone dosage forms are available and should be applied as directed to bite area three or four times daily for up to 7 days.

*Safety Considerations* Prolonged administration of hydrocortisone may cause epidermal atrophy, acneiform eruptions, irritation, folliculitis, and tightening and cracking of the skin.

Patients who suffer from scabies, fungal or bacterial infections, or candidiasis should be warned against using topical hydrocortisone. Not only may the underlying conditions be worsened, but hydrocortisone may also mask these disorders, thereby making accurate diagnosis difficult.

### Skin Protectants

Medications such as zinc oxide, calamine, and titanium dioxide are applied to insect bites mainly in the form of lotions, ointments, and creams. These agents act as protectants and tend to reduce inflammation and irritation. Zinc oxide and calamine also absorb fluids from weeping lesions.

FDA considers preparations with zinc oxide and calamine to be safe and effective in concentrations from 1% to 25% as nonprescription drugs. Titanium dioxide's mechanism of action is similar to that of zinc oxide, but FDA has not determined safety and effectiveness of this ingredient. These preparations should be applied to affected area as needed. They have minimal adverse effects and are recommended for adults, children, and infants.

### Product Selection Guidelines

Sensitization, specifically contact dermatitis, can occur with local anesthetics. If these agents are preferred, pramoxine and benzyl alcohol have a low incidence of adverse effects. Dibucaine and phenol have the most potential for adverse effects, especially if systemic absorption occurs from improper application.

Adverse effects and systemic absorption generally are not a concern with short-term use of the topical antihistamine diphenhydramine hydrochloride. However, its prolonged use can cause allergic or photoallergic contact dermatitis. Similarly, short-term use of hydrocortisone usually does not cause adverse effects or clinically significant systemic absorption, but patients with scabies, bacterial infections, or fungal infections should not use this agent without medical supervision. Hydrocortisone can worsen or mask these disorders, making accurate diagnosis difficult. Camphor-containing products can be very dangerous if ingested, making them an inappropriate choice for use in children.

Topical diphenhydramine's side effect profile makes it a suitable topical antipruritic to recommend. However, patients must understand that topical antipruritics and anesthetics should not be used longer than 7 days.

The patient's preference of dosage forms should also guide product recommendations. Creams, lotions, and sprays are the most commonly used dosage forms. Table 37-3 lists selected trade-name products.

## Assessment of Insect Bites: A Case-based Approach

The practitioner should first determine what type of insect inflicted the patient's injury. A primary care provider or dermatologist should evaluate bites from ticks and spiders because of the serious diseases or adverse effects associated with these bites. For other insect bites, the practitioner should evaluate the seriousness of the reaction before recommending a nonprescription product or nondrug measure. If a nonallergic reaction is present, the appropriate external analgesic for symptomatic relief should be recommended. The practitioner should explain proper use of the selected product as well as its possible adverse effects. If the patient is a child, recommendation of a skin protectant to prevent secondary bacterial infection is appropriate.

## Patient Counseling for Insect Bites

Counseling for insect bites includes an explanation of how to treat the injury as well as how to prevent recurrences. The practitioner should explain nondrug measures and/or proper use of recommended nonprescription products. The explanation should include potential adverse effects of these agents plus signs and symptoms that indicate the injury needs medical attention. Appropriate use of insect repellents to prevent further bites should also be discussed. The box Patient Education for Insect Bites lists specific information to provide patients.

## Evaluation of Patient Outcomes for Insect Bites

Follow-up should occur after 7 days of self-treatment. The patient should be advised to seek medical attention if symptoms such as redness, itching, and localized swelling worsen during treatment or if patient develops secondary infection, fever, joint pain, or lymph node enlargement. Medical attention is also necessary if symptoms persist after 7 days of treatment.

# INSECT STINGS

## Epidemiology of Insect Stings

As with insect bites, persons who work or spend time outdoors are at risk for insect stings. An estimated 0.5% of the population may show signs of significant systemic allergic reactions to insect stings, while 99% will have only local reactions. About 40 deaths caused by anaphylaxis as a result of insect stings are reported annually in the United States.[2,19]

## Etiology of Insect Stings

Venomous insects such as bees, wasps, hornets, yellow jackets, and fire ants belong to the order Hymenoptera. They attack their victims to defend themselves or to kill other insects. The injected venom contains allergenic proteins and pharmacologically active molecules. Since venom contents vary within the Hymenoptera order, venom is discussed in general terms.

### *Wild Honeybees, Wasps, Hornets, Yellow Jackets, and Africanized Bees*

Wild honeybees are most commonly found in the western and midwestern United States, and they usually nest in hollow tree trunks. Paper wasps, hornets, and yellow jackets

**TABLE 37-3 Selected External Analgesic Products for Insect Bites and Stings**

| Trade Name | Primary Ingredients |
|---|---|
| **Local Anesthetics** | |
| Americaine Anesthetic Spray | Benzocaine 20% |
| Foille Plus Aerosol | Benzocaine 5%; chloroxylenol 0.1% |
| Itch-X Gel/Pump Spray | Pramoxine HCl 1%; benzyl alcohol 10% |
| Lanacane Aerosol Spray | Benzocaine 20% |
| Nupercainal Ointment | Dibucaine 1% |
| Solarcaine Medicated First Aid Aerosol Spray | Benzocaine 20%; triclosan 0.13% |
| Unguentine Maximum Strength Cream | Benzocaine 5%; resorcinol 2% |
| **Topical Antihistamines** | |
| Di-Delamine Gel/Spray | Diphenhydramine HCl 1%; tripelennamine 0.5%, benzalkonium chloride 0.15%; menthol |
| Dermarest Gel | Diphenhydramine HCl 2%; resorcinol 2%; menthol |
| Maximum Strength Benadryl Cream/Spray | Diphenhydramine HCl 2% |
| **Counterirritants** | |
| Sarna Lotion | Camphor 0.5%; menthol 0.5% |
| **Corticosteroids** | |
| Cortaid with Aloe Cream/Ointment | Hydrocortisone 0.5%; aloe vera |
| Maximum Strength Cortaid Cream/Ointment | Hydrocortisone 1% |
| Cortizone-5 Cream | Hydrocortisone 0.5% |
| Cortizone-10 Ointment | Hydrocortisone 1% |
| Lanacort 10 Crème | Hydrocortisone 1% |
| **Combination Products** | |
| Aveeno Anti-Itch Cream/Lotion | Pramoxine HCl 1%; calamine 3%; camphor 0.3% |
| Benadryl Itch Stopping Maximum Strength Gel | Diphenhydramine HCl 2%; zinc acetate 1%; camphor |
| Caladryl Clear Lotion | Diphenhydramine HCl 1%; zinc oxide 2%; camphor |
| Campho-Phenique Gel | Camphor 11%; phenol 5%; eucalyptus oil |
| Medi-Quik Spray | Lidocaine 2%; benzalkonium chloride 0.2%; camphor |
| Sting-Eze Drops | Diphenhydramine HCl; camphor; phenol; benzocaine; eucalyptol |
| Sting-Kill Swabs | Benzocaine 19%; menthol 0.9% |

are found more commonly in the southern, central, and southwestern United States. Paper wasps tend to nest in high places, under eaves of houses, or on branches of high trees, whereas hornets prefer to nest in hollow spaces, especially hollow trees. Yellow jackets, considered the most common stinging culprits, usually nest in low places, such as burrows in the ground, cracks in sidewalks, or small shrubs. A species of "killer bees" or Africanized bees may be found in certain areas of the southwestern United States. These bees are known for their aggressive, swarming behavior and large number of stings.[20] Their venom is similar in potency to that of honeybees, but the large number of stings per individual causes an increased risk of severe allergic reaction. Deaths have been reported as the result of venom toxicity from massive numbers of stings.

### *Fire Ants*

Fire ants, imported from South America early in the 20th century, are now found in the southern and western United States, live in underground colonies, and form large raised mounds. Fire ants are considered a health hazard because of the severity of reactions to their bite.

## Pathophysiology of Insect Stings

Although small, many insects have venom as potent as that of snakes. However, whereas death from a snake bite is

## PATIENT EDUCATION FOR INSECT BITES

The objectives of self-treatment for insect bites are to (1) relieve swelling, pain, and itching, (2) prevent scratching that may lead to secondary bacterial infection, (3) monitor for infections transmitted by ticks, and (4) prevent future insect bites. For most patients, carefully following product instructions and the self-care measures listed here will help ensure optimal therapeutic outcomes.

### Nondrug Measures

- Apply ice pack promptly to bite area to reduce swelling, itching, and pain.
- Avoid scratching affected area; keep fingernails trimmed.
- Remove ticks with tweezers by grasping the tick's head and gently pulling; the head should be removed; keep the removed tick in a sealed container for future identification in case of systemic symptoms.
- Do not wear rough, irritating clothing over bite area.

### Preventive Measures

- To prevent exposure, cover skin as much as possible with clothing and socks.
- Avoid swamps, dense woods, and dense brush that harbor mosquitoes, ticks, and chiggers.
- Keep pets free of pests.
- Apply insect repellent according to package recommendations to repel biting insects (see Table 37-2); these repellents do not deter stinging insects.
- To prevent transmission of scabies, avoid close, physical contact with infected individuals.

### Nonprescription Medications

#### *External Analgesics*

- Use an external analgesic to relieve pain and itching of insect bites. Choice of medications includes local anesthetics, topical antihistamines, counterirritants, and hydrocortisone.
- These products can be applied to bite area three or four times daily. Do not use on children younger than 2 years. Do not use longer than 7 days.
- Note that local anesthetics can cause sensitization. If these agents are preferred, pramoxine and benzyl alcohol are less likely to cause adverse effects.
- Do not use dibucaine in large quantities, particularly over raw surfaces or blistered areas. Such use could cause myocardial depression, convulsions, or death.
- Do not apply phenol to extensive areas of the body or under compresses/bandages. Such application increases the possibility of skin damage or systemic absorption.
- Do not use topical diphenhydramine longer than the recommended 7 days. Prolonged use can cause hypersensitivity reactions or systemic effects.
- Do not use hydrocortisone on scabies, bacterial infections, or fungal infections without medical recommendation. Hydrocortisone can mask or worsen these disorders.
- Do not allow children to ingest camphor-containing products. Camphor is toxic when ingested.

#### *Skin Protectants*

- If needed to reduce irritation or inflammation, use a skin protectant such as zinc oxide or calamine.
- Apply protectant to affected area as needed up to four times daily.
- Protectants can be applied to skin of children younger than 2 years.
- Some insect bite products contain external analgesics and skin protectants.

⚠ Seek medical attention if the condition worsens during treatment or symptoms persist after 7 days of topical treatment.

usually caused by toxicity and quantity of injected venom, and occurs within 3 hours to several days, death from an insect sting usually is related to allergic hypersensitivity, which could lead to an anaphylactic reaction within 5 to 30 minutes after the sting. Simultaneous, multiple stings of 500 or more may cause death from toxicity. In the United States, more people die of insect stings than of bites from all poisonous animals combined.

Stinging insects inject venom into their victims through a piercing organ (stinger), a modified ovipositor delicately attached to the rear of the female's abdomen; males do not have an ovipositor and are stingless. The stinger consists of two lancets made of highly chitinous material and separated by the poison canal. The venom flows through the canal from the venom sac attached to the stinger's dorsal section. The tip of the stinger, which is directed posteriorly, may or may not be barbed, depending on the type of insect. Most species of bees and wasps have two types of venom glands under the last abdominal segment. The larger gland secretes an acidic toxin directly into the venom sac; the small one at the base of the sac secretes a less potent alkaline toxin. The injected venom is usually a mixture of the two toxins.

The honeybee stings by attaching itself firmly to skin with tiny, sharp claws at the tip of each foot, arching its abdomen, and immediately jabbing the barbed stinger into skin. The barbs firmly embed the stinger; when the honeybee pulls away or is brushed off, the entire stinging apparatus (stinger, appendages, venom sac, and glands) is detached from the bee's abdomen. The disemboweled bee later dies. The abandoned stinger, driven deeper into the skin by rhythmic contractions of the venom sac's smooth muscle wall, continues to inject venom.

The stinging mechanism of wasps, hornets, and yellow jackets resembles that of the honeybee, except their stingers are not barbed. Their stingers can be withdrawn easily after venom is injected, enabling these insects to survive and sting repeatedly.

The major antigenic proteins found in venom are the enzymes hyaluronidase and phospholipase A. Hyaluronidase breaks down hyaluronic acid, which is the binding agent in connective tissue. By altering tissue structure, hyaluronidase acts as a spreading factor, allowing for enhanced penetration of venom substances. Phospholipase A attacks phospholipids in cell membranes. It also contracts smooth muscle, causes hypotension, increases vascular permeability, and destroys mast cells. Other venom components include histamine, meletin, apamin, and mast cell–degranulating peptide, but of these components, only meletin is antigenic, and not all people make antibodies against it. Although these mediators do not contribute directly to insect sting anaphylaxis, they do affect the rate at which venom antigens become available to systemic circulation after a sting. These molecules have direct and indirect effects on mast-cell mediator release, vascular permeability, and smooth muscle contractions.

Some ants only bite, while others bite and sting simultaneously. Stinging ants (fire ants; *Solenopsis invecta*) use their mandibles to cling to their prey's skin; then they bend their abdomen to sting the flesh and empty the contents of the poison vesicle into the wound. Because these ants use their mandibles, it often is believed that the bite causes the reactions. Their alkaloid venom has inflammatory and necrotic characteristics;[2] fire ant stings cause intense itching, burning (hence the name), vesiculations, tissue necrosis, and anaphylactic reactions in hypersensitive persons. It appears that very limited or no cross-sensitivity exists between venom of fire ants and that of bees, wasps, hornets, and yellow jackets.

Intensity of allergic reactions to venomous insect stings varies significantly. The thrust of the stinger into flesh and the subsequent injection of venom cause a sharp pain. The reaction that follows depends on the person's sensitivity to the venom. Sensitivity develops from a previous exposure to the venom. The first sting is considered the sensitizing one. Systemic and local allergic manifestations usually occur in people who have been stung previously.

The venom may trigger a mild reaction or may precipitate anaphylaxis, a rapid allergic reaction that may affect more than one part of the body and, if severe, may result in death. After the initial sting, the antibody immunoglobulin E (IgE) is formed and binds to receptors on mast cells and basophils. Each subsequent sting produces more antibodies and intensifies allergic manifestations. When the allergen (venom) reaches IgE on mast cells, a reaction takes place, causing degranulation of the mast cells and release of chemical mediators such as histamine, prostaglandins, and leukotrienes. These inflammatory mediators are potent vasodilators and bronchoconstrictors. The vasodilation results in a rapid fall in blood pressure, as well as an increase in the permeability of the blood vessels, thus causing seepage of fluid into surrounding tissue and subsequent swelling (angioedema.) Severity of anaphylactic reactions depends largely on the amount of chemical mediators produced. The skin, respiratory, cardiovascular, and gastrointestinal systems most commonly are involved during anaphylaxis.

## Signs and Symptoms of Reactions to Insect Stings

Most people will complain of pain, itching, and irritation at the sting site but have no systemic effects. People who are allergic to insect stings may experience hives, itching, swelling, and burning sensations of the skin. Vasodilation and loss of fluid from blood vessels can cause a fall in blood pressure, and the person may experience light-headedness or even loss of consciousness. Obstruction of the nose and throat may occur, resulting in hoarseness and a choking sensation. Likewise, the bronchial tree may become constricted, causing chest tightness, dyspnea, and wheezing. Nausea, vomiting, abdominal cramps, and diarrhea are common. In women, uterine contractions may occur, resulting in pelvic cramps.

## Treatment of Insect Stings

Although labeling of nonprescription products for insect-related injuries mentions only "insect bites" as an indication, it is generally accepted that FDA had intended the term to also cover insect stings.

### *Treatment Goals*

The goal of self-treating insect stings is to relieve the itching and pain of cutaneous nonallergic reactions. Allergic reactions require evaluation and treatment by a primary care provider.

### *General Treatment Approach*

Removal of the stinger and application of an ice pack in 10-minute intervals[2] are the first steps in treating insect stings. Application of a local anesthetic, skin protectant, antiseptic, or counterirritant to the sting site is appropriate if the reaction is confined to the site and if none of the exclusions for self-treatment listed in Figure 37-2 applies.

Nonprescription systemic antihistamines can also be taken to alleviate itching. Figure 37-2 outlines the treatment of insect stings.

Avoiding future insect stings can prevent an individual from developing allergic reactions to stings. If symptoms of an allergic reaction develop, emergency treatment should be administered, and the patient should seek medical attention. Patients with severe allergic reactions might want to consider prophylactic treatment such as hyposensitization therapy. Such patients should be advised to wear a bracelet or carry a card identifying the nature of the allergy. They should also contact their primary care provider about carrying an injectable form of epinephrine.

### *Nonpharmacologic Therapy*

Prompt application of cold packs to the sting site in 10-minute intervals helps to slow absorption and reduce itching, swelling, and pain. It is important to remove the honeybee's stinger and venom sac, which are usually left in the skin. The patient should remove the stinger before all venom is injected; it takes approximately 2 to 3 minutes to empty all contents from the honeybee's venom sac. Current recommendations suggest immediate removal of

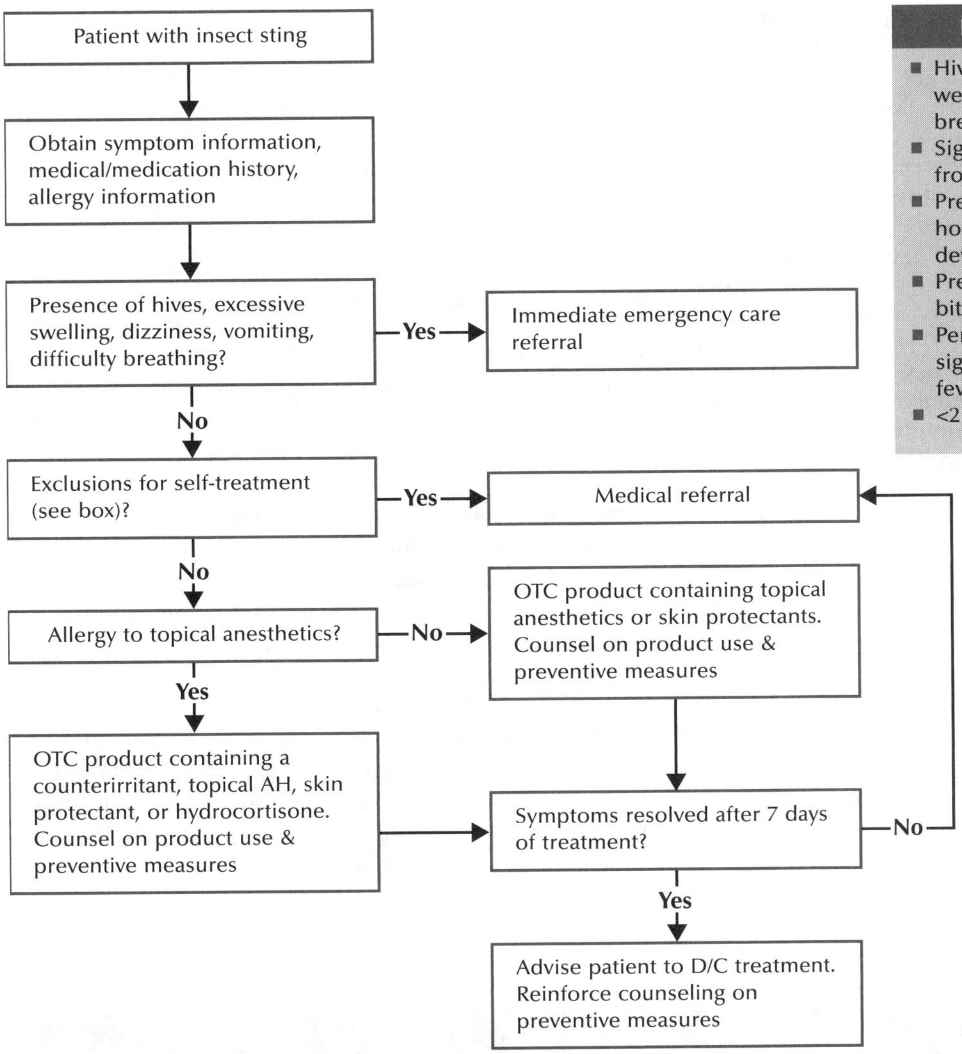


**Exclusions for Self-Treatment**

- Hives, excessive swelling, dizziness, weakness, nausea, vomiting, difficulty breathing
- Significant allergic response away from site of sting
- Previous sting by honeybee, wasp, or hornet (need to evaluate possible development of hypersensitivity)
- Previous severe reaction to insect bites
- Personal or family history of significant allergic reactions (e.g., hay fever)
- <2 years of age

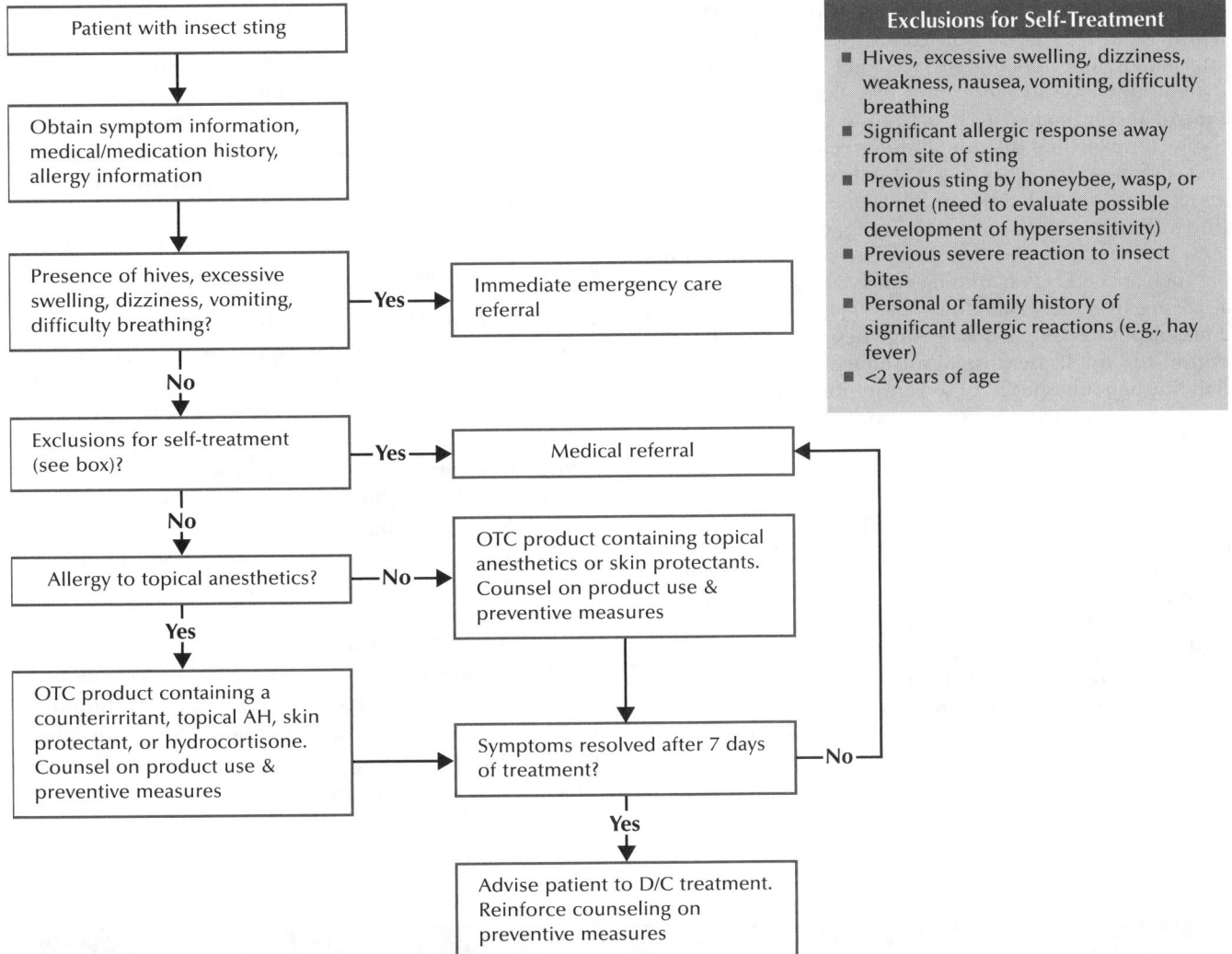

**FIGURE 37-2** Self-care of insect stings. Key: AH, antihistamine; D/C, discontinue; OTC, over-the-counter.

the stinger by any means.[2] Ideally, the patient should not squeeze the sac because rubbing, scratching, or grasping it releases more venom. Scraping away the stinger with a fingernail or edge of a credit card minimizes the venom flow. After the stinger is removed, an antiseptic, such as hydrogen peroxide or alcohol, should be applied.

To avoid attracting stinging insects, the patient should adhere to the following measures: avoid wearing perfume, scented lotions, and brightly colored clothes; control odors in picnic and garbage areas; change children's clothing if it becomes contaminated with summer foods such as fruits; wear shoes when outdoors; and destroy nests of stinging insects near homes.

### Pharmacologic Therapy

Treatment of Insect Bites discusses the following external analgesics approved for treatment of insect bites and, by inference, insect stings: local anesthetics, topical antihistamines, counterirritants, hydrocortisone, and skin protectants.

Product labels for systemic antihistamines do not include treatment of itching associated with insect stings as an indication even though these products are often used in this way.

### Complementary Therapies

Meat tenderizer has been used on insect stings to "break down" proteins in venom. Ammonia and baking soda have been used to "neutralize" venom in insect bites. These products may affect itching, but most reports of success are anecdotal and currently their effectiveness has not been determined.

### Emergency Treatment of Allergic Reactions

Epinephrine is the initial drug of choice for combating anaphylactic reactions precipitated by insect stings. Antihistamines often are used in conjunction with epinephrine hydrochloride and are given either orally or parenterally to relieve itching. Antihistamines alone are insufficient in life-threatening anaphylactic reactions.

Epinephrine is an $\alpha_1$-, and a $\beta_1$-, and $\beta_2$-agonist. Activation of $\alpha_1$-receptors, which constrict blood vessels in internal organs, mucosa surface, and skin, results in a systemic increase in blood pressure. Because β-receptors control the bronchial tree, activation of these receptors results in bronchial dilation, thereby relieving chest tightness, dyspnea, and wheezing. Patients who are allergic to insect stings should carry an injectable form of epinephrine with them to use only when stung; epinephrine is not used as a maintenance therapy. A prescription-only product such as the EpiPen autoinjector is available; it contains a 0.3 mg intramuscular dose of 1:1000 epinephrine in a 2 mL disposable single-dose syringe designed for self-injection in the thigh. Because of infrequent use and product stability, patients should observe the product for discoloration and regularly monitor the expiration date.

### *Prophylactic Treatment of Insect Stings*

Hymenoptera venom is used prophylactically to treat patients who have had reactions to stings. Venom immunotherapy is accomplished by subcutaneous injection of small amounts of venom at regularly scheduled intervals. The dose of the venom is gradually increased over many weeks until a predetermined maintenance dose is reached. The length of treatment is usually 3 to 5 years.[20] Benefits of immunotherapy appear to be greater the younger the age of the patient at the beginning of therapy, and can decrease the risk of reaction for up to 10 to 20 years after treatments are stopped.[19]

## Assessment of Insect Stings: A Case-based Approach

The critical determination in assessing a patient with an insect sting is whether the patient is allergic to the venom. Patients experiencing allergic reactions should be referred immediately for emergency medical attention. Case 37-1 illustrates assessment of a patient who has been stung by an insect.

## Patient Counseling for Insect Stings

The practitioner should advise the patient that local reactions to insect stings usually are transient and are experienced by the vast majority of the population, but that severe reactions to insect stings can occur if sensitization to the insect venom develops with repeated exposure. The symptoms of allergic reactions should be explained. The importance of consulting a primary care provider if such symptoms occur should also be emphasized. Patients who have a known hypersensitivity to insect stings should have epinephrine injection available at all times for emergency self-treatment.

For nonallergic reactions to stings, the practitioner should recommend one or more topical medications to manage immediate symptoms. The patient should be advised about adverse effects and any contraindications. The box Patient Education for Insect Stings lists specific information that should be provided.

**CASE 37-1**

| Relevant Evaluation Criteria | Scenario/Model Outcome |
|---|---|
| **Information Gathering** | |
| 1. Gather essential information about the patient's symptoms, including: | |
| a. description of symptom(s) (i.e., nature, onset, duration, severity, associated symptoms) | Patient presents with difficulty in breathing, nausea, and dizziness after being stung on the foot by a yellow jacket while walking barefoot on his lawn. His difficulty in breathing is becoming worse, and he must sit down to keep from falling. |
| b. description of any factors that seem to precipitate, exacerbate, and/or relieve the patient's symptom(s) | None |
| c. description of the patient's efforts to relieve the symptoms | Patient has applied ice to the affected area and has taken Benadryl 25 mg in an attempt to avoid local inflammation and redness. |
| 2. Gather essential patient history information: | |
| a. patient's identity | Bill Jeffries |
| b. age, sex, height, and weight | 25 y/o M, 5'10", 165 lb |
| c. patient's occupation | Financial advisor |
| d. patient's dietary habits | Normal diet |
| e. patient's sleep habits | 6-8 hours per night |

## CASE 37-1 (continued)

| Relevant Evaluation Criteria | Scenario/Model Outcome |
|---|---|
| f. concurrent medical conditions, prescription and nonprescription medications, and dietary supplements | Claritin (loratadine) 10 mg once daily as needed for seasonal allergies; albuterol spray 2 puffs as needed for wheezing when around cats |
| g. allergies | Cats and seasonal allergies; NKDA |
| h. history of other adverse reactions to medications | None |
| i. other (describe)_______ | None |
| **Assessment and Triage** | |
| 3. Differentiate the patient's signs/symptoms and correctly identify the patient's primary problem(s). | Bill is presenting with an anaphylactic-type reaction secondary to a yellow jacket sting; oral antihistamines are not sufficient. |
| 4. Identify exclusions for self-treatment (see Figure 37-2). | Difficulty breathing, dizziness, nausea, significant allergic response away from site of sting, personal history of allergic reactions |
| 5. Formulate a comprehensive list of therapeutic alternatives for the primary problem to determine if triage to a medical practitioner is required, and share this information with the patient. | Options include:<br>(1) Recommend self-care with nonprescription insect sting products.<br>(2) Refer Bill to a PCP.<br>(3) Recommend self-care until a PCP can be consulted.<br>(4) Take no action. |
| **Plan** | |
| 6. Select an optimal therapeutic alternative to address the patient's problem, taking into account patient preferences. | Any patient presenting with anaphylactic reaction needs to be transported to a nearby emergency room or urgent care facility for treatment, either by an EMT or by someone other than the patient; an EMT would be able to provide immediate support. |
| 7. Describe the recommended therapeutic approach to the patient. | You should go to an emergency facility immediately. |
| 8. Explain to the patient the rationale for selecting the recommended therapeutic approach from the considered therapeutic alternatives. | Anaphylactic reactions are potentially life threatening and are therefore best managed by emergency care providers. |
| **Patient Education** | |
| 9. When recommending self-care with nonprescription medications and/or nondrug therapy, convey accurate information to the patient, including: | Criterion does not apply in this case. |
| 10. Solicit follow-up questions from patient. | Do I need to ask my PCP for a prescription for emergency epinephrine injection (EpiPen) for future use? |
| 11. Answer patient's questions. | Yes, and you should keep an unexpired EpiPen on hand. Counseling on how to use the product will be necessary for both you and other family members in case you are unable to deliver the injection yourself. Identification in the form of wallet ID or bracelet ID is suggested in case an allergic reaction results in a loss of consciousness. Having an oral antihistamine such as diphenhydramine 25 mg available to take in conjunction with the epinephrine is appropriate, but it should not be taken in conjunction with loratadine nor as a replacement for the epinephrine injection. |

Key: EMT, emergency medical technician; ID, identification; NKDA, no known drug allergies; PCP, primary care provider.

## PATIENT EDUCATION FOR INSECT STINGS

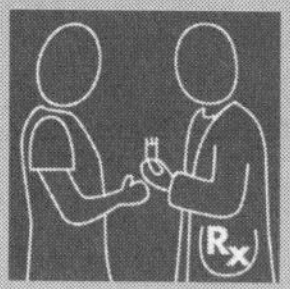

The objectives of self-treatment for insect stings are to (1) relieve swelling, pain, and itching of insect stings, (2) monitor any reaction to the sting to determine whether an allergic reaction is developing, and (3) prevent future insect stings. For most patients, carefully following product instructions and the self-care measures listed here will help ensure optimal therapeutic outcomes.

### Nondrug Measures

- For honeybee stings, it is important to remove the honeybee stinger immediately. Scraping the stinger away with the edge of a credit card is effective. Try not to squeeze or rub the stinger because these actions will actually release more venom.
- Apply an ice pack or a cold compress promptly to the sting site to help slow absorption of the venom. This action will reduce itching, swelling, and pain.
- Avoid scratching affected area; keep fingernails trimmed. Gloves or mittens may be used on small children during sleep to avoid unconscious scratching.
- To prevent stings, avoid wearing brightly colored clothing, as well as scented lotions or perfume/ cologne that attracts stinging insects.
- If you are hypersensitive to stings, wear a bracelet or carry a card showing the nature of the allergy.

### Nonprescription Medications

- For nonallergic stings, apply a topical nonprescription external analgesic such as a local anesthetic, topical antihistamine, counterirritant, or hydrocortisone to the affected site to relieve pain and itching.
- These products can be applied three to four times daily for up to 7 days.

⚠ If you have experienced previous severe reactions to insect stings, seek emergency medical care immediately. If a primary care provider has prescribed epinephrine and/or an oral antihistamine and you have it on your person, administer it according to the primary care provider's instructions.

⚠ Seek medical attention if symptoms of an allergic reaction, such as hives, excessive swelling, dizziness, vomiting, or difficulty breathing, develop.

⚠ Seek medical attention if the pain and itching worsen during treatment or if they do not improve after 7 days of topical treatment.

## Evaluation of Patient Outcomes for Insect Stings

Follow-up for nonallergic reactions to insect stings should occur within 7 days. The patient should be advised to seek medical attention if symptoms of pain, itching, and localized swelling worsen during the treatment period or persist after 7 days of treatment; symptoms of secondary infection or fever also warrant medical attention. Follow-up for patients who have allergic reactions should occur the same day, if possible; the need to have emergency epinephrine injection available for future situations should be emphasized.

# PEDICULOSIS

Pediculosis is lice infestation. Human lice are wingless parasites with well-developed legs for gripping hair shafts, but they do not jump or fly. They require frequent blood feedings.

## Epidemiology/Etiology of Pediculosis

Lice are irritating pests, and infestations in the United States are common. Three types of lice that infest humans are head lice (*Pediculus humanus capitis*), body lice (*P. humanus corporis*), and pubic lice (*Phthirus pubis*).

### *Head Lice*

Head lice are the most common cause of lice infestation, affecting 10 to 12 million Americans annually, with most cases involving children ages 3 to 12 years.[21] Outbreaks of lice infestation are common in places such as schools and day care centers; infestations are spread through close personal contact or sharing personal items such as caps, hairbrushes, combs, and so forth. Outbreaks usually peak after the opening of schools each year, between August and November.[21] All socioeconomic groups are affected, but the slightly lower incidence in the African American population probably is due to the unique oval structure of their hair shafts that make it more difficult for lice to attach to the hair.[21,22] Head lice create problem infestations, but they generally do not contribute to the spread of other diseases in the United States.[22]

### *Body Lice*

Body lice (or "cooties") live, hide, and lay their eggs in clothing, particularly in seams and folds of underclothes. They periodically attack body areas for blood feedings and can transmit infections such as typhus and trench fever.[2] Body lice are controlled easily by appropriate hygiene; therefore, infestations generally are hygiene related, occurring in individuals who do not shower or change clothing frequently, such as the homeless.[2] These insects are almost twice the size of head lice, and the female body louse lays more eggs, as many as 300 in a lifetime.

### Pubic Lice

Pubic lice or "crabs," referring to their crablike appearance, are generally transmitted through high-risk sexual contact, but may also spread by way of toilet seats, shared undergarments, or bedding. The lice usually are found in the pubic area but may infest armpits, eyelashes, mustaches, beards, and eyebrows.[2] They are smaller than head lice, approximately pin head-sized, and more rounded in appearance. During its life, a female adult pubic louse will deposit about 50 eggs.

## Pathophysiology of Pediculosis

Head lice usually infest the head and live on the scalp (see Color Plates, photographs 23A and B). The female deposits up to 150 eggs or nits in her 20- to 30-day life span; the grayish-white nits are found glued near the base of hair shafts, in close proximity to body heat, and hatch in 5 to 10 days. A nit is about 1 mm in diameter and has yellowish or grayish-white color. Once hatched, the louse must begin feeding within 24 hours or it dies. The nymph, or newly hatched, immature louse, resembles an adult and matures within 8 to 9 days. The nymph is active and tends to move about the head, whereas adults are less active. Without treatment, this cycle may repeat every 3 weeks.[22]

## Signs and Symptoms of Pediculosis

The bite of a louse causes an immediate wheal to develop around the bite, with a local papule appearing within 24 hours. Itching and subsequent scratching may result in secondary infection. Adult lice, which are about the size of a sesame seed, are often difficult to locate because they move, but nits and nit casings generally can be spotted at the base of hair shafts when hair is parted for physical inspection. Hair inspections should focus on the crown of the head, near ears, and at the base of the neck. The grayish nits blend in well with the hair, but nit casings (hatched nits) are a lighter color and more easily located; nits and nit casings may be differentiated from dandruff, dirt, and so forth, because of their firm attachment to the hair shaft. A lice comb may be beneficial in removing some nits and nit casings as part of the inspection. Evidence of lice feces, in the form of a dark powder or powder stains on linens or clothing, may also be present.[23]

## Treatment of Pediculosis

Nonprescription pediculicide agents, appropriate hair combing for nit removal, and home vacuuming/cleaning of personal items are primary treatments for lice infestation.[22] Awareness of the problem and appropriate actions by parents, as well as health and school officials, are also essential.

### *Treatment Goals*

The goal of treating pediculosis is to rid the infested patient of lice by killing adult and nymph lice, and removing nits from the patient's hair.

### *General Treatment Approach*

A pediculicide is applied to the infested body area for the designated amount of time to rid the patient of lice. The hair is then combed with a lice/nit comb to remove nits from the hair shaft; combing will also remove dead lice. Products containing formic acid or enzymes, used as secondary treatments, are purported to break down the substance cementing nits and eggs to hair shafts; these products may be used on the hair, before combing, to loosen lice eggs and facilitate their removal. Once rid of lice, patients should be instructed on how to avoid future infestations. Figure 37-3 outlines treatment of lice infestations and lists exclusions for self-treatment.

### *Nonpharmacologic Therapy*

Since none of the pediculicides kills 100% of lice eggs, careful visual inspection of the hair for nits and combing with a nit comb, such as the LiceMeister comb, to remove nits are helpful in treating and controlling head lice.[22,24] Direct physical contact with an infested individual should be avoided, and articles such as combs, brushes, towels, caps, and hats should not be shared. Clothing and bedding should be washed in hot water and dried in a clothes dryer to kill lice and their nits; an alternative to washing would be to seal contaminated items in a plastic bag for 2 weeks. Hair brushes and combs should be washed in very hot water. Carpets, rugs, and furniture should be vacuumed thoroughly and regularly.[22] Insecticidal sprays should be used on these items sparingly, if at all, because of the difficulty in controlling human exposure and because lice generally survive for less than 48 hours when not in contact with a host.[22,25] Given the increasing resistance to pediculicides, some patients are choosing to use nondrug therapy exclusively; these nondrug methods, specifically combing and vacuuming, can be effective but are labor intensive and tedious.[24] Complete head shaving has also been used as a lice treatment, but the social stigma involved makes this a questionable option.

### *Pharmacologic Therapy*

Two nonprescription pediculicide agents are available for treating pediculosis: permethrins and synergized pyrethrins. Patients should be warned about overusing these agents because of an apparent increasing trend of lice resistance to pediculicides, including the nonprescription products; the resistance may be due to overuse, improper use, or insufficient contact time.[21,25-28] Resistance is contributing to increased use of nonpharmacologic treatments.[24] A prescription-only topical malathion product has been shown to be the most effective pediculicide, and it shows less systemic toxicity and more effectiveness than the prescription product lindane.[26] The oral antibiotic sulfamethoxazole–trimethoprim has demonstrated effectiveness against head lice when used in conjunction with permethrin; the mechanism of action is not clearly defined, but may be due to direct toxicity of the antibiotic ingredients or possibly death of symbiotic bacteria in the gut of lice.[22,27]

#### Synergized Pyrethrins

Pyrethrins, oleoresins obtained from chrysanthemum flowers, are synergized by addition of piperonyl butoxide, a petroleum derivative.

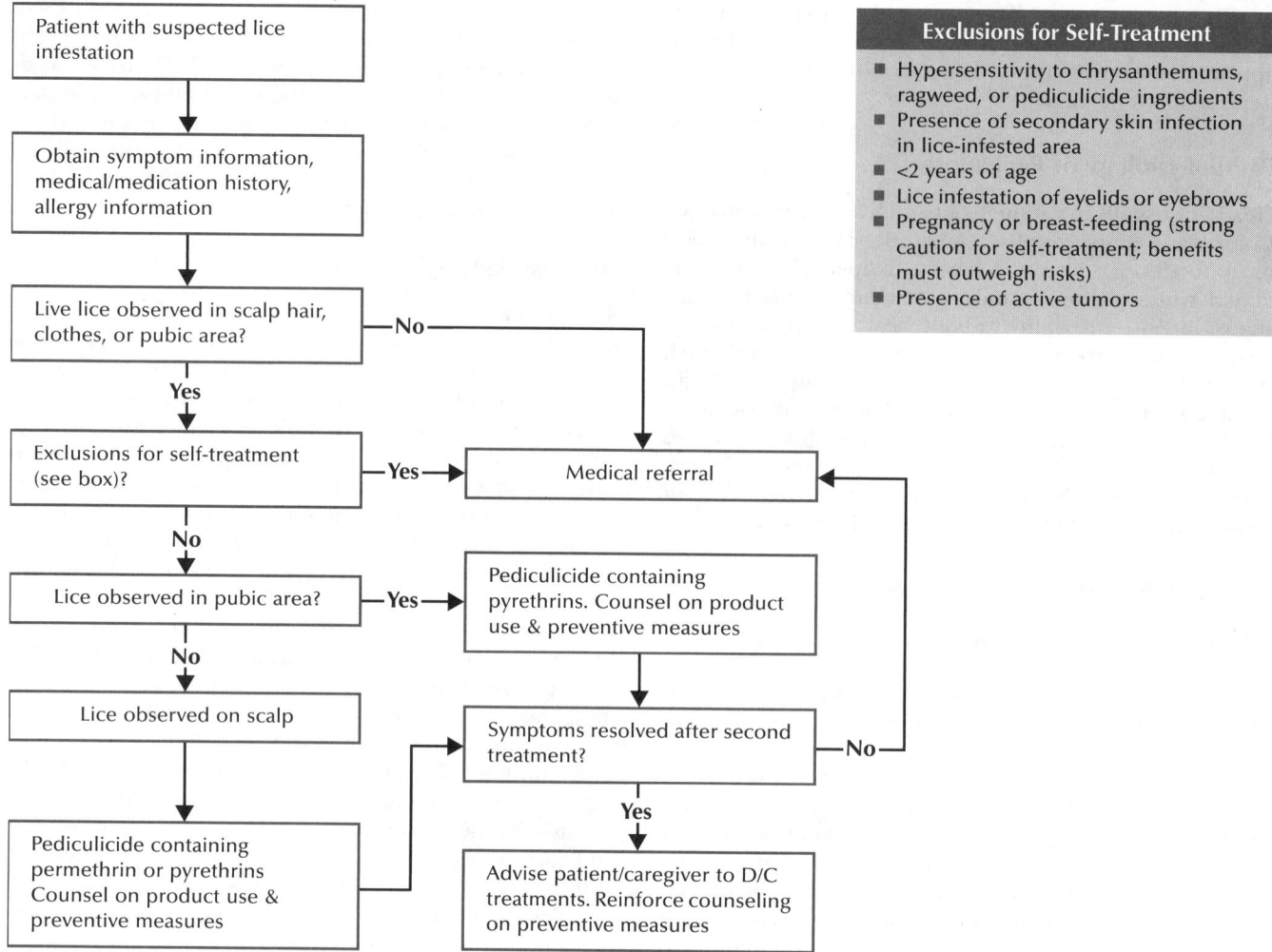

**Exclusions for Self-Treatment**

- Hypersensitivity to chrysanthemums, ragweed, or pediculicide ingredients
- Presence of secondary skin infection in lice-infested area
- <2 years of age
- Lice infestation of eyelids or eyebrows
- Pregnancy or breast-feeding (strong caution for self-treatment; benefits must outweigh risks)
- Presence of active tumors

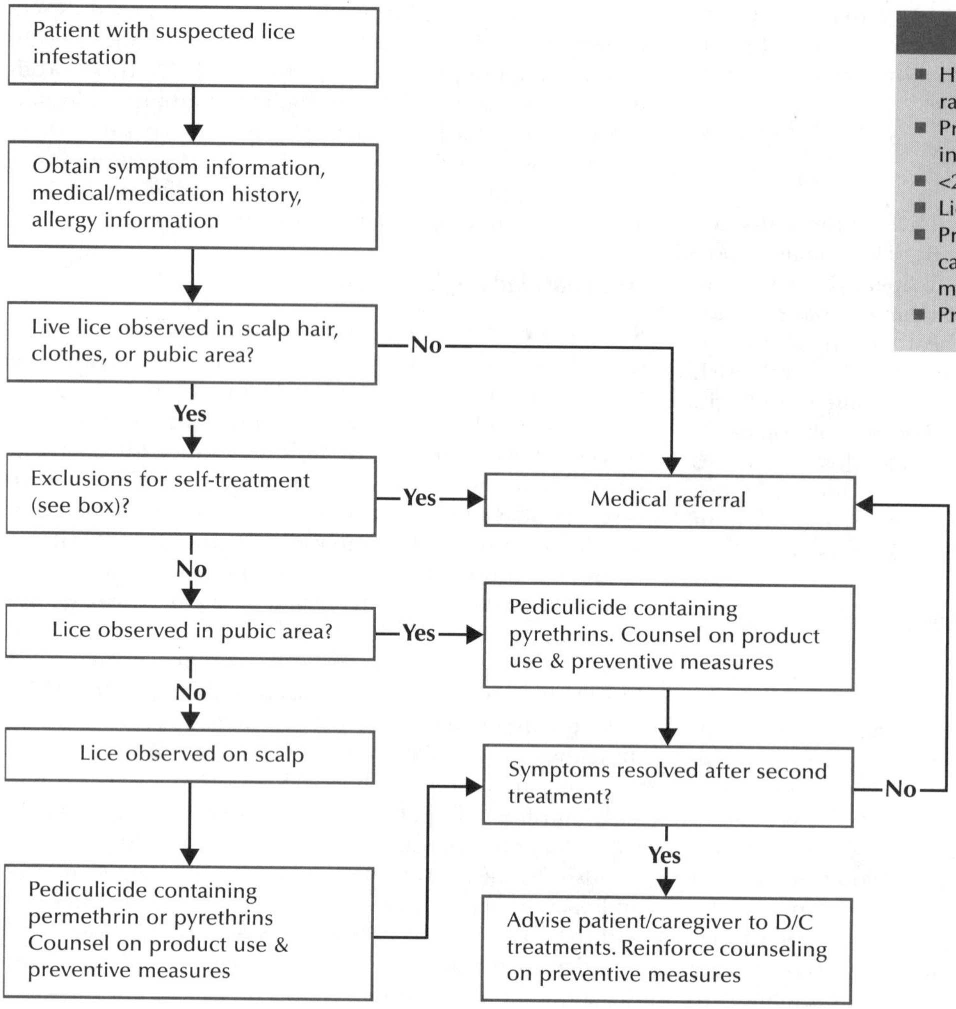


**FIGURE 37-3** Self-care of pediculosis. Key: D/C, discontinue.

*Mechanism of Action* Pyrethrins block nerve impulse transmission, causing the insect's paralysis and death. Addition of piperonyl butoxide to pyrethrins synergizes their insecticidal effect through inhibition of pyrethrin breakdown, increasing insecticide levels within the louse.[21,29]

*Pharmacokinetics* Excessive contact time or occlusion of scalp after product application may increase skin absorption of topical pyrethrins.

*Indications* Pyrethrins are approved for treating head and pubic lice.

*Dosage and Administration Guidelines* Pyrethrins, in concentrations ranging from 0.17% to 0.33%, generally are used in combination with 2% to 4% piperonyl butoxide. This combination is considered an effective pediculicide when applied topically as shampoos, foams, solutions, or gels. The medication is applied to affected area for 10 minutes, and then the treated area is rinsed or shampooed as recommended; combing with a lice comb should follow treatment. The treatment is repeated in 7 to 10 days to kill any remaining nits that have since hatched. The drug should not be applied more than twice in 24 hours.

*Safety Considerations* When applied according to directions, pyrethrins have a low order of toxicity. Most adverse reactions are cutaneous and include irritation, erythema, itching, and swelling.[22,30] Contact with eyes and mucous membranes should be avoided.

Individuals allergic to pyrethrins or chrysanthemums should not use this agent; ragweed-sensitive individuals risk cross-sensitivity. This agent should not be applied to eyelashes or eyebrows; upon recommendation of a health care professional, a nonmedicated ointment such as petrolatum can be applied to these areas to smother lice. (See discussion of lice infestation of the eyelid in Chapter 28.)

### Permethrin

Permethrin is a synthetic pyrethroid available as a nonprescription cream rinse for treating head lice.

*Mechanism of Action* Permethrin acts on the nerve cell membrane of lice. It disrupts the sodium channel, delaying repolarization and causing paralysis of the parasite.

TABLE 37-4 Selected Pediculicides

| Trade Name | Primary Ingredients |
|---|---|
| Nix Cream Rinse | Permethrin 1% |
| A-200 Lice Killing Shampoo | Piperonyl butoxide 3%; pyrethrins 0.33% |
| Pronto Lice Killing Shampoo | Piperonyl butoxide 4%; pyrethrins 0.33% |
| Maximum Strength RID Lice Killing Shampoo | Piperonyl butoxide 4%; pyrethrins 0.33% |
| Maximum Strength RID Mousse Foam | Piperonyl butoxide 4%; pyrethrins 0.33% |
| Tisit Gel | Piperonyl butoxide 2%; pyrethrins 0.3% |
| Tisit Shampoo | Piperonyl butoxide 4%; pyrethrins 0.3% |

*Pharmacokinetics* When permethrin is applied, an estimated less than 2% is absorbed, after which the agent is metabolized.

*Indication* Nonprescription permethrin is indicated for treating head lice only; prescription versions are used in treating scabies.

*Dosage and Administration Guidelines* The 1% cream rinse is applied in sufficient quantities to cover or saturate washed hair and scalp. It is left on the hair for 10 minutes before rinsing; the hair is then combed with a lice comb. The rinse has residual effects for up to 10 days; therefore, retreatment in 7 to 10 days is not required unless active lice are detected.

*Safety Considerations* Primary adverse effects include transient pruritus, burning, stinging, and irritation of the scalp. Contact with eyes and mucous membranes should be avoided

Permethrin is contraindicated in patients who are sensitive to pyrethrins or chrysanthemums. Permethrin should not be used on infants younger than 2 years.

### Pharmacotherapeutic Comparison

When treatment involves a single application of a pediculicide, permethrin is more effective than the pyrethrin and piperonyl butoxide combination. However, no significant difference exists in effectiveness of these agents when treatment consists of two applications.[23,26,31] Recent studies indicate a possible decline in effectiveness of both products related to increasing resistance.[28]

### Product Selection Guidelines

Preparations that contain pyrethrins may be used on infants and young children, but they should be used in pregnancy and lactation only if prescribed by a physician.

Pyrethrins may be recommended for treating pubic lice. For treatment of head lice, pyrethrins or permethrin may be selected on the basis of preferred dosage form, desire for single application, or patient allergies/sensitivities. Table 37-4 lists selected trade-name products containing these agents.

Body lice are controlled by appropriate body hygiene and frequent changing and appropriate laundering of clothing and bed linens.[2]

### *Complementary Therapies*

Products containing ingredients such as olive oil, eucalyptus oil, rosemary oil, and pennyroyal oil are being used as pesticide-free alternatives to traditional lice treatments with anecdotal reports of success.[21] Other oil-based products such as petroleum jelly and mayonnaise are also being used on the basis of the theory that they impair lice respiration; however, these products are not very effective and most likely only slow the movement of lice.[22,30] Tea tree oil, another alternative treatment, must be used with caution because of potential significant allergic reactions and possible liver toxicity.[32] Dangerous alternative treatments such as gasoline and kerosene should always be avoided because of their flammability and potential for toxicity.[24]

### Emerging Therapies

A new potential treatment under study is a class of products called DSP (Dry-on, Suffocation-based Pediculicide) lotions. Nuvo lotion, the first DSP product to be tested, is a nontoxic lotion that "shrink wraps" lice. It is applied to hair and dried with a hairdryer to form a shrink-wrap film over hair and lice. The lotion covers breathing holes, suffocating the louse. Nuvo Lotion must be applied for a second treatment 7 to 10 days later to kill lice that may have hatched since the first treatment.[30]

## Assessment of Pediculosis: A Case-based Approach

In many cases of pediculosis, visual inspection of the scalp will verify presence or absence of head lice or nits. Similarly, presence of body lice can be determined by identifying adult lice and nits in seams of clothing. If a patient does not want such inspection or if lice have not been confirmed by another health care professional, the practitioner should not recommend a pediculicide. When the disorder is confirmed, the practitioner should recommend the appropriate pediculicide according to the type of pediculosis and the patient's allergic history to chrysanthemums or ragweed. Case 37-2 illustrates assessment of a patient with pediculosis.

## CASE 37-2

| Relevant Evaluation Criteria | Scenario/Model Outcome |
|---|---|
| **Information Gathering** | |
| 1. Gather essential information about the patient's symptoms, including: | |
| a. description of symptom(s) (i.e., nature, onset, duration, severity, associated symptoms) | Patient complains of itching on her scalp, which provokes scratching and interferes with her sleep and studies. These symptoms began 2 weeks after she spent the night with a friend. |
| b. description of any factors that seem to precipitate, exacerbate, and/or relieve the patient's symptom(s) | Neither the patient nor her mother is aware of anything that worsens or relieves the symptoms. Regular shampooing has not helped. |
| c. description of the patient's efforts to relieve the symptoms | The mother has given the patient diphenhydramine 25 mg at bedtime to help her sleep and to help with the itching; it improved her daughter's sleep, but has not helped significantly with the itching. |
| 2. Gather essential patient history information: | |
| a. patient's identity | Blair Wexford |
| b. age, sex, height, and weight | 8 y/o F, 47", 45 lb |
| c. patient's occupation | Student |
| d. patient's dietary habits | Mother says Blair eats a well-balanced diet most of the time. |
| e. patient's sleep habits | 9 hours per night |
| f. concurrent medical conditions, prescription and nonprescription medications, and dietary supplements | None |
| g. allergies | Penicillin with cross-sensitivity to cephalosporins |
| h. history of other adverse reactions to medications | None |
| i. other (describe)_______ | Mother states Blair takes a shower and washes her hair daily. |
| **Assessment and Triage** | |
| 3. Differentiate the patient's signs/symptoms and correctly identify the patient's primary problem(s). | After closer examination of the patient's scalp and identification of nits, you realize that she is suffering from a lice infestation. |
| 4. Identify exclusions for self-treatment. | None |
| 5. Formulate a comprehensive list of therapeutic alternatives for the primary problem to determine if triage to a medical practitioner is required, and share this information with the caregiver. | Options include:<br>(1) Recommend self-care with nonprescription pediculicide products.<br>(2) Refer Blair to a PCP.<br>(3) Recommend self-care until a PCP can be consulted.<br>(4) Take no action. |
| **Plan** | |
| 6. Select an optimal therapeutic alternative to address the patient's problem, taking into account patient preferences. | The patient can be treated with an OTC lice product such as Nix Crème Rinse (permethrin) and a quality nit-removal comb. |
| 7. Describe the recommended therapeutic approach to the caregiver and patient. | Explain to Blair and her mother that permethrin has been very successful in ridding most patients of lice when used appropriately. The use of a lice comb to mechanically remove nits from hair stems has also been shown to help increase effectiveness of many lice products. |

CASE 37-2 (continued)

| Relevant Evaluation Criteria | Scenario/Model Outcome |
| --- | --- |
| 8. Explain to the patient and caregiver the rationale for selecting the recommended therapeutic approach from the considered therapeutic alternatives. | Many OTC lice products are effective in treating lice infestations, but many have begun to show decreased effectiveness related to increased lice resistance. Although some resistance to permethrin has been shown, it appears to be less than that of other products. Permethrin is a reliable option; it also has some residual effect that helps to kill lice eggs for up to 1 week after treatment. |
| **Patient Education** | |
| 9. When recommending self-care with nonprescription medications and/or nondrug therapy, convey accurate information to the patient and caregiver, including: | |
| a. appropriate dose and frequency of administration | See the box Patient Education for Pediculosis. |
| b. maximum number of days the therapy should be employed | See the box Patient Education for Pediculosis. |
| c. product administration procedures | See the box Patient Education for Pediculosis. |
| d. expected time to onset of relief | See the box Patient Education for Pediculosis. |
| e. degree of relief that can be reasonably expected | See the box Patient Education for Pediculosis. |
| f. most common side effects | See the box Patient Education for Pediculosis. |
| g. side effects that warrant medical intervention should they occur | See the box Patient Education for Pediculosis. |
| h. patient options in the event that condition worsens or persists | See the box Patient Education for Pediculosis. |
| i. product storage requirements | See the box Patient Education for Pediculosis. |
| j. specific nondrug measures | See the box Patient Education for Pediculosis. |
| 10. Solicit follow-up questions from patient and caregiver. | Are there any oral medications that can be used to treat lice infestations? |
| 11. Answer patient's and caregiver's questions. | There are no current oral drugs approved for treating lice infestations; however, the prescription drug sulfamethoxazole–trimethoprim has been shown to possibly increase the effectiveness of permethrin when they are used together. |

Key: OTC, over-the-counter; PCP, primary care provider.

## Patient Counseling for Pediculosis

Control of pediculosis requires both pharmacologic and nonpharmacologic intervention, as well as the patient's understanding of lice control. The practitioner should reassure parents of children with head lice that the condition is not the result of poor hygiene. Patients with confirmed head or pubic lice infestations should be counseled on which product is best for the situation and how to use the product properly; preventive measures should also be discussed.

## Evaluation of Patient Outcomes for Pediculosis

Follow-up of lice infestations should occur within 10 days. The practitioner should advise the patient to seek medical attention if signs of lice infestation persist after a second application of a pediculicide. Overuse of these products should be discouraged and nonpharmacologic control measures emphasized.[24]

## Key Points for Insect Bites and Stings and Pediculosis

- In people who are not hypersensitive, insect stings and bites cause local irritation, inflammation, swelling, and itching that provoke rubbing and scratching; a cold pack may be applied promptly to the bite area to reduce local symptoms.
- Topical nonprescription preparations that contain local anesthetics, antihistamines, hydrocortisone, or counterirritants are considered safe and effective in adults and children 2 years and older for relief of the itching and pain resulting from insect bites; oral antihistamines may also aid in the relief of local symptoms.

## PATIENT EDUCATION FOR PEDICULOSIS

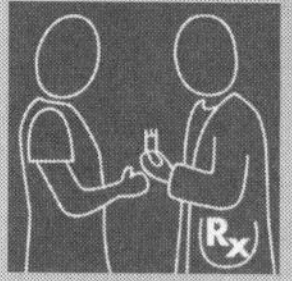

The objectives for self-treatment of pediculosis are to (1) rid the body of lice and nits and (2) implement measures to prevent future infestations. For most patients, carefully following product instructions and the self-care measures listed here will help ensure optimal therapeutic outcomes.

### Nondrug Measures

- Wash hairbrushes, combs, and toys of infested patients in water at a temperature of 130°F (39.4°C) or greater for 10 minutes.[22]
- Use water at a temperature of 130°F (39.4°C) or greater to wash the clothes, bedding, and towels of infested patients. Dry the items on the hottest dryer setting the fabric permits.[22]
- Objects or clothing that cannot be washed should be sealed in plastic bags for the length of the louse's life cycle (2 weeks) so it is unable to feed on a host.
- Avoid close, physical contact with an infested patient; do not share articles such as combs, brushes, towels, caps, and hats.
- Vacuum living areas thoroughly and regularly during treatment period.
- Visually inspect the hair and scalp before, during, and after treatment for evidence of lice or nits; use a nit comb diligently to remove nits; the hair should be combed in segments, and individual hairs can be trimmed if nit removal proves difficult.

### Nonprescription Medications

- Treatment of other family members should be determined on the basis of presence of lice or nits and the family members' level of contact with the infested individual; unnecessary treatment should be avoided.
- If using a pyrethrin shampoo, apply sufficient quantity to wet the dry hair and scalp; foams should also be applied to dry hair. Allow the treatment to remain for 10 minutes.
- Work the shampoo into a lather and then rinse thoroughly; foams should be removed with shampoo or soap and water. A nit comb should be used to remove dead lice and eggs by using the combing technique described previously.
- If using a permethrin cream rinse, shampoo with regular shampoo, rinse, and towel dry hair. Apply sufficient cream rinse to wet hair and scalp, and allow it to remain for 10 minutes; then rinse and towel dry. A nit comb then can be used as discussed previously.
- Avoid contact of the pediculicide with eyes and mucous membranes.
- The pediculicide can cause temporary irritation, erythema, itching, swelling, and numbness of the scalp; itching should be relieved in a few days.
- For pyrethrin products, repeat entire process in 7 to 10 days; permethrin products can be used again in 7 to 10 days if lice or nits are detected. Because of resistance, proper use of these products is required and overuse must be avoided.
- If desired, contact the National Pediculosis Association at www.headlice.org or 1-781-449-6487 for information about treatment of lice infestations.

⚠ Significant skin irritation or excessive exposure of eyes or mucous membranes to pediculicides warrants medical intervention.

⚠ Seek medical attention if symptoms of lice infestation persist after the second treatment.

- In hypersensitive people, anaphylactic reactions may pose serious emergency problems; immediate, active treatment such as administration of epinephrine hydrochloride is required; nonprescription products are of minimal value to hypersensitive patients.
- Suspected spider bites should be referred; nonprescription treatments are not appropriate.
- A tick should be removed by grasping it near the head with tweezers and gently pulling to cause the tick to release from the skin; the tick should be maintained in a sealed container for identification; the patient should be monitored for systemic effects such as Lyme disease and Rocky Mountain spotted fever.
- Preventive measures are an important component in prevention of bites from mosquitoes, ticks, and chiggers; appropriate use of insect repellents containing DEET will help in their prevention.
- Exposure to mosquito bites warrants patient monitoring for symptoms of West Nile virus.
- Lice infestation, especially in school-age children continues to be a significant problem; nondrug measures are an important component in treatment of lice infestation.
- Available nonprescription pediculicides contain either synergized pyrethrins or permethrin. Both agents are effective in treatment of head lice infestations, but only synergized pyrethrins are effective in treatment of pubic lice.
- Pediculicides are available in shampoo, cream rinse, and mousse formulations designed for initial treatment and retreatment in 7 to 10 days; hair combing with a nit comb after treatment is recommended; overuse should be avoided since resistance to pediculicides is a growing problem and impacts effectiveness.

## References


1. Paul J, Bates J. Is infestation with the common bedbug increasing? *BMJ* [serial online]. 2000;320:1141. Available at: letters@bmj.com. Accessed April 11, 2003.
2. Beers MH, Berkow R. *The Merck Manual.* 17th ed. West Point, Pa: Merck & Co; 1999:1053-4, 2649-54.
3. Statistics, Surveillance, and Control of West Nile Virus. Centers for disease Control and Prevention. Available at: http://www.cdc.gov/ncidod/dvbid/westnile/surv&controlCaseCount04_detailed.htm Accessed February 17, 2005.
4. Infectious disease. *Pharm Lett.* 2003;19:39.
5. Gea-Banacloche J, Johnson R, Bagic A, et al. West Nile virus: pathogenesis and therapeutic options. *Ann Inter Med.* 2004;140: 545-53.

6. Petersen L, Marfin A. West Nile virus: a primer for the clinician. *Ann Intern Med.* 2002;137: 173-9.
7. Nash D, Mostashari F, Fine A, et al. The outbreak of West Nile virus infection in the New York City area in 1999. *N Engl J Med.* 2001;344:1807-14.
8. Silverman A, Qu L, Low J, et al. Assessment of hepatitis B virus DNA and hepatitis C virus RNA in the common bedbug and kissing bug. *Am J Gastroenterol.* 2001;96:2194-8.
9. Gammons M, Salam G. Tick removal. *Am Fam Phys.* 2002; 66:643-44.
10. Steere AC. Lyme disease. *New Engl J Med.* 2001;345:115-25.
11. Hayes E, O'Leary D. West Nile virus infection: A pediatric perspective. *Pediatrics.* 2004;113:1375-81.
12. Fradin M, Day J. Comparative efficacy of insect repellents against mosquito bites. *N Engl J Med.* 2002;347:13-8.
13. Abramowicz M. Insect repellants. *Med Lett Drugs Ther.* 2003;45: 41-2.
14. US Environmental Protection Agency. Reregistration of the insect repellent DEET. April 1998. Available at: http:// www.epa.gov/pesticides/factsheets/chemicals/deet.htm. Accessed April 10, 2003.
15. Koren G, Matsui D, Bailey B. DEET-based insect repellants: safety implications for children and pregnant and lactating women. *CMAJ.* 2003; 169: 209-11.
16. Gennaro A. *Remington: The Science and Practice of Pharmacy.* 20th ed. Baltimore: Lippincott Williams & Wilkins; 2000:1045-6,1405-6.
17. McEvoy G. *AHFS Drug Information.* Betheseda, Md: American Society of Health-System Pharmacists; 2002:3444-5.
18. Killion K. *Drug Facts and Comparisons.* St. Louis: Facts and Comparisons; 2003:1599.
19. Golden D, Kagey-Sobotka A, Norman P, et al. Outcomes of allergy to insect stings in children, with and without venom immunotherapy. *N Engl J Med.* 2004;351:668-74.
20. Morrit J, Golden D, Reisman R, et al. Stinging insect hypersensitivity: a practice parameter update. *J Allergy Clin Immunol.* 2004; 114(4):869-86.
21. Stephens MB. Controlling head lice. *Patient Care.* September 15, 2000:99-107.
22. Frankowski B, Weiner L, Clinical report: head lice, guidance for the clinician in rendering pediatric care. *Pediatrics.* 2002;110:638-43.
23. DiNapoli JB, Austin RD, Englender SJ, et al. Eradication of head lice with a single treatment. *Am J Public Health.* 1998;78:978-80.
24. Pray S. Pediculicide resistance in head lice: a survey. *Hosp Pharm.* 2003;38:241-6.
25. Dawes M, Hicks NR, Fleminger M, et al. Treatment of head lice. *BMJ.* 1999;318:385.
26. Meinking T, Serrano L, Hard B, et al. Comparative in vitro pediculicidal efficacy of treatments in a resistant head lice population in the United States. *Arch Dermatol.* 2002;138:220-4.
27. Meinking T, Clineschmidt C, Chen C, et al. An observer-blinded study of 1% permethrin cream rinse with and without adjunctive combing in patients with head lice. *J Pediatr.* 2002;141:665-70.
28. Meinking T, Entzel P, Villar M, et al. Comparative efficacy of treatments for pediculosis capitis infestations. *Arch Dermatol.* 2001;137:287-91.
29. Burkhart C. Relationship of treatment-resistant head lice to the safety and efficacy of pediculicides. *Mayo Clin Proc.* 2004; 79:661-6.
30. Pearlman D. A simple treatment for head lice: dry-on, suffocation based pediculocide. *Pediatrics.* 2004;114:275-9.
31. Carson DS, Tribble PW, Weart CW. Pyrethrins combined with piperonyl butoxide (RID) vs 1% permethrin (NIX) in the treatment of head lice. *Am J Dis Child.* 1998;142:768-9.
32. Alternative treatments: what the NPA is saying about mayonnaise, Vaseline, and tea tree oil. Available at: http:// www.headlice.org/ faq/treatments/alternatives.htm. Accessed April 25, 2003.

CHAPTER 38

# Acne

*Karla T. Foster and Cynthia W. Coffey*

Acne vulgaris is a common chronic skin disease that affects millions of people. It remains one of the most prevalent disorders treated in a dermatologist's practice, accounting for over 20% of all visits.[1] Although acne is a common disorder, the physical and emotional impact of the disease should not be overlooked. Acne is associated not only with physical detriments such as disfigurement and scarring, but also with psychological consequences such as diminished self-esteem, social withdrawal resulting from embarrassment, and depression.[2]

There are a wide variety of treatment options available for acne vulgaris over the counter. The cost of nonprescription drugs for acne is $100 million annually.[1] Practitioners can be instrumental in assisting patients make informed choices about their selection of acne products. This interaction also represents an opportunity for clinicians to introduce a new group of consumers to the value of pharmaceutical care.

## Epidemiology of Acne

The incidence of acne is nearly universal; approximately 85% of all people between the ages of 15 and 24 years will develop it to some degree.[3] Acne typically develops in males from ages 12 to 18 years and in females from ages 15 to 17 years. Acne lesions may precede other signs of puberty and may be diagnosed as early as 8 years of age.[4] Papular lesions generally appear during the mid-teen years, and nodular lesions appear in the late teens (Table 38-1). Acne affects 40% to 54% of individuals over 25 years of age and 12% of women and 3% of men in their middle ages.[5] Acne may disappear spontaneously in adults for reasons that are not readily apparent.[6,7] Neonatal acne may also occur at 2 to 4 weeks of age and persist up to 6 months in response to maternal androgens.[4]

## Anatomy and Physiology of Skin

Acne vulgaris originates in the pilosebaceous units in the dermis (Figure 38-1A). These units, consisting of a hair follicle and associated sebaceous glands, are connected to the skin surface by a duct (infundibulum) lined with epithelial cells through which the hair shaft passes. The sebaceous glands produce sebum, which passes to the skin surface through the duct and then spreads over the skin to retard water loss and maintain about 10% hydration of the skin and hair.

**Editor's Note:** This chapter is based, in part, on the 14th edition chapter with the same title, which was written by Joye Ann Billow.

## Etiology of Acne

Although the precise cause of acne is not known, processes linked to the increase in androgens in both genders with the approach of puberty are closely correlated with acne development. These processes, discussed in detail in the next section, are (1) abnormal keratinization of cells in the infundibulum, (2) increased sebum production, (3) accelerated growth of *Propionibacterium acnes,* and (4) inflammation.[8]

Several factors contribute to the exacerbation of existing acne and cause periodic flare-ups of acne in some patients. Other factors widely assumed to cause acne have not been proven as etiologic factors.

### *Substantiated Exacerbating Factors for Acne*

#### Environmental and Physical Factors

Hydration decreases the size of the pilosebaceous duct orifice and prevents loosening of the comedone. Therefore, high-humidity environments or prolonged sweating can exacerbate acne. Occlusive clothing that prevents evaporation of skin moisture also increases skin hydration.

Acne symptoms may increase because of local irritation or friction from occlusive clothing, headbands, helmets, or other friction-producing devices (acne mechanica). Even resting the chin or cheek on the hand often or for long periods creates localized conditions conducive to lesion formation in acne-prone patients.

Exposure to dirt, vaporized cooking oils, or certain industrial chemicals, such as coal tar and petroleum derivatives, may cause occupational acne.

#### Cosmetic Use

Acne cosmetica is a mild form of acne on the face, cheek, and chin. It typically consists of closed, noninflammatory comedones and occurs as a result of using an oil-based product on the skin that causes occlusion of the pilosebaceous unit. Oil-based cosmetics may exacerbate acne or even induce it. Topical products, such as moisturizers and tanning oils, may contain comedogenic oils (e.g., lanolin, mineral oil, or cocoa butter). Pomade acne, most often seen in African Americans and manifested by comedones along the hairline on the forehead and temples, is caused by the long-term use of hair dressing that contains occlusive oils.

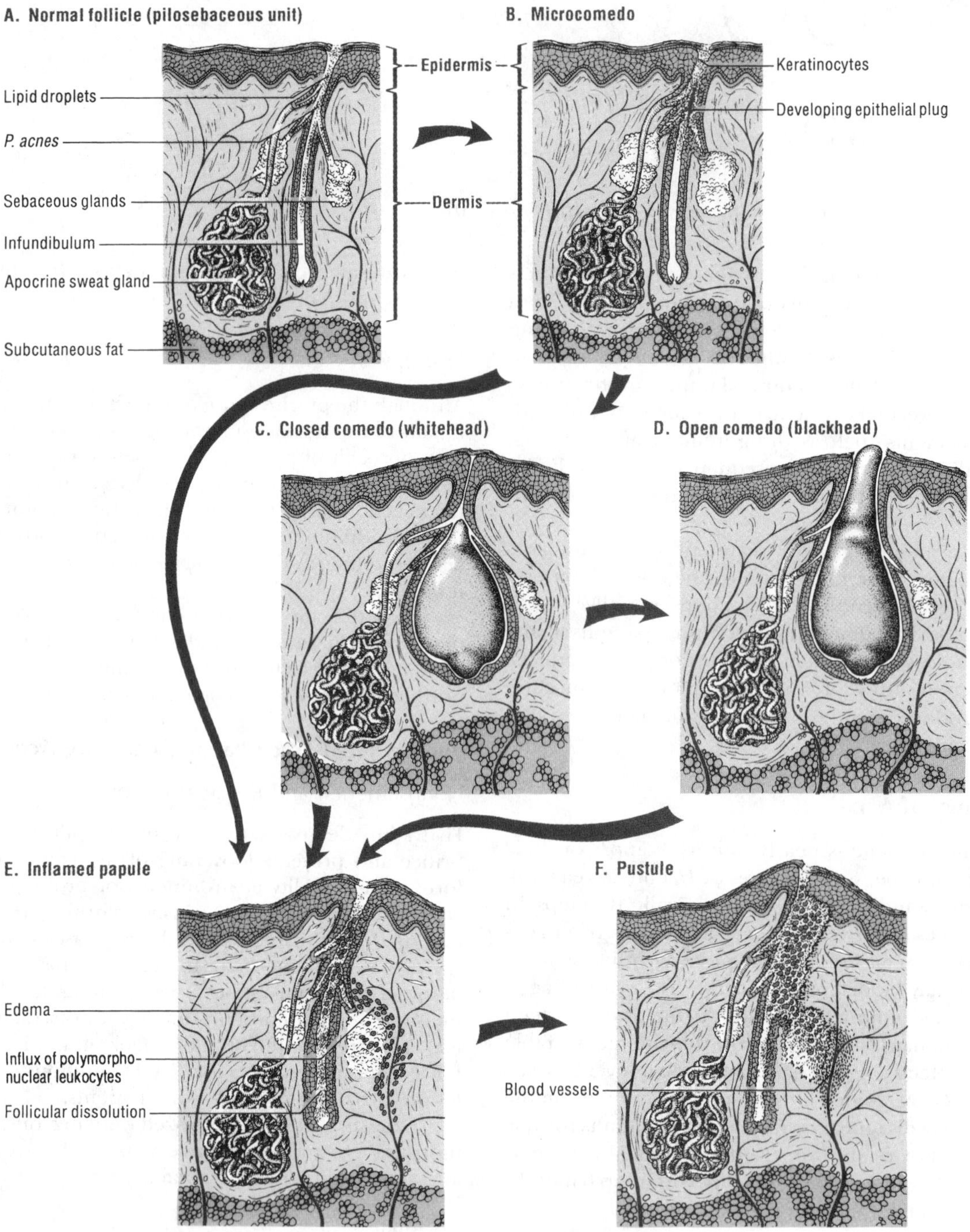


**FIGURE 38-1** Pathogenesis of acne. (Adapted with permission from Fulton JE, Bradley S. *Cutis.* 1976;7:560.)

## Emotional Factors

Severe or prolonged periods of stress or other emotional extremes may exacerbate acne. It has been hypothesized that stress may induce the expression of neuroendocrine modulators, which play a role in centrally and topically induced stress of the sebaceous glands. This expression may lead to the progression of acne.[9]

## Hormonal Factors

The onset of acne generally corresponds with menarche, however, the correlation between acne and menarche varies widely among women. Oral contraceptives with high-androgenic progestins have been implicated in the production of acne, whereas estrogen-dominant preparations have been postulated to improve preexisting acne.[9]

**TABLE 38-1 Assessment of Acne Severity[1,2]**

| Grade of Acne | Qualitative Description | Quantitative Description |
|---|---|---|
| **Comedonal** | | |
| I | Comedonal acne | Comedones only, <10 on face, none on trunk, no scars; noninflammatory lesions only |
| | Blackheads | Open comedo; dilated hair follicle with open orifice to skin |
| | | Dark color may be caused by oxidation of melanin, compacted epithelial cells, or presence of lipids may contribute |
| | Whiteheads | Closed comedo; dilated hair follicle filled with keratin, sebum, and bacteria with obstructed opening to the skin |
| **Papulopustular** | | |
| II | Papular acne | 10-25 papules on face and trunk, mild scarring; inflammatory lesions <5 mm in diameter |
| III* | Pustular acne | More than 25 pustules, moderate scarring; size similar to papules but with visible, purulent core |
| IV* | Severe/persistent pustulocystic acne | Nodules or cysts, extensive scarring; inflammatory lesions >5 mm in diameter |
| | Recalcitrant severe cystic acne | Extensive nodules/cysts |

* Some overlap with previous grade of acne.

**TABLE 38-2 Drugs That Exacerbate Acne[10]**

| | |
|---|---|
| P | Phenytoin |
| I | Isoniazid |
| M | Moisturizers |
| P | Phenobarbital |
| L | Lithium |
| E | Ethionamide |
| S | Steroids |

### Medication Use

Although medications can exacerbate preexisting acne vulgaris, medication-induced acne (acne medicamentosa) is not a true acne. A helpful mnemonic for drugs that exacerbate acne is PIMPLES (Table 38-2).[10] Other drugs that may exacerbate or cause acne include azithioprine, quinine, and rifampin.[11]

### Genetics

The patient may have control over exacerbating factors, such as environmental, physical, and emotional issues or cosmetic use. However, one predisposing factor, heredity, cannot be controlled. The chance of offspring developing acne is higher when both parents have had acne than when only one parent has had the disorder.[3,5,8,9] Bataille and colleagues, in a study evaluating acne in twins, found that 81% of acne cases are caused by genetic factors.[4]

### *Unsubstantiated Etiologic Factors*

Little evidence supports a direct relationship between diet and acne.[4] As a rule of thumb, people should be advised to avoid any particular food that seems to exacerbate their acne. Excessive scrubbing in an attempt to open blocked pores may exacerbate rather than improve acne.[4,12]

Because acne usually begins at puberty and sexual activity may begin in the same timeframe, some people conclude that the two events have a cause-and-effect relationship. There is no evidence that sexual activity causes or exacerbates acne.

## Pathophysiology of Acne

Abnormal keratinization (hyperkeratinization) of the cells shed in the infundibulum produces increased cohesiveness, resulting in obstruction of the follicle with impacted cells and sebum. This plug distends the follicle to form a microcomedo, the initial pathologic lesion of acne (Figure 38-1B). As more cells and sebum accumulate, the microcomedo enlarges and becomes visible as a closed comedo, or whitehead, a small, pale nodule just beneath the skin surface. This lesion is the precursor of other acne lesions.

Although the cause of hyperkeratinization is unknown, a deficiency of linoleic acid in the sebum has been implicated. Also, there is evidence that follicular keratinocytes release interleukin 1, which may stimulate comedone formation. Type 1-5$\alpha$-reductase is present in select sebaceous glands and, by converting testosterone to the more potent dihydroxytestosterone (DHT), may predispose persons to acne.[13]

The hair in the follicle may play a significant role in comedo development. If it is thin and small, the hair may become entrapped in the plug. The heavier hair of the scalp and beard push the developing plug to the surface, preventing comedo formation.

An open comedo or blackhead occurs when desquamated epithelial cells and sebum accumulate behind the plug and the orifice of the follicular canal becomes distended, allowing the plug to protrude. The tip of the plug may darken because of deposition of melanin, not dirt or oxidized fat.

The increase in circulating androgens stimulates production of sebum, which is prevented from reaching the skin surface by the obstructing plug. At the same time, *P. acnes* (a gram-positive anaerobic rod found on the skin) colonizes the pilosebaceous duct. Bacterial colony counts are higher in patients with acne than in those without acne. *P. acnes* is a major contributor to inflammatory acne lesions through the production of lipase, which causes the breakdown of sebum to highly irritating, free fatty acids. The resultant inflammation causes localized tissue destruction.[4]

Inflammatory acne begins with closed comedones that distend the follicle, causing the cellular lining of the walls to spread and become thin. Primary inflammation of the follicle wall develops with the disruption of the epithelial lining and lymphocyte infiltration. A severe inflammatory reaction results if the follicle wall ruptures spontaneously or is ruptured by picking, squeezing, or attempted expression with a comedo extractor. The contents are discharged into the surrounding tissue. At the worst, the results may be abscesses, which may cause scars or pits after healing. The pustules or purulent nodules of inflammatory acne are more likely to cause permanent scarring than those of noninflammatory acne.

## Signs and Symptoms of Acne

Acne is characterized by whiteheads, blackheads, acne pimples, and blemishes. Blemishes are characterized by an unesthetic alteration of the skin. Noninflammatory acne is characterized by the presence of closed or open comedones, also called whiteheads and blackheads, respectively (Figure 38-1C and D, and Color Plates, photograph 24).

Inflammatory acne is characterized by pimples (i.e., small, prominent, inflamed elevations of the skin), which may rupture to form a papule (Figure 38-1E). Papules are inflammatory lesions appearing as raised, reddened areas on the skin, which may enlarge to form pustules. Pustules appear as raised, reddened areas filled with pus (Figure 38-1F and Color Plates, photograph 25). More extensive penetration into surrounding and underlying tissue produces necrotic, purulent nodular lesions, previously designated as cysts, and may lead to pitting and scarring if left untreated.

The typical acne patient presents with a combination of lesions: comedones (open and closed), papules, and pustules. The lesions are usually found on the face, chest, and back where sebaceous glands are common, but they may also appear on the neck and upper arms.[6-9]

If acne lesions persist beyond the mid-20s or develop in the mid-20s or later, the symptoms may signal rosacea rather than acne vulgaris. A differential diagnosis is necessary because the treatment of rosacea, while similar to that for acne, has unique elements (Table 38-3).[14-18]

## Classification System for Acne

Various systems have been used to classify the severity of acne vulgaris. Table 38-1 presents a classification system in common use that assesses the severity of the acne from the mildest form (primarily comedones, often localized on one portion of the face) through the most severe form (consisting of necrotic, purulent nodules, often called cystic acne, nodulocystic acne, or acne conglobata, in which moderate to severe scarring is likely).[8,9] This approach also helps patients and practitioners select appropriate treatment regimens for the management of acne. Whiteheads and blackheads, although widespread, may be considered less severe than several large nodules because they are easier to clear. In other words, for selection of treatment, the lesion type is more important than the quantity.

## Treatment of Acne

In most cases, acne is self-limiting and can be controlled to varying degrees. Adherence to therapeutic regimens will reduce symptoms and minimize scarring. Because acne persists for long periods, treatment must be long-term, continuous, and consistent.

### *Treatment Goals*

The primary goal in self-treating acne is consistent, long-term use of methods to unblock pilosebaceous ducts, and thus keep the orifice open. Avoiding factors that exacerbate acne is another important goal in acne treatment. These two goals should aid in achieving the overall desired outcome—relieving the patient's physical and social discomfort.

### *General Treatment Approach*

Treatment of noninflammatory acne usually consists of using pharmacologic agents along with nonpharmacologic measures such as cleansing the skin to remove excess sebum and avoiding factors that may cause acne.[11] Irritants, such as nonprescription acne medications, also aid in unblocking the ducts. Low-dose oral contraceptives that are estrogen dominant and contain low-androgenic progestins, such as Ortho Tri-Cyclen (ethinyl estradiol, norgestimate) have been approved for acne treatment in women.[19] The chance of a positive outcome for noninflammatory acne is increased if the patient can avoid factors that exacerbate acne.

Treatment of inflammatory acne typically requires both nonprescription and prescription medication, such as oral and topical antibiotics and retinoids, as well as possible excision and drainage of inflammatory lesions. The effectiveness of oral antibiotics (e.g., erythromycin, clindamycin, minocycline, meclocycline, tetracycline, doxycycline, azithromycin, or clarithromycin) and topical antibiotics (e.g., tetracycline, erythromycin, or clindamycin) is a result of their ability to suppress the bacterial population

**TABLE 38-3 Differentiation of Acne and Rosacea[15-18,37]**

| Criterion | Acne | Rosacea |
|---|---|---|
| Etiology | Abnormal keratinization of cells in the infundibulum; increased sebum production; growth of *P. acne*; inflammation | Unknown; inflammatory process |
| Symptoms | Closed or open comedones; inflammatory acne characterized by pimples that may erupt to form pustules | Sensitivity to touch; symmetric reddening (telangiectasis) of face; ocular manifestations (intermittent conjunctivitis or blepharitis); late manifestations occur as solid red papules or pustule, rarely comedones |
| History | None | History of frequent facial flushing and blushing |
| Incidence | Nearly universal; affects 12% and 3% of middle-aged women and men, respectively | More common in women than men (3:1 ratio); primarily affects persons of northern or eastern European descent; may be overlooked in nonwhites, possibly causing delayed treatment and disproportionate ocular complications and late manifestations in this population |
| Onset | Usually ages 15-24 years | Usually ages 20-60 years |
| Location | Face, chest, and back; occasionally neck, and upper arms | Central portion of face (center of forehead, nose, chin) and eyes; if untreated, may extend to scalp and palmar surfaces |
| Aggravating factors | Cosmetic use; hormonal factors; emotional factors (stress, anxiety); physical factors (occlusive clothing); environmental factors (humidity); medication use | Temperature extremes, emotional influences (stress, anxiety); alcoholic beverages; smoking; hot or spicy foods and beverages; irritating skin products; systemic corticosteroids |
| Remitting factors | Cleanse skin; minimize aggravating factors | Minimize aggravating factors; use sunscreen products containing simethicone or cyclomethicone, which prevent irritation from other sunscreen ingredients |
| Treatment | See Treatment of Acne | Oral antibiotics (e.g., erythromycin, tetracycline), topical metronidazole gel (0.75%), oral isotretinoin, or topical azelaic acid cream (20%) for lesions of late stages; nonselective beta blockers for erythema and flushing |

of the sebaceous duct and reduce lipase activity. Notwithstanding, cleansing the skin and avoiding exacerbating factors are also beneficial.

Self-treatment is appropriate only for grade I acne (i.e., noninflammatory acne of mild to moderate severity; Table 38-1), presenting with open or closed comedones. Situations in which referral is appropriate are described as self-treatment exclusions (Figure 38-2). The treatment algorithm in Figure 38-2 outlines this approach to self-care by patients who have acne but none of the exclusions for self-treatment.

A primary care provider must direct suppressing or altering hormonal activity, correcting disfiguring effects, and using prescription drugs to treat acne. Furthermore, the patient should not add nonprescription medications to prescribed regimens unless recommended by the prescriber.

### *Nonpharmacologic Therapy*

Numerous products, medicated and nonmedicated, are available for cleansing the skin. Acne patients often need guidance in selecting the appropriate products for their special skin care needs.

#### Cleansing the Skin

Removing excess sebum from the skin by washing produces a mild drying of the skin and, perhaps, mild erythema. The affected areas should be thoroughly but gently washed at least twice daily (more frequently if skin is oily) with warm water, medicated or unmedicated soap, and a soft washcloth, then patted dry. Washing should not be excessively vigorous; it should cause barely noticeable peeling that can loosen comedones. Washing intensity and frequency should be reduced, and a mild facial soap should be considered if tautness occurs.

Facial soaps that do not contain moisturizing oils are usually satisfactory. Soaps containing antibacterial agents (such as triclosan) have no proven clinical value. Salicylic acid, sulfur, and sulfur-resorcinol combination soaps are of questionable effectiveness because little, if any, residue is left on the skin. Abrasive cleansers (containing pumice, polyethylene, or aluminum oxide particles) should be avoided because of their irritant effect on inflammatory acne, although they may be useful in noninflammatory acne. If it is inconvenient to wash during the day, the patient can use cleansing pads that contain an astringent.

#### Minimizing Exacerbating Factors

Minimizing factors that exacerbate acne can help prevent the condition. The patient should avoid wearing clothes or sports gear that cause friction; mechanical irritation may induce or exacerbate acne. Irritation also results from resting

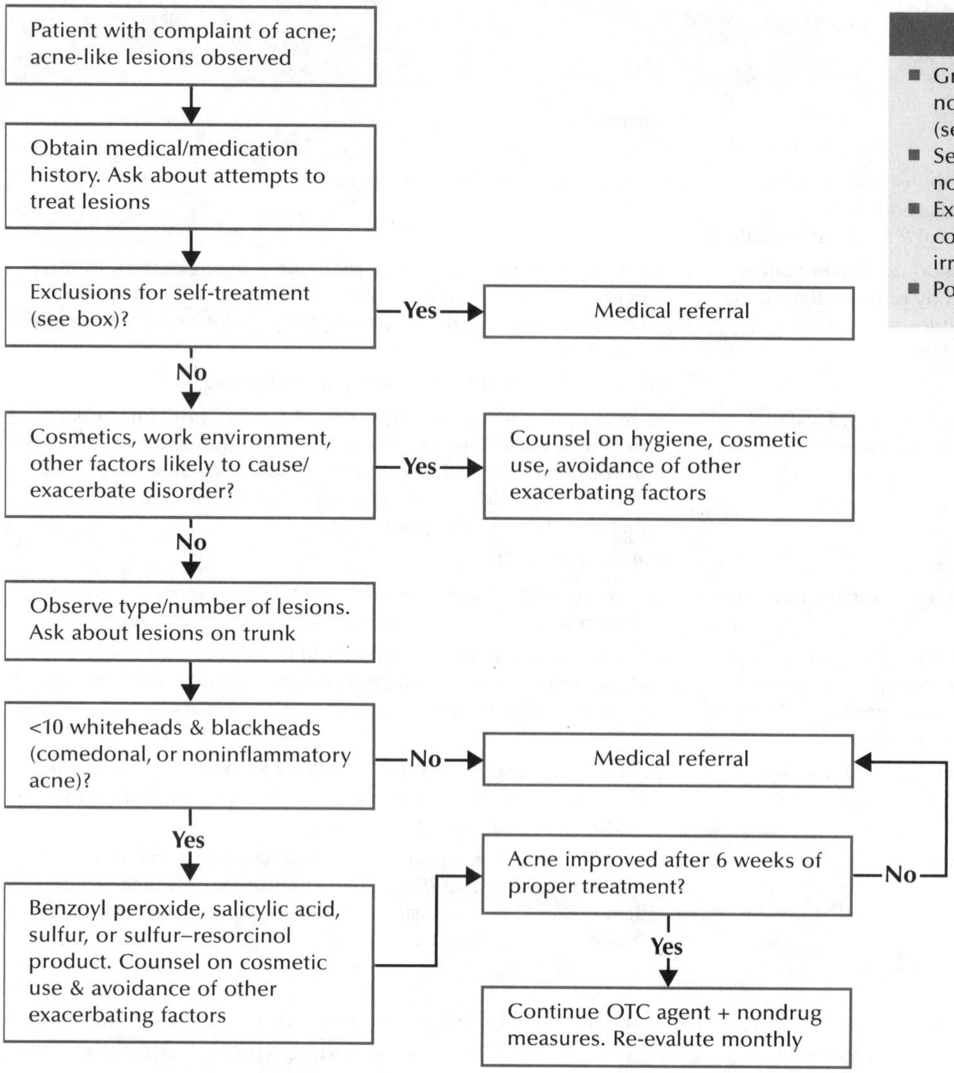


**Exclusions for Self-Treatment**

- Grades II-IV acne: papules, pustules, nodules, cysts and/or scarring (see Table 38-1)
- Severe, recalcitrant acne (extensive nodules/cysts)
- Exacerbating factors (e.g., comedogenic drugs, mechanical irritation)
- Possible rosacea

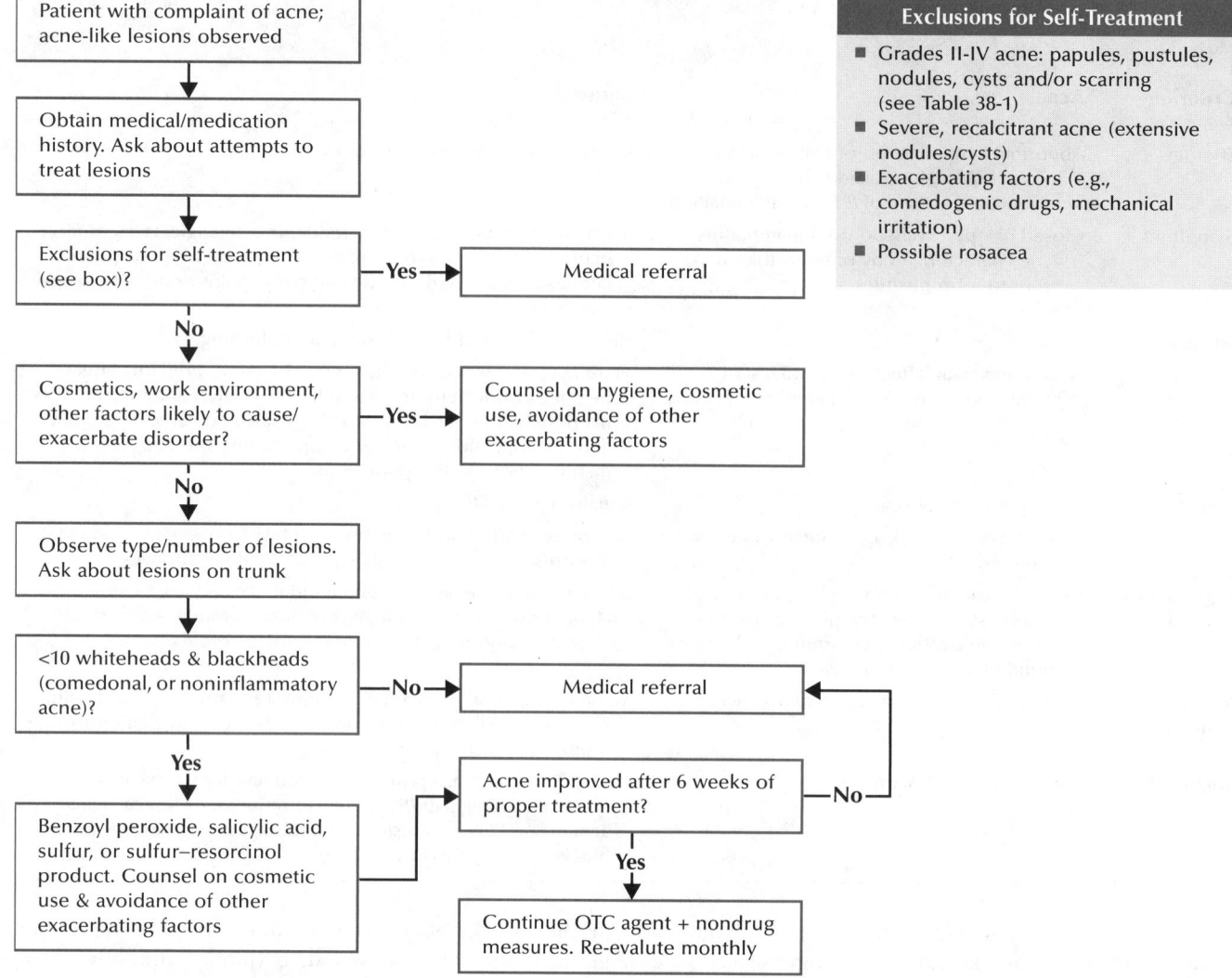

**FIGURE 38-2** Self-care of acne. Key: OTC, over-the-counter.

the face or chin on the hand and should be avoided or minimized.

The patient should use water-based cosmetic products and frequently wash oily hair with a water-based shampoo. Exposure to exacerbating environmental factors (e.g., dirt, dust, oil, or chemical irritants) should be minimized or avoided.

Acne lesions should not be picked or squeezed. Open comedones may be regarded as unsightly by the patient, but a dermatologist can easily express them, using a clean comedo extractor.

### *Pharmacologic Therapy*

Benzoyl peroxide is the most effective and widely used nonprescription medication currently available for treatment of noninflammatory acne. It is currently classified by the Food and Drug Administration (FDA) as Category III (i.e., more data needed to determine safety and use for "nonmonograph conditions") because of concern over its tumorigenic potential.

Category I (generally recognized as safe and effective) topical antiacne ingredients include salicylic acid 0.5% to 2%, sulfur 3% to 8%, and a combination of sulfur 3% to 8%, with either resorcinol 2% or resorcinol monoacetate 3%.[9]

In addition, after reviewing a time and extent application for triclosan as an active, topical acne agent, FDA determined the antibacterial agent is eligible for inclusion in the OTC topical acne drug products monograph. The agency announced December 5, 2005, that it is seeking safety and effectiveness information to determine whether the concentrations 0.2% to 0.5% and 0.3% to 1.0% are safe and effective in leave-on and rinse-off dosages, respectively.[38] March 6, 2006, is the deadline for comments. Some Clearasil products already contain triclosan.

#### Benzoyl Peroxide

Benzoyl peroxide is commonly available in concentrations of 2.5%, 5%, and 10% in such diverse dosage forms as lotions, gels, creams, cleansers, masks, and soaps. Benzoyl peroxide products in concentrations of 4%, 5.5%, and 20% are also available.

*Mechanism of Action* Benzoyl peroxide causes irritation and desquamation that prevent closure of the pilosebaceous duct. Its irritant effect causes an increased turnover rate of the epithelial cells lining the follicular duct, which then increases sloughing and promotes resolution of the comedones. Its oxidizing potential may contribute to antibacterial activity, decreasing the level of *P. acnes* and reducing the formation of irritating free fatty acids. It also has irritant, drying, and sensitizing effects. It currently is the nonprescription, topical treatment of choice.[16,20]

*Therapeutic Comparison of Dosage Forms* Clinical response to all concentrations is similar in reducing the number of inflammatory lesions. The different formulations are not equivalent. The drying effect of the alcohol gel base enhances benzoyl peroxide's effectiveness; therefore, this form is superior to a lotion of the same concentration. The gel products are available in assorted strengths (2.5%, 5%, 10%, and 20%) both with and without a prescription.[21] Washes and cleansers containing benzoyl peroxide, although widely used, have little or no comedolytic effect. A formulation of benzoyl peroxide in phospholipid liposomes (not commercially available) shows promise for improved topical treatment of papulopustular acne.[22,23]

*Dosage and Administration Guidelines* See Table 38-4 for instructions on the proper use of topical nonprescription benzoyl peroxide products.

*Safety Considerations* Excessive dryness, peeling, some skin sloughing, erythema, or edema indicates that lower concentrations should be used for shorter periods of time. Use of the drug may cause transient stinging and burning, and patients should not be alarmed unless these effects persist or become worse. Benzoyl peroxide may bleach hair, clothing, and bed linens. Care must be taken to avoid exposing these items to the product.

Other sources of irritation, such as sunlamps and excessive sun exposure, should also be avoided to prevent excessive burning and stinging. The drug should not be used concurrently with other topical products unless a primary care provider or clinician recommends concomitant use. Alcohol-based products, such as cleansers and after-shave lotions, may exacerbate the stinging and burning sensation.

Safety studies are ongoing to determine whether benzoyl peroxide enhances ultraviolet radiation-induced skin cancer. Meanwhile, the products remain on the market, but the FDA requires additional warning statements and directions on the label. While there are reports that benzoyl peroxide is a tumor promoter and progressor, it is neither an initiator nor a complete carcinogen. Thus, the FDA has not made a final determination of safety.[9]

An interim 52-week study by the Nonprescription Drug Manufacturers Association (NDMA; now called the Consumer Healthcare Product Association [CHPA]), filed with FDA on March 1, 1999, concluded that benzoyl peroxide "is not carcinogenic in the skin or in 'select internal organs' of mice and rats." A second 52-week study sponsored by NDMA indicates it "does not enhance photocarcinogenesis in mice."[24] At press time, FDA had not revised its 1991 final monograph for acne products.

**TABLE 38-4 Administration Guidelines for Benzoyl Peroxide**

- Using a nonmedicated soap, gently cleanse affected area and any area likely to be affected; pat dry.
- Smooth a small quantity of the preparation over the area once or twice daily.
- To determine sensitivity to the product, limit initial applications to one or two small areas at the 2.5% concentration.
- Leave initial application on the skin for only 15 minutes; then wash off.
- If no discomfort occurs, increase the time benzoyl peroxide is left on the skin in 15-minute increments as tolerance allows.
- Once the product is tolerated for 2 hours, leave it on overnight. The once-a-day application may be all that is needed. If sufficient improvement does not occur and the patient's face does not dry out or peel, applications may be gradually increased, over 2-3 days, to 2-3 times daily.
- For fair-skinned individuals, initiate therapy with the 2.5% strength and apply only once daily during the first few weeks of therapy.
- If treatment is well tolerated, but the problem persists, the strength may be increased to 5% after 1 week and to 10% after 2 weeks.
- Because it is highly irritating, use benzoyl peroxide with great care near the eyes, mouth, lips, and nose, as well as near cuts, scrapes, and other abrasions.
- Do not use this product concurrently with other topical products, unless a primary care provider or other practitioner recommends such use.
- If excessive dryness, marked peeling, some skin sloughing, erythema, or edema occur, use lower concentrations for shorter periods of time.
- If needed, apply cool compresses to relieve the discomfort of inflamed skin.
- Be aware that the product can bleach hair and fabrics.
- Do not be alarmed if transient stinging and burning occur unless the symptoms persist or become worse. If excessive stinging and burning occur after application, remove the preparation with soap and water; then wait until the next day to reapply.
- Avoid exposure to other sources of irritation, such as sunlamps or excessive time in the sun. If the patient will be exposed to the sun, allow the medication to dry and use a nonoil-based sunscreen with an SPF of 15 or greater.
- Recommended lifestyle modifications include washing the face in the morning and before bed, keeping cosmetic use to a minimum, switching to a noncomedogenic cosmetic, never opening whiteheads, and avoiding rubbing or touching the face throughout the day.
- Adhere to the treatment regimen for at least 4-6 weeks to see the full therapeutic effect.
- If improvement has not occurred after 6 weeks of treatment or if the adverse effects cause the patient to discontinue therapy, a medical referral should be made.
- Store product in a tightly closed container.

### Salicylic Acid

A mild comedolytic agent, salicylic acid is available in various nonprescription acne products in concentrations of 0.5% to 2%. It provides a milder, less effective alternative to the prescription agent tretinoin.[9] In cleansing preparations, salicylic acid is considered adjunctive treatment.

**TABLE 38-5 Comparison of Nonprescription Topical Acne Agents**

| | Benzoyl Peroxide | Salicylic Acid | Sulfur |
|---|---|---|---|
| Bactericidal | Yes | | |
| Keratolytic | | Yes | Yes |
| Comedolytic | | Yes | Yes |
| Concentration | 2.5%-20% | 0.5%-2% | 2%-10% |
| Frequency of use | 1-2 times daily | Used mainly as cleanser, then rinsed off | 1-3 times daily |
| Adverse effects | Bleached hair and clothing | Potent keratolytic at high concentration | Color, unpleasant odor |

*Source:* Adapted with permission from reference 12.

Pharmacologically, salicylic acid acts as a surface keratolytic.[3] Its safety, when used over large areas for prolonged periods of time (greater than 2 weeks), has been questioned; however, it presents minimal risk if gross skin disorders are not present.[17]

### Sulfur

Sulfur has met the criteria of FDA's Advisory Review Panel for Over-the-Counter Topical Acne Products, although the claim for its antibacterial effects was disallowed.[9] Sulfur, precipitated or colloidal, is included in acne products as a keratolytic and antibacterial in concentrations of 3% to 10%. It is generally accepted as effective in promoting the resolution of existing comedones, but, on continued use, may have a comedogenic effect. Alternative forms of sulfur, such as sodium thiosulfate, zinc sulfate, and zinc sulfide, are not recognized as safe and effective.

Sulfur-containing products are applied in a thin film to the affected area one to three times daily.[9] An esthetic consideration is that these products have a noticeable color and odor.

### Sulfur–Resorcinol Combination Products

Combinations of sulfur 3% to 8% with resorcinol 2%, which enhances the effect of the sulfur, are available in nonprescription acne products. The products function primarily as keratolytics, fostering cell turnover and desquamation. Resorcinol produces a reversible, dark brown scale on some darker-skinned individuals.

### Pharmacotherapeutic Comparison

See Table 38-5 for a comparison of the therapeutic properties among the major acne products.

### Product Selection Guidelines

Nonprescription medications for treating acne are applied topically. Because cosmetic appearance of the product may influence compliance, the patient's ability to adhere to long-term treatment is necessary for success.

Cleansing products (bars, liquids, suspensions, lotions, creams, gels, and pads/wipes) are not of much value because they leave little active ingredient residue on the skin. Lotions and creams with a low-fat content are intended to counteract drying (astringent effect) and peeling (keratolytic effect).[9] They are an acceptable alternative to the more effective gels and are recommended for dry or sensitive skin and for use during dry winter weather. Generally, gels are the most effective formulations because they are astringents and remain on the skin the longest. Nonfatty gels dry slowly if formulated in a completely aqueous base. Ethyl or isopropyl alcohol added to liquid preparations and gels hastens drying to a film. The drying effect of the volatile solvents may enhance effectiveness, but the greater irritant effect may be unacceptable to the patient.[9]

Solids in most preparations leave a film that is not noticeable and does not need coloring to blend in with the skin. Some products are intended to hide blemishes by depositing an opaque film of insoluble masking agents such as zinc oxide on the skin, but their tinting rarely produces a satisfactory color match.

In general, esthetic considerations of visibility suggest that cream formulations should be recommended for individuals with fair complexions and gels for those with dark complexions. Table 38-6 lists selected trade-name acne products in these and other formulations.

## *Complementary Therapies*

An interest in complementary and alternative medicine has given rise to many claims, and investigation continues into acne treatments not conforming to mainstream therapy. For example, topical nicotinamide (not commercially available) has been favorably compared as an alternative to topical clindamycin because it addresses concerns regarding the emergence of resistant microbial strains.[25] Acupuncture and hypnosis have also been reported to produce positive effects on select acne patients.[26-28]

With regard to herbal remedies, the Kampo formulations, or Japanese herbal medicines that are noncommercial combinations of powdered extracts of crude drugs, have received considerable attention as acne treatments. These products were found to have antibacterial activity against *P. acnes*.[28-30] Clinical trials of assorted Ayurvedic formulations showed a significant decrease in the number of acne lesions with the oral use of "Sunder Vati," a mixture of *Holarrhena antidysenterica, Emblica officinalis, Embelia ribes,* and *Zingiber officinale*.[29,32] Tea tree oil[28,32,33] and assorted other preparations derived from natural sources have also

**TABLE 38-6 Selected Acne Products**

| Trade Name | Primary Ingredients |
|---|---|
| **Benzoyl Peroxide Products** | |
| Benoxyl 5 Lotion | Benzoyl peroxide 5% |
| Clearasil Vanishing Acne Treatment Cream | Benzoyl peroxide 10% |
| Clear By Design Gel | Benzoyl peroxide 2.5% |
| Dryox Wash 10 Liquid | Benzoyl peroxide 10% |
| Oxy 10 Wash Solution | Benzoyl peroxide 10% |
| **Salicylic Acid Products** | |
| Clearasil Acne Defense Cleanser | Salicylic acid 2% |
| Clearasil Acne Defense Gel | Salicylic acid 2% |
| Clearasil Ice Wash Acne Fighting Gel | Salicylic acid 2% |
| PROPApH Acne Maximum Strength Cream | Salicylic acid 2% |
| Stri-Dex Alcohol Free Pads (Regular and Sensitive Skin) | Salicylic acid 0.5% |
| **Sulfur Products** | |
| Acne Lotion 10 | Sulfur 10% |
| Liquimat Lotion | Sulfur 4% |
| Sulmasque Mask | Sulfur 6.4% |
| Sulpho-Lac Acne Medication Cream | Sulfur 5% |
| Sulpho-Lac Soap | Sulfur 5% |
| **Combination Products** | |
| Acomel Cream | Sulfur 8%; resorcinol 2% |
| Dryox 10S 5 Gel | Benzoyl peroxide 10%; sulfur 5% |
| Dryox 20S 10 Gel | Benzoyl peroxide 20%; sulfur 10% |
| Stri-Dex Day and Night | Day gel, salicylic acid 2%; night lotion, benzoyl peroxide 2.5% |
| **Daily Skin Care Products** | |
| Clearasil Antibacterial Cleansing Soap | Triclosan 0.74% |
| Clearasil Daily Face Wash | Triclosan 0.3% |
| Stri-Dex Cooling Foaming Wash | Triclosan 1% |
| Stri-Dex Herbal Foaming Wash | Triclosan 1% |

been mentioned in recent literature.[34,35] (See Chapter 53 for further discussion of tea tree oil.)

Information and advice with respect to acne and its treatment is presented on Web sites such as www.holisticonline.com/Remedies/Acne.htm.[36]

## Assessment of Acne: A Case-based Approach

Patient assessment begins with asking questions to define the condition. Physical assessment, which involves observing the affected area and further questioning the patient, is the next step in evaluating the disorder. This evaluation helps determine whether the condition is acne vulgaris or another dermatologic condition with similar signs and symptoms. Physical assessment also determines whether the severity of the condition precludes self-treatment (Figure 38-2). Before self-care is recommended, an assessment of current medication use (prescription and nonprescription) is necessary to reveal prescribed treatments for the disorder or use of medications known to cause acne (Table 38-2). Cases 38-1 and 38-2 are provided to illustrate assessment of patients with acne.

## Patient Counseling for Acne

Before recommending self-treatment, the practitioner should evaluate the patient's maturity and willingness to comply with a skin care program that involves a continued daily regimen of washing affected areas and applying medication. The practitioner should clearly explain the basis for the recommended treatment. Comedonal and mild papular acne can usually be successfully self-treated. Patients who should not self-treat (Figure 38-2) should be

## CASE 38-1

| Relevant Evaluation Criteria | Scenario/Model Outcome |
|---|---|
| **Information Gathering** | |
| 1. Gather essential information about the patient's symptoms, including: | |
| a. description of symptom(s) (i.e., nature, onset, duration, severity, associated symptoms) | Patient has suffered from a skin disorder resembling noninflammatory acne that has worsened over the past year. Even though she has a dark complexion, her cheeks are red and rough with a number of lesions typical of closed comedones. Her face is sensitive to touch. Patient is self-conscious about appearance and would like to have a nonprescription acne product recommended. |
| b. description of any factors that seem to precipitate, exacerbate, and/or relieve the patient's symptom(s) | Symptoms seem to get worse before her menstrual period. She notices eye irritation about the same time. |
| c. description of the patient's efforts to relieve the symptoms | Washing regularly with soap and water has not helped to date. |
| 2. Gather essential patient history information: | |
| a. patient's identity | Claudia Smith |
| b. patient's age, sex, height, and weight | 34 y/o F, 5'6", 135 lb |
| c. patient's occupation | Financial advisor |
| d. patient's dietary habits | Balanced diet; occasional junk food and alcohol |
| e. patient's sleep habits | Averages 6-7 hours per night |
| f. concurrent medical conditions, prescription and nonprescription medications, and dietary supplements | Ortho Tri-Cyclen 1 tablet once daily beginning on day 1 of menstrual cycle; Tavist-D 1 tablet every 12 hours as needed stuffy nose. |
| g. allergies | NKA |
| h. history of other adverse reactions to medications | None |
| i. other (describe)______ | Claudia rarely had acne blemishes as a teenager. She uses makeup to cover the current blemishes. |
| **Assessment and Triage** | |
| 3. Differentiate the patient's signs/symptoms and correctly identify the patient's primary problem(s) (see Table 38-3). | Acnelike lesions that appear to be exacerbated by hormonal shift. Physical observation reveals a few small telangiectasias on patient's cheeks, which raises the possibility of rosacea. |
| 4. Identify exclusions for self-treatment (see Figure 38-2). | Onset well after adolescence and oral contraceptive use (may cause acne) |
| 5. Formulate a comprehensive list of therapeutic alternatives for the primary problem to determine if triage to a medical practitioner is required, and share this information with the patient. | Options include:<br>(1) Refer Claudia to a PCP or dermatologist for a differential diagnosis.<br>(2) Recommend an OTC acne product with lifestyle modifications.<br>(3) Take no action. |
| **Plan** | |
| 6. Select an optimal therapeutic alternative to address the patient's problem, taking into account patient preferences. | Refer the patient to a PCP or dermatologist for a differential diagnosis. |
| 7. Describe the recommended therapeutic approach to the patient. | N/A |

## CASE 38-1 (continued)

| Relevant Evaluation Criteria | Scenario/Model Outcome |
|---|---|
| 8. Explain to the patient the rationale for selecting the recommended therapeutic approach from the considered therapeutic alternatives. | You need to see a PCP or dermatologist is necessary because OTC acne therapy may not be appropriate. |
| **Patient Education** | |
| 9. When recommending self-care with nonprescription medications and/or nondrug therapy, convey accurate information to the patient. | Criterion does not apply in this case. |
| 10. Solicit follow-up questions from patient. | Is there an OTC medication that might work? |
| 11. Answer patient's questions. | No OTC medications are approved and/or appropriate to recommend without a definite diagnosis from a PCP or dermatologist. Patient also has a darker complexion and may have had rosacea for a longer period of time than suspected. Rosacea, left untreated, may cause delayed ocular complications. |

Key: N/A, not applicable; NKA, no known allergies; OTC, over-the-counter; PCP, primary care provider.

## CASE 38-2

| Relevant Evaluation Criteria | Scenario/Model Outcome |
|---|---|
| **Information Gathering** | |
| 1. Gather essential information about the patient's symptoms, including: | |
| a. description of symptom(s) (i.e., nature, onset, duration, severity, associated symptoms) | Patient has recently noticed five or so blackheads and red bumps around his lower jaw over the last few months. He shaves often and has not changed his shaving lotion, or his aftershave moisturizer products. He stated that he feels his skin is oily and dirty. He presents to your pharmacy for an OTC product that will help his acne problem. |
| b. description of any factors that seem to precipitate, exacerbate, and/or relieve the patient's symptom(s) | He started noticing the problem when the weather changed. It has been extremely hot and humid lately. |
| c. description of the patient's efforts to relieve the symptoms | Since he started to wash his face four times a day instead of twice a day, the problem has been getting worse. |
| 2. Gather essential patient history information: | |
| a. patient's identity | Barney Yarn |
| b. patient/s age, sex, height, and weight | 19 y/o M, 6'5", 200 lb |
| c. patient's occupation | Football player |
| d. patient's dietary habits | Balanced diet; occasional junk food and alcohol |
| e. patient's sleep habits | Averages 6 hours per night |
| f. concurrent medical conditions, prescription and nonprescription medications, and dietary supplements | Protein shake prior to practice |
| g. allergies | NKA |
| h. history of other adverse reactions to medications | None |

## CASE 38-2 (continued)

| Relevant Evaluation Criteria | Scenario/Model Outcome |
|---|---|
| i. other (describe)_______ | Barney notices that this is a seasonal problem, and his skin usually gets better during the winter. |
| **Assessment and Triage** | |
| 3. Differentiate the patient's signs/symptoms and correctly identify the patient's primary problem(s) (see Tables 38-1 and 38-3). | Acnelike lesions that appear to be exacerbated by environmental changes (heat and humidity). Patient is also a football player so it is very likely that he is outside often and may perspire during practice. |
| 4. Identify exclusions for self-treatment (see Figure 38-2). | None |
| 5. Formulate a comprehensive list of therapeutic alternatives for the primary problem to determine if triage to a medical practitioner is required, and share this information with the patient. | Options include:<br>(1) Refer Barney to a PCP or dermatologist for a differential diagnosis.<br>(2) Recommend an OTC acne product.<br>(3) Take no action. |
| **Plan** | |
| 6. Select an optimal therapeutic alternative to address the patient's problem, taking into account patient preferences. | Recommend an OTC product. |
| 7. Describe the recommended therapeutic approach to the patient. | Patient prefers sulfur-containing product because he has always used benzoyl peroxide and would like to try something different. |
| 8. Explain to the patient the rationale for selecting the recommended therapeutic approach from the considered therapeutic alternatives. | A PCP, that is, primary care provider, or dermatologist visit is not necessary because OTC acne therapy may be appropriate. |
| **Patient Education** | |
| 9. When recommending self-care with nonprescription medications and/or nondrug therapy, convey accurate information to the patient, including: | |
| a. appropriate dose and frequency of administration | See Table 38-5. |
| b. maximum number of days the therapy should be employed | If symptoms have not improved in 6 weeks, see PCP. |
| c. product administration procedures | Apply thin film to affected area. |
| d. expected time to onset of relief | 6 weeks |
| e. degree of relief that can be reasonably expected | Complete eradication of red papules may occur. Papules may reoccur, however, on continued long-term use and may have a comedogenic effect. |
| f. most common side effects | Noticeable color and odor |
| g. side effects that warrant medical intervention should they occur | With a sulfur-containing product, the patient may notice an odor and possibly dark brown scaling of the skin. |
| h. patient options in the event that condition worsens or persists | A PCP should be consulted if the condition does not improve or if irritation occurs. |
| i. product storage requirements | Store the product in a cool, dry place that is out of children's reach. |
| j. specific nondrug measures | Cleanse skin twice daily; avoid exacerbating factors; use oil-free products on hair and face; do not pick or squeeze the lesions. |
| 10. Solicit follow-up questions from patient. | Should I continue with my cleansing regimen? |

## CASE 38-2 (continued)

| Relevant Evaluation Criteria | Scenario/Model Outcome |
|---|---|
| 11. Answer patient's questions. | Since acne seemed to worsen with increased facial washing, it is best to reduce the frequency of washing to 2-3 times a day. Facial washing should be gentle with a mild soap. |

Key: NJA, no known allergies; OTC, over-the-counter; PCP, primary care provider.

## PATIENT EDUCATION FOR ACNE

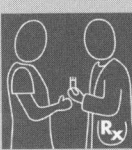


The goal of self-treatment is to control mild acne, thus preventing more serious forms from developing. Acne usually goes away on its own. Symptoms can usually be managed with diligent and long-term treatment. The best approaches to controlling acne are using cleansers and medications to keep the skin ducts and orifices open and avoiding situations that worsen acne. For most patients, carefully following product instructions and the self-care measures listed here will help ensure optimal therapeutic outcomes.

### Nondrug and Preventive Measures

- Cleanse skin thoroughly but gently at least twice daily to produce a mild drying effect that loosens comedones. Use a soft washcloth, warm water, and facial soap without moisturizing oils.
- To prevent or minimize acne flare-ups, avoid or reduce exposure to environmental factors, such as dirt, dust, petroleum products, cooking oils, or chemical irritants.
- To prevent friction or irritation that may cause acne flare-ups, do not wear tight-fitting clothes, headbands, or helmets; avoid resting the chin on the hand.To minimize acne related to cosmetic use, do not use oil-based cosmetics and shampoos.
- To prevent excessive hydration of the skin, which can cause flare-ups, avoid areas of high humidity and do not wear tight-fitting clothes that restrict air movement.
- Try to maintain a proper diet, although a link between diet and acne is unfounded.
- Avoid stressful situations. Stress may play a role in acne flare-ups, but it does not cause acne.
- Note that sexual activity plays no role in the occurrence or worsening of acne.

### Nonprescription Medications

- Keep all acne products away from eyes, eyelids, and mucous membranes.

#### *Benzoyl Peroxide*

- Benzoyl peroxide is the most effective and widely used nonprescription medication for treating acne. See Table 38-4 for administration guidelines and possible adverse effects.

#### *Salicylic Acid, Sulfur, and Sulfur–Resorcinol Combination Products*

- See Table 38-5 for administration guidelines and possible adverse effects of these agents.

encouraged to see a primary care provider, preferably a dermatologist.

Once the decision is made on which approach to recommend, the practitioner should explain acne as a medical condition, describe the treatment program, and correct any misconceptions the patient might have. The patient should be advised about scalp and hair care; the use of cosmetics; and, above all, the need for long-term, conscientious care. Also, the myths about acne being related to diet and sexual activity should be discounted. The box Patient Education for Acne lists specific information to provide patients. Because acne cannot be cured but only controlled, reassurance and emotional support are often necessary to reduce patient concern.

The Internet lists supplemental information about acne in lay language, including discussions of acne, nonprescription drugs used to treat it, and treatment expectations. Selected sites that appear to provide accurate information are listed in Table 38-7. If not copyrighted, these materials can be printed and given to the patient during the consultation. If the material is copyrighted, the practitioner should instead give the patient the Web site address.

**TABLE 38-7 Selected Web Sites for Acne Information**

www.aad.org
www.acne.org
www.derm-infonet.com/acnenet
www.facefacts.com
www.fda.gov
www.nlm.nih.gov/medlineplus/acne.html
www.rosacea.org
www.skincarephysicians.com/acnenet
www.holisticonline.com/Remedies/Acne.htm

## Evaluation of Patient Outcomes for Acne

Although the patient may expect complete resolution of the acne, an improvement in the disorder as defined by a decrease in both the number and severity of lesions is a more realistic expectation for effective self-treatment. The practitioner should determine whether patients whose acne shows no improvement after 6 weeks of self-treatment are following the recommended regimen. If they have been adherent, medical referral is appropriate. Patients who have not diligently followed the regimen should be encouraged to do so. The practitioner should again explain the expected results and the rigor with which treatment must be pursued. If some improvement is evident, the practitioner may suggest a monthly check on maintenance for improvement in the condition.

## Key Points for Acne

- Acne vulgaris occurs mainly in young adults from their early teens to their mid-20s and occasionally develops in prepubertal and older people.
- Acne cannot be cured, but it may be controlled enough to improve cosmetic appearance and prevent development of severe acne with resultant scarring.
- Minimizing environmental and physical factors that exacerbate acne can help prevent the condition.
- Patient pharmacologic and nonpharmacologic drug therapies should be individualized.
- Some people have chronic acne into adulthood and must care for their skin for a long time before improvement will occur.
- If given proper counseling, including empathy and reassurance, patients with acne may understand that the condition may not exist forever.

## References


1. Federman DG, Kirsner RS. Acne vulgaris: pathogenesis and therapeutic approach. *Am J Manage Care.* 2000;6:78-87.
2. Baldwin HE. The interaction between acne vulgaris and the psyche. *Cutis.*2002;70:133-9.
3. *Management of Acne.* Rockville, Md: Agency for Healthcare Research and Quality; 2001. AHRQ Pub No. 01-E018: Summary, evidence report/technology assessment: number 17.
4. Rudy SJ. Overview of the evaluation and management of acne vulgaris. *Pediatr Nurs.*2003;29:287-93.
5. Swanson JK. Antibiotic resistance of *Propionibacterium acnes* in acne vulgaris. *Dermatol Nurs.* 2003;15;359-62.
6. Cunliffe WJ, Holland DB, Clark SM, et al. Comedogenesis: some new aetiological, clinical and therapeutic strategies. *Br J Dermatol.* 2000;142:1084-91.
7. White GM. Recent findings in the epidemiologic evidence, classification, and subtypes of acne vulgaris. *J Am Acad Dermatol.* 1998; 39:S34-7.
8. Bello CE. Optimizing acne vulgaris treatment. *US Pharm.* April 2002;27:63-72.
9. Zouboulis CC, Bohm. Neuroendocrine regulation of sebocytes a pathogenic link between stress and acne. *Exp Dermatol.*2004; 13(suppl 4):31-5.
10. Burrall BA. Clinical Pearls from the Literature and Experience. Presented at: 59th Annual Meeting of the American Academy of Dermatology; March 2-7,2001; Washington, DC.
11. Allen LV. Secundum Artem. Available at: http://www.paddocklabs.com/secundum_artem.html. Accessed February 28, 2005.
12. Federman DG, Kirsner RS. Acne vulgaris: pathogenesis and therapeutic approach. *Am J Manage Care.* January 2000;6:78-87.
13. Thiboutot D. Acne 1991-2001. *J Am Acad Dermatol.* 2002;47:109-17.
14. National Rosacea Society. The faces of rosacea; Coping with rosacea. Available at: http://www.rosacea.org. Accessed March 3, 2003.
15. Blout BW, Pelletier AL. Rosacea: a common, yet commonly overlooked, condition. *Am Fam Phys.* August 1, 2002;66;435-40.
16. Johnson BA, Nunley JR. Topical therapy for acne vulgaris: how do you choose the best drug for each patient? *Postgrad Med.* 2000; 107:69-80.
17. Davis DA, Kraus AL, Thompson GA, et al. Percutaneous absorption of salicylic acid after repeated (14-day) in vivo administration to normal, acnegenic or aged human skin. *J Pharm Sci.* 1997; 86(8):896-9.
18. Nichols K, Desai N, Lebwohl MG. Effective sunscreen ingredients and cutaneous irritation in patients with rosacea. *Cutis.*1998;61: 344-6.
19. Koulianis GT. Treatment of acne with oral contraceptives: criteria for pill selection. *Cutis.* 2000;66:281-6.
20. Russell JJ. Topical therapy for acne. *Am Fam Phys.* 2000;6:357-66.
21. *Drug Facts and Comparisons.* St. Louis: Wolters Kluwer Health, Inc; 2003:1603-4.
22. Fluhr JW, Barsom O, Gehring W, et al. Antibacterial efficacy of benzoyl peroxide in phospholipid liposomes: a vehicle-controlled, comparative study in patients with papulopustular acne. *Dermatology.* 1999;198:273-7.
23. Patel VB, Misra AN, Marfatia YS. Preparation and comparative clinical evaluation of liposomal gel of benzoyl peroxide for acne. *Drug Dev Indust Pharm.* 2001;27:863-70.
24. Benzoyl peroxide carcinogenicity not shown in NDMA interim study results. *FDC Reports—The Tan Sheet.* 1999;7(11):13.
25. Livingstone C. Skin problems in pharmacy practice, part 2: acne. *Pharm J.* 1997;259:725-7.
26. Dai G. Advances in the acupuncture treatment of acne. *J Tradit Chin Med.* 1997;17:65-72.
27. Shenefelt PD. Hypnosis in dermatology. *Arch Dermatol.* 2000:136: 393-9.
28. Guyette JR, Rygwelski JM. Complementary or alternative medicine: therapies for common dermatologic conditions: atopic dermatitis, psoriasis, and acne. *Clin Fam Pract.* 2002;4:947-66.
29. Higaki S, Morimatsu S, Morohashi M, et al. Susceptibility of *Propionibacterium acnes,* Staphylococcus *aureus* and *Staphylococcus epidermidis* to 10 Kampo formulations. *J Int Med Res.* 1997;25:318-24.
30. Akamatsu H, Asada Y, Horio T. Effect of keigai-rengyo-to, a Japanese Kampo medicine, on neutrophil functions: a possible mechanism of action of keigyo-rengyo-to in acne. *J Int Med Res.* 1997;25:255-65.
31. *Sabinsa Corporation Newsletter.* January 2001. Available at: http://www.sabinsa.com/news/Jan2001.htm. Accessed July 12, 2003.
32. Combest WL. Tea tree. *US Pharm.* 24(4). Available at: http://www.uspharmacist.com/oldformat.asp?url=newlook/files/Alte/tea.cfm&pub_id+8&art. Accessed March 5, 2003.
33. Mantle D, Gok MA, Lennard TWJ. Adverse and beneficial effects of plant extracts on skin and skin disorders. *Adverse Drug React Toxicol Rev.* 2001:20:89-103.
34. Higaki S, Morimatsu S, Morohashi M, et al. The anti-lipase activity of shiunko on *Propionibacterium acnes. Int J Antimicrob Agents.* 1998;10:251-2.
35. Higaki S, Kitagawa T, Kagoura M, et al. Relationship between *Propionibacterium acnes* biotypes and Jumi-haidoku-to. *J Dermatol.* 2000;27:635-8.
36. Health Problems Knowledgebase. Conventional and holistic cures for acne. Available at: http://www.holisticonline.com/Remedies/Acne.htm. Accessed March 5, 2003.
37. Pray S, Pray J. Differentiating between rosacea and acne. *US Pharmacist.* 2004;29(4):11-12.
38. *Federal Register.* 2005;70:72447-8.

CHAPTER 39

# Prevention of Sun-induced Skin Disorders

*Dana G. Carroll and Kimberly M. Crosby*

Current research has demonstrated that exposure to ultraviolet radiation (UVR) is cumulative and can produce serious, long-term problems such as premature skin aging. In addition, cumulative exposure from childhood to adulthood, even without a serious sunburn, may predispose a person to develop precancerous and cancerous skin conditions. This fact is clear: avoiding excessive exposure to UVR will reduce the incidence of premature aging of the skin, skin cancer, and other long-term dermatologic effects.

The most common skin problem caused by UVR is sunburn. However, other conditions are either directly caused or exacerbated by UVR. These conditions include both drug and nondrug photosensitivity. Photodermatoses are idiopathic (self-originated) or exacerbated (photoaggravated) by radiation of varying wavelengths, including ultraviolet A (UVA) and some visible light. Ultraviolet B (UVB), however, is most often responsible for the reactions. More than 20 disorders are classified as photodermatoses (Table 39-1). Other UVR-induced disorders include premalignant actinic keratosis (which usually develops into squamous cell carcinoma if left untreated), keratoacanthoma, Kaposi's sarcoma, and malignant melanoma.

Along with the heightened awareness of the dangers of UVR has come a multitude of sunscreen (rather than suntan) products intended not only to help darken but also to protect the skin from the harmful effects of exposure to the sun. Applied properly, these products can block most of the sun's harmful UV rays. Unfortunately, the average consumer lacks sufficient understanding of both the process of tanning and the necessity of using sunscreens properly. There is a public health need for education about the safe and effective use of sunscreen and suntan products. To perform this function, health professionals should be aware of the hazards of UVR, as well as the criteria for selecting and properly using sunscreen products. Practitioners are encouraged to become involved in educational efforts to help minimize the morbidity and mortality associated with UVR exposure.

In 2000, the market for sun care products was $853 million, with sunscreen/sunblock products representing 65% of the total.[1] Although spending on sun care products continues to rise, there has been a slow but steady shift in sales from pharmacies to mass merchandisers.

**Editor's Note:** This chapter is based, in part, on the 14th edition chapter with the same title, which was written by Edward M. DeSimone II.

## Epidemiology of Sun-induced Skin Disorders

The four most common nondrug photodermatoses are polymorphous light eruption (PMLE), systemic lupus erythematosus (SLE), solar urticaria, and the porphyrias. PMLE appears to affect approximately 10% of the population, with a first occurrence usually before 30 years of age.[2] It affects women more often than men. In addition to the idiopathic photodermatoses, UVR can precipitate or exacerbate many photoaggravated dermatologic conditions, including herpes simplex labialis (cold sores), SLE and associated skin lesions, and chloasma, which may affect pregnant women and women taking oral contraceptives.

One of the other long-term hazards of UVR is premature photoaging of the skin.[3] It is now believed that 50% to 80% of all photodamage to the skin occurs by 20 years of age.[4]

Epidemiologic studies conducted since the 1950s demonstrate a strong relationship between chronic, excessive, and unprotected sun exposure and human skin cancer. Skin cancer is the most common type of cancer, accounting for approximately 50% of all malignancies.[5] About 80% of all skin cancers occur on the most exposed areas of the body, such as the face, head, neck, and back of the hands. It has been estimated that more than one million people are diagnosed with nonmelanoma skin cancer each year in the United States.[5]

The two most common types of nonmelanoma skin cancer (NMSC) are basal cell carcinoma (BCC) and squamous cell carcinoma (SCC). The majority of NMSCs break down into BCC (80%) and SCC (16%). These carcinomas grow and invade tissue relatively slowly (SCC is more likely to metastasize than BCC), and 95% to more than 99% are curable with early detection and treatment. In contrast, an estimated 59,600 new cases of malignant melanoma were expected to be diagnosed in 2005.[5] More than 70% of skin cancer-related deaths are from melanoma. It is estimated that 7800 deaths will be attributed to melanoma in the United States in 2005. Some of the risk factors for skin cancer include fair skin, a large number of melanocytic nevi (moles), large moles, a family history of moles, severe sunburns as a child, and excessive sun exposure or visits to a tanning salon.[5,6] One finding, also noted by Kricker and colleagues,[7] is the development of melanoma on any area of the body subjected to intense, intermittent sun exposure, such as the legs and trunk. It appears that an

**TABLE 39-1 Most Common Photodermatoses[2]**

| | |
|---|---|
| **Idiopathic Disorders** | |
| Actinic prurigo | Polymorphic light eruption |
| Chronic actinic dermatitis | Solar urticaria |
| **Photoaggravated Disorders** | |
| Acne vulgaris | Erythema multiforme |
| Atopic dermatitis | Herpes simplex labialis |
| Atopic eczema | Lichen planus |
| Bullous pemphigoid | Rosacea |
| Chloasma | Seborrheic dermatitis |
| Dermatomyositis | Systemic lupus erythematosus |
| Drug photosensitivity | |

increased (but modest) risk of developing melanoma exists if frequent sunburn episodes occur.

Research has shown that the type of skin cancer varies significantly according to the causes and contributing factors. For example, studies have shown conclusively that skin cancer occurs more often in light-skinned than dark-skinned individuals.[8] This is believed to occur because individuals with darker pigmentation have more melanin. Melanin absorbs UVR, thereby preventing the radiation from penetrating into the tissue. Accordingly, Gallagher and colleagues[9] reported the corroboration of other researchers in finding that individuals with blonde or red hair, a history of freckling, and light skin plus a tendency to burn rather than tan are at greater risk of developing SCC.

Another risk factor for developing skin cancer is a history of severe sunburn. Gallagher also reported that occupational sun exposure increases the risk of SCC, but only during the 10 years before the cancer develops. Another finding of this study—that lifetime or recreational UVR exposure had no effect—is contrary to current opinion. In a parallel study on BCC, however, Gallagher and others[10] reported an elevated risk from childhood (ages 5-15 years) sun exposure, but not from recreational exposure at other ages and no effect from occupational sun exposure. Freckling was shown to be a risk factor for both BCC and SCC. One implication from these data is that avoiding the sun as an adult may not alter the chances of developing BCC later in life. Kricker and others[7] reported no association between BCC and occupational sun exposure, but they did find an association with recreational exposure. Although follow-up studies need to be performed before a definitive relationship can be made between the type of sun exposure and the type of skin cancer, there is no question that skin cancer is linked to sun exposure.

Another factor affecting skin cancer has been generally accepted—its relationship to latitude. The incidence of skin cancer increases steadily in populations closer to the equator. The quantity of harmful UVR increases as the angle of the sun to the Earth approaches 90 degrees and the distance of the sun to Earth decreases.[11] People in the southern part of the United States are at greater risk from the harmful effects of UVR than are those in northern areas. A constant rate of increase in the incidence of skin cancer is found as one approaches the equator from north to south; the incidence approximately doubles for every 3 degree 48 minute decrease in latitude.[12] Also, the irradiance of UVB increases by 4% for every 1000 ft increase in altitude. This increase may be of particular concern to skiers and people who live and work in higher elevations.

## Etiology of Sun-induced Skin Disorders

Various bands of UVR cause or exacerbate sun-induced skin disorders. UVR is commonly referred to as UV light. However, *light* technically refers to only the visible spectrum; thus, the correct terminology in this context is *radiation.*

### *Bands of UVR*

The UV spectrum is divided into three major bands: ultraviolet C (UVC), UVB, and UVA.

#### UVC Radiation

The wavelength of UVC, also known as germicidal radiation, is within the 200 to 290 nm band. Little UVC radiation from the sun reaches Earth because it is screened out by the ozone layer of the upper atmosphere. However, UVC is emitted by some artificial sources of UVR, and most of the UVC that strikes the skin is absorbed by the dead cell layer of the stratum corneum.

#### UVB Radiation

The wavelength of the UVB band is between 290 and 320 nm. This is the most active UVR wavelength for producing erythema, which is why it is called sunburn radiation. The irradiance (i.e., intensity of the radiation reaching Earth) of UVB is most intense from 10 AM to 4 PM.

The only true therapeutic effect of UVB exposure is vitamin $D_3$ synthesis in the skin. Vitamin D deficiency does not seem to be a problem for infants who receive vitamin D-fortified milk. It may be a problem for chronic shut-ins or for persons of advanced age who spend little time outdoors if they do not receive adequate vitamin D in their diet or as a vitamin supplement, although a recent study casts doubt on this.[13] Vitamin D deficiency can be avoided in most individuals by 5 to 20 minutes of sunlight two to three times per week most months of the year.[14] Its therapeutic benefit notwithstanding, UVB is considered to be primarily responsible for inducing skin cancer, and its carcinogenic effects are believed to be augmented by UVA.[15] UVB is also primarily responsible for wrinkling, epidermal hyperplasia, elastosis, and collagen damage. However, UVA also contributes to premature aging of the skin.[16]

#### UVA Radiation

The wavelength of UVA radiation ranges from 320 to 400 nm. Although most concerns regarding the hazards of sun exposure to date have focused specifically on UVB, concern about the adverse effects of UVA has been slowly developing since the early 1980s. UVA radiation penetrates deeper into the skin than UVB, thereby having a greater effect on the dermis than on the epidermis. This deeper penetration can cause both histologic and vascular damage. Evidence suggests that subsequent UVA exposure may cause further and more serious acute and chronic damage to the underlying tissue than UVB exposure. In one study, UVA was found to cause sagging of the skin, thickening of the dermis and epidermis, and an increase in the activity of elastase.[17] It was believed previously that only UVB produced premature aging effects on the skin. Now UVA is believed to be involved in suppression of the immune system as well as in damage to DNA.[15,16] UVA radiation can trigger herpes simplex labialis. In addition, it can produce a photosensitivity reaction in patients who have ingested or applied photosensitizing agents.

The results of this research have caused some controversy about the relative importance of UVA effects on skin, compared with those of UVB. Although approximately 20 times more UVA than UVB reaches Earth at noon (30 times more in winter), erythemogenic activity is relatively weak in the UVA band, requiring up to 200 times more UVA energy than UVB energy.[18] In addition, the irradiance of UVA varies by a factor of 4 to 1 throughout the day and 3 to 1 from summer to winter; however, the significance of this variation is being debated.[18] UVA represents the wavelength in which most photosensitizing chemicals, such as 8-methoxypsoralen, are active. This activity is true throughout the UVA band, but especially above 360 nm.

### UVR in Tanning Booths and Sunbeds

Since 1980, manufacturers have shifted the composition of UVR emitted by tanning booths and sunbeds from UVB to UVA. The newer types of tanning devices use UVR sources consisting of more than 96% UVA and less than 4% UVB, a different mix of UVR than that obtained from natural sunlight.[19] Some tanning devices in commercial use emit UVA almost exclusively, although all of them contain a minimal amount of UVB, which is necessary to stimulate tanning. The emission spectrum of tanning devices varies significantly, and the user has no way of knowing the spectrum he or she is receiving.

UVA, if used properly, could generate a tan without producing an erythematous sunburn. However, a concern exists about the risk of skin cancer from sunlamp use. In addition, some UVA lamps produce more than five times as much UVA per unit of time than does sunlight.[20] A small but growing body of evidence suggests that the use of sunlamps (including tanning beds and booths) is related to the rising incidence of both malignant melanoma and nonmelanoma skin cancer worldwide.[21,22] Corroborating data may be insufficient because of a latent period between exposure and the development of skin cancer. In addition, consensus had not been reached on what biological endpoint should be used to assess the effects of sunlamps.[23] The effects of the transition to predominantly UVA sunlamps and sunbeds since 1980 may only now be surfacing.

Moreover, because UVA is less likely than UVB to produce erythema, patients may become complacent and forgo the use of eye goggles (although this is less likely today because of federal safety standards for commercial facilities). This practice will produce eye burns and may increase the risk of subsequently developing cataracts. In one study[24] on eye injuries from UV tanning devices, ophthalmologists treated 152 patients over a 12-month period for various ocular injuries, primarily of the cornea and retina. Only 24% of patients wore safety goggles while using the devices (see A Word about Sun-induced Ocular Damage in Chapter 28).The Food and Drug Administration (FDA) sets standards for sunlamp products and UV lamps.[25] These regulations deal with issues such as timers, exposure time, and device labeling, as well as the use of goggles with specified transmittance limits. Despite all FDA's precautions and warnings, however, its regulations do not include any specified limits on the amount of UVA and UVB emitted from tanning devices. The only requirement is that the ratio of UVB to UVA shall not exceed 0.05 (5%). Health care practitioners should advise patients that long-term hazards related to tanning devices have begun to surface and there are currently no accepted health benefits from these devices.

#### *Transmission/Reflection of UVR*

Contrary to popular opinion, cloud cover filters very little UVR. Seventy percent to 90% of UVR will penetrate clouds, depending on their density. Clouds tend to filter out the infrared radiation that contributes to the sensation of heat, creating a false sense of security against a burn.[26] Fresh snow reflects 85% to 100% of the light and radiation that strikes it, creating the need for sunglasses when skiing on a sunny day. This reflected radiation is also why a skier can receive a significant sunburn, even on a cloudy day, and thus should use a sunscreen. Similarly, sand and white-painted surfaces, although not as reflective as snow, reflect 10% to 15% of the radiation striking them.[27] A person sitting in the shade of a beach umbrella may still be bombarded by UVR reflecting off the sand. This reflection contributes to the overall radiation received, and a severe sunburn may result.

Water reflects no more than 5% of UVR, allowing the remaining 95% to penetrate and burn the swimmer. Therefore, time in the water, even if the swimmer is completely submerged, should be considered as part of the total time spent in the sun. In addition, although dry clothes reflect almost all UVR, wet clothes allow transmission of approximately 50% of UVR. However, if light passes through dry clothing when held up to the sun, UVR will also penetrate that clothing. Tightly woven material offers the greatest protection.

Although UVB does not penetrate window glass, UVA does.[28,29] A few automobile manufacturers have begun offering cars with glass that can reduce the amount of UVA penetration. This practice is not currently a standard for the industry. Therefore, patients sensitive to UVA (e.g., those with photodermatoses or those taking photosensitizing drugs) should use appropriate sunscreens even when driving with the window closed.

The Environmental Protection Agency (EPA) has developed a UV index that rates the amount of skin-damaging

**TABLE 39-2 Global Solar UV Index**[30]

| Rating Number | Interpretation of UVR Exposure Risk |
|---|---|
| 1-2 | Low |
| 3-5 | Moderate |
| 6-7 | High |
| 8-10 | Very high |
| 11+ | Extreme |

UVR reaching the Earth's surface at any instant in time. The higher the rating, the greater the risk of exposure (Table 39-2). UV index values in the United States are typically given for 12 noon, but it is important to remember that the UV index changes throughout the day. Factors that influence the UV index are time of day (midday has greater UVR exposure than early morning or late evening), ozone (a decreased ozone level increases UVR exposure), altitude (higher altitudes receive greater UVR exposure), season of year (UVR exposure is greater in spring and summer), surface (reflective surfaces increase UVR exposure), latitude (UVR exposure increases closer to the equator), and land cover (less tree cover increases UVR exposure).[30]

## Pathophysiology of Sun-induced Skin Disorders

### Sunburn and Suntan

The degree to which a person will develop a sunburn or a tan depends on several factors, including type and amount of radiation received, thickness of the epidermis and stratum corneum, skin pigmentation, skin hydration, and distribution and concentration of peripheral blood vessels.[31] Most UVR that strikes the skin is absorbed by the epidermis.

A sunburn involves a number of mediators, including histamine, lysosomal enzymes, kinins, and at least one prostaglandin. Such mediators produce peripheral vasodilatation as the UVR penetrates the epidermis; then an inflammatory reaction involving a lymphocytic infiltrate develops. Swelling of the endothelium and leakage of red blood cells from capillaries will also occur. Although the exact mechanism is not fully understood, it is believed that UVB radiation produces erythema by first damaging cellular DNA. The intensity of the UVB-induced erythema peaks at 12 to 24 hours after exposure.[31]

A tan is produced when UVR stimulates the melanocytes in the germinating skin layer to generate more melanin and UVR oxidizes the melanin already in the epidermis. Both processes serve as protective mechanisms by diffusing and absorbing additional UVR. Although UVB and UVA contribute to the tanning process, they induce pigmentation by different mechanisms. UVB acts by stimulating epidermal hyperplasia as well as shifting melanin up through the skin. UVA acts by increasing the total amount of melanin in the basal layer. Because of the location of melanin in each case, greater photoprotection from UVB-induced pigmentation is available than from UVA-induced pigmentation. UVA produces a tan through two processes. The first process is known as immediate pigment darkening, which involves photo-oxidation of existing melanin. It begins to be visible from 5 to 10 minutes after exposure and reaches its maximum effect in 60 to 90 minutes. The effects of immediate pigment darkening begin to fade quickly and may be gone within 24 hours. The second process is delayed tanning, or melanogenesis, which involves an increase in the number and size of melanocytes, as well as in the number of melanosomes or pigment granules produced by melanocytes. This delayed tanning contributes to the development of a slow natural tan.

### Drug Photosensitivity

Photosensitivity encompasses two types of conditions: photoallergy and phototoxicity. Drug photoallergy, a relatively uncommon immunologic response, involves an increased, chemically induced reactivity of the skin to UVR and/or visible light. UVR (primarily UVA) triggers an antigenic reaction in the skin. This reaction, which is not dose related, is usually seen after at least one prior exposure to the involved chemical agent or drug.

Phototoxicity is an increased, chemically induced reactivity of the skin to UVR and/or visible light. However, this reaction is not immunologic. It is often seen on first exposure to a chemical agent or drug, is dose related, and usually exhibits no drug cross-sensitivity. Some drugs associated with phototoxicity are tetracyclines (especially demeclocycline), sulfonamides, antineoplastics (e.g., 5-fluorouracil), hypoglycemics, thiazides, phenothiazines (especially chlorpromazine), and the psoralens (Table 39-3). This type of reaction is not limited to drugs but is also associated with plants, cosmetics, and soaps.

### Photodermatoses

Each of the more than 20 photodermatoses presents with a distinct morphology. The common factor in each of these is the development or exacerbation of signs and symptoms after exposure to UVR. This disorder usually occurs when the sap of plants (containing furanocoumarins) is bruised by high-speed weed-cutting machines (used by many homeowners), and gets on the skin; the skin is then struck by UVR. The only protection is to cover the skin with clothing before using such equipment.

### Photoaging

Photoaging, also known as premature skin aging, is genetically influenced. For example, whites are more susceptible than blacks. It is called photoaging because the obvious physical findings are similar to those seen in natural aging although there are significant histologic and biochemical differences.

### Skin Cancer

Basal cell carcinoma is often an aggressive, invasive disorder of the epidermis and dermis, and can cause serious damage to the skin and underlying tissue. However, it

**TABLE 39-3 Selected Groups of Medications Associated With Photosensitivity Reactions**

**Antidepressants**
Amitriptyline
Amoxapine
Bupropion
Citalopram
Clomipramine
Desipramine
Doxepin
Fluoxetine
Fluvoxamine
Imipramine
Maprotiline
Mirtazapine
Nefazodone
Nortriptyline
Paroxetine
Sertraline
Trazodone
Trimipramine
Venlafaxine

**Antihistamines**
Astemizole
Azatadine
Brompheniramine
Cetirizine
Chlorpheniramine
Cyproheptadine
Diphenhydramine
Loratadine
Promethazine
Terfenadine

**Antihypertensives**
Benazepril
Captopril
Diltiazem
Enalapril
Hydralazine
Labetalol
Lisinopril
Methyldopa
Minoxidil
Nifedipine
Ramipril
Sotalol
Quinapril

**Antipsychotics/Phenothiazines**
Alprazolam
Chlordiazepoxide
Chlorpromazine
Clozapine
Fluphenazine
Haloperidol
Loxapine
Olanzapine
Perphenazine
Prochlorperazine
Quetiapine
Risperidone
Thioridazine
Thiothixene
Trifluoperazine
Triflupromazine
Ziprasidone
Zolpidem

**Coal Tar and Derivatives**
Denorex Medicated Shampoo
DHS Tar Gel Shampoo
Doak Tar Shampoo
Estar Gel
Ionil T Plus Shampoo
Neutrogena T/Derm Body Oil
Neutrogena T/Gel Extra Strength Therapeutic Shampoo
Tegrin Shampoo
Zetar Shampoo

**Diuretics (Thiazides)**
Chlorothiazide
Chlorthalidone
Hydrochlorothiazide
Hydroflumethiazide
Indapamide
Methyclothiazide
Trichlormethiazide

**Diuretics (Other)**
Acetazolamide
Amiloride
Furosemide
Metolazone
Triamterene

**Estrogens/Progestins**
*Estrogens*
Chlorotrianisene
Diethylstilbestrol
Estradiol
Estrogens, conjugated
Estrogens, esterified
Estropipate
Ethinyl estradiol
Megestrol
*Progestins*
Medroxyprogesterone
Norethindrone
Norgestrel

**Hypoglycemics**
Acetohexamide
Chlorpropamide
Glimepiride
Glipizide
Glyburide
Tolazamide
Tolbutamide

**Nonsteroidal Anti-inflammatory Drugs**
Celecoxib
Diclofenac
Diflunisal
Etodolac
Fenoprofen
Flurbiprofen
Ibuprofen
Indomethacin
Ketoprofen
Meloxicam
Nabumetone
Naproxen
Oxaprozin
Piroxicam
Sulindac

**Psoralens**
Methoxsalen
Trioxsalen

**Sulfonamides**
Sulfadiazine
Sulfamethizole
Sulfamethoxazole
Sulfapyridine
Sulfasalazine
Sulfinpyrazone
Sulfisoxazole

**Dietary Supplements and Vitamins**
Bitter Orange
Chlorella
Dong Quai
Gossypol
Gotu Kola
St. Johns Wort
Vitamin A
Vitamin B

**Tetracyclines**
Doxycycline
Minocycline
Oxytetracycline
Tetracycline

**Other Agents**
*Anticancer Drugs*
Bexarotene
Capecitabine
Dacarbazine
Daunorubicin
Epirubicin
Fluorouracil
Flutamide
Interferon-α
Methotrexate
Pentostatin
Procarbazine
Thalidomide
Tretinoin
Vinblastine
*Anti-infectives (Other)*
Azithromycin
Capreomycin
Ceftazidime
Chlorhexidine
Ciprofloxacin
Dapsone
Flucytosine
Gemifloxacin
Gentamicin
Griseofulvin
Itraconazole
Ketoconazole
Levofloxacin
Metronidazole
Moxifloxacin
Nalidixic acid
Norfloxacin
Ofloxacin
Pyrazinamide
Ritonavir
Saquinavir
Sulfonamides
Trimethoprim
Trovafloxacin
Zalcitabine
*Antiparasitics*
Bithionol
Chloroquine
Quinine
Thiabendazole

**Sunscreens**
Aminobenzoic acid
Aminobenzoic acid esters
Benzophenones
Cinnamates
Homosalate
Menthyl anthranilate
Oxybenzone

**Miscellaneous**
Amiodarone (antiarrhythmic)
Benzocaine (local anesthetic)
Benzoyl peroxide
Carbamazepine (anticonvulsant)
Cyclobenzaprine (muscle relaxant)
Dantrolene (muscle relaxant)
Disopyramide (antiarrhythmic)
Etretinate (antipsoriatic)
Felbamate (anticonvulsant)
Fenofibrate (antihyperlipidemic)
Fluvastatin (antihyperlipidemic)
Gabapentin (anticonvulsant)
Gold salts (antiarthritic)
Isotretinoin (antiacne)
Lamotrigine (anticonvulsant)
Lovastatin (antihyperlipidemic)
Nabilone (antiemetic)
Phenytoin (anticonvulsant)
Pravastatin (antihyperlipidemic)
Quinidine sulfate (antiarrhythmic)
Selegiline (antiparkinsonism)
Simvastatin (antihyperlipidemic)
Sumatriptan (antimigraine)
Topiramate (anticonvulsant)
Valproic Acid (anticonvulsant)

*Source:* Albrant DH, ed. *The American Pharmaceutical Association Drug Treatment Protocols*. Washington, DC: American Pharmaceutical Association; 1999:417; *Med Lett*. 1993;37:946; *Medications That Increase Sensitivity to Light: A 1990 Listing*. FDA Pub No. 91-8280. Washington, DC: US Department of Health and Human Services, Public Health Service; 1995; *E Facts*. Wolters Kluwer Health, Inc: 2003-2004; *Prescriber's Lett*. 2004;20:200509; MICROMEDEX® Healthcare Series, Thomson MICROMEDEX, Greenwood Village, Colo.

rarely metastasizes. Squamous cell carcinoma is found in epithelial keratinocytes and grows very slowly. Melanoma exhibits a pathophysiology different from the NMSCs. Though most melanomas come from normal skin, about 30% arise from existing nevi. Initially, the melanoma grows horizontally across the skin. It then begins to grow vertically into deeper tissue, which explains the high percentage of metastasis associated with this condition. Because there are few melanocytes in the lips, they tend to burn rather than tan. Any growth on the lips should be suspected to be skin cancer.

## Signs and Symptoms of Sun-induced Skin Disorders

### *Sunburn*

Sunburn is, in fact, a burn. It is most often seen as a first-degree (superficial) burn, with a reaction ranging from mild erythema to tenderness, pain, and edema (see Color Plates, photograph 26). Severe reactions to excessive UVR exposure can sometimes produce a second-degree burn, with the development of vesicles (blisters) or bullae (many large blisters), as well as fever, chills, weakness, and shock. Shock caused by heat prostration or hyperpyrexia can lead to death. (See Chapter 41 for treatment of sunburn.)

### *Drug Photosensitivity*

Drug photoallergy presents like allergic contact dermatitis (e.g., poison ivy) and is characterized by pruritus with erythematous papules, vesicles, bullae, and/or urticaria (see Color Plates, photograph 27). Phototoxicity is most likely to appear as an exaggerated sunburn with pruritis.[2] Urticaria may also occur (see Color Plates, photograph 28).

### *Photodermatoses*

Each of these disorders has a unique morphology. PMLE, alone, can have multiple morphologic presentations of pruritus with papules, vesicles, plaques, and/or urticaria.

### *Photoaging*

This condition is characterized by wrinkling and yellowing of the skin. Conclusive evidence reveals that prolonged exposure to UVR results in elastosis (degeneration of the skin caused by a breakdown of the skin's elastic fibers). Pronounced drying, thickening, and wrinkling of the skin may also result.[4] Other physical changes include cracking, telangiectasia (spider vessels), solar keratoses (growths), and ecchymoses (subcutaneous hemorrhagic lesions).[3] (See Chapter 40 for measures for reversing photoaging.)

### *Skin Cancer*

Basal cell carcinoma is a translucent nodule with a smooth surface. It is usually firm to the touch and may be ulcerated or crusted. It is generally found as an isolated lesion on the nose or other parts of the face, although multiple lesions are sometimes found. Squamous cell carcinoma, on the other hand, is a slow-growing, isolated papule or plaque on sun-exposed areas of the body.

Self-examination for melanoma uses four factors ("A-B-C-D") for evaluation: *a*symmetric shape, *b*order irregularity or poorly defined border, *c*olor variation within the same mole or a change in color, and *d*iameter larger than 6 mm. A mole with these characteristics and any new growth or change in appearance of the skin (including the lips) should be evaluated by a dermatologist.

## Prevention of Sun-induced Skin Disorders

The short-term goals in preventing sun-induced skin disorders are relatively simple: avoiding or minimizing sunburn, photosensitivity reactions, and UVR-induced or exacerbated photodermatoses. The expected long-term outcomes are prevention of skin cancer and avoidance of photoaging of the skin.

UVR-induced skin disorders can be prevented by minimizing exposure to UVR and using sunscreen agents. The selection of a sunscreen product and the degree of protection varies, depending on the patient's intended use for the product, as well as the conditions under which the product will be used (Figure 39-1).

The greater the risk a patient has of developing a UVR-induced skin disorder, the greater the need to avoid sun exposure. However, most people do not spend warm, sunny July afternoons sitting inside, nor do they go to the beach or pool wearing lots of clothing. Practitioners can assist the patient in striking a balance between totally avoiding sun exposure, wearing protective clothing, and using sunscreen products. If, however, the patient suffers from a UVR-induced skin disorder, such as SLE, few options are available. In regard to preventing sunburn, the patient's natural skin type will be the primary factor in deciding the potency of the sunscreen product to be used. The lighter the natural skin color is (and the more quickly a burn develops), the higher the required potency of the sunscreen product.

### *Avoidance of Sun Exposure*

Complete avoidance of UVR, although unrealistic, is often the best approach for patients who have physical characteristics or history listed in Table 39-4. For patients who refuse to stay indoors or who must be outdoors for extended periods, the use of protective clothing such as a hat with a 4-inch brim, long pants, and a long-sleeved shirt should be recommended. In situations in which the patient is unwilling or unable to avoid the sun or to wear protective clothing, the next best choice is to use a sunscreen product.

### *Use of Sunscreens*

The Advisory Review Panel on Topical Analgesic, Antirheumatic, Otic, Burn, and Sunburn Prevention and Treatment Drug Products issued the advanced notice of proposal rule-making on over-the-counter (OTC) sunscreen agents in 1978.[32] Because of the number of responses and significant new developments in the area of photobiology,

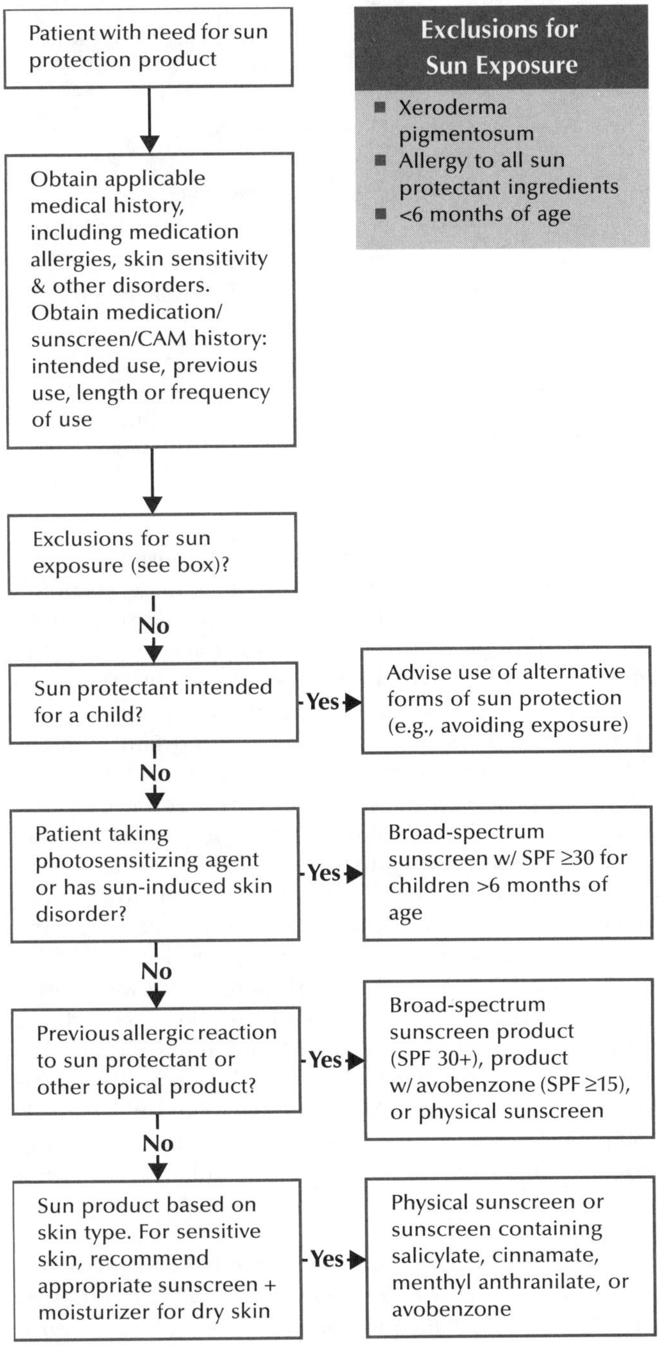


**FIGURE 39-1** Self-care for sun protection. Key: CAM, complementary and alternative medicine; SPF, sun protection factor.

the FDA delayed issuing guidelines on sunscreen products for 15 years. In May 1993, the FDA published the tentative final monograph.[33] The final monograph (FM) was published in 1999 with the new rules scheduled to become effective May 21, 2000 and May 21, 2001.[34] However, several key issues such as UVA protection factors and professional labeling were not addressed because they remain under review by the agency. On December 31, 2001, FDA stayed the implementation date until May 16, 2005.[35] In the September 3, 2004, issue of the *Federal Register,* FDA announced

**TABLE 39-4 Patient Risk Factors for Development of UVR-induced Problems**

| |
|---|
| Fair skin that always burns and never tans |
| A history of one or more serious or blistering sunburns |
| Blonde or red hair |
| Blue, green, or gray eyes |
| A history of freckling |
| A previous growth on the skin or lips caused by UVR exposure |
| The existence of a UVR-induced disorder |
| A family history of melanoma |
| Current use of an immunosuppressive drug |
| Current use of a photosensitizing drug |
| Excessive lifetime exposure to UVR, including tanning beds and booths |
| Xeroderma pigmentosum, a rare genetic disorder |

Key: UVR, ultraviolet radiation.

a delay in the May 16, 2005, implementation date of the drug facts rule as it applies to nonprescription sunscreen drug products. The agency intends to propose an amendment to the FM for sunscreen drug products to modify the labeling requirements; completion of the amendment process is projected to occur shortly after May 16, 2005.[36] The Cosmetic, Toiletry and Fragrance Association "strongly supports" FDA's indefinite extension of implementation date for drug facts labeling rule to avoid manufacturers having to make label changes twice in a short period. The delay in compliance date remains in effect until the amended FM is published providing a new compliance date or FDA issues further notice.[37] At the time of publication, FDA had not issued any notice for change or published an amendment.

### Labeled Uses

The FM allows only the term *uses*—not *indications*—on sunscreen labels and approves only two uses: protection (minimal/moderate/high) against sunburn and tanning. The degree of protection is related to the sun protection factor (SPF) of a sunscreen.

### Sunscreen Efficacy

Purchasers of sunscreens are usually familiar with SPF, one parameter for determining the effectiveness of sunscreens for UVB protection. Another parameter, minimal erythema dose (MED), is used to calculate the sunscreen's SPF. No comparable index of protection for UVA radiation has been developed.

*Minimal Erythema Dose* The MED is defined as the "minimum UVR dose that produces clearly marginated erythema in the irradiated site, given as a single exposure."[31] It is a dose of radiation and not a grade of erythema. Generally, 2 MEDs will produce a bright erythema, 4 MEDs a painful sunburn, and 8 MEDs a blistering burn.

**TABLE 39-5 Product Category Designations**

| SPF | Category Designation |
|---|---|
| 2 to ≤12 | Minimal sunburn protection |
| 12 to ≤30 | Moderate sunburn protection |
| 30+ | High sunburn protection |

Key: SPF, sun protection factor.
*Source:* Adapted from reference 34.

However, because of variations in thickness of the stratum corneum, different parts of the body may respond differently to the same MED. Further, the MED for heavily pigmented blacks is estimated to be 33 times higher than that for lightly pigmented whites.

*Sun Protection Factor* The important measure for sunscreens is the SPF, derived by dividing the MED on protected skin by the MED on unprotected skin. For example, if a person requires 25 mJ/cm$^2$ of UVB radiation to experience 1 MED on unprotected skin and requires 250 mJ/cm$^2$ of radiation to produce 1 MED after applying a given sunscreen, the product would be given an SPF rating of 10. The higher the SPF, the more effective the agent is in preventing sunburn. If it normally takes 60 minutes for someone to experience 2 MEDs (a bright erythematous sunburn), a sunscreen with an SPF of 6 will allow that person to stay in the sun six times longer (or 6 hours) before receiving this same sunburn (assuming the sunscreen is reapplied at the recommended intervals). The SPF is product specific because it is calculated on the basis of the final formulation of the product and cannot be determined on the basis of the active ingredient alone.

The FDA reduced the original five SPF categories to three (Table 39-5) and eliminated designation of a skin type for each category. Manufacturers use the classification system in Table 39-6 to select test subjects for general testing procedures for sunscreens. However, this system is not allowed on product labeling.

Setting a maximum SPF of 30 for all commercial sunscreen products will affect the greatest number of sunscreen uses; it is the most controversial change in the FM. Since 1978, SPFs have climbed to a high of 50, triggering debate about whether products with an SPF greater than 30 offer any advantage to users. For example, a product with an SPF of 15 blocks out 93% of UVB. Raising the SPF to 30 increases UVB protection to only 96.7%, and an SPF of 40 blocks out 97.5%.[31] A hypothetical SPF of 70 would increase UVB protection to only 98.6%.[33]

The small gain in protection made when SPF is increased from 30 to 40 may require up to 25% more sunscreen ingredients, which could increase the possibility of systemic and local adverse effects, as well as significantly increasing product cost. However, some researchers argue in favor of no SPF limits for medical reasons. Patients with SLE and other lupus-related disorders require a minimum SPF of 40 to prevent triggering the disease.[33] FDA has recognized that patients taking photosensitizing drugs may require an SPF of 45 to provide adequate protection.[33]

**TABLE 39-6 Sunburn and Tanning History***

| Skin Type | Sunburn/Tanning History |
|---|---|
| I | Always burns easily; never tans (sensitive) |
| II | Always burns easily; tans minimally (sensitive) |
| III | Burns moderately; tans gradually (normal) |
| IV | Burns minimally; always tans well (normal) |
| V | Rarely burns; tans profusely (insensitive) |
| VI | Never burns; deeply pigmented (insensitive) |

* Used for selection of test subjects for general testing procedures and is not to be used as part of any sunscreen label.
*Source:* Adapted from reference 34.

FDA responded that an SPF of 30 provides adequate protection for all skin types, including patients with UVR-induced disorders. When one determines protection from photosensitivity, the wavelength at which the product absorbs or reflects the UVR is more important than the SPF. For example, no evidence exists that an SPF of 40 will protect against photosensitivity if the reaction is triggered at 370 nm and if the product absorbs only up to 340 nm.

The question remains as to whether an SPF of 30 provides adequate protection for all individuals and whether the risks of higher SPF products outweigh the benefits. Because actinic keratoses can develop into SCCs, the implication is that regular sunscreen use will reduce the incidence of such cancers. FDA has acknowledged that a sunscreen with an SPF greater than 30 may be of some benefit. As a compromise for the time being, products with an SPF greater than 30 may be marketed but can have only "30 plus" or "30+" on the label. However, the FM labeling rules no longer allow use of the term "sunblock," although it has been a common labeling claim for many years.

*Measures of UVA Protection* With concern growing about the long-term adverse effects of UVA, the utility of the SPF value has been questioned. SPF provides a measure of a patient's erythemogenic response to UVB when using a sunscreen. However, UVA is at least 200 times less potent than UVB in producing erythema, and its effects on the skin are somewhat different from those produced by UVB.[18] Investigations have shown that sunscreens with similar SPFs demonstrate significant differences in their abilities to protect against UVR-induced immunologic injury to the skin.[38] Data suggest that high SPF products block significant amounts of UVA. However, among products of equal SPF, UVA blockage may vary considerably. SPF is not a reliable measure of UVA protection.[39,40] As a temporary measure, FDA has extended the rule that allows a product to make a claim of UVA protection as long as the ingredients have an absorption spectrum that extends to at least 360 nm.[33]

One area of considerable discussion and debate is how best to measure UVA protection. FDA received many comments and proposals in this regard. The key is to create an index of protection analogous to the SPF. FDA stated that the various UVA protection factors being proposed by sunscreen manufacturers are not yet "meaningful."[33] Although it has issued an FM on sunscreen products, FDA did not address the important issue of UVA, which will be dealt with in the future.

*Substantivity* The efficacy of a sunscreen is also related to its substantivity—that is, its ability to remain effective during prolonged exercising, sweating, and swimming. This property can be a function of the active sunscreen, the vehicle, or both. Generally speaking, products with cream-based (water in oil) vehicles appear more resistant to removal by water than those with alcohol bases, and will reduce desquamation of the skin. Also, part of a sunscreen's effectiveness may relate to the ability of the active agent to bind with constituents of the skin. This binding characteristic may be independent of the vehicle. Oil-based products have traditionally been the most popular and are easiest to apply. However, they tend to have lower SPF values.

FM requirements for sunscreen product substantivity related to sweating, perspiring, or participating in water activities are as follows:

- *Water resistant:* product retains its SPF for at least 40 minutes.
- *Very water resistant:* product retains its sun protection for at least 80 minutes.

The category of *very water resistant* is intended to replace *waterproof.* This terminology is one of the areas in which manufacturers do not agree with FDA (they prefer waterproof). The FM does not allow for the use of labeling that claims a specific number of hours of protection or "all-day protection." The only allowed labeling will be "Higher SPF gives more sunburn protection."

### Mechanism of Action

The mechanism of action of sunscreens is related to the definitions for the two therapeutic sunscreen types:[33]

1. *Sunscreen active ingredient:* An active ingredient absorbs at least 85% of the radiation in the UV range at wavelengths from 290 to 320 nm but may or may not allow transmission of radiation to the skin at wavelengths longer than 320 nm.
2. *Sunscreen opaque sunblock:* An opaque sunscreen active ingredient reflects or scatters all light in the UV and visible range at wavelengths from 290 to 777 nm, thereby preventing or minimizing suntan and sunburn.

### Types of Sunscreens

According to the therapeutic definitions, topical sunscreens can be divided into two major subgroups: chemical and physical. Chemical sunscreens work by absorbing and thus blocking the transmission of UVR to the epidermis. Physical sunscreens are generally opaque, and act by reflecting and scattering UVR rather than absorbing it.

The FM lists 14 chemical agents and two physical agents as safe and effective for use as sunscreens. Table 39-7 lists these agents, their UVR absorbance range, and their maximum concentrations. Because the SPF is product specific and does not depend on the sunscreen's active agent alone, the FM has eliminated a required minimum strength for sunscreens that contain a single active ingredient. (See Table 39-8 for examples of trade-name products.)

Two other agents may be approved for use in sunscreen products on the basis of time and extent applications. In the December 5, 2005, *Federal Register,* FDA requested safety and effectiveness data for bisoctrizole, up to 10%, and bemotrizinol, up to 10%, as single and combination active sunscreen ingredients.[41] FDA will evaluate submitted information to determine whether these agents can be generally recognized as safe and effective. March 6, 2006, is the deadline for comments. There also is a new ingredient for sunscreens, octyl triazone, that has not been approved by the FDA for use in the United States at the time of this publication. It is being used in other countries though. Octyl triazone is a polymer that is designed to enhance other sunscreen active ingredients capacity to protect against UVA and UVB radiation. Some studies have shown increases in SPF's by up to 70% when octyl triazone is added to other chemical sunscreen agents.[42]

*Aminobenzoic Acid and Derivatives* Because of the continuing confusion about the name of this sunscreen, the FM requires that product labels list it as aminobenzoic acid (formerly para-aminobenzoic acid [PABA]) and that each time this name appears on product labeling, it shall be followed by "(PABA)" so consumers know which chemical entity they are using. Aminobenzoic acid was once the most widely used sunscreen agent. Because it has been shown to be a major sensitizer, it has been replaced by other agents.

However, aminobenzoic acid is an effective UVB sunscreen, especially when formulated in a hydroalcoholic base (maximum of 50% to 60% alcohol). The SPF of such formulations increases proportionally as the concentration of aminobenzoic acid increases from 2% to 5%. One advantage of this agent is its ability to penetrate into the horny layer of the skin and provide lasting protection. It has significant substantivity on sweating skin, although not as much on skin that is immersed in water. The primary advantage of aminobenzoic acid derivatives over aminobenzoic acid itself is that the derivatives do not stain clothing. The only Category I derivative is padimate O.

The disadvantages of alcoholic solutions of aminobenzoic acid include contact dermatitis, photosensitivity, stinging and drying of the skin, and yellow staining of clothes on exposure to the sun. Patients who have experienced a photosensitivity reaction to a sunscreen product containing aminobenzoic acid or any of its derivatives should avoid using such products.

*Anthranilates* The anthranilates are ortho-aminobenzoic acid derivatives. Menthyl anthranilate, the menthyl ester of anthranilic acid, is a weak UV sunscreen with maximal absorbance in the UVA range. It is usually found in combination with other sunscreen agents to provide broader UV coverage.

**TABLE 39-7 Sunscreens Considered to Be Safe and Effective**

| Sunscreen Agent | Absorbance Range (Maximum Range) (nm) | Approved Maximum Concentration (%) |
|---|---|---|
| **ABA and Derivatives** | | |
| Aminobenzoic acid* | 260-313 (288.5) | 15 |
| Padimate O | 290-315 (310) | 8 |
| **Anthranilates** | | |
| Menthyl anthranilate (meradimate) | 260-380† (340†) | 5 |
| **Benzophenones** | | |
| Dioxybenzone | 260-380‡ (282§) | 3 |
| Oxybenzone | 270-350 (290‖) | 6 |
| Sulisobenzone | 260-375 (285¶) | 10 |
| **Cinnamates** | | |
| Cinoxate | 270-328 (310) | 3 |
| Octyl methoxycinnamate (octinoxate) | 290-320 (308-310) | 7.5 |
| Octocrylene | 250-360 (303) | 10 |
| **Dibenzoylmethane Derivatives** | | |
| Avobenzone# | 320-400 (360) | 3 |
| **Salicylates** | | |
| Octyl salicylate (octisalate) | 280-320 (305) | 5 |
| Homosalate | 295-315 (306) | 15 |
| Trolamine salicylate | 260-320 (298) | 12 |
| **Miscellaneous** | | |
| Phenyl benzimidazole sulfonic acid (ensulizole) | 290-320 (302) | 4 |
| Titanium dioxide** | 290-770 (—) | 25 |
| Zinc oxide** | 290-770 (—) | 25 |

Key: ABA, aminobenzoic acid.

* Formerly called para-aminobenzoic acid (PABA).

† Values are for concentrations higher than those normally found in nonprescription drugs.

‡ Values are achieved when used in combination with other sunscreen agents.

§ Second peak occurs at 217 nm.

‖ Second peak occurs at 329 nm.

¶ Second peak occurs at 324 nm.

\# Agent is currently marketed through a new drug application.

**Agent scatters, rather than absorbs, radiation in the 290 to 770 nm range.

*Source:* References 43-46; Shaath NA. Encyclopedia of UV absorbers for sunscreen products. *Cosmetic Toiletries*. 1987;102: 21-36.

*Benzophenones* Three agents are in the benzophenone group: dioxybenzone, oxybenzone (benzophenone-3), and sulisobenzone (benzophenone-4). As a group, these agents are primarily UVB absorbers, with maximum absorbance between 282 and 290 nm. However, their absorbance extends well into the UVA range, with oxybenzone up to 350 nm and dioxybenzone up to 380 nm. Because of the possibility of allergic reactions to aminobenzoic acid and its derivatives, many sunscreen products now contain benzophenones in their formulations because of the broader spectrum of action. Oxybenzone, also found in some cosmetic formulations, is a significant sensitizing agent among sunscreens.[47] There has been a rise in reports of sensitivity to the benzophenones as the use of these agents has increased.[43]

*Cinnamates* Cinnamates include cinoxate, octyl methoxycinnamate, and octocrylene. As shown in Table 39-7, cinoxate and octyl methoxycinnamate have similar absorbance ranges and maximum absorbances. Octocrylene, however, has an absorbance range of 250 to 360 nm, well into the UVA range. Octocrylene is currently found in more commercial sunscreen preparations than it was in the past, possibly reflecting its broader spectrum of absorbance.

Unfortunately, cinnamates do not adhere well to the skin and must rely on the vehicle in a given formulation for their substantivity.

*Dibenzoylmethane Derivatives* Avobenzone (butyl methoxydibenzoylmethane, originally known as Parsol 1789) is the first of a new class of sunscreen agents effective throughout the entire UVA range (320-400 nm; full spectrum). It has a maximum absorbance at approximately 360 nm. This agent entered the market through a new drug application and was officially approved in the published FM. Although avobenzone absorbs UVR through all the UVA spectrum, its absorbance falls off sharply at 370 nm. Therefore, reactions to photosensitive drugs and chemicals that are highly reactive in the 370 to 400 nm range could still occur. Avobenzone, however, offers the best protection in the UVA range compared with the other chemical sunscreens on the market.

*Salicylates* Salicylic acid derivatives are weak sunscreens and must be used in high concentrations. They do not adhere well to the skin and are easily removed by perspiration or swimming.

*Other Chemical Sunscreens* Phenylbenzimidazole sulfonic acid does not fit into any of the preceding classes. It is a pure UVB sunscreen with an absorbance range of 290 to 320 nm.

*Physical Sunscreens* Physical sunscreens scatter rather than absorb UVR and visible radiation (290-777 nm). They are most often used on small and prominently exposed areas by patients who cannot limit or control their exposure to the sun (e.g., lifeguards). A white or colored substance containing zinc oxide or titanium dioxide is often used to coat the nose and top of the ears. Manufacturers

**TABLE 39-8 Selected Sunscreen Products**

| Trade Name | SPF Value | Sunscreen Ingredients |
|---|---|---|
| Bain de Soleil All Day for Kids Lotion | 30 | Ethylhexyl p-methoxycinnamate; ethylhexylcyanodiphenylacrylate; oxybenzone; titanium dioxide |
| Bain de Soleil Orange Gelee Gel | 4 | Ethylhexylmethoxycinnamate; ethylhexyl salicylate |
| Blistex Ultra Protection Lip Balm | 30 | Octyl methoxycinnamate; oxybenzone; octyl salicylate; menthyl anthranilate; homosalate |
| Bullfrog Sunblock Gel | 30+ | Octocrylene; octyl methoxycinnamate; benzophenone-3 |
| ChapStick Sunblock 15 Lip Balm | 15 | Padimate; oxybenzone |
| Coppertone Kids Lotion | 30+ | Ethyl-hexyl p-methoxycinnamate (octyl methoxycinnamate); oxybenzone; ethylhexyl salicylate (octyl salicylate); homosalate |
| Coppertone Moisturizing Sunblock Lotion | 15 | Ethylhexyl methoxycinnamate; oxybenzone |
| Coppertone Moisturizing Sunscreen Lotion | 8 | Ethylhexyl p-methoxycinnamate (octyl methoxycinnamate); oxybenzone |
| Coppertone Suntan Lotion | 4 | Ethylhexyl methoxycinnamate; oxybenzone |
| Coppertone Oil-Free Lotion | 30 | Ethylhexyl p-methoxycinnamate (octyl methoxycinnamate); 2-ethylhexyl salicylate (octyl salicylate); oxybenzone; homosalate |
| Coppertone Shade Sunblock Lotion | 30+ | Ethylhexyl p-methoxycinnamate (octyl methoxycinnamate); 2-ethylhexyl salicylate; oxybenzone; homosalate |
| Coppertone Sport Lotion | 30+ | Ethylhexyl methoxycinnamate; oxybenzone; 2-ethylhexyl salicylate; homosalate |
| Coppertone Water Babies Lotion | 30+ | Ethylhexyl methoxycinnamate; 2-ethylhexyl salicylate; oxybenzone; homosalate |
| Coppertone Kids Spray n' Splash Spray | 30 | Ethylhexyl p-methoxycinnamate; oxybenzone; ethylhexyl salicylate; homosalate |
| Hawaiian Tropic Baby Faces Lotion | 30+ | Titanium dioxide; octyl methoxycinnamate; octocrylene; benzophenone 3; octyl salicylate |
| Hawaiian Tropic 15 Plus Sunblock Lotion | 15+ | Octyl methoxycinnamate; menthyl anthranilate; benzophenone |
| Hawaiian Tropic Protective Tanning Lotion | 6 | Titanium dioxide |
| Neutrogena No Stick Sunscreen Cream Lotion | 30 | Octyl methoxycinnamate; homosalate; octyl salicylate 5%; benzophenone-3 |
| Neutrogena Intensified Day Moisture Lotion | 15 | Octyl methoxycinnamate; phenylbenzimidazole; titanium dioxide; sulfonic acid |
| Neutrogena Chemical Free Sunblocker Skin Lotion | 17 | Titanium dioxide |
| Neutrogena Sunblock Stick | 25 | Octyl methoxycinnamate; octyl salicylate; benzophenone |
| PreSun Ultra Lotion | 30 | Oxybenzone; octyl methoxycinnamate; octyl salicylate; avobenzone |
| PreSun Active Gel | 30 | Octyl methoxycinnamate; oxybenzone; octyl salicylate; avobenzone |
| Shade UVAGuard Lotion | 30 | Ethylhexyl p-methoxycinnamate (octyl methoxycinnamate); oxybenzone; 2-ethylhexyl salicylate (octyl salicylate); homosalate |
| TI-Screen Lotion | 30 | Octyl methoxycinnamate; octocrylene; benzophenone-3 (oxybenzone); octyl salicylate |

Key: SPF, sun protection factor.
*Source:* Adapted from *E Facts*. Sunscreens Product List. Wolters Kluwer Health, Inc: 2003-2004.

have also developed a way to make titanium dioxide transparent while maintaining efficacy as a sunscreen. Their disadvantages are that they can discolor clothing and may occlude the skin to produce miliaria (prickly heat) and folliculitis. Because titanium dioxide increases the effective SPF of a product and extends the spectrum of protection well into the UVA range, the number of commercial products containing this agent has increased. The FM allows for zinc oxide to be used alone or combined with any of the other sunscreen agents except avobenzone because of a lack of data on effectiveness.

*Combination Products* FDA has not recommended limits on the number of sunscreen agents that may be used together. However, each sunscreen agent must contribute to the efficacy of a product and must not be included merely for marketing promotion purposes. Therefore, the FM requires that (1) each active ingredient contribute a minimum SPF of not less than 2, and (2) the finished product must have a minimum SPF of not less than the number of sunscreen active ingredients used in the combination multiplied by 2.

### Dosage and Administration Guidelines

The two major causes of poor sun protection with sunscreen use are application of inadequate amounts and infrequent reapplication. In a report on sunscreen application to eight areas of the face, the degree of complete coverage ranged from 8% periorbital and 18% ears to 80% forehead and 94% cheeks.[44] Although many sunscreen products that prevent burning of the lips (or nose) are available, the lips are often neglected. They differ in ingredients and in the UVA and UVB spectrum, but products for the lips carry most of the same labeling, including the SPF, as do sunscreen lotions. The SPF of products for lips is usually at least 15. Studies have shown that lip protection not only helps prevent drying and burning of the lips but also helps prevent the development of cold sores or fever blisters triggered by the herpes simplex virus in patients who are susceptible to recurrent outbreaks.

Sunscreens must be liberally applied to all exposed areas of the body and reapplied at least as often as the label recommends for maximum effectiveness. One recent study suggested that sunscreens be applied 15 to 30 minutes before UV exposure and every 15 to 30 minutes thereafter. The study also suggested reapplication after every episode of swimming, toweling dry, or excessive sweating.[45] Although these two factors drive up the cost of sunscreen use, the long-term benefits of proper sunscreen use outweigh the costs.

The FDA standard for application of sunscreens is 2 mg/cm$^2$ of body surface area. This standard means that, for sufficient protection, the average adult in a bathing suit should apply nine portions of sunscreen of approximately 1/2 tsp each, or approximately 4 1/2 tsp (22.5 mL) total. The sunscreen should be distributed as follows:

- *Face and neck:* 1/2 tsp
- *Arms and shoulders:* 1/2 tsp to each side of body
- *Torso:* 1/2 tsp each to front and back
- *Legs and top of feet:* 1 tsp to each side of body

Because of the cost of sunscreen products and the need to apply them often and in sufficient amounts, people may use far less sunscreen than is necessary to provide adequate protection. A study on sunscreen failure reported that men were significantly less likely to use sunscreens than women.[46] In addition, when men used sunscreens, they applied less to exposed skin than did women.

Outdoor exposure to UVR should be within the limits of the SPF value of the sunscreen. Another factor to consider is the time it takes the sunscreen to bind to the various skin constituents and become fully effective. For most sunscreen products, the interval is 15 to 30 minutes, although at least one product claims immediate effectiveness. Because this lag time varies from product to product, the FM allows each product to include its individual lag time on the label. Sunscreens should be reapplied as often as label instructions direct. Water-resistant products are reapplied every 40 minutes, whereas very water-resistant products are reapplied after every 80 minutes of water exposure.

If properly applied, products with an SPF of 15 to 30 allow an individual to stay out in the sun for long periods and to slowly develop a tan over several days to weeks. As an individual tans, a natural protection against burning also develops. Therefore, an individual who insists on tanning should begin the summer using a product with an SPF of at least 15 to 30 (depending on skin type and tanning history) and switch to a product with a lower SPF (e.g., 12, then 10, then 8, etc.) as the natural tan progresses. This change will allow a more rapid deepening of the tan while helping to build up natural protection in the skin. The individual can, however, continue to use the product with the higher SPF; it will simply take longer to achieve the desired tan.

Patients should be advised that, although tanning and thickening of the skin serve as protective mechanisms against future injury, peeling of the skin removes part of this protection. The amount of exposure to the sun as well as the SPF of the product being used must be reevaluated as tanning and peeling occur.

### Safety Considerations

The development of a rash, vesicles (blisters), hives, or an exaggerated sunburn is most likely a sign of either a photosensitivity or allergic reaction. Product labels must state the following: "Stop use if skin rash occurs." The patient should be referred to a primary care provider for evaluation of the situation. The degree of the reaction will determine what type of medical intervention (if any) is necessary.

Exercising in hot weather after applying a sunscreen product may increase the risk of overheating. Under hot, humid conditions, sweating increases, but evaporation is poor. When the humidity is low, overheating during exercise may still occur, possibly because the oily vehicle of the sunscreen may block the pores.

Although no evidence exists of significant effects from eye contact, FDA requires the warning label, "Keep out of eyes."

## Additional Product Considerations

*Sunscreens in Cosmetic Products* The FM addresses a gray area that has allowed the proliferation of cosmetics claiming to offer sun protection. It stipulates that sunscreen products will be classified as drugs rather than cosmetics because consumers expect that sunscreens will protect them from some of the sun's damaging effects. However, cosmetics that contain sunscreen agents will be classified as cosmetics as long as no therapeutic claims are made, and the sunscreen is intended for a nontherapeutic, nonphysiologic purpose. In addition, if the term "sunscreen" appears on the product labeling, a statement must appear that describes the cosmetic purpose of the sunscreen (e.g., "Contains a sunscreen—to protect product color").

*Suntan Products* Two types of products fall under the general heading of suntan products: those that contain a pigmenting agent and those that do not. Products that do not contain a pigmenting agent are formulated with oily vehicles (e.g., mineral oil) that tend to concentrate UVR onto the skin. Although they are also formulated with emollients, these products provide no protection whatsoever against the short- and long-term hazards of UVR exposure. The other type of suntan product contains the pigmenting agent, dihydroxyacetone (DHA). It may be formulated with or without an oily vehicle. DHA has been the major ingredient in products that claim to tan without the sun. DHA produces a reddish-brown color by binding with specific amino acids in the stratum corneum. The intensity of the tan is related to the thickness of the skin. If the product is not washed off the hands immediately after application, however, the palms may also develop this tan (turn orange). In addition, dry areas, such as elbows and kneecaps, will absorb the DHA more readily, resulting in uneven coloration. The color fades after 5 to 7 days with desquamation of the stratum corneum.

The FM issued new rules concerning suntan products. Products labeled for suntanning purposes cannot contain any sunscreen ingredients intended to provide protection from UVR. In addition, the product label must carry the following warning:

> Warning—This product does not contain a sunscreen and does not protect against sunburn. Repeated exposure of unprotected skin while tanning may increase the risk of skin aging, skin cancer, and other harmful effects to the skin even if you do not burn.

## Unapproved Suntan Agents

*Oral Pigmenting Agents* A number of products have claimed to be effective oral tanning compounds. Their active ingredients are the dyes canthaxanthin and β-carotene, chemically similar to one another. β-Carotene and canthaxanthin are both approved by FDA as color additives in foods and drugs, and β-carotene is also approved for use in cosmetics. Canthaxanthin is a synthetic dye that is similar to dyes found naturally in fruits, vegetables, and flowers. Both agents are used to enhance the appearance of foods such as pizza, barbecue and spaghetti sauces, soups, salad dressings, fruit drinks, baked goods, pudding, cheese, ketchup, and margarine.[48] However, the concentrations of these agents in food are lower (1/20 to 1/40) than those found in oral products that claim to produce tanning.

The dyes alter skin tone by coloring the fat cells under the epidermal layer. Because of variations in fat cells and epidermal thickness, the extent of the tan varies from person to person. Canthaxanthin is dosed by body weight. The promotional literature cautions the user that if the palms turn orange, too much of the product is being consumed.

According to the 1960 Color Additive Amendment, any new use of a color additive must be submitted to FDA for approval. FDA has not yet approved either β-carotene or canthaxanthin for artificial tanning. One major concern with these additives is the discoloration of the feces to brick red, which could mask gastrointestinal bleeding. A second concern is the long-term adverse effects that may be associated with the large doses recommended. Although β-carotene is used on a prescription basis to help prevent photosensitivity in patients with erythropoietic protoporphyria, no evidence documents the safety of canthaxanthin at the high doses found in oral tanning products. In fact, a case has been reported of fatal aplastic anemia associated with canthaxanthin ingestion from an oral tanning product. Reported cases of retinopathy as well as other medical problems associated with the use of oral tanning agents has prompted FDA to issue further warnings on such products.[44] Canada, which previously allowed the nonprescription sale of canthaxanthin for tanning purposes, has decided that there is insufficient evidence of its safety, and thus no longer allows such sales.

*Tan Accelerators* Tan accelerators are cosmetic products that claim to stimulate a faster and deeper tan. Their major ingredient is tyrosine, an amino acid necessary to produce melanin. Product literature recommends application of these products once daily for at least 3 days before sun exposure. However, there is currently no evidence that tan accelerators work. FDA recognizes this fact and has stated that "any product containing tyrosine or its derivatives and claiming to accelerate the tanning process is an unapproved new drug."[34]

*Melanotropins and Melanin Products* A hormone known as α-melanotropin or α-melanocyte–stimulating hormone (α-MSH) has been located within the human central nervous system. The role of α-MSH in humans, if any, has not yet been fully identified. However, this hormone is produced by the pituitary gland of numerous vertebrates and has been shown to affect skin color through its action on melanocytes.[49] α-Melanotropin is currently under investigation to determine whether it can affect skin tanning. Also, the FM states that melanin and artificial melanin ingredients are not recognized sunscreens, and that any products containing these agents and making sunscreen claims are new drugs and must be under a new drug application.

### Product Selection Guidelines

Two primary factors will determine the best product for a given patient: the intended use of the product and specific patient characteristics. The decision on which sunscreen product to use must be based on the information obtained from both categories.

*Intended Use* Some patients may want to use sunscreens to prevent sunburn or the photoaging effects of UVR or to protect themselves from skin cancer. Others may need protection from sun exposure because they are taking photosensitive drugs or they suffer from a photodermatosis.

The higher the SPF of the sunscreen product, the greater the protection it provides against sunburn and tanning. Studies have shown that sunscreens can protect against the long-term hazards of skin cancer.[50] Considerable research is currently being conducted on all aspects of ultraviolet radiation and its effects. However, there is a debate among experts about whether low SPF products protect individuals from UV skin damage or allow them to receive dangerously high levels of UVR over extended periods of time. Because of the known hazards associated with UVR, FDA and other organizations such as the American Academy of Dermatology recommend the use of sunscreen products of at least SPF 15. Any product in the SPF range of 15 to 30+ will significantly reduce the total amount of both UVB and some UVA radiation received compared with lower SPF products. Generally, if a product is to be used to prevent skin cancer, reduce the chances of a photosensitivity reaction, or reduce the risk of triggering a skin disorder induced or aggravated by UVR, a broad-spectrum 30+ SPF is best.

A number of commercial products claim to be broad spectrum; FDA allows such claims if the product contains ingredients that absorb or reflect UVB (290-320 nm) *and* absorb UVA up to 360 nm.[34] Products with equal SPFs may still differ significantly in total UVR protection, depending on the absorbances of the various sunscreens they contain. Most currently available broad-spectrum products have a minimum of two sunscreen ingredients, whereas many incorporate three or even four sunscreens.

No one generally accepted measure exists to evaluate the actual efficacy of a product that claims to provide UVA protection. The best recommendation would be to select a product that contains a combination of sunscreen agents that protect throughout the entire UVB range and across the widest possible UVA range. A product labeled as broad spectrum that contains avobenzone and has an SPF of at least 15 is an excellent choice for patients who have UVR-induced disorders or who are taking photosensitizing drugs. If the sunscreen product does not contain avobenzone, then a broad-spectrum sunscreen with an SPF of 30+ is recommended. A very broad spectrum of coverage can be obtained by using a sunscreen product containing padimate O with one of the benzophenones, octocrylene, or menthyl anthranilate. An increasing number of products have added micronized titanium dioxide to increase the SPF and provide a broad spectrum of coverage.

*Patient Factors* For patients not concerned with photosensitivity, photodermatoses, or prevention of skin cancer, product selection is much simpler. The following factors can serve as a guide in selecting products with the appropriate properties for a patient's particular situation.

Skin Type and Tanning History The most important factors in product selection are the individual's natural skin type and tanning history. An SPF product of 30+ should be used by people who always burn easily and tan minimally at best. The average person who uses sunscreen products does so to avoid getting burned while still obtaining a tan. For that individual, a product with an SPF of 12 to 30 is recommended, with the lower end for people who always tan well and the higher end for those who tan gradually. An SPF from 2 to 12 is recommended for people who are deeply pigmented or who tan easily. A higher SPF product can always be recommended, although tanning will occur at a slower than normal rate.

Physical Activity If the patient plans to swim, participate in vigorous activity (e.g., sand volleyball), or work outdoors, the sunscreen product must be able to adhere to the skin more substantially than if he or she just lies on the beach. The expected duration of the physical activity can also help to determine which sunscreen to use. Water-resistant products are usually effective for at least 40 minutes when used during the above activities, whereas very water-resistant products are labeled as effective for at least 80 minutes.

Adverse Reactions to Sunscreen Agents If a patient has had a prior reaction to a sunscreen product, the name of the product and the ingredients it contained should be identified, if possible. This action may be difficult because product formulations change frequently. Photosensitivity and contact dermatitis are more likely to occur with aminobenzoic acid and its esters, although the benzophenones, cinnamates, homosalate, avobenzone, and menthyl anthranilate have also been reported to produce both conditions. In a French study of contact dermatitis, 15.4% of patients were found to have an allergy to sunscreens with almost one half attributed to oxybenzone.[51] In addition, patients who are allergy prone and have allergies to various drugs (e.g., benzocaine, thiazides, sulfonamides) may also develop an allergic reaction to either aminobenzoic acid or its esters.

Cosmetic Considerations At least one third of the current commercial products are labeled noncomedogenic, fragrance-free, and hypoallergenic. Noncomedogenic products do not plug the pores and, therefore, do not exacerbate acne. This property is especially important for teenagers, who usually spend more time outdoors than other age groups and would generally prefer not to use comedogenic sunscreens. Regarding fragrance-free and hypoallergenic properties, many patients are sensitive to various ingredients, including fragrances, emulsifiers, and preservatives. In a randomized, placebo-controlled study of adverse reactions to sunscreens, 16% of subjects developed a local reaction to the topically applied product.[52]

Of these subjects, 53% agreed to be patch tested and photopatch tested. None of this subset showed an allergic sensitivity to the sunscreen agents. Instead, all the reactions were found to be caused by formulation ingredients such as fragrances and preservatives. This finding reinforces the belief that most sensitivity may be caused by nonsunscreen ingredients. Although it may not be possible to figure out what specific ingredient a patient is sensitive to, patients who have a history of sensitivity to certain types of ingredients would do well to use a fragrance-free, hypoallergenic product.

Some patients have normally dry skin. Sunbathing can further exacerbate this problem. These patients should avoid ethyl and isopropyl alcohols, which are included in a number of commercial sunscreen products and can further dry the skin.

Use in Young Children Absorptive characteristics of human skin in children younger than 6 months differ from those of adult skin. The metabolic and excretory systems of infants are not fully developed to handle any sunscreen agent absorbed through the skin. Therefore, only patients older than 6 months are considered to have skin with adult characteristics. FDA requires that sunscreen products be labeled with the statement "children under 6 months of age: ask a doctor." Caregivers should be extremely wary regarding sun exposure in children, especially infants. Although the evidence is not yet conclusive, researchers and clinicians agree that use of an SPF-15 product starting after age 6 months and continuing throughout one's lifetime can reduce the incidence of long-term skin damage from UVR. A product with an SPF of 30+ may result in even higher reductions in sunburn, photoaging, skin cancer, and other skin problems.

## Assessment of Sun-induced Skin Disorders: A Case-based Approach

The approach to UVR-induced skin disorders is different from that used in most self-care situations. Such disorders are addressed from a preventive rather than a treatment standpoint. According to FDA, the primary indication for sunscreen products is to protect against sunburn. A voluntary labeling "sun alert" may also advise that such products "may reduce the risks of skin aging, skin cancer, and other harmful effects of the sun."[53]

Consequently, assessment of the patient should focus on the *intended use* of the product. Two primary situations exist in which clinical practitioners intervene with patients. The first situation involves a request by the patient for the practitioner to recommend a sunscreen product to prevent a burn and/or to allow for developing a tan. The second situation is initiated by the practitioner when a patient is placed on a drug that can produce a photosensitivity reaction. In this second scenario, no real patient assessment is needed because prevention of exposure to UVR is the standard approach. Cases 39-1 and 39-2 illustrate the assessment of patients with sun-induced skin disorders.

### CASE 39-1

| Relevant Evaluation Criteria | Scenario/Model Outcome |
|---|---|
| **Information Gathering** | |
| 1. Gather essential information about the patient's symptoms, including: | |
| a. description of symptom(s) (i.e., nature, onset, duration, severity, associated symptoms) | Patient says her PCP suspects that she suffers from rosacea. Patient will be going on a work/vacation trip to Miami, Florida, for 4 weeks. She wants to spend as much time as possible outdoors while she is there. Patient suffers from erythema on her cheeks, nose, and forehead as well as inflammation in her eyes and lids. |
| b. description of any factors that seem to precipitate, exacerbate, and/or relieve the patient's symptom(s) | She recently went on a 2-week hiking trip in the Colorado Rockies and developed an erythematous rash over the bridge of the nose, chin, and forehead. She also was severely burned on her neck and arms after the first day of the hike, which was very sunny. |
| c. description of the patient's efforts to relieve the symptoms | Patient applies topical metronidazole as prescribed by her PCP. |
| 2. Gather essential patient history information: | |
| a. patient's identity | Debbie Smith |
| b. patient's age, sex, height, and weight | 30 y/o F, 5'5", 125 lb |
| c. patient's occupation | Computer engineer |
| d. patient's dietary habits | Normal healthy diet, eats fast food on occasion, but loves Chinese food and chocolate |

## CASE 39-1 (continued)

| Relevant Evaluation Criteria | Scenario/Model Outcome |
|---|---|
| e. patient's sleep habits | Normally sleeps 4-6 hours nightly; stress and work deadlines sometimes limit sleep to 3-4 hours nightly |
| f. concurrent medical conditions, prescription and nonprescription medications, and dietary supplements | Suspected rosacea; HCTZ 25 mg once daily for HTN; metronidazole 0.75% cream 2 times/day for rash |
| g. allergies | PCN (anaphylaxis) |
| h. history of other adverse reactions to medications | Cough related to captopril |
| i. other (describe)_______ | Debbie's PCP advised her to stay out of the sun and use sunscreen whenever she is outside since she started HCTZ. She did not realize that this included all sun exposure until she had the bad sunburn on her recent hiking trip. Debbie used to jog 2 miles three times per week and work out at the gym three times per week. Her work has forced her to cut back her exercise, but she plans to resume as soon as possible. |
| **Assessment and Triage** | |
| 3. Differentiate the patient's signs/symptoms and correctly identify the patient's primary problem(s). | Patient appears to be experiencing exacerbations of rosacea (see Chapter 38 for additional information) and photosensitivity reaction to HCTZ from UVR exposure. |
| 4. Identify exclusions for self-treatment (see Figure 39-1). | None |
| 5. Formulate a comprehensive list of therapeutic alternatives for the primary problem to determine if triage to a medical practitioner is required, and share this information with the patient. | Options include:<br>(1) Have Debbie follow up with her PCP.<br>(2) Recommend self-care with an appropriate sunscreen during exposure to UVR.<br>(3) Recommend avoidance of sun exposure.<br>(4) Recommend self-care until a dermatologist can be consulted on rosacea.<br>(5) Call Debbie's PCP and recommend change in HTN therapy to medication that less likely associated with photosensitivity.<br>(5) Take no action. |
| **Plan** | |
| 6. Select an optimal therapeutic alternative to address the patient's problem, taking into account patient preferences. | Avoidance of sun exposure and all UVR if at all possible; use of a broad-spectrum sunscreen and protective nondrug measures when exposure cannot be prevented |
| 7. Describe the recommended therapeutic approach to the patient. | Avoidance of UVR is the best way to prevent your symptoms from getting worse. When you must be outdoors, wear protective clothing and apply a sunscreen to exposed areas. |
| 8. Explain to the patient the rationale for selecting the recommended therapeutic approach from the considered therapeutic alternatives. | If the sunscreen and nondrug protective measures fail to prevent exacerbation of symptoms, a visit to a dermatologist for further assessment may be appropriate. |
| **Patient Education** | |
| 9. When recommending self-care with nonprescription medications and/or nondrug therapy, convey accurate information to the patient, including: | |
| a. appropriate dose and frequency of administration | See the box Patient Education for Protection from Sun Exposure. |
| b. maximum number of days the therapy should be employed | See the box Patient Education for Protection from Sun Exposure. |

## CASE 39-1 (continued)

| Relevant Evaluation Criteria | Scenario/Model Outcome |
|---|---|
| c. product administration procedures | See the box Patient Education for Protection from Sun Exposure. |
| d. expected time to onset of relief | See the box Patient Education for Protection from Sun Exposure. |
| e. degree of relief that can be reasonably expected | Complete prevention of exacerbations from UVR is possible. |
| f. most common side effects | See the box Patient Education for Protection from Sun Exposure. |
| g. side effects that warrant medical intervention should they occur | See the box Patient Education for Protection from Sun Exposure. |
| h. patient options in the event that condition worsens or persists | If rosacea flares even with sunscreen use, you should see a dermatologist. Hydrochlorothiazide is a photosensitizing drug. You may need a different medication for hypertension if photosensitivity continues to occur with sunscreen use. |
| i. product storage requirements | See the box Patient Education for Protection from Sun Exposure. |
| j. specific nondrug measures | See the box Patient Education for Protection from Sun Exposure. |
| 10. Solicit follow-up questions from patient. | I spent 4 hours per day for 2 days canoeing with my friends and used a whole bottle (8 oz) of SPF 30+ sunscreen. Am I applying too much? |
| 11. Answer patient's questions. | Not at all. Eight ounces of "very water resistant/waterproof" sunscreen should provide protection for about 10 hours. This means you are applying it correctly. |

Key: HCTZ, hydrochlorothiazide; HTN, hypertension; PCP, primary care provider; SPF, sun protection factor; UVR, ultraviolet radiation.

## CASE 39-2

| Relevant Evaluation Criteria | Scenario/Model Outcome |
|---|---|
| **Information Gathering** | |
| 1. Gather essential information about the patient's symptoms, including: | Patient plans to lifeguard for his summer job as well as maintain a lawn care business in his neighborhood on his off days. He is not too concerned about burning but his mom is because his dad died of skin cancer earlier this year at the age of 42. He has type II skin (see Table 39-6). He and his mom want advice on selection and use of a sunscreen. |
| a. description of symptom(s) (i.e., nature, onset, duration, severity, associated symptoms) | Patient burns every time soccer season starts in the spring until he "gets my base tan," which typically takes at least 8 weeks. The burns seem to get less severe except for his face and chest as the summer progresses. |
| b. description of any factors that seem to precipitate, exacerbate, and/or relieve the patient's symptom(s) | Sometimes he wears a hat. He isn't too concerned about burning or skin cancer, but he does want to keep his mom happy. His doctor has recommended using a sunscreen and wearing protective clothing as applicable, especially a broad-rim hat. |
| c. description of the patient's efforts to relieve the symptoms | |
| 2. Gather essential patient history information: | |
| a. patient's identity | Jarod Baker |
| b. patient's age, sex, height, and weight | 16 y/o M, 6'3", 180 lb |
| c. patient's occupation | Junior in high school |
| d. patient's dietary habits | Skips breakfast and eats fast food for lunch. He eats a nutritious dinner; consumes 2 L of soda a day. |
| e. patient's sleep habits | Normally sleeps 10 hours nightly |
| f. concurrent medical conditions, prescription and nonprescription medications, and dietary supplements | Diphenhydramine 25-50 mg 2 times/day for seasonal allergies |

## CASE 39-2 (continued)

| Relevant Evaluation Criteria | Scenario/Model Outcome |
|---|---|
| g. allergies | NKDA |
| h. history of other adverse reactions to medications | None |
| i. other (describe)_______ | Jarod plays soccer two for four times per week in the spring and golf two to three times per week in the fall. His summer jobs will have him in the sun 7 days per week, 8-10 hours per day. |
| **Assessment and Triage** | |
| 3. Differentiate the patient's signs/symptoms and correctly identify the patient's primary problem(s). | Jarod experiences frequent sunburns for several weeks till his "tan starts" in late spring/early summer. |
| 4. Identify exclusions for self-treatment (see Figure 39-1). | None |
| 5. Formulate a comprehensive list of therapeutic alternatives for the primary problem to determine if triage to a medical practitioner is required, and share this information with the patient. | Options include:<br>(1) Refer Jarod to a dermatologist.<br>(2) Recommend self-care with an appropriate sunscreen during exposure to UVR.<br>(3) Recommend avoidance of sun exposure.<br>(4) Recommend self-care until a dermatologist can be consulted.<br>(5) Take no action. |
| **Plan** | |
| 6. Select an optimal therapeutic alternative to address the patient's problem, taking into account patient preferences. | Jarod should use a sunscreen and protective nondrug measures to minimize sun exposure. Since Jarod is taking diphenhydramine, a potential photosensitizing agent, he should use a broad-spectrum sunscreen agent. |
| 7. Describe the recommended therapeutic approach to the patient. | You should wear long sleeves and pants when weather permits. Always wear a hat. Always use sunscreen. |
| 8. Explain to the patient the rationale for selecting the recommended therapeutic approach from the considered therapeutic alternatives. | Because of your skin type, burning will always be a problem. Although some tanning does develop as the summer progresses, the UVR damage to the skin has already been done. |
| **Patient Education** | |
| 9. When recommending self-care with nonprescription medications and/or nondrug therapy, convey accurate information to the patient, including: | |
| a. appropriate dose and frequency of administration | See the box Patient Education for Protection from Sun Exposure. |
| b. maximum number of days the therapy should be employed | See the box Patient Education for Protection from Sun Exposure. |
| c. product administration procedures | See the box Patient Education for Protection from Sun Exposure. |
| d. expected time to onset of relief | See the box Patient Education for Protection from Sun Exposure. |
| e. degree of relief that can be reasonably expected | Complete prevention of sunburn is possible. Further development of actinic keratoses may not be significantly retarded at this stage in your life regardless of sunscreen use. |
| f. most common side effects | See the box Patient Education for Protection from Sun Exposure. |
| g. side effects that warrant medical intervention should they occur | See the box Patient Education for Protection from Sun Exposure. |

## CASE 39-2 (continued)

| Relevant Evaluation Criteria | Scenario/Model Outcome |
|---|---|
| h. patient options in the event that condition worsens or persists | Play golf and soccer and work in lawn care business before 10 AM or after 3 PM. Have a shady shelter to stand or sit under while serving as a life guard at the pool this summer. Use a higher SPF sunscreen. You should see your primary care provider or a dermatologist if you continue to burn severely or continue to burn throughout the summer. |
| i. product storage requirements | See the box Patient Education for Protection from Sun Exposure. |
| j. specific nondrug measures | See the box Patient Education for Protection from Sun Exposure. |
| 10. Solicit follow-up questions from patient. | This product says "all day protection and very water resistant." Do I still need to apply it every 80 minutes? |
| 11. Answer patient's questions. | Yes. The current FDA standard for "very water resistant" products is reapplication every 80 minutes to guarantee full and complete protection from UVR. |

Key: FDA, Food and Drug Administration; NKDA, no known drug allergies; SPF, sun protection factor; UVR, ultraviolet radiation.

## Patient Counseling for Sun-induced Skin Disorders

Health care practitioners can provide a great service by counseling consumers about the suntanning process and properly selecting and using sunscreens. One study of Italian teenagers reported that "young people are aware of the risks associated with sunbathing, but they continue to expose themselves without taking precautions."[50] An American study[51] reported that 13% of children and 9% of adults participating had a sunburn during the previous week, and there was a relationship between sunburn and a parental attitude that tanning is healthy.

One simple way to find out if a patient is using a sunscreen properly is to ask how long the current bottle has lasted. When applied properly, according to the suggested dosing guidelines and in accordance with the appropriate substantivity of the product, a sunbather could easily use about 1 oz every 80 to 90 minutes. This use would amount to several ounces a day and several bottles per week. Incredibly, many frequent sunbathers use only one bottle in an entire season. This diminished usage demonstrates the importance of patients receiving adequate counseling to get the protection they desire. The box Patient Education for Protection from Sun Exposure lists specific information to provide patients.

## Evaluation of Patient Outcomes for Sun-induced Skin Disorders

The short-term outcomes for sunscreen use are readily apparent. Twenty-four hours after use, there will be no obvious sunburn, photosensitivity reaction, or eruption of photodermatosis. This success indicates that the appropriate sunscreen agents and/or SPF were used. However, the long-term effects of UVR (e.g., skin cancer, premature aging of the skin) may take up to 20 to 30 years to become evident.

## Key Points for Sun-induced Skin Disorders

- Ultraviolet radiation (UVA and UVB) triggers a variety of photodermatoses, and causes sunburn, photosensitivity, skin cancer, premature aging of the skin, cataracts, and a variety of other medical problems.
- The effects of UVR are cumulative over one's lifetime.
- The best protection against UVR is avoidance. The next best approach is to wear a hat, long sleeves, and pants, and wear UV-protective sunglasses.
- Maximum protection is provided by using a sunscreen of SPF 30+.
- A broad-spectrum sunscreen, because of its added UVA protection, is the best type to use regardless of the patient's history to prevent long-term effects.
- Most people regard sunscreen products as cosmetics, making good patient counseling even more important.
- When recommending a sunscreen product, it is important to identify the patient's skin type as well as to understand the intended use of the product.

## References


1. The U.S. Market for Suncare and Lipcare Products. MarketResearch.com. March 1, 2001. Available at: http://www.marketresearch.com/map/prod/222308.html. Accessed April 20, 2003.
2. Hawk JL, Norris PG. Abnormal reactions to ultraviolet radiation: idiopathic. In: Freedberg IM, Eisen AZ, Wolff K, et al., eds. *Fitzpatrick's Dermatology in General Medicine.* 5th ed. New York: McGraw-Hill, Inc; 1999:1573-89.
3. Yaar M, Gilchrest BA. Aging of skin. In: Fitzpatrick TB, Eisen AZ, Wolff K, et al., eds. *Fitzpatrick's Dermatology in General Medicine.* 5th ed. New York: McGraw-Hill, Inc; 1999:1697-706.
4. Robinson JK, Rigel DS, Amonette RA. Summertime sun protection used by adults for their children. *J Am Acad Dermatol.* 2000; 42(5 pt 1):746-53.
5. *Skin Cancer Facts.* American Cancer Society. April 2003. Available at: www.cancer.org/docroot/PED/content/ped_7_1_What_You_Need_. Accessed January 16, 2005.

## PATIENT EDUCATION FOR PROTECTION FROM SUN EXPOSURE

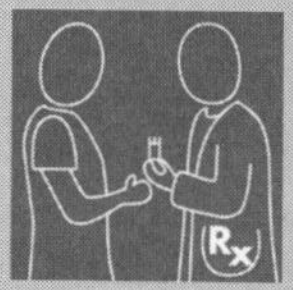

The objectives of self-care depend on a patient's specific goal or health status. Protection from sun exposure can prevent sunburn or tanning as well as photosensitivity reactions in susceptible persons or exacerbation of sun-induced photodermatoses. The primary long-term benefits are to prevent skin cancer and photoaging of the skin. For most patients, carefully following product instructions and the self-care measures listed here will help ensure optimal therapeutic outcomes.

### Avoiding/Minimizing Sun Exposure

- Avoid exposure to the sun and other sources of ultraviolet radiation (UVR) such as tanning beds/booths and sunlamps.
- The rays of the sun are the most direct and damaging between 10 AM and 4 PM. Avoid sun exposure during this time of day as much as possible.
- Sunburn can occur on a cloudy or overcast day; 70% to 90% of UVR penetrates clouds.
- Wear protective clothing such as long pants, a long-sleeved shirt, and a hat with a brim. Tightly woven fabrics that do not allow light to pass through will provide the most protection.
- Use a beach umbrella or other protection to reduce UVR.
- Wet clothing and water allow significant transmission of UVR. Consider time in the water, even if the body is completely submerged, as part of the total time spent in the sun.

### Use of Sunscreens

- An SPF of 30+ provides the greatest protection against sunburn and other UVB-induced skin problems.
- A broad-spectrum sunscreen product (e.g., avobenzone used in combination with padimate O and/or one of the benzophenones, octocrylene, menthyl anthranilate, or titanium dioxide) provides optimal protection against UVA and UVB sun exposure. This type of sunscreen is especially recommended if you have a sun-induced disorder or are taking photosensitizing drugs, or if you just want to reduce sun exposure as much as possible to prevent long-term effects.
- Apply first dose 15 to 30 minutes before exposure.
- Apply approximately 1 oz of sunscreen evenly to each exposed area of the body. Avoid contact with the eyes.
- Use the most substantive sunscreen available (very water-resistant).
- Reapply the sunscreen according to the label instructions, usually every 40 minutes for water-resistant sunscreens or 80 minutes for very water-resistant sunscreens.
- Higher altitudes and lower latitudes increase the amount of UVR to which an individual is exposed. Take proper precautions, including use of a sunscreen with a high SPF, to protect skin from UVR.
- Snow and sand reflect UVR. Take proper precautions, such as wearing sunglasses and using high SPF sunscreens, to protect exposed skin.
- Keep sunscreen out of direct sun to avoid reduction in potency.
- Continue to use a sunscreen as long you are taking a photosensitizing drug or exhibit signs and symptoms of photodermatitis.
- Avoid sunscreens containing aminobenzoic acid esters, benzophenones, cinnamates, or menthyl anthranilate if you have had a prior allergic reaction to a sunscreen product.

⚠ Stop using the sunscreen if redness, itching, rash, or exaggerated sunburn occurs.


6. Skin Cancer Fact Sheet. American Academy of Dermatology. 2004. Available at: www.aad.org/aad/Newsroom/skincancerfact.htm. Accessed January 16, 2005.
7. Kricker A, Armstrong BK, English DR, et al. A dose-response curve for sun exposure and basal cell carcinoma. *Int J Cancer.* 1995;60:482-8.
8. Armstrong BK, Kricker A. The epidemiology of UV-induced skin cancer. *J Photochem Photobiol B.* 2001;63:8-18.
9. Gallagher RP, Hill GB, Bajdik CD, et al. Sunlight exposure, pigmentation factors, and risk of nonmelanocytic skin cancer, II: squamous cell carcinoma. *Arch Dermatol.* 1995;131:164-9.
10. Gallagher RP, Hill GB, Bajdik CD, et al. Sunlight exposure, pigmentary factors, and risk of nonmelanocytic skin cancer, I: basal cell carcinoma. *Arch Dermatol.* 1995;131:157-63.
11. Urbach F, O'Beirn S, Judge P, et al. The influence of environment and genetic factors on cancer of the skin in man [abstract]. *Tenth International Cancer Congress.* Philadelphia: JB Lippincott; 1970:109-10.
12. Averbach H. Geographic variation in incidence of skin cancer in the United States. *Public Health Rep.* 1961;76:345-8.
13. Moloney FJ, Collins S, Murphy GM. Sunscreens: safety, efficacy and appropriate use. *Am J Clin Dermatol.* 2002;3:185-91.
14. Holick MF. Sunlight "D"elimma: risk of skin cancer, bone disease and muscle weakness. *Lancet.* 2001; 357:4-6.
15. Moyal DD, Fourtanier AM. Effects of UVA radiation on an established immune response in humans and sunscreen efficacy. *Exp Dermatol.* 2002;11(suppl 1):28-32.
16 Brenneisen P, Sies H, Scharffetter-Kochanek K. Ultraviolet-B irradiation and matrix metalloproteinases: from induction via signaling to initial events. *Ann NY Acad Sci.* 2002;973:31-43.
17. Motoyoshi K, Ota Y, Takuma Y, et al. Wrinkles from UVA exposure. *Cosmetic Toiletries.* 1998;113:51-6, 58.
18. Urbach F. Ultraviolet A transmission by modern sunscreens: is there a real risk? *Photodermatol Photoimmunol Photomed.* 1993;9:237-41.
19. Mutzhas MF, Cesarini JP. Risk-benefit calculations for UV tanning devices. In: Passchier WF, Bosnjakovic BFM, eds. *Human Exposure to Ultraviolet Radiation: Risk and Regulations.* Amsterdam, The Netherlands: Elsevier Science; 1987:345-52.
20. National Institutes of Health. *Consensus Development Conference Statement on Sunlight, Ultraviolet Radiation, and the Skin.* Bethesda, Md: National Institutes of Health; May 8-10, 1989.
21. Karagas MR, Stannard VA, Mott LA, et al. Use of tanning devices and risk of basal cell and squamous cell skin cancers. *J Natl Cancer Inst.* 2002;94:224-6.
22. Wang SQ, Setlow R, Berwick M, et al. Ultraviolet A and melanoma: a review. *J Am Acad Dermatol.* 2001;44(5): 837-46.
23. Office of Science and Technology. *Annual Report 2001.* Rockville, MD: US Department of Health and Human Services, Public Health Service, FDA Center for Devices and Radiological Health; July 10, 2002.
24. Injuries associated with ultraviolet tanning devices—Wisconsin. *MMWR Morb Mort Wkly Rep.* 1989;38:333-5.
25. Sunlamp products and ultraviolet lamps intended for use in sunlamp products. *21 CFR 1040.* 1992;20:519-22.

26. Pathak MA, Nghiem P, Fitzpatrick TB, et al. Acute and chronic effects of the sun. In: Freedberg IM, Eisen AZ, Wolff K, et al., eds. *Fitzpatrick's Dermatology in General Medicine.* 5th ed. New York: McGraw-Hill, Inc; 1999:1598-607.
27. *The Burning Facts.* Washington, DC: U.S. Environmental Protection Agency; May 2001. EPA430-01-015.
28. Johnson JA, Fusaro RM. Broad-spectrum protection: the roles of tinted auto windows, sunscreens, and browning agents in the diagnosis and treatment of photosensitivity. *Dermatology.* 1992; 185:237-41.
29. Kimlin MG, Parisi AV. Ultraviolet radiation penetrating vehicle glass: a field based comparative study. *Phys Med Biol.* 1999;44:917-26.
30. *A Guide to the UV Index.* Washington, DC: U.S. Environmental Protection Agency; May 2004. EPA30-F-04-020.
31. McGregor JM, Hawk JL. Acute effects of ultraviolet radiation on the skin. In: Freedberg IM, Eisen AZ, Wolff K, et al., eds. *Fitzpatrick's Dermatology in General Medicine.* 5th ed. New York: McGraw-Hill, Inc; 1999:1555-61.
32. *Federal Register.* 1978;43:38206-69.
33. *Federal Register.* 1993;58:28194-302.
34. *Federal Register.* 1999;64:27666-93.
35. *Federal Register.* 2001;66:67485-7.
36. *Federal Register.* 2004; 69: 53801-04.
37. *F-D-C Reports—The Tan Sheet.* 2004;12(52).[In Brief]
38. Moyal DD, Fourtanier AM. Efficacy of broad-spectrum sunscreens against the suppression of elicitation of delayed-type hypersensitivity responses in humans depends on the level of ultraviolet A protection. *Exp Dermatol.* April 2003;12:153-9.
39. Stege H, Budde M, Grether-Beck S, et al. Sunscreens with high SPF values are not equivalent in protection from UVA induced polymorphous light eruption. *Eur J Dermatol.* 2002;12:IV-VI.
40. Fourtanier A, Gueniche A, Compan D, et al. Improved protection against solar-simulated radiation-induced immunosuppression by a sunscreen with enhanced ultraviolet A protection. *J Invest Dermatol.* 2000;114:620-7.
41. *Federal Register.* 2005;70:72449-50.
42. Extending the benefits of UVA absorption. Rhom and Hass. Available at: http://www.rhomhaas.com/rhcis/whats_new/incos03-paper.pdf. Accessed July 7, 2005.
43. Journe F, Marguery MC, Rakotondrazafy J, et al. Sunscreen sensitization: a 5-year study. *Acta Derm Venereol.* 1999;79:211-3.
44. Loesch H, Kaplan DL. Pitfalls in sunscreen application. *Arch Dermatol.* 1994;130:665-6.
45. Diffey BL. When should sunscreens be reapplied? *J Am Acad Dermatol.* 2001;45:882-5.
46. Wright MW, Wright ST, Wagner, RF. Mechanisms of sunscreen failure. *J Am Acad Dermatol.* 2001;44:781-4.
47. Berne N, Ros AM. 7 years experience of photopatch testing with sunscreen allergens in Sweden. *Contact Dermatitis.* 1998;38:6-14.
48. Food and Drug Administration. *Tanning Pills.* Rockville, Md: Center for Food Safety and Applied Nutrition, Office of Cosmetics and Colors Fact Sheet. October 18, 2000; revised June 14, 2001. Available at: http://www.cfsan.fda. gov/~dms/cos-tan2.html. Accessed May 1, 2003.
49. Brown DA. Skin pigmentation enhancers. *J Photochem Photobiol B.* 2001;63:148-61.
50. Dummer R, Maier T. UV protection and skin cancer. *Recent Results Cancer Res.* 2002;160:7-12.
51. Journe F, Marguery MC, Rakotondrazafy J, et al. Sunscreen sensitization: a 5-year study. *Acta Derm Venereol.* 1999;79:211-3.
52. Foley P, Nixon R, Marks R, et al. The frequency of reactions to sunscreens: results of a longitudinal population-based study on the regular use of sunscreens in Australia. *Br J Dermatol.* 1993; 128:512-8.
53. Monfrecola G, Fabbrocini G, Posteraro G, et al. What do young people think about the dangers of sunbathing, skin cancer and sunbeds? A questionnaire survey among Italians. *Photodermatol Photoimmunol Photomed.* 2000;16:15-8.

CHAPTER 40

# Skin Hyperpigmentation and Photoaging

*Kimberly M. Crosby and Dana G. Carroll*

Many patients consider skin hyperpigmentation and photoaging cosmetically unacceptable.[1] Photoaging of the skin is related directly to exposure to ultraviolet (UV) radiation. Although sun exposure often is not the cause of hyperpigmentation, such exposure during or after treatment may negate the therapeutic effects. This chapter focuses on ameliorating the effects of hyperpigmentation and photoaging once they have occurred. Nonprescription products used to minimize sun exposure are discussed in Chapter 39.

α-Hydroxy acids (AHAs) play a role in treating both disorders. Hydroquinone, a skin bleaching agent, can be used alone or in combination with an AHA for self-treatment of hyperpigmentation. AHAs, β-hydroxy acids (BHAs), and *N*-furfuryladenine are promoted as nonprescription treatments for photoaging.

## SKIN HYPERPIGMENTATION

Hyperpigmentation, manifested as increased or more intense skin color, is usually a benign phenomenon, but may occasionally represent a sign of systemic disease. Hyperpigmentation may be perceived by the patient as disfigurement, especially when it occurs on the face and neck. Thus, agents that can reduce pigmentation when applied topically are used worldwide, especially when hyperpigmented skin is in noticeable contrast to surrounding normal skin color. Although these products serve a cosmetic function, it is important to emphasize that they are drugs with potential toxicity and side effects.

### Etiology of Skin Hyperpigmentation

Systemic as well as localized skin diseases may cause pigment cells to become overactive (resulting in skin darkening) or to become underactive (resulting in skin lightening). Endocrine imbalances caused by Addison's disease, Cushing's disease, hyperthyroidism, and pregnancy are capable of altering skin pigmentation. Metabolic alterations affecting the liver and certain nutritional deficiencies can be associated with diffuse melanosis. Inflammatory dermatoses (e.g., contact dermatitis from poison ivy) or physical trauma to the skin (e.g., thermal burn) may cause prolonged postinflammatory hyperpigmentation. Also, certain drugs (Table 40-1) have an affinity for melanin and may cause hyperpigmentation. Skin hyperpigmentation resulting from these conditions may occur as a result of increased melanin, increased melanocytes, or deposits in the skin of other darkening chemicals.[2]

### Pathophysiology of Skin Hyperpigmentation

Melanocytes (pigment cells) produce melanosomes, pigment granules that contain a complex protein called melanin, a brown-black pigment. These cells can be viewed as tiny one-celled glands with long projections used to pass pigment particles into the keratinocytes, which migrate upward to the skin surface. Melanocytes are also present in hair bulb cells that pass pigment granules to the hair.

There are about 800 to 1000 melanocytes per square millimeter of human epidermis. The number of melanocytes is the same in equivalent body sites in light and dark skin, but the rate of production of pigment and its distribution are different. It is believed that the function of the melanocyte is to provide protection from ultraviolet radiation (UVR). Dark skin usually has more active melanocytes than light skin, which explains why UVR-induced skin cancers of all types are less common in dark skin than in light skin.[3]

Freckles are spots of uneven skin pigmentation that first appear in childhood and are exacerbated by the sun. Melasma (also called chloasma), a condition in which macular hyperpigmentation appears, usually on the face or neck, is often associated with pregnancy ("the mask of pregnancy") or the use of oral contraceptives, as well as with sun exposure. Lentigines, hyperpigmented macules that may appear at any age anywhere on the skin or mucous membranes, are caused by an increased deposition of melanin and an increased number of melanocytes. These macules are not known to be induced by UVR. However, solar or "senile" lentigines (age spots or liver spots) appear on exposed skin surfaces, particularly in fair-skinned people, and are induced by UVR.

### Signs and Symptoms of Skin Hyperpigmentation

Depending on the etiology of hyperpigmentation, patients can present with varying signs and symptoms. Most notably, patients complain of persistent macular discoloration on the face or other sun-exposed areas. Discoloration typically

**Editor's Note:** This chapter is based, in part, on the 14th edition chapter with the same title, which was written by John S. Esterly, Lee E. West, and Dennis P. West.

**TABLE 40-1 Medications That May Cause Hyperpigmentation**

| |
|---|
| Amiodarone |
| Amitriptyline |
| Antimalarial agents (chloroquine, hydroxychloroquine) |
| Antineoplastic agents (cyclophosphamide, daunorubicin, doxorubicin, fluorouracil, busulfan) |
| Clofazimine |
| Heavy Metals (gold compounds, arsenic, mercury, silver, bismuth) |
| Hormone replacement therapy |
| Minocycline |
| Oral contraceptives |
| Phenothiazines (chlorpromazine, thioridazine, imipramine, clomipramine) |
| Phenytoin |
| Zidovudine |

Adapted from references 2 and 41.

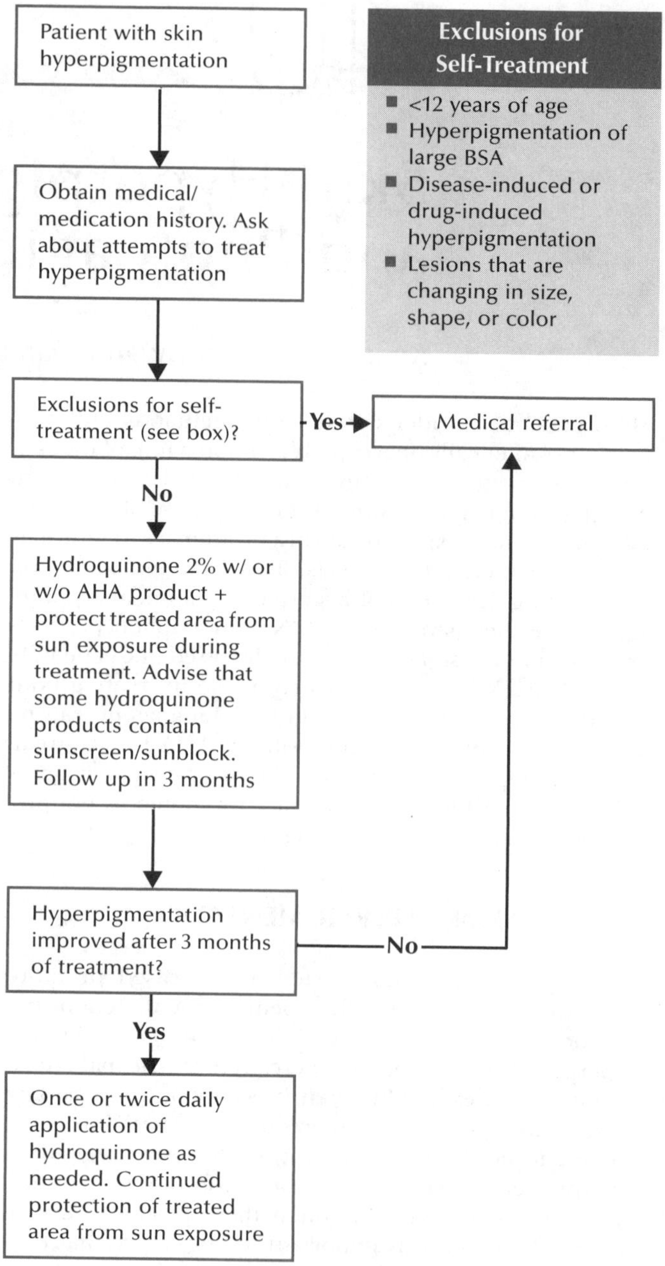


**FIGURE 40-1** Self-care of skin hyperpigmentation. Key: AHA, α-hydroxy acid; BSA, body surface area.

consists of a more intense brown coloration than that of surrounding normal skin; the discoloration may range from dark to faint in appearance.[4] As noted earlier, some hyperpigmentation can occur in areas of trauma or inflammation. Clinical evidence of hyperpigmentation and photoaging, as well as response to treatment, is not easily quantifiable by standard light photography or by routine clinical evaluation. Fluorescence photography is used to detect subtle but significant decreases in diffuse and mottled hyperpigmentation after topical treatment to clinically evaluate and effectively assess efficacy of topical products.[5]

## Treatment of Skin Hyperpigmentation

### *Treatment Goals*

The goal of treating skin hyperpigmentation is to diminish the degree of pigmentation of affected areas so the skin tone of these areas is consistent with surrounding normal skin.

### *General Treatment Approach*

Several types of hyperpigmentation, including freckles, melasma, and lentigines, are amenable to self-treatment with topical nonprescription skin-bleaching agents.[6] They diminish hyperpigmentation by inhibiting melanin production within skin.[7] Many treatments are available for melasma, but the combination of a bleaching agent (e.g., hydroquinone) with an exfoliant (e.g., an AHA) is considered efficacious (see Treatment of Photoaging), giving patients acceptable outcomes with minimal adverse effects.[8,9]

To prevent negating the effects of treatment, patients must avoid even minimal exposure to UVR and must use sunscreen agents and protective clothing on an indefinite, ongoing basis, even after discontinuing the bleaching agent. The algorithm in Figure 40-1 outlines the self-treatment of skin hyperpigmentation.

Management of hyperpigmentation directed by a primary care provider may include topical prescription agents composed of ingredients known to cause lightening of the skin, such as tretinoin (retinoic acid), azelaic acid, hydroquinone, and a corticosteroid, or even laser therapy. A combination of ingredients may sometimes be effective for postinflammatory hyperpigmentation that is resistant to nonprescription treatment.[10]

### *Pharmacologic Therapy*

Historically, a number of topical agents have been used in skin-bleaching preparations (fading creams).[11] These agents have included hydroquinone, monobenzyl and monomethyl ethers of hydroquinone, ammoniated mercury,

**TABLE 40-2 Selected Skin-bleaching/Fading Products**

| Trade Name | Primary Ingredients |
|---|---|
| Eldopaque | Hydroquinone 2% |
| Esoterica Facial | Hydroquinone2%; octyl dimethyl PABA 3.3%; benzophenone-3, 2.5% |
| Esoterica Regular | Hydroquinone 2% |
| NeoStrata Skin Lightening | Hydroquinone 2% |
| Nadinola Skin Discoloration Fade Cream Deluxe for Oily Skin | 2-Ethyl hexyl salicylate3%; hydroquinone 2% |
| Porcelana Skin Discoloration Fade Cream Night Time Formula | Hydroquinone 2%; octyl methoxycinnamate 2.5% |
| Solaquin | Hydroquinone 2% |

ascorbic acid, peroxides, and kojic acid. However, only preparations containing hydroquinone were submitted to the Advisory Review Panel on Over-the-Counter Miscellaneous External Drug Products of the Food and Drug Administration (FDA). Pigment disorders may present with both hypo- and hyperpigmented skin or skin that may appear mottled. Nonprescription skin-staining products such as Dy-O-Derm or Chromelin Complexion Blender, which contain dihydroxyacetone (the active ingredient in self-tanning products), may be used to adjust color in lightened skin areas to approximate natural darker tones in mixed hypo- and hyperpigmented disorders.[12] Once the desired skin color is attained, applications are decreased from daily to every fourth to seventh day to maintain the desired outcome. Since this product has a higher concentration of active ingredient than that found in self-tanning products, it is not intended for widespread application.

### Hydroquinone

FDA has recommended that hydroquinone (*p*-dihydroxybenzene) in concentrations of 1.5% to 2.0% be available for nonprescription use,[6] and the safety of bleaching creams containing hydroquinone has been separately reviewed in the literature.[13] Table 40-2 lists selected tradename products.

*Mechanism of Action* Hydroquinone and its derivatives act by reducing conversion of tyrosine to dopa and subsequently to melanin by inhibiting the enzyme tyrosinase. Other possible mechanisms of action include destruction of the melanocyte or melanosomes.[8,14] Topical preparations of hydroquinone 2% to 5% are effective in producing cutaneous hypopigmentation. The 2% concentration is safer and produces results equivalent to those of higher concentrations.[13] Exfoliants such as topical glycolic acid (an AHA) or topical tretinoin are sometimes combined with hydroquinone to enhance hydroquinone's absorption and effect.[15]

Monobenzone, the monobenzyl ether of hydroquinone, is a prescription medication, whose use usually is restricted to depigmenting remaining areas of normally pigmented skin in patients with extensive vitiligo (a condition resulting in patches of depigmentation, often with hyperpigmented borders).

*Dosage and Administration Guidelines* Hydroquinone is dosed as a thin topical application of a 2% concentration, rubbed gently but thoroughly into affected areas twice daily. The agent should be applied to clean skin before application of moisturizers or other skin care products. It should not be applied to damaged skin or near the eyes. If no improvement is seen within 3 months, its use should be discontinued and a primary care provider should be consulted.[7] Once the desired benefit is achieved, hydroquinone can be applied as often as needed in a once- or twice-daily regimen to maintain lightening of the skin. Because of the lack of safety data, hydroquinone is not recommended for children younger than 12 years, except under the supervision of a primary care provider.

*Safety Considerations* Adverse effects, such as tingling or burning on application, are mild with low concentrations of topical hydroquinine.[16] If desired, patients can apply the agent to a small test area and check for signs of irritation after 24 hours. Higher concentrations frequently irritate the skin and, if used for prolonged periods, may cause side effects including epidermal thickening, pitch-black pigmentation, and colloid milium (yellowish papules associated with colloid degeneration).[17]

The effectiveness of hydroquinone varies among patients, and treatment must usually be maintained on an indefinite basis to retain lightening once it has been achieved. Results are best on lighter skin and lighter lesions. In dark skin, the response to hydroquinone depends on the amount of pigment present. Hyperpigmented areas fade more rapidly and completely than surrounding normal skin. Although treatment may not lead to complete disappearance of hypermelanosis, the results are often satisfactory enough to reduce self-consciousness. A disadvantage of treatment with hydroquinone is that it tends to overshoot the intended degree of hypopigmentation and may produce treated areas that are lighter than the surrounding normal skin color. Therefore, the patient must carefully observe the degree of lightening as the treatment progresses and must subsequently decrease applications when sufficient lightening has occurred.

A decrease in skin color usually becomes noticeable in about 4 weeks; however, the time of onset varies from 3 weeks to 3 months. Hypopigmentation lasts for 2 to 6 months, but is reversible upon UVR exposure. Although sunscreens may help to prevent repigmentation, even visible light may cause some darkening. Thus, a sunscreen containing opaque ingredients, such as zinc oxide or titanium dioxide, is preferable for sun protection.[18] Some nonprescription hydroquinone products are formulated to include a sunscreen.

In some cases, lesions become slightly darker before fading. A transient inflammatory reaction may develop after the first few weeks of treatment. Inflammation makes subsequent lightening more likely although inflammation can occur without the development of hypopigmentation. Mild inflammation is not an indication to stop therapy except when the reaction increases in intensity at which point a patch test can be done for allergy to hydroquinone although most reactions are irritant rather than allergic in nature. Topical hydrocortisone may be used temporarily to alleviate the inflammatory reaction. Contact with eyes should be avoided. Accidental ingestion of hydroquinone seldom produces serious systemic toxicity. However, oral ingestion of 5 to 15 g has produced tremor, convulsions, and hemolytic anemia.[13] Reversible brown discoloration of nails has been reported occasionally after application of hydroquinone 2% to the back of the hand.[19] Discoloration is probably caused by formation of oxidation products of hydroquinone.

*Product Considerations* Hydroquinone is readily oxidized in the presence of light and air. Discoloration or darkening of the cream indicates product deterioration as well as a possible decline in the strength of available hydroquinone. Thus, the preferable method of packaging is in small, closed dispensing containers such as squeeze tubes.

### Hydroquinone Adjuvants and Combinations

Because hydroquinone is oxidized by contact with air, antioxidants such as sodium bisulfite may be added to the formulation. Hydroquinone is incompatible with alkali or ferric salts.[18] The inclusion of a sunscreen agent is rational and appropriate, provided that combination products are intended primarily as skin-bleaching agents with added sunscreen.

### Other Agents

Kojic acid, a product derived from certain species of fungus (e.g., Acetobacter, Aspergillus, Penicillum), can be found in cosmetic products promoted for the treatment of hyperpigmentation. This product is usually found in combination with AHAs with or without hydroquinone. Kojic acid works by inhibiting the production of tyrosinase. Adverse effects associated with this product include contact dermatitis and erythema. One study comparing the combination of kojic acid and glycolic acid to hydroquinone and glycolic acid demonstrated similar results between the two therapies.[2,8,20]

### Product Selection Guidelines

Product selection should be based on a suitable dosage form (i.e., cream, lotion, gel) for the patient's skin type (dry, normal, oily) and anatomic site (face, neck). For example, an emollient cream-based product may be more suitable for dry skin, whereas a gel-based preparation may be preferable for an oily skin type.

## Assessment of Skin Hyperpigmentation: A Case-based Approach

The practitioner should evaluate the affected areas to determine whether they are characteristic of freckles, melasma, or lentigines. The patient's medication history and health status are important factors in pinpointing possible causes of the hyperpigmentation. Case 40-1 gives an example of the assessment of patients with skin hyperpigmentation.

**CASE 40-1**

| Relevant Evaluation Criteria | Scenario/Model Outcome |
|---|---|
| **Information Gathering** | |
| 1. Gather essential information about the patient's symptoms, including: | |
| a. description of symptom(s) (i.e., nature, onset, duration, severity, associated symptoms) | Patient complains of "brown spots" covering the malar area of the face, bilaterally for about 2 years, gradually increasing in intensity and enlarging over time. She has no other symptoms. |
| b. description of any factors that seem to precipitate, exacerbate, and/or relieve the patient's symptom(s) | Patient is Hispanic with moderate pigmentation in noninvolved facial areas. She does not use a sunscreen and does not avoid prolonged sun exposure. |
| c. description of the patient's efforts to relieve the symptoms | None |

## CASE 40-1 (continued)

| Relevant Evaluation Criteria | Scenario/Model Outcome |
|---|---|
| 2. Gather essential patient history information: | |
| a. patient's identity | Patricia |
| b. age, sex, height, and weight | 28 y/o F |
| c. patient's occupation | Attorney |
| d. patient's dietary habits | N/A |
| e. patient's sleep habits | N/A |
| f. concurrent medical conditions, prescription and nonprescription medications, and dietary supplements | Ortho Tri-Cyclen 1 tablet once daily for the past 2 years |
| g. allergies | Ampicillin (skin rash) |
| h. history of other adverse reactions to medications | None |
| i. other (describe)_______ | None |
| **Assessment and Triage** | |
| 3. Differentiate the patient's signs/symptoms and correctly identify the patient's primary problem(s). | Patricia has bilateral large hyperpigmented macules over large areas of the cheek. |
| 4. Identify exclusions for self-treatment (see Figure 40-1). | None |
| 5. Formulate a comprehensive list of therapeutic alternatives for the primary problem to determine if triage to a medical practitioner is required, and share this information with the patient. | Options include:<br>(1) Recommend self-care with OTC fading cream such as hydroquinone 2% to lighten the area gradually, in combination with avoidance of prolonged sun exposure and use of sunscreen.<br>(2) Refer Patricia to a PCP for other treatment options.<br>(3) Recommend use of sunscreens with SPF 15 or greater and avoidance of prolonged sun exposure until PCP can be consulted.<br>(4) Take no action. |
| **Plan** | |
| 6. Select an optimal therapeutic alternative to address the patient's problem, taking into account patient preferences. | The patient prefers self-treatment with an OTC fading cream and sun avoidance. |
| 7. Describe the recommended therapeutic approach to the patient. | Apply a nonprescription fading cream with hydroquinone 2% up to twice daily. It is also important to apply sunscreen before any exposure to the sun. Use facial moisturizer as needed if treated skin becomes dry. |
| 8. Explain to the patient the rationale for selecting the recommended therapeutic approach from the considered therapeutic alternatives. | Sun exposure is probably causing the brown spots. Even if the fading cream lightens the darker skin areas, the hyperpigmentation will return if you do not protect your skin from sun exposure. |
| **Patient Education** | |
| 9. When recommending self-care with nonprescription medications and/or nondrug therapy, convey accurate information to the patient, including: | |
| a. appropriate dose and frequency of administration | Hydroquinone 2% cream should be applied to the entire hyperpigmented area of both cheeks daily to begin, increasing to two times daily as tolerated. Sunscreen should also be applied in adequate amounts (see Chapter 39). |

## CASE 40-1 (continued)

| Relevant Evaluation Criteria | Scenario/Model Outcome |
|---|---|
| b. maximum number of days the therapy should be employed | Indefinite application of hydroquinone and sunscreen to maintain lightening effect |
| c. product administration procedures | Dot a pea-sized amount of product over the involved areas of both cheeks, apply thinly and evenly. Use care not to apply to eyes or mucous membranes. |
| d. expected time to onset of relief | Optimal response may take up to 3 months. |
| e. degree of relief that can be reasonably expected | Hyperpigmented facial skin (brown spots) will become less visible; the degree of response may vary. |
| f. most common side effects | Mild tingling or burning may occur when the cream is applied. |
| g. side effects that warrant medical intervention should they occur | Excessive dryness or irritation warrants concurrent moisturizer application. Erythema, burning, and pruritus may represent allergic contact dermatitis, If this occurs, the product should be discontinued, and you should see your health care provider. |
| h. patient options in the event that condition worsens or persists | If there is no response or if cosmetically desirable response is not obtained after 3 months, you should see your health care provider for further treatment options. |
| i. product storage requirements | Store at room temperature, and keep container tightly closed. |
| j. specific nondrug measures | Use a sunscreen and daily moisturizers to minimize dry skin (especially in dry, cold climates) and maintain skin-lightening effect. |
| 10. Solicit follow-up questions from patient. | What do I do if my skin gets irritated? |
| 11. Answer patient's questions. | You may adjust the frequency of application (maximum twice daily) to reduce irritation as fading progresses. |

Key: N/A, not applicable; OTC, over-the-counter; PCP, primary care provider; SPF, sun protection factor.

## Patient Counseling for Skin Hyperpigmentation

The clinician should explain which types of hyperpigmentation are self-treatable while stressing the importance of avoidance of sun exposure during and after treatment. To ensure a successful therapeutic outcome, the practitioner should review the product instructions with the patient. The boxes Patient Education for Photoaging and Patient Education for Skin Hyperpigmentation list specific information to provide patients.

## PATIENT EDUCATION FOR SKIN HYPERPIGMENTATION

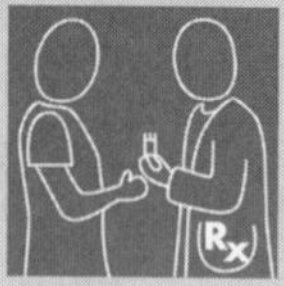


The objective of self-treatment with skin-bleaching products is to diminish the degree of pigmentation in affected areas. For most patients, carefully following product instructions and the self-care measures listed here will help ensure optimal therapeutic outcomes:

- Use hydroquinone to lighten only limited areas of hyperpigmented skin that show brownish discoloration.
- Do not use these products on nevi (moles), or reddish or bluish areas, such as port wine discoloration.
- Time to initial response averages 6 to 8 weeks, but it may take up to 3 months to see noticeable results.
- Test for possible irritant reactions to the product by applying it to a small test area and by checking the area for redness, itching, or swelling after 24 hours.
- Do not apply the product near the eyes or to damaged skin.
- Apply a thin layer of the product to clean, dry skin in the affected area only. Rub into the skin gently but thoroughly.
- If moisturizers or other topical agents are being used at the same time, apply the hydroquinone first.
- When you are outdoors for even a short time, apply an opaque sunblock or broad-spectrum sunscreen (see Chapter 39) to the affected area after applying the hydroquinone, if the product does not already contain a sunscreen in the formulation.
- Once the desired lightening of skin is reached, apply the hydroquinone once or twice daily to prevent hyperpigmentation from recurring. Continue to protect the treated area from sun exposure.

Consult a primary care provider if:

- No improvement is seen after 3 months of using hydroquinone.
- Skin pigmentation becomes darker during treatment with hydroquinone.

## Evaluation of Patient Outcomes for Skin Hyperpigmentation

The clinician should check on the patient's progress after 3 months of therapy. Follow-up can be achieved through a telephone call or a scheduled visit to the practitioner. If the pigmented area shows no improvement, the patient should consult a primary care provider. If the desired outcome has been achieved, the patient should continue applying the hydroquinone once or twice daily to maintain lightening of the skin.

# PHOTOAGING

Photoaging, or dermatoheliosis, is the pattern of characteristic skin changes associated with sun exposure. Most fair-skinned Americans will have some signs of photodamaged skin by 50 years of age. A variety of therapies are available for treatment of photodamaged skin, which range from surgical procedures such as face lifts and laser resurfacing to less invasive topical products and cosmetics.[22] Although some products are available only by prescription, many others are nonprescription, with AHAs being widely used to combat photoaged skin. A 1996 report indicated sales of approximately $300 million per year for AHA products.[23]

## Etiology/Pathophysiology of Photoaging

Aging skin results from a combination of extrinsic and intrinsic factors. Clinical and histologic changes that intrinsically occur include genetically controlled skin and muscle changes, expression lines, sleep lines, and hormonal changes. The second component, extrinsic aging, relates to environmental influences such as UVR, smoking, wind, and chemical exposure.[24,25] Medications known to induce photosensitivity can contribute to photoaging by making the skin sensitive to UVR (see Chapter 39).

Prematurely aged facial skin, with creases and wrinkles, dry texture, and blotchy hyperpigmentation, is largely attributed to cumulative UVR, or photoaging.[26] Exposure to UVB (290-320 nm) is primarily responsible for photoaging although the longer UVA (320-400 nm) wavelengths also contribute to damage. UVA is present in 10-fold greater amounts in sunlight than UVB, which allows for greater amounts of skin exposure. UVA can penetrate into the deeper dermal layer and can work synergistically with UVB to cause photodamage and skin cancers.[27]

Microscopically, sun-damaged skin shows dysplasia (abnormal tissue development), atypical keratinocytes, and occasional cell necrosis. Irregularity of epidermal cell alignment is also common. Deeper in the dermal layer is a loss of collagen and elastin.[22]

## Signs and Symptoms of Photoaging

Clinical signs of photoaging include changes in color, surface texture, and functional capacity (Table 40-3). Photoaged skin may have a sallow yellow color with discoloration and may show telangiectasias (visible distended capillaries). Textural changes include loss of smoothness, loss of subcutaneous tissue around the mouth, and epidermal thinning around the lip. As sebaceous glands hypertrophy, the skin begins to show coarse texture with increased pore size. In addition, fine vellus hairs can develop into unwanted terminal hairs. Other manifestations of photoaged skin may include development of precancerous (actinic keratosis) and cancerous (basal cell, squamous cell, and melanoma) tumor development.[22,28] Cosmetically, patients notice freckling, discolorations, or "crow's feet" (small parallel lines around the eyes). In contrast, postmenopausal skin is susceptible to reduced estrogen receptor stimulation of dermal metabolism and undergoes significant changes in collagen and moisture content. This leads to signs of skin aging evidenced by diminished elasticity and wrinkles.[29]

**TABLE 40-3 Classification of Photoaging**

| | |
|---|---|
| Type I (Mild) | No wrinkles; early photoaging; mild pigment changes<br>20-30 years of age |
| Type II (Moderate) | Wrinkles in motion; early to moderate photoaging; keratoses palpable<br>30-40 years of age |
| Type III (Advanced) | Wrinkles at rest; advanced photoaging; obvious dyschromia and keratoses<br>≥50 years of age |
| Type IV (Severe) | Only wrinkles; severe photoaging; yellow-gray skin<br>≥60 years of age |

*Source:* Glogau RG. Aesthetic and anatomic analysis of the aging skin. *Semin Cutan Med Surg.* 1996;15:134-8.

## Treatment of Photoaging

### *Treatment Goals*

The first goal is to prevent or minimize the likelihood of skin photoaging by appropriate sun protection, including sunscreens.[30] The goals of treating photoaging are to (1) reverse cumulative skin damage with prescription and nonprescription products and (2) maintain the skin and protect it from further extrinsic damage by making lifestyle changes and, most importantly, protecting the skin from further and prolonged sun exposure

### *General Treatment Approach*

The first step in preventing and treating photoaged skin is for the patient to commit to daily sun protection. Broad-spectrum sunscreens (UVA & UVB coverage) with a sun protection factor (SPF) of 15 or greater can minimize further photodamage during UVR exposure (see Chapter 39).[31]

Proper cleansing of the skin removes bacteria, dirt, desquamated keratinocytes, cosmetics, sebum, and perspiration. However, excessive use of soap leads to xerosis, eczematous dermatitis, and other skin conditions.[32] Use of AHAs enhances skin water retention and repairs damaged skin by improving the skin's elasticity.[33]

TABLE 40-4 Selected Products for Photoaged Skin

| Trade Name | Active Ingredients |
|---|---|
| **α-Hydroxy Acid Products** | |
| AmLactin 12% Moisturizing Lotion | Lactic acid 12% |
| Aqua Glycolic Hand & Body Lotion | Glycolic acid 14% |
| Alpha Hydrox Creme Enhanced*† | Glycolic acid 10% |
| Cetaphil Moisturizing Lotion* | Citric acid |
| Dermal Therapy Body Lotion Extra Strength | Urea 10%; lactic & malic acids 5% |
| Eucerin Dry Skin Therapy Plus Intensive Repair Lotion With Alpha Hydroxy | Sodium lactate; urea; panthenol |
| Lac-Hydrin Five Lotion* | Lactic acid |
| Nutraderm 30 Lotion | Lactic acid; malic acid |
| WellSkin Body Lotion with SPF 15 | Octyl methoxycinnamate 7.5%; octyl salicylate 5%; oxybenzone 3%; glycolic acid |
| **Other Products** | |
| Kinerase Lotion/Cream | *N*-Furfuryladenine 0.1% |
| Olay Age Defying Daily Renewal Cream, Beta Hydroxy Complex | Salicylic acid |

*Fragrance-free; †oil-free.

## *Pharmacologic Therapy*

Within the vast array of available nonprescription products for skin care, the division of categories is blurred. Cosmetics and moisturizers are not pharmaceuticals, whereas antiperspirants and sunscreens are considered nonprescription pharmaceuticals. Although "cosmeceuticals" are an undefined category of products recognized by practitioners and dermatologists, no final regulatory guidance currently is available for these products from FDA. Many cosmeceutical ingredients, such as AHAs, function as active pharmaceuticals that are known to penetrate and alter the stratum corne um.[34]

Various topical products are being used to treat aging skin. Nonprescription products include vitamin C and vitamin K products, *N*-furfuryladenine (Kinerase), and AHAs and BHAs.

### α-Hydroxy Acids

AHAs have generated much interest in the treatment of aging skin.[8] The AHAs are used in various concentrations, with a wide array of available products. Most AHAs are sold as cosmeceuticals, whereas others are sold as cosmetics, and yet others are sold as pharmaceuticals through a primary care provider. These products range in concentration from 2% to 20% (as nonpeeling AHAs) and act as peeling agents (as used by estheticians or dermatologists) in concentrations above 20%.

Of the available nonprescription products, AHAs currently play a major role in reliably reversing and cosmetically improving aging skin.[8,35] Many types of AHAs are available, with the most common being lactic and glycolic acids (Table 40-4). Other AHAs that are not as widely used include malic acid, citric acid, and tartaric acids. Although termed a *cosmeceutical* by industry, FDA has not yet defined AHAs as either cosmetics or drugs.[36]

The Cosmetic Ingredient Review Expert Panel, the cosmetic industry self-regulatory body, concluded that use of AHAs in cosmetic products is safe if (1) concentrations are less than or equal to 10%, (2) final pH is greater than or equal to 3.5, and (3) product is formulated with a sunscreen or directions to use a sunscreen are included.[36]

*Mechanism of Action* Used appropriately, AHA products act as exfoliants by causing detachment of keratinocytes, resulting in a smoother, nonscaly skin surface with eventual normalization of keratinization. The product's pH is important because products with a lower pH produce greater results, but may carry an increased risk of irritation.[24,31]

By improving skin elasticity, AHAs have been shown to make skin more flexible and less vulnerable to cracking and flaking. Long-term use has led to an increase in skin collagen and elastin.[8,23] Regular application of AHAs results in smoother skin texture, lessening of fine lines, and normalization of pigmentation.[37]

*Indications* Current labeling on AHA cosmetic products includes recommendations for melasma, acne, solar lentigines, and fine wrinkling of photoaging.[8]

*Dosage and Administration Guidelines* Guidelines for treatment with AHAs include identification of patient factors such as medications, prior procedures, and medical history, all of which may affect treatment outcome and realistic patient expectations.[38] Care should be taken to apply AHAs to completely dry skin, with an estimated wait time of 10 to 15 minutes after cleansing the face. It is also prudent to begin application gradually, starting every other night for approximately 1 week and then increasing as tolerated to a maximum of twice-daily application. AHA products may make the skin more sensitive to sun exposure. Patients should be advised to use daily sunscreen or sunblock with an SPF of 15 or greater during use of AHAs and after their discontinuation.[31]

*Safety Considerations* Common adverse effects include mild, transient stinging, burning, pruritus, skin lightening, and dryness. Many of these effects can be ameliorated if products are used with caution and proper counseling. Patients should also note that other topically applied products, both medications and cosmetics, may contain active ingredients (e.g., AHA, BHA, hydroquinone) capable of exacerbating irritation.

### Product Selection Guidelines

Skin type should determine the vehicle chosen. Creams are appropriate for drier skin types, lotions are best for combination or normal skin, and gels or solutions are useful for oilier skin. Use of products with higher concentrations and a lower pH may produce faster results. However, the patient should be warned that these products may also cause greater skin irritation.

AHAs are not contraindicated in pregnancy.[39]

### Other Agents

There is little scientific information to support mechanism of action for other agents used in photoaging treatment. However, the indications, dosage, and adverse events are similar to AHAs.

*β-Hydroxy Acids* Of the BHAs, salicylic acid is used widely even as a chemical peel for resurfacing moderately photodamaged facial skin.[40] Compared with AHA products, BHAs are less soluble and unstable in water and demonstrate keratolytic effects. Although BHAs are now marketed as cosmetics, they have been used to treat skin conditions such as dermatitis and psoriasis for quite some time. Products containing BHAs as the active ingredients may be beneficial to acne-prone skin.

*N-Furfuryladenine* Kinerase (N-furfuryladenine 0.1%) is an "antiwrinkle" compound marketed as a cream or lotion to reduce wrinkles, blotchiness, and dryness. Support exists for its use as a moisturizer to improve blotchiness and skin roughness, but efficacy in reversing photodamage, compared with available prescription products, is not yet established. Kinerase may be recommended for patients with sensitive skin or for those who choose not to obtain prescription therapy for photodamaged skin.

## Assessment of Photoaging: A Case-based Approach

If visual inspection of the patient's skin causes the clinician to suspect photoaging, the patient should be questioned about his or her history of UVR (sunlight as well as artificial light) exposure. Knowing whether the patient's current occupational or recreational habits require excessive exposure is useful not only in determining the cause of the skin disorder but also in developing a treatment plan. It is important to assess for a history of diseases or medications that may predispose the patient to premature photodamage or photosensitivity. The patient's health status, lifestyle practices, and daily skin maintenance regimen are other pertinent assessment criteria.[22] Case 40-2 gives an example of the assessment of a patient with photoaging.

**CASE 40-2**

| Relevant Evaluation Criteria | Scenario/Model Outcome |
|---|---|
| **Information Gathering** | |
| 1. Gather essential information about the patient's symptoms, including: | |
| a. description of symptom(s) (i.e., nature, onset, duration, severity, associated symptoms) | Patient complains of "crow's feet" around the eyes and fine wrinkles above her top lip. In the last few months her skin has been noticeably drier. |
| b. description of any factors that seem to precipitate, exacerbate, and/or relieve the patient's symptom(s) | Patient has fair skin which burns easily. She likes to regularly spend times outdoors especially in the summer months. She does not apply sunscreen regularly. |
| c. description of the patient's efforts to relieve the symptoms | None |
| 2. Gather essential patient history information: | |
| a. patient's identity | Kelly |
| b. age, sex, height, and weight | 44 y/o F |

## CASE 40-2 (continued)

| Relevant Evaluation Criteria | Scenario/Model Outcome |
|---|---|
| c. patient's occupation | Waitress |
| d. patient's dietary habits | N/A |
| e. patient's sleep habits | N/A |
| f. concurrent medical conditions, prescription and nonprescription medications, and dietary supplements | None |
| g. allergies | NKA |
| h. history of other adverse reactions to medications | None |
| i. other (describe)______ | N/A |
| **Assessment and Triage** | |
| 3. Differentiate the patient's signs/symptoms and correctly identify the patient's primary problem(s). | Patient has dry, aging skin aggravated by constant, unprotected sun exposure on fair skin. |
| 4. Identify exclusions for self-treatment. | None |
| 5. Formulate a comprehensive list of therapeutic alternatives for the primary problem to determine if triage to a medical practitioner is required, and share this information with the patient. | Options include:<br>(1) Recommend steps to minimize sun exposure such as: daily topical sunscreen application, protective clothing, and avoidance of mid-day sun.<br>(2) Recommend self-care with an OTC AHA topical product to exfoliate and minimize wrinkles and/or daily moisturizing care for dry skin.<br>(3) Refer Kelly to a PCP. Recommend self-care until a PCP can be consulted.<br>(4) Take no action. |
| **Plan** | |
| 6. Select an optimal therapeutic alternative to address the patient's problem, taking into account patient preferences. | Self-care with sunscreens to protect the skin from further sun exposure and an OTC AHA and/or moisturizer to minimize the wrinkles is appropriate. The patient prefers this option. |
| 7. Describe the recommended therapeutic approach to the patient. | Apply a nonprescription topical exfoliating product containing glycolic acid 10% up to twice daily. Use sun protection measures (see Chapter 39) and moisturizers regularly. |
| 8. Explain to the patient the rationale for selecting the recommended therapeutic approach from the considered therapeutic alternatives. | Daily use of a sunscreen will protect your skin from further damage. The glycolic acid product can improve the elasticity of your skin and diminish the appearance of the wrinkles. The moisturizer may also help to diminish the appearance of the wrinkles. |
| **Patient Education** | |
| 9. When recommending self-care with nonprescription medications and/or nondrug therapy, convey accurate information to the patient, including: | |
| a. appropriate dose and frequency of administration | Begin applying the product once every other day at bedtime for 1 week, increasing gradually to twice-daily application as tolerated. |
| b. maximum number of days the therapy should be employed | Indefinite application to maintain antiphotoaging effect. |
| c. product administration procedures | Apply a pea-sized amount of the glycolic acid product to dry skin 10-15 minutes after cleansing face. |
| d. expected time to onset of relief | Results should be seen within a 2-month period of time. |

## CASE 40-2 (continued)

| Relevant Evaluation Criteria | Scenario/Model Outcome |
|---|---|
| e. degree of relief that can be reasonably expected | Photoaged skin (fine wrinkles) will become less visible. |
| f. most common side effects | Mild and transient stinging, itching or burning may occur when the cream is applied. Dryness of the skin may also occur. |
| g. side effects that warrant medical intervention should they occur | Excessive dryness or irritation warrants concurrent moisturizer application or decreased application of product. Severe burning, itching, redness or drying of the skin may require you discontinue the product. If symptoms do not resolve with product discontinuation, see your health care provider. |
| h. patient options in the event that condition worsens or persists | If no response within 2 months, you may consider more potent alpha hydroxy acids, such as those in chemical peels. |
| i. product storage requirements | Store at room temperature, and keep container tightly closed. |
| | Alpha hydroxy acid products may make your skin more susceptible to photodamage. Daily use of a sunscreen will protect your skin. Use daily moisturizers (especially in dry, cold climates) to minimize dry skin. |
| 10. Solicit follow-up questions from patient. | What do I do if my skin gets too irritated? |
| 11. Answer patient's questions. | You should decrease the frequency of application of the alpha hydroxy acid until skin irritation lessens. As tolerated by your skin increase dosing to the maximum of twice-daily application. |

Key: AHA, α-hydroxy acid; N/A, not applicable; NKA, no known allergies; OTC, over-the-counter; PCP, primary care provider.

## Patient Counseling for Photoaging

The practitioner should advise patients that premature wrinkling, creases, dry texture, and blotchy hyperpigmentation are not inevitable.[26] The practitioner should be proactive in identifying and recommending products that are appropriate for a specific patient.

## Evaluation of Patient Outcomes for Photoaging

Patients treated with nonprescription products for photoaging should set a reasonable goal. Obviously, these preparations cannot "erase wrinkles." The practitioner should monitor the progress of the treatment and be sensitive to issues that may require intervention by a primary care provider.

## PATIENT EDUCATION FOR PHOTOAGING

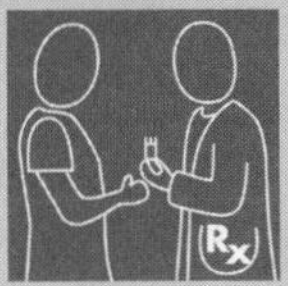


The objectives of self-treatment are to (1) reverse skin damage by using available nonprescription products and (2) protect the skin from further damage by making lifestyle changes and protecting skin from sun exposure. For most patients, carefully following product instructions and the self-care measures listed here will help ensure optimal therapeutic outcomes.

- Protect the skin from sun exposure by covering the skin with clothing. The FDA recommends advising patients to wear long-sleeved clothing and hats with brims of at least 4 inches. Patients should also use a sunblock or sunscreen product with an SPF of 15 or greater during use of alpha hydroxy acids (AHAs) and regularly in the future to prevent further damage.
- To prevent dry skin, cleanse the skin with a mild soap or a soap-free liquid cleanser. Do not cleanse skin more often than twice daily. Apply a pea-sized amount of an alpha hydroxy acid product to clean, dry skin.
- To minimize transient mild tingling and stinging, wait 10 to 15 minutes after cleansing the face to apply an AHA product.
- Excessive skin dryness or irritation warrants decreased application.
- Note that AHA products contain an active ingredient and that the use of other products, including cosmetics, could result in skin irritation, including mild stinging, burning, or erythema.
- Do not apply the product too close to the eyes or mucous membranes.
- Begin applying this product once at bedtime every other day for approximately 1 week. Gradually increase application to twice a day.
- Use a daily moisturizer with sunscreen after applying the AHA product to minimize dry skin and maintain the antiphotoaging effect.
- Store this product in a cool dry place out of the reach of children.

⚠ Discontinue the AHA product if severe irritation, such as redness or excessive dryness, or a rash occurs.

## KEY POINTS FOR SKIN HYPERPIGMENTATION AND PHOTOAGING

- Photoaging and hyperpigmentation are cosmetically unacceptable skin conditions. Patients who have reasonable expectations should be able to achieve even skin tone and minimize appearance and occurrence of fine wrinkling with the use of nonprescription products.
- Hydroquinone is the only FDA-approved nonprescription skin-bleaching product. Advise patients to apply a 2% concentration to skin twice daily.
- Patients younger than 12 years, those with large areas of hyperpigmentation, or disease- or drug-induced hyperpigmentation, or those with lesions that have changed in size, shape or color should consult their primary care provider.
- Patients should be referred to a primary care provider if no improvement occurs within 3 months or if skin darkens during treatment of hyperpigmentation.
- Patients should avoid applying hydroquinone-containing products near the eye area or on damaged skin areas.
- Patients using AHAs to reduce photoaging should be advised to apply AHAs up to twice daily to dry skin. Patients who do not see a desired improvement in skin appearance in 2 months or who experience excessive irritation or drying of the skin should contact their primary care provider.
- Patients who use products to prevent photoaging or hyperpigmentation should be instructed to protect their skin from daily sun exposure by using a sunscreen with SPF 15 or greater to maintain results.

## References


1. Taylor SC. Cosmetics problems in skin of color. *Skin Pharmacol Appl Skin Physiol.* 1999;12:139-43.
2. Stulberg DL, Clark N, Tovey D. Common hyperpigmentation disorders in adults, Part 1: Diagnostic approach, café au lait macules, diffuse hyperpigmentation, sun exposure and phototoxic reactions. *Am Fam Physician.* 2003;68:1955-60.
3. Nordlund JJ, Boissy R. The biology of melanocytes. In: Freinkel R, Woodley D, eds. *The Biology of the Skin.* New York: Parthenon; 2001:117.
4. Habif TP, Campbell JL, Quitadamo MJ, et al. *Skin Disease: Diagnosis and Treatment.* St. Louis: Mosby; 2001:318-9.
5. Kollias N, Gillies R, Cohen-Goihman, et al. Fluorescence photography in the evaluation of hyperpigmentation in photodamaged skin. *J Am Acad Dermatol.* 1997;36:226-30.
6. *Federal Register.* 1982;47:39108-17.
7. Briganti S, Camera E, Picardo M. Chemical and instrumental approaches to treat hyperpigmentation. *Pigment Cell Res.* 2003; 16:101-10.
8. Halder RM, Richards GM. Topical agents used in the management of hyperpigmentation. *Skin Ther Lett.* 2004;9:1-3.
9. Amer M, Metwalli M. Topical hydroquinone in the treatment of some hyperpigmentary disorders. *Int J Dermatol.* 1998;37:433-53.
10. Piamphongsant T. Treatment of melasma: a review with personal experience. *Int J Dermatol.* 1998;37:897-903.
11. Bleehan SS. Disorders of skin color. In: Champion RH, Burton JL, Burns DA, eds. *Textbook of Dermatology.* 6th ed. Oxford, England: Blackwell Science; 1998:1794-5.
12. Brown DA. Skin pigmentation enhancers. *J Photochem Photobiol.* 2001;63:148-61.
13. Fisher AA. The safety of bleaching creams containing hydroquinone. *Cutis.* 1998;61:303-4.
14. Kasraee B, Handjani F, Aslani FS. Enhancement of the depigmenting effect of hydroquinone and 4-hydroxyoxyanisole by all-TRANS-retinoic acid (tretinoin): the impairment of glutathion-dependent cytoprotection? *Dermatology.* 2003; 206:289-91.
15. Draelos ZD. Cosmetic therapy. In: Wolverton SE, ed. *Comprehensive Dermatologic Drug Therapy.* Philadelphia: WB Saunders; 2001:695.
16. Perez-Bernal A, Munoz-Perez MA, Camacho F. Management of facial hyperpigmentation. *Am J Clin Dermatol.* 2000;1:261-8.
17. Levin CY, Maibach H. Exogenous echronosis: an update on clinical features, causative agents and treatment options. *Am J Clin Dermatol.* 2001;2:213-7.
18. Arndt KA, Bowers KE. *Manual of Dermatologic Therapeutics.* 6th ed. Philadelphia: Lippincott Williams & Wilkins; 2002: 118-24.
19. Ozluer SM, Muir J. Nail staining from hydroquinone cream. *Australas J Dermatol.* 2000;41:255-6.
20. Garcia A, Fulton JE. The combination of glycolic acid and hydroquinone or kojic acid for the treatment of melasma and related conditions. *Dermatol Surg* 1999;22:443-7.
21. Stratigos AJ, Katsambas AD. Optimal management of recalcitrant disorders of hyperpigmentation in dark-skinned patients. *Am J Clin Dermatol* 2004;5:161-68.
22. Drake L, Dinehart S, Farmer E, et al. Guidelines of care for photoaging/photodamage. *J Am Acad Dermatol.* 1996;35:462-4.
23. Stiller MJ, Bartolone J, Stern R, et al. Topical 8% glycolic acid and 8% L-lactic acid creams for the treatment of photodamaged skin. *Arch Dermatol.* 1996;132:631-6.
24. Holck DE. Facial skin rejuvenation. *Curr Opin in Opthalmol.* 2003; 14:246-252.
25. Gendler EC. Topical treatment of the aging face. *Dermatol Clin.* 1997;15:561-7.
26. Kligman AM. Topical treatments for photoaged skin. *Postgrad Med.* 1997;102:115-26.
27. Yarr M, Gilchrest B. Aging of Skin. In: Freedberg IM, Eisen AZ, Wolff K, et al., eds. *Fitzpatrick's Dermatology in General Medicine.* 6th ed. New York: McGraw-Hill; 2003:1386-98.
28. Hashizume H. Skin aging and dry skin. *J Dermatol.* 2004;31:603-9.
29. Raine-Fenning N, Brincat M, Muscat-Baron Y. Skin aging and menopause: implications for treatment. *Am J Clin Dermatol.* 2003; 4:371-8.
30. Levy SB. Sunscreens. In: Wolverton SE, ed. *Comprehensive Dermatologic Drug Therapy.* Philadelphia: WB Saunders; 2001:632-46.
31. Stern RS. Treatment of photoaging. *N Eng J Med.* 2004;350:1526-34.
32. Draelos ZD. Therapeutic skin care in the mature patient. *Clin Plastic Surg.* 1997;24:369-77.
33. Rawlings AV, Davies A, Carlomusto M, et al. Effect of lactic acid isomers on kerotinocyte ceramide synthesis, stratum corneum lipid levels and stratum corneum barrier function. *Arch Dermatol Res.* 1996;288:383-90.
34. Draelos ZD, Jegasothy SM. Should cosmeceuticals be regulated by the FDA? *Skin Aging.* 1999;7:52-4.
35. Clark CP 3rd. New directions in skin care. *Clin Plast Surg.* 2001; 28:745-50.
36. US Food and Drug Administration, Guidance for Industry. Labeling for topically applied cosmetic products containing alpha hydroxy acids as ingredients. Dec 2, 2002. Available at: www.cfsan.fda.gov/~dms/ahaguide.html. Accessed December 2004.
37. Lewis AB. Alpha-hydroxy acids. In: Wolverton SE, ed. *Comprehensive Dermatologic Drug Therapy.* Philadelphia: WB Saunders; 2001:659-70.
38. Tung RC, Bergfeld WF, Vidimos AT, et al. Alpha-hydroxy acid-based cosmetic procedures: guidelines for patient management. *Am J Clin Dermatol.* 2000;1:81-8.

39. Cosmetic ingredient review. Final report on the safety assessment of glycolic acid, ammonium, calcium, potassium, and sodium glycolates, methyl, ethyl, propyl, and butyl glycolates, and lactic acid, ammonium, calcium, potassium, sodium, and TEA-lactates, methyl, ethyl, isopropyl, and butyl lactates, and lauryl, myristyl, and ceryl lactates. *Int J Toxicol.* 1998;17(suppl 1):1-242.
40. Kligman D, Kligman AM. Salicylic acid peels for the treatment of photoaging. *Dermatol Surg.* 1998;24:325-8.
41. Elias SS, Patel NM, Cheigh NH. Drug-induced skin reactions. In: Dipiro JT, Talbert RL, Yee GC, et al., eds. *Pharmacotherapy: A Pathophysiologic Approach.* 5th ed. New York: McGraw-Hill, Inc; 2002:1705-15.

CHAPTER 41

# Minor Burns and Sunburn

*John D. Bowman*

Approximately 1.4 million persons in the United States sustain burns each year; of these, an estimated 54,000 to 108,000 are hospitalized.[1] Over 95% of these patients can be managed as outpatients. A substantially greater number of minor burns and sunburns occur and are self-treated with nonprescription products. Because deep burn injuries can lead to scarring and nonhealing wounds, it is important to accurately assess the injury and determine whether self-care or referral for further evaluation is appropriate.

## Epidemiology of Minor Burns and Sunburn

In 1995, approximately 3600 deaths and 18,600 injuries were attributed to residential fires.[2] Burn deaths occur more often in patients younger than 5 years or older than 64 years.[2] During 1991, residential fires were the second leading cause of injury deaths (after motor vehicle injuries) among children 1 to 9 years of age and the sixth leading cause of injury deaths among those 65 years of age and older.[3] Sunburn, in comparison, occurs at all ages.

More than 80% of minor burns occur in the home. Among household burns, 63% are on the hands and arms, and 34% are on the face and legs. Of the minor burns that occur outside the home, sunburn is the most common. The incidence and significance of sunburn have been underrated, and the injury goes unreported in most burn surveys because the public often does not consider sunburn in the same context as thermal, electrical, and chemical burns.

## Anatomy and Physiology of Skin

The skin is the largest organ of the human body, accounting for approximately 17% of the body weight of an average person. The skin performs a number of vital physiologic functions. It protects the body from injury and serves as a barrier against microorganisms. By synthesizing melanin, the skin protects underlying tissues from certain forms of irradiation. In addition, the skin is a sense organ, receiving sensory input (especially touch and temperature) from the proximal environment. Cholecalciferol (vitamin $D_3$), which is involved in calcium regulation, is produced in the skin through exposure to ultraviolet (UV) radiation. The skin plays a major role in thermoregulation because cutaneous blood flow and perspiration are vital in maintaining core body temperature at a normal level and also help maintain body water balance. Sebaceous glands produce oil, which lubricates and prevents excessive drying of the skin.

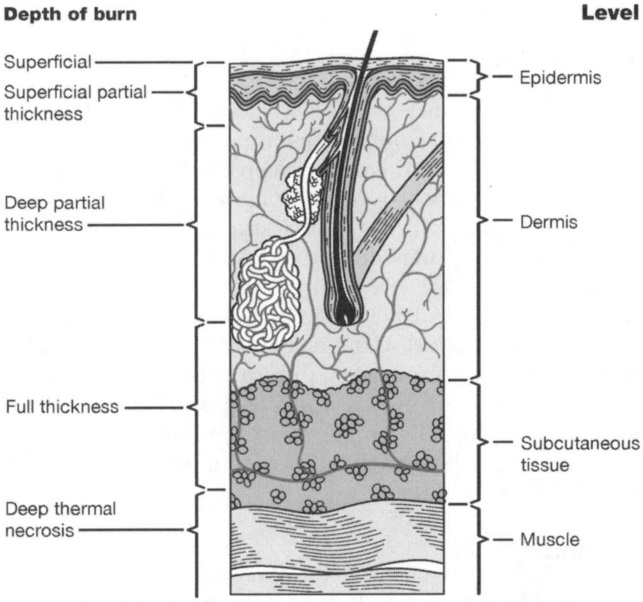


**FIGURE 41-1** Cross-section of skin showing depth of burns.

Figure 41-1 shows a cross-section of the anatomy of the skin and the depths of injury caused by thermal burns. (See Chapter 33 for further discussion of skin anatomy and physiology.)

## Etiology/Types of Burns

Burns are tissue injuries caused by thermal, electrical, chemical, or UV radiation exposure. Excluding sunburns, most burns occur in the home and are usually thermal burns.

### *Thermal Burns*

Thermal burns result from skin contact with flames, scalding liquids, or hot objects (e.g., irons, oven broiler elements, hot pans, curling irons, radiators) or from the inhalation of smoke or hot vapors. The leading causes of thermal burns in children are playing with fire ignition sources, such as matches, faulty or misused heating devices, and faulty or misused electrical sources. Among persons of advanced age, the leading causes are careless smoking, faulty or misused heating devices, and faulty or misused electrical sources.[3] Most fire-related deaths occur in December through February. The increased occurrence of deaths during the winter months reflects the seasonal use of space heaters, portable heaters, fireplaces, and Christmas trees.

Thermal damage to the respiratory tract from exposure to steam or hot gases can cause immediate upper airway obstruction as well as obstruction of the lower bronchioles caused by slowly developing edema. Smoke inhalation produces extensive lung damage because of toxic particles. Resultant injury to small airway alveolar capillaries can cause progressive respiratory failure. If smoke or heated gas inhalation has occurred, emergency services personnel should quickly transport the patient to a hospital emergency room.

### *Electrical Burns*

There are two types of electrical burns: flash electrical burns, which result from a high-temperature arc of current close to the skin, and contact electrical burns, which are caused by contact with a high-voltage source. Contact electrical burns generally have entry and exit sites, and tissue at every depth along the current's path can be injured, including bone. Electrical burns result from exposure to heat of up to 9000°F (5000°C). Electrical burns always injure the skin because the electrical energy is dissipated as heat. For the same reason, they can also cause extensive damage to underlying tissues. Progressive necrosis and sloughing are usually greater than the initial lesion indicates. The clinician should refer such injuries to a specialized burn care center.

### *Chemical Burns*

Chemical burns can result from skin contact with acids or alkalis contained in household products or from substances used in the workplace. Chemical burns can be partial or full thickness (see Classification of Burns). If not properly treated, chemical burns may continue to damage tissue for several hours after exposure. Thus, all efforts should be made to remove the chemical to prevent further injury, including removal of exposed clothing. The clinician should refer such patients to the emergency department of a hospital.

### *Sun Exposure*

Sunburn is caused by acute overexposure of the skin to UV radiation for periods that overcome the ability of melanin, skin thickness and hydration, and vascular supply to protect the skin from injury (see Color Plates, photograph 26). Sunburn from natural sunlight is mainly caused by ultraviolet band B (UVB).[4] Tanning beds can also cause sunburn and corneal burns. (See Chapter 39 for a discussion of UV radiation bands.)

Photosensitive reactions (photoallergy and phototoxicity) to sun exposure have signs and symptoms similar to those of sunburn. Photoallergy is relatively uncommon, usually caused by topical agents, and is characterized by an intensely pruritic eczematous dermatitis that may evolve into thickened leathery changes in sun-exposed skin[5] (see Color Plates, photograph 27). Phototoxicity usually appears as an exaggerated erythema, relative to the time of exposure, that quickly desquamates (peeling of the skin) within several days.[6] Edema, vesicles (blisters), and bullae (large blisters) may occur. Sun-exposed skin is the only area of involvement (see Color Plates, photograph 28). This reaction occurs more often with systemic rather than topical medications.

Cosmetics that contain fragrances such as musk ambrette, sandalwood oil, and bergamot oil are the most likely to cause a photoallergic reaction. A number of medications may cause photoallergy or phototoxicity reactions (see Chapter 39).

## Pathophysiology of Minor Burns and Sunburn

The extent of thermal injury to the skin is a function of the temperature generated and the duration of exposure. The skin can tolerate temperatures up to 104°F (40°C) for relatively long periods of time before injury. Temperatures above this produce a logarithmic increase in tissue destruction. Cell damage occurs as a result of protein denaturation. This damage is reversible unless temperatures exceed 113°F (45°C). At this temperature, protein denaturation exceeds the capacity for cellular repair. The pathophysiologic processes associated with the specific depths of burns are discussed in Classification of Burns.

## Signs and Symptoms of Minor Burns and Sunburn

### *Classification of Burns*

The traditional classification of burns as first, second, or third degree is obsolete and has been replaced by the terms *superficial, superficial partial thickness, deep partial thickness,* and *full thickness,* related to the depth of injury to the skin. Sunburn is discussed separately.

Skin burns are classified primarily according to depth of injury (see Figure 41-1). This pathophysiologic criterion is used to determine whether a burn patient needs emergency medical care. A second system developed by the American Burn Association (Injury Severity Grading System) classifies burn injuries as minor, moderate, and major.[5] Table 41-1 lists the criteria for these burn injury classifications, which incorporate the percentage of affected body surface area (BSA), depth of injury, location of burn, and cause of burn. This system is used by burn care treatment centers for major burn injuries.

Minor burns can often be managed in an outpatient environment if the eyes, ears, face, or perineum (genitalia) are not involved.[5] Either system can be used to assess a patient's burn; this chapter uses the depth of injury classification.

#### Superficial Burns

Superficial burns usually result from a brief exposure to low heat, causing a painful area of erythema similar to sunburn but without significant damage to epithelial cells. Superficial burns involve only the epidermis. In most circumstances, no blistering occurs. Redness, warmth, and slight edema are present. The burn may be painful because the sensory nerve endings are intact. Avoidance of additional injury and symptomatic relief of pain and fever are

**TABLE 41-1 American Burn Association Injury Severity Grading System**

| Type of Burn | Criteria |
|---|---|
| Minor | 15% BSA superficial and superficial partial-thickness burn in an adult<br>10% BSA superficial and superficial partial-thickness burn in a child<br>2% BSA deep partial-thickness or full-thickness burn in a child or adult not involving the eyes, ears, face, or genitalia |
| Moderate | 15%-25% BSA superficial partial-thickness burn in an adult<br>10%-20% BSA superficial partial-thickness burn in a child<br>2%-10% BSA deep partial-thickness or full-thickness burn in a child or adult not involving the eyes, ears, face, or genitalia |
| Major | 25% BSA superficial partial-thickness burn in an adult<br>20% BSA superficial partial-thickness burn in a child<br>All deep partial-thickness or full-thickness burns greater than 10% BSA<br>All burns involving the eyes, ears, face, or genitalia<br>All inhalation injuries<br>Electrical burns<br>Complicated burn injuries involving fractures or other major trauma<br>All poor-risk patients (preexisting condition such as closed head injury, cerebrovascular accident, psychiatric disability, emphysema or lung disease, cancer, or diabetes) |

*Key:* BSA, body surface area.
*Source:* Adapted from reference 5

usually the only treatment required. Sunburn is classified most often in this category. The majority of superficial burns can be managed through self-care or ambulatory care centers and will heal within 3 to 6 days.

## Superficial Partial-thickness Burns

Higher levels of heat or longer exposures than those involved in superficial burns will damage the outer epidermal layers and produce painful blistering, causing a superficial partial-thickness burn. If the damage does not involve the deeper proliferating area of the epidermis, rapid regeneration of a normal epidermis usually results. Superficial partial-thickness burns are often moist and weeping, and they blanch with pressure (lighten in color when pressed with a finger). They are painful and sensitive to temperature and air. They often occur from a splash or spill of hot liquid, a brief contact with a hot object, or a flash ignition. Healing is generally spontaneous, occurring within 2 to 3 weeks, with minimal or no scarring. If this type of burn occurs in a child or in a patient with multiple medical problems, or covers more than 10% BSA, fluid restoration may be required, and the patient should be transported to a hospital emergency room. Lesser degrees of superficial partial-thickness burn injuries can often be managed in an ambulatory setting; small burns (1% to 2% BSA) can usually be managed through self-care.

## Deep Partial-thickness Burns

Deep partial-thickness burns result from more extensive heat exposure than that involved in superficial partial-thickness burns. The heat damages deeper layers of the skin including the dermis, resulting in a blanched rather than moist erythematous wound. Such burns result from a spill of scalding liquid, contact with a hot object, flash ignition, and chemical contact, as well as from flame exposure. Such wounds can resurface because of surviving nests of epithelial cells that line the hair follicles and sweat glands. In this case, healing may be slow and scarring is likely to occur. In addition, these injuries are prone to infection because of the loss of barrier function and the loss of vasculature. Infection will worsen the severity of a burn injury, its depth, or both.

Deep partial-thickness burns involve the entire depth of the epidermis and may extend into the dermis. The appearance may be a patchy white to red area, and large blisters may be present. Blanching indicates loss of blood vessels to the area. Pain may be more intense than in superficial burns because of the irritation to nerve endings although some areas may lack sensation. More of the dermis is involved than in superficial partial-thickness burns, so these burns take longer to heal (up to 6 weeks) and may cause thick scar formation (hypertrophic scarring or cheloid) as well as contractures of the skin and underlying tissues that can affect use of the affected areas. Itching and hypersensation of the scar often occur when deep partial-thickness wounds are allowed to heal without skin grafting. Patients with deep partial-thickness burns should be examined in a hospital's emergency room. Such burn injuries can convert to full-thickness injuries if not properly and promptly managed.

## Full-thickness Burns

Even more extensive heat exposure than that involved in deep partial-thickness burns will cause death of the full thickness of skin in the affected area, resulting in a dry, leathery area that is painless and insensate. These full-thickness burns result from immersion in scalding liquid, flame exposure, electricity, and chemical contact, and are considered serious. The body attempts to heal these wounds by sloughing off the dead layer and contracting the wound. If the wounds are not surgically managed, significant scarring may result, as well as failure to completely heal.

Full-thickness burns destroy both the dermis and epidermis and may extend into underlying tissues. Initially, the wound may appear red, but will fade to white over 24 hours. Healing occurs slowly over months, and grafting is often required to achieve wound closure. Scarring usually results, and severe contractures may occur if physical therapy is not undertaken. Hospitalization is normally required for treatment of full-thickness burns, and patients should seek emergency care as soon as possible.

#### Sunburn

Sunburn causes a superficial burn injury, characterized by erythema and slight dermal edema resulting from an increase in blood flow to the affected skin. The increased blood flow begins approximately 4 hours after exposure, and peaks between 12 and 24 hours following exposure. Severe sunburn can lead to blistering (partial-thickness injury), fever, vomiting, delirium, and shock. If blisters occur, they will desquamate or "peel" over a period of several days. There is a slight chance of bacterial infection because of the loss of the outer skin barrier (see Color Plates, photograph 26). With mild exposure, erythema with subsequent scaling and exfoliation ("peeling") of the skin occurs. Pain and low-grade fever may accompany the erythema. More prolonged exposure causes pain, edema, skin tenderness, and possibly blistering. Systemic symptoms similar to those of thermal burn, such as fever, chills, weakness, and shock, may be seen in patients in whom a large portion of the BSA has been affected. Following exfoliation and for several weeks thereafter, the skin will be more susceptible than normal to sunburn.

## Complications of Minor Burns and Sunburn

A specialist should promptly examine patients who have received burns to the ear or eye, because loss of function in these structures may be devastating. Facial burns may be associated with respiratory injuries caused by inhalation, and intubation for airway protection may be required. Burns that are deeper than superficial may result in permanent scarring of the face.

Hand burns can result in scarring and loss of range of motion, leading to major functional problems. Feet burns are often slow to heal, particularly in adults, and may become infected. Perineal burn victims are often chair-bound patients of advanced age or patients who are paraplegic suffering spill scalds. Such wounds are difficult to dress and are readily infected by fecal organisms. Patients who are immunocompromised or otherwise at high risk for infection, such as those of advanced age and with diabetes, can develop serious infections without specialized care of the burn injuries. These patients should be referred for further evaluation.

Injuries deeper than superficial may require specialized care at a burn center. If treatment is delayed or not performed at all, incomplete wound healing, hypertrophic scarring, or abnormal pigmentation may occur.

Repeated sunburns are a risk factor for melanoma, particularly in children. Excessive unprotected exposure to the sun can also cause photoaging and ocular damage (see Chapter 39).[4]

## Treatment of Minor Burns and Sunburn

Superficial and some superficial partial-thickness burn injuries are the only types suitable for self-treatment. Deeper burns are referred for medical or hospital care.

### *Treatment Goals*

The goals in treating superficial and superficial partial-thickness burns are to (1) relieve pain associated with the burn, (2) provide physical protection, and (3) provide a favorable environment for healing that minimizes the chances of infection and scarring.

### *General Treatment Approach*

The treatment of a burn depends on its depth and severity. When a patient with burns presents for treatment, it is critical to assess the extent and depth of the injury, both initially and again in 24 to 48 hours. If appropriate and the patient has not already done so, the clinician should administer first aid. If the patient has none of the exclusions for self-treatment listed in Figure 41-2, the clinician should treat the patient (or guide the patient's treatment) using the treatment approach outlined in the algorithm.

Superficial burns are not likely to become infected and do not pose a problem with exudates. Physical protection for comfort can be provided by a number of dressings and skin protectants that are currently marketed (see Chapter 42).

Superficial partial-thickness burns in which the epithelium is lost and the surface is weeping are prone to surface infection. Blisters should not be disturbed because blister fluid protects the skin below. Once debrided (dead skin removed), a blistered area may become infected and should be cleansed periodically. For ambulatory care or self-care, cleansing and/or the use of first-aid antiseptics or topical antibiotics are sufficient. Dressings and skin protectant agents should be used to protect the injured area.

Most patients with superficial or superficial partial-thickness burns complain of pain. Therapeutic strategies include topical cold compresses, skin protectants, external anesthetics, topical corticosteroids, and oral nonprescription analgesics.

Generally, if the burned area is 2% of BSA or larger and consists of superficial partial-thickness or greater injury, medical attention is needed. The inflammatory response to a burn injury evolves over the first 24 to 48 hours; thus, the initial appearance of the injury often leads to an underestimation of its actual severity. As a rule, the patient should return after that period for reevaluation of the injury. Figure 41-3 illustrates the "rule-of-nine" method for estimating the percentage of BSA burned.

Some medications can cause a photosensitivity reaction (see Chapter 39). Such reactions require further referral.

### *First-aid Measures*

First-aid measures are described in Figure 41-2. The initial treatment of superficial and superficial partial-thickness thermal burns is to cool the affected area in cool tap water (no ice) for 10 to 30 minutes. This phase of treatment does not apply when the depth or extent of the burn or both are serious, because such action would delay emergency treatment. Cool immersion decreases cutaneous vasodilation and has been shown to decrease the area of redness, and thus edema, associated with tissue surrounding the

**Exclusions for Self-Treatment**

- Burn to BSA of 2% or more
- Burns involving eyes, ears, face, hands, feet, or perineum
- Chemical burns (use first-aid measures then seek medical attention)
- Electrical or inhalation burns
- Persons of advanced age
- Patients with DM or multiple medical disorders
- Immunocompromised patients

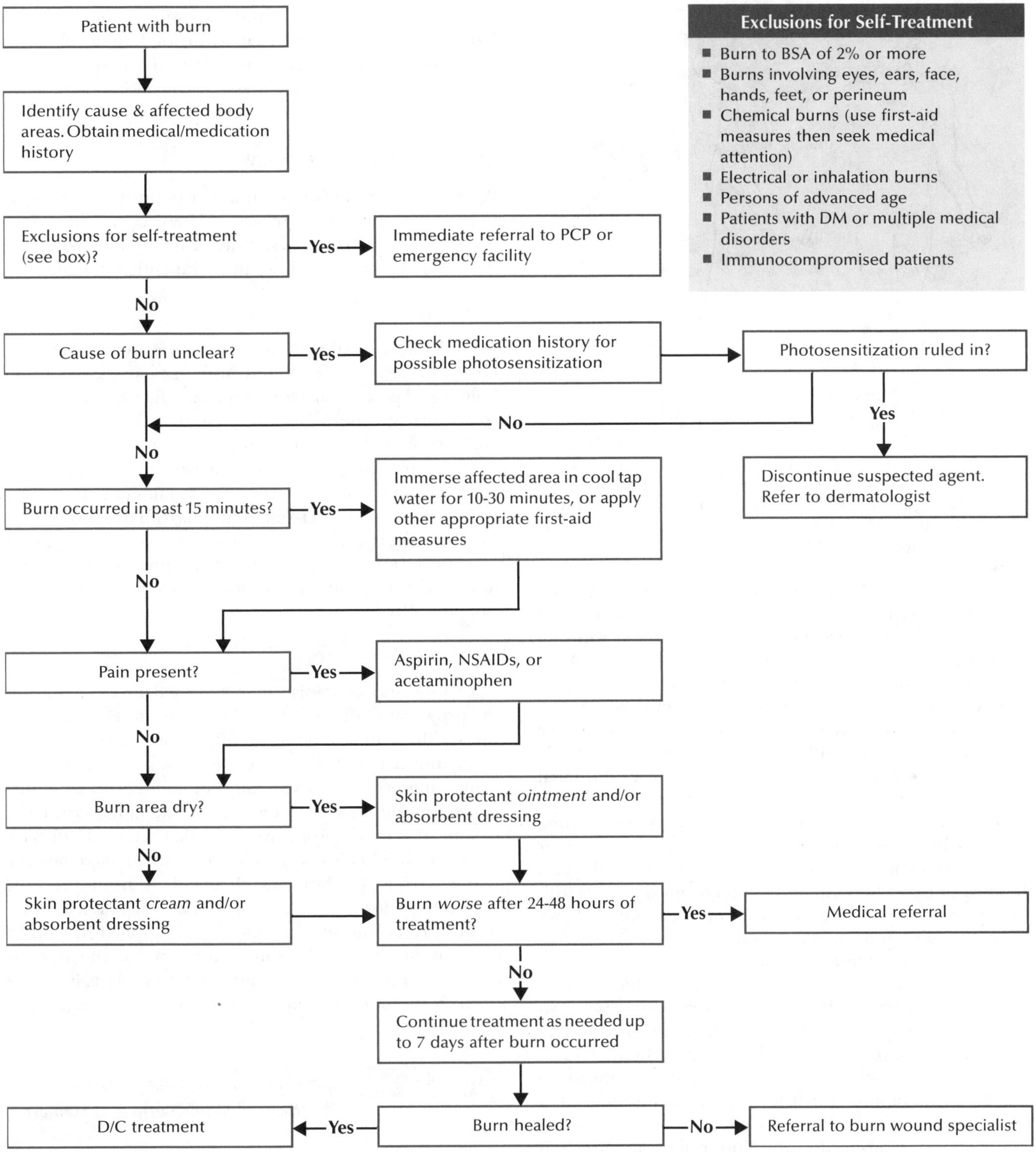


FIGURE 41-2 Self-care of minor burns and sunburn. Key: BSA, body surface area; D/C, discontinue; DM, diabetes mellitus; NSAID, nonsteroidal anti-inflammatory drug; PCP, primary care provider.

burn. This treatment may help prevent blister formation. An internal analgesic drug product such as aspirin, nonsteroidal anti-inflammatory drugs (NSAIDs), or acetaminophen can be given to reduce pain (see Chapter 5).

Patients with deep partial-thickness or full-thickness injuries should be transported to an emergency center promptly. If some delay is anticipated before emergency care can be initiated, the patient should drink water, if possible, to replace vascular losses. An oral analgesic drug product such as aspirin or an NSAID can be given to reduce pain if the patient is conscious. In inhalation injuries, edema of the larynx or other structures may obstruct breathing, and emergency intubation for airway protection may be required.

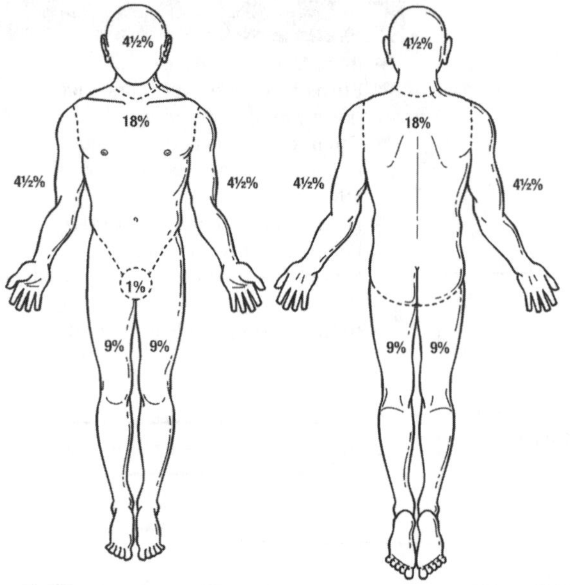


FIGURE 41-3 Rule-of-nine method for quickly establishing the percentage of adult body surface burned. (Adapted with permission from *The Guide to Fluid Therapy.* Deerfield, Ill: Baxter Laboratories; 1969:111.)

In the case of chemical burns, the patient should immediately remove any clothing on or near the affected area. The affected area should then be washed with tap water for anywhere from 15 minutes to 2 hours until the offending agent has been removed. Such treatment should not delay transport to a hospital emergency department.

If the eye is involved, the eyelid should be pulled back and the eye irrigated with tap water for at least 15 to 30 minutes. The irrigation fluid should flow from the nasal side of the eye to the outside corner to prevent washing the contaminant into the other eye. When the offending agent is identified, the area poison information center should be contacted immediately for treatment guidelines. In most cases of chemical burns and chemical contact with the eye, referral for further evaluation is encouraged and should be sought as soon as possible.

No attempt should be made to counteract or neutralize a chemical burn. Such action may produce an exothermic (heat-generating) chemical reaction, which can damage the injured area more than the original offending agent. For example, treating a burn caused by an acid by applying a base such as sodium bicarbonate is inappropriate. It should be noted that for certain chemicals, even a small area of contact can produce serious or lethal injury. For example, exposure to hydrofluoric acid, an industrial chemical, can result in life-threatening hypocalcemia.[7]

Electrical contact burns should receive emergency treatment because the depth of injury can be much greater than that suggested by the size of the entry or exit wounds. In an unconscious patient, other injuries may not be immediately apparent.

Initial treatment for minor sunburn is to get out of the sunlight and avoid further exposure. Minor sunburn can be relieved to some extent with cool compresses or a cool bath.

Heat stroke may occur with excessive exposure to sunlight in an environment that is hot or humid, or both. Because of complications from heat stroke, patients exhibiting fever, confusion, weakness, or convulsions should be referred for further evaluation immediately.

## *Nonpharmacologic Therapy*

Preventing or reducing the number of burn injuries is an important public health measure. However, if a burn does occur, nondrug measures such as cleansing and protecting the burned area are important therapeutic modalities.

### Preventive Measures

Several public health strategies are effective in reducing burn injuries. People should install smoke alarms in all homes and periodically test them. Families should develop escape plans; remove fire ignition sources from homes with children; and teach children not to play with matches, lighters, and the like. People should inspect electrical cords and portable heaters, clean chimneys periodically, and use fire screens in front of fireplaces. They should also use the correct fuel (not gasoline) in kerosene heaters.[2,3]

Sunburn can be prevented by avoiding overexposure to sunlight and using appropriate sunscreen agents (see Chapter 39).

### Cleansing Procedures

After applying cool moisture to a burned area to help stop the progression of the burn injury (refer to First-aid Measures), the patient should gently cleanse the area with water and a bland soap, such as a baby wash. Alcohol-containing preparations should not be used because they dehydrate the area and cause pain to denuded skin (skin missing the outer protective epithelial layer). Hydrogen peroxide should also be avoided as it will damage healthy tissue. After the burn is cleansed, a nonadherent, hypoallergenic dressing may be applied if the area is small. A skin protectant or lubricant may be applied instead of or in addition to a dressing, particularly if the burn is extensive or in an area that cannot be dressed easily (Table 41-2). If the burn is weeping, soaking it in cool tap water

**TABLE 41-2 Skin-protectant Ingredients Used in Treatment of Minor Burns and Sunburn**

| Ingredient | Proposed Concentrations (%) |
|---|---|
| Allantoin | 0.5-2 |
| Cocoa butter | 50-100 |
| Petrolatum | 30-100 |
| Shark liver oil | 3 |
| White petrolatum | 30-100 |

*Source:* Adapted from reference 8.

three to six times a day for 15 to 30 minutes will provide a soothing effect and diminish the weeping. Minor burns usually heal without additional treatment. For blistering burns in which blisters are no longer intact, cleansing once or twice daily to remove dead skin is recommended. Patients should be advised not to pull at loose skin or peel off burned skin because viable skin may be removed in the process, thereby delaying healing.

### Protective Measures

Sterile, nonadherent gauze dressings are the most convenient means of covering a small burn on a body area that is easily bandaged, such as the arm or leg. For superficial burns, films that are self-adhesive, waterproof, and semipermeable provide a protective barrier that is transparent and permits wound inspection without dressing changes (e.g., OpSite or Tegaderm).[9] Pressure points (the sacrum, heels, elbows) should be covered with self-adherent hydrocolloid dressings such as Duoderm or Comfeel.

Newer dressings have been designed to incorporate the desirable characteristics of exudate absorption with occlusiveness (e.g., DuoDERM, Vigilon, Viasorb) (see Chapter 42). Blistering burns should be dressed with these absorbent hydrocolloid dressings. If the dressing remains dry and intact, it may be left in place for 5 days.

## *Pharmacologic Therapy*

Various products are useful in treating minor burns and sunburn. Some agents relieve pain, swelling, and/or inflammation. Others either protect the burn from infection or aid in healing the skin.

### Skin Protectants

The Food and Drug Administration (FDA) has recognized the skin protectants in Table 41-2 as safe and effective for the temporary protection of minor burns and sunburn.

Skin protectants benefit patients with minor burns by making the wound area less painful. They protect the burn from mechanical irritation caused by friction and rubbing, and they prevent drying of the stratum corneum. Rehydrating the stratum corneum helps relieve the symptoms of irritation and permits normal healing to continue. Skin protectants provide only symptomatic relief. FDA has proposed revised labeling for the indications of skin protectants as follows: "For the temporary protection of minor cuts, scrapes, burns, and sunburn."[8] In selecting a skin protectant for burns, the clinician should choose products that prevent dryness and provide lubrication. Accordingly, FDA has proposed that bismuth subnitrate, boric acid, sulfur, and tannic acid not be considered safe or effective when used as skin protectants. FDA has also proposed that products with labeling claims of "cures any irritation" or "prevents formation of blisters" should not be generally recognized as safe and effective and should not be included in the proposed skin protectant monograph. FDA has not accepted claims that certain substances (e.g., allantoin, live yeast cell derivatives, or zinc acetate) contained in skin protectants are safe and effective in accelerating wound healing.

Liver oils have been used for many years as folk remedies for wound healing. Shark liver oil contains a high concentration of vitamin A and is proposed as a skin protectant. Vitamin A and D ointment has been used to treat minor skin burns and abrasions. FDA recommends that the restriction preventing the use of skin protectants on children younger than 2 years of age be waived, except for products containing live yeast cell derivatives, shark liver oil, and zinc acetate.

Generally, the patient with minor burns may apply a skin protectant as often as needed. If the burn has not improved in 7 days or if it worsens during or after treatment, the patient should consult a primary care provider promptly.

### Systemic Analgesics

An initial step in treating the patient with a minor burn is to recommend short-term administration of an internal analgesic, preferably one with anti-inflammatory activity, such as the NSAIDs (aspirin, naproxen, ketoprofen, or ibuprofen). As prostaglandin inhibitors, NSAIDs may decrease erythema and edema in the burned area. NSAIDs may be especially beneficial in the patient with mild sunburn, especially in the first 24 hours after overexposure to UV radiation. Their use has been shown to decrease inflammation caused by exposure to UV radiation. However, this effect has been found to last only about 24 hours,[10] possibly because the initial inflammation of sunburn is mediated by prostaglandins, whereas the later inflammation is associated primarily with leukocytes. For patients who cannot tolerate NSAIDs, acetaminophen can provide pain relief although it is a weak prostaglandin inhibitor and is not an anti-inflammatory agent. (See Chapter 5 for discussion of dosages and safety considerations for systemic analgesics.)

### Topical Anesthetics

The pain of minor burns and sunburn can be attenuated by the judicious use of topical anesthetics. Agents proposed as safe and effective in providing temporary relief of pain associated with minor burns are listed in Table 41-3.

*Mechanism of Action* Topical anesthetics relieve pain by inhibiting the transmission of pain signals from pain receptors. Relief is short lived, lasting only 15 to 45 minutes.

*Dosage and Administration Guidelines* Benzocaine (5% to 20%) and lidocaine (0.5% to 4%) are the two anesthetics most often used in nonprescription drug preparations. Dibucaine (0.25% to 1%), tetracaine (1% to 2%), butamben (1%), and pramoxine (0.5% to 1%) are also found in external anesthetic preparations. The higher concentrations of the topical anesthetics are appropriate for burns in which the skin is intact. Lower concentrations are preferred when the skin surface is not intact because absorption is enhanced. They should be applied only to small areas to avoid systemic toxicity.

Topical anesthetics should be applied no more than three or four times daily. Because their duration of action

**TABLE 41-3 Topical Analgesic Ingredients for Treatment of Minor Burns and Sunburn**

| Agent | FDA-approved Concentrations (%) |
|---|---|
| **Amine and Caine-type Local Anesthetics** | |
| Benzocaine | 5-20 |
| Butamben picrate | 1 |
| Dibucaine | 0.25-1 |
| Dibucaine hydrochloride | 0.25-1 |
| Dimethisoquin hydrochloride | 0.3-0.5 |
| Dyclonine hydrochloride | 0.5-1 |
| Lidocaine | 0.5-4 |
| Lidocaine hydrochloride | 0.5-4 |
| Pramoxine hydrochloride | 0.5-1 |
| Tetracaine | 1-2 |
| Tetracaine hydrochloride | 1-2 |
| **Antihistamines** | |
| Diphenhydramine hydrochloride | 1-2 |
| Tripelennamine hydrochloride | 0.5-2 |

*Source:* Federal Register. 1983;48:6820-33.

is short, continuous pain relief cannot be obtained with these agents. Increasing the number of applications increases the risk of a hypersensitivity reaction and, more important, the chance for systemic toxicity.

*Safety Considerations* Benzocaine produces a hypersensitivity reaction in about 1% of patients, a higher incidence than that seen with lidocaine. In a patch test study of 4000 patients with dermatitis, 9% were sensitive to benzocaine, and only neomycin was more sensitizing (10%).[11] In contrast, benzocaine is essentially free of systemic toxicity, whereas the systemic absorption of lidocaine can lead to a number of side effects. However, systemic toxicities caused by lidocaine are rare if the product is used on intact skin, on localized areas, and for short periods.

### Topical Hydrocortisone

Although not FDA-approved for use in treating minor burns, topical hydrocortisone 1% is often used in the first-aid treatment of minor burns covering a small area.

Hydrocortisone, an anti-inflammatory agent, should be used with caution if the skin is broken, because it may allow infections to develop. Topical corticosteroid treatment with high-potency agents has been shown to decrease collagen synthesis and delay reepithelialization in dermal wounds, whereas low-potency hydrocortisone 1% ointment does not interfere with resurfacing of the skin (see Chapter 34).[12] A randomized trial comparing topical methylprednisolone aceponate 0.1% milk and hydrocortisone 17-butyrate 0.1% emulsion in 24 healthy sunburned volunteers demonstrated efficacy in reducing erythema, edema, burning, and itching, compared with untreated areas.[13]

### Antimicrobials

For major burns, the topical prescription preparations silver sulfadiazine and mafenide are often used.[14] However, for minor burns, nonprescription first-aid antibiotic or antiseptic products are of limited value, especially on burns in which the skin is intact. These preparations may be used on minor burns when the skin has been broken. Chapter 42 discusses preparations that may be used to help prevent infection in minor burns or sunburn. The petrolatum base present in some first-aid products, such as triple-antibiotic ointment, is a skin protectant that can provide symptomatic relief.

### Vitamins

Vitamin supplements are commonly used by burn centers for severe burn injuries. Although the benefits of vitamin supplementation for minor burns are not known, a frank deficiency of vitamin C (ascorbic acid) or vitamin A will impair wound healing. No scientific evidence suggests that vitamin dosages beyond the normal daily requirements will accelerate wound healing. However, vitamin C does play a key role in healing wounds because it is required for collagen synthesis. Because vitamin C is not stored in the body, it is reasonable to recommend up to 2 g of vitamin C daily from the time of injury until healing is complete.

Animal studies indicate that vitamin A enhances healing in a variety of wounds. Following serious injury, the patient may have an increased requirement for vitamin A. In addition, deficiency states are associated with increased infections. Because vitamin A is stored in large amounts in the liver, supplemental vitamin A should not be used for long periods. Minor burn injuries will probably not benefit from supplemental oral vitamin A, but topical vitamin A (fish or shark liver oil–based products) may be helpful.

Deficiency of B vitamins may retard wound healing, so B vitamins should be supplemented if nutritional status is poor. Excess vitamin E may delay wound healing and does not play a role in burn injury. Vitamin D is not significantly involved in healing wounds.

Administering zinc is beneficial only in people who are zinc deficient. Iron-deficiency anemia can decrease the oxygen supply to the healing area and should be corrected if present. Copper deficiency may impair healing and can be corrected through normal dietary intake.

Oral supplementation with vitamins E and C, as well as dietary fish oil, may reduce sunburn.[15,16] β-Carotene supplementation, however, does not alter sunburn reactions.[17]

In summary, burned patients with good nutritional status may not benefit from vitamin or mineral supplementation. However, patients whose dietary intake is suboptimal will not be harmed by, and could benefit from, temporary supplementation with standard multivitamin or mineral preparations. Assurance of adequate vitamin C intake is recommended during healing from burn injury.

### Counterirritants

Although counterirritants such as camphor, menthol, and ichthammol are currently proposed for use in minor burn treatment, FDA is still evaluating them. They generally should not be used for burns. Even though these agents do reduce pain by stimulating sensory nerve fibers, they increase blood flow to the area, causing further development of edema. They also irritate the already sensitized and damaged skin.

### Miscellaneous Agents

The ability of topical forms of aloe vera and vitamin E to aid in the healing of minor burns and sunburn has not been substantiated, so FDA has not approved these agents as healing aids.

Topical nitrofurantoin and some petrolatum-containing products have been shown to retard epithelial healing, whereas an oil-in-water cream, triple-antibiotic ointment, silver sulfadiazine cream, and benzoyl peroxide lotion 10% and 20% have increased the rate of healing.[12]

### Combination Products

Rarely will a product intended to treat minor burns contain only one ingredient. FDA proposed that two or more of the skin-protectant ingredients listed in Table 41-2 may be combined, provided that each ingredient in the combination is within the concentration range in the proposed monograph.[8]

### Product Selection Guidelines

If a topical anesthetic or hydrocortisone is to be used, the clinician should recommend the most appropriate product formulation. Such products are available as ointments, creams, solutions (lotions), and sprays (aerosols).

Ointments are oleaginous-based preparations. They provide a protective film to impede the evaporation of water from the wound area, which helps keep the skin from drying. However, if the skin is broken, an ointment may not be appropriate because of its impermeability. The presence of excessive moisture trapped beneath the application may promote bacterial growth or maceration of the skin, thus delaying healing. Ointments are more appropriate for minor burns in which the skin is intact. Creams are emulsions that allow some fluid to pass through the film and are best for broken skin. Generally, creams are easier to apply and remove than are ointments. To prevent contaminating the preparation, the patient should not apply ointments and creams directly onto the burn from the container.

Lotions spread easily and are easier to apply when the burn area is large. However, lotions that produce a powdery cover should not be used on a burn because they tend to dry the area, are difficult (and possibly painful) to remove, and provide a medium for bacterial growth under the caked particles.

Generally, aerosol and pump sprays are more costly than other topical dosage forms. Sprays offer the advantage of precluding the need to physically touch the injured area, so there is less pain associated with applying the medication. Proper application requires holding the container approximately 6 in. from the burn and spraying for 1 to 3 seconds. This method decreases the chances of chilling the area. However, sprays are not usually protective in that the aerosol is typically water- or alcohol-based and will evaporate.

Table 41-4 lists selected trade-name topical products appropriate for treating minor burns and sunburn.

## *Complementary Therapies*

Therapy for minor burns and sunburn is largely empirical, with little scientific study. The use of complementary preparations such as herbals is also empirical, but in some societies such remedies have been used for many generations. Plants such as *Calendula, Aloe vera, Garcinia morella,* and *Datura metol* are said to have healing properties.[18] In fact, the traditional way of treating lightning burns in southern India involves smearing coconut oil on plantain (banana) leaves and dressing wounds with them. Externally applied extracts of *Picrorrhiza kurrea, Cassia fistula, Emblica officinalis, Euphorbia thymifolia,* and *Curcuma longa* have antimicrobial effects, whereas *Allium sativum, Boerhaevia diffusa, Curcuma longa,* and *Ricinus communis* possess anti-inflammatory properties.[18] (See Chapter 53 for further discussion of these types of remedies.)

Aloe gel has been widely used externally for its wound-healing properties although the effectiveness of commercial preparations compared with fresh aloe gel is controversial.[19] Differences in the extraction and processing techniques may be related to variable results in artificial cell culture systems for processed aloe gel. A few small clinical studies suggest the effectiveness of fresh aloe gel and some prepared products in skin ulcers, burn wounds, frostbite injuries, and psoriasis. Aloe gel's effects may result from inhibition of the pain-producing substance bradykinin. Aloe gel may also inhibit thromboxane and prostaglandins, and may have antibacterial and antifungal properties. FDA does not recognize aloe gel as safe and effective for treating any condition because of insufficient evidence. Nonetheless, aloe gel products are widely used for burns and sunburns, and freshly prepared aloe gel may be worth considering for self-care of minor burns.

Comfrey consists of the leaves or root of *Symphytum officinale* and has been used to treat various wounds.[19] However, variability in species used and inherent toxic alkaloids raise concerns about its safety. Internal use or any use of the plant's root should be avoided. Only mature leaves should be applied externally and then only to unbroken skin for a limited time. The levels of carcinogenic pyrrolizidine alkaloids in American products are unknown. The potential benefit of comfrey may be a result of its constituent allantoin, discussed under Skin Protectants.

Tea tree oil is prepared from the leaves of an Australian tree, *Melaleuca alternifolia.*[19] It has antimicrobial activity, and has been used for treating cuts, abrasions, burns, insect bites, other skin infections, and vaginal infections.

The dried flower heads of *Arnica montana* have been prepared as hydroalcoholic extracts and creams.[19] Arnica has been shown to have antimicrobial, antiedema, and anti-inflammatory properties. The German Commission E

**TABLE 41-4 Selected Topical Products for Minor Burns and Sunburn**

| Trade Name | Primary Ingredients |
|---|---|
| **Skin Protectants** | |
| A + D Ointment With Zinc Oxide | Zinc oxide 10%; cod liver oil (contains vitamins A and D) |
| A + D Original Ointment | Petrolatum 80.5%; lanolin 15.5%; cod liver oil (contains vitamins A and D) |
| Zinc oxide, Desitin Ointments | Zinc oxide 20 or 25%; white petrolatum |
| **Skin Protectants/Antiseptics** | |
| Unguentine Antiseptic Ointment | Phenol 2.5% |
| Vaseline First Aid Anti-Bacterial Petroleum Jelly | Petrolatum 98.3%; chloroxylenol 0.53%; phenol |
| **Local Anesthetics** | |
| Americaine Aerosol, Ointment | Benzocaine 20% |
| ELA-Max 4% | Lidocaine 4% |
| Dermoplast Pain-Relieving Spray | Benzocaine 20%; menthol 0.5% |
| Dibucaine Topical Ointment | Dibucaine 1% |
| Itch-X Spray, Gel | Pramoxine HCl 1%; benzyl alcohol 10% |
| Solarcaine Aloe Extra Burn Relief Gel/Spray | Lidocaine 0.5% |
| Tronothane Cream, Tronolane Cream | Pramoxine HCl 1% |
| Xylocaine Ointment | Lidocaine 2.5% |
| **Local Anesthetics/Antiseptics** | |
| Bactine First Aid Antiseptic Spray | Lidocaine HCl 2.5%; benzalkonium chloride 0.13% |
| Dermoplast Antibacterial Spray | Benzocaine 20%; benzethonium chloride 0.2% |
| Foille Plus Aerosol | Benzocaine 20%; benzethonium chloride 0.15% |
| Foille Medicated First Aid Spray/Ointment | Benzocaine 5%; chloroxylenol 0.1% |
| Lanacane Anti-Bacterial First Aid Spray | Benzocaine 20%; benzethonium chloride 0.2% |
| Lanacane Anti-Itch Creme | Benzocaine 6%; resorcinol 2% |
| Lanacane Maximum Strength Anti-Itch Cream | Benzocaine 20%; benzethonium chloride 0.1% |
| Solarcaine Medicated First Aid Spray | Benzocaine 20%; SD alcohol 40, 35%; triclosan 0.13% |
| Unguentine Maximum Strength Cream | Benzocaine 5%, resorcinol 2% |

has approved arnica for external application because of its anti-inflammatory, analgesic, and antiseptic properties.

One prospective randomized trial of honey versus silver sulfadiazine for superficial burns demonstrated that honey dressings resulted in faster healing and fewer infections than did the silver sulfadiazine dressings;[20] however, honey dressings are not advocated by burn centers.

A home remedy to relieve sunburn is to brew a quart of strong tea (e.g., orange pekoe or black tea) with no additives, then chill it until cold. The patient dips washcloths in the tea, wrings them out, and gently lays the cloths over the sunburned area(s) until the cloths feel warm to the touch. Applications are repeated until the pain is relieved.

## Assessment of Minor Burns and Sunburn: A Case-based Approach

When a patient presents with a burn, the practitioner should immediately assess the severity of the burn by determining the depth of the injury and the percentage of BSA involved. The percentage of the adult body that has been burned can be estimated by the rule of nines (Figure 41-3). The total BSA is divided into 11 areas, each accounting for 9% or a multiple of 9. An easy way to estimate the percentage of burned BSA is to use the back of the hand as 1% of BSA. The rule of nines is reliable for adults but inaccurate for children and patients with small body surfaces. Table 41-5 illustrates how the BSA of the head, extremities, and other parts of the body changes with age. Case 41-1 gives an example of the assessment of a patient with sunburn, and Case 41-2 illustrates the assessment of a patient with a minor burn.

## Patient Counseling for Minor Burns and Sunburn

Once a burn is assessed as self-treatable, the clinician should address the patient's immediate concern: relieving the pain and swelling. Some patients may not realize the

TABLE 41-5 Age-related Changes in BSA (%)

| | Age | | | | | |
|---|---|---|---|---|---|---|
| Surface | Birth | 1 year | 5 years | 10 years | 15 years | Adult |
| Head | 19 | 17 | 13 | 11 | 9 | 7 |
| Neck | 2 | 2 | 2 | 2 | 2 | 2 |
| Trunk (anterior) | 13 | 13 | 13 | 13 | 13 | 13 |
| Trunk (posterior) | 13 | 13 | 13 | 13 | 13 | 13 |
| Buttocks | 5 | 5 | 5 | 5 | 5 | 5 |
| Perineum | 1 | 1 | 1 | 1 | 1 | 1 |
| Arms | 8 | 8 | 8 | 8 | 8 | 8 |
| Forearms | 6 | 6 | 6 | 6 | 6 | 6 |
| Hands | 5 | 5 | 5 | 5 | 5 | 5 |
| Thighs | 11 | 13 | 16 | 17 | 18 | 19 |
| Legs | 10 | 10 | 11 | 12 | 13 | 14 |
| Feet | 7 | 7 | 7 | 7 | 7 | 7 |

## CASE 41-1

| Relevant Evaluation Criteria | Scenario/Model Outcome |
|---|---|
| **Information Gathering** | |
| 1. Gather essential information about the patient's symptoms, including: | |
| a. description of symptom(s) (i.e., nature, onset, duration, severity, associated symptoms) | Patient has suffered sunburn in conjunction with several visits to a tanning salon over the past week. She has bright red erythema on her face, and erythema on her arms, neck, and legs. She anticipates an upcoming social event and regrets overusing the tanning booths. She says her face "feels like it is on fire." No blistering is noted. |
| b. description of any factors that seem to precipitate, exacerbate, and/or relieve the patient's symptom(s) | The patient uses benzoyl peroxide 5% lotion at bedtime and cleanses her face with alcohol-based swabs during the day. She does this to minimize acne. These measures seem to further irritate sunburned areas. |
| c. description of the patient's efforts to relieve the symptoms | The patient has tried a commercial aloe vera gel product without relief. |
| 2. Gather essential patient history information: | |
| a. patient's identity | AF |
| b. patient's age, sex, height, and weight | 16 y/o F, 5'3", 115 lb |
| c. patient's occupation | High school student |
| d. patient's dietary habits | Overall healthy eating habits |
| e. patient's sleep habits | Normally sleeps well, but sunburn has made sleep difficult |
| f. concurrent medical conditions, prescription and nonprescription medications, and dietary supplements | Benzoyl peroxide 5% lotion |
| g. allergies | NKA |
| h. history of other adverse reactions to medications | None |
| i. other (describe)______ | The patient is very fair-skinned, with freckling; she uses makeup on face to cover up freckles. |

## CASE 41-1 (continued)

| Relevant Evaluation Criteria | Scenario/Model Outcome |
|---|---|
| **Assessment and Triage** | |
| 3. Differentiate the patient's signs/symptoms and correctly identify the patient's primary problem(s). | Patient has experienced sunburn caused by overuse of tanning salon. The burn is worse on her face because of the use of topical benzoyl peroxide and alcohol cleaning procedures. |
| 4. Identify exclusions for self-treatment (see Figure 41-2). | None |
| 5. Formulate a comprehensive list of therapeutic alternatives for the primary problem to determine if triage to a medical practitioner is required, and share this information with the patient. | Options include:<br>(1) Recommend self-care with nonprescription products and/or nondrug measures.<br>(2) Refer AF to an appropriate PCP.<br>(3) Recommend self-care until an appropriate PCP can be consulted.<br>(4) Take no action. |
| **Plan** | |
| 6. Select an optimal therapeutic alternative to address the patient's problem, taking into account patient preferences. | Because the sunburn is minor, self-care with nonprescription products and nondrug measures is an appropriate option. |
| 7. Describe the recommended therapeutic approach to the patient. | You should avoid benzoyl peroxide and any skin cleansing products that contain alcohol or astringent agents. Apply topical vitamin A and D ointment as often as possible to affected areas as thin applications. Do not go out into the sunlight; use a sunscreen if you must be in the sun. |
| 8. Explain to the patient the rationale for selecting the recommended therapeutic approach from the considered therapeutic alternatives. | By avoiding further sun damage and stopping the use of antiacne agents, your face will heal more rapidly. Vitamin A and D ointment will protect the skin and prevent drying, thus aiding healing. Further use of tanning salons is inadvisable since it is unlikely you will develop a tan. The use of cosmetics to conceal freckles will not likely decrease your acne. |
| **Patient Education** | |
| 9. When recommending self-care with nonprescription medications and/or nondrug therapy, convey accurate information to the patient, including: | |
| a. appropriate dose and frequency of administration | Apply vitamin A and D ointment to affected areas as often as needed to keep the skin moist. Cleanse the face with mild soaps prior to reapplication. |
| b. maximum number of days the therapy should be employed | Continue use of vitamin A and D ointment and/or hydrocortisone cream until sunburn symptoms are tolerable, but not more than 1 week. |
| c. product administration procedures | See the box Patient Education for Minor Burns and Sunburn. |
| d. expected time to onset of relief | Symptomatic relief will occur on application. |
| e. degree of relief that can be reasonably expected | The discomfort will be reduced but will not be completely eliminated until the burned areas heal. |
| f. most common side effects | See the box Patient Education for Minor Burns and Sunburn. |
| g. side effects that warrant medical intervention should they occur | See the box Patient Education for Minor Burns and Sunburn. |
| h. patient options in the event that condition worsens or persists | See the box Patient Education for Minor Burns and Sunburn. |
| i. product storage requirements | See the box Patient Education for Minor Burns and Sunburn. |
| j. specific nondrug measures | Avoid further sun exposure, and discontinue use of benzoyl peroxide and alcohol swabs until the burned areas heal. |
| 10. Solicit follow-up questions from patient. | What can I do to speed up healing? |

## CASE 41-1 (continued)

| Relevant Evaluation Criteria | Scenario/Model Outcome |
|---|---|
| 11. Answer patient's questions. | Your skin has been burned and will require several days to regenerate. It is possible that supplemental vitamin C 2000 mg daily by mouth may help. You are likely to suffer recurrences because your skin type is not conducive to tanning, so you should avoid prolonged sun exposure and tanning salons in the future. |

Key: NKA, no known allergies; PCP, primary care provider.

## CASE 41-2

| Relevant Evaluation Criteria | Scenario/Model Outcome |
|---|---|
| **Information Gathering** | |
| 1. Gather essential information about the patient's symptoms, including: | |
| a. description of symptom(s) (i.e., nature, onset, duration, severity, associated symptoms) | The patient burned her right hand and forearm when hot oil from a frying pan splashed onto her. She quickly rinsed these areas with cool water. Now she has patchy areas of erythema on her hand and forearm that "burn and sting." |
| b. description of any factors that seem to precipitate, exacerbate, and/or relieve the patient's symptom(s) | None |
| c. description of the patient's efforts to relieve the symptoms | Other than the use of cool water, patient has not used any treatment for her burn. |
| 2. Gather essential patient history information: | |
| a. patient's identity | WR |
| b. patient's age, sex, height, and weight | 39 y/o F, 5'6", 150 lb |
| c. patient's occupation | Housewife |
| d. patient's dietary habits | Generally healthy dietary habits |
| e. patient's sleep habits | Sleeps well |
| f. concurrent medical conditions, prescription and nonprescription medications, and dietary supplements | She takes calcium supplements and a vitamin/mineral product. |
| g. allergies | NKA |
| h. history of other adverse reactions to medications | None |
| i. other (describe)______ | N/A |
| **Assessment and Triage** | |
| 3. Differentiate the patient's signs/symptoms and correctly identify the patient's primary problem(s). | Patient was burned while cooking and received superficial burns to her right hand and forearm in several small areas. |
| 4. Identify exclusions for self-treatment (see Figure 41-2). | None |
| 5. Formulate a comprehensive list of therapeutic alternatives for the primary problem to determine if triage to a medical practitioner is required, and share this information with the patient. | Options include:<br>(1) Recommend self-care with nonprescription products and/or nondrug measures.<br>(2) Refer WR to an appropriate PCP.<br>(3) Recommend self-care until an appropriate PCP can be consulted.<br>(4) Take no action. |

CASE 41-2 (continued)

| Relevant Evaluation Criteria | Scenario/Model Outcome |
|---|---|
| **Plan** | |
| 6. Select an optimal therapeutic alternative to address the patient's problem, taking into account patient preferences. | Topical skin protectant, dressings, and oral analgesics are appropriate measures. |
| 7. Describe the recommended therapeutic approach to the patient. | Apply a skin protectant such as vitamin A and D ointment to the affected areas and cover them with an occlusive, transparent dressing. Take ibuprofen (see Chapter 5) as needed for pain relief. |
| 8. Explain to the patient the rationale for selecting the recommended therapeutic approach from the considered therapeutic alternatives. | The burns appear to be mild superficial injuries amenable to self-treatment. However, you should reassess the injury in 24 to 48 hours since the initial appearance of burn injuries can underestimate their severity. |
| **Patient Education** | |
| 9. When recommending self-care with nonprescription medications and/or nondrug therapy, convey accurate information to the patient, including: | |
| a. appropriate dose and frequency of administration | Vitamin A and D ointment may be applied as often as desired. If a transparent occlusive dressing is used, it should remain in place for up to 5 days. |
| b. maximum number of days the therapy should be employed | See the box Patient Education for Minor Burns and Sunburn. |
| c. product administration procedures | See the box Patient Education for Minor Burns and Sunburn. |
| d. expected time to onset of relief | Symptomatic relief will occur on application of the A and D ointment and within an hour following ingestion of ibuprofen. |
| e. degree of relief that can be reasonably expected | The discomfort will be reduced but will not be completely eliminated until the burned areas heal. |
| f. most common side effects | See the box Patient Education for Minor Burns and Sunburn. |
| g. side effects that warrant medical intervention should they occur | See the box Patient Education for Minor Burns and Sunburn. |
| h. patient options in the event that condition worsens or persists | See the box Patient Education for Minor Burns and Sunburn. |
| i. product storage requirements | See the box Patient Education for Minor Burns and Sunburn. |
| j. specific nondrug measures | Avoid sun exposure to the burned areas. |
| 10. Solicit follow-up questions from patient. | Should I use hydrogen peroxide or topical antibiotics? |
| 11. Answer patient's questions. | Hydrogen peroxide should not be used, as it will damage healthy tissue. Topical antibiotics are not needed because the skin is not broken; they can also cause contact dermatitis. |

Key: N/A, not applicable; NKA, no known allergies; PCP, primary care provider.

potential complications of even minor burns; therefore, advice on how to protect the injury is vital in preventing possible infection and scarring.

Using a 24- to 48-hour follow-up evaluation of the burn, the clinician should either recommend continuation of self-treatment or refer the patient for further evaluation. If self-treatment continues, the patient needs to know how long healing of the burn will take, as well as the signs and symptoms that indicate worsening of the injury. The box Patient Education for Minor Burns and Sunburn lists specific advice for successful treatment of these injuries.

## Evaluation of Patient Outcomes for Minor Burns and Sunburn

Burn wounds should be reassessed after 24 to 48 hours, because the full extent of skin damage may not be initially apparent. If the burn has progressed or worsened, the

## PATIENT EDUCATION FOR MINOR BURNS AND SUNBURN

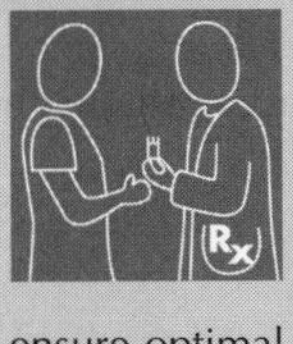

The objectives of self-treatment are to (1) relieve the pain and swelling, (2) protect the burned area from further physical injury, and (3) avoid infection and scarring of the burned area. For most patients, carefully following product instructions and the self-care measures listed here will help ensure optimal therapeutic outcomes.

### Nondrug Measures

- Treat superficial burns with no blistering as follows:
  - Immerse the affected area in cool tap water for 10 to 30 minutes.
  - Cleanse the area with water and a mild soap.
  - Apply a nonadherent dressing or skin protectant to the burn.
- For small burns with minor blistering, follow the first two steps above, but use a hydrocolloid dressing to protect the burn.
- If possible, avoid rupturing blisters.
- For sunburns, avoid further sun exposure and follow the previous procedures according to whether blistering is present.

### Nonprescription Medications

- For superficial burns (including sunburn) with unbroken skin, treat the affected area with thin applications of skin protectants or topical anesthetics using a tissue to reduce the risk of infection from the fingertips.
- If the skin is broken, use topical antibiotics to prevent infection.
- If nutritional status is poor, take supplements for vitamins A, B, and C.
- Do not apply camphor, menthol, or ichthammol to the burn.
- For temporary relief of pain, take aspirin, acetaminophen, ibuprofen, naproxen, or ketoprofen (see Chapter 5 for dosage guidelines and safety considerations).

⚠ If a skin rash, weight gain, swelling, or blood in the stool occurs while taking pain relievers, report these side effects to a primary care provider.

⚠ Report immediately to a primary care provider any redness, pain, or swelling that extends beyond the boundaries of the original injury.

⚠ If the burn seems to worsen or is not healed significantly in 7 days, see a primary care provider for further treatment.

patient should be referred to an appropriate health care professional for further evaluation.

The burn wound should exhibit decreased redness during healing. Signs of cellulitis or tissue infection, such as increasing redness, pain, and swelling that extend beyond the boundaries of the original wound, or signs of contact dermatitis from topical treatment suggest the need for further evaluation.

Burned skin is more susceptible to sunburn for several weeks after initial injury, so avoiding sun exposure and using sunscreen agents during this period are recommended.

## Key Points for Minor Burns and Sunburn

- Minor burns and sunburn can often be treated with self-care. However, deeper burn injuries or burns affecting more than 1% to 2% of BSA require medical attention.
- Burn injuries may increase in severity over the first 24 to 48 hours, so reassessment is always necessary.
- Patient complaints usually focus on pain. Skin protectants and dressings should be recommended, and aspirin or NSAIDs are often helpful. The type of dressing or skin protectant used depends on whether the wound is dry or weeping. Blisters should not be ruptured. Topical hydrocortisone or anesthetics may provide additional relief in some patients, but should be used sparingly on broken skin. Counterirritants should be avoided.
- Vitamins, whether systemic or topical, are generally of no value unless the patient is malnourished.
- Photosensitization reactions can often be assessed by history and must be distinguished from ordinary sunburns.

## References


1. Occupational burns among restaurant workers—Colorado and Minnesota. *MMWR Morb Mortal Wkly Rep.* 1993;42:713-6.
2. Deaths resulting from residential fires and the prevalence of smoke alarms—United States, 1991-1995. *MMWR Morb Mortal Wkly Rep.* 1998;47:803-6.
3. Deaths resulting from residential fires—United States, 1991. *MMWR Morb Mortal Wkly Rep.* 1994;43:901-4.
4. Rapaport MJ, Rapaport V. Preventive and therapeutic approaches to short- and long-term sun damaged skin. *Clin Dermatol.* 1998;16:429-39.
5. Mertens DM, Jenkins ME, Warden GD. Outpatient burn management. *Nurs Clin North Am.* 1997;32:343-64.
6. Bickers DR. Photosensitivity and other reactions to light. In: Fauci AS, ed. *Harrison's Principles of Internal Medicine.* 14th ed. New York: McGraw-Hill, Inc; 1998:1254-62.
7. Sheridan R, Tompkins RG. Evaluation and management of the thermally injured patient. In: Freedberg IM, Eisen AZ, Wolff K, et al., eds. *Fitzpatrick's Dermatology in General Medicine.* 5th ed. New York: McGraw-Hill, Inc; 1999:1505-14.
8. Federal *Register.* 1983;48:6820-33.
9. Judson R. Minor burns—modern management techniques. *Aust Fam Physician.* 1997;26:1023-6.
10. McGregor JM, Hawk JLM. Acute effects of ultraviolet radiation on the skin. In: Freedberg IM, Eisen AZ, Wolff K, et al., eds. *Fitzpatrick's Dermatology in General Medicine.* 5th ed. New York: McGraw-Hill; 1999:1555-61.
11. Bandmann HJ, Calnan CD, Cronin E, et al. Dermatitis from applied medicaments. *Arch Dermatol.* 1972;106:335-7.
12. Eaglestein WH, Mertz BA, Alvarez OM. Effect of topically applied agents on healing wounds. *Clin Dermatol.* 1984;2:112-5.
13. Duteil L. A randomized, controlled study of the safety and efficacy of topical corticosteroid treatments of sunburn in healthy volunteers. *Clin Exp Dermatol.* 2002;27:314-8.
14. Kaye ET, Kaye KM. Topical antibacterial agents. *Infect Dis Clin North Am.* 1995;9:547-61.
15. Fuchs J, Kern H. Modulation of UV-light-induced skin inflammation by D-alpha-tocopherol and L-ascorbic acid: a clinical study using solar simulated radiation. *Free Radical Biol Med.* 1998;25:1006-12.

16. Rhodes LE, Durham BH, Fraser WD, et al. Dietary fish oil reduces basal and ultraviolet B-generated PGE2 levels in skin and increases the threshold to provocation of polymorphic light eruption. *J Invest Dermatol.* 1995;105:532-5.
17. Garmyn M, Ribaya-Mercado JD, Russel RM, et al. Effect of beta-carotene supplementation on the human sunburn reaction. *Exper Dermatol.* 1995;4:104-11.
18. Sai KP, Babu M. Traditional medicine and practices in burn care: need for newer scientific perspectives. *Burns.* 1998;24:387-8.
19. Robbers JE, Tyler VE. *Tyler's Herbs of Choice.* New York: The Haworth Herbal Press; 1999:215-24.
20. Subrahmanyam M. A prospective randomised clinical and histological study of superficial burn wound healing with honey and silver sulfadiazine. *Burns.* 1998;24:157-61.

CHAPTER 42

# Minor Wounds and Secondary Bacterial Skin Infections

*Daphne B. Bernard*

Wound care management can be quite resource intensive, with much of the cost related to the expense of the medications and supplies used for wound healing. Annual worldwide expenditures on wound care are estimated to be approximately $7 billion;[1] in fact, $1 billion is spent worldwide on wound dressings alone.[2] Since patients commonly use self-care in wound management and, in light of these statistics, a thorough knowledge of wounds and how they heal is essential. Although the skin is well adapted to heal minor wounds over time, proper dressing and the appropriate use of antiseptics and antibiotics will facilitate healing as well as prevent scar formation and secondary bacterial skin infections.

Common concepts of wound care have changed drastically from earlier times and go against conventional wisdom, which encouraged "drying out" a wound and promoting the formation of a scab. Occlusive dressings were expressly avoided because it was believed that the moist, warm environment they created promoted bacterial colonization. This approach was challenged in the mid-1960s when experiments were conducted to determine the possible benefit of a moist environment in wound healing. Today, there is clear evidence to support the benefits of a moist wound-healing environment. In many circumstances, practitioners should now recommend newer synthetic products that provide a moist environment in place of the traditional gauze dressings that promote dehydration of the wound.

One of the primary goals of this chapter is to provide practitioners with current information to enable them to properly advise consumers on wound care and product selection. Principles of the moist wound-healing method and its proper implementation through the use of selected first-aid products are covered. In addition, the chapter's goals are realized with a thorough review of skin anatomy and function, the physiology of wound healing, the classifications, types, and complications of wounds, wound management through the use of drugs and/or dressings, and a schematic approach to triaging wounds. This integrated information should enable practitioners to communicate effectively with primary care providers on issues related to care of wounds and secondary bacterial infections, as well as to provide a firm foundation for effective patient counseling on the processes and treatments of these disorders.

## Epidemiology of Wounds

Each year nearly 25 million persons are afflicted with various acute and chronic wounds in need of intervention. Almost 11 million lacerations are treated annually in emergency departments in the United States, and this number is likely growing.[3]

## Anatomy and Physiology of Skin

The skin is a versatile, multifunctional organ whose intricate workings depend on a delicate balance between structure and function. When a wound alters or disturbs this balance, prompt restoration is required to ensure body homeostasis. Restoration of homeostasis is accomplished through the process of wound healing, a complex cascade of localized biochemical and cellular events regulated by the immune system and orchestrated by the skin.

The skin is composed of two anatomic layers, the epidermis and the dermis, and supported by a variably thick subcutaneous layer called the hypodermis (see Table 42-1 and Figure 33-1 in Chapter 33). The epidermis, the most superficial layer of the skin, is normally in direct contact with the outside environment. Approximately 0.04 mm thick and avascular, it consists of five layers of stratified squamous epithelium (keratinocytes). This keratinized layer provides a tough, resistant, waterproof covering for the skin. Aside from its protective function, the epidermis also serves several other functions, as it contains the cell types necessary for immune regulation (Langerhans' cells), skin color (melanocytes), and proprioception (Merkel's tactile cells). Skin appendages, including the sweat glands and hair follicles, are also derived from the epidermis.

The dermis is the layer directly below the epidermis. It is approximately 0.5 mm thick and contains a rich vascular supply, multiple nerve endings, lymphatics, collagen proteins, and connective tissue. It also contains two main cell types: fibroblasts and macrophages. The main function of fibroblasts is to produce collagen, a structural support protein necessary for scar formation. Macrophages, however, are multifunctional cells that are vital for wound repair. They serve as both immune regulators and growth regulators; these functions are necessary for the sterilization, debridement, and eventual healing of the wound. The dermis also contains the basilar projections of epidermally derived sweat glands and hair follicles.

**TABLE 42-1 Structure and Function of the Skin**

**Epidermis**

- Thickness of 0.04 mm
- No blood supply
- Composed of epithelium
- Resident flora
- Five layers (two are stratum corneum and stratum germinativum, or basement layer)

**Dermis**

- Thickness of 0.5 mm
- Main support structure
- Contains nerve endings, lymphatics, vasculature
- Normally moist
- Appendages: hair follicles, sebaceous glands, sweat glands

**Subcutaneous Tissue (Hypodermis)**

- Variable thickness
- Reservoir for fat storage
- Temperature insulator
- Shock absorber
- Stores calories

*Source:* Adapted with permission from Bryant R. Wound repair: a review. *J Enterostomal Ther.* 1987;14:262-3.

The subcutaneous tissue contains mostly adipocytes and is the origination site for dermal blood vessels. Its major function is to provide insulation, padding, and protection against mechanical injury. It also stores calories in the form of fat and provides the skin with a moderate degree of mobility, protecting it against friction and shear-related injury.

The skin has five basic functions: protection, sensation, thermoregulation, immunomodulation, and production of vitamin D. The skin has several other specialized features. Its surface is inhabited by bacteria (skin flora), including *Staphylococcus epidermidis* and *S. aureus*, as well as the fungus *Candida albicans*.[4] The skin flora serves to protect against invasion by other pathogenic bacteria. The pH of the skin is acidic (between 4.2 and 5.6),[4] which allows it to regulate the number and activity of skin flora. This feature is important, as the normal flora can become pathogenic under certain conditions.

## Physiology of Wound Healing

Wound healing begins immediately after injury and consists of three overlapping stages: inflammatory, proliferative, and maturation (remodeling).[4,5]

### *Inflammatory Phase*

The inflammatory phase is the body's immediate response to injury. This phase, which lasts approximately 3 to 4 days, is responsible for preparing the wound for subsequent tissue development and consists of two primary parts: hemostasis and inflammation.

In the initial portion of the inflammatory phase, hemostasis is initiated by the release of thromboplastin from injured cells. Thromboplastin, in turn, activates the body's intrinsic clotting system to form a clot within the first several hours. The newly formed clot stops the bleeding and allows healing to progress. The recruited platelets are crucial to the initial phases of healing because they release cytokines such as platelet-derived growth factor (PDGF) and transforming growth factor (TGF). These cytokines stimulate chemotaxis of polymorphonuclear neutrophil (PMN) leukocytes, monocytes, and fibroblasts. Cytokines will also subsequently promote mitogenesis and collagen synthesis.[6]

After hemostasis is achieved, an active inflammatory phase begins, cleansing the wound. PMN leukocytes are recruited during the first 24 to 48 hours to phagocytize debris and bacteria in the wound. Platelets release bradykinin, histamine, and prostaglandins into the wound during this time, thereby initiating an intense vasodilatation of the surrounding vessels and then flooding the wound in a rinsing action with water, plasma proteins, electrolytes, antibodies, and complement.[6] As a result, the wound becomes erythematous and edematous.

After the first 24 hours, blood monocytes are recruited into the wound by released chemotactic factors and become tissue macrophages. Macrophages function as phagocytes, releasing more chemotactic factors and, most important, releasing growth factors that stimulate epithelial mitogenesis and endothelial angiogenesis. They also induce fibroblasts to synthesize collagen, which provides a healthy bed of granulation tissue for future epithelial cells.

The final portion of the inflammatory phase involves epithelial migration into the wound. Epithelial cells from the stratum germinativum migrate from the intact wound edges and epithelial appendages to cover the denuded area of the wound. The successful migration and adherence of epithelial cells to the wound requires a clean, healthy bed of granulation tissue. Once the epithelial cells become established on their granulation bed, they provide the initial (one cell thick) layer of new skin for the wound. Epithelial cells can migrate under the clot and eschar (scab) in the wound, but in doing so they delay healing time and promote scar formation.

### *Proliferative Phase*

In the next phase of healing, the proliferative phase, the wound is filled with new connective tissue and covered with new epithelium. This phase starts on about day 3 and continues for about 3 weeks. It involves the formation of granulation tissue, which is a collection of new connective tissue (fibroblasts and newly synthesized collagen), new capillaries, and inflammatory cells. The formation of this matrix involves several key coexisting and ongoing processes, including neoangiogenesis (capillary formation) and collagen synthesis.

Collagen synthesis by fibroblasts is directed by cytokines produced by stimulated macrophages, including

PDGF, TGF-α and TGF-β, fibroblast growth factor, monocyte- and macrophage-derived growth factor, and interleukin-2.[6] Collagen synthesis also requires oxygen, zinc, iron, and vitamin C. As granulation tissue is being laid down, epithelial cells, which began to migrate during the inflammatory phase, resurface the wound defect. It is important to remember that epithelial cells do not migrate across a dry or necrotic surface. The final portion of this phase involves the action of cytokine-recruited smooth muscle cells, which begins the process of wound contraction. This process involves the mobilization and pulling together of the wound edges.

### Maturation Phase

The final phase of healing is known as the maturation or "remodeling" phase. This is the longest phase, beginning at about week 3, when the wound is completely closed by connective tissue and resurfaced by epithelial cells. It can continue for approximately 2 years after the injury. It involves a continual process of collagen synthesis and breakdown, replacing earlier, weak collagen with high-tensile-strength collagen. The result is a scar with approximately 70% to 80% of the original strength of the skin it replaced.

## Factors Affecting Wound Healing

Several local and systemic factors can affect how efficiently and to what extent a wound will heal. Only the most important systemic factors that can affect the healing process will be discussed.

### Tissue Perfusion and Oxygenation

Poor vascularization delays wound healing. The resultant poor oxygenation leads to impaired leukocyte activity, decreased production of collagen, decreased epithelialization, and reduced resistance to infection. Common disorders that may cause decreased perfusion include diabetes, severe anemia, hypotension, peripheral vascular disease and congestive heart failure.[7]

### Nutrition

Adequate nutrition provides the building blocks for wound repair. Protein, carbohydrates, vitamins, and trace elements are needed for collagen production and cellular energy.[8,9] Vitamins A and C promote wound integrity. Vitamin A enhances the synthesis of collagen and stimulates epithelialization by causing rapid cell turnover. Vitamin C is necessary to maintain proper cellular membrane integrity and further enhance collagen synthesis and cross-linkage. Zinc may enhance wound healing by promoting cell proliferation. Many practitioners recommend supplements of these and other complementary therapies for promotion of wound healing, despite the lack of substantial clinical evidence of their benefit.

### Age and Weight

Aging can cause a delayed inflammatory response and is associated with increased capillary fragility, reduced collagen synthesis, and neovascularization. Aging is also associated with slow epithelialization.[10,11] Patients who are obese have problems with poor perfusion (adipose tissue lacks vascular tissue) and tend to have delayed wound healing.[12]

### Infection

All traumatic wounds are contaminated with bacteria to some degree; such contamination is usually restrained by phagocytic action. However, an infection will develop if the following factors are present: (1) a high level of bacterial contamination (e.g., $>10^5$ bacteria per gram of wound tissue), (2) a compromised tissue microenvironment (e.g., eschar, necrosis), (3) systemic conditions (e.g., age, steroid therapy, malnutrition), and (4) immunoincompetence.[7,13]

Localized infection in the wound delays collagen synthesis and epithelialization and prolongs the inflammatory phase, causing additional tissue destruction. The most common bacteria implicated in community-acquired wound infections include gram-positive *Staphylococcus aureus*, *Streptococcus pyogenes*, and *Enterococcus faecalis*. Gram-negative *Escherichia coli*, *Pseudomonas aeruginosa*, and *Klebsiella* species are often associated with hospital-acquired or chronic wounds. Anaerobic organisms, such as *Bacteroides* species, are associated with necrotic or poorly perfused wounds.[13]

The classic signs and symptoms of a local wound infection include erythema, edema, induration, pain, crepitation, and the presence of purulent or odorous exudate in the affected area. Fever, flulike symptoms, and leukocytosis are frequently associated with systemic infections. Appropriate wound cultures should be taken to identify the infecting organisms when the classic clinical signs of infection are present.[13]

### Coexisting Diabetes Mellitus

Poorly controlled diabetes is usually associated with reduced collagen synthesis, impaired wound contraction, delayed epidermal migration, and reduced PMN leukocyte chemotaxis and phagocytosis. Strict professional attention should be given to wounds in patients with diabetes because of these inherent difficulties.[14]

### Medications

Practitioners can play a key role in identifying potential detriments to proper wound closure. Certain medications, for example, can act directly to impede healing through their interaction at various stages of the healing process. Corticosteroids suppress inflammation, resulting in a decrease in angiogenesis, collagen synthesis, and phagocytosis. Antineoplastic drugs and radiation therapy interfere with the cellular division necessary for fibroblast function and reepithelialization. Anticoagulants may interfere early in the inflammatory phase.[15] Patients who are taking these medications should be carefully followed by a wound care specialist to ensure that proper healing occurs.

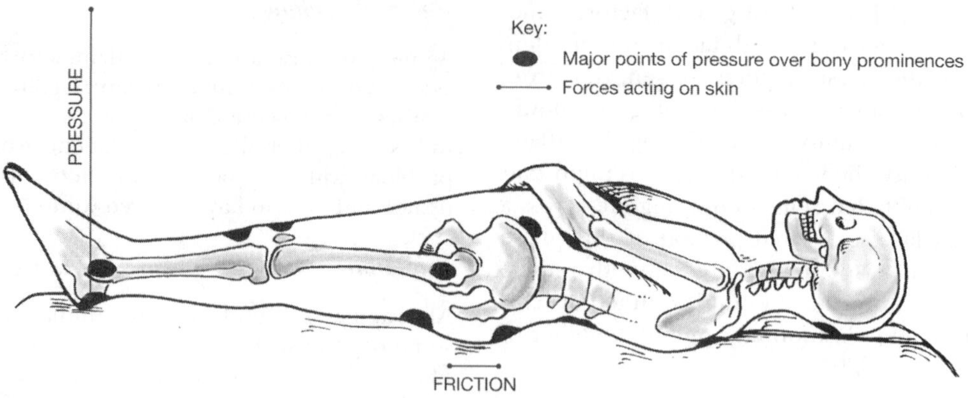


**FIGURE 42-1** Stresses on skin.

### *Wound Characteristics*

Local features that may impair wound closure include the presence of necrotic tissue, eschar, or foreign bodies (e.g., glass, dirt); the lack of moisture; and the presence of infection.[1,3,16] Practitioners who are aware of and can recognize problems with such local factors can, through careful counseling, do their part to ensure proper wound healing.

## Classification of Wounds

Classification of wound type is necessary for implementing proper and specific wound therapy; hence, it is imperative that practitioners who are recommending outpatient first-aid products be aware of these classifications. Wounds can be classified according to their acuity and/or depth.

### *Classification by Acuity*

Using the acuity classification, wounds can be either acute or chronic.

#### Acute Wounds

Acute wounds include abrasions, punctures, lacerations, and burns and usually result from injury. They take approximately 1 month to heal in healthy individuals. Burns are discussed in Chapter 41. *Abrasions* usually result from a rubbing or friction injury to the epidermal portion of the skin and extend to the uppermost portion of the dermis. *Punctures* usually result from a sharp object that has pierced the epidermis and lodged in the dermis or deeper tissues. *Lacerations* result from sharp objects cutting through the various layers of the skin.[12] Self-treatment of acute wounds such as abrasions and puncture wounds not extending beyond the dermis is generally deemed appropriate.

#### Chronic Wounds

Chronic wounds include pressure, arterial, and venous ulcers. These wounds do not proceed through the three phases of wound healing in a timely manner. Usually some underlying disease such as diabetes or external factors such as pressure contribute to poor wound healing.[12] All chronic wounds should be referred for further medical evaluation.

*Pressure Ulcers* A pressure ulcer results from unrelieved pressure that damages the skin and underlying tissue. Pressure ulcers are commonly referred to as pressure sores, bed sores, or decubitus ulcers and can range in severity from mild, with minor skin reddening, to severe, with deep crater formation that may extend to the bone or muscle. Pressure ulcers usually occur over bony prominences such as the sacrum, elbow, and heel (Figure 42-1). Sixty percent or more of all pressure ulcers are thought to occur during hospitalization, whereas 18% develop in nursing homes. Patients of advanced age and those who are immobile because of such circumstances as prolonged hospitalization, bedrest, paralysis, or paresis constitute the majority of patients affected by pressure ulcers. Other risk factors include obesity, malnutrition, and incontinence.[17]

Pathophysiology of Pressure Ulcers Four key factors are involved in skin breakdown: pressure, shearing forces, friction, and moisture. Tiny blood vessels that supply the skin with nutrients and oxygen are constricted by unrelieved pressure on the skin. Tissue death with ulcer formation results from the skin's prolonged deprivation of oxygen and nutrients.[17] These localized areas of tissue necrosis tend to occur when soft tissue is compressed between a bony prominence and an external surface for a prolonged period of time. Shearing forces result from adjacent structures sliding against one another, such as when a seated patient slides down. This stretching of subcutaneous tissue with the sacral skin remaining stationary causes occlusion of the subcutaneous blood vessels, resulting in ischemia. Friction can occur when an external object moves against the skin, such as when bedsheets are moved across the skin. Moisture often results from perspiration and incontinence and can lead to tissue maceration, which facilitates skin breakdown when any of the other factors are present.[18]

Classification of Pressure Ulcers Pressure ulcers may be classified on the basis of color and exudate formation. Red wounds are in an active healing state with cell proliferation, collagen synthesis, and the formation of granulation tissue. This newly formed tissue is quite fragile and requires a constant supply of oxygen and nutrients as well as protection from external elements and a moist environment to continue its healing process. Yellow wounds may contain

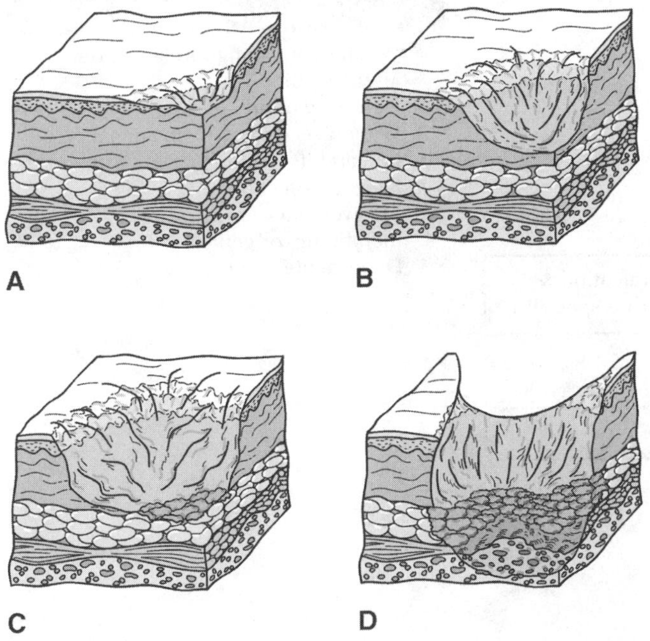


FIGURE 42-2 Stages of wounds. **Stage I,** Nonblanchable erythema of intact skin with warmth and redness. **Stage II,** Superficial lesions with partial-thickness skin loss involving the epidermis with or without the dermis involved. **Stage III,** Full-thickness skin loss with damage to subcutaneous tissue. **Stage IV,** Full-thickness skin loss with extensive tissue necrosis and damage to underlying muscle, tendon, and bone.

a portion of necrotic tissue and/or purulent drainage and generally extend through the dermis. A black wound indicates nonviable necrotic tissue, which must be removed before healing can occur.[19]

*Arterial and Venous Ulcers* Arterial and venous ulcers are the second form of chronic wounds. Arterial ulcers are usually secondary to severe peripheral vascular occlusive disease.[20] Commonly encountered in the lower extremities, they are painful. Venous ulcers result from dysfunctional valves. To assist in blood flow, the leg veins contain one-way valves that facilitate flow up the leg and prevent flow back down the vein. These valves are not very effective in some people or can be damaged by thrombosis (clots) or edema in the veins. Incompetent valves can result in "backward" flow down the veins, resulting in high pressure in the veins when the patient is standing up. This abnormally high pressure in the veins damages the skin and leads to the ulcers.[19, 20] Some ulcers occur as a result of both arterial and venous disease, representing ulcers of mixed etiologies.[21]

### *Classification by Wound Depth*

Wound depth classification (Figure 42-2) is used primarily by health care personnel and is based on the extent or number of skin layers damaged during the wound-initiating process. This classification has been divided, for simplicity's sake, into four descriptive stages. Stage I does not involve loss of any skin layers and consists primarily of reddened, nonblanching unbroken skin. Stage II includes blister or partial-thickness skin loss involving all the epidermis and part of the dermis. Stage III, full-thickness skin loss, includes damage to the entire epidermis, dermis, and dermal appendages, and may involve subcutaneous tissue. Stage IV is an extension of stage III but further involves the subcutaneous tissue and underlying muscle, tendon, and bone.[18] Understanding these stages helps in selecting appropriate dressings for proper wound closure.

## Treatment of Minor Wounds and Secondary Bacterial Infections

### *Treatment Goals*

The goal in treating wounds is to promote healing by protecting the wound from infection and further trauma and to minimize scarring. Treatment should include a stepwise approach that involves cleansing the wound, selectively using antiseptics and antibiotics, and creating closure with an appropriate dressing. Figure 42-3 lists exclusions for self-treatment.

### *General Treatment Approach*

Uncontaminated acute wounds at stages I and II (Figure 42-2) such as minor cuts, scrapes, and burns require only basic supportive measures, including irrigation with saline or bottled water for proper cleansing and using a wound dressing to prevent entry of bacteria into the affected area. Topical nonprescription antibiotic and antiseptic preparations can also be useful in preventing secondary infection, but these agents should be viewed as extensions of supportive treatment. Figure 42-3 outlines the triage and treatment of acute wounds.

More serious or deeper tissue injury (e.g., animal or human bites, puncture wounds, severe burns) requires primary care provider consultation to assess the need for systemic or topical prescription antibiotics as well as for a tetanus booster. The current Centers for Disease Control and Prevention recommendations for tetanus booster is 0.5 mL intramuscularly once every 10 years if the initial series has been completed. The basic instructions for treating acute wounds may not apply to chronic wounds. For that reason, patients with chronic wounds should seek medical advice concerning wound care. These patients should also do the following:

- Consult a primary care provider about any slow-healing wound, because the underlying defect in healing probably requires systemic treatment as well as local wound care.
- Prevent pressure ulcers by repositioning the body often and using pressure-relieving devices.
- Watch for early signs of skin redness over bony prominences as prompt intervention can prevent skin breakdown.

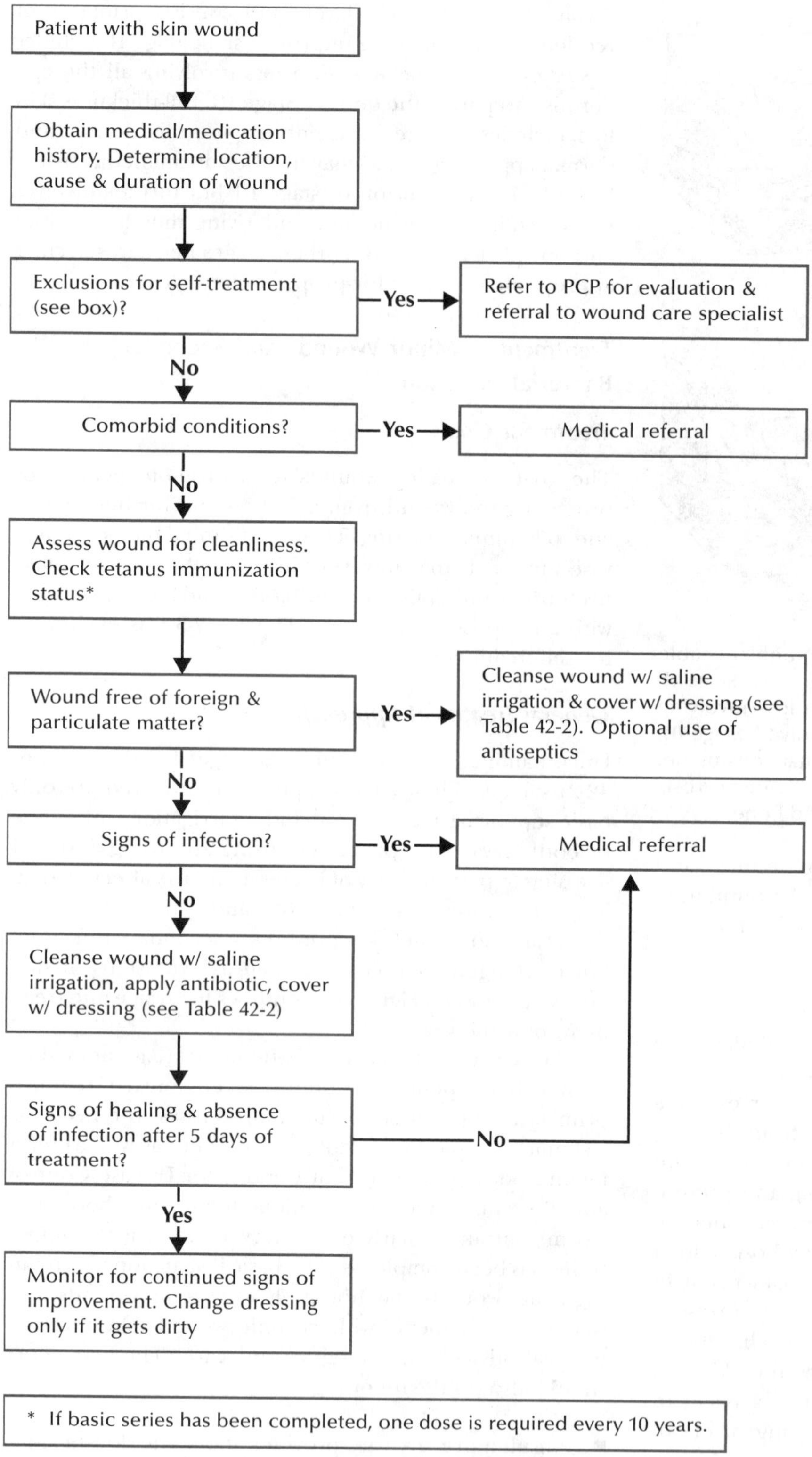


**Exclusions for Self-Treatment**

- Wound containing foreign matter after irrigation
- Chronic wound
- Wound secondary to an animal or human bite
- Signs of infection
- Involvement of face, mucous membrane, or genitalia
- Deep, acute wound

**FIGURE 42-3** Self-care of acute skin wounds. Key: PCP, primary care provider.

### *Nonpharmacologic Therapy (Wound Dressings)*

Traditional wound management involves leaving the wound open to air or covering it with a nonocclusive textile dressing (gauze). However, this type of management leads to eschar formation, which impedes reepithelialization of wounds and creates unwanted scars (Figure 42-4A). It may also lead to wound dehydration with delayed healing and increased risk of bacterial entry into the wound. Removal of gauze dressings often tears away not only the eschar but also the new tissue under the eschar. These cumulative

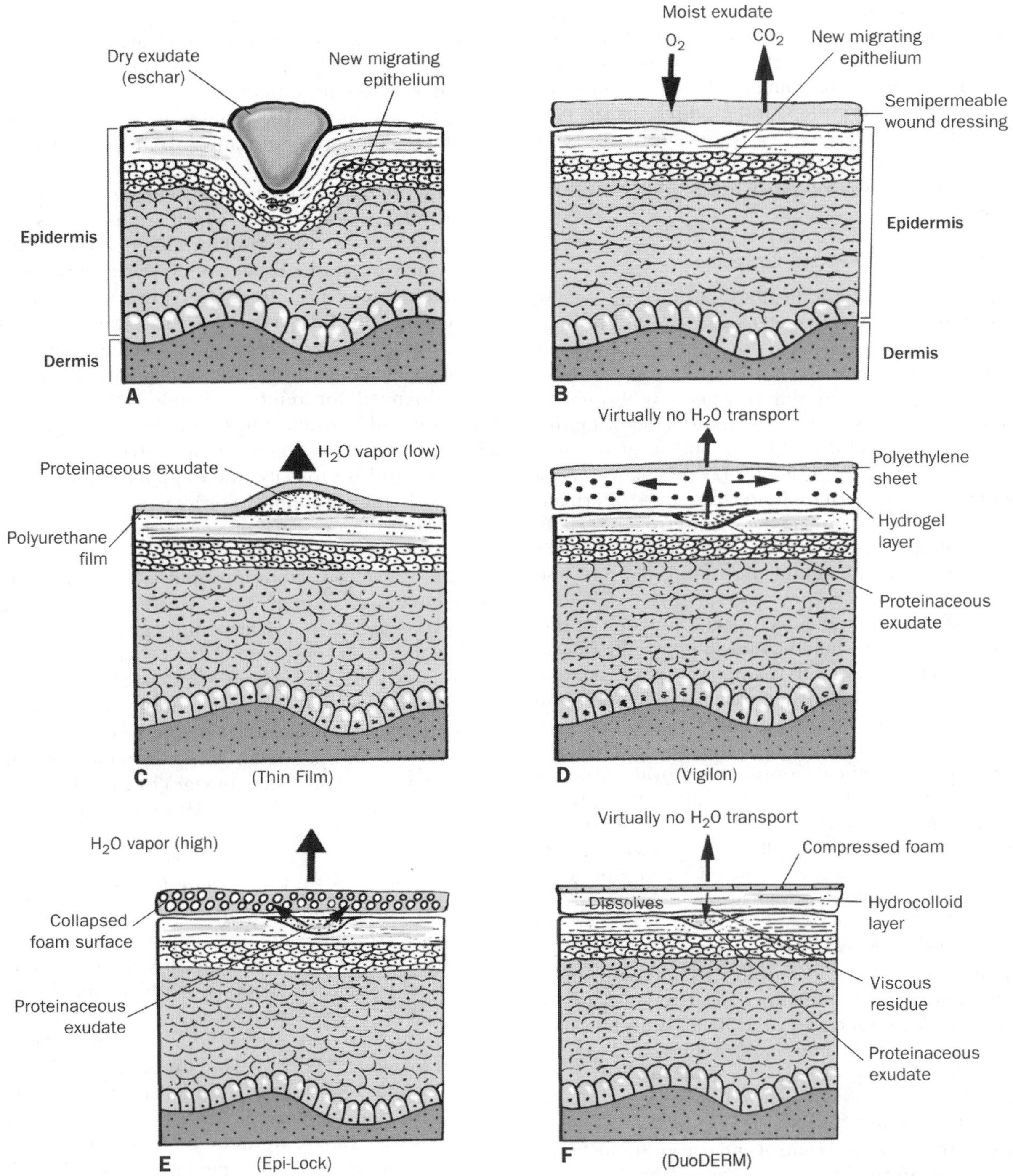


FIGURE 42-4 Mechanisms by which semipermeable wound dressings create a moist environment for wound healing. **A,** Regenerating epidermal cells are forced to "tunnel" below the dry wound eschar to attain wound closure. This tunneling delays wound closure. **B,** Semipermeable wound dressings prevent formation of eschar by maintaining optimal moisture level at the wound bed. Unhindered by the presence of a dry eschar, migrating epithelial cells are able to migrate and close the wound. **C,** Mechanism of water vapor transmission in thin films. **D,** Mechanism of action of a hydrogel wound dressing (Vigilon). **E,** Mechanism of action of a hydrophilic polyurethane foam dressing (Epi-Lock). **F,** Mechanisms of action of a hydrocolloid wound dressing (DuoDERM). (Adapted with permission from Syzcher M, Lee SJ. Modern wound dressings: a systemic approach to wounds. *J Biomater Appl.* 1992;7:142-213.)

problems have led primary care providers and nurses to develop new treatment strategies on the basis of creating a moist wound environment (Figure 42-4B). Such an environment prevents eschar development, removes excess exudate without dehydration, and prevents bacterial invasion of the wound. A moist environment, created by the use of semipermeable dressings, preserves exudates that contain white blood cells, growth factors, and other special enzymes and hormones that promote cell growth. It also prevents dressings from adhering to the wound and damaging the fragile tissue when the dressing is removed.[22] Practitioners should still recommend the use of gauze and gauze-type adhesive dressings; for example, gauze pads may be used with more advanced semiocclusive dressings such as foams for better exudate absorption. In addition, gauze-type adhesive bandages may be used for minor cuts and abrasions.

### Selection Criteria for Wound Dressings

The primary goal in wound healing is to heal the wound quickly with minimal scarring, deformity and loss of function. Scarring is closely related to the type of dressing used; occlusive dressings cause less scarring than gauze dressings. The timing of the dressing placement is also important; immediate occlusion leads to resurfacing of epithelium faster than delayed occlusion. The ideal dressing should (1) remove excess exudate, (2) maintain a moist environment, (3) be permeable to oxygen, (4) thermally insulate the wound, (5) protect the wound from infection, (6) be free of particulate or toxic contaminants, and (7) be able to be removed without disrupting delicate new tissue.[23]

Understanding the potential use and function of specific wound dressings should guide the practitioner in proper product selection. It is important to note that wound dressing requirements may change depending on the healing phase. In terms of promoting moist wound healing, the wound dressing may be used to absorb excess moisture, maintain optimal moisture, or provide moisture where it is lacking. Table 42-2 and Figure 42-5 (which provide guidelines for selection of dressings developed by Jeter and Tintle[24]) describe and illustrate the major categories of wound care products available today and provide an overview of their indications, advantages, and disadvantages.

*Abrasions and Lacerations* Most superficial wounds (minor abrasions and lacerations) that practitioners encounter may simply require the application of adhesive gauze-type bandages such as regular Band-Aid Brand bandages. Recognition of the importance of the moist wound-healing method has led to the development and marketing of more hydrocolloid-based bandages (Band-Aid Advanced Healing and New Skin), which meet the need for moisture retention and control and may promote faster healing.[25] For individuals with hypersensitive skin, hypoallergenic and latex-free tape (First-Aid Hurt Free Tape) may be less irritating and will not tear the skin or hair on removal. Patients with latex allergies who have generally developed dermatologic problems from synthetic latex exposure may benefit from using dressings containing natural rubber latex (Band-Aid Gentle Care and Curad Sensitive Skin); however, these products may still cause allergic reactions.

In selecting medicated bandages such as those with pads containing benzalkonium chloride (Band-Aid Antibacterial), which claim to "kill germs and prevent infection," benzocaine (Band-Aids Pain & Itch), which claim to decrease wound "pain and itch," calcium alginate (Band-Aids Quick Stop), which claim to "help blood clot faster," and ionic sliver (Actocoat; Silverderm), which are promoted as having antibacterial properties, it is important to evaluate whether the application of these agents is even necessary. Evidence supporting the benefits of these more expensive products compared with more traditional dressings is lacking.

Alternatives to conventional bandages are liquid adhesive bandages (Liquiderm), which are used for small cuts and abrasions and preferred for either cosmetic purposes (i.e., when a wound is located on the face) or when a more flexible dressing product is need (i.e., when a wound is located on the finger or elbow).[26] Cyanoacrylate tissue adhesives offer many advantages: patient comfort, resistance to bacterial growth, and one-time rapid application with no need for removal. Randomized clinical trials involving children and adults demonstrate that tissue adhesives offer long-term cosmetic outcomes as good as sutures[27] and no toxicity when applied topically for skin closure.[28] These products polymerize via an exothermic reaction in the presence of skin moisture or tissue fluid; therefore, a strong bond is formed with the skin.[28]

More extensive abrasions and lacerations should be inspected by a primary care provider, debrided, and flushed; tetanus prophylaxis is also important to consider. If they are clean, the wounds can be sutured to facilitate their contracture. If they are grossly contaminated by foreign particles or inorganic matter or show evidence of early infection, the wounds should not be sutured but cleaned and covered with a sterile, semipermeable nonadhering gauze-type (i.e., Band-Aid bandage) or hydrocolloid dressing (Band-Aid Brand Advanced Healing Strips) to facilitate healing.[4,16]

*Puncture Wounds* It is important for a primary care provider to inspect puncture wounds to ensure that no foreign bodies are retained and update tetanus prophylaxis, if necessary. If no debris is present, the wound should then be cleansed with either water or sterile saline. The wounds should be left open and soaked with soapy water for 30 minutes at least four times a day initially, to allow for proper healing.[4,16] Hydrocolloid dressings (i.e., Johnson & Johnson Brand Advanced Healing Pads) are indicated for punctures that produce light exudates while hydrogel dressings (i.e., Biolex Wound Gel) that absorb more exudates may be indicated for punctures extending deeper into the dermis and deeper tissues.

*Pressure Ulcers* Pressure ulcers deserve special attention because they often require intense supervision and professional aid to heal properly. A key objective is to remove dead tissue, debris, and excess exudate to enable optimal wound healing.[17] Offloading and relief of the inciting pressure is also required. (See Figure 42-5 for selection of dressings on the basis of wound depth [ulcer stage].) Close attention should be given to alleviating the cause of these wounds, and practitioners should counsel patients that the management of pressure ulcers should be closely supervised by individuals trained to treat such wounds.

**TABLE 42-2 Options in Wound Dressing**

| Description (Trade Name)* | Uses/Indications | Advantages | Disadvantages |
|---|---|---|---|
| **Gauze Dressings** | | | |
| Nonocclusive fiber dressing with loose, open weave (e.g., Kerlex Rolls and Sponges, Band-Aid Brand Bandages, Nexcare Comfort Bandages) | Stages II-IV<br>Minimal to heavy exuding wounds/topicals<br>Infected wounds<br>Debridement<br>Wound rehydration | Readily available<br>Deep wound packing<br>May use with infected wounds/ topicals<br>Mechanical debridement<br>Nonocclusive<br>Conformable | Wound bed may desiccate if dressing is dry<br>Nonselective debridement<br>May cause bleeding/pain on removal<br>Need secondary dressing<br>Frequent dressing changes |
| **Nonadherent (Gauze-type) Dressings** | | | |
| Nonadherent, porous dressings. Lightly coated dressings allow exudate to flow through (e.g., Adaptic, Telfa, Sofsorb Wound Dressing, Vaseline Gauze, CarraGauze) | Skin donor sites<br>Stage II, shallow stage III<br>Staple/suture lines<br>Abrasions<br>Lacerations<br>Punctures | Readily available<br>Less adherent than plain gauze | Need secondary dressing<br>May have traumatic/painful dressing removal<br>Some impregnated dressings may delay healing<br>May require frequent dressing changes<br>Some may cause exudate pooling |
| **Foams** | | | |
| Semipermeable, nonwoven, absorptive, inert polyurethane foam dressings (e.g., EPIGARD, Lyofoam, Hydrasorb, Allevyn, VigiFOAM; see Figure 42-4 E) | Stage II, shallow-stage III<br>Minimal to moderate drainage<br>Autolysis<br>First- and second-degree burns<br>Contraindicated in third-degree burns | Most are nonadhesive<br>Some can be used with infected wounds/topicals<br>Thermal insulation<br>Reduce pain<br>Nonocclusive<br>Moist environment<br>Conformable<br>Less frequent dressing changes<br>Trauma-free removal<br>Absorbent | Most require secondary dressing<br>May require cutting<br>May cause wound desiccation<br>May be difficult to determine wound contact surface |
| **Alginates** | | | |
| Hydrophilic, nonwoven dressings composed of calcium-sodium (percentages vary) alginate fibers. Alginates are processed from brown seaweed into pad or twisted fiber form. Exudate transforms fibers to gel at wound interface (e.g., Band-Aid Brand Quick Stop Adhesive Bandages, Kaltostat, Sorbsan, AlgiDERM, Algosteril) | Light to heavy exuding wounds<br>Stages II, III, IV<br>Autolysis<br>Skin donor sites | Absorptive<br>Reduce pain<br>Nonocclusive<br>Moist environment<br>Conformable<br>Easy, trauma-free removal<br>Can use on infected wounds<br>Accelerate healing time<br>Less frequent dressing changes<br>Potential to aid in control of minor bleeding | Require secondary dressing<br>Characteristic odor<br>May need wound irrigation<br>May desiccate<br>May promote hypergranulation |
| **Carbon-impregnated (Odor-control) Dressings** | | | |
| Dressings with an outer layer of carbon for odor control (e.g., Lyofoam "C," Carboflex, Odor) | Malodorous wounds | Control odor | Require appropriate seal or odor may escape<br>Carbon is inactivated when it becomes wet |

**TABLE 42-2 Options in Wound Dressing (continued)**

| Description (Trade Name)* | Uses/Indications | Advantages | Disadvantages |
|---|---|---|---|
| **Composite/Island Dressings** | | | |
| Nonadherent, absorptive center barrier with adhesive at perimeter (e.g., Nu-Derm, Airstrip, Viasorb, Allevyn island, Lyofoam "A, AcryDerm") | Stages II, III<br>Moderate to heavy exuding wounds | Nonadherent over wound<br>Semiocclusive<br>Autolysis<br>Suture/staple lines<br>Protective<br>Reduce pain<br>No secondary dressing required<br>Impermeable to fluids/bacteria | May cause periwound trauma on removal |
| **Hydrocolloids** | | | |
| Wafer dressings composed of hydrophilic particles in an adhesive form covered by a water-resistant film or foam (e.g., Band-Aid Brand Advanced Healing Strips, Comfeel, DuoDERM CGF Dressing, ULTEC, Cutinova, Tegasorb; see Figure 42-4 F) | Stages I, II, and shallow stage III<br>Clean, granular wounds<br>Autolysis<br>Minimal to moderate exuding<br>Can use with absorption products and alginates | Occlusive<br>Manage exudate by particle swelling<br>Autolysis<br>Long wear time<br>Self-adherent<br>Impermeable to fluids/bacteria<br>Conformable<br>Protective<br>Thermal insulation<br>Reduce pain<br>Moist environment | For uninfected wounds only<br>May cause periwound trauma on removal<br>Difficult wound assessment<br>Characteristic odor<br>Impermeable to gases<br>Some may leave residue on skin or in wound |
| **Transparent Adhesive Films** | | | |
| Semiocclusive, translucent dressings with partial or continuous adhesive composed of polyurethane or copolyester thin film (e.g., BIOCLUSIVE, ACU-derm, Op-Site, Blisterfilm, CarraFilm, Tegaderm; see Figure 42-4C) | Stages I, II, shallow stage III<br>Clean granular wounds<br>Minimally exuding wounds<br>Autolysis<br>Can use with absorption products and alginates<br>Can be used in conjunction with some enzymatic debriders | Semiocclusive<br>Gas permeable<br>Easy inspection<br>Autolysis<br>Protection<br>Impermeable to fluids/bacteria<br>Comfortable<br>Self-adherent<br>Reduce pain<br>Moist environment<br>Resist shear | For uninfected wounds only<br>Not absorptive<br>May cause periwound trauma on removal<br>With continuous adhesive, may reinjure wound on removal<br>With large amounts of exudate, maceration may occur |
| **Hydrogels/Gels** | | | |
| Nonadherent, nonocclusive dressings with high moisture content that come in the form of sheets and gels (e.g., New Skin Burn Relief Dressings; Elasto-Gel, Bioflex Wound Gel, Vigilon, 2nd Skin; see Figure 42-4D) | Stages II, III, some approved for stage IV<br>Granular or necrotic wound beds<br>Autolysis<br>Some used on partial- and full-thickness burns<br>Punctures | Nonadherent<br>Most are nonocclusive<br>Trauma-free removal<br>Varying absorption capabilities<br>Conformable<br>Some can be used in conjunction with topicals<br>Thermal insulation<br>Reduce pain<br>Moist environment | Most require secondary dressings<br>May macerate periwound skin<br>Some products may dehydrate<br>Slow to minimal absorption rate in most<br>Most require frequent/daily dressing change |

* The trade names listed for each type of wound dressing are given as examples of available products; however, these do not constitute an all-inclusive list of available wound-dressing products.

*Source*: Adapted with permission from an unpublished document prepared by McIntosh A, Raher E. Silver Cross Hospital, Joliet, Ill; 1991.

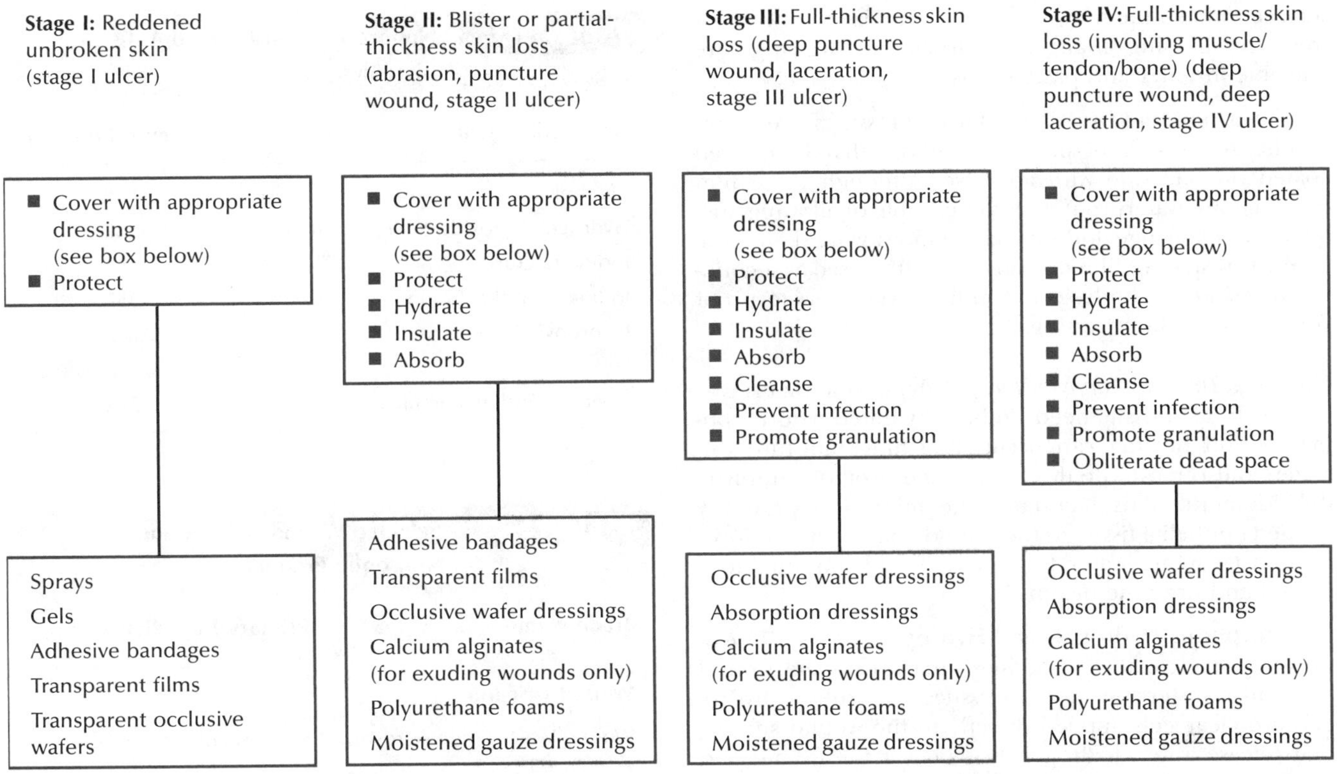
Stage I: Reddened unbroken skin (stage I ulcer)
Stage II: Blister or partial-thickness skin loss (abrasion, puncture wound, stage II ulcer)
Stage III: Full-thickness skin loss (deep puncture wound, laceration, stage III ulcer)
Stage IV: Full-thickness skin loss (involving muscle/tendon/bone) (deep puncture wound, deep laceration, stage IV ulcer)
■ Cover with appropriate dressing (see box below) ■ Protect
■ Cover with appropriate dressing (see box below) ■ Protect ■ Hydrate ■ Insulate ■ Absorb
■ Cover with appropriate dressing (see box below) ■ Protect ■ Hydrate ■ Insulate ■ Absorb ■ Cleanse ■ Prevent infection ■ Promote granulation
■ Cover with appropriate dressing (see box below) ■ Protect ■ Hydrate ■ Insulate ■ Absorb ■ Cleanse ■ Prevent infection ■ Promote granulation ■ Obliterate dead space
Sprays / Gels / Adhesive bandages / Transparent films / Transparent occlusive wafers
Adhesive bandages / Transparent films / Occlusive wafer dressings / Calcium alginates (for exuding wounds only) / Polyurethane foams / Moistened gauze dressings
Occlusive wafer dressings / Absorption dressings / Calcium alginates (for exuding wounds only) / Polyurethane foams / Moistened gauze dressings
Occlusive wafer dressings / Absorption dressings / Calcium alginates (for exuding wounds only) / Polyurethane foams / Moistened gauze dressings

**FIGURE 42-5** Guidelines for product selection on the basis of wound severity. (Adapted with permission from reference 24.)

## Types of Wound Dressings

Ideal dressings should be able to absorb excess moisture (foams, alginates, etc.), maintain moisture (hydrocolloid and transparent film dressings), or provide moisture where it is lacking (hydrogels).

*Dressings That Absorb Moisture* Early in the inflammatory phase of healing, the wound tissue may be overly moist as a result of the accumulation of fluid evaporated by exposed damaged tissue, as well as blood and serous drainage. A wound that is "too wet" may result in maceration of the tissue. Exudate is the fluid composed of serum, white blood cells, and fibrin that escapes from blood vessels into the exposed wound area or the area of inflammation. A wound that exudes moderate to high levels of drainage requires an absorbent dressing (foam, alginates, carbon-impregnated, and composite dressings). These dressings offer the benefit of requiring fewer dressing changes than nonabsorbent dressings enabling undisturbed wound healing.[29]

Foam Dressings These dressings usually consist of polyurethane or other polymer material that has been "foamed" by introducing air bubbles to create tiny open pockets capable of filling with and holding fluids to remove drainage from the wound's surface. The "fluid-filled" foam dressing covers the wound to create a humid environment to further promote healing. Care must be taken not to dehydrate a wound by using a foam dressing when there is minimal exudate release. Foam dressings vary in thickness, have different absorbance capacities, and may have adhesive borders and/or waterproof coating on one side. A secondary adhesive dressing is required for those that are nonadhesive. Foam dressings are generally not indicated for deep cavities because of their nonconformational design.

Alginate Dressings These dressings are made of soft tan fibers derived from a product of brown seaweed (alginic acid) and are considered more conformable than foam dressings. The fibers are compressed in flat sheets and have a high absorbance capacity; the fibers swell and gel on exposure to fluids, creating a moist mass over the top of the wound. A secondary dressing is required to prevent alginate dressings from drying out, and most require an adhesive dressing to hold them in place.

Carbon-impregnated Dressings These dressings absorb exudates as well as wound odor.

Composite Dressings These dressings contain several functional layers, including an absorptive layer to absorb heavy wound exudate.[29]

*Dressings That Maintain Moisture* The need for dressing absorbance because of drainage decreases as healing moves to the proliferative phase with the formation of new connective tissue. Dressings that maintain natural moisture are then preferred.[29]

Hydrocolloid Dressings These dressings are generally waterproof and have minimal absorption capacity. They also contain adhesive material that covers the entire dressing surface to keep them in place and minimize the need for frequent dressing changes. Hydrocolloid dressings are available in wafer and paste forms.

Transparent Film Dressings These dressings are transparent thin sheets of polymer material that have been coated on one side with adhesive. Although these film dressings are waterproof, they are capable of allowing adequate gas exchange and maintain a moist wound environment. Transparent film dressings are often used as secondary dressings to both secure and provide a waterproof covering for other dressings.[29]

*Dressings That Provide Moisture* A dry wound that is covered with dead tissue needs to be rehydrated before optimal wound healing can occur. Providing moisture will soften and remove the dead tissue and promote autolytic debridement. This facilitates the migration of newly formed epithelial tissue to the wound bed. A wound dressing must contain water to effectively add moisture to a wound and promote healing.[29]

Amorphous Hydrogels and Hydrogel Sheets These dressings are capable of adding moisture to the wound bed and transferring water to tissues. Amorphous hydrogels are clear gels applied directly to the wound surface that release water; hydrogel sheets cover the wound and gradually release water that has been cross-linked in a polymer network to give form. The sheets also provide a cooling effect that soothes the skin and are recommended for painful or inflamed wounds.[29]

### *Pharmacologic Therapy*

#### Wound Irrigants (Normal Saline)

Wound irrigation is often necessary to clean the wound surface by removing dirt and debris. Normal saline or bottled water is sufficient for irrigation; however, mechanical removal with clean gauze is sometimes appropriate. For noninfected granular wounds, low-pressure cleansing using normal saline and a bulb or piston syringe is recommended.[30] Aerosolized normal saline (e.g., Wound Wash Saline) for wound irrigation is also commercially available.[31]

#### First-aid Antiseptics

Antiseptics are chemical substances designed for application to intact skin up to the edges of a wound, for disinfection purposes. When effective antisepsis is combined with proper wound care technique, including gentle handling of tissue, the infection rate is low. Ideally, antiseptics should exert a sustained effect against all microorganisms without causing tissue damage. However, even therapeutic concentrations of antiseptics can harm tissue. Therefore, antiseptics should be used only to disinfect intact skin after the removal of all organic matter.

Antiseptic active ingredients recognized as safe and effective for use include ethyl alcohol (48% to 95%), isopropyl alcohol (50% to 91.3%), iodine topical solution USP, iodine tincture USP, povidone-iodine complex (5% to 10%), hydrogen peroxide topical solution USP, and camphorated phenol (Tables 42-3 and 42-4).

**TABLE 42-3 Nonprescription First-aid Antiseptic Ingredients**

| Antiseptic Agents | Concentration (%) |
|---|---|
| Alcohol | 48-95 |
| Hydrogen peroxide topical solution | USP |
| Iodine tincture | USP |
| Iodine topical solution | USP |
| Isopropyl alcohol | 50.0-91.3 |
| Phenol | 0.5-1.5 |
| Povidone-iodine complex | 5-10 |

**TABLE 42-4 Selected Wound Irrigant and Antiseptic Products**

| Trade Name | Primary Ingredients |
|---|---|
| **Wound Irrigants** | |
| Wound Wash Saline Aerosol | Sodium chloride 0.9% |
| **Antiseptics** | |
| Betadine Skin Cleanser Liquid | Povidone-iodine 7.5% |
| Campho-Phenique Gel/Liquid | Camphor 10.8%; phenol 4.7% |
| Unguentine Ointment | Phenol 1% |

*Hydrogen Peroxide* Hydrogen peroxide 3% topical solution USP is a widely used antiseptic. Enzymatic release of oxygen occurs when the hydrogen peroxide comes in contact with the skin, causing an effervescent cleansing action. The duration of action is only as long as the period of active oxygen release. Hydrogen peroxide should be used where released gas can escape; therefore, it should not be used in abscesses, nor should bandages be applied before the compound dries. Using hydrogen peroxide on intact skin is of minimal value because the release of nascent oxygen is too slow, and the reliance on the effervescent quality of hydrogen peroxide to mechanically debride wounds may come at the expense of tissue toxicity. Because of the limited bactericidal effect and the risk of tissue toxicity, hydrogen peroxide has little benefit over soapy water for antisepsis.

*Ethyl Alcohol* Alcohol has good bactericidal activity in a 20% to 70% concentration. Caution must be used, however, when applying it to the intact skin surrounding the wound because direct application of alcohol to the wound bed can cause tissue irritation. Alcohol usually contains denaturants that will dehydrate the skin when applied topically at high concentrations. It is also highly flammable and must be kept away from fire or flame. Alcohol wash may be used one to three times daily, and the wound may be covered with a sterile bandage after the washed area has dried.

*Isopropyl Alcohol* Isopropyl alcohol 70% aqueous solution, which has somewhat stronger bactericidal activity and lower surface tension than ethyl alcohol, is generally used for its cleansing and antiseptic effects on intact skin. It should not be used to clean open wounds because of possible cytotoxic effects and higher reported infection rates.[32] Denaturants are not added because isopropyl alcohol itself is not potable. However, isopropyl alcohol has a greater potential for drying the skin (astringent action) because its lipid solvent effects are stronger than those of ethyl alcohol. Like ethyl alcohol, it is flammable and must be kept away from fire or flame.

*Iodine* Iodine's broad antimicrobial spectrum against bacteria, fungi, virus, spores, protozoa, and yeast is attributed to its ability to oxidize microbial protoplasm.[33] An iodine solution USP of iodine 2% and sodium iodide 2.5% is used as an antiseptic for superficial wounds. An iodine tincture USP of iodine 2%, sodium iodide 2.5, and alcohol about 50% is less preferable than the aqueous solution because it is irritating to the tissue. Strong iodine solution (Lugol's) must not be used as an antiseptic. In general, bandaging should be discouraged after iodine application to avoid tissue irritation. Iodine solutions stain skin, may be irritating to tissue, and may cause allergic sensitization in some people. Iodine products are recommended if patients have chlorhexidine allergy.[34]

*Povidone–Iodine* Povidone–iodine is a water-soluble complex of iodine with povidone. It contains 9% to 12% available iodine, which is what accounts for its rapid bactericidal activity. Reduced concentration of povidone-iodine at 0.001% (e.g., vaginal douches) has been shown to be less toxic to leukocytes than to bacteria, so this antiseptic not only reduces bacterial counts but also allows for normal immune responses that promote wound maturation.[33] Povidone–iodine is nonirritating to skin and mucous membranes.

When used as a wound irrigant, povidone–iodine is absorbed systemically; the extent of iodine absorption is related to the concentration used and the frequency of application. Final serum level also depends on the patient's intrinsic renal function. When severe burns and large wounds are treated with povidone–iodine, iodine absorption through the skin and mucous membranes can result in excess systemic iodine concentrations and cause transient thyroid dysfunction, clinical hyperthyroidism, and thyroid hyperplasia. If renal function is normal, the absorbed iodine is rapidly excreted, and signs of hyperthyroidism do not develop. However, the association between the dose of iodine administered and thyroid dysfunction remains controversial. Detergents formed by the combination of surfactants with povidone–iodine have been found to damage wound tissue and potentiate infection. Therefore, these combination products are not recommended for scrubbing wounds.[34]

*Camphorated Phenol* Oily solutions of phenol and camphor are often used as nonprescription first-aid antiseptics. Such products contain relatively high concentrations of phenol (4%) and must be used with caution. If oleaginous phenolic solutions are applied to moist areas, the phenol is partitioned out of the vehicle into water, resulting in caustic concentrations of phenol on the skin. To avoid such damaging effects, these products should be applied only to dry skin. Wounds treated with camphorated phenol should not be bandaged because the moisture would result in damage.

In summary, sterile saline is the preferred choice for effective wound irrigation. The issue of which antiseptic solution is best remains unresolved. When choosing an antiseptic product, one must consider tissue toxicity and costs of the different ingredients.

### First-aid Antibiotics

Topical nonprescription antibiotic agents (e.g., the combination of bacitracin, neomycin, and polymyxin B sulfate) help prevent infection in minor cuts, wounds, scrapes, and burns. When applied to dirty, contaminated wounds up to 4 hours after insult, topical antibiotic combinations have been demonstrated to reduce the likelihood of wound infection by (1) removing the cause of tissue breakdown (infection and inflammation), (2) preventing the development of necrotic tissue, the presence of which delays healing, (3) assisting in wound closure, and (4) fostering the healing process.[35] Topical and, in some cases, oral antibiotics are indicated in contaminated wounds that have a moderately high risk of infection. However, clean wounds have a low infection rate and do not warrant the use of prophylactic antibiotics. A primary care provider should be consulted if questions arise concerning the degree of contamination and the need for oral antibiotics.

Topical antibiotic preparations should be applied to the wound bed after cleansing and before applying a sterile dressing. Special caution should be taken when applying these preparations to large areas of denuded skin, however, because the potential for systemic toxicity can increase. Prolonged use of these agents may result in the development of resistant bacteria and secondary fungal infection. If healing does not occur within 5 days, the patient should consult a primary care provider.

First-aid antibiotics available without a prescription in the United States consist of the active ingredients (Category I): bacitracin, neomycin, and polymyxin B sulfate (Table 42-5).[36]

*Bacitracin* Bacitracin is a polypeptide bactericidal antibiotic that inhibits cell wall synthesis in several gram-positive organisms. The development of resistance in previously sensitive organisms is rare. Minimal absorption occurs with topical administration. The frequency of allergic contact dermatitis (erythema, infiltration, papules, edematous, or vesicular reaction) is approximately 2%. Topical nonprescription preparations usually contain 400 to 500 U/g of ointment and are applied one to three times a day.

*Neomycin* Neomycin is an aminoglycoside antibiotic; it exerts its bactericidal activity by irreversibly binding to the 30S ribosomal subunit to inhibit protein synthesis in

**TABLE 42-5 Selected Antibiotic Products**

| Trade Name | Primary Ingredients |
|---|---|
| Betadine Brand First Aid Antibiotics + Moisturizer Ointment | Polymyxin B sulfate 10,000 U/g; bacitracin zinc 500 U/g |
| Mycitracin Ointment | Polymyxin B sulfate 10,000 U/g; bacitracin zinc 500 U/g; neomycin sulfate 5 mg (equivalent to neomycin base 3.5 mg) |
| Mycitracin Plus Ointment | Polymyxin B sulfate 10,000 U/g; bacitracin zinc 500 U/g; neomycin sulfate (equivalent to neomycin base 3.5 mg) |
| Neosporin Ointment | Polymyxin B sulfate 5000 U/g; bacitracin zinc 400 IU/g; neomycin base 3.5 mg/g |
| Neosporin Plus Maximum Strength Cream/Ointment | Polymyxin B sulfate 10,000 U/g; neomycin base 3.5 mg/g; pramoxine HCl 10 mg |
| Polysporin Ointment/Powder | Polymyxin B sulfate 10,000 U/g; bacitracin zinc 500 IU/g |

gram-negative organisms and some species of *Staphylococcus*. Neomycin has been demonstrated to decrease the severity of clinical infection 48 hours after treatment in tape-stripped wounds.[35] Resistant organisms may develop. Neomycin applied topically produces a relatively high rate of hypersensitivity; reactions occur in 3.5% to 6% of patients. Some patients with positive results to neomycin on skin tests will also react to bacitracin. Because the two agents are not chemically related, such responses apparently represent independent sensitization rather than cross-reactions. Although neomycin is not absorbed when applied to intact skin, application to large areas of denuded skin may cause systemic toxicity (ototoxicity and nephrotoxicity).

Neomycin is available in cream and ointment forms, alone or in combination. It is most frequently used in combination with polymyxin and bacitracin to prevent the development of neomycin-resistant organisms. The association of neomycin as a common cause of allergic contact dermatitis has led some practitioners to recommend products with the combination of bacitracin and polymyxin B sulfate over those containing neomycin as a precaution.[35] However, triple-antibiotic ointment preparations containing neomycin are regularly used by consumers without significant complications. The concentration of neomycin commonly used in nonprescription products is 3.5 mg/g. Applications are made one to three times a day.

*Polymyxin B Sulfate* Polymyxin B sulfate is a polypeptide antibiotic effective against several gram-negative organisms because it alters the bacterial cell wall permeability. However, its effect on healing is unknown; it also is a rare sensitizer. Concentrations of 5000 U/g and 10,000 U/g are available in nonprescription combination preparations. Applications are usually made one to three times a day.[37]

*Tetracyclines* Tetracycline, chlortetracycline, and oxytetracycline are broad-spectrum antibiotics that exert their bacteriostatic effects by binding to the 30S ribosomal subunit to inhibit bacterial protein synthesis. Tetracycline derivatives have activity against gram-positive and most gram-negative bacteria except *Proteus* and *Pseudomonas* species.[37] Because of the high incidence of bacterial resistance, topical tetracycline and chlortetracycline are often ineffective for treating primary bacterial infection. Toxicity is rare when applied topically; however, hypersensitivity reaction may be triggered in allergic patients even by topical application. If redness, irritation, swelling, or pain persists or increases in the applied area, use of tetracycline should be discontinued. Because tetracycline products oxidize in the presence of light on human skin, they may turn the skin a reversible yellow-brown color and may stain clothing.

Currently, 3% ointments of tetracycline and chlortetracycline are available as nonprescription agents. In its monograph for nonprescription first-aid antibiotics, FDA included oxytetracycline only in combination with polymyxin B sulfate in ointment or powder form. These products are usually applied one to three times per day and may be covered with a sterile bandage afterward.

In summary, topical antibiotics are effective in eradicating bacteria and producing faster wound healing when combined with appropriate cleansing and the use of proper dressings.

### Complementary Therapies

The benefits of vitamins and complementary therapies for wound care remain questionable as little reliable scientific data exist to substantiate their enhancement of healing. Animal studies have provided some insight on the role of complementary therapies in wound healing, but more reliable human studies are needed to support such claims. Vitamins A and C are believed to enhance collagen synthesis, whereas the antioxidant properties of vitamins C and E may decrease cell destruction by oxygen free radicals. Zinc supplements used to speed wound healing may enhance cell proliferation. Honey is believed to have antibacterial properties and improve healing, and aloe vera's watery composition is thought to increase the migration of epithelial cells to improve wound healing. Practitioners should use their clinical judgment when considering recommending these agents.[38]

## Assessment of Minor Wounds: A Case-based Approach

The pharmacist should assess the type, depth, location, and degree of contamination of a wound. Visual inspection of the affected area usually provides an accurate evaluation of these factors. The wound should also be assessed for signs of infection. Because noninfectious processes, including drug-induced eruptions, could be involved, the patient's health status and current medication use should also be determined. Antimicrobial agents should generally be recommended when secondary infection is present or might occur. Cases 42-1 and 42-2 give examples of the assessment of patients with minor wounds.

### CASE 42-1

| Relevant Evaluation Criteria | Scenario/Model Outcome |
|---|---|
| **Information Gathering** | |
| 1. Gather essential information about the patient's symptoms, including: | |
| a. description of symptom(s) (i.e., nature, onset, duration, severity, associated symptoms) | Patient has an injury on his right shoulder resulting from a fall on the basketball court 12 hours earlier. Currently, the wound is about 1 1/2 in. long, and contains a small amount of dirt particles only. Mild inflammation is noted around the wound edges, and the patient reports mild pain. No oozing is noted, and the patient has a normal temperature |
| b. description of any factors that seem to precipitate, exacerbate, and/or relieve the patient's symptom(s) | Symptoms appeared after the patient sustained an injury from falling on concrete basketball court. |
| c. description of the patient's efforts to relieve the symptoms | No attempt to treat the wound has been taken. |
| 2. Gather essential patient history information: | |
| a. patient's identity | John Wellington |
| b. patient's age, sex, height, and weight | 21 y/o M, 6'1", 150 lb |
| c. patient's occupation | College student |
| d. patient's dietary habits | Vegetarian |
| e. patient's sleep habits | Stays up late but manages to get about 5 hours of sleep most nights |
| f. concurrent medical conditions, prescription and nonprescription medications, and dietary supplements | None |
| g. allergies | NKA |
| h. history of other adverse reactions to medications | None |
| i. other (describe)_______ | None |
| **Assessment and Triage** | |
| 3. Differentiate the patient's signs/symptoms and correctly identify the patient's primary problem(s) (see Figure 42-5). | Wound appears to be a mild abrasion with injury to the epidermal portion of the skin and slight extension to the uppermost portion of the dermis. No puncture or multilayer skin involvement noted. |
| 4. Identify exclusions for self-treatment (see Figure 42-3). | None |
| 5. Formulate a comprehensive list of therapeutic alternatives for the primary problem to determine if triage to a medical practitioner is required, and share this information with the patient. | Options include:<br>(1) Recommend self-care management (wound irrigant, antiseptic, antibiotic, and wound dressing).<br>(2) Refer John to his PCP.<br>(3) Recommend self-care management until John's PCP can be contacted.<br>(4) Take no action. |

## CASE 42-1 (continued)

| Relevant Evaluation Criteria | Scenario/Model Outcome |
|---|---|
| **Plan** | |
| 6. Select an optimal therapeutic alternative to address the patient's problem, taking into account patient preferences. | The patient prefers to self-treat the wound with normal saline, an antibiotic, and wound dressing. |
| 7. Describe the recommended therapeutic approach to the patient. | Irrigate the wound with normal saline to remove dirt and debris and apply a topical antibiotic such as Neosporin (see Table 42-5). Cover with a transparent film dressing such as ACU-derm to maintain moisture (see Table 42-2). If frequent dressing changes are required because of excessive fluid release, a more absorbent dressing (i.e., Johnson & Johnson First Aid Brand Advanced Healing Pads) may be necessary. |
| 8. Explain to the patient the rationale for selecting the recommended therapeutic approach from the considered therapeutic alternatives. | Seeking a PCP, that is, primary care provider, may not be necessary if you keep the wound covered and continue to apply a topical antibiotic to prevent infection. |
| **Patient Education** | |
| 9. When recommending self-care with nonprescription medications and/or nondrug therapy, convey accurate information to the patient, including: | |
| a. appropriate dose and frequency of administration | See the box Patient Education for Acute Wounds. |
| b. maximum number of days the therapy should be employed | See the box Patient Education for Acute Wounds. |
| c. product administration procedures | See the box Patient Education for Acute Wounds. |
| d. expected time to onset of relief | See the box Patient Education for Acute Wounds. |
| e. degree of relief that can be reasonably expected | Complete closure of wound without infection. |
| f. most common side effects | See the box Patient Education for Acute Wounds. |
| g. side effects that warrant medical intervention should they occur | See the box Patient Education for Acute Wounds. |
| h. patient options in the event that condition worsens or persists | A PCP should be consulted if the condition does not improve after 5-7 days or if increased pain or pus at the site develops. |
| i. product storage requirements | See the box Patient Education for Acute Wounds. |
| j. specific nondrug measures | See the box Patient Education for Acute Wounds. |
| 10. Solicit follow-up questions from patient. | Wouldn't it be better to leave the wound uncovered and let it dry out? |
| 11. Answer patient's questions. | No. Providing a moist environment with the use of an appropriate dressing provides a more optimal wound-healing environment. |

Key: NKA, no known allergies; PCP, primary care provider.

## CASE 42-2

| Relevant Evaluation Criteria | Scenario/Model Outcome |
|---|---|
| **Information Gathering** | |
| 1. Gather essential information about the patient's symptoms, including: | |

## CASE 42-2 (continued)

| Relevant Evaluation Criteria | Scenario/Model Outcome |
|---|---|
| a. description of symptom(s) (i.e., nature, onset, duration, severity, associated symptoms) | Patient has an ulcer on left heel that he first noticed 3 weeks ago. He has been keeping it covered with a piece of gauze, but it seems to have gotten worse. The wound bed is red, with a slightly yellowish exudates. The margins appear red and inflamed. |
| b. description of any factors that seem to precipitate, exacerbate, and/or relieve the patient's symptom(s) | Walking has become difficult as it causes more pain at the ulcer site. It has also become difficult to wear regular shoes because of friction rubbing against the ulcer. |
| c. description of the patient's efforts to relieve the symptoms | No relief has been noticed despite keeping the wound covered with gauze. |
| 2. Gather essential patient history information: | |
| a. patient's identity | Benjamin Harper |
| b. patient's age, sex, weight, and height | 69 y/o M, 5'6", 150 lb |
| c. patient's occupation | Retired |
| d. patient's dietary habits | Balanced diet; likes sweets |
| e. patient's sleep habits | Averages 8 hours per night |
| f. concurrent medical conditions, prescription and nonprescription medications, and dietary supplements | HCTZ 25 mg once daily, atenolol 50 mg once daily, metformin 500 mg 2 times/day |
| g. allergies | NKA |
| h. history of other adverse reactions to medications | None |
| i. other (describe)_______ | None |
| **Assessment and Triage** | |
| 3. Differentiate the patient's signs/symptoms and correctly identify the patient's primary problem(s). | Wound appears to be a pressure ulcer classified as stage II with partial-thickness skin loss involving all of the epidermis and part of the dermis. The yellowish oozing exudates and significant pain suggest possible injection. |
| 4. Identify exclusions for self-treatment (see Figure 42-3). | Onset well after 7 days and antidiabetic medication use |
| 5. Formulate a comprehensive list of therapeutic alternatives for the primary problem to determine if triage to a medical practitioner is required, and share this information with the patient. | Options include:<br>(1) Refer Benjamin to a PCP or podiatrist for wound care.<br>(2) Recommend Benjamin use an alginate wound dressing such as Sorbsan while waiting to see his PCP.<br>(3) Take no action. |
| **Plan** | |
| 6. Select an optimal therapeutic alternative to address the patient's problem, taking into account patient preferences. | Refer the patient to a PCP or podiatrist for a differential diagnosis. |
| 7. Describe the recommended therapeutic approach to the patient. | Use appropriate wound dressing while waiting to see your PCP, that is, primary care provider. |
| 8. Explain to the patient the rationale for selecting the recommended therapeutic approach from the considered therapeutic alternatives. | Seeing a PCP or dermatologist because pressure ulcers require closely supervised medical management. |

## CASE 42-2 (continued)

| Relevant Evaluation Criteria | Scenario/Model Outcome |
|---|---|
| **Patient Education** | |
| 9. When recommending self-care with nonprescription medications and/or nondrug therapy, convey accurate information to the patient. | Criterion does not apply in this case. |
| 10. Solicit follow-up questions from patient. | Is there an OTC medication that might work? |
| 11. Answer patient's questions. | No OTC medications are appropriate without medical supervision. You may require a prescription medication for more appropriate wound treatment. |

Key: HCTZ, hydrochlorothiazide; N/A, not applicable; NKA, no known allergies; OTC, over-the-counter; PCP, primary care provider.

## PATIENT EDUCATION FOR ACUTE WOUNDS

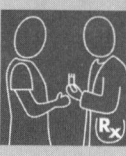


The objective of self-treatment is to promote healing by protecting the wound from infection or further trauma. For most patients, carefully following product instructions and the self-care measures listed here will help ensure optimal therapeutic outcomes.

- Position the wound above the level of the heart to slow bleeding and relieve throbbing pain.
- If the wound is dirty, irrigate it with normal saline solution, which is not toxic to cells. Use antiseptic solutions selectively and cautiously. Any inflammation should subside within 12 to 24 hours.
- When cleansing with soapy water, wash hands, apply mild liquid soap (e.g., Dove soap) to a wet cotton ball, and gently wash the wound area; rinse under running warm water and gently pat the area dry.
- Cover the wound with a dressing that will keep the wound site moist. Make sure the dressing is the appropriate size and contour for the affected body part.
- Continue using a wound dressing until the wound bed has firmly closed and signs of inflammation in surrounding tissue have subsided. This usually takes 2 to 3 weeks. Failure to keep the wound covered may delay healing.
- Avoid disrupting the dressing unnecessarily; change it only if it is dirty or is not intact. Most dressings should be changed every 3 to 5 days. Frequent changes may remove resurfacing layers of epithelium and slow the healing process. Change dressing if excessive fluid is released.
- Use a mild analgesic to control pain.
- All wound dressings should be kept in their original packaging and stored away from moisture.
- Observe the wound for signs of infection. Redness, swelling, and exudate are a normal part of healing; foul odor is not.

⚠ Consult a primary care provider if infection is suspected or the wound does not show signs of healing after 5 days of self-treatment.

### Patient Counseling for Minor Wounds

Assess the wound type, remembering that minor cuts and abrasions may be self-treated, while more severe acute and chronic wounds or those that appear infected should first be evaluated by a primary care provider (see Classification of Wounds and Figure 42-3). Irrigation with soapy water or normal saline is generally recommended if a wound is dirty. Patients should be instructed to change the dressing only when it is dirty or not intact. The practitioner should ensure that the patient understands the basic steps in wound care, especially the selection of appropriate wound dressings. An explanation of basic skin physiology and the wound-healing process will enhance patient compliance. The box Patient Education for Acute Wounds lists specific information to provide patients. The patient should consult a primary care provider if the wound does not show signs of healing after 5 days of self-treatment.

### Evaluation of Patient Outcomes for Minor Wounds

The practitioner should check the patient's progress after 5 days. Visual inspection, if possible, is the best method of assessing the healing process; therefore, a scheduled visit to see the practitioner is preferable. If the wound shows no signs of healing or has worsened (i.e., foul odor, worsened inflammation, etc.), the patient should see a primary care provider for more aggressive therapy.

## Key Points for Minor Wounds

- Self-treatment of minor acute wounds is appropriate.
- First-aid antibiotics are used to prevent infection.
- Moist wound healing is now considered the standard of care.
- Proper selection of first-aid products, including appropriate wound dressing, is key.

## References


1. Lait ME, Smith LN. Wound management: a literature review. *J Clin Nurs.* 1998;7:11-7.
2. *F-D-C-Reports—The Tan Sheet.* 2001;9(6):12.
3. Hollander JE, Singer AJ. Laceration management. *Ann Emerg Med.* 1999;34:356-67.
4. Cho CY, Lo JS. Dressing the part. *Dermatol Clin.* 1998; 16:25-47.
5. Hunt TK. Hopf H, Hussain Z. Physiology of wound healing. *Adv Skin Wound Care.* 2000;13(suppl 2):6-11.
6. Chen WY, Rogers AA, Hutchinson JJ, et al. Further characterization of biological properties of wound fluids' mitogenic and chemotactic properties. *J Investig Dermatol.* 1999;96:566.
7. Stotts NA, Wipke-Tevis D. Co-factors in impaired healing. In: Krasner D, Kane D, eds. *Chronic Wound Care: A Clinical Source Book for Healthcare Professionals.* 2nd ed. Wayne, Pa: Health Management Publications, Inc; 1997:64-72.
8. Dabrowski GP, Rombeau JL. Practical nutritional management in the trauma intensive care unit. *Surg Clin North Am.* 2000;8:921-32.
9. Green S, McLaren S. Nutrition and wound healing. *Community Nurse.* 1998;4:29-32.
10. Partridge C. Influential factors in surgical wound healing. *J Wound Care.* 1998;7:350-3.
11. Lenhardt R, Hopf HW, Marker E, et al. Perioperative collagen deposition in elderly and young men and women. *Arch Surg.* 2000;135:71-4.
12. Wilson JA, Clark JJ. Obesity: impediment to wound healing. *Crit Care Nurs Q.* April-June 2003;26:119-32.
13. Parker L. Applying the principles of infection control to wound care. *Br J Nurs.* 2000;9:394-6,398,400.
14. Silhi N. Diabetes and wound healing. *J Wound Care.* 1998; 7:47-51.
15. Phillips SJ. Physiology of wound healing and surgical wound care. *ASAIO J.* 2000:46(suppl 6): S2-5.
16. Pearson AS, Wolford RW. Management of skin trauma. *Dermatology.* 2000;27:475-91.
17. Life Sciences Education and Health Literacy. Understanding your body: what are pressure ulcers? August 2000. Agency for Healthcare Research and Quality, Rockville, Md. Available at http://www.ahrq.gov/consumer/bodysys/edbody6.htm. Accessed July 10, 2005.
18. Geriatric Medicine Community Internal Medicine Division, Mayo Clinic Rochester. Pressure ulcers: prevention and management. 2001. Available at: http://www.mayo. edu/geriatrics-rst/PU.html. Accessed July 10, 2005.
19. Richardson J, Prentice D, Rivers S. Clinical management extra: skin care pathway. Developing an interdisciplinary evidence-based skin care pathway for long term care. *Adv Skin Wound Care.* 2001;14:197-205.
20. Millington J, Thomas MD, Norris TW. Effective treatment strategies for diabetic foot wounds. *J Fam Pract.* 2000; 49(suppl 1): S40-8.
21. Ruckley CV. Caring for patients with chronic leg ulcer. *BMJ.* 1998; 316:407-8.
22. Wiechula R. The use of moist healing dressings in the management of split-thickness skin graft donor sites: a systemic review. *Int J Nurs Pract.* April 2003;9(suppl 2):S9-17.
23. Mionelli GT, Lawrence WT. *Surg Clin North Am.* 2003;83:617.
24. Jeter KF, Tintle TE. Wound dressings of the nineties: indications and contraindications. *Clin Podiatr Med Surg.* 1991;8:799-816.
25. *F-D-C-Reports—The Gray Sheet.* 2001;27(12):22.
26. *F-D-C-Reports—The Tan Sheet.* 2001;27(23):25.
27. Quinn JV, Wells G, Sutcliffe T, et al. Tissue adhesive versus suture wound repair at 1 year: randomized clinical trial correlating early, 3-month, and 1-year cosmetic outcome. *Ann Emerg Med.* 1998;32:645-9.
28. Osmond MH. Pediatric wound management: the role of tissue adhesives. *Pediatr Emerg Care.* 1999;15:137-40.
29. Ovington LG. The well-dressed wound: an overview of dressing types. *Wounds.* Jan/Feb 1998:10(suppl A):1A-11A.
30. Pontieri-Lewis. Principles for selecting the right wound dressing. *Medsurg Nurs.* 1999;8:267-70.
31. Newton GD, Pray WS, Popovich NS. New OTC drugs and devices 2000: a selective review. *J Am Pharm Assoc.* 2001;41: 273-82.
32. Harkavy KL. A topical topic: toxicity of antiseptics? *J Pediatr.* 1998; 133:309-10.
33. Mimoz O, Karim A, Mercat A, et. al. Chlorhexidine compared with povidone-iodine as skin preparation before blood culture: a randomized, controlled trial. *Ann Intern Med.* December 7, 1999;131:834-7.
34. Gouin S, Patel H. Office management of minor wounds. *Can Fam Physician.* 2001;47:769-74.
35. Bolton L, Fattu AJ. Topical agents and wound healing. *Clin Dermatol.* 1994;22:95-120.
36. *Federal Register.* 1996;61:58471.
37. Sanford JP. *Guide to Antimicrobial Therapy.* Dallas: Antimicrobial Therapy; 2001.
38. MacKay D, Miller AL. Nutritional Support for Wound Healing. *Altern Med Rev* 2003;8: 359-77.

CHAPTER 43

# Fungal Skin Infections

Gail D. Newton and Nicholas G. Popovich

Fungal skin infections, or dermatomycoses, are among the most common cutaneous disorders.[1] They are often referred to as ringworm because their characteristic lesions are ring-shaped with clear centers and red, scaly borders. However, these lesions can vary from the ring form and may present as single or multiple lesions ranging from mild scaling to deep granulomas (inflamed, nodular-size lesions).

Fungal infections are usually superficial and can involve the hair, nails, and skin. The term *tinea* refers exclusively to dermatophyte infections. Most often, tinea infections are named on the basis of the area of the body that is affected (i.e., scalp [tinea capitis], groin [tinea cruris), body [tinea corporis), feet [tinea pedis), and nails [tinea unguium]). They are generally caused by three genera of fungi: *Trichophyton*, *Microsporum*, and *Epidermophyton*. Species of *Candida* and other yeasts may also be involved.[2] However, currently available nonprescription antifungals are not indicated for self-management of cutaneous infections secondary to the latter microorganisms.[3]

## Epidemiology of Fungal Skin Infections

Although many pathogenic fungi exist in the environment, the overall prevalence of actual superficial fungal infections is remarkably low. An estimated 10% to 20% of the U.S. population suffer from a tinea infection at any one time.[4,5] Many degrees of susceptibility, from instantaneous "takes" by a single spore to severe trauma with massive exposure, produce a clinical infection. It appears, however, that trauma to the skin, especially that which produces blisters (e.g., from wearing ill-fitting footwear), may be significantly more important to the occurrence of human fungal infections than is simple exposure to the offending pathogens.[5] Other predisposing factors for the development of tinea infections include diabetes mellitus and other debilitating diseases associated with immune system depression, use of immunosuppressive drugs, impaired circulation, poor nutrition and hygiene, trauma, occlusion of the skin, and warm, humid climates.[5,6]

The most prevalent cutaneous fungal infection in humans is tinea pedis (dermatophytosis of the foot, or athlete's foot). Tinea pedis afflicts approximately 26.5 million people in the United States every year—of every 10 sufferers, 7 are male. Tinea pedis is rare among blacks but common in whites, particularly those who live in urban tropical areas.[7] An estimated 70% of people will be afflicted with athlete's foot in their lifetime and that approximately 45% will suffer with it episodically for more than 10 years. When exposure to infectious environments is equal, the incidence of tinea infections in women approaches that in men.[4,5,8,9] Although tinea pedis may occur at all ages, it is more common in adults, presumably because of their increased opportunities for exposure to pathogens.[5]

Individuals who use public pools or bathing facilities are at greater risk for the development of tinea pedis than the general population. However, tinea pedis may be acquired in the home if one or more members of the household are already infected. High-impact sports, such as long-distance running, that cause chronic trauma to the feet also predispose athletes to tinea pedis.[10-12] This trauma affords infecting fungi the opportunity to invade the outer layers of the skin. The problem is exacerbated because these individuals wear socks and shoes that impede the dispersion of heat and the evaporation of moisture, both of which facilitate fungal growth. In contrast, individuals who most often wear footwear that allows the feet to remain cool and dry (e.g., sandals) are less likely to develop tinea pedis.

Tinea unguium, also called ringworm of the nails or onychomycosis, is sometimes associated with tinea pedis. More than 2.5 million Americans are treated annually for tinea unguium. However, because many cases go untreated, the actual incidence of this infection is probably much higher.[13] Onychomycosis cannot be managed with topical nonprescription antifungals. Rather, the affected nail must be treated with systemic drug therapy (e.g., terbinafine or itraconazole) or removed surgically to rid the area of the offending fungus.

The next two most common infections are tinea corporis and tinea cruris. Tinea corporis, also called ringworm of the body, is most common in prepubescent individuals. It is frequently transmitted among children in day care centers. However, it is also more common in adults and children who live in hot, humid climates. Individuals who are under stress or overweight are also at increased risk for the development of tinea corporis.[14,15]

Tinea cruris, or jock itch, is most common during warm weather but can occur at any time of the year when the skin in the groin area is kept warm and moist for long periods of time. For example, sweating or prolonged contact with wet clothing provides an ideal environment for the growth of fungi. Tinea cruris occurs more often in men than in women and rarely affects children. Several reasons exist for more frequent infections in males than females: (1) males wear more occlusive clothing, (2) scrotal skin may increase occlusion of the groin area, (3) men generally are more active than women, and (4) men have a greater incidence of other tinea infections that may serve as a reservoir for generating new cases of tinea cruris.[14] Close indirect or direct physical contact between infected males and noninfected females does not negate the increased prevalence of tinea cruris in males.[5] For example, females who live in the same household with infected males do not develop infections at the same rate as noninfected males in the same household.

Although the true incidence is unknown, tinea capitis, or ringworm of the scalp, occurs most often in children because children are more likely to have contact with infected individuals and because they are less attentive to personal hygiene than are adults. Black female children are infected more often than black males and white children, possibly because of the hair care products and practices (e.g., occlusive hair dressings, tight braiding) that are unique to this population.[5,14]

Tinea capitis can be spread by direct contact with an infected person but is often spread by contact with infected fomites (e.g., using infected combs, hats, toys or telephones; wearing infected clothing; using infected towels; or sleeping on infected linens). In some instances, tinea capitis is spread through contact with other infected individuals or with infected cats or dogs.[16]

## Etiology of Fungal Skin Infections

Tinea infections are caused by three genera of pathogenic fungi: *Trichophyton, Microsporum,* and *Epidermophyton.* Tinea pedis and tinea cruris are caused by species of *Epidermophyton* and *Trichophyton.* Species of *Trichophyton* and *Microsporum* cause ringworm of the scalp. All species of the three genera can cause tinea corporis.[5] Fungal transmission can occur through contact with infected people, animals, soil, or fomites. Dermatophytes are classified on the basis of their habitat: anthropophilic (humans), zoophilic (animals), and geophilic (soil). Most tinea infections are caused by person-to-person contact with individuals infected with anthropophilic dermatophytes.[14]

In addition to specific fungi, other environmental factors contribute to the disease's development, such as climate and social customs. Footwear is a key variable, as illustrated by the incidence of tinea pedis in any population that wears occlusive footwear, especially in the summer and in tropical or subtropical climates. Nonporous shoe material increases temperature and hydration of the skin, which interferes with the barrier function of the stratum corneum. Similarly, sweating or wearing wet clothing for long periods of time can predispose individuals to the development of tinea corporis and tinea cruris.

Chronic health problems and medications that weaken or suppress the immune system can also increase the risk for development of tinea infections. For example, patients with diabetes and persons of advanced age taking medications such as glucocorticoids should be instructed to monitor themselves for the signs and symptoms of tinea infections. They should also be instructed about the importance of proper hygiene and diet for the prevention of tinea infections as well as other health problems.

## Pathophysiology of Fungal Skin Infections

After inoculation of a dermatophyte into the skin under suitable conditions, a tinea infection progresses through several stages. These stages include periods of incubation and then enlargement, followed by a refractory period and a stage of involution.

During the incubation period, the dermatophyte grows in the stratum corneum, sometimes with minimal signs of infection. After the incubation period and once the infection is established, two factors appear to play a role in determining the size and duration of the lesions: the growth rate of the organism and the epidermal turnover rate.[17] The fungal growth rate must equal or exceed the epidermal turnover rate, or the organism will be quickly shed.

Dermatophytid infestations remain within the stratum corneum. This resistance to the spread of infection seems to involve both immunologic and nonimmunologic mechanisms. For example, the presence of a serum inhibitory factor (SIF) appears to limit the growth of dermatophytes beyond the stratum corneum. SIF is not an antibody but a dialyzable, heat-labile component of fresh sera. It appears that SIF chelates the iron that dermatophytes need for continued growth.[17] Once in the stratum corneum, dermatophytes produce keratinases and other proteolytic enzymes that cause allergic reactions when they reach living epidermis.[5]

The major immunologic defense against fungal skin infections is the type IV delayed-hypersensitivity response. The refractory period precedes complete development of this cell-mediated immunity. The fungal growth rate typically exceeds epidermal turnover, and inflammation and pruritus are at their peak. After development of an adequate immune response, symptoms of superficial fungal infections diminish, and the infection may clear spontaneously during the involution period. Patients with chronic infections typically present with much less inflammation. This presentation may be due to a suppressed hypersensitivity response, which in turn reduces the inflammatory response.[2]

## Signs and Symptoms of Fungal Skin Infections

The clinical spectrum of tinea infections ranges from mild itching and scaling to a severe, exudative inflammatory process characterized by denudation, fissuring, crusting, and/or discoloration of the affected skin. Atopic individuals (i.e., those experiencing their first tinea infection) and patients with infections secondary to zoophilic fungi tend to present with greater inflammation.[14] Table 43-1 summarizes key differences between fungal skin infections and contact dermatitis.

### *Tinea Pedis*

Clinically, there are four accepted variants of tinea pedis; two or more of these types may overlap. The most common is the chronic, intertriginous type,[5] characterized by fissuring, scaling, or maceration in the interdigital spaces, malodor, pruritus, and/or a stinging sensation on the feet (see

**TABLE 43-1 Differentiation of Fungal Skin Infections and Skin Disorders With Similar Presentation**

| Criterion | Fungal Skin Infections | Contact Dermatitis | Bacterial Skin Infection |
|---|---|---|---|
| Location | On areas of the body where excess moisture accumulates such as the feet, groin area, scalp, and under the arms | Any area of the body exposed to the allergen/irritant; hands, face, legs, ears, eyes, anogenital area involved most often | Anywhere on the body |
| Signs | Presents either as soggy malodorous, thickened skin; acute vesicular rash; or fine scaling of affected area with varying degrees of inflammation; cracks and fissures may also be present | Presents as a variety of lesions from raised wheals to fluid filled vesicles or both | Presents as a variety of lesions from macules to pustules to ulcers with redness surrounding the lesion, which often are warmer than surrounding, unaffected skin |
| Symptoms | Itching and pain | Itching and pain | Irritation and pain |
| Quantity/severity | Usually localized to one region of the body but can spread | Affects all areas of exposed skin but does not spread | Usually localized to one region of the body but can spread |
| Timing | Variable onset | Variable onset from immediately after exposure to 3 weeks after contact | Variable onset |
| Cause | Superficial fungal infection | Exposure to skin irritants or allergens | Superficial bacterial infection |
| Modifying factors | Treated with OTC astringents, antifungals, and nondrug measures to keep the area clean and dry | Treated with topical antipruritics, skin protectants, astringents and nondrug measures to avoid reexposure | Treated with prescription antibiotics |

Color Plates, photograph 29). Typically, the infection involves the lateral toe webs, usually between the fourth and fifth or third and fourth toes. From these sites, the infection may spread to the sole or instep of the foot but rarely to the dorsum. Warmth and humidity aggravate this condition; consequently, hyperhidrosis (excessive sweating) becomes an underlying problem and must be treated along with the dermatophyte infestation.[5]

Normal resident aerobic diphtheroids may become involved in the athlete's foot process. After initial invasion of the stratum corneum by dermatophytes, enough moisture may accumulate to trigger a bacterial overgrowth. Increased moisture and temperature then lead to the release of metabolic products, which diffuse easily through the underlying horny layer already damaged by fungal invasion. In more severe cases, gram-negative organisms intrude and may exacerbate the condition, causing skin maceration, white hyperkeratosis, or erosions with increased patient symptomatology.[5]

The second variant of athlete's foot is known as the chronic, papulosquamous pattern.[5] It is usually found on both feet and is characterized by mild inflammation and diffuse, moccasinlike scaling on the soles of the feet. Tinea unguium (i.e., ringworm of the nails, or onychomycosis) of one or more toenails may also be present and may continue to fuel the infection. The toenails must first be cured with oral drug therapy, such as itraconazole, ketoconazole, or terbinafine, or must be removed surgically to rid the area of the offending fungus.

The third variant of tinea pedis is the vesicular type, usually caused by *T. mentagrophytes* var. *interdigitale*.[5] Small vesicles or vesicopustules are observed near the instep and on the mid-anterior plantar surface. Skin scaling is seen on these areas as well as on the toe webs. This variant is symptomatic in the summer and is clinically quiescent during the cooler months.

The acute ulcerative type is the fourth variant of tinea pedis. It is often associated with macerated, denuded, weeping ulcerations on the sole of the foot. Typically, white hyperkeratosis and a pungent odor are present. This type of infection, which is complicated by an overgrowth of opportunistic, gram-negative bacteria such as *Proteus* and *Pseudomonas*, has been called dermatophytosis complex, and it may produce an extremely painful, erosive, purulent interspace that can impede the patient's ability to walk.[5]

### *Tinea Unguium*

Nails affected by tinea unguium gradually loose their normal, shiny luster and become opaque. If left untreated, the nails become thick, rough, yellow, opaque, and friable. The nail may separate from the nail bed if the infection progresses secondarily to subungual hyperkeratosis. Ultimately, the nail may be lost altogether. Subungual debris also provides an excellent medium for the growth of opportunistic bacteria and other microorganisms, which can lead to further, infectious complications.[5]

### Tinea Corporis

Tinea corporis may have a diverse clinical presentation. Most often, the lesions, which involve glabrous (smooth and bare) skin, begin as small, circular, erythematous, scaly areas. They spread peripherally, and the borders may contain vesicles or pustules. Infected individuals may also complain of pruritus.[18]

Tinea corporis can occur on any part of the body. However, the location of the infection can provide clues to the type of infecting dermatophyte. For example, zoophilic dermatophytes often infect areas of exposed skin such as the neck, face, and arms. In contrast, infections secondary to anthropophilic dermatophytes often occur in occluded areas or in areas of trauma.[5]

### Tinea Cruris

Tinea cruris occurs on the medial and upper parts of the thighs and the pubic area and is more common in males. The lesions have well-demarcated margins that are elevated slightly and are more erythematous than the central area; small vesicles may be seen, especially at the margins. Acute lesions are bright red, and chronic cases tend to have more of a hyperpigmented appearance; fine scaling is usually present. This condition is generally bilateral with significant pruritus; however, the lesions usually spare the penis and scrotum. This can help to distinguish this infection from candidiasis, which does cause lesions in these areas.[19] Pain may also be present during periods of sweating or when the skin becomes macerated or infected by a secondary microorganism.[4,5]

### Tinea Capitis

Clinically, tinea capitis may present as one of four variant patterns, depending on the causative dermatophyte. In noninflammatory tinea capitis, lesions begin as small papules surrounding individual hair shafts. Subsequently the lesions spread centrifugally to involve all hairs in their path. Although there is some scaling of the scalp, little inflammation is present (see Color Plates, photograph 30). Hairs in the lesions are a dull gray color (because they are coated with arthrospores) and usually break off above scalp level.[5]

The inflammatory type of tinea capitis produces a spectrum of inflammation, ranging from pustules to kerion formation. Kerions are weeping lesions whose exudate forms thick crusts on the scalp.[8] Individuals with this type of tinea capitis also may complain more about pruritus in addition to fever and pain. Regional lymph nodes may also be enlarged.[5]

The black dot variety of tinea capitis was named for the appearance of infected areas of the scalp. The location of arthrospores on the hair shaft causes hairs to break off at the level of the scalp, leaving black dots on the scalp surface. Hair loss, inflammation, and scaling with this type of tinea capitis range from minimal to extensive. Thus, this variant is especially challenging to diagnose.[5,20,21]

The favus variant of tinea capitis typically presents as patchy areas of hair loss and yellowish crusts and scales known as scutula. Ultimately, these lesions can coalesce to involve a major portion of the scalp. If left untreated, this condition can lead to scalp atrophy, scarring, and permanent hair loss.[5]

## Complications of Fungal Skin Infections

Complications ranging from secondary infections to permanent hair loss or scarring may occur if tinea infections are not effectively treated.

## Treatment of Fungal Skin Infections

### Treatment Goals

The goals in treating fungal skin infections are to (1) provide symptomatic relief, (2) eradicate existing infection, and (3) prevent future infections.

### General Treatment Approach

In many instances, patients can self-treat effectively tinea pedis, tinea corporis, and tinea cruris with nonprescription topical antifungals and nonpharmacologic measures. However, individuals with tinea unguium or tinea capitis should be referred to a primary care provider for treatment. Patients who want to improve the appearance of the nail during prescription treatment can use Fungal Nail Revitalizer to reduce nail discoloration and to smooth out the thick, rough nail. This product contains calcium carbonate (a strong alkali) and urea (a protein denaturant) to debride nail tissue. The patient should apply the cream over the entire surface of the infected nail, scrub this area for at least 1 minute with the provided nailbrush, and then wash and dry the nail completely. For optimum results, this procedure should be performed daily for 3 weeks.

Before recommending therapy, the practitioner must be reasonably sure that the lesions are consistent with a tinea infection. Their appearance should conform to the descriptions provided in Signs and Symptoms of Fungal Skin Infections, and the color plates of the tinea lesions should be consulted for comparison. Further, the lesions should not resemble any other skin conditions covered in this text. When in doubt about the true cause of a condition, the patient should be advised to consult a primary care provider or dermatologist. Figure 43-1 outlines the appropriate self-treatment options for fungal skin infections as well as exclusions for self-treatment.

A number of topical antifungals are available in a variety of dosage forms for self-treatment of fungal skin infections. The selection of a particular product depends on the type of infection and on individual patient characteristics and preferences. For example, in acute, inflammatory tinea pedis, characterized by reddened, oozing, and vesicular eruptions, the inflammation must be counteracted with solutions of astringent aluminum salts before antifungal therapy can be instituted.

A critical determinant of the outcome of therapy is the patient's ability to comply with the recommended therapy for the appropriate length of time. Compliance may be difficult because these conditions may take between 2 and 4 weeks to resolve. Patients may be tempted to terminate

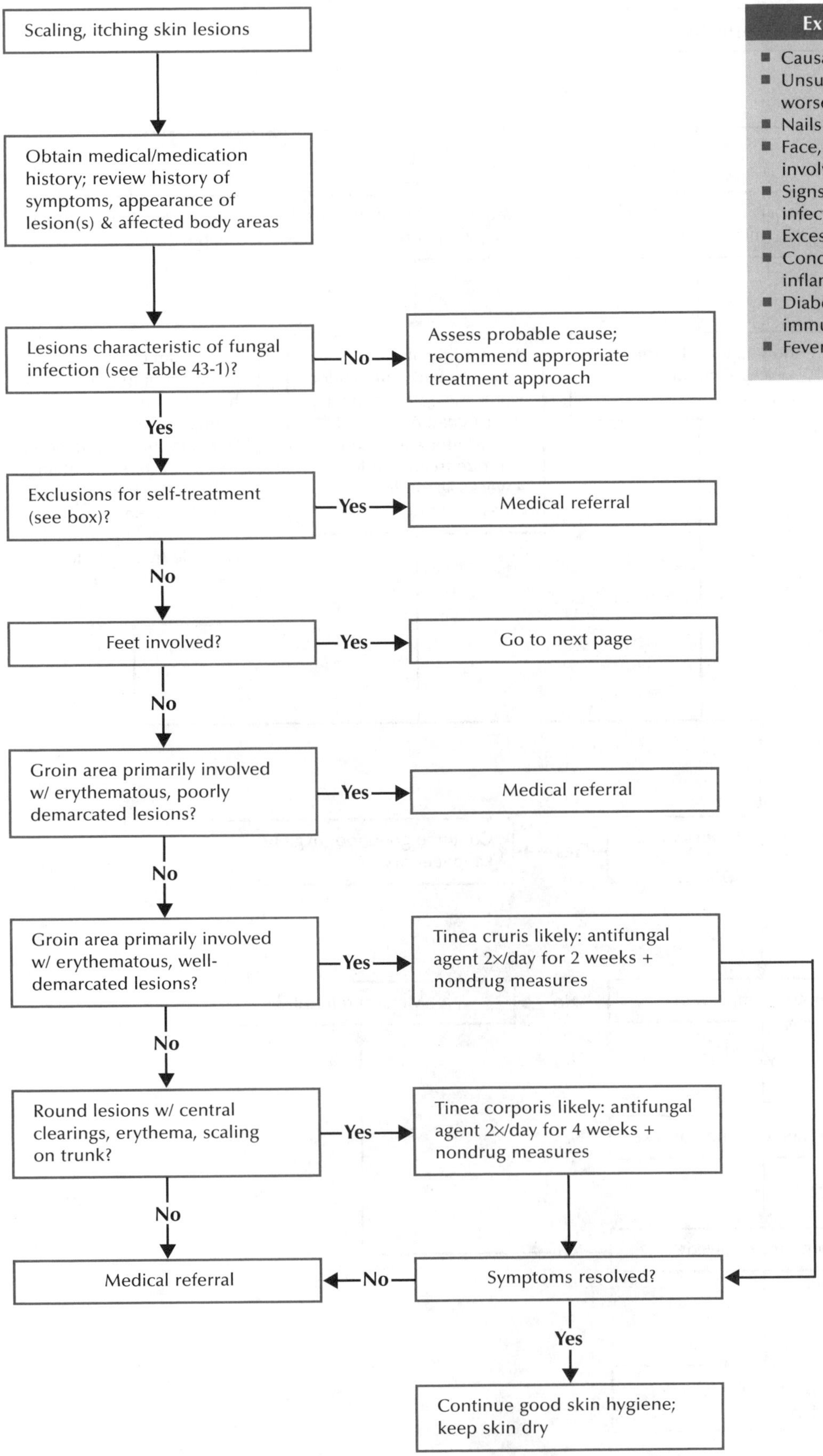

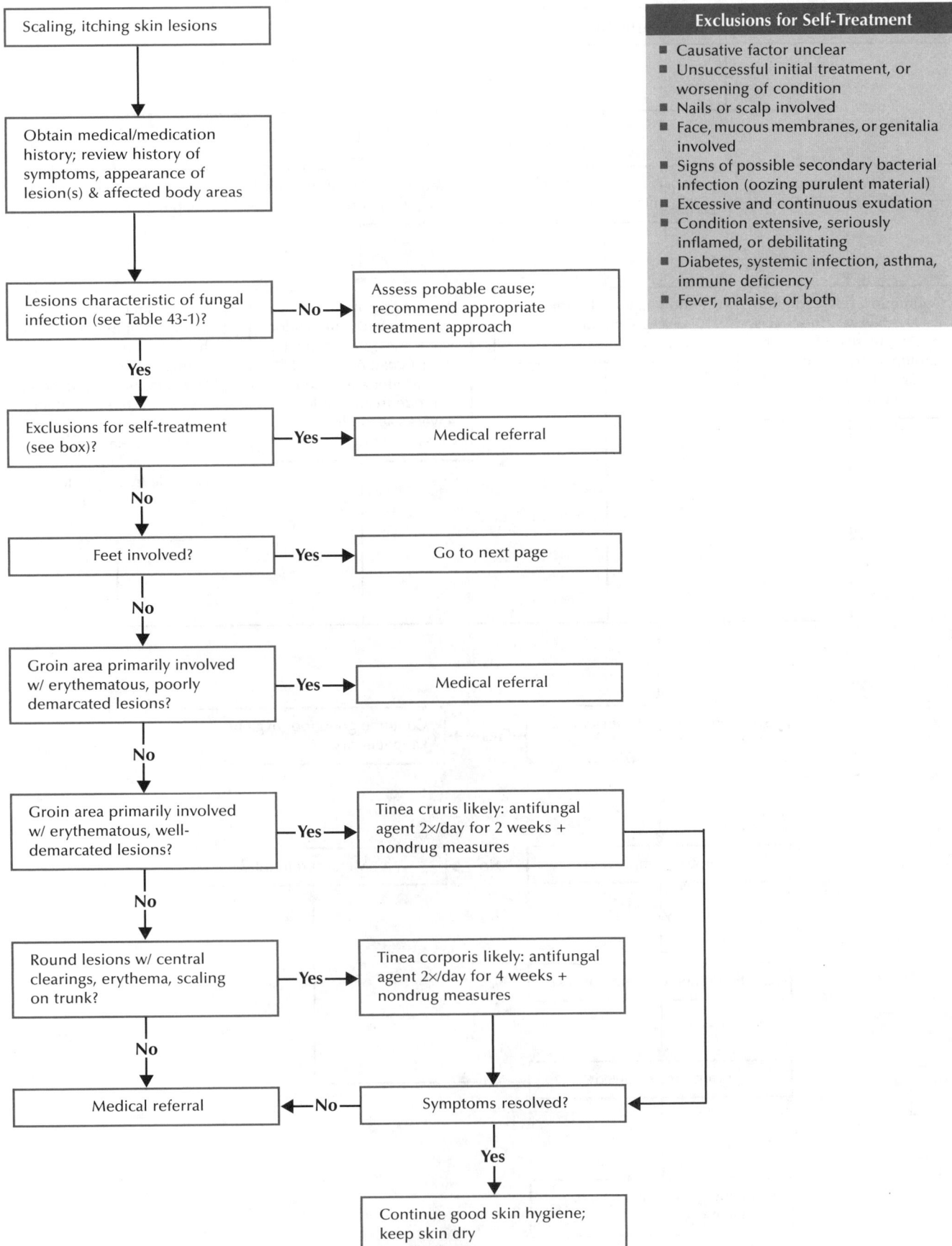

FIGURE 43-1 Self-care of fungal skin infections.

### Exclusions for Self-Treatment

- Causative factor unclear
- Unsuccessful initial treatment, or worsening of condition
- Nails or scalp involved
- Face, mucous membranes, or genitalia involved
- Signs of possible secondary bacterial infection (oozing purulent material)
- Excessive and continuous exudation
- Condition extensive, seriously inflamed, or debilitating
- Diabetes, systemic infection, asthma, immune deficiency
- Fever, malaise, or both

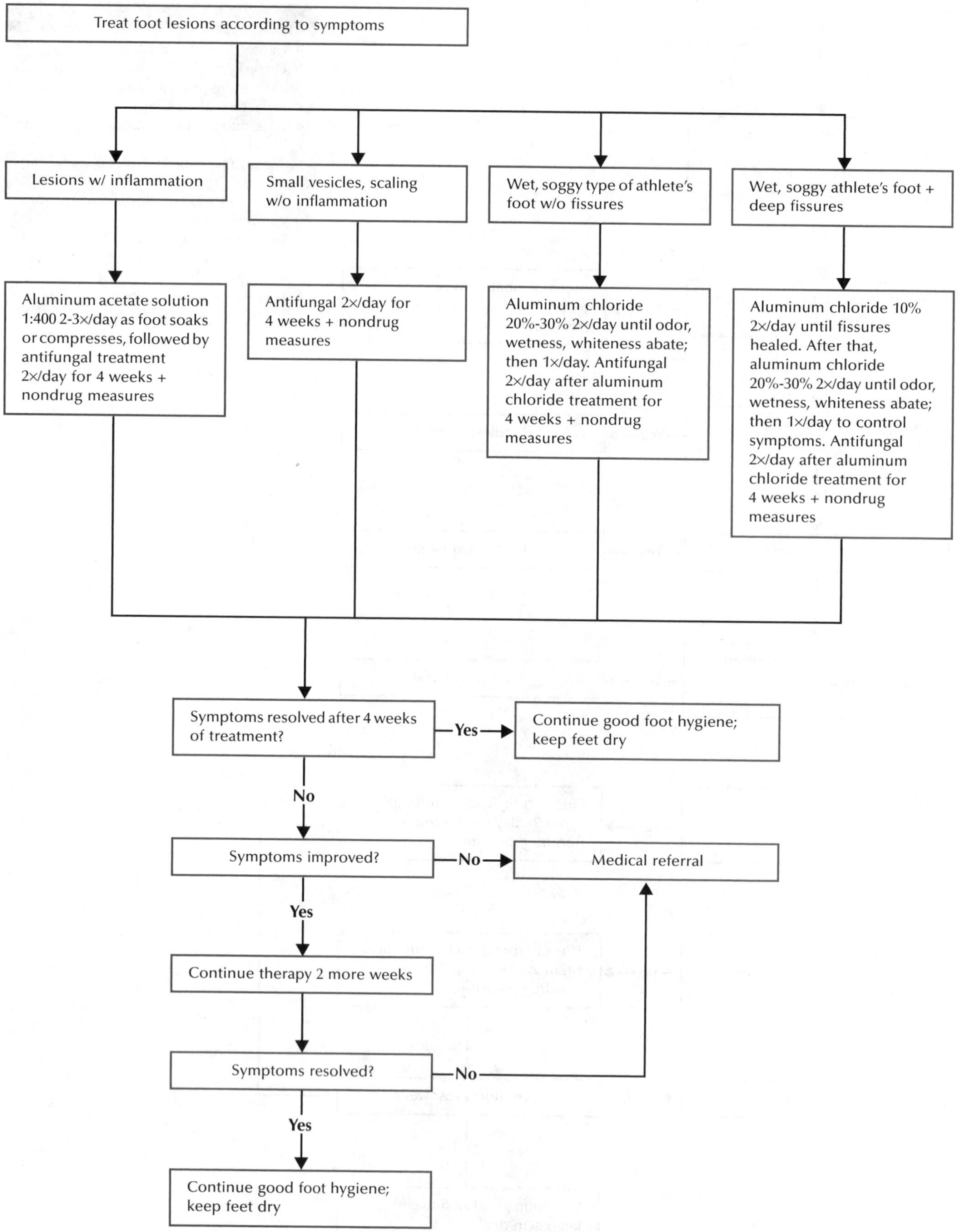


**FIGURE 43-1 (continued)** Self-care of fungal skin infections.

therapy when their symptoms subside but before the infection has been eradicated. Another determinant of therapeutic outcome relates to the patient's compliance with the nonpharmacologic measures intended to complement the effects of nonprescription antifungals and to prevent future infections. These measures include keeping the skin clean and dry, avoiding the sharing of personal articles, and avoiding contact with persons who have a fungal infection or contact with infected fomites.

### *Nonpharmacologic Therapy*

The box Patient Education for Fungal Skin Infections located at the end of the chapter describes nonpharmacologic measures intended to complement the effects of nonprescription antifungals and to prevent future infections. The patient should follow these measures during and after treatment of the infection.

### *Pharmacologic Therapy*

An antifungal ingredient must have at least one well-designed clinical trial demonstrating its effectiveness in treating athlete's foot before the Food and Drug Administration (FDA) will classify it as Category I (Table 43-2).[22] Butenafine hydrochloride, clioquinol, clotrimazole, haloprogin, miconazole nitrate, povidone–iodine, terbinafine hydrochloride, tolnaftate, and various undecylenates are considered to be safe and effective for nonprescription use in the treatment of fungal skin infections.[3] Except for povidone–iodine, these agents are labeled for treatment of athlete's foot, jock itch, and body ringworm. Although considered safe and effective for treating fungal skin infections, povidone–iodine products do not carry an indication for these infections. Recommended treatment period is a minimum of 2 to 4 weeks.

**TABLE 43-2 FDA-approved Nonprescription Topical Antifungal Drugs**

| Drug | Concentration (%) |
|---|---|
| Butenafine hydrochloride | 1 |
| Clioquinol | 3 |
| Clotrimazole | 1 |
| Haloprogin | 1 |
| Miconazole nitrate | 2 |
| Terbinafine hydrochloride | 1 |
| Tolnaftate | 1 |
| Povidone–iodine | 10 |
| Undecylenic acid and its salts | 10-25 |

*Source:* Reference 3 and Center for Drug Evaluation Research Approval Package for: Lotrimin Ultra (Butenafine Hydrochloride) Cream. Company: Schering-Plough HealthCare Products Application No.: 21-307 Approval date:12/7/2001. Available at http://www. fda.gov/cder/foi/nda/2001/21-307_Lotrimin.htm.

#### Clioquinol

Clioquinol, formerly called iodochlorhydroxyquin, has both antifungal and antibacterial properties. Its antibacterial properties have been used to treat cutaneous infections such as pyoderma, folliculitis, and impetigo; its antifungal properties have been used to treat mucocutaneous mycotic conditions such as superficial fungal infections and moniliasis.[23] Clioquinol 3% is available for nonprescription use in treating fungal infections.

Evaluations of clioquinol used alone and in combination with hydrocortisone indicate the following relative effectiveness: a clioquinol–hydrocortisone combination is greater than clioquinol alone, which is greater than hydrocortisone alone and greater than placebo. Such a combination product is not available for nonprescription use, however.

*Mechanism of Action* Clioquinol's mechanism of action is unknown.

*Indications* FDA classified clioquinol as Category I in treating tinea pedis, tinea cruris, and tinea corporis.

*Administration Guidelines* A thin layer of clioquinol is applied to the affected area two times daily for 4 weeks to treat tinea pedis and tinea corporis. Only 2 weeks of therapy is required for tinea cruris.

*Safety Considerations* Clioquinol has a low incidence of side effects; however, it may cause itching, redness, and irritation. If these symptoms persist, the patient should discontinue using the product. With general, nonocclusive application, the possibility of its percutaneous absorption is low. Clioquinol may also stain skin, hair, and nails yellow with its application and/or inadvertent contact with fabrics. Clothing stained by clioquinol should be washed in bleach, or the stain will become permanently set.

An adverse reaction known as subacute myelo-optic neuropathy that can result in permanent vision loss has occurred with oral use of clioquinol. FDA requires the following special warning statements: "Do not use on children under 2 years of age" and "Do not use for diaper rash."[3] The concern is that enough of the drug could be absorbed through an infant's skin to initiate this reaction.

If clioquinol is applied with an occlusive dressing, absorption can be rapid and extensive and may be sufficient to interfere with thyroid function tests. Thus, patients undergoing such tests must be questioned carefully to assess their prior use of iodine-containing clioquinol. Guidelines recommend discontinuing clioquinol for at least 1 month before performing certain thyroid function determinations (e.g., protein-bound iodine, butanol-extractable iodine, radioactive iodine uptake).

#### Clotrimazole and Miconazole Nitrate

Clotrimazole and miconazole nitrate are imidazole derivatives that demonstrate fungistatic/fungicidal activity (depending on concentration) against *T. mentagrophytes, T. rubrum, E. floccosum,* and *Candida albicans.*

*Mechanism of Action* These agents act by inhibiting the biosynthesis of ergosterol and other sterols, and by damaging the fungal cell wall membrane and altering its permeability, resulting in the loss of essential intracellular elements. These drugs have also been shown to inhibit oxidative and peroxidative enzyme activity, which results in intracellular buildup of toxic concentrations of hydrogen peroxide; this toxicity may then contribute to the degradation of subcellular organelles and to cellular necrosis. In C. albicans, such drugs have been shown to inhibit the transformation of blastospores into the invasive mycelial form that causes infection.

*Indications* FDA classified clotrimazole and miconazole nitrate as safe and effective for topical nonprescription use in treating tinea pedis, tinea cruris, and tinea corporis.

*Administration Guidelines* Clotrimazole and miconazole nitrate are suggested for application twice daily, once in the morning and once in the evening for up to 4 weeks.

*Safety Considerations* Rare cases of mild skin irritation, burning, and stinging have occurred with their use. No drug–drug interactions have been reported with topical use of clotrimazole and miconazole nitrate for up to 4 weeks.

### Haloprogin

Although FDA has approved haloprogin 1% for nonprescription use, no commercially available nonprescription topical antifungals currently contain this agent.

### Terbinafine Hydrochloride

Topical terbinafine hydrochloride 1% was reclassified as a nonprescription medication in 1999 under the trade name Lamisil AT. This product is available as a cream and as a spray.

*Mechanism of Action* This antifungal agent inhibits squalene epoxidase, a key enzyme in fungi sterol biosynthesis. This action results in a deficiency in ergosterol and a corresponding accumulation of squalene within the fungal cell, and it causes fungal cell death.

*Indications* Terbinafine hydrochloride is indicated for interdigital tinea pedis, tinea cruris, and tinea corporis caused by *E. floccosum, T. mentagrophytes,* and *T. rubrum.*

*Administration Guidelines* Similar to miconazole and clotrimazole, terbinafine hydrochloride should be applied sparingly to the affected area twice daily.

This drug is the only nonprescription topical antifungal available for which clinical trials demonstrated it could cure athlete's foot with 1 week of treatment. However, complete resolution of symptoms may require up to 4 weeks of treatment.

*Safety Considerations* Clinical trials to date have demonstrated a low incidence of side effects for terbinafine hydrochloride. These side effects include irritation (1%), burning (0.8%), and itching/dryness (0.2%).[24,25] No drug–drug interactions have been reported with topical use of terbinafine hydrochloride.

### Butenafine Hydrochloride

Topical butenafine hydrochloride 1% was reclassified as a nonprescription medication in 2001 under the trade name Lotrimin Ultra. This product is available as a cream.

*Mechanism of Action* Like terbinafine, this antifungal agent is a squalene epoxidase inhibitor. This action results in a deficiency in ergosterol, a corresponding accumulation of squalene within the fungal cell, and cell death.

*Indications* Butenafine hydrochloride is indicated as a cure for athlete's foot between the toes, jock itch, and ringworm caused by *E. floccosum, T. mentagrophytes,* and *T. rubrum.* Similar to other antifungals, it also relieves the itching, burning, cracking and scaling that can accompany these conditions. Effectiveness on the bottom or sides of the foot is unknown.

*Administration Guidelines* Patients suffering from athlete's foot should be advised to apply a thin film to affected skin between and around toes twice daily for 1 week, once a day for 4 weeks, or as directed by a primary care provider. Patients with jock itch or ringworm should apply a thin film to the affected area once daily for 2 weeks or as directed by a primary care provider.

Effective treatment rates for interdigital tinea pedis with 1-week and 4-week application durations are reported to be approximately 38% and 74%, respectively. In clinical trials Lotrimin Ultra kept users free of athlete's foot for up to 3 months.[26]

*Safety Considerations* To date, clinical trials demonstrate a low incidence of side effects. No drug–drug interactions have been reported with topical use of butenafine hydrochloride.

### Tolnaftate

Tolnaftate has demonstrated clinical efficacy since its commercial introduction in the United States in 1965. In addition, it was the standard against which the efficacy of other topical antifungals was compared for many years.

*Mechanism of Action* Although tolnaftate's exact mechanism of action has not been reported, it is believed that tolnaftate distorts the hyphae and stunts the mycelial growth of the fungi species.

*Indications* Tolnaftate is the only nonprescription drug approved for both preventing and treating athlete's foot.[3] It acts on fungi typically responsible for tinea infections, including *T. mentagrophytes, T. rubrum,* and *E. floccosum.*

Tolnaftate is valuable primarily in the dry, scaly type of athlete's foot. Superficial fungal infection relapse has occurred after tolnaftate therapy has been discontinued. Relapse may be caused by inadequate duration of treatment, patient noncompliance with the medication, or use of tolnaftate when an oral antifungal should have been used.

*Dosage Forms* As a cream, tolnaftate is formulated in a polyethylene glycol 400–propylene glycol vehicle. The 1% solution is formulated in polyethylene glycol 400 and may be more effective than the cream. The solution solidifies when exposed to cold, but will liquefy with no loss in potency if allowed to warm. These vehicles are particularly advantageous in superficial antifungal therapy because they are nonocclusive, nontoxic, nonsensitizing, water miscible, anhydrous, easy to apply, and efficient in delivering the drug to the affected area.

The topical powder formulation of tolnaftate uses cornstarch–talc as the vehicle. This vehicle not only is an effective drug delivery system but also offers a therapeutic advantage because the two agents absorb water. The topical aerosol formulation of tolnaftate includes talc, alcohol, and the propellant vehicle.

*Administration Guidelines* Tolnaftate (1% solution, cream, gel, powder, spray powder, or spray liquid) is applied sparingly twice daily after the affected area is cleaned thoroughly. Effective therapy usually takes 2 to 4 weeks, although some individuals (patients with lesions between the toes or on pressure areas of the foot) may require treatment lasting 4 to 6 weeks. When medication is applied to pressure areas of the foot, where the horny skin layer is thicker than normal, concomitant use of a keratolytic agent (e.g., Whitfield's ointment) may be advisable. Neither keratolytic agents nor wet compresses, such as aluminum acetate solution (Burow's solution), which promote the healing of oozing lesions, interfere with the efficacy of tolnaftate. If weeping lesions are present, the inflammation should be treated before tolnaftate is applied.

*Safety Considerations* Tolnaftate is well tolerated when applied to intact or broken skin, although it usually stings slightly when applied. Delayed hypersensitivity reactions to tolnaftate are extremely rare. As with all topical medications, however, discontinuation is warranted if irritation, sensitization, or worsening of the skin condition occurs.

No drug–drug interactions have been reported with topical use of tolnaftate.

### Undecylenic Acid

Combination undecylenic acid and undecylenate salts have been used widely and may be effective for various mild superficial fungal infections, excluding those involving nails or hairy parts of the body. It is fungistatic and effective in mild chronic cases of tinea pedis.

*Mechanism of Action* Compound undecylenic acid ointment (USP XXI) contains 5% undecylenic acid and 20% zinc undecylenate in an ointment base. It is believed that zinc undecylenate liberates undecylenic acid (the active antifungal entity) on contact with perspiration. In addition, zinc undecylenate has astringent properties because of the presence of the zinc ion; this astringent activity can help to decrease the irritation and inflammation of the infection.

*Indications* FDA approved undecylenic acid and its derivatives (10% to 25% total undecylenate content) as Category I for treating athlete's foot.[3]

*Dosage Forms* The vehicle in compound undecylenic acid ointment has a water-miscible base, which makes it nonocclusive, removable with water, and easy to apply. The powder uses talc as its vehicle and is absorbent. The aerosol contains menthol, which serves as a counterirritant and antipruritic. The solution contains 25% undecylenic acid in an isopropyl alcohol vehicle and is available with either an applicator or in a spray pump container. The foam dosage form contains 10% undecylenic acid.

*Administration Guidelines* The product is applied twice daily after the affected area is cleansed. When the solution is sprayed or applied to the affected area, the area should be allowed to air dry; otherwise, water may accumulate and further macerate the tissue. The usual period required for therapeutic results depends on the severity of the infection. However, if improvement does not occur in 2 to 4 weeks, the condition should be reevaluated and an alternative medication used.

*Safety Considerations* Applied to the skin as an ointment, diluted solution, or dusting powder, the combination of undecylenic acid–zinc undecylenate is relatively nonirritating, and hypersensitivity reactions are rare. The relatively high alcohol concentration in undecylenic acid solutions may cause some burning; the strong odor of undecylenic acid can be objectionable to some patients, possibly promoting patient noncompliance. Caution must be exercised to ensure that such ingredients do not come into contact with the eye or that the powder formulation is not inhaled.

### Salts of Aluminum

Because these drugs do not have any direct antifungal activity, aluminum salts were not included in the FDA final monograph for topical antifungal drug products. Rather, they are approved for the relief of inflammatory conditions of the skin, such as athlete's foot. However, their effectiveness as astringents and their possible use in treating athlete's foot merit their inclusion in this chapter. Historically, aluminum acetate has been the foremost astringent used for both the acute, inflammatory type and the wet, soggy type of tinea pedis. Aluminum chloride is also used to treat the wet, soggy type of infection.

Aluminum salts do not cure athlete's foot entirely but are useful when combined with other topical antifungal drugs. Application of aluminum salts merely shifts the disease process back to the simple dry type of athlete's foot, which can then be controlled with other agents such as tolnaftate or an azole.

*Mechanism of Action* The action and efficacy of aluminum salts appear to be two-pronged. First, these compounds act as astringents. Their drying ability probably involves the complexing of the astringent agent with proteins, thereby altering the proteins' ability to swell and hold water. Astringents decrease edema, exudation, and inflammation by reducing cell membrane permeability and by hardening the cement substance of the capillary epithelium. Second, aluminum salts in concentrations greater than 20% possess antibacterial activity. Aluminum chloride solution (20%) may exhibit that activity in two ways: by directly killing bacteria and by drying the interspaces. Solutions of 20% aluminum acetate and 20% aluminum chloride demonstrate equal in vitro antibacterial efficacy.

*Administration Guidelines* Aluminum acetate for use in tinea pedis is generally diluted with about 10 to 40 parts of water. Depending on the situation, the patient may immerse the whole foot in the solution for 20 minutes up to three times a day (every 6 to 8 hours) or may apply the solution to the affected area in the form of a wet dressing.

For patient convenience, aluminum acetate solution (Burow's solution) or modified Burow's solution is available for immediate use in solution or in forms (powder packets, powder, and effervescent tablets) to be dissolved in water.

Aqueous solutions of 20% to 30% aluminum chloride have been the most beneficial for the wet, soggy type of athlete's foot.[7] Twice-daily applications are generally used until the signs and symptoms (odor, wetness, and whiteness) abate. After that, once-daily applications may control the symptoms. In hot, humid weather, the original condition may return within 7 to 10 days after the application is stopped.

*Safety Considerations* Because aluminum salts penetrate the skin poorly, their toxicity, like that of aluminum chloride, is low. However, a few cases of irritation have been reported in patients with deep fissures. Thus, the use of concentrated aluminum salt solutions is contraindicated on severely eroded or deeply fissured skin. In such a case, the salts must be diluted to a lower concentration (10% aluminum chloride) for initial treatment.

Solutions of aluminum acetate or aluminum chloride have a potential for misuse (accidental childhood poisoning by ingesting the solutions or the solid tablets), and precautions must be taken to prevent this occurrence. Products containing these ingredients are intended for external use only and should not be applied near the eyes. Prolonged or continuous use of aluminum acetate solution may produce tissue necrosis. In the acute inflammatory stage of tinea pedis, this solution should be used for less than 1 week. The practitioner should instruct the patient to discontinue its use if inflammatory lesions appear or worsen.

## Pharmacotherapeutic Comparison

All the topical antifungals approved for treating cutaneous fungal infections have been demonstrated to be effective. The allure of butenafine hydrochloride and terbinafine hydrochloride is their demonstrated ability to cure athlete's foot in some patients after 1 week. However, a close analysis of the data demonstrates that the number of patients achieving complete resolution of the problem is low and that the effectiveness of these agents parallels that of other antifungals (e.g., clotrimazole, miconazole nitrate) previously approved for nonprescription use.[27]

Controlled studies have demonstrated the efficacy of clotrimazole and miconazole nitrate for athlete's foot, as well as for other kinds of fungal skin infections (see Chapter 8). Both would be expected to demonstrate efficacy comparable to that of tolnaftate for tinea infections. If patient factors (e.g., noncompliance or improper foot hygiene) can be ruled out as a cause of treatment failure, both can be suggested as alternative treatment modalities.

## Product Selection Guidelines

Cutaneous antifungals are available as ointments, creams, powders, and aerosols (Table 43-3). Creams or solutions are the most efficient and effective dosage forms for delivery of the active ingredient to the epidermis. Sprays and powders are less effective because often they are not rubbed into the skin. They are probably more useful as adjuncts to a cream or a solution or as prophylactic agents in preventing new or recurrent infections.

Patient compliance is influenced by product selection. Therefore, the practitioner should recommend a drug and product form that is likely to cause the least interference with daily habits and activities without sacrificing efficacy. For example, patients of advanced age may require a preparation that is easy to use; obese patients, in whom excessive sweating may contribute to the disease, should use topical talcum powders as adjunctive therapy. Under certain circumstances, it may be necessary for the practitioner to instruct the caregiver rather than the patient in the proper use of foot products.

Before recommending a nonprescription product, the practitioner should review the patient's medical history. For example, patients with diabetes should have their blood glucose levels moderately controlled because increased glucose in perspiration may promote fungal growth. Patients with allergic dermatitides usually have a history of asthma, hay fever, or atopic dermatitis and thus are extremely sensitive to most oral and topical agents. By acquiring a good history, the practitioner may be able to distinguish a tinea infection from atopic dermatitis and thus avoid recommending a product that may cause further skin irritation.

The practitioner should bear in mind that prescription drugs may sometimes be more beneficial than nonprescription products. If the patient has soggy, macerated athlete's foot complicated by bacterial infection, broad-spectrum antifungal agents (e.g., econazole nitrate) are preferable to both tolnaftate and prescription-strength haloprogin.

**TABLE 43-3 Selected Topical Antifungal Products**

| Trade Name | Primary Ingredients |
|---|---|
| Aftate Aerosol Spray Liquid/Aerosol Spray Powder | Tolnaftate 1% |
| Cruex Aerosol Spray Powder | Total undecylenate 19% (as undecylenic acid and zinc undecylenate) |
| Cruex Cream | Total undecylenate 20% (as undecylenic acid and zinc undecylenate) |
| Cruex Prescription Strength Aerosol Spray Powder | Miconazole nitrate 2% |
| Cruex Prescription Strength AF Cream | Clotrimazole 1% |
| Cruex Squeeze Powder | Calcium undecylenate 10% |
| Desenex Max Antifungal Cream | Terbinafine hydrochloride 1% |
| Desenex Prescription Strength AF Aerosol Spray Powder/Aerosol Spray Liquid | Miconazole nitrate 2% |
| Desenex Prescription Strength AF Cream | Clotrimazole 1% |
| Lamisil AT Cream | Terbinafine HCl 1% |
| Lotrimin AF Lotion/Solution/Cream | Clotrimazole 1% |
| Lotrimin AF Powder/Aerosol Spray Liquid/Aerosol Spray Powder | Miconazole nitrate 2% |
| Lotrimin Ultra Cream | Butenafine 1% |
| Micatin Jock Itch Cream/Aerosol Spray Powder | Miconazole nitrate 2% |
| Micatin Powder/Cream/Aerosol Spray Powder/Aerosol Spray Liquid | Miconazole nitrate 2% |
| Tinactin Aerosol Spray Liquid/Aerosol Spray Powder/Cream | Tolnaftate 1% |
| Tinactin Jock Itch Cream | Tolnaftate 1% |

The practitioner should also be aware that product line extensions carrying the same brand name do not necessarily have the same active ingredient(s). For example, the cream and solution formulations of Lotrimin AF contain clotrimazole 1%, whereas the topical spray and powder formulations contain miconazole nitrate 2%. Indeed, Lotrimin Ultra, the newest line extension, contains butenafine hydrochloride. It would have been prohibitively expensive for the manufacturer to pursue the new drug application necessary to market these products with clotrimazole 1% or butenafine hydrochloride 1% as their active ingredient. It was more economically prudent to develop them with an active ingredient that had already received FDA approval. Similarly, Desenex spray liquid and spray powder formulations contain miconazole nitrate 2%, whereas these products formerly contained undecylenic acid and zinc undecylenate in a 25% concentration. Likewise, Desenex Max Antifungal Cream now contains 1% terbinafine.

### *Complementary Therapies*

Research results suggest that twice-daily application of 100% tea tree oil solution for 6 months can eradicate fungus from infected toenails in about 18% of patients. It also improves nail appearance and symptoms in about 56% of patients after 3 months and 60% of patients after 6 months of treatment. However, lower concentrations of tea tree oil do not seem to be as effective.[28]

## Assessment of Fungal Skin Infections: A Case-based Approach

Fungal skin infections must be differentiated from bacterial infections, as well as from noninfectious dermatitis. If possible, the practitioner should examine the affected area to determine whether the disorder's manifestation is typical of a fungal infection (Table 43-1).[29]

The only true determinant of a fungal infection is a clinical laboratory evaluation of tissue scrapings from the affected area. This process involves a potassium hydroxide mount preparation of the scrapings and cuttings on a special growth medium to show the actual presence and specific identity of fungi. The procedure can be ordered and performed only at the direction of a primary care provider, and microscopic confirmation is probably possible only in the dry, scaly type of tinea infections. The recovery of fungi for diagnosis decreases as the infection becomes progressively more severe. In typical cases of dermatophytosis complex, fungus recovery rates are only about 25% to 50%.

The practitioner should question the patient thoroughly regarding the condition and its characteristics to determine symptoms, extent of disease, previous patient compliance with medications, and any compounding disorders (e.g., diabetes or obesity) that might render the patient susceptible. Patients with diabetes, for example, may present with a mixed dermatophytid and monilial infection. In general, it is appropriate to inspect the area if privacy and sanitary conditions allow, and it is especially appropriate for patients with diabetes. See Cases 43-1 and 43-2 for examples of assessing a patient with a fungal skin infection.

## CASE 43-1

| Relevant Evaluation Criteria | Scenario/Model Outcome |
|---|---|
| **Information Gathering** | |
| 1. Gather essential information about the patient's symptoms, including: | |
| a. description of symptom(s) (i.e., nature, onset, duration, severity, associated symptoms) | Patient complains of a burning, itching sensation between the toes of his left foot. The symptoms are becoming worse each day and are quite bothersome, particularly at bedtime. He says the area between the toes is very red and seems to become worse after showering. He describes his toenails as normal in appearance; the toenail beds show no apparent discoloration or brittleness. |
| b. description of any factors that seem to precipitate, exacerbate, and/or relieve the patient's symptom(s) | Patient is not aware of anything that worsens or relieves his symptoms. |
| c. description of the patent's efforts to relieve the symptoms | Patient has used Lotrimin AF cream intermittently for the past week. He says it seems to help a little. |
| 2. Gather essential patient history information: | |
| a. patient's identity | Anwar Bhor |
| b. age, sex, height, and weight | 21 y/o M |
| c. patient's occupation | College student |
| d. patient's dietary habits | Eats a lot of fried foods |
| e. patient's sleep habits | 7 hours per night |
| f. concurrent medical conditions, prescription and nonprescription medications, and dietary supplements | None |
| g. allergies | None |
| h. history of other adverse reactions to medications | None |
| i. other (describe)_______ | Anwar showers every day in his residence hall and at the gymnasium after his varsity baseball team's workout. He also reports that his feet sweat a lot. |
| **Assessment and Triage** | |
| 3. Differentiate patient's signs/symptoms and correctly identify the patient's primary problem(s) (see Table 43-1). | Anwar is suffering from athlete's foot that he likely contracted from a public shower. |
| 4. Identify exclusions for self-treatment (see Figure 43-1). | None |
| 5. Formulate a comprehensive list of therapeutic alternatives for the primary problem to determine if triage to a medical practitioner is required and share this information with the patient. | Options include:<br>(1) Refer Anwar to an appropriate health care professional.<br>(2) Recommend self-care with a nonprescription antifungal and nondrug measures.<br>(3) Recommend self-care until Anwar can see an appropriate health care professional.<br>(4) Take no action. |
| **Plan** | |
| 6. Select an optimal therapeutic alternative to address the patient's problem, taking into account patient preferences. | Anwar should use a nonprescription antifungal and nondrug measures to treat his problem. |
| 7. Describe the recommended therapeutic approach to the patient. | Regular use of any of the commercially available nonprescription antifungals in any dosage form, except a spray or powder, should alleviate the problem. However, to be optimally effective, you will have to take several measures to keep your feet clean and dry. |

## CASE 43-1 (continued)

| Relevant Evaluation Criteria | Scenario/Model Outcome |
|---|---|
| 8. Explain to the patient the rationale for selecting the recommended therapeutic approach from the considered therapeutic alternatives. | Athlete's foot can be effectively managed with nonprescription antifungals and nondrug measures (keeping the feet clean and dry) as long as there is no toenail involvement, evidence of secondary infection, or preexisting medical condition that would preclude self-treatment, as in your case. Sprays and powders are less effective, because they often are not rubbed into the skin. |
| **Patient Education** | |
| 9. When recommending self-care with nonprescription medications and/or nondrug therapy, convey accurate information to the patient, including: | |
| a. appropriate dose and frequency of administration | See the box Patient Education for Fungal Skin Infections. |
| b. maximum number of days the therapy should be employed | See the box Patient Education for Fungal Skin Infections. |
| c. product administration procedures | See the box Patient Education for Fungal Skin Infections. |
| d. expected time to onset of relief | Itching may be relieved somewhat within a few days, but eradication of the causative microorganism may take up to 4 weeks. |
| e. degree of relief that can be reasonably expected | Athlete's foot can be cured if you use the antifungal properly. |
| f. most common side effects | See the box Patient Education for Fungal Skin Infections. |
| g. side effects that warrant medical intervention should they occur | See the box Patient Education for Fungal Skin Infections. |
| h. patient options in the event that condition worsens or persists | See the box Patient Education for Fungal Skin Infections. |
| i. product storage requirements | Store the product in a cool, dry place out of children's reach. |
| j. specific nondrug measures | See the box Patient Education for Fungal Skin Infections. |
| 10. Solicit follow-up questions from patient. | Do I need to purchase another product, or can I just keep using the Lotrimin AF? |
| 11. Answer patient's questions. | You can use Lotrimin AF as long as you follow the product instructions and nondrug measures. |

## CASE 43-2

| Relevant Evaluation Criteria | Scenario/Model Outcome |
|---|---|
| **Information Gathering** | |
| 1. Gather essential information about the patient's symptoms, including: | |
| a. description of symptom(s) (i.e., nature, onset, duration, severity, associated symptoms) | Patient complains of a red, itchy rash on the intertriginous skin beneath both breasts. The rash has spread to the space between the fingers on both hands; she speculates that this occurred when she started scratching the original lesions.<br>Inspection of the lesions on the patient's hands reveals red, macerated patches of skin between each finger on the right hand and between the thumb and index finger on the left hand. Vesicopustules appear scattered around the red, pea-sized lesions.<br>Upon questioning, the patient reports that the lesions under her breasts are similar in appearance but are much larger. The problem began a little over a week ago and has progressively worsened. |

## CASE 43-2 (continued)

| Relevant Evaluation Criteria | Scenario/Model Outcome |
|---|---|
| b. description of any factors that seem to precipitate, exacerbate, and/or relieve the patient's symptom(s) | Patient is not aware of anything that worsens or relieves her symptoms and could not associate the onset of her rash with any new medication or with the use of new clothing, soaps, or toiletries. |
| c. description of the patient's efforts to relieve the symptoms | Patient has not tried anything other than scratching to relieve her symptoms. |
| 2. Gather essential patient history information: | |
| a. patient's identity | Florence Johnson |
| b. age, sex, height, and weight | 54 y/o F, 5'0", 175 lb |
| c. patient's occupation | She has been totally disabled for 5 years due to emphysema. |
| d. patient's dietary habits | Eats mostly frozen dinners |
| e. patient's sleep habits | 6 hours per night |
| f. concurrent medical conditions, prescription and nonprescription medications, and dietary supplements | Theophylline and albuterol to manage her emphysema; glyburide for Type 2 diabetes mellitus; allopurinol for gout; acetaminophen for osteoarthritis; and famotidine for gastroesophageal reflux disease |
| g. allergies | None |
| h. history of other adverse reactions to medications | None |
| i. other (describe)_______ | Florence is a resident at a nearby apartment complex for older people and people with disabilities, but she does not yet require assistance from the resident staff. |
| **Assessment and Triage** | |
| 3. Differentiate the patient's signs/symptoms and correctly identify the patient's primary problem(s) (see Table 43-1). | Florence is suffering from tinea corporis. |
| 4. Identify exclusions for self-treatment (see Figure 43-1). | History of diabetes |
| 5. Formulate a comprehensive list of therapeutic alternatives for the primary problem to determine if triage to a medical practitioner is required, and share this information with the patient. | Options include:<br>(1) Refer Florence to an appropriate health care professional.<br>(2) Recommend self-care with a nonprescription antifungal and nondrug measures.<br>(3) Recommend self-care until Florence can see an appropriate health care professional.<br>(4) Take no action. |
| **Plan** | |
| 6. Select an optimal therapeutic alternative to address the patient's problem, taking into account patient preferences. | Florence should be referred to her PCP for treatment. |
| 7. Describe the recommended therapeutic approach to the patient. | Only your primary care provider can prescribe treatment for your condition. |
| 8. Explain to the patient the rationale for selecting the recommended therapeutic approach from the considered therapeutic alternatives. | Fungal skin infections cannot be self-treated in patients with other conditions that predispose them to infectious disease, such as diabetes (see Figure 43-1). Infections in such patients require prescription medication and supervision by a primary care provider. |
| **Patient Education** | |
| 9. When recommending self-care with nonprescription medications and/or nondrug therapy, convey accurate information to the patient, including: | Criterion does not apply in this case. |

**CASE 43-2 (continued)**

| Relevant Evaluation Criteria | Scenario/Model Outcome |
|---|---|
| 10. Solicit follow-up questions from patient. | Can I do anything to keep from getting this condition again once it has cleared? |
| 11. Answer patient's questions. | Yes. See the box Patient Education for Fungal Skin Infections. |

The most common complaint of patients with a cutaneous fungal infection is pruritus. However, if fissures are present, particularly between the toes, painful burning and stinging may also occur. If the area is abraded, denuded, or inflamed, weeping or oozing may be present in addition to pain. Some patients may merely remark on the bothersome scaling of dry skin, particularly if the infection involves the soles of the feet. In other instances, small vesicular lesions may combine to form a larger bullous eruption marked by pain and irritation, or the only symptoms may be brittleness and discoloration of a hypertrophied nail.

The practitioner should seek to distinguish a tinea infection from diseases with similar symptoms, such as a bacterial infection, dermatitis, allergic contact dermatitis, and atopic dermatitis. For that reason, the manifestation of these disorders is briefly discussed here. In children, peridigital dermatitis or atopic dermatitis is more common than tinea pedis. Shoe dermatitis is perhaps the most common form of allergic contact dermatitis from clothing. Thus, the practitioner should inquire about the type of footwear worn by the patient and about recent footwear changes. Since 1950, the increased use of rubber and adhesives in footwear has paralleled the increase in reports of shoe dermatitis in the dermatologic and podiatric literature. Contact allergy to accelerators—the chemical compounds used to speed the processing of rubber used in sponge-rubber insoles for tennis shoes—has also been reported.[30] In addition to accelerators, antioxidants have been implicated as major chemical allergens, and various phenolic resins used in adhesives are also troublesome. The patient is usually unaware that his or her footwear may be causing the problem.

Hyperhidrosis of interdigital spaces and of the sole of the foot is common, as is infection of the toe webs by gram-negative bacteria. In hyperhidrosis, tender vesicles cover the sole of the foot and toes and may be quite painful. The skin generally turns white, erodes, and becomes macerated. This condition is accompanied by a foul foot odor. A soggy wetness of the toe webs and the immediately adjacent skin characterizes infection by gram-negative bacteria; the affected tissue is damp and softened. The last toe web (adjacent to the little toe) is the most common area of primary or initial involvement because it is deeper and extends more proximally than the Web between the other toes. Furthermore, abundant exocrine sweat glands, a semiocclusive anatomic setting, and the added occlusion provided by footwear enhance development of the disease at this site. The practitioner must be careful not to confuse this condition with soft corns, which also appear between the fourth and fifth toes.

## Patient Counseling for Fungal Skin Infections

The practitioner should describe the proper application technique for topical antifungals to the patient to prevent over- or undermedication. The patient should be told the expected duration of therapy and to apply the medication regularly throughout a complete course of therapy. In addition to information about product use, the practitioner may provide information that will help to control or eradicate the infection and will minimize the likelihood of recurrent infections. Such information should address proper care of the infected skin site, appropriate laundry techniques and products, minimal use of occlusive clothing, and avoidance of habits or behavior that may lead to recurring infections. The patient should also be told which conditions indicate a need to consult a primary care provider (e.g., the development of a secondary bacterial infection). The box Patient Education for Fungal Skin Infections lists specific information to provide patients.

## Evaluation of Patient Outcomes for Fungal Skin Infections

In general, the patient should begin to see some relief of the itching, scaling, and/or inflammation within 1 week. If the disorder shows improvement within this time frame, recommend continuing treatment for 1 to 3 more weeks (depending on the type of tinea infection). If the disorder has not improved or has worsened, refer the patient to a primary care provider for more aggressive therapy. Recurrent skin infections may be a sign of undiagnosed diabetes, immunodeficiency, or another organic problem that requires medical evaluation.

## Key Points for Fungal Skin Infections

- Historically, the nonprescription drug of choice to treat tinea corporis, tinea cruris, and tinea pedis has been tolnaftate. Other agents, such as clioquinol, clotrimazole, miconazole nitrate, terbinafine hydrochloride, butenafine hydrochloride, and undecylenic acid and its derivatives, are also efficacious for this purpose.
- The effectiveness of topical antifungals will be limited, however, unless the patient eliminates other predisposing factors to tinea infections.
- These drugs are effective in all their delivery vehicles, but the powder forms should be reserved only for extremely mild conditions or as adjunctive therapy.
- Because solutions and creams are spreadable, they should be used sparingly.

## PATIENT EDUCATION FOR FUNGAL SKIN INFECTIONS

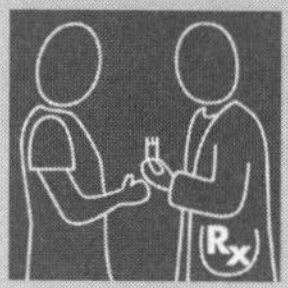


The objectives of self-treatment are to (1) relieve itching, burning, and other discomfort, (2) inhibit the growth of fungi and cure the disorder, and (3) prevent recurrent infections. For most patients, carefully following product instructions and the self-care measures listed here will help ensure optimal therapeutic outcomes.

### Nondrug Measures

- To prevent spreading the infection to other parts of the body, either use a separate towel to dry the affected area or dry the affected area last.
- Do not share towels, clothing, or other personal articles with family members, especially when an infection is present.
- Launder contaminated towels and clothing in hot water to prevent spreading the infection.
- Cleanse the skin daily with soap and water, and thoroughly pat dry to remove oils and other substances that promote growth of fungi.
- If possible, do not wear clothing or shoes that cause the skin to stay wet. Wool and synthetic fabrics prevent optimal air circulation.
- If needed, allow shoes to dry thoroughly before wearing them again. Dust shoes with medicated or nonmedicated foot powder to help keep them dry.
- If needed, place odor-controlling insoles (e.g., Odor Attackers, Sneaker Snuffers) in casual or athletic shoes. These insoles also provide some support and cushioning for the feet. Change insoles routinely every 3 to 4 months or more often if their condition warrants, and take care that the shoe fit is not compromised by the insoles.
- Avoid contact with people who have fungal infections. Wear protective footwear (e.g., rubber or wooden sandals) in areas of family or public use such as home bathrooms or community showers.

### Nonprescription Medications

- Ask a practitioner for assistance in picking the appropriate antifungal agent and dosage form for your infection.
- Available agents include butenafine, clioquinol, clotrimazole, miconazole nitrate, terbinafine, tolnaftate, and undecylenic acid–zinc undecylenate.
- It usually takes 2 to 4 weeks to cure tinea infections. Some cases may require 4 to 6 weeks of treatment.
- Apply the antifungal to the clean, dry, affected area in the morning and the evening. Massage the medication into the area. Note that creams and solutions are easier to work into the skin and thus are probably more effective treatment forms.
- Avoid getting the product in your eyes.
- Wash hands thoroughly with soap and water after applying the product.
- Topical antifungals themselves may cause itching, redness, and irritation.
- Clioquinol may interfere with thyroid function tests and also should not be used on children younger than 2 years of age.
- Note that clioquinol may cause transient stinging or itching, as well as a rash. If these symptoms persist, stop using the product.
- Tolnaftate may sting slightly upon application.
- An undiluted solution of undecylenic acid–zinc undecylenate may cause temporary stinging when applied to broken skin because of its isopropyl alcohol content.
- When medication is applied to pressure areas of the foot, where the horny skin layer is thicker than normal, apply a keratolytic agent (e.g., Whitfield's ointment) initially to the affected area to help the antifungal penetrate the skin.
- If oozing lesions are present, apply aluminum acetate solution (1:40) to the area before applying the antifungal:
  - Soak the area in an aluminum acetate solution for 20 minutes up to three times a day (every 6 to 8 hours), or apply the solution to the affected area in the form of a wet dressing.
  - Note that aluminum acetate solution (Burow's solution) or modified Burow's solution is available for immediate use in solution or in forms (powder packets, powder, and effervescent tablets) to be dissolved in water.
  - Avoid getting the product in your eyes.
  - To avoid skin damage, use the solution for no more than 1 week. Discontinue use of the solution if inflammatory lesions appear or worsen.
- For the wet, soggy type of athlete's foot, apply to or soak foot in aluminum acetate solution (1:40) before applying the antifungal:
  - Soak feet with aluminum acetate solution (1:40) twice daily until the odor, wetness, and whiteness abate. After that, soak once daily to control the symptoms.
  - If deep fissures are present in the skin, use a more dilute solution of aluminum acetate for initial treatment.

⚠ Discontinue use of the product and contact a primary care provider if itching or swelling occurs, or if the infection worsens.

⚠ Consult a primary care provider if the infection worsens or persists beyond the recommended length of therapy.

- When recommended for suspected or actual dermatophytosis, these drugs should be used twice daily (morning and night). Treatment should be continued for 2 to 4 weeks, depending on the symptoms. After that time, the patient and practitioner should evaluate the effectiveness of the therapy.
- To minimize noncompliance, the practitioner should advise patients that alleviation of symptoms will not occur overnight. Patients should also be cautioned that frequent recurrence of any of these problems is an indication that they should consult a primary care provider.
- Immunocompromised patients and those with diabetes or circulatory problems should be treated by a primary health care provider.

## References


1. Hay RJ, Roberts SOB, MacKenzie DWR. In: Campion RH, Burton JL, Ebling FJG, eds. *Textbook of Dermatology.* 5th ed. Oxford, England: Blackwell Scientific Publications;1992:1127-216.
2. Freeberg IM, Eisen AZ, Wolff K, et al., eds. *Dermatology in General Medicine.* 5th ed. New York: McGraw-Hill, Inc; 1999.
3. Federal Register. 1993;58:49890-9.

4. Drake LA, Dinehart SM, Farmer ER, et al. Guidelines for care of superficial mycotic infections of the skin: tinea corporis, tinea cruris, tinea faciei, tinea manuum and tinea pedis. *J Am Acad Dermatol.* 1996;34(2 pt 1):282-6.
5. Fitzpatrick TB, Eisen AZ, Wolf K, et al., eds. *Dermatology in General Medicine.* 4th ed. New York: McGraw-Hill, Inc; 1993.
6. Lesher J, Levine N, Treadwill P. Fungal skin infections. *Patient Care.* 1994;28:16-44.
7. Shrum JP, Millikan LE, Bataineh O. Superficial fungal infections in the tropics. *Dermatol Clin.* 1994;12:687-93.
8. Bergus GR, Johnson JS. Superficial tinea infections. *Am Fam Physician.* 1993;48:259.
9. Evans EG. Tinea pedis: clinical experience and efficacy of short treatment. *Dermatology.* 1997;194(suppl 1):3-6.
10. Aly R. Ecology and epidemiology of dermatophyte infections. *J Am Acad Dermatol.* 1994;31(3 pt 2):S21.
11. Auger P, et al. Epidemiology of tinea pedis in marathon runners: prevalence of occult athlete's foot. *Mycoses.* 1993;36:35-43.
12. Griffin LY. Common sports injuries of the foot and ankle seen in children and adolescents. *Orthop Clin North Am.* 1994;25:83-93.
13. Your podiatric physician talks about fungal nails. Available at: http://www.apma.org/topics/fungal.htm. Accessed July 2, 2001.
14. Noble SL, Forbes RC, Stam PL. Diagnosis and management of common tinea infections. *Am Fam Physician.* 1998;58:163-74,177-8.
15. Odom R. Pathophysiology of dermatophyte infections. J Am Acad Dermatol. 1993;28(5 pt 1):S2-7.
16. Pray SW. *Nonprescription Product Therapeutics.* Philadelphia: Lippincott Williams & Wilkins; 1999:543.
17. Dahl MV. Dermatophytosis and the immune response. *J Am Acad Dermatol.* 1994;31(3 pt 2):S34-41.
18. Pray, SW. Ringworm: easy to recognize and treat. Available at: http://www.uspharmacist.com. Accessed May 14, 2001.
19. Weinstein A, Berman B. Topical treatment of common superficial tinea infections. *Am Fam Physician.* 2002;65:2095-102.
20. Elewski BE, Silverman RA. Clinical pearl: diagnostic procedures for tinea capitis. *J Am Acad Dermatol.* 1996;34:498-9.
21. Drake LA, Dinehart SM, Farmer ER, et al. Guidelines for care of superficial mycotic infections of the skin: tinea capitis and tinea barbae. *J Am Acad Dermatol.* 1996;34(2 pt 1):290.
22. *Federal Register.* 1982;47:12480-566.
23. Chan ES, Benza RL. Minor wounds and skin infections. In: Allen LV, Berardi, RR, DeSimone EM, et al. *Handbook of Nonprescription Drugs.* 12th ed. Washington, DC: American Pharmaceutical Association; 1996:753-80.
24. Savin RC. Treatment of chronic tinea pedis (athlete's foot type) with topical terbinafine. *J Am Acad Dermatol.* 1990;23:786-9.
25. Savin RC, Zaias N. Treatment of chronic moccasin-type tinea pedis with terbinafine: a double-blind, placebo-controlled trial. *J Am Acad Dermatol.* 1990;23:804-7.
26. Center for Drug Evaluation and Research Approval Package for: Application Number: 020663, Trade Name: MENTAX CREAM 1%, Generic Name: Butenafine HCl Cream, Sponsor: Penederm, Inc., Approval Date: December 31, 1996. Available at http://www.fda.gov/cder/foi/nda/96/020663ap.pdf. Accessed November 11, 2002.
27. Gupta AK, Einarson TR, Smmerbell RC, et al. An overview of topical antifungal therapy in dermatomycoses: a North American perspective. Drugs. 1998:55;645-74.
28. Buck DS, Nidorf DM, Addino JG. Comparison of two topical preparations for the treatment of onychomycosis: Melaleuca alternifolia (tea tree) oil and clotrimazole. *J Fam Pract.* 1994;38:601-5.
29. Bruinsma W, ed. *A Guide to Drug Eruptions.* 6th ed. Amsterdam, The Netherlands: Free University Press; 1995.
30. Jung JH, McLaughlin JL, Stannard J, et al. Isolation, via activity-directed fractionation, of mercaptobenzothiazole and dibenzothiazyl disulfide as 2 allergens responsible for tennis shoe dermatitis. *Contact Dermatitis.* 1988;19:254-9.

CHAPTER 44

# Warts

*Nicholas G. Popovich and Gail D. Newton*

Warts, or verrucae, are common viral infections of the epidermis and mucous membranes.[1] Treatments described in this chapter apply to common warts on self-treatable areas of the body.

## Epidemiology of Warts

Approximately 7% to 10% of people have warts, and approximately 24% of the cases involve plantar warts (i.e., warts located on the sole of the foot).[2] Between 4% and 20% of school-age children will have a wart at some time.[3] The peak incidence of warts occurs between the ages of 12 and 16 years. As many as 10% of school-age children younger than 16 years have one or more warts. Warts usually are not permanent; approximately 30% clear spontaneously in 6 months, 65% clear in 2 years, and most warts clear in 5 years.[4] The mechanism of spontaneous resolution is not fully understood.

## Etiology of Warts

Warts are caused by human papillomaviruses (HPVs), which contain DNA composed of about 8000 base pairs.[5] Since the 1990s, immunologic techniques in conjunction with DNA purification and restrictive endonuclease digestion have identified at least 80 HPV subtypes; the actual number of subtypes may exceed 150.[5] Each subtype has its own characteristic histopathology and cytopathology.

Three criteria must be met for an individual to develop a wart. First, the papillomavirus must be present. Second, an open avenue, such as an abrasion, must exist through which the virus can enter the skin. Finally, the individual's immune system must be susceptible to the virus (probably the key reason that certain individuals develop warts and others do not). Indeed, immunodeficient patients (e.g., those maintained on systemic or topical glucocorticoids), once infected, can develop widespread and highly resistant warts.[6]

Warts may spread by direct person-to-person contact, autoinoculation to another body area, or indirect exposure to fomites through public shower floors or swimming pools. It is believed that swimming, especially in warm water with a pH greater than 5, swells and softens the horny skin layer cells on the sole of the foot. The abrasive surface of the pool and diving board also contribute to tissue debridement. Scrapings of the horny layer of plantar warts contain virus particles. Therefore, it is conceivable that the heavy traffic area of a pool can be contaminated easily by one person with a plantar wart, making inoculation in that area around the pool likely. In fact, athletes have a high incidence of plantar warts, and those who use communal and public showers are at high risk.[7] The incubation period after inoculation is 1 to 24 months, with an average of 3 to 4 months.

## Pathophysiology of Warts

Studies[5] have shown that common warts are caused by HPV-2, HPV-4, HPV-27, and HPV-29, whereas HPV-6 and HPV-11 are responsible for anogenital warts. The latter strains differ from other HPVs in serologic molecular hybridization. Often, flat warts are associated with types HPV-3, HPV-10, HPV-28, and HPV-49. Digital warts often found in butchers display subtype HPV-7. These findings prompted the belief that HPV type dictates the kind of wart and that these viruses are confined to specific body locations. Evidence now suggests that HPV types are not restricted to a specific site, but that, for unknown reasons (perhaps epithelial cell receptor specificity), viral particles function in keratinocytes only in specific locations and will induce warts only in these locations.[8] Different types may infect cornified stratified squamous epithelium of the skin or uncornified mucous membranes. Environmental and host factors besides the viral subtype also influence the lesion appearance.[9] (See Chapter 33 for discussion of anatomy and physiology of the skin.)

Papillomavirus particles assemble in the nuclei of upper-layer keratinocytes and are subsequently released into the milieu within the stratum corneum. It has been demonstrated that HPVs do not bud from the cell membrane and thus lack a thermosensitive lipid envelope like that found in the herpes viruses and the human retroviruses. It is believed that the presence of a heat-stable protein coat allows the HPV to remain infectious outside the host cells for substantial periods of time.[8]

## Signs and Symptoms of Warts

Common warts are recognized by their rough, cauliflowerlike appearance. They are slightly scaly, rough papules or nodules that appear alone or grouped. They can be found on any skin surface although they most often appear on the hands (see Color Plates, photograph 31). Warts begin as minute, smooth-surfaced, skin-colored lesions that enlarge over time. Repeated irritation causes them to continue enlarging. Plantar warts, hyperkeratotic lesions generally associated with pressure, are usually asymptomatic when small and may not be noticed.

However, if they are large or occur on the heel or ball of the foot, they may cause severe discomfort and limitation of function as the otherwise raised lesion is pushed inward secondary to pressure caused by walking. The lesion then impinges on the surrounding sensory nerve endings, causing discomfort or pain.

Warts are defined according to their location. Common warts (verruca vulgaris) usually are found on the hands and fingers, but may also occur on the face. Periungual and subungual warts occur around and underneath the nail beds, especially in nail biters and cuticle pickers. Juvenile, or flat, warts (verruca plana) usually occur on the face, neck, and dorsa of the hands, wrists, and knees of children. Typically, venereal warts (condyloma lata and condyloma acuminata) occur near the genitalia and anus; however, the penile shaft is the most common site of lesions in men. Plantar warts (verruca plantaris) are common on the soles of the feet (see Color Plates, photograph 32).

Plantar warts are more common in older children, adolescents, and adults. They may be confined to the weight-bearing areas of the foot (the sole of the heel, the great toe, the areas below the heads of the metatarsal bones, and the ball), or they may occur in non–weight-bearing areas of the sole of the foot. Plantar warts, if located on weight-bearing portions of the foot, are under constant pressure and usually are not raised above the skin surface. The wart itself is in the center of the lesion and is roughly circular, with a diameter of 0.5 to 3.0 cm. The surface is usually grayish and friable, and the surrounding skin is thick and heaped. Several warts may coalesce and fuse, giving the appearance of one large wart (mosaic wart).

Calluses are also commonly found on weight-bearing areas of the foot. Because of their smooth keratotic surfaces, calluses may resemble isolated plantar warts. Therefore, the visual distinction between a wart and a callus is sometimes unclear. However, unlike a callus, a plantar wart is tender with pressure and interrupts the footprint pattern. Optimally, a podiatrist or dermatologist will assess the condition and make the differential diagnosis. To make this assessment, the primary care provider may shave away the outer keratinous surface to expose thrombosed capillaries in the papilloma, which appear as black dots or seeds. In instances in which the results of this procedure are inconclusive, a skin sample can be sent to a clinical laboratory to confirm or refute the presence of HPV.

Warts occasionally may be confused with more serious conditions, such as squamous cell carcinoma (SCC) and deep fungal infections. An SCC may develop rapidly, attaining a diameter of 1 cm within 2 weeks. The lesion generally appears as a small, red, conical, hard nodule that quickly ulcerates. Subungual verrucae, which occur under the nail plate, may exist in conjunction with periungual verrucae. A long-standing subungual verruca may be difficult to differentiate from an SCC, especially in patients of advanced age.

## Treatment of Warts

No specific effective therapy for curing warts is available although topical agents and procedures can relieve pain and sometimes help in removing warts. No single treatment is 100% effective, and different types of therapies may be combined.[10] However, self-care therapies should not be combined by the patient or his/her caregiver. Clinical presentation and response to treatment are used to guide therapy. Typically, warts will regress spontaneously in 2 to 3 years, so a valid management option is to do nothing if this is acceptable to the patient. However, the decision to treat is based on the desire for treatment; painful, bleeding, disfiguring, or disabling lesions; prevention of spread; and presence of warts in immunocompromised patients that could develop into SCC.[5]

### *Treatment Goals*

The goals in treating warts are to (1) remove the wart with no recurrence, (2) leave no scars, and (3) prevent autoinoculation or transmission of the HPV to other people.

### *General Treatment Approach*

Many practitioners believe that early and vigorous treatment of warts is best. The urgency for treatment is based on considerations such as the cosmetic effect (facial warts), the number of warts present in an area, the site of the wart (weight-bearing area of the foot), the age of the patient, financial considerations, and available treatment modalities. Prolonged treatment with nonprescription products may increase the chance of autoinoculation. Figure 44-1 outlines the treatment of warts and lists exclusions for self-treatment.

### *Nonpharmacologic Therapy*

To avoid the spread of warts, which are contagious, patients should wash their hands before and after treating or touching wart tissue. A specific towel should be used for drying only the affected area after cleaning. Patients should not probe, poke, or cut the wart tissue. If warts are present on the sole of the foot, patients should not walk in bare feet unless the wart is securely covered.

### *Pharmacologic Therapy*

#### Salicylic Acid

Topical salicylic acid in three different vehicles has been recognized as the only drug that is safe and effective for self-treatment of common or plantar warts: salicylic acid 12% to 40% in a plaster vehicle, salicylic acid 5% to 17% in a collodionlike vehicle, and salicylic acid 15% in a karaya gum–glycol plaster vehicle (Table 44-1).[11] (See the section Salicylic Acid in Chapter 45 for a discussion of this agent's properties.)

The Food and Drug Administration (FDA) recommends that topical salicylic acid products be labeled for treating only common and plantar warts. It excluded the other wart types from self-therapy because of the difficulty in recognizing and treating them without supervision by a primary care provider.[11] Indeed, painful plantar warts—as well as the other wart types listed in Figure 44-1—should all be treated by a primary care provider.[5,9,12]

**Exclusions for Self-Treatment**

- Face, toenails or fingernails, anus and/or genitalia involved
- Extensive warts at one body site
- Painful plantar warts
- One or more chronic, debilitating diseases (e.g., diabetes, peripheral vascular disease), which contraindicate use of foot care products
- Physical or mental impairments that make following product directions difficult
- Immunosuppressive medications or other medications (e.g., other salicylates) that contraindicate use of salicylic acid

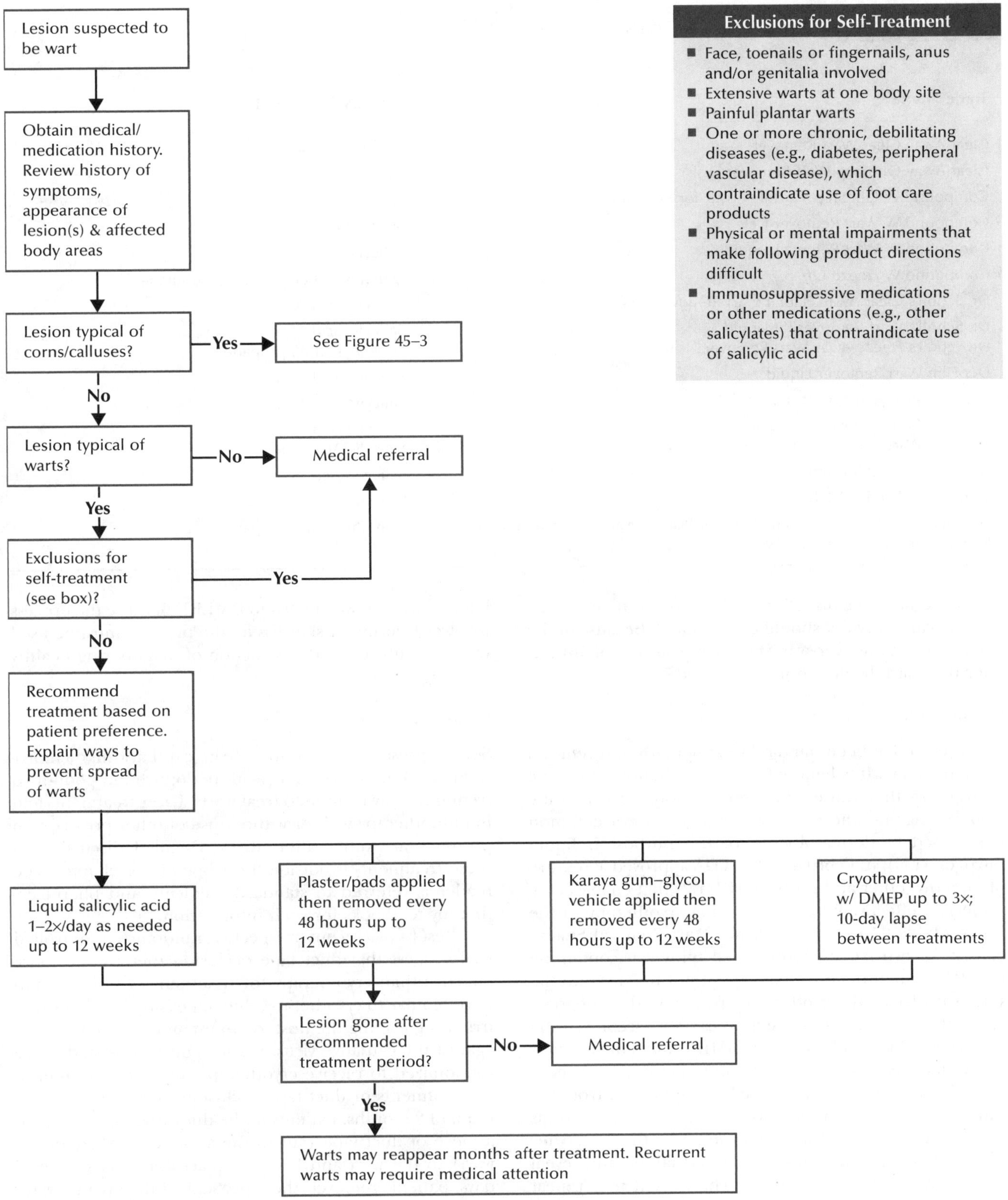

Lesion suspected to be wart
Obtain medical/ medication history. Review history of symptoms, appearance of lesion(s) & affected body areas
Lesion typical of corns/calluses?
Yes
See Figure 45–3
No
Lesion typical of warts?
No
Medical referral
Yes
Exclusions for self-treatment (see box)?
Yes
No
Recommend treatment based on patient preference. Explain ways to prevent spread of warts
Liquid salicylic acid 1–2×/day as needed up to 12 weeks
Plaster/pads applied then removed every 48 hours up to 12 weeks
Karaya gum–glycol vehicle applied then removed every 48 hours up to 12 weeks
Cryotherapy w/ DMEP up to 3×; 10-day lapse between treatments
Lesion gone after recommended treatment period?
No
Medical referral
Yes
Warts may reappear months after treatment. Recurrent warts may require medical attention

**FIGURE 44-1** Self-care of warts. Key: DMEP, dimethyl ether and propane.

In self-treatment of warts, patients should notice visible improvement within the first or second week of treatment; removal should be complete within 4 to 12 weeks of product use. Thus, selection of regular and convenient times to apply the product and adherence to the dosage regimen are important. Table 44-2 provides guidelines for using wart removal products that contain salicylic acid.

TABLE 44-1 Selected Products for Warts

| Trade Name | Primary Ingredient |
|---|---|
| Clear Away Clear Wart Remover | Salicylic acid 40% |
| Clear Away OneStep Wart Remover Disk | Salicylic acid 40% |
| Compound-W OneStep Wart Remover for Kids Pad | Salicylic acid 40% |
| Compound-W Wart Remover Gel | Salicylic acid 17% |
| Compound-W Wart Remover Liquid | Salicylic acid 17% |
| Compound W *Freeze Off* | Dimethyl ether; propane; isobutane |
| Dr. Scholl's Clear Away Plantar Wart Remover Disk | Salicylic acid 40% |
| Dr. Scholl's Wart Remover Kit Liquid | Salicylic acid 17% |
| Dr. Scholl's *Freeze Away* Wart Remover | Dimethyl ether, propane |
| DuoFilm Wart Remover Liquid | Salicylic acid 17% |
| DuoFilm Wart Remover Patch for Kids | Salicylic acid 40% |
| OFF-Ezy Wart Remover Kit Liquid | Salicylic acid 17% |
| Tinamed Wart Remover | Salicylic Acid 17% |
| Trans-Ver-Sal Adult Patch | Salicylic acid 15% |
| Trans-Ver-Sal Pedia Patch | Salicylic acid 15% |
| Wartner Wart Removal System; Wartner Plantar Wart Removal System, Kids Wartner Wart Removal System | Dimethyl ether; propane |

If the wart remains after a full course of treatment, a primary care provider should be consulted. Because of the latency factor, however, warts may reappear several months after they have been considered "cured."

## Cryotherapy

Cryotherapy has been standard treatment for wart removal for many years. It is believed to cause irritation and tissue destruction that causes the host to mount an immune response against the causative virus. The most common agent used by dermatologists for this purpose is liquid nitrogen (LN). In February 2002, FDA approved a mixture of dimethyl ether and propane (DMEP) that enables consumers to effectively treat warts using cryotherapy in the home (Table 44-1).[13] The Wartner Wart Removal System consists of two parts: a pressurized spray can containing the DMEP mixture and a foam applicator that fits into the spray can. To use the product, the patient pushes the foam applicator into the end of the spray can for 3 seconds using the provided key. Subsequently, DMEP enters the applicator, which becomes very cold (55°C [−131°F]). After 3 seconds, the patient removes the foam applicator from the can and holds it on the wart for no more than 20 seconds to freeze the wart. A blister will form under the wart. After about 10 days, the frozen skin and wart fall off and reveal newly formed skin underneath. The patient may repeat the process after 10 days using one of the remaining nine foam applicators. A persistent wart can be treated only three times. The spray can contains enough DMEP for 10 treatments.[14] Table 44-3 provides guidelines for using the Wartner Wart Removal system. Similar guidelines with minor procedural differences exist for other cryotherapy products. Studies have shown little difference in treatment effectiveness between LN and DMEP.[15] Because the process involves freezing of skin tissue, the product must be used very carefully to avoid destruction of neighboring healthy tissue.

## Other Therapies

Several prescription products (e.g., cantharidin, dichloroacetic acid, trichloroacetic acid, podophyllum, podofilox, tretinoin) may be used to treat warts. Laser treatments and immunotherapy with or without use of other prescription products are other alternatives. Detailed discussion of these treatments is outside the scope of this chapter. The reader is referred to standard medicine and pharmacotherapy textbooks for such information.[16-18]

Results of a recent prospective, randomized controlled trial suggest that duct tape occlusion therapy was more effective than cryotherapy for treatment of the common wart. Similar to cryotherapy, duct tape is believed to cause irritation, leading the host to mount an immune response against the causative virus. Participants in this study were randomized to receive cryotherapy up to a maximum of six treatments or duct tape occlusion therapy for a maximum of 2 months. Patients in the duct tape group applied a piece of duct tape (cut to the approximate size of the wart) to the wart and left it in place for 6 days. After 6 days, patients removed the tape, soaked the area in water and gently debrided the wart with a pumice stone. They then left the tape off overnight and reapplied it the following morning. Treatment was continued until the wart was removed or up to a maximum of 2 months. At the conclusion of the study, 85% of patients in the duct tape group had complete resolution of their warts. In contrast, only 60% of patients who received cryotherapy realized

**TABLE 44-2 Guidelines for Treating Warts With Salicylic Acid Products**

- Wash and dry affected area before applying the salicylic acid product.

**Salicylic Acid 5%-17% in Collodion Vehicle**

- Apply product to wart no more often than twice daily. Morning and evening are usually the most convenient times.
- Apply solution 1 drop at a time until affected area is covered. Do not overuse the product.
- If the medication touches healthy skin, wash it off immediately with soap and water.
- Allow the solution to harden so that it does not run. Repeat this procedure as needed for up to 12 weeks.
- After use, cap the container tightly to prevent evaporation and the active ingredients from assuming a greater concentration.
- Store product in an amber or light-resistant container away from direct sunlight or heat.

**Salicylic Acid 12%-40% Plaster/Pads**

- If using plaster, trim it to follow the contours of the wart. Apply plaster to the skin, and cover it with adhesive occlusive tape.
- If using disks with pads, apply appropriately sized disk directly on the affected area, and cover disk with the pad.
- Apply and remove plasters and pads every 48 hours as needed for up to 12 weeks.

**Salicylic Acid 15% in Karaya Gum–Glycol Vehicle**

- Apply plaster to wart at bedtime, and leave it on for at least 8 hours.
- Remove and discard plaster in the morning.
- Repeat this procedure every 24 hours as needed for up to 12 weeks.

complete resolution, a statistically significant difference ($p \leq .05$) Noncompliance and adverse effects were also less common in patients who received duct tape occlusion therapy.[19]

The use of oral cimetidine for treatment of warts remains controversial.[5] No studies have demonstrated its efficacy although there was a trend of efficacy in younger patients in one study. However, the best response to cimetidine was observed in younger patients who received 40 mg/kg/day. However, this dose may exceed the FDA-approved maximum of 2400 mg/day, and FDA does not recommend cimetidine use in children younger than 16 years.[5]

## Assessment of Warts: A Case-based Approach

When assessing a patient with warts, the practitioner should inspect the lesion, if possible, to determine its suitability for self-treatment. The patient's age, health status (especially immunologic status), and use of medications for other disorders should be factored into the choice of treatment. The practitioner should ask whether and how the patient has self-treated the disorder. The answers to

**TABLE 44-3 Guidelines for Treating Warts With Wartner Wart Removal System**

- Hold foam applicator on blue section between thumb and index finger and squeeze until a small opening appears.
- Remove holder from bag of applicators. Slide opening of foam applicator over the stick of the holder until the stick is no longer visible.
- Place holder with foam applicator in opening on top of cap so that foam applicator is no longer visible.
- Place aerosol spray can on a table or sturdy surface. CAUTION! Do not hold the spray can near your face or over parts of your body or clothing!
- Holding can firmly at the bottom, press down valve strongly for 2 to 3 seconds. You will hear a hissing sound.
- Remove holder with foam applicator from valve. Foam applicator is saturated with cold liquid and condensation will form. This condensation is harmless.
- Leave foam applicator on holder and then lightly place tip of foam applicator on the wart that is to be frozen. Apply foam applicator to area for no more than 20 seconds. Adjust the exact time depending on size of the wart and thickness of the skin. There will be an aching, stinging sensation. Discard foam applicator after a single use.
- Do not use this system to remove skin growths other than common warts. Do not use on genital warts, or warts on mucous membranes, face, nose, lips, ears, or near eyes. Do not use on warts on thin skin such as armpits, breasts, buttocks, or genitals, or on warts in places that you cannot see well, such as your back.
- Do not use on warts in children younger than 4 years, pregnant or breast-feeding women, or patients with diabetes or poor blood circulation.

these questions will help in evaluating expected compliance with self-treatment of the wart. Other important considerations before initiating treatment are the pain, inconvenience, and risk of scarring from the treatment. Table 44-4 illustrates differentiation of warts from other disorders with similar presentation. Cases 44-1 and 44-2 provide examples of assessment of patients with warts.

## Patient Counseling for Warts

Patients must understand that, unlike corns and calluses, warts are contagious and can spread to other parts of the body unless proper precautions are taken. The practitioner should point out differences in salicylic acid products used to treat warts and their proper application. Practitioners should stress contraindications, warnings, and precautions for topical salicylic acid to prevent the wart from progressing to a more serious disorder. The box Patient Education for Warts lists specific information to provide patients.

## Evaluation of Patient Outcomes for Warts

Because wart removal can take from 4 to 12 weeks, the practitioner should schedule the first follow-up on the patient's progress after 4 weeks of treatment. If the wart is still present, the patient should be reminded of proper administration procedures and advised to continue the

**TABLE 44-4 Differentiation of Corns, Calluses, and Warts**

| Criterion | Corns | Calluses | Warts |
|---|---|---|---|
| Location | Usually over bony prominences of fourth and fifth toes with hard corns occurring on tops of toes and soft corns in toe webs | Usually over weight-bearing areas of foot | Anywhere virus can gain entry into skin |
| Signs | Raised, sharply demarcated, hyperkeratotic lesion with central core; hard corns are shiny and soft corns are white | Raised, yellowish lesions with irregular margins and diffuse thickening of skin; may be broad based or have central core; no disruption of normal skin ridges | Slightly scaly, rough papules or nodules, cauliflowerlike in appearance; may occur alone or in groups; plantar warts disrupt normal skin ridges |
| Symptoms | Pain | Pain | Pain if warts appear on weight-bearing areas of foot |
| Quantity/severity | Varies from few millimeters to 1 cm | Varies from few millimeters to several centimeters | Varies from few millimeters to 3 cm |
| Timing | Variable onset; lesions may progressively enlarge | Variable onset; lesions may progressively enlarge | 1- to 24-month incubation period after inoculation, with average of 3-4 months |
| Cause | Friction from tight-fitting hosiery/shoes | Friction from tight- fitting hosiery/shoes; walking barefoot; structural biomechanical problems | Human papilloma viruses |
| Modifying factors | Well-fitted hosiery/footwear relieve signs and symptoms | Well-fitted hosiery/footwear relieve signs and symptoms | Cryotherapy or salicylic acid; proper hygiene |

**CASE 44-1**

| Relevant Evaluation Criteria | Scenario/Model Outcome |
|---|---|
| **Information Gathering** | |
| 1. Gather essential information about the patient's symptoms, including: | |
| a. description of symptom(s) (i.e., nature, onset, duration, severity, associated symptoms) | The patient points to a growth on her right upper arm and asks if she can buy a medication to treat the problem. She goes on to say she first noticed the wart about a month ago. She says it really does not bother her, but she is concerned it may be serious. The lesion consists of a single papule, roughly 0.5 cm in diameter. The lesion is flesh colored and has a rough, scaly surface. No inflammation, discharge, or bleeding is present. |
| b. description of any factors that seem to precipitate, exacerbate, and/or relieve the patient's symptom(s) | The patient cannot think of anything that improves or worsens the condition. |
| c. description of the patient's efforts to relieve the symptoms | The patient has been attempting to clear the lesion with Polysporin Antibiotic Ointment for the past 4 days. However, the ointment does not appear to be working. |
| 2. Gather essential patient history information: | |
| a. patient's identity | Courtney Minor |
| b. age, sex, height, and weight | 20 y/o F |
| c. patient's occupation | College student; part-time medical assistant |

## CASE 44-1 (continued)

| Relevant Evaluation Criteria | Scenario/Model Outcome |
|---|---|
| d. patient's dietary habits | Generally healthy |
| e. patient's sleep habits | 6-8 hours per night |
| f. concurrent medical conditions, prescription and nonprescription medications, and dietary supplements | One-A-Day Women's Formula vitamin tablet each morning |
| g. allergies | NKA |
| h. history of other adverse reactions to medications | None |
| i. other (describe)_______ | Courtney is putting herself through nursing school and is on an extremely tight budget. She lives alone in a mobile home she inherited when her aunt died, but she sometimes has trouble even paying for utilities. |
| **Assessment and Triage** | |
| 3. Differentiate the patient's signs/symptoms and correctly identify the patient's primary problem(s) (see Table 44-4). | Courtney is suffering from an uncomplicated common wart secondary to infection with a human papillomavirus. |
| 4. Identify exclusions for self-treatment (see Figure 44-1). | None |
| **Plan** | |
| 5. Formulate a comprehensive list of therapeutic alternatives for the primary problem to determine if triage to a medical practitioner is required, and share this information with the patient. | Options include:<br>(1) Refer Courtney to an appropriate health care professional.<br>(2) Recommend self-care with a nonprescription wart removal product and nondrug measures.<br>(3) Recommend self-care until Courtney can consult an appropriate health care professional.<br>(4) Take no action. |
| 6. Select an optimal therapeutic alternative to address the patient's problem, taking into account patient preferences. | Because of her financial constraints, Courtney prefers to simply observe the lesion for any growth or changes until it resolves on its own. |
| 7. Describe the recommended therapeutic approach to the patient. | Observe the wart for changes in size, texture, and color over the next several months, and take steps to prevent spreading the virus to other parts of the body. See the box Patient Education for Warts. |
| 8. Explain to the patient the rationale for selecting the recommended therapeutic approach from the considered therapeutic alternatives. | This option is superior to treatment with an expensive nonprescription wart removal product for the following reasons. Almost all warts resolve spontaneously over a period of 6 months to 5 years. The wart is in an inconspicuous area and is not causing distress. You live alone, so the risk of spreading the wart to other individuals is minimal. Your tight budget would be spared the extra expense of the wart removal product. |
| **Patient Education** | |
| 9. When recommending self-care with nonprescription medications and/or nondrug therapy, convey accurate information to the patient, including: | Criterion does not apply in this case. |
| 10. Solicit follow-up questions from patient. | What should I do if the wart changes in color or size? |
| 11. Answer patient's questions. | Consult your primary care provider as soon as possible. |

Key: NKA, no known allergies.

## CASE 44-2

| Relevant Evaluation Criteria | Scenario/Model Outcome |
|---|---|
| **Information Gathering** | |
| 1. Gather essential information about the patient's symptoms, including: | |
| a. description of symptom(s) (i.e., nature, onset, duration, severity, associated symptoms) | Patient asks for something to get rid of a callus on the bottom of his foot that has become increasingly painful. The callus started out about the size of a pencil eraser 6 months ago, but has enlarged to the size of a quarter. The pain has prevented him from participating in pick-up basketball games at the gym for the past week. He describes the pain as "constantly walking with a large stone in my shoe." The lesion is on the ball of the foot and is flat, whitish, and approximately 1 in. in diameter. It also appears to be a coalescence of four smaller lesions; the normal pattern of skin ridges is interrupted within the lesion. No inflammation, discharge, or bleeding is present. |
| b. description of any factors that seem to precipitate, exacerbate, and/or relieve the patient's symptom(s) | Patient cannot think of anything that improves or worsens the condition. |
| c. description of the patient's efforts to relieve the symptoms | Patient attempted to shave off part of the lesion with a razor blade, but that only seemed to cause the lesion to enlarge. |
| 2. Gather essential patient history information: | |
| a. patient's identity | Bryan Hammond |
| b. age, weight, sex, and height | 37 y/o M |
| c. patient's occupation | Sales representative |
| d. patient's dietary habits | High carbohydrate |
| e. patient's sleep habits | 7 hours per night |
| f. concurrent medical conditions, prescription and nonprescription medications, and dietary supplements | Dyazide 50 mg once daily for mild hypertension; Imitrex tablets 25mg as needed for migraine relief |
| g. allergies | NKA |
| h. history of other adverse reactions to medications | None |
| i. other (describe)_______ | Recently, Brian was divorced. Until a few months ago, he played basketball at the gym 4 times each week and used the public shower at the gym afterward. |
| **Assessment and Triage** | |
| 3. Differentiate the patient's signs/symptoms and correctly identify the patient's primary problem(s) (see Table 44-4). | Brian is suffering from multiple, debilitating plantar warts secondary to infection with human papillomavirus that he likely contracted in the gym shower. |
| 4. Identify exclusions for self-treatment (see Figure 44-1). | None |
| **Plan** | |
| 5. Formulate a comprehensive list of therapeutic alternatives for the primary problem to determine if triage to a medical practitioner is required, and share this information with the patient. | Options include:<br>(1) Refer Brian to an appropriate health care professional.<br>(2) Recommend self-care with a nonprescription wart removal product and nondrug measures.<br>(3) Recommend self-care until Brian can consult an appropriate health care professional.<br>(4) Take no action. |
| 6. Select an optimal therapeutic alternative to address the patient's problem, taking into account patient preferences. | Brian should consult a health care professional to treat his problem because the multiple warts seem to have coalesced into one. |

## CASE 44-2 (continued)

| Relevant Evaluation Criteria | Scenario/Model Outcome |
|---|---|
| 7. Describe the recommended therapeutic approach to the patient. | You should consult a health care professional for treatment. |
| 8. Explain to the patient the rationale for selecting the recommended therapeutic approach from the considered therapeutic alternatives. | This option is superior because you have multiple warts that are causing symptoms that interfere with your normal activity. |
| **Patient Education** | |
| 9. When recommending self-care with nonprescription medications and/or nondrug therapy, convey accurate information to the patient, including: | Criterion does not apply in this case. |
| 10. Solicit follow-up questions from patient. | Is there anything else I can do to keep from getting this condition? |
| 11. Answer patient's questions. | Yes. See the box Patient Education for Warts. |

Key: NKA, no known allergies.

## PATIENT EDUCATION FOR WARTS

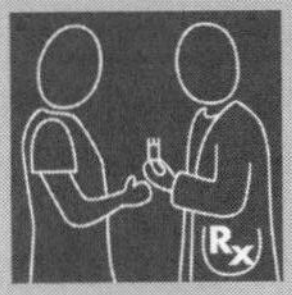

The objectives of self-treatment are to (1) remove the wart with no recurrence, (2) leave no scars, (3) induce lifelong immunity, and (4) prevent spread of warts to other parts of the body or other people. For most patients, carefully following product instructions and the self-care measures listed here will help to ensure optimal therapeutic outcomes.

### Nondrug Measures

- To avoid spreading warts, wash your hands before and after treating or touching warts.
- Use a specific towel for drying only the affected area after cleansing. Use a separate towel to dry other parts of the body.
- Do not probe, poke, or cut the wart.
- If warts are present on the sole of the foot, do not walk in bare feet unless the wart is securely covered.

### Nonprescription Medications

- Be sure to use only topical salicylic products that are labeled for use on warts (see Table 44-1). Table 44-2 describes proper methods for applying the products.
- Treat only common or plantar warts with these agents. Ask your practitioner or primary care provider to identify the type of wart if you are unsure. Do not apply the medication to warts on the face, genitals, toenails, or fingernails, or around the anus.
- Do not use this product on irritated skin or on any area that is infected or reddened.
- Do not use this product if you have diabetes or poor circulation.
- Salicylic acid is caustic. Do not allow it to come in contact with the mouth, and keep it out of children's reach.
- Note that the medication sloughs off skin and initially leaves an unsightly pinkish tinge to the skin.
- Expect to see visible improvement within the first or second week of treatment; expect to see complete removal of the wart within 4 to 12 weeks of product use.
- Note that warts may reappear months after the initial treatment.

⚠ Stop treatment and consult a primary care provider or podiatrist if swelling, reddening, or irritation of the skin occurs, or if pain occurs immediately when applying the product.

⚠ If the wart remains after 12 weeks of treatment, consult a primary care provider.

treatment. Reevaluation every 4 weeks is appropriate for persistent warts. The practitioner should refer the patient to a primary care provider for any warts that persist after 12 weeks of self-treatment.

## Key Points for Warts

- Historically, the nonprescription drug of choice to treat common and plantar warts was salicylic acid in a collodionlike vehicle or plaster product form, whichever is more convenient.

- Plantar warts should be treated with a higher concentration of salicylic acid (up to 40%); warts on thin epidermis require a lower concentration (up to 17%).
- Because warts are usually self-limiting, treatment should be conservative; vigorous therapy with salicylic acid may scar tissue.
- To minimize noncompliance, the practitioner should advise patients that alleviation of the symptoms should not be expected to occur overnight.
- Patients should also be cautioned that frequent recurrence of any of these problems indicates they should consult a podiatrist or primary care provider.
- The introduction of DMEP products enables consumers to effectively treat common and plantar warts using cryotherapy in the home.
- Consumers should be careful and follow directions when using these products as injury to normal, adjacent skin can occur with product misuse.
- Patients with diabetes, circulatory problems, immunodeficiencies, and/or arthritis should not to self-medicate with any topical nonprescription drug without first checking with their primary care provider, podiatrist, or other health care practitioner.

## References


1. Rothman KF, Bernhard JD. Warts. In: Gorbach SL, Bartlett JG, Zorab R, et al., eds. *Infectious Diseases.* Philadelphia: WB Saunders; 1998:1329-33.
2. Wanek EL, Pray WS. Warts: more than a minor nuisance. *US Pharm.* 1996;21:122-7.
3. Williams HC, Pottier A, Strachan D. The descriptive epidemiology of warts in British schoolchildren. *Br J Dermatol.* 1993;128: 504-11.
4. Janniger CK. Childhood warts. *Cutis.* 1992;50:15-6.
5. Berman B, Weinstein A. Treatment of warts. *Dermatologic Therapy.* 2000;13:290-304.
6. Melton JL, Rasmussen JE. Clinical manifestations of human papillomavirus infection in nongenital sites. *Dermatol Clin.* 1991;9: 219-33.
7. Johnson LW. Communal showers and the risk of plantar warts. *J Fam Pract.* 1995;40:136-8.
8. Bolton RA. Nongenital warts: classification and treatment options. *Am Fam Pract.* 1991;43:2049-56.
9. Sterling JC, Handfield-Jones S, Hudson PM. Guidelines for the management of cutaneous warts. *Br J Dermatol* 2001;144:4-11.
10. Gibbs S, Harvey I, Sterling J, et al. Local treatments for cutaneous warts: systematic review. *BMJ* 2002;325:461-9.
11. *Federal Register.* 1990;55:33246-56.
12. Goldfarb MT, Gupta AK, Gupta MA, et al. Office therapy for human papillomavirus infection in nongenital sites. *Dermatol Clin.* 1991;9:287-96.
13. Center for Drug Evaluation and Research New Device Clearance for: Application Number: K011708, Trade Name: Wartner Wart Removal System, Sponsor: Wartner Medical Products, Approval Date: February 20, 2002. Available at: http://www.fda.gov/cder/pdf/K011708.pdf. Accessed April 24, 2003.
14. Wartner Medical Products. Available at: http://www.wartner.com. Accessed April 24, 2003.
15. Caballero MF, Plaza NC, Perez CC, et al. Cutaneous cryosurgery in family medicine: dimethyl ether-propane spray *versus* liquid nitrogen. *Aten Primaria.*1996;18:211-6.
16. DiPiro JT, Talbert RL, Yee GC, eds. *Pharmacotherapy: A Pathophysiologic Approach.* 4th ed. Stamford, Conn: Appleton & Lange; 1999.
17. Conn F, ed. *Current Therapy.* Philadelphia: W.B. Saunders; 1997.
18. Fauci AS, Braunwald E, Isselbacher J, eds. *Harrison's Principles of Internal Medicine.* 14th ed. New York: McGraw-Hill Health Professions Division; 1998.
19. Focht DR, Spicer C, Fairchiok MP. The efficacy of duct tape vs cryotherapy in the treatment of verruca vulgaris (the common wart). *Arch Pediatr Adolesc Med.* 2002;156: 971-4.

CHAPTER 45

# Minor Foot Disorders

*Cynthia W. Coffey and Karla T. Foster*

On average, a person walks 115,000 miles in a lifetime, which is equivalent to circling the world nearly four times. Approximately 80% of Americans will have some type of foot disorder during their lifetime.[1] Sales of foot care products in the United States currently exceed $500 million per year. The five most common groups of foot disorders are heel/arch pain; corns, calluses, and plantar warts; athlete's foot (see Chapter 44); tired, aching feet; and ingrown toenails. Historically, Americans have used more than just commercially available products for foot disorders, including such harmful self-care practices as scraping or cutting corns and calluses, opening blisters or removing the skin cover, improperly trimming toenails, and (among patients with diabetes) inappropriately using hot water to clean and bathe/soak the feet. Thus, a significant need exists to educate patients about foot care, including appropriate self-treatment measures. The prevalence of foot problems increases as people age because of the lack of proper care. One of the primary causes of decreased mobility in persons of advanced age is damage of the legs and feet, which may be prevented with proper care.[2]

Instruction in proper foot care, including the selection of well-fitting footwear, should begin at an early age when good health habits can be nurtured. Health care practitioners can serve as a valuable resource in this regard.[2,3]

In some instances, foot disorders or inappropriate foot care practices may be life threatening to patients with diabetes, severe arthritis, and impaired circulation[4] (see box A Word About Chronic Diseases and Foot Disorders). Foot disorders may indicate serious underlying conditions. For most patients, however, such problems cause only a substantial measure of discomfort and impaired mobility.

## EPIDEMIOLOGY OF FOOT DISORDERS

Three distinct groups of patients often encounter foot problems. First are children with a congenital malformation or deformity or a specific disease that affects the foot (e.g., juvenile arthritis). These patients need special shoes and foot care overseen by an orthopedic surgeon or podiatrist. Second are adolescents who experience rapid growth. Growth plates in their feet may become stressed and irritated. Athletic activity at this age can also contribute to problems, especially if associated injuries to the feet are not properly treated. Osteoarthritis, for example, can occur secondary to a foot injury. The third group is made up of older patients who encounter foot problems because of aging (as the foot assumes its final shape) and disease. In particular, diabetes mellitus and arthritis can cause secondary foot problems.

An estimated 15% to 20% of the 16 million patients with diabetes will be hospitalized with a foot complication during the course of their disease.[5] Foot problems such as ulceration and infection can ultimately lead to gangrene, amputation of the foot/ankle, and even death. These problems are the leading causes of hospitalization for patients with diabetes. Diabetes contributes to 50% of nontraumatic lower-extremity amputations. Treating a patient with a foot ulcer can cost $28,000 without amputation and up to $34,000 in a patient requiring amputation.[6]

Individuals who exercise regularly are also at risk for foot disorders. Since the 1980s, society's attitude toward physical fitness and body awareness has changed dramatically. Millions of people exercise every day; jogging, running, and aerobic exercising are methods used most often to remain or get "in shape." Without adequate precautions, however, problems can arise, particularly involving the feet. Women are four times more likely than men to experience foot disorders. This is a result of chronically wearing improperly fitting shoes and dress shoes with high heels.

## ANATOMY AND PHYSIOLOGY OF THE FOOT

At birth, an infant's foot has 33 joints, 19 muscles, 107 ligaments, and cartilage that will develop into 26 bones. These small components continue to develop and mature until age 14 to 16 years for females and age 15 to 21 years for males. Women will generally begin to notice changes in their feet in their 40s; men, in their 50s.[9] After years of bearing the body's weight, the feet tend to broaden and flatten, thus stretching ligaments and causing bones to shift positions. These changes subject the feet to stress, which is compounded by prolonged standing. An estimated 40% of the U.S. population spends about 75% of their workday on their feet, increasing the potential for painful foot conditions.

**Editor's Note:** This chapter is based, in part, on the 14th edition chapter with the same title, which was written by Gail D. Newton and Nicholas G. Popovich.

## A WORD ABOUT
## Chronic Diseases and Foot Disorders

Some chronic diseases predispose certain patients to foot complications. Patients who have diabetes often have poor circulation and diminished limb sensitivity, and are especially vulnerable to infectious foot problems. Other susceptible patients include those with peripheral circulatory disease or arthritis. The practitioner can identify such patients by asking about daily medication use or reviewing the patient's drug profile. Typical drug-use patterns for high-risk patients include insulin, oral antidiabetic drugs (e.g., glipizide, glyburide, metformin, acarbose, nateglinide), drugs for circulation (e.g., cyclandelate, isoxsuprine, papaverine, and pentoxifylline), drugs used for neuropathic pain (e.g., gabapentin and duloxetine), and drugs for arthritic conditions (e.g., aspirin and NSAIDs).

Self-treatment with nonprescription products, if not properly supervised in patients with impaired circulation, may induce more inflammation, ulceration, or even gangrene, particularly in cases of vascular insufficiency in the foot. Patients with diabetes and those with peripheral circulatory impairments are particularly susceptible to gangrene. In addition, simple lesions may mask more serious abscesses or ulcerations. If left medically unattended, such lesions may lead to such conditions as osteomyelitis, which may require hospitalization and aggressive parenteral antibiotic therapy. If exostoses associated with corns are not excised by a primary care provider or podiatrist, the corns will persist.

### Diabetes Mellitus

Patients who have poorly controlled diabetes are at greater risk for lower extremity complications, which results in increased health care costs as well as decreased quality of life and increased morbidity.[7] Two major causes of foot ulcerations are peripheral neuropathy, which results in loss of injury perception, and excessive plantar pressure, which contributes to decreased mobility and foot deformities.[6] Patients with diabetes also contribute to foot complications by poor foot hygiene such as extreme hot water soaks, inappropriate footwear, and lack of daily foot self-exams. Patients with diabetes need to be educated on proper foot care such as appropriate toenail trimming, avoidance of creams/lotions between the toes, keeping socks clean and dry, and foot examinations at home and at the health care provider's office. (See Chapter 47 for further discussion of proper foot care and for potentially serious foot disorders in patients with diabetes.)

### Peripheral Vascular Disease

Patients with peripheral vascular disease often have poor circulation of the feet and legs. Because of decreased blood flow and low oxygen perfusion, ulcerations and decreased wound heeling may be problematic.[8] They may complain of persistent and unusual feelings of cold, numbness, tingling, burning, or fatigue. Other symptoms may include discolored skin, dry skin, absence of hair on the feet or legs, or a cramping or tightness in the leg muscles. The clinician should also palpate for pedal pulses. The most discriminating questions that a practitioner can ask this type of patient are (1) Do you experience aching in your calves when you walk? and (2) Do you have to hang your feet over the edge of the bed during sleep to relieve the soreness in your calves? A "yes" response to either question warrants referring the patient to a primary care provider or podiatrist.

Localized redness or unilateral coldness may indicate a possible blockage (a clot) of circulation to the foot. Sometimes the involved foot or lower leg will appear physically larger than the other, may be red or waxy in appearance, may have no hair growth on the toes, and will exhibit thickened nails. If the patient's medication history does not indicate the use of medications intended to relieve such symptoms, the practitioner should advise the patient with suspected circulatory problems to consult a primary care provider or podiatrist for evaluation immediately.

A daily footbath is a simple measure to assist these patients. After the foot is patted dry, an emollient foot cream can be applied to aid in retaining moisture and pliability. The footbath will also soften brittle toenails for clipping and filing. The feet should be kept warm and moderately exercised every day.

### Arthritis

Osteoarthritis is a noninflammatory, degenerative joint disease that occurs primarily in older people. Degeneration of the articular cartilage and changes in the bone result in a loss of resilience and a decrease in the skeleton's shock-absorption capability. This condition, however, is also experienced by individuals in their late teens and early 20s as a secondary complication of a previous athletic injury. This condition might be evidenced by the development of hallux limitus or rigidus of the big toe (i.e., a stiff toe or painful flexion or extension of the big toe because of stiffness and spur formation in the metatarsophalangeal joint). Subsequently, these patients have a lot of difficulty with their shoes not fitting properly. They may also develop an osteoarthritic condition in the ankle joint. Referral for further evaluation is appropriate.

Most patients with rheumatoid arthritis eventually have foot involvement. The major forefoot deformities in these patients are painful metatarsal heads, hallux valgus, and clawfoot. Corrective surgical procedures are often indicated to reduce pain and improve function and mobility. Little evidence exists that conventional nonsurgical therapy (e.g., orthopedic shoes, metatarsal inserts, conventional arch supports, and metatarsal bars) is effective in such cases.

Proper palliative foot care is especially important for arthritic patients. They should wear properly fitted shoes, pad their shoes with insoles to protect their feet from the shock of hard surfaces, and undergo regular podiatric or medical examinations. (See Chapter 7 for use of topical or systemic nonprescription analgesics for osteoarthritis.)

## CORNS AND CALLUSES

Although corns and calluses are common foot disorders, they should not be ignored. They may indicate a biomechanical problem in the feet or lead to serious complications in predisposed patients.

### Etiology/Pathophysiology of Corns and Calluses

Under normal conditions, the cells in the skin's basal cell layer undergo mitotic division at a rate equal to the continual surface cellular desquamation, leading to complete replacement of the epidermis in approximately 1 month.

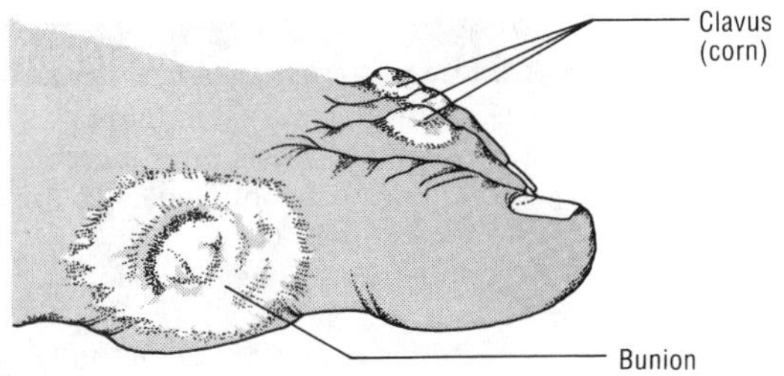


FIGURE 45-1 Disorders affecting top of foot.

During corn or callus development, however, friction and pressure increase mitotic activity of the basal cell layer, leading to the migration of maturing cells through the prickle cell (stratum spinosum) and granular (stratum granulosum) skin layers. This migration produces a thicker stratum corneum (hyperkeratosis) as more cells reach the outer skin surface, which is a natural protective mechanism of the skin surface. This process may signal a biomechanical problem and cause abnormal weight distribution in a particular area of the foot. In this case, a podiatric examination is warranted to determine whether an imbalance is present. When friction or pressure is relieved, mitotic activity returns to normal, causing remission and disappearance of the lesion.

## Signs and Symptoms of Corns and Calluses

Corns and calluses are similar in one respect: both produce a marked hyperkeratosis of the stratum corneum. Besides this one feature, however, there are marked differences. Table 44-4 in Chapter 44 differentiates the signs and symptoms of warts, corns, and calluses.

### *Corns*

A corn (clavus) is a small, raised, sharply demarcated, hyperkeratotic lesion with a central core caused by pressure from underlying bony prominences (Figure 45-1). The central core of the corn differentiates it from a wart (see Chapter 44, Table 44-4). Misidentification of warts and corns is common. A clinician can identify a corn by shaving the central core. A corn has a hard center and a wart will bleed because of multiple capillary loops.[10] Corns are yellowish gray with diameters ranging from a few millimeters to 1 cm or more. The base of the corn is on the skin surface; its apex points inward and presses on the nerve endings in the dermis, causing pain.

There are two types of corns—hard and soft. Hard corns (heloma durum) are most prevalent, usually occurring on the surface of the fourth or fifth toes, and appear shiny, dry, and polished. Soft corns (heloma molle) are whitish thickenings of the skin and may be extremely painful. Accumulated perspiration macerates the epidermis, giving the corn a soft appearance. Soft corns may occur between any adjacent toes, but are most frequently found between the fourth and fifth toe because the fifth metatarsal is much shorter than the fourth, and the Web between these toes is deeper and extends more proximally than the webs between the other toes.[9,11]

A bony spur, or exostosis (a bony tumor in the form of an ossified muscular or ligamentous attachment to the bone surface), nearly always exists between long-lasting hard and soft corns. Corns are the lesions usually located over non–weight-bearing bony prominences or joints, the bulb of the great toe, the dorsum of the fifth toe, or the tips of the middle toes.[9]

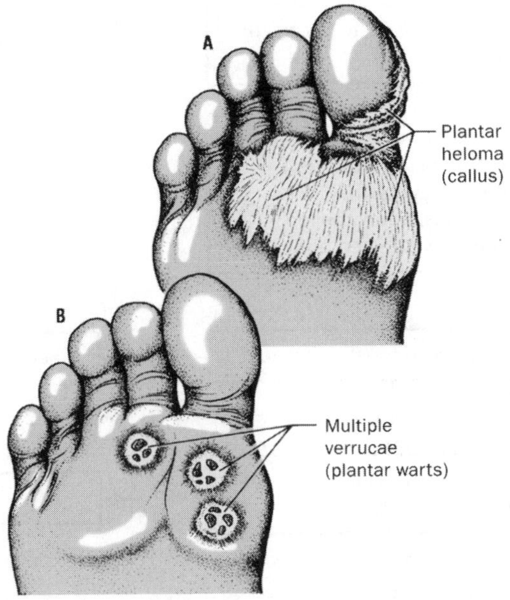


FIGURE 45-2 Disorders affecting sole of foot. **A,** Plantar tyloma (callus). **B,** Multiple verrucae (plantar wart).

Pressure from inappropriate, tight-fitting shoes is the most frequent cause of pain from corns. As narrow-toed or high-heeled shoes crowd toes into a narrow toe box, the most lateral toe, the fifth, sustains the most pressure and friction and is the usual site of a corn. The resultant pain may be severe and sharp (when downward pressure is applied) or dull and discomforting. Consumer research approximates that 82% of women ages 35 to 54 years suffer moderate to intense pain from corns and that 35% are consequently limited or restricted in their activities.

### *Calluses*

A callus has a broad base with relatively even thickening of skin generally found on the bottom of the foot in areas such as the heel, ball of the foot, toes, and sides of the foot (Figure 45-2). It has indefinite borders and ranges from a few millimeters to several centimeters in diameter. The indefinite borders help clinicians differentiate calluses from well-circumscribed margins of corns. It is usually raised and yellow, and it has a normal pattern of skin ridges on its surface. Calluses form on joints and weight-bearing areas of the hands and feet (see Color Plates, photograph 33).[11-13]

Friction (caused by loose-fitting shoes or tight-fitting hosiery), walking barefoot, and structural biomechanical problems contribute to the development of calluses. Structural problems include improper weight distribution, pressure, and development of bunions with age. Calluses can be symptomatic and protective.

Diffuse-shearing and discrete-nucleated are two types of calluses. The discrete-nucleated callus is smaller and has a localized translucent center; this type of callus is painful

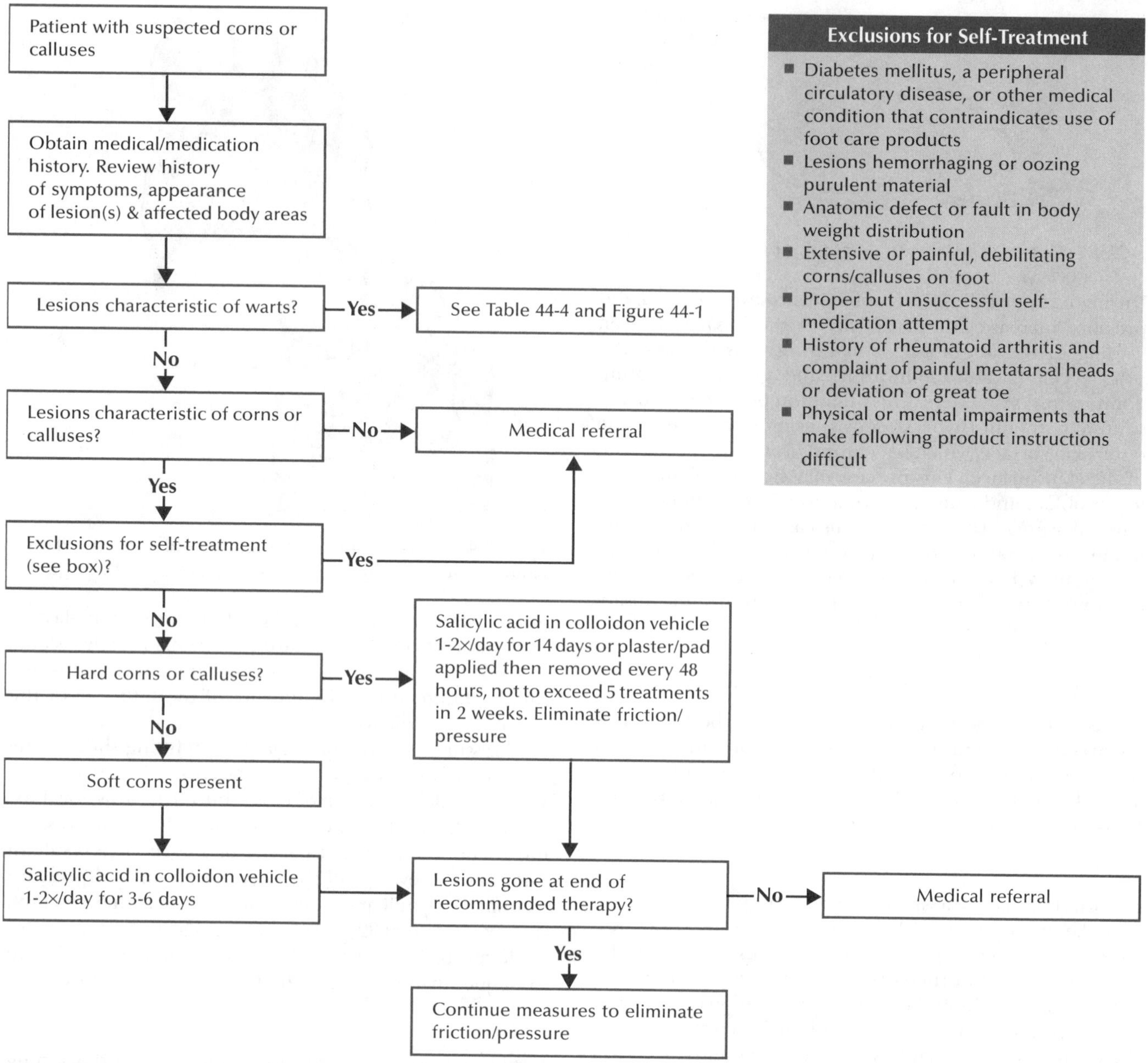


**FIGURE 45-3** Self-care of corns and calluses.

with applied pressure. The diffuse-shearing callus covers a larger surface area and does not have a central core.[11,12]

## Treatment of Corns and Calluses

### *Treatment Goals*

The goals of self-treatment are to (1) provide symptomatic relief, (2) remove corns and calluses, and (3) prevent their recurrence by correcting underlying causes.

### *General Treatment Approach*

Although effective nonprescription products are available for removing corns and calluses, ultimate success depends on eliminating the causes such as pressure and friction. The algorithm in Figure 45-3 outlines self-treatment of corns and calluses and lists exclusions for self-treatment.

### *Nonpharmacologic Therapy*

Nondrug adjunctive measures include daily soaking of the affected area throughout treatment for at least 5 minutes in warm (not hot) water to assist in removal of dead tissue. Dead tissue should be removed gently rather than forcibly after normal washing to avoid further damage. A rough towel, callus file, or pumice stone effectively accomplishes this purpose. These instruments for removing dead skin should be kept clean to avoid autoinoculating oneself at another body focus. Sharp knives or razor blades should not be used because they may cause bacterial contamination and infection.

To relieve painful pressure emanating from inflamed underlying tissue and irritated or hypertrophied bones directly underneath a corn or callus, patients may use a pad such as a Dr. Scholl's with an aperture for the corn or callus. If the skin can tolerate pads, they may be used for up to 1 week or longer. However, some podiatrists recommend that patients change the pads every day. Their concern stems from the fact that the pad adhesive can macerate the skin, leading to infection. To prevent the pads from adhering to hosiery, patients may cover the pads with paraffin wax and then powder them daily with a hygienic foot powder or cover them with an adhesive bandage. If, despite these measures, friction causes the pads to peel up at the edge and stick to hosiery, the practitioner may recommend that patients cover their toes with the forefoot of an old stocking or panty hose before putting on hosiery.

Many of the disadvantages associated with older pads have been overcome with the introduction of a new cushioning material. Cushlin, manufactured by Dr. Scholl's, is a soft polymer that provides a protective cushion without leaving a sticky residue. When applied to the skin, it molds to the shape of the foot and adheres to the skin without the adhesive properties found in other products. In addition, its smooth outer surface prevents snags and runs in socks and hosiery.

Practitioners should advise patients that if the pad begins to cause itching, burning, or pain at any time, it should be removed immediately and a primary care provider or podiatrist should be consulted. Patients should also be advised that these pads will provide only temporary relief and rarely cure a corn or callus. Practitioners may also recommend silicone toe sleeves for the toes affected by corns. The toe sleeves are lined with silicone, which is impregnated with mineral oil. The mineral oil is slowly released to soften the skin. The sleeves also protect and cushion the corn area. A foam spacer or lamb's wool may be used to provide relief in areas of soft corns. Placement of a metatarsal pad may help relieve pain and pressure from a diffuse-shearing callus.[14]

Eliminating the pressure and friction that induces corns and calluses entails using well-fitting, nonbinding footwear that evenly distributes body weight (Table 45-1). For anatomic foot deformities, orthopedic corrections must be made. These measures relieve pressure and friction, allowing normal mitosis of the basal cell layer to resume and the stratum corneum to normalize after total desquamation of the hyperkeratotic tissue secondary to the use of topical products. Orthotics (i.e., custom-molded arch supports) may have to be employed to help compensate for deformities by redistributing the mechanical forces. Ultimately, surgical correction of toe deformities and resection of the underlying bone may be necessary.

**TABLE 45-1 Selection of Properly Fitted Footwear**

- Buy shoes in the proper size (width and length). To obtain an accurate measurement, ask a trained salesperson to measure your feet. Recheck shoe size every 2 years.
- Base shoe length on the longest toe of your longest foot. Make sure the toes do not bump into the front of the shoe. There should be approximately a half-inch between the tip of shoe and longest toe.
- For proper arch length, choose a shoe in which the first metatarsal head of the foot fits the metatarsal break of the shoe.
- For proper shoe width, choose a shoe that feels comfortable at the first metatarsal joint (toes do not feel cramped in the toe box) and snug at the heel (with the shoes unlaced if a laced shoe is chosen).
- Once the shoe size is determined, choose a shoe shaped to match the shape of the foot. For example, choose a shoe shaped inward if the feet are shaped inward like a pigeon's. Choose a shoe shaped outward if the feet are shaped outward like a duck's.
- Choose a shoe with a heel less than 1 inch.
- If you have abnormalities of the toes (e.g., hammer toes) or use orthotics or padding in your shoes, select a shoe with adequate depth (vertical height) of the toe box to prevent friction of the tops of the toes. A wide toe box will help relieve pressure between toes.
- Make sure the heel support fits snugly and helps hold the foot straight.
- If you are physically active, make sure the shoe's midsole provides adequate cushioning and support.
- Try on both shoes at the time of purchase, preferably wearing a pair of socks or stockings of the type that will be worn normally with the new pair of shoes.
- If your feet tend to swell, select shoes at the end of the day.

### Pharmacologic Therapy

#### Salicylic Acid

Salicylic acid, the oldest of the keratolytic agents, is formulated in many strengths (0.5%-40%), depending on its intended use and dosage form. For the self-treatment of corns and calluses, the approved concentration ranges are 12% to 40% in a plaster vehicle and 12% to 17.6% in a collodionlike vehicle.[15]

*Mechanism of Action* Salicylic acid is believed to act on hyperplastic keratin in two ways: (1) it decreases keratinocyte adhesion, and (2) it increases water binding, which leads to hydration of keratin. Because of the latter effect, the presence of moisture was believed to be an important component of salicylic acid's therapeutic efficacy, and soaking the area in a warm water bath for 5 minutes before applying salicylic acid was recommended. However, evidence submitted to FDA indicated that presoaking produced no significant positive effects for any efficacy parameter assessed.[16] In its final rule, FDA proposed allowing manufacturers of these products to state as an optional direction to the consumer: "May soak corn/callus (or wart) in warm water for 5 minutes to assist in removal."

*Indications* The Food and Drug Administration (FDA) advisory review panel evaluated more than 20 agents for the treatment of corns and calluses. Of these agents, only salicylic acid in plaster, pad, disk, or collodion vehicle is approved as safe and effective for nonprescription marketing for the removal of corns and calluses (Table 45-2). FDA recognized that the term "plaster" includes disks and pads because these dosage forms are similar.[15]

*Dosage Form* Salicylic acid is usually applied to a corn, callus, or common wart in a collodion or collodionlike vehicle. These vehicles contain pyroxylin and various

**TABLE 45-2 Selected Corn and Callus Products**

| Trade Name | Primary Ingredients |
|---|---|
| Curad Mediplast Corn, Callus & Wart Remover | Salicylic acid 40% |
| Dr. Scholl's Callus Remover Disk | Salicylic acid 40% |
| Dr. Scholl's Corn/Callus Remover Liquid | Salicylic acid 12.6% |
| Dr. Scholl's Cushlin Gel Callus Remover Disk | Salicylic acid 40% |
| Dr. Scholl's Cushlin Gel Corn Remover Disk | Salicylic acid 40% |
| Dr. Scholl's One Step Callus Remover Disk | Salicylic acid 40% |
| Dr. Scholl's One Step Corn Remover Strip | Salicylic acid 40% |
| Freezone Corn and Callus Remover Liquid | Salicylic acid 17.6% |
| Freezone One Step Callus Remover Pads | Salicylic acid 40% |
| Freezone One Step Corn Remover Pads | Salicylic acid 40% |
| Mosco Corn & Callus Remover Liquid | Salicylic acid 17.6% |
| OFF-Ezy Corn and Callus Remover Kit Liquid | Salicylic acid 17% |

combinations of volatile solvents such as ether, acetone, or alcohol, or a plasticizer, which is usually castor oil. Pyroxylin is a nitrocellulose derivative that remains on the skin as a water-repellent film after the volatile solvents have evaporated.

The advantages of collodions are that they form an adherent flexible or rigid film and prevent moisture evaporation. These qualities aid penetration of the active ingredient into the affected tissue and result in sustained local action of the drug. The systems are largely water insoluble, as are most of their active ingredients such as salicylic acid. They are also less apt to run onto surrounding skin than are aqueous solutions.

The liquid form is often the easiest for the patient to apply. However, this treatment mode requires patience and persistence because it takes longer to resolve the problem.

Other disadvantages of collodions are that they are extremely flammable and volatile and that, by occluding normal water transport through the skin, they may be mechanically irritating. Also, the collodion's occlusive nature allows systemic absorption of some drugs. Some patients may abuse these vehicles by sniffing their volatile aromatic solvents.

Salicylic acid may be delivered to the skin through the use of a plaster, disk, or pad. This delivery system provides direct and prolonged contact of the drug with the affected area. Salicylic acid plaster is a uniform solid or semisolid adhesive mixture of salicylic acid in a suitable base, spread on appropriate backing material (e.g., felt, moleskin, cotton, plastic), which may be applied directly to the affected area. The usual concentration of salicylic acid in the base is 40%. A small piece of the 40% plaster may be cut to the size of the corn or callus and held in place by waterproof tape. More convenient, however, are corn or callus pads that have small salicylic acid disks for direct application to the skin. The patient selects the appropriately sized disk, places it directly on the affected area, and then covers it with the pad.

*Administration Guidelines* See Table 45-3.

*Safety Considerations* Significant percutaneous absorption may occur when salicylic acid is applied over large body areas, for example, during therapy for extensive psoriasis on the face, trunk, or extremities. Absorbed salicylic acid is largely metabolized in the liver and excreted in the urine. Patients with impaired liver or kidney function are, therefore, predisposed to accumulation and salicylate toxicity. However, although occlusive vehicles can enhance the percutaneous absorption of salicylic acid, it is highly unlikely that salicylism will result during corn, callus, or wart therapy with recommended dosages.

Because some patients will not use salicylic acid products properly or misapply it, topical salicylic acid therapy is not preferred by some podiatrists (see A Word About Chronic Diseases and Foot Disorders). In the past, packaging and labeling for corn and callus products warned patients with diabetes or peripheral vascular disease not to use the products, except under direct supervision of a primary care provider. This warning was included because any acute inflammation or ulcer formation caused by the topical salicylic acid could be dangerous. In its final monograph, FDA determined that the warning should be stronger and should directly caution against using the product under certain conditions, rather than including an "except under" condition for use. Consequently, the revised warning is as follows:

> Do not use this product on irritated skin, any area that is infected or reddened, moles, birthmarks, warts with hair growing from them, genital warts, warts on the face, or warts on the mucous membranes, such as inside the mouth, nose, anus, genitals, or lips. Do not use if you are diabetic, or if you have poor blood circulation.[16]

Petroleum jelly need not be applied to healthy skin surrounding the affected area before corrosive products are applied. However, this precaution should be suggested to patients with poor eyesight or other conditions that increase the likelihood of misapplication or accidental spillage of a salicylic acid product.

**TABLE 45-3 Guidelines for Treating Corns and Calluses with Salicylic Acid Products**

- Wash and dry the affected area thoroughly before applying any product.

**Salicylic Acid 12%-17.6% in Collodionlike Vehicle**

- Apply product no more than twice daily. Morning and evening are usually the most convenient times.
- Do not let adjacent areas of normal healthy skin come in contact with the drug. If they do, wash off the solution immediately with soap and water.
- Apply one drop at a time directly to the corn or callus until the affected area is well covered. Do not overuse the product.
- Allow the drops to dry and harden so the solution does not run.
- For hard corns and calluses, the solution is applied once or twice daily for up to 14 days.
- For soft corns between the toes, hold the toes apart until the solution has dried; then apply a dressing. Treat these corns for 3-6 days.
- After use, cap the container tightly to prevent evaporation and to prevent the active ingredients from assuming a greater concentration.
- Soak the affected foot in warm water for 5 minutes. Then remove the macerated, soft white skin of the corn or callus by scrubbing gently with a rough towel, pumice stone, or callus file. Do not debride the healthy skin.
- Store the product in an amber or light-resistant container away from direct sunlight or heat.

**Salicylic Acid 12%-40% Plasters/Pads**

- If using plaster, trim the plaster to follow the contours of the corn or callus. Apply the plaster to the affected skin, and cover it with adhesive occlusive tape.
- If using disks with pads, apply the appropriately sized disk directly on the affected area, and then cover it with the pad.
- Remove the plaster/pad and occlusive tape within 48 hours.
- Soak the foot and remove the macerated skin by scrubbing gently with a rough towel, pumice stone, or callus file. Do not debride the healthy skin.
- Reapply the plaster after removing the softened skin.
- Repeat every 8 hours as needed over a 2-week period.

### Nonmonograph Agents

Nonmonograph ingredients listed in the final monograph include acetic acid, glacial acetic acid, allantoin, ascorbic acid, benzocaine, lactic acid, menthol, and zinc chloride,[15] to name a few. Such ineffective drugs are no longer approved for self-treatment of corns and calluses, and cannot be marketed for use in this regard unless they are the subject of a specifically approved new drug application.

## Assessment of Corns and Calluses: A Case-based Approach

For corns, calluses, and other foot disorders, the practitioner should consider providing a private area where patients can be comfortable removing their shoe(s) to permit direct inspection of the foot. Direct inspection enables the practitioner to accurately assess the nature and extent of the problem.

Before recommending a course of action, the practitioner must identify not only the disorder but also its possible causes. The patient's health status and use of medications should be determined. The patient should be asked whether and how he or she has self-treated the disorder, as well as how successful the attempts were. This information should be recorded and regularly updated in the patient's medication profile. Case 45-1 illustrates the assessment of patients with corns or calluses.

## Patient Counseling for Corns and Calluses

Remission of corns and calluses can take several days to several months. Patients suffering from corns and calluses should understand that effective treatment and maintenance depends on eliminating predisposing factors that contributed to the foot problem in the beginning. It is important to discuss the need for appropriately fitting footwear, which will allow for plenty of width and length. Recommendations also can be made on types of padding to reduce pressure and shearing, which may predispose them to corns and calluses.

**CASE 45-1**

| Relevant Evaluation Criteria | Scenario/Model Outcome |
|---|---|
| **Information Gathering** | |
| 1. Gather essential information about the patient's symptoms, including: | |
| a. description of symptom(s) (i.e., nature, onset, duration, severity, associated symptoms) | Patient complains of an increasingly painful area on the top of her fourth toe on her left foot. She has been experiencing the pain for 2 months. The area has begun to be hard and reddish. The discomfort from the area has made if difficult for her to wear dress shoes to work. She finds it most painful to stand long hours and walk rapidly. |
| b. description of any factors that seem to precipitate, exacerbate, and/or relieve the patient's symptom(s) | The patient gets relief once she is off her feet and can wear her tennis shoes. She typically wears dress shoes with heels to work, which really exacerbates the pain. |

## CASE 45-1 (continued)

| Relevant Evaluation Criteria | Scenario/Model Outcome |
|---|---|
| c. description of the patient's efforts to relieve the symptoms | She has begun to wrap her toe in band aides, which helps relieve some of the pressure. Patient has also been taking ibuprofen 400 mg twice a day on busy workdays for temporary relief. |
| 2. Gather essential patient history information: | |
| a. patient's identity | Sally Hickson |
| b. patient's age, sex, height, and weight | 29 y/o F, 5'7", 130 lb |
| c. patient's occupation | Fine dining waitress |
| d. patient's dietary habits | Generally eats on the go between shifts. |
| e. patient's sleep habits | 5-7 hours per night |
| f. concurrent medical conditions, prescription and nonprescription medications, and dietary supplements | Ortho Tri-Cyclen 1 tablet once daily; MVI 1 tablet once daily; calcium supplement 500 mg 1 tablet at bedtime; Zyrtec 10 mg 1 tablet at bedtime for allergies; Flonase 2 sprays in each nostril at bedtime for allergies |
| g. allergies | Penicillin and sulfa |
| h. history of other adverse reactions to medications | Codeine upsets stomach. |
| i. other (describe)_______ | Sally is very particular about her appearance and is not willing to wear nonstylish shoes. |
| **Assessment and Triage** | |
| 3. Differentiate the patient's signs/symptoms and correctly identify the patient's primary problem(s) (see Chapter 44, Table 44-4). | Sally is suffering from a hard corn secondary to wearing high-heeled, snug-fitting dress shoes. |
| 4. Identify exclusions for self-treatment (see Figure 45-3). | None |
| 5. Formulate a comprehensive list of therapeutic alternatives for the primary problem to determine if triage to a medical practitioner is required, and share this information with the patient. | Options include:<br>(1) Refer Sally to an appropriate health care professional.<br>(2) Recommend self-care with a nonprescription corn removal product.<br>(3) Recommend appropriate footwear and corn cushions to prevent future irritation.<br>(4) Recommend self-care until Sally can see an appropriate health care professional.<br>(5) Take no action. |
| **Plan** | |
| 6. Select an optimal therapeutic alternative to address the patient's problem, taking into account patient preferences. | Sally prefers to use a nonprescription corn removal product and nondrug measures to treat her problem. |
| 7. Describe the recommended therapeutic approach to the patient. | Regular use of any commercially available nonprescription corn removal product in any dosage form should alleviate the problem. The plaster/disk form, will remain in place while at work and will remove the corn sooner (see Table 45-3). You may also use a silicone toe sleeve to reduce the pressure on the affected toe. However, for the best results, you also must change the type of shoes you wear at work (see Table 45-1). |
| 8. Explain to the patient the rationale for selecting the recommended therapeutic approach from the considered therapeutic alternatives. | Hard corns can be effectively managed with a nonprescription corn removal product and properly fitted, nonbinding footwear as long as there is no evidence of secondary infection or preexisting medical condition that would preclude self-treatment, as is the case with you. The toe sleeves will be useful when the plaster disk is not applied to soften the skin and reduce pressure on the toe. |

**CASE 45-1 (continued)**

| Relevant Evaluation Criteria | Scenario/Model Outcome |
|---|---|
| **Patient Education** | |
| 9. When recommending self-care with nonprescription medications and/or nondrug therapy, convey accurate information to the patient, including: | |
| a. appropriate dose and frequency of administration | See the box Patient Education for Corns and Calluses. |
| b. maximum number of days the therapy should be employed | See the box Patient Education for Corns and Calluses. |
| c. product administration procedures | See the box Patient Education for Corns and Calluses. |
| d. expected time to onset of relief | Symptoms may be relieved somewhat within a few days but complete removal of the corn may take up to 14 days. |
| e. degree of relief that can be reasonably expected | Complete removal of the corn is possible with proper use of the product along with removal of offending causes. |
| f. most common side effects | See the box Patient Education for Corns and Calluses. |
| g. side effects that warrant medical intervention should they occur | See the box Patient Education for Corns and Calluses. |
| h. patient options in the event that condition worsens or persists | See the box Patient Education for Corns and Calluses. |
| i. product storage requirements | Store the product in a cool, dry place that is out of children's reach. |
| j. specific nondrug measures | See the box Patient Education for Corns and Calluses. |
| 10. Solicit patient's follow-up questions. | Can't I just buy an adhesive corn pad to wear with my high-heeled shoes? |
| 11. Answer patient's questions. | This approach not only will not alleviate the problem, it will increase pressure over the affected toes and could actually cause more discomfort. |

Key: MVI, multivitamin.

The practitioner should counsel the patient or caregiver on how to use nonprescription medications that remove corns and calluses. Because many products contain corrosive materials, they must be applied only to the corn or callus. Practitioners should alert patients that products containing collodions are poisonous when taken orally and these products, as well as all other medications, should be stored out of children's reach. Collodion-containing products are volatile, have an odor similar to that of airplane glue, and may be subject to abuse by inhalation.

Nonprescription products for corns and calluses are not recommended for patients with diabetes or circulatory problems. Practitioners should reinforce contraindications, warnings, and precautions with all patients to avoid the inadvertent use of such products by individuals who have such conditions.

The box Patient Education for Corns and Calluses lists specific information to provide to patients.

## Evaluation of Patient Outcomes for Corns and Calluses

The progress of patients with hard corns or calluses should be checked after 14 days of treatment. If these conditions are still present, the patient should consult a primary care provider or podiatrist for evaluation.

# BUNIONS

## Epidemiology of Bunions

An estimated 3% of Americans (mainly women) and 7% of those older than 65 years have bunions. Women are ten times more likely to develop bunions than men. Often, several family members suffer from this disorder. However, despite a positive family history, aggravating circumstances (e.g., wearing tight shoes) must also be present for a bunion to actually develop.[9,17]

## Etiology/Pathophysiology of Bunions

The hallux, or great toe, along with the inner side of the foot, provides the elasticity and mobility needed to walk or run. Thus, the hallux is a dynamic body part. However, this mobility causes several anatomic disorders associated with the foot, such as hallux valgus in which there is a deviation of the great toe, or main axis of the toe, toward the outer toes or lateral side of the foot. Prolonged pressure

## PATIENT EDUCATION FOR CORNS AND CALLUSES

The objectives of self-treatment are to (1) provide symptomatic relief, (2) reduce and/or remove corns or calluses, and (3) prevent their recurrence by correcting underlying causes. For most patients, carefully following product instructions and the self-care measures listed here will help ensure optimal therapeutic outcomes.

### Nondrug Measures

- To avoid autoinoculating oneself at another body site, keep the instruments used to remove dead skin clean (see Table 45-3).
- Do not use sharp knives or razor blades to remove dead skin of corns and calluses. Such instruments may cause bacterial contamination and infection.
- If you have trouble applying the product to only the affected area because of poor eyesight or other conditions, apply petroleum jelly to healthy skin surrounding the affected area before applying the corn and callus remover.
- For temporary relief of painful pressure from the area under a corn or callus, cover the affected area with a pad such as Cushlin, which has an opening for the corn or callus. Use the pad for up to 1 week or longer unless it causes itching, burning, or pain.

Consult a primary care provider or podiatrist if the symptoms described previously occur.

### Preventive Measures

- To eliminate the pressure and friction that cause corns and calluses, wear well-fitting, nonbinding footwear that evenly distributes body weight (see Table 45-1).
- For anatomic foot deformities, consult a podiatrist about orthopedic corrections.

### Nonprescription Medications

- To remove corns and calluses, use a salicylic acid product labeled for use on these types of lesions (see Table 45-3).
- Do not use this product on irritated, infected, or reddened skin.
- Do not use this product if you are diabetic or have poor blood circulation.
- Salicylic acid is poisonous. Do not allow it to come in contact with the mouth, and keep it out of children's reach.
- Note that the medication sloughs off skin and may leave an unsightly pinkish tinge to the skin.

Stop treatment and consult a primary care provider or podiatrist if swelling, reddening, or irritation of the skin occurs, or if pain occurs immediately on applying the product.

associated with external shoe irritation over the prominent, angulated metatarsophalangeal joint of the great toe may result in painful inflammation, swelling, and/or exostosis over the involved bony joint structure (Figure 45-4). This process may result in bunion formation, as shown in Figure 45-1.

Bunions can be caused by various conditions. Pressure on the metatarsal head of the great toe may result from the manner in which a person sits, walks, or stands. In women, pressure from high-heeled shoes and/or too narrow or too shallow toe boxes force the side of the toe inward and can aggravate the condition. Friction on the toes from bone malformations (wide heads or lateral bending) is also a major factor in bunion production, as are biomechanical defects. Vigorous exercise such as running can cause bunions or exacerbate existing bunions and increase the severity of hallux valgus deformity itself.

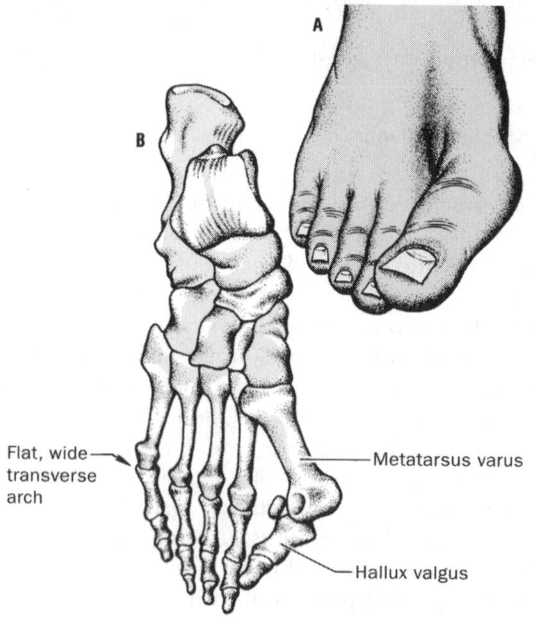


**FIGURE 45-4** Two views of hallux vagus. **A,** Gross representation of hallux valgus. **B,** Bone structure of hallux valgus.

## Signs and Symptoms of Bunions

Bunions are usually asymptomatic but may become quite painful, swollen, red, and tender. Pain is caused by pressure from shoes on the medial aspect of the first metatarsal head. The bunion itself is usually covered by an extensive keratinous overgrowth. Patients may experience increased pain or decreased movement of the great toe.

## Treatment of Bunions

Corrective steps to alleviate bunions often depend on the degree of discomfort. In some cases, corrective surgery is necessary.

### *Treatment Goals*

The goals in self-treating bunions are to decrease irritation of the affected area and prevent worsening of the condition by correcting the cause.

### *General Treatment Approach*

Bunions are not amenable to topical drug therapy, and the routine, chronic use of oral nonprescription analgesics, particularly ibuprofen, is not suggested. Management of the bunion should address the cause, such as tight-fitting or high-heeled shoes, excessive pronation of the foot, or a previous injury. Thus, self-treatment includes avoiding high-heeled shoes, using protective padding (e.g., bunion pads), and taking oral anti-inflammatory drugs on a short-term basis. Self-treatment only relieves the swelling caused by shoe friction; therefore, well-fitted shoes with a wide toe box should be worn at all times to prevent subsequent flares of inflammation. If shoe adjustments fail to alleviate pain, referral to a properly trained health care professional is indicated. Physical therapy may be beneficial to provide relief from pain and inflammation. Orthotics may help control irregularities of the foot movement.[18]

Patients with diabetes complaining of bunions should be immediately referred to an endocrinologist and a podiatrist. The presence of a discharge or bleeding from the bunion also precludes self-treatment.

### *Nonpharmacologic Therapy*

#### Selection of Footwear

See Table 45-1.

#### Bunion Pads/Cushions

Topical nonprescription padding (e.g., moleskin) can be helpful and may be all that is necessary to decrease the irritation of footwear. Eventually, padding can help to decrease inflammation around the bunion area. Before the protective pad is applied, the foot should be bathed and thoroughly dried. The pad is then cut into a shape that conforms to the bunion. If the intention is to relieve the pressure from the center of the bunion area, the pad should be cut to surround the bunion. Precut pads are available for immediate patient use. To minimize the risk of skin maceration and ulceration, constant skin contact with adhesive-backed pads should be avoided, unless such use is recommended by a podiatrist or primary care provider.

For patients who are allergic to adhesives, a non-medicated, self-adhesive bunion cushion (i.e., Bunion Guard) is commercially available. One advantage of this product is that it protects the bunion and can be easily removed before showering. The cushion, made of a soft polymer gel, can then be reapplied onto the bunion after showering for up to 3 months. Another advantage of Bunion Guard is that it does not contain an adhesive backing, which can be irritating to skin. The outer surface is smooth and not prone to snagging socks or hosiery.

Larger footwear may be necessary to compensate for the space taken up by the pad; in fact, not increasing shoe size appropriately may cause pressure in other areas. Also, protective pads should not be used on bunions when the skin is broken or blistered. Abraded skin should receive palliative treatment before pads are applied. If symptoms persist, these patients should consult a podiatrist or orthopedist.

## Assessment of Bunions: A Case-based Approach

Measures discussed in Assessment of Corns and Calluses: A Case-based Approach are also appropriate for evaluating bunions. Specific information the practitioner needs to obtain from the patient includes where the lesion is located, how long it has been a problem, whether it occurs with specific footwear, and how painful it is. It is also important to inquire about methods used to relieve symptoms (shoes, pads, and NSAIDs).

## Patient Counseling for Bunions

The practitioner should stress to the patient that effective, long-term "treatment" of bunions is to remove the source of irritation. Patients who do not achieve permanent relief by changing footwear should consult a podiatrist or orthopedist to determine whether anatomic defects are causing bunions. The practitioner should explain the proper short-term use of bunion pads and cushions to patients who want to use them. The box Patient Education for Bunions lists specific information to provide to patients.

## Evaluation of Patient Outcomes for Bunions

Depending on the severity of the irritation, bunions that are not caused by biomechanical defects of the foot may take a few weeks to resolve. The practitioner should follow up after 2 to 3 weeks to determine whether wearing new shoes and/or using bunion cushions or pads have eliminated the discomfort. If the patient is still experiencing discomfort, medical referral is appropriate.

# TIRED, ACHING FEET

With every step taken (8000 to 10,000 steps each day), gravity-induced pressure of up to twice the body's weight bears down on each foot, releasing powerful shocks of energy that the foot's natural padding must struggle to absorb. In an unpadded shoe, the shock as the foot strikes the ground is absorbed throughout the foot, ankle, leg, and back. This shock can fatigue muscles, resulting in tired, aching feet and/or back pain.

## Epidemiology of Tired, Aching Feet

An estimated two thirds of Americans suffer from tired, aching feet (the most common foot problem). In addition, 21 million adults are estimated to suffer from heel pain. People simply do not realize the daily abuse their feet must endure.

## Etiology/Pathophysiology of Tired, Aching Feet

Aching feet can be caused by increased frequency of standing and/or walking (especially on hard surfaces), age-related erosion of the fat padding on the bottom of the foot, circulatory or neurologic disorders, and poor-fitting/inappropriate footwear.

## PATIENT EDUCATION FOR BUNIONS

The objective of self-treatment is to decrease irritation of the bunion until the cause is corrected. For patients whose bunions are not related to anatomic defects of the foot, carefully following product instructions and the self-care measures listed here will help ensure optimal therapeutic outcomes.

- To help prevent footwear from rubbing the feet, make sure footwear fits properly (see Table 45-1).
- To decrease inflammation around existing bunions, apply adhesive-backed moleskin padding or a polymer gel cushion (e.g., Bunion Guard) to the bunion.
- If the skin of the bunion is broken or blistered, treat the abraded skin and wait until it heals before applying bunion pads.
- Before applying the protective pad, bathe and thoroughly dry the foot.
- Cut the pad into a shape that conforms to the bunion. Cut the pad large enough to surround the bunion.
- Note that constant exposure to the adhesive of moleskin pads may macerate and irritate the skin. If such irritation occurs, stop wearing the pads.
- When using Bunion Guard, remove the cushion before showering and reapply afterward. The cushion can be worn for up to 3 months.
- Note that larger footwear may be needed to compensate for the space taken up by the pad or cushion.
- Applying ice several times daily may reduce inflammation and pain.[17]

If the irritation persists after 2 to 3 weeks of implementing self-treatment measures, consult a podiatrist or orthopedist about the problem.

Because the cause of heel pain is difficult to determine, treatment can often be prolonged and expensive. The two most common types of heel pain are heel spurs (i.e., bony growths on the underside of the heel bone) and plantar fasciitis (strain on the connective tissue that attaches the arch to the front of the heel). Heel spurs are the result of strained foot muscles and the wearing away of the fat tissue surrounding the heel bone. Incorrect walking or running technique, excessive running, poor-fitting shoes, being overweight or experiencing a rapid weight gain, and aging are common contributors to this condition. Heel pain can be an early sign of systemic arthritis.[14]

Plantar fasciitis is often caused by high arches, flat feet, repetitive foot stress during athletic activity, or prolonged standing. This disorder can be determined by the patient's description of the pain and its occurrence. Usually, the pain occurs from the first moment the person gets out of bed in the morning or when standing up after sitting resulting from tissue contraction. The sensation on the bottom of the heel is quite painful, and the patient may complain of a burning sensation.[19,20]

## Treatment of Tired, Aching Feet

### *Treatment Goals*

The goal in self-treating tired, aching feet is to provide additional support and shock absorbance for the feet to reduce foot pain and fatigue.

### *General Treatment Approach*

The first measure to avoid tired, aching feet is to use well-fitted footwear that has sufficient padding and cushioning (Table 45-1). Wearing sport-specific shoes with good arch support (e.g., running/jogging shoes) is an excellent measure for preventing heel pain. People should purchase shoes carefully to ensure a proper fit. Although there are fewer specialty shoe stores now than in the past, patients prone to foot problems should seek out the advice of a competent shoe salesperson.

Active people or those who must stand for prolonged periods during the day may need to take additional measures. Some active individuals prefer to wear stylish rather than orthopedic shoes. Unfortunately, many stylish shoes are not built to provide adequate support and cushioning; however, various shoe inserts are available to enhance the comfort of most well-fitting shoes. Other self-treatment measures include replacing worn shoes or heel pads, using a night splint, strapping or taping the arch, decreasing the amount of weight-bearing activity, and, if necessary, entering a weight-reduction program.[21] Oral anti-inflammatory treatment, including ice applications, is also appropriate (see Cryotherapy). Athletes will use Epsom salt soaks to assist with decreasing fatigue and pain in feet and legs caused by inflammation and muscle cramps. Commonly adding 2 cups of Epsom salt to a warm bathtub and soaking for approximately 12 minutes will prove beneficial. When self-treatment fails, patients should be referred to an appropriate health care professional for evaluation of possible bony malalignments and possible orthotic therapy.

### *Nonpharmacologic Therapy*

#### Full-shoe Inserts

Full-shoe inserts, which can provide cushioning and absorb shock, are available in various sizes and thicknesses to accommodate most individuals. Commercially available shoe inserts assist in absorbing shock, decreasing the incidence of lower back pain associated with the impact from walking. The patient must select an insert that conforms to the type of shoe worn. Thus, because a thick shoe insert may alter the fit of a woman's pump, a thin insole would be preferable.

#### Partial Insoles

Partial insoles are preferred when cushioning or support is desired in a certain portion of the shoe. For example, metatarsal arch supports, which fit into the ball-of-foot region of a woman's shoe, help lift the arch behind the toes to alleviate pain associated with the spreading of the

## PATIENT EDUCATION FOR TIRED, ACHING FEET

The objectives of self-treatment are to (1) reduce impact on the feet by providing additional support and shock absorbance, and (2) relieve foot discomfort. For most patients, carefully following product instructions and the self-care measures listed here will help ensure optimal therapeutic outcomes.

- To reduce friction of the feet and impact on weight-bearing parts of the feet, wear well-fitted footwear that has sufficient padding and cushioning (see Table 45-1).
- Consider other measures to further decrease impact on the feet, such as decreasing the length of time you stand or exercise, switching to exercises that have less effect on the feet and, if necessary, losing weight.
- To relieve swelling or discomfort, apply an ice bag or cold wrap to the affected area (see Table 45-5).
- To improve circulation, select a compression stocking with mild to moderate compression.
- Choose a full-shoe insert when the entire foot aches. Make sure the insert conforms to the shoe. For example, choose a thin insole for a woman's pump and a thicker insole for a sneaker.
- Use partial insoles to cushion or support a certain portion of the foot, such as the ball of the foot, the arch, or the toes.
- Use a heel cushion for pain confined to the bottom of the heel.
- Use a heel cup when the pain is widespread and diffuse.

If discomfort or swelling continues after 1 week of implementing appropriate self-care measures, consult a podiatrist or primary care provider.

foot, a condition that occurs with increasing age. For women who wear high-heeled shoes, inserts (i.e., Toe Squish Preventer cushions) are available to prevent the toes from becoming cramped in the pointed toe box. Finally, the arch support insert is intended to cushion and support painful longitudinal arches.

#### Heel Cups/Cushions

Depending on the location and extent of the pain, a heel cup or heel cushion may be indicated. For example, a heel cushion might be appropriate when the pain is confined to the bottom of the heel. The cushion can support the entire heel as it elevates the sensitive area to prevent further irritation. Alternatively, when the pain is widespread and diffuse, a heel cup might be more appropriate. Heel cups help relieve the pain caused by the breakdown of the heel's natural padding or intense athletic activity. Heel cups and cushions should be made of a lightweight, nonslip material that easily fits into any shoe, including athletic shoes.

Caution should be used when selecting shoe inserts. If an insole affects the patient's gait, referral to a podiatrist is recommended. Insoles should be used only to cushion the foot, not to correct malformation, which requires a specialist's attention.

Compression stockings are also options to enhance support for those who spend many hours on their feet. Compression stockings are available without a prescription for compressions ranging from 15 to 40 mm Hg. This will decrease inflammation by improving circulation, thereby reducing fatigue of the feet, legs, and back.

### Assessment of Tired, Aching Feet: A Case-based Approach

Measures discussed in Assessment of Corns and Calluses: A Case-based Approach are appropriate for triage of a patient who complains of tired, aching feet. In addition, the practitioner must determine whether the pain affects the soles of the feet, the heels, or the entire foot. The practitioner must also evaluate lifestyle factors (e.g., occupation, daily exercise, footwear), underlying pathology (e.g., circulatory or neurologic disorders), the possibility of an aggravating event, and the walking/working surface. If underlying pathology is suspected, the practitioner should refer patients to a primary care provider or podiatrist for initial evaluation.

### Patient Counseling for Tired, Aching Feet

The practitioner can play an integral role in counseling patients on preventing and treating foot disorders caused by friction and excessive impact. The cornerstone of preventing such disorders is selecting the appropriate footwear. If the disorder still persists, the practitioner can help patients select in-shoe supports and advise them of other measures to reduce weight-bearing activities. The box Patient Education for Tired, Aching Feet lists specific information to provide patients.

### Evaluation of Patient Outcomes for Tired, Aching Feet

Resolution of pain in the soles or heels of the feet depends on the patient and the longevity of the foot problem. The practitioner should follow up after a few weeks to determine whether the use of new shoes and/or in-shoe supports has eliminated the discomfort. If the symptoms persist, the patient should consult a podiatrist for evaluation.

## EXERCISE-INDUCED FOOT INJURIES

The practitioner should be aware of the problem of exercise-induced foot injuries, particularly those caused by running, jogging, or other high-impact physical activities (Figure 45-5) as well as acute injury management techniques (Table 45-4). Often, individuals fail to take certain precautions and dive head first into a strenuous exercise program. Yet jogging, aerobic dance, and running are not without risk. One study documented that several exercise enthusiasts have died from heart attacks while jogging.[22] Some people, especially those older than 35 years, should consult a primary care provider before embarking on a fitness program, and so should patients with high blood pressure

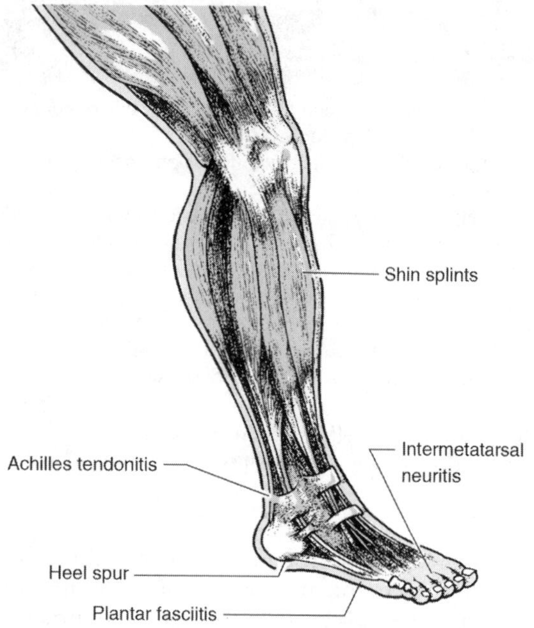


**FIGURE 45-5** Selected foot and leg injuries associated with excessive impact shock.

or a family history of heart disease or diabetes. Ultimately, a vigorous walking program may be a more prudent form of exercise for middle-aged, unconditioned individuals than jogging or running. Walking may minimize the potential orthopedic problems described here that can result from more strenuous forms of exercise.

## Types of Exercise-induced Injuries

### Shin Splints

The term *shin splint* is used generically to describe all the pain emanating from below the knee and above the ankle. Shin splints are an overuse phenomenon that occurs in runners or walkers who use hard surfaces. This condition may also occur from not stretching out properly before running, running on a banked track or the sloped shoulder of a road, wearing improper footwear, or overstriding.

The typical complaint of a runner with shin splints is pain in the medial lower third of the shin that seems to increase gradually with exercise. This pain is caused by excessive pronation, which causes weakness and strain on the posterior tibialis tendon. The tendon may pull away from the periosteum that lines the shinbone. The patient may admit that soreness begins after running; with a continual running program, the pain will eventually occur during and after running. Complaints of pain when walking or climbing stairs may indicate a serious case of shin splints. If the discomfort is located on the anterior lateral aspect of the shin and is described as a cramping, burning tightness, and repeatedly occurs at the same distance or time during a run, then referral to a primary care provider, podiatrist, or physical therapist is appropriate.[23,24]

Rest, ice (e.g., ice bag or cold compression wrap; Table 45-5), compression, and elevation (RICE) therapy to the painful area is good initial treatment. Some practitioners also treat sprains with PRICE therapy, which includes protection, such as supporting or immobilizing the area to prevent further injury. For mild sprains, an elastic bandage or tape can be used. For a more vulnerable sprain, immobilizing and use of a cane or crutch minimize the effusion.[25] Aspirin or ibuprofen can be used to relieve pain and reduce tissue inflammation. However, the use of analgesics to suppress pain or increase endurance during a workout is not recommended. A semirigid orthotic with a wedge can also be recommended to prevent shin splints.[24]

### Stress Fracture

Exercise-induced stress fractures account for 50% of stress fractures in men and 64% in women.[26] Stress fracture, also known as march, army, or fatigue fracture, may be encountered in runners, especially those who run repetitively on hard, inflexible surfaces. This injury usually involves the long bones of the foot or leg. It is not an overt break of the bone, but rather an alteration in the architecture of the normal bone in which the outer cortex of the bone cracks. Stress fractures also occur in car salespersons and individuals who climb stairs and/or ladders numerous times during the day.

Rapid increase in physical activity, running, jumping, hormonal disturbances (estrogen deficiency), nutritional deficiencies, obesity, inappropriate footwear, and poor flexibility are some of the risk factors associated with stress fractures. The onset of pain is typically associated with runners who drastically change aspects of their training routine (e.g., running surface, speed, or distance). Although the pain begins insidiously, the individual with a stress fracture will often complain of deep pain in the lower leg with an area of extreme tenderness. A misconception among runners is that they can "work out" the problem by continuing to jog. Runners must be instructed that pain is the body's communication mechanism to indicate that enough is enough and something is abnormal. Symptoms patients may experience are dull pain that worsens with exercise or applying weight, and swelling. The defining symptom is tenderness with applied pressure to the site of injury.[26] Treatment for stress fractures is complete rest from running, sometimes for 4 to 6 weeks, or longer if the tibia is involved. Conservative therapy includes application of ice and use of an oral nonsteroidal anti-inflammatory drug (NSAID) to relieve pain and inflammation.

### Achilles Tendonitis

Running on hills or on the beach, wearing improper footwear (e.g., running and jogging in shoes designed for racquet sports), and moving with excessive pronation (i.e., rolling in of the feet) are common causes of Achilles tendonitis. However, running by itself does not cause this condition. It may be an early sign of arthritis or rupture of a tendon; the exact cause of the problem is difficult to distinguish. Thus, patients with Achilles tendonitis should be referred to a primary care provider, podiatrist, or physical therapist.

TABLE 45-4 Differentiation of Exercise-induced Foot Injuries

| Type of Injury | Common Causes | Pathophysiology | Signs/Symptoms | Recommendations |
|---|---|---|---|---|
| Shin splints | Overzealous workout; inappropriate stretching; running/ walking on sloped or hard surfaces; wearing ill-fitting footwear; overstriding | Excessive pronation weakens/strains posterior tibialis; anterior tibial muscle stretches away from periosteum that lines shinbone | Pain in medial lower third of shin, or below knee and above ankle; pain worsens with exercise; cramping, burning, and tightness on anterior lateral section of shin | PRICE or RICE therapy; acetaminophen or ibuprofen; shoe orthotic |
| Stress fracture | Running on hard, rigid surfaces; rapid increase in physical activity; jumping; estrogen deficiency; nutritional deficiencies; obesity; ill-fitting footwear | Outer cortex of long bones of leg or foot cracks from alternation in tensile forces sent by ligaments, tendons, and muscles | Deep pain in lower leg; tender to touch; pain worsens with exercise; swelling | Complete rest; NSAID therapy |
| Achilles tendonitis | Running on hills or in sand; ill-fitting footwear; excessive pronation; arthritis | Inflammation of Achilles tendon; rupture of tendon | Posterior heel pain; tenderness; swelling | Referral to PCP |
| Blisters | Repetitive movement; ill-fitting footwear; tight hosiery | Continual friction on small surface of foot separates stratum corneum and stratum lucidum skin layers, causing space between layers to fill with fluid | Accumulation of fluid beneath stratum corneum; may be painful | Do not remove blister; protect with topical bandage; see PCP for drainage |
| Ankle sprains | Ankle rotating outside acceptable range | Lateral ligament damage | Pain; bruising; tenderness; difficulty walking | PRICE or RICE therapy |
| Intermetatarsal neuritis | Small toe box space | Inflammation of nerves from compression of or entanglement between metatarsal heads and digital bases | Pain and numbness between toes | Proper footwear |
| Toenail loss | Long, thick toenails in small toe box space; friction and pressure from running in "stop and go" sports, such as tennis | Fluid beneath nail plate pushes toenail from nail bed | Dark discoloration from blood underneath nail plate; pain at toe; nail loss | Referral to podiatrist or PCP |
| Runner's bunion | Pressure from ill-fitting footwear; friction on toes from bone abnormalities; heredity; overzealous exercise | Prolonged pressure causing metatarsophalangeal joint of big toe to form an angle, resulting in swelling of bursa and/or outgrowth of bone on joint | Pain, swelling, and tenderness on inside of foot near big toe joint; excessive skin covering over bunion; big toe positioned laterally | Correction of cause; referral to podiatrist or PCP |
| Heel pain | Prolonged standing; walking on hard surfaces; ill-fitting footwear; excessive running; obesity; rheumatoid arthritis; gout; flat feet; high arches; age-related loss of fat padding at base of foot; straining of foot muscles | Degeneration of collagen | Painful or burning sensation | Heel cups or cushions; decreased standing time |

Key: NSAID, nonsteroidal anti-inflammatory drug; PCP, primary care provider; PRICE, protection, rest, ice, compression, elevation; RICE, rest, ice, compression, elevation.

**TABLE 45-5 Guidelines for Applying Cold Compresses**

**Ice Bag Method**

- Fill the ice bag to one half to two thirds of capacity with crushed or shaved ice, if possible. These forms of ice will ensure greater contact with the injured body part.
- If needed, break ice into walnut-sized pieces with no jagged edges. An overfilled bag will be difficult to apply because it will not rest on the contour of the body area.
- After filling the bag, squeeze out trapped air. Then dry the outside of the bag and check for leaks.
- Bind the injured body part with a wet elastic wrap, and then apply the ice bag. The wet wrap aids transfer of cold to the injured area.
- If the ankle is being treated, keep it in a dorsiflexed position (foot toward the nose) when it is wrapped in the elastic bandage.
- Apply the ice bag to the specific body part.
- To avoid tissue damage, apply the ice bag for 10 minutes and then remove it for 10 minutes. If the bag is not cloth covered, wrap injured area or the ice bag in a thin towel to prevent tissue damage.
- Follow this procedure three to four times a day.
- For most injuries, continue the cryotherapy until swelling decreases or for a maximum of 12-24 hours. Depending on the severity of the injury, application of ice may be necessary for up to 48-72 hours. (For example, the maximum swelling of ankle injuries may occur up to 48 hours after the injury.)
- Before storing the ice bag, drain it and allow it to air dry. If possible, turn it inside out for more efficient drying. Cap the bag, and store it in a cool, dry place.

**Cold Wraps**

- To activate a single-use cold pack, squeeze the middle of the pack to burst the bubble. This action initiates an endothermic reaction of ammonium nitrate, water, and special additives.
- For a reusable cold wrap (cold pack or gel pack), store it in the freezer for 2 hours. Do not put the cloth cover in the freezer.
- Remove the cold wrap from the freezer, insert it in the cloth cover, and apply it to the injured body part.
- If the cold wrap is uncomfortable, remove it for a minute or 2 and then reapply it.
- Alternate application of the cold wrap (10 minutes on; 10 minutes off) three to four times a day for 24-48 hours.
- After use, store the cold wrap in the freezer.
- Although some gel packs are nontoxic, keep all cold wraps out of the reach of children.

By definition, Achilles tendonitis is a painful inflammation involving the Achilles tendon. However, the classic signs of inflammation, such as pain, erythema, increased skin temperature, or swelling may not be observed. Typical symptoms are posterior heel pain, which is worse in the morning when getting out of bed, at the beginning of an exercise session, and when walking after prolonged sitting.[24] No rupture, a partial rupture, or complete rupture of the tendon can produce this manifestation. Caution is advised when counseling these patients about self-care. If there is any possibility of a rupture, the patient should consult a primary care provider or podiatrist.

The best treatment is prevention with careful progression of training, including appropriate stretching exercises, and replacement of worn footwear. Bony malalignments leading to excessive pronation should be treated with orthotic therapy. An orthotic device approximately positions the foot. The properties of shoe inserts (e.g., flexible or rigid) vary; the choice of insert should be based on specific treatment objectives. Shoe inserts can be custom made or purchased off the shelf. Arch supports are intended to provide buttressing for the foot.

Symptomatic self-treatment after podiatric consultation may consist of rest, new shoes, ice applications (Table 45-5), appropriate oral NSAID use, temporary heel lifts prescribed by a primary care provider, reduction in mileage and hill running, and careful calf-stretching exercises.

### *Blisters*

Blisters occur on the heel or sole of the foot following repeated shearing forces moving across the skin. This results in midepidermal cell death between the stratum corneum and stratum lucidum. Heat, sweat, and skin maceration all increase the risk of blistering. Frequently, this occurs in an individual who overzealously reinitiates an exercise program. Ill-fitting footwear and inappropriate hosiery can also cause or contribute to the development of blisters. Fluid quickly accumulates at this site, often on the heel, the ball of the foot, and the ends or tops of the toes. Running barefoot can also cause blisters.

Appropriate care for large, symptomatic blisters includes sterile incision and drainage, carefully leaving the blister roof in place to assist in healing. Subsequent protection of the wound is accomplished with the use of doughnut moleskin or nonadherent hydrocolloid (e.g., Tegasorb, Cutinova hydro) dressings. The patient should not attempt to remove the blister roof for fear of subsequent topical infection.

Properly fitting footwear and synthetic insoles to absorb frictional force are preventive measures against blisters. Cotton or woolen socks are preferred for running. Acrylic or thin polyester socks under a thick, dense outer sock will help draw the moisture away from the foot and decrease the amount of shearing. Some individuals with soft skin will continue to develop blisters until their skin toughens enough to withstand friction during running. Application of compound tincture of benzoin or a flexible collodion product (e.g., New Skin) will help toughen the skin. Applying topical antibiotics to broken skin can prevent secondary bacterial infection (see Chapter 42).[27]

Application of 20% aluminum chloride hexahydrate antiperspirant preparations may also prove beneficial in reducing blistering. The antiperspirants have shown benefit in studies, but the incidence of secondary skin irritation was significant.[28]

### *Ankle Sprains*

Sprains account for 75% of ankle injuries. Approximately one million patients seek medical assistance related to acute injuries of the ankle each year.[29] Lateral ligament injury to the ankle is caused by rotation of the body over the fixed foot. This injury occurs most often in contact sports in which the foot remains stationary while the body is unintentionally rotated. The incidence of ankle sprains during jogging and running is low because runners usually do not take sharp diagonal cuts. However, stepping on an unnoticed stone or curb edge may result in an ankle sprain.

Diagnosis includes inquiring about the cause of the injury and the history of past injuries and physical examination of the affected area. The differential diagnosis of an ankle fracture from a sprained ankle is impossible without an X-ray. RICE or PRICE therapy is well accepted as the most appropriate immediate treatment for an ankle sprain.[25] It remains controversial whether cold application (Table 45-5) without elevation is helpful or harmful. Regardless, treatment for a sprained ankle should be initiated as soon as possible. Sometimes even trained professional athletes perceive an ankle sprain as a minor problem and neglect to treat it appropriately. The severity of ligament damage can vary widely, however, and an extensive ligament rupture that has been given insufficient treatment may result in a permanently unstable ankle.

### Intermetatarsal Neuritis

Pain and numbness between the toes, most often within the third interspace, characterize intermetatarsal neuritis. The cause is linked to the foot jamming forward into the shoe without enough space to accommodate it. Nerves become inflamed when compressed or caught in the area between the metatarsal heads and digital bases.

The solution is properly fitting shoes (Table 45-1) with the addition of a metatarsal pad or orthotic device. Lacing of the shoe can be modified by skipping the bottom two eyelets, which will provide additional room for the ball of the foot. If the pain persists or worsens after these measures are taken, the patient should consult a podiatrist. Worsening of the pain could indicate development of a neuroma.

### Toenail Loss

Blisters under the toenail occur as a result of the interaction between the toenail and the interior toe box of the shoe. Overgrown, thickened toenails and poorly fitted shoes can produce this problem. Long toenails catch on the sock or inside the shoe toe box, particularly when the individual is running downhill and in "stop and go" sports such as tennis. Friction and pressure produce fluid beneath the nail plate, causing it to separate from the nail bed. In some instances, blood also accumulates under the nail plate, causing a distinct dark coloration. This condition is very painful and can result in the temporary loss of the toenail. The patient should be referred to a podiatrist.

### Runner's Bunion

See Bunions.

### Heel Pain

See Tired, Aching Feet.

## Treatment of Exercise-induced Injuries

### Treatment Goals

The goals in self-treating exercise-induced foot problems are to (1) relieve pain if present, (2) prevent secondary bacterial infection if the skin is broken, and (3) institute measures to prevent further injury.

### General Treatment Approach

Measures to prevent exercise-induced injuries entail using suitable footwear that fits properly (Table 45-1), running on the proper surface, using correct posture (i.e., running erect), and stretching muscles before exercising. Most running injuries can be successfully treated with measures for shoe modifications, inserts, and in-shoe supports as discussed in Treatment of Tired, Aching Feet. Measures to correct leg length discrepancies and modified training methods may also be needed.

Some runners believe that the more mileage logged per week, the better their running ability, but the incidence of acquired injuries among runners increases dramatically after 25 to 30 miles per week. An increased injury rate is also observed in runners who increase mileage too rapidly. Continuous days of high-intensity workouts cause accumulated fatigue and microtrauma; to avoid this, the body must be allowed to recuperate after vigorous exercise. A good training program entails a schedule of both "hard" and "easy" days, with extended mileage on 3 or 4 days per week and light workouts on the remaining days.

If the runner or jogger has an injured leg or foot, activity must usually be interrupted to allow the injured leg or foot to rest. Relative rest (i.e., avoiding activities that produce the symptoms) is often indicated, but some runners resist this suggestion. When an injury occurs, the practitioner should encourage alternative exercise modes, such as swimming, rowing, and/or bicycling (stationary or outdoor), which will allow the serious runner to maintain aerobic conditioning.

If the injury warrants it, the practitioner can instruct the patient on selecting and using nonprescription accessories (e.g., cryotherapy, a compression ice wrap, ice bags, compression bandages, arch supports, heel cushions) that will alleviate injuries or problems. Systemic analgesics can also relieve the pain and inflammation of minor foot injuries (see Chapter 5). Exercise-induced injuries that are excluded from self-treatment include Achilles tendonitis, shin splints, stress fractures, and intermetatarsal neuritis. Patients with diabetes, peripheral vascular disease, or arthritis who suffer any type of foot injury should be referred to a primary care provider or podiatrist.

### Nonpharmacologic Therapy

#### Athletic Footwear

Shoes can be a powerful tool for manipulating human movement and can greatly influence the healing of injured tissues in both positive and negative ways. The importance of appropriate footwear has been reported by McPoil and coworkers.[30] These authors demonstrated that a well-designed shoe, even without an orthotic, can favorably alter the center-of-pressure recordings in individuals with foot deformities. Conversely, inappropriate shoes may be problematic, as observed by Frey and others,[31] who reported that most women surveyed indicated they wore shoes too small for their feet and had foot pain with deformity.

A motto of the fitness shoe industry and the sports medicine community for decades has been that "good shoes can prevent injuries." Identifying the right shoe store and finding a knowledgeable salesperson can ease the task of selecting proper footwear (Table 45-1). The owners or managers of independently owned and operated shoe stores are more likely to offer this kind of expertise. Although shopping at such stores may cost more, individuals with special needs should seek special service when searching for shoes. The Pedorthic Footwear Association in Columbia, Maryland, has a certification process for shoe sales personnel (pedorthist) and can provide a list of members.

Shoe manufacturers offer various types of shoes for different activities (e.g., running, walking, racquetball sports). Injuries and problems often develop when sport-specific shoes are used for a different activity; for example, the heel on tennis shoes is too low for jogging. Cross-training shoes are an attempt to provide features generic to many athletic activities. Practitioners should advise individuals to use proper equipment to prevent sport-related injuries. Although the depth of the toe box in extra-depth shoes and comfort shoes is similar to that of athletic shoes, only athletic shoes should be used for exercise activities.

Shoes are designed to provide stability and cushioning and decrease friction. Thus, shoes should be replaced as soon as they become worn. Studies on running shoes have demonstrated that the midsole of the shoe, which helps reduce the impact on the foot by cushioning or absorbing shock, is the part of the shoe that fatigues first. In the past, midsoles constructed of ethyl vinyl acetate or polyurethane lost 50% of their ability to attenuate force in as little as 250 to 500 miles of running. Individuals with a history of stress fractures, osteoarthritis, or rigid high arches should not wait until the outer sole wears through before replacing shoes. It is wise to replace shoes early and often.

## The Running Surface

Convenience, safety, and the preferences of the runner often dictate the running surface (e.g., concrete sidewalk, grassy surface, dirt shoulder of roads). Because hard surfaces have no give and provide little shock-absorbing capacity, they cause intense shock to the legs, feet, and back. Grassy surfaces, however, are often irregular, and the runner can easily incur a sprained ankle. Running on a sloping or banked surface may cause the foot to rotate excessively, and thus place additional stress on the tendons and ligaments of the leg and foot. Uphill running places a strain on the Achilles tendon and muscles of the lower back; downhill running places a lot of impact on the heel. The ideal running surface is relatively smooth, level, and resilient.

The ideal surface for a walker should also be relatively smooth, level, and resilient. Hard, inflexible surfaces should be avoided as much as possible. A walker who wants to increase energy expenditure may try walking on dirt or sand; such surfaces can boost energy expenditure by as much as one third. Similarly, walking on a mild, 14-degree slope requires more muscle power than walking on a straight, flat surface. However, walkers who become overzealous on these surfaces can encounter the same problems (e.g., sprained ankle) that runners encounter.

**TABLE 45-6 Application Guidelines for Compression Bandages**

- Choose the appropriate size of bandage for the injured body part. Purchase a product designed for the appropriate body part if you are unsure of the size.
- Unwind about 12-18 in. of bandage at a time, and allow the bandage to relax.
- If ice is also being applied to the injured area, soak the bandage in water to aid the transfer of cold (see Table 45-5).
- Wrap the injured area by overlapping the previous layer of bandage by about one third to one half of its width.
- Tightly wrap the point most distal from the injury. For example, if the ankle is injured, begin wrapping just above the toes.
- Decrease the tightness of the bandage as you continue to wrap. (Follow package directions on how far to extend the bandage past the injury.) If the bandage feels tight or uncomfortable or if circulation is impaired, remove the compression bandage and rewrap it. Cold or swollen toes and fingers indicate a bandage is too tight.
- After using the bandage, wash it in lukewarm, soapy water; do not scrub it. Rinse the bandage thoroughly and allow to air dry on a flat surface.
- Roll up the bandage to prevent wrinkles, and store it in a cool, dry place. Do not iron the bandage to remove wrinkles.

## Compression Bandages

Typically, a compression bandage (e.g., Ace Bandages) is used for an ankle or knee sprain. If a compression bandage is to be used, the width of bandage needed depends on the injury site. For example, a foot or an ankle requires a 2.5- to 3-in. bandage. Table 45-6 describes the proper method of applying this type of bandage.

## Cryotherapy

Applying cold compresses to an injury such as a muscle sprain anesthetizes the area and decreases the pain and inflammation. Ice bags or cold wraps are useful for cold application. If an ice bag is used, the English type, which is identified by its commercial cloth material, is preferred because the patient does not have to wrap a towel around it to protect the skin. Cold packs are available as either single-use (e.g., Faultless Instant Cold Pack) or multiple-use products. Another simple, inexpensive method is to prepare ice applications by freezing water in small paper cups, placing ice cubes in a resealable sandwich bag, or using a frozen bag of peas. Table 45-5 describes the proper method of cold application to injuries.

## Contrast Bath Soaks

For acute injury, cold application is beneficial in decreasing resultant inflammation. After the acute injury, some podiatrists advocate the use of alternating applications of cold therapy and warm therapy for chronic, nagging pain. Specifically, the cold therapy is intended to decrease inflammation. The warm therapy attempts to bring increased blood flow to the affected area and effect smooth muscle relaxation.

## Assessment of Exercise-induced Injuries: A Case-based Approach

The practitioner may be called on to play a triage role in treating an exercise-induced injury to the foot. Finding out the location of the pain will help determine the type and extent of the injury. Asking about the nature and duration of the pain will help in determining whether the injury is self-treatable. Case 45-2 illustrates assessment of patients with exercise-induced injuries.

## Patient Counseling for Exercise-induced Injuries

Although a sports enthusiast may resist such advice, the practitioner should encourage the patient to rest an injured foot or limb, allowing it to heal. The practitioner should also explain measures to prevent recurrences of the patient's particular injury. When rest alone does not relieve foot discomfort, the proper use of oral analgesics, compression bandages, and cryotherapy should be explained. The practitioner should review with the patient the correct procedure for wrapping, which is also described on the bandage package. If there is reason to believe the patient may cause further injury through inappropriate use of a compression bandage, the practitioner should recommend simply elevating the body part and applying an ice pack or, if warranted by the severity of the injury, consulting a primary care provider. The box Patient Education for Exercise-induced Injuries lists specific information to provide patients.

### CASE 45-2

| Relevant Evaluation Criteria | Scenario/Model Outcome |
|---|---|
| **Information Gathering** | |
| 1. Gather essential information about the patient's symptoms, including: | |
| a. description of symptom(s) (i.e., nature, onset, duration, severity, associated symptoms) | A patient who frequents the pharmacy is excited to tell you about the exercise program that he has begun. He expresses that he has already lost 5 lb just after 2 weeks of intense running. He points out that he has been experiencing pain in the shin area, especially while exercising. He feels a little stiff before running, but seems to loosen up after about 20 minutes of running. |
| b. description of any factors that seem to precipitate, exacerbate, and/or relieve the patient's symptom(s) | The pain grows gradually with increased exercise. The stiffness goes away on the one day a week that he does not run. |
| c. description of the patient's efforts to relieve the symptoms | Aspirin 325 mg (1-2 tablets, 3-4 times/day) with some relief. He also occasionally applies ice to the area, but has such a busy life it is almost impossible to do it regularly. |
| 2. Gather essential patient history information: | |
| a. patient's identity | Evan Baker |
| b. patient's age, sex, height, and weight | 37 y/o M, 6'1", 234 lb |
| c. patient's occupation | Local delivery driver |
| d. patient's dietary habits | Eats fast food while on the road. Now trying to modify diet to salads and grilled chicken sandwiches. |
| e. patient's sleep habits | 8 hours per night |
| f. concurrent medical conditions, prescription and nonprescription medications, and dietary supplements | Lipitor 10 mg 1 tablet at bedtime for hypercholesterolemia |
| g. allergies | NKA |
| h. history of other adverse reactions to medications | None |
| i. other (describe)_______ | Evan has begun an intense exercise program. He has been running for 1 hour on the treadmill and riding his bike 5-10 miles a day. He has been told that managing his weight will help him reduce his cholesterol. His father had a heart attach 2 weeks ago, which prompted the new exercise effort. He has not been actively involved in an exercise routine since high school. |

## CASE 45-2 (continued)

| Relevant Evaluation Criteria | Scenario/Model Outcome |
|---|---|
| **Assessment and Triage** | |
| 3. Differentiate the patient's signs/symptoms and correctly identify the patient's primary problem(s) (see Table 45-4). | Evan may be suffering from shin splints caused by lack of stretching and inappropriate initiation of exercise program. |
| 4. Identify exclusions for self-treatment. | If pain intensifies or worsens, he should seek assistance from a PCP. |
| 5. Formulate a comprehensive list of therapeutic alternatives for the primary problem to determine if triage to a medical practitioner is required, and share this information with the patient. | Options include:<br>(1) Refer Evan to an appropriate health care professional.<br>(2) Recommend self-care with a nonprescription analgesic and nondrug measures.<br>(3) Recommend self-care until Evan can see an appropriate health care professional.<br>(4) Take no action. |
| **Plan** | |
| 6. Select an optimal therapeutic alternative to address the patient's problem, taking into account patient preferences. | Evan should be instructed to seek medical advice before continuing an intense exercise program. Counseling Evan on the importance of gradually increasing distance and intensity will prevent shins splints. Proper stretching before and after exercise is necessary. Recommend RICE or PRICE therapy (see Tables 45-5 and 45-6) and use of aspirin or ibuprofen after exercise will help decrease inflammation. |
| 7. Describe the recommended therapeutic approach to the patient. | Only a PCP, podiatrist, or orthopedist can properly diagnose and prescribe treatment for your condition. Take a break from intense exercise until condition improves. Then begin a gradual exercise program and diet recommended by your doctor. Remember to thoroughly stretch before beginning any physical activity. |
| 8. Explain to the patient the rationale for selecting the recommended therapeutic approach from the considered therapeutic alternatives. | A gradual increase of exercise and proper stretching will prevent strain on the tendons and injuries. If the pain intensifies, cramps, burns, or remains constant, you should seek medical attention. Applying ice and taking an anti-inflammatory will decrease inflammation. |
| **Patient Education** | |
| 9. When recommending self-care with nonprescription medications and/or nondrug therapy, convey accurate information to the patient, including: | |
| a. appropriate dose and frequency of administration | Taking ibuprofen or aspirin appropriate for short term to relieve pain, but do not use to suppress pain or increase endurance during physical activity. |
| b. maximum number of days the therapy should be employed | See Chapter 5. |
| c. product administration procedures | See Chapter 5. |
| d. expected time to onset of relief | The ibuprofen or aspirin will begin working in approximately 20 minutes after ingestion. |
| e. degree of relief that can be reasonably expected | The ibuprofen or aspirin will only temporarily relieve the discomfort. Seek medical advice if pain persists or increases. |
| f. most common side effects | Upset stomach, nervousness, fatigue, rash |
| g. side effects that warrant medical intervention should they occur | See your PCP if you have severe abdominal pain or notice blood in your stool. |
| h. patient options in the event that condition worsens or persists | A PCP should be consulted if the condition does not improve or if irritation worsens. |
| i. product storage requirements | Store the product in a cool, dry place that is out of children's reach. |

## CASE 45-2 (continued)

| Relevant Evaluation Criteria | Scenario/Model Outcome |
|---|---|
| j. specific nondrug measures | Gradually increase the intensity of your workout. Remember that thorough stretching before exercise can help decrease injuries. |
| 10. Solicit patient's follow-up questions. | Does this problem have something to do with my weight? |
| 11. Answer patient's questions. | No. It is actually a result of lack of conditioning, poor stretching, hard running, and wearing improper footwear (e.g., running and jogging in worn-out shoes or shoes designed for racquet sports), and moving with excessive pronation (i.e., rolling in of the feet), which are common causes of shin splints. |

Key: NKA, no known allergies; PCP, primary care provider; PRICE, protection, rest, ice, compression; elevation; RICE, rest, ice, compression; elevation.

## PATIENT EDUCATION FOR EXERCISE-INDUCED INJURIES

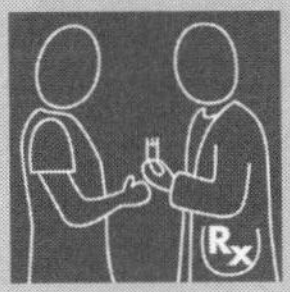

The objectives of self-treatment are to (1) rest the injured foot or limb to allow healing, (2) relieve discomfort, and (3) take measures to prevent further injury. For most patients, carefully following product instructions and the self-care measures listed here will help ensure optimal therapeutic outcomes.

- When a leg or foot injury occurs, rest the injured limb. If desired, perform other types of exercise, such as swimming or bicycling (stationary or outdoor), that do not put a great deal of force on the feet.
- Take the following actions to prevent exercise-induced injuries:
  - Stretch muscles before exercising.
  - Choose sport-specific shoes with good arch support for athletic activities.
  - Run or walk on a relatively smooth, level, and resilient surface.
  - Keep the back straight when running.

### Shin Splints

- Rest the feet, and apply an ice bag or a cold wrap to the painful area (see Table 45-5).
- If desired, take aspirin or ibuprofen to relieve pain and reduce tissue inflammation.
- Do not use analgesics to suppress pain or to increase your endurance during a workout.

⚠ Seek medical attention if the discomfort becomes a cramping, burning tightness that repeatedly occurs at the same distance or time during a run.

### Blisters

- To prevent blisters during running, wear cotton or woolen socks. If desired, wear two pairs of socks with ordinary talcum powder sprinkled between them. Using an acrylic sock will assist in drawing moisture from the foot.
- Apply compound tincture of benzoin or a flexible collodion product (e.g., New Skin) to help toughen the skin.
- Apply an antiperspirant containing 20% aluminum chloride to decrease incidence of blisters.
- If blisters break, apply a first-aid antibiotic to the broken skin to prevent secondary bacterial infection.
- Cover blistered area with moleskin to protect surface.

### Ankle Sprains

- Although maximum swelling will not occur for 48 hours, begin treatment as soon as possible.
- Stay off the injured foot, wrap a compression bandage around the ankle, apply ice, and elevate the ankle. (See Tables 45-5 and 45-6 for guidelines on applying ice and compression bandages.)
- Seek medical attention if swelling persists more than 72 hours.

### Toenail Blisters/Loss

- To prevent blisters under the toenail, keep toenails trimmed and run in properly fitted shoes.
- Should a blister develop, do not disturb or puncture the blister roof.

⚠ If the toenail separates from the skin or is lost, consult a primary care provider or podiatrist for proper treatment.

## Evaluation of Patient Outcomes for Exercise-induced Injuries

The practitioner should follow up with patients with shin splints or ankle sprains 7 days after the use of compression bandages, cryotherapy, or other anti-inflammatory therapy is begun to find out whether the symptoms are resolved. If symptoms of swelling and/or pain persist, referral to a podiatrist or primary care provider is appropriate. Patients with blisters of the feet or under the toenail should also be reevaluated after 7 days of the recommended therapy. If signs of infection are present or if the toenail has separated from the nail bed, medical referral is appropriate.

# INGROWN TOENAILS

## Etiology of Ingrown Toenails

The most frequent cause of ingrown toenails, onychocryptosis, is incorrect trimming of the nails. The correct method is to cut the nail straight across without tapering the corners in any way. Wearing pointed-toe or tight shoes or hosiery that is too tight has also been implicated. Other causes are hyperhidrosis, improper-fitting footwear, trauma, obesity, and excessive pressure. In such instances, direct pressure can force the lateral or medial edge of the nail into the soft tissue, and the embedded nail may then continue to grow. This results in swelling and inflammation of the nail fold.[32]

Bedridden patients may develop ingrown toenails because tight bedcovers press the soft skin tissue against the nails. Nail curling, which can be hereditary or secondary to incorrect nail trimming, onychomycosis, or a systemic, metabolic disease, can also result in ingrown toenails. The presence of psoriatic arthritis may also be demonstrated in the nail.

## Pathophysiology of Ingrown Toenails

An ingrown toenail occurs when a section of nail presses into the soft tissue of the nail groove. The nail curves into the flesh of the toe corners and becomes embedded in the surrounding soft tissue of the toe, causing pain. This process results in microtears of the skin that, when coupled with invasion by opportunistic resident foot bacteria, can cause a superficial infection. Swelling, inflammation, and ulceration are secondary complications that can arise from this condition.

## Treatment of Ingrown Toenails

### *Treatment Goals*

The goals of self-treating ingrown toenails are to (1) relieve pressure on the toenails, (2) relieve pain, and (3) prevent reoccurrence.

### *General Treatment Approach*

Education is probably the best means of preventing the development of ingrown toenails. In the early stages of development, therapy is directed at providing adequate room for the nail to resume its normal position adjacent to soft tissue. This therapy is accomplished by relieving the external source of pressure. Warm water soaks will help soften the area and topical antiseptics can be applied to prevent possible opportunistic infections. The patient should be referred to a podiatrist or primary care provider if the condition is recurrent or gives rise to an oozing discharge, pain, or severe inflammation. Sometimes surgery is warranted and, even with subsequent systemic antibiotic therapy, the toe may take up to 3 to 4 weeks to heal.

### *Pharmacologic Therapy*

In its final rule for ingrown toenail relief products, FDA did not propose any nonprescription active ingredient as safe and effective and not misbranded.[33] Thus, two previously approved drugs, tannic acid and sodium sulfide,[34] were classified as Category III and withdrawn from the market. Tannic acid was not proven to harden the skin and shrink the soft tissue surrounding the ingrown toenail. Sodium sulfide has considerable adverse side effects that made it unacceptable for nonprescription use.[33]

The practitioner, however, must be aware of tradename product reformulations to accommodate this rule. For example, Outgro Pain-Relieving Formula, which formerly contained tannic acid for treating ingrown toenails, now contains benzocaine 20% to relieve pain associated with ingrown toenails. Patients must be cautious because inappropriate use of this product can result in superficial burns on skin adjacent to the toenail. Further, this product does not treat the underlying problem.

Patients with ingrown toenails often fail to realize they may be helped by oral medication intended to allay pain and inflammation. Provided no contraindications exist for use by a particular patient, the practitioner may recommend oral aspirin, ibuprofen, ketoprofen, or naproxen, which are four proven analgesics with anti-inflammatory activity (see Chapter 5).

# FROSTBITE

Frostbite, a less frequent but nonetheless potentially serious condition that often involves the feet, is another area in which practitioners can educate patients and consumers about preventive measures. Frostbite is defined as the actual freezing of tissues by excessive exposure to low temperatures. To maintain normal core temperature in cold weather, the body reflexively reduces the flow of blood to the skin surface and the extremities. Therefore, frostbite usually involves areas of the body (e.g., feet, hands, earlobes, nose, cheeks) that are farthest from deep organs or large muscles. Minor frostbite may cause only blanching of the skin; severe frostbite may result in the loss of fingers and toes. With minor frostbite, the skin may have clear blisters when the skin is warmed and severe frostbite will produce hemorrhagic blisters.

Predisposing factors to developing frostbite include homelessness; diabetes mellitus; alcohol ingestion; motor vehicle problems in severe, wintry weather; mental illness; and/or a previous cold injury. Additional predisposing factors to the development of frostbite include the following:[35]

- Low temperatures (especially with high winds)
- Long periods of exposure to cold
- Lack of proper clothing
- Wet clothing
- Poor nutrition, exhaustion, dehydration, and/or smoking
- Circulatory disease
- Immobility
- Direct contact with metal or petroleum products at low temperatures
- Individual susceptibility to cold

Frostbite is not amenable to therapy with nonprescription drug products. The frostbitten part should be promptly and thoroughly rewarmed in water heated to 100°F to 108°F (45.6°C to 47.8°C). The water should *not* be hot to a normal hand at room temperature and should *not* be tested with the frozen part. The container of water should be large enough for the frozen part to move freely without bumping against the sides. Rewarming should be continued until a flush returns to the most distal tip of the thawed part. This process usually takes about 20 to 30 minutes. It is important not to rub or apply pressure to the skin to prevent tissue damage. Do not attempt to remove socks or other clothing that may be frozen to the skin. Immerse frozen clothing along with the affected body part.[36] Dry heat (e.g., a heating pad) should be avoided because it is difficult to control the temperature and rewarm the frozen part evenly. Overapplication of radiant heat (e.g., wood fire, stove heat) could actually burn the skin without the patient being aware. Once the injured part has been properly warmed, it should be soaked for about 20 minutes in a whirlpool bath once or twice daily until the healing process is complete. Blisters are left intact. Antibiotics are used only if the tissue is infected. Tetanus prophylaxis is indicated.

The best treatment for frostbite is prevention; practitioners should be able to provide a few simple rules to follow:

- Dress to maintain body warmth, taking into account the face, neck, and head, as well as the extremities.
- Avoid exposure to cold during times of sickness or exhaustion.
- Do not exceed the body's tolerance to cold exposure.
- Avoid tight-fitting garments; dress with layered clothing.
- Wear clothing that allows ventilation and prevents perspiration buildup (water enhances heat loss).
- Wear insulated boots or shoes and socks (preferably wool) that fit snugly but are not tight in spots.
- Wear mittens instead of gloves in severe cold; the thumb should be with the rest of the fingers and not by itself.
- Never touch objects (especially cold metal or petroleum products) that facilitate heat loss.
- Think twice about traveling by automobile in inclement, wintry weather in which one can be marooned (e.g., on an interstate highway). This activity can be especially disastrous for a patient with poor peripheral blood circulation.

When given the opportunity, the practitioner should seek to correct a few misconceptions. It is dangerous to rub the affected area with ice or snow even though it seems to provide warmth; this action can result in prolonged contact with the cold, and the ice crystals may lacerate cells. In addition, people should refrain from drinking alcohol for "antifreeze" purposes. Alcohol can induce a loss of body heat even though it may give the individual a feeling of warmth when ingested. Finally, frostbite victims should avoid smoking. Nicotine can induce peripheral vasoconstriction and further reduce the blood supply to the frostbitten extremity. It would also seem prudent to forewarn patients who want to stop smoking and are using a nicotine-containing smoking cessation product (e.g., gum, lozenge, inhaler) or one of the topical transdermal nicotine patches (e.g., Habitrol, Nicoderm, Nicotrol, or ProStep) that they should avoid excessive exposure to the cold (see Chapter 50).

## KEY POINTS FOR MINOR FOOT DISORDERS

- The nonprescription drug of choice to treat corns and calluses is salicylic acid in a collodionlike vehicle or plaster product form.
- Predisposing factors responsible for corns and calluses must be corrected.
- Patients should also be cautioned that frequent recurrence of any of these problems is an indication that they should consult a podiatrist or primary care provider.
- Patients with diabetes, circulatory problems, and/or arthritis should be counseled to avoid self-medicating with any topical or oral nonprescription drug without first checking with their primary care provider, podiatrist, or pharmacist.
- OTC products are powerful drugs and may exacerbate certain conditions; the practitioner must monitor patient progress carefully and be attuned to patient comments that might indicate the occurrence of drug-related problems.
- Be prepared to educate and assist patients who develop athletic injuries.
- Most running injuries can be treated with shoe modifications, in-shoe supports, modified training methods, ice applications, and stretching exercises.
- Maintaining good foot hygiene is an important component of overall health care.
- Talking with patients about proper foot hygiene is an important aspect of caring for the patient as a whole.[37]

## References

1. Georgia Podiatric Medical Association. Available at: http://www.gapma.com/FootFacts.htm. Accessed January 31, 2005.
2. Deaconess Associations Incorporated. Caring for the aging foot. Available at: http://www.deaconess-healthcare.com/cftaf.html. Accessed January 31, 2005.
3. Gorter K, de Poel S, de Melker R, et al. Variation in diagnosis and management of common foot problems by GPs. *Fam Pract.* 2001;18:569-73.
4. Plummer ES, Albert SG. Foot care assessment in patients with diabetes: a screening algorithm for patient education and referral. Diabetes *Ed.* 1995;21:47-51.
5. Frykberg RG. Diabetic foot ulcers: current concepts. *J Foot Ankle Surg.* 1998;37:440-6.
6. Singh N, Armstrong DG, Lipsky BA. Preventing foot ulcers in patients with diabetes. *JAMA.* 2005;293:217-28.
7. Hunt D. Using evidence in practice foot care in diabetes. *Endocrinol Metab Clin North Am.* 2002;31:306-611.
8. emedicine. Foot infections. Available at: http://www.emedicine.com/orthoped/topic601.htm. Accessed January 31, 2005.
9. Martin RW, Martin KS, Popovich NG. Podiatry and pharmacy: working together. *Drug Topics.* 2001;145(12):43-52.

10. Bedinghaus JM, Niedfeldt MW. Over-the-counter foot remedies. *Am Fam Physician.* 2001;64:791-96.
11. Freeman DB. Corns and calluses resulting from mechanical hyperkeratosis. *Am Fam Physician.* 2002;65:2277-80.
12. Singh D, Bentley G, Trevino SG. Fortnightly review: callosities, corns, and calluses. *BMJ.* 1996;312:1403-06.
13. Department of Surgery at University of Colorado Health Sciences Center. Available at: http://www.uschsc.edu/sm/surgery/podiatry.html. Accessed June 21, 2005.
14. Bedinghaus JM, Niedfeldt MW. Information from your family doctor. Over-the-counter remedies for common foot problems. *Am Fam Physician.* 2001;64:791-804.
15. *Federal Register.* 1990;55:33258-62.
16. *Federal Register.* 1990;55:33246-56.
17. Staying one step ahead of foot problems. *Consumer Rep Health.* January 1992;4(1):4.
18. American Podiatric Medical Association. Available at: http://www.apma.org/s_apma/doc.asp?TRACKID=&CID=146&DID=9388. Accessed January 31, 2005.
19. Adams SB, Theodore GH. Extracorporeal Shock Wave Therapy for Treatment of Plantar Fasciitis. *OJHMS Online.* Available at: http://orthojournalhms.org/volume5/manuscripts/ms13.htm. Accessed February 5, 2005.
20. Are you taking good care of your feet? *Tufts University Health and Nutrition Letter.* September 2002:6.
21. Wapner KL, Sharkey PF. The use of night splints for treatment of recalcitrant plantar fasciitis. *Foot Ankle.* 1991;12:135-7.
22. Thompson PD, Stern MP, Williams P, et al. Death during jogging or running. *JAMA.* 1979;242:1265-7.
23. American Podiatric Medical Association. Available at: http://www.apma.org/s_apma/doc.asp?TRACKID=&CID=25&DID=9122. Accessed January 31, 2005.
24. Goodman A. Foot orthoses in sports medicine. *South Med J.* 2004;97:867-70.
25. Safran MR, Zachazewski JE, Benedetti RS, et al. Lateral ankle sprains: a comprehensive review Part 2: treatment and rehabilitation with an emphasis on the athlete. *Med Sci Sports Exerc.* 1999;31:S438-47.
26. Sanderlin BW, Raspa RF. Common Stress Fractures. *Am Fam Physician.* 2003;68:1527-32.
27. Freiman A, Barankin B, Elpern DJ. Sports dermatology part 1: common dermatoses. *CMAJ.* 2004;171:851-3.
28. Knapik JJ, Reynolds KL, Barson J. The influence of antiperspirants on foot blister incidence during prolonged cross-country hiking 1337. *Med Sci Sports Exerc.* 1997;29:234.
29. Wolfe MW. Management of ankle sprains. *Am Fam Physician.* 2001;63:93-112.
30. McPoil TG, Adrian M, Pidcoe P. Effects of foot orthotics on center of pressure patterns in women. *Phys Ther.* 1989;69:149.
31. Frey C, Thompson F, Smith J, et al. American Orthopaedic Foot and Ankle Society women's shoe survey. *Foot Ankle.* 1993;14:79-81.
32. Zuber TJ. Ingrown toenail removal. *Am Fam Physician.* 2002;65:2547-50.
33. *Federal Register.* 1993;58:47602-6.
34. *Federal Register.* 1982;47:39120-5.
35. Biem J, Koehncke N, Classen D, et al. Out of the cold: management of hypothermia and frostbite. *CMAJ.* 2003;168(3):305-11.
36. Bourg P. When your patient has frostbite. Your quick action may save life and limb. *Nursing87.* 1987.
37. Howell M, Thirlaway S. Integrating foot care into the everyday clinical practices of nurses. *BJN.* 2004;13:470-3.

# CHAPTER 46

# Hair Loss

*Michael D. Hogue*

Significant numbers of both men and women experience either thinning hair or hair loss. Often hair loss is secondary to trauma, medication use, acute or chronic illness, dietary changes, and/or hormonal changes. Regardless of the cause, hair loss can have a significant psychologic and social impact on individuals' lives. Thus, patients spend millions of dollars each year on products and procedures both proven and unproven to treat hair loss.

Although only a few causes of hair loss account for the vast majority of cases, many causes and types of baldness exist. Hair loss is broadly categorized as nonscarring or scarring alopecia. Androgenetic alopecia (AGA or pattern hereditary hair loss), alopecia areata, anagen effluvium (rapid shedding of growing hairs), telogen effluvium (rapid shedding of resting hairs), cosmetic hair damage, and trichotillomania (a compulsive pulling out of one's own hair) are common forms of nonscarring alopecia. Of these causes, only androgenic alopecia is effectively treated by nonprescription products. Other types of nonscarring hair loss should be referred for medical evaluation to determine cause and proper treatment. Scarring alopecia may be related to conditions such as discoid lupus erythematosus, syphilis, sarcoid, or lichen planus and should also be referred for medical evaluation.[1]

## Epidemiology of Hair Loss

Androgenetic alopecia is the most common form of hair loss, affecting about one third of the U.S. male population and about one sixth of the female population. It is characterized by progressive, patterned hair loss from the scalp. By age 30, about 30% of white men have androgenetic alopecia, with the incidence increasing to 50% by age 50. White men are four times more likely than black men to develop premature hair loss.[2]

Alopecia areata (autoimmune hair loss) affects men and women of all races equally and occurs in 2% of the U.S. population. Most cases (60%) are in children and young adults.[3]

Telogen effluvium is a common condition internationally, but its exact prevalence has not been determined. Telogen effluvium has no racial bias and can occur at any age. Episodes are common in the first months of life. An episode can occur in either gender, but because postpartum hormonal changes are a frequent cause, the condition is believed to affect women more often than men. The chronic form of this disease has been reported mainly in women.[4]

## Anatomy and Physiology of Hair Growth

A strand of hair is a cylinder of tightly keratinized cells that grows at the base of the follicle (see Figure 33-1 in Chapter 33).[5] The hair follicle, which anchors the hair strand to the skin, contains cells that produce new hairs. These germinative cells, located at the base of the follicle next to the dermal papilla, make up the follicular matrix; the matrix cells eventually keratinize to form hair.

Hair follicle activity is cyclic. In the growing phase (anagen), the follicle lengthens, the dermal papilla enlarges, and a new hair is formed. During the catagen phase—a transition phase between the growing and resting phases—cell proliferation ceases, the hair follicle shortens, and a bulbous enlargement forms at the base of the hair. The resting phase (telogen) has an unpigmented, club-shaped root that is embedded in a shortened follicle. Telogen, or terminal, hairs are loosely held in place. Duration of the anagen phase in any individual normal scalp follicle is genetically determined and ranges from 2 to 5 years, with an average duration of 1000 days.[6] The average rate of human scalp hair growth is 0.37 mm per day. The average duration of the telogen phase, however, is only 100 days, resulting in a ratio of anagen to telogen hairs of 12:1. Typically, 100 to 150 hairs are lost from the scalp each day as telogen hairs are shed.

The type of hair growth depends on follicle location and the person's age and gender. Vellus hair is soft, fine, usually unpigmented, and less than 2 cm long (e.g., abdominal hair), whereas terminal hair is coarse, longer, and pigmented (e.g., scalp hair).

The human scalp contains approximately 100,000 to 150,000 hair follicles, which are evenly distributed.[7] These follicles have sebaceous glands whose oily secretions lubricate the scalp. Blondes apparently have greater than the usual number of follicles, and redheads, fewer. By the third decade of life, density of hair follicles usually decreases to one half that found in a newborn.[7]

Hair follicles and their sebaceous glands produce enzymes (δ-5-3 β-hydroxysteroid hydrogenase, 17 β-hydroxysteroid hydrogenase, and 5-α-reductase type I) that convert weak androgens (such as dehydro-3-epiandrosterone and 4-androstenedione) to testosterone and dihydrotestosterone (DHT). Testosterone and DHT stimulate production of growth factors and proteases, effect vascularization of the follicle and the composition of basement membrane

**Editor's Note:** This chapter is based, in part, on the 14th edition chapter with the same title, which was written by John S. Esterly, Lee E. West, and Dennis P. West.

proteins, and alter the amounts of cofactors required for follicle metabolism. Another enzyme (aromatase) found in the lower portion of the outer root sheath converts androgens (4-androstenedione and testosterone) to estrogens. These enzymes are believed to maintain androgen balance in the follicle, thereby regulating the hair cycle. Testosterone and DHT apparently bind to receptor proteins in bulbar dermal papilla cell nuclei. The complex then attaches to a DNA site that regulates the manufacture of messenger RNAs responsible for hair protein synthesis. In a scalp hair follicle, the complex downregulates synthesis, whereas the opposite occurs in a hair follicle on the face.[8]

## Etiology/Pathophysiology of Hair Loss

### *Androgenetic Alopecia*

In androgenetic alopecia, the hair follicle undergoes a stepwise miniaturization and change in growth dynamics. With each successive cycle, the anagen (growing) phase becomes shorter and the telogen (resting) phase becomes longer. Consequently over time, the anagen-to-telogen ratio decreases from 12:1 to 5:1. Because telogen hairs are more loosely anchored to follicles, their presence in increased numbers manifests eventually by increased shedding. Also, the catagen phase (the intermediate phase between anagen regrowth and telogen shedding) increases, reducing the number of hairs. As telogen hairs are shed, they are gradually replaced by velluslike (short and fine) hairs[9] (mean diameter reduced from 0.08 mm to less than 0.06 mm) or anagen hairs that are too short to reach the surface. Although miniaturization of the follicle may be an abrupt process, pharmacologic treatment may, likewise, trigger development of enlarged anagen follicles in a fast, one hair-cycle response.[10]

The site-specific effects on hair growth are paradoxical. Pubic, axillary, chest, and face hair follicles respond to androgens by growing into terminal hair, whereas scalp follicles respond by growing vellus hair (resembling peach fuzz). The androgen DHT, which is converted from testosterone by 5-α-reductase, is believed to be a primary repressor of hair growth by the mechanism mentioned in the previous section. This androgen also binds five times more readily than testosterone to androgen receptors. Although two forms of the 5-α-reductase are found in the scalps of bald men, the amount of DHT formed locally (in scalp hair) is small compared with what is available systemically (produced by the prostate gland). The relative contributions of local and systemic DHT to balding are still not known.

Increased 5-α-reductase–mediated conversion of testosterone to DHT in the balding areas of women with androgenetic alopecia also supports the contention that DHT is important to this process. Women with this disease rarely lose all their hair, not only because they have less 5-α-reductase but also because they have more aromatase that converts testosterone into estradiol.[11] In addition, women are more likely to have follicles with fewer localized androgen receptors and, therefore, are more likely to retain actively growing hair.[12]

Hair loss has also been noted as a marker of other abnormal physiologic processes and conditions. One study reported that prostate size, and hence the presence of benign prostate hyperplasia (BPH), directly correlates to the rate of AGA. Men with prostate size greater than 30 $cm^3$ and a diagnosis of BPH had a significantly higher rate of AGA than those with prostate size less than 30 $cm^3$ and no diagnosis of BPH. It is unclear whether BPH therapies reduce the prevalence of AGA or vice versa.[13]

Additionally, alopecia in women has been shown to be present in women diagnosed with polycystic ovary syndrome (PCOS). PCOS is perhaps one of the most common endocrine-related disorders in females of reproductive age, associated with many acute and chronic illnesses, including diabetes, cardiovascular disease, and several reproductive disorders.[14] Generally, the disorder is that of androgen excess. At least one study documented androgenic alopecia as a significant clinical finding in PCOS.[15]

The rate of progression and the pattern of hair loss appear to be genetically determined; however, premature hair loss is not always manifested because of variability in gene expression.[16] The possibility of a different model of gene expression, such as polygenic inheritance, has not been excluded. In this model, baldness would depend on the number of baldness genes.[17]

### *Alopecia Areata*

Alopecia areata is a disease marked by an autoimmune attack on an unidentified target within the hair follicle. Cytotoxic T cells are believed to attack an autoantigen that is normally sequestered. The result is arrested hair growth. Triggers believed to increase gene expression in alopecia areata include microtrauma, neurogenic inflammation, and microbial antigens.[18] Genetic factors may increase susceptibility to this condition.[19] The first hair loss gene for alopecia areata has been mapped. The gene was identified because it was missing from a family suffering from the most severe form of alopecia areata—alopecia universalis, a rare disorder that causes total body hair loss.[20] This scientific development has important implications for the future (perhaps genetic) treatment of this problem.

The pathophysiologic process of alopecia areata generally follows a course beginning with one or more small patches of concentric hair loss, followed by progression to total scalp hair loss. Complete loss of all body hair (alopecia universalis) is also possible. Onset is typically sudden, and both males and females can be affected by this disorder. The psychological impact of alopecia areata is significant, and patients should be referred to support groups, such as those offered through the National Alopecia Areata Foundation (www.naaf.org).

The more severe forms of alopecia areata can occur at any age but are most likely with initial hair loss at an early age that is very severe. Alopecia areata is also more likely in individuals with preexisting eczema or asthma. Patients with alopecia areata are more likely to have thyroid disease, vitiligo (patches of unpigmented skin), insulin-dependent diabetes, and other autoimmune diseases.[21] Moreover, the incidence of alopecia areata in patients with Down syndrome is high.[22]

**TABLE 46-1 Selected Drugs Known to Cause Hair Loss[23-26]**

| | |
|---|---|
| Anorexiants | Hydroxyurea |
| Antineoplastic agents | Idarubicin HCl |
| Benzodiazepines | Irinotecan HCl |
| β-Adrenergic blockers | Ketoconazole |
| Bromocriptine | Leuprolide acetate |
| Buspirone | Levodopa |
| Calcium channel blockers | Mefloquine |
| Capecitabine | Mesalamine |
| Carbamazepine | Methylphenidate HCl |
| Clomiphene citrate | Mexiletine HCl |
| Colchicine | Nonsteroidal anti-inflammatory drugs |
| Cyclosporine | Octreotide acetate |
| Danazol | Paclitaxel |
| Dexmethylphenidate HCl | Pentostatin |
| Didanosine | Retinoids |
| Doxorubicin | Selegiline |
| Eflornithine HCl | Selenium sulfide |
| Estrogens and estrogenic compounds (including those used for birth control) | Serotonin 5-$HT_1$ receptor agonists |
| Follitropins | Tamoxifen citrate |
| Gemcitabine HCl | Terbinafine |
| Gold compounds | Thyroid hormones and antithyroid agents |
| Guanethidine | Valproic acid and derivatives |
| | Vincristine sulfate |

### *Nonhereditary Hair Loss*

Nonhereditary alopecias (such as telogen effluvium) have no characteristic pattern of hair loss, and the baldness may be asymmetric. The cause is believed to be physiologic stress because this ailment can be a complication or result of the following:

- Acute illness involving fever; severe viral, fungal, or protozoan infection; major surgery; or severe trauma, with hair loss occurring for anywhere from a week to several months
- Chronic illness, such as cancer (especially lymphoproliferative cancer), systemic lupus erythematosus (SLE), end-stage renal disease, or liver disease
- Hormonal changes during and following a pregnancy (both mother and child can be affected), and endocrine disorders such as hypothyroidism and discontinuation of estrogen-containing medication
- Dietary changes leading to anorexia; excessive ingestion of dietary heavy metals, such as selenium, arsenic, and thallium; or severe nutritional deficiencies, such as low protein intake, chronic iron deficiency (runners sometimes develop anemia that leads to hair loss), or deficiencies of essential fatty acids, zinc, or biotin
- Use of certain drugs (Table 46-1) that trigger hair loss[23-26]

Antimitotic drugs, such as chemotherapy drugs used to treat cancer and antimitotics used to inhibit lactation (e.g., bromocriptine), can cause narrowing of the hair shaft, which may fracture the hair or stop hair growth. This condition is referred to as anagen alopecia or anagen effluvium (when referring to the shedding of anagen hairs). Another disease also marked by loose anagen hairs is "loose anagen syndrome." This uncommon disorder may be transmitted by autosomal dominant inheritance and is predominantly found in fair-haired girls ages 2 to 9 years.[27]

Certain diseases, hair care products, and hair-grooming methods associated with scarring or burns on the scalp may result in scarring alopecia. Traction alopecia is seen primarily in children who braid their hair tightly every day. Braiding traumatizes the hair follicles, causing hairs to loosen and break. Patients who use oily moisturizers to make hair more manageable and stop the scalp from flaking may develop folliculitis and resultant hair loss. Hot combs used to straighten hair may cause scalp inflammation and resultant scarring alopecia.[28]

Chronic papulosquamous diseases of the scalp, such as psoriasis and seborrheic dermatitis, may also lead to scarring alopecia.

Untreated, or improperly treated, tinea capitis may lead to hair loss. This disease, most commonly caused by *Trichophyton tonsurans* (a fungus), must be treated with systemic antifungals to eradicate it from the hair. The illness appears as black dots where the hair breaks off at the scalp's skin surface.[28] Other superficial dermatophytes may infect hair and cause hair loss.

Psychologic stress may potentiate several types of hair loss, although the literature on this subject is conflicting. High stress levels may depress the immune system and lead to symptoms such as hair loss.

## Signs and Symptoms of Hair Loss

The scalp of a patient with androgenetic alopecia shows no signs of inflammation or scarring. Hair loss is gradual, and the number of hairs coming out during brushing or shampooing does not suddenly increase, in contrast to other alopecias. Typically, male androgenetic hair loss is insidious in onset and usually does not start until after puberty. Progression fluctuates considerably, with 3 to 6 months of accelerated loss followed by 6 to 18 months of no loss. Most men take 15 to 25 years to lose their hair. Male pattern hair loss and/or gradual hair thinning usually occurs at the top rear of the head (vertex), the frontal hairline, and the occipital regions. The loss begins with a recession of the frontal hairline and continues with thinning at the vertex until all that is left is a fringe of hair at the occipital and temporal margins.

In women with androgenetic alopecia, hair loss is typically more diffuse. There is a characteristic retention of the frontal hairline. Later, diffuse thinning is seen over the entire crown. Hair density remains normal but hair length does not. The woman's scalp will show a high density of hair, but the hairs will be thinner than normal, short, and tapered (rather than blunt, as seen when hair is damaged by breakage).

Androgenetic alopecia in women is a cause for suspicion of hyperandrogenism—an excess of androgen, which commonly accompanies significant acne, hirsutism (hairiness in other parts of the body), menstrual irregularities, and infertility. Topical eflornithine cream is marketed as a prescription agent to treat facial hirsutism.[29] Eflornithine is an irreversible inhibitor of ornithine decarboxylase, an enzyme that produces polyamines in the hair follicle that are essential for anagen hair growth.[30] It is conceivable that a patient with pattern hair loss may be using a hair regrowth treatment agent on the scalp while using an antihirsute agent to remove excess hair on the face. Androgen excess may indicate serious metabolic disturbances, such as cardiovascular disease, diabetes mellitus, and endometrial cancer.[31]

Autoimmune hair loss (alopecia areata) has three stages: sudden loss of hair in patches, enlargement of the patches, and regrowth. The cycle may take months, sometimes years, and can occur in any hair-bearing area. Axillary, pubic, and other body hairs are often not affected. However, the eyebrows and eyelashes can be lost and sometimes may be the only sites affected.[32] Up to 5% of patients lose all their scalp hair (alopecia totalis), and 1% of patients lose all their body and scalp hair (alopecia universalis). Hair loss may accompany or be preceded by nail pitting or other nail abnormalities, as well as by itching, tingling, burning, or other painful sensations in the patch of hair loss.

A diagnostic criterion for alopecia areata is the presence of exclamation point hairs, which are shorter than normal and have a frayed distal end and a narrowed root end, making them look like exclamation points when viewed under a dissecting microscope. This characteristic is often used to distinguish trichotillomania (in which hair has blunt ends) from alopecia areata.

Telogen effluvium (also known as diffuse alopecia) is characterized by nonscarring, diffuse hair loss usually caused by metabolic or hormonal disturbances or medications. The acute form is defined by shedding that lasts less than 6 months; the chronic form lasts longer than 6 months. The metabolic or physiologic disturbance usually precedes shedding by 1 to 6 months, but identifying a specific causal event is often difficult, if not impossible.

Hair loss may be quantified by a gentle hair-pull test, a wash test, and a daily count test.[33] A primary care provider will confirm a diagnosis of telogen effluvium if the hair-pull test (the gentle forced extraction of 10 to 20 hairs from the scalp) reveals that more than 25% of the pulled hairs are in telogen phase. (Telogen hairs have a white bulb but no gelatinous hair sheath. Anagen hairs have both.[23])

Anagen alopecia is marked by loss of primarily anagen hairs, although some telogen hairs may also be removed by the gentle hair-pull test. Anagen hairs stop growing or will not grow long. In other ways, the disease is very similar to telogen effluvium.

## Treatment of Hair Loss

### Treatment Goals

The goal in self-treating hair loss is to restore the patient's appearance by recommending (1) cosmetic camouflage and, if applicable, (2) the use of topical minoxidil to stimulate hair growth.

### General Treatment Approach

Currently, only topical minoxidil 2% and 5% are approved for self-treatment of androgenetic alopecia. Treatment is specifically for loss of vertex but not frontal hair. If the patient's baldness is clearly androgenetic, treatment with topical minoxidil 2% for women and 5% for men can be recommended. Otherwise, patients should be referred to their primary care provider for diagnosis. The algorithm in Figure 46-1 outlines the self-treatment of hair loss and lists specific exclusions for self-treatment.

### Nonpharmacologic Therapy

Thinning hair can be camouflaged by using wigs (hair pieces) and hair weaves, which are cosmetically more appealing than they were a decade ago. Hair loss that is dramatic and extensive can be emotionally distressing. Although some people may need counseling to recover their self-image and regain self-confidence, an attractive wig may ease the problem. Treatment of less severe hair loss can be approached by using hair sprays, gels, colorants, perms, and topical hair-building products in moderation; these products can create an illusion of fullness without decreasing hair loss.

Scalp massage, frequent shampooing, and electrical stimulation have been proposed as treatments for hair loss; however, such remedies are considered ineffective.[34]

Acute telogen effluvium usually resolves spontaneously, and treatment is limited to comforting and reassuring the patient. Chronic telogen effluvium is slower to resolve, but the patient still needs comfort and reassurance. When a primary care provider has determined that the patient's hair loss is caused by poor diet or iron deficiency, the patient may benefit from consulting a dietitian. In deficiency states, increasing protein intake or providing iron supplements, and eliminating the intake of large amounts of vitamin A may be simple solutions to reversing hair loss seen in these situations.

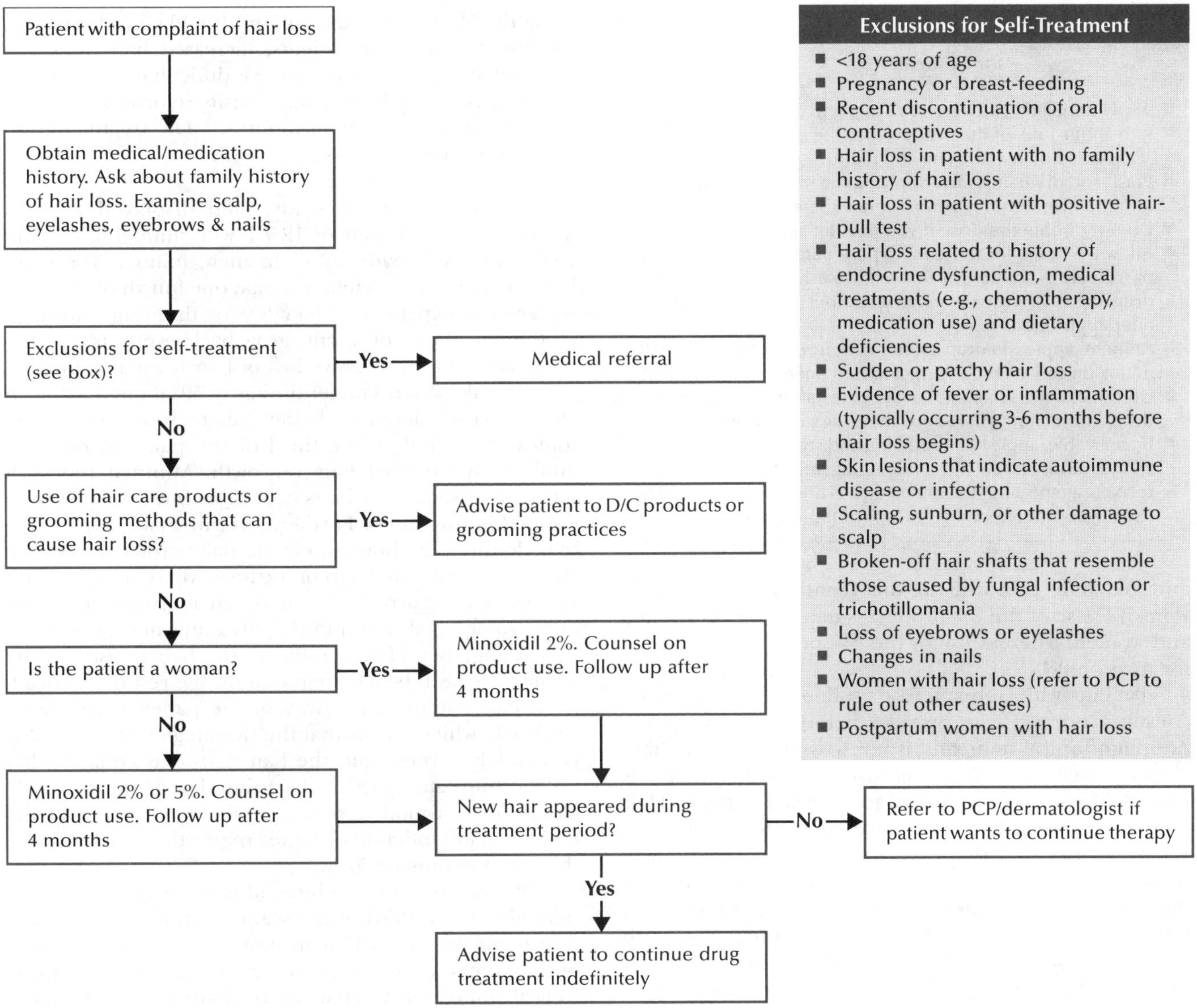


**Exclusions for Self-Treatment**

- <18 years of age
- Pregnancy or breast-feeding
- Recent discontinuation of oral contraceptives
- Hair loss in patient with no family history of hair loss
- Hair loss in patient with positive hair-pull test
- Hair loss related to history of endocrine dysfunction, medical treatments (e.g., chemotherapy, medication use) and dietary deficiencies
- Sudden or patchy hair loss
- Evidence of fever or inflammation (typically occurring 3-6 months before hair loss begins)
- Skin lesions that indicate autoimmune disease or infection
- Scaling, sunburn, or other damage to scalp
- Broken-off hair shafts that resemble those caused by fungal infection or trichotillomania
- Loss of eyebrows or eyelashes
- Changes in nails
- Women with hair loss (refer to PCP to rule out other causes)
- Postpartum women with hair loss

**FIGURE 46-1** Self-care of hair loss. Key: D/C, discontinue; PCP, primary care provider.

Hair loss that occurs as a result of trauma, such as braiding the hair (traction alopecia), using oils (inflammatory folliculitis), and compulsively pulling hair (trichotillomania), can all be reversed by abandoning these practices. Patients with inflammatory folliculitis may also benefit from the use of antibacterial shampoos.

Surgical transplantation of terminal hair follicles from another anatomic site is another alternative, nonpharmacologic approach to hair loss. This method may be useful in frontal hair loss as well as vertex hair loss.

## Pharmacologic Therapy

### Minoxidil

Minoxidil 2% and extra-strength topical minoxidil 5%, as hydroalcoholic solutions, are the only nonprescription agents currently approved by the Food and Drug Administration (FDA) for use in regrowing hair.

*Mechanism of Action* Minoxidil is a potassium channel opener and vasodilator (when used orally to control hypertension). The drug appears to act by increasing cutaneous blood flow directly to hair follicles, which increase in size after treatment,[35] and promotes and maintains vascularization of hair follicles in alopecia.[36] Minoxidil, which has been shown to directly stimulate follicular hypertrophy and prolong the anagen phase,[37] may transform resting (telogen phase) hair follicles into active (anagen phase) hair follicles. Another study, which used a higher-than-marketed concentration of minoxidil, reported an increase in mean hair shaft diameter.[38] After up to 12 months of therapy, a subset of these same patients also revealed a reduction in the percentage of telogen hairs.

*Indications* Androgenetic alopecia in men and women is amenable to topical minoxidil treatment. Treatment is indicated for baldness at the crown of the head in men

**TABLE 46-2 Administration Guidelines for Minoxidil[43,44]**

- Apply minoxidil to clean, dry scalp and hair.
- Rub about 1 mL of the product into the affected area of the scalp twice daily (morning and night).
- Wash and dry hands after applying the medication. If it gets into the eyes, mouth, or nose, rinse these areas thoroughly.
- Do not double the dose if you miss an application.
- Allow 2-4 hours for the drug to penetrate the scalp. Do not participate in any activity that might wash away or dilute the drug (e.g., bathing or swimming without a cap) for 2-4 hours after application.
- At night, apply the drug 2-4 hours before bedtime because minoxidil can stain clothing and bed linen if not fully dry.
- Do not dry the scalp with a hair dryer after applying the drug. This action will reduce the drug's effectiveness.
- If applicable, apply hair grooming and styling products (e.g., sprays, mousses, gels) or coloring agents, permanents, or relaxing agents after the minoxidil has dried. These products usually do not affect the efficacy of topical minoxidil.

and for hair thinning at the frontoparietal area in women.[39] Use of the 2% product is indicated in both men and women, whereas use of the 5% product is indicated for men only.

Patients with nonpattern or sudden hair loss should consult a primary care provider before using minoxidil. Although topical minoxidil is not well proven in treating alopecia areata or telogen effluvium, this medication is reported by some to be useful for selected patients. Hair often regrows spontaneously in patients with mild alopecia areata. Patients with persistent alopecia areata may respond to combination therapy in which topical minoxidil is one of the medications used. Several combination therapies including topical minoxidil in conjunction with anthralin, topical steroids, or topical retinoids have been used, with some therapeutic advantage, for treating severe alopecia areata.[40] Topical minoxidil only slightly inhibits the amount of hair loss caused by anagen effluvium and may therefore offer less potential benefit.[41]

For men undergoing hair transplantation, when hair follicles may be viable but not optimally functioning in the area to be transplanted, topical minoxidil can increase hair density, speed regrowth in transplanted follicles and complement the surgical outcome by minimizing the likelihood of progression of hair loss.[42]

*Dosage and Administration Guidelines* Minoxidil can be applied using various methods (Table 46-2), depending on the applicator (spray, extended spray tip, dropper, and/or rub-on assembly).[43,44]

It may take approximately 4 months for topical minoxidil 2% and approximately 2 months for topical minoxidil 5% to stimulate increased hair growth, which is usually colorless, soft, and short. As treatment progresses, the hairs gradually mature and begin to look like existing terminal hairs. If increased hair density fails to appear by 12 months for men and 8 months for women after using the 2% product, the patient should consider ending treatment. If increased hair density fails to appear by 4 months after using the 5% product, the patient should consider ending treatment. For many patients, increased hair density is minimal and treatment response is difficult to assess. Once the drug is discontinued, hair density returns to pretreatment levels in a matter of months.[45] The treatment also slows or inhibits hair loss.

*Efficacy* In a 48-week study, men displayed a mean increase in hair density of 12.7% with minoxidil 2% and 18.6% with minoxidil 5%.[41] In men, minoxidil is more likely to be effective when less than one fourth of the scalp surface has experienced hair loss or thinning. Although all the hair does not usually grow back, even with continued treatment, progressive loss of hair is usually slowed.

Of male patients under the age of 50, about one fourth experience moderate or better hair regrowth after using topical minoxidil.[39] One third of the patients, however, attain only minimal hair regrowth. Minimal regrowth means that some new hairs are visible but not enough to cover thinning areas. Furthermore, in treated areas, the hair density (i.e., how closely the hairs grow) is less than that on the untreated part of the head where no significant hair loss has occurred. With moderate regrowth, hairs may cover some or all the thinning area and may grow more closely together. However, again, the hair density in the treated area will be less than that on the rest of the head.

In one study, a minority of the patients had dense regrowth, which means that the thinning areas are almost completely covered and the hair density is equal to that on the untreated part of the head. The placebo vehicle also showed a modest response: about one tenth of the patients had moderate or better regrowth, and about one third had minimal regrowth.[39]

In women, topical minoxidil is more effective if less than about one third of the scalp is thinning. Study data for women ages 18 to 45 years indicate that about one fifth of the women experienced moderate regrowth after using topical minoxidil, whereas more than one third experienced only minimal regrowth. In comparison, the placebo vehicle showed a 7% response rate for moderate regrowth and a 33% response rate for minimal regrowth.[39]

No differences in side effects or other problems were demonstrated in a limited number of older patients up to age 65 years. In short, those most responsive to topical minoxidil treatment are younger patients who have limited hair loss that has existed for a relatively short period of time.[39]

Topical minoxidil solution 2% has also been investigated in combination with oral finasteride 1 mg. The outcomes of this combination treatment indicate a higher percentage of responders than with either agent alone. It is inferred that efficacy may be enhanced by the two-drug regimen that acts on multiple androgenetic alopecia etiologies.[46]

*Safety Considerations* The most common side effect associated with minoxidil—local itching or irritation at the site of application—may be related to the hydroalcoholic/propylene glycol vehicle. Rare side effects include acne at the site of application, increased hair loss, inflammation (soreness) of the hair roots, reddened skin, swelling of the face, and allergic dermatitis.[44]

The most common side effect of long-term use is transient hypertrichosis (excessive hair growth), usually on the forehead and cheeks. Occasionally, patients may notice hypertrichosis on the chest, back, forearms, and ear rims, which could indicate that the product has been applied excessively.[47] A few patients will notice increased hair loss in the first few weeks of use. Most likely, this loss represents a displacement of telogen by new anagen hairs.

Minoxidil is absorbed through the skin in relatively low concentrations, and documented systemic side effects are rare. In the unlikely event of an accidental ingestion, the patient should seek emergency medical attention. Symptoms may involve low blood pressure (dizziness, confusion, fainting, lightheadedness); blurred vision or other changes in vision; headache or chest pain; irregular heart rate; sudden unexplained weight gain; swollen hands or feet; flushing of the skin; and numbness or tingling of the face, hands, or feet.[44] Although hemodynamic changes have not been detected in most controlled clinical studies, patients with cardiovascular disorders may have an increased risk of cardiotoxicity.[48]

The use of topical minoxidil is not associated with any known drug interactions. However, the concurrent use of guanethidine could potentiate orthostatic hypotension, and the concurrent use of oral minoxidil could increase its systemic levels and enhance its effects. The application to the scalp of topical corticosteroids, petrolatum, or tretinoin (e.g., Retin-A) with minoxidil may increase the minoxidil absorption and the risk of side effects. Minoxidil should not be used for 24 hours before or after application of a permanent, a hair color, or a relaxant.[43]

Patients who are allergic to minoxidil or to any component of the preparation should avoid this medication, as should patients with scalp damage from psoriasis, severe sunburn, or abrasions, which may increase minoxidil absorption. Patients should take additional precautions if corticosteroids or any agents known to increase cutaneous absorption of a drug are used concurrently with this product.

Topical minoxidil has a Pregnancy Category C rating, which means it is not known whether the drug can harm an unborn baby. Similarly, the effect on nursing babies is not known. Therefore, pregnant women and women who are breast-feeding their babies should be advised not to use the product without first consulting a primary care provider.

The use of the 5% product by women is contraindicated because the results with 2% and 5% are not measurably different, and because the risk of facial hair growth is greater with the 5% product.

The product is alcohol based and will burn or irritate eyes, mucous membranes, or abraded skin. When spraying the product, the patient should avoid inhaling it. If the product gets into the eyes, mouth, or nose, the patient should thoroughly rinse these areas. Patients should wash and dry their hands after using the product. These precautions also are intended to prevent the systemic entry of minoxidil by alternate routes. Products containing minoxidil should not be used on any other part of the body.[44]

Researchers have found little evidence of a potential effect of minoxidil on systemic endocrine functions.[49] Measurement of plasma testosterone as well as excretion of urinary hydroxysteroids and ketosteroids in hypertensive patients who have been treated with oral minoxidil has not revealed any effects. Moreover, although serum cortisol, testosterone, and thyroid indexes are apparently unchanged by topical minoxidil, modification of follicular testosterone metabolism does occur.[50] However, unstable cardiac patients should not use the product unless supervised by a primary care provider because of potential hemodynamic alterations seen with minoxidil.

Safety and efficacy of the product in children (younger than 18 years) or in older adults (older than 65 years) have not been established, so the use of minoxidil in these populations is contraindicated.

**TABLE 46-3 Selected Hair Regrowth Products**

| Trade Name | Primary Ingredient |
|---|---|
| Equate Hair Regrowth Treatment, Extra Strength for Men | Minoxidil 5% |
| HealthGuard Minoxidil Topical Solution for Men | Minoxidil 2% |
| HealthGuard Minoxidil Topical Solution for Women | Minoxidil 2% |
| Minoxidil Topical Solution 2% for Men Hair Regrowth Treatment (ProGuard, Walgreens) | Minoxidil 2% |
| Minoxidil Topical Solution 2% for Women (ProGuard Hair System, Walgreens) | Minoxidil 2% |
| Minoxidil Extra Strength for Men Hair Regrowth Treatment (Kirkland Signature, Rite Aid, Walgreens) | Minoxidil 5% |
| Minoxidil Topical Solution 5% for Men (Alpharma) | Minoxidil 5% |
| Rogaine Extra Strength Solution for Men | Minoxidil 5% |
| Rogaine for Men Solution | Minoxidil 2% |
| Rogaine for Women Solution | Minoxidil 2% |

*Product Selection Guidelines* The 2% formulation should normally be recommended for use by women; however, men are usually advised to use the 5% concentration. Patient preference for method of application is another criterion in product selection. Table 46-3 lists examples of commercially available products. Patients with impaired vision or physical dexterity may find the rub-on method of application preferable to using sprays or droppers.

### Nonmonograph Products

In 1980 and then again in 1989, an FDA advisory panel proposed removing from the market a number of ingredients that were known to be safe for external use but claimed to prevent hair loss or promote hair growth. The false claims have generally disappeared from the market, but many of these ingredients are still available today in nonprescription lotions and shampoos. These ingredients include amino acids, aminobenzoic acid, B vitamins, hormones, jojoba oil, lanolin, polysorbates 20 and 660, sulfanilamide, tetracaine hydrochloride, urea, and wheat germ oil.[51]

## Assessment of Hair Loss: A Case-based Approach

In addition to recommending treatment for hair loss, the practitioner should first identify any possible underlying medical cause. To assess alopecia areata or telogen effluvium, the practitioner can direct the patient to perform a gentle hair-pull test (see Signs and Symptoms of Hair Loss). The removal of 25% or more of the pulled hairs may indicate that the patient's hair loss is an active process (as in alopecia areata or telogen effluvium) and the patient should be referred to a dermatologist. However, the test may be falsely negative if the patient's hair has been recently combed, brushed, or shampooed.[52] If pathology-induced and active hair loss are ruled out, the practitioner should determine whether the balding fits the criteria for androgenetic alopecia. Case 46-1 illustrates the assessment of patients with hair loss.

### CASE 46-1

| Relevant Evaluation Criteria | Scenario/Model Outcome |
|---|---|
| **Information Gathering** | |
| 1. Gather essential information about the patient's symptoms, including: | |
| a. description of symptom(s) (i.e., nature, onset, duration, severity, associated symptoms) | Patient has had gradual hair loss, which he recently noticed has increased. There are no signs of inflammation or scarring on scalp. |
| b. description of any factors that seem to precipitate, exacerbate, and/or relieve the patient's symptom(s) | None |
| c. description of the patient's efforts to relieve the symptoms | None |
| 2. Gather essential patient history information: | |
| a. patient's identity | Mike |
| b. patient's age, sex, height, and weight | 24 y/o M |
| c. patient's occupation | Graduate student |
| d. patient's dietary habits | N/A |
| e. patient's sleep habits | N/A |
| f. concurrent medical conditions, prescription and nonprescription medications, and dietary supplements | Patient in good health; takes no medications |
| g. allergies | None |
| h. history of other adverse reactions to medications | None |
| i. other (describe)______ | Father and maternal uncles suffer from male pattern baldness. Mike is concerned about the side effects of systemic therapy and prefers to use a topical treatment. |
| **Assessment and Triage** | |
| 3. Differentiate the patient's signs/symptoms and correctly identify the patient's primary problem(s). | Androgenetic alopecia. The patient has had gradual hair loss, and recently noticed increased hair loss. No signs of inflammation or scarring on scalp. |
| 4. Identify exclusions for self-treatment (see Figure 46-1). | None |
| 5. Formulate a comprehensive list of therapeutic alternatives for the primary problem to determine if triage to a medical practitioner is required, and share this information with the patient. | Options include:<br>(1) Recommend self-care using OTC minoxidil topical treatment and/or camouflage measures.<br>(2) Refer Mike to a PCP for treatment.<br>(3) Recommend self-care until a PCP can be consulted.<br>(4) Take no action. |

**CASE 46-1 (continued)**

| Relevant Evaluation Criteria | Scenario/Model Outcome |
|---|---|
| **Plan** | |
| 6. Select an optimal therapeutic alternative to address the patient's problem, taking into account patient preferences. | Topical minoxidil solution |
| 7. Describe the recommended therapeutic approach to the patient. | Apply approximately 1 mL of minoxidil 5% topical solution twice daily to a clean, dry scalp. |
| 8. Explain to the patient the rationale for selecting the recommended therapeutic approach from the considered therapeutic alternatives. | The most effective nonsystemic therapy is topical minoxidil 5% solution. |
| **Patient Education** | |
| 9. When recommending self-care with nonprescription medications and/or nondrug therapy, convey accurate information to the patient, including: | |
| a. appropriate dose and frequency of administration | See Table 46-2. |
| b. maximum number of days the therapy should be employed | See the box Patient Education for Hair Loss. |
| c. product administration procedures | See Table 46-2. |
| d. expected time to onset of relief | See the box Patient Education for Hair Loss. |
| e. degree of relief that can be reasonably expected | Progressive hair loss will be slowed in those with early thinning of hair. |
| f. most common side effects | See the box Patient Education for Hair Loss. |
| g. side effects that warrant medical intervention should they occur | See the box Patient Education for Hair Loss. |
| h. patient options in the event that condition worsens or persists | See the box Patient Education for Hair Loss. |
| i. product storage requirements | See the box Patient Education for Hair Loss. |
| j. specific nondrug measures | Minimize exposure to agents that may trigger hair loss. |
| 10. Solicit patient's follow-up questions. | How can I tell if I am responding to treatment? |
| 11. Answer patient's questions. | Hair density will increase if the treated area involves early thinning. Look for fine, short hairs as a first response. |

Key: N/A, not applicable; OTC, over-the-counter; PCP, primary care provider.

## Patient Counseling for Hair Loss

Patients should be advised that most treatment regimens for hair loss do not alter its progression, especially if the hair loss has gone on for a prolonged period of time. Some patients might instead be interested in hair transplants or surgical interventions. The practitioner should inform patients who want to use nonprescription minoxidil that the longer the hair thinning or loss has continued, the less likely it is that treatment will elicit a regrowth response. If the patient still wants to use minoxidil, the practitioner should review product instructions with the patient, making sure that the patient understands the possible adverse effects and the signs and symptoms that indicate the need for medical attention. The box Patient Education for Hair Loss lists specific information to provide patients.

## Evaluation of Patient Outcomes for Hair Loss

Patients should use minoxidil for the minimum recommended periods. If new hair growth does not occur after using minoxidil 2% or 5% for 4 months, the patient should consider ending treatment. If new hair does appear within

## PATIENT EDUCATION FOR HAIR LOSS

The objectives of self-treatment are to restore the appearance of the hair by (1) camouflaging thinning hair and/or (2) using minoxidil to regrow hair. For most patients, carefully following product instructions and the self-care measures listed here will help ensure optimal therapeutic outcomes.

### Nondrug Measures

- If desired, use wigs to cover severe hair loss until hair is regrown.
- For less severe hair loss, use hair sprays, gels, colorants, permanents, or hair-building products in moderation to create the illusion of full hair. These cosmetics will not increase the rate of hair loss.
- Avoid the use of oily hair products that can cause folliculitis.
- Avoid hair styles such as tight braids that pull on the hair.

### Nonprescription Medications

- Note that use of minoxidil must be continuous and indefinite to maintain regrowth. It may take up to 4 months to see any results. If treatment is interrupted, regrowth will typically be lost within 4 months or less, and progression of hair loss will begin again.
- If you are pregnant, breast-feeding, or become pregnant while using this product, consult a primary care provider about the appropriateness of such use. Minoxidil is not recommended for use in this population.
- See Table 46-2 for instructions on how to use this product.
- Do not apply the product more than twice daily. More frequent applications will not achieve better regrowth or a faster response, but may increase side effects.
- Do not apply the product to damaged or inflamed areas of the scalp, including patients with active scalp psoriasis or eczema lesions.
- Note that local itching or irritation at the site of application may occur. More rarely, allergic contact dermatitis or transient hypertrichosis (unwanted facial hair growth) may occur.
- Keep product containers in a cool, dry place, and avoid refrigeration
- Keep the product out of the reach of children. Ingestion of minoxidil is potentially hazardous and individuals should contact their poison control center immediately.[49]
- Product is flammable. Keep away from fire or flame.
- Do not use on infants or children aged 18 years or younger.
- Do not use if you have heart disease except under supervision of a primary care provider.

If hair fails to appear despite consistent use of the product within the time specified on the product (generally 4 to 6 months), consider stopping the treatment and seeing your primary care provider for further evaluation.

the recommended periods, the practitioner should advise the patient to continue the drug treatment indefinitely.

## Key Points for Hair Loss

- Minoxidil is suppressive, not curative, and is not effective for everyone.
- Offering cosmetic solutions may also be helpful.
- Patients, particularly women, are seeking treatment not only for hair loss but also for lost self-esteem resulting from the association of hair loss with illness and advanced age.
- Practitioners and primary care providers should dispense medication with a measure of emotional support and should make clear the limitations of existing treatment.

## References


1. Sperling LC, Mezebish DS. Hair diseases. *Med Clin North Am.* 1998;82:1155-69.
2. Sinclair R. Male pattern androgenetic alopecia. *BMJ.* 1998;317: 865-9.
3. Reiman P. Alopecia areata labeled autoimmune disease. *Dermatol Times.* 1999;20:43-4.
4. Camacho F. Alopecias due to telogenic effluvium. In: Camacho F, Montagna W, eds. *Trichology: Diseases of the Pilosebaceous Follicle.* Madrid: Aula Medica Group; 1997:403-11.
5. Lavker RM, Bertolino AP, Freedberg IM, et al. Biology of hair follicles. In: Freedberg IM, Eisen AZ, Wolff K, et al., eds. *Dermatology in General Medicine.* 5th ed. New York: McGraw-Hill, Inc; 1999:230-8.
6. Earhart RN, Ball J, Nuss DD, et al. Minoxidil-induced hypertrichosis: treatment with calcium thioglycolate depilatory. *South Med J.* 1977;70:442-3.
7. Messenger AG, Dawber RPR. The physiology and embryology of hair growth. In: Dawber R, ed. *Diseases of the Hair and Scalp.* Oxford: Blackwell Scientific Publications; 1997:1-22.
8. Sawaya ME. Biochemistry and control of hair growth. In: Arndt KA, LeBoit PE, Robinson JK, et al., eds. *Cutaneous Medicine and Surgery.* Philadelphia: WB Saunders; 1996: 1248-9.
9. Diseases of the skin appendages. In: Odom RB, James WD, Berger TG, eds. *Andrew's Diseases of the Skin—Clinical Dermatology.* Philadelphia: WB Saunders; 2000:947-9.
10. Whiting DA. Possible mechanisms of miniaturization during androgenetic alopecia or pattern hair loss. *J Am Acad Dermatol.* 2001;45(3 suppl):S81-6.
11. Sawaya ME, Price VH. Different levels of 5 alpha-reductase type I and II, aromatase, and androgen receptor in hair follicles of women and men with androgenetic alopecia. *J Invest Dermatol.* 1997;109:296-300.
12. Randall VA, Hibberts NA, Thornton MJ, et al. The hair follicle: a paradoxical androgen target organ. *Horm Res.* 2000;54:243-50.
13. Chen W, Yang C, Chen G, et al. Patients with a large prostate show a higher prevalence of androgenetic alopecia. *Arch Derm Res.* 2004;296:245-9.
14. Knochenhauer ES, Key TJ, Kahsar-Miller M, et al. Prevalence of the polycystic ovary syndrome in unselected black and white women of the southeastern United States: a prospective study. *J Clin Endocrinol Metab.* 1998;83:3078-82.
15. Hashemipour M, Faghihimani S, Zolfaghary B, et al. Prevalence of polycystic ovary syndrome in girls aged 14-18 years in Isfahan, Iran. *Horm Res.* 2004;62:278-82.
16. Simpson NB, Barth JH. Hair patterns: hirsuties and androgenetic alopecia. In: Dawber R, ed. *Diseases of the Hair and Scalp.* Oxford: Blackwell Science; 1997:67-122.
17. Birch MP, Messenger AG. Genetic factors predispose to balding and non-balding in men. *Eur J Dermatol.* 2001;11:309-14.

18. Sehgal VN, Jain S. Alopecia areata: clinical perspective and an insight into pathogenesis. *J Dermatol.* 2003;30:271-89.
19. McDonagh AJ, Tazi-Ahnini R. Epidemiology and genetics of alopecia areata. *Clin Exp Dermatol.* 2002;277:405-9.
20. Ahmad W, Faiyaz ul Haque M, Brancolini V, et al. Alopecia universalis associated with a mutation in the human hairless gene. *Science.* 1998;279:720-4.
21. Papadopoulos AJ, Schwartz RA, Janniger CK. Alopecia areata: pathogenesis, diagnosis, and therapy. *Am J Clin Dermatol.* 2000;1:101-5.
22. Sinclair R, DeBerker D. Hereditary and congenital alopecia and hypertrichosis. In: Dawber RPR, ed. *Diseases of the Hair and Scalp.* Oxford: Blackwell Science; 1997:168-9.
23. Pillans PI, Woods DJ. Drug-associated alopecia. *Int J Dermatol.* 1995;34:149-59.
24. Look on eBay for drugs that cause hair loss. E-Facts (online). Available at: http://www.e-facts.com. Accessed February 2005.
25. Marse H, Van Cutsem E, Grothey A, et al. Management of adverse events and other practical considerations in patients receiving capecitabine (Xeloda). *Eur J Oncol Nurs.* 2004;8 (suppl 1):S16-30.
26. Fiedler VC. Alopecia areata and other nonscarring alopecias. In: Arndt KA, LeBoit PE, Robinson JK, et al., eds. *Cutaneous Medicine and Surgery.* Philadelphia: WB Saunders; 1996:1274-8.
27. DeBerker D, Sinclair R. Defects of the hair shaft. In: Dawber RPR, ed. *Diseases of the Hair and Scalp.* Oxford: Blackwell Science; 1997:296-7.
28. Talsma J. Hair disorders pose problem for African Americans. *Dermatol Times.* 1999;20:42-5.
29. Hickman JG, Huber F, Palmisano M. Human dermal safety studies with eflornithine HCl 13.9% cream (Vaniqa), a novel treatment for excessive facial hair. *Curr Med Res Opin.* 2001;16:235-44.
30. Balfour JA, McClellan K. Topical eflornithine. *Am J Clin Dermatol.* 2001;2:197-201.
31. Birch MP, Lalla SC, Messenger AG. Female pattern hair loss. *Clin Exp Dermatol.* 2002;27:383-8.
32. Messenger AG, Simpson NB. In: Dawber RPR, ed. *Diseases of the Hair and Scalp.* Oxford: Blackwell Science; 1997:356-7.
33. Guarrera M, Semino MT, Rebora A. Quantitating hair loss in women: a critical approach. *Dermatology.* 1997;194:12-6.
34. Orentreich D, Orentreich N. Androgenetic alopecia and its treatment, a historical view. In: Unger WP, ed. *Hair Transplantation.* 3rd ed. New York: Marcel Dekker; 1995:1-33.
35. Otomo S. Hair growth effect of minoxidil. *Nippon Yakurigaku Zasshi.* 2002;119:167-74.
36. Lachgar S, Charveron M, Gall Y, et al. Minoxidil upregulates the expression of vascular endothelial growth factor in human hair dermal papilla cells. *Br J Dermatol.* 1998;138:407-11.
37. Kurata S, Uno H, Allenhoffmann BL. Effects of hypertrichotic agents on follicular and nonfollicular cells in vitro. *Skin Pharmacol.* 1996;9:3-8.
38. Price VH. Treatment of hair loss. *N Engl J Med.* 1999;341:964-73.
39. Minoxidil. In: *Drug Facts and Comparisons.* St. Louis: Facts and Comparisons; 2000:1674-4a.
40. Shapiro J, Price VH. Hair regrowth: therapeutic agents. *Dermatol Clin.* 1998;16:341-56.
41. Duvic M, Lemak NA, Valero V, et al. A randomized trial of minoxidil in chemotherapy-induced alopecia. *J Am Acad Dermatol.* 1996;35:74-8.
42. Avram MR, Cole JP, Gandelman M, et al. The potential role of minoxidil in the hair transplantation setting. *Dermatol Surg.* 2002;28:894-900.
43. Men's Rogaine Extra Strength and Women's Rogaine. *Physicians' Desk Reference for Nonprescription Drugs and Dietary Supplements.* Montvale, NJ: Thomson PDR; 2003:749-50.
44. USP DI (Volume I). Minoxidil. *Drug Information for the Health Care Professional.* 23rd ed. Greenwood Village, Colo: Micromedex; 2003:1914-7.
45. Price VH, Menefee E, Strauss PC. Changes in hair weight and hair count in men with androgenetic alopecia, after application of 5% and 2% topical minoxidil, placebo, or no treatment. *J Am Acad Dermatol.* 1999;41:717-21.
46. Khandpur S, Suman M, Reddy BS. Comparative efficacy of various treatment regimens for androgenetic alopecia in men. *J Dermatol.* 2002;29:489-98.
47. Peluso AM, Misciali C, Vincenzi C, et al. Diffuse hypertrichosis during treatment with 5% topical minoxidil. *Br J Dermatol.* 1997;136:118-20.
48. Satoh H, Morikaw S, Fujiwara C, et al. A case of acute myocardial infarction associated with topical use of minoxidil (RiUP) for treatment of baldness. *Jpn Heart J.* 2000;41:519-23.
49. Nguyen KH, Marks JG Jr. Pseudoacromegaly induced by the long-term use of minoxidil. *J Am Acad Dermatol.* 2003;48:962-5.
50. Sato T, Tadokoro T, Sonoda T, et al. Minoxidil increases 17 beta-hydroxysteroid dehydrogenase and 5 alpha-reductase activity of cultured human dermal papilla cells from balding scalp. *J Dermatol Sci.* 1999;19:123-5.
51. Hanover L. Hair replacement. *FDA Consumer.* 1997;31:7-10.
52. Kligman AM. Pathologic dynamics of human hair loss. *Arch Dermatol.* 1961;83:175-98.

SECTION IX

# Other Medical Disorders

CHAPTER 47

# Diabetes Mellitus

*Mitra Assemi and Candis M. Morello*

As defined by the American Diabetes Association (ADA), diabetes mellitus is a group of metabolic diseases characterized by hyperglycemia resulting from defects in insulin secretion, insulin action, or both.[1] Chronic hyperglycemia results in long-term damage, dysfunction, and potential failure of various organs, including the eyes, nerves, heart, blood vessels, and kidneys. Several types of diabetes are recognized. Types 1 and 2 account for the majority of cases and are the focus for this chapter. Type 1 diabetes mellitus results from a cellular-mediated autoimmune destruction of the pancreatic β-cells. These cells produce insulin, the hormone that facilitates glucose metabolism. To survive, patients with type 1 diabetes mellitus must receive daily and lifelong exogenous insulin to maintain their blood glucose (BG) levels within normal limits. Thus, type 1 diabetes mellitus is defined as absolute insulin deficiency. In type 2 diabetes mellitus, the metabolic defects include insulin resistance, β-cell dysfunction, and increased hepatic glucose production. Table 47-1 lists distinguishing features of these two types of diabetes.

Another type (1%-5% of all cases) represents all other factors that may induce glucose intolerance, such as specific genetic conditions (e.g., maturity-onset of diabetes in the young or MODY; leprechaunism), medications (e.g., glucocorticoids), and illnesses.[1,2] Gestational diabetes mellitus (GDM) develops in 4% of all pregnancies and can pose health risks for both mother and fetus.[1] GDM first becomes apparent after 24 to 28 weeks of pregnancy but usually wanes after delivery. Women who develop GDM have a 20% to 50% chance of developing type 2 diabetes later in life.

The tangible and intangible costs of diabetes care and treatment to both individuals and society are staggering. In 2002, combined direct and indirect costs were estimated at $132 billion.[3] Put another way, 19% of total health care costs in the United States were incurred by only 4% of the population. In the same year, the average health care cost for a person with diabetes was $13,243 versus $2560 for a person without diabetes. Annual costs are projected to continue rising, approaching $156 billion by 2010 and $192 billion by 2020. Since most health care expenditures are related to treatment of long-term diabetes complications, practitioners are focusing on prevention, early diagnosis, and metabolic control.

Regardless of type, self-care is integral to the effective management of diabetes. Practitioners can assist patients with diabetes by cultivating a relationship that will allow them to assess the patient's capability for self-care, identify gaps in the patient's knowledge of diabetes care, teach patients proper self-care strategies, and monitor self-care measures. The practitioner should be part of an interprofessional network of health care providers engaged in coordinating the patient's health care. Practitioners should also be a patient's resource for information on glucose monitors and other devices, self-monitoring of blood glucose (SMBG), medical nutrition therapy (MNT), physical activity, and drugs used in diabetes management and treatment.

## Epidemiology of Diabetes Mellitus

More than 18.2 million people in the United States, or 6.3% of the population, have diabetes.[2] These numbers are projected to more than double by 2050, because of both improved diagnostic criteria and the growing impact of a hypercaloric, sedentary lifestyle on our population. More than one million of these patients, including one out of every 400 to 500 children and adolescents, have type 1 diabetes. Although type 1 diabetes is most commonly diagnosed in childhood, it may present at any age in life. Risks for developing type 1 diabetes include genetic, autoimmune, and environmental factors that remain poorly defined.[1] Whites appear to be at higher risk than other ethnicities.

In contrast to other types of diabetes, the incidence of type 2 is reaching epidemic proportions in the United States. More than 16 million people, including 5.2 million undiagnosed individuals, currently have type 2 diabetes.[2] Its prevalence is higher among certain minority populations, including Hispanic Americans (1.9 times higher), African Americans (1.9 times higher), Asian Americans (1.6 times higher), and Native Americans/Alaska Natives (1.8 times higher, although prevalence rates vary across tribes).[4] Obesity and a sedentary lifestyle are widely recognized as risk factors, especially as a growing number of children and adolescents are being diagnosed with this disease. Overweight patients with type 2 diabetes likely have an increased distribution of body fat in the abdominal area. Other risk factors include a family history of type 2 diabetes, prior history of GDM, and age over 45 years.[1] Comorbid conditions commonly associated with type 2 diabetes include hypertension and dyslipidemia.

---

**Editor's Note:** This chapter is based on the 14th edition chapter with the same title, written by Robert W. Bennett and Cynthia P. Koh-Knox. Drs. Assemi and Morello contributed equally to this chapter.

**TABLE 47-1 Differentiation of Type 1 and Type 2 Diabetes Mellitus**

| Characteristics | Type 1 | Type 2 |
|---|---|---|
| **Demographics and Related Information** | | |
| Older Terminology | Type I diabetes, insulin-dependent diabetes mellitus (IDDM), juvenile-onset diabetes mellitus | Type II diabetes, non–insulin-dependent diabetes mellitus (NIDDM), adult onset diabetes mellitus |
| Percentage of people with diabetes | 5%-10% | 90%-95% |
| Family history of diabetes | Frequently negative | Commonly present |
| Age of onset | Usually <30 years, during childhood or adolescence | Frequently >40 years (although becoming more prevalent in obese children and younger adults) |
| **Symptoms** | | |
| Initial clinical presentation | Abrupt onset, moderate to severe symptoms of polyuria, polydipsia, fatigue, sudden weight loss, possible ketoacidosis | Usually gradual onset, possibly mild symptoms of polyuria, polydipsia, fatigue; often diagnosed when diabetic complications such as retinopathy, candidiasis, erectile dysfunction, and delayed wound healing are identified |
| Typical body habitus | Usually thin | Usually obese (central, intra-abdominal obesity) |
| Proneness to ketosis | Frequent, especially with insufficient insulin | Uncommon, except in the presence of unusual stress or moderate to severe sepsis |
| Macrovascular, microvascular, and neuropathy complications | Infrequent until diabetes has been present for ~5 years | Frequent, even at diagnosis |
| Plasma insulin (endogenous) | Negligible to zero | Plasma insulin secretion may be increased, normal, or decreased |
| **Possible Etiologies** | | |
| Primary cause | Autoimmune-mediated pancreatic β-cell destruction, usually leading to absolute insulin deficiency | Insulin resistance, impaired insulin secretion, and/or increased hepatic glucose production |
| Heredity | Associated with specific HLA tissue types, but only 40%-50% concordance in twins | 95%-100% concordance in twins, but not associated with specific HLA tissue types |
| Autoimmune disease | Positive; 50%-80% circulating islet cell antibodies | Negative; <10% circulating islet cell antibodies |
| **Treatment** | | |
| Medical nutrition therapy | Necessary in all patients; premeal insulin dose is determined by the carbohydrate content of the meal | Necessary in all patients, particularly for weight loss or maintenance and cardiovascular health |
| Physical activity | Very important in all patients for glycemic control and cardiovascular fitness | Very important in all patients to manage BG excursions and weight loss or maintenance to increase or enhance insulin sensitivity |
| Insulin | Necessary for all patients, usually in lower doses (0.5 units/kg/day) | Necessary for many patients, higher doses often required (0.7-2 units/kg/day) |
| Oral agents | Not indicated | Often efficacious |
| Glucose monitoring | Daily SMBG required and quarterly A1C | Frequent to daily SMBG very important for self-management and quarterly A1C |

Key: SMBG, self-monitoring of blood glucose; A1C, glycosylated hemoglobin.

## Physiology of Glycoprotein Metabolism

Working in conjunction with counterregulatory hormones (glucagon, epinephrine, norepinephrine, growth hormone, cortisol, and somatostatin), endogenous insulin (the glucoregulatory hormone) maintains normal BG levels between 60 and 100 mg/dL. Insulin and glucagon, the major hormones that control and balance glucose metabolism, are made and stored by the pancreatic β- and α-cells, respectively. The pancreatic β-cells release insulin into the portal vein in response to elevated plasma glucose, where the liver rapidly utilizes the hormone. Insulin action has two main effects on fuel metabolism: (1) promotes storage (anabolic) and (2) prevents breakdown (anticatabolic). Insulin stimulates glucose uptake and storage as glycogen in muscle and liver cells. It converts excess glucose in the blood to fatty acids and triglycerides and promotes their storage in adipose tissue. Insulin also decreases hepatic glucose output, inhibits lipolysis (breakdown of fat) and production of ketone bodies, and enhances incorporation of amino acids into proteins.

While insulin's main effect is fuel storage, glucagon antagonizes the physiologic actions of insulin by increasing fuel breakdown and use. Glucagon secretion is triggered by low BG or high amino acid levels, resulting in increased liver glycogenolysis (breakdown of glycogen into glucose) and a subsequent rise in BG. If both blood amino acids and glucose are high, the effect of glucose is dominant and glucagon secretion is suppressed.

## Etiology of Diabetes Mellitus

Diabetes mellitus is a syndrome consisting of a heterogenous group of metabolic disorders characterized by chronic hyperglycemia and associated with long-term consequences such as macrovascular and microvascular complications. While the causes of these metabolic disorders may be different, most cases fall into either type 1 or type 2 diabetes.

There are two categories of type 1 diabetes: immune-mediated and idiopathic diabetes. The first and most common form of type 1 diabetes is caused by autoimmune destruction of insulin-secreting pancreatic islet cells, usually leading to an absolute insulin deficiency. In the majority of cases, the autoimmune process can be identified by the presence of autoantibodies to islet cells, insulin autoantibodies, glutamic acid decarboxylase$_{65}$, and/or tyrosine phosphatases IA-2 and IA-2β.[5] This disease is also strongly associated with specific HLA tissue types, which may result in a protective or predisposing effect. Hence, not everyone with type 1 defects develops diabetes. Although genetics is a strong causal component, only a small percentage of defective genes are expressed. If both parents have type 1 diabetes, only 20% of their children can be expected to develop the disease. The exact etiology of idiopathic type 1 diabetes is unknown, but the cause is not autoimmune-mediated.

In contrast, patients with type 2 diabetes have functioning β-cells, which produce insulin. Muscles and peripheral tissues, however, are resistant to insulin effects. Patients who are overweight are at increased risk for insulin resistance. In these patients, insulin resistance may improve with weight reduction. Defects in postreceptor binding may also cause insulin resistance. In some individuals with type 2 diabetes, a decreased number of insulin receptors and postreceptor defects may coexist, resulting in hyperglycemia.[6]

In 1988, Reaven[7] proposed that insulin resistance leading to hyperinsulinemia directly contributes to the development of hypertension and the appearance of factors leading to cardiovascular disease and atherosclerosis (increased LDL-C, triglycerides, and plasminogen activator inhibitor-1; decreased HDL-C). This cluster of symptoms is known as metabolic syndrome (previously called syndrome X; also known as dysmetabolic syndrome). Patients with this syndrome have increased mortality and morbidity from cardiovascular disease.

Heredity is a major risk factor for type 2 diabetes mellitus. In identical twin studies, the chance of both twins having the disease if one twin has type 2 diabetes is nearly 100%. In contrast, if one twin has type 1 diabetes, there is a low likelihood for the second twin to develop this disease since the genes for type 1 and type 2 are on different chromosomes.

## Pathophysiology of Diabetes Mellitus

Pathophysiology of diabetes mellitus differs depending on the type. For a majority of people with type 1 diabetes, the distinguishing characteristic is selective cellular-mediated autoimmune pancreatic β-cell destruction. Islet cell and/or insulin antibodies are usually detectable on diagnosis of type 1 diabetes. Only a minority of type 1 patients (e.g., some patients of African or Asian descent) lack immunologic evidence for β-cell autoimmunity.[1] Destruction of β-cells results in a gradual decrease in insulin production, thus preventing peripheral tissues from effectively absorbing and utilizing glucose for energy. Initially, postprandial (after meal) glucose levels rise, usually undetected. Fasting hyperglycemia ensues once functional β-cell mass falls below 80% to 90%. As glucose remains trapped in the circulation, insulin-dependent cells perceive a glucose deficiency and signal for increased endogenous glucose production. Liver glycogen and amino acids are converted to glucose through glycogenolysis and gluconeogenesis, respectively. Because insulin production remains insufficient or absent, however, dependent tissues are unable to utilize glucose and hyperglycemia is pronounced.

These metabolic changes cause the onset of symptoms, which may vary in their rate and severity between children, adolescents, and adults with new-onset type 1 diabetes. As plasma glucose concentrations rise to exceed the normal renal threshold of 180 mg/dL, glycosuria produces an osmotic diuresis and potential dehydration. This diuresis manifests clinically as polyuria (frequent urination), especially at night (nocturia). Dehydration can progress to significant hypovolemia, electrolyte loss, and cellular dehydration, which manifests in symptoms of dry mouth and polydipsia (increased thirst). Because the lack of insulin prevents cells from utilizing circulating plasma glucose, the nervous system signals polyphagia (hunger accompanied by increased appetite). Eating subsequently promotes a further rise in plasma glucose level.

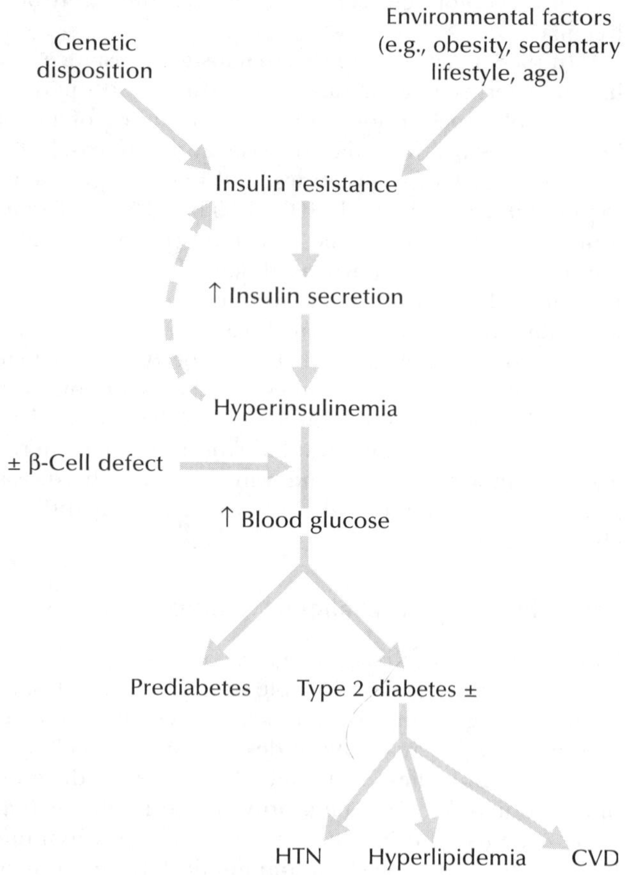


**FIGURE 47-1** Pathogenesis of type 2 diabetes mellitus. Key: CVD, cardiovascular disease; HTN, hypertension.

Over time, lack of insulin also stimulates protein and fat catabolism for energy, causing weight loss, which is more characteristic to type 1 diabetes. As excess free fatty acids are mobilized to the liver, they are metabolized to acidic ketone bodies, which can eventually induce a metabolic acidosis. Left untreated, systemic ketoacidosis is a life-threatening situation that can lead to coma and death.

In contrast, type 2 diabetes is often not accompanied by any symptoms early in the disease progression. Figure 47-1 provides an overview of the pathogenesis of this disorder.

Type 2 is caused by insulin resistance combined with a relative insulin deficiency. The degree of insulin resistance and/or β-cell deficiency varies among people with type 2 diabetes. The pancreas compensates for insulin resistance by increasing insulin release (hyperinsulinemia). When this compensation is not adequate (in the case of type 2 diabetes), however, hyperglycemia persists. The liver is resistant to insulin, causing increased hepatic glucose production. β-Cell function declines with increased duration of diabetes.

Hyperglycemia manifests in symptoms similar to those seen in type 1 patients: polyuria, polydipsia, and polyphagia. Because insulin is present, glucose is still transported into muscle and fat cells, resulting in a more gradual development of symptoms in type 2 patients. In addition, patients with type 2 diabetes seldom develop ketoacidosis, except during periods of significant stress. Dehydration caused by hyperglycemia in type 2 patients, however, may place them at risk for developing hyperosmolar hyperglycemic state (HHS). Although the acute management of this syndrome is similar to that of ketoacidosis in type 1 patients, diagnosis is often delayed because of nonspecific symptoms in elderly patients with type 2 disease.

Chronic hyperglycemia is associated with the development and progression of complications affecting major physiologic systems in all types of diabetes. Table 47-2 summarizes the pathophysiologic mechanisms for the long-term effects of uncontrolled BG on various organs and systems.

**TABLE 47-2** Pathophysiologic Mechanisms of Chronic Hyperglycemia on Various Organs and Systems

| Problem | Hyperglycemic Effects | Symptoms |
|---|---|---|
| **Eyes** | | |
| Retinopathy | Damage to retinal capillaries results in vascular leakage and edema. Capillary defects can lead to decreased profusion, damaging the macula. Proliferation of new but abnormally weak capillaries can lead to subsequent attachment to the posterior vitreous surface, causing retinal detachment or vitreal bleeding. | Visual changes (e.g., blurring)<br>Loss of central or peripheral vision |
| Cataract | Excessive glucose in the lens is metabolized by polyol pathway, resulting in increased fructose and sorbitol concentrations. Accumulation of sorbitol produces edema, eventually disrupting lens fiber membranes and protein deposits. | |
| **Mouth** | | |
| Gingivitis, dental caries, periodontal disease | Increased glucose concentrations in the saliva promote bacterial growth. | Gum inflammation; tooth pain or sensitivity, or loss |

**TABLE 47-2 Pathophysiologic Mechanisms of Chronic Hyperglycemia on Various Organs and Systems (continued)**

| Problem | Hyperglycemic Effects | Symptoms |
|---|---|---|
| **Nervous System** | | |
| Sensory, motor and autonomic neuropathy (e.g., peripheral neuropathy, increased risk of extremity and limb injury and infection, abnormal sweating, gastroparesis, orthostatic hypertension, bladder dysfunction, sexual dysfunction) | Excessive glucose metabolism via polyol pathway leads to increased sorbitol concentrations, causing edema and osmotic neuronal injury. Protein glycosylation and capillary changes caused by hyperglycemia may contribute to neuronal damage. Together, these mechanisms may contribute to segmental loss of myelin, resulting in decreased nerve conduction velocity. | Symmetrical sensory defects usually first affecting feet and hands, such as decreased sensation to touch, tingling, burning, numbness, and/or pain<br>Loss of ankle reflex, joint and gait abnormalities<br>Abnormal sweating on face and trunk<br>Dizziness<br>Low blood pressure<br>Slow, unresponsive heart rate<br>Nausea, bloating, anorexia, and reflux<br>Constipation<br>Fecal incontinence<br>Urinary incontinence<br>Erectile dysfunction in men and anorgasmia in women |
| **Vascular System** | | |
| Intermittent claudication<br>Accelerated atherosclerosis | Hemorheologic changes related to hyperglycemia lead to increased intermittent claudication.<br>Hyperglycemic damage to intimal cells of blood vessels initiating atherosclerotic lesions. | Difficulty and pain on walking<br>Heart attack, stroke, sudden cardiovascular death |
| **Kidneys** | | |
| Decreased renal function and progressive renal failure | Hyperglycemia activates protein kinase C-β, leading to increased production of vascular endothelial growth factor, which damages endothelium of small blood vessels, resulting in glomerular damage. Hyperglycemia and hypertension also cause intraglomerular hypertension and renal hyperfiltration, contributing to kidney damage. | Microalbuminuria<br>Increased serum creatinine<br>Renal failure |
| **Reproductive System** | | |
| Hyperglycemia and/or hypoglycemia interferes with normal fetal growth and development | Miscarriage, neonatal congenital malformations, and fetal macrosomia occur. | High-birth-weight babies<br>Congenital defects<br>Miscarriage<br>Still birth |
| **Immune System** | | |
| Skin infections<br>Bladder infections<br>Moniliasis (women) | Protein glycosylation may contribute to impairment of white blood cell phagocytic activity. | Severe skin infections progressing to amputation<br>Difficult or painful urination<br>Vulval and vaginal itching, discharge |
| **Skin** | | |
| Specific lesions such as diabetic bullae and lipodystrophies | Small blood vessel disease and increased serum lipids occur. | Physical changes and itching depending on diagnosis |

## Signs and Symptoms of Diabetes Mellitus

Prediabetes is diagnosed by an impaired fasting glucose (IFG), characterized by a fasting plasma glucose (FPG) level between 100 and 125 mg/dL, or an impaired glucose tolerance (IGT), characterized by a 2-hour plasma glucose level of 140 to 199 mg/dL following an oral glucose tolerance test (OGTT). Prediabetes is a risk factor for type 2 diabetes. Most patients with prediabetes or diabetes may be asymptomatic early in the course of the disease but typically experience polydipsia, dry mouth, tiredness, polyuria,

**TABLE 47-3 ADA Diagnostic Criteria for Diabetes Mellitus in Nonpregnant Patients***

| Testing Condition | Plasma Glucose (mg/dL) | Presence of Symptoms | Comments |
|---|---|---|---|
| Casual | ≥200 | + | Symptoms include polyuria, polydipsia, polyphagia, and unexplained weight loss. Casual is defined as any time of day without regard to time since last meal. |
| Fasting | ≥126 | +/- | Fasting is defined as no caloric intake for at least 8 hours. |
| 2-hour glucose during an OGTT | ≥200 | +/- | The test should be performed as described by World Health Organization, using a load of ~75 g anhydrous glucose dissolved in water for adults and 1.75 g/kg glucose dissolved in water for children. |

Key: OGTT, oral glucose tolerance test.

* In the absence of unequivocal hyperglycemia, these criteria should be confirmed by repeat testing on a different day.

nocturia, and polyphagia. Weight loss may also occur, especially in patients with type 1 disease. Onset of symptoms may be more rapid, especially following a stressful event, in type 1 than in type 2 diabetes. In addition, symptoms of long-term diabetes complications may appear before elevated plasma glucose is detected. These symptoms may include visual changes; numbness or pain in the feet, legs, and hands; dry, itchy skin; slowed healing of cuts and scratches; gingivitis and/or dental caries; frequent infections (e.g., dermal, vaginal, bladder); and impotence. For these reasons, patients with type 2 diabetes often remain undiagnosed for the first several years of the disease. Table 47-3 summarizes the diagnostic criteria for diabetes mellitus.

## Complications of Diabetes Mellitus

Long-term diabetes complications arising from poorly controlled glucose levels are responsible for significant morbidity and mortality. Diabetes is the sixth leading cause of death listed on death certificates in the United States in 2000.[2] Complications of diabetes are usually categorized as microvascular and macrovascular. Studies in patients with both type 1 and type 2 diabetes have clearly established a relationship between level of glycemic control and the risk for developing long-term microvascular and macrovascular complications.[8-11] For every 1% reduction of A1C (i.e., glycosylated hemoglobin), a marker for longer-term glycemic control, the risk of developing microvascular complications drops up to 40%. For this reason, glucose control forms the foundation of diabetes treatment and management.

### *Microvascular Complications*

Microvascular complications include retinopathy, neuropathy, and nephropathy. Among adults 20 to 74 years old in the United States, diabetes is the leading cause of new-onset blindness.[2] Maintaining glucose at euglycemic levels can decrease and halt the progression of retinopathy.[8-10] Patients with type 1 diabetes, however, may experience a transient worsening of retinopathy following initiation of intensive glycemic control.[8] This usually resolves within 18 months of tight metabolic control. Early detection and treatment of retinopathy and glaucoma can prevent progression to blindness. Drugs with parasympatholytic effects, such as anticholinergics, antihistamines, and ganglionic blockers, can alter the pupil and ciliary muscles, causing blurred vision. Because blurred vision is a symptom of hyper- and hypoglycemic episodes as well as retinopathy, the use of parasympathetic drugs in patients with diabetes should be avoided whenever possible.

More than 60% of patients with diabetes have some form of mild to moderate damage to their nervous system.[2] Severe neuropathy is a major contributor to lower-extremity amputations, with over 82,000 amputations performed in 2000 and 2001 secondary to diabetes-related complications in the foot and leg, such as gangrene. Lowering BG to normal levels can improve mild to moderate neuropathy symptoms.[8-10] Depending on the type of neuropathy, patients may be treated with medications that provide symptomatic relief (e.g., sensory pain, gastroparesis, incontinence, and sexual dysfunction).

Diabetes is the leading cause of end-stage renal disease in the United States.[2] More than 73% of people with diabetes also have hypertension, which further increases their risk for developing renal complications.[2,12] Studies have found that every 10 mm Hg reduction of systolic blood pressure results in a 12% reduction of risk for any complication related to diabetes.[2] Blood pressure control with diet, exercise, and medications therefore plays an important role in diabetes management. People with diabetes who have impaired renal function (e.g., as indicated by microalbuminuria) and/or hypertension are treated with angiotensin-converting enzyme inhibitors or angiotensin receptor blockers to prevent or slow the progression of nephropathy and end-stage renal disease.

### *Macrovascular Complications*

Macrovascular complications include atherosclerosis and arteriosclerosis, contributing to peripheral vascular disease (PVD). Symptoms of PVD include dry, callused skin, cold feet, decreased or absent foot pulses, leg pain, and difficulty walking (e.g., intermittent claudication). PVD, along with sensory-motor neuropathy, increases the risk for skin infections, gangrene, and subsequent amputation of extremities and limbs. Treatment includes reduction and elimination of risk factors (e.g., hyperglycemia, hypertension, hyperlipidemia, and smoking), proper foot self-care and exercise. Some patients may require antiplatelet therapy or vascular surgery.

Other macrovascular complications include cardiovascular disease and stroke. Heart disease is the leading cause of diabetes-related deaths.[2] People with diabetes have two to four times the risk for heart attack and stroke, compared with people without diabetes. Additional risk factors for cardiovascular disease include obesity, hypertension (blood pressure over 130/80 mm Hg), hyperlipidemia (LDL-C greater than 100 mg/dL, HDL-C less than 40 mg/dL in men and 50 mg/dL in women, and/or triglycerides greater than 150 mg/dL), and smoking.[13-16] Therefore, in addition to controlling BG and blood pressure, weight, and lipids with diet, exercise, and medications, smoking cessation plays a crucial role in reducing cardiovascular risk in patients with diabetes.

Rheologic changes also contribute to diabetes-related PVD and cardiovascular morbidity and mortality. Platelets in patients with diabetes are hypersensitive to platelet aggregants.[17] Studies have also found that type 2 patients with cardiovascular disease overproduce thromboxane, a potent vasoconstrictor and platelet aggregant. Smoking itself also causes changes in blood chemistry that contribute to cardiovascular disease. Evidence to date from both type 1 and 2 diabetes studies supports the use of low-dose aspirin (81-325 mg daily) as a primary or secondary prevention strategy to reduce the incidence of cardiovascular events.[17] Yet despite its proven efficacy, less than half of all patients qualifying for aspirin therapy actually take it.

### *Other Complications*

Patients with diabetes may have abnormalities in immune function that increase their morbidity and mortality from infection.[18] Immune cell function, such as polymorphonuclear leukocyte (PMNs) chemotaxis, is altered in these patients.[19] Uncontrolled hyperglycemia promotes glucose to bind to proteins, resulting in advanced glycation end products (AGEs). AGEs bind to immunoglobulin receptors on cells such as macrophages, stimulating the production of cytokines (e.g., tumor necrosis factor $\alpha$, interleukin $1\beta$, and interleukin 6) and other inflammatory response mediators. AGE binding on immune-related cells may alter collagen solubility. Together these factors may help explain observed slower rates of wound repair and increased risk of infection in persons with diabetes.

Studies have also demonstrated that people with diabetes, especially those with long-term complications, are at increased risk for complications, hospitalization, and death from influenza and pneumococcal disease.[18] For this reason, practitioners play a vital role in ensuring that these patients are up to date with their immunizations. People with diabetes should receive an annual influenza vaccination, as well as a pneumococcal vaccination. A one-time pneumococcal revaccination is recommended for patients greater than 64 years of age who were previously immunized more than 5 years earlier when they were less than 65 years of age. Finally, patients with diabetes should be able to demonstrate current immunization status for other vaccinations, such as tetanus-diphtheria, hepatitis A, and hepatitis B.

Poorly controlled diabetes is a risk factor for the development of oral and dental complications, including gingivitis, periodontitis, dental caries, oral mucosal diseases, oral infections, salivary dysfunction, and taste disturbances.[20] Patients with diabetes have higher rates of gingivitis, periodontitis, and associated alveolar bone loss than patients without diabetes.[19] Poor glycemic control and smoking increase the risk for periodontal diseases in these individuals. Maintaining glucose control and good dental hygiene, having regular checkups with a dentist, and smoking cessation can decrease the risk of developing oral and dental complications.

Unplanned pregnancies occur in about two thirds of women with diabetes.[21] Poorly controlled diabetes before conception and during the first trimester of pregnancy can cause miscarriage in 15% to 20% of pregnancies and major birth defects in 5% to 10% of births. Poor glycemic control during the second and third trimesters can result in excessively large babies (exceeding 10 lb), posing a risk to both mother and child. Patients with diabetes and complications and/or other comorbid conditions such as hypertension may be at additional risk for complications during pregnancy affecting both their own and fetal health. Preconception and prenatal care are therefore vital to a healthy pregnancy, healthy birth, and healthy infant. Practitioners should remember to screen all medications for teratogenicity and safety in women with diabetes who are planning to conceive, are pregnant, or are nursing.

Patients can reduce their risk for developing and/or decrease the progression of these complications by instituting self-care and other preventive measures (Table 47-4). Practitioners should educate patients about self-care and other preventive measures and serve as advocates for people with diabetes.

## Treatment of Diabetes Mellitus

Patients with diabetes should receive medical care from an interprofessional team with expertise and special interest in diabetes.[22] Team members may include, but are not limited to, the following practitioners: a physician, pharmacist, nurse educator or practitioner, physician assistant, dietitian, and mental health professionals. These types of practitioners may also become certified diabetes educators (CDE) specializing in the care of patients with diabetes. Effective diabetes management is patient-centered, taking into account patient-specific factors such as their health beliefs, attitudes, preferences, practices, health literacy, daily routine, and socioeconomic situation that may impact their self-care abilities. Collaborative diabetes management therefore includes patients, their families, and caregivers as active members of the team.

### *Treatment Goals*

Glycemic control is the cornerstone of diabetes management.[22] It includes preventing hypo- and hyperglycemic reactions. In conjunction with maintaining BG within normal

**TABLE 47-4 Self-Care and Other Preventive Measures for Diabetes Complications**

**SMBG**

- Determine frequency of BG testing (e.g., fasting, preprandial, postprandial, bedtime) with your health care provider.
- Keep track of low BG episodes by testing when you have symptoms and record the date, time, and BG value for discussion at next health care provider visit.

**Medical Nutrition Therapy**

- Work with health care providers (e.g., registered dietitian) to tailor nutrition and physical activity based on individual characteristics such as glycemic control and comorbid conditions.
- Maintain a healthy weight.
- Learn about SMBG and medication management before, during, and after exercise.
- Learn about proper management of hypoglycemic episodes.
- If you smoke, quit. Talk to a pharmacist or another practitioner about safe and successful strategies.

**Eye Care**

- Get an annual dilated eye exam.
- Do not use any topical eye preparations unless recommended or prescribed by health care provider.
- Seek medical attention immediately if changes in vision or eye irritation occur.

**Dental Care**

- Have teeth professionally cleaned and oral health checked by a dentist at least twice each year.
- Brush and floss teeth at least twice daily.
- Consult a dentist at the first sign of any gum abnormalities (e.g., bleeding).
- Use appropriate dental care products as recommended by your dentist.

**Skin Care**

- Bathe daily with mild soap and dry skin thoroughly.
- Inspect skin daily—head to toe—for signs of potential infection.
- Cleanse minor cuts and scratches promptly with soap and water.
- See a physician immediately for a serious cut, burn, or skin puncture.
- When needed, use nonprescription topical preparations only as recommended by a pharmacist and/or health care provider.
- Avoid topical drying agents (e.g., alcohol) or salicylic acid–containing products.

**Foot Care**

- Clean and inspect feet daily for any changes (e.g., corn, callus, open wound, fungal infection). If unable to do yourself, enlist the help of another household member or caretaker.
- Report any changes in foot appearance or tactile sensation to your health care provider.
- Trim nails carefully, preferably straight across and file them with an emery board to the contour of the toe.
- Do not walk barefooted.
- Wear soft cotton, synthetic blend, or wool socks to absorb moisture.
- Wear properly fitting, comfortable shoes and use caution when "breaking in" new shoes.
- Inspect shoes for foreign objects before inserting feet.
- Change socks and shoes periodically each day to keep toes dry and clean.
- Do not wear tight clothing and do not cross legs when seated.
- Get an annual foot exam from your health care provider or podiatrist.
- If you have neuropathy, remove shoes at each health care provider visit to have your feet visually inspected.

**Medication Adherence**

- Know what each of your prescribed medications is used for.
- Take your medications only as directed by your health care provider.
- Do not stop taking any of your medications unless you first discuss it with a pharmacist or your physician.
- Discuss taking a low-dose of aspirin daily to prevent heart attack and stroke with your health care provider.
- Do not start taking any nonprescription medications, herbal products, or supplements without first discussing them with your pharmacist or physician.
- Talk to your pharmacist about strategies to help you keep track of your medications and daily doses.
- Get a flu shot every fall.
- Make sure all your immunizations are up to date.

**Sick Day Management**

- Test BG and urine ketones frequently during acute illness.
- Continue taking your medications, including insulin, during acute illness.
- Stay well hydrated.

Key: BG, blood glucose; SMBG, self-monitoring of blood glucose.

levels, managing comorbid conditions such as overweight/obesity, hypertension, and hyperlipidemia also relieves and prevents the development and progression of symptoms related to long-term microvascular, macrovascular, and other complications. Treatment goals should be individualized, taking into account patient-specific factors such as age (e.g., children, adolescents, and the elderly), pregnancy status, and comorbid conditions. Table 47-5 summarizes the recommendations for nonpregnant adults with diabetes.

A diabetes care plan should include the following eight steps:

1. Assessment of the patient's knowledge, understanding, current care, and any factors (e.g., cultural, health literacy, and socioeconomic) that may impact patient care
2. Meal planning and healthy eating instruction
3. Physical activity recommendations
4. Self-monitoring of glucose and, when appropriate, ketone levels

**TABLE 47-5 ADA Treatment Goals for Nonpregnant Adults with Diabetes**

| | |
|---|---|
| **Glycemic Control** | |
| Hemoglobin A1C | <7.0%*† |
| Fasting plasma glucose | 90-130 mg/dL (5.0-7.2 mmol/L) |
| Postprandial plasma glucose‡ | <180 mg/dL (<10.0 mmol/L) |
| Body mass index | <25.0 kg/m² |
| Blood pressure | <130/80 mm Hg |
| **Lipids** | |
| Low-density lipoprotein | <100 mg/dL (< 2.6 mmol/L) (may be <70 mg/dL or 1.8 mmol/L in patients with overt cardiovascular disease) |
| Triglycerides | <150 mg/dL (<1.7 mmol/L) |
| High-density lipoprotein | |
| For men | >40 mg/dL (>1.1 mmol/L) |
| For women | >50 mg/dL (>1.15 mmol/L) |
| Immunizations | Flu vaccine annually<br>Pneumococcal<br>All other should be up to date (e.g., tetanus, hepatitis A/B) |

* Reference to a normal range for patients without diabetes of 4.0% to 6.0% using a Diabetes Control and Complications Trial–based assay.

† More stringent A1C goals (e.g., 6.0%) may be considered in individual patients.

‡ Postprandial plasma glucose measured 1-2 hours from the start of the meal, generally peak levels in patients with diabetes.

5. Drug therapy
6. Patient education
7. Assessment of adherence to SMBG, MNT, and other nondrug and drug therapy
8. Follow-up care to alter or adjust the plan as needed to achieve metabolic goals

### *General Treatment Approach*

Diabetes treatment focuses on maintaining glycemic control and preventing or delaying the progression of long-term diabetes-related complications. Patient education regarding the disease itself and appropriate self-care are the cornerstones of successful therapy. Strict adherence to MNT, encompassing a meal and physical activity plan, is important in glycemic control and achieving and maintaining a healthy weight. Patients with diabetes should also avoid unhealthy habits, such as smoking, which can impact their risk for developing diabetic complications as well as other comorbid conditions. Finally, patients must learn to SMBG to assess the effects of diet, physical activity, and medications on their BG. Not only does performing SMBG serve a clinical purpose, but it also gives the patient a sense of control over the disorder.

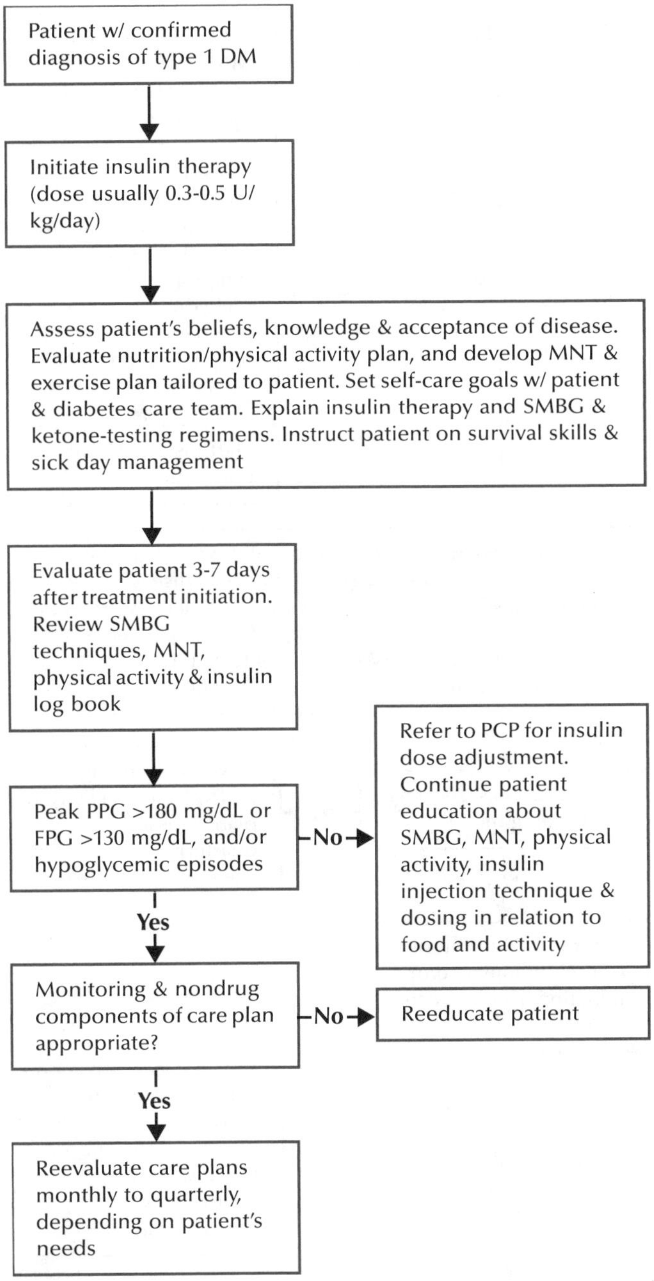


**FIGURE 47-2** General treatment of type 1 diabetes mellitus. Key: DM, diabetes mellitus; FPG, fasting plasma glucose; MNT, medical nutrition therapy; PCP, primary care provider; PPG, postprandial plasma glucose; SMBG, self-monitoring of blood glucose.

Pharmacologic treatment options for patients with type 1 are currently limited to insulin therapy delivered by self-injection or an insulin pump. Because they are unable to produce insulin, type 1 patients must inject themselves with insulin each day. Insulin therapy should be tailored to balance the effects of diet and physical activity. To achieve balance, patients must routinely self-monitor their BG levels. Hypo- and hyperglycemia are largely preventable once this balance is achieved. The algorithm in Figure 47-2 outlines a general treatment approach for type 1 diabetes.

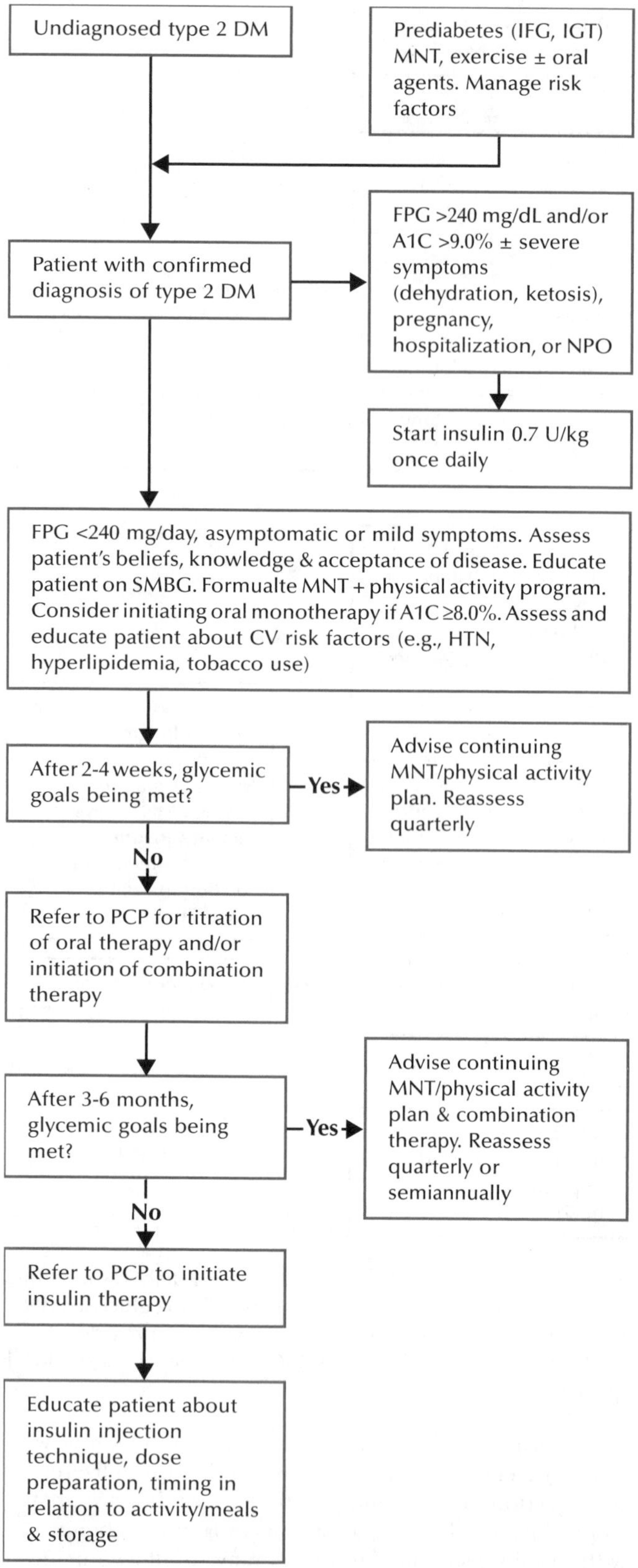


**FIGURE 47-3** General treatment of type 2 diabetes mellitus. Key: A1C, glycosylated hemoglobin; CV, cardiovascular; DM, diabetes mellitus; FPG, fasting plasma glucose; HTN, hypertension; IFG, impaired fasting glucose; IGT, impaired glucose tolerance; MNT, medical nutrition therapy; NPO, nothing by mouth; PCP, primary care provider; SMBG, self-monitoring of blood glucose.

Prediabetes may be detected in patients at risk for developing type 2 diabetes. Patients with prediabetes may be able to normalize their BG levels with diet, exercise, and weight loss alone. Patients with type 2 diabetes, however, often require MNT combined with pharmacologic intervention. Five classes of prescription oral agents (sulfonylureas, nonsulfonylurea secretagogues, α-glucosidase inhibitors, biguanides, thiazolidinediones) and two prescription injectable agents (amylinomimetics and incretin mimetics) are currently available to treat type 2 diabetes. Since most patients with type 2 demonstrate some degree of insulin resistance, oral agents from different classes that target different organs are often used in combination. In addition, oral and injectable agents may be combined with insulin therapy. Patient-specific factors, such as age, weight, liver and kidney function, and the presence of any comorbid conditions, determine the therapy of choice for a type 2 patient. At this time, only metformin has been tested for safety and efficacy in children and adolescents. Depending on the severity of hyperglycemia and/or age of the patient (e.g., children and adolescents) on diagnosis, some type 2 patients may initially require insulin therapy to lower BG before considering switching to orally available agents. Many type 2 patients show diminished insulin production over time, thus requiring supplemental insulin therapy for glycemic control. Figure 47-3 illustrates a general treatment algorithm for type 2 diabetes.

### *Nonpharmacologic Therapy*

#### Medical Nutrition Therapy

Coupled with regular physical activity, MNT is an essential nonpharmacologic component of diabetes care. Rather than focusing on the need to "diet" or "lose weight," the term "nutrition" is used to emphasize the importance of eating for a healthy lifestyle and achieving and maintaining metabolic goals.

Although the concepts of MNT are similar for patients with types 1 and 2 diabetes, different treatment goals exist. For patients with type 1 diabetes, the goals are to integrate insulin regimens into usual eating and physical activity habits and to ensure normal growth and development during childhood and adolescence. Since obesity and a sedentary lifestyle are key issues in type 2 diabetes, the main objectives are healthy eating habits (including caloric and fat restriction), moderate weight loss, and increased physical activity to achieve optimal metabolic goals.

Dietitians who specialize in diabetes care can help patients learn about and incorporate nutritional guidelines into their daily lives. Practitioners can support and reinforce all phases of MNT by encouraging patients to follow their meal plan and avoid fad diets or prolonged fasting. Moreover, patients need instruction in reading food product labels and interpreting nutritional values. Current ADA guidelines for meal planning represent a change from previous recommendations to a more individualized approach involving the patient in the decision-making process and taking into account personal and cultural preferences.[23,24]

The general recommended daily protein intake for most patients is up to 20% of total daily calories.[23] Protein intake is lower for patients with reduced renal function and higher for very active healthy individuals. The long-term consequences of high-protein and low-carbohydrate diets are not well-established in patients with diabetes.[25]

Less than 10% of the total daily caloric intake should come from saturated fats, with vegetable oils (converted to trans-fats) deemphasized in favor of monounsaturated oils (e.g., olive oil). Patients who are overweight or consume high amounts of fat, should decrease dietary fat intake. Consuming "light" or "fat-free" foods in which the fat has been replaced with a carbohydrate, however, may also contribute to obesity. For patients with near normal weight and lipid levels, carbohydrate and monounsaturated fat combined should provide 60% to 70% of daily calories.[24] Carbohydrates include starches (e.g., cereals, grains, starchy vegetables, legumes), sugars (e.g., glucose, fructose, sucrose, lactose), and fiber. Recommend a meal plan high in fresh fruits and vegetables and moderate in starches. High-fiber starches (e.g., whole grain breads and cereals with a goal of 20-35 g fiber per day), are preferred over low-fiber starches (e.g., mashed potatoes, pasta, rice). Some beverages such as regular sodas, juices (over 4 oz), and sports drinks contain excessive or "hidden" carbohydrates. These beverages should be replaced with "low-" or non–carbohydrate-containing alternatives such as water, diet sodas, or sugar-free flavored water drinks.

Carbohydrates do not all affect plasma glucose concentrations equally. Elevated glucose levels are determined by both the quality (glycemic index) and the total quantity of carbohydrates (glycemic load) consumed. Glycemic index (GI) is a system that ranks carbohydrates on a scale of 0% to 100%, on the basis of their potential to raise plasma glucose levels immediately after they are consumed. Carbohydrates with a high GI (70% or higher; e.g., doughnuts, most crackers, corn chips, dried fruits) break down quickly after ingestion, resulting in high and prolonged glucose levels. In contrast, carbohydrates that break down slowly during digestion have a low GI (55% or less; e.g., most fresh fruits and vegetables, beans, oatmeal, pasta) and raise glucose levels only modestly. Diets with low GI foods may improve glucose and lipid levels in people with diabetes. Glycemic load (GL) is the total glycemic response to a food or meal, on the basis of the grams of carbohydrates it contains. GL is calculated by multiplying the GI% by the total grams of carbohydrate per serving. Typical diets contain approximately 100 GL units per day.

Lifestyle changes, moderate daily physical activity, and portion-size control for carbohydrates, protein, and fats are the critical factors in controlling obesity in patients with diabetes. Sodium intake should be limited (less than 2400 mg/day), especially when hypertension is present.[13] All health professionals should encourage patients to keep a meal plan and physical activity log to track the effects of food, physical activity, and medication on BG.[23] In addition, patients should learn how to interpret these data and identify patterns to make a cause and effect relationship for glycemic control.[24]

*Use of Sweeteners* Both nutritive (caloric) and non-nutritive (noncaloric) alternative sweetening agents are available. The calories from nutritive sweeteners such as fructose (4 kcal/g; e.g., honey, fruits, vegetables) and sugar alcohols (2 kcal/g; e.g., sorbitol, mannitol, xylitol) should be counted in the carbohydrate total for meals and snacks.[25] Consuming large amounts of sugar alcohols may cause diarrhea, resulting from the laxative effects of polyols.

Currently the FDA has approved five non-nutritive sweeteners including saccharin (Sweet and Low), sucralose (Splenda), acesulfame potassium (Sweet One, Sunett), aspartame (Equal, NutraSweet), and neotame.[26] Although neotame has been approved for use in beverages and foods, no commercially available products are currently available in the United States. All non-nutritive sweeteners have undergone rigorous testing and are considered safe for consumption in moderate amounts, including by patients with diabetes and who are pregnant. All non-nutritive sweeteners except aspartame are heat stable and may be used in food preparation in a manner similar to sugar. In addition, aspartame contains phenylalanine in a high enough concentration that it should be avoided in patients with phenylketonuria. Stevia is a natural sweetening substance that is available as a dietary supplement.

*Use of Alcohol* Although alcohol consumption precautions for patients with diabetes are similar to those for the general population, some notable exceptions exist. Patients with diabetes must know that alcohol (1) is considered a fat (7 cal/g) in the nutrition plan; (2) alters insulin response; (3) changes manufacture, storage, and release of glycogen; (4) impairs judgment and coordination; and (5) produces chronic nerve toxicity. In addition, acute alcohol consumption can cause hypoglycemia, especially if consumed on an empty stomach. Some epidemiologic evidence suggests that adults with diabetes who chronically consume mild to moderate amounts of alcohol (5-15 g/day) have a reduced risk for coronary heart disease. Controlled trials are necessary to validate this observation.[27-29]

Adult patients choosing to drink should be advised as follows:[23]

- Limit daily intake to no more than two alcoholic beverages for men and one for women.
- One drink is considered 12 oz beer, 5 oz of wine, or 1.5 oz of distilled beverages (hard alcohol). Each contains 15 g of alcohol.
- Calories from alcoholic beverages and sugar-containing mixes must be included as an addition to the regular meal plan. No food should be omitted.
- To reduce hypoglycemia risk, consume alcohol with food and space drinks.
- Refrain from drinking if you are pregnant, overweight (adds calories), or have other medical problems such as pancreatitis, advanced neuropathy, severe hypertriglyceridemia, or alcohol abuse.

*Use of Caffeine* Patients with diabetes may respond differently to caffeine and consumption may need to be limited. Compared with placebo, acute caffeine doses of 375 mg/day (e.g., equivalent to over seven caffeinated carbonated beverages) have been shown to impair postprandial glucose metabolism in people with diabetes.[30] Thus, moderation is advised. Although the ADA does not provide specific guidelines, a conservative recommendation is for patients to consume no more than one to two caffeinated beverages per day.

*Use of Tobacco-related Products* Tobacco use is associated with an increased risk of mortality, macrovascular complications, and early microvascular complications and may predispose the user to developing type 2 diabetes.[22] Clinicians should encourage cessation of all tobacco-related products (e.g., cigarettes, cigars, cloves, bidis, chewing tobacco). Refer to Chapter 50 for a comprehensive approach to treating tobacco use and dependence.

*Physical Activity* Patients with diabetes benefit from an active lifestyle. The term *physical activity* is used because of the negative connotation of *exercise.* Regular physical activity can improve glycemic control (increased insulin sensitivity), facilitate weight loss (reduced body fat and increased muscle), reduce cardiovascular risk factors (reduce LDL-C and triglycerides; increase HDL-C with weight loss; improve blood pressure), and improve self-esteem.[24] Regular physical activity may even prevent the onset of type 2 diabetes.[31]

Before increasing physical activity, patients should undergo a thorough medical evaluation, including diagnostic studies to screen for any underlying diabetes-related complications that may limit certain activities.[32] The patient's lifestyle, preferences, metabolic goals, complications, and limitations should be accounted for to create an individualized fitness program.

In general, patients should engage in 30 minutes or more of moderate physical activity on most days of the week.[32] Patients of advanced age should start slowly (5-10 minutes/day) and increase the amount of time gradually as tolerated. Patients are encouraged to exercise the large muscle groups and participate in aerobic activities (e.g., walking, swimming, biking). Some modifications of physical activity are needed for patients with certain diabetes related-complications. For example, patients with moderate or worsening retinopathy should avoid activities that elevate blood pressure or are strenuous (e.g., heavy competitive sports, power weightlifting). Patients who have neuropathy with loss of protective sensation should avoid repetitive sports such as prolonged walking or jogging, although low-impact alternatives may be recommended by their physician with close follow-up.[32]

Effects of physical activity on BG vary in type 1 diabetes. Hyperglycemia results if insulin is inadequate when the patient begins the activity. In contrast, hypoglycemia may occur if the patient's BG concentration is normal or low just before physical activity. Generally speaking, only patients who use insulin need to consume extra carbohydrates and/or adjust insulin to account for the potential hypoglycemic effects of exercise. Because of a loss or delay of the counterregulatory response to low BG, patients with type 1 diabetes may experience hypoglycemia up to 8 to 15 hours after prolonged exercise. Preventive measures should be taken to avoid this complication. Occasionally type 2 patients taking sulfonylureas or nonsulfonylurea insulin secretagogues may experience hypoglycemia with exercise. The degree of hypoglycemia, however, is not as significant as in insulin users. Table 47-6 provides guidelines for the conscientious exerciser. Patients should be reminded to include their activity in their daily log.

**TABLE 47-6 Guidelines for Patients With Diabetes Who Exercise Conscientiously[32,33]**

- Wear properly fitted shoes and a diabetes identification bracelet or shoe tag.
- SMBG before and after physical activity. BG testing during exercise may be necessary for prolonged physical activity.
- Include a 5-10 minute, low-intensity, aerobic (e.g., walking or bicycling) warm-up (to prepare the muscles and heart) and cool-down (to bring heart rate down) period.
- Adjust insulin or carbohydrate intake if needed. For insulin users who engage in moderate exercise (e.g., 30-45 minutes of bicycling or jogging), reduce the preceding dose of regular or rapid-acting insulin by 30% to 50%.
- If glucose concentration is normal or low (e.g., <100 mg/dL) before exercise, consume a 10-15 g carbohydrate snack (e.g., 1 small apple, 6 oz cup of yogurt, or 4-6 whole-grain crackers) and have an additional snack available if needed after exercise.
- Avoid increased absorption of regular or rapid-acting insulin (and possible hypoglycemia) from exercise by injecting into the abdomen or exercising 30 minutes to 1 hour following insulin administration.
- Avoid physical activity if glucose concentration is greater than 250 mg/dL in the presence of ketosis, as this indicates severe insulin deficiency (particularly in type 1 patients) and may predispose patients to further hyperglycemia with exercise. Use caution if BG levels are over 300 mg/dL without ketosis.
- Monitor for postactivity, late-onset hypoglycemia (which can occur 8-15 hours following exercise, especially in patients with type 1 diabetes). If exercise occurs during the day, increase carbohydrate intake and SMBG during the night to identify nocturnal hypoglycemia. Individuals using insulin are more susceptible to hypoglycemia than those taking sulfonylureas or nonsulfonylurea insulin secretagogues. Type 2 patients treated only with MNT very rarely develop hypoglycemia.

Key: BG, blood glucose; MNT, medical nutrition therapy; SMBG, self-monitoring of blood glucose.

### *Pharmacologic Therapy (Insulin)*

Insulin is the primary medication used to treat type 1 and gestational diabetes. Insulin may also be used in the treatment of type 2 diabetes. Although primary care providers prescribe insulin therapy, other practitioners, especially pharmacists, are often consulted by both primary care providers and patients about insulin and the problems related to its use. Thus, practitioners should be knowledgeable about insulin products and pharmacotherapy.

The insulin molecule is composed of two amino acid chains, with the acidic A chain joined by a disulfide linkage to the basic B chain. Insulin formulations used in the treatment of diabetes are grouped by their species source and time-action profile. There are minor, but important,

**TABLE 47-7 Insulin Amino Acids**

| | A-Chain Position | | | B-Chain Position | | | | |
|---|---|---|---|---|---|---|---|---|
| **Sources/Types** | **A8** | **A10** | **A 21** | **B3** | **B28** | **B29** | **B30** | **B31 and B32** |
| Pork* | Thr | Ilc | Asn | | Pro | Lys | Ala | — |
| Human | Thr | Ilc | Asn | Asn | Pro | Lys | Thr | — |
| **Analogues** | | | | | | | | |
| Aspart | Thr | Ilc | Asn | Asn | Aspartic acid | Lys | Thr | — |
| Lispro | Thr | Ilc | Asn | Asn | Lys | Pro | Thr | — |
| Glulisine | Thr | Ilc | Asn | Lys | Pro | Glutamic acid | Thr | — |
| Glargine | Thr | Ilc | Gly | Asn | Pro | Lys | Thr | Arg |

Key: Ala, alanine; Arg, arginine; Asn, asparagine; Gly, glycine; Ilc, isoleucine; Lys, lysine; Pro, proline; Thr, threonine; Val, valine.

* Eli Lilly, the only manufacturer of pork insulin in the United States, announced on July 6, 2005, that it will cease production of pork insulin products by the end of 2005.

differences in the sequence of amino acids between pork, human, and analogue sources. Table 47-7 displays the differences in amino acid sequences for the available insulin sources.[34,35] All insulins except glargine have a neutral pH.

Insulins can be divided into four groups according to their pharmacodynamics or time-action profile: onset (e.g., rapid, short, intermediate, or long acting), peak, and duration of action after subcutaneous (SQ) injection. Lispro (Humalog), aspart (NovoLog), and glulisine (Apidra) are the most rapid-acting insulins. They differ from human regular insulin, a short-acting insulin, by substitution of amino acid residues (Table 47-7) in the insulin molecule. Rapid- and short-acting insulins are dosed according to carbohydrate content and provide mealtime insulin coverage. Their effects on BG are therefore measured by testing postprandial plasma glucose levels.

To sustain its action, human regular insulin can be bound to zinc alone or in combination with protein molecules. Both zinc and protamine slow insulin dissolution and absorption from the injection site. Neutral protamine Hagedorn (NPH) is an intermediate-acting insulin. NPH is an isophane insulin suspension, consisting of a complex mixture of human regular insulin, protamine, and some zinc, in which the ratio of insulin to protamine is equal. NPH insulin is typically dosed twice daily to supply basal insulin requirements. Another previously available intermediate-acting insulin, lente, was discontinued by its manufacturer, Eli Lilly, in 2005.

Insulin glargine (Lantus) and detemir (Levemir) are long-acting insulins. A previously available long-acting insulin, ultralente, was discontinued by its manufacturer, Eli Lilly, in 2005. Glargine is an insulin analogue whose amino acid sequence causes a shift in the isoelectric point, making it more soluble at an acidic pH.[36] On injection, glargine forms a microprecipitate in the subcutaneous tissue that is slowly absorbed. Detemir is similar in profile and action to glargine and is expected to reach the U.S. market sometime in late 2005/early 2006. Insulin glargine and detemir are usually dosed once daily to supply basal insulin needs. Some patients, however, may require administration of half the total daily dose of a long-acting insulin every 12 hours for better glycemic control. The effects of the intermediate and long-acting insulins on BG are primarily measured by testing fasting plasma glucose levels.

Information concerning the pharmacodynamic profiles of insulins is contained in Table 47-8.[34-36] Many factors, such as insulin type, site of injection, injection technique, insulin antibodies, and individual patient response, can affect the onset, peak, degree, and duration of insulin action on BG levels.[37] Thus, the values listed in Table 47-8 have some degree of variability.

Human insulin is available as nonprescription, whereas insulin analogues require a prescription. Most newly diagnosed patients with diabetes are started and maintained on human insulin and/or insulin analogues. Insulin is commercially available in concentrations of 100 units/mL (designated as U-100). Regular U-500 insulin (Humulin R, Lilly) is available by prescription only for hospital IV use and for insulin-resistant patients requiring greater than 100 to 200 units per injection.

Insulin is also available as fixed-dose mixtures. Mixtures of NPH and human regular insulin are available nonprescription in ratios of 70% NPH to 30% regular and 50% NPH to 50% regular. Mixtures containing insulin analogues are available with a prescription only in ratios of 75% lispro protamine to 25% lispro and 70% aspart protamine to 30% aspart. These formulations provide the rapid onset of lispro or aspart with the longer duration of action of a lispro or aspart protamine suspension, both of which are similar in action to human NPH. Table 47-9 summarizes the insulin formulations currently available in the United States. Patients who switch from one source, type, or formulation (e.g., mixture) of insulin to another require close medical supervision.

**TABLE 47-8 Select Insulin Pharmacodynamics[34,35,38]**

| Type | Source* | Onset of Action (hours) | Peak Action (hours) | Duration (hours) |
|---|---|---|---|---|
| **Rapid-acting** | | | | |
| Insulin lispro | Human analogue | 5-15 minutes | 0.5–1.5 | 3-4 |
| Insulin aspart | Human analogue | 5-15 minutes | 0.5–1.5 | 3-4 |
| Insulin glulisine | Human analogue | 5-15 minutes | 0.5-1.75 | 1-3 |
| **Short-acting** | | | | |
| Regular | Human | 0.5–1 | 2-3 | 3-6 |
| **Intermediate-acting** | | | | |
| NPH† | Human | 2-4 | 4-10 | 10-16 |
| **Long-acting** | | | | |
| Insulin glargine | Human analogue | 1.5 | No pronounced peak | 20-24 |

Key: NPH, neutral protamine Hagedorn.

* Human insulin is produced through recombinant DNA technology.

† These insulins are isophane suspensions.

## Mechanism of Action

Insulin is produced by pancreatic β-cells. It stimulates glucose uptake and storage as glycogen in muscles and the liver and fatty acid and triglyceride synthesis. Insulin decreases hepatic glucose output, lipolysis, and ketone production. It also enhances amino acid incorporation into proteins.

## Indications

Insulin is indicated for the treatment of all types of diabetes mellitus.

## Dosage Guidelines

The goal of insulin therapy in type 1 patients is to mimic physiologic pancreatic insulin secretion to maintain normal plasma glucose levels. Physiologic insulin therapy provides basal and prandial (mealtime) needs. Newly diagnosed patients are usually started on 0.3 to 0.5 units/kg of insulin daily.[39] Doses are adjusted according to age and other patient-specific variables (e.g., plasma glucose levels, growth, diet, activity, ketosis).

One half of the total daily dose is usually given as an intermediate or long-acting formulation to supply the basal metabolic needs. Depending on the insulin type and formulation used, this dose may be administered all at once daily or divided to be administered twice daily. For example, if the patient is using NPH to provide the daily basal insulin requirement, the total daily basal requirement is divided to be administered as two-thirds dose in the morning and one-third dose in the evening. If glargine is used, the estimated basal insulin dose is administered once daily, often at bedtime.

The other half of the estimated total daily insulin dose is given as a rapid- or short-acting formulation to supply the patient's prandial needs. For patients with type 1, practitioners often use the "500 Rule" to estimate the number of carbohydrate grams covered by 1 unit of rapid-acting insulin (500 divided by the total daily dose of insulin equals the number of carbohydrate grams covered).[39] As a general rule in newly diagnosed type 1 patients, 1 unit of rapid-acting insulin covers 10 to 15 g of carbohydrate. As part of MNT education, patients can be taught to estimate the total carbohydrates per meal to determine a prandial insulin dose. For patients who eat three meals a day, rapid- or short-acting insulin is dosed three times a day to be administered 0 to 30 minutes before meals, depending on the type used.

Insulin formulations are selected on the basis of patient-specific factors, such as diet, exercise, ease of use (e.g., vials versus delivery devices) and insurance status (e.g., formulary options available, affordability for uninsured patients). Dosing regimens are also tailored to patients' lifestyle and routine (e.g., number of daily meals and snacks, sleep, and work schedules). Insulin doses are adjusted on the basis of patient response to therapy as evidenced by trends in A1C, fasting, pre-, and postprandial plasma glucose levels and incidence of hypo- and hyperglycemia. Euglycemia can be achieved through intensive insulin therapy via multiple daily injections or an insulin infusion pump. Figure 47-4 depicts the glucose surges from three daily meals and the resultant insulin release from a healthy pancreas in response to prandial glucose. Patients can learn to manage and adjust their daily basal and prandial insulin requirements on the basis of plasma glucose levels, diet, and activity levels.

Insulin therapy in type 2 patients is therefore governed by level of glycemic control and duration of disease.

**TABLE 47-9 Selected Insulin Preparations Available in the United States (U-100 Concentration)[34,35,38]**

| Type* (Source) | Trade Name* | Manufacturer | How Supplied | Appearance |
|---|---|---|---|---|
| **Rapid-acting†** | | | | |
| Insulin lispro (human analogue) | Humalog | Lilly | 10 mL vials; 3mL disposable pen; 5 x 3 mL refill cartridges | Clear |
| Insulin aspart (human analogue) | Novolog | Novo Nordisk | 10 mL vials; 3mL FlexPen prefilled pens; 3 mL Penfill cartridges | Clear |
| Insulin glulisine (human analogue) | Apidra | Aventis | 10 mL vials | Clear |
| **Short-acting** | | | | |
| Regular (human) | Humulin R | Lilly | 10 mL vials | Clear |
| Regular (human) | Novolin R | Novo Nordisk | 10 mL vials; 3 mL prefilled disposable pens and 3 mL refill cartridges | Clear |
| **Intermediate-acting** | | | | |
| NPH‡ (human) | Humulin N | Lilly | 10 mL vials; 3 mL prefilled disposable pens and 3 mL refill cartridges | Cloudy |
| NPH‡ (human) | Novolin N | Novo Nordisk | 10 mL vials; 3 mL prefilled disposable pens and 3 mL refill cartridges | Cloudy |
| **Long-acting** | | | | |
| Insulin glargine (human analogue)† | Lantus | Aventis | 10 mL vials and 3 mL cartridges for OptiClik device | Clear |
| **Mixtures** | | | | |
| 75% NPL, 25% lispro (human analogues)† | Humalog Mix 75/25 | Lilly | 10 mL vials; 5 x 3 mL disposable pen | Cloudy |
| 70% protamine crystalline aspart, 30% aspart (human analogues)† | NovoLog Mix 70/30 | Novo Nordisk | 10 mL vials; 3 mL FlexPen prefilled pens; 3 mL Penfill cartridges | Cloudy |
| 70% NPH, 30% regular (human) | Humulin 70/30 | Lilly | 10 mL vials; prefilled disposable pens and refill cartridges | Cloudy |
| 70% NPH, 30% regular (human) | Novolin 70/30 | Novo Nordisk | 10 mL vials; prefilled disposable pens and refill cartridges | Cloudy |
| 50% NPH, 50% regular (human) | Humulin 50/50 | Lilly | 10 mL vials | Cloudy |

Key: NPH, neutral protamine Hagedorn; NPL, neutral protamine lispro.

* Human insulin is produced through recombinant DNA technology.

† These insulins are available with prescription only.

‡ These insulins are isophane suspensions.

Type 2 patients whose BG is not controlled with oral agents may require long-term supplemental insulin therapy to achieve glycemic goals. In some cases, newly diagnosed type 2 patients with severe hyperglycemia may be started on insulin therapy alone or in combination with other medications to rapidly reduce A1C and BG levels. Once BG levels stabilize, these patients are usually transitioned to oral therapeutic options for management.

Insulin formulation and dosing considerations in type 2 patients are based on patient-specific factors, such as overall glycemic control and presence and degree of insulin resistance. Total daily dosage of insulin in type 2 patients can vary, but typically range from 0.5 to 1.2 units/kg daily. Typically, type 2 patients starting insulin therapy are initiated on once- or twice-daily dosing of an intermediate- or long-acting insulin. Like type 1 patients, type 2 patients may require mealtime insulin therapy with a rapid- or short-acting formulation to minimize postprandial glucose excursions. Total daily insulin dose requirements are generally split between appropriate formulations to provide 50% as basal insulin and 50% as mealtime insulin. Dose is adjusted on the basis of patient response to therapy as

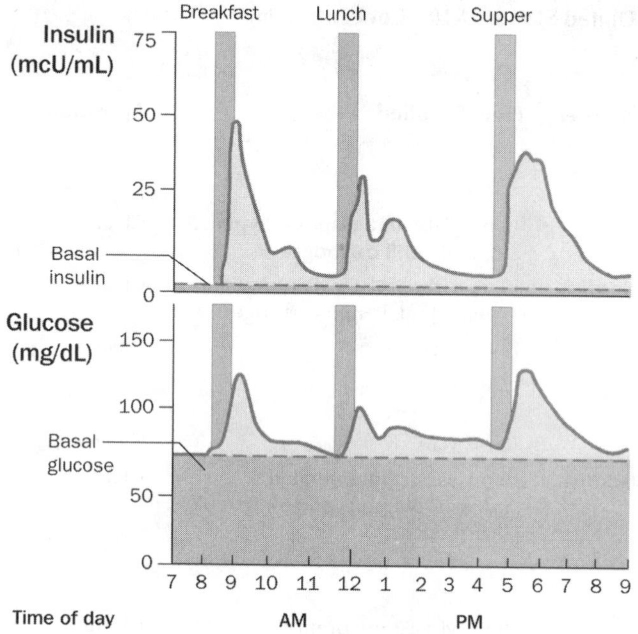


**Examples of some intensive insulin therapy regimens**

| | Fasting | Prelunch | Predinner | Bedtime |
|---|---|---|---|---|
| 1. 3 doses rapid or rapid & intermediate | Rapid & intermed. | Rapid | Rapid & intermed. | |
| 2. 3 doses rapid or long-acting | Rapid | Rapid | Rapid | Long-acting |

**FIGURE 47-4** Relationship between insulin and glucose.

evidenced by A1C trends, fasting and postprandial plasma glucose (FPG, PPG) trends, and hypoglycemic episodes.

Patients with other types of diabetes (e.g., gestational or drug-induced diabetes) or who receive parenteral nutrition may require insulin therapy to maintain normal glucose levels. Insulin therapy in these patients should be combined with appropriate modifications to both nutrition and physical activity. Insulin dose adjustments should be titrated to achieve euglycemia while preventing hypoglycemia, considering the patient's glycemic (FPG, PPG) goals.

## Administration Guidelines

Patients with diabetes self-administer insulin as a subcutaneous (SQ) injection. Unless a patient is too young or has physical and/or mental impairments that preclude self-injection, they should know (1) how to prepare their dose for injection, (2) the location of acceptable self-injection sites, and (3) proper injection technique. Advances from vials and syringes in the form of insulin-delivery devices, such as prefilled insulin pens, are now readily available. In addition to providing convenience, these devices can improve the accuracy of insulin administration and/or adherence in certain patients (e.g., visually or neurologically impaired). Table 47-10 describes the steps for preparing an insulin dose using a syringe and insulin vial or a prefilled insulin-delivery device.

*Injection Sites/Routes/Absorption Rates* Insulin injection site influences insulin absorption and thus therapeutic efficacy. Acceptable SQ injection sites include the abdomen, upper arms (deltoid region), thighs (anterior and lateral aspects), and buttocks (Figure 47-5).[37]

**TABLE 47-10 Guidelines for Preparing an Insulin Dose**

**Using a Vial and Syringe**

- Wash hands with soap and warm water.
- Check the insulin label on the vial to verify the type of insulin to be injected.
- Visually inspect the insulin vial for signs of contamination or degradation (e.g., white clumps, color changes).
- For all cloudy insulins (see Table 47-9), roll the vial gently back and forth between the hands to resuspend the insulin.
- Wipe the top of the vial off with an alcohol swab or cotton ball dipped in alcohol.
- Remove the protective coverings over the plunger and needle of the syringe.
- Taking care not to touch the needle, draw up air equal to the insulin dose to be administered into the syringe.
- Inject the air into the insulin vial.*
- With the syringe still inserted, invert the vial and withdraw the insulin dose.†
- Be sure to keep the hub of the needle below the surface of the insulin to prevent creating air bubbles within the syringe.
- If bubbles are present, gently tap the syringe to coax air to the top of the barrel where it can be injected back into the vial.
- Remove the syringe from the vial and self-inject dose, utilizing proper injection technique (see Table 47-11).

**Using a Prefilled Insulin Pen Delivery Device**

- Wash hands with soap and warm water.
- Check the insulin label on the device (e.g., pen) to verify the type of insulin to be injected.
- Remove the protective pen cap and visually inspect the insulin for signs of contamination or degradation.
- For all cloudy insulins (see Table 47-9), roll the device (e.g., pen) gently back and forth between the hands to resuspend the insulin.
- Wipe the rubber stopper with an alcohol swab.
- Attach needle onto device per manufacturer's directions.
- Remove the needle cap.
- Follow any manufacturer's recommendations for priming the device (e.g., 2-unit airshot).
- Making sure pen dose selectors are first set to zero, dial the insulin dose to be injected.
- Use proper injection technique (see Table 47-12).
- To deliver insulin when injecting, push down on the plunger button.
- Remove the needle from the device after injection to avoid allowing air into the insulin reservoir.

Key: NPH, neutral protamine Hagedorn.

* Patients mixing rapid- or short-acting insulin with NPH into the same syringe for injection should be instructed to inject air first into the NPH vial, then into the rapid- or short-acting vial.

† Patients mixing rapid- or short-acting insulin with NPH into the same syringe for injection should be instructed to withdraw the dose of the rapid- or short-acting insulin *before* the NPH.

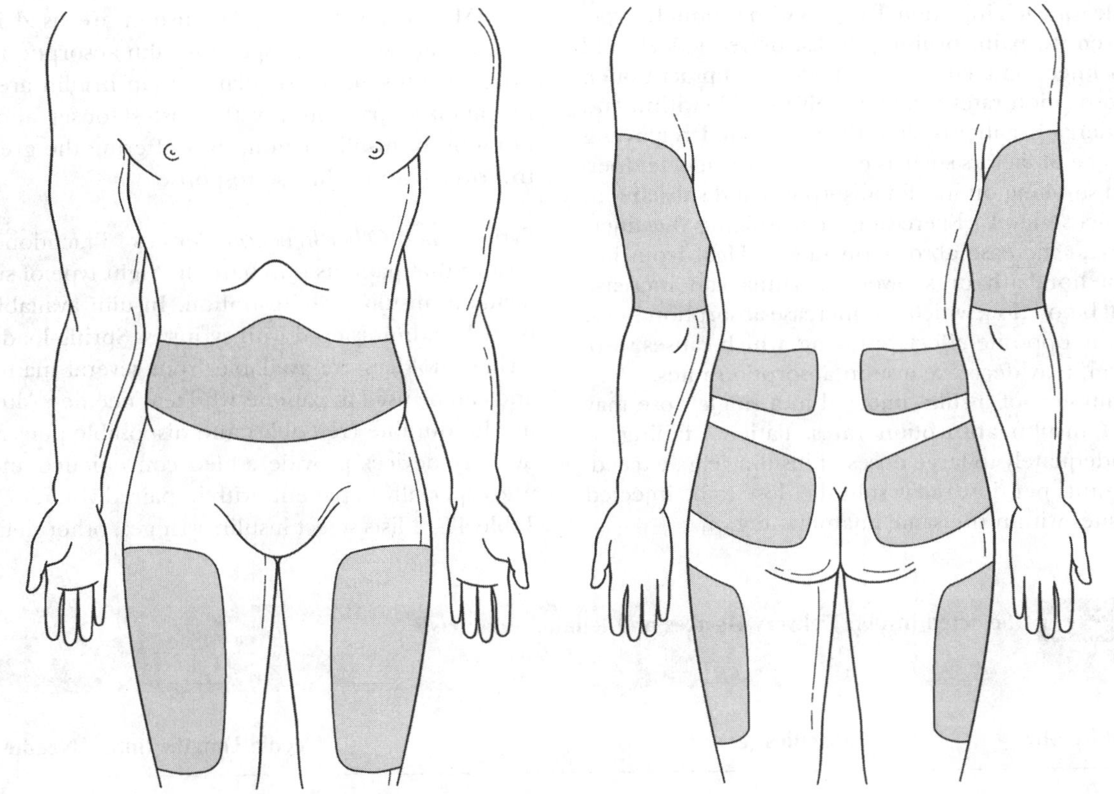

**FIGURE 47-5** Body map of subcutaneous insulin injection sites.

Different anatomic sites differ in their rates of absorption. To decrease dose-to-dose absorption, patients should select then stick to one anatomic injection site. The abdomen, the area of fastest absorption, is the preferred site for SQ injection of insulin. Patients should avoid the area within 2 in. around the navel. Rotation of injection sites within an anatomic area helps prevent lipohypertrophy or lipoatrophy.

Patients (and/or their families or caregivers) are taught to administer insulin via SQ injection (Figure 47-5). Proper SQ injection technique is depicted in Figure 47-6 and described step-by-step in Table 47-11.

Injection technique may need to be altered for certain patients (e.g., 45-degree injection angle for infants and thin individuals with minimal SQ fat). Pinching the skin provides a firm injection surface and lifts the fat off the muscle to avoid intramuscular (IM) or intravenous (IV) injection. Properly injected insulin leaves only the needle puncture dot to show the injection site. If insulin leakage is observed, patients should be instructed to apply pressure to the injection site for 5 to 10 seconds (without rubbing). BG monitoring should be done more frequently on any day that insulin leakage or blood is observed. Patients who routinely experience insulin leakage postinjection should have their injection technique evaluated. In some cases, a longer needle may be needed.

Injection pain can be reduced by injecting room-temperature insulin, keeping muscles relaxed before injection, ensuring air bubbles are not present in the syringe, penetrating the skin quickly, not changing direction of the needle during insertion and/or withdrawal, and using a

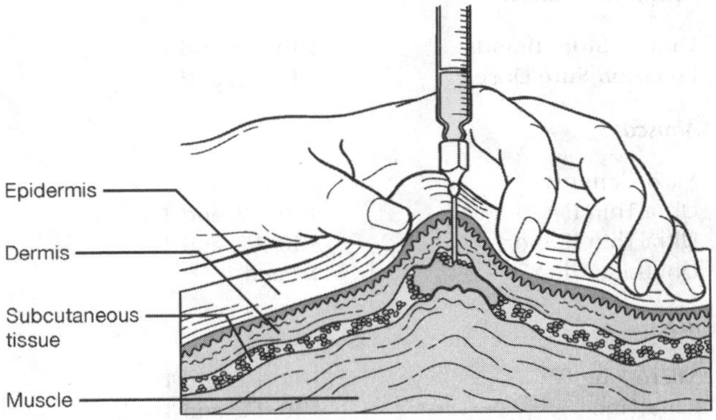


**FIGURE 47-6** Correct method of subcutaneous insulin injection; needle angle should be 90 degrees.

**TABLE 47-11 Insulin Subcutaneous Self-Injection Technique**

- Prepare insulin dose for administration (see Table 47-10).
- Pinch the area to be injected.
- Insert the needle at a 90-degree angle to the skin in the center of the pinched area (a 45-degree angle for insertion may be used in small children and very thin adults).
- Release the pinch.
- Press down on the syringe or device plunger to inject insulin.
- Hold the syringe or device in the area for 5-10 seconds to ensure full delivery of insulin.
- Remove the syringe or device.

new needle for each injection. Patients who routinely experience soreness, pain, bruising, welts, or redness should have their injection technique evaluated by a practitioner.

SQ absorption rates can be highly variable within and across patients.[39] Patients should be educated regarding the influence of factors such as exercise, massage, temperature, and smoking on insulin absorption and subsequent plasma glucose levels. Exercising or massaging the injection area can increase absorption rates.[39] Heat from hot weather, a hot bath or shower, or sauna can increase peripheral blood flow, which can increase absorption rates. Cold has the opposite effect. Smoking, which causes vasoconstriction, may decrease insulin absorption rates.

The amount of insulin injected in a single dose may also affect insulin absorption rates. Patients failing to respond adequately to large doses of insulin (e.g., exceeding 50-60 units per dose) may split the dose to be injected over two sites within the same anatomic region.

IM injections of regular insulin are used in certain patient care settings to speed insulin absorption. IV injections or infusions of regular human insulin are used for hospitalized patients for the fastest onset and shortest duration of insulin action, thus offering the greatest control over plasma glucose response.

*Syringes and Other Injection Devices* Practitioners should ensure that patients purchase the right type of supplies to facilitate insulin administration. Insulin available in vials must be administered with syringes. Spring-loaded plastic syringe holders are available from several manufacturers and can be used in patients who fear needles. Alternatively, insulin durable (reusable) and disposable pens and other delivery devices provide added convenience and ease of use, especially in patients with impaired vision or dexterity. Table 47-12 lists select insulin syringes, other delivery aids,

**TABLE 47-12 Selected Insulin Delivery Devices and Related Products[38]**

| Products (Grouped by Mfr) | Capacities (cc) | Needle Lengths (in.) | Needle Gauges |
|---|---|---|---|
| **Insulin Syringes with Needles*** | | | |
| ***Abbott Laboratories*** | | | |
| Various Store Brands | 3/10, 1/2, and 1 | 3/8 and 1/2 | 29, 30 |
| Precision Sure Dose | 3/10, 1/2, and 1 | 5/16 and 1/2 | 28, 29, 30 |
| ***Aimsco*** | | | |
| Maxi Comfort | 1/2 and 1 | 1/2 | 28 |
| Ultra Thin II | 3/10, 1/2, and 1 | 1/2 | 29 |
| Ultra Thin II Short | 3/10, 1/2, and 1 | 5/16 | 30 |
| Uni Body Ultra II | 1/2 and 1 | 1/2 | 28, 29 |
| ***BD*** | | | |
| Micro-Fine IV | 3/10, 1/2, and 1 | 1/2 | 28 |
| Ultra-Fine | 3/10, 1/2, and 1 | 1/2 | 30 |
| Ultra Fine II Short | 3/10 (available in 1/2 unit and full unit scales), 1/2 and 1 | 5/16 | 31 |
| SafetyGlide | 3/10,1/2, and 1 | 1/2 | 29 |
| Safety-Lok | 1 | 1/2 | 29 |
| ***Can-Am Care Corp*** | | | |
| Monoject Ultra Comfort Short | 3/10, 1/2, and 1 | 5/16 | 30 |
| Monoject Ultra Comfort 29 | 3/10, 1/2, and 1 | 1/2 | 29 |
| Monoject Ultra Comfort 28 | 1/2 and 1 | 1/2 | 28 |
| Various store brands | 3/10, 1/2, and 1 | 5/16 and 1/2 | 28, 29, 30, 31 |
| ***Medicore*** | | | |
| Medicore Lite Touch | 1/2 and 1 | 5/16 and 1/2 | 28, 29, 30 |
| ***UltiMed, Inc.*** | | | |
| UltiCare, UltiFine | 3/10, 1/2, and 1 | 1/2 | 29 |
| UltiCare, UltiSmooth | 1/2 and 1 | 1/2 | 28 |
| UltiCare, UltiThin Short | 3/10, 1/2, and 1 | 5/16 | 30 |
| UltiGuard, UltiFine UltiGuard, | 3/10, 1/2, and 1 | 1/2 | 29 |
| UltiThin Short | 3/10, 1/2, and 1 | 5/16 | 30 |

TABLE 47-12 Selected Insulin Delivery Devices and Related Products[38] (continued)

| Products (Grouped by Mfr) | Needle Lengths (in.) | Needle Gauges | Special Features |
|---|---|---|---|
| **Pen Needles** | | | |
| *BD* | | | |
| UltraFine Original Pen Needles | 1/2 | 29 | Can be used with BD, Lilly, and Novo insulin pens and dosers |
| UltraFine III Mini Pen Needles | 3/16 | 31 | Can be used with BD, Lilly, and Novo insulin pens and dosers |
| UltraFine III Short Pen Needles | 5/16 | 31 | Can be used with Aventis, BD, Lilly, and Novo insulin pens and dosers |
| *Novo Nordisk* | | | |
| NovoFine 30 | 5/16 | 30 | For use with Novo Nordisk line of insulin delivery systems |
| NovoFine 31 | 6 mm | 31 | |
| *Owen Mumford Inc.* | | | |
| Unifine Pentips Pen Needles | 6 mm, 5/16, and 12 mm | 29, 31 | Compatible with all brand name reusable and disposable cartridge pens |

| Products (Grouped by Mfr) | Insulin Capacity (mL) | Unit Increments of Insulin Delivered | Compatibility |
|---|---|---|---|
| **Insulin Injection Devices** | | | |
| *Aventis* | | | |
| OptiClik | 3.0 | 1-U | Large dialing window and audible clicks; may be dialed forward or backward; year lifetime for device. |
| *Lilly* | | | |
| Humalog Pen | 3.0 | 1-U | Magnified dose window; dosage knob can be dialed forward or backward for correction |
| Humulin N Pen | 3.0 | 1-U | |
| Humalog Mix 75/25 Pen | 3.0 | 1-U | |
| Humulin 70/30 Pen | 3.0 | 1-U | |
| *Novo Nordisk* | | | |
| Novolog FlexPen | 3.0 | 1-U | Large dialing window and audible clicks (except NovoPen 3 and NovoPen Junior) for each unit; for some devices, dosage knob may be dialed forward or backward for correction; dose scale of FlexPen and 70/30 FlexPen reset to zero after injection |
| NovoLog Mix 70/30 FlexPen | 3.0 | 1-U | |
| NovoPen Junior | 3.0 | 1/2-U | |
| NovoPen 3 | 3.0 | 2-70 U in 1-U | |
| InDuo | 3.0 | 1-70 U in 1-U | Combined OneTouch Ultra BG monitor and insulin delivery system |
| InnoLet | Prefilled disposable doser 3.0 | 1-50 U in 1-U | Large dial with easily read numbers for dose selection and audible clicks for each unit; dosage knob can be dialed forward or backward for correction |
| Innovo | 3.0 | 1-70 U in 1-U | Large display with memory function (timing and amount of last dose); 6-second countdown display from time of dose delivery to needle withdrawal |
| *Owen Mumford, Inc.* | | | |
| Autopen AN 3000 | 1.5 | 2-32 U in 2-U | Automatic side injection for delivery from 1.5 or 3.0 mL insulin cartridges; compatible with Lilly 3.0 mL cartridges |
| Autopen AN3100 | 1.5 | 1-16 U in 1-U | |
| Autopen AN3800 | 3.0 | 2-42 U in 2-U | |
| Autopen AN 3810 | 3.0 | 1-21 U in 1-U | |

**TABLE 47-12 Selected Insulin Delivery Devices and Related Products[38] (continued)**

| Product (Mfr) | Description | Syringe Type and Size Used | Needle Visible? | Adjustable Depth of Skin Penetration? |
|---|---|---|---|---|
| **Syringe Injection Aids** | | | | |
| BD inject-Ease Automatic injector (BD) | Spring-loaded plastic syringe holder positioned over skin; button activated | BD 3/10, 1/2, 1 mL syringes | No | Yes |
| Instaject (Medicool Inc.) | Combination blood lancet and syringe injection device; button activated | Most 3/10, 1/2, 1 mL syringes | No | Yes |
| NeedleAid (NeedleAid Ltd.) | Stabilizing guide for syringe or pen injection; broad base hides needle, masks sensation of needle entry, and ensures insulin injection at proper angle and depth; needle automatically withdrawn | Most 3/10, 1/2, and 1 mL syringes; Lilly and Novo Nordisk pens | No | No |
| NovoPen 3 PenMate (Novo Nordisk) | Attachment to conceal needle and reduce pain perception | NovoPen 3 and NovoPen Junior | No | No |
| Autoject (Owen Mumford Inc.) | Spring-loaded plastic syringe holder positioned over skin; button activated | Most 3/10, 1/2, and 1mL syringes | No | Yes |
| Autoject 2 (Owen Mumford Inc.) | Spring-loaded plastic syringe holder positioned over skin; button activated | Abbott Labs, BD, and Medisense 1/2 and 1 mL syringes | No | Yes |

| Product | Description |
|---|---|
| **Lancet and Needle Disposal** | |
| BD Home Sharps Container | For disposal of used lancets, pen needles, and syringes |
| BD Sharps Disposal by Mail | Container holding up to 300 used lancets or pen needles or 100 used syringes; comes with postage paid packing for returning full containers via mail; 1-888-232-2736 or www.Bddiabetes.com |
| BD Safe-Clip | Needle clipping and storage device; holds up to 1500 needles |
| UltiMed Inc UltiGuard Syringes and Dispoable Container Unit | Syringes sold with a disposable container unit |

Key: Mfr, manufacturer.

* Product features will vary by manufacturer's marketed line. Syringes usually packaged in quantities of 100.

and related products currently available in the United States. Insulin pumps are an alternative delivery device available for use in select patients. Patients using syringes and disposable needles with other delivery devices should properly dispose of them according to local regulations. Practitioners should be familiar with the sharps disposal programs available to patients within their geographic area.

*Types of Syringes* Insulin syringes are plastic, disposable syringes that come with very fine, well-lubricated needles. Recall that insulin is usually supplied as 100 units per milliliter (U-100). Insulin syringes are marked in insulin units. Depending on the syringe, marker increments may differ and therefore should be pointed out to patients. Depending on the manufacturer, insulin syringes are available in 0.3, 0.5, and 1 mL capacities which hold 30, 50, and 100 units, respectively. Syringes are usually packaged in quantities of 100. Patients should be reminded to purchase syringes closely matched to their individual insulin dose(s). For example, a patient taking 38 units of NPH twice daily should use 0.5 mL syringe to draw up insulin to the 38-unit mark.

Today's needles have virtually no "dead space" or air space at the hub of the needle, thus reducing a potential source of dosing error. Several needle lengths, including 1/2, 3/8, and 5/16 in., are available. The shortest needles are usually reserved for use in children or very thin adults. Needles come in a variety of gauges (e.g., 28-31). The higher the gauge, the finer the needle, reducing pain on injection. Silicone-coating eases insertion, also reducing pain.

Manufacturers currently do not recommend reusing disposable syringes and pen needles. Studies have investigated the reuse of insulin syringes. The ADA suggests that some patients may opt to reuse syringes or needles until the needle becomes dull, bent, or comes in contact with any surface other than the skin.[37] In practice, fine-gauge (e.g., 30 or 31) syringes and pen needles are more susceptible to bending and breaking on reuse, which could result in injury or other adverse effects. Syringes and needles to be reused should not be cleaned with alcohol, which removes the silicone coating. Syringes and needles to be reused must be safely recapped and stored at room temperature away from children and pets. Certain patients, such as those with poor hygiene, an acute illness, open wounds, decreased immunity, or poor dexterity and/or vision should not reuse syringes or needles. Practitioners should evaluate patients for syringe or needle reuse and instruct them on proper recapping and storage. Patients should be instructed to inspect injection sites and report any redness, swelling, or other symptoms of infection to their provider.

*Injection Devices/Aids* Several types of insulin injection aids and devices are available for patients who have an aversion to or difficulty with self-injection. Such products include syringe magnifiers, needle guides and vial stabilizers, syringe insertion aids, insulin pens, and jet injectors. Syringe magnifiers enlarge the marks on a syringe barrel, making them easier to see for visually impaired patients. Patients should be reminded that, depending on the manufacturer, magnifiers work only with specific syringe brands. Needle guides and vial stabilizers are available to help patients with limited dexterity safely insert syringes into vials and draw up accurate insulin doses.

Syringe insertion aids typically consist of a jacket that fits over a filled syringe. Most of these devices are spring-loaded and guide the insertion of an unseen needle into the skin. Insertion aids may vary in their compatibility with different syringe brands. Needle length may or may not be adjustable. Patients should familiarize themselves with the varying features of syringe insertion aids before selecting one for use. Table 47-12 lists select syringe insertion aids available in the United States.

Insulin pens, most of which resemble writing pens, use single-use or disposable cartridges filled with 150 or 300 units of human insulin. These devices may be ideal for children, adolescents, and any patient with visual or physical dexterity impairment. Depending on manufacturer, pens are available in a variety of insulin types and mixtures (e.g., lispro, aspart, NPH, glargine, NPL/lispro 75/25, and aspart protamine/aspart 70/30). Pen needles should be selected on the basis of their compatibility with the device. "Dose gauges" are available that allow doses to be dialed in or have audible dose selectors. Patients should be reminded to roll suspension formulations of insulin (i.e., NPH) between their hands before injection. Table 47-12 lists select insulin pen delivery devices and pen needles currently available in the United States.

Jet injectors force a tiny pressurized liquid stream of insulin through the skin without using a needle. The injected insulin disperses into a very thin spray as it enters the subcutaneous tissue. The jet injector must be held firmly against the skin to deliver the exact dose. Short-acting (e.g., regular) insulin may be absorbed more rapidly when administered via jet injector versus traditional SQ injection.[37] First-time users may have to adjust the insulin dose because the increased tissue contact may cause faster insulin absorption. As with any device, improper use can result in dose errors. Jet injector devices may cause less lipoatrophy and inflammation but more bruising than standard needle injections.

*Insulin Pumps* Intensive insulin therapy to achieve tight glycemic control in either type 1 or type 2 diabetes requires multiple daily injections (MDIs). An alternative to MDIs for certain patients is an insulin pump. Insulin pump therapy comes closest to mimicking endogenous normal insulin secretion. It also requires intensive patient training to ensure optimal and safe insulin delivery and BG levels. For these reasons, only patients who are extremely motivated, responsible, have demonstrated appropriate health literacy about diabetes care and monitoring, and have proven consistent ability to adhere to SMBG, MNT, and insulin therapy recommendations are appropriate candidates for insulin pump therapy. Medicare currently covers insulin pumps and related supplies for patients with types 1 and 2 diabetes who meet its eligibility requirements.[38]

Insulin pumps are computerized, battery-driven portable devices smaller than a pager that can be worn on the belt loop, in a pocket, or attached to undergarments. The computer is programmed to deliver a continuous insulin infusion (usually 0.5–1.0 U/hour) to meet basal requirements and bolus doses for mealtime, snack, and exercise requirements. Both basal and bolus rates can be programmed to fluctuate or be manually adjusted, on the basis of SMBG results. Human regular, lispro, aspart, or glulisine insulin is delivered from a reservoir via a computer-controlled plunger through tubing to an SQ implanted catheter that must be changed regularly (usually every 2-3 days) to prevent irritation, lipodystrophy, and infection. The infusion line can be disconnected from the syringe when the patient is swimming, showering, or engaged in intimate activities or when the infusion line is occluded.

Currently available pumps are open-loop systems in that they do not automatically test BG and regulate insulin dosing accordingly. They therefore do not function as an artificial pancreas. Some pumps also have BG monitors attached for the patient to access easily. Patients must learn how to insert and change catheters and tubing and monitor for signs and symptoms of cutaneous infection. In addition, they must learn to program and trouble-shoot the device. Finally, patients must still SMBG frequently, monitor for signs and symptoms of hypoglycemia, count carbohydrates, and predict the effects of exercise to determine the dose of basal and bolus insulin to be programmed into the device.

Several U.S. manufacturers make insulin pumps, including Amigo (Nipro Diabetes Systems), Animas IR 1200 (Animas Corp), DANA Diabecare II (DANA Diabecare USA), Deltec CozMore Insulin Technology System (Smiths Medical MD, Inc.), and the Medtronic Minimed 512/712 (Medtronic Minimed). Pump features (such as a low battery, low insulin reservoir, or line occlusion alarms; the ability to program multiple patient-specific insulin delivery profiles; and basal delivery ranges) vary depending

**TABLE 47-13 Mixing Insulins**[34,35,37,39]

| Mixture | Proportion | Pharmacodynamics | Stability |
|---|---|---|---|
| Lispro + NPH | Any | Slight decrease in absorption rate but not total bioavailability of lispro; postprandial BG response of lispro unaffected | Prepare mixture and inject immediately |
| Aspart + NPH | Any | Slight decrease in absorption rate but not total bioavailability of aspart; postprandial BG response of aspart unaffected | Prepare mixture and inject immediately |
| Glulisine + NPH | Any | No significant change in bioavailability or time to maximum concentration versus glulisine alone | Prepare mixture and inject immediately |
| Regular +NPH | Any | No change in onset or duration of action of either insulin when administered in mixture | May be premixed into syringe, to be stored under refrigeration up to 7 days |
| Regular + normal saline | Any | N/A | Use within 2-3 hours of preparation |

Key: N/A, not applicable.

on the device. Patients must also learn to select and stock appropriate pump supplies, such as batteries, battery rechargers, infusion tubing, catheters, tape, and insulin on the basis of their specific device.

## Mixing Insulins

Depending on the type of insulin, patients may mix two formulations together in a single syringe to limit the number of injections required. Table 47-13 summarizes the compatibility of various insulin mixtures.

Aspart in mixture with crystalline intermediate (e.g., NPH) has not been studied to date.[39] Glulisine has been studied to date only in mixture with NPH and therefore should not be mixed with other long-acting insulins.[35] Glargine should not be mixed with any other form of insulin because of its low pH.

Patients using insulin pumps should be aware of insulin-pump compatibility and preparation. Lispro, aspart, and glulisine should not be diluted or mixed with other insulins when used in an insulin pump.[34]

## Safety Considerations

The most common side effect of insulin therapy is hypoglycemia. Many other factors (e.g., a decrease or inconsistency in mealtime carbohydrate content, exercise, and alcohol intake) can also contribute to hypoglycemic episodes. For this reason, practitioners must carefully assess the relationship between insulin dose and timing and patient BG trends, including hypoglycemic or hyperglycemic episodes, when adjusting insulin therapy. Patients with comorbid conditions, such as gastroparesis caused by neuropathy or compromised renal function, may be at increased risk for hypoglycemia. In such cases, insulin doses should be adjusted accordingly.

Weight gain is another common side effect. It is usually caused by increased efficiency of glucose and fat storage resulting from insulin therapy. Hypoglycemic episodes, which stimulate appetite, also contribute to weight gain.

Some patients experience local reactions on insulin injection, including pain, redness, bruising, burning, stinging, or irritation. Using a new syringe or pen needle with each injection or an injection aid may help minimize or alleviate pain associated with injections. Reminding patients to inject room temperature insulin minimizes burning and stinging associated with cold insulin injections. Glargine has been associated with a higher incidence of pain/stinging at injection sites than other currently marketed neutral pH insulin preparations.[34] Most patients, however, tolerate glargine well. Proper insulin injection technique minimizes redness, swelling, and bruising. Good hygiene and proper use and storage of syringes and other delivery devices minimize the risk for infection. Practitioners should stress the importance of rotating/alternating injection sites within an anatomic area to limit local irritation, tissue reactions, and lipodystrophy.

Newly diagnosed patients are usually started on human and/or analogue insulin, which are highly purified. Sensitivity and hypersensitivity reactions with human and analogue insulins are rare. Allergic reactions attributed to insulin additives (e.g., metacresol, phenol, methylparaben) are also rare. Insulin resistance secondary to insulin-blocking antibodies with human or analogue insulins are exceedingly rare. Patients demonstrating adherence to therapy yet requiring more than 200 units of insulin daily may be evaluated for the presence of insulin antibodies.

Table 47-14 contains a partial list of drugs that can alter BG levels, especially when taken in combination with oral hypoglycemic agents or insulin. Patients receiving hypoglycemic agents or insulin in combination with any of these medications should continue to SMBG frequently and have their insulin dose-adjusted as needed.

Patients who have had systemic allergic reactions (e.g., hives, angioedema, or anaphylaxis) to any insulin should be skin tested with each new preparation before initiating its use. Situations such as growth, puberty, menses, and acute illness can alter glycemic control. Patients with decreased

**TABLE 47-14 Selected Drugs That May Cause Clinically Significant Hypoglycemia or Hyperglycemia[34,39]**

| Hypoglycemia | Hyperglycemia |
|---|---|
| Alcohol (acute) | Alcohol (chronic) |
| Anabolic steroids | Antimicrobials (pentamidine, rifampin) |
| β-Adrenergic blockers | Asparaginase |
| $β_2$-Agonists | Atypical antipsychotics |
| Chloroquine | β-Adrenergic blockers |
| Clofibrate | Caffeine |
| Disopyramide | Calcitonin |
| Exenatide | Calcium-channel blockers |
| Guanethidine | Carbamazepine |
| Haloperidol | Cimetidine |
| Insulin | Corticosteroids |
| Lithium carbonate | Cyclosporine |
| Monoamine oxidase inhibitors | Diazoxide |
| Nateglinide | Didanosine |
| Norfloxacin | Diuretics, both loop and thiazides |
| Pentamidine | Encainide |
| Phenobarbital | Estrogens |
| Phenothiazines | Imipramine |
| Pramlintide | Interferon-α |
| Prazosin | Isoniazid |
| Propoxyphene | Lactulose |
| Quinine | Lithium |
| Quinolones | Marijuana |
| Repaglinide | Megestrol acetate |
| Salicylates in large doses | Niacin and nicotinic acid |
| Sulfonamides | Oral contraceptives |
| Sulfonylureas | Phenothiazines |
| Tricyclic antidepressants | Phenytoin |
| | Probenecid |
| | Protease inhibitors |
| | Quinolones |
| | Sympathomimetic amines |
| | Tacrolimus |
| | Thyroid preparations |

renal function may have decreased insulin clearance and should be closely monitored for hypoglycemic episodes. Patients undergoing hemodialysis may have fluctuating BG levels and should be closely monitored. Certain medications, such as β-blockers, can mask symptoms associated with hypoglycemia, such as tachycardia. Patients and their families/caregivers should be reminded to carefully monitor for other symptoms associated with hypoglycemia. Other medications, such as corticosteroids, can increase BG. In instances in which normal physiologic processes, comorbid conditions, or medications can affect BG levels, patients should have their insulin therapy adjusted on the basis of their BG trends.

### Contamination of Insulin

All insulins are produced at a near-neutral pH of 7.4 with the exception of glargine, which has a pH of 4. Lispro, aspart, glulisine, regular, and glargine insulins are clear aqueous fluids. If any of these products appears cloudy, flocculated, clumped, crystallized or tinted, it may be contaminated and should not be dispensed or used. Other insulins (NPH and insulin mixtures containing an intermediate-acting insulin such as NPH, NPL, or protamine crystalline aspart) are cloudy suspensions. If any of these types of insulin suspensions rapidly settles out, precipitates, clumps, flocculates, crystallizes, or discolors, it may be altered and should not be dispensed or used.

### Storage of Insulin

Insulin is a heat-labile protein, so all preparations must be stored carefully to maintain stability and maximum potency. Patients should inspect their insulin for visible changes in appearance before each injection. Color changes may be associated with protein denaturation and should be interpreted as evidence of potency loss. Clear insulins that become cloudy or precipitate can also signal chemical changes and degradation that could decrease insulin potency.

Unopened insulin vials and cartridges may be stored in the refrigerator (36°F-46°F [2°C-8°C]) up until the expiration date listed on the product. Insulin should never be frozen. The refrigerator door is usually a good storage location to ensure that insulin does not become frozen. The stability of unopened and in-use insulin vials or cartridges stored at room temperature (RT) varies depending on the product. Once opened (in-use), all insulin in vials may be stored away from heat sources and direct sunlight at RT (<77°F or 25°C for glulisine and <86°F or 30°C for all other insulins) for up to 28 to 30 days (in practice, ~1 month). In contrast, the stability of open insulin pens, refill cartridges, and other delivery devices varies depending on the product. Insulin pump cartridges, once opened, are generally stable for 48 hours. Table 47-15 summarizes the stability of open insulin at RT for select insulin products. Some delivery devices, such as the OptiClik, should not be refrigerated. Practitioners should contact individual manufacturers with specific questions regarding the stability of individual insulin products and devices under different storage or exposure conditions.

Patients who transport insulin regularly (e.g., to and from school or work, while running errands) should be reminded to insulate insulin from heat, direct sunlight, and excess agitation. Patients should never store insulin in the car. Insulin should be carried in an insulated pack by patients when traveling by bus, train, or air to ensure proper storage conditions.

## *Special Treatment Considerations*

### Hyperglycemia

Hyperglycemia can occur if an insulin dose is missed, the dose is insufficient to meet metabolic needs or excess carbohydrates are consumed. Symptoms of this adverse effect

**TABLE 47-15 Stability of Select Open (in-use) Insulin Devices and Refill Cartridges at Room Temperature[37,40,41]**

| Insulin Product (Mfr) | Stability at Room Temperature (<86°F [30°C]) |
|---|---|
| Humalog Pen (Lilly) | 28 days |
| Novolog FlexPen (Novo Nordisk) | 28 days |
| Humulin N Pen (Lilly) | 14 days |
| Novolin R InnoLet (Novo Nordisk) | 28 days |
| Novolin N InnoLet (Novo Nordisk) | 14 days |
| Humalog 75/25 Pen (Lilly) | 10 days |
| Humulin 70/30 Pen (Lilly) | 10 days |
| Novolog 70/30 FlexPen (Novo Nordisk) | 14 days |
| Novolin 70/30 InnoLet (Novo Nordisk) | 10 days |
| Glargine OptiClik (Aventis)* | 28 days |

Key: Mfr, manufacturer.

* OptiClik device is currently distributed to physicians only and therefore not available at pharmacies.

**TABLE 47-16 Fast-acting Carbohydrates for Treating Hypoglycemia (15 g)**

| Source (Mfr) | Quantity |
|---|---|
| Milk (low- or nonfat) | 8 oz (1 cup) |
| Fruit juice (e.g., apple, orange) | 4 oz (1/2 cup) |
| Soft drink (nondiet) | 4 oz (1/2 cup) |
| Sugar | 1 tbsp or 3 cubes |
| Raisins | 2 tbsp |
| Hard candies (e.g., Lifesavers, Brach's, Starbursts, Skittles, jelly beans) | 5-6 pieces |
| Glucose tablets | |
| B-D Glucose Tablets (BD) | 3 tablets (5 g per tablet, orange flavored) |
| DEX 4 (Iverness Medical) | 4 tablets (4 g per tablet, grape, lemon, orange, or raspberry flavored) |
| Glucose gels | |
| Glutose 15 (Paddock) | 1 tube (15 g per tube, natural lemon flavored) |
| Glutose 45 (Paddock) | 1/3 tube (45 g per reusable tube, natural lemon flavored) |
| Insta-Glucose (ICN Pharmaceuticals) | 2/3 tube (24 g per tube, cherry flavored) |

Key: Mfr, manufacturer.

—frequent urination, dehydration, thirst, increased appetite—usually occur at BG levels higher than 180 mg/dL. If ketosis develops, the patient's breath may have a fruity odor. Untreated hyperglycemia requires immediate medical attention as it could progress to diabetic ketoacidosis (mainly in type 1 diabetes) or HHS (in type 2 diabetes), followed by coma and death. SMBG allows patients to detect consistent upswings in BG levels and adjust the insulin therapy accordingly or to contact the medical provider for reevaluation of pharmacologic and nonpharmacologic management of diabetes.

Morning hyperglycemia may result from an asymptomatic nocturnal hypoglycemia (Somogyi effect) in patients who are otherwise well controlled on intensive insulin regimens. In response to hypoglycemia, the body secretes epinephrine, which induces hepatic glucose production and results in morning hyperglycemia. Another reaction that can present with a similar morning hyperglycemia is termed the "dawn phenomenon."[39] As part of the circadian rhythm, hormones such as growth hormone, cortisol, and epinephrine are released during the night. In response, the plasma glucose level rises in the early morning hours and insulin is released from the functioning pancreas. In people with diabetes, the insulin release may not occur, resulting in morning hyperglycemia. Thus, a Somogyi effect is caused by too much insulin whereas the dawn phenomenon is caused by too little insulin. Patients with morning hyperglycemia should monitor their plasma glucose level between 2 and 3 AM to determine if it is low (Somogyi effect) or normal/high (dawn phenomenon). They should record the results along with any changes in their diet and activities and be assisted in interpreting the results and adjusting therapy accordingly.

## Hypoglycemia

Several factors can contribute to hypoglycemia including insufficient caloric intake (e.g., skipping or delaying meals, vomiting), inaccurate insulin dose (e.g., too high, frequent adjustments, inadequate preparation, irregular timing), concomitant use of hypoglycemic drugs, drug interactions, very tight glycemic control, and physical activity. Although a BG concentration of less than 70 mg/dL indicates hypoglycemia, some patients experience symptoms at higher glucose levels.[42] Early warning symptoms may be both autonomic (e.g., trembling, shaking, sweating, palpitations, tachycardia) and neuroglycopenic (e.g., slow thinking, difficulty concentrating, slurred speech, uncoordinated, dizziness). Some patients may be hypoglycemic without experiencing any symptoms, a serious condition called hypoglycemic unawareness.

Mild hypoglycemic symptoms usually are rapidly relieved by glucose. As a preventive measure, people with diabetes should always carry a source of fast-acting carbohydrate (Table 47-16). At the onset of hypoglycemic symptoms, patients should check their plasma glucose. If the result is low, patients should apply the "Rule of 15" and consume 15 g of carbohydrates. If symptoms persist or BG concentrations are still below 70 mg/dL after 15 minutes, an additional 15 g of carbohydrates should be consumed. BG levels of less than 50 mg/dL may require 20 to 30 g of carbohydrates.[43] Foods high in fat (e.g., chocolate, potato chips, pizza) are poor choices for treating hypoglycemia, as fat delays carbohydrate absorption and add unnecessary calories.[23] Protein-rich foods do not increase BG or prevent further hypoglycemic episodes and thus do not need to be added to carbohydrates for treatment of hypoglycemia. Patients who take α-glucosidase inhibitors (acarbose, miglitol) cannot rapidly digest table sugar (sucrose) or sugar from juices (fructose) or sodas. These patients should treat hypoglycemia with glucose (tablets or gel) or milk. Once hypoglycemia is treated, if mealtime is not within 1 hour, a small snack (e.g., crackers, piece of fruit, small sandwich) should be consumed to prevent further hypoglycemia. BG should be monitored frequently to prevent recurrent hypoglycemia.

Severe hypoglycemia may result in unconsciousness, coma, seizures, and inability to swallow and should be treated with glucagon. All patients using insulin should have a glucagon emergency kit. Available by prescription, this kit contains a 1 mg ampule of glucagon, a syringe of diluent, and administration directions. Glucagon is indicated when a patient becomes unconscious because of hypoglycemia. For this reason, family members, other patient caregivers, and coworkers should be taught to mix and administer glucagon by SQ or IM injection. Encourage them to practice the process of glucagon administration ahead of time so they will be prepared if an emergency arises. The usual dose is 1 mg for adults and children over 10 years old, 0.5 to 1 mg for children 5 to 10 years old, and 0.25 to 0.5 mg for children less than 5 year old. Glucagon may cause vomiting, lasting up to 24 hours. Unconscious patients should therefore be turned on their side before glucagon is administered, to prevent choking. Glucagon usually works within 5 to 10 minutes, but the effects are short-lived. If no response is seen after 5 to 10 minutes, a second injection may be given. If this is ineffective, the caregiver should call 911 immediately. Once the patient is conscious and can swallow, the caregiver should give a carbohydrate liquid (e.g., juice, milk, nondiet soft drink) followed by a carbohydrate snack (small sandwich, crackers with peanut butter). For the next 24 hours, regular SMBG is necessary as well as adequate food intake to replenish hepatic glycogen stores. The primary care provider should be informed of the episode.

## Monitoring of Glycemic Control

Results of the Diabetes Control and Complications Trial and United Kingdom Prospective Diabetes Study demonstrated the benefits of attaining close to normal glucose concentrations in patients with types 1 and 2, respectively.[8,10] Regular monitoring of glycemic control is essential to achieving these goals. With knowledge of their glycemic status, patients are able to play a more integral role in managing and controlling their diabetes. Glycemic testing methods can be divided into two main categories; day-to-day glycemic measures (e.g., BG, urine glucose, blood ketones, urine ketones) and chronic glycemic control measures (e.g., glycosylated hemoglobin, glycated serum proteins). Home testing products for urine protein are also available.

Over the last decade SMBG has become the gold standard and most accurate method for day-to-day assessment of glycemic control. SMBG provides patients immediate feedback. Patients can recognize glucose patterns to track whether daily goals are being met, to prevent or detect hypoglycemia and to evaluate glycemic response to foods, physical activity, or medication changes. Health care providers use SMBG data to help patients make changes to their diabetes care plan.

Few patients with diabetes are not candidates for SMBG. The following patients should be strongly encouraged to self-test their BG:[44]

- All patients with type 1 diabetes
- All patients who use insulin
- Patients who use sulfonylureas or nonsulfonylurea insulin secretagogues to monitor for and prevent asymptomatic hypoglycemia
- All patients having difficulty recognizing symptoms of hypoglycemia
- Pregnant patients with type 1, type 2, or gestational diabetes

The ADA also suggests that SMBG "may be desirable in all patients not achieving glycemic goals."[44] Testing frequency and timing depends on patients' individual needs, yet should be sufficient to help patients reach target glycemic goals. More frequent monitoring may be necessary for patients prone to hypoglycemia and during illness, insulin or other diabetes medication dose changes, physical activity, diet changes, or travel.[37] SMBG improves glucose control only with proper use and application.[8] Thus, the patient must be trained in SMBG technique and given specific guidelines for therapy alterations.[44]

Cost of SMBG may be a factor for some patients. In 1997, Congress passed legislation that mandates access to SMBG to all Medicare recipients with diabetes. Since then most insurance companies and managed care organizations, under the provisions of major medical plans, reimburse patients for all or part of the cost of SMBG, including the cost of a glucose monitor.

Several factors play a role in SMBG product selection including costs of necessary supplies not covered by the medical plan and individual patient special considerations (e.g., manual dexterity, visual acuity). Although SMBG offers many benefits, some drawbacks include expense (both out-of pocket and time), possible invasive finger or skin punctures, and motivation and health literacy (e.g., cognition) required to perform SMBG and learn to interpret test results.

*BG Tests* There are two types of BG tests: A test that uses reagent strips and a BG monitor, and one that uses only reagent strips.

BG Tests Using Glucose Monitors A glucose monitor used in conjunction with reagent strips gives the specific BG level. Two types of monitors measure BG. Both are based on (oxidation) enzymatic activity. One type uses a photometric or reflectance measurement that is based on a dye-related reaction. The patient places a drop of blood on a reagent strip either before or after inserting the strip into a monitor, where it is read photometrically or colorimetrically. The other type of monitor measures BG with a biosensor that records an electronic charge produced by a chemical reaction. Reflectance monitors must be regularly cleaned, whereas monitors using biosensor technology do not generally require cleaning.

All monitors are calibrated and will generally analyze the BG level according to programmed data. All monitors provide a digital display of the BG level. Many have audio components or memories for later recall of recent BG levels and can print retained data. Patients who are blind or visually impaired may benefit from monitors with audio features (e.g., Accu-Chek Voicemate).

Many factors are used to determine the best monitor for an individual patient such as monitor size, size of display, blood sample size, alternate site testing capabilities, timing devices, calibration, accuracy, ease of use, effect of temperature on accuracy, memory/data management and print features, battery types, need for cleaning, accessories required, audio capabilities, and price. Several monitors are available, and Table 47-17 lists products and features that may influence patient selection. FDA has set specific allowable variances for the monitors.

Even when BG monitoring equipment is used properly, calibrated frequently, and interpreted correctly, however, accuracy can vary by up to 20%. Most glucose monitors report plasma glucose concentrations, while some report capillary (whole blood) glucose concentrations. Since plasma BG concentrations are typically 10% to 15% higher than whole blood, patients should know which results their monitors yield to determine their glycemic goals.[44]

Many BG monitors (Table 47-17) allow for alternate site blood sampling from the fleshy part of the palm, forearm, upper arm, thigh, and calf. Blood flow to the finger is faster than that to the forearm. Therefore, when glucose concentrations are rapidly fluctuating (e.g., after meals, during hypoglycemia, with increased physical activity level), a fingerstick will reflect the change in BG before the alternate sites.[45] Patients should be educated that alternate site testing is approved only for a fasting state, 2 hours after exercise, or 2 hours after meals.

Since drug therapy changes are made on the basis of results, accuracy is imperative. Tips for improving accuracy can be found in Table 47-18.

Finally, the BG monitoring method recommended to the patient must be flexible and capable of being easily incorporated into the patient's lifestyle or daily routine. Providers can help individual patients select the best monitor for home use.

Proper education in the methods for self-monitoring, the differences between individual monitors, the importance of multiple daily tests, and the interpretation and application of test results will encourage patients to perform SMBG consistently. Return demonstration by the patient is necessary to ensure patient understanding and correct any errors as they are observed. Patients should be encouraged to maintain accurate records of SMBG and return with their logbook, which should also contain records of medication use (e.g., name, dose, time taken), diet changes, activities, and body weight. Despite the memory and downloading capability of most monitors, these features do not replace the importance of a patient-maintained logbook. This patient documentation is invaluable for the patient and clinician to identify BG patterns and assess the outcome of behavior and lifestyle modifications and adjust treatment as necessary. In addition, computerized data-management systems accompanying monitors can be used at home and/or in the clinician's workplace. The programs include software for downloading monitor

**TABLE 47-17 Selected Blood Glucose Monitors***

| Name (Mfr) | Sample Size | Test Strip | Alternate Site | Test Time (seconds) | Touchable Strips | Ability to Reapply Blood to Strip | Provide Reading Only with Adequate Sample | Range (mg/dL) | Coding/Calibration | Battery | Memory (no. of BG tests) |
|---|---|---|---|---|---|---|---|---|---|---|---|
| Accu-Chek Active (Roche Diagnostics) | 1 μL | Active | Yes | 5 | Yes (out-of-monitor dosing) | Yes | No | 10-600 | Snap-in key | (2) CR2023 | 200 |
| Accu-Chek Advantage (Roche Diagnostics) | 4 μL | Comfort Curve† | No | 26 | Yes | Yes (up to 15 s) | No | 10-600 | Snap-in key | (2) 2032 Li 3V | 480 |
| Accu-Chek Compact (Roche-Diagnostics) | 1.5 μL | Compact 17-test drum | Yes | 8 | Yes | No | Yes | 10-600 | Automatic | (2) AAA | 100 |
| Accu-Chek Complete (Roche Diagnostics) | 4 μL | Comfort Curve† | No | 26 | Yes | Yes (up to 15 s) | No | 10-600 | Snap-in key | (2) AAA | 1000 |
| Ascensia Breeze (Bayer) | 2.5-3.5 μL | 10-test cartridge Ascensia Autodisc | Yes | 30 | Yes | No | No | 10-600 | Automatic | (1) Li 3V | 100 |

**TABLE 47-17 Selected Blood Glucose Monitors* (continued)**

| Name (Mfr) | Sample Size | Test Strip | Alternate Site | Test Time (seconds) | Touchable Strips | Ability to Reapply Blood to Strip | Provide Reading Only with Adequate Sample | Range (mg/dL) | Coding/Calibration | Battery | Memory (no. of BG tests) |
|---|---|---|---|---|---|---|---|---|---|---|---|
| Ascensia DEX 2 (Bayer) | 2.5-3.5 μL | 10-test cartridge Ascensia Autodisc | Yes | 30 | Yes | No | No | 10-600 | Automatic | (2) Li 3V | 100 |
| Ascensia Elite (Bayer) | 2 μL | Elite (individually wrapped) | Yes | 30 | Yes | No | No | 20-600 | Strip | (2) Li 3V | 20 |
| Ascensia Elite XL (Bayer) | 2 μL | Elite (individually wrapped) | Yes | 30 | Yes | No | No | 20-600 | Strip | (2) Li 3V | 120 |
| Asecencia Contour (Bayer) | 0.6 μL | Ascensia Microfill | Yes | 15 | Yes | No | Yes | 10-600 | Automatic | (2) Li 3V | 240 |
| BD Logic | 0.3 μL | BD | No | 5 | Yes | No | Yes | 20-600 | Button | (1) 2450 Li 3V | 250 (+250 insulin records) |
| FreeStyle (Abbott Diabetes Care) | 0.3 μL | FreeStyle | Yes | up to 15 | Yes | Yes (up to 60 s) | Yes | 20-500 | Button | (2) 2032 Li 3V | 250 |
| FreeStyle Flash (Abbott Diabetes Care) | 0.3 μL | FreeStyle | Yes | 7 | Yes | Yes (up to 60 s) | Yes | 20-500 | Button | (2) 2032 Li 3V | 250 |
| One Touch Basic (LifeScan) | 5 μL | One Touch Blue | No | 45 | No | No | No | 0-600 | Button | (2) AAA | 75 |
| One Touch SureStep (LifeScan) | 10 μL | SureStep | No | 15-30 | Yes (out-of-monitor dosing) | No | No | 0-500 | Button | (2) AAA | 150 |
| One Touch Ultra [FastTake-mail order only] (LifeScan) | 1 μL | Ultra | Yes | 5 | Yes | No | Yes | 20-600 | Button | (1) 2032 Li 3V | 150 |
| One Touch UltraSmart (Lifescan) | 1 μL | Ultra | Yes | 5 | Yes | No | Yes | 20-600 | Button | (2) AAA | 3000 (& electronic logbook) |
| Precision Xtra (Abbott) [measures ketones too] | 1.5 μL | Precision Xtra (individually wrapped) | Yes | 10 (30 for ketones) | Yes | Yes (up to 30 s) | Yes | 20-500 | Strip | (2) AAA or (1) CR2032 Li | 450 |
| Prestige IQ (Home Diagnostics) | 4 μL | Prestige Smart System | No | 10-50 | No (out-of-monitor dosing) | No | Yes | 25-600 | Strip | (1) AAA | 365 |
| ReliOn Ultima (Wal-Mart) | 2.5 μL | ReliOn Utlima (individually wrapped) | No | 20 | Yes | Yes (up to 30 s) | Yes | 20-500 | Strip | (2) AAA | 450 |
| TrueTrack Smart System (Home Diagnostics) | 1 μL | TrueTrack Smart System | Yes | 10 | Yes | No | Yes | 20-600 | Code chip | (1) CR2032 Li or (1) 3V Li | 365 |

Key: Mfr, manufacturer.

* List is not all-inclusive. Items may have been changed since time of publication. All monitors are plasma referenced except One Touch Basic and Surestep, which are whole blood.

† Takes Advantage strips also (blood glucose reading).

Adapted with permission from Glucose Monitor Comparison Table prepared by Lisa Kroon, PharmD, CDE, and Gloria Yee, RN, CDE, University of California at San Francisco.

**TABLE 47-18 Tips for Improving Accuracy of Fingerstick Technique[46]**

**Using Test Strips**

- Properly store test strips at room temperature in the original vial/container.
- Avoid exposing test strips to changes in temperature, humidity, and light as this may affect accuracy.
- Check expiration date on test strips.
- Code monitor for the batch of test strips. This is necessary for most monitors (e.g., manual coding, code strip).

**Using Glucose Monitor**

- Follow manufacturer's directions for calibrating monitor and using control solutions.
- Use control solutions to verify glucose monitor and test strips are working properly.
- Make sure monitor is clean.

**Obtaining an Adequate Blood Sample**

- Gather all necessary supplies (e.g., monitor, test strips, lancet, lancet device, tissue).
- Vigorously clean hands with warm soapy water to increase blood circulation.
- If alcohol must be used to clean hands, wait 1 minute to ensure alcohol has completely evaporated.
- Dry hands thoroughly.
- Hang hand below heart for 30-60 seconds to increase blood flow to fingers.
- Using the other hand, apply pressure on the finger from the base to the finger pad.

**Lancing the Finger**

- Use a lancet device with an adjustable puncture depth and adjust as needed to ensure adequate blood drop.
- Point fingers to the ground and lance the side of the fingertip.
- Avoid lancing finger pads since more nerves in these areas may cause pain.
- If lancing the index finger or thumb causes pain, avoid these areas as well.

**Applying the Drop of Blood**

- Ensure adequate size of blood drop is applied to test strip.
- If necessary, apply light pressure on the finger from the base to the finger pad to increase size of blood drop.
- Quickly place drop of blood on test strip. Method varies with monitor type. Refer to monitor instructions for proper technique.

information, modules for personal digital assistants (PDA), electronic logbooks, and Web-based programs to help patients track SMBG trends.

BG Tests Using Reagent Strips Reagent strips (e.g., Chemstrip bG, Glucostix, Select GT Strips, Supreme Strips) are used infrequently to test BG. Unlike glucose monitor readings, which provide a specific glucose concentration at the time of the test, reagent strips provide a visual glucose level *range*. The patient places a drop of blood on a strip impregnated with glucose oxidase. After 30 to 60 seconds, the blood is wiped or washed off the strip. The patient then waits another 60 seconds before comparing the color on the strip with the colors on a color chart. To improve accuracy, test strips should be stored at room temperature. Bottle caps should be replaced immediately and tightly after a strip is removed because most strips will react to moisture.

Accuracy can be achieved only when the blood is properly placed and when the correct amount of time has transpired. Few patients with visual impairments are able to match the strips accurately to the corresponding color chart, especially if lighting is poor. Those who perform the color match by using single-source direct lighting (e.g., a table lamp) are more accurate. No known medications cause false readings.

Lancets and Blood Sampling Equipment Most BG testing requires the use of lancets, lancet devices, and tissue. Several lancing devices are available and are often provided with BG monitors. These devices allow for a fingerstick with less associated pain, since most have an autoretractable needle, and the amount of skin penetration can be adjusted in some products. Getting an adequate blood sample is essential for test accuracy. Clinicians should instruct patients on proper techniques for improving accuracy (Table 47-18). Lancets should be disposed in a puncture-resistant disposable container (e.g., sharps containers or hard plastic detergent or fabric softener container, labeled and taped closed when full).

*Urine Glucose Tests* Although SMBG is the gold standard for testing glucose, urine glucose testing kits remain available. Disadvantages of urine glucose tests, compared with BG tests, are as follows: (1) retrospective glucose data provided; (2) inability to detect hypoglycemia; (3) many possible drug interferences; (4) patient variance with reference to renal threshold for glucose; (5) lack of correlation between urine and BG levels; (6) for some patients, difficulty in reading and performing tests; (7) more privacy required than in blood testing; and (8) inability to measure hyperglycemia. As a result of these limitations, urine glucose should not be used to assess glycemic control.

*Urine Ketone Tests* The development of home blood ketone monitoring is revolutionizing the process of detecting or predicting ketoacidosis. When the body does not have sufficient insulin, BG levels rise and the body's cells become energy deprived. During these times of low carbohydrate availability, the liver breaks down fat to produce ketone bodies (acetoacetate [AcAc], 3-β-hydroxybutyrate [3HB], and acetone [Ac]). A sufficient blood level of ketones can result in a diabetic ketoacidosis, a potentially fatal condition. Because ketones in the blood overflow into the urine, urinary ketone levels can be tested to detect whether metabolic changes leading to ketoacidosis are occurring. The basis for the urinary ketone testing is that sodium nitroprusside alkali turns lavender in the presence of acetone or acetoacetic acid. These tests require comparing the color change to a reference chart.

Acetest reagent tablets are specific for acetoacetic acid and acetone only. They will detect 10 mg of AcAc or Ac (but not 3HB) in 100 mL of serum, plasma, or whole blood. The Improved Ketostix Test only detects AcAc, and thus shows a false-negative result if the predominant ketone body is Ac or 3HB. Ketostix, Chemstrip K, and other tests will detect 5 to 10 mg of AcAc or Ac in 100 mL of urine. These tests are easier to perform than Acetest and require no dropper. However, if the predominant ketone body produced is 3HB, a false-negative result will be obtained. High 3HB production is not uncommon in diabetic ketoacidosis. Once treatment is initiated with fluids, electrolytes, and insulin, the 3HB will be metabolized to AcAc and Ac, then eventually to $CO_2$ and $H_2O$. In these instances, it may appear that the patient's ketosis is worsening when in actuality, proper therapy is energizing the body's metabolic mechanisms to eliminate the ketoacids.

Certain BG monitors, such as Precision Xtra, are capable of using test strips designed to detect 3HB levels in the blood. Unlike urine ketone tests, blood ketone tests provide a real-time picture. Another advantage of blood ketone testing over urine ketone and tablet testing is the lack of false positives in the presence of vitamin C or during exposure to ambient air.

Patients with type 1 diabetes should test for ketones when the plasma glucose is 240 mg/dL or greater. All patients with diabetes should check for ketones during times of stress or illness, during pregnancy, when the glucose level is over 300 mg/dL, or whenever ketoacidosis is suspected. In addition, patients should be counseled on the proper methods of testing for ketones in the urine and blood. Pregnant diabetes patients (type 1, type 2, gestational) are commonly instructed to test for ketones each morning and sometimes more often, to assess their metabolic status. The presence of ketones on two or more consecutive urine tests should be reported to the primary care provider.

*Urinary Microalbumin and Protein Tests* Detection of microalbuminuria (trace protein in the urine) is an early sign of kidney damage. The ADA recommends annual screening, although more frequent screening may be necessary in high-risk patients. Several home tests are available (e.g., AccuBase μAlb, Appraise Microalbumin Diabetes Monitoring System, KidneyScreen At Home), but urine specimens must be mailed to a laboratory for analysis and reporting. Large protein particles in the urine can be determined by using an array of products (e.g., Albustix, Chemstrip).

### Self-Monitoring of Glycosylated Hemoglobin and Glycated Protein

Compared with SMBG, glycosylated hemoglobin and glycated protein testing provide useful information about a patient's glycemic control over a longer time period. Traditionally, these tests were performed in a laboratory setting from venipuncture samples. New technology allows for home or clinic testing with smaller blood samples.

Plasma glucose binds to red blood cells. Glycosylated hemoglobin, referred to as A1C, is formed at a rate directly proportional to the BG concentration over the previous 120 days (lifespan of the average erythrocyte).[44] Since A1C levels correlate with mean plasma glucose values over the preceding 2 to 3 months, it may be used to asses overall glycemic control in patients with diabetes.

In general, the ADA recommends testing the A1C twice yearly in patients who are stable and meeting glycemic goals and every 3 months for patients not at goal or whose therapy has changed.[44] The exact testing frequency should be on the basis of clinical judgment. Normal nondiabetic A1C range is 4% to 6%. The goal for most people with diabetes is less than 7%. Several A1C kits are available for use at home (e.g., AccuBase A1c Glycohemoglobin Test Kit, A1c At Home, Appraise A1c Diabetes Monitoring System, BIOSAFE Hemoglobin A1c Test Kit).[38] Once a drop of blood is placed on a test strip, the patient mails the sample to a lab for analysis. Results are usually mailed or faxed back to the patient. A new monitor, Choice$_{DM}$ A1C Home Test (A1c Now), is a single-use device for home or office use that tests from a fingerstick sample and provides results in approximately 8 minutes. Patients should discuss the use and results of these home monitoring kits with their health care providers.

Glycated protein or fructosamine tests measure glycemic control over 2 to 3 weeks (the lifespan of serum albumin). Monitoring should not replace daily SMBG, but the once-weekly testing may be useful for evaluating recent changes in diabetes treatment. Normal fructosamine range is less than 285 μmol/L. Currently, all fructosamine testing must be completed in a laboratory. In 2002 the only device available for home use was removed from the market because of concerns about falsely high readings.

### Identification Tags

All persons with diabetes should wear a visible identification bracelet, necklace, or tag indicating the person has diabetes and takes medication. Patients can find information for MedicAlert, a reputable nationwide service available since 1956, at www.medicalert.org or 1-800-432-5378. Patients should also carry an identification card (e.g., in a wallet) including their name, address, and telephone number; the amount and type of medication used; and the name and telephone number of the patient's primary care provider. This information may be lifesaving if hypoglycemia or ketoacidosis occurs, requiring emergency services or hospitalization. Because a hypoglycemic reaction may be confused with drunkenness, hypoglycemic patients have been known to be jailed rather than given medical care.

### Travel Supplies and Preparations

Patients with diabetes planning travel should pack enough diabetes supplies for the entire trip, plus at least 1 extra week's worth. Advise patients to carry their supplies with them, not in checked luggage. The following is a travel checklist:

- Extra vials of U-100 insulin (only U-40 is available in some countries) or insulin pen(s)
- Extra supply of syringes and needles because access may be limited; patients should refrain from prefilling syringes for a trip because of potential for leakage
- Extra supply of all oral medications in their original prescription bottles
- Extra SMBG supplies (e.g., glucose monitor, test strips, control solutions, lancets and devices, batteries if needed)
- Written prescriptions for medications including insulin, in case of an emergency
- A written note from patient's primary care provider indicating the need for diabetes supplies (especially syringes and needles)
- A summary of the patient's current medical regimen and emergency contact phone numbers
- Identification cards and an identification bracelet, necklace or tag, indicating the person has diabetes
- Snacks and glucose tablets (and glucagon kit for insulin users) to be prepared for schedule changes or prevent hypoglycemia (refer to Table 47-16)
- If traveling abroad, the names of English-speaking primary care providers in each city and some cards with several key phrases (e.g., "I have diabetes"; "Please get me a doctor") to access care in the language of the country being visited

Travelers should monitor their caloric intake carefully and allow time for physical activity. If notified in advance, most airlines offer special-order meals for people with diabetes. Advise the patient to wear comfortable well-fitting shoes if the patient intends to walk more than usual during the trip.

Insulin users should know that time zone changes of 2 or more hours usually require insulin dose adjustments. Rapid-acting insulins offer the most flexibility to account for unpredictable mealtimes and should be adjusted as needed. When traveling across time zones, patients should adjust basal insulin on the day of travel to provide the same amount of insulin/hour that they normally take.[47] For westbound travel, basal insulin is increased proportionately for the number of hours gained. (i.e., if basal insulin rate is 0.5 units/hour and gained 3 hours, add an extra 1.5 units of long-acting insulin to basal insulin dose). For eastbound travel, basal insulin is decreased proportionately for the number of hours lost. After arriving at the final destination, advise patients to change their watch to the new time zone and continue with their normal insulin regimen. More frequent SMBG may be necessary.

### *Complementary Therapies*

More than one in three Americans has sought treatment for medical conditions from alternative sources, commonly in the form of natural products or dietary supplements.[48] Consumers spend more than $19.4 billion annually for these remedies.[49] People with diabetes are 1.6 times more likely to use some form of complimentary and alternative medicine, including herbal products or dietary supplements, than those without diabetes.[50] Several herbs and dietary products have been studied for their efficacy in treating diabetes. Table 47-19 lists several common herbs and dietary supplements and their potential interactions with diabetes therapy and management. To date, no herbal product or dietary supplement has been proven to be a safe and effective alternative to MNT and pharmacologic therapy of diabetes. To date the size and/or methodology of studies with various herbs and supplements often limit their clinical implications for efficacy and safety.

Reports of interactions between herbal and dietary supplements and FDA-approved products are often anecdotal and are based on theoretical pharmacologic effects from in vitro and animal studies and/or limited case reports. The clinical significance of potential effects and interactions therefore remains unknown. Practitioners should encourage patients to openly discuss herbal and dietary supplement use with them by asking and listening in a nonjudgmental manner. Information available to date regarding efficacy and safety should be shared with patients to help them make an informed decision regarding use of these products. Patients should also be reminded of the challenges to product selection in an environment of nonregulation. Patients choosing to continue to use herbal and dietary supplement should have their BG monitored regularly.

## Assessment of Diabetes Mellitus: A Case-based Approach

If a patient describes classic symptoms of diabetes, the practitioner should ask whether a primary care provider has made this diagnosis. If not, screening for diabetes is appropriate. ADA recommends that a laboratory-based glucose test should be considered in all individuals 45 years of age or older. If normal, patients should be tested every 3 years.[1] Patients with risk factors for diabetes should be considered for testing more frequently and at an earlier age. (Refer to Pathophysiology of Diabetes Mellitus.) Screening can start with the diabetes survey developed by ADA (Table 47-20). Adding the point values of the questions gives a person's relative risk for developing diabetes. Individuals with a high risk for the disease can then be tested by capillary BG (fingerstick). Test results should be compared with the diagnostic criteria in Table 47-3. High-risk patients, identified during screening, should be referred to a primary care provider for follow-up.

When working with a newly diagnosed patient, the practitioner should determine all medications and supplements the patient takes, any known drug allergies, any concurrent diseases or infections and relevant social history (e.g., tobacco use, alcohol use, payer status). Practitioners should sensitively assess the patient's beliefs, attitudes, and knowledge toward the disease and the impact of diabetes care on the patient's lifestyle. These assessments allow for development of a culturally sensitive diabetes education and care plan centered on the patient's expectations and needs. Practitioners should be prepared to negotiate treatment and adherence strategies, provide information and answer the patient's questions concerning diabetes and related conditions. Case 47-1 illustrates assessment of patients with type 1 diabetes mellitus.

**TABLE 47-19 Selected Complementary/Alternative Medicines That May Affect Blood Glucose Control*[51-53]**

| Agent | Possible Effect(s) on Blood Glucose |
|---|---|
| **Botanical Medicines (Scientific Name)** | |
| Aloe (*Aloe vera*) | May have hypoglycemic effects |
| Barley (*Hordeum vulgare; H. distychum*) | May slow gastric emptying |
| Bitter melon (*Momordica charantia*) | May have hypoglycemic effects |
| Cinnamon (*Cinnamomum aromaticum*) | Has hypoglycemic effects |
| Ephedra (*Ephedra sinica*) | May have hyperglycemic effects; FDA has banned ephedra sales (see Chapter 27) |
| Fig leaf (*Ficus carica*) | May have hypoglycemic effects |
| Fenugreek (*Trigonella foenugraecum*) | May have hypoglycemic effects |
| Garlic (*Allium sativum*) | May have hypoglycemic effects |
| Ginseng (American/Panax/Siberian) (*Panax quinquefolius/P. ginseng/Eleutherococcus senticosus*) | May have hypoglycemic effects |
| Gotu kola (*Centella asiatica*) | May have hyperglycemic effects |
| Guar gum (*Cyamopsis tetragonoloba*) | May inhibit gastric glucose absorption to lower blood glucose |
| Guarana (*Paullinia cupana*) | May have hyperglycemic effects |
| Gymnema (*Gymnema sylvestre*) | May stimulate insulin production and enhance insulin sensitivity |
| Holy basil (*Ocimum sanctum*) | May have hypoglycemic effects |
| Ivy gourd (*Coccinia indica*) | May have hypoglycemic effects |
| Milk thistle (*Silibum marianum*) | May reduce insulin resistance secondary to hepatic damage |
| Nopal, or prickly pear cactus (*Pountia streptacantha*) | May have hypoglycemic effects |
| Oat bran (*Avena sativa*) | Reduces postprandial blood glucose and insulin levels |
| Stevia (*Stevia rebaudiana*) | May lower postprandial blood glucose |
| **Nonbotanical Dietary Supplements** | |
| α-Lipoic acid | May have hypoglycemic effects |
| Chromium | Deficiency associated with impaired glucose tolerance |
| L-carnitine | May enhance insulin sensitivity |
| Vanadium | May enhance insulin sensitivity |

* Note: This table does not include all case reports or possible interactions.

For overweight patients diagnosed with type 2 diabetes, practitioners should also discuss weight loss issues (see Chapter 27). Education should focus on the link between obesity and type 2 diabetes and the importance of weight loss in controlling and possibly reversing the disease. The health benefits of weight reduction should also be discussed. Learning that weight loss and consistent physical activity may obviate the need for medications may motivate the patient to lose weight. Patients with both types 1 and 2 diabetes should be evaluated by a primary care provider before engaging in a physical activity program. Case 47-2 illustrates assessment of patients with type 2 diabetes mellitus.

## Patient Counseling for Diabetes Mellitus

Healthy eating and a realistic regular physical activity program are the biggest challenges for individuals with diabetes. All clinicians must continually help patients overcome barriers and provide encouragement and counseling on meal planning and physical activity. Each patient encounter is an opportunity for the practitioner to evaluate and educate patients. Asking simple questions such as "What are your glucose levels running these days?" or "What was your last A1C level?" are good ways to initiate conversation and help identify patient knowledge and commitment to self-care. If insulin has been prescribed, the practitioner should explain the various diabetes care products and teach the patient how to use the selected products. Patients should be encouraged to return for reevaluation of injection technique, use of glucose monitors and adherence to a prescribed self-care routine. Moreover, practitioners should be familiar with new medications and devices and should keep abreast of current practice guidelines for the care of people with diabetes. The box Patient Education for Diabetes Mellitus lists specific information to provide patients.

**TABLE 47-20 Diabetes Screening Questionnaire**

| Could You Be at Risk for Diabetes? | Point Values |
|---|---|
| 1. I am a woman who has had a baby weighing more than nine pounds at birth. | Yes 1 |
| 2. I have a sister or brother with diabetes. | Yes 1 |
| 3. I have a parent with diabetes. | Yes 1 |
| 4. My weight is equal to or above that listed in the chart below.* | Yes 5 |
| 5. I am under 65 years of age AND I get little or no exercise. | Yes 5 |
| 6. I am between 45 and 64 years of age. | Yes 5 |
| 7. I am 65 years old or older. | Yes 9 |
| Total† | ____ |

**At-risk Weight Chart Body Mass Index**

| Height (in feet and inches, without shoes) | Weight (in pounds, without clothing)‡ |
|---|---|
| 4' 10" | 129 |
| 4' 11" | 133 |
| 5' 0" | 138 |
| 5' 1" | 143 |
| 5' 2" | 147 |
| 5' 3" | 152 |
| 5' 4" | 157 |
| 5' 5" | 162 |
| 5' 6" | 167 |
| 5' 7" | 172 |
| 5' 8" | 177 |
| 5' 9" | 182 |
| 5' 10" | 188 |
| 5' 11" | 193 |
| 6' 0" | 199 |
| 6' 1" | 204 |
| 6' 2" | 210 |
| 6' 3" | 216 |
| 6' 4" | 221 |

* Chart does not discriminate between men and women.

† If you scored 3-9 points: You are probably at low risk for having diabetes now, but don't just forget about it. Keep your risk low by losing weight if you are overweight, being active most days and eating low fat meals that are high in fruits and vegetables and whole grain foods. If you scored ≥10 points: You are at high risk for having diabetes. Only your health care provider can determine if you have diabetes. At your next office visit, find out for sure.

‡ If you weigh the same as or more than the amount listed for your height, you may be at risk for diabetes.

*Source:* Diabetes Risk Test. Copyright © 2005 American Diabetes Association. From: http://www.diabetes.org/risk-test/text-version.jsp. Reprinted with permission from The American Diabetes Association.

## Evaluation of Patient Outcomes for Diabetes Mellitus

The ADA recommends specific therapeutic goals for people with diabetes (Table 47-3). If the patient is not achieving such outcomes, adherence to the care plan should be assessed. Nonadherent patients should be reevaluated and, if necessary, reeducated about the need for and benefits of the care plan. If nonadherence is not the problem, medical referral is appropriate. In addition, weight management should be closely monitored in patients with type 2 diabetes.

## CASE 47-1

| Relevant Evaluation Criteria | Scenario/Model Outcome |
|---|---|
| **Information Gathering** | |
| 1. Gather essential information about the patient's symptoms, including: | |
| a. description of symptom(s) (i.e., nature, onset, duration, severity, associated symptoms) | Patient asks about using an insulin pump. States that trying to incorporate insulin dosing into school, softball, and social schedule is very difficult.<br>She also wants to purchase Monistat. Her primary care provider has prescribed it twice for vaginal yeast infections over the last year (most recently 4 months ago). She recently started to have mild symptoms of itching and burning again. Denies presence of fever or back pain. |
| b. description of any factors that seem to precipitate, exacerbate, and/or relieve the patient's symptom(s) | Her BG levels before lunch have been elevated. A review of memory readings on her monitor shows a range of 140-160 mg/dL at 12 noon. Patient thinks she should drop her midmorning snack since she stopped working out regularly in the mornings. Other readings are generally normal. |
| c. description of the patient's efforts to relieve the symptoms | She started noticed yeast infection symptoms yesterday and decided to stop at the pharmacy today. She is busy with midterms and does not want to set up an appointment with her PCP. |
| 2. Gather essential patient history information: | |
| a. patient's identity | Ashley Stratton |
| b. patient's age, sex, height, and weight | 19 y/o F, 5'4", 120 lb, BMI 20.6 |
| c. patient's occupation | College student, plays on softball team; has a game or practice during the season every day except Sunday |
| d. patient's dietary habits | Eats a 2400-calorie ADA diet consisting of 3 meals and 3 snacks per day. |
| e. patient's sleep habits | Sleeps well; no nightmares, night sweats, or other symptoms of Somogyi effect |
| f. concurrent medical conditions, prescription and nonprescription medications, and dietary supplements | For her prandial insulin needs, she takes 6 units of insulin lispro at breakfast and lunch and 8 units at dinner. For her basal insulin, she takes 30 units of insulin glargine daily at bedtime. |
| g. allergies | NKA |
| h. history of other adverse reactions to medications | No previous reactions |
| i. other (describe)_______ | N/A |
| **Assessment and Triage** | |
| 3. Differentiate the patient's signs/symptoms and correctly identify the patient's primary problem(s) (see Table 47-3). | Repeat *Candida* vulvovaginitis. History of two previous infections in the past year treated successfully with Monistat.<br>High BG concentrations at the noon reading.<br>Concern about ability to administer insulin injections with busy, unpredictable schedule. Patient is interested in learning more about insulin pumps. |
| 4. Identify exclusions for self-treatment | None |
| 5. Formulate a comprehensive list of therapeutic alternatives for the primary problem to determine if triage to a medical practitioner is required, and share this information with the patient. | Options include:<br>(1) Recommend nonpharmacologic and/or nonprescription therapy for the *Candida* vaginal infection.<br>(2) Recommend discontinuing morning snack and monitoring BG levels between 10 AM and noon.<br>(3) Suggest steps to establish whether the breakfast lispro dose is sufficient for amount of carbohydrates being consumed at breakfast.<br>(4) Refer Ashley to her PCP to be evaluated for an insulin pump.<br>(5) Take no action. |

## CASE 47-1 (continued)

| Relevant Evaluation Criteria | Scenario/Model Outcome |
|---|---|
| **Plan** | |
| 6. Select an optimal therapeutic alternative to address the patient's problem, taking into account patient preferences. | Advise the patient to eat low-fat, sugar-free yogurt daily and use the same Monistat product that worked previously. Remind the patient of the carbohydrate content of yogurt and the need to adjust her daily carbohydrate intake appropriately.<br>Advise her to discontinue midmorning snack and subsequently monitor her BG between 10 AM and 12 PM every day for 7 days.<br>Identify insulin pump materials in pharmacy's library of manufacturers' materials and refer her to her PCP for evaluation. |
| 7. Describe the recommended therapeutic approach to the patient. | You should eat 8 oz of low-fat, sugar-free yogurt daily and use the same Monistat product you used before (see Chapter 8). I would suggest substituting the yogurt for another carbohydrate source during a regularly scheduled meal or snack.<br>Stop your midmorning snack and monitor your BG, that is, blood glucose, at 10 AM and 12 noon for 7 days. If your blood glucose level normalizes, continue without the snack. If your BG level stays elevated or drops too low, see your PCP, that is, primary care provider. Make sure you carry glucose tablets with you in case hypoglycemia occurs.<br>Please take copies of insulin pump brochures and the videotape. Your PCP can evaluate you for an insulin pump. |
| 8. Explain to the patient the rationale for selecting the recommended therapeutic approach from the considered therapeutic alternatives. | You should use the same Monistat product since it worked before and you are familiar with its use.<br>The midmorning snack is the likely cause of your hyperglycemia, but you must monitor your BG levels closely to make sure hyper- or hypoglycemia does not occur. |
| **Patient Education** | |
| 9. When recommending self-care with nonprescription medications and/or nondrug therapy, convey accurate information to the patient, including: | |
| a. appropriate dose and frequency of administration | One 8-oz serving of low-fat, sugar-free yogurt daily in place of another carbohydrate serving.<br>See Chapter 8 for information on Monistat.<br>Monitor BG between 10 AM and 12 noon daily for 7 days. |
| b. maximum number of days the therapy should be employed | See Chapter 8. |
| c. product administration procedures | See Chapter 8. |
| d. expected time to onset of relief | The itching and burning symptoms should improve within 2 days of starting treatment with Monistat.<br>The BG values should normalize by the following day. |
| e. degree of relief that can be reasonably expected | All symptoms of the yeast infection should resolve.<br>BG concentrations should fall in the target goal range. |
| f. most common side effects | See Chapter 8 for side effects of Monistat.<br>Since the insulin dosing is not being changed and a snack is being dropped, it is important to monitor for signs and symptoms of low blood glucose or hypoglycemia. If signs or symptoms occur, remember to check your BG and use glucose tablets as directed. Be sure to follow up with a snack. |
| g. side effects that warrant medical intervention should they occur | See Chapter 8.<br>If hyperglycemia does not abate or if hypoglycemia occurs, contact your PCP. |
| h. patient options in the event that condition worsens or persists | See Chapter 8. |
| i. product storage requirements | See Chapter 8. |
| j. specific nondrug measures | See Chapter 8. |

## CASE 47-1 (continued)

| Relevant Evaluation Criteria | Scenario/Model Outcome |
|---|---|
| 10. Solicit patient's follow-up questions. | I usually drink some juice or a soda when I feel low, but the tablets seem more convenient. I would like to buy some. How should I use them? |
| 11. Answer patient's questions. | The usual dose is to dissolve 3 tablets (15 g) in the mouth. Wait 15 minutes. If hypoglycemic symptoms are still present, take an additional 3 tablets. If these measures do not correct the hypoglycemia, seek medical attention. If the hypoglycemia is corrected, eat a small meal or snack (e.g., fruit and cheese, peanut butter and crackers) to prevent a recurrence of the attack. |

Key: BG, blood glucose; NKA, no known allergies; PCP, primary care provider.

## CASE 47-2

| Relevant Evaluation Criteria | Scenario/Model Outcome |
|---|---|
| **Information Gathering** | |
| 1. Gather essential information about the patient's symptoms, including: | |
| a. description of symptom(s) (i.e., nature, onset, duration, severity, associated symptoms) | Patient came to the pharmacy with a new prescription for Actos and to pick up strips for his BG monitor. BG concentrations at PCP's office were above 300 mg/dL. Today's A1C was 10%.<br>The PCP told him that he has to "start taking better care of himself," monitor his blood glucose more regularly, and take his medications as prescribed. The patient also has an appointment with a Certified Diabetes Educator registered dietitian for meal planning and weight loss. He asks if the new pill will help control his diabetes so he does not have to bother with changing his diet or regularly checking his BG, since money is tight for groceries and strips. |
| b. description of any factors that seem to precipitate, exacerbate, and/or relieve the patient's symptom(s) | N/A |
| c. description of the patient's efforts to relieve the symptoms | Patient checks his fasting BG in the mornings every few days. He has been fairly adherent with his prescription medications. His wife also makes him "special drinks" containing nopales and aloe vera. |
| 2. Gather essential patient history information: | |
| a. patient's identity | Francisco Perez |
| b. patient's age, sex, height, and weight | 52 y/o M, 5'5", 170 lb, BMI: 28.3 |
| c. patient's occupation | Farm laborer who works seasonally; married with 4 children, 2 of whom still live at home |
| d. patient's dietary habits | Primarily tortillas, potatoes, and beans when he is out of work. Other times has more access to chicken and fresh fruits and vegetables. Currently is unfamiliar with ADA dietary guidelines. |
| e. patient's sleep habits | Sleeps "like a baby" |
| f. concurrent medical conditions, prescription and nonprescription medications, and dietary supplements | Glipizide XL 10 mg before breakfast and metformin 500 mg mornings and evenings for type 2 diabetes; enalapril 20 mg daily for hypertension for past 2 years and diabetic nephropathy for past year, Lipitor 20 mg daily for dyslipidemia for past 2 years; his wife also makes him "special drinks" containing nopales and aloe vera |
| g. allergies | Penicillin (rash) |
| h. history of other adverse reactions to medications | None |

## CASE 47-2 (continued)

| Relevant Evaluation Criteria | Scenario/Model Outcome |
|---|---|
| i. other (describe)_______ | Type 2 diabetes diagnosed in Mexico 11 years ago. Resting BP taken at pharmacy is 140/90 mm Hg. Francisco says his cholesterol has been elevated.<br>Francisco is concerned about his health, as he is the primary income earner for his family. He does not have insurance coverage for diabetes supplies and medications. He currently obtains all of his prescription medications through various patient assistance programs available through your pharmacy. He "tries to remember to" take his medications as prescribed, and his wife helps him by reminding him at breakfast and dinner. His daughter translates the instructions on his prescription bottles from English into Spanish for him and his wife, which they are both able to read. He currently does not formally exercise daily. He ran out of monitor strips 2 days ago but was unable to make it to the pharmacy to pick up more. |
| **Assessment and Triage** | |
| 3. Differentiate the patient's signs/symptoms and correctly identify the patient's primary problem(s) (see Table 47-3). | Francisco's immediate self-care need is to obtain BG monitoring strips for his monitor.<br>Francisco also needs a great deal of education and support on the basics of diabetes, hypertension, and hyperlipidemia and self-care including SMBG, diet, exercise, and medication adherence. Based on his known medical diagnoses and comments, it would appear he has metabolic syndrome. |
| 4. Identify exclusions for self-treatment. | None |
| 5. Formulate a comprehensive list of therapeutic alternatives for the primary problem to determine if triage to a medical practitioner is required, and share this information with the patient. | Options include:<br>(1) Remind Francisco of the need for regular SMBG. Assess his beliefs and expectations regarding and commitment to monitoring. Negotiate a monitoring schedule that addresses his economic concerns and limitations, such as checking FBG and 2-hour PPG after dinner every other day to help him save money on strips.<br>(2) Work with him to identify resources for groceries and meals available within his community (e.g., charitable organizations) to access during periods when he is out of work. Suggest he bring his wife, who prepares all the meals, with him to his upcoming appointment with the dietitian.<br>(3) Discuss the safety and efficacy of nopales and aloe vera with him to ensure he is educated regarding their safety and effectiveness in diabetes.<br>(4) Counsel him on his new prescription for Actos and explain how this agent fits in with his glipizide and metformin. Explain the delay in time to onset of noticeable effects (e.g., lowered A1C). Review the dose and directions for Actos and discuss and negotiate adherence strategies (e.g., take at breakfast with his other morning medication doses). Educate him about monitoring for side effects of Actos. Explain the need to follow up with his physician and laboratory testing to monitor for efficacy and potential side effects related to his medications.<br>(5) Explore his attitudes and expectations for drug therapy and then discuss and negotiate strategies to help him adhere to therapy, such as Spanish labeling on prescription bottles and the use of a mediset to track daily medication doses.<br>(6) Ask him whether or not his PCP has recommended aspirin therapy for him. Screen him for aspirin allergy or contraindications. Discuss the risks and benefits of aspirin therapy as primary cardioprotection and recommend that he follow up with his PCP.<br>(7) Ask him whether his immunizations (e.g., influenza, *Pneumococcus*, tetanus) are up-to-date, and make recommendations for immunizations as appropriate.<br>(8) Ask him whether he uses tobacco and/or alcohol-related products and counsel him as appropriate.<br>(9) Take no action. |

**CASE 47-2 (continued)**

| Relevant Evaluation Criteria | Scenario/Model Outcome |
|---|---|
| **Plan** | |
| 6. Select an optimal therapeutic alternative to address the patient's problem, taking into account patient preferences. | Provide Francisco with strips and a list of community resources for groceries and meals. Counsel Francisco on his new and existing prescription medications. Discuss dosing, adherence strategies, and monitoring for side effects.<br>(After reviewing dietary supplements, practitioner concluded the patient may continue to drink nopales shakes but should eliminate aloe vera, which can cause diarrhea.)<br>Discuss the need for aspirin therapy with the patient. |
| 7. Describe the recommended therapeutic approach to the patient. | I recommend monitoring your BG, that is, blood glucose, in the morning before breakfast every other day and in the evening 2 hours after dinner every other day. This will help you save some money on strips and also provide your PCP, that is, primary care provider, with the information he or she needs to evaluate your diabetes and medications. Record the date, time, and value from your monitor into a logbook to share with your PCP at your regular visits.<br>Take your new medication, Actos, once daily in the morning with your other morning medications. Report any unusual symptoms, such as swelling of your feet or legs, difficulty breathing, or unusual tiredness to your doctor or pharmacist if they occur.<br>Take your wife with you to your appointment with the registered dietitian to discuss healthy meal planning tailored to your food preferences and budget. Follow up with resources in your community for groceries and meals as needed during the year to help you maintain a healthy, well-balanced diet.<br>(Patient says his wife is interested in knowing what foods he should and should not eat.) |
| 8. Explain to the patient the rationale for selecting the recommended therapeutic approach from the considered therapeutic alternatives. | The BG monitor will show you the effects of different foods, exercise, and medications on your BG. Your providers and you can use this information to plan your meals and activities and adjust your medications as needed. |
| **Patient Education** | |
| 9. When recommending self-care with nonprescription medications and/or nondrug therapy, convey accurate information to the patient. | Discuss the benefits and risk of aspirin therapy with the patient, counsel them on appropriate generic options available and dosing, and recommend that he follows up and discusses his need for aspirin therapy with his PCP at his next visit. |
| 10. Solicit patient's follow-up questions. | Can you help me interpret my blood glucose readings? |
| 11. Answer patient's questions. | Yes. If you carry the monitor with you, monitor your blood glucose levels as we discussed and record your meals and exercise. We can set an appointment to review and interpret the readings. |

Key: ADA, American Diabetes Association; BG, blood glucose; BP, blood pressure; BMI, body mass index; FBG, fasting blood glucose; N/A, not applicable; PCP, primary care provider; PPG, postprandial glucose; SMBG, self-monitoring of blood glucose.

## Key Points for Diabetes Mellitus

- Early detection, extensive patient education, and intensive glycemic control through medical nutrition therapy (MNT), physical activity, and pharmacologic therapy can prevent the development and progression of long-term complications, morbidity, and mortality associated with diabetes.
- Familiarity with the most current standards for diabetes screening and management imperative to reducing and eliminating health disparities associated with diabetes risk, outcomes, morbidity, and mortality and improving care for all patients with diabetes (Table 47-21).
- Patients must be educated about diabetes, the role of BG control in the prevention of long-term complications, self-care strategies (including SMBG and MNT), and pharmacologic therapy.
- Practitioners should be familiar with and help patients select BG monitoring devices and related supplies.

**TABLE 47-21 Online Resources Regarding Diabetes Care and Management for Practitioners**

| Organization | Web Address | Comments |
|---|---|---|
| American Diabetes Association (ADA) | www.diabetes.org | Information for both practitioners and patients regarding diabetes and its management; free access to a variety of information and tools including ADA guidelines to diabetes care and management (published annually in a supplement to *Diabetes Care*), recent research news and patient education materials (e.g., *Diabetes Forecast*); restricted access to a variety of resources including scientific journals for members |
| American Association of Clinical Endocrinologists (AACE) | www.aace.com | Free access to guidelines and practice standards; CME and other resources available for members |
| American Association of Diabetes Educators (AADE) | www.diabeteseducator.org | Information for both practitioners and patients |
| National Institute of Diabetes and Digestive and Kidney Disorders (NIDDK) | www.niddk.nih.gov | Statistics, health information, and research opportunities for practitioners |
| Centers for Disease Control (CDC) Diabetes Public Resource | www.cdc.gov/diabetes | Statistics, recommendations for the Task Force on Community Preventative Services for diabetes, and other resources for practitioners and patients |
| National Diabetes Education Program (NDEP) | www.ndep.nih.gov | Collaboration of the NIH and CDC providing information for practitioners and patients; patient education materials available that are designed for specific ethnic populations and in a variety of languages |
| American Pharmacists Association (APhA) Foundation | www.aphafoundation.org/MetabolicSyndrome/Metabolicresource.htm | National Clinical Issues Forum: Metabolic Syndrome Web pages providing information and links to care and treatment guidelines for diabetes and related comorbid conditions |
| Insulin Pumpers | www.insulin-pumpers.org | Support and information for children and adults with diabetes and insulin pump delivery devices |

- Patients using insulin therapy must be educated about insulin and related supplies, proper injection site and technique, insulin storage, potential adverse events, and their management.
- Practitioners and patients should negotiate adherence strategies tailored to patient-specific factors such as, but not limited to, food and activity preferences, sleep/mealtime/work schedules, insurance status, and income.
- Patients with diabetes should be educated regarding the safety and efficacy of nonprescription medications for self-care of limited acute conditions and complimentary and alternative medicines.

## References


1. American Diabetes Association. Diagnosis and classification of diabetes mellitus. *Diabetes Care.* 2005;28(suppl 1):S37-S42.
2. Centers for Disease Control and Prevention. National diabetes facts sheet: general information and national estimates on diabetes in the United States, 2002. Atlanta, Ga: US Department of Health and Human Services, Centers for Disease Control and Prevention; 2003.
3. American Diabetes Association. Economic costs of diabetes in the United States in 2002. *Diabetes Care.* 2003;26:917-32.
4. McNeely MJ, Boyko EJ. Type 2 diabetes prevalence in Asian Americans. *Diabetes Care.* 2004;27:66-9.
5. American Diabetes Association. Report of the expert committee on the diagnosis and classification of diabetes mellitus. *Diabetes Care.* 2003;26(suppl 1):S5-S20.
6. Nathan DM. Initial management of glycemia in type 2 diabetes mellitus. *N Engl J Med.* 2002;347:1342-9.
7. Reaven GM. Pathophysiology of insulin resistance in human disease. *Physiol Rev.* 1995;75:473-89.
8. The Diabetes Control and Complications Trial Research Group. The effect of intensive treatment of diabetes on the development and progression of long-term complications in insulin-dependent diabetes mellitus. *N Engl J Med.* 1993;329:977-86.
9. The Writing Team for the Diabetes Control and Complications Trial/Epidemiology of Diabetes Interventions and Complications Research Group. Sustained effect of intensive treatment of type 1 diabetes mellitus on development and progression of diabetic nephropathy. *JAMA.* 2003;290:2159-67.
10. UK Prospective Diabetes Study (UKPDS) Group. Intensive glycemic control with sulphonlyureas or insulin compared with conventional treatment and risk of complications in patients with type 2 diabetes (UKPDS 33). *Lancet.* 1998;352:837-53.
11. Stratton IM, Adler AI, Neil HAW, et al. Association of glycaemia with macrovascular and microvascular complications of type 2 diabetes (UKPDS 35): prospective observational study. *BMJ.* 2000;321:405-11.

## PATIENT EDUCATION FOR DIABETES MELLITUS

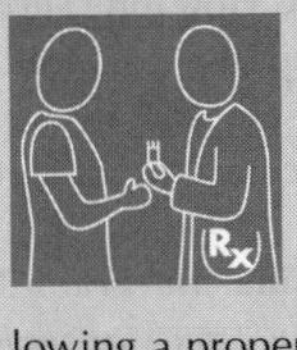

The primary objective of self-care is to achieve and maintain glycemic control. Secondary benefits of meeting metabolic goals are (1) preventing or reversing diabetes complications; (2) maintaining normal daily activities with maximum lifestyle flexibility; (3) avoiding weight gain by following a proper nutrition and physical activity plan; (4) avoiding infection; and (5) achieving a sense of well-being. For most patients, carefully following product instructions (including instructions on the proper use of insulin) and the self-care measures listed here will help ensure optimal therapeutic outcomes.

### Nondrug Measures

- Recognize that having diabetes requires lifestyle and behavioral changes.
- If newly diagnosed with diabetes, meet with your primary care provider, nurse, dietitian, or pharmacist to develop a nutrition plan and physical activity program that suits your lifestyle.
- Read food labels.
- Involve your entire family in your healthy lifestyle changes.
- Knowledge is power. Know your glycemic and other diabetes-related goals (see Table 47-5). Learn about your disease and the ways you can take control of your diabetes.
- SMBG regularly and know what makes your glucose go up and down (e.g., foods, activity, medications, stress).
- Use a logbook to document BG results, diet, physical activity, insulin, or other medication administration changes and bring it with you to every health care visit.
- Feeling like you have to tackle everything at once can be overwhelming. Set realistic, achievable goals. Make one or two specific changes at a time and recognize your accomplishments.
- If you have diabetes complications, consult a diabetes specialist. Practice the preventive measures listed in Table 47-4.
- For exercising conscientiously, follow the guidelines in Table 47-6.
- Monitor your BG several times each day. If a BG reading is above 240 mg/dL, check urine ketones. If your values indicate a problem, see your primary care provider for adjustments to your therapy.
- If you use tobacco products, it is strongly advised to quit. A tobacco cessation program is highly recommended (Chapter 50).
- If you have cuts or bruises that are not healing or appear infected, consult with your primary care provider.

### Nonprescription and Prescription Medications

- If applicable, follow your prescribed insulin regimen carefully.
- Inject your insulin at the proper sites and rotate your injection sites (see Figure 47-5).
- Follow the guidelines in Tables 47-10 and 47-11 for preparing and injecting insulin doses.
- Know the signs and symptoms related to low or high BG levels and appropriate monitoring and management strategies.
- Discuss taking a low dose of aspirin daily to prevent heart attack and stroke with your primary care provider.
- Do not start taking any nonprescription medications, herbal products or supplements without first discussing them with your pharmacist or primary care provider.
- Take your medications only as directed by your pharmacist or primary care provider.
- Do not stop taking any of your medications unless you first discuss it with a pharmacist or your primary care provider.
- Consult your pharmacist for safe over-the-counter medication options to treat self-limiting conditions such as allergies, cough, or upset stomach.
- Read the labels of nonprescription medications to identify sugar and alcohol content. Avoid medications that contain sugar or alcohol.
- Certain cold medications, such as pseudoephedrine, may raise blood glucose levels. Talk to your provider or pharmacist before selecting any allergy, cough, or cold preparations.
- Talk to your pharmacist about strategies to help you keep track of your medications and daily doses.

⚠ If you use insulin therapy and experience symptoms of hypoglycemia (e.g., sweating, hunger, rapid heart beat, confusion, tiredness), hyperglycemia (e.g., frequent urination, dehydration, thirst, increased appetite), or ketoacidosis (e.g., BG greater than 240 mg/dL + urine ketones and flulike symptoms, confusion, stupor), contact your primary care provider.


12. Adler AI, Stratton IM, Neil HAW, et al. Association of systolic blood pressure with macrovascular and microvascular complications in type 2 diabetes (UKPDS 36): a prospective observational study. *BMJ.* 2000;321:412-19.
13. Chobanian AV, Bakris GL, Black HR, et al. The seventh report of the joint national committee on prevention, detection, evaluation and treatment of high blood pressure: the JNC 7 Report. *JAMA.* 2003;289(19):2560-72.
14. American Diabetes Association. Hypertension management in adults with diabetes. *Diabetes Care.* 2004;27(suppl 1):S65-7.
15. American Diabetes Association. Dyslipidemia management in adults with diabetes. *Diabetes Care.* 2004;27(suppl 1):S68-S71.
16. Grundy SM, Cleeman JI, Merz CN, et al. The implications of recent clinical trials for the National Cholesterol Education Program Adult Treatment Panel III guidelines. *Circulation.* 2004;110: 227-39.
17. American Diabetes Association. Aspirin therapy in diabetes. *Diabetes Care.* 2004;27(suppl 1):S72-3.
18. American Diabetes Association. Influenza and pneumococcal immunization in diabetes. *Diabetes Care.* 2004;27(suppl 1):S111-3.
19. Ryan M, Carnu O, Kamer A. The influence of diabetes on the periodontal tissues. *JADA.* 2003;134(suppl):34S-40S.
20. Ship JA. Diabetes and oral health. *JADA.* 2003;134(suppl):4S-10S.
21. American Diabetes Association. Preconception care of women with diabetes. *Diabetes Care.* 2004;27(suppl 1):S76-8.
22. American Diabetes Association. Standards of medical care in diabetes [position statement]. *Diabetes* Care. 2005;28(suppl 1): S4-S36.
23. American Diabetes Association. Nutrition Principles and Recommendations in Diabetes [position statement]. *Diabetes Care.* 2004; 27(suppl 1);S36-S46.
24. Franz MJ. Medical nutrition therapy for diabetes. In: Franz MJ, ed. *A CORE Curriculum for Diabetes Education, Diabetes Management Therapies.* 5th ed. Chicago: American Association of Diabetes Educators; 2003.

25. Franz MJ, Bantle JP, Beebe CA, et al. Evidence-based nutrition principles and recommendations for the treatment and prevention of diabetes and related complications [Technical Review]. *Diabetes Care.* 2002; 25;148-98.
26. American Dietetic Association. Position of the American Dietetic Association: use of nutritive and nonnutritive sweeteners. *J Am Diet Assoc.* 2004;104:255-75.
27. Valmadrid CT, Klein R, Moss SE, et al. Alcohol intake and the risk of coronary heart disease mortality in persons with older-onset diabetes mellitus. *JAMA.* 1999;282:239-46.
28. Solomon CG, Hu FB, Stampfer MJ, et al. Moderate alcohol consumption and risk of coronary heart disease among women with type 2 diabetes mellitus. *Circulation.* 2000;102:494-9.
29. Ajani UA, Gaziano M, Lotufo PA, et al. Alcohol consumption and risk of coronary heart disease by diabetes status. *Circulation.* 2000;102:500-5.
30. Lane JD, Barkauskas CE, Surwit RS, et al. Caffeine impairs glucose metabolism in type 2 diabetes. *Diabetes Care.* 2004;27;2047-48.
31. The Diabetes Prevention Program Research Group. Reduction in the incidence of type 2 diabetes with lifestyle intervention or metformin. *N Engl J Med.* 2002;346:393-403.
32. American Diabetes Association. Physical activity/exercise and diabetes [position statement]. Diabetes *Care.* 2004;27(suppl 1): S58-62.
33. Mullooly CA, Chalmers KH. Physical activity/exercise. In: Franz MJ, ed. *A CORE Curriculum for Diabetes Education, Diabetes Management Therapies.* 5th ed. Chicago: American Association of Diabetes Educators; 2003.
34. Insulin monograph and product tables. eFacts [online database]. St. Louis: Facts and Comparisons; 2005. Accessed July 18, 2005.
35. Aventis pharmaceuticals. Apidra package insert. Available at: www.aventis.com. Accessed December 13, 2004.
36. DeWitt DE, Hirsch IB. Outpatient insulin therapy in type 1 and type 2 diabetes mellitus. *JAMA.* 2003;289:2254-64.
37. American Diabetes Association. Insulin administration [position statement]. *Diabetes Care.* 2004;27(suppl 1):S106-9.
38. American Diabetes Association. Resource Guide 2005. Products for testing glycohemoglobin. *Diabetes Forecast.* 2005;58:RGC16-RGC-35.
39. Carlisle BA, Kroon LA, Koda-Kimble MA. Diabetes mellitus. In: Koda-Kimble MA, Young LY, Kradjan WA, et al, eds. *Applied Therapeutics: The Clinical Use of Drugs.* 8th ed. Vancouver, Wash: Applied Therapeutics, Inc; 2004:50-1 to 50-86.
40. Grajower MM, Fraser CG, Holcombe JH, et al. How long should insulin be used once a vial is started? *Diabetes Care.* 2003;26:2665-9.
41. Holcombe JH, Daugherty ML, De Felippis MR. How long should insulin be used once a vial is started? Response to Molitch. *Diabetes Care.* 2004;27:1241-2.
42. Cryer PE, Davis SN, Shamoon H. Hypoglycemia in diabetes. *Diabetes Care.* 2003;26:1902-12.
43. Gonder-Frederick LA, Zrebiec J. Hypoglycemia. In: Franz MJ, ed. *A CORE Curriculum for Diabetes Education, Diabetes Management Therapies.* 5th ed. Chicago: American Association of Diabetes Educators; 2003.
44. American Diabetes Association. Tests of glycemia in diabetes [position statement]. *Diabetes Care.* 2004;27(suppl 1):S91-3.
45. McGarraugh G, Price D, Schwartz S, et al. Physiological influences on off-finger glucose testing. *Diabetes Technol Ther.* 2001;3: 367-76.
46. Peragalo-Dittko V. Monitoring. In: Franz MJ, ed. *A CORE Curriculum for Diabetes Education, Diabetes* Management *Therapies.* 5th ed. Chicago: American Association of Diabetes Educators; 2003.
47. Franz MJ. Medical Nutrition Therapy. In: Franz MJ, ed. *A CORE Curriculum for Diabetes Education, Diabetes* Management *Therapies.* 4th ed. Chicago: American Association of Diabetes Educators; 2001.
48. National Center for Complimentary and Alternative Medicine (NCCAM), National Institutes of Health (NIH). A new portrait of CAM use in the United States. *CAM at NIH.* Summer 2004; 11(3):1-4.
49. Consumer reports. Dangerous supplements still at large. *Consumer Reports.* May 2004.
50. Egede LE, Ye X, Zheng D, et al. The prevalence and pattern of complimentary and alternative medicine use in individuals with diabetes. *Diabetes Care.* 2002;25:324-9.
51. Yeh GY, Eisenberg DM, Kaptchuk TJ, et al. Systematic review of herbs and dietary supplements for glycemic control in diabetes. *Diabetes Care.* 2003;26:1277-94.
52. Rotblatt M, Ziment I, eds. *Evidence-Based Herbal* Medicine. Philadelphia: Hanley and Belfus Inc.; 2002.
53. McCarty MF. Nutraceutical resources for diabetes prevention—an update. *Medical Hypothesis.* 2005;64:151-8.
54. American Diabetes Association. Diabetes Risk Test. Pamphlet Item Code 5989-01; 03/04.

CHAPTER 48

# Insomnia

*Cynthia K. Kirkwood and Sarah T. Melton*

Insomnia is one of the most common patient complaints, ranking third behind headache and the common cold. Insomnia is a symptom with diverse etiologies and patient complaints and can progress to a disorder.[1,2] There is no ideal duration of sleep. The perceived sleep pattern and quality of daytime functioning can be more important to an individual than the duration of sleep. Thus, patients with insomnia feel that they sleep poorly at night, which adversely affects their daytime functioning.

Patients with other sleep disorders, such as sleep apnea, narcolepsy, and restless legs syndrome, also seek nonprescription sleep aids. Because these disorders can have significant clinical effects, patients with such disorders should, preferably, see a sleep specialist.

## Epidemiology of Insomnia

Although the average adult requires 8 or more hours of sleep nightly, the typical American gets 6.9 hours.[3] According to the 2005 National Sleep Foundation survey, about three fourths of all adult Americans reported one or more symptoms of insomnia during the past year.[3] About 33% of the U.S. population experienced insomnia almost every night. The use of sleep aids is prevalent. About 11% of adult Americans report using alcohol; 9%, a nonprescription sleep aid; 7%, a prescription hypnotic medication; and 2%, melatonin to manage insomnia.[3] Patients reporting medical conditions were the most likely to report sleep problems and to take sleep products. The following medical conditions were associated with complaints of sleep problems: hypertension (29%), arthritis (28%), heartburn or gastroesophageal reflux disease (19%), depression (18%), diabetes (11%), and heart disease (10%).[3]

The prevalence of sleep complaints is high among persons of advanced age, and more than half of this population reports at least one sleep complaint.[4] An estimated 35% of all hypnotic prescriptions are written for patients 65 years of age or older.[1] As many as 25% of these patients have reported self-medicating for sleep disturbances.[5] This group also has an increased incidence of sleep apnea and restless legs syndrome. Significant morbidity is associated with obstructive sleep apnea, which has been linked to 38,000 cardiovascular deaths annually.[6] For these reasons, complaints of insomnia in patients of advanced age should be carefully evaluated.

Despite these data, only a small percentage of patients with a sleep disorder actually verbalize their complaints to a health care provider.[7] Combined with the frequent misuse of hypnotics and the availability of nonprescription agents, this makes insomnia a disorder of significant concern.

## Physiology of Sleep

Physiologically, sleep can be categorized into different stages by using the sleeping electroencephalogram (EEG) in conjunction with electro-oculography and electromyography. Stage 1 sleep is a transitional stage, occurring as the patient falls asleep; the EEG resembles the waking state more than sleep. Stage 2 sleep, which comprises about 50% of sleep time, is light sleep. Stages 3 and 4, collectively known as deep sleep or delta sleep, are characterized by the patterns of delta waves, or slow-frequency waves, on the EEG. Rapid eye movement (REM) sleep is neither light nor deep, and the EEG manifests an increase in high-frequency waves. REM sleep is characterized by physiological activity compared with other sleep stages; skeletal muscle movement is inhibited. The eyes move rapidly from side to side, while blood pressure, heart rate, temperature, respiration, and metabolism are increased.[4,8]

Upon falling asleep, an individual progresses through the four stages of sleep, reaching the first REM period in about 70 to 90 minutes. The time from falling asleep to the first REM period is referred to as REM latency. The first REM period is of short duration—usually 5 to 7 minutes. The sleep cycle then repeats about every 70 to 120 minutes, with each progressive REM period becoming longer and the time spent in deep sleep becoming shorter.[4,8] The relative importance of medication effects in the different stages of sleep is unclear. However, prolonged suppression of REM sleep can result in psychologic and behavioral changes.

Sleep physiology changes with increasing age. Among persons of advanced age, the total duration of sleep is shorter, the number of nocturnal awakenings increases, and less time is spent in stage 4 and REM sleep. Sleep latency usually remains normal with increasing age. In spite of these changes, it cannot be assumed that this population requires less sleep.[4]

## Etiology of Insomnia

Insomnia can be classified as transient, short term, or chronic according to the duration of sleep disturbance. Transient insomnia is often self-limiting, lasting less than 1 week. Short-term insomnia usually lasts from 1 to

---

**Editor's Note:** This chapter is based, in part, on the 14th edition chapter with the same title, which was written by M. Lynn Crismon and Patricia Ludi Canales.

3 weeks.[1,2] Chronic, or long-term, insomnia lasts from more than 3 weeks to years and is often the result of medical problems, mental disorders, or substance abuse.[4,8]

Insomnia can also be classified on the basis of an identifiable cause. Primary insomnia is the term used to describe patients who have sleep difficulty that lasts at least 1 month, affects psychosocial functioning, and is not caused by another sleep disorder, general medical disorder, psychiatric disorder, or medication.[1] All underlying causes of insomnia must be identified and managed to relieve the sleep disturbance.[2]

Difficulty falling asleep is often associated with acute life stresses or medical illness, anxiety, and poor sleep habits. The severity of stressful situations can affect the length of insomnia. Travel, hospitalization, or anticipation of an important or stressful event can cause transient insomnia. However, if more severe stresses are present (e.g., the death of a loved one, recovery from surgery, the loss of a job, or divorce), transient insomnia can become short-term insomnia. Unless managed appropriately, short-term insomnia can progress to chronic insomnia.

Shift workers often complain of sleep disturbance and/or excessive sleepiness. Sleep problems occur more frequently in individuals who must rotate shifts. Some nighttime workers adjust to their change in sleep schedule, whereas others never do. Among night-shift workers with complaints of excessive sleepiness, the worst period of the day is between 3 and 5 AM.[6]

Sleep apnea is a common, undiagnosed cause of chronic insomnia. Patients with this disorder complain of daytime fatigue and sedation. Sleep apnea affects the quality of sleep of both the patient and family members because of the patient's gasping and snoring during sleep. Sleep apnea appears to be more common in men; the stereotypical patient is middle-aged, overweight, and hypertensive. Sleep apnea can be caused by an obstruction in the airway or central nervous system (CNS) mechanisms.[6]

Some individuals are extremely sensitive to the stimulant effects of caffeine and nicotine. Drinking caffeinated beverages in the late afternoon or evening hours can cause insomnia. Alcohol, if taken in excess, especially in the evening or on a chronic basis, can disturb sleep. Alcohol will often assist the individual in falling asleep but then result in frequent awakening and restless sleep throughout the night. Late-night exercise and late evening meals can also interfere with sleep, as well as environmental distractions (e.g., noise, lighting, uncomfortable temperatures, new surroundings.)[9]

Several general medical disorders, in addition to psychiatric disorders, are associated with chronic insomnia (Table 48-1). Chronic insomnia can also be secondary to use of medications or other substances, sleep-wake schedule disorders, or primary sleep disorders.[10] Early morning awakening is often associated with depression. Nonprescription hypnotics are generally not helpful in patients with chronic insomnia; medical referral is indicated.

Finally, medications—prescription and nonprescription—can either produce insomnia or withdrawal insomnia (Table 48-2). Antidepressants, antihypertensives, and sympathomimetic amines are the medication classes commonly associated with insomnia as an adverse effect.

**TABLE 48-1 Etiology of Chronic Insomnia**

| | |
|---|---|
| **General Medical Disorders** | **Psychiatric Disorders** |
| Arthritis | Anxiety disorders |
| Cancer | Bipolar disorder |
| Chronic pain syndromes | Dementia |
| Congestive heart failure | Depression |
| Gastroesophageal reflux disease | Personality disorders |
| Headaches | Psychosis |
| Nocturnal angina | Substance abuse |
| Peptic ulcer | |
| Postoperative pain | **Sleep Disorders** |
| | Delayed sleep phase syndrome |
| **Respiratory Disorders** | Drug-related insomnia |
| Asthma | Psychophysiologic insomnia |
| Bronchitis | Restless legs syndrome |
| Chronic obstructive pulmonary disease | Shift-work sleep disorder |
| | Sleep apnea |
| **Other Medical Conditions** | |
| Alzheimer's disease | |
| Arrhythmias | |
| Benign prostatic hyperplasia | |
| Constipation | |
| Diabetes mellitus | |
| Epilepsy | |
| Hyperthyroidism | |
| Irritable bowel syndrome | |
| Menopause | |
| Nocturia | |
| Parkinson's disease | |
| Pregnancy | |
| Renal insufficiency | |

Alcohol can cause insomnia after acute use and as a withdrawal effect after chronic use.

## Signs and Symptoms of Insomnia

Patients with insomnia can have any number of complaints, such as difficulty falling asleep, frequent awakening, early morning awakening and inability to fall back to sleep, disturbed quality of sleep with unusual or troublesome dreams, or just poor sleep in general. Their actual duration of sleep as determined by sleep laboratory studies may or may not differ from that of individuals who report normal sleep. However, these patients usually report that it takes them more than 30 minutes to fall asleep and/or that their duration of sleep is less than 6 to 7 hours nightly. Patients who complain of insomnia characterized by frequent nighttime awakenings or early morning awakenings with difficulty going back to sleep, or those with a duration of insomnia of 4 weeks or longer should be referred to their health care provider for further investigation.

## Complications of Insomnia

Sleep-deprived individuals are highly symptomatic, and their quality of life is negatively affected. Some impairment in daytime functioning is necessary for a diagnosis of

**TABLE 48-2 Drugs That Can Exacerbate Insomnia**

| Drugs That Can Cause Insomnia | Drugs That Can Produce Withdrawal Insomnia |
|---|---|
| Alcohol | Alcohol |
| Antidepressants | Antihistamines (first generation) |
| Bupropion | Barbiturates |
| Monoamine oxidase inhibitors (tranylcypromine) | Benzodiazepines |
| Selective serotonin reuptake inhibitors | Chloral hydrate |
| Serotonin-norepinephrine reuptake inhibitors (venlafaxine, duloxetine) | Monoamine oxidase inhibitors |
| Tricyclic antidepressants | Tricyclic antidepressants |
| Antihypertensives | Miscellaneous |
| β-Blockers (especially propranolol) | Amphetamines |
| Clonidine | Cocaine |
| Diuretics (at bedtime) | Marijuana |
| Methyldopa | Opiates |
| Reserpine | Phencyclidine |
| Hypnotic use (chronic) | |
| Nicotine | |
| Sympathomimetic amines | |
| Amphetamines | |
| Appetite suppressants | |
| β-Adrenergic agonists | |
| Caffeine | |
| Decongestants (e.g., pseudoephedrine, phenylephrine) | |
| Miscellaneous | |
| Anabolic steroids | |
| Anticonvulsants | |
| Antineoplastics | |
| Corticosteroids | |
| Histamine$_2$-receptor antagonists (e.g., cimetidine) | |
| Levodopa | |
| Oral contraceptives | |
| Phenytoin | |
| Quinidine | |
| Theophylline | |
| Thyroid preparations | |

insomnia, and a majority of untreated patients with insomnia report symptoms of fatigue, drowsiness, anxiety, irritability, depression, decreased concentration, and memory impairment. If left untreated, insomnia is associated with an increase in accidents and a rise in morbidity and mortality rates from general medical and psychiatric disorders (i.e., depression, anxiety, and substance abuse).[10]

## Treatment of Insomnia

### *Treatment Goals*

The optimal goal of treatment is to have a patient who reports normal sleep and awakes feeling rested, with no daytime fatigue or drowsiness.

### *General Treatment Approach*

For patients with transient or short-term insomnia but no underlying problems, reestablishing the normal sleep cycle with good sleep hygiene practices, with or without a nonprescription sleep aid, should help normalize sleep patterns (Figure 48-1). If diphenhydramine is recommended, it should be taken at bedtime only as needed. Patients who complain of continuing insomnia after 14 days of treatment with diphenhydramine combined with good sleep hygiene and those who experience side effects from this medication should be referred for a more thorough evaluation of the sleep disturbance and its etiology.[11] The algorithm in Figure 48-1 outlines the assessment and self-treatment of transient and short-term insomnia, and lists exclusions for self-treatment.

### *Nonpharmacologic Therapy*

The sleep hygiene measures in Table 48-3 are recommended for all patients with insomnia. In many patients with sleep disturbances, these measures should be tried before initiating pharmacotherapy. Patients should be encouraged to try one or two measures at a time.

### *Pharmacologic Therapy*

When the Food and Drug Administration (FDA) issued its final monograph on over-the-counter sleep aids in 1989, the antihistamine diphenhydramine (HCl and citrate salts) was the only Category I sleep aid listed.[13] Although the safety and efficacy of another antihistamine, doxylamine, have not been fully established, FDA has allowed it to remain on the market.[13] Minimal studies supporting the efficacy of doxylamine as a hypnotic are available.[5] Products containing pyrilamine maleate, potassium or sodium bromide, and scopolamine hydrobromide were removed from the U.S. market;[6] however, clinicians, particularly in the southwestern United States, may see these products imported from other countries.

#### Antihistamines

*Mechanism of Action/Pharmacokinetics* Both diphenhydramine and doxylamine are members of the ethanolamine group of antihistamines. Ethanolamines are thought to affect sleep through their affinity for blocking histamine$_1$ and muscarinic receptors.[13]

Selected clinical and pharmacokinetic properties of diphenhydramine and doxylamine are summarized in Table 48-4.[11,13,14] Both drugs are well absorbed from the gastrointestinal tract and have short to intermediate half-lives. Diphenhydramine is metabolized in the liver through two successive N-demethylations, and its apparent half-life can be prolonged in patients with hepatic cirrhosis.[11] Some, but not all studies have shown a positive relationship between diphenhydramine plasma concentrations and drowsiness and cognitive impairment. Significant drowsiness lasted from 3 to 6 hours after a single dose of diphenhydramine 50 mg.[15] However, next-morning hangover was reported after multiple nightly dosing for insomnia.

**Exclusions for Self-Treatment**

- Frequent nocturnal awakenings or early morning awakening
- Chronic insomnia (>3 weeks)
- Sleep disturbance occurring nightly for several days
- Sleep disturbance secondary to psychiatric or general medical disorders

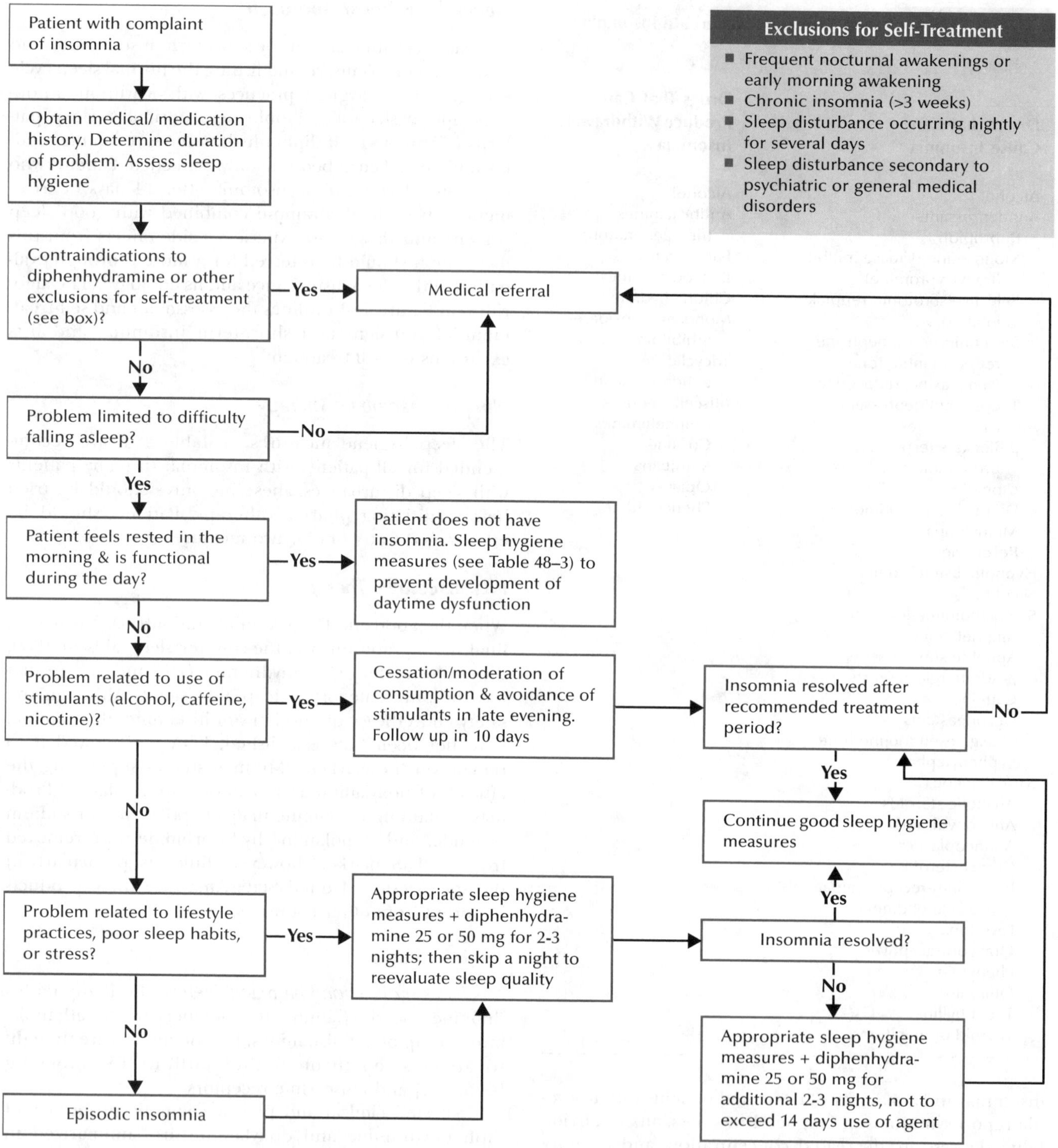


**FIGURE 48-1** Self-care of transient and short-term insomnia.

*Indications* The primary indication for diphenhydramine in insomnia is the symptomatic management of transient and short-term sleep difficulty, particularly in individuals who complain of occasional problems falling asleep. The evidence for the efficacy of diphenhydramine in patients with chronic insomnia is poor, and tolerance to the hypnotic effect was reported to develop with repeated use.[1,10] Diphenhydramine is not recommended to induce sleep in infants.[16]

*Dosage and Administration Guidelines* Although the usual optimal diphenhydramine dose is 50 mg nightly, some individuals benefit from a 25 mg dose. In patients over 65 years of age, diphenhydramine use should be

**TABLE 48-3 Principles of Good Sleep Hygiene** [7,12]

- Use bed for sleeping or intimacy only.
- Establish a regular sleep pattern: Go to bed and arise at about the same time daily, even on the weekends.
- Make the bedroom comfortable for sleeping. Avoid temperature extremes, noise, and light.
- Engage in relaxing activities before bedtime.
- Exercise regularly but not within 2-4 hours of bedtime.
- If hungry, eat a light bedtime snack, but avoid eating meals within 2 hours before bedtime.
- Avoid daytime napping.
- Avoid using caffeine, alcohol, or nicotine for at least 4-6 hours before bedtime.
- If unable to fall asleep, do not continue to try to sleep, but perform a relaxing activity until you feel tired.
- Do not watch the clock at night.

**TABLE 48-4 Selected Pharmacokinetic and Clinical Properties of Nonprescription Hypnotics**[11,13,14]

| | Diphenhydramine | Doxylamine |
|---|---|---|
| Time to maximum plasma concentration ($t_{max}$) | 1-4 hours | 2-3 hours |
| Maximum sedation | 1-3 hours | NA |
| Protein binding | 80%-85% | NA |
| Elimination half-life | 2.4-9.3 hours | 10 hours |
| Duration of sedation | 3-6 hours | 3-6 hours |
| Bioavailability | 40%-60% | NA |

Key: NA, not available.

avoided because of increased risk of anticholinergic side effects, dizziness, and cognitive impairment that can lead to falls.[13,17] The safety and effectiveness of diphenhydramine in children under 12 years of age has not been proven. In children between 2 and 12 years of age, a dosage of 1 mg/kg, not to exceed 50 mg, has been recommended.[13]

Tolerance to the hypnotic effects of diphenhydramine was poorly studied but appears to result with repeated use.[7] Intermittent use for 3 days with an "off" night to assess sleep quality without medication is suggested to reduce tolerance to the hypnotic effect. Diphenhydramine should be used for no more than 14 consecutive nights.[11]

Anticholinergic toxicity can result from excessive antihistamine dosages. Drug interactions, intentional overdosage, or individual sensitivity can lead to toxicity.[16,18] CNS anticholinergic toxicity is one of the primary presenting features of antihistamine excess. Patients can be anxious, excited, delirious, hallucinating, or stuporous; in more severe cases, coma or seizures may occur. Other physical signs of anticholinergic toxicity include dilated pupils, flushed skin, hot and dry mucous membranes, and elevated body temperature. Tachycardia and moderate QTc prolongation on the electrocardiogram are common. In severe cases, rhabdomyolysis, dysrhythmias, cardiovascular collapse, and death can occur.[19]

Anticholinergic toxicity is particularly common in children, in whom the symptoms are usually more severe. Diphenhydramine toxicity was reported in children using the topical application over large areas of their bodies, and in those using both the topical and oral preparations.[11] In December 2002, FDA issued a ruling that required a warning statement on all diphenhydramine-containing products (by December 6, 2004), not to be used in conjunction with any other preparations that contain diphenhydramine.[11]

In the case of diphenhydramine overdose, patients should be referred for emergency treatment, which includes gastric lavage and activated charcoal via gastric tube, and further symptomatic treatment. Syrup of ipecac should not be recommended.

*Safety Considerations* Sedation, the intended effect when diphenhydramine is used as a hypnotic, may be associated with next-morning hangover in susceptible individuals.[11] Other primary side effects of diphenhydramine and doxylamine are anticholinergic.[1,13] Dry mouth and throat, constipation, blurred vision, urinary retention, and tinnitus commonly occur. Patients of advanced age, patients with comorbid general medical disorders, and patients taking multiple medications are particularly susceptible to developing adverse effects. The most recent revision of the Beer's criteria recommends avoiding the use of anticholinergics in older patients,[20] and diphenhydramine has caused cognitive impairment in patients of advanced age.[5,17]

Additive sedation or anticholinergic effects occur when diphenhydramine is used in combination with other medications having these properties.[13] Diphenhydramine, an inhibitor of the hepatic enzyme CYP 2D6, causes more than a twofold decrease in the clearance of venlafaxine and metoprolol.[21,22] Diphenhydramine likely causes a significant decrease in the clearance of numerous medications metabolized by CYP 2D6 (e.g., codeine, desipramine, fluoxetine, nortriptyline, propranolol, risperidone, and quinidine). In patients on multiple medications, particularly patients of advanced age, these potential interactions should be carefully monitored.

Diphenhydramine has several contraindications. Male patients of advanced age with prostatic hyperplasia and difficulty urinating should not use diphenhydramine because of increased urinary retention. Because anticholinergics can increase intraocular pressure, narrow-angle (closed-angle) glaucoma is another contraindication. Patients with cardiovascular disease (e.g., angina or rhythm disturbance) may be particularly susceptible to the anticholinergic adverse effects of ethanolamine sleep aids, and therefore should not use these agents.[13] Anticholinergics tend to decrease cognition and increase confusion in patients with dementia; diphenhydramine is contraindicated in these patients as well.

Patients should be cautioned to avoid performing tasks that require their full attention or coordination (e.g., driving, cooking, operating equipment) until their

**TABLE 48-5 Selected Sleep Aid Products**

| Trade Name | Primary Ingredients |
|---|---|
| **Single-entity Antihistamine Products** | |
| Compoz Nighttime Sleep Aid Tablets/Gelcaps* | Diphenhydramine HCl 50 mg |
| Simply Sleep Nighttime Sleep Aid Caplets* | Diphenhydramine HCl 25 mg |
| Sominex Maximum Strength Caplets* | Diphenhydramine HCl 50 mg |
| Sominex Nighttime Sleep Aid Tablets* | Diphenhydramine HCl 25 mg |
| Unisom Nighttime Sleep Aid Tablets* | Doxylamine succinate 25 mg |
| Unisom Sleepgels* | Diphenhydramine HCl 50 mg |
| **Antihistamine–Analgesic Combination Products** | |
| Bayer PM Extra Strength Caplets | Diphenhydramine citrate 38.3 mg; aspirin 500 mg |
| Excedrin PM Geltabs/Caplets/Tablets* | Diphenhydramine citrate 38 mg; acetaminophen 500 mg |
| Goody's PM Powder* | Diphenhydramine citrate 38 mg; acetaminophen 500 mg |
| Tylenol PM Extra Strength Geltabs/Gelcaps/Caplets* | Diphenhydramine HCl 25 mg; acetaminophen 500 mg |
| **Melatonin Products** | |
| GNC Melatonin Tablets*†‡ | Melatonin 3 mg |
| Natrol Melatonin Liquid* | Melatonin 500 μg/2 droppersful |
| Nature's Bounty Melatonin Tablets* | Melatonin 1 mg |
| Nature's Way Melatonin Lozenges* | Melatonin 500 μg |
| Twin Lab Melatonin Controlled-Release Tablets* | Melatonin 2 mg |
| **Valerian Products** | |
| Nature's Way Valerian Nighttime Tablets* | Valerian root extract 160 mg, lemon balm 80 mg |
| Olympian Valerian Root Capsules*† | Valerian root extract 150 mg |

*Aspirin-free; †dye-free; ‡sodium-free.

response to diphenhydramine is known. They should be warned of the additive CNS depressant effects of alcohol and encouraged not to drink alcoholic beverages while taking diphenhydramine. Some patients can develop excitation from diphenhydramine and other highly anticholinergic antihistamines.[13] This paradoxical effect occurs more often in children, patients of advanced age, and patients with organic mental disorders. Symptoms include nervousness, restlessness, agitation, tremors, insomnia, delirium, and, in rare cases, seizures.

### Combination Products

Combination products containing diphenhydramine and acetaminophen (e.g., Excedrin PM, Tylenol PM) or aspirin (e.g., Bayer PM) are available,[13] though no published studies establish whether these products are of additive benefit in inducing sleep in patients who complain of insomnia caused by pain.

### Product Selection Guidelines

Because no published efficacy and safety studies document the value of doxylamine as a hypnotic, only diphenhydramine should be recommended to patients for such use at the present time. Nonprescription diphenhydramine is available as capsules, gelcaps, tablets, chewable tablets, solution, and elixir (Table 48-5), thus allowing various forms for different patient preferences.[14]

*Special Populations* The safety of antihistamines during pregnancy has not been clearly established.[13] Therefore, the benefit-risk ratio of using these drugs during pregnancy should be carefully evaluated. Doxylamine was formerly marketed as a prescription combination product for treating morning sickness during pregnancy. However, the manufacturer voluntarily removed this combination from the market in 1976 after allegations of teratogenicity. Although it is not possible to prove conclusively that doxylamine is not teratogenic, epidemiologic studies indicate that the possibility of such a relationship is remote.[13,14] Diphenhydramine is classified as Pregnancy Category B. Epidemiologic studies did not demonstrate increased risk of teratogenicity during the first trimester, but there are reports of cleft palate alone and with other fetal abnormalities associated with diphenhydramine use.[11] Nevertheless, rather than recommending a nonprescription product, pregnant women should be referred for further medical evaluation.

An increased risk of CNS side effects appears to occur with antihistamine use in neonates. For this reason and because such drugs may inhibit lactation, antihistamines are not recommended for use in nursing mothers.[11,13,14]

## Complementary Therapies

### Physiologic Agents

*Melatonin* Melatonin (5-acetyl-5-methoxytryptamine) is an endogenous hormone produced by the pineal gland, located behind the third ventricle in the brain. It is known to play a role in the regulation of the body's natural wake-sleep cycle (circadian rhythm).[23] Levels of melatonin increase with decreasing exposure to light. Known actions of melatonin include the shift of circadian rhythms, decreased body temperature, alteration of reproductive rhythm, enhanced immune function, and decreased alertness.[24] Commercially available melatonin can be isolated from the pineal glands of beef cattle or chemically synthesized.[23,24]

Wide variation in study methodology, including dose, time of administration, study population, and assessment parameters, has made it difficult to evaluate the efficacy of melatonin in insomnia. A comprehensive report on the safety and effectiveness of melatonin found that, although there is some evidence for the benefits of melatonin supplements, for most sleep disorders the evidence suggests limited or no benefits.[24] Melatonin may be effective in short-term treatment of delayed sleep phase syndrome.[24] In delayed sleep phase syndrome, the person's internal biologic clock is "out of sync," making it difficult to fall asleep until very late at night or to wake up early the next morning. Melatonin acts to reset the circadian rhythm by reducing sleep onset latency, but does not improve sleep efficiency in people with a primary sleep disorder. Overall, the evidence suggests that melatonin is not effective in treating most secondary sleep disorders with short-term use.[24] No evidence suggests that melatonin is effective in alleviating the sleep disturbance aspect of jet lag and shift-work disorders.

Although studies are not favorable for all types of insomnia, melatonin is used clinically to help people fall asleep. Often prescribed as a mild hypnotic in long-term care facilities, melatonin has the benefit of not causing dizziness or next-morning hangover, which can lead to falls in older adults.

Research on melatonin in children is lacking. Melatonin 5 mg improved the health status and advanced the sleep-wake rhythm in children ages 6 to 12 years with idiopathic chronic sleep-onset insomnia.[25] Studies in children with severe insomnia resulting from various neurologic disorders showed that administration of melatonin improved sleep patterns and sleep duration.[26] Parents reporting that their child has difficulty falling asleep should be instructed to contact the child's health care provider because insomnia in children can be related to various other conditions. Children appear to be sensitive to melatonin treatment, but its safety was poorly evaluated. A particular caution is that melatonin can exacerbate epilepsy and asthma.[27] Melatonin was effective as a mild sedative in children undergoing a magnetic resonance imaging procedure[28] and was as effective as midazolam in alleviating preoperative anxiety in children.[29]

The optimal dose and time of administration of melatonin for the treatment of insomnia have not been determined. The usual dose is 0.3 to 5 mg at bedtime.[26] Potential drug interactions, side effects, and toxicity, particularly with long-term use, are largely unknown. Until more information is available, melatonin should not be recommended in pregnant women or nursing mothers. Contaminants in commercial preparations of melatonin were reported.[22,23]

*L-Tryptophan and 5-Hydroxytryptophan* L-tryptophan was recalled by FDA in 1990 because of safety concerns linking the supplement to eosinophilia-myalgia syndrome (EMS) and death.[30] Many trace level impurities were discovered in the L-tryptophan involved in the EMS cases; however, the role of these impurities in EMS in not clear.[31] L-tryptophan in the United States is limited for use under medical supervision in special dietary products such as infant formulas, enteral products, and approved parenteral drug products. Given its questionable efficacy, concerns regarding contaminants, and known adverse effects, L-tryptophan should not be recommended as a sleep aid.

Since the withdrawal of L-tryptophan from the market, 5-hydroxytryptophan (5-HTP), the immediate precursor of serotonin, is being used to treat insomnia. Although there is concern that 5-HTP, like L-tryptophan, can cause EMS, to date there are no reported cases of EMS with 5-HTP. The efficacy of 5-HTP in insomnia is not proven and it should not be recommended as a sleep aid.

### Medicinal Herbs

*Valerian* Valerian (*Valeriana officinalis*) is a perennial plant native to Europe and Asia. Preparations of valerian marketed as dietary supplements are made from its roots and stems.[23] Dried roots are prepared as tinctures or teas, and dried plant materials are compounded into tablets and capsules.

*Mechanism of Action* Valerian causes sedation by increasing the amount of gamma aminobutyric acid (GABA) available in the synaptic cleft. Valerian reduces the time to sleep onset and improves subjective sleep quality.

*Indications* Valerian is used for sleep disturbances. The evidence for valerian as a treatment for insomnia is inconclusive. A comprehensive review of controlled trials of valerian used in insomnia found the studies were contradictory and inconsistent in the types of patients, experimental design, procedures, and methodological quality.[32]

*Dosage and Administration Guidelines* The optimum dose of valerian is unknown. Doses used in clinical studies ranged from 450 to 900 mg of an aqueous or aqueous-ethanolic extract (corresponding to 1.5-3 g of herb) taken 30 minutes to 2 hours before bedtime.[32] Traditionally valerian was ingested in the form of a tea (1.5-3 g of root steeped for 5 to 10 minutes in 150 mL of boiling water), although this formulation was not studied in clinical trials. Continuous nightly use for several days or weeks is required for effect, so valerian is not useful for acute insomnia.

*Safety Considerations* Migraines, dizziness, and gastrointestinal upset are the most common adverse effects reported with valerian.[32] Patients should be informed that the long-term effect of valerian on liver function is not known.

Patients using large doses of valerian over several years can experience severe benzodiazepinelike withdrawal symptoms and cardiac complications.[33] Therefore, valerian should be slowly tapered after extended use.

Compared with another agent, valerian 600 mg was equal to oxazepam 10 mg for improving sleep quality, duration of sleep, and feeling refreshed on awakening in a controlled 6-week study of 202 outpatients.[34] However, the oxazepam dose in this study is lower than that typically used.

*Kava* Kava (*Piper methysticum*) is a plant native to the islands of the South Pacific. Kava-containing supplements are advertised to promote relaxation (e.g., to reduce anxiety, stress, and tension), and for sleeplessness and menopausal symptoms.[35] In the South Pacific, kava often is used socially in a manner similar to alcohol use in Western cultures. There is little evidence to support the use of kava in insomnia. Kava was removed from the market in numerous countries (e.g., Australia, England, Germany, Switzerland, Canada) after reports of hepatotoxicity and hepatic failure requiring liver transplantation.[35] In the United States, kava was not removed from the market; however, many pharmacies stopped carrying it as a precautionary measure. Therefore, kava should not be recommended as a sleep aid.

#### Other Natural Products

Chamomile, ginseng, lavender, hops, lemon balm, and passionflower are being used to treat insomnia.[36] Inadequate evidence is available regarding their efficacy and safety in insomnia. Chamomile was reported to cause cross-reactions in individuals with ragweed allergy.[36] For further discussion of herbal and homeopathic sleep aids, see Chapters 53 to 55.

#### Ethanol

About 30% of patients with persistent insomnia report using alcohol to help fall asleep in the past year, with 67% reporting it was effective.[37] Ethanol initially improves sleep in nonalcoholics at both low and high doses, with disturbance in the second half of the night at high doses. However, tolerance quickly develops after the initial beneficial effects, often leading to the use of higher doses.[37] With heavy or continuous consumption, the patient usually begins to experience restless sleep, often awakening within 2 to 4 hours, and total sleep duration decreases.[37,38] Moreover, after alcohol is discontinued, rebound insomnia is likely to occur. Chronic alcoholics usually have marked disorganization of their sleep cycle with shortened REM periods and delta sleep.

Alcohol is present in some nonprescription combination cold products, such as Nyquil, which contains 10% alcohol by volume. Products of this type are marketed and sometimes recommended to induce sleep. Data are limited, however, regarding the efficacy and safety of these products as hypnotics. They contain multiple ingredients, which increases the risk of side effects and interactions with other drugs.

Alcohol has negative effects on patients with sleep apnea.[37] During wakefulness, ethanol is a mild respiratory depressant, but during sleep it can exacerbate obstructive sleep apnea and precipitate breathing disorders in those at risk.

### *Pharmacotherapeutic Comparisons*

Most published clinical trials indicate that diphenhydramine is effective in decreasing time to fall asleep (sleep latency) and in improving the reported quality of sleep for individuals with occasional sleep difficulty.[13] Patients who have never been treated with hypnotics tend to respond better to diphenhydramine than those who have been previously treated.[39] In general, diphenhydramine is not as efficacious as benzodiazepine hypnotics, and it should not be recommended in individuals with chronic sleep disturbance.[40]

Although valerian possesses mild sedative properties, the clinical significance of these effects is unclear. Valerian should not be used with other hypnotics or by pregnant or breast-feeding women. An additional consideration with the use of natural products is selecting a standardized and pure product. Unfortunately, not all manufacturers follow consistent standards in purity and potency, making the decision to use a particular product difficult. Consumers can be directed to select a dietary supplement that bears the United States Pharmacopoeia (USP) logo on the bottle. For these reasons, careful consideration should be given to the decision whether to recommend an herbal product for sleep. Recommendations for use of these agents should take place only after sleep hygiene measures are initiated.

### *Pharmacoeconomics*

Insomnia has a significant economic impact, accounting for $11 to $15 billion annually in direct medical costs.[41] The direct cost of insomnia estimated in 1995 includes costs for both prescription ($809.92 million) and nonprescription medications, including use of alcohol to promote sleep ($780.39 million), over-the-counter medications ($325.8 million), and melatonin ($50 million).[41,42] Insomnia is associated with increased health care use, impaired quality of life, and an increased rate of traffic accidents, depression, alcohol abuse, and mortality.[41]

The pharmacoeconomic effects of hypnotic treatment of insomnia are unknown. However, the high economic burden and impact on health-related quality of life attributable to insomnia suggest that treatment would be cost-effective.[41]

## Assessment of Insomnia: A Case-based Approach

In assessing whether to recommend a nonprescription sleep product, the practitioner should determine if use of such products is appropriate, what nondrug interventions should be recommended, and whether medical referral is indicated. Identifying acute precipitators of insomnia, poor sleep hygiene practices, or underlying medical disorders can assist the practitioner in making a recommendation. Cases 48-1 and 48-2 illustrate the assessment of patients with insomnia.

## Patient Counseling for Insomnia

Patients with sleep disorders should be encouraged to practice good sleep hygiene measures. For some patients, these measures alone will resolve the problem. If use of a nonprescription sleep aid is appropriate, the dosage guidelines and recommended duration of therapy should be reviewed with the patient. Potential adverse side effects, drug interactions, and any precautions or warnings should be carefully explained. In addition, patient education should include the signs and symptoms that indicate the need for further visits to the practitioner. Taking multiple products (i.e., prescription, nonprescription, herbal) concomitantly to treat insomnia should be discouraged, as this increases the risk of adverse effects. The box Patient Education for Insomnia lists specific information to provide patients.

## Evaluation of Patient Outcomes for Insomnia

Successful outcomes include decreased time to fall asleep, improved sleep quality, and decreased daytime fatigue and drowsiness. The patient should be advised to seek medical evaluation if sleep has not improved within 10 days.

### CASE 48-1

| Relevant Evaluation Criteria | Scenario/Model Outcome |
|---|---|
| **Information Gathering** | |
| 1. Gather essential information about the patient's symptoms, including: | |
| a. description of symptom(s) (i.e., nature, onset, duration, severity, associated symptoms) | Patient complains of difficulty sleeping for the past week. She feels drowsy and irritable during the day and occasionally falls asleep when she sits still. |
| b. description of any factors that seem to precipitate, exacerbate, and/or relieve the patient's symptom(s) | She typically sleeps well. |
| c. description of the patient's efforts to relieve the symptoms | She usually lies in bed and becomes more anxious when she cannot sleep. She says it is especially frustrating to watch the alarm clock, knowing that she will have to get up in just a few hours. Sometimes she will get up and read the newspaper. She prefers not to be drowsy during the daytime because this interferes with her studying. |
| 2. Gather essential patient history information: | |
| a. patient's identity | Andrea Walton |
| b. patient's age, sex, height, and weight | 25 y/o F, 5'1", 143 lb |
| c. patient's occupation | Graduate nursing student |
| d. patient's dietary habits | Vegetarian |
| e. patient's sleep habits | Often stays up late studying, especially when projects are due; sleeps late on the weekends often into the early afternoon. When asked about other sleep hygiene habits, such as napping, she admits to taking an afternoon nap several days during the past week. She drinks only decaffeinated drinks and exercises twice a week at noon. |
| f. concurrent medical conditions, prescription and nonprescription medications, and dietary supplements | Ortho Tri-Cyclen 1 tablet daily for contraception and Benadryl Dye-Free Allergy 25 mg every 4-6 hours as needed during the day for seasonal allergies to pollen and grass. |
| g. allergies | Sulfa drugs, azithromycin |
| h. history of other adverse reactions to medications | None |
| i. other (describe)_______ | Drinks 3-4 beers on weekend nights |

**CASE 48-1 (continued)**

| Relevant Evaluation Criteria | Scenario/Model Outcome |
|---|---|
| **Assessment and Triage** | |
| 3. Differentiate the patient's signs/symptoms and correctly identify the patient's primary problem(s). | Poor sleep, likely secondary to stress of graduate school and poor sleep hygiene; possible use of alcohol on weekends disrupting sleep |
| 4. Identify exclusions for self-treatment (see Figure 48-1). | None |
| 5. Formulate a comprehensive list of therapeutic alternatives for the primary problem to determine if triage to a medical practitioner is required, and share this information with the patient. | Options include:<br>(1) Refer Andrea to her PCP.<br>(2) Recommend diphenhydramine until Andrea can make an appointment with her PCP.<br>(3) Recommend diphenhydramine and good sleep hygiene, including limiting weekend alcohol use.<br>(4) Take no action. |
| **Plan** | |
| 6. Select an optimal therapeutic alternative to address the patient's problem, taking into account patient preferences. | Diphenhydramine 25 mg capsules and good sleep hygiene measures, as well as limited alcohol consumption. She prefers not to take an herbal sleep aid. |
| 7. Describe the recommended therapeutic approach to the patient. | Take 2 diphenhydramine 25 mg capsules 1/2-1 hour before anticipated bedtime every night for 3 nights. Skip 1 night and evaluate your ability to sleep. If no better, take medication for 3 more nights and reevaluate ability to sleep without it. If symptoms persist for 10 days, seek medical evaluation. Follow measures for positive sleep hygiene (see Table 48-3). Limit alcohol consumption to 2 cans of beer, or less, consumed no later than 2 hours before bedtime. Avoid daytime naps. |
| 8. Explain to the patient the rationale for selecting the recommended therapeutic approach from the considered therapeutic alternatives. | Seeking a PCP, that is, primary care provider, may not be necessary if you take the diphenhydramine and follow good sleep hygiene measures. Poor sleep practices are a common cause of insomnia. If these practices are continued, they can create a chronic sleep disturbance. A hypnotic such as diphenhydramine can facilitate falling asleep, but must be combined with measures of good sleep hygiene. Alcohol in more than modest quantities can disrupt sleep and make insomnia worse. Thus, alcohol consumption should be avoided before bedtime and limited at other times. |
| **Patient Education** | |
| 9. When recommending self-care with nonprescription medications and/or nondrug therapy, convey accurate information to the patient, including: | |
| a. appropriate dose and frequency of administration | Diphenhydramine 50 mg nightly for 3 nights, then reevaluate sleep for 1 night without the medication. Do not exceed this nightly dose. Always use sleep aids in combination with positive sleep hygiene measures. Never take hypnotics nightly for longer than 14 days without seeking medical evaluation. Alcoholic beverages should not be taken with diphenhydramine because of increased chances of sedation and negative effects of alcohol on sleep patterns. |
| b. maximum number of days the therapy should be employed | 14 days of continuous nightly use |
| c. product administration procedures | Take a half or a whole tablet before bedtime with a full glass of water. |
| d. expected time to onset of relief | Onset of sedation should occur within 1-2 hours. |
| e. degree of relief that can be reasonably expected | When combined with sleep hygiene measures, sleep should improve within 1-3 nights. |

## CASE 48-1 (continued)

| Relevant Evaluation Criteria | Scenario/Model Outcome |
|---|---|
| f. most common side effects | Sedation, next-morning hangover, and anticholinergic effects (e.g., dry mouth and throat, urinary retention, blurry vision, constipation) |
| g. side effects that warrant medical intervention should they occur | Hives, severe itching, shortness of breath |
| h. patient options in the event that condition worsens or persists | If insomnia persists beyond 10 days, see your PCP. |
| i. product storage requirements | Keep in a tightly closed container. Keep out of the reach of children and pets. |
| j. specific nondrug measures | See Table 48-3 for sleep hygiene measures. Limit alcohol intake. |
| 10. Solicit patient's follow-up questions. | (1) Could I repeat the dose if I do not fall asleep within 2 hours?<br>(2) Could I take diphenhydramine with my allergy medication? |
| 11. Answer patient's questions. | (1) No. Repeating the dose increases the risk of side effects, and likely will not improve sleep.<br>(2) No. The Benadryl Dye-Free Allergy contains diphenhydramine. Combining diphenhydramine as a sleep aid and products that contain diphenhydramine can lead to an excessive dose and increased side effects (e.g., sedation, drowsiness, blurred vision, constipation) or toxicity. |

Key: PCP, primary care provider.

## CASE 48-2

| Relevant Evaluation Criteria | Scenario/Model Outcome |
|---|---|
| **Information Gathering** | |
| 1. Gather essential information about the patient's symptoms, including: | |
| a. description of symptom(s) (i.e., nature, onset, duration, severity, associated symptoms) | Patient complains of sporadic difficulty sleeping for the past 3 months. He awakens around 4:00 AM and is not able to go back to sleep. He also complains of severe fatigue and a lack of interest in work or family activities. |
| b. description of any factors that seem to precipitate, exacerbate, and/or relieve the patient's symptom(s) | Sleep has been much worse since his divorce became final 2 months ago. Nothing really seems to improve the symptoms. |
| c. description of the patient's efforts to relieve the symptoms | He has tried to increase his exercise routine in the evenings, but he just lacks the energy and motivation to do this activity. |
| 2. Gather essential patient history information: | |
| a. patient's identity | Samuel Davidson |
| b. patient's age, sex, weight, and height | 45 y/o M, 5'8", 188 lb |
| c. patient's occupation | Lawyer |
| d. patient's dietary habits | Samuel indicates that he has felt very tired and sad for the past 2 months with a reduced appetite and weight loss of 15 lb. |
| e. patient's sleep habits | He usually goes to sleep around 11 PM, but finds that he awakes by 3:30 or 4 AM and has trouble going back to sleep. He estimates that he has only gotten 3 or 4 full nights of sleep in the past month. |
| f. concurrent medical conditions, prescription and nonprescription medications, and dietary supplements | Atenolol 50 mg daily for angina for 6 years, loratadine 10 mg daily for allergies for 3 years, Depakote-ER 500 mg daily for migraines for 1 year |
| g. allergies | NKA |
| h. history of other adverse reactions to medications | None |
| i. other (describe)_______ | Smokes 1/2 pack per day |

**CASE 48-2**

| Relevant Evaluation Criteria | Scenario/Model Outcome |
|---|---|
| **Assessment and Triage** | |
| 3. Differentiate the patient's signs/symptoms and correctly identify the patient's primary problem(s). | Chronic poor sleep, most likely secondary to depression. |
| 4. Identify exclusions for self-treatment (see Figure 48-1). | The symptoms that the patient complains of suggest an underlying cause (i.e., depression) for the insomnia that requires referral for evaluation. |
| 5. Formulate a comprehensive list of therapeutic alternatives for the primary problem to determine if triage to a medical practitioner is required, and share this information with the patient. | Options include:<br>(1) Refer Samuel to his PCP for evaluation.<br>(2) Recommend an OTC sleep aid and good sleep hygiene measures (see Table 48-3).<br>(3) Recommend an OTC sleep aid and refer for medical evaluation.<br>(4) Take no action. |
| **Plan** | |
| 6. Select an optimal therapeutic alternative to address the patient's problem, taking into account patient preferences. | Refer Samuel to his PCP. The underlying disorder(s) causing his insomnia needs to be addressed. Recommend measures for sleep hygiene. |
| 7. Describe the recommended therapeutic approach to the patient. | See your primary care provider as soon as possible for evaluation of your sleep disturbance. Follow measures of good sleep hygiene (see Table 48-3), including cessation of smoking. |
| 8. Explain to the patient the rationale for selecting the recommended therapeutic approach from the considered therapeutic alternatives. | You have described symptoms that may indicate a medical disorder that possibly is causing your sleep disturbance. This will need to be addressed if your sleep is to improve. OTC hypnotics are unlikely to help you. |
| **Patient Education** | |
| 9. When recommending self-care with nonprescription medications and/or nondrug therapy, convey accurate information to the patient. | Criterion does not apply in this case. |
| 10. Solicit patient's follow-up questions. | Would herbals help me sleep instead? |
| 11. Answer patient's questions. | No. Multiple complicating factors may be contributing to your insomnia. It is very important that all of these be thoroughly addressed if your sleep problems as well as other symptoms are to improve. Some herbal medications are helpful for occasional use for insomnia, but they are not effective in treating medical causes of insomnia. |

Key: N/A, not applicable; NKA, no known allergies; OTC, over-the-counter; PCP, primary care provider.

## Key Points for Insomnia

- Advise patients that diphenhydramine is the only antihistamine recommended as a sleep aid for occasional insomnia.
- Refer patients with chronic insomnia or sleep disturbance caused by an underlying disorder for medical evaluation.
- Counsel patients on the side effects of diphenhydramine and other sleep aids, particularly drowsiness and the additive CNS effects of alcohol and other sedating drugs.
- Counsel patients that nonprescription sleep aids can cause next-day hangover.

## PATIENT EDUCATION FOR INSOMNIA

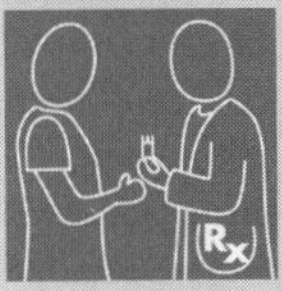

The objectives of self-treatment are to (1) improve duration and perceived quality of sleep, (2) decrease daytime fatigue and drowsiness, (3) improve daytime functioning, and (4) minimize adverse effects of treatment. For most patients, carefully following product instructions and the self-care measures listed here will help ensure optimal therapeutic outcomes.

### Nondrug Measures

- See Table 48-3 for nondrug measures to prevent insomnia.
- Note that principles of good sleep hygiene can help improve bad sleep habits and enhance quality sleep.
- If insomnia worsens or continues beyond 2 weeks, seek medical attention.

### Nonprescription Medications/Dietary Supplements

- Do not drive or operate machinery after taking sleep aids, including melatonin and valerian.

#### *Diphenhydramine*

- Establish a consistent bedtime and take diphenhydramine 30 to 60 minutes before you want to go to sleep. Do not take more than 50 mg of diphenhydramine each night.
- After two to three nights of improved sleep, skip taking the medication for one night to see if the insomnia is relieved.
- Do not take the medication for longer than 14 days. Longer use will cause tolerance to the medication's sleep-inducing effects but not necessarily to its side effects.
- Note that diphenhydramine can cause morning grogginess or excessive sedation, dry mouth, blurred vision, constipation, and urinary retention (particularly in older men).
- Do not take diphenhydramine with alcohol; alcohol can increase the effects of the medication on the central nervous system. Alcohol also disrupts the sleep cycle.
- Do not take diphenhydramine with prescription sleep aids in an attempt to improve sleep further.
- Consult your health care provider before taking diphenhydramine with other medications.

#### *Melatonin*

- If melatonin is being used, take it approximately 1 hour before the established bedtime. Bedroom should be dark. Somnolence may occur within 30 to 45 minutes after taking.
- Do not take more than 5 mg of melatonin each night.
- After taking melatonin, bedroom lights should be turned off.
- Sleep usually occurs within 30 to 45 minutes after taking the dose.

#### *Valerian*

- If valerian is being used, take it 1/2 to 2 hours before retiring to bed.
- It takes 2 to 4 weeks for optimal effects on sleep to occur.
- If you take valerian for several weeks or months, discontinue it slowly over several weeks to avoid withdrawal effects.

---

- Advise patients with self-treatable symptoms that if symptoms worsen or do not improve after 10 days, they should contact their primary care provider.
- Counsel patients with insomnia on nondrug measures such as good sleep hygiene (see Table 48-3).
- Refer children younger than 12 years or pregnant patients with insomnia to their primary care provider.
- Advise patients of the different dosage forms of sleep aids so they can select a product that is best suited for them.
- Advise patients of the advantages and disadvantages of complementary therapies so they can choose an agent.
- Advise patients not to take other oral medications that contain diphenhydramine with a nonprescription sleep aid that also contains diphenhydramine or to apply products that contain diphenhydramine topically.

## References


1. Roth T, Hajak G, Ustun TB. Consensus for the pharmacological management of insomnia in the new millennium. *Int J Clin Pract.* 2001;55:42-52.
2. Estivill E, Bov A, Garcia-Borreguero D, et al. Consensus on drug treatment, definition and diagnosis for insomnia. *Clin Drug Invest.* 2003;23:351-85.
3. National Sleep Foundation. 2005 Sleep in America Poll. Available at: http://www.sleepfoundation.org/_content/hottopics/2005_Summary_of_findings.pdf. Accessed August 18, 2005.
4. Neubauer DN. Sleep problems in the elderly. *Am Fam Physician.* 1999;59:2551-60.
5. Sproule BA, Busto UE, Buckle C, et al. The use of non-prescription sleep products in the elderly. *Int J Geriatr Psychiatry.* 1999; 14:851-7.
6. Moore CA, Williams RL, Hirshkowitz M. Sleep disorders. In: Sadock BJ, Sadock VA, ed. *Comprehensive Textbook of Psychiatry.* 7th ed. Philadelphia: Lippincott Williams & Wilkins; 2000:1677-700.
7. Benca RM. Diagnosis and treatment of chronic insomnia. *Psychiatric Serv.* 2005;56:332-43.
8. Jackson C, Curtis JL. Sleep disorders. In: DiPiro JT, Talbert RL, Yee GC, et al., eds. *Pharmacotherapy: A Pathophysiologic Approach.* 6th ed. New York: McGraw Hill, Inc; 2005:1321-32.
9. Epstein DR, Bootzin RR. Insomnia. *Nurs Clin North Am.* 2002;37: 611-31.
10. Sateia MJ, Pigeon WR. Identification and management of insomnia. *Med Clin North Am.* 2004;88:567-96.
11. STAT!Ref Online Electronic Medical Library [database online]. Diphenhydramine. In: McEvoy GK, ed. *AHFS Drug Information 2005.* Bethesda, Md: American Society of Health-System Pharmacists, Incorporated. Updated March 15, 2005.
12. Stepanski EJ, Wyatt JK. Use of sleep hygiene in the treatment of insomnia. *Sleep Med Rev.* 2003;7:215-25.

13. STAT!Ref Online Electronic Medical Library [database online]. Antihistamine drugs. In: McEvoy GK, ed. *AHFS Drug Information 2005*. Bethesda, Md: American Society of Health-System Pharmacists, Incorporated. Updated March 15, 2005.
14. STAT!Ref Online Electronic Medical Library [database online]. Doxylamine. In: McEvoy GK, ed. *AHFS Drug Information 2005*. Bethesda, Md: American Society of Health-System Pharmacists, Incorporated. Updated March 15, 2005.
15. Glass JR, Sproule BA, Herrmann N, et al. Acute pharmacological effects of temazepam, diphenhydramine, and valerian in healthy elderly subjects. *J Clin Psychopharmacol*. 2003;23:260-8.
16. Baker AM, Johnson DG, Levisky JA, et al. Fatal diphenhydramine intoxication in infants. *J Forensic Sci*. 2003;48:425-8.
17. Basu R, Dodge H, Stoehr GP, et al. Sedative-hypnotic use of diphenhydramine in a rural, older adult, community-based cohort: effects on cognition. *Am J Geriatr Psychiatry*. 2003;11:205-13.
18. Bockholdt B, Klug E, Schneider V. Suicide through doxylamine poisoning. *Forensic Sci Int*. 2001;119:138-40.
19. Zareba W, Moss AJ, Rosero SZ, et al. Electrocardiographic findings in patients with diphenhydramine overdose. *Am J Cardiol*. 1997;80:1168-73.
20. Fick DM, Cooper JW, Wade WE, et al. Updating the Beer's criteria for potentially inappropriate medication use in older adults. *Arch Intern Med*. 2003;163:2716-24.
21. Lessard E, Yessine MA, Hamelin BA, et al. Diphenhydramine alters the disposition of venlafaxine through inhibition of CYP2D6 activity in humans. *J Clin Psychopharmacol*. 2001;21:175-84.
22. Hamelin BA, Bouayad A, Methot J, et al. Significant interaction between the nonprescription antihistamine diphenhydramine and the CYP2D6 substrate metoprolol in healthy men with high or low CYP2D6 activity. *Clin Pharmacol Ther*. 2000;67:466-77.
23. National Center for Complementary and Alternative Medicine. Available at: http://nccam.nih.gov. Accessed July 20, 2005.
24. Buscemi N, Vandermeer B, Pandya R, et al. Melatonin for Treatment of Sleep Disorders. Summary. Evidence Report/Technology Assessment No. 108 (Prepared by the University of Alberta Evidence-based Practice Center, under Contract No. 290-02-0023.) AHRQ Publication No. 05-E002-1. Rockville, Md: Agency for Healthcare Research and Quality; November 2004.
25. Smits MG, van Stel HF, van der Heijden K, et al. Melatonin improves health status and sleep in children with idiopathic chronic sleep-onset insomnia: a randomized placebo controlled trial. *J Am Acad Child Adolesc Psychaitry*. 2003;42:1286-93.
26. Ross C, Davies P, Whitehouse W. Melatonin treatment for sleep disorders in children with neurodevelopmental disorders: an observational study. *Dev Med Child Neurol*. 2002;44:339-44.
27. Armour D, Paton C. Melatonin in the treatment of insomnia in children and adolescents. *Psychiatric Bull*. 2004;28:222-4.
28. Johnson K, Page A, Williams H, et al. The use of melatonin as an alternative to sedation in uncooperative children undergoing an MRI examination. *Clin Radiol*. 2002;57:502-6.
29. Samarkandi A, Naguib M, Riad W, et al. Melatonin vs. midazolam premedication in children: a double-blind, placebo-controlled study. *Eur J Anaesthesiol*. 2005;22:189-96.
30. US Food and Drug Administration Office of Health Affairs "Dear Colleague" Letter Regarding Research on Eosinophilia-mylagia Syndrome and Current Regulatory Status of L-tryptophan. September 3, 1992. Available at: http://www.cfsan.fda.gov/~dms/ds-ltr3.html. Accessed on August 24, 2005.
31. US Food and Drug Administration Center for Food Safety and Applied Nutrition Information Paper on L-Tryptophan and 5-hydroxy-L-Tryptophan. February 2001. Available at: http://www.cfsan.fda.gov/~dms/ds-tryp1.html. Accessed July 20, 2005.
32. Hadley S, Petry JJ. Valerian. *Am Fam Physician*. 2003;67:1755-8.
33. Ziegler-G, Ploch M, Miettinen-Baumann A, et al. Efficacy and tolerability of valerian extract LI 156 compared with oxazepam in the treatment of non-organic insomnia: a randomized, double-blind, comparative clinical study. *Eur J Med Res*. 2002;7:480-6.
34. Garges HP, Vana I, Doraiswamy PM. Cardiac complications and delirium associated with valerian root withdrawal. *JAMA*.1998; 280:1566-7.
35. US Food and Drug Administration Center for Food Safety and Applied Nutrition Consumer Advisory on Kava-Containing Dietary Supplements May Be Associated with Severe Liver Injury, March 25, 2002. Available at: http://www.cfsan.fda.gov/~dms/addskava.html. Accessed August 24, 2005.
36. Gyllenhaal C, Merritt SL, Peterson SD, et al. Efficacy and safety of herbal stimulants and sedatives in sleep disorders. *Sleep Med Rev*. 2000;4:229-51.
37. Roehrs T, Roth T. Sleep, sleepiness, sleep disorders and alcohol use and abuse. *Sleep Med Rev*. 2001;5:287-97.
38. Drake CL, Roehrs T, Roth T. Insomnia causes, consequences, and therapeutics: an overview. *Depression Anxiety*. 2003;18:163-76.
39. Kudo Y, Kurihara M. Clinical evaluation of diphenhydramine hydrochloride for the treatment of insomnia in psychiatric patients: a double-blind study. *J Clin Pharmacol*. 1990;30:1041-8.
40. Roehrs T, Zwyghuizen-Doorenbos A, Roth T. Sedative effects and plasma concentrations following single doses of triazolam, diphenhydramine, ethanol, and placebo. *Sleep*. 1993;16:301-5.
41. Martin SA, Aikens JE, Chervin RD. Toward cost-effectiveness analysis in the diagnosis and treatment of insomnia. *Sleep Med Rev*. 2004;8:63-72.
42. Walsh JK, Engelhardt CL. The direct economic costs of insomnia in the United States for 1995. *Sleep*. 1999;22(suppl 2):S386-93.

CHAPTER 49

# Drowsiness and Fatigue

*Robert J. Anderson and Diane Nykamp*

Drowsiness and fatigue can increase the risk of work-related or driving-related accidents, as well as adversely impact productivity. The U.S. National Highway Traffic Safety Administration estimates that a staggering 100,000 auto accidents annually are caused principally by drowsiness and fatigue; estimates of injuries resulting from driver fatigue are an additional 71,000 per year.[1] In fact, the negative impact of sleep deprivation on driving performance is equivalent to driving legally drunk.[2] A study of medical interns demonstrated a significant increase in both automobile accidents and near misses after working extended shifts in the hospital.[3] Caffeine is the most frequently used central nervous system (CNS) stimulant in the world. In this chapter its beneficial and harmful effects are discussed. In addition, several herbal medications, increasingly being used for "energy and alertness," are reviewed.

The primary sources of daily caffeine intake in the diet are coffee (50-130 mg/5 oz), tea (25-50 mg/5 oz), and soft drinks (30-60 mg/12 oz). The per capita consumption of caffeine from all sources is estimated to be 3 to 7 mg/kg/day[4] with a moderate intake generally defined as less than 300 mg/day. The average daily intake of caffeine in adults is 200 mg with the majority from coffee; children and young adults the average daily intake is 50 mg with the majority from tea or soft drinks.[5] Caffeine is an ingredient in many nonprescription, prescription, and herbal medications. Indeed, it is the sum total of our daily intake of caffeine from all sources that may lead to adverse effects, withdrawal reactions, or rarely, drug interactions.

## Etiology of Drowsiness and Fatigue

Daytime drowsiness and fatigue are often caused by inadequate sleep. Caffeine as a supplement, or in dietary form, is not a substitute for adequate sleep. Before recommending any caffeine-containing nonprescription product, the pharmacist should also rule out any drug-induced cause of daytime drowsiness and fatigue. Consumption of excessive amounts of caffeine in medications or dietary sources can paradoxically cause daytime drowsiness by impairing sleep.

## Treatment of Drowsiness and Fatigue

### *Treatment Goals*

The goal in treating daytime drowsiness and fatigue is to identify and eliminate the underlying cause to improve mental alertness and productivity. The algorithm in Figure 49-1 outlines the approach to self-treatment.

### *General Treatment Approach*

Many consumers use dietary sources of caffeine, such as coffee, tea, or carbonated soft drinks, to self-treat occasional symptoms of fatigue and drowsiness. If dietary sources are not available, or inconvenient to use, nonprescription caffeine-containing products may be used. However, if drowsiness and fatigue are chronic symptoms, especially with adequate sleep, a referral to a physician or specialist may be indicated. Medical conditions such as hypothyroidism (especially in women), anemia, and sleep apnea often present with similar symptoms.

### *Nonpharmacologic Therapy*

Good sleep hygiene principles should be emphasized (see Table 48-3 in Chapter 48).

### *Pharmacologic Therapy (Caffeine)*

#### Mechanism of Action and Pharmacokinetics

Caffeine is a xanthine derivative that acts as a nonselective competitive antagonist of A1 and A2A receptors of adenosine.[6] An increase in the concentration of adenosine in the brain, especially during prolonged wakefulness, is theorized to be the cause of early morning grogginess. By reversing the effects of adenosine, caffeine exerts its pharmacologic effect by increasing arousal, decreasing fatigue, and elevating mood. Secondary effects on other neurotransmitters may also increase alertness.

An oral dose of 1 mg/kg of caffeine (equivalent to 1 cup of coffee or a low nonprescription dose) results in a maximum peak plasma concentration of 1 to 2 mg/L. Caffeine is rapidly and completely absorbed, reaching a peak concentration within 30 minutes.[7] It is water soluble with a rapid and wide distribution to nearly every tissue in the body with an almost immediate effect on alertness. The elimination half-life is generally 3 to 5 hours; however, the metabolism of caffeine may be influenced by prior ingestion of caffeine, gender, smoking status, and other drugs.[8]

As a xanthine derivative, caffeine possesses weak bronchodilation action. Caffeine also stimulates the sympathetic nervous system resulting in the release of norepinephrine, epinephrine, and renin. In cardiac tissue, caffeine has a positive inotropic effect on the myocardium and a positive chronotropic effect on the sinoatrial node

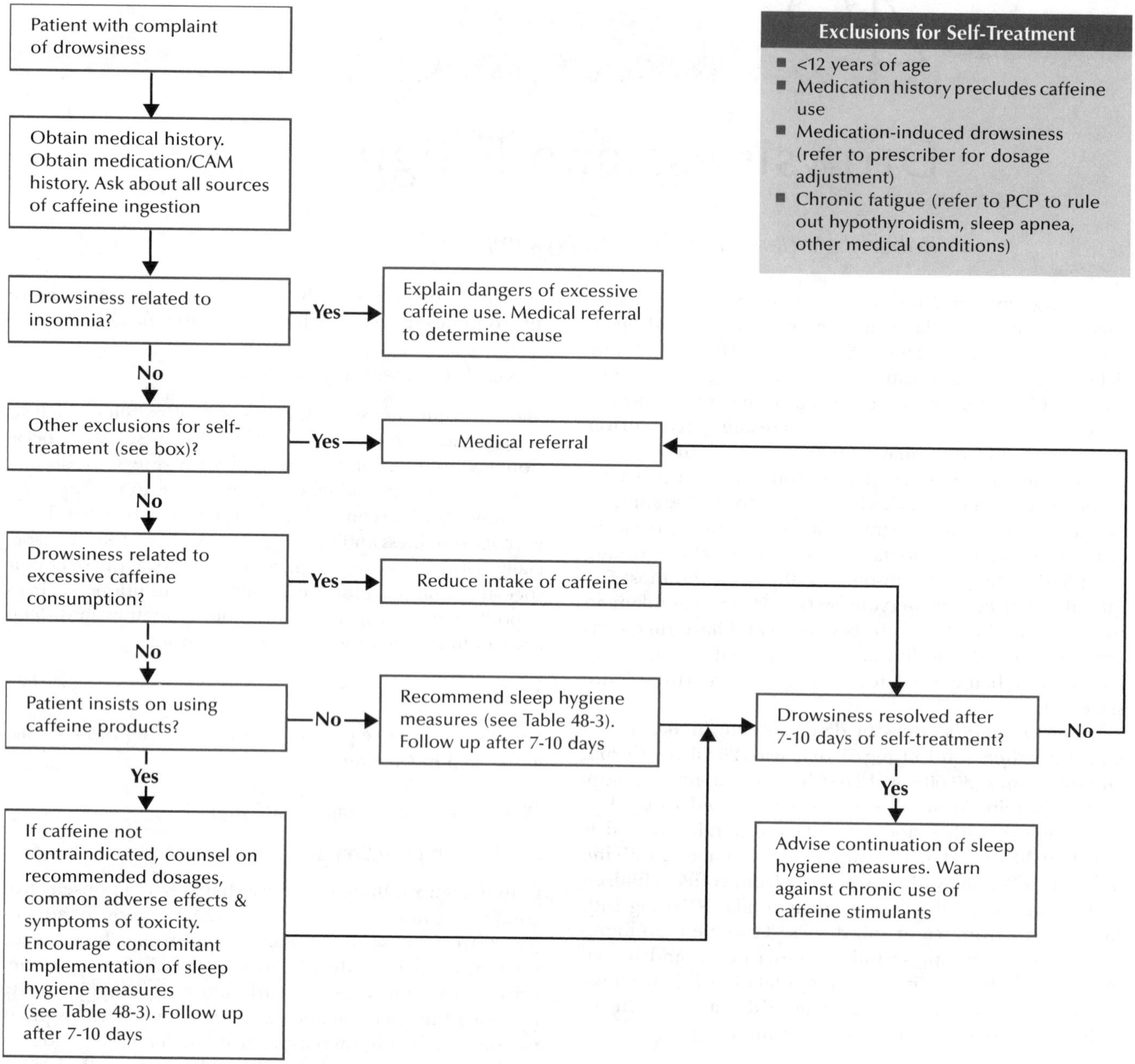


**FIGURE 49-1** Self-care of drowsiness and fatigue. CAM, complementary and alternative medicine; PCP, primary care provider.

that results in a transient increase in heart rate, force of contraction, and cardiac output. It can cause modest increases in blood pressure and may also increase the secretion of hydrochloric acid and pepsin, and relax the lower esophageal sphincter (LES), which could aggravate symptoms of peptic ulcer disease, gastric reflux, or esophagitis. Caffeine can increase sodium, calcium, and water excretion and exerts a mild diuretic effect. High intake and prolonged use of caffeine may increase the risk of calcium oxalate stone formation in patients with a history of kidney stones.[9]

## Indications and Dosage

Caffeine is the only nonprescription stimulant approved by the Food and Drug Administration (FDA) and is commonly available in doses of 200 mg. Table 49-1 lists selected trade-name caffeine-only products. The labeled dose of most nonprescription supplements is 100 to 200 mg every 3 to 4 hours as needed, to a maximum daily dose of 600 mg. Used as a CNS stimulant, caffeine is marketed to help fatigued patients to stay awake and restore mental alertness. Many consumers take caffeine to reduce fatigue or increase their alertness. Examples may include shift workers with irregular work patterns, overnight truck drivers, soldiers on active duty, medical residents on call at the hospital, or students studying late for an exam.

The effects of caffeine on daytime performance in alert individuals is unclear, and may depend on the type of task and prior state of alertness. Studies[10,11] suggest that regular use of caffeine in doses of 2 to 4 mg/kg/day is

**TABLE 49-1 Selected Caffeine Products**

| Trade Name | Caffeine Content (mg) |
|---|---|
| **Nonprescription Caffeine-only Products** | |
| Keep Alert | 200 |
| Keep Going | 200 |
| Maximum Strength NoDoz | 200 |
| Vivarin | 200 |
| **Nonprescription Combination Products** | |
| Anacin Caplets/Tab | 32 |
| Anacin Maximum Strength Tablet | 32 |
| BC Powder Arthritis Strength | 38 |
| BC Powder Original Formula | 33.3 |
| Excedrin ASA Free Caplets/Gel Tabs | 65 |
| Excedrin Extra Strength Gel Tabs/Tabs | 65 |
| Excedrin Migraine | 65 |
| Excedrin Quick Tabs | 65 |
| Goody's Extra Strength | 32.5 |
| Midol Maximum Strength Menstrual Caplets/Gelcaps | 60 |
| Vanquish Caplets | 33 |
| **Prescription Combination Products** | |
| Butalbital | 40 |
| Butalbital Compound | 40 |
| Cafergot | 100 |
| Darvon Compound 65 | 32.4 |
| Esqic | 40 |
| Esqic Plus | 40 |
| Fioricet | 40 |
| Fiorinal | 40 |
| Fioricet with Codeine | 40 |
| Synalgos-DC | 30 |
| Wigraine Tablets | 100 |

*Note:* Information is not all-inclusive. Products may have changed formulations or caffeine content since time of publication.

most effective in improving performance on simple, routine, repetitive tasks that require sustained attention when alertness is reduced, often because of inadequate sleep or excessive daily stress. The dose-related response is such that "high users" of caffeine exhibit a better response; however, this benefit is offset by an increase in the incidence of side effects. For example, in one study, a 70 mg dose of caffeine improved hand steadiness and reduced fatigue, but a 250 mg dose decreased hand steadiness and increased jitteriness.[12]

The effect of low doses of caffeine (12.5-100 mg) versus placebo on cognitive performance and mood was measured in consumers with low, moderate, and habitual caffeine intake.[13] All doses of caffeine affected cognitive performance favorably; tolerance was not found to have an effect on performance or mood in the regular users of caffeine.

The positive effect of caffeine on performance appears to be maintained throughout the day. A randomized crossover study compared the effects of 1 or 2 cups of tea (37.5 mg/cup) or coffee (75 mg/cup) versus water administered four times during the day.[14] At all doses, and regardless of source, caffeine improved cognitive and psychomotor performance throughout the day and evening. As expected, the higher doses significantly and negatively impacted the ability to sleep. Lower doses of caffeine found in tea provided benefits similar to coffee but without disrupting sleep patterns.

Can caffeine improve our alertness and performance to minimize traffic accidents? A double-blind study compared the effects of 200 mg of caffeine versus placebo on driving performance and sleepiness in a driving simulator during early morning hours.[15] After "restricted sleep," caffeine reduced early morning sleepiness for approximately 2 hours; after "no sleep," caffeine delayed sleep by only 30 minutes. Thus, it is important to counsel patients that caffeine cannot compensate for inadequate sleep.

A common antidote for excess alcohol ingestion is an increased intake of strong black coffee. How effective is caffeine in neutralizing alcohol-induced impairment of automobile driving? In a randomized, double-blind study the effect of caffeine (200 and 400 mg) versus placebo on driving performance was measured in a driving simulator in alcohol-impaired adults.[16] Both doses of caffeine were effective in counteracting "brake latency" but did not counteract other driving impairments caused by the alcohol.

What is the effect of caffeine on athletic performance? Caffeine in doses varying from 4 to 10 mg/kg has improved athletic performance in endurance events such as cycling,[17] tennis,[18] swimming,[19] and rowing[20] and may impact outcomes in competitions. The mechanism of action for caffeine may be enhanced muscle metabolism with an increase in free fatty acid concentrations as an energy source, and a delay in the utilization of glycogen stores.[21]

The International Olympics Committee has a maximum allowable level of urinary caffeine set at 12 mg/L, equivalent to approximately 3 to 6 cups of coffee. Above this level, caffeine is considered "doping." However, great interindividual variation in caffeine elimination exists, with the potential to cause some athletes to fail drug tests, especially if dietary sources are combined with prescription, nonprescription or diet supplements that also contain caffeine.

## Safety Considerations

Caffeine taken in higher doses (5-8 mg/kg) can cause both cardiovascular and CNS side effects that may be manifested as increases in heart rate and blood pressure, as well as headache, symptoms of anxiety and insomnia, and an increase in hand tremor. Excessive dietary intake of caffeine has been reported to produce frequent headaches in children and adolescents.[22]

Patients who are more likely to experience adverse effects include (1) those “naïve” to caffeine use,[23] (2) patients of advanced age,[24] (3) females, especially those who are “caffeine naive” and nonsmokers,[25] and (4) people prone to anxiety or panic attacks.[26] Pharmacists should counsel these patients to temper their use of caffeine-containing nonprescription products in combination with dietary sources or drugs that also contain caffeine (Table 49-1). The overuse of caffeine should be a part of the medication and dietary history in patients with persistent headache.

Rapid tolerance to the effects on respiratory and cardiovascular systems is common with caffeine even in low to moderate doses[27] possibly because of an upregulation of the adenosine receptors.[28] Habitual caffeine drinkers who routinely consume as little as 1 to 2 cups of coffee (or 80-160 mg caffeine per day) and abruptly discontinue may experience mild signs and symptoms of withdrawal. Common symptoms include a throbbing headache, fatigue, or anxiety that may start within 12 hours after cessation. Symptoms usually peak in 24 to 48 hours but may persist up to 7 days.[29] The etiology of rebound or migraine headaches is often caffeine withdrawal especially in adults or children with prolonged high-dose ingestion, and should be incorporated into the medication history.

In a preliminary study of prepubertal children, withdrawal and physical dependence-like symptoms were reported to occur if caffeine was consumed at 150 mg/day (or four times their normal intake) over a 2-week period of time.[30] Withdrawal symptoms in neonates have been reported after excessive (>800 mg/day) chronic maternal ingestion of caffeine.[31]

Caffeine is eliminated in the liver via the P450 CYP 1A2 isoenzyme[32]; the primary demethylated metabolite is paraxanthine, which predominantly exerts a sympathomimetic effect. An exaggerated pharmacologic effect can occur when nonprescription caffeine is combined with other sources commonly found in the diet, or with prescription or nonprescription medications that contain caffeine (Table 49-1). Caffeine may increase the absorption of aspirin, which explains the rationale for its use in many headache formulations. Medications for headache and pain often contain 30 to 100 mg of caffeine per dose.

A recent study by Nesher and others[33] suggests that caffeine may interfere with the anti-inflammatory effect of methotrexate in patients with rheumatoid arthritis. Patients who were taking lower doses of caffeine (<120 mg/day) had 30% more improvement in joint pain and morning stiffness than those on higher doses of caffeine (>180 mg/day). The caffeine effect as an adenosine receptor antagonist may interfere with the anti-inflammatory action of methotrexate. High caffeine intake from a social and medication history should be ruled out as a cause of treatment failure. Until more studies are completed, patients on methotrexate therapy for rheumatoid arthritis should be counseled to avoid routine use of nonprescription caffeine supplements and limit their daily dietary intake of caffeine.

The CYP 1A2 isoenzyme can be induced or inhibited by other drugs. The routine use of high doses of caffeine (>400 mg/day) may saturate the binding sites and increase the risk of interactions with drugs that share this metabolic pathway. For example, case reports indicated that higher doses of caffeine may competitively inhibit the metabolism of the atypical antipsychotic clozapine,[34,35] thus increasing its toxicity in some patients. Once stabilized on a clozapine dose, patients should be cautioned to avoid drastic changes in caffeine intake until more definitive information is available.

Cigarette smoking is a strong inducer of the CYP 1A2 isoenzyme. Smoking cessation will cause a decrease in the elimination of caffeine and a potential increase in caffeine side effects.[36] Conversely, oral contraceptives can inhibit the CYP 1A2 isoenzyme and may increase caffeine side effects.[37] This may be partially responsible for gender differences in caffeine sensitivity. Ciprofloxacin and fluvoxamine are examples of other drugs that strongly inhibit CYP 1A2. While the clinical significance of these interactions is unknown, at-risk patients should be cautioned to moderate their use of caffeine, and the pharmacist should monitor for signs of toxicity.

Patients with existing coronary heart disease, uncontrolled hypertension, or preexisting arrhythmias should be counseled to avoid nonprescription caffeine-containing preparations and to moderate their intake of dietary caffeine.

Several studies investigating the cardiovascular effects of caffeine intake in both healthy males[38] and females[39] have concluded that there was no increased risk for coronary artery disease, hypertension, myocardial infarction,[40] or cardiac arrythmias.[41] Even high caffeine intake (an average of 5.6 cups of coffee per day) in Finnish men did not increase the risk of coronary heart disease or death.[42]

A small increase in blood pressure has been demonstrated in healthy individuals and patients with hypertension after the consumption of caffeine.[43] Lane and others[44] found that a relatively high dose of 500 mg of caffeine in healthy, nonsmoking, habitual coffee drinkers significantly raised systolic blood pressure by 4 mm Hg, diastolic blood pressure by 3 mm Hg, and heart rate by 2 beats per minute. The increase in blood pressure is not clinically significant in healthy individuals without hypertension who may adapt to the cardiovascular effects possibly because of tolerance. An average caffeine intake of 2 cups per day (<200 mg/day) in a large physician group during a period of 33 years was not found to be a risk factor for the development of hypertension.[45]

Patients with a history of coronary heart disease, especially those of advanced age and those who are not daily consumers of caffeine, may be more susceptible to increases in blood pressure and heart rate. Though habitual users of caffeine may develop a tolerance to the cardiovascular effects, routine higher daily doses may cause an increase in blood pressure. The clinical significance of these physiological changes on the risk of cardiac complications is unknown.

Patients should be cautioned about excessive consumption of caffeine in energy sports drinks and/or diet weight loss supplements. Caffeine has replaced ephedra and ma huang in many weight-loss products. Natural caffeine, other methylxanthines and caffeine-containing herbs like guarana, green tea, mate and cola nut, are

**TABLE 49-2 Caffeine Content in Selected Dietary Supplements and Sports Energy Drinks**

| Trade Name | Caffeine Content (mg) per Serving |
|---|---|
| **Dietary Supplements** | |
| Dexatrim Natural | 50 |
| Dexatrim Max | 50 |
| Hydroxycut | 200* |
| Metabolift | 176† |
| Xenadrine NRG | 300‡ |
| Xtreme Lean | Unknown§ |
| **Sports Energy Drinks** | |
| Amp Energy | 77 |
| Full Throttle | 150 |
| KMX | 53 |
| Red Bull | 80 |
| SoBe Adrenalin Rush‖ | 79 |
| SoBe No Fear¶ | 158 |

* As determined by guarana extract content plus unlisted amount of caffeine anhydrous.

† Total amount of methylxanthines from natural sources.

‡ As determined by guarana extract content.

§ Contains bitter orange, methylxanthines, synephrine, and yerba mate.

‖ Also contains 50 mg Panax ginseng.

¶ Also contains 25 mg guarana and 25 mg Panax ginseng.

*Note:* Information is not all-inclusive. Products may have changed formulations or caffeine content since time of publication.

common ingredients in products that are marketed to the young consumer for energy or weight loss, but the caffeine content is often not listed on the label. Table 49-2 lists the amount of caffeine that is contained in both selected weight-loss dietary supplements and sports energy drinks. The amount of caffeine found in most products is usually equivalent to, or greater than, 1 cup of coffee, or more than twice the level of caffeine contained in a can of carbonated cola. Guarana contains an even more concentrated dose of caffeine (200 mg), which can more easily lead to adverse effects when consumed in high doses or combined with other sources of caffeine commonly found in the diet or in nonprescription or prescription medications.

## Product Selection Guidelines

*Special Populations* Table 49-3 lists the safe amount of daily caffeine intake for special populations.

Pregnant and Breastfeeding Patients Caffeine is classified in FDA Pregnancy Category B, and freely crosses the placenta. Does caffeine decrease fertility, increase the risk of miscarriage, or growth retardation to the fetus? A recent review of the literature has concluded that moderate caffeine consumption (<300 mg/day) has little or no effect on the ability to conceive among nonsmoking women.[46] Likewise there appears to be no association between caffeine consumption (up to 300 mg/day) and the risk of miscarriage,[47] though higher consumption has been associated with an increased risk.[48-50]

**TABLE 49-3 Guidelines on Safe Total Daily Intake of Caffeine in Special Populations**

| | |
|---|---|
| Pregnancy | <300 mg |
| Breast-feeding | 200-300 mg |
| Advanced age | <300 mg |
| Heart disease | <200 mg |

Recent studies[51,52] have not found an association between moderate caffeine consumption and reduced birth weight, gestational age, or fetal growth. High caffeine consumption (>300 mg/day) during pregnancy has been associated with a higher risk of fetal growth retardation,[53,54] especially during the third trimester.[55] It would be prudent to limit total daily caffeine intake to less than 300 mg during pregnancy. A nonprescription caffeine-containing product should not be recommended during pregnancy because combined with dietary sources it would likely increase the total daily intake to over the 300 mg maximum amount.

The American Academy of Pediatrics considers usual amounts of caffeine in the diet to be compatible with breast-feeding.[56] Caffeine is readily excreted into breast milk but does not affect milk production. The quantity of caffeine in breast milk after maternal ingestion of coffee has been estimated to be 1.5 to 3.0 mg/cup consumed.[57] The range of milk concentration of caffeine is thought to be related to the mother's ability to metabolize caffeine.[8] Peak caffeine concentration in breast milk occurs 1 hour after maternal consumption. Neonates eliminate caffeine very slowly.[23] Infants unable to metabolize caffeine or those who receive large quantities of caffeine via the breast milk may have symptoms of nervousness, increased heart rate, sleeplessness, poor feeding, and irritability. Women who breast-feed should be advised to consume caffeine in small to moderate amounts preferably after breast-feeding to minimize effects of caffeine on the neonate.

Children/Adolescents Children are more susceptible to the cardiovascular and CNS side effects of caffeine because of their lower body weight. For children and adolescents in the United States, the average caffeine intake is 0.7 mg/kg/day, with large individual variations.[4] Soft drink consumption in adolescents has more than tripled in the past three decades.[59] In a recent study[60] in adolescents, a dose of more than 100 mg of caffeine per day (approximately three to four cans of soda) significantly increased systolic pressure, especially in an African American group. The impact of caffeine from soft drinks on the development of hypertension (and obesity) at an early age requires further study.

Castellanos and others[61] completed a literature review on the behavioral effects of caffeine in children, concluding that the effects are modest at best. Based on available evidence to date, the maximum recommended daily intake of caffeine in children is less than 2.5 mg/kg/day.[62] nonprescription caffeine products are not indicated in children under age 12 years.

Patients of Advanced Age The elimination half-life of caffeine is prolonged in patients of advance age,[24] thus increasing their susceptibility to an exaggerated pharmacologic effect and interference with sleep. It is not recommended that these patients consume caffeine in the diet or as an ingredient in a medication after dinner.

Concerns have been expressed that chronic high doses of caffeine may reduce bone mineral density (BMD) in women and increase the risk of osteoporosis and fractures. The mechanism of action was thought to be a result of decreased absorption of calcium and/or increased calcium excretion. The results of studies discount the presence of a link between caffeine use and osteoporosis.[63-65] The effect of caffeine on calcium absorption is minimal, with no adverse effect on urinary calcium excretion.[66] High caffeine intake may be a surrogate marker for low calcium intake. No evidence exists that caffeine, even in high doses, decreases BMD in healthy patients taking daily recommended amounts of calcium.

Tea may be protective against osteoporosis. In addition to caffeine, tea contains fluoride and many beneficial nutrients such as flavonoids. Hegarty and others,[67] studying elderly females in the United Kingdom, found that those who consumed tea had higher BMD measurements than those who did not. A Taiwanese study of men and women over the age of 30 years determined that habitual tea drinkers had an increased BMD.[68]

## Complementary Therapies

### Ginseng

The Chinese herb, ginseng, is frequently used as an adaptogen or tonic to boost "physical and mental energy and a sense of well being." There are two species—*Panax ginseng,* which is the source plant for Asian ginseng (also sold as Chinese, Oriental, Korean, or Panax ginseng), and *Panax quinquefolius,* which is the source plant of American ginseng. Asian ginseng is more common and purported to have stronger "antifatigue" properties than American ginseng. The active ingredients are thought to be multiple ginsenosides, which are saponins, or triterpenoid glycosides. Different ginenosides appear to exert different pharmacologic effects.

As with most herbal products, quality control issues may adversely impact both efficacy and incidence of side effects. ConsumerLab[69] tested quality and purity of 12 Panax ginseng products and found that 10 met test criteria for quality, label claims, lack of contaminants, and disintegration. One product contained pesticide contaminants and the other "extra-strength" labeled product contained less than 10% of the expected ginsenoside.

A review of randomized controlled trials reveals weak and contradictory scientific evidence to support claims of enhanced mental and physical performance. Two months of Panax ginseng at either 200 or 400 mg/day in healthy men and women had no effect on mental outlook or mood.[70] Other studies using similar doses and duration of therapy showed minimal[71] or no differences[72] in mental performance. Ellis and others[73] compared the effect on quality of life of *P. ginseng* (200 mg/day) versus placebo in a randomized, double-blind study. At 4 weeks, the ginseng group demonstrated improved aspects of social functioning compared with placebo. However, these beneficial effects did not persist at 8 weeks, and the incidence of mild side effects was 33% with the herb versus 17% with the placebo.

The recommended dose for ginseng is 100 mg of an extract standardized to over 5% ginsenoside taken twice daily; the equivalent daily dose of the dried root is approximately 2 g.[74] Because of potential effects in animal studies on the hypothalamic-pituitary-axis, long-term continuous use for longer than 2 months is not recommended. Most side effects are mild and transient, and have been reported only at higher than recommended doses including skin rash, headache, nervousness, tachycardia, fever, sleep, and gastrointestinal disorders.

Ginseng possesses weak estrogenic activity, and may cause breast tenderness and vaginal bleeding in some women. Its use is contraindicated in pregnancy, during lactation, and in patients with hypertension and acute infections.

Ginseng may potentially interact with caffeine, warfarin, antidepressants, lithium, and oral hypoglycemics/insulin. Ginseng may inhibit thromboxane formation in vitro[75] and thus possesses a weak antiplatelet effect, increasing the risk of bleeding with concurrent use of warfarin. There are conflicting in vivo reports on a potential warfarin-ginseng interaction perhaps because of study design or type of ginseng. One study[76] in healthy volunteers demonstrated that American ginseng may lower international normalized ratio (INR) while another did not detect any adverse impact of Korean ginseng on warfarin pharmacokinetics or pharmacodynamics.[77] Until more definitive information is available, patients maintained on warfarin should avoid use of ginseng.

The Rb1 ginsenoside has psychoactive effects that may exacerbate mania when it is combined with monoamine oxidase (MAO) inhibitors, tricyclic antidepressants, and lithium. In one case, a young healthy male with no history of psychiatric illness took 500 to 750 mg of Chinese ginseng root daily for 2 months and developed mania; the manic symptoms slowly reversed with treatment.[78] It would appear prudent to avoid ginseng in patients with a history of any psychiatric illness.

Animal studies suggest that natural glycans found in both *Panax* species may exhibit hypoglycemic effects. Vuksan and others[79] reported their results in a small study of nine subjects with type 2 diabetes. They demonstrated administration of a very high dose of American ginseng (3 g) taken prior to or with a glucose challenge significantly decreased postprandial blood glucose. The mechanism is unknown, but the study results suggest that caution should be exercised with all high-dose ginseng products in people with diabetes.

## Assessment of Drowsiness and Fatigue: A Case-based Approach

When assessing a patient with a complaint of daytime drowsiness, the practitioner should determine the etiology of the patient's fatigue. Evaluating the patient's medical or psychiatric problems, current medication use, dietary caffeine consumption, sleep patterns, and lifestyle will help in determining the underlying cause. Given the paucity of data supporting the efficacy of caffeine, the side effects associated with recommended doses, and the effects of excessive doses of caffeine, practitioners should usually recommend improved sleep hygiene and lifestyle modifications or medical referral before recommending the use of a caffeine-containing product. Cases 49-1 and 49-2 provide examples of the assessment of patients with drowsiness and fatigue.

### CASE 49-1

| Relevant Evaluation Criteria | Scenario/Model Outcome |
|---|---|
| **Information Gathering** | |
| 1. Gather essential information about the patient's symptoms, including: | |
| a. description of symptom(s) (i.e., nature, onset, duration, severity, associated symptoms) | Patient picks up new prescription for ciprofloxacin and is also requesting an OTC stimulant to help stay awake during her 6-hour car ride for a business meeting for this weekend. She states that she gets very drowsy when she drives for long periods of time. |
| b. description of any factors that seem to precipitate, exacerbate, and/or relieve the patient's symptom(s) | On questioning, patient relates that it has been a long year with much travel and stress in her job and at home. |
| c. description of the patient's efforts to relieve the symptoms | Patient admits that she probably consumes too much caffeine in her usual intake of coffee and soft drinks. The caffeine seems to keep her awake but she would like to minimize her fluid intake (and restroom stops) for this trip. |
| 2. Gather essential patient history information: | |
| a. patient's identity | Fiona Ingols |
| b. patient's age, sex, height, and weight | 48 y/o female, 5'6", 130 lb |
| c. patient's occupation | Elementary educational consultant who frequently travels the region by car |
| d. patient's dietary habits | Healthy low-fat diet; consumes at least 2 cups of coffee in the morning and 3-4 colas in the afternoon |
| e. patient's sleep habits | Stays up late and sleeps an average of 5-6 hours per night as allowed by her schedule |
| f. concurrent medical conditions, prescription and nonprescription medications, and dietary supplements | Estrogen patch for hot flashes; iron tablets for anemia; Excedrin Migraine or naproxen for headache; methotrexate for rheumatoid arthritis; folic acid as supplement with methotrexate; ciprofloxacin (new prescription) for UTI; Protonix for GERD |
| g. allergies | Penicillin |
| h. history of other adverse reactions to medications | None |
| i. other (describe)_______ | Quit smoking 3 days ago (used to smoke ~5 cigarettes a day); hysterectomy 3 years ago |
| **Assessment and Triage** | |
| 3. Differentiate the patient's signs/symptoms and correctly identify the patient's primary problem(s). | Drowsiness and fatigue before and during a long road trip |
| 4. Identify exclusions for self-treatment (see Figure 49-1). | None |

## CASE 49-1 (continued)

| Relevant Evaluation Criteria | Scenario/Model Outcome |
|---|---|
| 5. Formulate a comprehensive list of therapeutic alternatives for the primary problem to determine if triage to a medical practitioner is required, and share this information with the patient. | Options include:<br>(1) Identify the source of the fatigue: stress, anemia, or other medical cause.<br>(2) Recommend resting before beginning the trip.<br>(3) Recommend taking an OTC stimulant to prevent drowsiness and fatigue while driving.<br>(4) Take no action. |
| **Plan** | |
| 6. Select an optimal therapeutic alternative to address the patient's problem, taking into account patient preferences. | Instruct patient to rest if possible prior to the long drive and to take an OTC caffeine product such as NoDoz or Vivarin 200 mg every 3-4 hours (see Table 49-1). |
| 7. Describe the recommended therapeutic approach to the patient. | A caffeine dose of 200 mg every 3-4 hours will act as a stimulant and not produce adverse effects of irritability or nervousness as seen with higher doses. |
| 8. Explain to the patient the rationale for selecting the recommended therapeutic approach from the considered therapeutic alternatives. | Drug-drug interactions are present and may be significant if you continue your dietary intake of caffeine in coffee and colas along with the OTC stimulants. |
| **Patient Education** | |
| 9. When recommending self-care with nonprescription medications and/or nondrug therapy, convey accurate information to the patient, including: | |
| a. appropriate dose and frequency of administration | NoDoz or Vivarin 200 mg every 3-4 hours to a maximum of 600 mg |
| b. maximum number of days the therapy should be employed | Only during the 12-hour trip |
| c. product administration procedures | As above |
| d. expected time to onset of relief | With usage of agent, improvement in alertness should be noticed in 30 minutes. Patient should be counseled that effect of caffeine stimulant is minimal with inadequate sleep and a subsequent increase in risk of motor vehicle accidents because of fatigue. |
| e. degree of relief that can be reasonably expected | Decrease in fatigue and increased alertness |
| f. most common side effects | Insomnia, nervousness, increase in pulse rate |
| g. side effects that warrant medical intervention should they occur | Chest pain or arrhythmias; combination of caffeine and ciprofloxacin (and perhaps estrogen) may cause adverse effects of caffeine such as increase in heart rate, anxiety, and fine hand tremor.<br>Combination of caffeine in the diet and OTC forms with methotrexate may reduce efficacy of methotrexate.<br>Combination of caffeine, iron, and naproxen may increase gastrointestinal distress.<br>Excessive caffeine may be aggravating GERD.<br>Patient's caffeine level from usual coffee and colas may be increased because of recent smoking cessation.<br>Headache may be caused by caffeine withdrawal. |
| h. patient options in the event that condition worsens or persists | Stop caffeine and see health care provider. |
| i. product storage requirements | Keep in original container. |
| j. specific nondrug measures | Patient should be advised to take frequent rest stops and exercise every 2 hours to increase circulation and mental alertness. |

## CASE 49-1 (continued)

| Relevant Evaluation Criteria | Scenario/Model Outcome |
|---|---|
| 10. Solicit patient's follow-up questions. | Could I double the dose of any of these products to get better more quickly? |
| 11. Answer patient's questions. | No. Doubling the dose will only increase your risk of experiencing unwanted side effects. |

Key: GERD, gastroesophageal reflux disease; OTC, over-the-counter; UTI, urinary tract infection.

## CASE 49-2

| Relevant Evaluation Criteria | Scenario/Model Outcome |
|---|---|
| **Information Gathering** | |
| 1. Gather essential information about the patient's symptoms, including: | |
| a. description of symptom(s) (i.e., nature, onset, duration, severity, associated symptoms) | Patient lacks energy and is easily fatigued. These symptoms have been chronic for the past 6 months. Patient has noticed recent onset of weight gain. Patient cannot take caffeine because of a history of GERD and requests a natural herbal energy booster as a substitute for her caffeine. |
| b. description of any factors that seem to precipitate, exacerbate, and/or relieve the patient's symptom(s) | On questioning, no factors seem to precipitate, exacerbate, or relieve Janet's symptoms. |
| c. description of the patient's efforts to relieve the symptoms | Patient has tried to exercise regularly and get an adequate amount of sleep. |
| 2. Gather essential patient history information: | |
| a. patient's identity | Janet Peers |
| b. patient's age, sex, height, and weight | 45 y/o F, 5'3", 145 lb |
| c. patient's occupation | Paralegal who works in a time-sensitive and pressured work environment |
| d. patient's dietary habits | Healthy diet |
| e. patient's sleep habits | Light sleeper who routinely gets 7-8 hours each night |
| f. concurrent medical conditions, prescription and nonprescription medications, and dietary supplements | Atrial fibrillation and mild depression; allergic rhinitis relieved by OTC Claritin as needed; warfarin (variable dose on alternate days); St. John's wort |
| g. allergies | NKDA |
| h. history of other adverse reactions to medications | Local anesthetics at dentist's office |
| i. other (describe)_______ | N/A |
| **Assessment and Triage** | |
| 3. Differentiate the patient's signs/symptoms and correctly identify the patient's primary problem(s). | Daytime drowsiness and fatigue with weight gain despite adequate sleep |
| 4. Identify exclusions for self-treatment (see Figure 49-1). | None |
| 5. Formulate a comprehensive list of therapeutic alternatives for the primary problem to determine if triage to a medical practitioner is required, and share this information with the patient. | Options include:<br>(1) Refer patient to PCP.<br>(2) Ask about recent INR results.<br>(3) Recommending a dietary supplement such as ginseng.<br>(4) Take no action. |

## CASE 49-2 (continued)

| Relevant Evaluation Criteria | Scenario/Model Outcome |
|---|---|
| **Plan** | |
| 6. Select an optimal therapeutic alternative to address the patient's problem, taking into account patient preferences. | Janet's fatigue is chronic and, therefore, requires a medical referral. |
| 7. Describe the recommended therapeutic approach to the patient. | Ginseng should not be used until the cause of your chronic fatigue is determined. |
| 8. Explain to the patient the rationale for selecting the recommended therapeutic approach from the considered therapeutic alternatives. | A medical referral is necessary. You have had long-term recurring symptoms with weight gain despite adequate diet and sleep. You may have hypothyroidism or even sleep apnea that may be causing a "restless" sleep. We need to reevaluate your ongoing need for St. John's wort and its possible interference with warfarin. |
| **Patient Education** | |
| 9. When recommending self-care with nonprescription medications and/or nondrug therapy, convey accurate information to the patient. | Criterion does not apply in this case. |
| 10. Solicit patient's follow-up questions. | Will a trial of ginseng be harmful to me? |
| 11. Answer patient's questions. | It is important to determine the cause of the fatigue and related symptoms such as weight gain and depression. Ginseng may increase the risk of bleeding if taken with warfarin. |

Key: GERD, gastroesophageal reflux disease; INR, international normalized ratio; N/A, not applicable; NKDA, no known drug allergies; OTC, over-the-counter; PCP, primary care provider.

## PATIENT EDUCATION FOR DROWSINESS AND FATIGUE

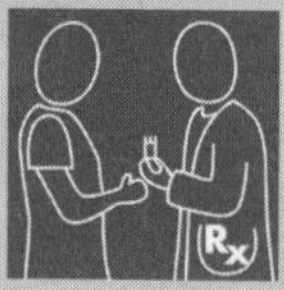

The objective of self-treatment is to maintain wakefulness. For most patients, improved sleep hygiene will help ensure optimal therapeutic outcomes. If the patient insists on taking a caffeine-containing product, carefully following product instructions and the self-care measures listed here will help ensure optimal therapeutic outcomes for most patients.

### Nondrug Measures

- Practice good principles of sleep hygiene. (See Table 48-3 in Chapter 48.)
- If drowsiness or fatigue persists or recurs, consult your primary care provider.

### Nonprescription Medications

- Do not exceed the recommended dose of 200 mg every 3 to 4 hours to a maximum daily dose of 600 mg. Note that higher doses of caffeine may cause side effects.
- Do not use caffeine tablets in combination with coffee or other caffeinated products including herbal products.
- Do not use if pregnant or breast-feeding.
- Do not use in children less than age 12.
- If you are taking methotrexate, clozapine, birth control pills, or ciprofloxacin, consult your pharmacist or primary care provider before using caffeine-containing products.
- If you have symptomatic gastroesophageal reflux disease (GERD) or a history of kidney stones, avoid caffeine supplements and minimize dietary intake.

⚠ If you have a history of peptic ulcer disease, psychiatric disorders, symptomatic heart disease, or uncontrolled hypertension, consult your primary care provider before using caffeine stimulants.

⚠ Seek medical attention immediately if symptoms of caffeine toxicity occur:

- Increases in heart rate and blood pressure
- Headache
- Symptoms of anxiety and insomnia
- Increase in hand tremor

## Patient Counseling for Fatigue and Drowsiness

Counseling on the treatment of drowsiness and fatigue should focus on practicing good sleep hygiene and eliminating factors that may interfere with normal sleep. If a caffeine product is indicated, the pharmacist should review dosage guidelines with the patient, and emphasize the adverse effects and drug interactions that can occur with its use. The patient should be counseled on symptoms of excessive caffeine ingestion such as irritability, tremor, rapid pulse, dizziness, or heart palpitations, especially in elderly patients with cardiac disease. Regular users of caffeine should also be counseled on withdrawal symptoms such as headache and anxiety, which can occur if caffeine from any source is stopped abruptly. The box Patient Education for Fatigue and Drowsiness lists information to provide to patients.

## Key Points for Fatigue and Drowsiness

- Caffeine in any form appears to be safe and effective in low to moderate doses in the diet and for occasional use as a nonprescription supplement while completing tasks of short duration when enhanced alertness is desired.
- Pregnant or breast-feeding patients, children less than age 12, patients with heart disease, or patients with anxiety or psychiatric disorders should limit their caffeine intake.
- Pharmacists should be aware of the various prescription, nonprescription, and diet supplements containing caffeine in addition to dietary consumption.
- Side effects are more likely to occur in occasional users and patients of advanced age while drug interactions can occur in those patients taking higher daily doses of caffeine with medications sharing a similar metabolic pathway.
- There is insufficient data for pharmacists to recommend the use of ginseng supplements for energy or fatigue.

## References


1. National Sleep Foundation Web site. Available at: www.sleepfoundation.org/activities/daafacts.cfm. Accessed December 13, 2004.
2. Williamson AM, Feyer AM. Moderate sleep deprivation produces impairments in cognitive and motor performance equivalent to legally prescribed levels of alcohol intoxication. *Occup Environ Med.* 2000;57:649-55.
3. Barger LK, Cade BE, Najib TA, et al. Extended work shifts and the risk of motor vehicle crashes among interns. *N Engl J Med.* 2005;352:125-34.
4. Barone JJ, Roberts HR. Caffeine consumption. *Food Chem Toxicol.* 1996;34:119-29.
5. International Food International Council. Questions and answers about caffeine and health. Available at: www.ific.ofr/publications/qa/caffqa.cfm. Accessed August 24, 2005.
6. Daly JW. Mechanism of action of caffeine. In: Garattini S, ed. *Caffeine, Coffee and Health.* New York: Raven Press Ltd.; 1993:97-150.
7. Mumford GK, Benowitz NL, Evans SM, et al. Absorption rate of methylxanthines following capsules, cola and chocolate. *Eur J Clin Pharmacol.* 1996;51:319-25.
8. Grant DM, Tang BK, Kalow W. Variability in caffeine metabolism. *Clin Pharmacol Ther.* 1983;33:591-602.
9. Massey LK, Sutton RA. Acute effects on urine composition and calcium kidney stone risk in calcium stone formers. *J Urol.* 2004;172:555-8.
10. Penetar D, Thorne DR. Caffeine reversal of sleep deprivation effects. *Sleep Res.* 1990;20:74.
11. Rosenthal L, Roehrs T, Zwyghhuizen-Doorenbos A, et al. Alerting effects of caffeine after normal and restricted sleep. *Neuropsychopharmacology.* 1991;4:103-8.
12. Richardson NJ, Rogers PJ, Elliman NA, et al. Mood and performance effects of caffeine in relation to acute and chronic caffeine deprivation. *Pharmacol Biochem Behav.* 1995;52:313-20.
13. Smit HJ, Rogers PJ. Effects of low doses of caffeine on cognitive performance, mood and thirst in low and higher caffeine consumers. *Psychopharmacologia.* 2000;152:167-73.
14. Hindmarch I, Rigney U, Stanley N, et al. A naturalistic investigation of the effects of day-long consumption of tea, coffee and water on alertness, sleep onset and sleep quality. *Psychopharmacologia.* 2000;149:203-16.
15. Reyner LA, Horne JA. Early morning driver sleepiness: effectiveness of 200 mg caffeine. *Psycholphysiology.* 2000;37: 251-6.
16. Liguori A, Robinson JH. Caffeine antagonism of alcohol-induced driving impairment. *Drug Alcohol Dependence.* 2001;63:123-9.
17. Bell DG, Jacobs I, Zamecnik J. Effects of caffeine, ephedrine and their combination on time to exhaustion during high intensity exercise. *Eur J Appl Physiol.* 1998;77:427-33.
18. Ferrauti A, Weber K, Struder, HK. Metabolic and ergogenic effects of carbohydrate and caffeine beverages in tennis. *J Sports Med Phys Fitness.* 1997;37:258-66.
19. MacIntosh, BR, Wright BM. Caffeine ingestion and performance of a 1,500-metre swim. *Can J Appl Physiol.* 1995;20:168-77.
20. Bruce CR, Anderson ME, Fraser SF, et al. Enhancement of 2000-m rowing performance after caffeine ingestion. *Med Sci Sports Exercise.* 2000;32:1958-63.
21. Costill DL, Coyle E, Dalsky G, et al. Effects of elevated plasma FFA and insulin on muscle glycogen usage during exercise. *J Appl Physiol.* 1977;43:695-9.
22. Hering-Hanit R, Gadoth N. Caffeine-induced headache in children and adolescents. *Cephalalgia.* 2003;23:332-5.
23. Benowitz NL. Clinical pharmacology of caffeine. *Annu Rev Med.* 1990;41:277-88.
24. Massey LK. Caffeine and the elderly. *Drugs Aging.* 1998;13:43-50.
25. Carrillo JA, Benitez J. CYP 1A2 activity, gender and smoking as variables influencing the toxicity of caffeine. *Br J Clin Pharmacol.* 1996;41:605-8.
26. Charney DS, Heninger GR, Jatlow PI. Increased anxiogenic effects of caffeine in panic disorders. *Arch Gen Psych.* 1985;42:233-43.
27. Daly JW, Fredholm BB. Caffeine: an atypical drug of dependence. *Drug Alcohol Dependence.* 1998;51:199-206.
28. Varani K, Portaluppi F, Merighi S, et al. Caffeine alters A2A adenosine receptors and their function in human platelets. *Circulation.* 1999;9:2499-502.
29. Schuh KJ, Griffiths RR. Caffeine reinforcement: the role of withdrawal. *Psychopharmacology.* 1977;132:320.
30. Bernstein GA, Carroll ME, Dean NW, et al. Caffeine withdrawal in normal school-age children. *J Am Acad Child Adoles Psychiatr.* 1998;37:858-65.
31. McGowan JD, Altman RE, Kanto WPJ. Neonatal withdrawal symptoms after chronic maternal ingestion of caffeine. *South Med J.* 1988;81:1092-4.
32. Tantcheva-Poor I, Zaigler M, Rietbrock S, et al. Estimation of cytochrome P-450 CYP 1A2 activity in 863 healthy Caucasians using a saliva-based caffeine test. *Pharmacogenetics.* 1999;9:131-44.

33. Nesher G, Mates M, Zevin S. Effect of caffeine consumption on efficacy of methotrexate in rheumatoid arthritis. *Arthritis Rheum.* 2003;48:571-2.
34. Odom-White A, de Lion J. Clozapine levels and caffeine (Letter). *J Clin Psychiatry.* 1996;57:175-6.
35. Hagg S, Spigset O, Mjorndal T, et al. Effect of caffeine on clozapine pharmacokinetics in healthy volunteers. *Br J Clin Pharmacol.* 2000;49:59-63.
36. Faber MS, Fuhr U. Time response of cytochrome P450 1A2 activity on cessation of heavy smoking. *Clin Pharmacol Ther.* 2004; 76:178-84.
37. Abernethy DR, Todd EL. Impairment of caffeine clearance by chronic use of low estrogen-containing oral contraceptives. *Eur J Clin Pharmacol.* 1985;28:425-8.
38. Grobbee DE, Rimm EB, Giovannucci E, et al. Coffee, caffeine, and cardiovascular disease in men. *N Engl J Med.* 1990;323:1026-32.
39. Willett WC, Stampler MJ, Manson JE, et al. Coffee consumption and coronary heart disease in women: a ten year follow-up. *JAMA.* 1996;275:458-62.
40. Myers MG, Basinski A. Coffee and coronary heart disease. *Arch Int Med.* 1992;152:1767-72.
41. Myers MG, Caffeine and cardiac arrhythmias. *Ann Int Med.* 1991; 114:147-50.
42. Kleemola P, Jousilahti P, Pietinen P, et al. Coffee consumption and the risk of coronary heart disease and death. *Arch Intern Med.* 2000;160:3393-400.
43. Jee SH, He J, Whelton PK, et al. The effect of coffee on blood pressure: a meta-analysis of controlled clinical trials. *Can J Cardiol.* 1997;13 (suppl B):36B.
44. Lane JD, Peiper CF, Phillips-Bute BG, et al. Caffeine affects cardiovascular and neuroendocrine activation at work and home. *Psychosomatic Med.* 2002;64:595-603.
45. Klag MJ, Wang NY, Meoni LA. Coffee intake and risk of hypertension: the Johns Hopkins precursors study. *Arch Int Med.* 2002; 162:657-62.
46. Leviton A, Cawan L. A review of the literature relating caffeine consumption by women to their risk of reproductive hazards. *Food Chem Toxicol.* 2002;40:1271-310.
47. Klebanoff MA, Levine RJ, DerSimonian R, et al. Maternal serum paraxanthine, a caffeine metabolite, and the risk of spontaneous abortion. *N Engl J Med.* 1999;341:1639-44.
48. Rasch V. Cigarette, alcohol and caffeine consumption: risk factors for spontaneous abortion. *Acta Obstet Gyn Scand.* 2003;82: 182-8.
49. Wisborg K, Kesmodel U, Bech BH, et al. Maternal consumption of coffee during pregnancy and stillbirth and infant death in first year of life: prospective study. *BMJ.* 2003;326:420-1.
50. Gianelli M, Doyle P, Roman E, et al. The effect of caffeine consumption and nausea on the risk of miscarriage. *Ped Perinal Epidemiol.* 2003;17(4):316-23.
51. Clausson B, Granath F, Ekbom A, et al. Effects of caffeine exposure during pregnancy on birth weight and gestational age. *Am J Epidemiol.* 2002;155:429-36.
52. Santos IS, Victora CG, Huttly S, et al. Caffeine intake and low birth weight: a population-based case-control study. *Am J Epidemiol.* 1998;147:620-7.
53. Fenster L, Eskenazi B, Windham GC, et al. Caffeine consumption during pregnancy and fetal growth. *Am J Public Health.* 1991;81: 458-61.
54. Bracken MB, Triche EW, Belanger K, et al. Association of maternal caffeine consumption with decrements in fetal growth. *Am J Epidemiol.* 2003;157:456-66.
55. Vik T, Bakketeig LS, Trygg KU, et al. High caffeine consumption in the third trimester of pregnancy: gender-specific effects on fetal growth. *Ped Perinatal Epidemiol.* 2003;17:324-31.
56. Committee on Drugs, American Academy of Pediatrics. The transfer of drugs and other chemicals into human milk. *Pediatrics.* 1994;93:137-50.
57. Tyrala EE, Dodson WE. Caffeine secretion into breast milk. *Arch Dis Child.* 1979;54:787-800.
58. Ryu JE. Caffeine in human milk and in serum of breast fed infants. *Dev Pharmacol Ther.* 1985;8:329-37.
59. St-Onge M-P, Keller KL, Heymsfield SB. Changes in childhood food consumption patterns: a cause for concern in light of increasing body weights. *Am J Clin Nutr.* 2003;78:1068-73.
60. Savoca MR, Evans CD, Wilson ME, et al. The association of caffeinated beverages with blood pressure in adolescents. *Arch Ped Adoles Med.* 2004;158: 473-7.
61. Castellanos FX, Rapoport JL. Effects of caffeine on development and behavior in infancy and childhood: a review of the published literature. *Food Chem Toxicol.* 2002;40:1235-42.
62. Nawrot P, Jordan S, Eastwood J, et al. Effects of caffeine on human health. *Food Additives Contaminants.* 2003;20:1-30.
63. Lloyd T, Rollings N, Eggli DF, et al. Dietary caffeine intake and bone status of postmenopausal women. *Am J Clin Nutr.* 1997;65: 1826-30.
64. Conlisk AJ, Galuska DA. Is caffeine associated with bone mineral density in young adult women? *Prevent Med.* 2000;31:562-8.
65. Lloyd T, Hohnson-Rollings N, Eggli DF, et al. Bone status among postmenopausal women with different habitual caffeine intakes: a longitudinal investigation. *J Am Coll Nutr.* 2000;19:256-61.
66. Heaney RP, Rafferty K. Carbonated beverages and urinary calcium excretion. *Am J Clin Nutr.* 2001;74:343-7.
67. Hegarty VM, May HM, Khaw KT. Tea drinking and bone mineral density in older women. *Am J Clin Nutr.* 2000;71:1003-7.
68. Wu-Hsing C, Yi-Ching Y, Wei-Jen Y, et al. Epidemiological evidence of increased bone mineral density in habitual tea drinkers. *Arch Int Med.* 2002;162:1001-6.
69. ConsumerLab Web site: Available at: http://www.consumerlab.com/results/ginseng.asp. Accessed December 6, 2004.
70. Cardinal, BJ, Engels HJ. Ginseng does not enhance psychological well being in healthy young adults: results of a double-blind, placebo-controlled, randomized clinical trial. *J Am Diet Assoc.* 2001;101:655-60.
71. D'Angelo L, Grimaldi R, Caravaggi M, et al. A double-blind placebo controlled clinical study on the effect of a standardized ginseng extract on psychomotor performance in healthy volunteers. *J Ethnophamacol.* 1986;16:15-22.
72. Sorenson H, Sonne JA. Double-masked study of the effects of ginseng on cognitive functions. *Curr Ther Res.* 1996;57:959-68.
73. Ellis JM, Reddy P. Effects of Panax ginseng on quality of life. *Ann Pharmacotherapy.* 2002;36:375-9.
74. Ginseng, Panax ginseng. *Clin Pharmacol.* Available at: www.cponline.gsm.com/. Accessed August 24, 2005.
75. Teng CM, Kuo SC, Ko FN, et al. Antiplatelet actions of panaxynol and ginsenosides isolated from ginseng. *Biochim Biophys Acta.* 1989;990:315-20.
76. Yuan CS, Wei G, Dey L, et al. American ginseng reduces warfarin's effect in healthy patients: a randomized, controlled trial. *Ann Int Med.* 2004;141:23-7.
77. Jiang X, Williams KM, Liauw WS, et al. Effect of St. John's wort and ginseng on the pharmacokinetics and pharmacodynamics of warfarin in healthy subjects. *Br J Clin Pharmacol.* 2004;57:592-9.
78. Engelberg D, McCutcheon A, Wiseman S. A case of ginseng-induced mania (letter). *J Clin Psychopharmacol.* 2001;21:535-7.
79. Vuksan V, Sievenpiper JL, Koo VY, et al. American ginseng (Panax quinquefolius L) reduces postprandial glycemia in nondiabetic subjects and subjects with Type II diabetes mellitus. *Arch Int Med.* 2000;160:1009-13.

CHAPTER 50

# Smoking Cessation

*Karen Suchanek Hudmon, Lisa A. Kroon, and Robin L. Corelli*

In 1982, the U.S. Surgeon General C. Everett Koop stated that cigarette smoking is the "chief, single, avoidable cause of death in our society and the most important public health issue of our time."[1] This statement remains true today, nearly 25 years later. Because the recommended treatment for tobacco dependence involves both behavioral counseling and pharmacotherapy,[2] health care providers are strategically positioned to make significant contributions toward reducing the prevalence of tobacco use. The U.S. Public Health Service's clinical practice guideline for treating tobacco use and dependence,[2] which summarizes more than 6000 published articles, indicates that clinicians can significantly increase patients' likelihood of quitting, even with brief interventions (less than 3 minutes). More intensive counseling, a greater number of counseling sessions, and teaming multiple types of clinicians (e.g., physicians, pharmacists, nurses, physician assistants, dental hygienists, and dentists) yields enhanced quit rates.[2]

While clinicians should address use of all forms of tobacco (smoked and smokeless), this chapter focuses on cigarette smoking, as it is the most commonly used form of tobacco in the United States and the only form for which nonprescription nicotine replacement therapy (NRT) products are indicated. This chapter provides an overview of currently available nonprescription medications for smoking cessation and outlines practical strategies clinicians that can use when assisting patients prior to and during a quit attempt.

## Epidemiology of Tobacco Use and Dependence

In the United States, cigarette smoking is the leading known cause of preventable death,[3] resulting in an estimated 437,902 deaths each year.[4] In addition to lives lost, the economic impact of smoking is enormous—for each of approximately 22 billion packs of cigarettes sold in 1999, the associated medical and lost productivity costs were $3.45 and $3.73, respectively, totaling $7.18 per pack and $157 billion overall.[5]

Because smoking initiation occurs primarily during adolescence,[6] tobacco-use trends among youth are key indicators of the overall health of our nation.[7] An estimated 89% of adult smokers smoked their first cigarette by age 18, and 71% of adult daily smokers initiated regular smoking by age 18.[6] Since 1999, the prevalence of smoking among adolescents has decreased—in 2004, an estimated 25% of 12th graders had smoked one or more cigarettes in the past 30 days.[8]

Despite the well-established and well-publicized negative effects of smoking, an estimated 20.9% of adult Americans (23.4% of males and 18.5% of females) continue to smoke; 81.3% of these persons smoke daily.[9] The prevalence of smoking among adult Americans varies by sociodemographic factors, including sex, race/ethnicity, education level, age, and socioeconomic status.[9] In 2004, the prevalence of smoking in the United States was highest among American Indian/Alaska Natives (33.4%) and next highest among non-Hispanic whites (22.2%), followed by non-Hispanic blacks (20.2%), Hispanics (15.0%), and Asians (11.3%).[9] Smoking also tends to be more common among persons of lower educational levels and those living below the U.S. threshold poverty level.[9] The median prevalence of smoking varies by state, with Utah exhibiting the lowest prevalence at 10.5% and Kentucky exhibiting the highest, at 27.6%.[10]

Although the overall prevalence of smoking in the United States has exhibited a fairly stable decline over the past two decades, annual reports from the Centers for Disease Control and Prevention suggest this downward trend has leveled in recent years. An estimated 70% of smokers want to quit,[11] and, in 2004, approximately 14.6 million (40.5%) of 36.1 million every-day, current smokers stopped smoking at least 1 day during the past year because they were trying to quit.[9] Yet, smoking cessation rates remain low, and much effort is needed if our nation is to reach the Healthy People 2010 goals of (a) an adult smoking prevalence of no more than 12% and (b) an adult smoking cessation attempt rate of 75%.[7]

## Etiology of Tobacco Use and Dependence

In 1988 the U.S. Surgeon General released a landmark report, concluding that tobacco products are effective nicotine delivery systems capable of inducing and sustaining chemical dependence. The primary criteria used to categorize nicotine as an addictive substance included its (1) psychoactive effects, (2) use in a highly controlled or compulsive manner, and (3) reinforcement of behavioral patterns of tobacco use. The underlying pharmacologic and behavioral processes associated with tobacco dependence are considered to be similar to those that determine addiction to drugs such as heroin and cocaine.[12]

As with other addictive substances (e.g., opiates, cocaine, amphetamines), nicotine stimulates the mesolimbic dopaminergic system in the midbrain inducing pleasant or rewarding effects that promote continued use of the drug.[13] Psychosocial and environmental factors also play an important role in establishing and maintaining dependence.[14] For example, smokers commonly associate smoking with specific activities such as driving, talking on the telephone, drinking coffee or alcohol, being around other smokers, or eating. Over time, the habitual use of cigarettes under these circumstances can lead to the development of smoking routines that can be difficult to break. Indeed, specific environmental situations can become powerful stimuli capable of triggering "automatic" smoking patterns. It is well established that tobacco is a detrimental substance,[15] and its use dramatically increases one's odds of dependence, disease, disability, and death. Cigarettes are carefully engineered and heavily marketed products—in 2003, the tobacco industry spent $15.15 billion advertising cigarettes in the United States.[16] It is the only marketed consumable product that, when used as intended, will kill half or more of its users.[17]

## Pathophysiology of Tobacco Use and Dependence

Cigarette smoke, which is classified by the Environmental Protection Agency as a Class A carcinogen (i.e., a carcinogen with no safe level of exposure for humans), is a complex mixture of an estimated 4800 compounds found in gaseous and particulate phases. Approximately 500 compounds are present in the vapor phase, including nitrogen, carbon monoxide, ammonia, hydrogen cyanide, and benzene. The remaining constituents of tobacco smoke, the most important of which is the alkaloid nicotine, are found in the particulate phase. The particulate fraction, excluding the nicotine and water components, is collectively referred to as tar. Numerous carcinogens, including polycyclic aromatic hydrocarbons and nitrosamines, have been identified in the tar fraction of tobacco smoke.[18]

Nicotine, the addictive component of tobacco, is distilled from burning tobacco and carried in tar droplets to the small airways of the lung, where it is absorbed rapidly into the arterial circulation and distributed throughout the body. Most U.S. cigarettes contain between 6 and 13 mg of nicotine, and the typical smoker absorbs between 1 and 3 mg of nicotine per cigarette, regardless of the nicotine-yields obtained during standardized machine testing conditions.[19] Nicotine readily penetrates the central nervous system and has been estimated to reach the brain within 11 seconds after inhalation.[20] Nicotine binds to receptors in the brain and other organs and stimulates the release of numerous neurotransmitters including norepinephrine, acetylcholine, dopamine, and others that induce a variety of predominantly stimulatory effects on the cardiovascular, endocrine, nervous, and metabolic systems.[20, 21] Pharmacodynamic effects associated with nicotine administration include increases in the heart rate, blood pressure, and force of myocardial contraction; vasoconstriction of coronary and peripheral blood vessels; pleasure, arousal, enhanced task performance; increases in the metabolic rate; and appetite suppression.[20]

## Signs and Symptoms of Tobacco Use and Dependence

The majority of chronic tobacco users develop tolerance to the effects of nicotine, and abrupt cessation precipitates symptoms of nicotine withdrawal, which include depression, insomnia, irritability/frustration/anger, anxiety, difficulty concentrating, restlessness, increased appetite and weight gain, and decreased heart rate. Typically, the physiologic nicotine withdrawal symptoms peak within 48 hours after tobacco cessation and gradually dissipate over the following 2 to 4 weeks.[20] For most individuals, withdrawal symptoms completely resolve within 1 month of quitting; however, increased appetite and weight gain can persist for 6 or more months. Multiple factors influence tobacco use behavior, including the desire to experience the pleasurable effects of nicotine, exposure to various environmental cues, and relief of nicotine withdrawal symptoms.

## Complications of Smoking

According to a report issued by the U.S. Surgeon General in 2004, smoking adversely affects nearly every organ system in the body and plays a causal role in the development of numerous diseases (Table 50-1).[15] Furthermore, the report concludes that smoking cigarettes with lower machine-measured yields of tar and nicotine (e.g., "light" cigarettes) provides no clear benefit to health.[15] In nonsmokers, passive exposure to secondhand smoke, which includes the smoke emanating from burning tobacco and that exhaled by the smoker, also increases the risk of lung cancer, cardiovascular disease, and chronic respiratory conditions.[15, 22]

### *Drug Interactions With Tobacco Smoke*

Many clinically significant interactions between tobacco smoke and medications have been identified. Tobacco smoke interacts with medications through pharmacokinetic or pharmacodynamic mechanisms that may lead to reduced therapeutic efficacy or, less commonly, increased toxicity.[23] The majority of pharmacokinetic interactions are the result of induction of hepatic cytochrome P-450 enzymes (primarily the CYP1A2 isozyme) by polycyclic aromatic hydrocarbons present in tobacco smoke.[23] Induction of the CYP1A2 enzyme can increase the hepatic metabolism of fluvoxamine (Luvox), olanzapine (Zyprexa), tacrine (Cognex), and theophylline, potentially resulting in a reduced therapeutic response or need for higher dosages in smokers; conversely, the dosages of these agents might need to be reduced in patients who quit smoking.[23] Similarly, the clearance of caffeine is significantly increased (by 56%) in smokers. Upon cessation, smokers who drink caffeinated beverages should be advised to decrease their usual caffeine intake to avoid higher levels of caffeine, which may induce symptoms similar to nicotine withdrawal.

A significant pharmacodynamic drug interaction occurs with tobacco smoke and oral contraceptives. Data indicate that cigarette smoking substantially increases the risk of serious adverse cardiovascular events (mainly stroke and myocardial infarction) in women using oral contraceptives.[24-29]

**TABLE 50-1 Health Consequences of Smoking[15]**

**Cancer**

Acute myeloid leukemia
Bladder
Cervical
Esophageal
Gastric
Kidney
Laryngeal
Lung
Oral cavity and pharyngeal
Pancreatic

**Cardiovascular Diseases**

Abdominal aortic aneurysm
Coronary heart disease (angina pectoris, ischemic heart disease, myocardial infarction)
Cerebrovascular disease (transient ischemic attacks, stroke)
Peripheral arterial disease

**Pulmonary Diseases**

Acute respiratory illnesses
- Upper respiratory tract (rhinitis, sinusitis, laryngitis, pharyngitis)
- Lower respiratory tract (bronchitis, pneumonia)

Chronic respiratory illnesses
- Chronic obstructive pulmonary disease
- Respiratory symptoms
- Poor asthma control
- Reduced lung function

**Reproductive Effects**

Reduced fertility in women
Pregnancy and pregnancy outcomes
- Preterm, premature rupture of membranes
- Placenta previa
- Placental abruption
- Preterm delivery
- Low infant birth weight

Infant mortality
- Sudden infant death syndrome

**Other Effects**

Cataract
Osteoporosis (reduced bone density in postmenopausal women, increased risk of hip fracture)
Periodontitis
Peptic ulcer disease
- (in patients infected with *Helicobacter pylori*)

Surgical outcomes
- Poor wound healing
- Respiratory complications

This risk is markedly increased in women who are 35 years of age or older and smoke 15 or more cigarettes per day.[28] Accordingly, most experts consider use of oral contraceptives to be a contraindication in this population, and an alternative form of contraception should be used.[25,29] Additional interactions, with corresponding underlying mechanisms for the interactions, are depicted in Table 50-2.

During the course of routine patient care, it is important to assess tobacco use status at each visit, assess for potential drug-smoking interactions, and make appropriate adjustments to the medication regimen. For patients who are preparing to quit smoking, dosage adjustments might be necessary for some medications.

### *Benefits of Smoking Cessation*

The 1990 Surgeon General's Report on the health benefits of smoking cessation outlines the numerous and substantial health benefits incurred when patients quit smoking.[31] Some health benefits are incurred shortly (e.g., within 2 weeks to 3 months) after quitting, and others are incurred over time (Figure 50-1). Recent findings show a clear picture of the risks associated with smoking. On average, cigarette smokers die approximately 10 years earlier than nonsmokers, and, of those who continue smoking, at least half will eventually die from a tobacco-related disease. Quitting at ages 30, 40, 50, and 60 results in a gain of 10, 9, 6, and 3 years of life, respectively.[17] Thus, although it is important to educate tobacco users that it is never too late to incur many of the benefits of quitting, there are significant benefits to quitting earlier in life.

## Smoking Cessation Treatment

### *Treatment Goals*

For most smokers, tobacco dependence is a chronic disease characterized by multiple failed attempts to quit before long-term cessation is achieved.[2] Because tobacco use is a complex, addictive behavior, helping a patient to quit and prevent relapse is best achieved by combining appropriate pharmacotherapy with behavioral counseling. For any patient who uses tobacco, the primary goal is complete, long-term abstinence from all nicotine-containing products. To increase the chances of quitting, smokers should be encouraged to adhere closely to pharmacotherapy regimens and to participate in tobacco cessation counseling throughout their quit attempt. In prescribing or dispensing pharmaceutical aids for quitting, clinicians can have a significant impact on a patient's likelihood of quitting by supplementing medication counseling with behavioral counseling, as described here.

### *General Treatment Approach*

Most quit attempts end in relapse. According to the Centers for Disease Control and Prevention, in 2000 only 4.7% of current smokers were able to quit and maintain abstinence for 3 to 12 months.[11] Although the majority of smokers quit without assistance,[32] typically after multiple attempts, decades of research demonstrate clearly that patients who receive assistance have increased odds of quitting. In 2000, the U.S. Public Health Service published a clinical practice guideline for treating tobacco use and dependence,[2] which presents evidence-based recommendations and effective strategies for clinician-facilitated tobacco cessation counseling. Although even brief advice from a clinician is associated with increased odds of quitting,[2,33] more intensive behavioral counseling (longer and

**TABLE 50-2 Drug Interactions with Tobacco Smoke**[23,30]

| Drug/Class | Mechanism of Interaction and Effects |
|---|---|
| Benzodiazepines (diazepam, chlordiazepoxide) | Pharmacodynamic: ↓ sedation and drowsiness, possibly caused by nicotine stimulation of CNS |
| β-Blockers | Pharmacodynamic: ↓ control of hypertensive and heart rate, possibly caused by nicotine-mediated sympathetic activation |
| Caffeine | ↑ Metabolism (induction of CYP 1A2); clearance ↑ 56%; possible ↑ caffeine levels after smoking cessation |
| Chlorpromazine | ↓ AUC (36%) and serum concentrations (24%); ↓ sedation and hypotension possible in smokers; smokers may need ↑ dosages |
| Clozapine | ↑ Metabolism (induction of CYP 1A2); ↓ plasma concentrations (28%) |
| Flecainide | ↑ Clearance (61%); ↓ trough serum concentrations (25%); smokers may need ↑ dosages |
| Fluvoxamine | ↑ Metabolism (induction of CYP 1A2); ↑ clearance (24%); ↓ AUC (31%); ↓ plasma concentrations (32%); dosage modifications not routinely recommended but smokers may need ↑ dosages |
| Haloperidol | ↑ Clearance (44%); ↓ serum concentrations (70%) |
| Heparin | Mechanism unknown but ↑ clearance and ↓ half-life observed; smokers may need ↑ dosages |
| Insulin | Possible ↓ insulin absorption secondary to peripheral vasoconstriction; possible release of endogenous substances that antagonize insulin's effects; interactions likely not clinically significant; smokers may need ↑ dosages |
| Mexiletine | ↑ Clearance (25%; via oxidation and glucuronidation); ↓ half-life (36%) |
| Olanzapine | ↑ Metabolism (induction of CYP 1A2); ↑ clearance (98%); ↓ serum concentrations (12%); dosage modifications not routinely recommended but smokers may need ↑ dosages |
| Opioids (propoxyphene, pentazocine) | Pharmacodynamic: unknown mechanism, ↓ analgesic effect; smokers may need ↑ dosages for pain relief |
| Oral contraceptives | Pharmacodynamic: ↑ risk of cardiovascular adverse effects (e.g., stroke and myocardial infarction) in women who smoke and use oral contraceptives; substantially ↑ risk in women at least 35 years of age who smoke at least 15 cigarettes per day |
| Propranolol | ↑ Clearance (77%; via side-chain oxidation and glucuronidation) |
| Tacrine | ↑ Metabolism (induction of CYP 1A2); ↓ half-life (50%); serum concentrations 3-fold lower; smokers may need ↑ dosages |
| Theophylline | ↑ Metabolism (induction of CYP 1A2); ↑ clearance (58%-100%); ↓ half-life (63%); levels should be monitored if smoking is initiated, discontinued, or changed; ↑ clearance with passive smoking (secondhand smoke); considerably ↑ maintenance doses in smokers |

Key: AUC, area under the curve; CNS, central nervous system.

*Source*: Adapted with permission from reference 30. 

more frequent counseling sessions, or greater overall contact time) and use of pharmacotherapy (excluding patients who should not self-treat, as listed in Figure 50-2) result in increased quit rates.[2] Three particularly effective types of counseling and behavioral therapies are practical counseling (problem solving and skills training), support from a health care provider, and support from others (family, friends, and coworkers).[2]

Clinicians can have an important impact on their patients' likelihood of achieving cessation. In a meta-analysis of 29 studies,[2] it was determined that patients who receive a tobacco cessation intervention from a nonphysician clinician or a physician clinician are 1.7 and 2.2 times as likely to quit (at 5 or more months postcessation), respectively, compared with patients who do not receive an intervention from a clinician. Self-help materials are only slightly better than no clinician intervention. Because the use of pharmacotherapy approximately doubles a patient's chances of quitting,[2,34,35] cessation interventions should combine pharmacotherapy with behavioral counseling, when feasible and not contraindicated.[2] Figure 50-2 outlines a self-treatment approach for smoking cessation.

## *Nonpharmacologic Therapy*

### Helping Patients Quit: Five Key Counseling Components (the "5 A's")

Five key components of comprehensive counseling for tobacco cessation are (1) asking patients whether they use tobacco; (2) advising tobacco users to quit; (3) assessing patients' readiness to quit; (4) assisting patients with quitting; and (5) arranging follow-up care. These steps are referred to as the "5 A's."[2]

TIME ELAPSED

**20 minutes after quitting:** Blood pressure drops to a level close to that before the last cigarette. Temperature of hands and feet increases to normal.

**8 hours after quitting:** Blood levels of carbon monoxide drop to normal.

**24 hours after quitting:** Chance of having a heart attack decreases.

**2 weeks to 3 months after quitting:** Circulation improves, and lung function improves by up to 30%.

**1 to 9 months after quitting:** Coughing, sinus congestion, fatigue, and shortness of breath decrease, and cilia regain normal function in the lungs, increasing the ability to handle mucus, clear the lungs, and reduce infection.

**1 year after quitting:** Excessive risk of coronary heart disease is half that of a smoker's.

**5 years after quitting:** Risk of stroke is reduced to that of a nonsmoker 5 to 15 years after quitting.

**10 years after quitting:** Lung cancer death rate is about half that of continuing smokers. Risk of cancer of the mouth, throat, esophagus, bladder, kidney, and pancreas also are lower than that of continuing smokers.

**15 years after quitting:** Risk of coronary heart disease is similar to that of a nonsmoker.

FIGURE 50-1 Health benefits of smoking cessation.[31]

*Ask* A key first step is asking about tobacco use. Because tobacco use is the primary known preventable cause of mortality in the United States, and because smoking interacts with multiple medications, screening for tobacco use is crucial and should be a routine component of care provided by all clinicians. The following question can be used to identify all types of tobacco use, even for infrequent users: "Do you ever smoke or use any type of tobacco?" Tobacco use status should be considered a vital sign, and collected routinely along with blood pressure, pulse, weight, temperature, and respiratory rate.[2] At a minimum, tobacco use status (current, former, never a user) and level of use (e.g., number of cigarettes smoked per day) should be documented in the medical record and reassessed periodically.

*Advise* All tobacco users should be advised to quit. The advice should be clear and compelling, yet delivered with sensitivity and a tone of voice that communicates concern for the patient and a willingness to assist the patient with quitting when he or she is ready. When possible, clinicians should personalize the messages by linking their advice to the patient's health status, current medication regimen, personal reasons for wanting to quit, and/or the impact of tobacco on others. For example, "Ms. Bettis, I see that you now are on two different inhalers for your emphysema. As your clinician, I need to tell you that quitting smoking is the single most important treatment for your emphysema. I strongly encourage you to quit, and I would like to help you."

*Assess* Because many patients will not be ready to quit in the near future, it is important for clinicians to gauge patients' readiness to quit before recommending a treatment regimen. Patients should be categorized as (1) not ready to quit in the next month; (2) ready to quit in the next month; (3) a recent quitter, having quit in the past 6 months; or (4) a former user, having quit more than 6 months ago.[2] This classification defines the clinician's next course of action, which is to provide counseling that is tailored to the patient's readiness to quit. As an example for a current smoker: "Mr. Ward, have you given any thought to quitting? Is this something that you might consider doing in the next month?" Counseling a patient who is ready to quit in the next month should be very different from counseling a patient who is not considering quitting in the near future.

*Assist* Important elements of the "assist" component of treatment include helping patients to make the decision and commitment to quit and setting an actual quit date. Clinicians should be sympathetic to the fact that quitting is a difficult process. As such, the goal is to help maximize patients' chances of success by designing an individualized treatment plan.

Except in the presence of special circumstances, all patients attempting to quit should be encouraged to use pharmacotherapy (described below) combined with some form of nonpharmacologic intervention (described below), as this combination will yield higher quit rates than either approach alone.[2,34] Nonpharmacologic methods, which focus on promoting behavior change, include tapering the number of cigarettes (e.g., setting a quit date and applying a scheduled, gradual reduction strategy), reading self-help materials, and entering a formal cessation program (face-to-face counseling, telephone counseling, or group program). Acupuncture and hypnosis also are common nonpharmacologic aids; however, limited data are available to support their effectiveness in promoting quitting.[2]

*Arrange* Because a patient's ability to quit increases substantially when multiple counseling interactions are provided, arranging follow-up counseling is an important, yet typically neglected, element of treatment for tobacco dependence. Follow-up contact should occur soon after the quit date, preferably during the first week. This does not have to be done in person and could be performed by telephone or e-mail. A second follow-up contact is recommended within the first month after quitting.[2] Periodically, additional follow-up contacts should occur, to monitor patient progress (including adherence with pharmacotherapy) and to provide ongoing support. Quit rates at 5 or more months postcessation are associated with the total number of contacts: 12.4% for 0 to 1 contact, 16.3% for 2 to 3 contacts, 20.9% for 4 to 8 contacts, and 24.7% for more than 8 contacts.[2]

### Counseling Interventions for Quitting

When counseling a patient, the goal is to facilitate forward progress in the process of change, assisting patients to develop "readiness" for permanent cessation. It is important that clinicians view quitting as a process that might take months or even years to achieve, rather than a "now or never" event.

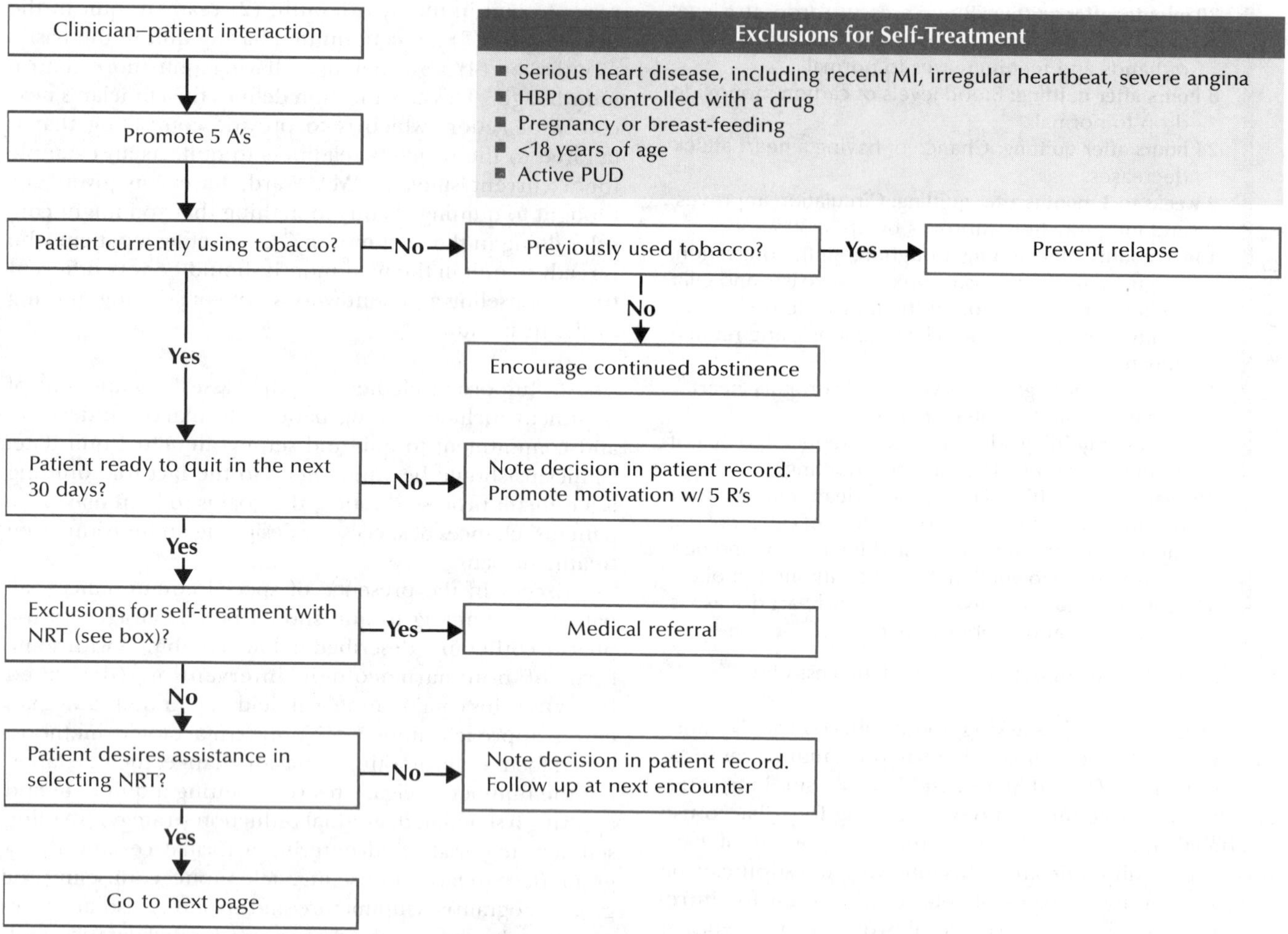


**FIGURE 50-2** Self-care of tobacco use and dependence. Key: 5 A's, ask, advise, assess, assist, arrange; 5 R's, relevance, risks, rewards, roadblocks, repetition; HBP, high blood pressure; MI, myocardial infarction; NRT, nicotine replacement therapy; OTC, over-the-counter; PUD, peptic ulcer disease; Rx, prescription; TMJ, temporomandibular joint.

*Counseling Patients Who Are Not Ready to Quit* When counseling patients who are not ready to quit, an important first step is to motivate the patient to start thinking about quitting and to consider making the difficult decision to quit sometime in the foreseeable future. Sometimes patients who are not ready truly do not understand the need to quit. In general, most smokers will recognize the need to quit but are not yet ready to make the commitment to quit. Many patients will have tried to quit multiple times and relapsed, and thus might feel too discouraged to try again.

Strategies for working with patients who are not ready to quit include increasing patient awareness of the available treatment options, having patients identify their reasons for smoking and for wanting to quit, and identifying barriers to quitting. Clinicians can motivate patients to begin thinking about quitting by raising awareness of specific drug interactions between medications and smoking (Table 50-2), and how tobacco use can induce or exacerbate medical conditions (e.g., COPD and coronary heart disease). While it may be useful to provide patients with information about the medications available for quitting, it is not appropriate to recommend a treatment regimen until a patient is ready to quit in the near future (e.g., within the next month). A treatment goal at this stage should be to promote motivation to quit, and this can be accomplished by providing tailored, motivational messages, applying what is referred to as the "5 R's."[2]

Relevance Encourage patients to think about why quitting is important to them. Because information has a greater impact if it takes on a personal meaning, counseling should be framed to relate to the patient's risk for disease or exacerbation of disease, other health concerns, family or social situation (e.g., having children with asthma), age, and other patient factors such as prior experience with quitting.

Risks Ask patients to identify negative health consequences of smoking, such as acute risks (e.g., shortness of breath, asthma exacerbations, pregnancy complications, infertility), long-term risks (e.g., cancer, cardiac and pulmonary disease), and environmental risks (e.g., effects of secondhand smoke on others, including children and pets, role modeling unhealthy behaviors around children and adolescents).

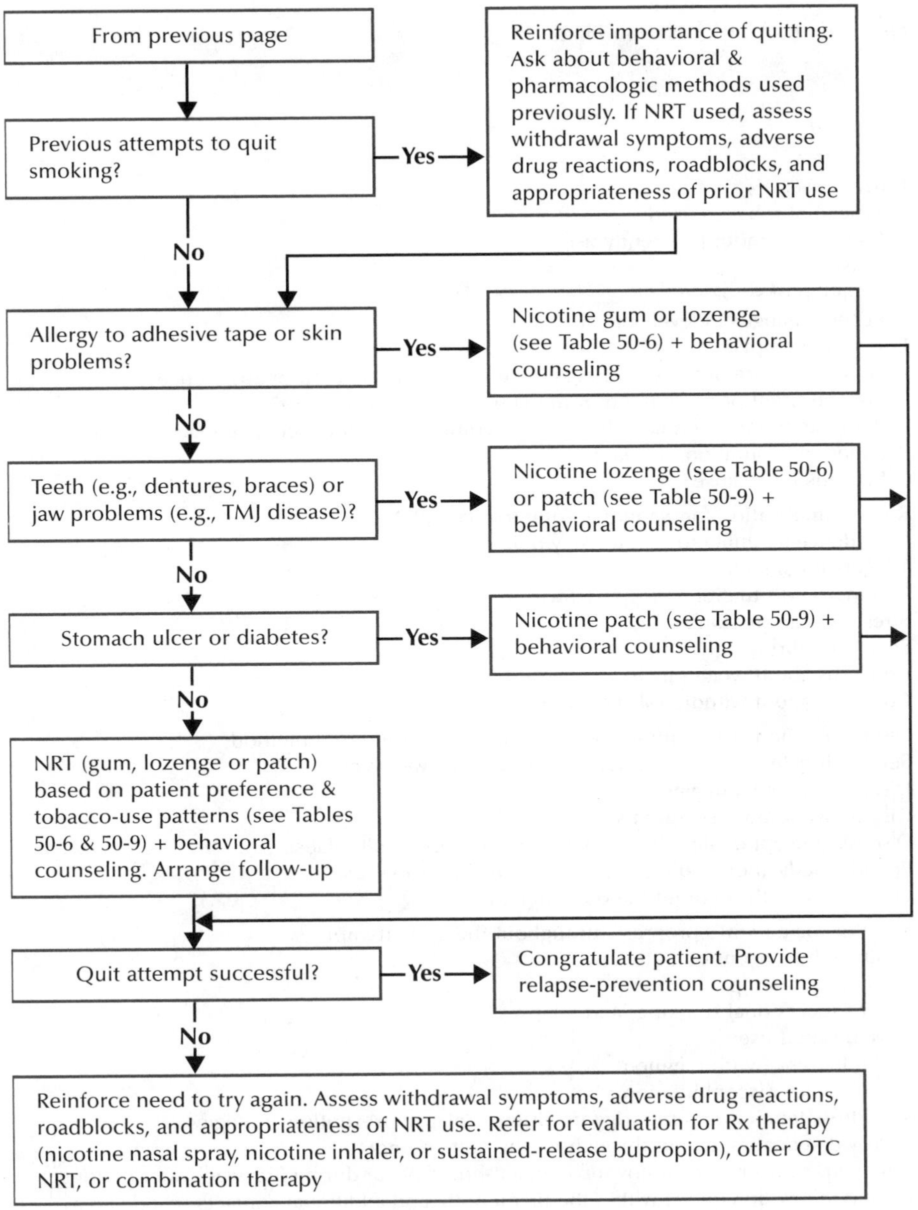


**FIGURE 50-2 (continued)**

Rewards Ask patients to identify specific benefits of quitting, such as improved health, enhanced physical performance, acuity of taste and smell, reduced expenditures for tobacco, less time wasted or work missed, reduced health risks to others (fetus, children, housemates), and reduced aging of the skin.

Roadblocks Help patients identify significant barriers to quitting, and assist in developing coping skills to address or circumvent each barrier. Common barriers include nicotine withdrawal symptoms, fear of failure, a need for social support while quitting, depression, concern about weight gain, and a sense of deprivation or loss.

Repetition Continue to work with patients who are either not motivated to quit or have been unsuccessful in quitting. Discussing circumstances in which smoking occurred will help identify triggers for relapse and should be viewed as part of the learning process. Repeat interventions whenever possible.

*Counseling Patients Who Are Ready to Quit* For patients who are ready to quit in the next month, clinicians can either provide comprehensive counseling or refer patients to local cessation programs or a toll-free telephone quitline.

The goal for patients who are ready to quit is to achieve cessation by providing an individualized treatment plan, addressing the key issues listed in Table 50-3. The first step is to discuss the patient's tobacco use history, inquiring about levels of smoking, number of years smoked, methods used previously for quitting, and reasons for previous failed quit attempts. Clinicians should understand fully the patient's preferences for the different pharmacotherapies

**TABLE 50-3 Key Topics for Individualized Smoking Cessation Plans**

| Topic | Description |
|---|---|
| Assess tobacco use history | ■ Current use:<br>– Type(s) of tobacco used<br>– Brand and amount currently used<br>■ Past use:<br>– Duration of smoking<br>– Recent changes in levels of use<br>■ Past quit attempts:<br>– Number of attempts, date of most recent attempt, duration of abstinence<br>– Previous methods: What did or didn't work? Why or why not?<br>– Prior experience with cessation pharmacotherapy: agent used, adequacy of dose, adherence, duration of treatment<br>– Reasons for relapse |
| Discuss key issues for the upcoming or current quit attempt | ■ Reasons/motivation for wanting to quit (or stay quit)<br>■ Confidence in ability to quit (or stay quit)<br>■ Triggers for smoking<br>■ Routines and situations associated with smoking<br>■ Stress-related smoking<br>■ Social support for quitting<br>■ Concerns about weight gain<br>■ Concerns about withdrawal symptoms |
| Facilitate the quitting process | ■ Discuss methods for quitting: pros and cons of the different methods<br>■ Set a quit date: more than 2 days but less than 2 weeks away<br>■ Discuss coping strategies<br>■ Discuss withdrawal symptoms<br>■ Discuss concept of slip (occasional smoking) versus full relapse<br>■ Provide medication counseling: adherence and proper use<br>■ Offer to assist throughout the quit attempt |
| Arrange and provide follow-up counseling | ■ Monitor the patient's progress throughout the quit attempt<br>■ Evaluate the current quit attempt<br>– Status of attempt<br>– Slips (occasional smoking) and relapses<br>– Medication use:<br>• Adherence with regimen<br>• Plans for discontinuation<br>– Address temptations and triggers; discuss relapse prevention strategies<br>– Provide encouragement throughout the quit attempt<br>■ Follow-up contacts: First follow-up contact should occur during first week after quitting, a second follow-up contact within the first month, and additional contacts scheduled as needed. Can occur face-to-face, by telephone, or by e-mail |

*Source*: Adapted with permission from reference 30. 

for quitting, and work with patients in selecting the quitting methods (e.g., medications, behavioral counseling programs). While it is important to recognize that pharmaceutical aids might not be desirable or affordable for all patients, clinicians should educate patients that medications, when taken correctly, can substantially increase the likelihood of quitting.

In general, patients should be encouraged to select a quit date that is more than 2 days but less than 2 weeks away. This time frame provides patients with ample time to prepare themselves and their environment prior to the actual quit date. This includes removing all tobacco products and ashtrays from the home, car, and workplace. Patients should be advised to discuss their desire to quit with their family, friends, and coworkers and request their support and assistance. It is helpful to have patients think about when and why they smoke; this information is useful for anticipating situations that might trigger a desire to smoke and contribute to relapse. Additional counseling strategies to address with patients during a quit attempt are listed in Table 50-4. Patients should be counseled on proper medication use (including administration), side effects, and adherence, and it is crucial to emphasize the importance of receiving behavioral counseling throughout the quit attempt.

When the clinician's or patient's time is limited, patients who are ready to quit can be referred to local tobacco cessation programs or a toll-free quitline. With the recent introduction of a national toll-free quitline number (1-800-QUIT-NOW), all Americans can receive tobacco cessation counseling at no cost. Counseling provided by telephone

**TABLE 50-4 Cognitive and Behavioral Strategies for Smoking Cessation[30]**

| | |
|---|---|
| Cognitive strategies focus on *retraining the way a patient thinks.* Often, patients mentally deliberate on the fact that they are thinking about a cigarette, and this leads to relapse. Patients must recognize that thinking about a cigarette does not mean they need to have one. | |
| Review commitment to quit, focus on the downside of tobacco | Remind oneself that cravings and temptations are temporary and will pass.<br>Announce, either silently or aloud, "I want to be a nonsmoker, and the temptation will pass." |
| Distractive thinking | Practice deliberate, immediate refocusing of thinking when cued by thoughts about tobacco use. |
| Positive self-talks, "pep-talks" | Say "I can do this" and remember previous difficult situations in which tobacco use was avoided with success. |
| Relaxation through imagery | Mentally focus on a scene, place, or situation that is peaceful, relaxing, and positive. |
| Mental rehearsal, visualization | Prepare for situations that might arise by envisioning how best to handle them. For example, envision what would happen if offered a cigarette by a friend, mentally craft and rehearse a response, and perhaps even practice it by saying it aloud. |
| Behavioral strategies involve *specific actions to reduce risk for relapse.* For maximal effectiveness, these should be considered prior to quitting, after determining patient-specific triggers for smoking. Below are some behavioral strategies for responding to several common cues or triggers for relapse. | |
| Stress | Anticipate upcoming challenges at work, at school, or in personal life. Develop a substitute plan for smoking during times of stress (e.g., deep breathing, take a break/leave the situation, call supportive friend or family member, self-massage, use nicotine replacement therapy). |
| Alcohol | Drinking alcohol can lead to relapse. Consider limiting/abstaining from alcohol during the early stages of quitting. |
| Other smokers | Quitting is more difficult when other smokers are around. This is especially difficult if there is another smoker in the household. Limit prolonged contact with individuals who are smoking during the early stages of quitting. Ask coworkers, friends and housemates not to smoke in your presence. |
| Oral gratification needs | Have nontobacco oral substitutes (e.g., gum, sugarless candy, straws, toothpicks, lip balm, toothbrush, nicotine replacement therapy, bottled water) readily available. |
| Automatic smoking routines | Anticipate routines that are associated with tobacco use and develop an alternative plan.<br>Examples:<br>■ *Smoking with morning coffee:* change morning routine, drink tea instead of coffee, take shower before drinking coffee, take a brisk walk shortly after awakening.<br>■ *Smoking while driving:* remove all tobacco from car, have car interior detailed, listen to a book on tape or talk radio, use oral substitute.<br>■ *Smoking while on the phone:* stand while talking, limit call duration, change phone location, keep hands occupied by doodling or sketching.<br>■ *Smoking after meals:* get up and immediately do dishes or take a brisk walk after eating, call supportive friend. |
| Postcessation weight gain | The majority of tobacco users gain weight after quitting. Most quitters will gain less than 10 lb, but there is a broad range of weight gain reported, with up to 10% of quitters gaining as much as 30 lb.[2] In general, attempting to modify multiple behaviors at one time is not recommended. If weight gain is a barrier to quitting, engage in regular physical activity and adhere to a healthy diet (as opposed to strict dieting). Carefully plan and prepare meals; increase fruit, vegetable, and water intake to create a feeling of fullness; and chew sugarless gum or eat sugarless candy. Consider use of pharmacotherapy that has been shown to delay weight gain (e.g., nicotine gum, bupropion). |
| Cravings for tobacco | Cravings for tobacco are temporary and usually pass within 5-10 minutes. Handle cravings through distractive thinking, taking a break, changing activities/tasks, taking deep breaths, or performing self-massage. |

*Source*: Adapted with permission from reference 30. 

quitlines has been shown to be effective in promoting quitting among users,[36,37] and even the busiest of clinicians can serve an important role by simply identifying tobacco users and referring them to the quitlines for more comprehensive counseling. All patients, whether counseled face-to-face by a clinician or referred to external sources of counseling, should be commended for making the important and difficult decision to quit.

**TABLE 50-5 Tobacco Cessation Withdrawal Symptoms Management**

| Symptoms | Cause | Duration | Relief |
|---|---|---|---|
| Chest tightness | Tightness is likely caused by tension created by the body's need for nicotine or may be caused by sore muscles from coughing. | A few days | Use relaxation techniques<br>Try deep breathing<br>Use of NRT might help |
| Constipation, stomach pain, gas | Intestinal movement decreases. | Up to 2 weeks | Drink plenty of fluids<br>Add fruits, vegetables, and whole grain cereals to diet |
| Cough, dry throat, nasal drip | The body is getting rid of mucus, which has blocked airways and restricted breathing. | A few days | Drink plenty of fluids |
| Craving for a cigarette | Nicotine is a strongly addictive drug, and abstinence causes cravings. | Frequent for up to 3 days; can happen for months or years | Avoid additional stress during first few weeks<br>Wait out the urge (which lasts only a few minutes)<br>Distract yourself<br>Exercise (take walks) |
| Difficulty concentrating | The body needs time to adjust to not having constant stimulation from nicotine. | A few weeks | Plan workload accordingly<br>Avoid additional stress during first few weeks |
| Dizziness | The body is getting extra oxygen. | 1-2 days | Use extra caution<br>Change positions slowly |
| Fatigue | Nicotine is a stimulant. | 2-4 weeks | Take naps<br>Do not push yourself<br>Use of NRT might help |
| Hunger | Cravings for a cigarette can be confused with hunger. Sensation may result from oral cravings, or the desire for something in the mouth. | Up to several weeks | Drink water or low-calorie liquids<br>Be prepared with low-calorie snacks |
| Insomnia | Nicotine affects brain wave function and influences sleep patterns. Coughing and dreams about smoking are common. | 1 week | Avoid caffeine after 12 PM<br>Use relaxation techniques |
| Irritability | The body's craving for nicotine can produce irritability. | 2-4 weeks | Take walks<br>Try hot baths<br>Use relaxation techniques |

*Source*: Adapted with permission from reference 30. 

*Counseling Patients Who Recently Quit* Patients who recently quit will face frequent, difficult challenges in countering withdrawal symptoms (Table 50-5) and cravings or temptations to use tobacco. It is important to help them identify situations that might trigger relapse and suggest appropriate coping strategies. Because smoking is a habitual behavior, patients should be advised to alter their daily routines. This helps to disassociate the behaviors from the tobacco.

Often, patients expect that they can change their behavior over a short period of time (weeks to months), yet experts believe patients must remain vigilant for at least 6 months before a new behavior is adopted or an old behavior is extinguished.[38] If a patient indicates he or she has quit smoking, it is important to ask *for how long* he or she has been abstinent. Many persons who quit using tobacco will experience cravings years and even decades after quitting. Thus, *relapse prevention* counseling should be part of every follow-up contact with patients who have recently quit smoking. Patients who slip and smoke a cigarette (or use any form of tobacco) or experience a full relapse back to habitual smoking should be encouraged to think through the scenario in which smoking first recurred and identify the trigger for relapse. Identifying triggers will provide valuable information for future quit attempts.

*Counseling Patients Who Are Former Smokers* Although patients who have been smoke-free for 6 or more months can be considered former smokers, many remain vulnerable to relapse. The strategies to be applied for former tobacco users are similar, but typically less intensive, than

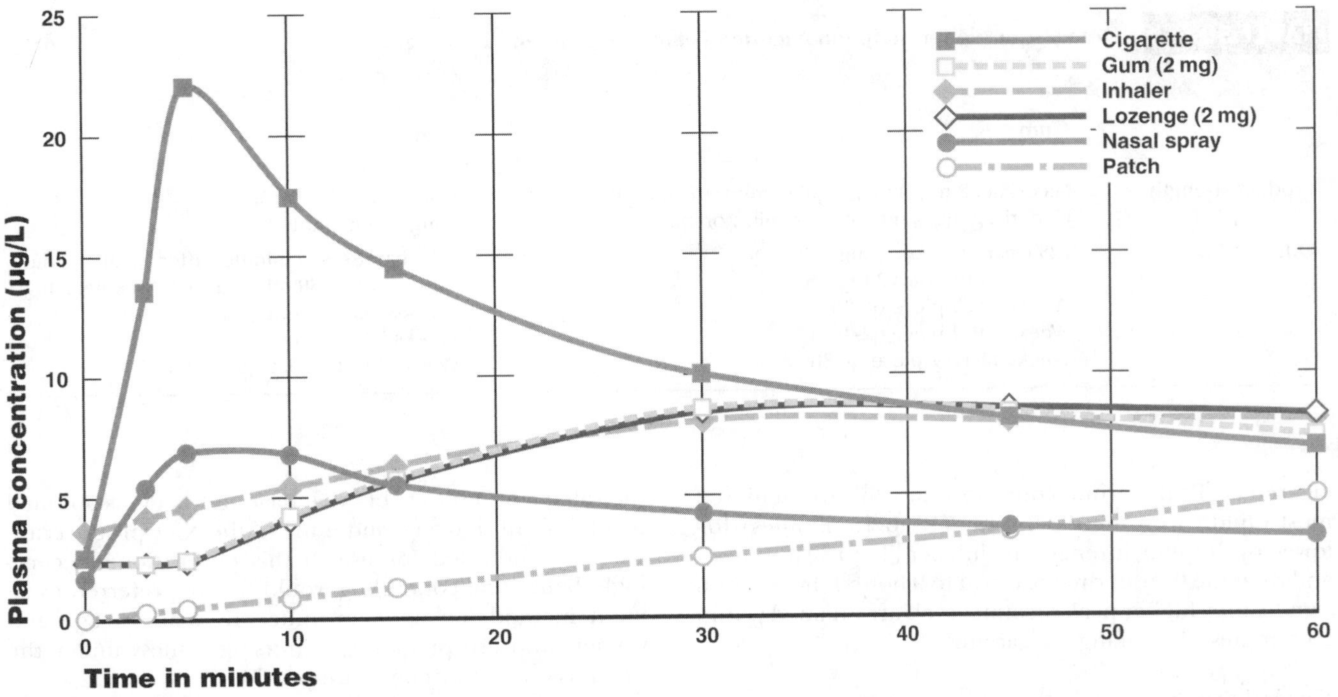


FIGURE 50-3 Plasma nicotine concentrations for various nicotine delivery systems. (Adapted with permission from reference 30. Copyright © 1999-2006 The Regents of the University of California, University of Southern California, and Western University of Health Sciences. All rights reserved.)

those to be applied for recent quitters. The goal for these patients is to remain tobacco-free for life. Clinicians should evaluate their patient's quit attempt and coping strategies—has the patient had any strong temptations to use tobacco, or any occasional use of tobacco products (even a puff)? Also, it is important to ensure that patients are appropriately terminating or tapering off of pharmacotherapy products. Patients who have been smoke-free should be congratulated for their enormous success.

### *Pharmacologic Therapy*

Although there are select situations in which pharmacotherapy should be used with caution or only while under the supervision of a primary care provider (see Safety Considerations), the vast majority of quitters should be advised to incorporate pharmacotherapy as a component of their treatment plan. Currently, there are six Food and Drug Administration (FDA)-approved, first-line[2] agents for smoking cessation, including five formulations of NRT and sustained-release bupropion. Three of the NRT formulations (gum, lozenge, and transdermal patch) are available without a prescription, whereas the nicotine inhaler, nicotine nasal spray, and bupropion require a prescription. Although nortriptyline and clonidine are considered as second-line agents and significantly increase long-term cessation rates compared with placebo, these medications require a prescription and currently do not have an FDA-approved indication for smoking cessation.

#### Nicotine Replacement Therapy

When nicotine gum and transdermal patches were originally approved, both were available only with a prescription. In 1996, these agents were switched to nonprescription status, enabling consumers to self-treat their tobacco dependence. The most recent NRT formulation to receive an FDA approval for smoking cessation is the nicotine lozenge, which was released directly to the nonprescription market in late 2002.

*Mechanism of Action/Pharmacokinetics* The main mechanism of action of NRT is thought to be stimulation of the nicotine receptors in the brain's ventral tegmental area, which results in release of dopamine into the nucleus accumbens. One rationale for using NRT during a quit attempt is that it provides smokers with a nontobacco source of nicotine, which lessens the severity of the symptoms of nicotine withdrawal. This assists quitters by allowing them to focus their efforts on breaking the behavioral habit of smoking. Because the onset of action for nicotine replacement therapy is not as rapid as that of nicotine obtained through smoking, patients who use NRT become less habituated to the nearly immediate, reinforcing effects of inhaled nicotine.[2]

Nicotine is well absorbed (Figure 50-3) from many sites, including the lung, skin, and nasal and buccal (oral) mucosa. Nicotine absorption is pH dependent, and lower systemic concentrations are achieved under acidic conditions. Nicotine also is well absorbed from the gastrointestinal tract (small intestine) but undergoes extensive first-pass hepatic metabolism resulting in negligible systemic levels of nicotine.[20]

The major difference between the various NRT formulations is the site and rate of nicotine absorption (Figure 50-3). All of the NRT formulations deliver nicotine less rapidly and achieve lower serum nicotine levels than do

**TABLE 50-6 Dosages for Nonprescription Nicotine Polacrilex Gum and Lozenge**

| | Gum | Lozenge |
|---|---|---|
| Product strength | Nicorette: 2 mg, 4 mg; regular, mint, fresh mint, orange<br>Generic: 2 mg, 4 mg; regular, mint, orange | Commit:<br>2 mg, 4 mg; mint |
| Dose | ≥25 cigarettes/day: 4 mg<br><25 cigarettes/day: 2 mg<br>Weeks 1-6: 1 piece q1-2h<br>Weeks 7-9: 1 piece q2-4h<br>Weeks 10-12: 1 piece q4-8h | 1st cigarette ≤30 minutes after waking: 4 mg<br>1st cigarette >30 minutes after waking: 2 mg<br>Weeks 1-6: 1 lozenge q1-2h<br>Weeks 7-9: 1 lozenge q2-4h<br>Weeks 10-12: 1 lozenge q4-8h |

cigarettes. Peak serum concentrations[19,39] are achieved most rapidly with the nasal spray (10 to 15 minutes) followed by the gum, lozenge, and inhaler (15 to 30 minutes), and then the transdermal patch (4 to 9 hours). In contrast, significantly higher peak nicotine levels are attained within 10 minutes of smoking a cigarette.

*General Safety Considerations*

Concomitant Use of Tobacco Patients should be instructed not to smoke cigarettes or use other forms of tobacco (e.g., snuff, chewing tobacco, cigars, pipes) while using NRT. Use of tobacco in combination with NRT may result in serum nicotine concentrations that are higher than those achieved from tobacco products alone, increasing the likelihood of nicotine-related adverse effects, including nausea, vomiting, hypersalivation, perspiration, abdominal pain, dizziness, weakness, and palpitations.

Patients With Severe Cardiovascular Disease NRT should be used with caution in patients with serious underlying cardiovascular disease, including those who have had a recent myocardial infarction (i.e., in the preceding 2 weeks), those with serious arrhythmias, and those with serious or worsening angina pectoris.[2] Nicotine may increase the myocardial workload by increasing the heart rate and blood pressure and may constrict coronary arteries, leading to cardiac ischemia.[40,41] While most experts believe the risks of NRT in patients with cardiovascular disease are small relative to the risks of continued smoking,[41,42] patients with serious underlying cardiovascular disease (as previously delineated) are advised to use NRT only while under the supervision of a primary care provider.

Use in Pregnant/Nursing Women and Adolescents Nicotine is classified by the FDA as Pregnancy Category D, meaning there is evidence of risk to the human fetus.[43] Although nicotine is excreted in breast milk, the nicotine levels produced by NRT are quite low and likely not hazardous to infants.[44] Despite potential risks, the use of NRT during pregnancy is probably safer than smoking,[44,45] and NRT might be warranted in selected patients who are unable to quit using nonpharmacologic methods alone, or in situations in which the increased likelihood of quitting outweighs the risks associated with NRT use.[2] Furthermore, the safety and efficacy of NRT have not been established in adolescent smokers, and none of the NRT products are currently indicated for use in this population.[2] Accordingly, behavioral counseling would be the preferred treatment method for smokers under 18 years of age and women who are pregnant or nursing, unless under the supervision of a primary care provider.

Patients Taking Prescription Medicine for Depression or Asthma The manufacturers of nicotine gum, lozenge, and patch recommend that patients taking a prescription medicine for depression or asthma speak with their doctor or pharmacist before using NRT. As indicated in Table 50-2, fluvoxamine and theophylline, both now used infrequently, are the only two agents for depression or asthma that have a known clinically significant interaction with smoking.

*Nicotine Polacrilex Gum* Nicotine polacrilex gum is a resin complex of nicotine and polacrilin in a sugar-free (0.8 cal/piece) chewing gum base. The product is available as 2 and 4 mg strengths, in regular (tobaccolike), mint, and orange flavors (Table 50-6). Recently, a second "fresh mint" formulation of the nicotine gum became available. This product differs from the previous formulations in that it is softer to chew and has a longer-lasting mint taste. All gum formulations contain buffering agents (sodium carbonate and sodium bicarbonate) to increase salivary pH, thereby enhancing absorption of nicotine across the buccal mucosa. When the 2 mg strength gum is used properly, approximately 1 mg of nicotine is absorbed from each dose.[19] Peak serum concentrations of nicotine are achieved approximately 30 minutes after chewing a single piece of gum and then slowly decline over 2 to 3 hours.[39]

Dosage Individuals who smoke fewer than 25 cigarettes per day should initiate therapy with the 2 mg strength, and heavier smokers should initiate with the 4 mg strength. Table 50-6 provides the manufacturer's recommended dosing schedule. During the initial 6 weeks of therapy, patients should use one piece of gum every 1 to 2 hours while awake. In general, this amounts to at least nine pieces of gum daily. Table 50-7 provides specific instructions for proper use of the nicotine gum. The "chew and park" method described in this table allows for the slow, consistent release of nicotine from the polacrilin

**TABLE 50-7 Usage Guidelines for Nicotine Polacrilex Gum**

- Do not smoke cigarettes or use other forms of tobacco (e.g., snuff, chewing tobacco, cigars, pipes) while on nicotine gum therapy.
- Note that nicotine gum is a nicotine delivery system, not a chewing gum.
- Proper administration technique is necessary when using this product. Nicotine from the gum is released using the "chew and park" method:
  - Chew each piece of gum *very slowly* several times.
  - Stop chewing at first sign of peppery, minty, or citrus taste or after experiencing a slight tingling sensation in the mouth. This usually occurs after about 15 chews, but varies.
  - "Park" the gum between the cheek and gum to allow absorption of nicotine across the lining of the mouth.
  - When the taste or tingling dissipates (generally after 1-2 minutes), slowly resume chewing.
  - When the taste or tingle returns, stop chewing and park the gum in a different place in the mouth. Parking the gum in different areas of the mouth will decrease the incidence of mouth irritation.
  - The chew/park steps should be repeated until most of the nicotine is gone, which is when the taste or tingle does not return after continued chewing. On average, each piece of gum lasts 30 minutes.
- To minimize withdrawal symptoms, use the nicotine gum on a scheduled basis rather than as needed.
- Follow the dosage regimen carefully; reduce the dosage at the recommended intervals and stop using the product after 12 weeks of treatment.
- Do not chew more than 24 pieces per day.
- Do not eat or drink 15 minutes before or while using the nicotine gum.
- If acidic drinks (e.g., fruit juices, cola drinks, coffee, wine) or foods (e.g., citrus fruits, tomatoes, vinegar-containing condiments) have been consumed, rinse the mouth with water before placing the gum in the mouth.
- Note that chewing the gum too quickly will result in an unpleasant taste caused by too much nicotine in the saliva and, if the nicotine is swallowed, may cause effects similar to those produced by excess smoking (e.g., nausea, throat irritation, lightheadedness, hiccups).
- Carry or have at least one full sleeve of nicotine polacrilex gum (12 pieces per sleeve) readily available at all times. Keep the nicotine gum in the same place you previously kept your cigarettes (e.g., shirt pocket, purse, or desk).
- Keep this product, including used pieces, out of the reach of children or pets.

resin. Patients can use additional pieces of gum (up to the daily maximum of 24 pieces per day) if cravings occur between the scheduled doses. In general, heavier smokers will need more pieces to alleviate their cravings.

It is important to emphasize that patients often do not use enough of the gum to derive its full benefit. Commonly, patients chew too few pieces per day or shorten the duration of treatment. For this reason, it is preferable to recommend a fixed schedule of administration, tapering over 1 to 3 months rather than using the gum "as needed" to control cravings.[2]

Safety Considerations The most common side effects associated with use of the nicotine gum include unpleasant taste, mouth irritation, jaw muscle soreness/fatigue, hypersalivation, hiccups, and dyspepsia. Many of these side effects can be minimized or prevented by using proper chewing technique. The nicotine polacrilin resin is more viscous than ordinary chewing gum and more likely to adhere to fillings, bridges, dentures, crowns, and braces. If excessive sticking or damage to dental work occurs, the patient should stop using the nicotine gum and consult a dentist. Patients should be warned that chewing the gum too rapidly may result in excessive release of nicotine, leading to lightheadedness, nausea, vomiting, irritation of the throat and mouth, hiccups, and indigestion.

The effectiveness of nicotine gum may be reduced by acidic beverages such as coffee, juices, wine, or soft drinks. These beverages transiently reduce the salivary pH, resulting in decreased absorption of nicotine across the buccal mucosa. Patients should be advised not to eat or drink for 15 minutes before or while using the nicotine gum.

Patients with severe cardiac disease, women who are pregnant or nursing, and adolescents under the age of 18 should use the nicotine gum only while under the supervision of a medical provider. Patients with active temporomandibular joint disease should not use the nicotine gum because the highly viscous consistency of the formulation and the need for frequent chewing may exacerbate this condition. Additionally, the manufacturer recommends that patients with stomach ulcers or diabetes contact their medical provider before use as these conditions are more serious and might require further monitoring.

*Nicotine Polacrilex Lozenge* The nicotine polacrilex lozenge is a resin complex of nicotine and polacrilin in a sugar-free (4 cal/lozenge), lightly mint-flavored lozenge (Table 50-6). The lozenges are available as 2 and 4 mg dime-sized tablets intended for use similar to other medicinal lozenges or troches (i.e., sucked and rotated within the mouth until it dissolves). The pharmacokinetics of the nicotine lozenge and gum formulations are comparable, but a nicotine lozenge delivers approximately 25% more nicotine than does an equivalent dose of nicotine gum because of complete dissolution of the dosage form.[46] Like nicotine gum, the lozenge also contains buffering agents (sodium carbonate and potassium bicarbonate) to increase salivary pH, enhancing the buccal absorption of nicotine.

Dosage Unlike other forms of NRT, which are dosed based on the number of cigarettes smoked per day, the recommended dosage of the nicotine lozenge is based on the "time to first cigarette" of the day. Some studies suggest that the best indicator of nicotine dependence is having a strong desire or need to smoke soon after waking.[46] Thus, patients who smoke their first cigarette of the day within 30 minutes of waking are likely to be more highly dependent on nicotine and require higher dosages than those who delay smoking for more than 30 minutes after waking (Table 50-6).

During the initial 6 weeks of therapy, patients should use 1 lozenge every 1 to 2 hours while awake. In general,

**TABLE 50-8 Usage Guidelines for Nicotine Polacrilex Lozenge**

- Do not smoke cigarettes or use other forms of tobacco (e.g., snuff, chewing tobacco, cigars, pipes) while using the nicotine lozenge.
- Proper administration technique is necessary when using the nicotine lozenge:
  - Place the lozenge in the mouth and allow it to dissolve slowly (20-30 minutes). As the nicotine is released from the lozenge, you may experience a warm, tingling sensation.
  - To reduce the risk of side effects (nausea, hiccups, heartburn), the lozenge should *not* be chewed or swallowed.
  - Occasionally rotate the lozenge to different areas of the mouth to decrease mouth irritation.
- To minimize withdrawal symptoms, use the nicotine lozenge on a scheduled, rather than an as-needed basis.
- Follow the dosage regimen carefully; reduce the dosage at the recommended intervals and stop using the product after 12 weeks of treatment.
- Do not use more than 5 lozenges in 6 hours, or more than 20 lozenges per day.
- Do not eat or drink 15 minutes before or while using the nicotine lozenge.
- If acidic drinks (e.g., fruit juices, cola drinks, coffee, wine) or foods (e.g., citrus fruits, tomatoes, vinegar-containing condiments) have been consumed, rinse the mouth with water before using the lozenge.
- Patients who use more than 1 lozenge at a time, continuously use 1 lozenge after another, or chew or swallow the lozenge are more likely to experience heartburn or indigestion.
- Carry or have at least one full sleeve of nicotine polacrilex lozenges (12 pieces per sleeve) readily available at all times. Keep the nicotine lozenge in the same place you previously kept your cigarettes (e.g., shirt pocket, purse, or desk).
- Keep this product out of the reach of children or pets.

this amounts to at least 9 lozenges daily. Table 50-8 provides further instructions for proper use of the nicotine lozenge. Patients can use additional lozenges (up to 5 lozenges in 6 hours or a maximum of 20 lozenges per day) if cravings occur between the scheduled doses.

Safety Considerations Side effects associated with the nicotine lozenge include mouth irritation, nausea, hiccups, cough, heartburn, headache, flatulence, and insomnia. Patients who use more than one lozenge at a time, continuously use one lozenge after another, or chew or swallow the lozenge are more likely to experience heartburn or indigestion.

The effectiveness of the nicotine lozenge may be reduced by acidic beverages such as coffee, juices, wine, or soft drinks. These beverages may transiently reduce the salivary pH, resulting in decreased absorption of nicotine across the buccal mucosa. Patients should be advised not to eat or drink for 15 minutes before or while using the nicotine lozenge.

Patients with severe cardiac disease, women who are pregnant or nursing, and adolescents under the age of 18 should use the nicotine lozenge only under the supervision of a medical provider. Additionally, the manufacturer recommends that patients with stomach ulcers or diabetes contact their medical provider before use as these conditions, which are more serious, may require further monitoring.

*Nicotine Transdermal Systems (Nicotine Patch)* Nicotine transdermal systems deliver continuous, low levels of nicotine across the skin over 16 or 24 hours. The patch consists of a waterproof surface layer, a nicotine reservoir, an adhesive layer, and a disposable protective liner. Currently, there are three marketed products (Table 50-9). Two of the products (Nicoderm CQ and the generic formulation) deliver the labeled dose of nicotine continuously over 24 hours. The Nicotrol formulation provides continuous nicotine delivery over 16 hours. This system, which more closely approximates typical smoking patterns, is applied in the morning and removed at bedtime.

Dosage The dosing schedules for the nicotine patches vary (Table 50-9). Before recommending a specific product and a dosing schedule, it is important to know how many cigarettes the patient smokes per day. In general, heavier smokers (e.g., more than 10 cigarettes per day) will require higher-strength formulations for a longer duration of therapy. Patients with strong morning cravings for cigarettes might consider a 24-hour patch, because some data suggest this formulation is more effective in reducing cravings in the morning and throughout the day, during the initial 2 weeks after quitting (21 mg, 24-hour patch compared to 15 mg, 16-hour patch).[47] Patients experiencing side effects such as dizziness, perspiration, nausea, vomiting, diarrhea, or headache should consider a lower dose. Eight weeks of nicotine patch therapy has been shown to be as effective as longer durations of therapy, and there is no evidence that dose tapering of the patch results in better quit rates than those seen with abrupt discontinuation.[34] Additional instructions for proper use of the nicotine patch are listed in Table 50-10.

Safety Considerations The most common side effects associated with the nicotine patch are local skin reactions (erythema, burning, and pruritus) at the application site. These reactions, which occur more commonly with the 24-hour products, are caused by skin occlusion or sensitivity to the patch adhesives. Skin reactions can be minimized or prevented by rotating the patch application site on a daily basis. Other less common side effects include vivid or abnormal dreams, insomnia, and headache. Sleep disturbances are more commonly reported in patients using the 24-hour formulations and may be the result of nocturnal nicotine absorption. If this side effect becomes troublesome, patients using the 24-hour products should consider the using the 16-hour Nicotrol patch or removing the 24-hour patch at bedtime.

Patients with severe cardiac disease, women who are pregnant or nursing, and adolescents under the age of 18 should use the nicotine patch only while under the supervision of a medical provider. Patients with dermatologic conditions (e.g., psoriasis, eczema, atopic dermatitis) or those with an allergy to adhesive tape are more likely to experience skin irritation and should not use the nicotine patch.

**TABLE 50-9 Dosages for Nonprescription Transdermal Systems (Nicotine Patch)**

| | Nicotrol Patch | Nicoderm CQ Patch (regular and clear) | Generic Patch (formerly Habitrol) |
|---|---|---|---|
| **Product strength** | 5, 10, 15 mg (16 hour) | 7, 14, 21 mg (24 hour) | 7, 14, 21 mg (24 hour) |
| **Dose** | >10 cigarettes/day: 15 mg/day × 6 weeks; 10 mg/day × 2 weeks; 5 mg/day × 2 weeks | >10 cigarettes/day: 21 mg/day × 6 weeks; 14 mg/day × 2 weeks; 7 mg/day × 2 weeks | >10 cigarettes/day: 21 mg/day × 4 weeks; 14 mg/day × 2 weeks; 7 mg/day × 2 weeks |
| | ≤10 cigarettes/day: *not* recommended | ≤10 cigarettes/day: 14 mg/day × 6 weeks; 7 mg/day × 2 weeks | ≤10 cigarettes/day: 14 mg/day × 6 weeks; 7 mg/day × 2 weeks |

## Prescription Medications for Smoking Cessation

*Nicotine Inhaler* The nicotine inhaler consists of a plastic mouthpiece and a nicotine-containing cartridge that delivers 4 mg of nicotine as an inhaled vapor, which is absorbed across the oropharyngeal mucosa. The inhaler reduces nicotine withdrawal symptoms and may give some degree of comfort by providing a hand-to-mouth ritual that emulates smoking. Side effects of the inhaler include mild mouth and throat irritation, cough, and rhinitis.

*Nicotine Nasal Spray* The nicotine nasal spray is an aqueous solution of nicotine for administration to the nasal mucosa. Each actuation delivers a 0.5 mg bolus of nicotine that is absorbed rapidly (within 10 to 15 minutes) across the nasal mucosa. Because of its rapid onset of action, the spray is a potential option for patients who prefer a medication to rapidly manage withdrawal symptoms. Initially, most patients will experience nose and throat irritation (peppery sensation), watery eyes, sneezing, or coughing when using this product. This product is to be administered without sniffing (i.e., not administered like standard allergy nasal sprays). With regular use, tolerance generally develops and after the first week, most patients have minimal difficulty tolerating the spray.

*Sustained-release Bupropion* Sustained-release bupropion is the only non-nicotine pharmaceutical aid approved for smoking cessation. This agent is thought to affect dopamine and norepinephrine levels, decreasing the cravings for cigarettes and symptoms of nicotine withdrawal.[2]

Therapy is initiated with a dose of 150 mg orally every morning for 3 days, followed by 150 mg twice daily for 7 to 12 weeks. Because steady-state levels are reached after approximately 7 days of therapy, patients set their quit date for 1 to 2 weeks after commencing therapy. Insomnia and dry mouth are the most common side effects reported with bupropion. Because seizures have been reported in approximately 0.1% of patients, bupropion is contraindicated in patients who (1) have a seizure disorder, (2) have a current or prior diagnosis of anorexia or bulimia nervosa, (3) are undergoing abrupt discontinuation of alcohol or sedatives (including benzodiazepines), (4) are currently using or have used a monoamine oxidase inhibitor within the past 14 days, or (5) are currently being treated with any other medications that contain bupropion. Other factors that might increase the odds of seizure and are classified as warnings for this medication include a history of head trauma or prior seizure, central nervous system tumor, the presence of severe hepatic cirrhosis, and concomitant use of medications that lower the seizure threshold. Bupropion can be used safely in combination with NRT and may be beneficial for use in patients with underlying depression.

## Pharmacotherapeutic Comparison

Currently, there are insufficient data to evaluate the relative effectiveness of the different agents for smoking cessation.[2] In general, all of the approved agents (Table 50-11) approximately double the long-term quit rates compared with placebo.[2,34,35] For the NRT products, the pooled abstinence rate is 17% at the longest available follow-up assessment point for all nicotine replacement therapy products, compared with 10% for placebo.[34] In a randomized controlled trial comparing four NRT formulations, all products exhibited similar efficacy, but compliance with therapy was higher with the patch, followed by the gum, which was higher than the inhaler and nasal spray.[48]

## Product Selection Guidelines

Little information is available to guide the selection of one form of pharmacotherapy over another for a given patient. The choice of therapy is therefore based largely on patient preference and tolerability of the available dosage forms.

*Patient Factors* When recommending a nonprescription agent for smoking cessation, it is essential to determine the patient's smoking patterns, lifestyle habits, and coexisting medical conditions. In general, higher levels of smoking will require higher dosages of NRT and longer treatment durations. Patients who smoke continuously throughout the day might have better success with the nicotine patches, because these provide a sustained, steady release of nicotine over 16 or 24 hours. Conversely, patients

**TABLE 50-10 Usage Guidelines for Nicotine Transdermal Systems (Nicotine Patch)**

- Do not smoke cigarettes or use other forms of tobacco (e.g., snuff, chewing tobacco, cigars, pipes) while using the nicotine patch.
- Apply the patch to a clean, dry, hairless area of the skin on the upper body or the upper outer part of the arm at approximately the same time each day.
- The patch should be applied to a different area of skin each day. To minimize the potential for local skin reactions, the same area should not be used again for at least 1 week.
- During application, apply firm pressure to the patch with the palm of the hand for 10 seconds. Be sure that the patch adheres well to the skin, especially around the edges; this is necessary for a good seal.
- Wash your hands after applying or removing the patch.
- The patch should not be left on the skin for more than 16 hours (Nicotrol) or 24 hours (Nicoderm CQ, generic patch) as this may lead to skin irritation.
- Any adhesive remaining on the skin after the patch removal may be removed with rubbing alcohol.
- Water will not reduce the effectiveness of the nicotine patch if it is applied correctly. You may bathe, swim, shower, or exercise while wearing the patch.
- Do not cut patches in half or into smaller pieces to adjust or reduce the nicotine dosage. Nicotine in the patch may evaporate from the cut edges and the patch may be less effective.
- Local skin reactions (itching, burning, and redness) are common with the nicotine patch. These reactions are generally caused by adhesives; they can be minimized by rotating patch application sites and, if they occur, treated with nonprescription hydrocortisone cream.
- Remove the nicotine patch prior to having a magnetic resonance imaging (MRI) procedure. Burns from nicotine patches worn during MRIs have been reported, and are likely caused by the metallic component in the backing of some patches.
- Individuals experiencing vivid dreams or other sleep disruptions should either use the 16-hour patch or remove the 24-hour patch after 16 hours (e.g., before bedtime).
- Discard the removed nicotine patch by folding it onto itself, completely covering the adhesive area.
- Keep new and used patches out of the reach of children and pets.

who smoke intermittently throughout the day or who smoke intensely for short periods of time followed by long periods of abstinence might prefer a relatively short-acting formulation such as nicotine gum or lozenges to more closely mimic their tobacco use patterns. For some quitters, frequent gum chewing may not be feasible or socially acceptable. The nicotine patch, which can be concealed under clothing, might be a reasonable choice for these individuals. Others may find nicotine lozenges, which can be used more discreetly, to be an acceptable alternative. Smokers with underlying dermatologic conditions (e.g., psoriasis, eczema, atopic dermatitis) are more likely to experience skin irritation and should not use the nicotine patch. The nicotine lozenge or patch is better suited for patients with temporomandibular joint disease or dentures. Finally, patients with serious cardiovascular disease, women who are pregnant or nursing, and adolescents should be referred for further evaluation before initiating self-treatment with NRT.

*Patient Preferences* Too often, clinicians are quick to "dispense" instructions or information without first eliciting the patient's preference and/or point of view. When assisting patients with quitting, it is particularly important to understand the patient's perceptions and expectations regarding pharmacotherapy, including the ability to comply with the regimen, previous experience with cessation medications, concern about weight gain, and other issues. Because NRT formulations require frequent dosing or nontraditional routes of administration, patient education regarding proper use of these products is essential. Patients who have difficulty taking multiple doses of medications throughout the day or those who want a simplified regimen might achieve greater success with the nicotine patch. In contrast, the gum or lozenge may be preferable for patients desiring the ability to titrate nicotine levels to manage withdrawal symptoms. This may include smokers who need a more flexible nicotine dosage form to avoid injury, such as transportation workers or persons who work with heavy machinery. Some quitters may find they need an oral substitute for tobacco; the oral gratification afforded by the nicotine gum, lozenge, or inhaler might be beneficial in these patients.

All smokers making a repeat quit attempt should be queried about their prior use of pharmacotherapy and their perceptions of the treatment options. For patients reporting a favorable past experience with a given product, retreatment with the same agent may be appropriate, with consideration given to increasing the dose, frequency, or duration of therapy. For patients reporting a negative experience with pharmacotherapy (e.g., poor adherence, side effects, palatability issues, and cost) a different regimen should be considered. For example, if a patient had short-term success with the 24-hour patch but discontinued therapy because of intolerable nightmares, he or she may quit again using the patch, but it should be worn only during the waking hours. A patient who is unable to tolerate nicotine gum because of jaw muscle ache may switch to the nicotine lozenge or patch. For patients expressing concern about postcessation weight gain, nicotine gum may be particularly helpful as this product has been shown to delay weight gain after quitting.[2] Because most health insurance plans do not cover the cost of pharmacotherapy, the out-of-pocket expense of NRT might be a barrier to treatment. For these patients, use of the generic formulations of the nicotine patch and gum may be preferable.

In recalcitrant quitters who have experienced numerous failed attempts using monotherapy, combination therapy might be appropriate. Combination therapy generally involves the use of a long-acting medication (nicotine patch or sustained-release bupropion) in combination with a short-acting formulation (nicotine gum, lozenge, inhaler, or nasal spray). The long-acting formulation, which delivers relatively constant levels of drug, is used to prevent the onset of severe withdrawal symptoms, whereas the short-acting formulation, which delivers nicotine more

**TABLE 50-11 Methods for Smoking Cessation: Estimates of Treatment Efficacy for First-line Agents**

| Pharmacotherapy Agent | Number of Studies | Estimated OR for Tobacco Abstinence, Compared with Control at ≥6 months (95% CI)* |
|---|---|---|
| Nicotine gum[34] | 52 | 1.66 (1.52-1.81) |
| Nicotine lozenge[34] | 4 | 2.05 (1.62-2.59)† |
| Nicotine transdermal patch[34] | 37 | 1.81 (1.63-2.02) |
| Nicotine oral inhaler[34] | 4 | 2.14 (1.44-3.18) |
| Nicotine nasal spray[34] | 4 | 2.35 (1.63-3.38) |
| Bupropion SR[35] | 19 | 2.06 (1.77-2.40) |

Key: CI, confidence interval; OR, odds ratio.

* Odds ratios also depend on the duration of therapy, intensity of additional support provided, and setting in which the NRT was offered.[34]

† Values include two studies conducted using the sublingual tablet, which currently is not available in the United States.

rapidly, is used "as needed" to control withdrawal symptoms that may occur during potential relapse situations (e.g., after meals, or when stressed or around other smokers). While research suggests that combination therapy may be somewhat (but not convincingly) more efficacious than monotherapy,[2,34] this approach should be reserved for patients who have failed with monotherapy, because of the increased risk of nicotine toxicity and lack of long-term safety data. Furthermore, patients considering combination NRT should be referred for further evaluation to ensure they are appropriate candidates for this more aggressive form of treatment.

### *Complementary Therapies*

Although a variety of herbal and homeopathic products are available to aid cessation, data are lacking to support their safety and efficacy. Many herbal preparations for cessation contain lobeline (*Lobelia inflata*), an herbal alkaloid with partial nicotinic agonist properties. A recent meta-analysis found no evidence to support the role of lobeline as an aid for smoking cessation.[49] Controlled trials to test the effects of other complementary therapies, including hypnosis and acupuncture, similarly have not been found to be effective treatments for smoking cessation.[2,50] Patients should be cautioned that "herbal" cigarettes are not safe alternatives; similar to cigarettes, these products also result in the inhalation of tar, carbon monoxide, and other harmful byproducts of combustion.

## Assessment of Smoking Cessation: A Case-based Approach

To help the smoker succeed at smoking cessation, the clinician must help patients evaluate how they smoke, what they have or have not tried in the past, and how willing they are to try different cessation therapies. Analysis of the patient's smoking patterns and the reasons for smoking helps the clinician work with the patient to develop an appropriate treatment plan. Cases 50-1 and 50-2 illustrate the assessment of patients who want to quit.

**CASE 50-1**

| Relevant Evaluation Criteria | Scenario/Model Outcome |
|---|---|
| **Information Gathering** | |
| 1. Gather essential information about the patient's symptoms, including: | |
| a. description of symptom(s) (i.e., nature, onset, duration, severity, associated symptoms) | Patient is interested in quitting smoking within the next month. He smokes approximately 1 pack per day and has been smoking for 25 years. |
| b. description of any factors that seem to precipitate, exacerbate, and/or relieve the patient's symptom(s) | He smokes during breaks at work; very few of his coworkers smoke. He likes to have 1 to 2 cigarettes before getting out of bed in the morning and then another 1 to 2 cigarettes shortly thereafter with his morning coffee. He smokes in the evenings after dinner and while watching TV. |

## CASE 50-1 (continued)

| Relevant Evaluation Criteria | Scenario/Model Outcome |
|---|---|
| c. description of the patient's efforts to relieve the symptoms | The patient has tried to quit several times. Last attempt was years ago when nonprescription nicotine gum first became available. He was successful for 1 week, but disliked the taste of the gum and felt it didn't work well (he experienced frequent withdrawal symptoms). He likes the idea of the nicotine patch, because he can put it on and not have to think about it for the rest of the day. |
| 2. Gather essential patient history information: | |
| a. patient's identity | Pat Maddox |
| b. patient's age, sex, height, and weight | 53 y/o M, 5'10", 220 lb |
| c. patient's occupation | High school chemistry teacher |
| d. patient's dietary habits | Recently (1 week ago) started the diet recommended by the American Diabetes Association |
| e. patient's sleep habits | Generally retires before 10 PM (sleeps ~8 hours night) |
| f. concurrent medical conditions, prescription and nonprescription medications, and dietary supplements | Hypertension well controlled on medication; dyslipidemia, recently diagnosed with type 2 diabetes; metformin 500 mg twice daily; ramipril 5 mg once daily; atorvastatin 10 mg once daily; aspirin 81 mg once daily |
| g. allergies | NKDA |
| h. history of other adverse reactions to medications | None |
| i. other (describe)_______ | Married with 2 teenage sons living at home. His wife also smokes (~1 pack daily). |
| **Assessment and Triage** | |
| 3. Differentiate the patient's signs/symptoms and correctly identify the patient's primary problem(s). | Current smoker. Pat would like to quit smoking as soon as possible. He has five cardiovascular risk factors (smoking, diabetes, hypertension, dyslipidemia, and age). |
| 4. Identify exclusions for self-treatment (see Figure 50-2). | None |
| 5. Formulate a comprehensive list of therapeutic alternatives for the primary problem to determine if triage to a medical practitioner is required, and share this information with the patient. | Work with Pat to set a quit date within the next 1-2 weeks.<br>Options include:<br>(1) Recommend nicotine gum; new flavors have become available since Pat last used it.<br>(2) Recommend nicotine transdermal patch.<br>(3) Recommend nicotine lozenge.<br>(4) Refer to medical provider for prescription pharmacotherapy (nicotine inhaler, nicotine nasal spray, or sustained-release bupropion).<br>(5) Take no action. |
| **Plan** | |
| 6. Select an optimal therapeutic alternative to address the patient's problem, taking into account patient preferences. | Pat has expressed interest in using a nicotine patch. Select a patch type and dose (see Table 50-9) based on the number of cigarettes smoked daily (20 per day). |
| 7. Describe the recommended therapeutic approach to the patient. | Behavioral counseling: See Tables 50-3, 50-4, and 50-5.<br>Pharmacologic therapy: Use of nicotine replacement therapy will help reduce nicotine withdrawal symptoms. The nicotine patch should be applied at approximately the same time each day. Duration of treatment is 6-10 weeks, depending on the specific patch selected. |
| 8. Explain to the patient the rationale for selecting the recommended therapeutic approach from the considered therapeutic alternatives. | You do not have any medical conditions in which nicotine replacement therapy should be used with caution (e.g., recent heart attack, serious arrhythmias, or angina). Your blood pressure is controlled with medication but should continue to be monitored while on NRT. Because you said you are interested in using the nicotine patch, this would be an appropriate agent for you. |

## CASE 50-1 (continued)

| Relevant Evaluation Criteria | Scenario/Model Outcome |
|---|---|
| **Patient Education** | |
| 9. When recommending self-care with nonprescription medications and/or nondrug therapy, convey accurate information to the patient, including: | |
| a. appropriate dose and frequency of administration | We have a choice of initiating step-down therapy with Nicoderm CQ 21 mg/day for 6 weeks; Nicotrol 15 mg/day for 6 weeks; or generic 21 mg/day for 4 weeks. See Table 50-9 for patch dosages for tapering schedule for Nicoderm CQ, Nicotrol, and the generic patch. |
| b. maximum number of days the therapy should be employed | Depending on the product we select, you should plan to use the patch for 8-10 weeks. Shorter treatment courses might increase the severity of nicotine withdrawal symptoms. |
| c. product administration procedures | See Table 50-10. |
| d. expected time to onset of relief | The level of nicotine in your body will gradually rise and level off within 4-9 hours, then remain steady with continued use of the patch. The blood nicotine levels are lower than those from smoking but should be sufficient to help control your nicotine withdrawal. |
| e. degree of relief that can be reasonably expected | Most patients find that nicotine withdrawal symptoms peak 24-48 hours after the last cigarette; withdrawal symptoms then gradually diminish over the next 2-4 weeks. Use of nicotine replacement therapy will help minimize these symptoms. |
| f. most common side effects | The most common side effects include skin reactions (redness, burning, itching) at the application site, sleep disturbances (vivid dreams, insomnia), and headaches. |
| g. side effects that warrant medical intervention should they occur | You should seek medical attention if you experience severe skin irritation (rash or redness of the skin that does not go away after 4 days, or if the skin swells); irregular heartbeats or palpitations; symptoms of nicotine overdose (nausea, vomiting, dizziness, weakness, or rapid heartbeat). |
| h. patient options in the event that condition worsens or persists | If you experience withdrawal symptoms or severe cigarette cravings you should contact your medical provider because you might need a higher dosage of nicotine. If you have side effects related to nicotine excess (see above), you should use the next lower patch dose. |
| i. product storage requirements | Store at room temperature. Keep unused patch in closed, protective pouch. After removing the patch from your skin, fold the adhesive ends together and discard. Keep both new and used patches out of the reach of children and pets. |
| j. specific nondrug measures | Think about ways to make your environment conducive to your quit attempt. Some coping strategies are shown in Table 50-4. It would be helpful if you and your wife quit together. Is she willing to quit smoking at this time, too? You should be very proud of your decision to quit. Let's talk again in 1 week to discuss how you are doing. |
| 10. Solicit patient's follow-up questions. | (1) Can I cut the patch in half when I decrease the dose?<br>(2) Can I swim with the patch on?<br>(3) Will the patch interact with any of my medications? |
| 11. Answer patient's questions. | (1) The patch should not be cut in half, because nicotine can evaporate rapidly from the cut edges, resulting in erratic or reduced delivery of nicotine from the patch.<br>(2) Exposure to water (e.g., swimming, showering, or bathing) for short periods of time should not affect the patch if it is applied correctly (see Table 50-10). The nicotine contained in the patch will not interact with any of the medications you are taking.<br>(3) Some medications may require dosage adjustment when a person quits smoking. However, none of the medications you are taking (aspirin, atorvastatin, metformin, ramipril) require dosage adjustment after quitting smoking. |

Key: NKDA, no known drug allergies; NRT, nicotine replacement therapy.

## CASE 50-2

| Relevant Evaluation Criteria | Scenario/Model Outcome |
|---|---|
| **Information Gathering** | |
| 1. Gather essential information about the patient's symptoms, including: | |
| a. description of symptom(s) (i.e., nature, onset, duration, severity, associated symptoms) | Patient would like information about the various nonprescription medications for smoking cessation. She would like to start a family in the next 6-12 months and wants to quit smoking soon. She has been smoking 1-1.5 packs per day for 10 years. She smokes her first cigarette of the day immediately after waking. She has not received any counseling from a clinician. |
| b. description of any factors that seem to precipitate, exacerbate, and/or relieve the patient's symptom(s) | Patient smokes during breaks at work, after meals, and when she is stressed. |
| c. description of the patient's efforts to relieve the symptoms | The patient tried to quit "cold turkey" last year but resumed smoking after 2 days. She would like to try a nonprescription medication during her next quit attempt. |
| 2. Gather essential patient history information: | |
| a. patient's identity | Cynthia Phelps |
| b. patient's age, sex, height, and weight | 28 y/o F, 5'8", 125 lb |
| c. patient's occupation | Postdoctoral research scientist in a biochemistry laboratory |
| d. patient's dietary habits | Reasonably healthy, low-fat diet |
| e. patient's sleep habits | Works long hours, so sleeps about 6 hours during work week |
| f. concurrent medical conditions, prescription and nonprescription medications, and dietary supplements | Eczema treated with Elocon (mometasone) cream 0.1% as needed for "flares" |
| g. allergies | NKDA |
| h. history of other adverse reactions to medications | None |
| i. other (describe)_______ | None |
| **Assessment and Triage** | |
| 3. Differentiate the patient's signs/symptoms and correctly identify the patient's primary problem(s). | Patient is a young smoker in reasonably good health who would like to quit smoking before trying to become pregnant. |
| 4. Identify exclusions for self-treatment (see Figure 50-2). | None |
| 5. Formulate a comprehensive list of therapeutic alternatives for the primary problem to determine if triage to a medical practitioner is required, and share this information with the patient. | Options include:<br>(1) Recommend nicotine gum.<br>(2) Recommend nicotine lozenge.<br>(3) Recommend nicotine transdermal patch.<br>(4) Refer Cynthia to her primary medical provider for prescription pharmacotherapy (nicotine inhaler, nicotine nasal spray, or sustained-release bupropion).<br>(5) Take no action. |
| **Plan** | |
| 6. Select an optimal therapeutic alternative to address the patient's problem, taking into account patient preferences. | Cynthia would like to use a nonprescription medication and therefore her options include the nicotine gum, the nicotine lozenge, and the transdermal nicotine patch. The transdermal patch is not recommended for use in patients with eczema because of an increased risk for developing skin reactions. Alternatives include the nicotine gum and lozenge. Cynthia indicates a preference for the nicotine lozenge. |

## CASE 50-2 (continued)

| Relevant Evaluation Criteria | Scenario/Model Outcome |
|---|---|
| 7. Describe the recommended therapeutic approach to the patient. | Behavioral counseling: Some coping strategies are listed in Tables 50-3, 50-4, and 50-5. Pharmacologic therapy: Use of the nicotine lozenge will help reduce the symptoms of nicotine withdrawal. The combination of pharmacotherapy and behavioral counseling will increase Cynthia's chances for quitting smoking. |
| 8. Explain to the patient the rationale for selecting the recommended therapeutic approach from the considered therapeutic alternatives. | Given you have eczema, I would not recommend the nicotine patch because patients with skin conditions are more likely to experience skin irritation with the patch. Other medications for smoking cessation that do not require a prescription include the nicotine gum or nicotine lozenge. You have expressed interest in the lozenge formulation (Cynthia further agrees, indicating that she is not a "gum chewer") and this is a reasonable choice. Because you smoke your first cigarette of the day immediately after waking, I would recommend the 4 mg strength lozenge. |
| **Patient Education** | |
| 9. When recommending self-care with nonprescription medications and/or nondrug therapy, convey accurate information to the patient, including: | |
| a. appropriate dose and frequency of administration | Nicotine lozenge 4 mg. See Table 50-6 for nicotine lozenge dosing. |
| b. maximum number of days the therapy should be employed | You should use this treatment for 12 weeks. A shorter treatment duration will increase your chances of experiencing withdrawal symptoms. |
| c. product administration procedures | See Table 50-8 for use of the nicotine lozenge. |
| d. expected time to onset of relief | The level of nicotine in your body will rise within 30 minutes after you take a lozenge. |
| e. degree of relief that can be reasonably expected | Most patients find that nicotine withdrawal symptoms peak 24-48 hours after the last cigarette; withdrawal symptoms then gradually diminish over the next 2-4 weeks. Use of nicotine replacement therapy, such as the nicotine lozenge, will help minimize these symptoms. |
| f. most common side effects | The most common side effects are mouth irritation, nausea, hiccups, cough, heartburn, headache, flatulence, and insomnia. |
| g. side effects that warrant medical intervention should they occur | You should seek medical attention if you experience severe mouth problems; persistent indigestion or severe sore throat; irregular heartbeats or palpitations; or symptoms of nicotine overdose (nausea, vomiting, dizziness, weakness, or rapid heartbeat). |
| h. patient options in the event that condition worsens or persists | During the initial stages of quitting you should use at least 9 lozenges daily. If you experience withdrawal symptoms or cigarette cravings, you may need additional lozenges (up to 5 lozenges in 6 hours or a maximum of 20 lozenges per day). If you have side effects related to nicotine excess (see above), you should use fewer lozenges per day. |
| i. product storage requirements | Store at room temperature. Protect from light. |
| j. specific nondrug measures | Some coping strategies are shown in Table 50-4. You should be very proud of your decision to quit. Women who smoke are more likely to have fertility problems and among those who become pregnant, smoking can cause serious health effects including pregnancy complications, premature birth, low birth weight infants, and sudden infant death. By quitting smoking now you will improve your health and increase your chances for having a healthy baby. |
| 10. Solicit patient's follow-up questions. | I don't want to gain weight after I quit. How many calories are in each lozenge? |
| 11. Answer patient's questions. | The nicotine lozenge is sugar-free and does not contain a significant number of calories (~4 calories per lozenge). See Table 50-4 for additional counseling points regarding postcessation weight gain. |

Key: NKDA, no known drug allergies.

## PATIENT EDUCATION FOR SMOKING CESSATION

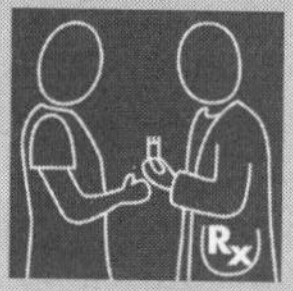

Tobacco use and dependence is a chronic medical condition optimally treated with a combination of behavioral counseling and medications. The primary objective of smoking cessation treatment is to attain complete, long-term abstinence from all nicotine-containing products. For most patients, carefully following product instructions and the self-care measures listed here will help ensure optimal therapeutic outcomes.

### Nondrug Measures

- Receiving counseling from a clinician will increase success of smoking cessation.
- A clinician can help develop a tailored smoking cessation treatment plan.
- Telephone quitlines (1-800-QUIT-NOW) are also available to provide comprehensive counseling services at no cost.

### Nonprescription Medications

#### *Nicotine Replacement Therapy*

- NRT helps relieve and prevent symptoms of nicotine withdrawal by partially replacing the high levels of nicotine your body is used to obtaining from cigarettes. Use of NRT helps you focus on changing your smoking routines and practice new coping skills while decreasing your withdrawal symptoms.
- NRT does not contain any of the harmful tars and other toxins present in tobacco smoke.
- Symptoms and management of nicotine withdrawal are listed in Table 50-5.
- Recommended daily dosages for NRT are shown in Tables 50-6 and 50-9.
- See Table 50-7 for guidelines for the use of nicotine gum, Table 50-8 for the nicotine lozenge, and Table 50-10 for the nicotine patch.
- Follow the dosage regimen of the selected product carefully. Failure to do so will increase the chance of having withdrawal symptoms.
- Use the selected product as recommended. Discontinue use of any form of NRT if you relapse back to smoking.
- Symptoms of nicotine excess include nausea, vomiting, dizziness, diarrhea, weakness, and rapid heartbeat.
- Do not eat or drink 15 minutes before or while using the nicotine gum or lozenge.
- Store NRT products at room temperature and protect from light.
- Keep new and used products out of the reach of children or pets.
- For all forms of NRT, consult your primary care provider before use if you have had a recent (in the past 2 weeks) heart attack, experience frequent pain caused by severe angina, have irregular heartbeats, are pregnant or breast-feeding, or are less than 18 years of age.
- Do not use more than one form of nicotine replacement medication (gum, lozenge, patch, inhaler, or nasal spray) at the same time unless directed by a primary care provider to use combination therapy.

⚠ For all forms of NRT, stop use and seek medical attention if irregular heartbeat or palpitations occur or if you have symptoms of nicotine overdose, such as nausea, vomiting, dizziness, diarrhea, and weakness.

⚠ *Nicotine gum*: stop use if mouth, teeth, or jaw problems develop.

⚠ *Nicotine lozenge*: stop use if mouth problems, persistent indigestion, or severe sore throat develop.

⚠ *Nicotine patch*: stop use if the skin swells, a rash develops, or skin redness caused by the patch does not go away after 4 days.

## Patient Counseling for Smoking Cessation

Smoking is the leading known cause of preventable morbidity and mortality in the United States. Substantial benefits of quitting can be realized at any age. While approximately 70% of adult smokers would like to quit,[11] few are able to do so on their own. Research has shown that tobacco cessation rates can be substantially improved with treatment that includes behavioral counseling and pharmacotherapy.[2] (See Nonpharmacologic Therapy for a detailed discussion of behavioral counseling.) Health care providers are in an ideal position to identify tobacco users and provide assistance throughout the quit attempt.

## Evaluation of Patient Outcomes for Smoking Cessation

Follow-up contact is an essential component of treatment for tobacco use and dependence.[2] At each follow-up contact, the clinician should assess the patient's tobacco use status and, if appropriate, assess and monitor pharmacotherapy use. If the patient has remained abstinent, congratulate success and provide encouragement to remain tobacco-free. If the patient has used tobacco, review the specific circumstances and reassess the commitment to abstinence. Encourage the patient to learn from his or her mistakes and identify strategies to prevent future lapses. Determine if the patient is experiencing nicotine withdrawal symptoms or adverse effects from the pharmacotherapy. Finally, offer ongoing support; if a practitioner is unable to provide the level of ongoing support a patient needs or desires, refer the patient to a specialist for more intensive treatment.

## Key Points for Smoking Cessation

- Clinicians should use the "5 A's" to provide smoking cessation counseling: ask, advise, assess, assist, and arrange.
- For a patient not ready to quit, provide brief counseling addressing the "5 R's": relevance, risks, rewards, roadblocks, and repetition.
- For a patient who is ready to quit, offer behavioral counseling and pharmacotherapy. If time is limited, refer patient to a toll-free quit line (1-800-QUIT-NOW).

- Effective medications are available to help patients quit smoking. Unless medically contraindicated, all patients who are trying to quit should be encouraged to use pharmacotherapy. Drug therapy should be combined with behavioral counseling to further increase the patient's chances for success.
- If a patient has exclusions to self-treatment with NRT, refer to primary care provider for further assessment.
- It is never too late to quit. Quitting smoking at any age has immediate as well as long-term benefits by reducing the risk for smoking-related diseases and improving health in general.

## REFERENCES


1. US Department of Health and Human Services. *The Health Consequences of Smoking: Cancer. A Report of the Surgeon General.* Rockville, Md: Public Health Service, Office on Smoking and Health; 1982. DHHS Publication No. (PHS) 82-50179.
2. Fiore MC, Bailey WC, Cohen SJ, et al. *Treating Tobacco Use and Dependence. Clinical Practice Guideline.* Rockville, Md: US Department of Health and Human Services, Public Health Service; June 2000.
3. Mokdad AH, Marks JS, Stroup DF, et al. Actual causes of death in the United States, 2000. *JAMA.* 2004;291:1238-45.
4. Centers for Disease Control and Prevention. Annual smoking-attributable mortality, years of potential life lost, and productivity losses—United States, 1997-2001. *MMWR Morb Mortal Wkly Rep.* 2005;54:625-8.
5. Centers for Disease Control and Prevention. Annual Smoking-Attributable Mortality, Years of Potential Life Lost, and Economic Costs—United States, 1995-1999. *MMWR Morb Mortal Wkly Rep.* 2002;51:300-3.
6. U.S. Department of Health and Human Services. *Preventing Tobacco Use among Young People: A Report of the Surgeon General.* Atlanta, Ga: US Department of Health and Human Services, Public Health Service, Centers for Disease Control and Prevention, National Center for Chronic Disease Prevention and Health Promotion, Office on Smoking and Health; 1994.
7. U.S. Department of Health and Human Services. *Healthy People 2010.* Washington, DC: US Department of Health and Human Services; 2000.
8. Johnston LD, O'Malley PM, Bachman JG, et al. *Monitoring the Future National Survey Results on Drug Use, 1975-2003. Volume I: Secondary school students.* Bethesda, Md: National Institute on Drug Abuse; 2004. NIH Publication No. 04-5507.
9. Centers for Disease Control and Prevention. Cigarette smoking among adults—United States, 2004. *MMWR Morb Mortal Wkly Rep.* 2005;54:1121-4.
10. Centers for Disease Control and Prevention. State-specific prevalence of cigarette smoking and quitting among adults—United States, 2004. *MMWR Morb Mortal Wkly Rep.* 2004;54:1124-7.
11. Centers for Disease Control and Prevention. Cigarette smoking among adults—United States, 2000. *MMWR Morb Mortal Wkly Rep.* 2002;51:642-5.
12. U.S. Department of Health and Human Services. *The Health Consequences of Smoking: Nicotine Addiction. A Report of the Surgeon General.* Washington, DC: Government Printing Office; 1988. DHHS Publication No. (PHS) 88-8406.
13. Melichar JK, Daglish MR, Nutt DJ. Addiction and withdrawal—current views. *Curr Opin Pharmacol.* 2001;1:84-90.
14. Benowitz NL. Cigarette smoking and nicotine addiction. *Med Clin North Am.* 1992;76:415-37.
15. US Department of Health and Human Services. *The Health Consequences of Smoking: A Report of the Surgeon General.* Bethesda, Md: US Department of Health and Human Services, Centers for Disease Control and Prevention, National Center for Chronic Disease Prevention and Health Promotion, Office on Smoking and Health; 2004.
16. Federal Trade Commission. Cigarette Report for 2003. Issued 2005. Available at: http://www.ftc.gov/reports/cigarette05/050809cigrpt.pdf. Accessed August 30, 2005.
17. Doll R, Peto R, Boreham J, et al. Mortality in relation to smoking: 50 years' observations on male British doctors. *BMJ.* 2004;328:1519-27.
18. National Cancer Institute. *Risks Associated with Low Machine-Measured Yields of Tar and Nicotine.* Smoking and Tobacco Control Monograph No. 13. Bethesda, Md: US Department of Health and Human Services, National Institutes of Health, National Cancer Institute; October 2001. NIH Publication No. 02-5074.
19. Fant RV, Owen LL, Henningfield JE. Nicotine replacement therapy. *Prim Care.* 1999;26:633-52.
20. Benowitz NL. Nicotine addiction. *Prim Care.* 1999;26:611-31.
21. Taylor P. Agents acting at the neuromuscular junction and autonomic ganglia. In: Hardman JG, Limbird LE, Gilman AG, eds. *Goodman and Gilman's The Pharmacological Basis of Therapeutics.* 10th ed. New York: McGraw-Hill, Inc; 2001.
22. National Cancer Institute. *Health Effects of Exposure to Environmental Tobacco Smoke: The Report of the California Environmental Protection Agency.* Smoking and Tobacco Control Monograph No. 10. Bethesda, Md: US Department of Health and Human Services, National Institutes of Health, National Cancer Institute; 1999. NIH Publication No. 99-4645.
23. Zevin S, Benowitz NL. Drug interactions with tobacco smoking. An update. *Clin Pharmacokinet.* 1999;36:425-38.
24. Seibert C, Barbouche E, Fagan J, et al. Prescribing oral contraceptives for women older than 35 years of age. *Ann Intern Med.* 2003;138:54-64.
25. World Health Organization. Low dose combined oral contraceptives. In: *Improving Access to Quality Care in Family Planning: Medical Eligibility Criteria for Contraceptive Use.* 2nd ed. Geneva: World Health Organization; 2000:1-12.
26. Burkman R, Schlesselman JJ, Zieman M. Safety concerns and health benefits associated with oral contraception. *Am J Obstet Gynecol.* 2004;190(4 suppl):S5-S22.
27. Rosenberg L, Palmer JR, Rao RS, et al. Low-dose oral contraceptive use and the risk of myocardial infarction. *Arch Intern Med.* 2001;161:1065-70.
28. Schwingl PJ, Ory HW, Visness CM. Estimates of the risk of cardiovascular death attributable to low-dose oral contraceptives in the United States. *Am J Obstet Gynecol.* 1999;180(1 pt 1):241-9.
29. Schiff I, Bell WR, Davis V, et al. Oral contraceptives and smoking, current considerations: recommendations of a consensus panel. *Am J Obstet Gynecol.* 1999;180(6 pt 2):S383-4.
30. *Rx for Change: Clinician-Assisted Tobacco Cessation.* San Francisco: University of California San Francisco, University of Southern California, and Western University of Health Sciences; 1999-2006.
31. US Department of Health and Human Services. *The Health Benefits of Smoking Cessation. A Report of the Surgeon General.* Bethesda, Md: US Department of Health and Human Services, Public Health Service, Centers for Disease Control and Prevention and Health Promotion, Office on Smoking and Health; 1990. DHHS Publication No. (CDC) 90-8416.
32. Zhu S, Melcer T, Sun J, et al. Smoking cessation with and without assistance: a population-based analysis. *Am J Prev Med.* 2000;18:305-11.
33. Silagy C, Stead LF. Physician advice for smoking cessation. *Cochrane Database Syst Rev.* 2001(2):CD000165.

34. Silagy C, Lancaster T, Stead L, et al. Nicotine replacement therapy for smoking cessation. *Cochrane Database Syst Rev.* 2004(3):CD000146.
35. Hughes J, Stead L, Lancaster T. Antidepressants for smoking cessation. *Cochrane Database Syst Rev.* 2004(4):CD000031.
36. Stead LF, Lancaster T, Perera R. Telephone counselling for smoking cessation (Cochrane Review). *Cochrane Database Syst Rev.* 2003(1):CD002850.
37. Zhu SH, Anderson CM, Tedeschi GJ, et al. Evidence of real-world effectiveness of a telephone quitline for smokers. *N Engl J Med.* 2002;347:1087-93.
38. Prochaska JO, DiClemente CC. The transtheoretical approach: crossing traditional boundaries of therapy. Homewood, Ill: Dow Jones-Irwin; 1984.
39. Schneider NG, Olmstead RE, Franzon MA, et al. The nicotine inhaler: clinical pharmacokinetics and comparison with other nicotine treatments. *Clin Pharmacokinet.* 2001;40:661-84.
40. Benowitz NL, Gourlay SG. Cardiovascular toxicity of nicotine: implications for nicotine replacement therapy. *J Am Coll Cardiol.* 1997;29:1422-31.
41. Benowitz NL. Cigarette smoking and cardiovascular disease: pathophysiology and implications for treatment. *Prog Cardiovasc Dis.* 2003;46:91-111.
42. Joseph AM, Fu SS. Safety issues in pharmacotherapy for smoking in patients with cardiovascular disease. *Prog Cardiovasc Dis.* 2003; 45:429-41.
43. Dempsey DA, Benowitz NL. Risks and benefits of nicotine to aid smoking cessation in pregnancy. *Drug Safety.* 2001;24:277-322.
44. Benowitz N, Dempsey D. Pharmacotherapy for smoking cessation during pregnancy. *Nicotine Tob Res.* 2004;6(suppl 2):S189-S202.
45. Coleman T, Britton J, Thornton J. Nicotine replacement therapy in pregnancy. *BMJ.* 2004;328:965-6.
46. Shiffman S, Dresler CM, Hajek P, et al. Efficacy of a nicotine lozenge for smoking cessation. *Arch Intern Med.* 2002;162:1267-76.
47. Shiffman S, Elash CA, Paton SM, et al. Comparative efficacy of 24-hour and 16-hour transdermal nicotine patches for relief of morning craving. *Addiction.* 2000;95:1185-95.
48. Hajek P, West R, Foulds J, et al. Randomized comparative trial of nicotine polacrilex, a transdermal patch, nasal spray, and an inhaler. *Arch Intern Med.* 1999;159:2033-8.
49. Stead LF, Hughes JR. Lobeline for smoking cessation. *Cochrane Database Syst Rev.* 2000(2):CD000124.
50. Villano LM, White AR. Alternative therapies for tobacco dependence. *Med Clin North Am.* 2004;88:1607-21.

SECTION X

# Home Medical Equipment

CHAPTER 51

# Home Testing and Monitoring Devices

*Wendy Munroe Rosenthal and Geneva Clark Briggs*

In 1977, Warner-Lambert introduced the first home pregnancy test kit—an event that had a dramatic effect on the home diagnostics market. Annual sales of home medical tests are predicted to be $389 million in 2005.[1] The market continues to grow, with an expanded array of products and more user-friendly versions of established ones. Several forces are driving growth in home diagnostics. First is the increased public interest in health, fitness, and preventive medicine: Testing and monitoring kits now allow patients to test themselves conveniently at home, which encourages active participation in their own health care. Second is a reduction in health care costs: Home tests help patients avoid unnecessary visits to health care providers or allow them to seek earlier treatment of a medical condition. Third is the increased number of available tests. Fourth, important advances in technology, such as monoclonal antibodies, have led to simplified tests that can be accurately and easily performed at home.

Home testing and monitoring kits are designed to detect presence or absence of a medical condition and to monitor disease therapy. The Food and Drug Administration (FDA) requires home tests to perform as well as the professional-use equivalent, but these products must be used properly to achieve accurate results.[2]

This chapter discusses home test kits that aid in detecting the following conditions: pregnancy, female fertility, male infertility, menopause, colorectal cancer (fecal occult blood tests), high cholesterol levels, urinary tract infections (UTIs), human immunodeficiency virus (HIV), and hepatitis C, as well as illicit drug use. This chapter also covers proper selection and use of blood pressure monitors. In addition, a table of miscellaneous tests is included. (See Chapter 13 and Chapter 47 for products used in self-monitoring asthma and diabetes mellitus, respectively.)

## SELECTION CRITERIA

With the variety of diagnostic and monitoring products available, deciding which test to recommend to patients is quite challenging. The major product variables to consider include the test's complexity, ease of reading results, presence of a control, and cost. Table 51-1 addresses these variables as well as the major patient assessment variables, which comprise three general areas:

1. Appropriateness of testing
2. Ability to accurately conduct the test and interpret the results
3. Potential interference with test results

**TABLE 51-1 Selection and Use of Home Tests/Devices**

- Always check the test kit's expiration date before purchase to ensure reagents are not outdated.
- Follow the manufacturer's instructions for storing the tests to ensure reagents remain stable.
- When selecting a test, consider simplicity of use. Simple tests are usually desirable because each step is a potential source of error.
- When considering cost, determine the cost per test unit and whether kits with multiple tests are needed. If available, generic or store-brand kits may cost significantly less.
- When possible, select a test that includes a control to ensure the test is functioning correctly.
- Read all instructions carefully and completely before attempting to perform a test.
- Note the time of day the test is to be conducted, the length of time required, and any necessary supplies or equipment; then schedule the best time and place to conduct the test.
- Follow instructions exactly as described and in sequence. If you have questions about the testing procedure or interpretation of the results, consult a health care professional or, if provided, call the test manufacturer's toll-free number for customer assistance.
- Use an accurate timing device that measures seconds to ensure that you wait the specified length of time between steps.
- If the selected test requires observation of a color change and you have color-defective vision or other visual impairment, ask someone with no vision problems to observe the color change and/or read the test results. Also, read the test in good lighting.
- If you have physical limitations that could interfere with performing the test, ask someone to help you perform the test.
- If the test requires a fingerstick and you have a medical condition or take medications that may cause excessive bleeding, ask your primary care provider to conduct the test.

## PREGNANCY DETECTION TESTS

In 2002, the birth rate in the United States was 13.9 live births per 1000 population.[3] The largest numbers of births are by women between ages 18 and 34 years. In the United States, one third of women who think they may be pregnant report using a home pregnancy test.[4] Early detection of pregnancy is desirable for many reasons, including allowing the woman to make decisions regarding prenatal care and lifestyle changes to avoid potential harm to the fetus.

### Physiology of the Female Reproductive Cycle

The female reproductive cycle, which is approximately 28 days long, is hormonally controlled. At the beginning of the cycle (day 1 through approximately day 12), low levels of circulating estrogen and progesterone cause the hypothalamus to secrete gonadotropin-releasing hormone (GnRH). GnRH stimulates release of follicle-stimulating hormone (FSH) and low levels of luteinizing hormone (LH) from the anterior pituitary gland. This combination of hormones promotes development of several follicles within an ovary during each cycle. One follicle is self-selected and continues to mature while the others regress. At midcycle (approximately day 14 or 15), circulating and urinary LH levels significantly increase and cause final maturation of the follicle. Ovulation (rupturing of the follicle and release of the ovum) occurs approximately 20 to 48 hours after the LH surge. Cells in the ruptured follicle then luteinize and form the corpus luteum, which begins to secrete progesterone and estrogen. For approximately 7 to 8 days after ovulation, the corpus luteum continues to develop and secrete estrogen and progesterone, which inhibits further secretion of FSH and LH.

Once ovulation occurs, the ovum remains viable for fertilization for only 12 to 24 hours. Because sperm may live up to 72 hours, the optimal days for sexual intercourse that will result in fertilization are the 2 days before ovulation, the day of ovulation, and the day after ovulation. For the greatest chance of achieving pregnancy, intercourse should take place within 24 hours after the LH surge.

If fertilization occurs, trophoblastic cells produce human chorionic gonadotropic (hCG) hormone. This hormone causes the corpus luteum to continue to produce progesterone and estrogen, forestalling the onset of menses while the placenta develops and becomes functional. As early as day 7 after conception, the placenta produces hCG, some of which is excreted in the urine. The concentration of hCG continues to increase during early pregnancy, reaching maximum levels of hCG 6 weeks after conception. hCG levels decline over the following 4 to 6 weeks, and then stabilize for the remainder of the pregnancy.

If fertilization does not occur during a cycle, the corpus luteum degenerates, circulating levels of progesterone and estrogen diminish, and menstruation occurs (days 1 to 5). Resulting low levels of progesterone and estrogen cause release of GnRH from the hypothalamus, and the hormonal cycle begins again.

### Usage Considerations

hCG, a hormone produced by the trophoblast of the fertilized ovum, is detectable in the urine within 1 to 2 weeks after fertilization. It is considered a diagnostic indicator of pregnancy. Numerous pregnancy tests with different reaction times and hCG sensitivity are available for home use. Table 51-2 lists some available products available that *Consumer Reports* tested for accuracy.

**TABLE 51-2 Selected One-step Pregnancy Tests**

| Trade Name | hCG Sensitivity* | Product Features |
|---|---|---|
| First Response Early Result | Excellent | 2 tests; uses test stick; best combination of sensitivity and reliability |
| Clear Choice | Excellent | 1 test; uses cup; some samples failed to work in Consumer Reports test |
| Answer Quick & Simple One-Step | Very good | 2 tests; uses test sticks; no wick protection; possibly messy to use |
| ClearBlue Easy One Minute | Good | 2 tests; uses test sticks; digital display |
| e.p.t. | Good | 1 or 2 tests; uses test sticks; e.p.t. Certainty has digital display |
| CVS, Equate (Wal-Mart), Target, Walgreens, Rite Aid, and Sav-On Osco house brand | Fair | 1 or 2 tests; use test sticks; some Equate samples failed to work in Consumer Reports test |
| Inverness Medical | Fair | 2 tests; uses test cassette |
| Confirm | Fair | 2 tests; uses test sticks; some samples failed to work in Consumer Reports test |

* *Consumer Reports'* ratings: "Excellent" is approximately equivalent to 6.25 IU/mL and fair 100 IU/mL. Values for "very good" and "good" were not given. For all tests rated "very good," "good," or "fair," waiting 10 minutes before reading test improved sensitivity.[5]

### Mechanism of Action

Home pregnancy tests are designed to detect the presence of hCG in urine. The tests use monoclonal or polyclonal antibodies in an enzyme immunoassay. The antibodies are bound to a solid surface such as a stick, bead, or filter. If urinary hCG is present, it will form a complex with the antibodies. Another antibody, one linked to an enzyme that will react with a chromogen to produce a distinctive color, is added. The hCG is "sandwiched" between the antibody linked to the enzyme and the antibodies bound to the solid surface. Washing or filtering within the testing device removes unbound substances; a chromogen then reacts with the enzyme causing a color change.

### Accuracy Rate

A pregnancy cannot be detected before implantation. Because of natural variability in the timing of ovulation, implantation does not necessarily occur before the expected onset of the next menses. One study found the highest possible screening sensitivity for an hCG-based pregnancy test conducted on the first day of a missed period is 90% because 10% of women may not have an implanted embryo at that point.[6] The authors estimate that the highest possible screening sensitivity of a home pregnancy test by 1 week after the first day of the missed period is 97%.[6] A test sensitivity for hCG of 12.4 mIU/mL is needed to detect 95% of pregnancies on the expected day of a missed period.[7] Although most pregnancy tests are advertised as 99% accurate, studies of consumer use of home pregnancy tests have found the actual accuracy rate to be 50% to 75% because the directions were not followed carefully.[4]

### Exclusions for Self-Testing

A false-positive result may occur if the woman has had a miscarriage or given birth within the previous 8 weeks because hCG may still be present in the body. Medications such as Pergonal (menotropins for injection) and Profasi (chorionic gonadotropin for injection) can produce false-positive results. Unreliable results may occur in patients with ovarian cysts or an ectopic pregnancy. Oral contraceptive use does not affect test results.

### Interferences

Because hCG levels are very low in early pregnancy and may be below the sensitivity of a particular test, false-negative results may occur with home pregnancy tests if they are performed on or before the first day of a missed period. Erroneous results may also result from refrigerated urine not allowed to warm to room temperature before testing, waxed cups used for collecting urine, or soap residue in household containers used for collecting urine.

### Usage Guidelines

See the box Patient Education for Pregnancy Tests.

### Product Selection Guidelines

Product labeling for most tests states women may use the test as early as the first day of a missed menstrual period. Some tests that can detect hCG levels at 25 IU/mL or less can be used 3 days before the missed period. The earlier a pregnancy test is used, the greater the likelihood of a false-negative result. Most pregnancy tests are one-step procedures. Some tests have clear test sticks that allow the woman to see the reaction occurring as a check that sufficient urine was absorbed by the stick. Other tests include two devices, which can be helpful if a negative test is obtained first. The newest tests are digital and display the results as "pregnant" or "not pregnant" instead of colored lines, which eliminates the need to interpret the results. The time to obtain test results varies from 1 to 5 minutes. Generic (store-brand) kits are available and are usually less expensive than the brand-name kits.

In a test of 18 pregnancy test kits, *Consumer Reports* found that First Response Early Result was the most sensitive and reliable test kit.[5] It detected hCG at concentrations as low as 6.5 IU/mL. Although many of the kits tested did not perform as well as the First Response Early Result, waiting 10 minutes (the maximum time allowed for each test) to read the results improved the performance for most of the tests.

## Assessment of Use of Pregnancy Tests: A Case-based Approach

The practitioner should first determine whether the patient used the appropriate timing for the pregnancy test. If product use is appropriate, the practitioner should ask about previous use of pregnancy tests and any difficulties the patient had with the tests. The practitioner must ask questions about medical disorders and medication use to determine whether inaccurate test results are possible or special measures may be required to protect the unborn child. Case 51-1 illustrates assessment of a patient who wishes to use a pregnancy test.

## Patient Counseling for Pregnancy Tests

When counseling a patient on the use of pregnancy tests, the practitioner should emphasize the importance of following package instructions carefully, especially the instruction for when to begin testing. Pregnancy tests are very sensitive; therefore, the patient should be advised of medical and environmental factors that can cause inaccurate test results. The box Patient Education for Pregnancy Tests lists specific information to provide patients.

## Evaluation of Patient Outcomes With Pregnancy Tests

If the pregnancy test result is positive, the woman should assume she is pregnant and contact her primary care provider or an obstetrician as soon as possible. Also, if the patient is taking teratogenic medications (e.g., Accutane, methotrexate) or any drugs for chronic conditions, advise her to discuss with her health care practitioners any possible effects the drugs may have on a fetus. If the test result

## CASE 51-1

| Relevant Evaluation Criteria | Scenario/Model Outcome |
|---|---|
| **Information Gathering** | |
| 1. Gather essential information relative to the patient's reason for testing including: | |
| a. description of symptom(s) (i.e., nature, onset, duration, severity, associated symptoms) | Patient has been attempting to get pregnant for 2 months. She states that her period is due in 3 days and wonders if she can go ahead and test. She has no pregnancy symptoms. |
| b. medical history, including family history | None relevant to testing |
| 2. Gather essential patient history information: | |
| a. patient's identity | Susan Wilson |
| b. age, sex, weight, and height | 33 y/o F, weight 128 lb (per patient), height 5'2" (per patient) |
| c. patient's occupation | N/A |
| d. patient's dietary habits | N/A |
| e. patient's sleep habits | N/A |
| f. concurrent medical conditions, prescription and nonprescription medications, and dietary supplements | Prenatal multivitamin with 0.8 mg folic acid |
| g. allergies | N/A |
| h. history of other adverse reactions to medications | N/A |
| i. prior use of diagnostic/monitoring test | Susan has used a home pregnancy test (store brand) in the past. Recently she has been testing on the day her period was due. |
| j. potential problems with performing/ interpreting test | Susan has had some difficulty deciding if the test was positive or negative when testing the past 2 months. She could not really decide if a line was present or not. She has no visual or physical impairments. |
| k. other (describe) ________ | N/A |
| **Assessment and Triage** | |
| *3. Determine if self-testing is appropriate. | Self-testing at this time is not appropriate. Although many tests are marketed for "early" testing, the possibility of an erroneous result and the need for repeat testing make it advisable to wait to test. |
| 4. Identify exclusions for self-testing (see section Exclusions for Self-Testing under Pregnancy Tests). | None |
| 5. Formulate a comprehensive list of therapeutic alternatives for the reason for testing to determine if triage to a medical practitioner is required and share this information with the patient. | Options include:<br>(1) Recommend waiting until at least the first day after a missed period.<br>(2) Recommend a test with lowest hCG detection level and advise patient to retest in 1 week if negative and period has not started.<br>(3) Take no action. |
| **Plan** | |
| 6. Select an optimal alternative to address the patient's problem, taking into account patient preferences. | The patient prefers testing now with a more sensitive test. |
| 7. Describe the recommended therapeutic approach to the patient. | N/A |
| 8. Explain to the patient the rationale for selecting the recommended therapeutic alternatives that were considered. | N/A |

## CASE 51-1 (continued)

| Relevant Evaluation Criteria | Scenario/Model Outcome |
|---|---|
| **Patient Education** | |
| 9. Describe the testing procedure to the patient, including: | |
| a. specific instructions | When you do perform the test, follow the instructions carefully (see box Patient Education for Pregnancy Tests). |
| b. how to avoid incorrect results | See the box Patient Education for Pregnancy Tests. Since she had difficulty in the past interpreting the results, suggest she use a test with a digital readout. |
| 10. Solicit follow-up questions from patient. | If I get a negative result on this test, does this mean I am definitely not pregnant? |
| 11. Answer patient's questions. | No. Because of the variable time of ovulation, implantation of a fertilized egg may not have occurred by the date of the expected period or the levels of hCG in the urine could be below the sensitivity of the test. Retest in 1 week if your period has not begun. |

Key: hCG, human chorionic gonadotropin; N/A, not applicable.

## PATIENT EDUCATION FOR PREGNANCY TESTS

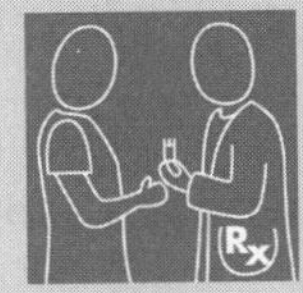

The obvious objective of self-testing is to determine whether a patient is pregnant. For most patients, carefully following package instructions and the self-care measures listed here will help ensure accurate test results.

### Avoidance of Incorrect Results

- The most accurate results will be obtained by waiting at least 1 week after the date of the expected period. Performing the test too early may produce false-negative results.
- Be sure to use the urine collection device provided in the kit. Wax particles in waxed cups can clog the test matrix, causing false results. Soap residue in household containers can also interfere with test results.
- Try to test the urine sample immediately after collection.
- If the sample must be tested later, store it in the refrigerator, but allow the sample to warm to room temperature for 20 to 30 minutes before testing. Chilled urine may produce false-negative results. Be careful not to redisperse any sediment present in the sample. Do not shake the sample.

### Usage Guidelines

- Unless package instructions specify otherwise, use the first morning urine because the levels of hCG, if present, will be concentrated at that time.
- If testing occurs at other times of the day, restrict fluid intake for 4 to 6 hours before urine collection.
- Remove test stick or cassette from packaging just before use. For test sticks, remove cap, if present, from absorbent tip.
- Apply urine to testing device using whichever of the following methods is specified in package instructions: (1) hold test stick in the urine stream for designated time, (2) urinate into testing well of test cassette, and/or (3) collect urine in a collection cup and dip the strip or use a dropper to apply the urine.
- After the urine is applied, lay the testing device on a flat surface. Wait the recommended time (1-5 minutes) before reading results. Waiting the maximum allowed time may improve the sensitivity of the test.
- After reading the results, discard the testing device. If the test result is negative, test again in 1 week if menstruation has not started.

⚠ If the second test is negative and menstruation has not begun, see a health care provider.

*Source:* References 5 and 8.

is negative, the woman should review the procedure and make sure she performed the test correctly. She should test again in 1 week if menstrual flow has not begun. If the results of the second test are negative and menses still has not begun, the woman should seek the advice of a health care provider.

## FERTILITY TESTS

Women who have difficulty becoming pregnant use various methods of predicting ovulation to allow them to detect ovulation so they can time sexual intercourse to coincide with optimal fertility. This section discusses the use of basal

**TABLE 51-3 Selected Ovulation Prediction Tests and Devices**

| Trade Name | Reaction Time | Product Features |
|---|---|---|
| Clearblue Easy Ovulation Test Pack (former name: ClearPlan Easy) | 3 minutes | 5-day kit. Uses urine test sticks; predicts ovulation within 24-36 hours; most sensitive product in *Consumer Reports* test; easy to read |
| Clearblue Easy Fertility Monitor (former name: ClearPlan) | 3 minutes | Reusable monitor. Uses urine test sticks; predicts 1-to-5-day window of peak fertility; easy to read; permits only one reading per day; tests for LH and E3G |
| Answer 1-Step Ovulation | 5 minutes | 5-day kit. Uses urine test sticks; predicts ovulation within 24-36 hours |
| Conceive Ovulation Test | 3 minutes | 5-day kit. Provides urine test cassette, dropper, plastic cup; predicts ovulation within 24-40 hours |
| First Response 1-Step Ovulation Predictor Test | 5 minutes | 5-day kit. Uses urine test sticks; predicts ovulation within 24-36 hours |
| OvuQUICK One Step | 4 minutes | 6-day or 9-day kit. Uses urine test pads; predicts ovulation within 24-40 hours |
| OvaCue Fertility Monitor | 3 seconds | Monitor, reusable saliva electrolyte sensor, and optional vaginal sensor. Predicts ovulation within 5-7 days; tracks cycle data; can upload results to free software for graphing |
| Mini-Microscope Saliva Ovulation Tester | 10-15 minutes | Reusable microscope. Uses saliva; lipstick size; predicts ovulation within 5-7 days |
| Ovulook Ovulation Tester | 5-20 minutes | Reusable microscope. Uses saliva; round compact-disk size device with 12 tracking disks; 31 days of samples per disk; battery-operated light |
| BD Basal Thermometer | 1 minute | Digital thermometer. Auto memory for last reading; continuous beep to indicate it is working; signals when done; large lighted display |
| Geratherm Basal Thermometer | 3 minutes | Mercury-free thermometer. Magnified case for easier reading |

thermometers, ovulation prediction test kits, and fertility microscopes. These tests and devices are also useful for women who want to be more aware of their time of ovulation. However, they are not a reliable means of birth control.

It may take several months for fertile women to become pregnant. In contrast, infertility is the medical inability to conceive after 1 year of unsuccessful attempts in women younger than 35 years and after 6 months in women older than 35 years.[8] Infertility is estimated to occur in 5.3 million American men and women.[8]

## Female Fertility Tests

### *Usage Considerations*

Available nonprescription products for ovulation prediction (Table 51-3) include basal thermometers, urine tests, and saliva tests. Each detection method has a different mechanism of action and method of use. Women should pick a method that best suits their lifestyle or philosophy of self-care. Because of the environmental concerns with mercury, digital basal thermometers are becoming more widely available.

#### Basal Thermometry

For many years, women have measured basal body temperature (BBT) to predict the time of ovulation. Resting BBT is usually below normal during the first part of the female reproductive cycle. After ovulation, it rises to a level closer to normal (i.e., 98.6°F [37°C]).

*Mechanism of Action* When using basal thermometry, women take their temperature (orally, rectally, or vaginally) with a basal thermometer each morning before arising. These temperature measurements are then plotted graphically. A rise in temperature signals that ovulation has occurred. When the increase occurs, women who want to become pregnant should have intercourse as soon as possible to maximize their chances of conception.

*Accuracy Rate* The only equipment necessary for monitoring BBT is a basal thermometer, which has smaller gradations than a regular thermometer. Although basal thermometry is a relatively simple method of ovulation prediction, recording and interpreting temperature data can be confusing. In addition, some women may have difficulty reading thermometers accurately. Because the temperature increase that follows ovulation is small (0.4°F to 1.0°F [0.2°C to 0.6°C]), women who have trouble reading a thermometer may miss the rise altogether. In this case, a digital model should be used.

*Interferences* Several factors, such as emotions, movements, and infections, can influence the basal metabolic temperature. Eating, drinking, talking, and smoking should be postponed until after each measurement is obtained.

*Usage Guidelines* See the box Patient Education for Ovulation Prediction Tests and Devices.

*Product Selection Guidelines* Basal digital thermometers are better environmental choices than mercury thermometers and do not require the patient to interpret the reading. The BD basal digital thermometer includes an FDA-approved fertility software program (Taking Charge of Your Fertility). Digital thermometers that track multiple temperature readings for the user are available although they are more expensive than digital thermometers without such a feature. Non–mercury-containing basal thermometers are now available.

### Urinary Hormone Tests

Ovulation prediction tests that use urine samples to estimate the time of ovulation are marketed to women who are having difficulty conceiving and need to pinpoint ovulation.

*Mechanism of Action* Urine-based ovulation prediction tests use monoclonal antibodies specific to LH to detect the surge in LH. An enzyme-linked immunosorbent assay (ELISA) elicits a color change indicating the amount of LH in the urine.[8] The LH surge is revealed by a difference in color or color intensity from that noted on the previous day of testing. The intensity of color on the test stick is directly proportional to the amount of LH in the urine sample. Generally, early morning collection of urine is recommended because the LH surge usually begins early in the day, and the urine concentration is relatively consistent at this time. Some products do not specify a time of day, requiring only that a consistent time of day be used.

Testing should begin 2 to 4 days before the estimated day of ovulation. The kit contains directions to determine when to begin testing according to the average length of the past three menstrual cycles. If the cycle varies by more than 3 to 4 days each month, the woman should use the shortest menstrual cycle to determine the starting date.

The Clearblue Easy Fertility Monitor increases the specificity of ovulation prediction by measuring both LH and E3G, a component of estrogen. E3G levels rise and fall in a similar pattern to LH. This product uses test sticks that the woman places in her urine stream and then inserts into a small, palm-size monitor with a light-emitting diode screen. The patient must establish a baseline with data about her hormone-level fluctuations to accurately predict ovulation. For the first month, she tests for 20 consecutive days, starting on approximately the sixth day after the beginning of menstruation. Using these data, the monitor calculates the time window during which the woman is most likely to conceive. After establishing her baseline, she tests for 10 to 20 days each month, depending on her cycle length. The results each day are displayed as low, high, or peak fertility.[9] A low result indicates a small chance of conception; accordingly, a high result indicates increased chance of conception. This reading is typically taken for 1 to 5 days leading up to peak fertility for each cycle. A "peak" reading indicates the highest chance of conception and is usually taken 2 days before ovulation.

*Exclusions for Self-Testing* Medications used to promote ovulation (e.g., menotropins) artificially elevate LH and may cause false-positive results in ovulation prediction tests that measure only LH. The true LH surge can be detected in patients receiving clomiphene as long as testing does not begin until the second day after drug therapy ends. Medical conditions associated with high levels of LH, such as menopause and polycystic ovary syndrome, may also cause false-positive results for ovulation. Pregnancy can give a false-positive result for ovulation. If the patient has recently discontinued using oral contraceptives, the start of ovulation may be delayed for one to two cycles. Thus, it would not be appropriate to use a home ovulation prediction test until fertilization has been attempted unsuccessfully for 1 to 2 months after discontinuation of the oral contraceptives.

Polycystic ovary syndrome, medications that affect the cycle (e.g., oral contraceptives, certain fertility treatments, estrogen containing medications), impaired liver or kidney function (which alters levels of E3G), breast-feeding, tetracycline (not oxytetracycline or minocycline), and perimenopause may produce false-positive results with the Clearblue Easy Fertility Monitor. Women who have recently been pregnant, stopped breast-feeding, or stopped using hormonal contraception should consider waiting until they have at least two natural menstrual cycles in a row (lasting 21 to 42 days) before using the Clearblue Easy Fertility Monitor.[9]

*Usage Guidelines* See the box Patient Education for Ovulation Prediction Tests and Devices.

*Product Selection Guidelines* The available ovulation prediction tests vary in the length of time needed to complete the test, method of applying urine to the test stick, and number of individual tests provided. Patients with longer cycles may benefit from purchasing kits that contain more testing sticks.

The Clearblue Easy Fertility Monitor does have some possible advantages over the standard ovulation prediction kits. The traditional kits identify the 24-to-48-hour window around ovulation, whereas the Clearblue Easy Fertility Monitor identifies a larger window of several days. This monitor needs no patient interpretation of color changes. It is effective for women with monthly cycle lengths of 21 to 42 days because the monitor calculates the fertility period on the basis of each woman's hormone levels.[9] In addition, it measures both LH and E3G, increasing the specificity of ovulation prediction. However, it has not been proven whether these possible advantages increase a woman's chance of accurately identifying ovulation and, ultimately, conceiving.

In a test of 11 ovulation prediction kits, *Consumer Reports* found that the ClearBlue Easy Ovulation Test Pack was the most sensitive and easiest to read.[10] The test also found that the Clearblue Easy Fertility Monitor was the second most sensitive test. The initial cost of the Clearblue Easy Fertility Monitor is higher than that of the traditional ovulation prediction kits that detect only LH, but it is reusable for an indefinite period with only the additional expense of more test sticks. *Consumer Reports* estimated that a user would need to test for ovulation for 8 months or longer to make this monitor price competitive.[10]

### Saliva Electrolyte Tests

Fertility microscopes are reusable devices that analyze crystallization of salts in saliva to predict ovulation. The OvaCue Fertility Monitor measures the concentration of electrolytes in the saliva to predict ovulation.

*Mechanism of Action* Fertility microscopes allow women to examine dried saliva ferning patterns using a lipstick-sized illuminated microscope. The hormonal changes that occur before, during, and after ovulation directly affect saliva electrolyte concentrations, which in turn affect dried saliva patterns. During fertile periods, sample patterns resemble fern leaves (straight lines with railroad track–like cross-hatches). Dotted or bubblelike structures appear during nonfertile periods. The characteristic fern pattern appears in samples approximately 3 to 4 days before ovulation and persists until 2 to 3 days after ovulation.[11] (See the box Patient Education for Ovulation Prediction Tests and Devices for illustrations of the fern patterns.)

A woman should track her cycle daily to get a clear picture of the changes that occur in saliva samples. Random use of the microscope can yield a misleading interpretation. Some women may notice an occasional day of light ferning before menstruation starts.[11]

The OvaCue monitor measures saliva electrolyte resistance.[12] Salivary resistance, a function of saliva electrolyte composition, appears to be altered by changes in adrenocorticotropic hormone (ACTH) or aldosterone throughout the menstrual cycle.[13] Salivary resistance rises a mean of 7.2 days (range 5 to 8 days) before ovulation. The monitor calculates the cycle length, reports a visual indicator of fertility status for each day, reports salivary resistance in ohms, and reports a projected date of peak fertility. If the patient is taking fertility medications, she programs this into the monitor. The monitor then considers this when determining ovulation. A vaginal sensor can also be purchased with the monitor to confirm ovulation by measuring electrolyte changes in the vaginal mucus. Data from the monitor can be charted by hand or transferred to a home computer for graphing with the use of software available from the manufacturer.

*Exclusions for Self-Testing* Patients should not use the microscopes if they have conditions such as polycystic ovary syndrome and perimenopause, which cause increased LH levels and may result in consistent ferning throughout the cycle.[11]

*Interferences* Smoking, alcohol consumption, anticholinergic medications such as antihistamines, or food consumption can affect the quality of saliva specimens.[11,12] The woman should not collect saliva samples within 2 hours of smoking, eating, drinking, or brushing teeth.

*Usage Guidelines* See the box Patient Education for Ovulation Prediction Tests and Devices.

*Product Selection Guidelines* Examining ferning patterns can identify a larger fertility window than traditional ovulation prediction kits, but identification of saliva ferning is subjective. In addition, testing must be done daily. Some products include an instructional videotape and/or a chart for daily recording of saliva sample interpretations to assist the woman in identifying changes.

The initial cost of fertility microscopes is higher than that of ovulation prediction kits that detect LH in the urine, but the microscopes are reusable indefinitely if the slide surface is cared for appropriately. The initial cost of a microscope is less than that of a Clearblue Easy Fertility Monitor.

The initial cost of the OvaCue fertility monitor is more than that of the Clearblue Easy Fertility Monitor. Unlike the Clearblue Easy Fertility Monitor, neither the microscopes nor the OvaCue has any ongoing costs. The saliva measurement devices may be more appealing to women who do not want to test urine.

## Assessment of Use of Female Fertility Tests

The practitioner should ask a patient privately about her reasons for using an ovulation prediction test. If the reason is difficulty in conceiving, the practitioner should find out whether the patient has consulted a health care provider about a possible fertility problem and whether she has previously used ovulation prediction tests or devices such as basal thermometers or fertility microscopes. Questions about other possible pathology and medication use are appropriate for determining possible interferences with test results or temperature measurements.

## Patient Counseling for Female Fertility Tests

To use ELISA-based ovulation prediction products effectively, a woman must know approximately when ovulation occurs or be willing to track three menstrual cycles to determine when it occurs. The practitioner should explain the hormonal fluctuations during the cycle and how they relate to the use of ovulation prediction tests, basal thermometers, and fertility microscopes. The practitioner should also explain the reason for the number of tests or measurements that must be performed with each type of product. The practitioner should emphasize that the woman must consistently use the products for at least 3 months. The box Patient Education for Ovulation Prediction Tests and Devices lists specific information to provide patients.

## Evaluation of Patient Outcomes with Female Fertility Testing

Ovulation prediction products should not be used for more than 3 months. If conception does not occur within this period, the woman should see a primary care provider.

# Male Fertility Tests

Sperm concentration is one of the many factors used to determine male fertility. Since many additional factors play

## PATIENT EDUCATION FOR OVULATION PREDICTION TESTS AND DEVICES

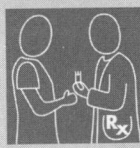

The objective of self-testing is to more accurately determine the time of ovulation to increase the chances of conception. For most patients, carefully following product instructions and the self-care measures listed here will help increase the chances of achieving this goal.

### Basal Thermometers

#### *Avoidance of Incorrect Results*

- Do not move while taking temperature measurements.
- Emotions can affect temperature measurements.
- If an infection is suspected, discontinue the measurements until the disorder is resolved. Begin taking temperatures again on the first day of menstruation of the cycle after resolution of the disorder.
- Do not eat, drink, talk, or smoke within 30 minutes before taking temperature measurements.

#### *Usage Guidelines*

- Read the instructions thoroughly before using the thermometer, and follow instructions carefully.
- Choose one method of taking temperatures (orally, vaginally, or rectally), and use that method consistently.
- Take temperature readings at approximately the same time each morning. Take temperatures just before rising each morning after at least 5 hours of sleep. If using a regular basal thermometer, plot the temperatures on a graph. A rise in temperature indicates that ovulation has occurred.

### Ovulation Prediction Tests Excluding Clearblue Easy Fertility Monitor

#### *Avoidance of Incorrect Results*

- Fertility medications, polycystic ovary syndrome, menopause, and pregnancy can cause false-positive results for ovulation.
- Recent pregnancy or discontinuation of oral contraceptives or breast-feeding will delay ovulation for one or two cycles. Start testing after two natural menstrual cycles have occurred.

#### *Usage Guidelines*

- Start using the test 2 to 3 days before ovulation is expected.
- Follow the manufacturer's specific directions regarding the timing of urine collection. If the first morning urine is not tested, restrict fluid intake for at least 4 hours before testing and avoid urinating until ready to test the urine, so the urine will not be diluted.
- Test the urine sample immediately after collection.
- If immediate testing is not feasible, refrigerate urine for the length of time specified in the directions for each product. Allow refrigerated sample to stand at room temperature for 20 to 30 minutes before beginning the test.
- Do not redisperse any sediment that may be present in the sample.
- If using a kit designed to be passed through the urine stream, either hold a test stick in the urine stream for the specified time, or collect urine in a collection cup and dip the stick in the urine.
- If using a kit not designed to be passed through the urine stream, collect urine in a collection cup, then place the urine in the testing well using the dropper provided.
- After the urine is placed on the testing device, read the results in 3 to 5 minutes, depending on the manufacturer's instructions.
- Watch for the test's first significant increase in color intensity, which indicates that the surge of luteinizing hormone (LH) has occurred and ovulation will occur within a day or 2.
- Once the LH surge is detected, discontinue testing. Remaining tests can be used later, if necessary.
- If the LH surge is not detected, carefully review the testing instructions to ensure they were performed properly.
- If the testing procedure was accurate, ovulation may not have occurred or testing may have occurred too late in the cycle. Consider testing for a longer period in the next cycle to increase the chances of detecting the LH surge.

### Clearblue Easy Fertility Monitor Test

#### *Avoidance of Incorrect Results*

- Fertility medications, polycystic ovary syndrome, menopause, and pregnancy can cause false-positive results for ovulation tests.
- Oral contraceptives, hormone replacement therapy, impaired liver or kidney function, breast-feeding, tetracycline (but not oxytetracycline or minocycline), and perimenopause can cause false-positive results with the Clearblue Easy Fertility Monitor.
- Recent pregnancy or discontinuation of oral contraceptives or breast-feeding will delay ovulation for one or two cycles. Start testing after two natural menstrual cycles have occurred.

#### *Usage Guidelines*

- For the first month, begin testing on the sixth day after beginning menstruation and test for 20 days.
- For subsequent months, test the number of days indicated by the monitor.
- Remove test stick or cassette from packaging just before use.
- Hold the test stick in the urine stream; insert stick in monitor.
- Discard test stick after use.

### Fertility Microscopes

#### *Avoidance of Incorrect Results*

- Do not smoke, drink, or eat within 2 hours of testing saliva.
- Medications with anticholinergic properties can decrease the quality of the saliva sample.
- Polycystic ovary syndrome and perimenopause may interfere with the test results.

#### *Usage Guidelines*

- Wash and dry hands. Place saliva on the slide area of the microscope eyepiece. Allow saliva to dry for 5 to 7 minutes.
- Compare the observed saliva pattern with drawing A (fertile period) and B (nonfertile period).

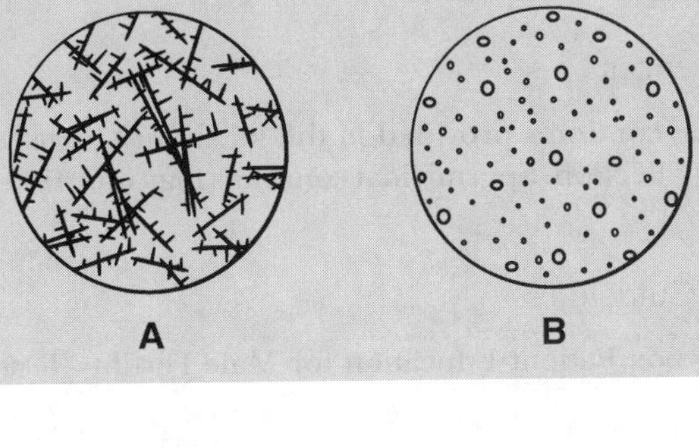

A B

## PATIENT EDUCATION FOR OVULATION PREDICTION TESTS AND DEVICES (continued)

- Clean the round slide surface after each use with a cotton swab soaked with water or alcohol. Be careful not to scratch the glass.
- Do not wash or soak the eyepiece because water may be trapped between the lens of the microscope and the slide.
- To improve accuracy in identifying the fertile period, combine saliva examination with basal thermometry or other fertility test.

**Saliva Electrolyte Monitor**

***Avoidance of Incorrect Results***

- Do not smoke, drink, brush teeth, or eat for 2 hours before testing saliva.
- Test at approximately the same time every morning.
- Avoid excessive sodium consumption. Recent excessive consumption can be identified by a reading that does not follow the existing pattern.

***Usage Guidelines***

- If using the oral sensor, place on the tongue for 3 seconds.
- If using the optional vaginal sensor, connect to monitor and insert into vagina for 5 seconds.
- Track daily readings on a chart or optional software to identify peak values, which indicate fertile period.

⚠ If pregnancy does not occur after 3 months of using these products, see a health care provider.

*Source:* References 8-12.

a role in male infertility, a positive test for sperm count is not a guarantee of fertility. Sperm production is influenced by physical, emotional, and psychologic factors. Factors such as concentration of hormones, stress, high fever, exercise, travel, surgery, medication, and changes in diet may result in a decreased sperm concentration.

### *Usage Considerations*

The male fertility test measures sperm concentration as either above or below the cutoff of 20 million sperm cells per milliliter, which is the World Health Organization (WHO) criterion for determining low sperm count. Two test results of fewer than 20 million cells per milliliter obtained at least 3 days but not more than 7 day apart may indicate male infertility.[14]

#### Mechanism of Action

The test works by staining cells in the sperm sample to produce a color. The intensity of the color is compared with a color reference on the test cassette. The color comparison identifies whether the sperm concentration in the test sample is above 20 million/mL (positive test) or below 20 million/mL (negative test). The test kit contains all the necessary supplies for two tests: test cassette, testing solution, plastic droppers, two liquefaction cups, and two nonspermicidal condoms.

#### Accuracy Rate

Testing performed by the manufacturer found the overall accuracy of the test was 78%.[14]

#### Interferences

Only the condoms provided in the kit should be used for semen collection. Spermicidal condoms may interfere with the test.

#### Usage Guidelines

See the box Patient Education for Male Fertility Tests.

#### Product Selection Guidelines

At this time, only one test kit is available for determining male fertility. The product is marketed as FertilMARQ or BabyStart male infertility test by the same company. Because this test requires the user to make a color comparison, patients with visual difficulties should seek assistance in interpreting the test results.

### *Assessment of Use of Male Fertility Tests*

The practitioner should ask a patient privately whether he has consulted a primary care provider about a possible fertility problem and whether the patient has used male fertility tests previously. Questions about possible pathology, medication use, stress, and physical activity are appropriate for determining possible interference with test results.

### *Patient Counseling for Male Fertility Tests*

Because physical, psychologic, and emotional factors can affect sperm concentration, the practitioner should explain the need for two tests to confirm a sperm count above or below 20 million cells per milliliter. The box Patient Education for Ovulation Prediction Tests/Devices lists specific information to provide patients.

### *Evaluation of Patient Outcomes with Male Fertility Tests*

With the male fertility test, the patient should contact his primary care provider or a fertility specialist if two negative tests are obtained. If one positive and one negative test are obtained, the test should be repeated in 10 weeks with a new test kit.

## FSH TESTS FOR MENOPAUSE

Menopause typically occurs between the ages of 40 and 55 years, but can occur as early as 35 years or as late as 60 years.[15] Menopause results from the decline and eventual cessation of estrogen production. As estrogen levels

## PATIENT EDUCATION FOR MALE FERTILITY TESTS

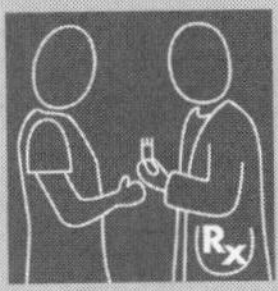

The objective of self-testing is to screen for low sperm levels in semen. For most patients, carefully following product instructions and the self-care measures listed here will help ensure accurate test results.

### Avoidance of Incorrect Results

- Use only the condoms provided in the kit for semen collection.
- Wait 3 days after last ejaculation before collecting a semen sample for testing.
- Use only thinned (liquefied) semen for testing. Some patients have high-viscosity semen, which will not properly liquefy. These patients cannot get accurate results with this test, but they cannot be identified until they attempt the test and discover the semen sample will not liquefy sufficiently to pass through the test cassette.
- Test within 12 hours of sample collection.
- If the sample or solutions take more than 5 minutes to drain through the test wells, the test is invalid.

### Usage Guidelines

- Semen sample can be collected in one of three ways:
  - By masturbation, directing semen into the liquefaction cup
  - By masturbation, using the supplied condom
  - During intercourse, using one of the supplied condoms
- Because freshly ejaculated semen is gel-like, the sample must be allowed to thin to a liquid consistency for testing. The liquefaction cups speed this process from 1 hour to 15 minutes.
- After collection, squeeze all the semen collected into a liquefaction cup and place cap on cup. Small flakes at the bottom of the liquefaction cup are normal.
- Swirl the cup gently at least 10 times.
- Allow the semen sample to liquefy for 15 minutes.
- The semen sample may be stored in the cup for up to 12 hours before testing.
- Swirl the cup again before beginning testing.
- The test cassette contains four wells labeled A, B, C, and D. Reference wells A and C are blue. Test wells B and D are white, and the liquefied semen sample is placed in these wells. The cassette contains enough wells to test two separate semen samples.
- The color of test well B or D is compared with the adjacent blue reference well.
- Fill dropper with semen and add one drop to test well B. Let the drop soak in for at least 1 minute.
- Add two drops of blue solution to test well B. Let the drops soak in for at least 1 minute.
- Add two drops of clear solution to test well B. Let the drops soak in at least 1 minute. Read results within 5 minutes.
- Compare the color in the test well with the color in the adjacent reference well A. A blue color as dark as or darker than the reference color is positive (sperm ≥20 million/mL). A blue color lighter than the reference color is negative (sperm ≤20 million/mL).
- Two separate semen samples should be tested before a complete interpretation of the results can be made. Collect and test the second sample at least 3 days, but not more than 7 days, after the first test was performed.
- When performing the second test, use test well D and reference well C.

⚠ If two negative tests are obtained, see a health care provider for evaluation and further testing.

*Source:* Reference 14.

decline, FSH levels increase. To most patients, menopause refers to a series of changes beginning with early menopause (perimenopause) and ending with the cessation of menstrual periods for a full 12 months (menopause). Symptoms of perimenopause and menopause may include irregular menstrual cycles, hot flashes, vaginal dryness, mood swings, insomnia, and fatigue. Many women find the symptoms of menopause interfere with their daily lives.

## Usage Considerations

At this time several home tests are being marketed for menopause. The urine-based tests for FSH are FDA-approved; the saliva tests are not.

### *Mechanism of Action*

Tests for menopause use monoclonal antibodies specific to FSH to detect the hormone in urine. An ELISA elicits a color change indicating the amount of FSH in the urine. A positive test indicates the presence of FSH at a concentration greater than 25 IU/L, which may indicate a woman is menopausal. Because FSH levels change during the menstrual cycle, the test should be done twice to confirm the results. The two tests should be performed 1 to 2 weeks apart.

### *Interferences*

Dilute urine can produce incorrect results. The patient should test the first morning urine, avoid drinking large amounts of fluids the night before testing, and not consume any fluids after midnight. Oral contraceptives, hormone replacement therapy, and estrogen supplements may affect the test and produce inaccurate results because of their estrogen content and effects on FSH levels.

### *Usage Guidelines*

See the box Patient Education for Menopause Tests. Table 51-4 lists selected menopause tests.

### *Product Selection Guidelines*

Urine-based tests consist of either sticks placed in the urine stream or cassettes to which collected urine is applied. Patient preference should dictate which product is selected. Most of the test kits come with two testing devices for the recommended repeat test.

**TABLE 51-4 FSH Tests for Menopause**

| Brand | Availability | Product Features |
| --- | --- | --- |
| Menocheck Menopause Indicator Test | www.menocheck.com<br>Select retail stores | 2 test sticks |
| Estroven Menopause monitor | www.testsymptomsathome.com<br>Select retail stores | 2 test cassettes, 2 droppers, 2 urine collection dishes |
| CARE Menopause Test | www.home-drugtest.com<br>Select retail stores | 2 test cassettes, 2 droppers, 2 urine collection dishes |
| RU25 Plus Home Menopause Test Kit | www.home-menopause-test.com<br>www.hormonecheck.com | 2 test sticks |

Saliva tests, which are mailed to a laboratory for analysis, measure numerous hormone levels; however, they are not FDA-approved.

### Assessment of Use of FSH Tests for Menopause

The practitioner should find out whether the patient is experiencing classic symptoms of perimenopause and has consulted her primary care provider about them. Questions about use of estrogenic medications are appropriate for determining possible interference with test results.

### Patient Counseling for FSH Tests for Menopause

The practitioner should emphasize that this is not a definitive diagnostic test for menopause. The diagnosis would need to be confirmed by the woman's primary care provider. The box Patient Education for Menopause Testing lists specific information to provide patients.[16,17]

### Evaluation of Patient Outcomes With FSH Tests for Menopause

While FSH is elevated during menopause (the 12-month period of menses cessation), FSH levels may be normal during the perimenopause period, which is when women often are most symptomatic. Thus, a negative test (FSH <25 IU/mL) does not indicate necessarily that the menopausal process has not begun. If a woman gets a negative result and is experiencing classic menopausal symptoms or obtains a positive result for elevated FSH, she should consult her primary care provider for symptom management and osteoporosis prevention.

## FECAL OCCULT BLOOD TESTS

Colorectal cancer, accounting for 15% of all cancers, is the second leading cause of cancer death in the United States.[18] This disorder may be hard to detect. One early and common symptom of colorectal cancer is rectal bleeding. Checking for hidden (occult) blood in the stool is an easy way to screen for a potential colon problem. Fecal occult blood tests (FOBTs) can be used as an adjunct to more invasive tests to detect colorectal cancer and other causes of gastrointestinal (GI) bleeding.

Colorectal cancer occurs most commonly in patients with a family history of colorectal cancer, intestinal polyps, or ulcerative colitis. The incidence of colorectal cancer increases with advancing age. Consumption of high amounts of animal fat and very low amounts of fruit and vegetable fiber is positively related to colorectal cancer.[19,20]

### Usage Considerations

Several nonprescription FOBTs are available. They fall into three categories: toilet tests (Accustat colorectal disease test and EZ-Detect Stool Blood Test), stool wipes (LifeGuard), and manual stool application device (ColonTest-Sensitive). They are all noninvasive and easy to use in the privacy of the home.

#### *Accuracy Rate*

One study found that a 3-day FOBT identified only 24% of colon lesions.[21] When a 3-day FOBT was combined with sigmoidoscopy, many more cancers were identified (75.8%).[21]

#### *Mechanism of Action*

The in-home tests detect blood in feces with a colorimetric assay for hemoglobin. The heme portion of hemoglobin acts as an oxidizing agent, catalyzing oxidation of the test reagent, tetramethylbenzidine, which produces a blue-green color. The appearance of this color indicates a positive test.[22-25]

Blood may be present on the surface or contained within the stool matrix. In general, matrix blood originates in the upper GI tract, whereas surface blood comes from the lower tract. The kits are more likely to detect blood from lower GI abnormalities. With the toilet and wipe tests, the reagent is sandwiched between two layers of biodegradable paper. The toilet tests are placed in the toilet bowl after a bowel movement. This type of kit is based on the premise that a significant amount of fecal blood will remain on the surface of the toilet bowl water after a bowel movement. In wipe tests, the stool sample is collected by using the test wipe to clean the anus after a bowel movement. With the stool application devices, stool is applied to two wells using a wooden stick.

## PATIENT EDUCATION FOR MENOPAUSE TESTS

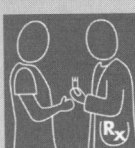

The objective of self-testing is to screen for high FSH levels in the urine. For most patients, carefully following product instructions and the self-care measures listed here will help ensure accurate test results.

### Avoidance of Incorrect Results

- Use first morning urine.
- Do not drink large amounts of fluids the night before performing test.
- Do not drink fluids after midnight before testing in the morning.

### Usage Guidelines

#### *Test cassettes*

- Remove test cassette from foil and place on flat, hard surface.
- Catch midstream urine in the collection cup.
- Urine can be stored in the refrigerator for up to 24 hours before testing. Bring sample to room temperature before testing.
- Fill plastic dropper with urine. Hold the dropper vertical to the test cassette and gently squeeze 4 full drops of urine into the round urine well on right side of cassette.
- Wait 15 minutes. Do not move cassette during this time.
- Read results in test window. Do not move the test cassette until results are checked.
- Repeat test in 7 days with a new test cassette. Each test cassette should be used only once.

#### *Test sticks*

- Open the protective sleeve and remove test stick.
- Remove the cap to expose the tip. Hold by the thumb grip and point the tip down while testing. Avoid touching the tip.
- Place the tip in urine stream for 5 seconds.
- Replace the cap and place on a flat surface with the test window facing up.
- Check in 5 minutes for color changes.
- Repeat test in 7 days with a new test stick. Each test stick should be used only once.

If result is positive or negative with symptoms, see a health care provider for evaluation and further testing.

*Source:* References 16 and 17.

### *Exclusions for Self-Testing*

Women who are menstruating should delay testing until menses has ceased. Menstrual blood present in the toilet bowl water or contaminating the stool sample can produce a positive result.

### *Interferences*

Blood in the stool can signify a number of conditions in addition to cancer of the colon and rectum, including ulcers, Crohn's disease, colitis, anal fissures, diverticulitis, and hemorrhoids. Any of these conditions can give a positive result for an FOBT.

Aspirin, nonsteroidal anti-inflammatory drugs (NSAIDs), steroids, and reserpine may cause sufficient gastric bleeding to produce positive results. These medications should be avoided for at least 2 to 3 days before testing as well as during the test period. A recent study found that aspirin and NSAIDs did not increase the risk of a false-positive FOBT.[26] The authors concluded there is little concern for a false-positive FOBT in patients who cannot safely discontinue aspirin or NSAIDS for specimen collection. Rectally administered medications should also be avoided. However, patients should always consult their primary care provider before discontinuing any prescribed medications.

Vitamin C ingestion in excess of 250 mg/day may interfere with the peroxidase action of hemoglobin, causing false-negative results in the Accustat, ColonTest-Sensitive, and LifeGuard tests.[22,24,25] FOBTs are not specific for human blood and may produce false-positive results if red meat is consumed. Toilet bowl cleaners may also produce false-positive results. The box Patient Education for Fecal Occult Blood Tests lists measures for avoiding inaccurate test results.

### *Usage Guidelines*

See the box Patient Education for Fecal Occult Blood Tests.

### *Product Selection Guidelines*

Patients who want to avoid restricting their diet or stopping vitamin C may prefer the EZ-Detect product, which does not require a diet or medication change. Some patients may prefer the wipe or toilet tests to the stool collection type. All the tests are similar in cost. All the products except ColonTest-Sensitive have a card for recording results to give to the primary care provider.

## Assessment of Use of Fecal Occult Blood Tests

Assessing the degree of risk a patient has for colorectal cancer is a major consideration in determining whether to recommend an FOBT. Patients with a personal or family history of colorectal cancer have a higher risk of developing the disease and would most likely benefit from testing. Patients with a family history should start testing annually at age 40 years; everyone should be tested yearly starting at age 50.19,27 Determining the potential for false test results is another important consideration. False-negative tests could delay necessary treatment, whereas false-positive tests could cause unwarranted anxiety.

## PATIENT EDUCATION FOR FECAL OCCULT BLOOD TESTS

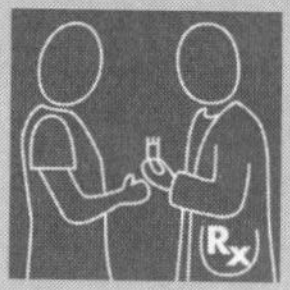

The objective of self-testing is to screen for blood in the stool. For most patients, carefully following product instructions and the self-care measures listed here will help ensure accurate test results.

### Avoidance of Incorrect Results

- Do not perform test during times of known bleeding, such as hemorrhoidal or menstrual bleeding.
- Increase dietary fiber intake for several days before testing. Roughage increases the accuracy of the test by stimulating bleeding from lesions that might not otherwise bleed.
- Because bleeding from cancerous lesions may be intermittent, perform the test on three consecutive bowel movements to increase the chance of detecting a possible lesion.
- Complete all three stool tests even if the first two produce negative results.
- Do not take nonprescription medications such as aspirin and NSAIDs for 2 to 3 days before testing and during testing.
- Some medications can cause bleeding and may need to be stopped before testing. Consult a primary care provider about which medications to stop before performing the test.
- Chemicals in the toilet can interfere with the test. Following the instructions carefully can prevent this problem.

### Usage Guidelines

- Do not eat red meat 2 to 3 days before testing and during the test period.
- Do not take more than 250 mg/day of vitamin C for 2 to 3 days before and during the test period.

#### *EZ-Detect and Accustat*

- Remove toilet tank cleansers or deodorizers and flush toilet twice before testing.
- Before testing, use one test pad to perform a water quality check. If any trace of blue appears in the cross-shaped area when the pad is placed in the toilet water, use another toilet to complete the testing. Perform a water quality check on the second toilet as well.
- Immediately after a bowel movement, place a pad in the toilet bowl, printed side up. After 2 minutes, check for the appearance of a blue cross on the test pad (positive result).
- Two control areas on the bottom of each Accustat pad indicate whether the test is functioning properly. Check that the left area has turned blue or green and that the right area did not change color. If color changes differ from these, discard the pad and repeat the test after the next bowel movement.
- Repeat the test on the next two bowel movements.
- If results are negative for all three tests, use remaining pad to perform a quality check of the test pads. Flush the toilet and empty the contents of the positive control chemical package into the bowl as it refills. Float the remaining test pad in the water, printed side up. After 2 minutes, check for a blue cross, which indicates the test pads were working properly. If the blue cross does not appear, call the assistance line provided with the product.

Notify a primary care provider if any of the three tests is positive.

#### *LifeGuard*

- Wipe with test pad after bowel movement.
- Peel and flush biodegradable tissue liner. Fold test in half to seal sample.
- Add 4 drops of developer to test pad. Observe for blue color change that indicates a positive result. Can wait up to 14 days to add the developer.
- Add one drop of developer between the positive and negative lines on the control side of pad. The controls should not be developed until after the stool sample is developed. If the positive control line (+ • + • +) turns blue and the negative control line (- • - • -) stays red, the test is working properly.
- Repeat the test on the next two bowel movements.

Notify a health care provider if any of the three tests is positive.

#### *ColonTest-Sensitive*

- Open test device lid. Apply stool sample to wells A and B.
- Close lid and press on "press last" space to break test ampule.
- Turn test device over and hold vertical for 15 seconds.
- Test is positive if wells are partially or completely blue. Test is negative if wells are beige or brown.
- Repeat the test on the next two bowel movements.

Notify a primary care provider if any of the three tests is positive.

*Source:* References 22-25.

## Evaluation of Patient Outcomes With Fecal Occult Blood Tests

A patient evaluating the results of an FOBT must remember that the test is a screening method and is not specific to a particular disease. A positive test result may indicate any medical condition that causes a loss of blood through the GI system. The primary value of FOBT is to alert patients and health care providers that a thorough workup may be needed. The kits are not intended to replace other diagnostic procedures. Patients should be advised to contact their primary care provider if a positive test result is obtained.

# CHOLESTEROL TESTS

Elevated cholesterol levels result from excessive production of cholesterol by the liver, deficient removal of the cholesterol from the bloodstream, and excessive intake of cholesterol-rich foods, such as eggs and red meat. Elevated low-density lipoprotein cholesterol (LDL-C) is the major cause of atherosclerotic heart disease, which can contribute to incidents of heart attack and stroke.[28] Although lowering LDL-C is the main target of therapy, raising levels of high-density lipoprotein cholesterol (HDL-C), which removes deposits from the blood vessels, and lowering triglycerides, which contribute to development of heart disease, are also important.[28]

**TABLE 51-5 Cholesterol Tests**

| Trade Name | Product Features |
|---|---|
| CholesTrak AccuMeter Home Cholesterol Test<br>Accustat Home Cholesterol Test<br>Home Access Instant Cholesterol Test | Measures total cholesterol; not reusable; includes test cassette, lancet, and chart for interpreting test results from a drop of blood; chart is specific for test cassette and should not be reused |
| Personal Cholesterol Monitor | Measures total cholesterol; stores results on smart card; reusable; all materials needed to conduct test packaged together in 6-unit quantities |
| CardioChek | Measures total cholesterol, HDL-C, and triglycerides; can also measure glucose and ketone; stores results; reusable; separate testing strip and corresponding color-coded memory chip required for each type of test; cholesterol strips available in vials of 6, 25, 50, and 100; HDL-C and triglyceride strips available in vials of 6 and 25; each vial contains memory chip |
| BIOSAFE Total Cholesterol | Total cholesterol results are obtained after mailing sample to laboratory; not reusable; contains lancet and sample collection card |
| BIOSAFE Total Cholesterol Panel | Lipid profile (total cholesterol, triglycerides, HDL-C, LDL-C) results are obtained after mailing sample to laboratory; not reusable; contains lancet and sample collection card |

Almost 19% of American adults have high cholesterol. Twenty-six percent of women and 16% of men ages 55 to 64 years have high cholesterol.[3] Because of these statistics, the National Cholesterol Education Program recommends that all adults have a lipid profile measured at least every 5 years, starting at age 20.[28] A home cholesterol test is one means of achieving this first critical step to minimize the risk for cardiovascular heart disease. However, this should not replace a complete lipid panel. Patients who are being treated for elevated cholesterol will require more frequent measurement.

Because elevated cholesterol is a chronic condition that requires lifestyle modification and, frequently, medication for treatment, adhering to a treatment plan can be difficult for patients. Home cholesterol tests can help monitor the efficacy of and adherence to diet, exercise, and medication plans.

## Usage Considerations

The majority of nonprescription cholesterol tests (Table 51-5) measure only total cholesterol. A few tests also measure LDL-C, HDL-C, and triglycerides. Persons with diabetes might want to consider the CardioChek, which measures glucose and ketone levels in addition to cholesterol and triglyceride levels. The CholesTrack, Accustat, and Home Access kits allow patients to measure their total blood cholesterol levels at home, whereas patients who use the Personal Cholesterol Monitor store their total cholesterol level results on a smart card to share with their primary care provider or other practitioner. BIOSAFE offers self-collected, laboratory-performed tests for total cholesterol or complete lipid profile.

### *Mechanism of Action*

With the total cholesterol test cassettes, cholesterol present in a blood sample is converted into hydrogen peroxide through a chemical reaction involving cholesterol esterase and cholesterol oxidase.[29,30] The peroxide then reacts with horseradish peroxidase and a dye to produce the color that rises along the cholesterol test's measurement scale. The test cassette has two separate indicator spots that change color to show that the test is functioning properly. One of the indicator spots also indicates completion of the test, signaling it is time to read the scale.

The CardioChek and the Personal Cholesterol Monitor are reflectance photometers that read the color intensity of the chemical test reaction.[31,32] Similar to a glucose meter, the results of the test are displayed on an LCD screen. BIOSAFE's total cholesterol and lipid profile tests are performed by a CLIA (Clinical Laboratory Improvement Act)–certified laboratory.[33]

### *Exclusions for Self-Testing*

Excessive bleeding from a fingerstick can occur in patients who have coagulation disorders or use anticoagulants. These patients should not self-test for cholesterol levels.

### *Accuracy Rate*

The accuracy rate of home cholesterol tests is debated. All of the products, except BIOSAFE which is mailed to a laboratory, are FDA-approved for home use, CLIA-waived devices, and rated substantially equivalent to a laboratory-based cholesterol test. A published study of the CholesTrak device found that untrained consumers obtained results well-correlated with a laboratory-based cholesterol reference method.[34] *Consumer Reports* tested the CholesTrak, Accustat (previously named First Check), Home Access, CardioChek, and BIOSAFE Total Cholesterol Panel kits. The first three, which are essentially the same device, gave results that varied no more than 15% from laboratory values. The CardioChek and BIOSAFE Total Cholesterol Panel yielded results that were "often wide of the mark."[35] The report gave no more specifics.

## PATIENT EDUCATION FOR CHOLESTEROL TESTS

One objective of self-testing is to screen for high total cholesterol levels, allowing patients with elevated levels to start making lifestyle changes that can prevent heart attack and stroke and to see a primary care provider for a full lipid profile and medical evaluation. Another objective is to monitor the effects of diet, exercise, or medication in patients with diagnosed hypercholesterolemia. For most patients, carefully following package instructions and the self-care measures listed here will help ensure achievement of accurate test results, which, in turn, can help patients achieve their medical goals with the assistance of a health care professional.

### Avoidance of Incorrect Results

- If two or three hanging drops of blood cannot be obtained or if it takes longer than 5 minutes to collect this amount of blood, do not perform the test.
- Do not excessively squeeze or milk the finger.
- If taking vitamin C in doses of 500 mg or more, do not take the dose within 4 hours of testing.
- Do not take standard doses of acetaminophen or naproxen within 4 hours of testing.

### Usage Guidelines

- Do not use cholesterol tests if you have hemophilia or take anticoagulants because of the risk of excessive bleeding from the fingerstick. Have a primary care provider perform the test.
- Before starting the test, wash your hands thoroughly with soap and warm water and dry them.
- To stabilize the cholesterol level, sit and relax for 5 minutes before performing the test.
- For the CardioChek test, insert the memory chip corresponding to the desired test into the meter and turn on the meter.
- Lance the outside of one fingertip and wipe away the first sign of blood with the gauze pad. Then apply blood to the testing device as quickly as possible. For the total cholesterol test cassettes, fill the well of the test cassette. For the CardioChek test and Personal Cholesterol Monitor, apply enough blood to cover the testing area of a strip. For either BIOSAFE test, place enough blood to fill each of the three rings on the test paper. Do not touch the area of the rings directly.
- For the total cholesterol test cassettes, wait at least 2 minutes but no more than 4 minutes before pulling the clear plastic tab on the right side of the cassette until it clicks into place and a red line appears. Use a timepiece with a second hand for accurate timing. After another 10 to 12 minutes, when the "END" indicator turns green, measure the height of the purple column against the scale printed on the cassette. Use the paper result chart included in the kit to interpret the reading.
- For the CardioChek test, insert the test strip into the meter either before or after the blood sample has been applied. The meter displays the test results in approximately 1 minute.
- For the Personal Cholesterol Monitor, insert the test strip into the meter either before or after the blood sample has been applied. The meter displays the test results in approximately 3 minutes.
- For either BIOSAFE test, allow blood to dry on the test paper. Complete your name and address on the test paper and place into the plastic container provided. Mail to BIOSAFE. Results will be mailed back to the patient in approximately 1 week.
- Dispose of the lancet in a puncture-resistant container because it is potentially biohazardous.

⚠ If the total cholesterol reading is 200 mg/dL or greater, HDL-C is 40 mg/dL or less, or triglycerides are 150 mg/dL or greater, see a primary care provider for evaluation and further testing.

*Source:* References 29-33.

### *Interferences*

Good fingersticking technique is necessary to avoid erroneous results with cholesterol tests. Two or three hanging drops of blood are needed, but excessive squeezing and milking of the finger will negatively affect the quality of the blood sample. If sufficient blood cannot be obtained from the first fingerstick, the patient should use a different finger. A low cholesterol value may result if the blood sample is too small or if it takes longer than 5 minutes to collect the necessary amount of blood.

The patient should avoid doses of 500 mg or more of vitamin C or standard doses of acetaminophen or naproxen for 4 hours before the test because they may cause an artificially low result.

### *Usage Guidelines*

See the box Patient Education for Cholesterol Tests.

### *Product Selection Guidelines*

Although significantly more expensive than individual total cholesterol test cassette kits, the CardioChek and the Personal Cholesterol Monitor are reusable with the purchase of additional testing materials and will store test results. The CardioChek has the ability to test for HDL-C and triglycerides, whereas the other home tests measure only total cholesterol. BIOSAFE provides total cholesterol or a lipid profile, but results are not immediately available.

## Assessment of Use of Cholesterol Tests: A Case-based Approach

Before recommending a cholesterol test, the practitioner should first determine whether the patient has been diagnosed with heart disease or has some reason to be concerned about hypercholesterolemia. Conscientious monitoring of cholesterol is imperative for patients with heart disease because elevated cholesterol levels have a significant impact on cardiovascular health. The practitioner should also ask about lifestyle and other factors that can affect test results. Case 51-2 gives an example of a cholesterol test assessment.

## CASE 51-2

| Relevant Evaluation Criteria | Scenario/Model Outcome |
|---|---|
| **Information Gathering** | |
| 1. Gather essential information relative to the patient's reason for testing including: | |
| a. description of symptom(s) (i.e., nature, onset, duration, severity, associated symptoms) | Patient is interested in knowing his cholesterol level. He has no symptoms of cardiac disease. |
| b. medical history, including family history | He has a family history of heart disease and has never had his cholesterol tested. His father died from a heart attack at 50 years of age. |
| 2. Gather essential patient history information: | |
| a. patient's identity | Blake Stevens |
| b. age, sex, weight, and height | 45 y/o M, weight 140 lb (per patient), height 5'6" (per patient) |
| c. patient's occupation | N/A |
| d. patient's dietary habits | He says he knows he has a pretty poor diet. |
| e. patient's sleep habits | N/A |
| f. concurrent medical conditions, prescription and nonprescription medications, and dietary supplements | Deep vein thrombosis 3 months ago, treated with warfarin 5 mg once daily |
| g. allergies | N/A |
| h. history of other adverse reactions to medications | N/A |
| i. prior use of diagnostic/monitoring test | He has never used a home monitoring test. |
| j. potential problems with performing/interpreting test | Blake is anticoagulated. He does not have any visual or physical impairment. |
| k. other (describe) _______ | N/A |
| **Assessment and Triage** | |
| 3. Determine if self-testing is appropriate. | Self-testing is not appropriate, because Blake is anticoagulated. Given his family history, he should have his cholesterol checked, but should not do it himself. |
| 4. Identify exclusions for self-testing (see section Exclusions for Self-Testing under Cholesterol Tests) | Anticoagulation |
| 5. Formulate a comprehensive list of therapeutic alternatives for the reason for testing to determine if triage to a medical practitioner is required and share this information with the patient. | Options include:<br>(1) Refer for cholesterol testing.<br>(2) Wait until he is not anticoagulated to perform self-test.<br>(3) Take no action. |
| **Plan** | |
| 6. Select an optimal alternative to address the patient's problem, taking into account patient preferences. | The patient thinks his PCP is planning to stop his warfarin at his next visit. He will discuss cholesterol testing with PCP. |
| 7. Describe the recommended therapeutic approach to the patient. | N/A |
| 8. Explain to the patient the rationale for selecting the recommended therapeutic alternatives that were considered. | Because the home cholesterol tests require a fingerstick, he is at risk for excessive bleeding from the fingerstick while anticoagulated. Although significant bleeding with a fingerstick is unlikely, the cautious approach is to refer him for laboratory testing. |

## CASE 51-2 (continued)

| Relevant Evaluation Criteria | Scenario/Model Outcome |
|---|---|
| **Patient Education** | |
| 9. Describe the testing procedure to the patient, including: | |
| a. specific instructions | N/A |
| b. how to avoid incorrect results | N/A |
| 10. Solicit follow-up questions from patient. | If the test I get at the laboratory shows a high level, does it mean I have high cholesterol? |
| 11. Answer patient's questions. | No. More than one test showing a high result is necessary for the diagnosis of high cholesterol. |

Key: N/A, not applicable; PCP, primary care provider.

### Patient Counseling for Cholesterol Tests

When counseling a patient about cholesterol tests, the practitioner should emphasize the importance of properly collecting blood samples and advise the patient to seek assistance with the fingerstick, if needed. To further ensure accurate test results, the practitioner should advise the patient of medical and lifestyle factors that can cause inaccurate test results. The box Patient Education for Cholesterol Tests lists specific information to provide patients.

### Evaluation of Patient Outcomes With Cholesterol Tests

Any patient who obtains a result of a total cholesterol of 200 mg/dL or greater, an HDL-C of 40 mg/dL or less, or triglycerides of 150 mg/dL or greater should see a primary care provider for a repeat measurement, full lipid profile, and appropriate medical workup. Patients should not adjust their cholesterol-lowering medications on the basis of a home test without consulting their primary care provider.

## URINARY TRACT INFECTION TESTS

Urinary tract infections (UTIs) are the cause for 4 million visits to primary care providers every year.36 Women have a shorter urethra than men and are therefore more likely to contract UTIs because of retrograde migration of bacteria from the skin. Men older than 50 years have a greater likelihood of contracting UTIs than women because of prostate problems. Conditions that increase risk of UTIs include pregnancy, diabetes, urinary stones, urinary obstructions such as those caused by an enlarged prostate, presence of urinary catheters, and a history of UTIs.[37]

The gram-negative bacterium *Escherichia coli* is responsible for 80% of UTIs.[36] Both gram-positive and gram-negative bacteria account for the other 20% of causative organisms. Symptoms of a UTI include pain on urination, sensation of an urgent need to urinate, frequent urination, blood in the urine, and lower abdominal pain or discomfort.

Two primary uses for UTI tests are (1) early detection of such infections in patients with a history of recurrent UTIs or risk factors associated with UTIs and (2) confirmation that an infection has been cured by antibiotic therapy.

### Usage Considerations

Two types of UTI tests are available. The mechanism of action is the primary difference between the two.

#### *Mechanism of Action*

One type of UTI test (TECO Nitrite Test and UTI Home Screening Test) detects nitrites in the urine on the basis of the principle that gram-negative bacteria reduce nitrate in the urine to nitrite.[38,39] The other type of test (AZO Strips) detects both nitrite and leukocyte esterase (LE), an enzyme unique to leukocytes (white blood cells).[40] White blood cells may be found in the urine when a UTI is present.

The nitrite strips detect only infections caused by gram-negative bacteria. In the strip, arsanilic acid reacts with urinary nitrite to form a diazonium compound, which in turn reacts with another chemical on the strip to produce a pink color. A positive test requires a bacterial concentration of $10^5$/mL of urine. Nitrite and LE-detecting strips identify infections caused by non–nitrate-reducing organisms on the basis of presence of white blood cells in urine.

#### *Interferences*

A strict vegetarian diet that provides insufficient urinary nitrates can cause false-negative nitrite results with a UTI test. Tetracycline may produce a false-negative reading for nitrites. False-negative results can also be caused by doses of vitamin C in excess of 250 mg, because ascorbic acid blocks the nitrite test reaction. The patient should allow 10 hours between the last dose of vitamin C and the test procedure. Doses of vitamin C in excess of 500 mg within

## PATIENT EDUCATION FOR URINARY TRACT INFECTION TESTS

The objective of self-testing is to detect UTIs in the early stages or to confirm that an infection was successfully treated. For most patients, carefully following the package instructions and the self-care measures listed here will help ensure achievement of accurate test results and allow prompt treatment of a detected UTI.

### Avoidance of Incorrect Results

- Persons on a strict vegetarian diet or tetracycline may not obtain accurate results.
- Certain dyes or drugs, such as phenazopyridine, may cause a false-positive result by changing the sensor pad to pink.
- If using TECO or UTI Home Screening Test, do not take 250 mg or more of vitamin C within 10 hours of testing.
- If using AZO Test Strips, do not take 500 mg or more of vitamin C within 24 hours of testing.
- Women should not use AZO Test Strips during menses because blood will cause a false-positive result.

### Usage Guidelines

- Clean the genital area thoroughly before collecting a urine sample.
- Test the first urine of the morning or, if tested later, urine held in the bladder for at least 4 hours.
- To improve sensitivity, test urine samples on 3 consecutive days.
- Depending on the test purchased, pass the test strip or stick through the urine stream.
- Do not touch the sensor pad because skin oils can interfere with the test reaction. If urine is collected in a cup, immerse the sensor pad into the cup for 1 second.
- Make sure urine completely covers the pad.
- Wait the indicated time (30-60 seconds); then compare the color on the sensor pad with the color chart provided. For TECO and UTI Home Screening Test, a pink color on the pad indicates a positive result. For AZO Test, a dark tan to purple color on the leukocyte pad indicates a positive result.
- Wait no longer than 3 minutes to read the test strip, and ignore any color changes that occur after that time.

If the test is positive, see a primary care provider immediately for evaluation and treatment.

If the test is negative but symptoms persist, see a primary care provider immediately for evaluation and treatment.

*Source:* References 38-40.

24 hours of testing may result in a false-negative result for the LE test.[40] Dyes or drugs such as phenazopyridine, commonly used by patients with UTIs, may cause a false-positive result by changing the sensor pad to pink.

### *Usage Guidelines*

See the box Patient Education for Urinary Tract Infection Tests.

### *Product Selection Guidelines*

The combination of nitrite and LE tests gives AZO Strips enhanced specificity and sensitivity. The UTI Home Screening Test is a test stick used like pregnancy tests that might be easier to hold in the urine stream than the AZO test strips. The TECO nitrite test strips are the least expensive per test but are available only on the Internet.

### Assessment of UTI Tests

Before recommending a UTI test, the practitioner should first determine the patient's reason for using the test. If the patient is testing for a suspected UTI, the practitioner should evaluate the patient's symptoms and risk factors for UTIs. If symptoms of a UTI are present, the patient should be referred to his or her primary care provider immediately for evaluation and treatment. If the patient is testing to find out whether a treated UTI has been cured, the practitioner should assess patient adherence to the therapy. The patient's diet and medication use are important factors to evaluate for possible interference with test results.

### Patient Counseling for UTI Tests

Counseling on the use of UTI tests should emphasize the importance of collecting a clean sample of midstream urine if the sensor pad is to be immersed in a cup of urine. The practitioner should advise a patient with visual difficulties to seek assistance in interpreting test results. To further ensure accurate test results, the pharmacist should advise the patient of medical and dietary factors that can cause inaccurate test results. The box Patient Education for Urinary Tract Infection Tests lists specific information to provide patients.

### Evaluation of Patient Outcomes With UTI Tests

Because tests will detect only about 90% of infections, the patient should contact a primary care provider if a negative result is obtained, but UTI symptoms persist.[38-40] If a positive result is obtained, the patient should contact a primary care provider immediately for evaluation and treatment.

## HIV-1 TESTS

An estimated 850,000 to 950,000 persons in the United States are living with human immunodeficiency virus (HIV), including 180,000 to 280,000 who do not know they are infected.[41] Home HIV-1 tests allow a person to test for HIV type 1 (HIV-1) in privacy. In a study describing the first year of availability of HIV-1 tests, nearly 60% of all users and 49% of those who tested positive had never been tested before.[42]

AIDS is an incurable disease caused by HIV-1 virus. The disease destroys the body's immune system. AIDS can be contracted by contact with infected body fluids such as blood or semen. People at risk for contracting the virus include those who (1) share needles or syringes for the purpose of injecting drugs, including steroids; (2) have sexual intercourse with a person infected with HIV-1, with someone who injects drugs, or with multiple partners; (3) had a blood transfusion anytime between 1978 and May 1985.

## Usage Considerations

Two test kits that use blood samples for HIV-1 detection currently are available: Home Access HIV-1 Test System and Home Access Express HIV-1 Test System.

### *Mechanism of Action*

The HIV-1 tests detect antibodies to the virus. Because 3 weeks to 6 months may be required to develop sufficient antibodies for detection, the time since possible exposure to the virus must be considered in determining when to perform the test.

After collection, the home HIV-1 test samples are mailed to a certified laboratory for processing with an ELISA. Positive samples are rescreened twice. Repeated positive samples are confirmed with an immunofluorescent assay.[43]

### *Interferences*

No factors are known to interfere with home HIV-1 tests.

### *Usage Guidelines*

See the box Patient Education for HIV-1 Tests.

### *Product Selection Guidelines*

The two available HIV-1 tests differ in price and turnaround time to obtain results. The first test, Home Access, takes approximately 7 business days to obtain the results. The second, Home Access Express, takes approximately 3 business days. The Home Access sample is sent to the testing laboratory by regular mail, whereas the Home Access Express sample is shipped by Federal Express. Consequently, the Home Access Express version costs more.

## Assessment of Use of HIV-1 Tests

Before recommending an HIV-1 test, the practitioner should first determine how much time has elapsed since the patient was possibly exposed to the HIV-1 virus. The patient may not know all the risk factors for HIV-1 infection; therefore, the practitioner should tactfully find out whether the patient has engaged in any activities that increase risk for contracting HIV-1. The patient should be asked about medical disorders that might rule out use of a fingerstick-based test such as anticoagulation or physical limitations that might interfere with performing the test.

## Patient Counseling for HIV-1 Tests

Counseling on the use of HIV-1 tests should emphasize the importance of applying enough blood on the specimen card to ensure an accurate reading. The practitioner should also advise the patient of the fragility of blood samples and not to delay mailing the specimen card. The practitioner should counsel infected patients on precautions to avoid infection of others. The box Patient Education for HIV-1 Tests lists specific information to provide patients.

## PATIENT EDUCATION FOR HIV-1 TESTS

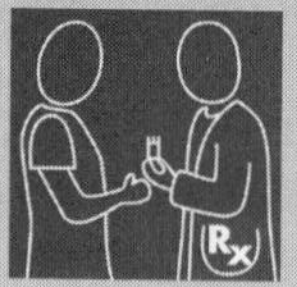


The objective of self-testing is to determine whether an HIV-1 infection is present. For most patients, carefully following package instructions and the self-care measures listed here will help ensure the achievement of accurate test results. Furthermore, self-testing will allow prompt treatment of a detected infection.

**Precautions**

- Do not share the test lancet with other individuals. Do not allow the blood being tested to contact other individuals.
- The lancet is a biohazard; dispose of it in a puncture-resistant container.

**Usage Guidelines**

- Call the product manufacturer's toll-free number to register and receive pretest counseling. The manufacturer's customer representative will ask for the confidential code included in the kit.
- With alcohol, clean the fingertip chosen for puncture.
- Prick the cleaned fingertip using the lancet provided, and place a few drops of blood on the blood specimen card. Fill the circle on the card completely to ensure a readable test. Examine the back of the card to ensure the blood soaked through. If it did not, place more blood on the front of the card. If a second fingerstick is needed, use the second lancet provided in the kit.
- Allow the card to air-dry for 30 minutes, place sample in specimen return pouch, and seal it in the prepaid and addressed shipping package. Be sure that the processing laboratory receives the specimen within 10 days of sampling.
- Call the manufacturer's toll-free number in 3 to 7 business days to obtain the results, depending on which test kit was used.

⚠ If the test is positive, see a primary care provider immediately for evaluation and treatment. Avoid activities that can result in transfer of blood or other body fluids to other individuals.

*Source:* Reference 43.

### Evaluation of Patient Outcomes With HIV-1 Tests

A patient with a positive result should see a primary care provider to be retested for confirmation of HIV-1 infection. Patients with negative results should confirm that sufficient time had passed since potential exposure before they tested themselves.

## HEPATITIS C TESTS

Hepatitis C is one of six identified hepatic viruses and is considered the most common cause of chronic viral hepatitis in the United States.[44] An estimated 3.9 million Americans have been infected with hepatitis C.[44] This infection accounts for approximately one third of all deaths caused by chronic liver disease each year and is a major reason for liver transplantation.[44]

Risk factors for hepatitis C are as follows:

- Injection use of illegal drugs
- Receipt of clotting factor concentrate produced before 1987
- Long-term hemodialysis
- Transfusion or organ transplant before 1992
- Sexual intercourse with multiple partners
- Previous history of a sexually transmitted disease
- Birth to a mother infected with hepatitis C
- Use of intranasal cocaine[44]

The Centers for Disease Control and Prevention estimate that injection drug use accounts for 60% of all new cases of hepatitis C.[44] Anyone who has or may have occupational exposure to blood, including health care workers and military personnel, are also at increased risk for developing hepatitis C.[44,45]

Hepatitis C induces liver damage by causing hepatic cell necrosis and inflammation, which over time may progress to fibrosis, cirrhosis, and hepatocellular carcinoma. Of people infected with hepatitis C, 85% are likely to progress to the chronic disease state.[45] Clinically, hepatitis C may go undetected for many years; liver disease may be advanced by the time symptoms arise.

### Usage Considerations

One test kit currently is available for hepatitis C detection, Hepatitis C Check. After collection, the test blood sample is mailed to a certified laboratory for processing.

#### *Mechanism of Action*

The kit tests for presence of antibodies to the hepatitis C virus, not the virus itself. The Hepatitis C Check uses an ELISA to test for antibodies, then confirms the results with a recombinant immunoblot assay.[46] Because 6 months may be required to develop sufficient antibodies for detection, the time since possible exposure to the virus must be considered in determining when to perform the test.

#### *Interferences*

Providing an inadequate blood sample (i.e., incompletely filling the circle on the blood sample card) may cause inaccurate results.

#### *Usage Guidelines*

See the box Patient Education for Hepatitis C Tests.

#### *Product Selection Guidelines*

Home Access Hepatitis C Check is a single-use test kit containing two lancets, a blood sample card, gauze pad, an adhesive bandage, and a postage-paid envelope. Each kit also includes a unique personal identification number, which the purchaser uses to register the kit and access test results.

### Assessment of Use of Hepatitis C Tests

A patient who recently has been infected may receive a false-negative result because antibodies to the virus have not had sufficient time to form. Clinical studies on file with the manufacturer report no false-positive results.[46] The patient may not know all the risk factors for hepatitis C; therefore, the practitioner should tactfully find out whether the patient has engaged in any activities that can cause the disease. The patient should be asked about medical disorders that might rule out use of a fingerstick-based test such as anticoagulation or physical limitations that could interfere with performing the test.

### Patient Counseling for Hepatitis C Tests

The practitioner should advise the patient of the fragility of blood samples and not to delay mailing the specimen card. The practitioner should counsel infected patients on precautions to avoid infection of others. These patients should also be advised to avoid alcohol and other drugs that may advance the progression of liver disease. The box Patient Education for Hepatitis C Tests lists specific information to provide patients.

### Evaluation of Patient Outcomes With Hepatitis C Tests

Patients who test positive should be referred to a primary care provider because treatment options are available only by prescription. These patients should also be vaccinated against other forms of hepatitis, such as the hepatitis A virus and hepatitis B virus.[45]

## ILLICIT DRUG USE TESTS

An estimated 13 million Americans use illicit drugs.[47] Drug abuse, in turn, leads to higher accident and absentee rates at work. Drug abuse in adolescents is often undiagnosed, only partially diagnosed, or diagnosed too late for proper intervention.[47] Illicit drug use is a problem in the United States regardless of socioeconomic status, gender, or race.

## PATIENT EDUCATION FOR HEPATITIS C TESTS

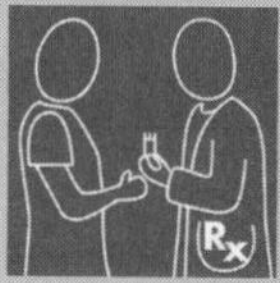

The objective of self-testing is to determine whether a hepatitis C infection is present. Self-testing will also allow prompt treatment of a detected infection. For most patients, carefully following package instructions and the self-care measures listed here will help ensure achievement of accurate test results.

### Precautions

- Do not share the test lancet with other individuals.
- Do not allow the blood being tested to contact other individuals.
- The lancet is considered a biohazard; dispose of it in a puncture-resistant container.

### Usage Guidelines

- Register the PIN with the manufacturer by calling the enclosed toll-free telephone number and following the automated directions.
- Remain seated during the testing process to prevent falling if dizziness occurs.
- Before starting the test, wash your hands thoroughly with soap and warm water and dry them.
- Date the blood sample card.
- Lance the side of one of the middle fingers.
- Apply a sufficient number of blood drops until both the front and back of the circular area on the testing card are saturated.
- Allow the sample to dry at least 30 minutes before sealing it in the pouch and mailing.
- After 4 to 10 business days, call the toll-free number provided, using the PIN number to access the test results. Test results are available for up to 1 year.
- Note that counseling is available 24 hours/day, for both negative and positive results, and is included in the cost of the testing unit.

⚠ If the test is positive, see a primary care provider immediately for evaluation and treatment. Avoid activities that can result in transfer of blood or other body fluids to other individuals.

*Source:* Reference 46.

**TABLE 51-6 Selected Home Drug Abuse Tests**

| Product | Time to Result | Body Site | Testing Location | Substances Detected |
|---|---|---|---|---|
| Dr. Brown's Home Drug Testing System | 5-7 days | Urine | Send away | Marijuana, cocaine, amphetamine, phencyclidine, codeine, morphine, heroin |
| Parent's Alert Home Drug Testing Service | 3-5 days | Urine | Send away | Marijuana, cocaine, opiates, methamphetamine, ecstasy, barbiturates, benzodiazepines, lysergic acid diethylamide (LSD) |
| Accustat Home Drug Test | 3-8 minutes for initial screen; 5-7 days for laboratory confirmation | Urine | Home and send away for confirmation | Panel 1: marijuana<br>Panel 2: marijuana, cocaine<br>Panel 3: marijuana, cocaine, methamphetamine<br>Panel 4: marijuana, cocaine, methamphetamine, morphine/opiates |
| Quick Screen Pro Multi-Drug Screening | 3-15 minutes for initial screen; 5-7 days for laboratory confirmation | Urine | Home and send away for confirmation | Amphetamine, cocaine, marijuana, opiates, phencyclidine |
| PDT-90 Personal Drug Testing Service | 5-7 days | Hair | Send away | Marijuana, cocaine, opiates, methamphetamine, amphetamine, phencyclidine, barbiturates, benzodiazepines |

The symptoms of illicit drug use are varied, but may include withdrawal from activities, fatigue, red eyes, drowsiness, slurred speech, and chronic cough.

Drug abuse tests may allow parents and caregivers to detect such use early enough to affect the course of addiction.

## Usage Considerations

Numerous products for detecting use of illicit drugs are available in retail stores and pharmacies, by telephone, and through the Internet. A number of the tests currently available are not FDA-approved for home use. FDA has proposed a policy (which it currently follows) that allows the marketing of non–FDA-approved home test kits if the specimen is mailed to a certified laboratory. Table 51-6 lists some example tests and the substances each test identifies.

Home drug tests are marketed primarily to parents as an aid for determining illicit drug use in their children. These tests are a means of obtaining results anonymously when drug use by a child is suspected. Home drug testing, however, is not a substitute for open communication between parents and children regarding drug use.

Samples of urine or hair are collected at home. The hair and some of the urine tests are mailed to a clinical laboratory. Results are obtained by telephone. Some of the urine tests have the user conduct a preliminary screening test in the home and then mail positive samples to a laboratory for confirmation. Other urine tests are performed only at home. Saliva tests are available, but are expensive and currently marketed only to drug testing programs and employers.

Some of the test kits include telephone counseling to (1) help parents recognize the signs of drug use, (2) assist in creating a family drug policy, and (3) emphasize that parents should use the test to develop trust and open communication within their families, rather than to intimidate with the threat of random testing. Some telephone counseling programs provide referrals to rehabilitation and counseling services in the family's community.

### Mechanism of Action

For the at-home urine tests, an immunochromatographic assay similar to the home pregnancy and ovulation tests is used for initial screening of a sample. Available testing devices include (1) a test cassette (Accustat home drug test) to which urine is applied and (2) a test device that is placed in the urine sample (QuickScreen Pro). In each test, a positive result for a particular drug is absence of a line next to the drug name in the testing area. For a negative test, a line appears by the drug name and in the control area.

Urine samples sent to clinical laboratories for testing are checked for evidence of adulteration before processing for the presence of illicit drugs.[48-51] Substances such as water or household chemicals can be added to urine samples in an attempt to mask drug use. The laboratories use an enzyme-multiplied immunoassay technique to detect illicit drugs in the urine samples. Gas chromatography–mass spectrometry is then used to identify the specific drug.

Home urine tests detect drug use that occurred from several hours before testing to within 2 to 3 days of testing. The amount of drug found in the urine is affected by the time since consumption, the amount taken, and the amount of water consumed before sampling. Test results are reported only as positive or negative for a drug. Quantity or route of ingestion is not determined.

Hair testing detects trace amounts of ingested drugs that become trapped in the core of the hair shaft as it grows at an average rate of 1/2 inch per month. Drug use over a 90-day period can be determined from a 1 1/2-inch hair sample.[52] The presence of drugs is determined by radioimmunoassay techniques, and then gas chromatography–mass spectrometry analysis identifies the specific substance. Hair tests report positive or negative results for a drug. Positive results are reported as a number indicating low, medium, or high levels of use for all drugs except marijuana.

### Usage Guidelines

See the box Patient Education for Drug Abuse Tests.

### Interferences

Ingestion of decongestants, antidiarrheals, or cough medicines containing codeine may cause false-positive results for home drug abuse tests. These items contain substances structurally related to certain drugs of abuse. Consumption of large quantities of poppy seeds or poppy seed paste may or may not cause a false-positive result, depending on the test's sensitivity. Sensitivity standards for opiates were raised in the year 2000 from 300 to 2000 ng/mL to eliminate the possibility of false-positive results.[51] Only the QuickScreen Pro lists the higher sensitivity standard in its package labeling.

### Product Selection Guidelines

The criteria for selecting one drug abuse test over another include the drugs that are suspected of being used, type of suspected use (i.e., casual versus chronic), length of time since last use, and possibility of the suspected drug user tampering with the sample. The list of drugs that may be identified with each kit varies (Table 51-6). In general, urine tests are better for detecting low-level, casual drug use. Urine testing detects drugs from several hours before testing to the previous 2 to 3 days. Hair testing detects drugs from 5 to 90 days of use. It takes at least 5 to 7 days for hair to grow long enough away from the scalp for testing purposes.

Urine samples are subject to tampering by adding chemicals, diluting with water, or substituting someone else's sample. Some of the test kits include a temperature strip on the urine collection cup to ensure the sample is at body temperature. Hair samples, if taken directly from the person being tested, are not subject to tampering. Parents should weigh the possibility of tampering when deciding which type of test to choose.

Information on FDA approval of a test for illicit drugs for home use is available at www.fda.gov/cdrh/ode/otclist.html.

## Assessment of Use of Drug Abuse Tests

To determine which type of drug abuse test to recommend, the practitioner should ask about the length of suspected drug use and the types of drugs that are suspected. The practitioner should also ask whether the suspected user is likely to tamper with urine samples. The practitioner should determine if the suspected user takes legal prescription or nonprescription medications.

## Patient Counseling for Drug Abuse Tests

When parents or caregivers ask for assistance in selecting a drug abuse test, the practitioner should be prepared to offer information about family counseling agencies as well as clinical advice. The practitioner should emphasize the limitations of the tests when confirming illicit drug use and, in the case of urine tests, when identifying anything

## PATIENT EDUCATION FOR DRUG ABUSE TESTS

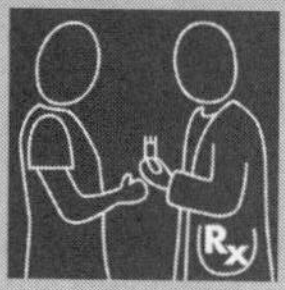

The objective of self-testing is to detect and identify abuse of illicit drugs. Self-testing will also allow prompt intervention to rehabilitate a confirmed drug user. For most patients, carefully following package instructions and the self-care measures listed here will help ensure achievement of accurate test results.

### Avoidance of Incorrect Results

- Urine samples can be tampered with by adding water or household chemicals, possibly giving false results.
- Drug tests on urine samples report only a positive or negative outcome. Neither the quantity of drug taken nor the method in which it was taken is determined.
- Drug tests on hair samples can report low, medium, or high level of drug use, but the use could have occurred as long as 90 days before testing.
- Cough medicines that contain codeine, decongestants, antidiarrheals, and possibly poppy seeds can cause false-positive test results.

### Usage Guidelines for Urine Drug Abuse Tests

- Collect urine using the collection device included with the test. Do not take urine from the toilet.
- Check the temperature of the urine sample immediately after collection using the temperature strip included in the package. If the sample is not between 90°F (32°C) and 100°F (38°C), adulteration may have occurred.

#### *QuickScreen Pro*

- Immerse the test card in the urine sample for 10 seconds or until visible migration across the test panels has occurred. Place device on flat surface or leave immersed in sample. Do not allow urine to exceed the "max line."
- Read the results when the "results ready" indicator changes to a pinkish red.
- Do not read results after 15 minutes or when the "results expired" indicator changes color.
- If no line appears in the control region, the test is invalid and should be repeated with a new card.

#### *Accustat*

- Fill the included dispenser to the line with urine from the sample cup.
- Dispense all of the urine into the test well one drop at a time.
- Allow the test to remain undisturbed until read. Read the result after 3 minutes but not after 8 minutes.
- Make sure the collection device is tightly closed. Put the device in the collection package as directed and mail the package to the laboratory.
- Results are available 2 to 7 business days after the laboratory receives the sample. To obtain the results, call the toll-free number provided in the kit and provide the code number accompanying the kit.

### Usage Guidelines for Hair Drug Abuse Tests

- Collect a hair sample that is 1/2 in. wide and one strand deep from the crown of the head, as close to the scalp as possible.
- Align the cut ends of the hair sample, and place the sample in the collection package as directed. Do not collect hair from a hairbrush, comb, or clothing because there is no guarantee the hair is actually from the person to be tested.
- Results are available approximately 5 days after receipt by the laboratory. To access results, call the toll-free number and provide the code number accompanying the kit.

⚠ If the test is positive, seek the services of a drug rehabilitation organization.

*Source:* References 48-52.

more than the type of drug that is being abused. The box Patient Education for Drug Abuse Tests lists specific information to provide patients.

## Evaluation of Patient Outcomes With Drug Abuse Tests

If a positive result is obtained with a drug abuse test, parents or caregivers need to consider potential problems with the test itself before concluding that drug use is confirmed. They must not assume that a negative result is accurate. Parents should also consider the testing window when evaluating results.

# BLOOD PRESSURE MONITORS

Hypertension, defined as either a systolic blood pressure greater than 140 mm Hg or a diastolic blood pressure greater than 90 mm Hg, is often an asymptomatic disease.[53]

**TABLE 51-7 Classification of Blood Pressure[53]**

| Category | Systolic BP (mm Hg) | | Diastolic BP (mm Hg) |
|---|---|---|---|
| Normal | <120 | and | <80 |
| Prehypertension | 120-139 | or | 80-89 |
| Hypertension, Stage 1 | 140-159 | or | 90-99 |
| Hypertension, Stage 2 | ≥160 | or | ≥100 |

Table 51-7 lists the classification of blood pressures from the most recent report of the Joint National Committee on Prevention, Detection, Evaluation and Treatment of High Blood Pressure (JNC 7).

Thirty-two percent of Americans 20 years of age and older have hypertension.[3] Thirty percent of people with hypertension are unaware of their condition; almost 40%

are not receiving treatment; and 66% have not achieved national goals for blood pressure control.[53] The reasons for the lack of adequate control are multiple, but a significant factor is lack of patient motivation to take steps to control blood pressure, especially if the patient is asymptomatic, which leads to nonadherence with treatment strategies.

The consequences of untreated hypertension are well documented. Longstanding elevations in blood pressure can lead to damage of the heart, kidney, lungs, eyes, and blood vessels, and to an increase in morbidity and mortality.

Treatment of high blood pressure often involves significant lifestyle changes (diet and exercise) and the institution of drug therapies. These measures inevitably produce side effects, so the patient who was without symptoms of disease may become symptomatic. Patient education and empowerment play a large role in improving patient adherence with antihypertensive efforts. Adherence, in turn, helps reduce morbidity and mortality, maintains or improves the patient's quality of life, and improves the patient's use of health care resources.

Teaching patients to take their own blood pressure at home is an excellent means of achieving these goals because home blood pressure monitoring gives patients a sense of control over their health, allows them to measure their progress toward a goal blood pressure level, and provides useful data on blood pressure values that occur away from the primary care provider's office. Three general advantages of measuring blood pressure outside the clinician's office are the ability to (1) distinguish sustained hypertension from "white-coat hypertension," (2) assess response to antihypertensive medication, and (3) improve patient adherence to treatment.

## Usage Considerations

Of the three categories of blood pressure monitors—mercury column, aneroid, and digital—aneroid and digital monitors are the most popular choices for home use.

### *Mechanism of Action*

Blood pressure readings include two types of pressures: systolic, which indicates pressure at the time of contraction of the heart cavities, and diastolic, which indicates pressure at the time of dilation of the heart cavities. Blood pressure is measured indirectly by two methods: auscultatory (measurement of sound) and oscillometric (measurement of vibration). Mercury and aneroid meters involve auscultation with the use of a stethoscope to detect Korotkoff's sounds, which are produced by the motion of the arterial wall in response to changes in arterial pressure. Oscillometric sensors, which are often used with digital meters, measure blood pressure by detecting blood surges underneath the cuff as it is deflated. The detection device, which is usually indicated on the cuff with a tab or other marking, is placed directly over the brachial artery. The brachial artery can be found by palpating 1 to 2 inches above and just to the inside of the antecubital space. As cuff pressure increases during the measurement procedure, the brachial artery is compressed and blood flow is obstructed. As cuff pressure is gradually released, blood flow is reestablished and Korotkoff's sounds can be heard in different phases. Phase I, which corresponds to systolic pressure, can be identified when at least two consecutive "beats" are heard as cuff pressure is decreased. The nature of the sounds changes over the next three phases. Diastolic pressure is identified as phase V, the disappearance of sound.

### *Interferences*

Stress, tobacco smoking, and ingestion of caffeine-containing beverages can increase blood pressure. Some medications such a pseudoephedrine may also increase blood pressure. Conversely, eating or taking a hot bath can lower blood pressure.

### *Usage Guidelines*

The actual measurement of blood pressure is a relatively simple procedure; however, many people consistently do it incorrectly. Blood pressure is naturally variable and can change in seconds. Thus, proper technique is essential to reduce measurement variability and improve the quality of results. The normal range for blood pressure is established with patients sitting in the resting state; thus, any variation from this setting can produce inaccurate results.

Using the appropriate size cuff is essential for accurately measuring a patient's blood pressure (Table 51-8). If the cuff is too small, blood pressure readings can be overestimated significantly by as much as 20 to 30 mm Hg. Several monitors are supplied with a large cuff; many others allow for purchase of a large cuff separately. For patients with arms too large for the largest size cuff, a wrist monitor may be a useful alternative. To obtain accurate readings with wrist cuffs, the patient must hold the wrist at heart level during the reading. Because these devices are also highly sensitive to changes in the wrist level, it is best to support the arm on a table with a pillow that will raise the wrist to the appropriate level. For the person who is doing the actual monitoring, following the steps outlined in the box Patient Education for Self-Monitoring of Blood Pressure will help improve the accuracy of blood pressure readings, regardless of whether they are taken in the primary care provider's office, the pharmacy, or the home by the patient.

**TABLE 51-8 Arm Circumferences for Determining Appropriate Cuff Size**

| Arm Circumference (adult)* | Cuff Size |
|---|---|
| <31 cm | Regular adult cuff |
| 31-40 cm | Large adult cuff |
| >40 cm | Thigh cuff† |

* Determine arm circumference by measuring around the midpoint of the upper arm. Remeasure the patient's arm periodically, especially if he or she has recently gained or lost significant weight.

† Consider a wrist monitor for patients whose arm circumference is >40 cm.

## PATIENT EDUCATION FOR SELF-MONITORING OF BLOOD PRESSURE

The objective of self-testing is to identify elevated blood pressure or monitor the efficacy of diet, exercise, or medication in managing hypertension. For most patients, carefully following product instructions and the self-care measures listed here will help ensure accurate blood pressure readings.

### Precautions/Avoidance of Incorrect Results

- Keep a log of blood pressure readings and any circumstances that might have affected the reading (e.g., nervous, late for work).
- If home readings are being performed for diagnostic purposes, take readings at different times throughout the day and under different circumstances.
- If readings are being done to determine adequacy of antihypertensive therapy, take the reading at the same time of day, preferably in the early morning soon after arising from bed.
- Allow plenty of time to relax before taking a blood pressure reading. Feelings of stress or pressure can elevate the blood pressure.
- Do not smoke tobacco or drink caffeine-containing beverages for at least 30 minutes before taking a measurement. These activities can increase blood pressure.
- Wait 10 to 15 minutes after a bath and 30 minutes after eating to take a measurement. These activities can lower blood pressure.
- Some medications such as oral decongestants may increase blood pressure. Be alert for possible changes in readings when starting or stopping medications.

### Usage Guidelines

- Make sure the room is at a comfortable temperature.
- Sit in a comfortable chair, with the back supported and the feet straight ahead and flat on the floor.
- If using an arm cuff, place the arm to be measured on a table, making sure the upper arm is at heart level. Remove restrictive clothing from the arm.
- If using a wrist cuff, place a pillow (or two pillows) under the arm to be measured to bring the wrist up to heart level.
- Place the cuff on the arm to be measured. The cuff should be snug but not tight enough to restrict blood flow. Use the guidelines in Table 51-8 for selecting cuff size.
- Rest for at least 5 minutes in this position.
- Measure the blood pressure as directed by the product instructions. If using a stethoscope, listen for the Korotkoff's sounds as defined:
  - Phase 1: Sound begins as a soft tapping. Record the systolic pressure at the point when two taps are heard in sequence.
  - Phase 2: Tapping sound gets louder and is accompanied by a swishing sound or murmur.
  - Phase 3: Tapping sounds persist, but the swishing or murmur sound stops.
  - Phase 4: Muffling or softening of tapping sounds.
  - Phase 5: Sound stops. Record the diastolic pressure at the point when sound stops.
- Take two to three measurements separated by at least 2 minutes using the same arm.
- Record the results, arm used, and the time and date of the measurement, as well as any medications, including antihypertensive medications, currently being taken plus the time of the last dose of each.

⚠ Do not adjust blood pressure medications based on home measurements unless specifically instructed to do so by a health care provider.

⚠ See a primary care provider immediately for evaluation and treatment if blood pressure values are high and you are having symptoms such as headache or blurred vision.

*Source:* References 53 and 55.

## *Product Selection Guidelines*

Of the three types of blood pressure measuring devices, no single one is best for every patient. The choice of device is individualized according to characteristics such as the patient's ability and willingness to learn, physical disabilities, patient preference, and the cost of the device. Mercury column devices are expensive and, as discussed in the next section, have other disadvantages for home use. In general, aneroid devices are the least expensive. Depending on the features, a digital device can cost as much as a mercury column device. A discussion of the pros and cons of all three types of devices follows.

### Mercury Column Devices

The mercury column blood pressure monitor is still the reference standard in blood pressure measurement. This monitor typically comes with a cuff and an inflation bulb. The tubing from the cuff is attached to a column of mercury encased in a glass gauge.

Although mercury monitors are the most accurate and reliable of the devices, their routine use for home measurement is discouraged because they are cumbersome and pose the risk of mercury toxicity should the glass tubing break. They also require good eyesight and hearing for effective use. If the mercury does not rest at zero when the cuff is lying flat and completely deflated, the device needs recalibration.

### Aneroid Devices

Next to mercury column monitors, aneroid devices are the most accurate and reliable. They are light, portable, and very affordable, and they pose no risk from mercury toxicity. They include several features that make patient teaching much easier. First, many devices now come with a stethoscope attached to the cuff, which frees the patient from having to hold the bell of the stethoscope in place. Second, a D-ring on the cuff allows a single user to place the cuff on the arm easily. Third, a few manufacturers offer a gauge attached to the inflation bulb, making it easier to manipulate the equipment because there are fewer pieces to control. Such monitors are considered the option of choice for home use, but they do require careful patient instruction and follow-up. Good eyesight and hearing are necessary for accurate readings with standard models. For patients with reduced visual capacity, however, devices with large-type print on the face of the gauge are available.

At the bottom of the face of each aneroid device is a small box. When the cuff is completely deflated and lying on the table, the needle of the gauge should rest in the box. If the needle is outside the box, the gauge needs recalibration. Many manufacturers sell recalibration tools to allow health care professionals to adjust the devices.

#### Digital Devices

With advancing technology, digital devices have become more accurate, reliable, and easy to use, and as a result have skyrocketed in popularity. Such devices include semi-automatic (manually inflating), fully automatic (autoinflating), wrist, and finger blood pressure monitors. Features such as printouts, pulse monitor, digital clock, automated inflation and deflation, memory, large display, and D-ring for the cuff differentiate many of the devices. These features significantly affect the price.

A major drawback to the digital monitors is the user's inability to determine whether the device is out of calibration. As a result, many clinicians recommend the aneroid devices over the easier-to-use digital products. A study comparing blood pressure devices found that only 34% of systolic and 48% of diastolic pressures measured with a digital monitor were within ±5 mm Hg of a mercury monitor.[54] Fifty-four percent of systolic and 58% of diastolic readings with an aneroid device were within 5 mm Hg of a mercury monitor. The JNC 7 report notes that home measurement devices should be checked regularly for accuracy;[53] therefore, patients should be advised to have their monitors checked at least yearly.

### Assessment of Self-Monitoring of Blood Pressure

The practitioner should first determine why a patient wants to use a blood pressure monitor. If the use is warranted, the practitioner should determine whether the patient has physical impairments that can interfere with proper use of the monitor. The practitioner should also evaluate the patient's ability to comprehend and follow instructions.

### Patient Counseling for Self-Monitoring of Blood Pressure

The practitioner should emphasize the importance of tracking blood pressure values to monitor control of hypertension. Regular self-monitoring of blood pressure will illustrate positive effects of proper diet, exercise, and medication use in controlling the disorder. Such reinforcement can improve patient adherence with prescribed therapies. The patient should be shown the proper technique for blood pressure monitoring and encouraged to return for a follow-up evaluation of the patient's technique. Because of white coat hypertension, patients measuring blood pressure at home usually obtain lower results than those taken at the doctor's office. In the home setting, a blood pressure greater than 135/85 mm Hg should be considered elevated.[53] The box Patient Education for Self-monitoring of Blood Pressure lists specific information to provide patients.

### Evaluation of Patient Outcomes for Self-Monitoring of Blood Pressure

Patients measuring blood pressure for diagnostic and monitoring purposes should be instructed on how to track values and discuss the values with a primary care provider. Patients monitoring their blood pressure should be cautioned not to adjust their medications unless instructed otherwise. Patients should be instructed to immediately contact their primary care provider if they are obtaining very high values and having any symptoms of high blood pressure such as headache or blurred vision. The practitioner can play a major role in aiding hypertensive patients by (1) motivating them to perform home BPM, (2) guiding them in product selection, (3) training them to use devices appropriately, and (4) facilitating communication between the patient, the patient's family, and the patient's primary care provider regarding any antihypertensive therapy.

## MISCELLANEOUS HOME TESTS

As the market for home test products and shopping over the Internet has exploded, new tests are becoming available with increasing frequency. Selected miscellaneous home tests are detailed in Table 51-9. Instructions for use are generally available from the manufacturer's Web site or an Internet site that sells the product. Following the general guidelines given in this chapter will also help patients obtain accurate results.

Not all available tests are FDA-approved for home use. The status of a particular test can be checked at www.accessdata.fda.gov/scripts/cdrh/cfdocs/cfIVD/Search.cfm.

## KEY POINTS FOR HOME TESTING AND MONITORING DEVICES

- To advise patients properly on selecting and using home testing or monitoring products, the practitioner must be familiar with the procedures for each available product.
- Manufacturers continually introduce new products and modifying current ones to provide more user-friendly versions. To keep up-to-date, the practitioner should request product information from manufacturers by calling their toll-free numbers, visiting their Web sites, or contacting their sales representatives.
- Patients who are using diagnostic tests should be encouraged to follow instructions carefully and to contact either the practitioner or the manufacturer's toll-free number for assistance, if needed.

**TABLE 51-9 Miscellaneous Home Tests**

| Test | Purpose | Testing Medium | Important Points | Comments |
|---|---|---|---|---|
| **In-home Tests** | | | | |
| Alcohol screening tests | Prevent inappropriate alcohol consumption | Breath (SAFE-Slim, BreathScan) Saliva (ALCO-Screen) | Put nothing in mouth for 15 minutes before or during the test; follow timing directions carefully and use a timing device | Semiquantitative BAC; saliva test strips can be used to detect alcohol in drinks |
| Visiderm | Monitor moles for changes over time | Skin | Use a transparent overlay to trace outline of individual moles; record color and other details; do subsequent examinations of each mole on same overlay | Includes transparent overlays, pen, color chart, instructions, and storage box |
| Breast Self-Examination Aid | Aid to make breast self-examination easier and more comfortable | | Examine breasts monthly; does not take place of mammogram and professional examination | Two-layer polyurethane breast shield or glove containing a small amount of silicone lubricant to reduce friction; some kits come with instructional video (Aware, Sensatouch) |
| TobacAlert | Detect tobacco use or exposure | Urine | Detects cotine, a metabolite of nicotine; detects use or exposure in previous 48-72 hours; dip strip in urine sample and read results in specified time (10-15 minutes) | Use of nicotine patch or gum can affect results; tobacalert.com |
| Early Alert Alzheimer's Home Screening Test | Screen for early stage of Alzheimer's disease | | Release 1 strip, sniff, and identify odor based on four suggested answers; do not use if nasal congestion or long-lasting loss of smell from other causes | Loss of smell among first signs of Alzheimer's disease; 12 microencapsulated, one-time use only odor strips; if ≥4 incorrect answers see a PCP for evaluation |
| My Allergy Test | Detect allergy to 10 most common allergens: dust mites, cat hair, mold (*Alternaria*), ragweed, mountain cedar (juniper), Timothy grass, Bermuda grass, egg white, milk, wheat | Blood (4-5 drops) | If negative result + symptoms, see PCP | Measures IgE antibodies; Only tests for 10 allergens; results available by e-mail in 10 days or regular mail; also a version that analyzes house dust for common allergens; immunetech.com |
| Proview Eye Pressure Monitor Kit | Monitor IOP in patients with glaucoma | Eye | Press device on partially closed eyelid until see the appearance of a pressure phosphene, usually described as a dark circle with a ring of light around the outside; does not replace in-office IOP measurement | Kit includes eye pressure monitor, log book, instructions, educational brochure, magnifier, and case; makes contact with the eyelid only no anesthetic required; can be used to increase patient involvement and track effect of medications; Bausch.com |

**TABLE 51-9 Miscellaneous Home Tests (continued)**

| Test | Purpose | Testing Medium | Important Points | Comments |
|---|---|---|---|---|
| **Mail-away Tests** | | | | |
| BIOSAFE Prostate Screen | Measure PSA | Blood (3 drops) | Men >50: have PSA checked annually; procedure same as BIOSAFE cholesterol test; does not substitute for rectal examination | Results are obtained by phone or mail; ebiosafe.com |
| BIOSAFE Thyroid Test | Measure TSH | Blood (3 drops) | Procedure same as BIOSAFE cholesterol test | Results obtained by phone or mail; patients with positive results or symptoms of thyroid disorder need to see PCP |

Key: BAC, blood alcohol concentration; Ig, immunoglobulin; IOP, intraocular pressure; PCP, primary care provider; PSA, prostate specific antigen; TSH, thyroid stimulating hormone.

- The practitioner should stress that the patient is self-testing, not self-diagnosing. Positive test results should be reported to a primary care provider immediately for definitive diagnosis and management. Negative test results should be questioned when the patient is experiencing symptoms of a suspected condition.
- If there is any question about the results, the patient should seek the advice of a health care provider.

## References


1. Levy S. The boom in home diagnostics. *Drug Topics.* 2003;3:33.
2. Food and Drug Administration. Assessing the Safety and Effectiveness of Home-Use in Vitro Diagnostics (IVDs) Guidance Regarding Premarket Submissions. Rockville, Md: Center for Devices and Radiological Health; 1998.
3. *Health, United States, 2004.* Hyattsville, Md: National Center for Health Statistics; 2004. Available at: www.cdc.gov/nchs/hus.htm.
4. Bastian L, Nanda K, Hasselblad V, et al. Diagnostic efficiency of home pregnancy test kits: a meta-analysis. *Arch Fam Med.* 1998; 7:465-9.
5. When the test really counts. Part one: earliest pregnancy detection. *Consumer Reports.* February 2003:45-7.
6. Wilcox AJ, Baird DD, Dunson D, et al. Natural limits of pregnancy testing in relation to the expected menstrual period. *JAMA.* 2001;286:1759-61.
7. Cole L, Khanlian S, Sutton J, et al. Accuracy of home pregnancy tests at the time of a missed menses. *Am J Obstet Gynecol.* 2004; 190:100-5.
8. Quattrocchi E, Hove I. Ovulation and pregnancy home testing products. *US Pharm.* 1998;23:54-63.
9. Clearblue Easy Fertility Monitor product information. New York: Unipath Diagnostics; 1999.
10. When the test really counts. Part two: the fertility window. *Consumer Reports.* February 2003:48-50.
11. Ovulook product information. Kapaau, Hawaii: Ovulook, LLC. Available at: http://www.ovulationtester.com. Accessed February 8, 2005.
12. OvaCue product information. Aurora, Colo: Zetek, Inc. Available at: http://www.zetek.net. Accessed February 8, 2005.
13. Fehring RJ. A comparison of the ovulation method with the CUE ovulation predictor in determining the fertile period. *J Am Acad Nurse Pract.* 1996;8:461-6.
14. FertilMARQ product information. Wilmington, Mass: Embryotech Laboratories. Available at: http://www.embryotech.com. Accessed February 8, 2005.
15. The American College of Obstetricians and Gynecologists Web site. The menopause years. Available at: http://www.acog.org. Accessed February 8, 2005.
16. Estroven product information. Bloomfield, Conn: Amerifit Nutrition, Inc. Available at: http://testsymptomsathome.com. Accessed February 8, 2005.
17. Menocheck Menopause Indicator product information. Media, Pa: Synova Healthcare. Available at: http://www.menocheck.com. Accessed February 8, 2005.
18. Jamal A, Thomas A, Murray T, et al. Cancer statistics 2002. *CA Cancer J Clin.* 2002;52:23-47.
19. Read TE, Kodner IJ. Colorectal cancer: risk factors and recommendations for early detection. *Am Fam Physician.* 1999;59:3083-92.
20. Terry P, Giovannucci E, Michels KB, et al. Fruit, vegetables, dietary fiber, and risk of colorectal cancer. *J Natl Cancer Inst.* 2001; 93:525-33.
21. Lieberman DA, Harford WV, Ahnen DJ, et al. One-time screening for colorectal cancer with combined fecal occult blood testing and examination of the distal colon. *N Engl J Med.* 2001; 345(8):555-60.
22. Accustat colorectal disease test product information. Lake Forest, Calif: WorldWide Medical Corporation. Available at: http://www.wwmed.com. Accessed February 10, 2005.
23. EZ-Detect product information. Newport Beach, Calif: Biomerica, Inc. Available at: http://www.ezdetect.com. Accessed February 8, 2005.
24. ColonTest-Sensitive product information. Las Vegas, Nev: Diagnostica Corporation. Available at: http://www.testsymptomsathome.com. Accessed February 8, 2005.
25. LifeGuard product information. Durham, NC: MedTek,LLC. Available at: http://www.orderlifeguard.com. Accessed February 8, 2005.

26. Kahi CJ, Imperiale TF. Do aspirin and nonsteroidal anti-inflammatory drugs cause false-positive fecal occult blood test results? A prospective study in a cohort of veterans. *Am J Med.* 2004; 117(11):837-41.
27. Walsh JME. Terdiman JP. Colorectal cancer screening: scientific review. *JAMA.* 2003;289:1288-96.
28. National Institutes of Health. Executive summary. In: Third Report of the National Cholesterol Education Program (NCEP) Expert Panel on Detection, Evaluation, and Treatment of High Blood Cholesterol in Adults (Adult Treatment Panel III). Bethesda, Md: National Institutes of Health; May 2001. NIH Publication No. 01-3670.
29. CholesTrak product information. Vista, Calif: Accutech. Available at: http://www.accutech.llc.com. Accessed February 8, 2005.
30. Accustat Cholesterol Test product information. Lake Forest, Calif: WorldWide Medical Corporation. Available at: http://wwmed.com. Accessed February 8, 2005.
31. Cardiochek product information. Indianapolis: Polymer Technology Systems. Available at: http://www.ptspanels.com. Accessed February 8, 2005.
32. Personal Cholesterol Monitor product information. Post Falls, Idaho: Lifestream Technologies; 2000.
33. BIOSAFE Total Cholesterol and Total Cholesterol Panel product information. Lincolnshire, Ill: BIOSAFE. Available at: http://www.ebiosafe.com. Accessed February 8, 2005.
34. McNamara JR, Warnick GR, Leary ET, et al. Multicenter evaluation of a patient-administered test for blood cholesterol measurement. *Prev Med.* 1996;25:583-92.
35. Do home cholesterol tests work? *Consumer Reports.* August 2003:9.
36. CDC. Urinary tract technical information. Available at: http://www.cdc.gov/ncidod/dbmd/diseaseinfo/urinarytractinfections_t.htm. Accessed February 8, 2005.
37. Bass PF, Jarvis JA, Mitchell CK. Urinary Tract Infections. *Primary Care.* 2003;30:41-61.
38. Teco Urine Reagent Strips product information. Anaheim, Calif: Teco Diagnostics. Available at: http://www.tecodiag.com. Accessed February 8, 2005.
39. UTI Home Screening Test product information. Redmond, Wash: Consumers Choice Systems. Available at: http://www.womanswellbeing.com. Accessed February 8, 2005.
40. AZO test strips product information. Woburn, Mass: PolyMedica Health. Available at: http:// www.azoproducts.com/strips/stripes.asp. Accessed February 8, 2005.
41. Division of HIV/AIDS Prevention, National Center for HIV, STD and TB Prevention, Centers for Disease Control & Prevention. *Basic Statistics.* Available at: http://www.cdc.gov/hiv/stats.htm. Accessed February 8, 2005.
42. Branson BM. Home sample collection tests for HIV infection. *JAMA.* 1998;280:1699-701.
43. Home Access Express HIV-1 test system product information. Hoffman Estates, Ill: Home Access Health Corporation. Available at: http://www.homeaccess.com. Accessed February 8, 2005.
44. CDC. Hepatitis fact sheet. Available at: http://www.cdc.gov/nci-dod/diseases/hepatitis/c/fact.htm. Accessed February 15, 2005.
45. Agency for Healthcare Research and Quality. *Management of Chronic Hepatitis C. Summary, Evidence Report/Technology Assessment: Number 60.* Rockville, Md: Agency for Healthcare Research and Quality; June 2002. Publication No. 02-E030. Available at: http://www.ahrq.gov/clinic/epcsums/hepcsum.htm. Accessed May 15, 2005.
46. Home Access Hepatitis C Check product information. Hoffman Estates, Ill: Home Access Health Corporation. Available at: http://www.homeaccess.com. Accessed February 8, 2005.
47. Hogan MJ. Diagnosis and treatment of teen drug use. *Med Clin North Am.* 2000;84:927-66.
48. Dr. Brown's Home Drug Testing System product information. Available at: http://www.drbrowns.com. Accessed February 12, 2005.
49. Parent's Alert Home Drug Test Service product information. Atlanta, Ga: Parents Alert, Inc. Available at: http://www.parentsalert.com. Accessed February 10, 2005.
50. Accustat Home Drug Test Kit product information. Lake Forest, Calif: WorldWide Medical Corporation. Available at: http://www.wwmed.com. Accessed February 10, 2005.
51. Quick Screen Pro product information. Vista, Calif: Craig Medical Distribution. Available at: http://www.craigmedical.com. Accessed February 10, 2005.
52. PDT-90 Personal Drug Testing Service product information. Cambridge, Mass: Psychemedics Corp. Available at: http://www.hairtestingfordrugs.com. Accessed February 10, 2005.
53. US Department of Health and Human Services. JNC 7 Express: The Seventh Report of the Joint National Committee on the Detection, Evaluation, and Treatment of High Blood Pressure (JNC-VII). Bethesda, Md: U.S. Department of Health and Human Services. Available at: http://www.nhlbi.nih.gov/guidelines/hypertension/jncintro.htm. Accessed February 10, 2005.
54. Johnson KA, Partsch DJ, Gleason P, et al. Comparison of two home blood pressure monitors with a mercury sphygmomanometer in an ambulatory population. *Pharmacotherapy.* 1999;19:333-9.
55. Pickering TG. Principles and techniques of blood pressure measurement. *Cardiol Clin.* 2002;20:207-23.

CHAPTER 52

# Adult Urinary Incontinence and Supplies

*Christine K. O'Neil*

Urinary incontinence (UI) is defined as the involuntary loss of urine that is sufficient to be a problem. Although often mistakenly thought of as a problem of aging, UI affects persons of all ages, socioeconomic backgrounds, and ethnicities. UI is twice as common in women, but men also suffer from the symptoms.[1] An estimated 17 million people in the United States are affected by UI, while another 34 million may suffer from overactive bladder (OAB).[2]

UI is an underdiagnosed and underreported condition with major psychosocial and economic effects on society. Feelings of embarrassment, denial, and misinformation prevent many people from seeking help, which may lead to anxiety, depression, and, possibly, social isolation. Severe UI usually results in a loss of self-esteem and the ability to maintain an independent lifestyle, and it is generally recognized as a major cause of institutionalization of older people. Direct costs associated with UI include the expenses for diagnosis, specific treatment, routine care, rehabilitation, and hospital and nursing home admissions. The direct costs of treating UI and OAB in men and women of all ages was estimated at 19.5 billion and 12.6 billion, respectively, in 2000.[2]

Despite the high prevalence of UI, less than half of community-dwelling persons with UI consult with their health care professional.[3] Many accept the symptoms as a natural part of aging and use self-care strategies with little or no health professional guidance. Although they are reluctant to talk about UI, Americans spend $1.1 billion annually on disposable incontinence products (e.g., pads, shields, guards, undergarments, and briefs).[4]

## Epidemiology of Urinary Incontinence

Several studies have determined the prevalence of UI in nursing homes and the community.[5,6] The reported prevalence rates are approximately 50% for people in nursing homes and range between 2% and 55% for adults living in the community, depending on the definition of UI, population characteristics, and methodologic approach.[7] Among adults 30 to 60 years of age, the prevalence of UI ranges from 12% to 42% for women and from 3% to 5% for men. For older people (>60 years of age), prevalence rates from 17% to 55% have been reported for women and from 11% to 34% for men.

## Anatomy and Physiology of the Urinary Tract

Urination is a complex process, involving a coordinated effort by the bladder, urethra, muscular components of the lower urinary tract (detrusor muscle, internal sphincter, and external sphincter), brain, and spinal cord.[8,9] Urine produced by the kidneys passes through the ureters to the bladder. The detrusor muscle, the smooth muscle layer of the bladder, gives tone to the bladder, relaxing as the bladder fills with urine and contracting during urination. The bladder neck, which joins the bladder and the urethra, is surrounded by smooth muscle, referred to as the internal sphincter, which either constricts to hold urine in the bladder or relaxes, permitting urine flow through the urethra. Voluntary control of micturition is maintained by contraction of the external sphincter, a striated muscle located at the proximal end of the urethra around the bladder. When relaxed, the urethra, surrounded by both smooth and striated muscle, allows urine to leave the body.

The bladder and the internal sphincter are innervated by the autonomic nervous system, and the external sphincter is innervated by the somatic or voluntary nervous system. Parasympathetic and sympathetic nerves innervate the smooth muscle of the bladder and urethra. Both α-adrenergic and β-adrenergic receptors are present in the urinary structures. The α-receptors are located in the base of the bladder and the proximal urethra, and the β-receptors are found primarily in the body of the bladder detrusor. Stimulation of the α-receptors causes contraction of the smooth muscles in the bladder neck and urethra, thus closing the bladder outlet. Stimulation of the β-receptors results in smooth muscle relaxation and allows the bladder to fill. Thus, sympathetic stimulation causes the bladder to retain urine. Parasympathetic cholinergic receptors are located throughout the bladder. Stimulation of these receptors causes the detrusor to contract, emptying the bladder. The sacral center, lying between vertebrae S2 and S4, acts as the relay center for information to and from the bladder, pelvic floor, and brain.

The capacity of the bladder is approximately 400 to 500 mL. When the bladder fills, stretch receptors in the detrusor wall transmit signals to the brain through the spinal cord, initiating the urge to urinate when the bladder is approximately half full. Under normal circumstances, adults can delay voiding for 30 to 60 minutes as a result of the short sacral reflex, which diminishes the urge to urinate by increasing contraction of the external sphincter

**TABLE 52-1 Risk Factors for Urinary Incontinence**

| | |
|---|---|
| Immobility/chronic degenerative disease | High-impact physical activities |
| Impaired cognition | Diabetes |
| Medications (Table 52-2) | Stroke |
| Metabolic disorders (hyperglycemia, hypercalcemia) | Neurologic disorders (spinal cord injury, neuropathy) |
| Obesity: moderate to morbid | Estrogen depletion |
| Smoking | Pelvic floor muscle weakness |
| Fecal impaction | Childhood nocturnal enuresis |
| Delirium | Caucasian race |
| Low fluid intake (leading to concentrated urine and bladder irritation that worsens symptoms) | Pregnancy/vaginal delivery/episiotomy |
| Environmental barriers | BPH/TURP/ prostatectomy |

Key: BPH, benign prostatic hyperplasia; TURP, transurethral resection of the prostate.

*Source:* Adapted from references 1 and 11-13.

**TABLE 52-2 Reversible Conditions That Cause or Contribute to Urinary Incontinence[1,21]**

**Conditions Affecting the Lower Urinary Tract**

Urinary tract infections, atrophic vaginitis/urethritis, pregnancy/vaginal delivery/episiotomy, prostatectomy, stool impaction

**Drug Side Effects**

Polyuria, frequency, urgency: caffeine, diuretics, alcohol, acetylcholinesterase inhibitors

Urinary retention: anticholinergics, antidepressants, hypnotics/sedatives, antipsychotics, narcotics, muscle relaxants, antihypertensives (calcium-channel blockers), β-adrenergic agonists, α-adrenergic agonists

Urethral relaxation: α-adrenergic blockers

Cough: ACE inhibitors

**Increased Urine Production**

Metabolic disorders (hyperglycemia, hypercalcemia), excessive fluid intake, volume overload, venous insufficiency with edema

**Impaired Ability or Willingness to Reach a Toilet**

Dementia, delirium, chronic illness/injury that interferes with mobility, psychologic conditions

and relaxing the detrusor muscle of the bladder. Bladder emptying is initiated voluntarily, causing relaxation of the external sphincter and contraction of the detrusor. Normal urination results in complete emptying of the bladder, with little or no residual urine (50 mL or less). Any disruption in the integration of musculoskeletal and neurologic function can lead to loss of control of normal bladder function and UI.[10]

## Etiology/Types of Urinary Incontinence

UI is a symptom that can be caused by anatomic, physiologic, and pathologic factors affecting the urinary tract, as well as external factors.[1,11-13] In many cases, multiple and interacting factors contribute to UI. The risk of UI is strongly associated with aging. Additional risk factors for UI, some at least partially reversible, have been identified (Table 52-1). Identification of the cause(s) of UI is essential for the assessment and successful management of UI.

UI can be described broadly as transient or chronic. Transient UI is usually of sudden onset and secondary to acute illness (e.g., urinary tract infections) or to any disease that causes acute confusion (e.g., respiratory disease, myocardial infarction, or septicemia) or immobility, preventing the person from reaching a toilet independently or in time. Many other conditions and medications can cause or contribute to transient UI (Table 52-2). Managing these conditions may resolve UI in some patients, but in others only reduce the severity of symptoms. Chronic UI is often related to neurologic or other chronic conditions, such as benign prostatic hyperplasia (BPH), cystocele, or uterine prolapse. UI can be classified as OAB, stress incontinence, mixed incontinence (OAB plus stress incontinence), overflow incontinence, or functional incontinence, depending on the underlying etiologies.

## Pathophysiology/Signs and Symptoms of Urinary Incontinence

Recognition of signs and symptoms of UI is an essential first step in providing treatment advice. Patients often delay discussion or do not seek medical evaluation for UI with their primary care provider. Therefore, it is important for practitioners to inquire about potential UI symptoms when such conditions are suspected on the basis of clinical evidence or patient inquiries. Open-ended questions such as "What problems are you having, if any, with your bladder?" and "How often do you experience urine leakage?" can be used to begin this dialogue. An awareness of signs such as the odor of urine or appearance of wetness is also necessary to identify potential patients suffering from UI. In most cases, observed and reported symptoms can be correlated with the types of UI (Table 52-3).

### *Overactive Bladder*

Overactive bladder occurs in both men and women, and its incidence increases with age. This condition is characterized by sudden and profound urinary urgency (strong desire to void), frequency (urinating more than eight times daily), nocturia (two or more awakenings at night to pass urine), or enuresis and is often, but not always, accompanied by urge incontinence (involuntary urine leakage with

**TABLE 52-3 Common Signs/Symptoms of Urinary Incontinence, by Type**

| Classification of UI | Signs/Symptoms |
|---|---|
| Urge | Urgency<br>Frequency<br>Large amount of urine loss<br>Nocturia or nocturnal incontinence (enuresis)<br>Inability to reach toilet following urge to void |
| Stress | Urine leakage during physical activity, lifting coughing, sneezing<br>Small to moderate urine loss depending on level of activity<br>Able to reach toilet in time to complete void<br>Occasional urgency<br>Nocturia and enuresis are rare |
| Overflow | Sensation of bladder or abdominal fullness<br>Sensation of incomplete bladder emptying<br>Hesitancy<br>Straining to void<br>Decreased or incomplete urine stream; dribbling<br>Frequency common<br>Urgency common |

urgency).[1,9,10,14] Overactive bladder is usually, but not always, attributable to uninhibited contractions of the detrusor muscle, referred to as detrusor instability. Other terms describing detrusor instability are detrusor hyperreflexia, detrusor hyperactivity with impaired bladder contractility, and bladder instability.

Neurogenic causes of detrusor instability include dementia, stroke, Parkinson's disease, suprasacral spinal cord injury, multiple sclerosis, and medullary lesions. Detrusor instability of neurologic origin is referred to as hyperreflexia. Nonneurogenic causes of detrusor instability include bladder irritation caused by infection or interstitial cystitis, obstruction (e.g., BPH), bladder stones, and tumors. Some therapeutic agents (e.g., diuretics and alcohol) can exacerbate symptoms of urge incontinence as a result of increased filling of the bladder. Bethanechol can also lead to urge incontinence through cholinergically mediated bladder smooth-muscle contraction.

### *Stress Incontinence*

Stress incontinence is the most frequently encountered type of UI in women, except in the very old (more than 75 years of age), in whom OAB is most common. Symptoms of stress incontinence may occur in some men after transurethral resection of the prostate and radical prostatectomy.[10] Stress incontinence is characterized by involuntary leakage of urine with sudden increases in abdominal pressure associated with sneezing, laughing, coughing, exercising, and lifting, and during pregnancy. This involuntary leakage is believed to be caused by hypermobility of the bladder neck or weakness of the urethral sphincter and pelvic floor muscles. Hypermobility refers to displacement of the bladder neck and urethra during physical exertion, and it occurs when the supporting pelvic muscles have been weakened as a result of vaginal childbirth and aging. The weakening of the urethral sphincter can be secondary to vaginal or urologic surgery, trauma, aging, or inadequate estrogen, or it may be neurologic in etiology.[14]

Drug-related causes of stress incontinence include α-adrenergic antagonists such as prazosin, terazosin, doxazosin, tamsulosin, and alfuzosin, which cause urethral relaxation (Table 52-2).

### *Mixed Incontinence*

Mixed incontinence, most common in women, consists of the combination of OAB and stress incontinence.[1,15] While the term mixed UI is generally applied to women, men with outlet obstruction resulting from BPH may exhibit mixed symptoms of OAB and overflow incontinence. Men may also exhibit mixed symptoms as a result of stress UI attributable to radical prostatectomy or transurethral resection of the prostate combined with OAB.

### *Overflow Incontinence*

Overflow incontinence, an involuntary urine loss associated with overdistention of the bladder, is observed in 7% to 11% of incontinent older patients.[1,15] Symptoms include dribbling, reduced force and caliber of urinary stream, urgency, and a sensation of incomplete voiding. The two main causes are outlet obstruction and/or an underactive bladder (detrusor) muscle. Outlet obstruction can be caused by BPH, urogenital tumors, pelvic organ prolapse, or previous anti-incontinence surgery. Dysfunctional bladder contractility can result from diabetic or alcoholic neuropathy, lower spinal cord injury, radical pelvic surgery, or medications with anticholinergic properties, such as antihistamines, antipsychotics, narcotics, tricyclic antidepressants, and muscle relaxants. These medications can cause overflow incontinence by blocking cholinergically mediated bladder contractions, thus inhibiting normal bladder function.

### *Functional Incontinence*

Functional incontinence is described as urine loss caused by factors such as physical or cognitive impairment, which interfere with a person's ability to reach toilet facilities in time or to perform toileting tasks.[1,9] Causes of this type of UI are many and include stroke, diminished mobility, impaired cognitive function or perception, environmental barriers, use of sedative and hypotensive agents, poorly controlled severe pain, and psychologic unwillingness to release urine in the proper place. Because many functionally impaired people may have other types of UI, functional incontinence should be a diagnosis of exclusion.

### *Age-related Physiologic Changes Affecting Micturition*

Age-related changes in the bladder and urinary tract may contribute to an older person's vulnerability to UI. With age, the kidney's ability to concentrate urine diminishes, resulting in larger urine volumes. In addition, age-related hypotrophic changes in bladder tissue lead to frequent urination and nocturia, whereas decreased muscle tone of the bladder, as well as the bladder sphincters and pelvic muscles, contributes to the potential for reduced urine control. This loss of control, combined with diminished mobility and reaction time, predispose older people to UI.[15,16]

In women, the loss of estrogen with age causes a decrease in bladder outlet and urethral resistance, as well as a decline in pelvic musculature—all of which increase the likelihood of UI. In addition, estrogen loss results in atrophic changes in the vaginal and urethral mucosa, disrupting the vaginal flora and leading to atrophic vaginitis and chronic urethritis. These conditions, in turn, may cause urinary frequency and urgency, dysuria, urinary tract infections, and UI. The woman's short urethra exerts less resistance to intravesicular pressure than the longer male urethra. Childbirth, gynecologic procedures, and obesity also weaken the woman's pelvic floor muscles, thereby decreasing support for the bladder. As a consequence, the anatomy of the bladder becomes distorted, resulting in cystocele, rectocele, or uterine prolapse. These conditions may result in chronic obstruction of the bladder, again leading to UI.

Older men often have prostatic enlargement, which results in urethral obstruction, leading to decreased urinary flow rates, increased residual volumes, detrusor instability, and overflow incontinence. Paradoxically, prostatectomy to relieve symptoms related to BPH can result in stress incontinence caused by incidental injury to the internal sphincter.

## Complications of Urinary Incontinence

The consequences of UI are considerable. Many people are embarrassed by such a condition and refrain from discussing their urinary problems with their primary health care providers. Some people with UI believe it is a normal consequence of aging, rather than a symptom of underlying disease or anatomic change. Social isolation occurs because the incontinent patient avoids social interaction to prevent the embarrassment and rejection that often accompany UI. In turn, social isolation leads to depression. Intimate contact and sexual activity with the patient's partner can also decrease. Attempts to limit episodes of involuntary urine loss by restricting fluid intake can cause dehydration and hypotension, whereas skin irritation and ulceration caused by long exposure to urine results in "diaper rash" and possibly pressure ulcers.[1]

The caregivers of incontinent older patients are under stress because of the tedious and time-consuming care needed to deal with the problems at home. Often, the loss of urine control leads to a drastic reduction in quality of life, nursing home placement, or elder abuse.[1,17] Falls and fractures can result from urinary incontinence and with urgency symptoms in the absence of incontinence.

## Treatment of Adult Urinary Incontinence

### *Treatment Goals*

The goals of treatment of UI are to reduce the severity of symptoms, avoid complications, and improve the patient's quality of life. When incontinence aids are used as part of self-management in UI, additional goals are to control or treat skin breakdown (diaper rash), control the odor of leaked urine, and contain urine in the undergarment.

### *General Treatment Approach*

After medical evaluation, treatment is individualized for the type of UI. The three major categories of intervention are behavioral, pharmacologic, and surgical. Figure 52-1 outlines the self-management of adult UI.

### *Behavioral Therapy*

Behavioral techniques decrease the frequency of UI in most patients, have no reported side effects, and do not limit future therapies.[1] To be most successful, they generally require patient and/or caregiver involvement and continued practice. Three types of behavioral techniques, listed in order of increasing need for patient involvement, are toileting assistance, bladder training, and pelvic floor muscle training. Behavioral techniques are now the accepted first-line therapy in treating all forms of UI except overflow incontinence.[9] Practitioners should educate patients about the role of behavioral therapy in the management of UI.

Toileting assistance includes routine/scheduled toileting performed at fixed, regular intervals (every 2 to 4 hours); habit training, which is toileting scheduled to match voiding patterns in those who have natural voiding patterns; and prompted voiding. In prompted voiding, patients are trained to void only if the need is voiced on direct questioning. They are checked for wetness and praised for maintaining continence and trying to toilet.

Bladder training consists of education, scheduled voiding with systematic delay, and positive reinforcement. Patients are taught to delay voiding when the urge occurs and to use tactics to increase urine volume and the interval between voids. Bladder training is recommended for urge, stress, or mixed incontinence, but is often difficult to achieve in cognitively impaired or frail older people.

Pelvic floor muscle training, also known as Kegel exercises or pelvic floor exercises, is designed to strengthen the voluntary periurethral and perivaginal muscles, giving the patient more control of micturition and reducing UI.[1] These exercises have been used successfully for stress and OAB; they are performed by squeezing the pelvic muscles as if to stop the flow of urine. These contractions should be held for about 10 seconds, then released for 10 seconds; 3 to 4 sets of 10 contractions per day are generally recommended.[1,18] It is important to advise patients that the response to pelvic muscle exercises is delayed. The exercises may be augmented by the use of vaginal weights or biofeedback techniques. Biofeedback can facilitate learning of pelvic muscle exercises. Direct electrical stimulation of the pelvic floor muscles with vaginal or anal probes or

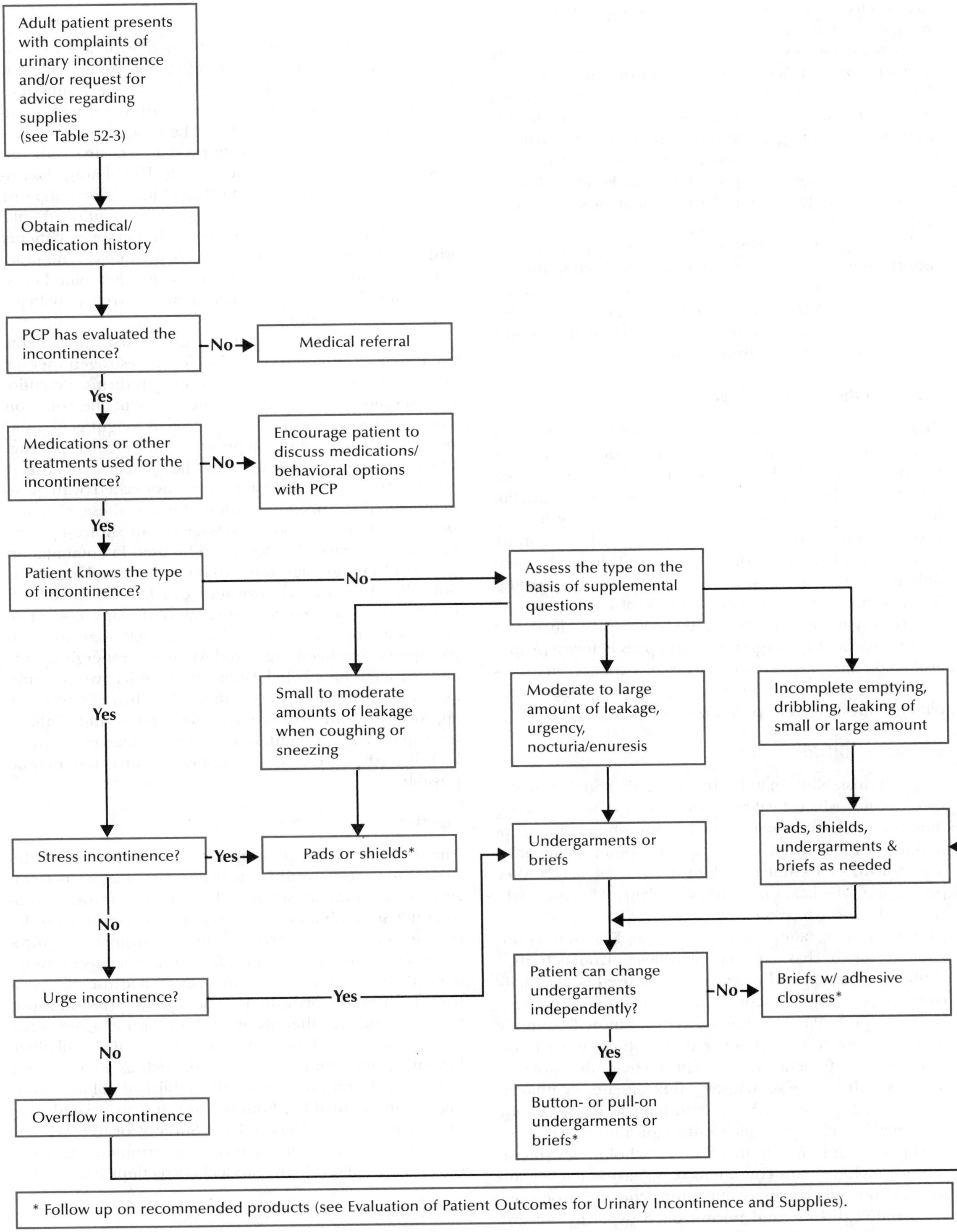


FIGURE 52-1 Self-care of adult urinary incontinence. Key: PCP, primary care provider.

surface electrodes has been used with limited success in stress, urge, and mixed UI.

A relatively new option available only through a primary care provider's office is the NeoControl Pelvic Floor Therapy System.[19] This is a pulsating magnetic chair that uses directed magnetic fields to induce pelvic muscle contractions. Patients generally require treatments twice a week for about 20 to 30 minutes for a total of 8 weeks or more. This option is approved by the Food and Drug Administration (FDA) for the treatment of stress, OAB, and mixed UI.

Although the technique is unproven, anecdotal reports suggest that crossing legs before coughing or sneezing prevents urine leakage in women with stress incontinence. Volitional precontraction to prepare the pelvic floor for an impending challenge has demonstrated the capacity to reduce stress incontinence.[20]

### *Type-specific Pharmacologic Treatment*

The type of UI influences the choice of treatments. For that reason, an overview of the pharmacologic measures for specific types of UI is presented here. Most medications used to treat these disorders are prescription products, but in some cases nonprescription medications may be suggested. Nonprescription medications for UI are considered an off-label indication, however, and should be used only after a thorough evaluation by a primary care provider has determined the cause and/or type of UI. Inappropriate use of systemic nonprescription products and incorrect use of absorbent undergarments and pads before a proper evaluation may result in unnecessary expense, inappropriate treatment, and possibly unnecessary changes in the patient's lifestyle and psychologic well-being.

#### Overactive Bladder

Detrusor instability may be treated with anticholinergic medications, which facilitate urine storage by decreasing uninhibited detrusor contractions. Most often, a prescription medication such as tolterodine, trospium, solifenacin, darifenacin, or oxybutynin chloride, is used first. Other prescription medications with less evidence of clinical efficacy and concerns about risk of side effects include propantheline, imipramine, and nifedipine. Flavoxate is not effective on the basis of four placebo-controlled trials.[21] Diphenhydramine and dicyclomine are used occasionally (see Chapter 12).[22] Practitioners should counsel patients about the potential side effects that occur more frequently with diphenhydramine than with the other prescription products. Sedation, dry mouth (a problem for denture use, patients with gastroesophageal reflux disease, dysphagia, or stroke), constipation, and confusion can be significant problems in older patients. Contraindications to the use of diphenhydramine (and other anticholinergic medications) include many conditions (e.g., narrow-angle glaucoma, peptic ulcer, urinary tract obstruction, gastroesophageal reflux disease, and uncontrolled hyperthyroidism) that occur more often in older patients than in other patients.

#### Stress Incontinence

Stress incontinence is often treated with agents that increase outflow resistance through α-receptor stimulation that enhances contraction of the bladder neck muscles.[1] A commonly recommended nonprescription drug is pseudoephedrine (see Chapter 12). The dose of pseudoephedrine is 15 to 30 mg three times daily, starting with the lowest dose, especially in older people. Use of nonprescription medications for UI is an off-label indication and must be approved by a primary care provider. Caution should be used, however, when initiating such therapy in patients with hypertension and/or cardiac arrhythmias. The practitioner should advise patients to monitor their blood pressure and pulse, and to report any new occurrences of heart palpitations or fainting.

In women, estrogen therapy may be used, and benefits are usually seen in 4 to 6 weeks. Topical estrogen therapy is useful for underlying vaginitis and urethritis. Practitioners should counsel female patients about the common side effects of estrogen therapy, such as weight gain, fluid retention, increased blood pressure, and vaginal spotting. In light of recent concerns about the complications (heart attack, stroke, and breast cancer) associated with postmenopausal estrogen/progestin therapy, these products should be used in the lowest dosage for the shortest period of time (3-5 years). Estrogen can be used in combination with α-adrenergic agonists; however, the combination is only slightly more effective and can be associated with more adverse effects and increased therapy cost. The antidepressant imipramine, which also acts as an adrenergic agonist, has been suggested when α-adrenergic agents and estrogens have failed. Duloxetine, a selective serotonin and norepinephrine reuptake inhibitor currently approved for the treatment of depression and diabetic neuropathy, is moderately effective in managing stress UI.[23] If medical treatment fails, surgical correction may be possible.

#### Overflow Incontinence

The treatment of overflow incontinence is directed by the underlying cause. In BPH, α-adrenergic antagonists (terazosin, doxazosin, tamsulosin, alfuzosin, or prazosin) or 5-α-reductase inhibitors (finasteride or dutasteride) can be used to reduce the degree of outlet obstruction. α-Adrenergic antagonists have a much faster onset of effect (several days) than do 5-α-reductase inhibitors. Because of a relatively high rate of orthostatic hypotension, prazosin is not recommended for therapy of UI. Prescription agents such as bethanechol chloride may be initiated if the bladder has insufficient contractile strength such as after general anesthesia. Its efficacy is not well established in long-standing hypotonic bladder, however, and it is associated with potentially serious adverse effects. Surgery for BPH is often necessary. Catheterization, usually intermittent, is a last resort when medical and surgical corrections have failed.

#### Functional/Iatrogenic Incontinence

Treatment of functional and iatrogenic incontinence requires evaluating the patient's entire medical status and medication history. UI resulting from medications can be resolved by initiating alternative treatments. Underlying dysfunctions such as pain related to rheumatoid arthritis and decreased mobility can be remedied by medical and environmental changes that make using the toilet possible or easier within the limitations of the patient's functional status. Often an assessment by physical or occupational therapists can be useful in enhancing physical function.

### Other Interventions

Other devices that have been used for UI, include elevating devices to support the bladder neck (pessary, tampon, or prosthesis), urethral occlusive devices (urethral plug, expandable urethral devices, or urethral shields), external collection systems (condom catheters), penile compression devices, and catheterization (intermittent, indwelling, or suprapubic).[1] Although most of these external or occlusive devices require a prescription or primary care provider supervision, an adhesive foam patch was approved for nonprescription use in 1998. The patch has an adhesive coating on one side and, when placed over the urinary opening, helps reduce urine leakage in stress incontinence. Information on the availability of nonpharmacologic UI products, particularly the urethral occlusive devices and the incontinence patch, is limited and some devices may no longer be available.

### Surgical Treatment

Surgery is uncommon in the treatment of OAB; however, both stress and overflow incontinence can be treated successfully by surgery. Surgery is an option when other nonpharmacologic and pharmacologic therapies have failed or the patient wants definitive treatment. The aims of continence surgery are to elevate the bladder neck, support the urethra, and increase urethral resistance.[1,24] Some surgical options include urethral bulking agents (collagen), sling operation, tension-free vaginal tape, artificial sphincter insertion, needle bladder neck suspension, retropubic suspension, urinary diversion, and bladder denervation.

### Use of Urinary Incontinence Supplies

Absorbent undergarments and pads are used to protect clothing, bedding, and furniture while allowing the patient to have independence and mobility. Although absorbent products are beneficial, they should be used only after a thorough and complete physical examination. Prematurely initiating the use of absorbent protective products, relieves the discomfort and obscures the cause of UI. Because correction of the cause may be possible, the premature acceptance of UI may have significant financial, social, and psychologic consequences.

#### Product Selection Guidelines

The type of absorbent product selected depends on several factors:[1]

- Type and severity of UI
- Functional status
- Sex
- Availability of caregivers
- Patient preference
- Cost
- Convenience

The clinician needs to discuss these factors with patients and their caregivers when helping them select absorbent garments and pads, which are available as reusable or disposable products (Table 52-4). This is particularly important for low-income patients who often do not have the economic flexibility to purchase absorbent products; they may be forced to resort to toilet paper, an ineffective substitute. The disposable product market has been a multimillion-dollar industry since the 1990s. These products work in the same manner as children's disposable diapers. They are designed to absorb urine; provide a moisture barrier to protect clothes, bedding, and furniture; and minimize skin contact with urine. Urine is jelled in the matrix of the absorbent layer, minimizing its contact with skin.

The capacity of each disposable product corresponds to the needs of the patient:

- *Guards/shields:* 2 to 12 oz (60-360 mL), light to heavy capacity.
- *Undergarments:* 12 to 18 oz (360-540 mL), moderate to heavy capacity.
- *Briefs:* 28 to 36 oz (840-1100 mL), moderate to heavy capacity.

Patients with small amounts of leakage (e.g., dribbling), as occurs in stress or overflow incontinence and after urologic surgical procedures, may require only a pad or shield.[25,26] If larger amounts of urine are lost with UI, as often occurs with detrusor instability, products with a larger capacity would be more appropriate. Many products designed for overnight (heavy) use tend to have the largest capacities.

Another important issue is the functional capacity of the patient. If the patient needs assistance with absorbent garments, the caregiver may find that briefs or diapers with "roll-on" bed application and adhesive closures are useful. Securing the product may be an important issue. Close-fitting underwear is recommended. Some garments or shields have adhesive strips or belts to hold them in place. The use of belts may require assistance from a caregiver. Of course, comfort and leg security from urine leakage are important. Many product lines offer elastic legs or contoured shapes. Caregivers and patients should consider products designed for the differences between male and female anatomy when selecting large-capacity products.[25,26]

Protective underpads are often used in conjunction with briefs and undergarments for extended duration activities, such as sleeping and sitting. Both bed and chair pads are available, and the practitioner should inquire about the need for additional protection. The underpad should have a known capacity, a waterproof duration of several hours, and an ability to remain intact when wet. Bed pads are available in sizes from 16 by 24 in. to 30 by 36 in. For chairs, a 16 by 18-in. pad should be used.[26]

**TABLE 52-4 Selected Adult Incontinence Products**

| Trade Name | Product Features*† |
|---|---|
| Assurance Slip-On Protective Undergarment‡ | For moderate/heavy leakage; one-size, one-piece design; no buttons or tapes |
| Attends Briefs | For heavy leakage; sizes Y, S, M, L; refastenable tapes |
| Attends Briefs w/ Waistband | For heavy leakage; sizes M, L |
| Attends Guards Super Absorbency | For light/moderate leakage; curved fit |
| Attends Pads | For light leakage; medium-, extra-, superabsorbency |
| Attends Undergarments Super Absorbency | For moderate leakage; reusable elastic belts |
| Conveen Drip Collector | For dribbling/light leakage; 3 oz and 4 oz capacity; adheres to underwear; designed for men |
| Depend Underwear Extra & Super Plus Absorbency | For heavy leakage; S/M & L; feels and wears like underwear |
| Depend Refastenable Underwear Extra & Super Plus Absorbency | For heavy leakage; S/M & L/XL; feels and wears like underwear; four refastenable tabs |
| Depend Fitted Briefs Regular & Overnight Absorbency | For heavy leakage; sizes M, L; six refastenable tapes plus elastic leg and waist; wetness indicator; overnight absorbency absorbs 30% more urine than regular absorbency |
| Depend Guards for Men | For light/moderate leakage; one size; anatomic design with elasticized pouch and cuplike fit |
| Depend Undergarments Easy Fit Elastic Leg/Adjustable Straps Regular & Extra Absorbency | For moderate leakage; soft, clothlike outer cover; one size; reusable hook and loop strap tabs; fits hip sizes up to 65 in. |
| Depend Undergarments Elastic Leg/Button Straps Regular & Extra Absorbency | For moderate leakage; soft, clothlike outer cover; one size; reusable button strap tabs; fits hip sizes up to 65 in. |
| Depend Undergarments Elastic Leg Extra Absorbency | For moderate leakage; soft, clothlike outer cover; one size; reusable button strap tabs |
| Poise Pantiliners | Very light absorbency; 6 1/2 in. long |
| Poise Extra Coverage Pantiliners | Very light absorbency; 7 1/2 in. long |
| Poise Thin Pads Light Absorbency | For light leakage; 8 1/2 in. long; elasticized sides |
| Poise Pads Regular Absorbency | For light leakage; 8 1/2 in. long; elasticized sides |
| Poise Pads Extra Absorbency | For light leakage; 9 1/2 in. long; elasticized sides, one end wider |
| Poise Pads Extra Plus Absorbency | For light/moderate leakage; 11 in. long; elasticized sides, one end wider |
| Poise Pads with Side Shields Ultra Absorbency | For light/moderate leakage; 11 in. long |
| Poise Pads with Side Shields Ultra Plus Absorbency | For moderate leakage; 13 in. long; padlike comfort with guardlike absorbency; one end wider |
| Prevail Underwear | For heavy leakage; S,M, L; for men and women; look and feel like underwear; pull-on |
| Serenity/TENA Dry Active Liners | For extra light leakage |
| Serenity/TENA Thin Pads Light | For light leakage |
| Serenity/TENA Pads Slender | For light leakage |
| Serenity/TENA Pads Extra | For moderate leakage |
| Serenity/TENA Pads Extra Plus | For moderate leakage |
| Serenity/TENA Pads Ultra | For heavy leakage |
| Serenity/TENA Pads Ultra Plus Night and Day | For heavy leakage; longest pad |
| Serenity/TENA Guards Super Absorbency | For moderate/heavy leakage |
| Serenity Guards Super Plus Absorbency | For heavy leakage |
| TENA Briefs | For heavy leakage; Y, S, M, L; refastenable tabs |

* Y = youth, S = small, M = medium, and L = large.

† Products change often; refer to Web sites for current product availability (i.e., www.depend.com, www.poise.com, www.serenity.com).

‡ Manufacturer markets other products similar to the Depend line but offers a lower price point.

TABLE 52-5 Botanical Medicines Used to Treat Incontinence Related to BPH[33–35]

| Herb (Scientific Name) [Trade Name] | Dosage | Side Effects and Risks | Effectiveness for Incontinence Comments |
|---|---|---|---|
| Pygeum (*Prunus africana*) [Pronitol, Provol, Tadenan] | 100–200 mg in divided doses | Mild diarrhea, indigestion. No contraindications are known. No reported drug interactions | 3-month symptomatic improvement in BPH,* commonly used in France and Italy |
| Saw palmetto (*Serenoa repens* [LSESR], *Sabal serrulata*) [Permixin, Propalmex, Strogen] | 160 mg 2 times/ day | Headache, hypertension, abdominal pain, constipation, diarrhea, nausea, decreased libido, dysuria, impotence, urine retention, and back pain. Avoid in pregnancy and women of childbearing age | Use supported by in vitro, animal, and human clinical studies;† use only in diagnosed BPH: PSA and size of prostate not affected |

Key: BPH, benign prostate hyperplasia; LSESR, lipidosterolic extract of *Serenoa repens*; PSA, prostate-specific antigen.

* Trials included 12 double-blind, placebo-controlled trials; 34 open-label trials; no comparative trials.

† Studies showed saw palmetto was more effective than placebo and as effective as finasteride, and time to maximum effect is delayed for several months; more comparative studies with α-blockers are needed.

## Complications From Absorbent Products

Because the use of absorbent products increases the risk of skin irritation and maceration, such products should be checked every 2 hours. With continual urine loss, it is recommended that the absorbent material be changed every 2 to 4 hours. The use of skin protectants (barrier creams and ointments), as in diaper rash, is appropriate. If a rash occurs, the same treatment is indicated as that described for infants in Chapter 36.

Urine odor is an embarrassing problem. Nonprescription products containing chlorophyll (e.g., Derifil, Pals, Nullo) can be recommended to help decrease urine odor. However, frequent checks and changes are preferable to efforts to mask the odor.

The healing of skin wounds may be delayed in the patient with skin wetted by urine. Any skin breakdown needs to be reported to the primary care provider. This serious complication should not be treated with nonprescription products without medical supervision.

UI products not available from the pharmacy or specialty supply store may be obtained by contacting the National Association for Continence, PO Box 8310, Spartanburg, SC 29305-8310; 1-864-579-7900, 1-800-BLADDER; fax: 1-864-579-7902; or www.nafc.org.

### *Complementary Therapies*

Nutritional deficiencies of protein, calcium, vitamin C, zinc, magnesium, and vitamin $B_{12}$ have been proposed as possibly contributing to the development of UI.[27] Of these, the relationship between vitamin $B_{12}$ deficiency and UI has been established.[28] A $B_{12}$ deficiency may lead to diminished neurosensory input regarding bladder fullness or to inappropriate neurologic stimulation of the bladder, causing detrusor instability. Many factors such as spicy and acidic foods (caffeine, alcohol, and tobacco), dyes (Food Drug and Cosmetic yellow dye no. 5), food preservatives, and sugar substitutes (i.e., aspartame) may cause urinary frequency and urgency with the potential for UI. Several herbal treatments have been suggested for UI (Table 52-5), among them phytoestrogens (soybean, flaxseed), saw palmetto and pygeum or African plum, St. John's wort, and bearberry (uva-ursi) teas (see Chapter 53).[27] With the exception of the use of saw palmetto and pygeum for overflow incontinence related to BPH, evidence is lacking for their effectiveness.

Evidence from a recent meta-analysis of 18 randomized controlled trials suggests that saw palmetto improves urologic symptoms and urine flow measures.[29] Saw palmetto produces similar improvement in urinary symptoms and urinary flow compared with finasteride and was associated with fewer side effects. The most frequently reported dosage in the analysis was 160 mg twice daily. Adverse effects included erectile dysfunction and gastrointestinal problems, which were generally mild and comparable to those of placebo. Duration of studies ranged from 4 to 48 weeks with a mean of 9 weeks. Further research is needed to determine long-term efficacy, ability to prevent BPH complications, and comparative efficacy with α-adrenergic antagonists. Subsequent meta-analyses have supported these findings.[30]

Pygeum extract, derived from the bark of the African plum tree, is the most popular treatment of BPH in France and has been fairly well researched. A 1995 review of pygeum therapy for BPH examining 32 open-label studies and 12 placebo-controlled trials reported that pygeum extract improved symptoms and objective measures of BPH.[31,32] The recommended dosage of pygeum is 100 mg to 200 mg per day, given in divided doses. Adverse effects are rare with gastrointestinal complaints listed as most common at 3%. While, pygeum appears to have some efficacy, more studies are needed to provide conclusive evidence and define the role of pygeum in BPH.

It should be stressed that dietary supplements are not FDA approved or regulated. Therefore, product purity and potency cannot always be ensured. In addition, the cost of such products typically is not covered by insurance providers, and their use without physician knowledge of the problem can delay appropriate diagnosis and initiation of optimum therapy (e.g., underlying prostate cancer).

## Assessment of Adult Urinary Incontinence and Supplies: A Case-based Approach

Because of the public's general lack of sufficient medical knowledge about the different types of UI, some patients (or their caregivers) may attempt self-diagnosis and treatment without consulting their primary care providers. Self-diagnosis obviously could lead to inappropriate assessment and treatment. Therefore, it is imperative that practitioners inquire about a proper medical evaluation before recommending nonprescription products, including absorbent products. A primary care provider must recommend use of nonprescription medications for off-label indications.

Armed with the patient's history and proper diagnosis, the practitioner can answer questions appropriately and help in the selection and proper use of devices and medications for treating this disorder. Cases 52-1 and 52-2 illustrate the assessment of adult patients with UI.

### CASE 52-1

| Relevant Evaluation Criteria | Scenario/Model Outcome |
|---|---|
| **Information Gathering** | |
| 1. Gather essential information about the patient's symptoms, including: | |
| a. description of symptom(s) (i.e., nature, onset, duration, severity, associated symptoms) | Patient complains of "urine release." The first incident occurred after the birth of her third child. As a result, she has refrains from step dancing, an activity that she once enjoyed. Patient pleads for help, exclaiming, "I'm so embarrassed. I'm too young to have these problems." |
| b. description of any factors that seem to precipitate, exacerbate, and/or relieve the patient's symptom(s) | The "leakage" occurs when she lifts her children, coughs, sneezes, or laughs. No leakage at any other times. |
| c. description of the patient's efforts to relieve the symptoms | I have been using panty liners, but they don't seem to protect my clothes. |
| 2. Gather essential patient history information: | |
| a. patient's identity | Carol Otter |
| b. age, sex, height, and weight | 34 y/o F, 5'4", 170 lb |
| c. patient's occupation | Teacher |
| d. patient's dietary habits | 4-5 cans of diet cola per day; social alcohol use |
| e. patient's sleep habits | No nighttime awakenings |
| f. concurrent medical conditions, prescription and nonprescription medications, and dietary supplements | Occasional use of ibuprofen for migraine headaches |
| g. allergies | Latex |
| h. history of other adverse reactions to medications | None |
| i. other (describe)______ | Lives with husband and 4 children |
| **Assessment and Triage** | |
| 3. Differentiate the patient's signs/symptoms and correctly identify the patient's primary problem(s) (see Table 52-3). | Characteristics of Carol's urine leakage are consistent with stress incontinence. |

## CASE 52-1 (continued)

| Relevant Evaluation Criteria | Scenario/Model Outcome |
|---|---|
| 4. Identify exclusions for self-treatment (see Figure 52-1). | None; however, Carol should be encouraged to seek a diagnosis for her UI before relying on incontinence products. |
| 5. Formulate a comprehensive list of therapeutic alternatives for the primary problem to determine if triage to a medical practitioner is required, and share this information with the patient. | Options include:<br>(1) Refer Carol to her PCP/gynecologist for evaluation of stress incontinence.<br>(2) Recommend a pad or shield for light urine leakage.<br>(3) Advise Carol that weight loss may help.<br>(4) Suggest pelvic floor strengthening exercises.<br>(5) Avoid frequent use of caffeine.<br>(6) Take no action. |
| **Plan** | |
| 6. Select an optimal therapeutic alternative to address the patient's problem, taking into account patient preferences. | See Figure 52-1. Carol should be referred for medical evaluation before she uses an incontinence product. |
| 7. Describe the recommended therapeutic approach to the patient. | Once you have seen your primary care provider, a pad or shield may be appropriate for persistent symptoms. |
| 8. Explain to the patient the rationale for selecting the recommended therapeutic approach from the considered therapeutic alternatives. | Medical evaluation is necessary to determine the type of incontinence and the need for prescription medication. |
| **Patient Education** | |
| 9. When recommending self-care with nonprescription medications and/or nondrug therapy, convey accurate information to the patient, including: | |
| a. appropriate dose and frequency of administration | See the box Patient Education for Adult Urinary Incontinence and Supplies. |
| b. maximum number of days the therapy should be employed | See the box Patient Education for Adult Urinary Incontinence and Supplies. |
| c. product administration procedures | See the box Patient Education for Adult Urinary Incontinence and Supplies. |
| d. expected time to onset of relief | N/A |
| e. degree of relief that can be reasonably expected | See the box Patient Education for Adult Urinary Incontinence and Supplies. |
| f. most common side effects | Skin irritation, rash, maceration, and breakdown |
| g. side effects that warrant medical intervention should they occur | You should check for skin irritation every 2 hours. See the box Patient Education for Adult Urinary Incontinence. |
| h. patient options in the event that condition worsens or persists | If urine loss is continual, change absorbent undergarments every 2-4 hours. See your primary care provider for further follow-up. |
| i. product storage requirements | N/A |
| j. specific nondrug measures | See the box Patient Education for Adult Urinary Incontinence and Supplies for behavioral measures to reduce and improve incontinence symptoms. Pelvic floor exercise may be beneficial in stress incontinence. |
| 10. Solicit follow-up questions from patient. | What if the incontinence product does not provide enough protection? |
| 11. Answer patient's questions. | You may select another absorbent product on the basis of the amount of urine leakage (see Table 52-4). |

Key: N/A, not applicable; PCP, primary care provider; UI, urinary incontinence.

## CASE 52-2

| Relevant Evaluation Criteria | Scenario/Model Outcome |
|---|---|
| **Information Gathering** | |
| 1. Gather essential information about the patient's symptoms, including: | |
| a. description of symptom(s) (i.e., nature, onset, duration, severity, associated symptoms) | Patient wants to use an herbal product for recent problem of "dribbling and a feeling of a full bladder." He wants to use something natural since he is concerned about side effects from prescription medications. He complains of daytime fatigue since he must wake up several times during the night to urinate. |
| b. description of any factors that seem to precipitate, exacerbate, and/or relieve the patient's symptom(s) | The "leakage" and "full bladder" sensations occur throughout the day. He often wakes up 2-3 times per night to urinate. |
| c. description of the patient's efforts to relieve the symptoms | Frequent trips to the bathroom; drinking less water and other beverages. |
| 2. Gather essential patient history information: | |
| a. patient's identity | John James |
| b. age, sex, height, and weight | 56 y/o M, 5'7", 150 lb |
| c. patient's occupation | College professor |
| d. patient's dietary habits | Likes spicy food, no caffeine-containing beverages; social alcohol use |
| e. patient's sleep habits | Frequent nighttime awakenings to urinate |
| f. concurrent medical conditions, prescription and nonprescription medications, and dietary supplements | Atenolol 50 mg once daily for hypertension; HCTZ 25 mg once daily for hypertension |
| g. allergies | Ragweed |
| h. history of other adverse reactions to medications | None |
| i. other (describe)_______ | Single, lives alone |
| **Assessment and Triage** | |
| 3. Differentiate the patient's signs/symptoms and correctly identify the patient's primary problem(s) (see Table 52-3). | John 's urine leakage is consistent with symptoms of BPH. However, John should be evaluated by a PCP or urologist before starting any herbal or other nonprescription treatment. |
| 4. Identify exclusions for self-treatment (see Figure 52-1). | None, however John should be encouraged to seek a diagnosis for his UI before relying on incontinence products. |
| 5. Formulate a comprehensive list of therapeutic alternatives for the primary problem to determine if triage to a medical practitioner is required, and share this information with the patient. | Options include:<br>(1) Refer John for further evaluation for BPH.<br>(2) Suggest a dietary supplement such as saw palmetto or pygeum.<br>(3) Recommend a guard for urine leakage.<br>(4) Take no action. |
| **Plan** | |
| 6. Select an optimal therapeutic alternative to address the patient's problem, taking into account patient preferences. | See Figure 52-1. John should see a PCP for further evaluation before using any nonprescription medication or incontinence product. A thorough work-up to eliminate the diagnosis of prostate cancer is necessary. |
| 7. Describe the recommended therapeutic approach to the patient. | Once your urinary incontinence has been evaluated, a guard may be appropriate for persistent symptoms. Prescription medication or a dietary supplement may be suggested by your primary care provider. |
| 8. Explain to the patient the rationale for selecting the recommended therapeutic approach from the considered therapeutic alternatives. | Medical evaluation is necessary to rule out the presence of a more serious condition and determine the need for prescription medication. Regular screening for prostate cancer is recommended for men in your age group. |

**CASE 52-2 (continued)**

| Relevant Evaluation Criteria | Scenario/Model Outcome |
|---|---|
| **Patient Education** | |
| 9. When recommending self-care with nonprescription medications and/or nondrug therapy, convey accurate information to the patient, including: | |
| a. appropriate dose and frequency of administration | See the box Patient Education for Adult Urinary Incontinence and Supplies. |
| b. maximum number of days the therapy should be employed | See the box Patient Education for Adult Urinary Incontinence and Supplies. |
| c. product administration procedures | See the box Patient Education for Adult Urinary Incontinence and Supplies. |
| d. expected time to onset of relief | N/A |
| e. degree of relief that can be reasonably expected | See the box Patient Education for Adult Urinary Incontinence and Supplies. |
| f. most common side effects | Skin irritation, rash, maceration, and breakdown |
| g. side effects that warrant medical intervention should they occur | Patients should check for skin irritation every 2 hours. See the box Patient Education for Adult Urinary Incontinence and Supplies. |
| h. patient options in the event that condition worsens or persists | If urine loss is continual, change absorbent undergarments every 2-4 hours. See your primary care provider for further evaluation. |
| i. product storage requirements | N/A |
| j. specific nondrug measures | See the box Patient Education for Adult Urinary Incontinence and Supplies for behavioral measures to reduce and improve incontinence symptoms. |
| 10. Solicit follow-up questions from patient. | What if the incontinence product does not provide enough protection? |
| 11. Answer patient's questions. | You can always select another absorbent product on the basis of the amount of urine leakage (see Table 53-4). |

Key: BPH, benign prostatic hyperplasia; HCTZ, hydrochlorothiazide; N/A, not applicable; PCP, primary care provider; UI, urinary incontinence.

## Patient Counseling for Adult Urinary Incontinence and Supplies

The clinician's role in self-treatment of UI includes educating patients about UI; recommending medical evaluation, as appropriate, on the basis of an initial evaluation of signs and symptoms; assisting patients and caregivers in selecting products to manage the overflow of urine; and avoiding aggravating factors. Patients should be provided with information to help them understand UI. The box Patient Education for Adult Urinary Incontinence and Supplies lists specific information to provide patients regarding the use of incontinence supplies.

## Evaluation of Patient Outcomes for Adult Urinary Incontinence and Supplies

At follow-up, the clinician should find out whether the recommended incontinence product is comfortable and easy to use, and whether leakage from the undergarment or odor is a problem. If leakage is occurring, the absorbency and/or type of product should be reassessed. Patients who have problems with odor may need to use deodorizers. The patient or caregiver should also be asked whether the skin, especially in the perivaginal and perianal areas, is being checked for breakdown. Redness or skin fissures call for the use of skin protectants. Questioning about occurrence of urinary tract or vaginal infections is also appropriate. Such infections may indicate a need to change undergarments more often or to use another type of incontinence product. These measures will prevent prolonged skin contact with urine. In addition, the practitioner should monitor the effectiveness of other prescription medication and behavioral therapies for UI. The patient should be asked about side effects on the basis of the medication he or she may be prescribed.

Practitioners should also evaluate whether the use of incontinence products and other treatments has allowed the patient to resume his or her normal lifestyle and social interactions. If these objectives are not being met after an adequate duration of any pharmacotherapy, the medication dose and type of should be reviewed. Alternative absorbent products should also be considered. The patient should be encouraged to seek further advice from his or her primary care provider on treatment options.

## PATIENT EDUCATION FOR ADULT URINARY INCONTINENCE AND SUPPLIES

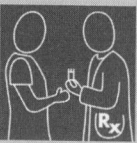

The objectives of self-treatment are to (1) reduce or eliminate symptoms of urinary incontinence (UI), (2) control or treat skin irritation caused by contact with urine, (3) control the odor of urine leaked from the bladder, (4) control leakage of urine from undergarments, and (5) prevent other complications such as falls and social isolation. For most patients, carefully following product instructions and the self-care measures listed here will help to ensure optimal therapeutic outcomes.

- Consult a primary care provider for a thorough examination before using absorbent undergarments or shields. Many cases of urinary incontinence are reversible with treatment.
- These products are designed to absorb urine; to provide a moisture barrier to protect clothes, bedding, and furniture; and to minimize skin contact with urine.
- Base selection of absorbent products on the amount of leaked urine:
  - Guards/shields: 2 to 12 oz (60-360 mL), light to heavy capacity
  - Undergarments: 12 to 18 oz (360-540 mL), moderate to heavy capacity
  - Briefs: 28 to 36 oz (840-1000 mL), moderate to heavy capacity
- Choose briefs or diapers with roll-on bed application and adhesive closures for patients who are unable to change themselves.
- If additional protection is needed during sleeping and sitting, select absorbent bed or chair pads to use with absorbent undergarments.
- Check skin for irritation or maceration every 2 hours, even when absorbent garments are used.
- If urine loss is continual, change absorbent undergarments every 2 to 4 hours and consult your primary care provider if UI symptoms worsen.
- If desired, use skin protectants labeled for diaper rash to protect the patient's skin.
- If desired, use products containing chlorophyll, such as Derifil, Pals, and Nullo, to help decrease odor. However, continue frequent skin checks and frequent changes of absorbent undergarments.
- If pressure ulcers (open sores) occur in an immobile patient, consult a primary care provider. Do not attempt to treat the ulcers with nonprescription products.
- Identify and eliminate foods, liquids, or other substances that can irritate the bladder (e.g., coffee, tea, soda, alcohol, chocolate, acidic juices, tomato-based sauces, spicy food, artificial sweeteners, and nicotine).
- Avoid products that irritate the urethra and bladder. Use cotton underwear, avoid scented powders or bath products, and use white toilet paper.
- Follow instructions for behavioral therapy and medications for incontinence if prescribed by your primary care provider.

## Key Points for Adult Urinary Incontinence and Supplies

- UI is a common treatable condition that is often cured or improved with therapy.
- Because the cause of UI may be multifactorial, the patient should receive a comprehensive medical evaluation before planning therapy.
- A variety of treatment options are available, including drug therapy, behavioral therapies, devices, incontinence aids, and surgery.
- Incontinence aids are designed to absorb urine; to provide a moisture barrier to protect clothes, bedding, and furniture; and to minimize skin contact with urine.
- The selection of absorbent products is based on the amount of urine leakage.
- Practitioners can play an important role in patient education about UI, perform assessment and triage to medical evaluation, counsel on the selection and appropriate use of prescription and nonprescription incontinence products and the avoidance of aggravating factors, and follow-up on patient response.

## References


1. Fantl AJ, Newman DK, Lolling L, et al. *Urinary Incontinence in Adults: Acute and Chronic Management, Clinical Practice Guideline.* Rockville, Md: US Department of Health and Human Services, Public Health Service, Agency for Health Care Policy and Research; 1996. Pub No. 96-0682.
2. Hu T-W, Wagner TH, Bentkover JD, et al. Costs of urinary incontinence in the United States: a comparative study. *Urology.* 2004;63:461-5.
3. Burgio KL, Ives DG, Locher JL, et al. Treatment seeking for urinary incontinence in adults. *J Am Geriatr Soc.* 1994;42:208-12.
4. Lee SY, Phanumus D, Fields SD. Urinary incontinence: a primary care guide to managing acute and chronic symptoms in older adults. *Geriatrics.* 2000;55:65-72.
5. Brandeis GH, Baumann MM, Hossain M, et al. The prevalence of potentially remediable urinary incontinence in frail older people: a study using the Minimum Data Set. *J Am Geriatr Soc.* 1997;45:179-84.
6. Roberts RO, Jacobsen SJ, Rhodes T, et al. Urinary incontinence in a community-based cohort: prevalence and health care-seeking. *J Am Geriatr Soc.* 1998;46:467-72.
7. Thom D. Variation in estimates of urinary incontinence prevalence in the community: effects of differences in definition, population characteristics, and study type. *J Am Geriatr Soc.* 1998; 46:473-80.
8. de Groat WC, Yoshimura N. Pharmacology of the lower urinary tract. *Annu Rev Pharmacol Toxicol.* 2001;41: 691-721.
9. Busby-Whitehead J, Johnson TM. Urinary incontinence. *Clin Geriatr Med.* 1998;14:285-96.
10. Couture JA, Valiquette L. Urinary incontinence. *Ann Pharmacother.* 2000;34:646-55.
11. Holroyd-Leduc JM, Strauss SE. Management of urinary incontinence in women. *JAMA.* 2004;291: 986-95.
12. Grodstein F, Fretts R, Lifford K, et al. Association of age, race, and obstetric history with urinary symptoms among women in the Nurses' Health Study. *Am J Obstet Gynecol.* 2003;189:428-34.
13. Sampselle CM, Harlow SD, Skurnick J, et al. Urinary incontinence predictors and life impact in ethnically diverse perimenopausal women. *Obstet Gynecol.* 2002;100:1230-8.
14. Culligan PJ, Heit M. Urinary incontinence in women: evaluation and management. *Am Fam Physician.* 2000;62:2433-44.

15. Chutka DS, Fleming KC, Evans MP, et al. Urinary incontinence in the elderly population. *Mayo Clin Proc.* 1996;71:93-101.
16. Resnick NM, Yalla SV. Geriatric incontinence and voiding dysfunction. In: Walsh PC, Retik AB, Vaughan ED, Wein AJ, eds. *Campbell's Urology.* 7th ed. Philadelphia: WB Saunders; 1998:1044-58.
17. Jackson S. The patient with an overactive bladder: symptoms and quality of life issues. *Urology.* 1997;50(suppl 6A):18-22.
18. Culligan PJ, Neit M. Information from your family doctor: exercising your pelvic muscles. *Am Fam Physician.* 2000;62:2447.
19. NeoControl® Pelvic Floor Therapy System. Available at: http://www.neocontrol.com. Accessed June 9, 2005.
20. Miller JM, Aston Miller JA Delancey JO. A pelvic muscle precontraction can reduce cough-related urine loss in selected women with mild SUI. *J Am Geriatr Soc.* 1998;46:470-4.
21. Anderson KE. Drug therapy for urinary incontinence. *Baillieres Best Pract Res Clin Obstet Gynaecol.* 2000;14:291-313.
22. Malone DC, Okano GJ. Treatment of urge incontinence in Veterans Affairs medical centers. *Clin Ther.* 1999;21:867-77.
23. McCormick PL, Keating GM. Duloxetine: in stress urinary incontinence. *Drugs.* 2004;64:2567-73.
24. Thakar R, Stanton S. Regular review: management of urinary incontinence in women. *BMJ.* 2000;321:1326-31.
25. Smith DA. Devices for continence. *Nurse Pract Forum.* 1994;5:186-9.
26. Brink CA. Absorbent pads, garment, and management strategies. *J Am Geriatr Soc.* 1990;38:368-73.
27. Bottomley JM. Complementary nutrition in treating urinary incontinence. *Top Geriatr Rehab.* 2000;16:61-77.
28. Rana S, D'Amico F, Merenstein JH. Relationship of vitamin B12 deficiency with incontinence in older people. *J Am Geriatr Soc.* 1998;46:931-2.
29. Wilt TJ, Ishani A, Stark, G, et al. Saw palmetto extracts for treatment of benign prostatic hyperplasia: a systematic review. *JAMA.* 1998;280:1604-9.
30. Boyle R, Robertson C, Lowe F, et al. Updated Meta-analysis of clinical trials of *Serenoa repens* extract in the treatment of symptomatic benign prostatic hyperplasia. *BJU Internatl.* 2004;93:751-6.
31. McQueen CE, Bryant PJ. Pygeum. *Am J Health-Syst Pharm.* 2001; 58:120-3.
32. Andro M-C, Riffaud J-P. *Pygeum africanum* extract for the treatment of patients with benign prostatic hyperplasia: a review of 25 years of published experience. *Curr Ther Res.* 1995;56:796-817.
33. Gordon AE, Shaughnessy AF. Saw palmetto for prostate disorders. *Am Fam Physician.* 2003;67:1281-3.
34. Dvorkin L, Song KY. Herbs for benign prostatic hyperplasia. *Ann Pharmacother.* 2002;36:1443-52.
35. Wilt TJ, Ishani A, Rutks I, et al. Phytotherapy for benign prostatic hyperplasia. *Public Health Nutr.* 2000;3(4A):459-72.

SECTION XI

# Complementary and Alternative Medicine

# Introduction to Botanical and Nonbotanical Natural Medicines

*Cydney E. McQueen and Anne Lamont Hume*

Complementary and alternative medicine (CAM) has been defined as "a group of diverse medical and health care systems, practices and products that are not presently considered to be part of conventional medicine."[1] Complementary medicine is used with conventional treatment, while alternative medicine is a substitute for Western medical care.[1] Chapters 53 and 54 address botanical and nonbotanical medicines, also known as dietary supplements, which are one type of CAM.

In 2002, an estimated 36% of 31,044 adults ages 18 years and older reported the use of at least one form of CAM, according to the National Institutes of Health/National Center for Complementary and Alternative Medicine (NIH/NCCAM) National Health Interview Survey. Prayer, natural products, and deep breathing exercises were commonly used CAM therapies. Almost 19% of adults reported the use of dietary supplements during one year (2002), with echinacea (40.3%), ginseng (24.1%), ginkgo (21.1%), and garlic (19.9%) use frequently.[2] CAM therapies are utilized by women more than men, and its use increased with higher income levels.[2,3] Many consumers reported they believed that CAM provided additional benefit to conventional medicine. CAM was used by 26% because a conventional medical professional had recommended the therapy.[2] Estimates have indicated that approximately $36 billion to $47 billion was spent on CAM therapies by American consumers in 1997, with $5 billion spent on herbal products.[1]

The growth rate in the use of dietary supplements has plateaued, perhaps because of continuing concerns about product quality and safety issues.[4,5] Manufacturers are challenged to ensure the quality of raw materials and of the extraction, formulation, and manufacturing processes that are critical to the safety and efficacy of botanical products. As a result, the American Botanical Council has developed new initiatives such as the Safety Assessment Program for the dietary supplement industry to provide current safety information in formulating new products, as well as in preparing labels and marketing materials.[6]

Clinicians must be knowledgeable and open to discussing the use of dietary supplements. In a national survey, 63% of participants had not informed their primary care provider about their use of CAM.[7] An estimated 16% of individuals taking prescription medications also were using herbal and other supplements in 1999.[8] With many consumers now seeking information about supplements on the Internet, the risk of adverse reactions and interactions may be significant if clinicians are unaware of an individual's use of natural products.

This section includes chapters on botanical medicines, nonbotanical natural medicines, and homeopathic medicines. This introduction focuses on issues common to both botanical and nonbotanical medicines. These chapters were developed by identifying the best quality data and by adhering to the principle of doing no harm when definitive information was not available. Data on drug and natural medicine interactions and contraindications may be based on potential concerns to alert clinicians to possible problems.

## Evidence on Natural Medicines

The chapters in this section discuss the existing scientific evidence for a product's safety and efficacy. While research on dietary supplements is increasing, clinicians should recognize common problems with published studies of CAM. Many studies have small sample sizes, a short duration, improperly controlled study populations, variably processed and standardized botanicals, and inappropriate dosage regimens. Small, poorly controlled studies can detect benefits of treatment that are not supported by later, higher-quality trials. Conversely, if a study does not find benefit with a natural product, the product may simply have lacked the active components. This issue is less common with studies sponsored by government or independent funding that use standardized botanical medicines whose content is confirmed independently. At times, lack of efficacy may be due to the inability of the formulation used to have the bioavailability to achieve meaningful plasma concentrations of active components. Comparisons of standardized natural products to drugs in clinical trials occasionally have been demonstrated to contain subtherapeutic doses.[9] Another consideration is that standardized formulations that are effective in clinical trials in other parts of the world often may not be commercially available in the United States. In addition, few pharmacoeconomic and outcome studies of natural products are available. As a result, even when several trials of a supplement for a particular indication exist, the safety, efficacy, and place in therapy may still be difficult to determine.

The scientific literature for CAM includes meta-analyses of botanical and nonbotanical medicines. A meta-analysis should combine well-conducted clinical trials with similar methodologies. Many meta-analyses use the Jadad scale for evaluating the quality of studies. This scale assigns points to a study on the basis of the presence of explicit criteria for randomization, blinding, dropouts, and withdrawals.[10] Some meta-analyses of natural products are of poor quality; some include trials inappropriately or use inappropriate statistical methods for analysis of data.[11] Although a high-quality meta-analysis may contribute important information, it is not a substitute for a randomized controlled trial (RCT) with long-term outcomes.

## Research on Natural Medicines

Patient care recommendations always should be based on quality research whenever possible. Information regarding the safety and efficacy of natural products continues to emerge from RCT. Several governmental agencies are involved with sponsoring research relevant to ongoing issues with CAM.

### National Institutes of Health

Two sections of the National Institutes of Health (NIH) primarily are involved with supporting and disseminating research findings related to natural products. The Office of Dietary Supplements (ODS) was created as part of the Dietary Supplement and Health Education Act (DSHEA) of 1994. The ODS has identified five goals for its 2004-2009 strategic plan, which include (1) evaluating the role of dietary supplements in the prevention of disease and in physical and mental health performance, (2) exploring cellular effects of dietary supplements across the life cycle, (3) improving scientific methodology in the study of dietary supplements, and (4) educating scientists, health care providers, and the public about the risks and benefits of dietary supplements.[12]

The National Center for Complementary and Alternative Medicine (NCCAM) is one of the 27 institutes and centers of NIH. The mission of NCCAM is to support rigorous CAM research including natural products, to educate and train researchers, to provide education and outreach to consumers and health professionals, and to encourage integration of scientifically proven CAM approaches into conventional medical practice.[13] Similarly, the Office of Cancer Complementary and Alternative Medicine (OCCAM) was established to increase the activities of the National Cancer Institute (NCI) in CAM with a focus on the treatment of cancer, cancer-related symptoms, and side effects of conventional treatments.[14] Recently, OCCAM developed the NCI Best Case Series Program to provide guidance to practitioners who wish to document the benefit from CAM therapies in cancer. The goal of the program is to gain adequate information in order to determine if further research is indicated on the value of a potential CAM therapy.

### Institute of Medicine

The Institute of Medicine is a part of the National Academies of Science and is recognized as an authority on challenges confronting health care. In 2005, the Institute of Medicine published a two-year comprehensive study of the major scientific and policy issues related to the use of CAM in the United States.[3] The report provided a broad overview of the use of CAM by the American public and identified scientific, policy, and practice issues related to CAM research.[3]

## Regulation of Natural Medicines

The DSHEA became law in recognition that many consumers believe that dietary supplements have health benefits. The law represented a balance between consumer access to dietary supplements and the authority of the Food and Drug Administration (FDA) to withdraw dangerous products and to address false and misleading claims. (Chapter 4 discusses the law and the resulting regulations in detail.)

The Federal Trade Commission (FTC) is responsible for monitoring the advertisement of dietary supplements. This includes print and broadcast ads, infomercials, catalogs, Internet promotions, and direct marketing materials. Advertisements must be truthful, and be supported by adequate evidence for the claims. Working closely with FTC, FDA has responsibility for claims on product labeling, including packaging, inserts, and other promotional materials distributed at the point of sale.[15]

## Quality Issues

Several quality issues are present with botanical and nonbotanical medicines. Studies of supplement quality by independent researchers have revealed that many brands do not contain the quantity of product listed on the label.[16] Contaminants of various types, both accidental or intentional, also are found frequently in dietary supplements. (See Nongovernmental Evaluation of Dietary Supplements.) Accidental contamination could result from misidentification of plants processed for use in a supplement, while intentional contamination could include knowingly substituting one substance (usually less costly) for another or deliberating adulterating a product with a pharmaceutical drug.

"Standardization" is a concept relevant to botanical medicines and means that one component, not necessarily the therapeutic substance, in a botanical extract is assured to be present in a specific amount. For example, St. John's wort is commonly standardized to either 0.3% hypericin or 5% hyperforin. These products contain both constituents, among many others, but in the first case, hypericin content will be a known quantity, while the content of hyperforin, pseudohypericin, pseudohyperforin, and other constituents may vary from batch to batch. In the second case, hyperforin content is known, but hypericin and other constituent content is not. Standardization is used generally in two instances. The first is when one chemical constituent has been identified as probably having the associated pharmacologic action of the product. Standardization also is used when one component is serving as a marker compound (i.e., an extract with a certain level of one chemical has been associated with therapeutic success), even if that constituent has not been determined to be the most necessary for pharmacologic action. Not all botanical medicines are used in standardized form, often because components primarily responsible for activity have not been identified.

Standardization usually does not apply to nonbotanical medicines, which generally consist of a single ingredient. Quality problems with nonbotanical medicines frequently concern contaminants of various types. Some categories of supplements are associated with specific risks. For example, supplements from ocean sources (e.g., coral, fish, seaweeds, or seawater) are at risk for clinically significant levels of mercury, arsenic, or other heavy metals, if production or collection areas are contaminated, or if the supplement source is known to biologically concentrate heavy metals from normal levels in the organism's environment. Clinicians should be aware of potential purity concerns and be able to appropriately guide product selection or refer patients to reliable sources for that information (see Nongovernmental Evaluation of Dietary Supplements).

Another quality-related issue with nonbotanical products is possible contamination in animal-origin products. Several products discussed in Chapter 54 can be derived from animal sources, primarily cattle, pigs, sheep, or goats. Any animal product can be contaminated, whether from diseased animals or lack of cleanliness in processing, but the actual clinical risk is unknown. Many of the concerns with contamination are theoretical and not based on actual occurrences. For example, the transmission of bovine spongiform encephalopathy, also known as "mad cow disease" is a theoretical, but serious, concern with nonsynthetic melatonin, as well as any "glandular" preparations. To date, no cases of transmission from glandular supplements have been reported and most commercially available melatonin is synthetic in origin. Although the risk may be minimal, the safest approach is to avoid any dietary supplements of bovine origin.

## Nongovernmental Evaluation of Dietary Supplements

Several organizations have established programs to develop analytical reference standards and to certify the composition of dietary supplements. These organizations can assure consumers that the product contains the substance(s) stated on the label. This assurance does not extend to a guarantee of safety or efficacy.

### *AOAC INTERNATIONAL*

AOAC INTERNATIONAL is a scientific association that facilitates the development, use and harmonization of validated analytical methods.[17] Its methods serve as the "gold standard" for diverse governmental organizations ranging from the Department of Homeland Security to the FDA. In September 2001, AOAC began a 5-year project to validate analytical methods for common dietary supplements. Most recently, AOAC has requested that scientists submit analytical methods for coenzyme Q10, kava kava, garlic, yohimbe, cranberry, eleuthero, and echinacea.[17] The FDA and the NIH jointly fund the program.

### *U.S. Pharmacopeia Dietary Supplement Verification Program*

In 2002, the U.S. Pharmacopeia (USP) initiated a voluntary Dietary Supplement Verification Program.[18] The purpose of the program is to provide consumers with a method for identifying dietary supplements that have passed rigorous standards for purity, accuracy of ingredient labeling, and good manufacturing practices. Products earning USP certification use a distinctive mark on the product label. These products are certified to contain the listed ingredients in the indicated amounts, to be bioavailable, to be free of contaminants and to have been manufactured under appropriate conditions. As of October 1, 2004, 730 dietary supplements have been verified through the program. USP will periodically conduct audits of certified products to ensure continuing adherence to quality standards. Approved products can be found at http://www.usp.org/USPVerified/dietarySupplements/supplements.html.

### *Consumerlab.com's Seal of Approval*

Consumerlab.com, LLC, is an independent company that tests products relating to health, wellness, and nutrition such as botanical medicines, vitamins, and minerals.[16] Products are tested on the basis of identity, purity, and consistency to the labeled ingredients. The test results are posted on its Web site (http://www.consumerlab.com/aboutcl.asp) with new results available every 4 to 6 weeks. Manufacturers whose products "pass" the review are allowed to license the CL Seal of Approval for that product. The site openly displays names of a few products in each category that have passed testing on a freely accessible basis, while names of products that fail testing are available only to subscribers (subscription currently costs about $25 per year). The company is not affiliated with manufacturers of health and nutrition products.

### *NSF International*

NSF International (http://www.nsf.org/consumer) is an independent, nonprofit organization that provides certifications of dietary supplements, as well as of food and water quality. The organization verifies that the product contains the labeled ingredients and that contaminants and unlisted ingredients are not present.[19]

## Information Resources on Natural Medicines

Ten to 15 years ago, only a few evidence-based resources were available on the safety and efficacy of natural products. In 2005, many studies, meta-analyses and review articles have been published on all types of CAM therapies. Well-known journals indexed in major indexing services such as Medline or EMBASE are increasing publication of clinical trials of natural medicines and other CAM modalities. In the last decade, many tertiary resources have become available, in both electronic and print formats, and provide evidence-based information and specific recommendations.

The most important point to remember when consulting any tertiary resource on natural medicines is that all resources may have errors and inconsistencies. All information should be confirmed in more than one resource.

### *Electronic Resources*

#### Cochrane Database[20]

The Cochrane Database is accessible through Medline and offers evidence-based analyses on the use of a therapy for a specific disease state. Multiple analyses of CAM therapies also have been completed. These reports provide detailed information on trials that were included and excluded from the analysis, and on the methodology used. An advantage is that statements in support or in refute of use of the agent in question are very clearly expressed. A disadvantage is that many practitioners may have difficulty understanding the style and arrangement of the information that document the reasoning for supporting the analyses.

#### Natural Medicines Comprehensive Database[21]

The Natural Medicines Comprehensive Database (NMCD) is produced by Therapeutics Faculty, Inc., which also publishes *The Pharmacists Letter* and *The Prescribers Letter*. The database is a comprehensive source in that both botanical and nonbotanical medicines are reviewed. Many combination products also are listed, with lists of ingredients and links to the individual monographs for those ingredients. Each monograph has an accompanying patient handout. The database includes a drug-supplement checker. Print and PDA-based versions also are available, as well as a patient information version. An online subscription costs approximately $100 per year and is updated frequently.

#### Natural Standard[22]

The Natural Standard is an electronic database, produced by an international research collaboration of primarily academic MD, PhD, and PharmD professionals. Professional level monographs are highly detailed and descriptive of all available evidence. Recommendations are graded to reflect the type and quality of the clinical evidence on which they are based. The number of products included in Natural Standard currently is fewer than some other resources, primarily because of the length of time required to prepare such detailed reviews. In addition to reviews of supplements, the database also includes monographs on other CAM modalities and a dictionary of terms. This resource costs approximately $100 per year.

#### Consumerlab.com[16]

In addition to the services described earlier (see Nongovernmental Evaluation of Dietary Supplements), this site provides access to a Natural Products Encyclopedia. The information in this encyclopedia is not as comprehensive or as thorough as other resources, but can be useful for basic information. A subscription to consumerlab.com is approximately $25 per year.

### *Print Resources*

#### *Professional's Handbook of Complementary & Alternative Medicines* (3rd edition)[23]

This resource offers the advantage of quick access to bottom-line information for more than 325 products. Although only monographs on the most popular supplements have a detailed discussion, information and recommendations for all products are based on available clinical and scientific evidence. There are several minor limitations. For example, in the index, "yellowroot" directs readers to the goldenseal (*Hydrastis canadensis*) monograph, because yellowroot is also a common name for that plant. However, there is no caution about possible confusion with another plant called yellowroot (*Coptis chinensis*). Overall, this reference, which costs about $40, is an appropriate option when used with another tertiary resource.

#### *Evidence-based Herbal Medicine*[24]

This reference includes monographs on botanical medicines and selected nonbotanical supplements, such as glucosamine and melatonin. It includes an extensive discussion of the quality of available clinical evidence and also offers clear-cut summaries of the value of the product in practice. The primary disadvantages are the limited number of products included (65) and that pregnancy and lactation information is not addressed consistently. It is an excellent resource for practitioners who want to learn about the commonly used supplements and costs approximately $35.

## Counseling Issues With Natural Medicines

The main consideration in counseling on natural medicines is to recognize the importance of respecting the person's beliefs and values so that a trusting, nonjudgmental relationship can develop. The person must feel comfortable fully sharing with the clinician any use of natural medicines. Clinicians must be able to provide evidence-based recommendations regarding botanical and nonbotanical natural medicines. When evidence is not available, the risk of adverse effects versus the potential for positive effects must be weighed and the process of decision making clearly explained to patients. Clinicians should discourage the use of unsafe products and practices. Pharmacists, in particular, should ensure that the pharmacy itself does not carry dangerous natural medicines. However, health care professionals do not control access to dietary supplements; patients may choose to use any available supplement. Many times practitioners may be in the position of educating patients on supplements whose use they have discouraged. These are the situations in which complete counseling on expectations and adverse events is essential. For example, educating a patient on the early signs of a serious toxicity will enable the patient to recognize a problem and discontinue the supplement soon enough to minimize any harm. Consumers always should be advised to seek medical care for serious conditions and should be counseled to tell all health care providers, including dentists and surgeons, about their use of natural medicines.

Patients should be taught to read labels carefully and to ask questions. *Thymus* is an example of a term that might be dangerous if misunderstood. On a supplement label, "*Thymus extract*" may refer to an extract of the herbs thyme, Spanish thyme, or wild thyme, products with relatively few adverse events when used in small doses, while "thymus extract" may refer to a preparation made from animal thymus gland, a product with considerable quality concerns.

In addition to these broad counseling issues, the following points should be emphasized. First, clinicians should emphasize that most self-care with natural medicines should be for a limited period of time. If a problem persists, the consumer should seek medical care. Second, consumers should not take botanical or nonbotanical medicines for a condition that also is being treated with a prescribed medication without informing their primary care provider. Third, consumers should be informed that FDA does not control the quality of botanical and nonbotanical natural medicines. Some products may or may not contain the listed ingredients.

Reputable manufacturers do follow appropriate manufacturing guidelines and are willing to provide documentation to that effect. Despite the regulatory environment (see Chapter 4) that allows marketing of poor-quality supplement products, there are a few "rules of thumb" that will help patients choose a quality product. The following points should be used in counseling patients who wish to use a supplement product:

- Purchase products that have a seal of quality through a program such as United States Pharmacopeia's DSVP or Consumerlab.com.
- Check specific products through third-party evaluators such as Consumerlab.com.
- Purchase from large, reputable companies. These companies are at higher risk of litigation if they produce a poor product and may be more likely to follow quality assurance procedures. Companies that also manufacture regulated prescription or nonprescription medications (e.g., Bristol-Meyers-Squibb, American Home Products, drugstore chain store brands) already have good manufacturing practices in place and are more likely to follow these procedures when producing dietary supplements. Some reputable dietary supplement companies do follow good manufacturing and quality-control standards even though they may not participate in a quality seal program.
- Once a quality supplement has been selected, patients should continue to purchase and use the same brand and formulation. Although this approach does not guarantee a lack of potential quality issues, as variability between production lots can occur, it does increase the likelihood of a consistent product and dose. Because of the likelihood of variable quality, clinicians working with patients who have not had positive results with a dietary supplement product should consider a trial of a different brand of the supplement before making a determination that the supplement is ineffective for that patient.

"If you don't know exactly where it's from or what it is, don't put it in your mouth!" This motherly advice is very applicable to supplements. Product labels do not always identify ingredients in a straightforward manner. If a substance or ingredient cannot be clearly and completely identified, the product should be avoided.

## Considerations for Special Populations

The following sections provide a brief overview of issues regarding the use of botanical medicines by different patient populations. The lack of data on safety and efficacy in these populations, as well as the current regulatory issues, underscore the need for comprehensive assessment of the patient's health status and knowledgeable counseling on botanical products.

### *Patients of Advanced Age*

An estimated 17.6% of Americans older than 65 years have used at least one herbal supplement in their lifetime, with 12.9% having used an herbal product in 1 year (2002).[25] Although many older people are healthy and living independently, other individuals may have a significant burden of disease. Many may have age- and disease-related physiologic declines such as in renal function. Older individuals may be chronically taking multiple prescription and nonprescription medications. A thorough medication and dietary supplement history is essential. The potential for interactions between drugs/foods and botanical products, age-related functional declines, and concomitant diseases should be considered in counseling older patients about dietary supplements. Older patients should be counseled specifically to avoid botanical medicines with antiplatelet properties such as garlic and ginkgo if they are currently taking aspirin, warfarin, or similar drugs. Given the significance and scope of interactions with St. John's wort, the practitioner should ask specifically about use of this product.

### *Pediatric Patients*

Precise estimates of the use of CAM in children are not available and have ranged from 1.8% to more than 12%.[26,27] A recent survey of 505 pediatric patients with chronic illnesses reported that dietary supplement use varied among medical conditions. Almost 50% of individuals with solid tumors used a dietary supplement, while approximately one third of children with cystic fibrosis, rheumatologic diseases, and neurobehavioral conditions used these products.[28] Use of botanical medicines by children presents unique challenges. Under the age of 2 years, the child's renal function is less developed than that of an adult. The central nervous system of a child may be uniquely sensitive to many drugs and chemicals. Very little research is available regarding the safe and effective use of botanical medicines in children, making evidence-based recommendations difficult. Also from a practical perspective, an appropriate dose of a botanical product for a child cannot be determined if the content of the product is unknown. Finally, dietary supplements should have safety closures, as accidental ingestions may occur in young children.[29]

### *Pregnant Patients*

The prevalence of dietary supplement use during pregnancy is unknown. A Norwegian study of 400 postpartum women reported that over one third of individuals had used an herbal preparation during their pregnancy.[30] Many herbs including ginger, chamomile, dandelion root, and wild yam have been used during pregnancy either as supplements or as part of herbal teas. The use of botanical medicines by a woman who is either planning to become pregnant or who is pregnant presents several significant dilemmas. Throughout the world, botanical medicines have been used to maintain health during pregnancy, prevent miscarriages, and induce labor. In the United States, concern has focused on minimizing fetal exposures to prescription, nonprescription, or botanical medicines. While many botanicals have been used in pregnancy, very little data exist to document their safety on the developing embryo and fetus. Blue cohosh, a traditional approach used to induce delivery, has been associated with the development of heart failure in a neonate.[31] The Teratology Society and other groups have emphasized that these products should not be assumed to be safe.[32] As part of standard preconception care, a woman should be asked about her use of botanical medicines, especially if it might affect her nutritional status at the time of conception or her ability to become pregnant. Many Web sites and personnel of health food stores willingly offer advice, based on limited evidence, regarding the use of herbs during pregnancy and lactation.[33] The most important issue in use of botanical medicines during pregnancy is simply not knowing the exact content in any given batch or brand of an herbal product. At the present time, clinicians should advise women to limit their use of dietary supplements to those that are proven to be safe and effective during pregnancy.

### Patients With Renal Disease

Many Americans have chronic renal insufficiency (CRI) or failure attributable to systemic diseases, such as diabetes mellitus, as well as to exposure to nephrotoxic chemicals. Chronic renal insufficiency presents many challenges to the safe use of many prescription and nonprescription drugs. Most commonly, the individual may be unable to eliminate the drug appropriately, potentially resulting in toxic concentrations. This also is true for hepatically metabolized drugs with active, renally eliminated metabolites. When CRI is severe enough to require dialysis, the absorption, distribution, and hepatic metabolism of drugs also may be altered. Although evidence is limited, these concerns also are potentially applicable to botanical medicines. In addition, many herbs possess antiplatelet properties that might increase the risk of bleeding in renal patients.

### Surgical Patients

Patients who use botanical medicines and are undergoing surgical procedures present special challenges. This is primarily because little evidence regarding potential adverse effects and drug interactions is available. Many botanical medicines, including garlic, ginkgo, and ginseng, possess antiplatelet effects that may or may not increase the risk of bleeding from surgery. Hypoglycemia has been reported with ginseng and this may be important if a patient is fasting prior to surgery. Interactions between anesthetics and botanical medicines such as valerian may be possible. Also, St. John's wort has a broad range of drug interactions that may be important in the surgical patient. In addition, the effect of discontinuing botanicals before surgery is unknown. Every individual scheduled to have surgery must have as part of their preoperative history a detailed review of their use of herbal medicines to minimize potential adverse outcomes.[34]

## References


1. National Center for Complementary and Alternative Medicine. What is complementary and alternative medicine (CAM)? May 2002. Available at: http://nccam.nih.gov/health/whatiscam. Accessed May 18, 2005.
2. Barnes PM, Powell-Griner E, McFann K, Nahin RL. Complementary and alternative medicine use among adults: United States, 2002. *Adv Data.* 2004;343:1-19.
3. Committee on the Use of Complementary and Alternative Medicine by the American Public. *Complementary and Alternative Medicine in the United States.* Washington, DC: The National Academies Press; 2005.
4. Kelly JP, Kaufman DW, Kelley K, et al. Recent trends in use of herbal and other natural products. *Arch Intern Med.* 2005;165: 281-286.
5. Cardellina JH. Challenges and opportunities confronting the botanical dietary supplement industry. *J Nat Prod.* 2002;65: 1073–84.
6. American Botanical Council. Safety Assessment Program. Available at: http://www.herbalgram.org/default.asp?c=sap. Accessed February 12, 2005.
7. Eisenberg DM, Kessler RC, Van Rompay MI, et al. Perceptions about complementary therapies relative to conventional therapies among adults who use both: results from a national survey. *Ann Intern Med.* 2001;135:344–51.
8. Kaufman DW, Kelly JP, Rosenberg L, et al. Recent patterns of medication use in the ambulatory adult population of the United States. The Slone Survey. *JAMA.* 2002; 287:337–44.
9. Linde K, Ramirez G, Mulrow CD, Pauls A, Weidenhammer W, Melchart D. St John's wort for depression–an overview and meta-analysis of randomised clinical trials. *BMJ.* 1996;313:253-8.
10. Jadad AR, Moore A, Carroll D, et al. Assessing the quality of reports of randomized clinical trials: is blinding necessary? *Control Clin Trials.* 1996;17:1–12.
11. McAlindon TE, LaValley MP, Gulin JP, Felson DT. Glucosamine and chondroitin for treatment of osteoarthritis. A systematic quality assessment and meta-analysis. *JAMA.* 2000;283:1469-75.
12. NIH Office of Dietary Supplements. Strategic Plan for the Office of Dietary Supplements 2004-2009. Available at: http://ods.od.nih.gov/strategicplan2004. Accessed February 12, 2005.
13. National Center for Complementary and Alternative Medicine. 2002. Available at: http://nccam.nih.gov/about. Accessed February 12, 2005.
14. Office of Cancer Complementary and Alternative Medicine of the National Cancer Institute. 2005. Available at: http://www3.cancer.gov/occam/about.html. Accessed February 12, 2005.
15. US Federal Trade Commission. Dietary supplements: an advertising guide for industry. April 2001. Available at: http://www.ftc.gov/bcp/conline/pubs/buspubs/dietsupp.htm. Accessed February 12, 2005.
16. Consumer Lab, LLC. 2003. Available at: http://www.consumerlab.com/aboutcl.asp. Accessed May 18, 2005.
17. AOAC INTERNATIONAL. Call for methods for coenzyme Q10, echinacea, garlic, eleuthero, kava kava, yohimbe, and cranberry. Available at: http://www.aoac.org. Accessed May 18, 2005.
18. USP's Dietary Supplement Verification Program Overview. Available at: http://www.usp.org/USPVerified. Accessed May 18, 2005.
19. NSF International. NSF consumer information: the importance of dietary supplement certification. Available at: http://www.nsf.org/consumer. Accessed May 18, 2005.
20. The Cochrane Database of Systemic Reviews [electronic resource]. Chichester, West Sussex, UK: Wiley; 2004.
21. Jellin JM, et al, eds. *Natural Medicines Comprehensive Database.* Stockton, Calif: Therapeutic Research Faculty; 2005. Available at www.naturaldatabase.com. Accessed May 18, 2005.

22. Basch E, Ulbricht C, eds. *Natural Standard.* Cambridge, Mass; Natural Standard; 2003. Available at www.naturalstandard.com.
23. Fetrow CW, Avila JR, eds. *Professional's Handbook of Complementary and Alternative Medicines.* 3rd ed. Philadelphia: Lippincott; 2004.
24. Rotblatt M, Ziment I, eds. *Evidence-Based Herbal Medicine.* Philadelphia: Hanley and Belfus, Inc; 2002.
25. Bruno JJ, Ellis JJ. Herbal use among US elderly: 2002 National Health Interview Survey. *Ann Pharmacother.* 2005;39:643-8.
26. Davis MP, Darden PM. Use of complementary and alternative medicine by children in the United States. *Arch Pediatr Adolesc Med.* 2003;157:393–6.
27. Sawni-Sikand A, Schubiner H, Thomas RI. Use of complementary/alternative therapies among children in primary care pediatrics. *Ambul Pediatr.* 2002;2:99–103.
28. Ball SD, Kertesz D, Moyer-Mileur LJ. Dietary supplement use is prevalent among children with a chronic illness. *J Am Diet Assoc.* 2005;105:78-84.
29. Palmer ME, Haller C, McKinney PE, et al. Adverse events associated with dietary supplements: an observational study. *Lancet.* 2003;361:101–6.
30. Nordeng H, Havnen GC. Impact of socio-demographic factors, knowledge and attitude on the use of herbal drugs in pregnancy. *Acta Obstet Gynecol Scand.* 2005;84:26-33.
31. Jones TK, Lawson BM. Profound neonatal congestive heart failure caused by maternal consumption of blue cohosh herbal medication. *J Pediatr.* 1998;132:550-2.
32. Marcus DM, Snodgrass WR. Do no harm: avoidance of herbal medicines during pregnancy. *Obstet Gynecol.* 2005;105:1119-22.
33. Buckner KD, Chavez ML, Raney EC, Stoehr JD. Health food stores' recommendations for nausea and migraines during pregnancy. *Ann Pharmacother.* 2005;39:274-9.
34. Ang-Lee ML, Moss J, Yuan CS. Herbal medicines and perioperative care. *JAMA.* 2001;286:208–16.

CHAPTER 53

# Botanical Medicines

*Anne Lamont Hume and Kathryn Michele Strong*

In a 2002 national survey, almost one in every five adults in the United States reported use of a natural product at least once during the previous 12 months.[1] Echinacea (40.3%), ginseng (24.1%), ginkgo (21.1%) and garlic (19.9%) were the most commonly used products.[1] This chapter focuses on natural products of botanical origin and takes an organ system approach. Botanicals were selected on the basis of their widespread use and some evidence of their efficacy and safety. Some of the information on individual botanicals is adapted from an earlier version of this chapter.[2]

## CARDIOVASCULAR SYSTEM

Botanical supplements such as garlic, ginkgo, and horse chestnut seed extract commonly are used to prevent and treat vascular and nonvascular diseases. This section reviews common botanical medicines for cardiovascular disorders.

### Garlic

Garlic is derived from dried or fresh bulbs of *Allium sativum* L. of the lily family Liliaceae.

#### *Therapeutic Uses*

Garlic supplements have been used to treat hyperlipidemia, hypertension, peripheral arterial disease, and type 2 diabetes mellitus. Garlic has also been used orally to prevent stomach, colorectal, prostate, and breast cancer.[3,4]

#### *Physiologic Activity*

Garlic bulbs contain an odorless sulfur-containing amino acid derivative alliin (S-allyl-L-cysteine sulfoxide). When the bulb is crushed, the enzyme allinase is released. This enzyme converts alliin in adjacent cells to the pungent allicin. This compound is the main component of garlic's volatile oil. Allicin is the primary active compound, but other organosulfur-containing substances are produced in the plant and by aging and may also exert pharmacologic effects. In animal and in vitro models, garlic possesses hypotensive, hypolipidemic, antiplatelet, antioxidant, and anti-infective properties. Ajoene, a component of the volatile oil, has been shown to have antiplatelet effects and antibacterial activity.[3]

#### *Dosage and Administration Guidelines*

Garlic supplements in divided doses between 600 and 1200 mg daily have been used for hyperlipidemia and hypertension. Clinical trials have used garlic powder extracts standardized to alliin 1.3%.[4] Currently, the equipotent doses of fresh whole garlic cloves, dried garlic powder, and garlic powder extracts are not known.

#### *Safety Considerations*

Garlic may cause gastrointestinal (GI) side effects including nausea, vomiting, and heartburn. Bad breath and body odor may also occur. Allergic reactions have been reported with the use of oral garlic on rare occasions.[4] Topical applications of garlic cloves and concentrates have been associated with the development of burns, especially in children.[6] Garlic supplements should be stopped at least 7 to 10 days before any surgical procedure because of their antithrombotic effects.[7,8] As a general warning, patients taking warfarin and other platelet-active drugs and natural products such as ginkgo should use garlic bulbs or supplements with caution because of potential risk for bleeding.[7-9] The effect of garlic supplements on drugs metabolized through cytochrome P450 (CYP) isoenzymes is unclear. Garlic has been reported to decrease the peak and trough concentrations of saquinavir by approximately 50%.[9,10] The mechanism for this interaction may involve induction of CYP 3A4. A recent study involving 14 health volunteers failed to find an interaction between garlic tablets (Kwai) and substrates for either CYP 3A4 or CYP 2D6.[11] Of note, the authors found that, although the tablets were intended to produce 600 μg of allicin per 600 mg tablet, only 300 μg actually was detected in an in vitro dissolution test.[11] Currently, a small clinical trial is examining the effect of garlic on elimination of docetaxel in patients with breast cancer.[12]

#### *Administration and Product Issues*

A product review by Consumer Labs has found that some garlic preparations may not release sufficient amounts of allicin despite claims to being "allicin-rich." The recommended yield of allicin should be at least 3000 μg of allicin per gram of dried garlic.[13] Odorless, aged preparations of garlic have reduced amounts of alliin (the more stable precursor of allicin) compared with fresh garlic, which is approximately 1% alliin.[4] Dried forms of garlic should be enteric coated to prevent further destruction of alliin by gastric acid.

### Summary of Clinical Evidence

Garlic supplements slightly reduce total and low-density lipoprotein (LDL) cholesterol concentrations.[4,14,15] The effect is modest, with the most rigorous studies showing the smallest benefit. A meta-analysis has indicated that garlic's effect on cholesterol is present for the first few months and is reduced at 6 months.[14] Garlic supplements vary significantly in their chemical composition, which may contribute to the negative findings of research studies in lipid disorders. A new clinical trial is studying the comparative effect of fresh garlic, dried powdered garlic tablets, and aged garlic extracts on serum cholesterol concentrations in adults.[12] Garlic has not been demonstrated to be effective in hypertension and peripheral arterial disease.

Garlic, aged garlic extracts, and related plants may have a role in preventing some cancers. The available evidence is based primarily on epidemiologic and animal studies, not on clinical trials with garlic supplements.[16] A review of epidemiologic studies suggests that high dietary intake of raw and/or cooked garlic is inversely related to the development of stomach and colorectal cancer.[17]

## Ginkgo

*Ginkgo biloba* L. is a tree and the only living member of the family Ginkgoaceae.

### Therapeutic Uses

Ginkgo has been used for many conditions including Alzheimer's disease (AD), vascular dementias, intermittent claudication (IC), tinnitus, and acute mountain sickness.[18,19]

### Physiologic Activity

The extract or tincture from leaves is used primarily for medicinal purposes. The standardized *Ginkgo biloba* L. concentrated (50:1) leaf extract contains diterpene lactones such as ginkgolides (A, B, C, and M) and the sesquiterpene bilobalide. These constituents may be responsible for neuroprotective properties reported with the leaf extract. Ginkgolide B is also a potent platelet-activating factor (PAF) antagonist. The extract also contains bioflavonoids and flavone glycosides such as quercetin, 3-methyl quercetin, and kaempferol. The flavonoid fractions have been shown to possess antioxidant and free radical scavenger effects.[3]

### Dosage and Administration Guidelines

Recommended doses for dementias and IC range between 120 and 240 mg daily of ginkgo leaf extract in two to three divided doses. *Ginkgo biloba* L. is available as capsules or tablets containing 40, 60, or 120 mg of a concentrated (50:1) leaf extract.[19]

### Safety Considerations

Ginkgo is generally well tolerated.[18,19] In a Cochrane systematic review, ginkgo was similar to placebo in terms of its safety in clinical trials of cognitive impairment and dementia.[18] Mild GI side effects, headache, dizziness, and allergic skin reactions have been reported. Ginkcolic acids are similar to poison ivy allergens and may increase the risk of allergic reactions. Seizures and bleeding associated with ginkgo have also been described in case reports.[20,21] A recent in vitro study indicated that ginkgolides in standardized ginkgo products have minimal effect on PAF and are unlikely to cause bleeding.[22] As a general warning, however, patients taking warfarin and other platelet-active drugs and natural products such as garlic should use ginkgo with caution because of the potential risk for bleeding.[7-9] The use of ginkgo should also be stopped at least 7 to 10 days before any surgical procedure.[7,8] A recent study involving 12 health volunteers failed to find an interaction between ginkgo and substrates for either CYP 3A4 or CYP 2D6.[23] On the basis of a single case report involving an 80-year-old woman with AD, a drug interaction may exist between trazodone and ginkgo.[24] A loss of antihypertensive efficacy has also been reported between ginkgo and thiazide diuretic.[19]

### Administration and Product Issues

Ginkgo preparations should contain 24% ginkgo flavone glycosides and 6% terpenoids. Products should be free of ginkgolic acid.[3,19] Egb 761 is the standardized *Ginkgo biloba* L. extract used in many clinical trials. Commercially available ginkgo supplements may contain subtherapeutic amounts of ginkgolides and bilobalide.

### Summary of Clinical Evidence

Ginkgo has been used to treat both vascular and nonvascular conditions. Its most common use is in AD and vascular dementias. In a Cochrane systematic review, ginkgo was better than placebo on selected measures of cognition and functioning in clinical trials of patients with dementia or cognitive impairment.[18] The underlying severity of dementia may influence clinical response to ginkgo. Greater improvement in symptoms may occur in patients with mild cognitive impairment. Older studies showing benefit with ginkgo have been criticized on the basis of methodologic and statistical issues. Overall, the benefit from ginkgo is modest at best. A review of placebo-controlled trials using either ginkgo or cholinesterase inhibitors such as donepezil has suggested similar benefits in patients with dementia.[25] Rigorous clinical trials directly comparing ginkgo and cholinesterase inhibitors in mild to moderate AD are needed to determine the relative value of these therapies. A clinical trial of 230 older adults with normal cognitive function failed to demonstrate a benefit from ginkgo (Ginkoba) 40 mg three times daily on enhancing memory.[26]

Research into the potential benefits of ginkgo for its other uses is limited. A meta-analysis of eight randomized, double-blind, placebo-controlled trials of IC indicated that ginkgo has a modest benefit and is more effective than placebo.[27] Direct comparisons with other interventions are not available. A study of 978 patients with tinnitus without other symptoms of cerebral insufficiency did not demonstrate any benefit from 50 mg of *Ginkgo biloba* L. extract

(LI 1370) three times daily, compared with placebo.[28] A recent meta-analysis has also failed to identify a benefit from ginkgo in patients with tinnitus.[29] Recently, a study of 614 participants compared ginkgo, acetazolamide, and ginkgo and acetazolamide with placebo for prevention of acute mountain sickness. Ginkgo was similar to placebo and inferior to acetazolamide in decreasing incidence and severity of acute mountain sickness.[30] The design and results of this study differ from those of earlier reports since treatments were given after participants were already at a high elevation. Other studies with ginkgo biloba extract in the treatment of asthma and short-term memory loss after electroconvulsive therapy are ongoing.[12]

## Grape Seed/Pine Bark

Grape seed extract is derived from seeds of *Vitis vinifera*, a member of the family Vitaceae. Pine bark extract is derived from bark of the French maritime coastal pine *Pinus nigra* Arnold var. *maritima* (also known as *Pinus maritima* Lam.) from the family Pinaceae.

### *Therapeutic Uses*

Grape seed and pine bark extracts have been used to treat chronic venous insufficiency, atherosclerosis, diabetic retinopathy, erectile dysfunction, and cardiac or cerebral infarction.[31]

### *Physiologic Activity*

Both grape seed and pine bark extracts contain oligomeric proanthocyanidins and are potent antioxidants. Pine bark extract, commonly known as pycnogenol, contains water-soluble flavonoids, procyanidins, and phenolic acids.

### *Dosage and Administration Guidelines*

Pycnogenol has been used in dosages of 100 mg two to three times daily in clinical trials of chronic venous insufficiency.[32,33]

### *Safety Considerations*

Grape seed and pine bark extracts are well tolerated. Theoretically, pycnogenol may interact with immunosuppressant drugs because of its immune-stimulating properties.[3] In addition, pycnogenol may potentially interact with some chemotherapeutic agents such as cisplatin and doxorubicin.[3]

### *Administration and Product Issues*

There are no product issues.

### *Summary of Clinical Evidence*

In a 6-week study of 25 healthy subjects, pycnogenol 150 mg daily was shown to increase antioxidant capacity of plasma, decrease LDL cholesterol, and increase high-density lipoprotein (HDL) cholesterol in two thirds of subjects.[34] A study compared pycnogenol with horse chestnut seed extract in 40 patients with chronic venous insufficiency (CVI). Pycnogenol improved both objective and subjective measures to a greater degree than horse chestnut seed extract. Lipid and lipoprotein measurements also improved.[32]

## Hawthorn

Hawthorn trees are members of the family Rosaceae; *Crataegus laevigata* (Poiret) DC, *C. monogyna* Jacq., and, less often, *C. pentagyna* Waldst. Et Kit are used.

### *Therapeutic Uses*

Hawthorn supplements have been used for cardiovascular diseases including mild heart failure, hypertension, and coronary heart disease.

### *Physiologic Activity*

Flowers and leaves contain mixtures of chlorogenic acid and flavonoids such as quercin, hyperoside (quercetin 3-galactoside), vitexin, and vitexin 4-rhamnoside. Other major constituents are triterpenoids (e.g., oleanolic acid, ursolic acid, crataegus acid) with anti-inflammatory and hypolipidemic properties.

### *Dosage and Administration Guidelines*

The dosage of standardized hawthorn extract has ranged from 160 to 1800 mg in published randomized, double-blind clinical trials of heart failure.[35] Larger studies of heart failure have used standardized extracts of hawthorn leaves with flowers (WS 1442) 900 to 1800 mg daily in divided doses.[36,37]

### *Safety Considerations*

Hawthorn is generally well tolerated. Nausea and other GI symptoms occur, as well as palpitations, dizziness, and nervousness.[35] Interactions may be possible with herbs or drugs that have similar physiologic cardiovascular effects such as antihypertensive and antiarrhythmic agents.[3,5,9] A multidose study involving eight healthy volunteers did not show a pharmacokinetic interaction with the use of 900 mg of a standardized hawthorn extract and digoxin 0.25 mg.[38]

### *Administration and Product Issues*

Standardized hawthorn extracts used in clinical trials have included WS 1442 and LI 132. Hawthorn extracts are prescription products in some countries such as Germany. Heart failure should never be self-treated by patients.

### *Summary of Clinical Evidence*

Short-term studies have suggested that hawthorn is useful in managing mild heart failure. A meta-analysis of eight randomized, double-blind, placebo-controlled trials was published.[35] The reviewed studies primarily evaluated the effect of hawthorn on maximal workload in patients with New York Heart Association (NYHA) Class I to III heart failure. A total of 632 patients were in the studies with duration of the trials ranging from 3 to 16 weeks. Hawthorne was used as an adjunct to standard treatments for heart failure. The actual concomitant drugs for heart failure were not specified in most of the studies. The findings of the meta-analysis indicated that symptoms such as dyspnea and fatigue improved with use of hawthorn as an adjunctive therapy, compared with placebo.[35] A 2-year, randomized, double-blind, placebo-controlled trial is investigating the effects of hawthorn in up to 2300 patients with NYHA Class II and III heart failure. The primary outcome variable is the combined endpoint of cardiac death, nonfatal myocardial infarction, and hospitalization related to progression of heart failure. Patients enrolled in the study will be maintained on standard therapy consisting of diuretics, digoxin or digitoxin, β-blockers, and angiotensin-converting enzyme (ACE) inhibitors.[36] The results of this study have yet to be published, but may be important because the primary and some of the secondary outcomes represent the current standard for heart failure studies. No clinical trials have shown that hawthorn decreases morbidity and mortality in heart failure. A small multicenter, observational cohort study has demonstrated the noninferiority of a homeopathic hawthorn preparation, compared with standard treatment with an ACE inhibitor and diuretic in patients with NYHA Class II heart failure.[39] This study design, however, is not a substitute for a large randomized controlled trial directly comparing the two interventions.

### Horse Chestnut Seed Extract

Horse chestnut trees (*Aesculus hippocastanum* L.) are members of the family Hippocastanaceae. The seeds, leaf, flower, and branch bark are used medicinally.

#### *Therapeutic Uses*

Horse chestnut seed extract (HCSE) has been used to treat CVI, including varicose veins and hemorrhoids.[40]

#### *Physiologic Activity*

Horse chestnut seeds contain complex mixtures of triterpenoid saponins called aescin that may reduce venous capillary permeability and have anti-inflammatory effects. Aescin may also have very weak diuretic properties. Flavonoids such as quercetin and kaempferol are also present. Aesculin may increase bleeding time.[3]

#### *Dosage and Administration Guidelines*

The usual dose of HCSE is 300 mg twice daily, but regimens vary according to the individual product.

#### *Safety Considerations*

HCSE is generally well tolerated, but can cause nausea and vomiting.[3,40] Horse chestnut may lower blood glucose, but the evidence is limited. HCSE preparations containing aesculin may potentially interact with warfarin or platelet-active drugs or herbs to increase risk of bleeding.[3,9]

#### *Administration and Product Issues*

Clinical trials have used HCSE standardized to aescin 16% to 20%. HCSE should not contain aesculin.[3]

#### *Summary of Clinical Evidence*

CVI has few effective treatments and is limited to use of leg compression stockings and limb elevation. In a recent update of a Cochrane review of seven randomized controlled trials of CVI, leg pain and leg volume were reduced by HCSE in six studies. HCSE was reported to have modest efficacy in the available short-term studies.[40] As mentioned earlier, pycnogenol may be more effective than HCSE for CVI.[32]

## DIGESTIVE SYSTEM

Botanicals are commonly used for digestive system disorders with ginger and peppermint among the top 10 natural products reported in a national survey of adults.[1] This section reviews common botanical medicines for digestive system disorders.

### Chamomile

Two common forms of chamomile are Roman or common chamomile (*Chamaemelum nobile* L. All., *Anthemis nobilis* L.) and German or Hungarian chamomile (*Matricaria recutita* L., *Chamomilla recutita* L.) Rauchert. Both herbs are from the family Asteraceae. Indigenous natives and Spanish-speaking people of the Americas have used dog fennel, a member of the genus *Anthemis*, as "chamomile."

#### *Therapeutic Uses*

German chamomile has been used for motion sickness, as well as many GI, inflammatory, and dermatologic diseases including those in children. Chamomile has been used to decrease mucositis after some types of chemotherapy including methotrexate.[3] It has also been used for anxiety, insomnia, and gastrointestinal spasms, especially as an herbal tea. Topically, chamomile has been used for hemorrhoids and inflammation of skin and mucous membranes.

#### *Physiologic Activity*

Chamomile contains volatile oil 0.3% to 2.0%. The oil contains α-bisabolol, sesquiterpene α-bisabolol, which have anti-inflammatory and antibacterial activity. Important flavonoids have been identified in German chamomile, including apigenin, luteolin, and quercetin. Apigenin is believed to affect central neurotransmitter systems, including serving as a benzodiazepine (BZDP)-receptor–binding ligand.[41] Dog fennel contains a higher concentration of anthecotulid, a sesquiterpene lactone.

### Dosage and Administration Guidelines

German chamomile may be prepared as a 3 g infusion. The dosage of the liquid extract (1:1 in alcohol 45%) is 1 to 4 mL taken three times daily.

### Safety Considerations

Chamomile generally is safe. Allergic reactions have been reported with a frequency of 1.7%[42] and may be more common than previously thought.[43] Patients with an allergy to ragweed and related plants in the family Asteraceae should avoid chamomile.[3] Theoretically, patients taking warfarin and platelet-active drugs or herbs should use chamomile with caution. Also, patients taking sedatives might experience additive effects if chamomile is also used. Little evidence supports these potential interactions. In vitro and animal studies suggest that chamomile extracts and tea infusions may decrease activity of CYP 1A2, CYP 2E1, and CYP 3A4.[9,44] The evidence should be considered preliminary because significant interactions have not been reported.

### Administration and Product Issues

Chamomile products containing dog fennel may have a higher rate of allergic reactions attributed to the concentration of anthecotulid and should be avoided.

### Summary of Clinical Evidence

Evidence of chamomile's effectiveness from clinical trials is limited. A study of the effect of chamomile tea on recurrent abdominal pain from functional bowel disorders in children is currently ongoing.[12]

## Ginger

Ginger (*Zingiber officinale* Roscoe) is a perennial from the Zingiberaceae family whose rhizomes and roots are used medicinally.

### Therapeutic Uses

The primary use of ginger has been as an antiemetic agent to relieve nausea and vomiting associated with many conditions, including pregnancy, motion sickness, chemotherapy, and surgery. Ginger has also been used for indigestion, colic, and arthritis.[3]

### Physiologic Activity

Ginger rhizomes possess volatile oil (1% to 3%) containing sesquiterpene hydrocarbons, including zingiberene and α-curcumene. Lesser amounts of farnesene, β-sesquiphellandrene, and β-bisabolene are present. An oleoresin (4% to 7.5%) is also present with nonvolatile pungent components, including gingerol, shogaols, and zingerone. Shogaol and gingerol have antiemetic activity.[3] Galanolactone, a diterpenoid isolated from ginger, has been shown to have anti-5-hydroxytriptamine activity and may also contribute to the antiemetic activity of ginger preparations.[3]

### Dosage and Administration Guidelines

For morning sickness, dried ginger 250 mg four times daily has been used. For motion sickness, a typical dose is two 500 mg capsules of dried powdered ginger root taken 30 minutes before beginning travel, followed by one or two more 500 mg capsules as needed every 4 hours.

### Safety Considerations

Ginger is safe and well tolerated. Heartburn and dermatitis have been reported with ginger. Belching was also identified in a clinical trial comparing the botanical with pyridoxine.[45] In overdosages of ginger, central nervous system (CNS) depression and arrhythmias have occurred.[3] Ginger has been used during pregnancy, and a recent clinical trial found no differences in pregnancy outcomes between ginger and pyridoxine.[45] A cohort study evaluating pregnancy outcomes through the Canadian Motherisk Helpline reported that exposure to ginger between the fourth and 14th week of pregnancy did not increase risk of major malformations.[46] Of note, 49% of women used ginger capsules with the remainder using ginger teas, cookies, candies, and other products.[46] Ginger may alter platelet function, depending on the dose and the specific formulation.[3] Fresh ginger root and ginger teas may have greater likelihood of interactions than dried ginger in patients taking warfarin and platelet-active drugs or herbs.[3,9,47]

### Administration and Product Issues

There are no product issues.

### Summary of Clinical Evidence

A meta-analysis evaluated ginger in the management of nausea and vomiting.[48] The Jadad scale was used to rate the quality of the six randomized, controlled trials. Although the studies received a quality score of 3 out of 5 points, all had a small sample size. Ginger appeared to be at least equivalent to metoclopramide although the dosage of the latter may have been too low.[48] The study with the strongest design failed to find a difference between ginger and placebo.[48] This meta-analysis provides evidence of a modest benefit from ginger in the management of nausea and vomiting. A recent systematic review evaluated six randomized controlled clinical trials and one observational study of ginger in the treatment of pregnancy-induced nausea and vomiting.[49] Five of the six clinical trials were of high quality. The evidence indicated that ginger was more effective than placebo and similar to pyridoxine in early pregnancy.[49] Of note, the effectiveness of ginger for the more severe form of nausea and vomiting in pregnancy, hyperemesis gravidarum, is unknown and ginger should not be recommended as a therapy for this condition without further research. An ongoing study is evaluating the role of ginger as an addition to conventional antiemetics in the management of nausea and vomiting secondary to cisplatin or adriamycin.[12]

## Licorice

Licorice (*Glycyrrhiza glabra* L.) is in the family Fabaceae (formerly Leguminosae). Its below-ground parts contain the active ingredients.

### Therapeutic Uses

Derivatives of licorice have been used to treat gastric and duodenal ulcers, chronic gastritis, constipation, and hepatitis C.

### Physiologic Activity

Licorice contains a sweet triterpene glycoside, glycyrrhizin (GL), at 2% to 14% of the dried root and rhizome. GL may bind to diverse groups of receptors in the body including glucocorticoid, mineralocorticoid, and estrogen.[3] GL is partially hydrolyzed by hepatic glucuronidase to its aglycone glycyrrhetinic acid (GA). GL and GA inhibit two enzymes that control breakdown of prostaglandins in the gastric mucosa. Many compounds with antioxidant activity have been isolated from the dried roots. In vitro, GA may induce apoptosis in human cells infected with latent Kaposi sarcoma-associated herpesvirus.[50]

### Dosage and Administration Guidelines

The usual dose of licorice is GL 200 to 600 mg daily for a maximum of 4 to 6 weeks. A tea can be made by adding 1 to 4 g dried or freshly grated licorice roots to a cup of hot water.[2]

### Safety Considerations

High doses or chronic use of licorice may result in sodium and water retention. Hypokalemia, increased blood pressure, lethargy, muscle pain, and paralysis can occur.[3,51] Patients with cardiovascular or renal disease should avoid licorice. An observational study of women who had a premature delivery suggests that heavy use of licorice is a risk factor for prematurity.[52] In vitro studies have suggested that licorice may decrease the activity of CYP 3A4.[9,44] Documented interactions with licorice are rare. Patients taking digoxin should avoid licorice because of the risk of hypokalemia and digoxin toxicity.[3] Because licorice and its derivatives may possess diverse hormonal effects, concomitant use with other drugs should be discouraged.

### Administration and Product Issues

Many commercial licorice products and foods actually contain anise flavoring, which lacks triterpene glycosides. Clinical trials have used deglycyrrhizinated licorice to decrease potential side effects.[3]

### Summary of Clinical Evidence

Licorice and its derivatives have traditionally been used for treatment of peptic ulcer disease. Current research with licorice has concentrated on the potential benefits of GL and GA in the treatment of viral hepatitis. A systematic review of complementary therapies for hepatitis C concluded that further research is needed before recommending these approaches, including licorice in the treatment of hepatitis C.[53] A recent study has reported that glycyrrhizin may inhibit replication of the coronavirus associated with severe acute respiratory syndrome (SARS).[54]

## Milk Thistle

Milk thistle (*Silybum marianum* (L.) Gaertn.) is a member of the aster family Asteraceae (formerly Compositae).

### Therapeutic Uses

Milk thistle has been used in Europe to treat poisoning by the mushroom *Amanita phalloides* (death cap). Milk thistle has been used as a protective agent after the liver was exposed to alcohol, acetaminophen, and carbon tetrachloride. A recent study of 500 veterans with hepatitis C reported that milk thistle was the most commonly used herbal therapy.[55] Silybin is undergoing phase 1 clinical trial for prostate cancer.[56]

### Physiologic Activity

The seeds and, to a lesser extent, the leaves and stems contain several compounds collectively referred to as silymarin (4% to 6% in seeds). Silymarin is composed primarily of silybin, along with isosilybin, dehydrosilybin, silydianin, and silychristin. These biologically active compounds may have antioxidant, antifibrotic, anti-inflammatory activity, as well as other beneficial effects such as regulation of cell permeability and inhibition of mitochondrial injury.[57,58] The antioxidant properties of silymarin are believed to be the primary beneficial effects of the botanical product.

### Dosage and Administration Guidelines

The average daily dose is 12 to 15 g (equivalent to silymarin 200 to 400 mg). Silybin has been reported to be hepatoprotective when administered within 24 to 48 hours of ingestion of a toxic mushroom.[58]

### Safety Considerations

Milk thistle is generally well tolerated. GI effects have been reported including nausea, abdominal fullness, and diarrhea.[57] Allergic reactions have been reported with milk thistle. Patients who have an allergy to ragweed and other members of the Asteraceae family should be cautioned not to use milk thistle although documented cases of cross-sensitivity are rare.[3] The potential effects of milk thistle on major CYP isoenzymes are unlikely to be clinically important according to healthy volunteer studies.[59] A study in healthy volunteers failed to find an interaction between milk thistle and indinavir, which is metabolized through CYP 3A4.[60]

### Administration and Product Issues

Milk thistle capsules contain varying amounts of a concentrated seed extract, standardized to flavonolignans 70% to

80% calculated as silybin.[2] Milk thistle is marketed in the United States most often in a capsule that contains 140 mg of silymarin. Most importantly, liver disease resulting from alcohol, acetaminophen, and other drugs or chemicals is potentially fatal, and patients should be cautioned against self-treatment.

### *Summary of Clinical Evidence*

A systematic review conducted by the Agency for Healthcare Research and Quality identified 16 prospective studies of milk thistle in varying types of liver disease. Milk thistle was demonstrated to improve aminotransferase levels and other measures of liver function in four of six studies of alcoholic liver disease. The effect of milk thistle on survival is unknown.[57] A recent Cochrane systematic review of 13 randomized controlled studies of the effect of milk thistle on liver disease caused by alcohol or hepatitis B or C viral infection did not find a reduction in mortality or development of hepatic complications.[61] A panel of experts on milk thistle and liver disease has emphasized the need for new clinical trials using standardized products. In addition, the effects of milk thistle on the progression, regression, or stabilization of hepatic fibrosis, and not solely on liver enzymes, should be evaluated.[62]

## Peppermint

Peppermint (*Mentha piperita* L.) is a member of the mint family Lamiaceae. It has been cultivated for its fragrant volatile oil, which is extracted primarily from its leaves.

### *Therapeutic Uses*

Both peppermint leaf and oil have been used for many purposes including treatment of irritable bowel syndrome (IBS).

### *Physiologic Activity*

The biological activity of peppermint may be a result of its essential oil (0.5% to 4%, average 1.5%). The oil or leaf preparations should be standardized to contain not less than 44% menthol. Menthol stereoisomers are also present, including d-neomenthol (3%), as well as other monoterpenes such as menthone, menthofuran, eucalyptol, and limonene. The mechanism of action of peppermint involves direct relaxation of GI smooth muscle.

### *Dosage and Administration Guidelines*

The usual dosage of peppermint oil is 0.2 to 0.4 mL (enteric-coated capsules) three times daily between meals.

### *Safety Considerations*

Peppermint oil is generally well tolerated. Heartburn in some patients may be attributed to relaxation of the lower esophageal sphincter. Patients who have severe preexisting GI disease should avoid use of peppermint oil. Peppermint leaf tea should be used with caution in infants and small children because of possible laryngeal and bronchial spasms from volatilized menthol. The oil may also irritate mucous membranes. In vitro and in vivo studies suggest that peppermint tea and peppermint oil may decrease activity of some CYP isoenzymes, including CYP 3A4.[63] The evidence should be considered preliminary since significant interactions have not been reported. The ingestion of peppermint may decrease absorption of iron.[9]

### *Administration and Product Issues*

Enteric-coated preparations may reduce risk of heartburn.

### *Summary of Clinical Evidence*

A meta-analysis evaluating peppermint oil and other alternative therapies in the treatment of IBS concluded that peppermint oil has modest efficacy.[64] The reviewed studies had significant flaws including small sample sizes, short durations of therapy, and crossover designs. In a study of 42 children with IBS, 75% experienced a reduction in severity of their abdominal pain with the use of pH-dependent, enteric-coated peppermint oil capsules.[65]

## Plantago (Plantain, Psyllium Seed)

Plantago (*Plantago arenaria* Waldst. et Kit.), from the family Plantaginaceae, is also known as plantain or psyllium seed. Products generally consist of the cleaned, dried, ripened seeds of psyllium.

### *Therapeutic Uses*

Plantago is used to treat chronic constipation and IBS, as well as weight loss. Dietary supplements containing psyllium seed husk may carry a health claim indicating that their use may reduce the risk of coronary heart disease.[66]

### *Physiologic Activity*

Plantago seeds contain insoluble fiber up to 80% and a hydrocolloid soluble fiber 10% to 30%. The hydrocolloid consists of acidic and neutral polysaccharide fractions. On hydrolysis, L-arabinose, D-galactose, D-galacturonic acid, L-rhamnose, and D-xylose are released. Plantago or psyllium seed is a bulk-forming laxative that binds fluid and swells, increasing the volume of intestinal content and causing physical stimulation of the gut wall. The bowels are lubricated by the seeds' mucilage, achieving accelerated transit through the colon.

### *Dosage and Administration Guidelines*

The dosage of psyllium seed is between 7 and 40 g per day taken with adequate amounts of fluid 30 to 60 minutes after a meal or after administration of other drugs.

### *Safety Considerations*

Plantago is generally well tolerated. Allergic reactions to plantago have been reported in patients and in individuals involved with either its production or administration.[67] Plantago should not be used in the presence of an obstruction of the GI tract.[68,69] Cases of choking and esophageal obstruction have been reported with psyllium and other laxative products.[69] Concurrent administration with other drugs may alter their absorption.

### Administration and Product Issues

There are no product issues.

### Summary of Clinical Evidence

The ingestion of psyllium 10.2 g/day has been studied as an adjunct to a low-fat diet. Reductions in total and LDL cholesterol concentrations of 4% and 7%, respectively, have resulted. HDL cholesterol concentrations remained unchanged.[70] The addition of 6 g of psyllium to orlistat therapy for obesity resulted in a significant reduction in GI side effects.[71] The use of psyllium improved glucose control in 125 patients with type 2 diabetes mellitus, but did not result in weight loss.[72] Psyllium may improve constipation caused by IBS, but abdominal pain is not decreased.[73]

## Senna

Alexandria senna (*Cassia acutifolia* Delile) and Tinnevelly senna (*C. augustifolia* Vahl), both of which are also referred to as *Senna alexandrina,* are shrubs or herbaceous perennials. Members of the family Fabaceae, their leaves and fruits contain the active ingredients.

### Therapeutic Uses

Senna has been used as a laxative to treat constipation.

### Physiologic Activity

Dianthrone glycosides, particularly sennosides A, $A_1$, B, C, D, and G, are present with various other anthraquinone derivatives. Sennosides increase motility of the colon. Chloride secretion is also stimulated, which increases the colon's water and electrolyte content.

### Dosage and Administration Guidelines

The usual dose of senna is hydroxyanthracene derivatives (sennoside B) 15 to 30 mg.

### Safety Considerations

Patients may experience cramping and other abdominal discomfort. Use of stimulant laxatives should not continue beyond 1 to 2 weeks, except under medical supervision. Chronic abuse or overdose can result in fluid and electrolyte losses. Anatomic changes caused by either neuronal injury or damage to the musculature of the colon have been associated with use of stimulant laxatives. Severe diaper rash and blisters have been reported in young children who ingested senna laxatives.[74] Cases of choking and esophageal obstruction have been reported with senna and other laxative products.[69] Senna should not be used in the presence of acute inflammatory bowel disease, appendicitis, or other serious intestinal diseases. Theoretically, chronic abuse or overdosage can result in potassium loss and a potential increase in adverse effects from digoxin; however, these effects have not been documented.

### Administration and Product Issues

Senna products should not be used chronically.

### Summary of Clinical Evidence

None is available.

# IMMUNE STIMULANTS AND PERFORMANCE ENHANCERS

Botanical medicines classified as immune stimulants are used to prevent and treat upper respiratory tract infections including the common cold. Performance-enhancing botanicals are used to improve physical and mental functioning.

## Andrographis ("Indian Echinacea")

*Andrographis paniculata* (Burm f.) Nees from the family Acanthaceae is an annual shrub that grows in Asia and is cultivated in northern India.

### Therapeutic Uses

Andrographis is typically used as an immune stimulant to prevent and treat common viral respiratory infections including the common cold and influenza.

### Physiologic Activity

Andrographolide and deoxyandrographolide found in the leaf and rhizome are the active components.[75] Preliminary evidence suggests that andrographis may have both anti-inflammatory and immunostimulating properties. Administration may increase antibody activity and phagocytosis by macrophages, as well as inhibit PAF-induced platelet aggregation.[75,76]

### Dosage and Administration Guidelines

On the basis of clinical trials, the recommended dosage for treating the common cold is 400 mg of the andrographis dried extract three times daily. For prevention of colds, 200 mg andrographis dried extract once daily has been suggested.

### Safety Considerations

Andrographis is well tolerated. Patients may experience headache, fatigue, rash, diarrhea, and vomiting with high doses. Animal studies have suggested andrographis may decrease male and female fertility. These findings have not been confirmed. Safety data for use of andrographis is limited to 3 months. Because of its proposed effect on PAF, andrographis may inhibit platelet aggregation. Patients taking warfarin and other platelet-active drugs or herbs should use this botanical with caution. Given its potential for immune stimulation, andrographis should not be taken with immunosuppressive agents. No reports of this interaction have been documented.

### *Administration and Product Issues*

Commercial products are typically standardized to contain between 4% and 6% andrographolide. Andrographis is often evaluated in clinical trials with a single-ingredient product containing only andrographis. However, andrographis is more commonly available in multi-ingredient cold formulas containing other "immune stimulants."

### *Summary of Clinical Evidence*

Clinical studies of andrographis often use visual analogue scales and rely on patients' subjective assessments to determine improvement in symptoms. In a systematic review of safety and efficacy, andrographis was superior to placebo in improving subjective symptoms of uncomplicated upper respiratory tract infections. The botanical may also reduce the frequency of coldlike infections if taken chronically.[77] Patients with human immunodeficiency virus (HIV) infection taking high doses of andrographolide have experienced increases in CD4+ counts.[78]

## Echinacea

Echinacea, or purple coneflower, was the most commonly used natural product according to a recent national survey.[1] Nine species of echinacea, a member of the Asteraceae family, are found in North America. *Echinacea* species typically used in clinical trials include *E. purpurea* (L.) Moench, *E. angustifolia* (DC.) Heller, and *E. pallida* (Nutt.) Britt. The roots, leaves, and flowers of echinacea are the medicinally active parts of the plant.

### *Therapeutic Uses*

Echinacea has been used as an immune stimulant to prevent and treat colds and other respiratory infections.

### *Physiologic Activity*

Although the specific mechanism of action of echinacea remains unclear, components that target the nonspecific cellular immune system have been identified. These include alkylamides, caffeic acid derivatives (chicoric acid, chlorogenic acid, and cynarin), flavonoids, glycoproteins, isobutylamides, polyenes, and polysaccharides.[79] Newer research has questioned echinacea's ability to stimulate the immune system and suggests its effect may actually be from possible anti-inflammatory action.[80]

### *Dosage and Administration Guidelines*

Dosing recommendations for echinacea are lacking because preparations are not typically standardized to one active constituent. Echinacea is available in single- and multiple-ingredient formulations such as teas, tinctures, extracts, juices, capsules, and tablets. Each product has its own dosing regimen. Echinacea appears to work best when started at the onset of cold symptoms. Most people report 10 to 14 days of therapy adequate to treat acute illnesses.

### *Safety Considerations*

Echinacea products are well tolerated. Adverse effects may include mild GI discomfort, tingling sensation of the tongue, and headache. Patients with allergies to plants in the Asteraceae family, as well as those with a history of asthma, atopy, and allergic rhinitis should avoid echinacea. Patients with severe systemic illnesses including HIV/AIDS, multiple sclerosis, tuberculosis, and autoimmune disorders including rheumatoid arthritis should also avoid the use of echinacea. Evidence supporting this concern is limited to case reports.[81] Avoidance of immune suppressants such as azathioprine, cyclophosphamide, and cyclosporine may be advisable although no interactions have been documented. In vitro analyses have implicated echinacea as a potential inhibitor of CYP 3A4 isoenzymes.[44] This interaction has not been reported in humans.

### *Administration and Product Issues*

Products labeled "echinacea" may be chemically different plants or plant parts.

### *Summary of Clinical Evidence*

Several studies evaluating the efficacy of echinacea-containing products for the acute treatment of the common cold and other upper respiratory infections have demonstrated that echinacea may decrease modestly the severity and duration of coldlike symptoms in adults if treatment is started at first appearance of symptoms.[80,82-84] Other studies have shown no benefit.[79,85] A recent randomized controlled trial evaluating the use of echinacea in treating upper respiratory tract infections in children ages 2 to 11 years found no benefit.[86] Although the study methodology has been questioned, it is promising to see evaluation of use in children begin. Evidence does not support chronic use of echinacea to prevent or reduce frequency of respiratory infections.[87]

## Eleuthero

*Eleutherococcus senticosus* from the Araliaceae family is often referred to as Siberian ginseng. The plant is not a genus of *Panax*, as are Asian and American ginseng. *Eleutherococcus* is found in eastern Siberia, northeastern China, Korea, and Hokkaido Island.

### *Therapeutic Uses*

Eleuthero is considered an "adaptogen," an agent used for increasing resistance to environmental and psychological stressors. Other uses for eleuthero include treatment of herpes simplex type II infections, normalization of blood pressure, including hypotension and hypertension, prevention of atherosclerosis, and normalization of blood glucose in diabetes mellitus.

### Physiologic Activity

The active compounds of eleuthero are derived primarily from the root and leaf and are referred to as eleutherosides (subtypes A-M). Flavonoids, hydroxycinnamates, and other constituents such as sesamin, B-sitosterol, hedarasaponin B, and isofraxidin may also have biological activity.[88] Animal studies and in vitro analysis suggest these compounds may have antiplatelet, immunostimulant, and antioxidant properties.

### Dosage and Administration Guidelines

Siberian ginseng products are available in many forms with varying recommended doses. Commercial products are often standardized to eleutheroside B and/or eleutheroside E content. Siberian ginseng extract standardized to contain eleutheroside E 0.3% in doses of 400 mg/day was used in the herpes simplex type II study.[89]

### Safety Considerations

Both drowsiness and stimulant effects have been reported with eleuthero. Because of its variable effects on blood pressure, eleuthero should be avoided in patients with hypertension. Theoretically, patients with diabetes mellitus should be monitored for hypoglycemia. Eleuthero is recommended only for short-term use because the herb allegedly has estrogenic effects, although clinical evidence is lacking.[90] In patients taking digoxin, eleuthero may produce falsely elevated plasma digoxin concentrations, depending on the assay used.[91] Eleuthero does not affect activity of CYP 2D6 and CYP 3A4.[88]

### Administration and Product Issues

In the past, eleuthero has been adulterated with other plants, such as silk vine (*Periploca graeca*) that contain cardiac glycosides, or with caffeine to enhance its stimulant effects.[90]

### Summary of Clinical Evidence

Well-designed, randomized clinical trials documenting the safety and efficacy of eleuthero are lacking. Studies using standardized preparations of eleuthero are required to determine the actual benefit of eleuthero. In a small 6-month study, *Eleutherococcus* extract taken once daily demonstrated a beneficial effect on frequency, severity, and duration of herpes simplex type II infections.[89]

## Ginseng

The root and rhizome of Asian ginseng (*Panax ginseng* C.A. Meyer) and North American ginseng (*P. quinquefolius* L.) are from the family Araliaceae. The Asian product is exported primarily from Korea and China. The North American species is cultivated primarily in the United States, Canada, and China.

### Therapeutic Uses

Asian and American ginseng, classified as adaptogens, have been used to treat mental and physical stress, anemia, diabetes mellitus, insomnia, impotence, and fever.

### Physiologic Activity

The constituents most responsible for ginseng's activity are triterpenoid saponins, including ginsenosides. At least 30 ginsenosides, also referred to as panaxosides, have been identified. Additional constituents include carbohydrates, B vitamins, and flavonoids. Advances in isolation and testing of ginseng's chemical constituents are revealing differences in the content of both Asian and North American ginseng as well as in the physiologic activity of individual ginsenosides. While the study of individual effects is beneficial, the overall interplay of all constituents is most important to patient outcomes.

### Dosage and Administration Guidelines

Most studies of ginseng used dosages of standardized extracts between 200 and 600 mg/day.[92] Doses as high as 3 g have been used. Raw herb in doses of 1 to 2 g has also been used.

### Safety Considerations

Side effects include insomnia, headache, blood pressure changes, anorexia, rash, and unusual vaginal bleeding. Large doses may cause gastric upset and CNS stimulation. Ginseng should be used with caution in patients with cardiovascular disease, including hypertension, or diabetes mellitus and in the presence of acute illness. Treatment duration with ginseng should be limited to 3 months because of the possibility of hormonelike effects although clearly defined support for this effect is lacking. In the late 1970s a "ginseng-abuse syndrome" was described in long-term ginseng users. This report has since been discredited because the study was poorly controlled. Ginseng's effect on anticoagulant and antiplatelet therapy is not predictable, warranting caution in concomitant use.[9] Evidence suggests that American ginseng but not Asian ginseng may reduce warfarin's effect.[93,94] The concomitant use of ginseng with psychotropic agents including phenelzine and corticosteroids, as well as with large amounts of stimulants including caffeine-containing beverages, should be avoided.[9]

### Administration and Product Issues

Ginseng products may contain adulterants.

### Summary of Clinical Evidence

Both American and Asian ginseng may lower blood glucose levels in people with type 2 diabetes mellitus.[95,96] Small studies and poorly controlled large studies from the former Soviet Union have shown that Asian ginseng may improve memory and mathematical skills, and resistance to stress and common respiratory infections.[97,98]

## Green Tea

Leaves from the tea shrub *Camellia sinensis* (L.) Kuntze provide green tea. This plant belongs to the family Theaceae. Native to southeastern Asia, tea leaves are heated immediately after harvesting, then mechanically rolled and crushed before drying to produce green tea. From the same plant as green tea, black tea is produced by allowing the leaves to wilt before they are rolled and left in a humid environment for several hours. This process promotes enzymatic changes (fermentation) and a gradual change in color to reddish-brown. Oolong, another commonly available tea, is a partially fermented tea.

### *Therapeutic Uses*

Green tea is considered a performance enhancer because of the stimulant effect from caffeine. Green tea has also been used to protect against development of many diseases, including cardiovascular disease, cancer, and liver disorders.

### *Physiologic Activity*

In addition to caffeine, green tea contains polyphenolic compounds including flavonols (also known as catechins), flavonoids, and phenolic acids. The most prevalent flavonols include epicatechin, epicatechin-3-gallate, epigallocatechin, and epigallocatechin-3-gallate (EGCG).[99]

### *Dosage and Administration Guidelines*

Doses of green tea in epidemiologic studies vary between 1 and 10 cups daily. On average, the dose commonly consumed in Asian countries is about 3 cups per day. Ingestion of 10 cups or more of green tea has shown benefit in reducing cholesterol concentrations. Green tea extract supplements standardized to polyphenol content retain similar effects to that of green tea while reducing exposure to caffeine.[100]

### *Safety Considerations*

Ingestion of large quantities of green tea can cause adverse GI symptoms as well as CNS and cardiac stimulation attributed to the caffeine content. Green tea (1 bag) has 20 mg of caffeine on average, with a range of 8 to 30 mg. In comparison, black tea (1 bag) has 40 mg of caffeine on average, with a range of 25 to 110 mg, and Oolong tea (1 bag) has 30 mg of caffeine on average, with a range of 12 to 55 mg.[101] Green tea should be avoided if other stimulating medications including theophylline are being ingested. Conversely, green tea may oppose the action of sedating medications, including BZDPs. Green tea in large doses may antagonize the effects of warfarin, although brewing destroys most of its vitamin K content.[102]

### *Administration and Product Issues*

Green, black, and Oolong teas are different products with varying amounts of caffeine. Research into their health benefits has focused primarily on green tea.

### *Summary of Clinical Evidence*

Epidemiologic evidence suggests that daily consumption of green tea may protect against cardiovascular disease as well as liver disorders.[103] Japanese men older than 40 years who consumed green tea daily had decreased serum concentrations of total cholesterol, triglyceride, and increased HDL cholesterol. However, another study of men and women who smoked cigarettes found no effect of green tea on lipids and lipoproteins.[104] A randomized controlled trial of theaflavin-enriched green tea extract demonstrated mild reductions in LDL cholesterol in patients on diets low in saturated fats.[105] Human and animal studies suggest that consumption of green tea may reduce the incidence of a variety of cancers including breast, bladder, esophageal, pancreatic, and head and neck cancers.[106] High levels of green tea consumption may reduce the risk of gastric cancer. Evidence suggests low to moderate consumption of green tea did not reduce the risk of developing gastric cancer.[107]

## Combination Formulas

While the preceding section addressed individual products used for boosting immunity or improving performance, botanicals are often found in formulas containing multiple ingredients. This is especially true for formulations aimed at preventing colds or general immune stimulation. Efficacy and safety data may be available for ingredients such as andrographis and echinacea but completely lacking for others such as astragalus, propolis, and goldenseal. Formulations may also include nonbotanical ingredients purported to have immune effects, such as vitamin A, vitamin C, vitamin E, and zinc. The ingredients should be closely analyzed to ensure that the total daily dose of individual ingredients is neither sub- nor supratherapeutic. This may be difficult for supplements lacking formal dosage ranges.

# KIDNEY, URINARY TRACT, AND PROSTATE DISORDERS

Botanicals have been used to prevent and treat urinary tract and prostate disorders such as benign prostatic hyperplasia (BPH). This section reviews four botanical medicines.

## African Plum

African plum is derived from the bark of *Prunus africana* (Hook f.) Kalkman (syn. *Pygeum africanum* Hook f.), a member of the Rosaceae family.

### *Therapeutic Uses*

African plum tree bark has been used to treat BPH.

### *Physiologic Activity*

Pygeum bark contains phytosterols, pentacyclic triterpenes, including ursolic and oleanic acids, and ferulic acid esters, including docosanol and tetracosanol.[108] Phytosterols may inhibit prostaglandin synthesis in the prostate. Triterpenes may also have anti-inflammatory properties. Ferulic acid esters reduce prolactin levels and prostate cholesterol levels, a precursor to testosterone synthesis.[108] Pygeum reduces excitability of the detrusor muscle, increases prostatic secretions, and possibly may decrease proliferation of fibroblasts within the prostate.[109]

### *Dosage and Administration Guidelines*

In products standardized to contain 14% triterpenes and 0.5% n-docosanol, the average dosage is 50 to 100 mg twice daily.[108]

### *Safety Considerations*

Pygeum is generally well tolerated. Most adverse effects reported in clinical trials involve GI complaints, including diarrhea, constipation, and gastric pain.[3] All men presenting with prostate symptoms should be counseled to contact their primary care provider before starting pygeum to rule out prostate cancer. It is unclear whether pygeum affects prostate specific antigen (PSA) levels.

### *Administration and Product Issues*

Pygeum products are often standardized to contain triterpenes 14% and n-docosanol 0.5%.[3] In 1998 the demand for pygeum extract was so high that it caused the African plum tree to become a threatened species, with current international trade being monitored under the Convention on International Trade in Endangered Species of Wild Fauna and Flora.[109]

### *Summary of Clinical Evidence*

While clinical trials are limited, pygeum has demonstrated improvements in urinary flow, void volumes, residual volumes, nocturia, daytime frequency, and subjective symptom assessments of BPH.[108]

## Cranberry

Cranberry (*Vaccinium macrocarpon* Ait.) is an evergreen bush native to North America belonging to the family Ericaceae.

### *Therapeutic Uses*

Cranberry has been used to prevent and treat urinary tract infections (UTI).

### *Physiologic Activity*

Cranberry contains condensed tannins called proanthocyanidins. Epicatechin is the primary proanthocyanidin found in cranberry extracts. The exact mechanism is unknown, but evidence suggests that cranberry blocks bacteria, *Escherichia coli* in particular, from adhering to bladder, kidneys, and urethra.[110] Fructose found in cranberry juice may also alter bacterial adhesion. Cranberry was once thought to stop growth of bacteria by acidifying urine. While this is no longer believed to be true, cranberry's ability to slightly lower urinary pH may retard degradation of urine by *E. coli* and reduce the urinary odor of incontinent patients.

### *Dosage and Administration Guidelines*

The ideal dosage of cranberry has not been well defined. For prevention of UTI, the dosage is cranberry juice 1 to 10 ounces per day, whereas the dosage for treating UTI is 10 to 32 ounces per day. Cranberry juice cocktail is approximately 30% pure cranberry juice. Three ounces of cranberry juice cocktail is equal to 1 ounce of cranberry juice. Encapsulated cranberry formulations are administered in a dosage of 300 to 400 mg twice daily. Fresh or frozen cranberries may also be used although the bitter taste makes this method unpopular.

### *Safety Considerations*

Evidence suggests that regular use of cranberry concentrate tablets might increase risk of kidney stones.[111] Patients may experience diarrhea with very large daily doses. Theoretically, cranberry juice may alter excretion of weakly alkaline drugs or botanicals such as uva-ursi. Case reports have emerged suggesting cranberry may cause bleeding in patients taking warfarin.[112] Cranberry may be a CYP 2C9 inhibitor although only the warfarin interaction has been reported.

### *Administration and Product Issues*

The exact formulation or product is less important than ingesting the equivalent amount of cranberry juice used in the studies. While 100% cranberry juice may be available, its bitter taste may be unpalatable.

### *Summary of Clinical Evidence*

Clinical trials suggest that daily consumption of cranberry juice may help prevent UTI. A study of 153 elderly women compared the effect of cranberry juice and placebo on the frequency of bacteriuria with pyuria and showed that cranberry juice reduced the frequency.[113] The clinical significance of these findings is unknown because many elderly women have asymptomatic bacteriuria that does not progress to an actual infection requiring treatment. An open, randomized, controlled trial of 150 women compared the effects of ingesting either cranberry-lingonberry juice concentrate 50 mL daily for 6 months, a probiotic drink 5 days per week for 1 year, and no intervention.[114] Regular use of cranberry-lingonberry juice reduced the rate of UTI, compared with the other two groups. Cranberry does not prevent UTIs in patients with neurogenic bladder.[115] Evidence does not support its use in treating UTIs; patients should be referred to their health care provider.

## Saw Palmetto

Saw palmetto (*Serenoa repens* [Michx.] G. Nichols), a dwarf palm tree from the Arecaceae family, is native to the southeast coastal region of the United States.

### Therapeutic Uses

Saw palmetto has been used to treat BPH.

### Physiologic Activity

The lipophilic extracts from the ripened fruit contain saturated and unsaturated fatty acids and plant sterols. Although the active compounds responsible have not been identified, they are likely present in the lipophilic extract. Saw palmetto may inhibit 5-α-reductase, the enzyme responsible for conversion of testosterone to dihydrotestosterone. Saw palmetto may also inhibit cytosolic androgen receptor binding and have local antiestrogenic and anti-inflammatory effects on the prostate.[116]

### Dosage and Administration Guidelines

The dosage used in clinical studies is 160 mg twice daily or 320 mg once daily. For whole berries, 1 to 2 g is usually recommended.

### Safety Considerations

Saw palmetto is well tolerated. GI complaints from saw palmetto have been reported. One report exists of a 54-year-old man taking saw palmetto who had intraoperative hemorrhage during surgery.[117] Saw palmetto should be used with caution in patients taking any drug or natural product that might prolong bleeding. Men with prostate symptoms should contact their provider before starting saw palmetto to rule out prostate cancer.

### Administration and Product Issues

Saw palmetto products should contain at least 85% standardized fatty acids.

### Summary of Clinical Evidence

In a systematic review, saw palmetto provided mild to moderate improvement in urinary symptoms and flow measures in men with BPH.[118] Improvements were similar to those seen with finasteride, and saw palmetto was associated with fewer adverse effects. Typical study durations range from 4 to 48 weeks. Long-term data on the efficacy and safety of saw palmetto are lacking. Saw palmetto does not alter prostate volume or PSA levels.

## Uva-Ursi

Uva-ursi, or bearberry (*Arctostaphylos uva-ursi* (L.) Spreng.), is an evergreen shrub from the Ericaceae family that grows throughout the Northern hemisphere. The leaves, and not the berries, are used therapeutically.

### Therapeutic Uses

Uva-ursi is an ingredient in many kidney and bladder tea formulations. It is often included in botanical weight-loss products and nonprescription products as a diuretic.

### Physiologic Activity

Uva-ursi contains the phenol arbutin, tannins, and small amounts of the free aglycone hydroquinone, in addition to flavonoids and gallic and ellagic acid. The urinary antiseptic constituent is arbutin, which is hydrolyzed to hydroquinone in alkaline urine.[119]

### Dosage and Administration Guidelines

Uva-ursi is available in dried herb, teas, and fluid extracts. It is often available in multiple-ingredient products for kidney and bladder health. Uva-ursi administered in a tea is taken up to three or four times a day; liquid extract 1.5 to 4.0 mL or tincture 2 to 4 mL are administered three times daily.[120] Uva-ursi should be taken with meals.

### Safety Considerations

Hydroquinone can cause nausea, vomiting, tinnitus, cyanosis, and convulsions. Large doses are toxic and hydroquinone possesses hepatotoxic, mutagenic, and carcinogenic effects. Uva-ursi should be avoided during pregnancy or lactation, by children younger than 12 years, or by persons with severe liver or kidney disease. Uva-ursi may be toxic to the retina with prolonged use because of its ability to inhibit melanin synthesis.[121] Uva-ursi should not be combined with urinary acidifiers such as cranberry juice. The botanical may decrease absorption of iron.[9]

### Administration and Product Issues

Uva-ursi should be taken with food, including fruits, vegetables, and milk, that will alkalinize the urine to enhance the antiseptic effect of arbutin. Uva-ursi should not be taken for more than 1 week.

### Summary of Clinical Evidence

Proof of clinical effect is limited to case reports and observational studies. Given its potential toxicities, uva-ursi should be avoided until more evidence on safety and efficacy exist.

# NERVOUS SYSTEM DISORDERS

Many botanicals have been used to treat CNS disorders because of the perceived lack of effective therapies or the presence of significant side effects from conventional medications. This section reviews the common and emerging botanicals for these disorders.

## Butterbur

*Petasites hybridus* (L.) Gaertner, Meyer & Scherb, also referred to as butterbur, is native to marshy areas in northern Asia,

Europe, and parts of North America. It is a member of the Asteraceae family.

### Therapeutic Uses

Butterbur is used to prevent migraines as well as treat allergic rhinitis and asthma.

### Physiologic Activity

The sesquiterpenes petasin and isopetasin are isolated from the plant's rhizomes, roots, and leaves.[122] Extracts also contain volatile oils, tannins, flavonoids, and pyrrolizidine alkaloids. Petasin may reduce spasms in smooth muscle and vascular walls and inhibit leukotriene synthesis. Isopetasin reduces prostaglandin synthesis, thereby reducing inflammation. Both compounds have an affinity for cerebral blood vessels.

### Dosage and Administration Guidelines

For migraine prevention, studies use standardized extracts containing a minimum of petasin 7.5 mg and isopetasin 7.5 mg per 50 mg tablet of the crude drug. Dosages of standardized crude drug ranging from 50 to 100 mg twice daily are administered for 4 to 6 months, then tapered until migraine incidence increases.[122] Standardized petasin (Ze 339) 8 mg were administered four times daily for allergic rhinitis.[123]

### Safety Considerations

Pyrrolizidine alkaloids (PAs) are a minor, highly toxic compound in butterbur extract. PAs with an unsaturated pyrrolizidine alkaloid nucleus can cause serious damage to the liver and carcinogenesis. Germany and Switzerland license butterbur products only after they are certified to provide less than 1 μg of PAs in a daily dose.[124] Use of butterbur should be avoided in pregnancy and lactation. Patients should also avoid the use of butterbur if they are allergic to plants in the Asteraceae family.

### Administration and Product Issues

Butterbur products should be free of pyrrolizidine alkaloids.

### Summary of Clinical Evidence

Studies have shown the ability of butterbur to reduce migraine frequency, decrease associated symptoms, and reduce duration and intensity of migraine pain.[122,125] The effect may be dose-related, with higher doses (i.e., 75 mg twice daily) having a greater effect. Preliminary studies also suggest butterbur extract may be as effective as cetirizine and fexofenadine for symptoms associated with allergic rhinitis.[123,126]

## Feverfew

Feverfew (*Tanacetum parthenium* [L.] Schultz-Bip.) is a member of the family Asteraceae. The plant is native to the Balkans.

### Therapeutic Uses

Feverfew has been used to prevent migraines as well as treatment of dysmenorrhea, arthritis, and psoriasis.[3]

### Physiologic Activity

The actual "active" components of feverfew for preventing headaches are unknown. The sesquiterpene lactone, parthenolide, is the most abundant and best studied component. However, a study using an alcoholic extract of feverfew standardized to parthenolide content was found to be ineffective in the prevention of migraines.[127] Chrysanthenyl acetate, an essential oil of feverfew, may inhibit prostaglandin synthetase and possess analgesic properties. Melatonin has been identified in small quantities in commercial feverfew products and leaf samples.[128] Feverfew may have pharmacologic effects on prostaglandin synthesis, platelet aggregation, serotonin release, macrophage function, and vascular smooth muscle contraction. Extracts may also inhibit pain transmission.

### Dosage and Administration Guidelines

Clinical studies have used feverfew extract in doses of 50 to 100 mg daily.

### Safety Considerations

GI side effects may result from ingestion of feverfew. Oral ulcers may occur from chewing fresh leaves. "Postfeverfew syndrome" may occur after abrupt withdrawal from chronic use and may result in anxiety, headaches, insomnia, and muscle stiffness. Patients should avoid use of feverfew if they are allergic to plants in the Asteraceae family. Feverfew may possess antiplatelet effects, and patients taking warfarin and other platelet-active drugs or herbs should use it with caution.[9]

### Administration and Product Issues

Standardization of a feverfew product to its parthenolide content does not appear necessary. Feverfew must be taken continuously to be effective for migraine prophylaxis. The botanical is not effective for treatment of acute migraine attacks.

### Summary of Clinical Evidence

After an analysis of the clinical evidence supporting the use of feverfew for migraine prevention, the 2000 U.S. Headache Consortium ranked it as a second-line therapy for the prevention of migraines.[129] However, a systematic review of feverfew in preventing migraine found insufficient evidence from randomized, double-blind trials to suggest an effect.[130]

## Huperzine

Huperzine A is derived from the Chinese club moss (*Huperzia serrata* [Thumb.] Trev.) and is a member of the Lycopodiaceae family. It is approved as a treatment for AD in China.

### Therapeutic Uses

Huperzine A has been used to treat dementia, increase memory, and enhance learning. Huperzine A is considered a protective agent against organophosphate chemical-warfare agents and a treatment for myasthenia gravis.

### Physiologic Activity

Huperzine A is an unsaturated sesquiterpene compound of which only the levorotatory isomer is pharmacologically active. Huperzine A is a potent peripherally and centrally acting reversible acetylcholinesterase inhibitor, which crosses the blood brain barrier.[131]

### Dosage and Administration Guidelines

The dosages used to treat AD range from 50 to 200 μg of huperzine A twice daily.[131]

### Safety Considerations

Adverse effects are primarily cholinergic and include sweating, blurred vision, nausea, vomiting, diarrhea, dizziness, bradycardia, and loss of appetite. Theoretically, huperzine should be avoided in patients with bradycardia, peptic ulcer disease, and increased gastric acid secretion. Concurrent use of anticholinergic drugs such as atropine and benztropine may decrease the effectiveness of huperzine A. Additive cholinergic effects may occur if taken with other acetylcholinesterase inhibitors such as donepezil or cholinergic agents such as bethanechol. In addition, huperzine A may have additive effects in the presence of other medications that may cause bradycardia, including β-blockers.

### Administration and Product Issues

Huperzine A is derived from a moss, and lead has been detected in some products. In an effort to develop more selective acetylcholinesterase inhibitors, chemical hybrids of huperzine A and tacrine or huperzine A and donepezil are being investigated. The huperzine A and tacrine hybrid is also referred to as huprine X.[132]

### Summary of Clinical Evidence

Huperzine A may have efficacy against common neuronal problems associated with AD, including decreased acetylcholine levels in the brain and glutamate-induced neuronal death.[131] Clinical studies of patients with AD and multi-infarct dementias treated with huperzine A have demonstrated significant improvements on memory, cognitive, and behavioral function scales.[131] More rigorous trials need to be performed to confirm the role of huperzine A in dementia.

## Kava

Kava is derived from the rhizome and roots of *Piper methysticum* G. Forster. A member of the black pepper family (Piperaceae), it is widely used by Pacific Islanders as a social and ceremonial tranquilizing beverage. The emergence of safety concerns has placed kava under intense scrutiny worldwide.

### Therapeutic Uses

Kava is used to treat mild anxiety.

### Physiologic Activity

The pharmacologically active constituents of kava are the fat-soluble lactones, also referred to as kavalactones and kavapyrones. The mechanism of action includes interacting with dopaminergic transmission, inhibiting central monoamine oxidase-B (MAO-B), and modulating gamma-aminobutyric acid-B (GABA-B) receptors.[133] Kava may also inhibit uptake of noradrenaline and have antithrombotic activity.

### Dosage and Administration Guidelines

The usual dose of kava preparations is equivalent to 60 to 120 mg of kavapyrones. In trials using extracts standardized to 70% kavalactones, the recommended dosage is 100 mg two to three times a day.

### Safety Considerations

Kava is fairly well tolerated with dizziness and drowsiness most commonly reported. Mouth ulceration and numbness may occur if the raw plant is chewed. The use of kava is discouraged when operating machinery or motor vehicles. Acute overdoses with kava may result in impaired mental status and ataxia similar to alcohol intoxication.[134] A dry, scaly rash primarily on the palms, soles, forearms, shins, and back can occur in patients chronically using high-dose kava teas, tablets, or the native plant.[135] In March 2002, the Center for Food Safety and Nutrition issued a warning advising consumers and professionals of the risk of severe liver injury associated with kava-containing supplements. Several countries, including Germany, Switzerland, Canada, Australia, and France, have restricted the sale of kava products in response to case reports of liver failure associated with kava use.[136] As of 2004, at least 78 cases of hepatotoxicity have been associated with kava ingestion. Of these, four are probably linked to kava and another 23 are potentially linked.[136] Thrombocytopenia, leukopenia, and hearing impairment have also been reported with kava.[135] Kava potentially may interact with anticoagulants and drugs that increase the risk of bleeding.[9] Concomitant use of kava with alcohol and other CNS depressants such as BZDPs, anticonvulsants, opioids, and valerian could increase sedation. In vitro analyses reveal the potential of kava for causing pharmacokinetic drug interactions by inhibiting the CYP 450 enzyme system. The potential link between this inhibition and the development of liver failure in some patients is currently under investigation.[137]

Kava should not be taken with other hepatotoxic medications, natural products, or alcohol. Kava may interfere with dopamine transmission, resulting in an interaction with levodopa or worsening of symptoms of parkinsonism;[138] therefore, parkinsonian patients should not use kava.

### *Administration and Product Issues*

Kava-containing products have limited availability because of ongoing concerns about the risk of liver disease.

### *Summary of Clinical Evidence*

Several small studies have reported kava extracts to be superior to placebo for short-term treatment of anxiety. Many botanical references currently recommend against use of kava until its full potential for hepatotoxicity is completely understood.

## St. John's Wort

*Hypericum perforatum* L. is a perennial with more than 400 species that grows wild throughout Europe, Asia, North America, and South America. The yellow flowers and the leaves contain the highest levels of medicinally useful compounds. St. John's wort (SJW) is classified in the Clusiaceae family, but may also be listed under the Hypericaceae family.

### *Therapeutic Uses*

SJW is used to treat depression, pain, anxiety, insomnia, and premenstrual syndrome.[3]

### *Physiologic Activity*

Antidepressant activity originally was attributed to hypericin; however, current evidence suggests hyperforin is responsible.[139] Other potential biologically active constituents include flavonoids, tannins, volatile oils, and phenols. SJW may modulate serotonin, dopamine, and norepinephrine. In vitro analysis suggests SJW may also have an affinity for sigma receptors and acts as a receptor antagonist at adenosine, BZDP, GABA, and inositol triphosphate receptors.[139,140]

### *Dosage and Administration Guidelines*

The recommended dosage for adults with mild to moderate depression is hypericum extract 500 to 1050 mg/day.[140] The product should be taken in divided doses with meals.

### *Safety Considerations*

An analysis of randomized trials found rates of adverse effects in patients taking SJW similar to those for placebo. In addition, rates for SJW were much lower, compared with older antidepressants, and slightly lower, compared with selective serotonin receptor inhibitors (SSRIs).[141] The most frequently reported adverse effects included paresthesias, headache, nausea, dry mouth, agitation, and skin reactions. SJW should be avoided in patients with psychiatric illnesses including bipolar disorder and schizophrenia. Photosensitivity reactions in fair-skinned people have also been reported although this may be a dose-related phenomenon. Similar to SSRIs, SJW may cause sexual dysfunction. Abrupt discontinuation after chronic use of SJW may result in withdrawal symptoms similar to those of conventional antidepressants. Unlike many herb-drug interactions discussed in this chapter, interactions with SJW are well documented and clinically significant. SJW contains many compounds that may influence activities of major human drug-metabolizing enzymes, resulting in multiple pharmacokinetic interactions. The specific enzymes, the degree of influence of hypericin versus hyperforin, and in vitro analysis versus clinical outcomes are still under debate. SJW is recognized to be a potent inducer of CYP 3A4, resulting in significantly lower concentrations of drugs metabolized through this pathway. SJW may also induce p-glycoprotein transport proteins that result in lower serum concentrations of drugs such as digoxin.[9] Additional evidence suggests possible induction of CYP 1A2 and CYP 2C9—although to a lesser extent than CYP 3A4.[9] Many drug interactions are based on extrapolating across drug class or metabolic pathway. SJW may also increase the risk of developing serotonin syndrome if taken concurrently with other serotonergic drugs or natural products.

### *Administration and Product Issues*

As with prescription antidepressant agents, therapeutic effects of SJW are not experienced for several weeks. In many cases, depression is not appropriate for self-diagnosis or self-treatment. Patients should be counseled to seek appropriate medical care for this potentially life-threatening condition. Until the significance of potential photosensitivity with SJW is clearly established, patients should limit their exposure to the sun and apply sunscreen.

### *Summary of Clinical Evidence*

Many clinical trials evaluating use of SJW have been published. Comparisons have been made to placebo, light therapy, and traditional antidepressants. Efficacy evaluations also vary from study to study, with rankings of "less than" to "as effective" as traditional agents to treat various degrees of depression (i.e., mild, moderate, severe). In 2000 the American College of Physicians/American Society of Internal Medicine published a critique of newer drug therapies for depression. This review included SJW as a therapeutic option for short-term treatment of mild to moderate depression and suggested that SJW is less likely to cause side effects than commonly prescribed antidepressants.[142] A recent Cochrane review evaluated 26 clinical trials comparing SJW with placebo and 14 studies comparing SJW with standard antidepressants. The authors concluded that withdrawal rates with SJW are lower than those with older antidepressants and similar to those of SSRIs. In addition, the authors indicate that the results vary significantly between studies, with some demonstrating minimal efficacy, while others suggest similar benefits with SJW and traditional antidepressants.[143] A recent study of 251 adults with moderate to severe major depression has reported similar outcomes on the 17-item Hamilton Depression Scale between a standardized extract of hypericum 900 to 1800 mg daily versus paroxetine 20 to 40 mg daily.[144] Research is ongoing on the use of SJW in seasonal affective disorder, alcoholism, somatoform disorders, and wound healing.

## Valerian

Native to Europe and Asia, valerian grows in most parts of the world. More than 200 plant species belong to the genus *Valeriana.* The most common plant used for medicinal purposes is *Valeriana officinalis* L. from the Valerianaceae family.

### Therapeutic Uses

Valerian is used for its sedative properties in alleviating insomnia and anxiety.

### Physiologic Activity

The CNS activity of valerian may be a result of valepotriates and sesquiterpene constituents of the volatile oils.[145] Major sesquiterpenes are valerienic acid, valerenone, and kessyl glycol. Aqueous extracts lacking valepotriates and sesquiterpenes have similar effects, indicating other unidentified, active components may also be involved. Data suggest that sedation from valerian extracts results from interaction with $GABA_A$ receptors in the brain.[146] Valerian may also have barbituratelike CNS depressant effects.

### Dosage and Administration Guidelines

Most clinical trials using valerian for insomnia studied the botanical in a dosage of valerian root extract 400 to 900 mg, administered 30 to 60 minutes before bedtime. Teas can be prepared from dried roots 2 to 3 g (1 tsp) per cup of boiling water.

### Safety Considerations

Valerian products containing little or no valepotriates are generally well tolerated. Side effects may include headache, excitability, and paradoxical insomnia. Cardiac disturbances and BZDP-like withdrawal symptoms have been reported during valerian withdrawal.[147] Residual daytime sedation has been reported with higher doses. *V. officinalis* preparations are considered safe despite the known in vitro cytotoxic activity of valepotriates. Pregnant women should not use valerian because of its potential to induce uterine contractions. Chronic administration of valerian has been linked to hepatotoxicity. Valerian can potentiate the effects of other CNS depressants such as alcohol, opiates, barbiturates, and BZDPs; they should not be taken concomitantly.

### Summary of Clinical Evidence

Small studies from the late 1970s to early 1990s demonstrated a decrease in sleep latency and an increase in sleep quality in patients taking 270 to 1200 mg of valerian per day.[145] While recent evidence suggests *Valerian edulis* improved sleep in intellectually impaired children, an evaluation in older adults found *V. officinalis* to be inferior to temazepam or diphenhydramine.[148,149]

# RESPIRATORY TRACT DISORDERS

Botanicals used for respiratory tract disorders alleviate symptoms of the common cold or improve airway function. Products such as licorice or peppermint are often available in preparations used to soothe cough and sore throat. Butterbur, discussed elsewhere in this chapter, is also commonly used for allergic rhinitis and asthma.

In previous editions of this chapter, ephedra was reviewed in this section because of its decongestant and bronchodilatory properties. In February 2004 the FDA issued a final regulation declaring dietary supplements containing ephedrine alkaloids as adulterated under the Federal Food, Drug and Cosmetic Act.[150] The determination was based on the review required by the Dietary Supplement Health and Education Act, and included information about ephedrine's pharmacology, clinical evidence of safety and effectiveness, and public comments. The FDA concluded that "dietary supplements containing ephedrine alkaloids pose a risk of serious adverse events, including heart attack, stroke, and death, and that these risks are unreasonable in light of any benefits that may result for the use of these products."[150] In April 2005, the U.S. District court in Utah ruled against FDA's withdrawal of ephedra, stating that the agency had not proven the herbal was unsafe in low doses.[151] As of August 2005, the status of ephedra remains uncertain. This section no longer includes a review of ephedra, but instead has added a botanical product considered to be an "ephedra alternative."

## Bitter Orange

*Citrus aurantium* L. is a member of the Rutaceae family. This small tree produces citrus fruit considered too bitter for casual consumption.

### Therapeutic Uses

Bitter orange was originally used for digestive disorders in Asian medicine. It is also now used as a nasal decongestant and weight-loss agent.

### Physiologic Activity

Bitter orange contains many active constituents including synephrine, octopamine, and methyltyramine.[152] Similar to phenylephrine, these compounds act as a decongestant by stimulating the $\alpha$-adrenergic receptors, which causes vasoconstriction and decreases vascular leakage into the sinuses. Bitter orange may act as an indirect $\beta$-agonist, causing an increased heart rate and possibly minor bronchodilation.[152]

### Dosage and Administration Guidelines

There are no dosage recommendations for bitter orange as a decongestant or weight-loss agent. One clinical trial assessing a multi-ingredient product's effect on weight loss included a daily dose of 975 mg bitter orange extract in combination with SJW and caffeine.[153] The amount of bitter orange in commercial products range between 50 and 500 mg per dosage unit.

### *Safety Considerations*

The adverse effects from bitter orange products may be similar to those of other adrenergic stimulants, including cardiovascular and CNS stimulation resulting in hypertension, myocardial infarction, seizure, and stroke. One report has been published of a myocardial infarction occurring in a patient with no history of cardiac disease who took a supplement containing 300 mg bitter orange in addition to other stimulants such as guarana and green tea.[152] The Seventh Report of the Joint National Committee of Prevention, Detection, Evaluation and Treatment of High Blood Pressure lists bitter orange as a possible cause of resistant hypertension.[154] Photosensitivity is also a possible adverse effect. Bitter orange juice may inhibit intestinal CYP 3A4 isoenzymes in a manner similar to that of grapefruit juice, resulting in elevated drug levels and adverse effects. Concomitant use with other stimulant drugs including pseudoephedrine and caffeine may increase risk of adverse cardiac and CNS events. Patients using monoamine oxidase inhibitors should also avoid bitter orange-containing products.

### *Administration and Product Issues*

Bitter orange products range in concentration from 1% to 6% synephrine. There have been reports of some manufacturers increasing the concentration of synephrine to 30%. Bitter orange is often found with other stimulant- or caffeine-containing herbs including cola nut, green tea, and guarana. These combinations may increase the risk of stimulant-related adverse effects.

### *Summary of Clinical Evidence*

Clinical trials evaluating the use of bitter orange in respiratory conditions are not available.

## Slippery Elm

A member of the Ulmaceae family, slippery elm is also known as *Ulmus rubra* Muhl. or *Ulmus fulva* Michx. and is obtained from the reddish-brown inner bark of the sweet elm, a deciduous tree that grows in North America.

### *Therapeutic Uses*

Slippery elm is used to soothe sore throats. Other uses include soothing of and prophylaxis against stomach and duodenal ulcers, gastritis, and colitis. Topically, slippery elm has been used as a treatment for burns, wounds, chapped lips, and toothaches. It is also found in some baby foods and adult nutritional supplements.

### *Physiologic Activity*

The inner bark of slippery elm is high in mucilage, primarily consisting of a water-soluble polysaccharide, bioflavonoids, vitamin E, starch, and small amounts of tannins. The mucilage polysaccharides contribute to the demulcent and emollient properties of slippery elm.

### *Dosage and Administration Guidelines*

Slippery elm is available in lozenges, to be used as needed.

### *Safety Considerations*

Most common adverse effects are allergic reactions and possible contact dermatitis. There are no known drug interactions although theoretically slippery elm may slow absorption of oral medication by means of its "coating" action.[3]

### *Administration and Product Issues*

Commercially prepared lozenges and troches are the preferred products because they provide sustained exposure of the mucilage to the throat. Patients should be aware of additional ingredients present in combination products. Additional botanicals in these products include marshmallow root, Icelandic moss, mullein flowers, mallow leaf and flower, and plantain. Herbal expectorants may also include licorice and white horehound.

### *Summary of Clinical Evidence*

The herb is considered safe and effective for soothing sore throats although clinical studies of the safety and efficacy of slippery elm products are not available.

# SKIN AND MUCOUS MEMBRANE CONDITIONS

Botanicals have been used to treat skin and mucous membrane conditions for many years. Many botanicals continue to be used as part of combination products.

## Aloe Vera Gel (Topical)

Aloe vera gel is obtained from the center of the leaf of *Aloe vera* (L.) N. L. Burm., a member of the lily family Liliaceae.

### *Therapeutic Uses*

Topically aloe vera is used for burns and wound healing, inflammation, itching, and arthritis. Orally, aloe vera products have been used for digestive disorders, mucositis secondary to radiation, diabetes, and immune stimulation.

### *Physiologic Activity*

The mucilaginous gel obtained from the inner leaf consists primarily of several types of polysaccharides that may be responsible for antiviral, antibacterial, and antifungal properties. Carboxypeptidase and salicylate components of the gel may inhibit bradykinin and reduce pain, whereas magnesium lactate may inhibit histamine and reduce itching. Aloe may also inhibit formation of thromboxane.[155]

### Dosage and Administration Guidelines

Aloe gel is applied topically, as necessary.

### Safety Considerations

No precautions are noted when aloe is used externally. Adverse effects may include allergic responses, contact dermatitis, and urticaria. Aloe is contraindicated in patients with allergies to plants in the *Liliaceae* family. Application of aloe vera gel with topical steroids may increase their absorption.

### Administration and Product Issues

Controversy exists as to whether aloe retains its skin-soothing properties during storage.

### Summary of Clinical Evidence

Evidence suggests that application of aloe vera may not be effective for treating sunburn and may actually impair healing of more severe burns and wounds.[156,157] A 0.5% aloe vera extract cream applied three times daily for 4 weeks improved mild to moderate psoriasis, compared with placebo. The benefits persisted for almost a year after treatment was stopped.[158] A similar cream formulation applied three times daily for 5 days reduced lesion healing time in genital herpes.[159]

## Goldenseal

Goldenseal is from the plant *Hydrastis canadensis* L. From the Ranunculaceae family, it is most famous for its rumored ability to mask the presence of illicit drugs in urine. This belief is based on a novel written by a pharmacist in 1900.[160]

### Therapeutic Uses

Goldenseal has been used orally to treat the common cold, gastritis, diarrhea, urinary tract infections, hemorrhoids, and fever. The botanical is used topically as a mouthwash for sore gums and mouth, skin rashes, ulcers, wound infections, itching, eczema, acne, dandruff, ringworm, and herpes blisters.

### Physiologic Activity

Goldenseal contains berberine, hydrastine, canadine, canadaline, hyrastidine, and berberastine. These compounds are isolated most often from the rhizome and root. The alkaloids isolated from goldenseal have weak antimicrobial activity and antioxidant properties.[161]

### Dosage and Administration Guidelines

The most commonly used oral dosage is dried root 0.5 to 2 g three times daily. As a mouthwash or other topical agent, goldenseal can be prepared by boiling 6 g of the dried herb in 150 mL of water for 5 to 10 minutes. Infusions should be used within 24 hours and not stored in the refrigerator longer.

### Safety Considerations

Goldenseal can cause nausea, anxiety, depression, paralysis, and seizures.[161] It may also increase sensitivity to sunlight. Topical doses can cause irritation and ulceration of the mucous membranes. Pregnant women should avoid goldenseal because of its possible oxytocic activity. Goldenseal may inhibit CYP 3A4 and CYP 2D6 isoenzymes according to an in vivo study in healthy volunteers.[162] Goldenseal may interact with antihypertensives, CNS depressants, and antiarrhythmics.[9]

### Administration and Product Issues

Goldenseal products are expensive and often adulterated because of the scarcity of goldenseal.

### Summary of Clinical Evidence

No clinical trials documenting goldenseal's ability to treat any of the conditions mentioned here have been published.

## Melissa (Lemon Balm)

Melissa is derived from the plant *Melissa officinalis* L. of the family Lamiaceae.

### Therapeutic Uses

Melissa is used commonly as a topical cream for cold sores (herpes labialis) and orally for relaxation, AD, insomnia, or nervous stomach. It is inhaled as a part of aromatherapy.

### Physiologic Activity

Melissa's effects may be a result of volatile oils extracted from the plant's leaves that are believed to have sedative, antioxidant, and antiviral effects. Preliminary research suggests orally administered lemon balm may have acetylcholine receptor activity.[163]

### Dosage and Administration Guidelines

For herpetic lesions, studies have used a cream or ointment containing 1% of a 70:1 lyophilized aqueous extract, which is applied two to four times daily at first sign of symptoms until after all lesions heal. If a topical product is not available, a tea can be made by steeping 2 to 3 tsp of crushed leaf in 150 mL of boiling water and applied with a cotton ball.

### Safety Considerations

Hypersensitivity reactions have been associated with topical application. Theoretically, concomitant use of herbs and medications with sedating properties should not be combined with oral ingestion of lemon balm.

#### Administration and Product Issues

Treatment of herpes with melissa does not alter the ability to transmit the infection to others.

#### Summary of Clinical Evidence

In the treatment of oral herpes, application of melissa cream produced significant benefits by reducing the intensity of discomfort as well as the number and size of lesions. Long-term follow-up suggested that chronic application also delays the time to the next herpes flare-up.[164,165] Orally administered lemon balm is also being investigated for use in AD.[166]

### Tea Tree Oil

Tea tree oil is derived from leaves of the tree, *Melaleuca alternifolia* (Maiden & Betche) Cheel from the family Myrtaceae.

#### Therapeutic Uses

Tea tree oil has been used as an antiseptic and anti-infective.

#### Physiologic Activity

Tea tree leaves contain about 2% of volatile oil, with more than 100 monoterpenenoid, sesquiterpenoid, and alcohol compounds. The primary constituent is terpinen-4-ol, which is active against pathogenic bacteria and fungi.

#### Dosage and Administration Guidelines

The oil is applied topically once or twice daily in solution concentrations of 0.4% to 100%, depending on the condition and area of treatment. For acne, a 5% concentration is applied daily. For athlete's foot, tea tree oil 10% cream is applied daily for as many as 4 to 8 weeks. For fungal toenail infections, tea tree oil 100% has been used twice daily for 6 months.

#### Safety Considerations

Skin irritation may occur in sensitive patients. Although the oil can be safely used on oral mucosa, it should not be swallowed because ingesting even small amounts may cause confusion, ataxia, and systemic contact dermatitis that resolve very slowly.

#### Administration and Product Issues

The tea tree is not related to the plant that is used to make black and green teas.

#### Summary of Clinical Evidence

Preliminary studies have found that tea tree oil may be an effective treatment for athlete's foot and other fungal infections of the skin and nails.[167] In the treatment of acne, daily application of a tea tree oil gel 5% for 3 months appeared to reduce the average number of lesions at a rate similar to that of benzoyl peroxide 5% but with less irritation.[168] Tea tree oil may be effective in the treatment of *Candida* vaginal infections.

### Witch Hazel

Witch hazel (*Hamamelis virginiana* L.), a deciduous shrub native to North America, is commercially cultivated in Europe. In the United States, distilled witch hazel extract is available, whereas in Europe the hydroalcoholic extracts are commonly used. The shrub is a species of the Hamamelidaceae family.

#### Therapeutic Uses

Witch hazel has been used both externally and internally although it is currently recommended only for external use. It has been taken internally for diarrhea, colitis, and tuberculosis, among other uses.

#### Physiologic Activity

Witch hazel leaves and bark contain various tannins. Although tannins may be responsible for the astringent and styptic properties, the distilled product contains almost no active tannins. Alcohol provides the astringent effect. When applied to broken skin or mucous membranes, witch hazel tannins induce protein precipitation that tightens up superficial cell layers and shrinks colloidal structures. This action, in turn, causes capillary vasoconstriction, thereby decreasing vascular permeability and inflammation. The astringent action on tissues provides a less than favorable environment for bacterial growth.

#### Dosage and Administration Guidelines

Witch hazel preparations are applied topically, as needed for the described disorders.

#### Safety Considerations

Oral use might cause stomach irritation and liver damage. Topical use may result in contact dermatitis.

#### Administration and Product Issues

Most commercially available witch hazel preparations are a mixture of alcohol 14% in water with only a trace amount of the volatile water.

#### Summary of Clinical Evidence

Little clinical trial data are available. Witch hazel's astringent effects are useful for treating minor skin injuries and relieving the itch, irritation, and pain of hemorrhoids and after anal surgery.

## WOMEN'S HEALTH

Women are more likely than men to use complementary and alternative medicine.[1] The botanical medications are commonly used for treatment of premenstrual and menopausal symptoms. A population-based survey reported over 75% of women used an alternative therapy for their menopausal symptoms.[169] Black cohosh, evening primrose oil, and phytoestrogens are among the most common botanicals used for vasomotor symptoms.[170]

## Black Cohosh

Black cohosh is made from the dried rhizome and roots of *Cimicifuga racemosa* (L.) Nutt., formerly *Actaea racemosa.* It is a member of the Ranunculaceae family.

### *Therapeutic Uses*

Traditionally black cohosh has been used to treat the symptoms of premenstrual syndrome (PMS), dysmenorrhea, menopause, and rheumatoid arthritis.[3]

### *Physiologic Activity*

The primary active components of black cohosh rhizomes are triterpene glycosides, including acetein and cimicifugoside (cimigoside). Isoflavones such as formononetin may be present although they may be absent from commercial products.[3] Other constituents include isoferulic and salicylic acids, tannins, resin, starch, and sugars. Although the issue is controversial, black cohosh probably does not exhibit estrogenic activity.[171]

### *Dosage and Administration Guidelines*

Black cohosh, as a standardized extract, is usually administered in two 20 mg tablets twice daily.[172]

### *Safety Considerations*

Black cohosh is well tolerated. Side effects are mild, with GI complaints, headache, rash, and weight gain occurring occasionally. Hepatitis, seizures, and cardiovascular disease have been reported in patients taking multiple herbal products including black cohosh.[173] A case report of autoimmune hepatitis associated with black cohosh was published recently.[174] The use of black cohosh longer than 6 months is not recommended because of the lack of long-term safety studies. Clinical data on drug interactions with black cohosh is limited. Preliminary evidence suggests that the botanical may have additive effects with tamoxifen and may increase the toxicity of doxorubicin and docetaxel.[3] A recent review identified potential interactions with iron, digoxin, and antihypertensive agents.[9]

### *Administration and Product Issues*

The most commonly used commercial preparation is Remifemin. The preparation is standardized to 20 mg of the root per tablet, consisting of 1 mg of terpene glycosides.[172]

### *Summary of Clinical Evidence*

Since publication of the Women's Health Initiative, interest in black cohosh as a "natural" alternative to estrogen replacement therapy (ERT) has increased.[175] Remifemin has been used in small, short-term clinical trials for menopausal symptoms. The use of validated outcome measures has varied. A 6-month study of 150 peri- and postmenopausal women showed that 40 mg daily provided the same symptom relief as 120 mg daily. Although symptoms were relieved in 70% of the subjects regardless of dose, the study was not placebo controlled. No evidence of estrogenic effects from the product was detected.[176] A more recent randomized placebo-controlled study by the same investigators enrolled 304 women and demonstrated symptomatic relief of vasomotor symptoms, especially in women earlier in the peri- and postmenopausal period. The study used 40 mg daily of a standardized isopropanolic extract of black cohosh root.[177] The safety and efficacy of black cohosh in women who have had breast cancer remain controversial.[3,171] A study of breast cancer survivors failed to find a difference between black cohosh and placebo in reducing the number or intensity of hot flashes. Levels of follicle-stimulating hormone and luteinizing hormone were similar in the two groups.[178] The North American Menopause Society recommends a trial of nonprescription products such as black cohosh for mild vasomotor symptoms. Their position statement acknowledges that the clinical trial data are insufficient, but supports short-term use because of the overall safety profile.[179] The long-term effects of black cohosh on cardiovascular disease, osteoporosis, and breast cancer are unknown.

## Chastetree Berry

Chastetree (*Vitex agnus-castus* L.), commonly referred to as vitex, is a member of the Verbenaceae family. The dried ripe fruits or berries and the leaves are the medicinally useful parts of the plant.

### *Therapeutic Uses*

Chastetree berry has been used to treat symptoms of PMS, dysmenorrhea, mastalgia, and menopausal symptoms.

### *Physiologic Activity*

The fruits contain various flavonoids including casticin, orientin, and quercetagetin. Progesterone-related compounds may be present.[3] The dried fruits also contain an essential oil (up to 1.22%).

### *Dosage and Administration Guidelines*

The dosage of chastetree berry is variable and depends on the individual product.

### *Safety Considerations*

Chastetree berry is generally well tolerated, with GI complaints occurring occasionally. Other symptoms include headache, rashes, itching, and agitation.[3] Chastetree berry potentially may interact with dopamine antagonists such as haloperidol and oral contraceptives, but this has not been documented.[3]

### Administration and Product Issues

No issues are known.

### Summary of Clinical Evidence

Chastetree berry has some efficacy in improving symptoms associated with PMS. A double-blind study of 170 women with PMS compared the effect of chastetree berry extract daily with placebo on mood, breast fullness, and other symptoms over three menstrual cycles. The results indicated that chastetree berry extract improved the main symptom scores and had a significantly greater overall response rate than placebo. Symptoms improved in 24% of women taking placebo compared with 52% of women taking the botanical.[180] This study was well designed, with a placebo group, a large number of women with PMS using established diagnostic criteria, descriptive data on the study groups at baseline, and a method of scoring symptoms.

## Evening Primrose Oil, Black Currant Oil, Borage Seed Oil

Evening primrose (*Oenothera biennis* L.) is a member of the primrose family Onagraceae and is used for its high content of essential fatty acids. The seed oils of black currant (*Ribes nigrum* L.) and borage (*Borago officinalis* L.) are also used for similar purposes.

### Therapeutic Uses

Evening primrose oil (EPO) has been used for mastalgia, symptoms of PMS and menopause, preeclampsia, diabetic neuropathy, and chronic fatigue syndrome.

### Physiologic Activity

The oil from evening primrose seeds consists of at least 85% to 92% unsaturated fatty acids. Most of the polyunsaturated fatty acids are the essential *cis*-linoleic acid (LA) and the rare *cis*-gamma-linolenic acid (GLA) forms. The seed oil contains smaller amounts of palmitic, oleic, and stearic acids, as well as steroids, including campesterol and β-sitosterol.

### Dosage and Administration Guidelines

For symptoms of PMS, daily doses of EPO 2 to 4 g have been used.

### Safety Considerations

EPO is generally well tolerated, with headache, nausea, diarrhea, and abdominal pain occurring occasionally.[3] Use of EPO for cervical ripening during labor may be associated with adverse pregnancy outcomes including prolonged rupture of membranes and vacuum extraction.[181] EPO products may possess antiplatelet effects, and patients taking warfarin and other platelet-active drugs or herbs should use this botanical with caution.[3] Concurrent use with phenothiazines potentially may result in seizures.[3]

### Administration and Product Issues

Depending on the brand, the oil contains a minimum of 8% to 12% GLA.

### Summary of Clinical Evidence

Despite its widespread use, study results with EPO for PMS have been contradictory and inconsistent. A recent study of 120 women with severe mastalgia failed to demonstrate a difference between EPO and its control oil on the number of days with breast pain.[182]

## Phytoestrogens

Unlike other botanicals, phytoestrogens are derived from many different plants.

### Therapeutic Uses

Phytoestrogens, including soy and red clover products, have been used primarily for symptoms associated with menopause. Preliminary evidence suggests that phytoestrogens may have a role in preventing prostate cancer

### Physiologic Activity

Phytoestrogen supplements have been derived primarily from soy (*Glycine max* [L.] Merrill) and red clover (*Trifolium pratense* L.). Soy-based phytoestrogens may include isoflavones such as genistein, daidzein, and glycitein. Red clover-based products may include biochanin, genistein, daidzein, and formononetin.[3] These compounds have multiple complex effects including estrogenic, antiestrogenic, antioxidant, and anticancer activity.

### Dosage and Administration Guidelines

A recommended dose of "phytoestrogen" has not been established. Products contain varying amounts and types of isoflavones.

### Safety Considerations

Phytoestrogen products derived from soy or red clover are generally well tolerated. GI complaints, headaches, and allergic reactions may occur.[3] The long-term safety of phytoestrogens is unknown, especially with respect to the risk of estrogen-dependent cancers and thromboembolic disease. The safety of phytoestrogen supplements in women with estrogen-receptor-positive breast cancer is unknown, and the supplements should be avoided.[3,183] Coumestans in red clover may increase the risk of bleeding, especially if warfarin and similar drugs are taken concomitantly, although evidence of an interaction is limited. Genistein may counteract the beneficial effect of tamoxifen in slowing breast cancer growth.[184] Daidzein may inhibit the activity of CYP 1A2.[3,9]

### Administration and Product Issues

Products derived from soy and red clover sources may have different effects. The benefits from soy are primarily from dietary sources, not from supplements.

### Summary of Clinical Evidence

Publication of the Women's Health Initiative has suggested that the risks of ERT may outweigh its benefits in some women.[175] Research into safety and efficacy of soy isoflavones is in a period of rapid growth. The purported benefits of phytoestrogens, especially soy-based products, are based on population-based observational studies of dietary patterns in different parts of the world. It is simplistic to think that the lifetime risk of any given disease is related solely to the presence or absence of one dietary component such as isoflavones. A second critical factor is the recognition that the phytoestrogen content in foods, especially of the biologically active isoflavones, will vary significantly even in soy foods, let alone various supplements.

The effect of phytoestrogens on prevention and treatment of breast cancer is unknown. The potential effect likely will depend on the specific isoflavone and whether the cancer is estrogen-receptor positive or negative.[183] Recent animal studies using implanted human breast cancer cells have shown that genistein can support tumor growth.[185]

The ingestion of at least 25 g of soy protein daily as part of a diet low in saturated fat and cholesterol may reduce the risk of coronary heart disease. The effect of phytoestrogen dietary supplements on the risk of myocardial infarction is unclear.

The effect of soy isoflavones on the risk of osteoporosis remains controversial, with contradictory study findings. A recent study of Chinese women indicated that soy may be more beneficial in maintaining bone mineral density, especially in older women and those with lower calcium intake.[186]

The most common use of phytoestrogens is for managing vasomotor symptoms. A recent systematic review that included soy foods and extracts, as well as red clover-based products, reported that hot flushes and other symptoms were not improved.[187] A 3-month study compared two red clover products with placebo in 252 women experiencing at least 35 hot flashes per week. One product contained a higher content of biochanin A and genistein (Promensil), while the other had higher amounts of formononetin and daidzein (Rimostil). The two active products were similar to placebo in reduction of mean daily hot flash count.[188]

## ASSESSMENT OF BOTANICAL MEDICINE USE: A CASE-BASED APPROACH

The clinician should determine a patient's reasons for purchasing a botanical medicine. The appropriateness of supplements for a child, a pregnant woman, or a person of advanced age must be determined. If a medically diagnosed condition is being treated, the clinician should encourage the patient to involve the primary care provider in the use of the supplement, if its use is appropriate. Information about possible allergies to plant materials, current conventional medication use, and comorbidity will help identify possible contraindications to use of the botanical medicine.

If self-treatment with a botanical supplement is appropriate, the clinician should review the length of therapy and recommended dosages with the patient. The efficacy of different dosage forms should also be explained. Cases 53-1 and 53-2 give examples of the assessment of patients who are considering use of a botanical medicine.

### CASE 53-1

| Relevant Evaluation Criteria | Scenario/Model Outcome |
|---|---|
| **Information Gathering** | |
| 1. Gather essential information about the patient's symptoms, including: | |
| a. description of symptom(s) (i.e., nature, onset, duration, severity, associated symptoms) | Patient reports coldlike symptoms including runny nose, sneezing, congestion, and headache. Onset occurred this morning. Symptoms are not very severe at this time but patient has a history of asthma that is usually exacerbated by even mild colds and is looking for something to help prevent this. She has noticed an increase in shortness of breath and need for rescue inhaler (albuterol) in last day or two. |
| b. description of any factors that seem to precipitate, exacerbate, and/or relieve the patient's symptom(s) | She just finished finals and admits to not taking care of herself. Her roommate had a cold about a week ago, so she probably caught it from her. |
| c. description of the patient's efforts to relieve the symptoms | Patient has not taken anything yet. Past efforts of treating symptoms with OTC agents (decongestants, cough suppressants, expectorants, and antihistamines) have not decreased exacerbation of her asthma secondary to her cold symptoms. |

**CASE 53-1 (continued)**

| Relevant Evaluation Criteria | Scenario/Model Outcome |
|---|---|
| 2. Gather essential patient history information: | |
| a. patient's identity | Nancy Harvey |
| b. age, sex, height, and weight | 23 y/o F, 5'1", 122 lb |
| c. patient's occupation | College student |
| d. patient's dietary habits | Normal healthy diet with recent increase in junk food because of final exams |
| e. patient's sleep habits | Stays up late studying and sleeps in according to her class schedule. Recently, she has been missing a lot of sleep while studying for finals. |
| f. concurrent medical conditions, prescription and nonprescription medications, and dietary supplements | Asthma since childhood; triggers: ragweed, daisies, sinusitis, URTIs; multiple hospitalizations, no intubations; albuterol inhaler 1 to 2 puffs 3 times/day as needed asthma; cetirizine (Zyrtec) 1 tablet once daily for allergies |
| g. allergies | NKDA |
| h. history of other adverse reactions to medications | Drinking chamomile tea precipitated severe asthma attack (hospitalization, no intubation). |
| i. other (describe)______ | Nancy says she plans to take echinacea on a daily basis to treat this cold and then continue use chronically to prevent future colds, thus reducing asthma exacerbations.<br>Her last severe asthma exacerbation was about 1 month ago precipitated by allergies. She was on oral steroids for 5 days. PCP also prescribed inhaled steroid, but it didn't help her breath better right away so she stopped using it. |
| **Assessment and Triage** | |
| 3. Differentiate the patient's signs/symptoms and correctly identify the patient's primary problem(s), | Onset of common cold with symptoms of runny nose, sneezing, congestion, and headache; history of URTIs as precipitating factor for worsening of asthma symptoms; lack of compliance with prescribed asthma medications |
| 4. Identify exclusions for self-treatment. | Acute asthma exacerbation not responsive to rescue therapy; evidence of bacterial sinusitis, bronchitis, severe headache or high fever |
| 5. Formulate a comprehensive list of therapeutic alternatives for the primary problem to determine if triage to a medical practitioner is required, and share this information with the patient. | Options include:<br>(1) Refer Nancy to her PCP or campus' health clinic.<br>(2) Suggest classic OTC agents for symptoms in addition to lifestyle modifications.<br>(3) Counsel/discuss effect of using steroid inhaler on preventing the worsening of her asthma symptoms.<br>(4) Assist patient in selecting an echinacea or other botanical immune-boosting product.<br>(5) Take no action. |
| **Plan** | |
| 6. Select an optimal therapeutic alternative to address the patient's problem, taking into account patient preferences. | Suggest classic OTC agents for symptoms. Discuss regular use of the steroid inhaler to prevent worsening of her asthma symptoms, particularly when she has a cold. |
| 7. Describe the recommended therapeutic approach to the patient. | You should use OTC cold products for your specific symptoms (i.e., antihistamines for sneezing and runny nose, decongestant for congestion, and acetaminophen for headache). Lifestyle modifications include proper rest, adequate fluids, and balanced diet. Wash your hands frequently and/or use antibacterial lotions/gels to reduce transmission of cold viruses. Begin using your steroid inhaler as directed by your primary care provider; use it regularly as it is the cornerstone of asthma therapy. Return for reassessment in 1-2 weeks or sooner if symptoms worsen. |
| 8. Explain to the patient the rationale for selecting the recommended therapeutic approach from the considered therapeutic alternatives. | OTC agents for specific symptoms will help with the most bothersome symptoms. Proper use of control medications (i.e., steroid inhaler) will help prevent asthma exacerbations and reduce the need for albuterol. Given your history of seasonal allergies and dramatic reaction to chamomile tea, you should avoid botanical products. Chronic use of echinacea will not reduce frequency of colds and may be dangerous for you. You may need to see your primary care provider if your asthma worsens despite recommended treatment. |

## CASE 53-1 (continued)

| Relevant Evaluation Criteria | Scenario/Model Outcome |
|---|---|
| **Patient Education** | |
| 9. When recommending self-care with nonprescription medications and/or nondrug therapy, convey accurate information to the patient, including: | |
| a. appropriate dose and frequency of administration | See instructions for individual OTC ingredients. |
| b. maximum number of days the therapy should be employed | Take OTC products for cold symptoms for only 7-10 days as needed. Use steroid inhaler on a regular basis. Apply lifestyle modifications daily. |
| c. product administration procedures | Proper inhaler technique |
| d. expected time to onset of relief | With usage of medication and proper lifestyle modifications, you should see noticeable improvement in your cold symptoms within the next few days. The steroid inhaler will take at least 2 weeks for full effect. |
| e. degree of relief that can be reasonably expected | Complete relief from symptoms, no asthma exacerbations |
| f. most common side effects | See instructions for individual OTC ingredients. |
| g. side effects that warrant medical intervention should they occur | Worsening asthma symptoms. Also see side effects concerning specific cold products. Oral thrush can develop from improper steroid inhaler technique. |
| h. patient options in the event that condition worsens or persists | Consult your primary care provider if the condition does not improve or asthma worsens. |
| i. product storage requirements | Keep all products in appropriate storage area away from heat and out of children's reach. |
| j. specific nondrug measures | Rinse mouth after using steroid inhaler. Drink plenty of fluids. |
| 10. Solicit follow-up questions from patient. | What might happen if I take an echinacea product anyway? |
| 11. Answer patient's questions. | You could have a hypersensitivity reaction that may cause severe exacerbation of your asthma. |

Key: OTC, over-the-counter; URTI, upper respiratory tract infection; NKDA, no known drug allergies; PCP, primary care provider.

## CASE 53-2

| Relevant Evaluation Criteria | Scenario/Model Outcome |
|---|---|
| **Information Gathering** | |
| 1. Gather essential information about the patient's symptoms, including: | |
| a. description of symptom(s) (i.e., nature, onset, duration, severity, associated symptoms) | Patient presented to physician (urologist) complaining of symptoms consistent with BPH, including increased urination frequency, nocturia, and reduced flow/weak urinary stream. After much testing, patient was diagnosed with BPH. Patient is interested in botanical product for BPH. |
| b. description of any factors that seem to precipitate, exacerbate, and/or relieve the patient's symptom(s) | N/A |
| c. description of the patient's efforts to relieve the symptoms | N/A |
| 2. Gather essential patient history information: | |
| a. patient's identity | John Adcock |
| b. age, sex, height, and weight | 65 y/o M, 5'9", 218 lb |

| CASE 53-2 (continued) | |
|---|---|
| **Relevant Evaluation Criteria** | **Scenario/Model Outcome** |
| c. patient's occupation | Newly retired |
| d. patient's dietary habits | Regular low fat, low sodium |
| e. patient's sleep habits | Gets up multiple times during the night to urinate |
| f. concurrent medical conditions, prescription and nonprescription medications, and dietary supplements | None at this time; takes one multivitamin per day |
| g. allergies | NKDA |
| h. history of other adverse reactions to medications | None |
| i. other (describe)_______ | John has heard many bad things about prescription medications for BPH, and his friend successfully used saw palmetto for his BPH. John's physician said he could try a botanical product. |
| **Assessment and Triage** | |
| 3. Differentiate the patient's signs/symptoms and correctly identify the patient's primary problem(s). | Symptomatic BPH as diagnosed by urologist |
| 4. Identify exclusions for self-treatment. | Urinary symptoms without evaluation by doctor or urologist |
| 5. Formulate a comprehensive list of therapeutic alternatives for the primary problem to determine if triage to a medical practitioner is required, and share this information with the patient. | Options include:<br>(1) Refer John back to physician for prescription medication.<br>(2) Assist John in selecting a proper botanical product.<br>(3) Take no action. |
| **Plan** | |
| 6. Select an optimal therapeutic alternative to address the patient's problem, taking into account patient preferences. | Assist with selection of reputable saw palmetto product. |
| 7. Describe the recommended therapeutic approach to the patient. | Take product twice daily. Pay attention to symptoms and follow up with physician as directed. |
| 8. Explain to the patient the rationale for selecting the recommended therapeutic approach from the considered therapeutic alternatives. | You can try saw palmetto because you have already been assessed by a physician and other potential genitourinary problems have been ruled out. The physician approved treatment with a botanical product. |
| **Patient Education** | |
| 9. When recommending self-care with nonprescription medications and/or nondrug therapy, convey accurate information to the patient, including: | |
| a. appropriate dose and frequency of administration | 160 mg saw palmetto extract taken twice daily with morning and evening meal to minimize side effects |
| b. maximum number of days the therapy should be employed | Use product continuously while being monitored by physician or other health care provider. |
| c. product administration procedures | Whenever possible, always purchase products from the same manufacturer. |
| d. expected time to onset of relief | May take up to 10 weeks to see full effect |
| e. degree of relief that can be reasonably expected | Potentially could achieve complete resolution of symptoms |

## CASE 53-2 (continued)

| Relevant Evaluation Criteria | Scenario/Model Outcome |
|---|---|
| f. most common side effects | Nausea, diarrhea, and vomiting may occur. |
| g. side effects that warrant medical intervention should they occur | Severe GI complaints, intractable vomiting, skin rash |
| h. patient options in the event that condition worsens or persists | Try another herbal product (African plum) or return to physician and try prescription medication. |
| i. product storage requirements | Cool dry place out of reach of children or animals |
| j. specific nondrug measures | Avoid drinking fluids close to bedtime. |
| 10. Solicit follow-up questions from patient. | Can this product have sexual side effects? |
| 11. Answer patient's questions. | Clinical studies have shown that saw palmetto had a lower rate of sexual side effects, compared with finasteride, a prescription treatment commonly used for BPH. Never be afraid to discuss these concerns with your physician or other health care provider. |

Key: BPH, benign prostatic hyperplasia; N/A, not applicable; NKDA, no known drug allergies.

## PATIENT COUNSELING FOR BOTANICAL MEDICINES

The use of botanical medicines has continued to grow over the last 10 to 15 years, presenting many challenges and opportunities for clinicians, especially in the ambulatory care setting. The most important issue is to encourage a culture of respect for the patient's beliefs and values so that a trusting, nonjudgmental relationship can develop. Patients must feel comfortable sharing their use of botanical and other natural products with the clinician. (For a complete discussion of counseling issues, refer to the introductory section for Chapters 53 and 54.) With botanical medicines, clinicians should also be aware of the potential for interactions with prescription or OTC medications (Table 53-1) and for cross-sensitivity reactions in patients with ragweed allergy (Table 53-2).

**TABLE 53-1 Selected Herb–Drug Interactions**

| Herb | Interaction/Results | Theoretical Interactions/Results |
|---|---|---|
| Aloe vera gel | Topical steroids: possible increased absorption of steroids | |
| Andrographis | | Possible additive effects if taken with other platelet-active drugs or herbs; possible interaction with immunosuppressant drugs related to herb's immunostimulating properties |
| Bitter orange | Decongestants: additive stimulant effects<br>Dextromethorphan: increased DM levels<br>Felodipine: increased felodipine levels | Intestinal CYP 3A4 inhibitor similar to grapefruit juice; possible hypertensive crisis if taken with MAOIs |
| Chamomile | | Reported anaphylaxis possibly more common than previously thought; clinical significance of preliminary evidence suggesting decreased CYP 1A2 and 3A4 activity unknown |
| Chastetree berry | | Minimal evidence for possible interference with hormonal contraceptives |
| Cranberry | | Possible increased INR and risk of bleeding in people on warfarin; possible CYP 2C9 inhibition |
| Echinacea | | Possible interaction with immunomodulating therapies; clinical support lacking for in vitro analysis suggesting CYP 3A4 inhibition |
| *Eleutherococcus* (Siberian ginseng) | Digoxin: possible false elevation in plasma levels (assay dependent) | SMBG recommended in patients taking antihyperglycemic medications |

**TABLE 53-1 Selected Herb–Drug Interactions (continued)**

| Herb | Interaction/Results | Theoretical Interactions/Results |
|---|---|---|
| Evening primrose oil | | Possible additive effects if taken with other platelet-active drugs or herbs; seizure possible if taken with phenothiazines |
| Feverfew | | Possible additive effects if taken with other platelet-active drugs or herbs |
| Garlic | Warfarin: increased INR in case reports; 50% decrease in levels of saquinavir | Contradictory evidence regarding induction of drugs metabolized through CYP 3A4 and 2D6 |
| Ginger | Platelet-active drugs: possible additive effect | |
| Ginkgo | Platelet-active drugs: possible additive effect<br>Trazodone: case report of coma in patient taking low-dose trazodone | Ingestion associated with seizures; avoid in patients with a history of seizures or on drugs that may lower seizure threshold; clinical impact of preliminary evidence suggesting ginkgo leaf extract may affect CYP 1A2, 2D6, and 3A4 has not been determined |
| Ginseng | Glucose-lowering medications: possible lowered BG levels in type 2 DM; careful monitoring of BG levels required<br>Phenelzine: possible headache, tremor, and mania in case report; cause of effect (herb or other factors) unclear | Unpredictable effect on concurrent anticoagulant and antiplatelet therapy |
| Goldenseal | | Possible inhibition of CYP 3A4 and 2D6, per in vivo studies |
| Grape seed/ pine bark | | Possible interaction with immunosuppressant drugs related to pycnogenol's immunostimulating properties |
| Green tea | Decongestants: additive stimulant effects | Possible antagonism of warfarin's effect; possible antagonism of concurrent sedatives related to caffeine content |
| Hawthorn | Cardiac medications: possible interactions herbs or drugs that contain cardiac glycosides (digoxin) | Possible interference with digoxin levels |
| Horse chestnut | Platelet-active drugs: possible additive effects if taken with other platelet-active drugs or herbs | Limited available evidence supports concern HCSE may lower blood glucose |
| Huperzine A | | Possible decreased effectiveness if taken with anticholinergic drug such as benztropine; possible additive cholinergic effects if taken with other acetylcholinesterase inhibitors (donepezil) or cholinergic agents (bethanechol); additive effects if taken with drugs causing bradycardia |
| Kava | Levodopa: reduced efficacy of levodopa; concern over kava's possible hepatotoxic effect contraindicates use with other drugs and herbs that damage liver | Possible increased sedative effect with alcohol and other CNS depressants; possible additive effects with other platelet-active drugs or herbs |
| Licorice | | Significance of in vitro studies suggesting possible decreased activity of CYP 1A2, 2D6, and 3A4 unknown; possible licorice-induced hypokalemia increases risk for digoxin toxicity; efficacy of antihypertensive agents possibly reduced by sodium and water retention; possible increased potassium loss and risk of potassium depletion if taken with potassium-depleting drugs |
| Melissa | | Concomitant use of oral lemon balm and sedating herbs and drugs contraindicated |
| Milk thistle | | Effect on activity of CYP 3A4 and 2C9 in vitro unclear |
| Peppermint | Decreased absorption of iron salts; premature dissolution of enteric-coated peppermint oil by drugs that increase gastric pH | Significance of decreased activity of CYP 3A4 in vitro and in vivo studies unknown |
| Phytoestrogen | | Possible increased risk of bleeding in patients taking warfarin with red clover–based products |
| Plantago | | Concurrent ingestion with medications may alter absorption of other drugs and minerals |

**TABLE 53-1 Selected Herb–Drug Interactions (continued)**

| Herb | Interaction/Results | Theoretical Interactions/Results |
|---|---|---|
| Slippery elm | | Concurrent ingestion with medications may alter absorption of drugs because of coating action |
| St. John's wort | Alprazolam: ↓ drug effect<br>Amitriptyline: possible ↓ serum levels of amitriptyline and nortriptyline<br>Antidepressants: ↑ risk of serotonin syndromes with nefazodone, sertraline, and paroxetine<br>Cyclosporine: ↓ blood levels of immunosuppressant, including case reports of transplant graft rejection<br>Digoxin: ↓ serum levels<br>Imatinib: ↓ serum levels<br>Irinotecan: ↓ blood levels<br>Morphine: ↑ narcotic-induced sleep time in animal studies<br>Nifedipine: >50% ↓ in serum concentration of nifedipine<br>Oral contraceptives: breakthrough bleeding and reported unplanned pregnancies, possibly resulting from this interaction<br>Simvastatin: ↓ drug levels<br>Tacrolimus: ↓ therapeutic levels<br>Theophylline: possible ↓ levels<br>Protease inhibitors and nonnucleoside reverse transcriptase inhibitors: possible ↓ serum levels<br>Warfarin: possible ↓ effect related to subtherapeutic INR | Possible ↑ risk of serotonin syndrome if taken with 5-$HT_1$ agonists ("triptans"), DM, meperidine, pentazocine, and tramadol; interaction possibly similar to conventional antidepressants and MAOIs with ↑ potential for hypertension, hyperthermia, agitation, and coma; possible ↓ levels and effect of amiodarone; monitoring for fexofenadine toxicity recommended if taken concomitantly; use with other photosensitizing agents contraindicated |
| Uva-ursi | | Conversion of herb to the active hydroquinone inhibited by urinary acidifiers, possible loss of efficacy |
| Valerian | | Possible ↑ sedative effect if taken with alcohol or other CNS depressants (BZDPs, opioids, kava) |

Key: BG, blood glucose; BZDP, benzodiazepine; CNS, central nervous system; CYP, cytochrome P450; DM, dextromethorphan; 5-$HT_1$, 5-hydroxytryptamine$_1$; HCSE, horse chestnut seed extract; INR, international normalized ratio; MAOI, monoamine oxidase inhibitor; SMBG, self-monitoring of blood glucose.

**TABLE 53-2 Selected Herbs With Potential Cross-sensitivity in Patients With Ragweed Allergy**

| | |
|---|---|
| Arnica | Milk thistle |
| Calendula | Mugwort |
| Dandelion | Pyrethrum |
| Echinacea | Stevia |
| Feverfew | Tansy |
| German chamomile | Wormwood oil |
| Goldenrod | Yarrow |
| March blazing star | |

## KEY POINTS FOR BOTANICAL MEDICINES

- Use of botanical medicines has increased significantly over the last 10 to 15 years.
- Clinical research has compared botanical medicines with prescription drugs for prevention and treatment of common conditions.
- Some botanicals, such as ginger and saw palmetto, have evidence of safety and efficacy, while others, including huperzine A, demonstrate promise.
- Botanical medicines have also demonstrated significant adverse effects and drug interactions.
- Concerns remain regarding commercial availability of the studied product to the typical American consumer.

- Patients and clinicians must communicate clearly to ensure safe use of these products.
- Patients must recognize that "natural" does not always mean "safe." Clinicians must take advantage of the fact that patients use botanicals because they want greater involvement in their own health care and are increasingly interested in health promotion and disease prevention.
- Safe and effective use of botanical products, especially in patients taking prescription and nonprescription drugs for chronic diseases, requires a partnership between patients and clinicians.

## References


1. Barnes PM, Powell-Griner E, McFann K, et al. Complementary and alternative medicine use among adults: United States, 2002. *Adv Data.* 2004; 343:1-19.
2. Nemecz G, Combest WL. Herbal remedies. In: Allen LV, Berardi RR, DeSimone EM, et al., eds. *Handbook of Nonprescription Drugs.* 12th ed. Washington, DC: American Pharmaceutical Association; 2001:953-82.
3. Memorial Sloan Kettering website. Available at: http://www.mskcc.org/mskcc/html/11570.cfm. Accessed June 6, 2005.
4. Garlic effects on cardiovascular risks and disease, protective effects against cancer, and clinical adverse effects. Summary, evidence report/technology assessment: number 20. Rockville, Md: Agency for Healthcare Research and Quality; October 2000. AHRQ Publication No. 01-E022.
5. Brinker F. *Herb Contraindications and Drug Interactions.* 2nd ed. Sandy, Ore: Eclectic Medical Publications; 1998: 145-6.
6. Rafaat M, Leung AK. Garlic burns. *Pediatr Dermatol.* 2000;17:475-6.
7. Ciocon JO, Ciocon DG, Galindo DJ. Dietary supplements in primary care. Botanicals can affect surgical outcomes and follow-up. *Geriatrics.* 2004;59:20-4.
8. Ang-Lee ML, Moss J, Yuan CS. Herbal medicines and perioperative care. *JAMA.* 2001;286:208-16.
9. Boullata J. Natural health product interactions with medication. *Nutr Clin Pract.* 2005;20:33-51.
10. Piscitelli SC, Burstein AH, Welden N, et al. The effect of garlic supplements on the pharmacokinetics of saquinavir. *Clin Infect Dis.* 2002;34:234-8.
11. Markowitz JS, Devane CL, Chavin KD, et al. Effects of garlic (*Allium sativum* L.) supplementation on cytochrome P450 2D6 and 3A4 activity in healthy volunteers. *Clin Pharmacol Ther.* 2003; 74:170-7.
12. National Institutes of Health. ClinicalTrials.gov 2005. Available at: http://www.clinicaltrials.gov. Accessed May 18, 2005.
13. Consumer Labs. Available at: http://www.consumerlabs.com/results/. Accessed May 18, 2005.
14. Stevinson C, Pittler MH, Ernst E. Garlic for treating hypercholesterolemia. A meta-analysis of randomized clinical trials. *Ann Intern Med.* 2000;133:420-9.
15. Superko HR, Krauss RM. Garlic powder, effect on plasma lipids, postprandial lipemia, low density lipoprotein particle size, high density lipoprotein subclass distribution and lipoprotein (a). *J Am Coll Cardiol.* 2001;35:321-6.
16. Thomson M, Ali M. Garlic [Allium sativum]: a review of its potential use as an anti-cancer agent. *Curr Cancer Drug Targets.* 2003;3:67-81.
17. Fleischauer AT, Arab L. Garlic and cancer: a critical review of the epidemiologic literature. *J Nutr.* 2001;131:1032-40.
18. Birks J, Grimley EV, van Dongen M. Ginkgo biloba for cognitive impairment and dementia. *Cochrane Database Syst Rev.* 2002; CD003120.
19. Sierpina VS, Wollschlaeger B, Blumenthal M. Ginkgo biloba. *Am Fam Physician.* 2003;68:923-6.
20. Granger AS. *Ginkgo biloba* precipitating epileptic seizures. *Age Ageing.* 2001;30:523-5.
21. Matthews MK. Association of *Ginkgo biloba* with intracerebral hemorrhage. *Neurology.* 1998;50:1933.
22. Koch E. Inhibition of platelet activating factor (PAF)-induced aggregation of human thrombocytes by ginkgolides: considerations on possible bleeding complications after oral intake of *Ginkgo biloba* extracts. *Phytomedicine.* 2005;12:10-6.
23. Markowitz JS, Donovan JL, DeVane CL, et al. Multiple-dose administration of *Ginkgo biloba* did not affect cytochrome P-450 2D6 or 3A4 activity in normal volunteers. *J Clin Psychopharmacol.* 2003;23:576-81.
24. Galluzzi S, Zanetti O, Binetti G, et al. Coma in a patient with Alzheimer's disease taking low dose trazodone and *Ginkgo biloba. J Neurol Neurosurg Psychiatry.* 2000;68: 679-80.
25. Wettstein A. Cholinesterase inhibitors and ginkgo extracts—are they comparable in the treatment of dementia? Comparison of published placebo-controlled efficacy studies of at least six months' duration. *Phytomedicine.* 2000;6:393-401.
26. Solomon PR, Adams F, Silver A, et al. Ginkgo for memory enhancement: a randomized controlled trial. *JAMA.* 2002;288: 835-40.
27. Pittler MH, Ernst E. *Ginkgo biloba* extract for the treatment of intermittent claudication: a meta-analysis of randomized trials. *Am J Med.* 2000;108:276-81.
28. Drew S, Davies E. Effectiveness of *Ginkgo biloba* in treating tinnitus: double-blind, placebo controlled trial. *BMJ.* 2001;322:73.
29. Rejali D, Sivakumar A, Balaji N. Ginkgo biloba does not benefit patients with tinnitus: a randomized placebo-controlled double-blind trial and meta-analysis of randomized trials. *Clin Otolaryngol.* 2004;29:226-31.
30. Gertsch JH, Basnyat B, Johnson W, et al. Randomised, double-blind, placebo controlled comparison of ginkgo biloba and acetazolamide for prevention of acute mountain sickness among Himalayan trekkers: the prevention of high altitude illness trial (PHAIT) *BMJ.* 2004;328:797.
31. Rohdewald P. A review of the French maritime pine bark extract (Pycnogenol): a herbal medication with a diverse clinical pharmacology. *Int J Clin Pharmacol Ther.* 2002;40:158-68.
32. Koch R. Comparative study of Venostasin and Pycnogenol in chronic venous insufficiency. *Phytother Res.* 2002;16:1-5.
33. Petrassi C, Mastromarino A, Spartera C. Pycnogenol in chronic venous insufficiency. *Phytomedicine.* 2000;7:383-8.
34. Devaraj S, Vega-Lopez S, Kaul N, et al. Supplementation with a pine bark extract rich in polyphenols increases plasma antioxidant capacity and alters the plasma lipoprotein profile. *Lipids.* 2002;37:931-4.
35. Pittler MH, Schmidt K, Ernst E. Hawthorne extract for treating chronic heart failure: meta-analysis of randomized trials. *Am J Med.* 2003;114:665-74.
36. Holubarsch CJ, Colucci WS, Meinertz T, et al. Survival and prognosis: investigation of *Crataegus* extract WS 1442 in congestive heart failure (SPICE)—rationale, study design and study protocol. *Eur J Heart Fail.* 2000;2:431-7.
37. Tauchert M. Efficacy and safety of crataegus extract WS 1442 in comparison to placebo in patients with chronic stable New York Heart Association class-III heart failure. *Am Heart J.* 2002;143: 910-5.
38. Tankanow R, Tamer HR, Streetman DS, et al. Interaction study between digoxin and a preparation of hawthorn (*Crataegus oxyacantha*). *J Clin Pharmacol.* 2003;43:637-42.

39. Schroder D, Weiser M, Klein P. Efficacy of a homeopathic Crataegus preparation compared with usual therapy for mild (NYHA II) cardiac insufficiency: results of an observational cohort study. *Eur J Heart Fail.* 2003;5:319-26.
40. Pittler MH, Ernst E. Horse-chestnut seed extract for chronic venous insufficiency. *Cochrane Database Syst Rev.* 2004;CD003230.
41. Viola H, Wasowski C, Levi de Stein M, et al. Apigenin, a component of Matricaria recutita flowers, is a central benzodiazepine receptors-ligand, with anxiolytic effects. *Planta Med.* 1995;61:213-6.
42. Robbers JE, Tyler VF. *Tyler's Herbs of Choice: The Therapeutic Use of Phytomedicine.* New York: Haworth Herbal Press; 1999:70.
43. Reider N, Sepp N, Fritsch P, et al. Anaphylaxis to chamomile: clinical features and allergic cross-reactivity. *Clin Exp Allergy.* 2000;30:1436-43.
44. Budzinski JW, Foster BC, Vandenhoek S, et al. An in vitro evaluation of human cytochrome P450 3A4 inhibition by selected commercial herbal extracts and tinctures. *Phytomedicine.* 2000;7: 273-82.
45. Smith C, Crowther C, Willson K, et al. A randomized controlled trial of ginger to treat nausea and vomiting in pregnancy. *Obstet Gynecol.* 2004;103:639-45.
46. Portnoi G, Chng LA, Karimi-Tabesh L, et al. Prospective comparative study of the safety and effectiveness of ginger for the treatment of nausea and vomiting in pregnancy. *Am J Obstet Gynecol.* 2003;18:1374-7.
47. Lesho EP, Saullo, Udvari-Nagy S. A 76 year-old woman with erratic anticoagulation. *Cleveland Clin J Med.* 2004;71:651-6.
48. Ernst E, Pittler MH. Efficacy of ginger for nausea and vomiting: a systematic review of randomized clinical trials. *Br J Anaesth.* 2000;84:367-71.
49. Borrelli F, Capasso R, Aviello G, et al. Effectiveness and safety of ginger in the treatment of pregnancy-induced nausea and vomiting. *Obstet Gynecol.* 2005;105:849-56.
50. Curreli F, Friedman-Kien AE, Flore O. Glycyrrhizic acid alters Kaposi sarcoma-associated herpesvirus latency, triggering p53-mediated apoptosis in transformed B lymphocytes. *J Clin Invest.* 2005;115:591-3.
51. Lin SH, Yang SS, Chau T, et al. An unusual cause of hypokalemic paralysis: chronic licorice ingestion. *Am J Med Sci.* 2003;325:153-6.
52. Strandberg TE, Andersson S, Jarvenpaa AL, et al. Preterm birth and licorice consumption during pregnancy. *Am J Epidemiol.* 2002;156:803-5.
53. Coon JT, Ernst E. Complementary and alternative therapies in the treatment of chronic hepatitis C: a systematic review. *J Hepatol.* 2004;40:491-500.
54. Cinati J, Morgensterm B, Bauer G, et al. Glycyrrhizin, an active component of liquorice roots, and replication of SARS-associated coronavirus. *Lancet.* 2003;361:2045-6.
55. Siddiqui U, Weinshel EH, Bini EJ. Prevalence and predictors of herbal medication use in veterans with chronic hepatitis C. *J Clin Gastroenterol.* 2004;38:605-10.
56. Singh RP, Agarwal R. Prostate cancer prevention by silibinin. *Curr Cancer Drug Targets.* 2004;4:1-11.
57. Milk thistle: effects on liver disease and cirrhosis and clinical adverse effects. Summary, Evidence Report/Technology Assessment: Number 21, September 2000. Agency for Healthcare Research and Quality, Rockville, Md. Available at: http://ahrq.gov/clinic/epcsums/milktsum.htm. Accessed February 25, 2005.
58. *PDR for Herbal Medicines.* 2nd ed. Montvale, NJ: Medical Economics Co; 2000.
59. Gurley BJ, Gardner SF, Hubbard MA, et al. In vivo assessment of botanical supplementation on human cytochrome P450 phenotypes: *Citrus aurantium, Echinacea purpura,* milk thistle, and saw palmetto. *Clin Pharmacol Ther.* 2004;76:428-40.
60. DiCenzo R, Shelton M, Jordan K, et al. Coadministration of milk thistle and indinavir in healthy subjects. *Pharmacotherapy.* 2003; 23:866-70.
61. Rambaldi A, Jacobs B, Iaquinto G, Gluud C. Milk thistle for alcoholic and/or hepatitis B or C virus liver diseases. *Cochrane Database Syst Rev.* 2005;(2):CD003620.
62. Digestive Diseases Interagency Coordinating Committee. Silymarin as therapy of liver disease. March 22, 2004. Available at: http://www.niddk.nih.gov/federal/ddicc/Final-March-22-Summary.pdf. Accessed February 25, 2005.
63. Dresser GK, Wacher V, Wong S, et al. Evaluation of peppermint oil and ascorbyl palmitate as inhibitors of cytochrome P450 3A4 activity in vitro and in vivo. *Clin Pharmacol Ther.* 2002;72:247-55.
64. Spanier JA, Howden CW, Jones MP. A systematic review of alternative therapies in the irritable bowel syndrome. *Arch Intern Med.* 2003;163:265-74.
65. Kline RM, Kline JJ, DiPalma J, et al. Enteric-coated, pH dependent peppermint oil capsules for the treatment of irritable bowel syndrome in children. *J Pediatr.* 2001;138:125-8.
66. Center for Food Safety and Nutrition. Health claim for psyllium. Available at: http://www.cfsan.fda.gov/~lrd/cf101-77.html. Accessed February 25, 2005.
67. Khalili B, Bardana EJ, Yunginger JW. Psyllium-associated anaphylaxis and death: a case report and review of the literature. *Ann Allergy Asthma Immunol.* 2003;91:579-84.
68. Shulman LM, Minagar A, Weiner WJ. Perdiem causing esophageal obstruction in Parkinson's disease. *Neurology.* 1999;52:670-1.
69. Karwoski CB. Esophageal obstruction and choking. OPDRA Post-marketing safety review. May 15, 2002. Available at: http://www.fda.gov/ohrms/dockets/dailys/03/Aug03/081503/78n-0036l-bkg0004-06-tab8-vol1.pdf. Accessed February 25, 2005.
70. Anderson JW, Allgood LD, Lawrence A, et al. Cholesterol-lowering effects of psyllium intake adjunctive to diet therapy in men and women with hypercholesterolemia: meta-analysis of 8 controlled trials. *Am J Clin Nutr.* 2000; 71:472-9.
71. Cavaliere H, Floriano I, Medeiros-Neto G. Gastrointestinal side effects of orlistat may be prevented by concomitant prescription of natural fibers (psyllium mucilloid). *Int J Obes Relat Metab Disord.* 2001;25:1095-9.
72. Rodriguez-Moran M, Guerrero-Romero F, et al. Lipid- and glucose-lowering efficacy of Plantago psyllium in type II diabetes. *J Diabetes Complications.* 1998;12:273-8.
73. American College of Gastroenterology Functional Gastrointestinal Disorders Task Force. Evidence-based position statement of the management of irritable bowel syndrome in North America. *Am J Gastroenterol.* 2002;97:1-5.
74. Spiller HA, Winter ML, Weber JA, et al. Skin breakdown and blisters from senna-containing laxatives in young children. *Ann Pharmacother.* 2003;37:636-9.
75. Panossian A, Hovhannisyan A, Mamikonyan G, et al. Pharmacokinetic and oral bioavailability of andrographolide from *Andrographis paniculata* fixed combination Kan Jang in rats and humans. *Phytomedicine.* 2000;7: 351-64.
76. Puri A, Saxena R, Saxena RP, et al. Immunostimulant agents from *Andrographis paniculata. J Nat Prod.* 1993;56:995-9.
77. Coon JT, Ernst E. Andrographis paniculata in the treatment of upper respiratory tract infections: a systematic review of safety and efficacy. *Planta Med.* 2004;70:293-8.
78. Calabrese C, Berman SH, Babish JG, et al. A phase I trial of andrographolide in HIV positive patients and normal volunteers. *Phytother Res.* 2000;14:333-8.
79. Grimm W, Muller HH. A randomized controlled trial of the effect of fluid extract of Echinacea purpurea on the incidence and severity of colds and respiratory infections. *Am J Med.* 1999; 106:138-43.

80. Schwarz E, Metzler J, Diedrich JP, et al. Oral administration of freshly expressed juice of Echinacea purpurea herbs fail to stimulate the nonspecific immune response in healthy young men: results of a double-blind, placebo-controlled crossover study. *J Immunother.* 2002;25:413-20.
81. Lee A, Werth V. Activation of autoimmunity following use of immunostimulatory herbal supplements. *Arch Dermatol.* 2004; 140:723-7.
82. Giles JT, Cuthbert TP, Chien SH, et al. Evaluation of echinacea for treatment of the common cold. *Pharmacotherapy.* 2000;20:690-7.
83. Lindenmuth GF, Lindenmuth ED. The efficacy of Echinacea compound herbal tea preparation on the severity and duration of upper respiratory and flu symptoms: a randomized, double-blind placebo-controlled study. *J Altern Complement Med.* 2000;6: 327-34.
84. Goel V, Lovlin R, Barton R, et al. Efficacy of a standardized echinacea preparation (Echinilin) for treatment of the common cold: a randomized double-blind, placebo-controlled trial. *J Clin Pharm Ther.* 2004;29:75-83.
85. Yale S, Liu K. Echinacea purpurea therapy for the treatment of the common cold. *Arch Intern Med.* 2004;164:1237-41.
86. Taylor J, Weber W, Standish L, et al. Efficacy and safety of echinacea in treating upper respiratory tract infections in children: a randomized controlled trial. *JAMA.* 2003;290:2824-30.
87. Melchart D, Walther E, Linde K, et al. Echinacea root extracts for the prevention of upper respiratory tract infections: a double-blind placebo controlled randomized trial. *Arch Fam Med.* 1998; 7:541-5.
88. Donovan JL, DeVane CL, Chavin KD, et al. Siberian ginseng (*Eleutherococcus senticosus*) effects on CYP2D6 and CYP3A4 activity in normal volunteers. *Drug Metab Dispos.* 2003;31:519-22.
89. Williams M. Immunoprotection against herpes simplex type II infection by eleutherococcus root extract. *Int J Altern Complement Med.* 2001;13:9-12.
90. Waller DP, Martin AM, Farnsworth NR, et al. Lack of androgenicity of Siberian Ginseng. *JAMA.* 1992;267:2329.
91. Dasgupta A, Wu S, Actor J, et al. Effect of Asian and Siberian ginseng on serum digoxin measurement by five digoxin immunoassays. *Am J Clin Path.* 2003;119:289-303.
92. Blumenthal M, Goldberg A, Brinckmann J, eds. *Herbal Medicine: Expanded Commission E Monographs.* Atlanta, Ga: Integrative Medicine Communications; 1999.
93. Yuan C, Wei G, Dey L, et al. American ginseng reduces warfarin's effect in healthy patients: a randomized, controlled trial. *Ann Intern Med.* 2004;141:23-7.
94. Jiang X, Williams K, Liauw W, et al. Effect of St John's Wort and ginseng on the pharmacokinetics and pharmacodynamics of warfarin in healthy subjects. *Br J Clin Pharmcol.* 2004;57:592-9.
95. Vuksan V, Stavro MP, Sievenpiper JL, et al. Similar postprandial glycemic reductions with escalation of dose and administration time of American ginseng in type 2 diabetes. *Diabetes Care.* 2000; 23:1221-6.
96. Sotaniemi E, Haapakowski E, Rautio A. Ginseng therapy in non-insulin dependent diabetic patients. *Diabetes Care.* 1995;18:1373-5.
97. Scaglione F, Cattaneo G, Alessandra, et al. Efficacy and safety of the standardized ginseng extract G115 for potentiating vaccination against the influenza syndrome and protection against the common cold. *Drugs Exp Clin Res.* 1996;22:65-72.
98. Volger BK, Pittler MH, Ernst E. The efficacy of ginseng: a systematic review of randomized clinical trials. *Eur J Clin Pharmacol.* 1999;55:567-75.
99. Mukhtar H, Ahmad N. Tea polyphenols: prevention of cancer and optimizing health. *Am J Clin Nutr.* 2000;71(suppl):1698-702.
100. Henning S, Niu Y, Lee N, et al. Bioavailability and antioxidant activity of tea flavanols after consumption of green tea, black tea, or green tea extract supplement. *Am J Clin Nutr.* 2004;80:1558-64.
101. The Stash Tea Company. Caffeine information on tea. Available at: http://www.stashtea.com/caffeine.htm. Accessed January 28, 2005.
102. Heck A, DeWitt B, Lukes A. Potential interactions between alternative therapies and warfarin. *Am J Health-Syst Pharm.* 2000;57: 1221-30.
103. Imai K, Nakachi K. Cross sectional study of effects of drinking green tea on cardiovascular and liver disease. *BMJ.* 1995;310:693-6.
104. Princen HM, Duyvenvoorde W, Buytenhek R, et al. No effect of consumption of green and black tea on plasma lipid, on antioxidant levels and on LDL oxidation in smokers. *Arterioscler Thromb Vasc Biol.* 1998;18:833-41.
105. Maron D, Lu G, Cai N, et al. Cholesterol lowering effect of a theaflavin-enriched green tea extract: a randomized controlled trial. *Arch Intern Med.* 2003;163:1448-53.
106. Bushman J. Green tea and cancer in humans: a review of the literature. *Nutr Cancer.*1998;31:151-9.
107. Yoshitaka T, Yoshikazu N, Shoko K, et al. Green tea and the risk of gastric cancer in Japan. *N Engl J Med.* 2001;344: 632-6.
108. Pygeum africanum (*Prunus africana*) (African plum tree). *Altern Med Rev.* 2002;7:71-4.
109. McQueen C, Bryant P, Pepping J. Alternative therapies: pygeum. *Am J Health-Syst Pharm.* 2001;58:120-3.
110. Howell AB, Der Marderosian A, Foo LY. Inhibition of the adherence of P-fimbriated *Escherichia coli* to uroepithelial-cell surfaces by proanthocyanidin extracts from cranberries. *N Engl J Med.* 1998;339:1085-6.
111. Terris MK, Issa MM, Tacker JR. Dietary supplementation with cranberry concentrate tablets may increase the risk of nephrolithiasis. *Urology.* 2001;57:26-9.
112. Suvarna R, Pirmohamed M, Henderson L. Possible interaction between warfarin and cranberry juice. *BMJ.* 2003;327:1454.
113. Avorn J, Monane M, Gurwitz J, et al. Reduction of bacteriuria and pyuria after ingestion of cranberry juice. *JAMA.* 1994;271: 751-4.
114. Kontiokari T, Sundqvist K, Nuntinen M, et al. Randomised trial of cranberry-lingonberry juice and Lactobacillus GG drink for the prevention of urinary tract infections in women. *BMJ.* 2001; 322:1-5.
115. Linsenmeyer T, Harrison B, Oakley A, et al. Evaluation of cranberry supplement for reduction of urinary tract infections in individuals with neurogenic bladders secondary to spinal cord injury. A prospective, double-blinded, placebo-controlled, crossover study. *J Spinal Cord Med.* 2004;27:29-34.
116. Gerber GS, Zabaja GP, Bales GT, et al. Saw palmetto in men with lower urinary tract symptoms: effect on urodynamic parameters and voiding symptoms. *Urology.* 1998; 51:1003-7.
117. Cheema P, El-Mefty O, Jazieh AR. Intraoperative haemorrhage associated with the use of extract of Saw Palmetto herb: a case report and review of literature. *J Intern Med.* 2001;250:167-9.
118. Wilt T, Ishani A, Mac Donald R. *Serenoa repens* for benign prostatic hyperplasia. *Cochrane Database Syst Rev.* 2002;(2):CD001423.
119. Schindler G, Patzak U, Brinkhause B, et al. Urinary excretion and metabolism of arbutin after oral administration of Arctostaphylos uvae ursi extract as film-coated tablets and aqueous solution in healthy humans. *J Clin Pharm.* 2002;42:920-7.
120. Locock R. Bearberry. *Can Pharm J.* 2000;133:38-40.
121. Wang L, Del Priore L. Bull's-eye maculopathy secondary to herbal toxicity from uva ursi. *Am J Ophthalmol.* 2004;137:1135-7.
122. Grossmann W, Schmidramsl H. An extract of *Petasites hybridus* is effective in prophylaxis of migraine. *Int J Clin Pharm Ther.* 2000; 38:430-5.
123. Schapowal A. Randomised controlled trial of butterbur and cetirizine for treating seasonal allergic rhinitis. *BMJ.* 2002;321:1-4.
124. Hasler A, Passafaro A, Meier B. Trace analysis of pyrrolizidine alkaloids b GC-NPD of extracts from the roots of *Petasites hybridus. Pharmaceutica Acta Helvetiae.* 1998;72:367.

125. Lipton R, Gobel H, Einhaupl K, et al. *Petasites hybridus* root (butterbur) is an effective preventative treatment for migraine. *Neurology.* 2004;63:2240-4.
126. Lee D, Gray R, Robb F, et al. A placebo-controlled evaluation of butterbur and fexofenadine on objective and subjective outcomes in perennial allergic rhinitis. *Clin Exp Allergy.* 2004;34:646-9.
127. de Weerdt CJ. Herbal medicines in migraine prevention. Randomized double-blind placebo-controlled crossover trial of feverfew preparation. *Phytomedicine.* 1996;3: 225-30.
128. Murch S, Simmons C, Saxena P. Melatonin in feverfew and other medicinal plants. *Lancet.* 1997;350:1598-9.
129. Ramadan NM, Silberstein SD, Freitag FG, et al. Evidence-based guidelines for migraine headache in the primary care setting: pharmacological management for the prevention of migraine. Available at: http://www.aan.com. Accessed February 18, 2005.
130. Pittler M, Ernst E. Feverfew for preventing migraine (Cochrane Review). In: *The Cochrane Library,* Issue 3; 2004. Chichester, UK: John Wiley and Sons, Ltd.
131. Pepping J. Huperzine A. *Am J Health-Syst Pharm.* 2000;57:530-4.
132. Camps P, Cusack B, Mallender W, et al. Huprine X is a novel high-affinity inhibitor of acetylcholinesterase that is of interest for treatment of Alzheimer's disease. *Mol Pharm.* 2000;57:409-17.
133. Cagnacci A, Arangino S, Renzi A, et al. Kava-kava administration reduces anxiety in perimenopausal women. *Maturitas.* 2003;44: 103-9.
134. Perez J, Holmes JF. Altered mental status and ataxia secondary to acute Kava ingestion. *J Emerg Med.* 2005;28:49-51.
135. Clouatre D. Kava kava: examining new reports of toxicity. *Toxicol Lett.* 2004;150:85-96.
136. Centers for Disease Control and Prevention. Hepatic toxicity possibly associated with kava-containing products - United States, Germany, and Switzerland, 1999-2002. *MMWR Morb Mortal Wkly Rep.* 2002;51:1065-7.
137. Matthews J, Etheridge A, Black S. Inhibition of human cytochrome P450 activities by kava extract and kava lactones. *Drug Metab Disp.* 2002;30:1153-7.
138. Meseguer E, Taboada R, Sanchez V, et al. Life threatening parkinsonism induced by kava-kava. *Mov Disord.* 2002;17:195-6.
139. Barnes J, Anderson L, Phillipson J. St. John's wort (*Hypericum perforatum L.*): a review of its chemistry, pharmacology and clinical properties. *J Pharm Pharmacol.* 2001;53:583-600.
140. *Hypericum perforatum. Altern Med Rev.* 2004;9:318-25.
141. Knuppel L, Linde K. Adverse effects of St. John's wort: a systematic review. *J Clin Psychiatry.* 2004;65:1470-9.
142. Snow V, Lascher S, Mottur-Pilson C. Pharmacologic treatment of acute major depression and dysthymia. American College of Physicians-American Society of Internal Medicine. *Ann Intern Med.* 2000;132:738-42.
143. Linde K, Mulrow C, Berner M, Egger M. St. John's wort for depression. *Cochrane Database Syst Rev.* 2005;(2):CD000448.
144. Szegedi A, Kohnen R, Dienel A, et al. Acute treatment of moderate to severe depression with hypericum extract WS5570 (St. John's wort): randomized controlled double blind non-inferiority trial versus paroxetine. *BMJ.* 2005; 330:503.
145. Pepping J. Valerian: *Valeriana officinalis. Am J Health-Syst Pharm.* 2000;57:328-35.
146. Wagner J, Hening W. Beyond benzodiazepines: alternative pharmacologic agents for the treatment of insomnia. *Neuropsychiatry.* 1998;32:680-91.
147. Garges HP, Varia I, Doraiswamy PM. Cardiac complications and delirium associated with valerian root withdrawal. *JAMA.* 1998; 280:1566-7.
148. Francis A, Dempster R. Effect of valerian, *Valeriana edulis,* on sleep difficulties in children with intellectual deficits: randomized trial. *Phytomedicine.* 2002;9:273-9.
149. Glass J, Sproule B, Herrmann N, et al. Acute pharmacological effects of temazepam, diphenhydramine, and valerian in healthy elderly subjects. *J Clin Psychopharmacol.* 2003;23:260-8.
150. Center for Food Safety and Applied Nutrition, U.S. Food and Drug Administration,Department of Health and Human Services. Final Rule Summary: Dietary Supplements Containing Ephedrine Alkaloids. Available at: http://www.cfsan.fda.gov/~dms/ds-ephed.html. Accessed February 20, 2005.
151. U.S. District Court for the District of Utah ruling in *Nutraceutical Corp. and Solaray Inc. v. Lester Crawford, DVM, et al.* Available in: (www.utd.uscourts.gov/reports/204cv409-28.pdf).
152. Nykamp D, Fackih M, Compton A. Possible association of acute lateral-wall myocardial infarction and bitter orange supplement. *Ann Pharmacotherapy.* 2004;38:812-16.
153. Colker CM, Kalman D, Torina GC, et al. Effects of *Citrus aurantium* extract, caffeine, and St. John's wort on body fat loss, lipid levels, and mood states in overweight healthy adults. *Curr Ther Res.* 1999;60:145-53.
154. Chobanian A, Bakris G, Black H, et al. The seventh report of the joint national committee of prevention, detection, evaluation, and treatment of high blood pressure. *JAMA.* 2003:289: 2560-72.
155. Klein AD, Penneys NS. Aloe vera. *J Am Acad Derm.* 1988;18:714-20.
156. Crowell J, Penneys N. The effects of aloe vera on cutaneous erythema and blood flow following ultraviolet B (UVB) exposure. *Clin Res.* 1987;35:676A.
157. Schmidt JM, Greenspoon JS. *Aloe vera* dermal wound gel is associated with a delay in wound healing. *Obstet Gynecol.* 1991;78:115-7.
158. Syed TA, Ahmad SA, Holt AH, et al. Management of psoriasis with *Aloe vera* extract in a hydrophilic cream: a placebo-controlled, double-blind study. *Trop Med Int Health.* 1996;1:505-9.
159. Syed T, Afzal M, Ashfaq A, et al. Management of genital herpes in men with 0.5% Aloe vera extract in a hydrophilic cream: a placebo-controlled double-blind study. *J Dermatol Treat.* 1997;8: 99-102.
160. Lloyd JU. *Stringtown on the Pike.* New York: Dodd, Mead & Co.; 1901.
161. Bedard M. Goldenseal: high on promises, low on evidence. *Can Pharm J.* 2002;135:44-8.
162. Gurley BJ, Gardner SF, Hubbard MA, et al. In vivo effects of goldenseal, kava kava, black cohosh, and valerian on human cytochrome P450 1A2, 2D6, 2E1, and 3A4/5 phenotypes. *Clin Pharmacol Ther.* 2005;77:415-26.
163. Kennedy D, Scholey A, Tildesley N, et al. Modulation of mood and cognitive performance following acute administration of *Melissa officinalis. Pharmcol Biochem Behav.* 2002;72:953-64.
164. Wolbling RH, Leonhardt K. Local therapy of herpes simplex with dried extract from *Melissa officinalis. Phytomedicine.* 1994;1:25-31.
165. Koytchev R, Alken RG, Dundarov S. Balm mint extract for topical treatment of recurring Herpes labialis. *Phytomedicine.* 1999;6:225-30.
166. Akhondzadeh S, Noroozian M, Mohammadi M, et al. *Melissa officinalis* extract in the treatment of patients with mild to moderate Alzheimer's disease: a double blind randomized, placebo controlled trial. *J Neurol Neurosurg Psychiatry.* 2003;74:863-6.
167. Buck DS, Nidorf DM, Addino JG. Comparison of two topical preparations for the treatment of onychomycosis: *Melaleuca alternifolia* (tea tree) oil and clotrimazole. *J Fam Pract.* 1994;38: 601-5.
168. Bassett IB, Pannowitz DL, Barnestson RSC. A comparative study of tea-tree oil versus benzoyl peroxide in the treatment of acne. *Med J Aust.* 1990;153:455-8.
169. Newton KM, Buist DS, Keenan NL, et al. Use of alternative therapies for menopause symptoms: results of a population-based survey. *Obstet Gynecol.* 2002;100:18-25.

170. Fugate SE, Church CO. Nonestrogen treatment modalities for vasomotor symptoms associated with menopause. *Ann Pharmacother.* 2004;38:1482-99.
171. Lupu R, Mehmi I, Tsai MS, et al. Black cohosh, a menopausal remedy, does not have estrogenic activity and does not promote breast cancer cell growth. *Int J Oncol.* 2003;23:1407-12.
172. Kligler B. Black Cohosh. *Am Fam Physician.* 2003;68:114-6.
173. Huntley A, Ernst E. A systematic review of the safety of black cohosh. *Menopause.* 2003;10:58-64.
174. Cohen SM, O'Connor AM, Hart J, et al. Autoimmune hepatitis associated with the use of black cohosh. *Menopause.* 2004;11:575-7.
175. Writing Group for the Women's Health Initiative Investigators. Risks and benefits of estrogen plus progestin in healthy postmenopausal women: principal results from the Women's Health Initiative. Randomized controlled trial. *JAMA.* 2002;288:321-33.
176. Liske E, Hanggi W, Henneicke-von Zepelin HH, et al. Physiological investigation of a unique extract of black cohosh (*Cimicifuga racemosa rhizoma*): a 6-month clinical study demonstrates no systemic estrogenic effect. *J Womens Health Gend Based Med.* 2002; 11:163-74.
177. Osmers R, Friede M, Liske E, et al. Efficacy and safety of isopropanolic black cohosh extract for climacteric symptoms. *Obstet Gynecol.* 2005;105:1074-83.
178. Jacobson JS, Troxel AB, Evans J, et al. Randomized trial of black cohosh for the treatment of hot flashes among women with a history of breast cancer. *J Clin Oncol.* 2001;19:2739-45.
179. North American Menopause Society. Treatment of menopause-associated vasomotor symptoms: position statement of the North American Menopause Society. *Menopause.* 2004;11:11-33.
180. Schellenberg R. Treatment for the premenstrual syndrome with *Agnus castus* fruit extract: prospective, randomized, placebo controlled study. *BMJ.* 2001;322:134-7.
181. Dove D, Johnson P. Oral evening primrose oil: its effect on length of pregnancy and selected intrapartum outcomes in low-risk nulliparous women. *J Nurse Midwifery.* 1999;44:320-4.
182. Blommers J, de Lange-De Klerk ES, Kuik DJ, et al. Evening primrose oil and fish oil for severe chronic mastalgia: a randomized double-blind, controlled trial. *Am J Obstet Gynecol.* 2002;187: 1389-94.
183. Duffy C, Cyr M. Phytoestrogens: potential benefits and implications for breast cancer survivors. *J Womens Health.* 2003;12:617-31.
184. Ju YH, Doerge DR, Allred KF, et al. Dietary genistein negates the inhibitory effect of tamoxifen on growth of estrogen-dependent human breast cancer (MCF-7) cells implanted in athymic mice. *Cancer Res.* 2002;62:2474-7.
185. Ju YH, Allred CD, Allred KF, et al. Physiologic concentrations of dietary genistein dose-dependently stimulate growth of estrogen-dependent human breast cancer (MCF-7) implanted in athymic nude mice. *J Nutr.* 2001;131:2957-62.
186. Chen YM, Ho SC, Lam SS, et al. Beneficial effect of soy isoflavones on bone mineral content was modified by years since menopause, body weight, and calcium intake. *Menopause.* 2004; 11:246-41.
187. Krebs EE, Ensrud KE, MacDonald R, et al. Phytoestrogens for treatment of menopausal symptoms: a systematic review. *Obstet Gynecol.* 2004;104:824-36.
188. Tice JA, Ettinger B, Ensrud K, et al. Phytoestrogen supplements for the treatment of hot flashes: the Isoflavone Clover Extract (ICE) study. *JAMA.* 2003;290:207-14.

CHAPTER 54

# Nonbotanical Natural Medicines

*Cydney E. McQueen*

In addition to the information about individual supplements discussed in this chapter, decisions regarding a patient's use of a supplement should take into account other factors that affect supplement choice. (See the "Introduction to Botanical and Nonbotanical Natural Medicines" for discussion of issues such as product quality concerns, research concerns, regulations, and tips on counseling patients.) The products discussed in this chapter are included because they (1) have evidence to support their use, (2) are widely promoted alone or in combination products with or without evidence supporting their use, or (3) present known or theoretical safety concerns.

## GASTROINTESTINAL SYSTEM

### Chitosan

#### *Therapeutic Uses*

Chitosan is a mucopolysaccharide component of chitin found in the exoskeleton of marine organisms such as shrimp and crabs. As a dietary supplement, it is primarily marketed for losing weight and lowering cholesterol.

#### *Physiologic Activity*

Many dietary supplement references include the explanation that chitosan's positively charged amino groups bind negatively charged groups on fatty acids and bile acids, preventing fat absorption and increasing fecal fat excretion. This does occur, but the lipid of greatest concern to most patients, cholesterol, does not have negatively charged groups and therefore might not be bound. In addition, despite animal studies that support an increase in fecal fat excretion, at least three studies in healthy adults did not find changes in fat excretion.[1-3] More studies are needed to elucidate any possible mechanisms of action.

#### *Dosage and Administration Guidelines*

See Table 54-1 for dosing information.

#### Safety Considerations

Side effects of chitosan are mild and consist primarily of mild GI distress such as nausea.[4,9-12] Patients with allergies to shellfish may experience allergic reactions. Pregnant and lactating women should not use chitosan because of the lack of information on its effects. Patients should be counseled to avoid taking chitosan within 2 to 3 hours of taking prescription medications because positively charged groups on the chitosan molecule could bind some drugs and prevent absorption.

#### Administration and Product Issues

Shellfish chitin can be contaminated with clinically significant levels of heavy metals.

#### Summary of Clinical Evidence

To date, several fairly small clinical trials have examined chitosan's efficacy for cholesterol management.[13-20] Although methodologic limitations in the majority of trials prevent definitive conclusions about efficacy, six trials reported mild to moderate benefits on total cholesterol, low-density lipoprotein (LDL), and triglyceride levels in healthy patients, with decreases of about 3% to 6%.[20,21] Similar reductions in total cholesterol and LDL levels (–4.4% and –6.5%) were seen in a small crossover trial in diabetic patients.[9] However, a larger study in healthy middle-aged patients found no changes in plasma lipids or glucose levels.[10] A study in patients on chronic hemodialysis demonstrated average decreases in total cholesterol of 42%.[11] Further studies in lipid management in this and the general population are needed to clarify whether benefits of chitosan treatment are clinically significant.

Trials examining efficacy for weight loss do not support chitosan's use without a concomitant program of calorie reduction and exercise.[21] Even in conjunction with other weight-loss efforts, benefits seen have been slight and generally clinically insignificant.[12] This conclusion was also reached by a recent systematic review, which combined chitosan trials for weight loss with trials examining effects on cholesterol.[22]

### Probiotics

#### *Therapeutic Uses*

Probiotics are strains of microorganisms normally present in the human gut. These are taken as supplements to improve digestion, prevent recurrence of vaginal yeast infections, and treat conditions that involve alteration of normal intestinal flora, such as infectious diarrhea, antibiotic-associated diarrhea, inflammatory and functional bowel conditions, and traveler's diarrhea. The three types discussed here are *Lactobacillus*, *Bifidobacterium*, and *Saccharomyces*. Of the *Lactobacillus* species, *Lactobacillus reuteri* is the most common strain found in the body. Supplements

**TABLE 54-1 Product Dosage and Administration Guidelines**

| Product | Product Quality Considerations | Dosage and Comments |
|---|---|---|
| Chitosan | Contamination with shellfish allergens very likely; contamination with heavy metals possible. | Dosing not well established; trials used 1-6 g once daily. Because products differ, following manufacturer recommendations is advised. Take 2-3 hours apart from prescription or OTC medications. |
| *Lactobacillus, Bifidobacterium* | Many products contain other *Lactobacillus* strains or fewer live cells than stated; buy from company with high QC standards.<br>Do not use in immunocompromised patients, due to case reports of pathogenic colonizations, including death. | Adults: 1-10 billion CFU/day in 3-4 divided doses, for infectious and antibiotic-induced diarrhea<br>Infants/children: 1-10 billion CFU/day in 3-4 divided doses<br>Some *Lactobacillus* strains may be used at much higher doses in children, such as *Lactobacillus reuteri* at 100 billion CFU once daily. |
| *Saccharomyces* | As fungemia is of theoretical concern, avoid use in immunocompromised patients. | 250-500 mg 2 to 4 times/day<br>Infants/children: 250 mg 2 to 4 times/day |
| Coenzyme Q10 | | 100-200 mg once daily for most cardiovascular indications. Doses >100 mg daily should be divided into 2-3 doses. Higher doses are sometimes used in mitochondrial dysfunction diseases. Research in Parkinson's disease patients has used doses as high as 2400 mg. |
| Melatonin | Synthetically produced melatonin is preferred and most common. Melatonin extracted from bovine pineal glands is occasionally available. These products carry a possible risk of bacterial contamination; faint risk of BSE contamination. | Insomnia: 0.3-5 mg 30 minutes before bedtime<br>Jet lag: 2-5 mg on evening of departure and at bedtime for following 2-5 days. See text for discussion of dosing range. Low doses (0.3-0.5 mg) may be as effective as larger doses for insomnia. |
| (S-adenosyl-L-methionine) | SAMe is expensive; depending on the dose used, treatment could range from $80 to $220 per month. Use of enteric-coated preparations and dose titration may help minimize GI side effects. | Depression: 800-1600 mg/day in 3-4 divided doses<br>Osteoarthritis: 400-800 mg/day in 2-4 divided doses; most commonly 200 mg 3 times/day<br>Doses above 800 mg/day should be discouraged because of association with mania/hypomania. |
| 5-HTP (5-hydroxy-trytophan) | 5-HTP or a common contaminant may be associated with eosinophilia myalgia syndrome. | Depression: 150-300 mg once daily |
| DMAE (2-dimethyl-aminoethanol) | | 300-500 mg once daily, generally titrated from a beginning dose of 100 mg once daily. Clinical studies have used doses of up to 2000 mg once daily. |
| Lecithin | Lecithin products contain varying amounts of phosphatidylcholine, phosphatidylethanolamine, phosphatidylserine, and phosphatidylinositol. | 1.2-2.4 g once daily for FDA-approved indications. Up to 45 g once daily has been used in studies for Alzheimer's disease. |
| Phosphatidylserine | | 100 mg 3 times/day for memory or dementia |
| Phosphatidylcholine | | 10-25 g once daily; optimum dose is not well-characterized because of variability of study data. |
| DHEA (dehydro-epiandrosterone) | Counsel patients to purchase synthetically manufactured, rather than animal-based, products to avoid risks of contamination association.<br>Patients should not use wild yam extracts, which are often falsely promoted as DHEA precursors. | 25-50 mg once daily<br>Due to the greater frequency of adverse events associated with doses of 50 mg and higher, patients should use only lower doses unless use of higher doses is supervised by a primary care provider. |
| α-Lipoic acid | | 1200 mg daily in 1 or 2 doses or 1800 mg daily, divided in 2 or 3 doses.<br>Take on empty stomach for better absorption. |
| Bovine colostrum | An animal product, so it has possible risk of bacterial or viral disease; faint risk of BSE contamination. | Powder: 20-60 g once daily. Trials have used a wide variety of doses and formulations. Optimum dose and formulation are unknown. |

**TABLE 54-1 Product Dosage and Administration Guidelines (continued)**

| Product | Product Quality Considerations | Dosage and Comments |
|---|---|---|
| Thymus gland extract | An animal, usually bovine, product, so has possible risk of bacterial or viral disease; faint risk of BSE contamination.<br>Because preparations vary in type and quality, following manufacturer recommendations is advised. | Doses are not well established. |
| Glucosamine sulfate | Other salt forms are not currently recommended. May be manufactured from shellfish chitin, so patients allergic to shellfish should avoid. Often found in combination with chondroitin; see cautions below. | 1500 mg once daily or 500 mg 3 times/day<br>Dose is well established. Counsel patients regarding the delay in onset of effects. |
| Chondroitin sulfate | An animal product; usually produced from bovine cartilage; possible risk of bacterial or viral disease, or faint risk of BSE contamination. | 400 mg 3 times/day or 1200 mg once daily<br>Trials have used 800-1200 mg daily.<br>Counsel patients regarding the delay in onset of effects. |
| MSM (methyl-sulfonyl-methane) | | Not currently recommended<br>Documented doses range from 250 to 3000 mg once daily. Up to 5200 mg once daily has been used in a clinical trial. |
| Proteolytic enzymes (bromelain, papain) | Many products are combinations that may contain bromelain, papain, trypsin, chymotrypsin, or other enzymes in varying percentages. For combination products, follow manufacturer's directions. | Bromelian: 80-320 mg 2 to 3 times/day<br>Dosing is not well established, as doses used in trials varied widely.<br>Papain: for postsurgical or trauma, use 1500 mg once daily. |
| Cetyl myristoleate | Often found in products that include other ingredients. | Dosing cannot be established. Use is not recommended, but patients who choose to use this product should be counseled to not exceed the manufacturer's dose recommendations. |
| Shark cartilage | Products are often reported to have very bad taste and smell. It is unknown if this is related to contamination. Some methods of processing may inactivate proteins/peptides that could be responsible for activity. | Dosing is not well established and use is not recommended. Patients who choose to use shark cartilage should be counseled to not exceed the manufacturer's dose recommendations. |

Key: BSE, bovine spongiform encephalitis; CFU, colony-forming unit, OTC, over-the-counter; QC, quality control.

*Source*: Dosing is compiled from clinical trials cited in text and references 4-8.

may contain *L. rhamnosus, reuteri, acidophilus, bulgaricus,* or *fermentum.* Clinical trials have primarily used *L. rhamnosus* GG. *Bifidobacterium* strains seen in supplements may include *B. longum, bifidum, breve, infanti,* or *lactis,* whereas *S. boulardii,* a yeast, is the only *Saccharomyces* species used as a supplement.[4] Many alternative medicine practitioners use bacterial probiotics to treat overgrowth of *Candida* and other yeasts.

### Physiologic Activity

Normal gastrointestinal (GI) flora have several functions in the gut: prevention of colonization by pathogenic bacteria, production of vitamins B and K, breakdown of food, and absorption of nutrients. Various conditions, such as infectious diarrhea, and medications such as antibiotics alter these effects. Normalization of the flora aids in resolving symptoms such as diarrhea. Probiotics are associated with a wide variety of activities, including competition with pathogens for binding sites on intestinal mucosa, reduction of intestinal permeability, alteration of intestinal pH, and direct antimicrobial action against some pathogens.[23-26] Probiotics, especially *Lactobacillus,* are also associated with immune-modulating and anti-inflammatory activities such as reduction of tumor necrosis factor and stimulation of immunoglobulin and transforming growth factor-β production.[27,28]

### Dosage and Administration Guidelines

See Table 54-1 for dosing information. Doses of antibiotics and probiotics should be separated by several hours.

### Safety Considerations

Oral probiotics are generally well tolerated. Side effects can include mild bloating and flatulence, which generally subside with continued use. Diarrhea has been reported in children.[4] Immunocompromised patients should not use probiotics because of reports of systemic infection.[29] Although information is limited, no harmful effects have been observed in women in late-stage pregnancy or in breast-feeding infants during long-term use.[30] Concurrent administration with antibiotics or antifungal agents is not recommended. Doses of antimicrobials should be separated by several hours.

### *Administration and Product Issues*

Studies of purchased probiotic products have demonstrated many problems with quality and loss of activity. Practitioners should recommend purchase of products from reputable companies experienced with pharmaceuticals. (See the "Introduction to Botanical and Nonbotanical Natural Medicines" for more details about product quality.) In addition, refrigerated products may be more likely to have higher levels of active microorganisms. The *Lactobacillus rhamnosus* GG strain, often used in clinical trials, is widely available.

### *Summary of Clinical Evidence*

Numerous studies support the efficacy of probiotic treatment of infectious diarrhea, especially rotaviral diarrhea in pediatric patients.[31-33] Such patients are often hospitalized and therefore not regularly encountered in the community or ambulatory care setting. Practitioners are most likely to see probiotics used for the prevention or treatment of antibiotic-associated diarrhea or traveler's diarrhea. With a few exceptions, several trials to date strongly support use for these indications.[34-36] Clinical trials of probiotics in prevention of antibiotic-associated diarrhea have documented efficacy in 79% to 100% of patients.[34]

Preliminary evidence from three trials indicates that *Lactobacillus,* particularly the *plantarum* species, may be useful for decreasing flatulence, abdominal pain, and possibly bowel frequency in irritable bowel syndrome (IBS).[37-39] However, one crossover trial found no significant differences in most symptoms.[40] A recent review concluded that preliminary evidence suggests symptoms of inflammatory bowel disease (i.e., ulcerative colitis, Crohn's disease) may also be reduced with *L. rhamnosus* GG and *S. boulardii,* although further research is needed to make stronger recommendations.[41] An additional small study found reduction of pain and symptoms with two specific combinations, one containing *L. plantarum* and *Bifidobacterium breve* and the other *L. plantarum* and *L. acidophilus.*[42] More research is needed before efficacy for inflammatory bowel disease can be determined and the best species or combination of species identified.

Probiotics have also been investigated for treatment of atopic eczematous dermatitis. One placebo-controlled crossover study of 43 children found a significant decrease in the extent of eczema in favor of the *Lactobacillus* treatment ($p = .02$). Significantly more treated patients had self-evaluations of improvement of symptoms ($p = .001$), but SCORAD (scoring atopic dermatitis) scores were not different from those of placebo.[43] A smaller study ($n = 27$) of *Lactobacillus* in infants demonstrated a significant ($p = .008$) decrease in SCORAD scores compared with placebo.[44] More study is needed to determine if some subpopulations may response more favorably to treatment; a recent trial in infants with allergy to cow's milk found benefit in infants who were IgE-sensitized, but none in those infants not IgE-sensitized.[45]

A potential use of probiotics is to reduce the risk of eczematous dermatitis related to atopic conditions or in infants at high risk (i.e., those whose mothers have atopy or are from families with atopy). One study examined 159 pregnant women who received *Lactobacillus* or placebo for 4 weeks prior to birth. Infants of mothers in the treatment group had a lower risk of developing chronic relapsing atopic eczema (15% versus 47%; $p = .0098$).[30] Although research is promising, more trials are needed to determine the efficacy, safety, and effectiveness of probiotics for use in prevention or treatment of atopy.

A common use of probiotics is in the treatment or prevention of vulvovaginal candidiasis or bacterial infections. Although orally administered probiotics have been shown to result in vaginal colonization, the clinical evidence regarding their efficacy for treatment or prevention of candidiasis or bacterial infections is both scarce and inconsistent.[46,47] One small study using *L. acidophilus* administered in yogurt noted a decrease in bacterial vaginosis, whereas a recent trial examining efficacy for prevention of postantibiotic vulvovaginal yeast infections in 235 women found no benefit.[48,49] That trial tested both orally and vaginally administered probiotics against placebos.

# CARDIOVASCULAR SYSTEM

## Coenzyme Q10

### *Therapeutic Uses*

Coenzyme Q10 (CoQ10) is endogenous and found in every cell of the human body, primarily in the mitochondria. Originally extracted from bovine heart tissue, it is now manufactured using a beet and sugarcane fermentation process.[50] The chemically reduced form is called ubiquinone; this name is occasionally used in supplement labeling and reference books. CoQ10 is usually taken as a general antioxidant and for cardiovascular health.

### *Physiologic Activity*

CoQ10 exists in greatest concentrations in the mitochondria of the heart, liver, pancreas, and kidneys.[51] It is a cofactor in many functions associated with energy production and is the rate-limiting cofactor in mitochondrial adenosine triphosphate (ATP) formation. A powerful antioxidant itself, it is also involved with regeneration of other antioxidants such as vitamin E. CoQ10 stabilizes membranes and may have vasodilatory and inotropic effects.[52,53] One dosage form of CoQ10 has Food and Drug Administration (FDA) orphan drug status for the treatment of encephalomyopathies associated with mitochondrial dysfunction.[54]

Hydroxymethyl glutaryl coenzyme A reductase inhibitors, or "statins," lower serum levels of CoQ10, but possibly not levels within muscle tissue.[55-58] The decrease could be a result of decreased production of mevalonic acid, a direct precursor to CoQ10. Despite some evidence to the contrary, this lowering is believed to be a class effect, but may be dose-related or differ in extent among drugs.[59,60] Clinical relevance is not well-understood, as is also true for the less extensive lowering effects noted with other drugs such as β-blockers.[61]

### Dosage and Administration Guidelines

See Table 54-1 for dosing information. CoQ10 products that meet USP guidelines are available.

### Safety Considerations

Side effects of CoQ10 are rare. Those reported in trials include nausea, GI distress, anorexia, headache, irritability, and dizziness in fewer than 1% of patients.[4] Pregnant and lactating women should not use CoQ10 because of the lack of information about its effects.

The CoQ10 structure is similar to that of menaquinone, a synthetic vitamin K, which theoretically may have some vitamin K–like procoagulant effects.[62] There are case reports of decreases in warfarin effectiveness attributed to concomitant CoQ10 use, although one placebo-controlled crossover study noted no differences in international normalized ratio (INR) values in patients stable on warfarin doses.[62-65] CoQ10 may provide protection from doxorubicin-associated cardiotoxicity without decreasing clinical effectiveness, although more research is needed to characterize effects.[50,66] CoQ10 may increase the effectiveness of some chemotherapy agents, and may or may not have the same effect on radiation therapy. Animal studies have shown decreases in effectiveness of radiation therapy with large doses, but not with doses that would be equivalent to approximately 700 mg in a human being.[67] Information on interactions changes rapidly. Chemotherapy patients interested in using CoQ10 should discuss interactions with their oncologist.

### Administration and Product Issues

Patients on warfarin therapy should discuss CoQ10 with their primary care provider prior to use. If the decision is made to use CoQ10, monitor the patient's INR more frequently until effects are determined.

### Summary of Clinical Evidence

Early clinical trials demonstrated promise for the use of CoQ10 in congestive heart failure (CHF).[68,69] More recent well-designed studies, using doses of 100 to 200 mg daily in patients with New York Heart Association (NYHA) Class II to IV CHF, have not clearly shown a significant benefit in outcomes such as ejection fraction or oxygen consumption.[70,71] A trial in patients on a heart transplant waiting list found significant improvements in multiple symptoms, especially the 6-minute walk test, and NYHA class, but with no difference in measurements of cardiac efficiency on echocardiography.[72] At this time, although extent of efficacy is still being debated, CoQ10 is being used as an adjunctive therapy in some patients because of the favorable side effect profile. More research is needed to clearly define its benefit in CHF treatment.

Preliminary trials with small sample sizes have investigated CoQ10 for use in cardiomyopathy and ischemic heart disease. Some benefit was noted in parameters such as high-density lipoprotein (HDL) and lipoprotein in patients with ischemic heart disease, but overall risk reduction for death or secondary cardiac events was minimal.[73,74] Additional trials suggest lipid reduction and decreased insulin resistance in patients with coronary artery disease; however, the clinical significance of these changes on long-term outcomes is unknown.[75,76] Future research may find benefit in secondary protection in patients who have had a myocardial infarction. A 1-year trial comparing CoQ10 (120 mg/day) with a B vitamin capsule in 144 post-myocardial infarction patients reported a significantly lower rate of cardiac events (24.6% versus 45%; $p < .02$) in the CoQ10 group.[77]

Beneficial effects on blood pressure have been documented in some trials; additionally, one placebo-controlled trial of CoQ10 120 mg/day in 76 patients with isolated systolic hypertension documented a significant reduction in blood pressure compared with placebo (-17.8 mm Hg versus -1.7 mm Hg; $p < .01$) at 12 weeks.[78] This trial had methodologic limitations, so more evidence is needed to accurately determine the extent of effect on hypertension.

Various doses of CoQ10 have also been investigated for Parkinson's disease, Huntington's disease, breast cancer, and migraine headaches. Although some of the evidence looks very promising, at this point, conclusions regarding efficacy cannot be made.[79-82]

The clinical significance of statin-induced reduction of CoQ10 levels is not well characterized. Although some clinicians recommend CoQ10 supplementation for patients experiencing statin-associated fatigue, the effectiveness of this treatment remains unstudied and the clinical benefit unknown.

# CENTRAL NERVOUS SYSTEM

## Melatonin

### Therapeutic Uses

Melatonin, or N-acetyl-5-methoxytryptamine synthesized from tryptophan via a serotonin pathway, is an endogenous hormone produced by the pineal gland. Melatonin has FDA orphan drug status for treatment of sleep disorders in blind patients.[83] As a dietary supplement, it is primarily used for treatment of insomnia and prevention of "jet lag" in air travelers.[84]

### Physiologic Activity

Melatonin regulates sleep and circadian rhythms and also has hormonal effects. Release of melatonin is induced by darkness and suppressed by light; exogenous administration of melatonin increases endogenous levels and stimulates sleep regulation mechanisms. When taken for insomnia near bedtime, melatonin does not generally cause a feeling of drowsiness; rather, it may make a patient's attempt to sleep more successful. A swifter adjustment of the circadian rhythm may be responsible for melatonin's use for prevention and treatment of "jet lag." Melatonin has regulatory effects on sexual development and ovulation (high doses have been studied as a contraceptive), has effects on the immune system, and is also a very potent antioxidant.[84-86]

### Dosage and Administration Guidelines

See Table 54-1 for dosing information. The ideal dose for occasional insomnia remains unclear. For measurable supraphysiologic levels, as little as 0.3 mg is required and may be more effective than higher doses.[87,88] To reduce the risk of side effects, not more than 5 mg is recommended on an occasional basis.

### Safety Considerations

Melatonin is generally very well tolerated. Reported side effects include nausea and vomiting, headache, tachycardia, irritability, dysthymia and worsening of depressive symptoms, and a morning "hangover" effect.[4,84] Long-term administration of this hormone is not recommended unless under the direct supervision of a primary care provider.

It is unclear whether all use, or only long-term or high-dose use, should be avoided in children and adolescents, because of hormonal effects. Any use should be first discussed with a primary care provider. Pregnant and lactating women should not use melatonin because of possible hormonal effects on the fetus.

Several interactions with melatonin are known, although clinical significance is not well understood. Fluvoxamine, monoamine oxidase inhibitors (MAOIs), and tricyclic antidepressants may increase endogenous melatonin levels, whereas benzodiazepines and sodium valproate decrease nighttime levels.[89,90] Oral contraceptives and caffeine have variable effects on melatonin levels in women depending on the phase of the reproductive cycle.[91] Verapamil may also decrease levels by increasing melatonin excretion.[89] The clinical significance of the preceding interactions is not well-defined. However, melatonin's effect on nifedipine delivered via the GI therapeutic system (GITS) is clinically significant.[92] The drug's effectiveness is reduced, but whether melatonin affects the drug or the delivery system is unknown because no studies examining its impact on the effectiveness of immediate-release nifedipine have been conducted.

Because melatonin is known to have some stimulatory effects on the immune system, concomitant use with immunosuppressant therapy is not recommended. Like coenzyme Q10, melatonin may help to reduce toxicities of some cancer chemotherapy agents such as doxorubicin and cisplatin.[93] As information on effects on chemotherapy changes rapidly, all patients receiving cancer treatment should be advised to discuss melatonin use with their oncologist.

### Administration and Product Issues

See Bovine Source Precautions and Table 54-1.

### Summary of Clinical Evidence

Clinical evidence to date for treatment of insomnia is not definitive. Increases in rapid eye movement sleep, slightly faster sleep onset, increased duration of sleep, decreased daytime somnolence, and more "normal" patterns of time in sleep stages have been demonstrated in healthy insomniacs and in females with asthma.[84,94,95] A recent meta-analysis of 17 studies, conducted primarily in healthy, normal patients and insomniacs, supports the claim that melatonin has small but clinically significant benefits.[87] Observed clinical benefits, however, are variable; not all patients report feeling more rested, and some report better sleep even when no increases in sleep time are documented. More benefits may occur in patients whose natural sleep patterns are disrupted for physical reasons, such as ill health, although one study in patients with Alzheimer's disease found no difference from placebo.[96]

The clinical evidence for jet lag prevention is slightly more consistent than that for insomnia, although not definitive. Some studies have found no clinically significant benefits.[97] Although insomnia resulting from the circadian rhythm disruption caused by shift work may seem similar to insomnia associated with jet lag, current evidence does not support use of melatonin for this indication.[98] An Agency for Healthcare Research and Quality review concluded that more research of a higher technical quality is needed, and evidence to date is insufficient to support use for any of the preceding conditions.[99]

Melatonin's use in pediatric patients with insomnia has been sufficiently studied only in patients with neurologic disorders or blindness.[4,88] These patients should take melatonin as prescribed by a primary care provider. Use of dietary supplement melatonin products in children with occasional insomnia is not recommended (see Adverse Effects/Precautions/Contraindications).

Melatonin has also been tested for use to facilitate discontinuation of benzodiazepines by long-time users and for a variety of other CNS conditions, including tardive dyskinesia. Current evidence is insufficient to recommend these uses.[100,101]

## S-adenosyl-L-methionine

### Therapeutic Uses

S-adenosyl-L-methionine (SAMe) is an endogenous substance formed from L-methionine and ATP that is also manufactured as a dietary supplement. This product has two unrelated common uses: for depression and osteoarthritis.

### Physiologic Activity

SAMe is produced primarily in the liver. Liver disease and low levels of $B_{12}$ and folate may decrease SAMe levels.[102] SAMe donates methyl groups to a variety of endogenous substances, including neurotransmitters and catecholamines. It crosses the blood-brain barrier and increases brain neurotransmitter levels, including norepinephrine, dopamine, and serotonin.[105] Low activity of methionine-adenosyl transferase, the enzyme responsible for SAMe production, has been documented in depressed and schizophrenic patients, whereas high activity of this enzyme may be associated with mania.[105] For osteoarthritis, SAMe's true mechanism of action is unknown. It may serve as a source of sulfur required for cartilage growth and repair, and to stimulate proteoglycan production. Some anti-inflammatory and analgesic effects may also exist, but whether these effects are extensive enough to have clinical significance is unknown. Animal studies have demonstrated an increase in endogenous glucocorticoid levels with SAMe administration, so this may be related to anti-inflammatory effects.[103]

### Dosage and Administration Guidelines

See Table 54-1 for dosing information. Because of the possibility of side effects that may be dose-related, patients using SAMe should be encouraged to take the lowest dose that provides relief of osteoarthritis symptoms.

### Safety Considerations

The most common side effects reported for SAMe include nausea, diarrhea, and heartburn.[5,102-103] Less frequently, dry mouth, vomiting, headache, dizziness, nervousness, insomnia, cognitive impairment, and a switch to manic state in bipolar patients have also been reported.[102,104-106] In addition, SAMe has been associated with the development of hypomania or severe mania in subjects who had no personal or family history of mania or bipolar disease.[107-109] At least one report of mixed mania was associated with suicidal ideation within 2 weeks.[102] SAMe has been noted in several trials to be associated with significantly increased homocysteine levels and changes in plasma levels of related compounds, such as 5-methyltetrahydrofolate.[102,109,110] At least two studies, however, have not found such changes and, although elevated homocysteine levels are known to be a risk factor for cardiovascular disease, the clinical relevance of levels elevated by an exogenous substance is controversial.[102,111] Until more is known, it may be wise to avoid use in patients with existing hyperhomocysteinemia and to monitor levels, especially in patients with cardiac risk factors.

Researchers have postulated that some effects may be dose related (Table 54-1), as mania/hypomania has not been reported in any of the trials in patients with osteoarthritis using lower doses of 400 to 800 mg/day. More research is needed to determine if this association is accurate. Until more is known, it is a reasonable precaution to avoid use and especially higher doses. Long-term safety issues have yet to be determined. Although one study of intravenous SAMe in pregnant women noted no adverse outcomes, SAMe should not be used in pregnant or lactating women until more is known about possible fetal effects.[103]

SAMe should not be taken in conjunction with other serotonergic agents, such as antidepressants or 5-hydroxytryptamine$_1$ (5-HT$_1$)-agonists for migraine, because of an increased risk of serotonin syndrome. Avoid concomitant use of SAMe and corticosteroids until more is known about the extent of glucocorticoid increases.

### Administration and Product Issues

Depression is not self-treatable. Because of the potential for serious psychologic adverse events, patients should be counseled to avoid the use of SAMe for this indication unless treatment is recommended and monitored by a licensed mental health professional. Use of lower doses for osteoarthritis may be warranted, although patients should be encouraged to use therapy options with greater evidence of efficacy and safety, such as glucosamine sulfate (see Musculoskeletal System).

### Summary of Clinical Evidence

Clinical trials of oral SAMe in depression to date have been of small sample sizes, with many methodologic limitations. Results are often reported as mean response rates, rather than mean changes on a depression rating scale, with a wide range of response rates documented.[112] One meta-analysis suggested clinical benefits may be comparable to tricyclic antidepressants.[112] Symptom improvement occurs more rapidly than standard antidepressant treatment. Changes have been seen as early as 1 to 2 weeks, although those responses were observed in trials using intravenous doses or intravenous and oral dose combinations.[5] Comparisons with selective serotonin reuptake inhibitors (SSRIs), needed to characterize the effectiveness of SAMe treatment, have not been done to date.

A few small trials focused on depression associated with fibromyalgia noted an improvement in pain and other physical and psychologic symptoms.[113-115] Although evidence is very limited, the dearth of effective prescription therapies for fibromyalgia may lead primary care practitioners to attempt SAMe therapy in refractory patients.

Clinical trial evidence for use of SAMe in osteoarthritis is not definitive. Many early trials that reported symptom improvement used injectable dosage forms, did not diagnose patients with standard criteria, and were limited in length.[5] Several literature reviews and a meta-analysis have concluded that, even though included trials possessed many limitations, SAMe performed significantly better than placebo and similarly to NSAIDS in restoring functionality and decreasing pain, though with a slower onset of action.[101,116,117] Similar results were seen in a comparison to a selective cyclooxygenase 2 (COX2) inhibitor.[116] More research is needed to clarify the extent of SAMe's effects in osteoarthritis and the incidence of adverse events.

## 5-Hydroxytryptophan

### Therapeutic Uses

5-Hydroxytryptophan (5-HTP) is used for depression, anxiety, and insomnia. It is marketed as a safer alternative to tryptophan, a supplement banned after greater than 1500 case reports of eosinophilia myalgia syndrome (and 38 deaths) were reported in 1989. The cases were later linked to widespread product contamination with peakX (4,5-tryptophan-dione) during the manufacturing process.[118] However, 5-HTP may not actually be safer in this regard; peakX has also been found in samples of 5-HTP, including products tested after being associated with cases of an eosinophilia myalgialike illness and purchased from stores.[119-122]

### Physiologic Activity

5-HTP crosses the blood-brain barrier and is converted to serotonin, although much of it is broken down in the periphery.[123] Increased serotonin levels may result in serotonergic effects within the central nervous system (CNS).

### Dosage and Administration Guidelines

See Table 54-1 for dosing information.

### Safety Considerations

Reported side effects include GI effects such as nausea, vomiting, diarrhea, anorexia, belching, and flatulence.[4,123,124] It should not be used by pregnant or lactating women because of the lack of information regarding its effects. 5-HTP may increase the risk of serotonergic side effects (e.g., serotonin syndrome) and should not be used with other serotonergic agents, such as SSRIs, $5HT_1$-agonists, tramadol, and dextromethorphan.[123] Carbidopa, which decreases peripheral metabolism of 5-HTP, may increase its risk of side effects.[125]

### Administration and Product Issues

Patients should be encouraged to avoid 5-HTP because of safety concerns. Additional counseling points should center on the issue that depression and serious anxiety and panic disorders are not self-treatable conditions. Encourage patients to discuss their symptoms with a primary care provider.

### Summary of Clinical Evidence

Clinical evidence for use in depression is very preliminary, as trials performed to date are small and have shortcomings that limit their usefulness in decision making.[124] 5-HTP's use in anxiety and insomnia has not been well studied. One study examining treatment of night terrors in pediatric patients noted substantial benefit, but more evidence is needed before this use can be recommended.[126] Use in panic attacks is also being investigated, but research to date is limited to chemically induced attacks in healthy patients in a laboratory setting.[127,128]

## 2-Dimethylaminoethanol (DMAE)

### Therapeutic Uses

2-Dimethylaminoethanol (DMAE, or deanol) is a version of a former prescription medication called Deaner (deanol acetamidobenzoate) removed from the U.S market in 1983 because of lack of efficacy.[4] Dietary supplement DMAE is most commonly found as the bitartrate salt. It is promoted for treatment of attention-deficit hyperactivity disorder, Alzheimer's disease, Huntington's chorea, and tardive dyskinesia. DMAE is also marketed as an "antiaging" supplement. DMAE is often seen in small amounts in widely available combination products marketed for a variety of purposes. By itself, it is not commonly found in retail stores, but is easily available for purchase on the Internet.

### Physiologic Activity

DMAE is a precursor to choline and, to a much smaller extent, acetylcholine, a primary neurotransmitter. Decreases in brain acetylcholine levels, or reduced cholinergic activities, are observed in some neurologic conditions such as Huntington's chorea, and this provides the rationale for use of DMAE in these conditions. Whether administration of DMAE actually results in an increase in brain acetylcholine levels is still controversial because of contradictory study results.[129]

### Dosage and Administration Guidelines

See Table 54-1 for dosing information. Because of the lack of evidence of efficacy and the risk of CNS-associated adverse events, patients inquiring about DMAE should be counseled to avoid use unless they are closely monitored by their primary care provider.

### Safety Considerations

Adverse events reported for DMAE include CNS symptoms of confusion, drowsiness, depression, insomnia, and manic behavior, with depression and hypomania being reported more often in patients with previous psychiatric histories.[6,130,131] Other side effects include itching, increased blood pressure, diarrhea, and constipation.[130] One case report exists of tardive dyskinesia developing in a patient treated with DMAE for essential tremor.[132] DMAE may worsen schizophrenia symptoms and, despite being investigated in the past for mood elevation, is contraindicated in depression.[130,131] DMAE should not be used by pregnant or lactating women because of the lack of information about its effects. Because of reported cholinergic effects such as rhinorrhea and sialorrhea, it should not be used in conjunction with anticholinergic drugs, nor in patients with Parkinson's disease.[6,133]

### Administration and Product Issues

No product issues have been identified.

### Summary of Clinical Evidence

Most clinical research on DMAE is 25 to 50 years old. Although there are anecdotal reports of response in individuals, use of DMAE for treatment of tardive dyskinesia is not supported by clinical research findings.[130,131,134-138] One clinical trial in patients with Alzheimer's disease demonstrated no benefit and a high incidence of side effects.[6] Efficacy in Huntington's chorea is not supported by controlled trials.[139] Although some improvement in symptoms has been observed in small trials in children with attention-deficit/hyperactivity disorder (ADHD), the demonstrated lack of efficacy resulting in Deaner's discontinuation is still overriding.[140-142]

## Lecithin, Phosphatidylserine, and Phosphatidylcholine

### *Therapeutic Uses*

Lecithin is a phospholipid composed of other phospholipids, including phosphatidylcholine, phosphatidylserine, phosphatidylethanolamine, and phosphatidylinositol. Lecithins from animal versus plant sources vary in percentages of each component.[143] As dietary supplements, they are used to improve memory and treat dementia.

### *Physiologic Activity*

Lecithin, phosphatidylserine, and phosphatidylcholine are promoted as precursors to the neurotransmitter acetylcholine. The extent to which these actually raise brain levels of acetylcholine, either serving as choline sources or affecting release, is still undetermined.[143,144]

### *Dosage and Administration Guidelines*

See Table 54-1 for dosing information.

### *Safety Considerations*

The side effect profiles of these phospholipids are similar. GI side effects include nausea, diarrhea, and abdominal distress. These are common with lecithin and less so for phosphatidylserine and phosphatidylcholine. Large doses (≥600 mg) of phosphatidylserine may be associated with insomnia.[145] These supplements should not be used in pregnant and lactating women because of the lack of information about effects. No interactions have been identified.

### *Administration and Product Issues*

No product issues have been identified.

### *Summary of Clinical Evidence*

Multiple clinical trials using various doses and a recent meta-analysis by the Cochrane Collaboration of 12 trials with a total of 376 patients have concluded that there is no significant benefit in the use of lecithin for patients with Alzheimer's disease, parkinsonian dementia, or unclassified memory impairment.[146-150] A small benefit in Alzheimer's patients was observed in one trial of lecithin used in conjunction with tacrine, which was deemed to be separate from the benefit achieved by tacrine alone.[151] No memory benefit has been found in healthy subjects.[152]

Phosphatidylserine may slightly improve memory in patients with Alzheimer's disease, although this evidence can be considered preliminary.[153] Studies have found no improvement of memory or cognition in age-related memory impairment.[154,155]

One study with a small sample size, using a lecithin preparation with greater than 90% phosphatidylcholine, noted improvements in learning and mental symptom test scores in Alzheimer's patients.[156] A study of a single dose in healthy subjects found slight improvements in memory scores, which were attributed to learning responses.[157] A meta-analysis of studies of a closely related form of choline, cytidinediphosphocholine, found a limited, short-term improvement in memory function for individuals with cognitive impairment from several cerebrovascular disorders.[158]

Overall, individual acetylcholine precursors may have some slight beneficial effects in patients with neurologic disorders, although the clinical significance of benefit is not well-characterized. Healthy individuals, however, are unlikely to benefit from supplementation.

# ENDOCRINE SYSTEM

## Dehydroepiandrosterone

### *Therapeutic Uses*

Dehydroepiandrosterone (DHEA) is a steroid hormone secreted by the adrenal cortex; its levels normally decline with advancing years. DHEA is marketed primarily to treat sexual dysfunction or improve sexual performance, to combat symptoms of aging, and to enhance athletic performance or increase muscle mass. Although the FDA banned "designer steroids" in 2004 from having dietary supplement status, DHEA was exempted from this ban.[159]

### *Physiologic Activity*

DHEA circulates in its sulfate storage form, dehydroepiandrosterone sulfate. DHEA is a precursor for male and female sex hormones and does not bind directly to estrogen or androgen receptors.

Exogenous administration causes gender-dependent changes in a number of hormones. In women, DHEA increases testosterone levels more than estrogen levels. In men, estrogen increases, but not testosterone.[160] The extent to which androgen and estrogen transformation occurs depends partly on the patient's baseline hormone levels.

### *Dosage and Administration Guidelines*

See Table 54-1 for dosing information. Studies have often used doses of 50 to 100 mg daily; however, the fairly serious side effects that have been reported seem to occur at doses of 50 mg/day or greater.[161-164] It may be prudent to caution patients not to use these higher doses unless their physician recommends them and their blood levels are monitored. If hormone-associated effects appear (see Safety Considerations), the patient should discontinue the supplement. Women must be warned that voice changes caused by increased testosterone levels are generally irreversible. Although DHEA levels decline with age as endogenous production decreases, patients under the age of 40 are unlikely to need supplementation.

### *Safety Considerations*

Side effects are sex hormone related. Women may experience hirsutism, voice deepening, increased acne, and menstrual changes, while men have reported gynecomastia. Other side effects include increased HDL and liver function enzymes, headache, congestion, and insomnia.

At least four case reports of severe mania requiring hospitalization and treatment exist.[161-164] DHEA should be avoided in patients with bipolar disorder and is contraindicated in pregnant and lactating women because of the possibility of hormonal effects on the fetus or nursing child. Because it is a hormone precursor, DHEA should not be taken in conjunction with any other hormonal or hormone-blocking medications, or in patients with a history of breast, prostate, cervix, or endometrial cancer. One study noted increased levels of 5α-androstane-3α-17β-diol glucuronide (ADG) with DHEA supplementation in healthy young men. Because ADG may function as a prostate growth factor, high doses and long-term use may have negative effects on prostate health.[165]

### Administration and Product Issues

No product issues have been identified.

### Summary of Clinical Evidence

Some clinicians currently recommend DHEA supplementation for patients with documented DHEA deficiencies. An example is in women with adrenal failure, (i.e., who do not produce sufficient quantities of endogenous adrenal hormones). One study found that when DHEA 50 mg/day was added to the standard hydrocortisone treatment regimen, patients showed significant improvement in general well-being, sexual function, and lipid profiles.[160] Another study using a 25 mg/day dose, however, did not observe any benefits.[166] True efficacy of DHEA in this population remains unclear. In healthy pre- or postmenopausal women, DHEA does not improve sexual function.

In postmenopausal women greater than 70 years of age, one clinical trial noted a decrease in serum phosphate (a marker of bone turnover), increase in epidermal thickness and sebum production, and improvement of libido and sexual dysfunction as measured on a nonvalidated questionnaire.[167] Improvement of skin was also noted in a trial in men of advanced age.[168] Two additional trials in postmenopausal women noted improvements in scores on the Kupperman index, a validated measurement of postmenopausal vasomotor and psychological symptoms.[169,170] No improvement was found, however, in two trials specifically evaluating sexual arousal/function in healthy premenopausal and postmenopausal women.[171,172]

In a study of healthy men and women between the ages of 50 and 65, DHEA supplementation resulted in slight body composition benefits in men, but not in women.[173,174] Studies in healthy older men and women do not show any benefit in general well-being, memory, or cognition.[175-178] Preliminary evidence suggests that DHEA supplementation in the elderly may decrease abdominal fat and increase insulin sensitivity.[179] Clinical evidence for efficacy in men with erectile dysfunction is very preliminary. Significant improvement has been noted in men with erectile dysfunction from hypertension or unknown causes, but not for diabetes-induced or neurologically induced dysfunction.[168,180] Even in those populations, the newer prescription treatment options should be first-line therapy unless contraindicated.

Studies using up to 100 mg daily in young healthy men have shown no increases in strength or lean body mass or improvements in athletic performance.[181,182]

## α-Lipoic Acid

### Therapeutic Uses

α-Lipoic acid, also known as thioctic acid, is a lipophilic and hydrophilic endogenous substance promoted as a supplement for diabetic patients. In Europe, intravenous α-lipoic acid is an approved treatment for diabetic peripheral neuropathy.[4]

### Physiologic Activity

α-Lipoic acid is a cofactor for several enzymes involved in glucose metabolism. α-Lipoic acid levels are reduced in diabetic animals that have decreased glucose uptake in muscle tissue. Supplementation theoretically would increase the activity of enzymes responsible for glucose uptake. Human studies have shown improvement in a variety of measurements of glucose metabolism, and animal studies have noted improvements in nerve blood flow and distal conduction.[183-188] α-Lipoic acid is a chelating agent, and, along with its metabolite, dihydrolipoic acid, is an antioxidant.[4,189]

### Dosage and Administration Guidelines

See Table 54-1 for dosing information. Because bioavailability is approximately 30%, an 1800 mg oral dose should be comparable to an intravenous dose of 600 mg, the dose used in most European trials.[190] Diabetic patients who wish to add α-lipoic acid to their current medication regimen should discuss this therapy with their primary care provider. Patients must understand the increased risk of hypoglycemia and frequently monitor their glucose levels. If glucose levels improve, dose adjustment of other medications by a primary care provider may be necessary.

### Safety Considerations

Oral α-lipoic acid is generally well tolerated. Reported side effects include headache, nausea, and allergic rash.[191,192] Reductions in mineral stores are possible because of chelating activity, although the dose at which this becomes clinically significant is unknown.[193]

α-Lipoic acid may interfere with conversion of thyroxine to triiodothyronine. Patients with thyroid conditions should be cautioned to avoid use.[194] Additive glucose-lowering effects may occur when used with antidiabetic medications. Administration concurrently with food decreases bioavailability.[195] α-Lipoic acid is a chelating agent, therefore doses should be separated by 2 to 3 hours from doses of antacids or other mineral-containing supplements.

### Administration and Product Issues

Patients on high doses of α-lipoic acid may be at risk for thiamin deficiency.[4,192] This is likely to be clinically significant only in those patients already at risk for deficiency, such as alcoholics. Use of a daily multivitamin containing thiamin is advisable in these populations. α-Lipoic acid should be taken on an empty stomach for better absorption.

### Summary of Clinical Evidence

A recent review concluded that parenteral α-lipoic acid has demonstrated sufficient benefit, especially in light of its limited side effects profile, to be considered as a treatment option for diabetic neuropathy.[191] Evidence for reduction of neuropathy symptoms by oral α-lipoic acid is promising, but not definitive. A 2-year study of 600 and 1200 mg doses found improvements in nerve conduction, but not neuropathy symptoms.[196] One 3-month uncontrolled study of 600 mg daily (n = 20) found improvement in both nerve conduction and clinical symptoms.[197] Two placebo-controlled trials, one of 1800 mg daily for 3 weeks (n = 24) and the other of 600 mg daily for 8 weeks (n = 61), noted improvements in symptoms such as pain, numbness, paresthesia, and burning sensation.[198,199] A long-term investigation of oral α-lipoic acid is underway. Recent development of an oral sustained-release dosage form may improve future research methodology and patient compliance.[200]

Despite improvement in laboratory measurements of glucose uptake and metabolism, clinical trials to date do not document improvement in glucose and glycosylated hemoglobin levels.[201,202] Future research is needed to determine if long-term supplementation with α-lipoic acid will aid glucose control or reduce disease complications.

## PERFORMANCE ENHANCERS/IMMUNE SYSTEM

### Colostrum

### Therapeutic Uses

Colostrum is the thin, white fluid produced by mammary glands immediately after birth prior to milk production. In addition to treatment of diarrhea of various etiologies, colostrum is marketed for general well-being, improved athletic performance, and immune system stimulation. Patients interested in colostrum for "staying healthy" during cold and flu season should be advised that this benefit is unlikely.

### Physiologic Activity

Colostrum is rich in antibodies, immunoglobulins A and E, and growth factors. It provides passive immunity against many pathogens until the newborn is able to produce sufficient antibodies. Hyperimmune bovine colostrum is collected from cows inoculated with pathogens to induce production of specific antibodies and immunoglobulins and has FDA-approved orphan drug status for AIDS-related diarrhea. Dietary supplement bovine colostrum is generally not collected from inoculated cows. Serum levels of insulinlike growth factor (IGF) increase after colostrum administration in humans, and it is theorized that better utilization of glucose could improve athletic performance.[4,203]

### Dosage and Administration Guidelines

General dosing guidelines are given in Table 54-1, but because of the variety of available concentrations and dosage forms, following the manufacturer's listed dosing is recommended.

### Safety Considerations

Colostrum is generally well tolerated. Reported side effects include increased liver function enzymes in AIDS patients.[204] Because of the animal source, extra caution is needed to ensure a quality product (see Quality Issues in the "Introduction to Botanical and Nonbotanical Natural Medicines"). Patients allergic to milk should not use colostrum. Pregnant or lactating women should avoid use because of the lack of information about effects. No interactions are known.

### Administration and Product Issues

Because of its animal origin, the possibility of contamination of colostrum from diseased cattle must be considered.

### Summary of Clinical Evidence

Colostrum sold as a dietary supplement in the United States is marketed primarily for two purposes: to "strengthen the immune system" and to improve athletic performance. These products are not the FDA-approved hyperimmune colostrums, which have evidence of efficacy for indications such as infectious diarrhea.[205,206] To date, no studies have examined the immune-stimulating or illness-preventing effects of dietary supplement colostrums available in the United States.

Use of hyperimmune colostrum to improve athletic performance has been heavily investigated; overall, studies do not demonstrate any improvement in strength or endurance.[207-211] Dietary supplement colostrum products have not been clinically investigated, and so there is no support for the marketing claims of "building muscle, not fat."[211]

### Thymus Extract

### Therapeutic Uses

The thymus gland, a two-lobe gland lying above the heart and below the thyroid gland, is involved in immune function. The gland reaches peak size at about 1 year of age and then begins to decline in function and size. Thymus extracts are not approved for use in the United States, but purified, concentrated preparations (i.e., thymodulin and thymostimulin) are used in Europe and South America and are discussed here because of possible availability through Internet sources. These compounds have been used to treat several congenital immune deficiency syndromes. They have also been studied for immune-related conditions, allergies, and viral hepatitis, and as an adjunct to cancer chemotherapy and radiation therapy.[212-217]

### Physiologic Activity

Thymus gland extracts contain several polypeptide types with varying stimulatory effects on β-cells, maturation of T-cells, macrophage function, and activity and number of several subtypes of T-cells.[4,212]

### Dosage and Administration Guidelines

See Table 54-1 for dosing information. Optimum and safe dosing of thymus extracts remains unknown.

### Safety Considerations

Thymus extracts are generally not associated with adverse events.[4,215] Patients with autoimmune disorders (including HIV/AIDS) and those receiving immune-suppressing therapy should avoid the use of thymus extract until more safety information becomes available.

Although thymus is often promoted for patients with autoimmune diseases, its use could be dangerous in this patient population because of the lack of knowledge about supplement-disease interactions. In the future, thymus extracts may prove to be of benefit in HIV and AIDS patients, but the possibility of contamination with pathogens prevents recommendations for current use.

### Administration and Product Issues

See Bovine Source Precautions and Table 54-1.

### Summary of Clinical Evidence

Only one clinical trial has examined a "dietary supplement" thymus extract, as opposed to a purified prescription product. The product included many standard vitamins and minerals, herbs, amino acids, "thymus enzymatic polypeptide fractions" 1100 mg, "thymus extract, and raw spleen, lymph, bone marrow, and pituitary extracts" 100 mg.[218] The product was compared with placebo for 3 months in 38 patients with hepatitis C who had previously failed interferon therapy. No differences were observed between the treatment and placebo groups in the 3-month study period or in the following 6-month open-label period.[215]

## MUSCULOSKELETAL SYSTEM

## Glucosamine

### Therapeutic Uses

Glucosamine is one of the more well-researched nonbotanical supplements. A substance used by the body to make cartilage, it is primarily promoted for osteoarthritis.

### Physiologic Activity

Glucosamine is an endogenous mucopolysaccharide used in the synthesis of cartilage. Exogenous administration of glucosamine increases the "building blocks" available for cartilage production. Because sulfur is essential for glycosaminoglycan bonds within cartilage, the sulfate salt form may also provide important activity.[219] In addition, glucosamine stimulates chondrocyte cartilage production and synoviocyte synovial fluid production, inhibits matrix metalloproteinase, and modulates activities of collagenase and cytokines involved in stress reactions.[220-224] A recent study demonstrated greater effectiveness of glucosamine in patients with high cartilage turnover rates, as indicated by increased levels of collagen Type II.[225] More research is needed to determine if results of this assay could be used to predict a successful or unsuccessful response to glucosamine therapy.

### Dosage and Administration Guidelines

See Table 54-1 for dosing information. Patients interested in using glucosamine should be counseled regarding the proper dose (1500 mg/day), regimen options (three times/day or once daily), use of the appropriate sulfate salt (see Administration and Product Issues), side effects, and contraindications. Patients should be counseled strongly that glucosamine will not provide pain relief as quickly as NSAIDs or acetaminophen might. Effects may not be experienced for 6 to 8 weeks, with full benefit not evident for several months.

Some topical preparations containing glucosamine among other ingredients known to be topically effective for osteoarthritis are currently marketed. Only one small trial with severe methodologic limitations has been conducted.[226] Although one recent study found that glucosamine is absorbed transdermally, additional confirmation and clinical trials are needed before this route of administration can be recommended.[227]

### Safety Considerations

Glucosamine is generally well tolerated. Nausea, stomach upset, constipation, and diarrhea are the most common side effects.[4] Taking divided doses with meals may help alleviate these effects. Drowsiness, headache, and skin reactions have been infrequently reported. Glucosamine can be manufactured from shellfish (crab, lobster, shrimp) chitin as well as produced synthetically. Because source materials may not remain consistent, even for a particular manufacturer, patients with shellfish allergy should avoid this product. One report has documented exacerbation of previously well-controlled asthma, which resolved completely on discontinuation of a glucosamine-chondroitin product.[228]

Preliminary in vitro and animal studies indicate that intravenous glucosamine may increase blood glucose levels and insulin resistance. Because of glucosamine's glucose-based chemical structure, there was concern over the possibility of hyperglycemia and increased insulin resistance in both normoglycemic and diabetic patients. Two 3-year studies monitored glucose levels.[229,230] No changes in glycemic indicators were observed, however, the authors did not report the percentage of diabetic subjects in the study. A recent placebo-controlled trial evaluated the effects of a glucosamine hydrochloride and chondroitin combination on glycosylated hemoglobin in diabetic patients.[231] No changes were observed. Diabetic patients initiating glucosamine therapy should be aware of the possibility of an effect on glucose levels, but use is not contraindicated. Increased monitoring of glucose levels is advised until levels are noted to be stable.

Although anecdotal reports of cholesterol elevations in patients using glucosamine are being discussed among health care professional, no published case reports exist and no indication of changes in lipid status has been observed in any long-term clinical trials.[229,230] Lipid monitoring is recommended. Pregnant or lactating women should avoid glucosamine because of the lack of information about its effects. There are no known interactions.

### *Administration and Product Issues*

To date, the vast majority of trials demonstrating efficacy and safety have used the sulfate form of glucosamine. Two studies have examined efficacy of the hydrochloride form. One study observed effects similar to placebo, whereas in a more recent study of 46 patients using 2000 mg/day, 81% of glucosamine patients reported an improvement in pain compared with 17% of placebo patients.[232,233] Although in vitro studies have observed similar activities for the hydrochloride form, until further clinical trials of it and other salt forms have clearly established efficacy and safety, the sulfate form is recommended.[220]

Glucosamine sulfate is available in timed-release formulations, however, the bioavailability and kinetics of only one of those formulations has been compared to immediate-release glucosamine.[234] Because glucosamine may be taken in one daily dose, a time-release preparation may not offer any compliance advantage to offset higher costs.

### *Summary of Clinical Evidence*

Several clinical trials have compared glucosamine against placebo and/or standard treatments such as NSAID therapy. The majority had positive results for symptoms, showing greater benefit than placebo and similar efficacy in symptom relief to NSAID treatment, but most trials were small with methodologic limitations in study design.[235,236] Two large ($n = 202, 212$), well-designed 3-year studies in patients with knee osteoarthritis demonstrated significant efficacy and safety.[229,230] Patients with knee osteoarthritis treated with glucosamine sulfate for 3 years had significant ($p = .05$ and $.013$) reduction of knee cartilage loss and some experienced increased cartilage growth compared with placebo patients.

Meta-analyses of randomized, controlled trials concluded that glucosamine sulfate is safe and effective for the treatment of osteoarthritis, though the full extent of effectiveness is not completely characterized.[235-237] However, not all well-designed trials have had positive results; the benefits of glucosamine compared with other drug therapies should be investigated further.

## Chondroitin Sulfate

### *Therapeutic Uses*

Chondroitin sulfate (CS) is a glucosaminoglycan made from glucuronic acid and galactosamine present in animal cartilage. CS, in combination with hyaluronic acid, is an FDA-approved product for ophthalmic indications, such as preserving corneas for transplant and as a viscoelastic agent for use in cataract surgery. As a dietary supplement, CS is often combined with other supplements in products for osteoarthritis and joint health and has primarily been studied for knee and hip osteoarthritis.

### *Physiologic Activity*

There may be some truth to the layperson's explanation that "glucosamine builds up cartilage, and chondroitin keeps it from being broken down." Similar to glucosamine, CS serves as building material for cartilage production as well as inhibiting leukocyte elastase, an enzyme that is involved in cartilage degradation.[238] CS may also stimulate chondrocytes to produce more cartilage components.[239] Some evidence does suggest that chondroitin might be considered a disease-modifying agent, with beneficial effects lasting beyond dates of use.[240]

### *Dosage and Administration Guidelines*

See Table 54-1 for dosing information. Because so many products include both glucosamine and chondroitin, patients need to know that chondroitin, the ingredient with less evidence of efficacy, is also the more expensive ingredient. A patient concerned about cost could be advised to begin treatment with glucosamine sulfate monotherapy. If after 4 to 5 months some significant benefit is seen but symptoms are still bothersome, a CS product may be added. If no additional benefit is readily apparent after 3 to 5 months, the CS should be discontinued. Patients should be counseled to take CS with food if nausea or GI upset occurs.

### *Safety Considerations*

CS is generally well tolerated. Common side effects include mild GI upset and nausea. During clinical trials, allergic reactions, edema, diarrhea, constipation, nausea, heartburn, and hair loss were reported infrequently.[239-241] One report has documented exacerbation of previously well-controlled asthma, which resolved completely on discontinuation of the glucosamine-chondroitin product.[228] Use in pregnant or lactating women should be avoided because of the lack of information about effects.

Some animal studies have shown intravenous CS to have antithrombotic properties.[242] Theoretically, CS could increase bleeding risk when used with anticoagulants or antiplatelet agents, although there are currently no reports of increased bleeding in humans. Patients taking antiplatelet agents or anticoagulants should be reminded to report any bleeding to their primary care provider.

### Administration and Product Issues

Because CS is an animal product, concern about contamination is always present. Often, CS is still produced from bovine trachea, so BSE cautions apply (see Quality Issues in the "Introduction to Botanical and Nonbotanical Natural Medicines"). Product quality remains a concern as many CS supplements have been shown to contain little actual chondroitin.[243]

### Summary of Clinical Evidence

Because many trials combined CS with glucosamine sulfate, there is far less evidence for the efficacy of CS monotherapy in osteoarthritis, although this difference is shrinking with publication of more CS research. Several chondroitin trials are published in non-English journals and so are often not included in reviews or meta-analyses because of language barriers. Meta-analyses have concluded that CS therapy may provide moderate benefit in osteoarthritis, especially in combination with NSAID therapy. Trials reviewed, however, were limited in size, design, and methodology.[239,244] A 2001 trial comparing CS with placebo found differences between the groups that did not reach statistical significance in favor of CS.[241] This trial used a 1000 mg/day dose, which is lower than the usually recommended 1200 mg/day dose. A recent trial comparing CS (800 mg/day) and naproxen (500 mg/day) to naproxen alone for osteoarthritis of the hands noted a reduced progression of joint erosion in the CS-treated patients ($p < .05$).[245] In addition, a 1-year trial in which patients received 800 mg/day for months 1 to 3 and then months 6 to 9 noted statistically and clinically significant improvement in pain and function index scores during both active treatment and the 3 months of no treatment, supporting claims of disease-modifying activity.[240] More research is needed to further characterize findings and determine an optimal dose range.

## Methyl-sulfonyl-methane

### Therapeutic Uses

Methyl-sulfonyl-methane (MSM), also known as dimethylsulfone, is a naturally occurring compound found in foods such as vegetables and milk. MSM has become a popular ingredient in dietary supplements for use in arthritis and allergies despite lack of clinical study. It is a major metabolite of dimethylsulfoxide (DMSO) and was developed as a therapy in an attempt to avoid the toxicity and unpleasant side effects of DMSO[246] (Table 54-2[4,8,247-253]).

### Physiologic Activity

MSM is a source of sulfur, released on breakdown by intestinal bacteria. The sulfur is then incorporated into amino acids such as cysteine and methionine. The mechanism for activity in osteoarthritis is unclear, although sulfur is essential for bonding in cartilage and animal studies have found lower levels of sulfur in arthritic cartilage.[254] One study did find a decrease in joint disease in a rheumatoid arthritis mice model.[255] Promoters often make claims of proven anti-inflammatory effects, but with little scientific support. Much of the touted evidence is for DMSO, rather than MSM. The two products have many different properties.[246]

### Dosage and Administration Guidelines

Table 54-1 lists dosing ranges used in trials. Patients should be counseled on treatment choices with greater evidence, especially for osteoarthritis. If a patient chooses to use MSM, counseling should include expected side effects.

### Safety Considerations

MSM is generally well tolerated. The rarely reported side effects include headache, pruritus, and GI symptoms of nausea and diarrhea.[256] A recent 90-day high-dose study in rats demonstrated no toxicities.[257] Use in pregnant and lactating women should be avoided because of lack of information. No known interactions are known.

### Administration and Product Issues

MSM can be destroyed by water or excessive heat in manufacture or storage. Purchasing from a large, well-known company with good quality assurance measures is vital. Proper storage away from excessive heat and moisture will preserve supplement quality.

### Summary of Clinical Evidence

One 12-week clinical trial of 118 subjects comparing MSM with glucosamine sulfate, placebo, and the combination of MSM and glucosamine sulfate found statistically significant improvement in pain and functioning in all groups but placebo. Improvement was greater in the combination group than with either MSM or glucosamine sulfate alone.[258] One open-label clinical trial (n = 55) explored MSM use in seasonal allergic rhinitis.[256] Researchers reported significant ($p < .005$) reductions in allergy symptom (e.g., sneezing, rhinorrhea, and nasal itching) questionnaire scores during the trial month and in a 2-week follow-up period. Current clinical evidence is of interest, but insufficient to support use for any indication; more research is needed to confirm and fully characterize benefits.

# PROTEOLYTIC ENZYMES

## Bromelain and Trypsin

### Therapeutic Uses

Proteolytic enzymes most commonly used in dietary supplements include bromelain, a combination enzymatic extract from pineapple, and trypsin, an enzyme endogenous to the human small intestine. Proteolytic enzymes are used for treatment of osteoarthritis, fibromyalgia, muscular injuries such as sprains and strains, and reduction of postoperative pain and swelling. Trypsin is an active ingredient in an FDA-approved product (Granulex, Granulderm) indicated for debridement of wounds and decubitus ulcers.[259]

**TABLE 54-2 Unsafe Nonbotanical Substances**

| Product | What Is It? | Side Effects/Adverse Events | Summary and Evidence of Efficacy |
|---|---|---|---|
| Hydrazine | Organic substance used as industrial solvent and fuel in rocket engines. Inhibits enzyme involved in gluconeogenesis.<br>Not generally available in retail stores, but still promoted in some alternative cancer clinics and available for purchase on the Internet. | Orally: N/V/D, CNS depression, neuropathy, lethargy, irregular breathing, hypo- or hyperglycemia, violent behavior, restlessness, seizures, coma, hepatic and renal toxicity; carcinogenic and fetotoxic<br>Topically or inhaled: irritation, burning, permanent damage to eyes or mucous membranes, pulmonary edema, death | Any possible benefits are greatly outweighed by safety concerns.<br>Clinically tested in the 1960s and 1970s for cancer treatment and cancer-related cachexia. Promising preliminary results, but later studies demonstrated poor outcomes, especially in patients on certain chemotherapy regimens. |
| Tiratricol | Triiodothyroacetic acid, structurally related to T3 and a metabolite of T4 | Severe diarrhea and weight loss, fatigue, lethargy, CV events, hyperthyroidism; possible events include pseudohypothyroidism, hypothyroidism, paralysis of eye muscles, and hepatotoxicity | FDA determined to be unapproved new drug. Products recalled and should not be available; however, at least one incidence reported of product for sale at a discount outlet after recall.<br>Trials in thyroid cancer do not support benefit. Evidence from small studies and case reports for treatment of pituitary resistance to thyroid hormone is promising, but preliminary. |
| Colloidal silver | Inorganic silver in a suspending agent. Mechanisms to produce silver solutions at home are available. Inorganic silver has antimicrobial action; used in topical prescription products | Argyria (permanent blue-gray skin discoloration), damage to renal tissue, neurologic damage; photograph of patient with argyria available at http://homepages.together.net/~rjstan/ | Argyria can occur after only a few months of use with any available salt forms. Intake from food and water sources can come close to levels of daily safe intake.<br>No trials support efficacy. |
| DMSO (dimethyl sulfoxide) | High-polarity industrial solvent commercially prepared from waste products of paper manufacture. A 50% solution is FDA approved for treatment of bladder conditions by intravesical instillation. Other clinical use disallowed because of vision damage found in animal studies; excellent transdermal absorption. | Topically: irritation and burning, blisters, scaly rash, HA, drowsiness, N/V/D, sedation, constipation, anorexia, eosinophilia, respiratory symptoms such as cough, dyspnea, sore throat, flulike symptoms, offensive garlic-oyster body/breath odor<br>*Note:* ALL events could be experienced with topical or intravesical use. Patients with body/breath odor have triggered transient respiratory irritation and headache in other people. | Industrial- and veterinary-grade products likely to contain contaminants and are not for human use.<br>Although may provide some symptomatic relief, high rates of adverse events and risks of serious toxicities outweigh limited and inconsistent benefits seen in trials. |
| Canthaxanthin | A carotenoid without vitamin A activity; used in "sunless tanning" dietary supplements. No clinical trials have assessed this use. | Fatal aplastic anemia, crystalline retinal deposits and decreased vision, orange discoloration of skin and body fluids, GI distress | Use should be discouraged. Although some skin color change is usually apparent, it is commonly uneven, i.e., streaks of dark orange rather than a "golden glow."<br>Used in combination with other carotenoids for treatment of protoporphyria and other photosensitivity diseases. |

**TABLE 54-2 Unsafe Nonbotanical Substances (continued)**

| Product | What Is It? | Side Effects/Adverse Events | Summary and Evidence of Efficacy |
|---|---|---|---|
| Androstenedione | An endogenous precursor to both androgens and estrogens | Increased lipids (decreased HDL), increased platelet aggregation, aggressive behavior, mood swings, acute mania, increases in LFTs, hepatic failure<br>Men: acne, testicular atrophy, and gynecomastia<br>Women: hirsutism, amenorrhea, male pattern baldness, clitoral hypertrophy, and deepening of voice | Three trials found no benefit over placebo for strength, performance, or muscle mass.<br>Although men use to increase testosterone, this does not occur; instead, estrogen levels generally increase, while in women, androgen levels increase.<br>Manufacture and distribution banned by the FDA, but products are still available from many Internet sources. |

Key: LFTs, liver function tests (serum hepatic transaminases); N/V/D, nausea/vomiting/diarrhea; T3, triiodothyronine; T4, thyroxine; CV, cardiovascular; HA, headache.

*Source:* Table compiled from references 4, 8, and 247-253.

Poultices or preparations made from meat tenderizers containing bromelain or papain are commonly recommended and used in home remedies for fire ant, bee, or jellyfish stings, but clinical trial evidence has shown no benefit in reducing pain or swelling.[260,261]

### Physiologic Activity

Both bromelain and trypsin may decrease symptoms of inflammatory conditions by decreasing inflammatory prostaglandin levels, reducing adhesion molecules, increasing fibrinolytic activity, and decreasing bradykinin, a pain mediator.[262,263] Some of bromelain's anti-inflammatory activity may be a result of effects on the migration, adhesion, and possibly activation, of immune system cells such as leukocytes and monocytes.[264] The amount of orally administered bromelain to survive degradation and reach the bloodstream intact is very small, as little as 10 μg after a 1 g dose.[265]

### Dosage and Administration Guidelines

See Table 54-1 for dosing information. Because of the variety of dosages and combination products available, observing manufacturers' listed doses is recommended. For acute pain and arthritic conditions, symptomatic response should be rapid. If a patient is not noting substantial symptom relief within 2 to 3 weeks, discontinue the enzymes.

### Safety Considerations

Adverse events reported for bromelain and trypsin products include mild GI symptoms of nausea and diarrhea. Allergic reactions are possible for both enzymes, with contact dermatitis (cheilitis) being reported for bromelain.[266] Bromelain has cross-sensitivity documented with carrots, celery, fennel, pawpaw, and wheat flour.[266-268] Persons allergic to members of the Asteraceae family (echinacea, ragweed, daisies, chrysanthemums) could potentially experience reactions to bromelain, although the extent and severity of this sensitivity is unknown.[267] Topically used trypsin can result in irritation, a burning sensation, and pain.[259]

Because animal studies have shown bromelain may stimulate production of prostaglandin $E_1$–like compounds that can inhibit platelet activity, there is a theoretical possibility of increased risk of bleeding when it is used in conjunction with anticoagulant or antiplatelet therapy.[269,270] Because of possible antiplatelet activity, as well as lack of information on other effects, pregnant and lactating women should not use bromelain in greater amounts than found in foods.

### Administration and Product Issues

No product issues have been identified.

### Summary of Clinical Evidence

The clinical evidence supporting proteolytic enzyme use in osteoarthritis and acute joint pain is limited. Many trials have used combination products, making determinations of individual component efficacy difficult. Efficacy and safety of two bromelain doses were examined in a 2002 open-label trial in 77 volunteers with acute knee pain who completed self-assessment questionnaires by mail. After 1 month, pain scores decreased by 44.6% and 58.2% in the 200 and 400 mg dose groups, respectively ($p < .0001$).[263] Additional bromelain evidence dates from the 1960s and consists of small trials with major methodologic limitations. A 1975 trial using a trypsin and chymotrypsin product for sprained ankles found no benefit compared with placebo.[271]

Phlogenzym (made by Mucos Pharma) combines bromelain with trypsin and rutin. Rutin serves as a source of quercetin, a citrus bioflavonoid antioxidant and anti-inflammatory. Two clinical trials have compared it with standard doses of diclofenac sodium for knee osteoarthritis.[262,272] Both studies found equivalent and clinically significant, 30%

to 80%, reductions in pain and improvements in range of movement. A similar dietary supplement, Wobenzym (made by Mucos Pharma), containing smaller amounts of bromelain and trypsin plus additional ingredients (chymotrypsin, pancreatin, and papain), is available for sale in the United States. Two studies have compared Wobenzym to diclofenac sodium for knee osteoarthritis and noted similar outcomes, but the quality of those trials cannot be evaluated as one is unpublished and the other not published in English.[273]

In addition to the musculoskeletal uses, bromelain is sometimes recommended for digestive disorders, despite the lack of evidence for this use. One case report describes two patients with ulcerative colitis who experienced improvement or resolution of symptoms, with endoscopy demonstrating healed mucosa in one patient and "quiescent disease" in the other.[274] At this time, bromelain is not recommended for any GI disorders.

## Papain

### Therapeutic Uses

Another proteolytic enzyme, papain, is a mixture of enzymes found in papaya fruit. Papain has many industrial uses and is the functional ingredient in meat tenderizer. As a supplement or home remedy, papain or combination products containing papain are promoted for treatment of inflammation and edema from injury, herpes zoster (shingles), and chronic diarrhea, and as first aid for insect bites and jellyfish stings.[275-282]

### Physiologic Activity

The proteolytic activities of papain include fibrinolysis, which may be responsible for decreasing swelling and improved blood flow in injured areas. Preparations of multiple enzymes have been shown to induce release of cytokines such as tumor necrosis factor and interleukins.[279,280]

### Dosage and Administration Guidelines

See Table 54-1 for dosing information. Patients wishing to use papain should be counseled not to take more than the manufacturer's recommended amount for a specific product. Use should be discontinued if stomach pain or heartburn occurs.

### Safety Considerations

Cross-sensitivity with kiwi and figs may occur and allergic reactions can be severe. Other side effects include severe gastritis and blisters, pruritus, and irritation with topical use.[4] Use in pregnant and lactating women should be avoided because of lack of information. According to a 5-year toxicologic study, papain may increase the activity of warfarin.[281] Case reports on the use of "large amounts" (unspecified) of papain for the treatment of meat impaction in the esophagus noted the occurrence of esophageal perforation and gastric ulcer, although causation was not determined.[282] Theoretically, release of tumor necrosis factor and interleukins may be problematic in patients with autoimmune diseases or HIV; until more is known about effects, use should be avoided in these patients.

### Administration and Product Issues

No product issues have been identified.

### Summary of Clinical Evidence

The majority of papain research is published in non-English journals. Determining efficacy for many conditions is therefore challenging. Further research is needed for use in herpes zoster and pharyngitis symptom reduction before any recommendation for use can be made. The evidence does not support use of papain from meat tenderizer in home remedies for insect or jellyfish stings.[275,277]

## Cetyl Myristoleate

### Therapeutic Uses

Cetyl myristoleate (CM) was identified when an NIH researcher toiled in his home laboratory to solve a mystery. Why could arthritis be induced with a trigger substance (desiccated *Mycobacterium butyricum* or bovine type II collagen) in rats, but not in mice? The substance isolated from those resistant mice was identified as CM, a fatty acid cetyl ester easily synthesized from cetyl alcohol and myristoleic acid. When rats were injected with CM prior to a trigger substance, they did not develop arthritis.[283-285] A recent animal study confirmed similar protective effects in mice using both injected and oral CM; it is promoted for use in both osteoarthritis and rheumatoid arthritis.[286]

### Physiologic Activity

It is unknown whether effects are related to CM as a whole or its myristoleic acid component; a reasonable hypothesis since other fatty acids have been shown to have anti-inflammatory activity.[286,287] Speculations about other modes of action include increased production of immunoglobulins and prostaglandins, and surfactant activity.[286,287] Changes in neutrophil counts and markers of inflammation have been noted in clinical trials.[287]

### Dosage and Administration Guidelines

See Table 54-1 for dosing information. Until more is known about CM, patients desiring a dietary supplement for arthritis should be directed to other products with more evidence of safety and efficacy, such as glucosamine sulfate.

### Safety Considerations

Side effects reported include undefined "GI symptoms."[287] Adverse events possibly associated with CM include pruritic skin rash, headaches, severe muscle spasms, nausea, abdominal bloating, and severe indigestion.[288] Use in pregnant and lactating women should be avoided because of the lack of information about effects. No interactions have been identified.

### Administration and Product Issues

Although CM was originally isolated from animals, production is now synthetic, so animal source precautions do not apply. CM is available as a single product, but is more commonly found in combination products marketed for osteoarthritis.

### Summary of Clinical Evidence

Very little clinical evidence on CM is available to date. Three small trials using primarily CM in combination with other products for osteoarthritis or fibromyalgia have reported improvements in symptoms but all had severe methodologic limitations.[288-289] Topical use of a CM cream versus placebo in osteoarthritis patients noted significant benefit in several test parameters, particular stair-climbing activity.[290] Further CM trials are needed to establish efficacy before it can be recommended for use.

## Shark Cartilage

### Therapeutic Uses

Cartilage from sharks is touted for a variety of conditions: osteoarthritis and joint problems, cancer, and psoriasis. Shark cartilage is composed of proteins, glycosaminoglycans such as chondroitin, and calcium. Although dietary supplements of shark cartilage are promoted with the idea that sharks have a "natural immunity to cancer," this statement is egregiously false.[291]

### Physiologic Activity

Shark cartilage components may decrease angiogenesis in a variety of ways, such as inhibition of endothelial cell proliferation and matrix metalloproteinase activity.[292] Purified anti-angiogenesis factors are being studied for cancer treatment.[293]

### Dosage and Administration Guidelines

See Table 54-1 for dosing information. Counseling patients on shark cartilage should stress the lack of clinical studies for efficacy in osteoarthritis or cancer. The concentrated extract that may have benefit for psoriasis is currently not available in the United States. Patients need to understand the risk of hypercalcemia and hepatitis. Symptoms such as fever, fatigue, jaundice, and discoloration of urine and feces should be reported immediately to a primary care provider. The greatest danger in using shark cartilage for cancer treatment is substitution of an ineffective treatment for treatments that have been shown to be beneficial.

### Safety Considerations

Side effects reported for shark cartilage include nausea, vomiting, constipation, diarrhea, dizziness, and hepatitis.[292] Hyperglycemia, transient hypotension, and hypercalcemia may also be associated with shark cartilage.[292] Patients at risk for hypercalcemia, such as those with renal disease, should avoid shark cartilage because of its high calcium content.

Angiogenesis is necessary for normal growth and repair. Shark cartilage should be avoided in children, pregnant and lactating women, cardiac patients, and patients with healing wounds. No interactions have been identified.

### Administration and Product Issues

Many shark cartilage products have been reported to have a bad smell or taste. Patients should be educated regarding the difference between the purified anti-angiogenesis factors being studied in clinical trials and the whole shark cartilage found in dietary supplements.

### Summary of Clinical Evidence

Investigation of shark cartilage for osteoarthritis arose from observations of improved arthritic symptoms in cancer patients enrolled in a shark cartilage trial. Although chondroitin, a component of shark cartilage, has been studied for osteoarthritis (see chondroitin sulfate), no trials examining the efficacy of shark cartilage for osteoarthritis have been published to date.[292]

The clinical evidence for shark cartilage in cancer treatment is poor and inconclusive. A case series reporting on patients who used shark cartilage often in combination with standard treatment such as radiation, noted improvement or disease stabilization.[294] These are balanced by reports from uncontrolled trials ranging from increased survival, to disease stability over the study period, to worsening of disease and death. The most rigorously designed study found no effect of shark cartilage at a dose of 1 g/kg for 12 weeks.[293] Further studies of shark cartilage are being conducted.

One non–placebo-controlled study has examined efficacy of differing doses of a liquid extract of shark cartilage (unavailable in the United States) in patients with plaque psoriasis.[294] Improvement of at least 20% on the Psoriasis Area and Severity Index was noted in 30.6% of all patients, with up to 50% improvement noted in the two patients in the highest-dose (240 mL/day) group. More studies are needed to examine efficacy and adverse events.

# UNSAFE NONBOTANICAL NATURAL MEDICINES

Several substances that carry an unacceptable risk of toxicity or adverse events are still often advertised and recommended in the lay media (Table 54-2). They are often touted as "medical miracles" being repressed by the government or health care industry. These products are easily available through mail order over the Internet. The most likely to be encountered are colloidal silver and dimethyl sulfoxide (DMSO), but health care professionals should have a basic familiarity with each of the products listed in the table.

## ASSESSMENT OF USE OF NONBOTANICAL NATURAL MEDICINES: A CASE-BASED APPROACH

A recent survey regarding patients' beliefs about regulation of dietary supplements reinforced the idea that many consumers and patients do not understand much about the supplements they take and believe labels are required to carry warnings about side effects and other safety issues.[295] This lack of understanding underscores the importance of educating patients who use supplements about the safety issues that must be considered before they decide to take a supplement.

We also know that most patients who use supplements do not tell their physicians, pharmacists, or other health care providers about their supplements.[296] Reasons for this are many and varied. Often, a patient may think that health care professionals will automatically have a negative attitude toward all supplements. Because the patient does not wish to be told to stop taking a chosen supplement, he or she simply does not tell the provider. Obtaining complete information about a patient's supplements and OTC medications is vital to monitoring for side effects and efficacy and preventing interactions.

To gain the most accurate information about a patient's medications and supplements, all health care providers must specifically inquire about the use of both supplements and prescription medications at every visit. Questions must be phrased in an open, nonthreatening manner that encourages a patient to share this information. For example, a patient in a diabetes clinic could be told, "Many of my patients are taking some herbal medications to help control their blood sugar. Have you tried any supplements?" That open question is more likely to establish a rapport with the patient than "Are you taking any herbs?" This question does not specifically indicate openness or real interest and may simply produce an inaccurate negative response. Cases 54-1 and 54-2 illustrate the assessment of patients who wish to use a nonbotanical natural medicine.

### CASE 54-1

| Relevant Evaluation Criteria | Scenario/Model Outcome |
|---|---|
| **Information Gathering** | |
| 1. Gather essential information about the patient's symptoms, including: | |
| a. description of symptom(s) (i.e., nature, onset, duration, severity, associated symptoms) | Patient reports joint pain in knees and right elbow that has slowly worsened over a 4-year period from an occasional discomfort to constant pain he describes as mild. His PCP has told him that he has osteoarthritis. |
| b. description of any factors that seem to precipitate, exacerbate, and/or relieve the patient's symptom(s) | The pain is aggravated by walking for extended periods, so he is using a cart while golfing, has limited his walking exercise, and has taken up swimming instead. |
| c. description of the patent's efforts to relieve the symptoms | He has been taking acetaminophen 500 mg 3 times/day on a daily basis for at least 6 months with moderate benefit; he states that the drug dulls the pain, but does not eliminate it. He has tried ibuprofen at both moderate and maximum doses with good relief, but cannot tolerate the GI side effects. |
| 2. Gather essential patient history information: | |
| a. patient's identity | John N. Sellers |
| b. patient's age, sex, height, and weight | 68 y/o M, 6'1", 186 lb |
| c. patient's occupation | Retired building contractor |
| d. patient's dietary habits | Low-fat, low-cholesterol diet |
| e. patient's sleep habits | Usually gets 7-8 hours of sleep per night; has insomnia 4-5 times per year |
| f. concurrent medications and medical conditions | Mild hypertension, well controlled on HCTZ 12.5 mg once daily; borderline elevated cholesterol, controlled with diet and exercise; Centrum Silver once daily |
| g. allergies | NKDA |
| h. history of other adverse reactions to medications | Intolerant of erythromycin (severe nausea and vomiting requiring change in antibiotic); no food allergies |

## CASE 54-1 (continued)

| Relevant Evaluation Criteria | Scenario/Model Outcome |
|---|---|
| i. other (describe)_______ | John has been reading about glucosamine products and has a friend who had used a glucosamine product in the past with good results. He is considering a product with the following ingredients: glucosamine hydrochloride 250 mg; chondroitin sulfate 100 mg; methyl-sulfonyl-methane (MSM) 10 mg; and manganese 15 mg. Instructions are to take 2 capsules 3 times/day. John wants to know if this is a good product and if it will interfere with his blood pressure medication. |
| **Assessment and Triage** | |
| 3. Differentiate patient's signs/symptoms and correctly identify the patient's primary problem(s). | History of joint discomfort slowly worsening to constant pain consistent with diagnosis of osteoarthritis with inadequately treated pain; patient lacks education regarding appropriate dietary supplement. Secondary problems include hypertension (controlled) and hyperlipidemia (controlled). |
| 4. Identify exclusions for self-treatment. | None for primary problem |
| 5. Formulate a comprehensive list of therapeutic alternatives for the primary problem to determine if triage to a medical practitioner is required and share this information with the patient. | Options include:<br>(1) Refer John to his PCP.<br>(2) Suggest maximizing his dose of acetaminophen.<br>(3) Guide John to an appropriate glucosamine supplement and provide education on its use.<br>(4) Take no action. |
| **Plan** | |
| 6. Select an optimal therapeutic alternative to address the patient's problem. | Guide John to an appropriate glucosamine supplement and provide counseling. |
| 7. Describe the recommended therapeutic approach to the patient. | You should start with a glucosamine sulfate single-ingredient product. You also should continue your low-fat diet and regular swimming exercise for control of hyperlipidemia and hypertension. |
| 8. Explain to the patient the rationale for selecting the recommended therapeutic alternatives that were considered. | Research evidence shows that glucosamine sulfate is more effective than the hydrochloride salt form. The studies supporting the other ingredients in this product are much more limited. In addition, the doses of MSM and manganese are inappropriate; the MSM dose (60 mg/day) is lower than recommended dose range of 100-300 mg/day, and the amount of manganese (90 mg/day) is higher than the safe upper limit for this element. |
| **Patient Education** | |
| 9. When recommending self-care with over-the-counter medications, convey accurate information to the patient, including: | |
| a. appropriate dose and frequency of administration | Glucosamine sulfate 1500 mg daily in single or divided doses |
| b. maximum number of days the therapy should be employed | Glucosamine sulfate will be a chronic or long-term medication because of slow onset of action. |
| c. product administration procedures | Take with meals if any GI upset should occur. |
| d. expected time to onset of relief | You may experience some slight reduction in pain or greater ease of movement within 2-4 weeks, but maximum benefit will not occur for 4-6 months. |
| e. degree of relief that can be reasonably expected | Symptom resolution is highly individual. Complete resolution of pain is probably not to be expected. |
| f. most common side effects | Nausea, diarrhea, or constipation |
| g. side effects that warrant medical intervention should they occur | There have been isolated reports of increases in lipid levels with glucosamine use. You should have your cholesterol checked in 3-4 months and continue your low-fat, low-cholesterol diet and regular exercise. |

## CASE 54-1 (continued)

| Relevant Evaluation Criteria | Scenario/Model Outcome |
|---|---|
| h. patient options in the event that condition worsens or persists | If no benefit has been noted after 6 months of use, you should stop using glucosamine and see your primary care provider for further evaluation. |
| i. product storage requirements | Keep product in an appropriate storage area away from excessive heat and moisture and out of reach of children and pets. |
| j. specific nondrug measures | After choosing an appropriate, high-quality product, maintain therapy with that same product. |
| 10. Solicit patient's follow-up questions. | Does it matter what brand I buy? |
| 11. Answer patient's questions. | Some products may not contain the stated amount of glucosamine sulfate. It is a good idea to buy a product that has a quality assurance seal of approval or that is listed on www.consumerlab.com as having passed tests to confirm appropriate amounts. |

Key: GI, gastrointestinal; HCTZ, hydrochlorothiazide; NKDA, no known drug allergy; OTC, over-the-counter; PCP, primary care provider.

## CASE 54-2

| Relevant Evaluation Criteria | Scenario/Model Outcome |
|---|---|
| **Information Gathering** | |
| 1. Gather essential information about the patient's symptoms, including: | |
| a. description of symptom(s) (i.e., nature, onset, duration, severity, associated symptoms) | Patient reports that despite several adjustments to her diabetes medications since she was diagnosed 8 months ago, she still has not been able to gain close control over her glucose levels. She reports occasional postprandial glucose spikes of 260-280 mg/dL and has had several episodes of hypoglycemia. She is frustrated and wants to try an $\alpha$-lipoic acid supplement. |
| b. description of any factors that seem to precipitate, exacerbate, and/or relieve the patient's symptom(s) | Patient states that sometimes when she is not feeling well, and thinks she may be hypoglycemic, her glucose levels are actually high. She states that on weeks when she is able to walk 3 or 4 days out of the week, she does feel a little better overall. Overall, her energy level has been lower than usual for 2-3 months. |
| c. description of the patent's efforts to relieve the symptoms | She tried an herbal blend supplement a month ago, but did not feel it helped her glucose at all and her blood pressure was higher than usual when she monitored it at home. She cannot remember any of the ingredients except for *Panax ginseng*. |
| 2. Gather essential patient history information: | |
| a. patient's identity | Louise J. Millerton |
| b. patient's age, sex, height, and weight | 59 y/o F, 5'5", 193 lb |
| c. patient's occupation | CPA |
| d. patient's dietary habits | Follows ADA diet "most of the time" but admits to eating many fast-food meals during tax season |
| e. patient's sleep habits | Generally 6-7 hours per night, although she frequently awakes at night and has not felt rested over the last 2 months |
| f. concurrent medications and medical conditions | Glipizide XL 5 mg, 1 tablet in morning, 2 tablets at evening meal, and metformin 500 mg 3 times/day for type 2 DM; HCTZ 25 mg once daily and lisinopril 40 mg once daily for HTN (not at goal); levothyroxine 0.125 mg once daily for hypothyroidism; atorvastatin 40 mg at bedtime; Allegra 180 mg once daily as needed for seasonal allergic rhinitis |
| g. allergies | NKDA |

## CASE 54-2 (continued)

| Relevant Evaluation Criteria | Scenario/Model Outcome |
|---|---|
| h. history of other adverse reactions to medications | None |
| i. other (describe)_______ | Louise has difficulty remembering to take her noon dose of metformin, but she is compliant with other medications. |
| **Assessment and Triage** | |
| 3. Differentiate patient's signs/symptoms and correctly identify the patient's primary problem(s). | Diabetes mellitus, glucose levels not at goal; hypertension, not at goal; hyperlipidemia, at goal on treatment<br>Potential supplement-disease state interaction (lipoic acid and thyroid disorder)<br>Potential for future noncompliance secondary to frustration with lack of success in controlling disease state<br>Lack of knowledge regarding appropriate dietary supplement use |
| 4. Identify exclusions for self-treatment. | N/A |
| 5. Formulate a comprehensive list of therapeutic alternatives for the primary problem to determine if triage to a medical practitioner is required and share this information with the patient. | Options include:<br>(1) Refer Louise to her PCP for evaluation.<br>(2) Help Louise select another dietary supplement that has evidence of some benefit to reduce blood glucose levels.<br>(3) Tell Louise that people with diabetes mellitus should never use dietary supplements to help control blood glucose levels.<br>(4) Prevent the immediate potential supplement-disease state interaction, refer Louise to PCP for evaluation and optimization of prescription medications, and discuss the possibility of trying a dietary supplement option in the future after her disease state is more stable.<br>(5) Take no action. |
| **Plan** | |
| 6. Select an optimal therapeutic alternative to address the patient's problem, taking into account patient preferences. | Prevent the immediate potential supplement-disease state interaction. Address Louise's frustration with current problems and refer her to her PCP for evaluation and optimization of prescription medications. Minimize future drug-supplement or supplement-disease state interaction by educating Louise on safety issues with supplement use and encouraging an open relationship. Let Louise know that if she chooses to use supplements as adjunctive therapy to control her diabetes, you will work with her to find products that might benefit her without interfering with her prescription medications. |
| 7. Describe the recommended therapeutic approach to the patient. | Although many diabetic patients use lipoic acid safely, it is contraindicated in patients with thyroid conditions and so is not safe for you.<br>Many diabetics also have difficulty in finding an optimum medication regimen. By working closely with your PCP, that is, primary care provider, and your pharmacist, you should be able to gain better control over your glucose levels. Use a blood glucose diary, and monitor and document your blood sugar 3-4 times a day for 1 week prior to your appointment so that your PCP will have an accurate picture of your levels at different times during the day. This will allow more appropriate adjustments to your medications to achieve successful control of your blood sugars. An extended-release version of metformin is available that may help you take it more regularly; you should discuss that with your PCP.<br>The herbal product containing ginseng could have been responsible for your increased blood pressure. It may also have affected your blood sugar levels; you should avoid it in the future. Because of your diabetes and thyroid disorder, there are many dietary supplements that you will not be able to use safely. You should discuss any supplements with me or your PCP prior to use. After your prescription medication has been adjusted, if you still want to try a dietary supplement, I will help you investigate any possible supplements to determine if they interact with your medications or disease states. |

**CASE 54-2 (continued)**

| Relevant Evaluation Criteria | Scenario/Model Outcome |
|---|---|
| 8. Explain to the patient the rationale for selecting the recommended therapeutic alternatives that were considered. | Because of the lack of knowledge regarding the interaction of many supplements with other drugs and because of safety concerns, patients with conditions such as diabetes, hypertension, and thyroid disorders need to be especially careful when deciding to take supplements.<br>Before you try to use any supplements, all your prescription medications should be optimized and your conditions should be stable. This will allow for easier recognition of any adverse events resulting from use of a supplement. |
| **Patient Education** | |
| 9. When recommending self-care with over-the-counter medications convey accurate information to the patient. | Criterion does not apply in this case. |
| 10. Solicit patient's follow-up questions. | I realize now that I have to be careful about what I take, but aren't there any supplements that I can try now to help control my blood sugar? |
| 11. Answer patient's questions. | As we discussed, you need to make sure that your prescription medications are at optimum doses first. The only supplement that I might consider trying right now is adding a psyllium fiber supplement. This may help slow absorption of food and slightly lower the postprandial glucose peaks; it may also help slightly decrease your cholesterol levels. Because this supplement may also interfere with the absorption of your medications, you will have to be careful about timing your doses. If your PCP changes your metformin to an extended-release form so that you aren't taking any medications at lunchtime, we can try adding a dose of psyllium then. |

Key: ADA, American Diabetes Association; CPA, certified public accountant; DM, diabetes mellitus; HCTZ, hydrochlorothiazide; HTN, hypertension; NKDA, no known drug allergy; PCP, primary care provider.

## PATIENT COUNSELING FOR NONBOTANICAL NATURAL MEDICINES

See the "Introduction to Botanical and Nonbotanical Natural Medicines" for a discussion of important counseling issues and tips.

## References


1. Gades MD, Stern JS. Chitosan supplementation does not affect fat absorption in healthy males fed a high-fat diet, a pilot study. *Int J Obes Relat Metab Disord.* 2002;26:119-22.
2. Gades MD, Stern JS. Chitosan supplementation and fecal fat excretion in men. *Obes Res.* 2003;11:683-8.
3. Guerciolini R, Radu-Radulescu L, Boldrin R, et al. Comparative evaluation of fecal fat excretion induced by orlistat and chitosan. *Obes Res.* 2001;9:364-7.
4. Natural Medicines Comprehensive Database. Stockton, Calif: Therapeutic Research Faculty, Inc.; 2003. Available at: http://www.naturaldatabase.com. Accessed March, 2005.
5. Fetrow CW, Avila JR. Efficacy of the dietary supplement S-adenosyl-L-methionine. *Ann Pharmacother.* 2001;35:1414-25.
6. Fisman M, Mersky, Helmes E. Double-blind trial of 2-dimethylaminoethanol in Alzheimer's disease. *Am J Psychiatry.* 1981;138:970-2.
7. Sauder DN, DeKoven J, Champagne P, et al. Neovastat (Æ-941), an inhibitor of angiogenesis: randomized phase I/II clinical trial results in patients with plaque psoriasis. *J Am Acad Dermatol.* 2002;47:535-41.
8. Rosenstein ED. Topical agents in the treatment of rheumatic disorders. *Rheum Dis Clin North Am.* 1999;25:899-918.
9. Tai T-S, Sheu WH-H, Lee W-J, et al. Effect of chitosan on plasma lipoprotein concentrations in type 2 diabetic subjects with hypercholesterolemia. *Diabetes Care.* 2000; 23:1703-4.
10. Metso S, Ylitalo R, Mikkila M, et al. The effect of long-term microcrystalline chitosan therapy on plasma lipids and glucose concentrations in subjects with increased plasma total cholesterol: a randomised placebo-controlled double-blind crossover trial in healthy men and women. *Eur J Clin Pharmacol.* 2003;59:741-6.
11. Jing SB, Li L, Ji D, et al. Effect of chitosan on renal function in patients with chronic renal failure. *J Pharm Pharmacol.* 1997;49:721-3.
12. Schiller RN, Barrager E, Schauss AG, et al. A randomized, double-blind, placebo-controlled study examining the effects of a rapidly soluble chitosan dietary supplement on weight loss and body composition in overweight and mildly obese individuals. *J Am Nutraceutical Assoc.* 2001;4:42-9.
13. Wuolijoki E, Hirvela T, Ylitalo P. Decrease in serum LDL cholesterol with microcrystalline chitosan. *Methods Find Exp Clin Pharmacol.* 1999;21:357-61.
14. Maezaki Y, Tsuji K, Nakagawa Y, et al. Hypocholesterolemic effect of chitosan in adult males. *Biosci Biotech Biochem.* 1993;57:1439-44.

15. Ho SC, Tai ES, Eng PHK, et al. In the absence of dietary surveillance, chitosan does not reduce plasma lipids or obesity in hypercholesterolaemic obese Asian subjects. *Singapore Med J.* 2001;42:6-10.
16. Sciutto AM, Colombo P. Lipid-lowering effect of chitosan dietary integrator and hypocaloric diet in obese subjects. *Acta Toxicol Ther.* 1995;16:215-30.
17. Veneroni G, Veneroni F, Contos S, et al. Effect of a new chitosan dietary integrator and hypocaloric diet on hyperlipidemia and overweight in obese patients. *Acta Toxicol Ther.* 1996;16:53-70.
18. Colombo P, Sciutto AM. Nutritional aspects of chitosan employment in hypocaloric diet. *Acta Toxicol Ther.* 1996;16:287-302.
19. Macchi G. A new approach to the treatment of obesity: chitosan's effect on body weight reduction and plasma cholesterol levels. *Acta Toxicol Ther.* 1996;16:303-20.
20. Bokura H, Kobayashi S. Chitosan decreases total cholesterol in women: a randomized, double-blinded, placebo-controlled trial. *Eur J Clin Nutr.* 2003;57:721-5.
21. Pittler MH, Abbot NC, Harkness EF, et al. Randomized, double-blind trial of chitosan for body weight reduction. *Eur J Clin Nutr.* 1999;53:379-81.
22. Ni Mhurchu C, Dunshea-Mooj C, Bennet D, et al. Effect of chitosan on weight loss in overweight and obese individuals: a systemic review of randomized controlled trials. *Obesity Rev.* 2005; 6:35-42.
23. Macfarlane FT, Cummings JH. Probiotics and probiotics: can regulating the activities of intestinal bacteria benefit health? *BMJ.* 1999;318:999-1003.
24. Macfarlane FT, Cummings JH. Probiotics, infection and immunity. *Curr Opin Infect Dis.* 2002;15:501-6.
25. Liévin V, Peiffer I, Hudault S, et al. Bifidobacterium strains from resident infant human gastrointestinal microflora exert antimicrobial activity. *Gut.* 2000;47:646-52.
26. Holzapfel WH, Haberer P, Snel J, et al. Overview of gut flora and probiotics. *Int J Food Microbiol.* 1998;41:85-101.
27. Isolauri E, Arvola T, Sütas Y, et al. Probiotics in the management of atopic eczema. *Clin Exp Allergy.* 2000;30:1604-10.
28. Schultz M, Linde HJ, Lehn N, et al. Immunomodulatory consequences of oral administration of *Lactobacillus rhamnosus* strain GG in healthy volunteers. *J Dairy Res.* 2003;70:165-73.
29. MacGregor G, Smith AJ, Thakker B, et al. Yoghurt biotherapy: contraindicated in immunosuppressed patients? *Postgrad Med.* 2002;78:366-7.
30. Rautava S, Kalliomäki M, Isolauri E. Probiotics during pregnancy and breastfeeding might confer immunomodulatory protection against atopic disease in the infant. *J Allergy Clin Immunol.* 2002; 109:119-21.
31. Van Niel CW, Feudtner C, Carrison MM, et al. Lactobacillus therapy for acute infectious diarrhea in children: a meta-analysis. *Pediatrics.* 2002;109:678-84.
32. Isolauri E, Juntunen M, Rautanen T, et al. A human Lactobacillus strain (*Lactobacillus casei* sp strain GG) promotes recovery from acute diarrhea in children. *Pediatrics.* 1991;88:90-7.
33. Rosenfeldt V, Michaelsen KF, Jakobsen M, et al. Effect of probiotic *Lactobacillus* strains on acute diarrhea in a cohort of nonhospitalized children attending day-care centers. *Pediatr Infect Dis J.* 2002;21:417-9.
34. D'Souza AL, Rajkumar C, Cooke J, et al. Probiotics in prevention of antibiotic associated diarrhea: meta-analysis. *BMJ.* 2002;324:1361-4.
35. Thomas MR, Litin SC, Osmon DR, et al. Lack of effect of *Lactobacillus* GG on antibiotic-associated diarrhea: a randomized, placebo-controlled trial. *Mayo Clin Proc.* 2001;76:883-9.
36. Scarpignato C, Rampal P. Prevention and treatment of traveler's diarrhea: a clinical pharmacological approach. *Chemotherapy.* 1995;41(suppl 1):48-81.
37. Sen S, Mallun MM, Parker TJ, et al. Effect of *Lactobacillus plantarum* 299v on colonic fermentation and symptoms of irritable bowel syndrome. *Dig Dis Sci.* 2002;47:2615-20.
38. Nobaek S, Johansson M-L, Molin G, et al. Alteration of intestinal microflora is associated with reduction in abdominal bloating and pain in patients with irritable bowel syndrome. *Am J Gastroenterol.* 2000;95:1231-8.
39. Niedzielin K, Kordecki H, Birkenfeld B. A controlled, double-blind, randomized study on the efficacy of Lactobacillus plantarum 299V in patients with irritable bowel syndrome. *Eur J Gastroenterol Hepatol.* 2001;13:1143-7.
40. O'Sullivan MA, O'Morain CA. Bacterial supplementation in the irritable bowel syndrome: a randomized double-blind placebo-controlled crossover study. *Dig Liver Dis.* 2000;32(4):294-301.
41. Jonkers D, Stockbrügger R. Probiotics and inflammatory bowel disease. *J R Soc Med.* 2003;96:167-71.
42. Saggioro A. Probiotics in the treatment of irritable bowel syndrome. *J Clin Gastroenterol.* 2004;38(suppl 2):S104-6.
43. Rosenfeldt V, Benfeldt E, Dam Nielsen S, et al. Effect of probiotic *Lactobacillus* strains in children with atopic dermatitis. *J Allergy Clin Immunol.* 2003;111:389-95.
44. Majamaa H, Isolauri E. Probiotics: a novel approach in the management of food allergy. *J Allergy Clin Immunol.* 1997;99:179-85.
45. Viljanen M, Savilahti E, Haahtela T, et al. Probiotics in the treatment of atopic eczema/dermatitis syndrome in infants: a double-blind placebo-controlled trial. *Allergy.* 2005;60:494-500.
46. McQueen CE. *Sigler's Dietary Supplement Drug Cards* (probiotics monograph). 1st ed. Lawrence, Kan: SFI Medical Publishing; 2004.
47. Morelli L, Zonenenschain D, Del Piano M, et al. Utilization of the intestinal tract as a delivery system for urogenital probiotics. *J Clin Gastroenterol.* 2004;38(suppl 2):S107-10.
48. Shalev E, Battino S, Weiner E, et al. Ingestion of yogurt containing *Lactobacillus acidophilus* compared with pasteurized yogurt as prophylaxis for recurrent candidal vaginitis and bacterial vaginosis. *Arch Fam Med.* 1996;5:593-6.
49. Pirotta M, Gunn J, Chondros Patty, et al. Effect of lactobacillus in preventing post-antibiotic vulvovaginal candidiasis: a randomized controlled trial. *BMJ Online.* doi:10.1136/bmj.38210.494977.DE (published August 27, 2004).
50. Roffe L, Schmidt K, Ernst E. Efficacy of coenzyme Q10 for improved tolerability of cancer treatments: a systematic review. *J Clin Oncol.* 2004;22:4418-24.
51. Overvad K, Diamant B, Holm L, et al. Coenzyme $Q_{10}$ in health and disease. *Eur J Clin Nutr.* 1999;53:764-70.
52. Turunen M, Olsson J, Dallner G. Metabolism and function of coenzyme Q. *Biochim Biophys Acta.* 2004;1660(1-2):171-90.
53. Crane FL. Biochemical functions of coenzyme Q10. *J Am Coll Nutr.* 2001;20:591-8.
54. Food and Drug Administration. List of orphan product designations for 1999. Available at: http://www.fda.gov/ohrms/dockets/dailys/00/jan00/010500/lst0092.pdf. Accessed May 2005.
55. De Pinieux G, Chariot P, Ammi-Said M, et al. Lipid-lowering drugs and mitochondrial function: effects of HMG-CoA reductase inhibitors on serum ubiquinone and blood lactate/pyruvate ratio. *Br J Clin Pharmacol.* 1996;42:333-7.
56. Ghirlanda G, Oradei A, Manto A, et al. Evidence of plasma CoQ10-lowering effect by HMG-Co-A reductase inhibitors: a double-blind, placebo-controlled study. *J Clin Pharmacol.* 1993;33:226-9.
57. Rundek T, Naini A, Sacco R, et al. Atorvastatin decreases the coenzyme Q10 level in the blood of patients at risk for cardiovascular disease and stroke. *Arch Neurol.* 2004;61:889-92.
58. Laaksonen R, Jokelainen K, Sahi T, et al. Decreases in serum ubiquinone concentrations do not result in reduced levels in muscle tissue during short-term simvastatin treatment in humans. *Clin Pharmacol Ther.* 1995;57:62-6.

59. Bleske BE, Willis RA, Anthony M, et al. The effect of pravastatin and atorvastatin on coenzyme Q10. *Am Heart J.* 2001;142:e2.
60. Mortenson SA, Leth A, Agner E, et al. Dose-related decrease of serum coenzyme Q10 during treatment with HMG-CoA reductase inhibitors. *Mol Aspects Med.* 1997;18(suppl):S137-44.
61. Kishi T, Watanabe T, Folkers K. Bioenergetics in clinical medicine XV. Inhibition of coenzyme Q10-enzymes by clinically used adrenergic blockers of beta-receptors. *Res Commun Chem Pathol Pharmacol.* 1977;17:157-64.
62. Landbo C, Almdal TP. Interaction between warfarin and coenzyme Q10 [abstract]. *Ugeskr Laeger.* 1998;160:3226-7.
63. Spigset O. Reduced effect of warfarin caused by ubidecarenone. *Lancet.* 1994;334:1372-3.
64. Heck AM, DeWitt BA, Lukes AL. Potential interactions between alternative therapies and warfarin. *Am J Health-System Pharm.* 2000;57:1221-30.
65. Engelsen J. Effect of coenzyme $Q_{10}$ and *Ginkgo biloba* on warfarin dosage in stable, long-term warfarin treated outpatients. A randomized, double-blind, placebo-crossover trial. *Thromb Haemost.* 2002;87:1075-6.
66. Conklin KA. Dietary antioxidants during cancer chemotherapy: impact on chemotherapeutic effectiveness and development of side effects. *Nutr Cancer.* 2000;37:1-18.
67. Lund EL, Quistorff B, Span-Thomsen M, Kristjansen PE. Effect of radiation therapy on small-cell lung cancer is reduced by ubiquinone intake. *Folia Microbiol.* 1998;43:505-6.
68. Rengo F, Abete P, Landino P, et al. Role of metabolic therapy in cardiovascular disease. *Clin Investig.* 1993;71:S124-8.
69. Morisco C, Trimarco B, Condorelli M. Effect of coenzyme $Q_{10}$ therapy in patients with congestive heart failure: a long-term multicenter randomized study. *Clin Investig.* 1993;71:S134-6.
70. Khatta M, Alexander B, Krichten C, et al. The effect of coenzyme Q10 in patients with congestive heart failure. *Ann Intern Med.* 2000;132:636-40.
71. Watson PS, Scalia GM, Galbraith A, et al. Lack of effect of coenzyme Q10 on left ventricular function in patients with congestive heart failure. *J Am Coll Cardiol.* 1999;33:1549-52.
72. Berman M, Erman A, Ben-Gal T, et al. Coenzyme Q10 in patients with end-stage heart failure awaiting cardiac transplantation: a randomized, placebo-controlled study. *Clin Cardiol.* 2004;27:295-9.
73. Langsjoen PH, Vadhanavikit S, Folkers K. Response of patients in classes III and IV of cardiomyopathy to therapy in a blind and crossover trial with coenzyme Q10. *Proc Natl Acad Sci USA.* 1994; 15:S287-94.
74. Permanetter B, Rossy W, Klein G, et al. Ubiquinone (coenzyme Q10) in the long-term treatment of idiopathic dilated cardiomyopathy. *Eur Heart J.* 1992;13:1528-33.
75. Singh RB, Niaz MA, Rastogi SS, et al. Effect of hydrosoluble coenzyme Q10 on blood pressures and insulin resistance in hypertensive patients with coronary artery disease. *J Hum Hypertens.* 1999;13:203-8.
76. Singh RB, Niaz MA. Serum concentration of lipoprotein(a) decreases on treatment with hydrosoluble coenzyme Q10 in patients with coronary artery disease: discovery of a new role. *Int J Cardiol.* 1999;68:23-9.
77. Singh RB, Neki NS, Kartikey K, et al. Effect of coenzyme Q10 on risk of atherosclerosis in patients with recent myocardial infarction. *Mol Cell Biochem.* 2003;246(1-2):75-82.
78. Burke BE, Neuenschwander R, Olson RD. Randomized, double-blind, placebo-controlled trial of Coenzyme Q10 in isolated systolic hypertension. *South Med J.* 2001;94:1112-7.
79. Shults C, Oakes D, Kieburtz K, et al. Effects of Coenzyme $Q_{10}$ in early Parkinson's disease. *Arch Neurology.* 2002;59:1541-50.
80. Huntington Study Group. A randomized, placebo-controlled trial of coenzyme Q10 and remacemide in Huntington's disease. *Neurology.* 2001;57:397-404.
81. Lockwood K, Moesgaard S, Yamamoto T, et al. Progress on therapy of breast cancer with vitamin Q10 and the regression of metastases. *Biochem Biophys Res Comm.* 1995;212:172-7.
82. Sándor PS, Di Clemente L, Coppola G, et al. Efficacy of coenzyme Q10 in migraine prophylaxis: a randomized controlled trial. *Neurology.* 2005;64:713-5.
83. *Drug Facts and Comparisons.* St. Louis: Wolters Kuwer Health; 2005:KU-14b.
84. Dennehy CE, Tsourounis C. Botanicals ("herbal medications") and nutritional supplements. In: Katzung BG, ed. *Basic and Clinical Pharmacology.* 9th ed. New York: Lange/McGraw Hill; 2004: 1088-9.
85. Luboshitzky R, Lavie P. Melatonin and sex hormone interrelationships—a review. *J Ped Endocrinol.* 1999;12:355-62.
86. Reiter RJ. Melatonin and human reproduction. *Ann Med.* 1998; 30:103-8.
87. Brzezinski A, Vangel MG, Wurtman RJ, et al. Effect of exogenous melatonin on sleep: a meta-analysis. *Sleep Med.* 2005;9:41-50.
88. Zhdanova IV. Melatonin as a hypnotic: pro. *Sleep Med.* 2005;9:51-65.
89. Claustrat B, Brun J, Chazot G. The basic physiology and pathophysiology of melatonin. *Sleep Med.* 2005;9:11-24.
90. Djeridane Y, Touitou Y. Chronic diazepam administration differentially affects melatonin synthesis in rat pineal and Harderian glands. *Psychopharmacology.*2001;154:403-7.
91. Wright KP Jr, Myers BL, Plenzler SC, et al. Acute effects of bright light and caffeine on nighttime melatonin and temperature levels in women taking and not taking oral contraceptives. *Brain Res.* 2000;873:310-7.
92. Lusardi P, Piazza E, Fogari R. Cardiovascular effects of melatonin in hypertensive patients well controlled by nifedipine: a 24-hour study. *Br J Pharmacol.* 2000;49:423-7.
93. Lissoni P, Barni S, Mandala M, et al. Decreased toxicity and increased efficacy of cancer chemotherapy using the pineal hormone melatonin in metastatic solid tumour patients with poor clinical status. *Eur J Cancer.* 1999;35:1688-92.
94. Andrade C, Srihari BS, Reddy KP, et al. Melatonin in medically ill patients with insomnia: a double-blind, placebo-controlled study. *J Clin Psychiatry.* 2001;62:41-5.
95. Campos FL, da Silva-Júnior FP, de Bruin VMS, et al. Melatonin improves sleep in asthma. A randomized, double-blind, placebo-controlled study. *Am J Resp Crit Care Med.* 2004;170:947-51.
96. Singer C, Tractenberg RE, Kaye J, et al. A multicenter, placebo-controlled trial of melatonin for sleep disturbance in Alzheimer's disease. *Sleep.* 2003;26:893-901.
97. Spitzer RL, Terman M, Williams JBW, et al. Jet lag: clinical features, validation of a new syndrome-specific scale, lack of response to melatonin in a randomized, double-blind trial. *Am J Psychiatry.* 1999;156:1392-6.
98. Burstein AH. Melatonin for shift-work insomnia. *Pharmacist's Diet Suppl Alert.* 2000;1:33-6.
99. Buscemi N, Vandermeer B, Pandya R, et al. Melatonin for treatment of sleep disorders. Summary, Evidence Report/Technology Assessment Number 108. Prepared by the University of Alberta Evidence-based Practice Center, under Contract No. 290-02-0023. AHRQ Publication No. 05-E002-1. Rockville, Md: Agency for Healthcare Research and Quality; November 2004.
100. Nelson LA, McGuire JM, Hausafus SN. Melatonin for the treatment of tardive dyskinesia. *Ann Pharmacother.* 2003;37(1-2):1128-31.
101. Garfinkel D, Zisapel N, Wainstein J, et al. Facilitation of benzodiazepine discontinuation by melatonin. *Arch Intern Med.* 1999; 159:2456-60.
102. Gorēn JL, Stoll AL, Damico KE, et al. Bioavailability and lack of toxicity of S-adenosyl-L-methionine (SAMe) in humans. *Pharmacotherapy.* 2004;24:1501-7.

103. Fetrow CW, Avila JR, eds. *Professional's Handbook of Complementary & Alternative Medicines*. 34rd ed. Springhouse, Pa: Lippincott Williams & Wilkins; 2004.
104. Brown RP, Gerbarg P, Bottiglieri T. S-adenosylmethionine (SAMe) for depression. *Psychiatric Ann.* 2002;1:29-44
105. Berger R, Nowak H. A new medical approach to the treatment of osteoarthritis: report of an open phase IV study with ademethionine (Gumbaral). *Am J Med.* 1987;83:84-4.
106. Lipinski JF, Cohen BM, Frankenberg F, et al. An open trial of S-adenosyl methionine for treatment of depression. *Am J Psychiat.* 1984;141:448-50.
107. Carney MWP, Martin R, Bottiglieri T, et al. Switch mechanism in affective illness and S-adenosyl methionine. *Lancet.* 1983;1:820-1.
108. Carney MWP, Edeh J, Bottiglieri T, et al. Affective illness and S-adenosyl methionine: a preliminary report. *Clin Neuropharmacol.* 1986;9:379-85.
109. Kagan BL, Sultzer DL, Rosenlicht N, et al. Oral S-adenosylmethionine in depression: a randomized, double-blind, placebo-controlled trial. *Am J Psychiat.* 1990;147:591-5.
110. Carrieri PB, Indaco A, Gentile S, et al. S-adenosylmethionine treatment of depression in patients with Parkinson's disease. A double-blind, crossover study versus placebo. *Curr Therapeut Res.* 1990;48:154-60.
111. Fetrow CW. S-Adenosyl-L-methionine (SAMe) and depression. *Pharmacist's Dietary Suppl Alert.* 2000;1:1-8.
112. Bressa GM. S-adenosyl-l-methionine (SAMe) as antidepressant: meta-analysis of clinical studies. *Acta Neurol Scand Suppl.* 1994; 154:7-14.
113. Tavoni A, Vitali C, Bombardieri S, et al. Evaluation of S-adenosylmethionine in primary fibromyalgia. *Am J Med.* 1987;83(suppl A):107-10.
114. Jacobsen S, Danneskiold-Samsøe B, Bach Andersen R. Oral S-adenosylmethionine in primary fibromyalgia. Double-blind clinical evaluation. *Scand J Rheum.* 1991;20:294-302.
115. Tavoni A, Jeracitano G, Cirigliano G. Evaluation of S-adenosylmethionine in secondary fibromyalgia: a double-blind study. *Clin Exp Rheum.* 1998;16:106-7.
116. Najm WI, Reinsch S, Hoehler F, et al. S-adenosyl methionine (SAMe) versus celecoxib for the treatment of osteoarthritis symptoms: a double-blind cross-over trial. *BMC Musculoskeletal Disord.* 2004;5:6. Available at: http://www.biomedcentral.com/1471-2474/5/6.
117. Soeken KL, Lee W-L., Bausell RB, et al. Safety and efficacy of S-adenosyl methionine (SAMe) for osteoarthritis: a meta-analysis. *J Fam Pract.* 2002;51:425-30.
118. FDA Talk Paper. Impurities confirmed in dietary supplement 5-hydroxy-L-tryptophan. Available at: http://vm.cfsan.fda.gov/~lrd/tp5htp.html. Accessed June 2005.
119. Klarskov K, Johnson KL, Benson LM, et al. Structural characterization of a case-implicated contaminant, "peak X," in commercial preparations of 5-hydroxytryptophan. *J Rheumatol.* 2003;30: 89-95.
120. Klarskov K, Johnson KL, Benson LM, et al. Eosinophilia-myalgia syndrome case-associated contaminants in commercially available 5-hydroxytryptophan. *Adv Exp Med Biol.* 1999;467:461-8.
121. Michelson D, Page SW, Casey R, et al. An eosinophilia-myalgia syndrome related disorder associated with exposure to L-5-hydroxytryptophan. *J Rheumatol.* 1994;21:2261-5.
122. Williamson BL, Klarskov K, Tomlinson AJ, et al. Problems with over-the-counter 5-hydroxy-L-tryptophan. *Nature Med.* 1998;4: 983.
123. Birdsall TC. 5-Hydroxytryptophan: a clinically-effective serotonin precursor. *Altern Med Rev.* 1998;3:271-80.
124. Shaw K, Turner J, Del Mar C. Tryptophan and 5-hydroxytryptophan for depression. *Cochrane Database Syst Rev.* 2002;(1): CD003198.
125. Gijsman HJ, van Gerven JM, de Kam ML, et al. Placebo-controlled comparison of three dose-regimens of 5-hydroxytryptophan challenge test in healthy volunteers. *J Clin Psychopharmacol.* 2002;22:183-9.
126. Bruni O, Ferri R, Miano S, et al. L-5-hydroxytryptophan treatment of sleep terrors in children. *Eur J Ped.* 2004;163:402-7.
127. Schruers K, van Diest R, Overbeek T, et al. Acute L-5-hydroxytryptophan administration inhibits carbon dioxide-induced panic in panic disorder patients. *Psychiatry Res.* 2002;113:237-43.
128. Maron E, Tõru I, Vasar V, et al. The effect of 5-hydroxytryptophan on cholecystokinin-4-induced panic attacks in healthy volunteers. *J Psychopharmacol.* 2004;18:194-9.
129. Tamminga CA, Smieth RC, Ericksen SE, et al. Cholinergic influences in tardive dyskinesia. *Am J Psych.* 1977;134:769-74.
130. Casey DE. Mood alterations during deanol therapy. *Psychopharmacology.* 1979;62:187-91.
131. De Montigny C, Chouinard G, Annable L. Ineffectiveness of deanol in tardive dyskinesia: a placebo controlled study. *Psychopharmacology.* 1979;65:219-23.
132. Haug BA, Holzgraefe M. Orofacial and respiratory tardive dyskinesia: potential side effects of 2-dimethylaminoethanol (deanol). *Eur Neurol.* 1991;31:423-5.
133. Nesse R, Carroll BJ. Cholinergic side-effects associated with deanol. *Lancet.* 1976;2:50-1.
134. Penovich P, Morgan JP, Kerzner B, et al. Double-blind evaluation of deanol in tardive dyskinesia. *JAMA.* 1978;239:1997-8.
135. Davis KL, Berger PA, Hollister LE. Deanol in tardive dyskinesia. *Am J Psychiatry.* 1977;134:807.
136. De Silva L, Huang CY. Deanol in tardive dyskinesia. *BMJ.* 1975; 3:466.
137. Jus A, Villeneuve A, Gautier, et al. Deanol, lithium and placebo in the treatment of tardive dyskinesia. A double-blind crossover study. *Neuropsychobiology.* 1978;4:14-9.
138. George J, Pridmore S, Aldous D. Double blind controlled trial of deanol in tardive dyskinesia. *Aust NZ J Psychiatry.* 1981;15:68-71.
139. Caraceni TA, Girotti F, Celano I, et al. 2-Dimethylaminoethanol (Deanol) in Huntington's chorea. *J Neurol Neurosurg Psychiatry.* 1978;41:1114-8.
140. Oettinger L Jr. Pediatric psychopharmacology. A review with special reference to deanol. *Dis Nerv System.* 1977;38(12 Pt 2):25-31.
141. Lewis JA, Young R. Deanol and methylphenidate in minimal brain dysfunction. *Clin Pharmacol Ther.* 1975;17:534-40.
142. Coleman N, Dexheimer P, DiMascio A, et al. Deanol in the treatment of hyperkinetic children. *Psychosomatics.* 1917:68-72.
143. Sweetman SC, ed. *Martindale: The Complete Drug Reference.* 34th ed. London: Pharmaceutical Press; 2005:1706.
144. Katzung BG. Introduction to Autonomic Pharmacology. In: Katzung BG, ed. *Basic and Clinical Pharmacology.* 9th ed. New York: Lange/McGraw Hill; 2004:78.
145. Pepping J. Phosphatidylserine. *Am J Hosp Pharm.* 1999;56; 2038,2043-4.
146. Etienne P, Dastoor D, Gauthier S, et al. Alzheimer disease: lack of effect of lecithin treatment for 3 months. *Neurology.* 1981;31: 1552-4.
147. Weintraub S, Mesulan MM, Auty R, et al. Lecithin in the treatment of Alzheimer's disease. *Arch Neurol.* 1985;40:527-8.
148. Fisman M, Merskey H, Helmes E, et al. Double blind study of lecithin in patients with Alzheimer's disease. *Can J Psychiatry.* 1981;26:426-8.
149. Little A, Levy R, Chuaqui-Kidd P, et al. A double-blind, placebo controlled trial of high-dose lecithin in Alzheimer's disease. *J Neurol.* 1985;48:736-42.
150. Higgins JPT, Flicker L. Lecithin for dementia and cognitive impairment. *Cochrane Database Syst Rev.* 2005;(2):CD001015.

151. Holford NH, Peace K. The effect of tacrine and lecithin in Alzheimer's disease. A population pharmacodynamic analysis of five clinical trials. *Eur J Clin Pharmacol.* 1994;47:17-23.
152. Harris CM, Dysken MW, Fovall P, et al. Effect of lecithin on memory in normal adults. *Am J Psychiatry.* 1983;140:1010-2.
153. Crook TH, Petrie W, Wells C, et al. Effects of phosphatidylserine in Alzheimer's disease. *Psychopharmacol Bull.* 1992;28:61-6.
154. Crook TH, Tinklenberg J, Yesavage J, et al. Effects of phosphatidylserine in age-associated memory impairment. *Neurology.* 1991; 41:644-9.
155. Jorissen BL, Brouns F, Van Boxtel MP, et al. The influence of soy-derived phosphatidylserine on cognition in age-associated memory impairment. *Nutr Neurosci.* 2001;4:121-34.
156. Levy R, Little A, Chuaqui P, et al. Early results from double-blind, placebo-controlled trial of high dose phosphatidylcholine in Alzheimer's disease. *Lancet.* 1983;1:987-8.
157. Ladd SL, Sommer SA, LaBerge S, et al. Effect of phosphatidylcholine on explicit memory. *Clin Neuropharmacol.* 1993;16:540-9.
158. Fioravanti M, Yangi M. Cytidinediphosphocholine (CDP choline) for cognitive and behavioral disturbances associated with chronic cerebral disorders in the elderly. *Cochrane Database Syst Rev.* 2003;(1):CD000269.
159. Blumenthal M. President signs new law banning designer steroids dietary supplements: DHEA exempted from ban. *HerbalGram.* 2005;65:58-9.
160. Arlt W, Callies F, van Vlijmen JC, et al. Dehydroepiandrosterone replacement in women with adrenal insufficiency. *N Engl J Med.* 1999;341:1013-20.
161. Vacheron-Trystram MN, Cheref S, Gauillard J, et al. A case report of mania precipitated by use of DHEA [French]. *Encephale.* 2002; 28(6 pt 1):563-6.
162. Dean CE. Prasterone (DHEA) and mania. *Ann Pharmacother.* 2000;34:1419-22.
163. Kline MD, Jaggers ED. Mania onset while using dehydroepiandrosterone. *Am J Psychiatry.* 1999;156:971.
164. Markowitz JS, Carson WH, Jackson CW. Possible dehydroepiandrosterone-induced mania. *Biol Psychiatry.* 1999;45:241-2.
165. Acacio BD, Stanczyk FZ, Mullin P, et al. Pharmacokinetics of dehydroepiandrosterone and its metabolites after long-term daily oral administration to healthy young men. *Fertil Steril.* 2004; 81:595-604.
166. Løvås K, Gebre-Medhin G, Trovik TS, et al. Replacement of dehydroepiandrosterone in adrenal failure: no benefit for subjective health status and sexuality in a 9-month, randomized, parallel group clinical trial. *J Clin Endocrinol Metab.* 2003;88:1112-8.
167. Bauleiu EE, Thomas G, Legrain S, et al. Dehydroepiandrosterone (DHEA), DHEA sulfate, and aging: contribution of the DHEAge study to a sociobiomedical issue. *Proc Nat Acad Sci USA.* 2000;97:4279-84.
168. Reiter WJ, Pycha A, Schatzl, et al. Dehydroepiandrosterone in the treatment of erectile dysfunction: a prospective, double-blind, randomized, placebo-controlled study. *Urology.* 1999;53: 590-4.
169. Stomati M, Rubino S, Spineti A, et al. Endocrine, neuroendocrine and behavioral effects of oral dehydroepiandrosterone sulfate supplementation in postmenopausal women. *Gynecol Endocrinol.* 1999;13:15-25.
170. Stomati M, Monteleone P, Casarosa E, et al. Six-month oral dehydroepiandrosterone supplementation in early and late postmenopause. *Gynecol Endocrinol.* 2000;14:342-63.
171. Meston CM, Heiman JR. Acute dehydroepiandrosterone effects on sexual arousal in premenopausal women. *J Sex Marital Ther.* 2002;28:53-60.
172. Hackbert L, Heiman JR. Acute dehydroepiandrosterone (DHEA) effects on sexual arousal in postmenopausal women. *J Womens Health Gend Based Med.* 2002;11:155-62.
173. Morales AJ, Haubrich RH, Hwang JY, et al. The effect of six months treatment with a 100 mg daily dose of dehydroepiandrosterone (DHEA) on circulating sex steroids, body composition and muscle strength in age-advanced men and women. *Clin Endocrinol.* 1998;49:421-32.
174. Percheron G, Hogrel JY, Deont-Ledunois S, et al. Effect of 1-year oral administration of dehydroepiandrosterone to 60-to 80 year-old individuals on muscle function and cross-sectional area. *Arch Intern Med.* 2003;163:720-7.
175. Wolf OT, Naumann E, Hellhammer DH, et al. Effects of dehydroepiandrosterone replacement in elderly men on event-related potentials, memory, and well-being. *J Gerontol.* 1998; 53A(5):M385-90.
176. van Niekirk JK, Huppert FA, Herbert J. Salivary cortisol and DHEA: association with measures of cognition and well-being in normal older men, and effects of three months of DHEA supplementation. *Psychoneuroendocrinology.* 2001;26:591-612.
177. Wolf OT, Kudielka BM, Hellhammer DH, et al. Opposing effects of DHEA replacement in elderly subjects on declarative memory and attention after exposure to a laboratory stressor. *Psychoneuroendrocrinology.* 1998;23:617-29.
178. Hirshman E, Wells E, Wierman ME, et al. The effect of dehydroepiandrosterone (DHEA) on recognition memory decision processes and discrimination in postmenopausal women. *Psychonomic Bull Rev.* 2003;10:125-34.
179. Villareal DT, Holloszy JD. Effect of DHEA on abdominal fat and insulin action in elderly women and men. *JAMA.* 2004;292:2243-8.
180. Reiter WJ, Schatzl G, Mark I, et al. Dehydroepiandrosterone in the treatment of erectile dysfunction in patients with different organic etiologies. *Urol Res.* 2001;29:278-81.
181. Wallace MB, Lim J, Cutler A, et al. Effects of dehydroepiandrosterone vs androstenedione supplementation in men. *Med Sci Sports Exerc.* 1999;31:1788-92.
182. Brown GA, Vukovich MD, Sharp RL, et al. Effect of oral DHEA on serum testosterone and adaptations to resistance training in young men. *J Appl Physiol.* 1999;87:2274-83.
183. Jacob S, Henriksen EJ, Schiemann AL, et al. Enhancements of glucose disposal in patients with type 2 diabetes by alpha-lipoic acid. *Arzneimittelforschung.* 1995;45:872-4.
184. Jacob S, Henriksen EJ, Tritschler HJ, et al. Improvement of insulin-stimulated glucose-disposal in type 2 diabetes after repeated parenteral administration of thioctic acid. *Exp Clin Endocrinol Diabetes.* 1996;104:284-8.
185. Konrad T, Vicini P, Justerer K, et al. Alpha-lipoic acid treatment decreases serum lactate and pyruvate concentrations and improves glucose effectiveness in lean and obese patients with type 2 diabetes. *Diabetes Care.* 1999;22:280-7.
186. Jacob S, Ruus P, Hermann R, et al. Oral administration of rac-a-lipoic acid modulates insulin sensitivity in patients with type-2 diabetes mellitus: a placebo-controlled pilot trial. *Free Radical Biol Med.* 1999;27(3-4):309-14.
187. Nagamatsu M, Nickander KK, Schmelzer JD, et al. Lipoic acid improves nerve blood flow, reduces oxidative stress, and improves distal nerve conduction in experimental diabetic neuropathy. *Diabetic Care.* 1995;18:1160-7.
188. van Dam PS, van Asbeck BS, Van Oirschot JF, et al. Glutathione and alpha-lipoate in diabetic rats: nerve function, blood flow and oxidative state. *Eur J Clin Invest.* 2001;31:417-24.
189. Scott BC, Aruoma OI, Evans PJ, et al. Lipoid and dihydrolipoic acids as antioxidants: a critical evaluation. *Free Radical Res.* 1994; 20:119-33.
190. Tiechert J, Kern J, Tritschler HJ, et al. Investigations on the pharmacokinetics of alpha-lipoic acid in healthy volunteers. *Intl J Clin Pharmacol Ther.* 1998;36:625-8.

191. Ziegler D, Nowak H, Kempler P, et al. Treatment of symptomatic diabetic polyneuropathy with the antioxidant α-lipoic acid: a meta-analysis. *Diabetic Med.* 2004;21:114-21.
192. Alpha-lipoic acid. *Altern Med Rev.* 1998;3:308-10.
193. Halat KM, Dennehy CE. Botanical and dietary supplements in diabetic peripheral neuropathy. *J Am Board Fam Pract.* 2003;16: 46-57.
194. Segermann J, Hotze A, Ulrich H, et al. Effect of alpha-lipoic acid on the peripheral conversion of thyroxine to triiodothyronine and on serum lipid-, protein- and glucose levels. *Arzneimittelforschung.* 1991;41:1294-8.
195. Gleiter CH, Schug BS, Hermann R, et al. Influence of food intake on the bioavailability of thioctic acid enantiomers. *Eur J Clin Pharmacol.* 1996;50:513-4.
196. Reljanovic M, Reichel G, Rett K, et al. Treatment of diabetic polyneuropathy with the antioxidant thioctic acid (α-lipoic acid): a two year multicenter randomized double-blind placebo-controlled trial (ALADIN II). *Free Radical Res.* 1999;31:171-9.
197. Negrisanu G, Rosu M, Bolte B, et al. Effects of 3-month treatment with the antioxidant alpha-lipoic acid in diabetic peripheral neuropathy. *Rom J Int Med.* 1999;37:297-306.
198. Ruhnau K-J, Meissner HP, Finn J-R, et al. Effects of 3-week oral treatment with the antioxidant thioctic acid (alpha-lipoic acid) in symptomatic diabetic polyneuropathy. *Diabetic Med.* 1999;16; 1040-3.
199. Hahm JR, Kim, BJ, Kim KW. Clinical experience with thioctacid (thioctic acid) in the treatment of distal symmetric polyneuropathy in Korean diabetic patients. *J Diab & Its Complications.* 2004; 18:79-85.
200. Bernkop-Schnürch A, Reich-Rohrwig E, Marschütz M, et al. Development of a sustained release dosage form for α-lipoic acid. II. Evaluation in human volunteers. *Drug Develop Indust Pharm.* 2004;30:35-42.
201. Ziegler D, Schatz H, Conrad F, et al. Effects of treatment with the antioxidant (alpha-lipoic acid on cardiac autonomic neuropathy in NIDDM patients: a 4-month randomized controlled multicenter trial (DEKAN Study). *Diabetes Care.* 1997;20:369-73.
202. Ziegler D, Hanefeld M, Ruhnau K-J, et al. Treatment of symptomatic diabetic polyneuropathy with the antioxidant alpha-lipoic acid: a 7-month multicenter randomized controlled trial (ALADIN III Study). *Diabetes Care.* 1999;22(8):1296-301.
203. Mero A, Kahkonen J, Nykanen T, et al. IGF-I, IgA, and IgG responses to bovine colostrum supplementation during training. *J Appl Physiol.* 2002;93:732-9.
204. Greenberg PD, Cello JP. Treatment of severe diarrhea caused by Cryptosporidium parvum with oral bovine immunoglobulin concentrate in patients with AIDS. *AIDS Hum Retrovirol.* 1996;13:348-54.
205. Sarker SA, Casswall TH, Mahalanabis D, et al. Successful treatment of rotavirus diarrhea in children with immunoglobulin from immunized bovine colostrum. *Pediatr Infect Dis J.* 1998;17: 1149-54.
206. Huppertz H-I, Rutkowski S, Busch DH, et al. Bovine colostrum ameliorates diarrhea in infection with diarrheagenic Escherichia coli, Shiga toxin-producing E. coli, and E. coli expressing intimin and hemolysin. *J Pediatr Gastroenterol Nutr.* 1999;29:452-6.
207. Coombes JS, Conacher M, Austen SK, et al. Dose effects of oral bovine colostrum on physical work capacity in cyclists. *Med Sci Sports Exerc.* 2002;34:1184-8.
208. Hofman Z, Smeets R, Verlaan G, et al. The effect of bovine colostrum supplementation on exercise performance in elite field hockey players. *Int J Sport Nutr Exerc Metab.* 2002;12:461-9.
209. Brinkworth GD, Buckley JD, Bourdon PC, et al. Oral bovine colostrum supplementation enhances buffer capacity but not rowing performance in elite female rowers. *Int J Sport Nutr Exerc Metab.* 2002;12:349-65.
210. Buckley JD, Abbott MJ, Brinkworth GD, et al. Bovine colostrum supplementation during endurance running training improves recovery, but not performance. *J Sci Med Sport.* 2002;5:65-79.
211. Antonio J, Sanders MS, Van Gammeren D. The effects of bovine colostrum supplementation on body composition and exercise performance in active men and women. *Nutrition.* 2001;17:243-7.
212. Cunningham-Rundles S, Harbison M, Guirguis S, et al. New perspectives on use of thymic factors in immune deficiency. *Ann N Y Acad Sci.* 1994;730:71-83.
213. Marzari R, Mazzati P, Cazzola P, et al. Perennial allergic rhinitis. Prophylaxis of acute episodes using thymomodulin [Italian]. *Minerva Med.* 1987;78:1678-81.
214. Cavagni G, Piscopo E, Rigoli E, et al. Food allergy in children: an attempt to improve the effects of the elimination diet with an immunomodulating agent (thymodulin). A double-blind clinical trial. *Immunopharmacol Immunotoxicol.* 1989;11:131-42.
215. Raymond RS, Fallon MB, Abrams GA. Oral thymic extract for chronic hepatitis C in patients previously treated with interferon. A randomized, double-blind, placebo-controlled trial. *Ann Intern Med.* 1998;129:797-800.
216. Iaffaioli RV, Frasci G, Tortora G, et al. Effect of thymic extract 'thymostimulin' on the incidence and myelotoxicity during adjuvant chemotherapy for breast cancer. *Thymus.* 1988-89;12:69-75.
217. Mustacchi G, Pavesi L, Milani S, et al. High-dose folinic acid (FA) and fluorouracil (FU) plus or minus thymostimulin (TS) for treatment of metastatic colorectal cancer: results of a randomized multicenter clinical trial. *Anticancer Res.* 1994;14(2B):617-9.
218. Preventative Therapeutics, Inc. Dr. Burgstiner's Complete Thymic Formula. Product information. Available at: http://thymic.com/thymicformula.php. Accessed March 22, 2005.
219. Hoffer LJ, Kaplan LN, Hamadeh MJ, et al. Sulfate could mediate the therapeutic effect of glucosamine sulfate. *Metab Clin Exp.* 2001;50:767-70.
220. Nakamura H, Shibakawa A, Tanaka M, et al. Effects of glucosamine hydrochloride on the production of prostaglandin E2, nitric oxide and metalloproteases by chondrocytes and synoviocytes in osteoarthritis. *Clin Exp Rheumatol.* 2004;22:293-9.
221. Piperno M, Reboul P, Hellio Le Graverand MP, et al. Glucosamine sulfate modulates dysregulated activities of human osteoarthritic chondrocytes in vitro. *Osteoarth Cart.* 2000;8:207-12.
222. Byron CR, Orth MW, Venta PJ, et al. Influence of glucosamine on matrix metalloproteinase expression and activity in lipopolysaccharide-stimulated equine chondrocytes. *Am J Vet Res.* 2003;64:666-71.
223. Lippiello L. Glucosamine and chondroitin sulfate: biological response modifiers of chondrocytes under simulated conditions of joint stress. *Osteoarth Cart.* 2003;11:335-42.
224. Largo R, Alvarez-Soria MA, Diez-Ortega I, et al. Glucosamine inhibits IL-1beta-induce NFkappaB activation in human osteoarthritis chondrocytes. *Osteoarth Cart.* 2003;11:290-8.
225. Christgau S, Henrotin Y, Tankó LB, et al. Osteoarthritic patients with high cartilage turnover show increased responsiveness to the cartilage turnover show increased responsiveness to the cartilage protecting effects of glucosamine sulphate. *Clin Exp Rheumatol.* 2004;22:36-42.
226. Cohen M, Wolfe R, Mai T, et al. A randomized, double blind, placebo controlled trial of a topical cream containing glucosamine sulfate, chondroitin sulfate, and camphor for osteoarthritis of the knee. *J Rheumatol.* 2003;30:523-8.
227. Kanwischer M, Kim SY, Kim JS, et al. Evaluation of the physiochemical stability and skin permeation of glucosamine sulfate. *Drug Devel Indust Pharm.* 2005;31:91-7.
228. Tallia AF, Cardone DA. Asthma exacerbation association with glucosamine-chondroitin. *J Am Board Fam Pract.* 2003;15:481-4.

229. Reginster JY, Deroisy R, Rovati LC, et al. Long-term effects of glucosamine sulphate on osteoarthritis progression: a randomized, placebo-controlled clinical trial. *Lancet.* 2001;357:251-6.
230. Pavelka K, Gatterová J, Olejarová M, et al. Glucosamine sulfate use and delay of progression of knee osteoarthritis. *Arch Intern Med.* 2002;162:2113-23.
231. Scroggie DA, Albright A, Harris MD. The effects of glucosamine-chondroitin supplementation on glycosylated hemoglobin levels in patients with type 2 diabetes mellitus. *Arch Intern Med.* 2003; 163:1587-90.
232. Houpt JB, McMillan R, Wein C, et al. Effect of glucosamine hydrochloride in the treatment of pain of osteoarthritis of the knee. *J Rheumatol.* 1999;26:2423-30.
233. Braham R, Dawson B, Goodman C. The effect of glucosamine supplementation on people experiencing regular knee pain. *Br J Sports Med.* 2003;37:45-9.
234. Basak M, Joseph S, Joshi S, et al. Comparative bioavailability of a novel timed release and powder-filled glucosamine sulfate formulation—a multi-dose, randomized, crossover study. *Intl J Clin Pharmacol Therapeutics.* 2004;42:597-601.
235. Kayne SB, Wadeson K, MacAdam A. Is glucosamine an effective treatment for osteoarthritis? A meta-analysis. *Pharm J.* 2000;265: 759-63.
236. Richy F, Bruyere O, Ethgen O, et al. Structural and symptomatic efficacy of glucosamine and chondroitin and knee osteoarthritis. A comprehensive meta-analysis. *Arch Int Med.* 2003;163:1514-22.
237. Towheed TE, Anastassiades TP, Shea B, et al. Glucosamine therapy for treating osteoarthritis. *Cochrane Database Syst Rev.* 2001; (1):CD002946.
238. Morreale P, Manopulo R, Galati M, et al. Comparison of the anti-inflammatory efficacy of chondroitin sulfate and diclofenac sodium in patients with knee osteoarthritis. *J Rheumatol.* 1996; 23:1385-91.
239. Leeb BF, Schweitzer H, Montag K, et al. A meta-analysis of chondroitin sulfate in the treatment of osteoarthritis. *J Rheumatol.* 2000;27:205-11.
240. Uebelhart D, Malaise M, Marcolongo R, et al. Intermittent treatment of knee osteoarthritis with oral chondroitin sulfate: a one-year, randomized, double-blind, multicenter study versus placebo. *Osteoarthritis Cartilage.* 2004;12:269-76.
241. Mazieres B, Combe B, Phan Van A, et al. Chondroitin sulfate in osteoarthritis of the knee: a prospective, double-blind, placebo-controlled multicenter clinical study. *J Rheumatol.* 2001;28:173-81.
242. Morrison LM, Rucker PG, Ershoff BH. Prolongation of thrombus-formation time in rabbits given chondroitin sulfate A. *J Atheroscler Res.* 1968;8:319-27.
243. Consumerlab.com. White Plains, NY: Consumerlab.com, LLC. Available at: http://www.consumerlab.com. Accessed January 2005.
244. McAlindon TE, LaValley MP, Gulin JP, et al. Glucosamine and chondroitin for treatment of osteoarthritis: a systematic quality assessment and meta-analysis. *JAMA.* 2000;283:1469-75.
245. Rovetta G, Monteforte P, Molfetta G, et al. A two-year study of chondroitin sulfate in erosive osteoarthritis of the hands: behavior of erosions, osteophytes, pain and hand dysfunction. *Drugs Exp Clin Res.* 2004;30:11-16.
246. Ely A, Lockwood B. What is the evidence for the safety and efficacy of dimethyl sulfoxide and methylsulfonylmethane in pain relief? *Pharmaceutical J.* 2002;269:685-7.
247. Abt L, Hammerly M, eds. AltMedDex System. Greenwood Village, Colo: MICROMEDEX; edition expires June 2005.
248. Jimenez RAH, Willkens RE. Dimethyl sulfoxide: a perspective of its use in rheumatic diseases. *J Lab Clin Med.* 1982;100(4):489.
249. King DS, Sharp RL, Vukovich MD, et al. Effect of oral androstenedione on serum testosterone and adaptations to resistance training in young men. *JAMA.* 1999;281:2020-8.
250. Ballantyne CS, Phillips SM, MacDonald JR, et al. The acute effects of androstenedione supplementation in healthy young males. *Can J Appl Physiol.* 2000;25:68-78.
251. Rasmussen BB, Volpi E, Gore DC, et al. Androstenedione does not stimulate muscle protein anabolism in young healthy men. *J Clin Endocrinol Metab.* 2000;85:55-9.
252. Broeder CE, Quindry J, Brittingham K, et al. The andro project. Physiological and hormonal influences of androstenedione supplementation in men 35 to 65 years old participating in a high-intensity resistance training program. *Arch Int Med.* 2000;160: 3093-104.
253. McQueen CE. *Sigler's Dietary Supplement Drug Cards.* 1st ed. Lawrence, Kan: SFI Medical Publishing; 2004; canthaxanin monograph.
254. Rizzo R, Grandolfo M, Godeas C, et al. Calcium, sulfur, and zinc distribution in normal and arthritic articular equine cartilage: a synchrotron radiation-induced X-ray emission (SRIXE) study. *J Exp Zoology.* 1995;273:82-6.
255. Moore RD, Morton JI. Diminished inflammatory joint disease in MRL/1pr mice ingesting dimethylsulfoxide (DMSO) or methylsulfonylmethane (MSM). *Federation Proc.* 1985;44:530,692.
256. Barrager E, Veltmann JR Jr., Schauss AG, et al. A multi-centered, open-label trial on the safety and efficacy of methylsulfonylmethane in the treatment of seasonal allergic rhinitis. *J Altern Complement Med.* 2002;8:167-73.
257. Horvath K, Noker PE, Somfai-Relle S, et al. Toxicity of methylsulfonylmethane in rats. *Food Chem Toxicol.* 2002;40:1459-62.
258. Usha PR, Naidu MUR. Randomised, double-blind, parallel, placebo-controlled study of oral glucosamine, methylsulfonylmethane and their combination in osteoarthritis. *Clin Drug Invest.* 2004;24:353-63.
259. *Drug Facts and Comparisons.* St. Louis: Facts and Comparisons, Inc; January 2005.
260. Ross EV Jr., Badame AJ, Dale SE. Meat tenderizer in the acute treatment of imported fire ant stings. *J Am Acad Dermatol.* 1987; 16:1189-92.
261. Thomas CS, Scott SA, Galanis DJ, et al. Box jellyfish (*Carybdea alata*) in Waikiki. The analgesic effect of sting-aid, Adolph's meat tenderizer and fresh water on their stings: a double-blinded, randomized, placebo-controlled clinical trial. *Hawaii Med J.* 2001; 60:205-7.
262. Klein G, Kullich W. Short-term treatment of painful osteoarthritis of the knee with oral enzymes. *Clin Drug Invest.* 2000;19:15-23.
263. Walker AF, Bundy R, Hicks SM, et al. Bromelain reduces mild acute knee pain and improves well-being in a dose-dependent fashion in an open study of otherwise healthy adults. *Phytomedicine.* 2002;9:681-6.
264. Hale LP. Greer PK, Sempowski GD. Bromelain treatment alters leukocyte expression of cell surface molecules involved in cellular adhesion and activation. *Clin Immunol.* 2002;104:183-90.
265. Castell JV, Friedrich G, Kuhn C-S, et al. Intestinal absorption of undegraded proteins in men: presence of bromelain in plasma after oral intake. *Am J Physiol.* 1997;273(1 pt 1):G139-46.
266. Raison-Peyron N, Roulet A., Guillot B, et al. Bromelain: an unusual cause of allergic contact cheilitis. *Contact Dermatitis.* 2003;49:218-9.
267. Nettis E, Napoli G, Ferrannini A, et al. IgE-mediated allergy to bromelian. *Allergy.* 2001;56(suppl 65):257-8.
268. Tanabe S, Tesaki S, Watanabe M, et al. Cross-reactivity between bromelain and soluble fraction from wheat flour [Japanese]. *Arerugi.* 1997;46:1170-3.
269. Metzig C, Grabowska E, Eckert K, et al. Bromelain proteases reduce human platelet aggregation in vitro, adhesion to bovine endothelial cells and thrombus formation in rat vessels in vivo. *In Vivo.* 1999;13:7-12.

270. Felton GE. Fibrinolytic and antithrombotic action of bromelain may eliminate thrombosis in heart patients. *Med Hypoth.* 1980;6: 1123-33.
271. Craig RP. The quantitative evaluation of the use of oral proteolytic enzymes in the treatment of sprained ankles. *Injury.* 1975;6:313-6.
272. Tilwe GH, Beria S, Turakhia NH, et al. Efficacy and tolerability of oral enzyme therapy as compared to diclofenac in active osteoarthritis of knee joint: an open randomized controlled clinical trial. *J Assoc Physicians India.* 2001;49:617-21.
273. Brien S, Lewith G, Walker A, et al. Bromelain as a treatment for osteoarthritis: a review of clinical studies. *Evidence-based Comp Altern Med.* 2004;1:251-7.
274. Kane S, Goldberg MJ. Use of bromelain for mild ulcerative colitis [letter]. *Ann Intern Med.* 2000;132:680.
275. Thomas CS, Scott SA, Galanis DJ, et al. Box jellyfish (Carybdea alata) in Waikiki. The analgesic effect of sting-aid, Adolph's meat tenderizer and fresh water on their stings: a double-blinded, randomized, placebo-controlled clinical trial. *Hawaii Med J.* 2001; 60:205-7,210.
276. Billigmann P. Enzyme therapy—an alternative in treatment of herpes zoster. A controlled study of 192 patients [German]. *Fortschritte der Medizin.* 1005;113:43-8.
277. Ross EV Jr, Badame AJ, Dale SE. Meat tenderizer in the acute treatment of imported fire ant stings. *J Am Acad Dermatol.* 1987; 16:1189-92.
278. Nomura JT, Sato RL, Ahern RM, et al. A randomized paired comparison trial of cutaneous treatments for acute jellyfish (Carybdea alata) stings. *Am J Emerg Med.* 2002;20:624-6.
279. Desser L, Rehberger A, Paukovits W. Proteolytic enzymes and amylase induce cytokine production in human peripheral blood mononuclear cells in vitro. *Cancer Biother.* 1994;9:253-63.
280. Zavadova E, Desser L, Mohr T. Stimulation of reactive oxygen species production and cytotoxicity in human neutrophils in vitro and after oral administration of a polyenzyme preparation. *Cancer Biother.* 1995;10:147-52.
281. Shaw D, Leon C, Kolev S, et al. Traditional remedies and food supplements: a 5-year toxicological study (1991-5). *Drug Safety.* 1997;17:342-56.
282. Walker-Renard P. Update on the medicinal management of phytobezoars. *Am J Gastroenterol.* 1993;88:1663-6.
283. Cochran C, Dent R. Cetyl myristoleate—a unique natural compound valuable in arthritis conditions. *Townsend Lett Doctors Patients.* 1997;168:70-4.
284. Diehl HW, May EL. Cetyl myristoleate isolated from Swiss albino mice: an apparent protective agent against adjuvant arthritis in rats. *J Pharm Sci.* 1994;83:296-9.
285. Tibbets D. Use of cetyl myristoleate for arthritis and tendonitis in holistic veterinary medical practice. *J Am Holistic Vet Med Assoc.* 1999;18:27-31.
286. Hunter KW, Gault RA, Stehouwer JS, et al. Synthesis of cetyl myristoleate and evaluation of its therapeutic efficacy in a murine model of collagen-induced arthritis. *Pharmacol Res.* 2003;47:43-7.
287. Siemandi H. The effect of cis-9-cetyl myristoleate (CMO) and adjunctive therapy on arthritis and auto-immune disease: a randomized trial. *Townsend Lett Doctors Patients.* Aug/Sept 1997; 169/170.
288. Edwards AM. CMO (Cerasomol-cis-9-cetyl myristoleate) in the treatment of fibromyalgia: an open pilot study. *J Nutr Environ Med.* 2001;11:105-11.
289. Hesslink R Jr, Armstrong D III, Nagendran MV, et al. Cetylated fatty acids improve knee function in patients with osteoarthritis. *J Rheumatol.* 2002;29:1708-12.
290. Kraemer WJ, Ratamess NA, Anderson JM, et al. Effect of a cetylated fatty acid topical cream on functional mobility and quality of life of patients with osteoarthritis. *J Rheumatol.* 2004;31:767-74.
291. Borucinska JD, Harshbarger JC, Bogicevic T. Hepatic cholangiocarcinoma and testicular mesothelioma in a wild-caught blue shark, *Prionace glauca* (L.). *J Fish Disease.* 2003;26:43-9.
292. National Cancer Institute. Cartilage (bovine and shark) monograph. Available at: http://www.cancer.gov/cancertopics/pdq/cam/cartilage. Accessed March 2005.
293. Miller DR, Anderson GT, Stark JJ, et al. Phase I/II trial of the safety and efficacy of shark cartilage in the treatment of advanced cancer. *J Clin Oncol.* 1998;16: 3649-55.
294. Milner M. Follow-up of cancer patients using shark cartilage. *Altern Comple Therapies.* 1996;2:99-109.
295. Taylor H, Leitman R, eds. Widespread ignorance of regulation and labeling of vitamins, minerals and food supplements. *Health Care News.* 2002;2:1-4. Harris Interactive. Available at: http://www.harrisinteractive.com/news/newsletters/healthnews/HI_HealthCareNews2002Vol2_Iss23.pdf. Accessed March 2005.
296. Eisenberg DM, Kessler RC, van Rompay MI, et al. Perceptions about complementary therapies relative to conventional therapies among adults who use both: results from a national survey. *Ann Intern Med.* 2001;135:344-51.

CHAPTER 55

# Homeopathic Medicines

*June E. Riedlinger and Begabati Lennihan*

Homeopathy is a distinct system of medicine with its own pharmacopoeia and principles of practice that differ from those of phytopharmacy and conventional medicine (CM). Homeopathic medicines are commonly referred to as remedies, a term practitioners also use for herbal therapies. Therefore, when a plant-based product is referred to, patients and clinicians should make sure to designate which form of a plant-derived drug (herbal or homeopathic remedy) they are using, recommending, or assessing.

The term *homeopathy* comes from the two Greek words *homoios* (similar) and *pathos* (suffering or disease). The National Center for Complementary and Alternative Medicine (NCCAM) classifies homeopathy under alternative medical systems, describing it as an unconventional Western system based on the principle of "like cures like" (i.e., the same substance that in large doses produces the symptoms of an illness can cure it in very minute doses), in which the more attenuated a homeopathic medicine, the greater its potency. The practice uses small doses of specially prepared plant extracts and minerals to stimulate the body's defense mechanism and healing process in the treatment of illness.[1] The practitioner should keep in mind that NCCAM's definition of homeopathy is simplified and not meant to be a full or detailed explanation of the practice. For example, homeopathic medicines are also prepared from zoologic specimens and pharmacologic agents, and the potency of a homeopathic drug depends not only on its dilution but also on a dynamization process called succussion (shaking with impact), which is performed along with each dilution. The principle of like cures like, also called the law of similars, has many ramifications that are not apparent without a full understanding of the principle and its application.

To fully implement the law of similars, the professional homeopathic practitioner must have excellent patient communication skills to obtain the detailed description of a patient's illness needed to determine a therapeutic homeopathic drug specific (individualized) for that patient. Individualization is a fundamental principle of homeopathy, as it is with other alternative and complementary medical (CAM) practices. Many years of study and specialized training in paradigms of healing unique to homeopathy are required to achieve proficiency in individualizing homeopathic therapy (especially for patients with chronic/complex diseases).

Most experts on homeopathy would agree that using a single drug is optimal in all cases and especially important when treating serious, complex, or chronic conditions. Combination products, which include several single homeopathic drugs, may provide another option for otherwise healthy individuals with common, mild to moderate, self-limiting illness who desire to use homeopathy but do not have enough knowledge or training to use single homeopathic drugs safely and effectively. Fortunately, in most cases, even if patients self-select one of these products and ingest an unneeded ingredient, most will not react adversely to the nonindicated drug.

Even though homeopathic medications are considered CAM therapies, they are not regulated under the Dietary Supplement Health and Education Act (DSHEA) of 1994, as are herbs and dietary supplements. In fact, the Food and Drug Administration (FDA) regulates the manufacture and distribution of homeopathic medicines as drugs. A homeopathic drug can be designated as a prescription drug similar to conventional pharmaceutical agents.

Nonprescription homeopathic medicines are available as single or combination drugs in familiar dosage forms (tablets, medicated pellets or globules, liquid attenuations, syrups, nasal sprays, lozenges, topical aerosols, creams, gels, ointments, and suppositories), and are commonly sold in natural pharmacies, chain drugstores, and health food stores. Pediatric and veterinarian formulations are also available. Single homeopathic drugs (prescription and nonprescription) are most commonly available as medicated pellets or globules. Homeopathic drug sales are estimated to represent 0.26% of the U.S. drug market. Consumer sales increased by $30 million from 1994 to 1999.[2] Chain drugstores are the primary retail outlets for homeopathic products in America, but in Europe and many other countries sales are primarily through pharmacies. Combination homeopathic nonprescription products, comparable in price, labeling, and packaging to conventional nonprescription products, are the fastest growing sector of the U.S. homeopathic drug market.

According to a 2002 National Health Interview Survey, 3.6% of the 31,044 adults (18 years or older) interviewed reported using homeopathy.[3] Even though the U.S. homeopathic market is much smaller than the pharmaceutical or herb and supplement markets, its growth is accelerating. Given the Centers for Disease Control and Prevention's (CDC's) recommendation to limit the indiscriminate use of antibiotics, homeopathy's ability to substitute effectively for the indiscriminant use of antibiotics for conditions ranging from childhood otitis media to prophylaxis in animal feed suggests that its use will continue to grow.[4,5] As this industry and profession expand, need for clinicians who can accommodate

**TABLE 55-1 Information Resources for Homeopathy**

**Patient/Introductory Texts**

Cummings S, Ullman D. *Everybody's Guide to Homeopathic Medicines*. New York: Tarcher/Putnam; 1997.

Hershoff A. *Homeopathic Medicines*. Garden City Park, NY: Avery/Putnam; 2000.

Jonas WB, Jacobs J. *Healing with Homeopathy: The Doctor's Guide*. New York: Warner Books, Inc; 1996.

Lansky A. *Impossible Cure: The Promise of Homeopathy*. Portola Valley, Calif: RL Ranch Press; 2003.

**Intermediate Professional Texts**

De Schepper L. *Hahnemann Revisited: A Textbook of Classical Homeopathy for the Professional*. Santa Fe, NM: Full of Life Publishing; 1999.

Kaplan B. *The Homeopathic Conversation: The Art of Taking the Case*. London: Natural Medicine Press; 1992.

Kayne S. *Homeopathic Pharmacy: An Introduction and Handbook*. Edinburgh: Churchill Kane; 1997.

Kruzel T. *Homeopathic Emergency Guide*. Berkeley, Calif: North Atlantic Books; 1992.

Skinner S. *Homeopathy in Primary Care*. Gaithersburg, Md: Aspen Publications; 2001.

**Professional Reference Books**

Kent JT. *Repertory of the Homeopathic Materia Medica*. New Delhi: B. Jain Publishers; 1993.

Morrison R. *Desktop Companion to Physical Pathology*. Albany, Calif: Hahnemann Clinic Publishing; 1998.

Morrison R. *Desktop Guide to Keynotes and Confirmatory Symptoms*. Albany, Calif: Hahnemann Clinic Publishing; 1993.

Schroyens F, ed. *Synthesis Repertorium Homeopathicum Syntheticum*. 9.1 ed. London: Homeopathic Book Publishers; 2004.

Vermeulen F. *Concordant Materia Medica*. 3rd ed. Haarlem, The Netherlands: Merlijn; 2001.

Vermeulen F. *Prisma*. Haarlem, The Netherlands: Emryss bv Publishers, 2002.

Yasgur J. *Yasgur's Homeopathic Dictionary and Holistic Health Reference*. Greenville, Pa: Van Hoy Publishers; 1998.

**Introductory Research Books**

Bellavite P, Signorini A. *The Emerging Science of Homeopathy: Complexity, Biodynamics and Nanopharmacology*. Berkeley, Calif: North Atlantic Books; 2002.

Dean ME. *The Trials of Homeopathy*. Essen, Germany: KVC Verlag; 2004

Ernst E, Hahn E. *Homeopathy: A Critical Appraisal*. Oxford, England: Butterworth/Heinemann; 1998.

Gray W. *Homeopathy: Science or Myth?* Berkeley, Calif: North Atlantic Books; 2000.

Schulte J, Endler PC. *Fundamental Research in Ultra High Dilution Homeopathy*. Dordrecht, The Netherlands: Kluwer Academic Publishers; 1998.

Ullman D. *Homeopathic Family Medicine* [eBook]. Berkley, Calif: Homeopathic Educational Services; 2005. Available at: www.homeopathic.com.

**U.S. Homeopathic Journals**

*American Journal of Homeopathic Medicine* (journal of the American Institute of Homeopathy)

*Homeopathy Today* (magazine of the National Center for Homeopathy)

*Simillimum* (journal of the Homeopathic Academy of Naturopathic Physicians)

**Web Sites**

www.homeopathic.org, National Center for Homeopathy (includes a review of research on homeopathy and a directory of practitioner)

www.homeopathicpharmacy.org, American Association of Homeopathic Pharmacists (booklist, recent articles, list of homeopathic manufacturers)

www.homeopathyhome.com (good basic information and many links for further information)

www.homeoint.org, Homeopathie Internationale (books and articles online including materia medicas and repertories)

patients choosing to use homeopathy and conduct research that supports its safety and efficacy will increase.

In a survey of American Pharmaceutical Association members, 24% of respondents reported having no knowledge or training in homeopathy, and only 16% reported having a sufficient level of knowledge to discuss homeopathy with patients.[6] This situation needs to be rectified, given the increased use of homeopathy by American consumers. Therefore, the aim of this chapter is to provide clinicians with a basic working knowledge of homeopathy that will assist them in integrating it into a patient care plan, communicate effectively with patients and practitioners who use it, and evaluate research involving its implementation. Some resources for information on homeopathy are listed in Table 55-1.

## Homeopathy Reconsidered

The concepts of like cures like and increased potency with increasing dilutions are counterintuitive, especially if they are examined superficially. However, homeopathy can offer patients valuable alternatives and adjuncts to CM when no effective CM option exists, when the patient has an illness and an underlying condition (e.g., pregnancy, renal or hepatic impairment) for which CM therapy may be toxic, when the side effect profile of the CM option is unacceptable, or when CM therapy fails to control escalation of a disease process.[7,8] As with any medical practice, use of homeopathy has limitations and benefits (Table 55-2).

Homeopathy plays a major role in health care systems of many countries around the world. An estimated one third of conventional doctors in France, the Netherlands, Belgium, and Germany use homeopathic drugs in their practice or refer patients to a homeopath.[9] Eighty-five percent of the general practitioners in Belgium offer homeopathy as a complementary therapeutic modality.[10] All 45 European member countries of the Council of Europe adopted a resolution on nonconventional therapies, which states that homeopathy is one of the four best-established CAM therapies in Europe, and the European Council for

**TABLE 55-2 Benefits and Limitations of Homeopathy**

**Benefits**

- Low cost: drugs average less than $1 per day in acute conditions and a few cents per day (sometimes a fraction of a cent) in chronic conditions.
- Minimal side effects, no toxicity, no addiction, no dependency, no withdrawal.
- Can work while patient is on prescription medication (e.g., in patients with asthma, diabetes, or other conditions in which medication cannot safely be withdrawn).
- No interaction with pharmaceuticals, because it works on a different (energetic) level.
- Patients can obtain good results when self-treating for many common acute conditions.
- Patients unable to use conventional pharmaceuticals because of side effects can often safely use homeopathic drugs.
- Patients often report improvement in overall energy, mood, quality of sleep, and digestion, and the disappearance of other symptoms apparently unrelated to the condition being treated with homeopathy.

**Limitations**

- Chronic conditions require professional homeopaths, and the United States currently has an insufficient number of trained homeopaths to meet the potential demand.
- Prescribing for acute conditions can be more complex than in allopathic (conventional) medicine because a single condition such as a cough or headache may require consideration of several dozen possible homeopathic drugs.
- There is a lack of homeopathic hospitals and medical schools in the United States.
- Limited research funds are available to conduct studies on the effectiveness of homeopathy because homeopathic drugs are not patentable; homeopathic pharmaceutical companies do not generate revenues from patent rights as do U.S. conventional drug manufacturers to support research, especially large, multicenter controlled trials.
- Some homeopaths ask patients to discontinue prescription medications before beginning homeopathic treatment, and to forgo coffee, mint, camphor, electric blankets, and dental treatments while under homeopathic care.
- Symptoms may initially worsen if the patient is extremely sensitive or the potency is too high.

Classical Homeopathy (ECCH) fully supports the Council of Europe's resolution.[11] Other countries that officially recognize homeopathy are Brazil, Ghana, India, Mauritius, New Zealand, Pakistan, United Arab Emirates, and Zimbabwe. Just as Europe has provided the bulk of research on herbal medicine, it plays a leading role in conducting research and establishing criteria for homeopathy education and practice today (see Research in Homeopathy).

Homeopathy, similar to other CAM systems (e.g., naturopathy, Ayurvedic, and Chinese medicine) is not opposed to the modern CM approach, but has its own pragmatic system of diagnosis and treatment. This system is based on the observation that the body has an inherent healing power (*vis medicatrix naturae*) and that the person is an integral whole composed of body, mind, and spirit.[12] This multifaceted approach produces highly individualized diagnoses and treatments and, as a consequence, uses information that is not commonly recognized by conventionally trained medical practitioners. Although the information collected by a homeopathic practitioner may be foreign to a clinician unfamiliar with homeopathic practice, individualizing therapy is consistent with pharmaceutical care tenets that stipulate drug therapy should be tailored to accommodate the patient's individual needs. By learning about the different approach used in homeopathy, clinicians have an opportunity to expand their ability to individualize therapy beyond CM parameters and sharpen their consultation skills.

The fact that homeopathy is not accepted by many conventionally trained health care professionals is understandable, given their belief that the action of drugs can be explained only by biochemical activity. Modern scientists are investigating the concept of bioenergy to describe actions of therapies such as homeopathy that are conceived to use the inherent healing powers or vital force of the human body.[12] It is worth keeping in mind that within CM, many drugs are used despite a lack of understanding of their precise mechanism of action.[13]

The clinician who wants to evaluate homeopathic research needs to understand that its principles of practice should not be compromised and that biochemical mechanisms of action are not applicable to high-potency homeopathic drugs. Homeopathic research along with evolving theories suggesting a mechanism of action for homeopathic medicines are discussed in more detail in the Research in Homeopathy section.

## Homeopathic Terms

The first challenge in becoming knowledgeable about homeopathy is mastering its "language." The following definitions of key terms, adapted from *Yasgur's Homeopathic Dictionary and Holistic Health Reference*,[14] are essential to understanding further discussion of the principles and implementation of homeopathic medicine.

- *Acute condition:* Disease state that is usually brief and self-limiting (i.e., the patient quickly recovers or, rarely, dies), as opposed to a chronic condition (lasting indefinitely).
- *Aggravation:* Transient reaction to the drug in which the patient feels worse, or symptoms are intensified. This is one possible scenario for a healing reaction from a drug, which occurs when the drug is correct but too strong.
- *Antidote:* Substance that can cancel the effects of a homeopathic drug. This can be another homeopathic drug such as Camphora, strong aromatic odors, or coffee.
- *Attenuation:* Potency or dilution.
- *Centesimal scale:* Dilution of 1 part drug substance in 99 parts solvent to give a 1:100 dilution. This is the most widely known and used potency scale, developed by Hahnemann; abbreviated as C. Two methods are used for making C potencies: the Hahnemann (multiple-vial) method, abbreviated as CH, and the Korsakovian (single-vial) method, abbreviated as K or CK.

- *Classical homeopathy:* Use of a single drug at a time, prescribed by the totality of the patient's symptoms, as opposed to variations such as the use of combination drugs.
- *Constitutional prescribing:* Prescribing for the totality of the patient's symptoms (mental, emotional, and physical) in a chronic case.
- *Decimal scale:* Dilution of 1 part drug substance in 9 parts solvent to give a 1:10 dilution; abbreviated as X in the United States and as D in Europe.
- *Hering's law* (of cure)*:* Fundamental principle of homeopathic healing, first observed by Constantine Hering, the first great American homeopath. Healing occurs from the inside out, from above to below, and from the most recent to the most chronic symptoms.
- *50-Millesimal scale:* Complex process used to make dilutions, abbreviated as LM or Q potencies (see Homeopathic Pharmaceutics for details).
- *Materia medica:* Reference work listing homeopathic drugs and their therapeutic actions; for examples, see Using the Repertory and Materia Medica.
- *Mother tincture:* The starting alcoholic liquid (1X dilution) from which subsequent botanical homeopathic potencies are made; abbreviated as MT or ∅.
- *Proving:* Determination of the medicinal/curative properties of a substance by administering it in homeopathic doses (or, less often, in crude form) to healthy volunteers who then observe and record any symptoms that develop.
- *Repertory:* Index/library of symptoms from provings and clinical/toxicologic data, organized in alphabetical order within chapters based on organs of the body; for an example, see Using the Repertory and Materia Medica.
- *Rubric:* Abbreviated symptom, which in the repertory is followed by a list of homeopathic drugs for the symptom.
- *Succussion:* Process of potentization. Consists of vigorously shaking the diluted drug with impact; may be done manually or, more recently, mechanically.
- *Totality:* All signs and symptoms of disease in a particular person.
- *Trituration:* Reduction of a crude substance to a minute state or division (in lactose) by means of long, continued rubbing or grinding using a mortar and pestle; used for drug substances insoluble in water or alcohol (e.g., minerals) and in the first stage of making LM potencies. After the third centesimal trituration, insoluble substances can be further attenuated using solvent.

## History and Basic Laws of Homeopathy

Homeopathy is a complete system of medicine. Its foundation is the work of German physician Samuel Hahnemann (1755–1843) and is contained in his *Organon of the Medical Art.*[15] Trained as a conventional doctor, Hahnemann gave up his medical practice and stopped using the toxic drugs, bleeding, and leeching procedures of his day because he felt he was only harming his patients. Instead, he translated medical texts from around the world and experimented with medicinal substances in the desire to learn a better way of healing.[15] While translating a text on herbal medicine by William Cullen, he questioned Cullen's statement that *Cinchona officinalis* bark's ability to cure malaria was based on its bitter and astringent properties. Knowing of many other herbs with these properties that were useless against malaria, Hahnemann decided to take some of the substance (also called China) to discover its antimalarial properties. After taking "twice a day four drachms of good China," he experienced the symptoms of malaria, which reappeared consistently with repeated administrations.[16] His experience with *Cinchona* most certainly led him to the Hippocratic principle of *similia similibus curantur* or "likes are cured by likes," which is the basis of the first principle of homeopathy, the law of similars.

Hahnemann's paradigm of healing may also have its roots in Ayurvedic or traditional Chinese medicine, in which he had a keen interest.[17] He believed that humans consist not only of a physical body but also an animating energy, which he called the vital force, similar to the concept of *chi* in Chinese medicine. He believed this life force is ultimately responsible for all homeostatic processes that sustain health and support the continuation of life. Hahnemann perceived that the measurable physical manifestations of illness (symptoms) could be the result of the changes (imbalances or disharmonies) in the energetic state of the vital force. Furthermore, in line with the law of similars, a substance that produced the same symptoms as the illness could be used as a homeopathic agent to rebalance the vital force and restore health.[16] The concept that each drug has a remedy picture or physical-mental-emotional "portrait" was further developed by Kent, the greatest American homeopath,[18] as well as many modern homeopaths, including George Vithoulkas of Greece and Rajan Sankaran of India.[16,19]

Hahnemann used his knowledge of medicine from around the world, his understanding of human nature, and keen powers of observation to design a clinical trial or proving to determine the symptom constellation for each substance he tested. Today, provings are still used to identify the symptom constellations of substances and are conducted as randomized, double-blind, placebo-controlled trials. (Table 55-3 summarizes a typical set of guidelines). The European Council for Classical Homeopathy has recommended guidelines for provings, which are available on their Web page at www.homeopathy-ecch.org/content/view/24/41. Similar guidelines are also published in the current *Homoeopathic Pharmacopoeia of the United States* (*HPUS*);[20] information on obtaining this text is available at www.hpus.com/ordfrm.htm.

With his great knowledge of chemistry and toxicology, Hahnemann began experimenting with different methods for making the newly proven substances into medicines that were as nontoxic as possible. It is not documented how he discovered the process of succussion (also called potentization or dynamization), but he reported that, when serially diluted, substances produced stronger effects if he struck the container holding them multiple times against a resilient surface (e.g., a leatherbound book) at each step of dilution. The more he succussed them, the more effective they became.[15] Thus, through extensive experimentation, he arrived at his second principle of homeopathy, the "minimum dose" or "infinitesimal dose"

**TABLE 55-3 Elements of A Proving Trial**

- The director is the principal investigator for the trial and ensures that the methods used conform to the highest scientific standards. This person is also responsible for keeping the randomization records and the identity of the substance being tested secret from the panel of experimenters and subjects or provers.
- Experimenters distribute test samples to the subjects, collect all information recorded by the subjects, and analyze the data.
- Subjects must be between 18 and 45 years of age and be in good physical and mental health. They must also lead a healthy lifestyle and be well acquainted with homeopathic methodology.
- During a 1-month period before subjects receive the test substance, they document any symptoms or slight discomforts they experience in a written diary that describes each symptom in detail, including the time of day when it occurred.
- Subjects take the test substance for up to 1 month or until symptoms occur. Subjects continue to document detailed descriptions of symptoms in their diaries for up to 3 months after the test substance has been discontinued.
- At conclusion of the experiment, the experimenter collects all dairies and determines which symptoms deviated from the subject's normal state. The experiment is then unblinded and symptoms generated by subjects given placebo are deleted from the other subject lists. Thus, only symptoms from the drug's influence are considered in the final analysis.

*Source:* Adapted from reference 20.

and devised a methodology for preparing these very dilute agents, discussed in Homeopathic Pharmaceutics.

Hahnemann also conducted verification trials to demonstrate the ability of potentized medication to cure the disorder it resembled. He gave homeopathic doses of the substance to subjects who had symptoms similar to those produced by the substance in its proving trial. When the substance demonstrated the ability to cure a particular disorder or constellation of symptoms, its therapeutic role was characterized and documented for future reference. Modern verification trials are conducted as case series, outcome studies, prospective observational studies, longitudinal data collection network studies, or randomized controlled trials (RCTs).[20] From the collective proving and verification studies that Hahnemann and his successors have conducted, the characteristic pattern of effects demonstrated by a considerable number of substances have been extensively documented and indexed in various homeopathic materia medicas and repertories. These essential tools are described in Selection of a Homeopathic Drug.

Another important principle adopted by Hahnemann is the individualization of therapy. It involves both versatility and specificity; a single drug can be useful across a variety of body systems and abnormal conditions, yet this drug must also be specific (have proving symptoms like the specific expression of the condition in the patient) to have a curative effect.[21] In the homeopathic method of individualization, drugs are chosen only after all the dimensions of the person have been considered in the analysis. Mental and emotional symptoms are at least as important as physical signs of illness. For example, if two children have otitis media, and one child is clingy, weepy, sweet, and needy of affection, while the other is nasty, irritable, cranky, and impossible to please, in CM both children are likely to receive the same antibiotic and analgesic. With homeopathic medicine, however, each child would be given a different drug (Pulsatilla and Chamomilla, respectively) because their mental and emotional symptoms are regarded as manifestations of the disease process, which help characterize distinctive individual cases of otitis media.

Hahnemann's principle of the single remedy involves using only one drug at a time, the one that is most closely individualized to the patient. Most classical homeopaths know the characteristics of hundreds of drugs, can access information on even more, and have developed the specialized case-taking skills necessary to determine the single correct homeopathic drug for an individual patient. Common, self-limiting conditions are more amenable to combination products, which are useful when one does not know how to find an individualized single drug.[22] The use of combination products are discussed further in books by Lansky and by Cummings and Ullman listed in Table 55-1.

## Homeopathic Training, Certification, and Licensure

Homeopathic education is becoming more accessible in North America, with at least 25 schools and many more occasional seminars to choose from although these programs are not yet accredited by the Department of Education. The Council on Homeopathic Education (CHE) is currently taking steps to change this by establishing professional standards of homeopathic education to be submitted for accreditation status in the future.[23] Information about accredited homeopathic programs, conferences, and agencies that presently certify homeopaths (Table 55-4) can be found on the Web site www.chedu.org.

The organizations have stringent prerequisites, including documented formal training in classical homeopathy (classroom and supervised practice instruction), acceptable written cases, and demonstrated knowledge of basic medical sciences. The Certificate in Classical Homeopathy (CCH) examination process includes a written and oral section, and is much like the board exams taken by conventional health care practitioners to achieve professional status. The organizations provide listings of certified homeopathic practitioners on their Web sites, which the clinician can use to identify qualified homeopaths throughout the United States.

Certification from the previously mentioned organizations is not recognized by any state as a license to practice homeopathy. However, three states—Arizona (since 1982), Connecticut (since 1892), and Nevada (since 1983)—do have licensing laws for homeopathic practitioners. They require that homeopaths be an MD or DO, or, in the case of Nevada and Arizona, an assistant working under the supervision of an MD or DO who is licensed as a homeopathic physician. Naturopaths (NDs) whose training includes homeopathy are licensed to practice in 14 states (Alaska, Arizona, California, Connecticut, Hawaii, Iowa,

**TABLE 55-4 Certification Organizations for Homeopathic Practitioners**

| Organization | Eligible Practitioners | Certification Credential |
|---|---|---|
| American Board of Homeotherapeutics (ABHT) | Doctor of Medicine (MD); Doctor of Osteopathy (DO) | DHt—Diplomate of Homeotherapeutics |
| Homeopathic Academy of Naturopathic Physicians (HANP) | Doctor of Naturopathy (ND)—graduate of an accredited Naturopathic College of Medicine | DHANP—Diplomate of the Homeopathic Academy of Naturopathic Physicians |
| Council for Homeopathic Certification (CHC) | Anyone with sufficient classroom and clinical/ supervision hours | CCH—Certified in Classical Homeopathy |
| North American Society of Homeopaths (NASH) | Anyone, with or without other medical licensure, who has passed the CCH exam and submitted an application | RSHom(NA)—Registered with the Society of Homeopaths (North America) |

Kansas, Maine, Montana, New Hampshire, Oregon, Utah, Vermont, and Washington) as well as in the District of Columbia, Puerto Rico, and the Virgin Islands. Health freedom acts in three states (California, Minnesota, and Rhode Island) protect the rights of professionals without medical licenses to practice homeopathy and other modalities that the state deems harmless. All other states lack specific regulatory language for homeopathy, which thus falls under the statutes regulating the practice of medicine.

## Regulation of Homeopathic Medications

Homeopathic drugs are regulated under the Food, Drug, and Cosmetic Act (FD&C Act), 21 U.S.C. § 201 *et seq.*, Section 201(g)(1) of the FD&C Act, 21 U.S.C. § 321(g)(1), which defines the term *drug* as articles recognized in official compendiums or pharmacopoeias of the United States. Section 201(j) of the act, 21 U.S.C. § 321(j), defines the term *official compendium* as the most current edition of the *HPUS*, the *National Formulary*, or the *United States Pharmacopeia*.[20] The drugs are also regulated under the Federal Trade Commission and Bureau of Tobacco, Alcohol, and Firearms because alcohol is used in the manufacturing process and is present in some dosage forms (e.g., cough syrups) of homeopathic products.[24]

The Homoeopathic Pharmacopoeia Convention of the United States (HPCUS), whose members include physicians, pharmacists, homeopaths, lawyers, biochemists, and botanists, defines eligibility criteria for homeopathic drugs and ensures that these criteria are met before the drug is added to *HPUS* revisions or supplements.[20] Eligibility for inclusion in *HPUS* involves compliance with specific criteria, as outlined in Table 55-5. For homeopathic agents, these criteria are accepted in place of FDA's New Drug Application procedures used for conventional pharmaceutical drug approval. According to Section 502 of the FD&C Act, a homeopathic product is considered unadulterated when manufactured in accordance with *HPUS* specifications and is not misbranded if labeled in accordance with the labeling provisions of *HPUS*. Clinicians interested in reimbursement for medical services related to homeopathy may be interested to know that homeopathic drugs are

**TABLE 55-5 Eligibility Criteria for Inclusion of Drugs in *HPUS***

To be eligible for inclusion in *HPUS*, the drug must meet criteria 1, 2, and 3 and at least one of 4, 5, 6, or 7, as set forth here:

1. HPCUS has determined the drug is safe and effective.
2. The drug must be prepared according to specifications of the General Pharmacy and relevant sections of *HPUS*.
3. The submitted documentation must be in an approved format, as set forth in relevant sections of *HPUS*, and must include any data relevant to toxicity.
4. Therapeutic use of a new and nonofficial homeopathic drug is established by a homeopathic drug proving and clinical verification acceptable to HPCUS. During the clinical verification period, the drug will be accepted for provisional review and should be available on a monitored basis. (See the Guideline for Homeopathic Drug Provings and the Guideline for Clinical Verification for more information.)
5. Therapeutic use of the drug is established through published documentation that the substance was in use before 1962. This documentation must include the symptom picture, including any subjective and/or objective symptoms. Such use and documentation may include, but not be limited to, medical literature of the following homeopathic authors: S. Hahnemann, C. Hering, T.F. Allen, H.C. Allen, J.H. Clarke, and J.T. Kent.
6. Therapeutic use of the drug is established by at least two adequately controlled, double-blind clinical studies using the drug as the single intervention. Each study is to be accompanied by adequate statistical analysis and adequate description of the symptom picture acceptable to HPCUS, which includes the subjective symptoms and, where appropriate, the objective symptomatology.
7. Therapeutic use of the drug is established by data gathered from clinical experience encompassing the symptom picture, pre- and posttreatment, including any subjective and/ or objective symptoms, or from data documented in the medical literature (all sources of medical literature may be considered on a case-by-case basis) subject to further verification (statistical and/or other forms of verification).

Key: *HPUS, Homoeopathic Pharmacopoeia of the United States;* HPCUS, Homeopathic Pharmacopoeia Convention of the United States.

**KALI PHOSPHORICUM** 5228 KAPH

NAME IN CONTEMPORARY USE: Potassium phosphate, dibasic

SYNONYMS: Latin: *Kalium phosphoricum, Dikalii phosphas*
English: Dibasic potassium phosphate, Dipotassium phosphate
French: Phosphate dipotassique
German: Dikaliumphosphat

CHEMICAL FORMULA AND MOLECULAR WEIGHT:

$K_2HPO_4$ 174.18

DESCRIPTION: White, amorphous, odorless masses, of a saline taste, somewhat hygroscopic. Very soluble in water, slightly soluble in alcohol. It melts readily at a low temperature and is converted into pyrophosphate by ignition.

PREPARATION AND CLASSIFICATION:

Solution 1:10 in distilled water (Class A).
Trituration (Class F).

MEDICATION: OTC: 1X
Ext. Use: 1X
Rx: N/A
HPN: N/A

**Quality Control Specifications**

[Standards & Controls Data is a draft standard open for public comment for a period of 2 1/2 years from the Standard & Controls revision date on this monograph. After this comment period, this Standards & Controls data will become official.]

**Starting Material:**

A. Macroscopic identification: To comply with monograph description.
B. General identification tests:
Criteria for identification; starting material must meet all of the identification tests for dibasic potassium phosphate USP.
C. Additional tests:
Starting materials must meet all of the tests for dibasic potassium phosphate USP.
D. Assay:
Starting material must meet the assay for dibasic potassium phosphate USP.

**FIGURE 55-1** Sample *HPUS* monograph. (Reprinted with permission from *The Homeopathic Pharmacopoeia of the United States*. Southeastern, Pa: The Homeopathic Pharmacopoeia Convention of the United States Revision Service; December 2001.)

covered by the Medicare/Medicaid statute, 42 U.S.C. § 1395x(t), which defines drugs to "include only such drugs…as are included (or approved for inclusion) in the United States Pharmacopeia, the National Formulary or the United States Homeopathic Pharmacopoeia."

The 2004 issue of the *HPUS* contains 1286 monographs such as the one shown in Figure 55-1 for potassium phosphate, dibasic (its name in contemporary use), or Kali phosphoricum (official homeopathic name). Basically, monographs specify the drug's nomenclature; origin; botanical, zoologic, or chemical description and classification; requirements for preparation; and medication status. The medication status designates the lowest potency at which a product can be sold as a prescription (Rx), nonprescription oral (OTC), topical (Ext Use), or pharmaceutical necessity (HPN). Homeopathic drugs are given prescription status for a variety of reasons (Table 55-6); however, most are nonprescription in commonly available potencies. Quality control tests, such as thin-layer chromatography for plant-based starting materials, are being added to the monographs as part of the ongoing revision process.

FDA guidelines on regulations for the manufacture and labeling of homeopathic prescription and nonprescription drugs differ in some respects from those for pharmaceutical medicine. FDA's Compliance Policy Guide 7132.15 (also known as 400.400) contains information outlining the conditions under which homeopathic drugs may be marketed. Labeling requirements under these guidelines are similar in many ways to those for conventional nonprescription and prescription products. With homeopathic agents, however, a medication's strength is not labeled in grams or milligrams but in homeopathic terms, and an expiration date is not required on the label.[25] FDA has waived the obligation to use English names on labels, allowing use of Latin names. In many cases, the Latin name is necessary to distinguish between drugs that are derived from a number of species within a particular genus. *HPUS* lists official short names that can be used in place of the longer Latin names. Because a single individual drug may have many indications, manufacturers are required to list at least one indication (not all of them) on single-drug products. Of the more than 3000 known homeopathic remedies, about 1286 remedies in historic use or extensive current use have been recognized by the HPCUS, as identified by "HPUS" on the label; the others lack the necessary verification data or have not yet been submitted for approval. (For more details about the differences and similarities in homeopathic and conventional pharmaceutical labeling, see Table 55-7.)

## Homeopathic Pharmaceutics

Medicines used in homeopathy are derived from a multitude of substances including botanical, zoologic (e.g., insect, reptile, or animal/human material or byproducts), mineral, and pharmaceutical substances. These substances are serially diluted and successed (or triturated) to increase the strength or potency of the medication. This process is called attenuation or potentization. After each attenuation step, the preparation is given a higher number, so a substance that was attenuated four times would be designated as 4X, 4C, or LM4, depending on the dilution factor. The decimal (1:10 dilutions) and centesimal (1:100 dilutions) scales of attenuation are used to make X and C potencies, respectively, as illustrated in Figure 55-2.[14,15] The letter M is also used in potency terminology and means 1000C, not the use of 1:1000 dilution in the attenuation process.

**TABLE 55-6 Homeopathic Prescription Drugs**

| Examples of Drugs | Reason for Prescription Status |
|---|---|
| Cannabis, Opium, Cocainum, Phenobarbitalum | Drugs are made from a controlled substance, Schedules I-IV. |
| Tuberculinum, Syphilinum, Medorrhinum, Bacillinum | Drugs are made from disease substance tissue and exudates (also called nosodes). (Note: Even though pathogens are killed and sterilized before the homeopathic process, they still require a prescription.) |
| Lachesis mutus ≤6X, Naja tripudians ≤6X | Low potencies of possibly toxic substances (in these cases, snake venoms) are prescription; higher potencies, greater than 6X, are usually considered safe for OTC use. |
| Crataegus oxyacantha, Digitalis purpurea, Digitalinum, Digitoxinum | Drugs are indicated for a condition (e.g., a cardiac condition) not amenable to self-treatment. (Note: Crataegus or hawthorn is used in herbal medicine as a tonic for the heart muscle; thus, herbal tinctures of Crataegus can be sold OTC.) |

Key: OTC, over-the-counter.

**TABLE 55-7 Information Found on Label of Homeopathic Products**

| Label Information | Comments |
|---|---|
| Ingredients | Latin name for natural substances; otherwise, the established common name or abbreviation of each drug in the product. "HPUS" appears after the name if the drug is in *HPUS*. |
| Potency or strength | The common OTC potencies are 6, 12, and 30 C or X. The letter X or D stands for the use of decimal dilutions of 1:10 for each step of the attenuation process. C stands for the centesimal potency, where 1:100 dilutions are used instead. K, CK, or CH indicate if a single-vial or multiple-vial method was used to make the C potency, respectively; the M and LM potencies are not found in products marked for consumer use. |
| Indication(s) | Most OTC combination products are labeled for common, self-limiting conditions. Single-drug products are required to have one or more indications. Because the same drug can be used for many conditions, space limitation prevents listing all of them on the label. For example, Lachesis can be used for headache or sore throat even though these indications are not listed on the package. |
| Directions for use | Combination OTC products should be taken as directed on the label. For single homeopathic drugs, the dosage required by a patient may deviate from labeled guidelines. The size of the label limits listing all possible dosing regimens, depending on the acuteness and severity of the condition being treated, or a patient's sensitivity to homeopathic drugs. |
| HPUS | This designation indicates the drug was made in accordance with FDA standards. |
| Conventional pharmaceutical label information | This information includes manufacturer name and address, NDC number, UPC code, and lot or control number; declaration of net contents, warnings, tamper-evident statement, storage instructions, prescription-only statement if the drug and/or potency is designated as such in *HPUS*. |
| Exceptions to conventional pharmaceutical label information | FDA waives the requirement for an expiration date with homeopathic drugs because most homeopathic drugs on the market are diluted beyond the point at which the deterioration of contents can be measured with current technology. However, many homeopathic manufacturers provide an expiration date on their product packages even though it is not required. Because homeopathic drugs are FDA regulated, they are not required to display a supplement facts box or disclaimer statement as required for herbs and supplements regulated under DSHEA. They may opt to use the "drug facts box." |

Key: *HPUS, Homoeopathic Pharmacopoeia of the United States;* OTC, over-the-counter; FDA, Food And Drug Administration; NDC, National Drug Code; UPC, Universal Product Code; DSHEA, Dietary Supplement Health and Education Act.

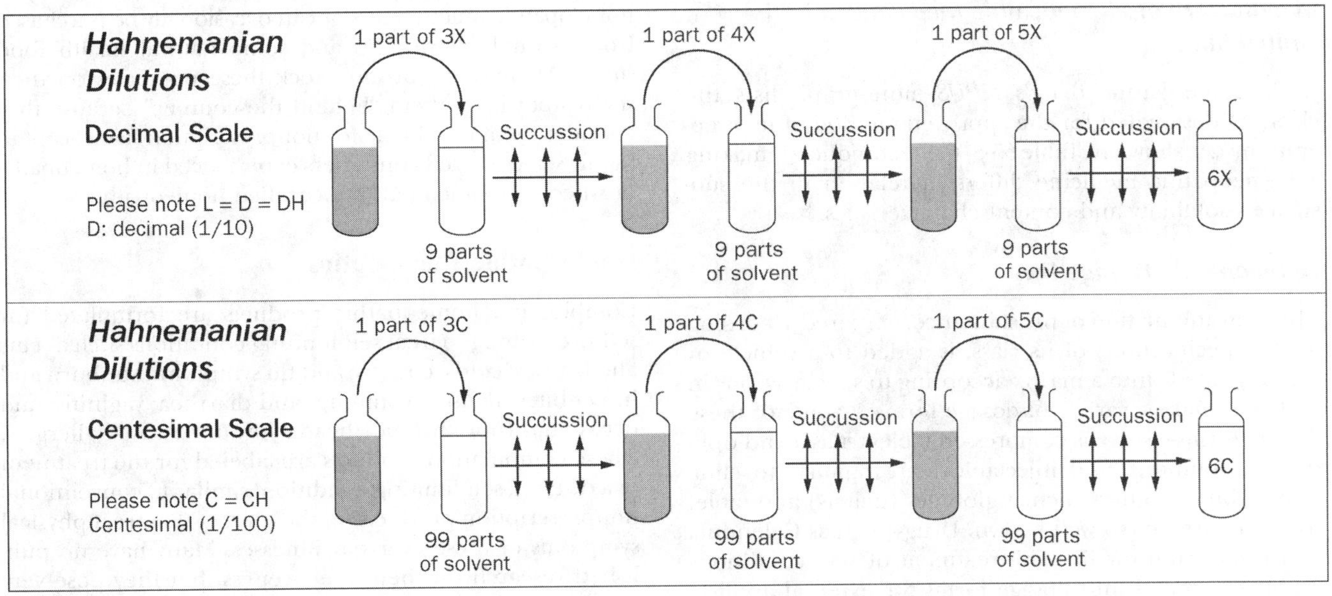


**FIGURE 55-2** Method for making X and C potencies. Decimal scale, designated by an X or D, involves dilutions of 1:10 for each attenuation (dilution with succussion) step taken to make the desired X potency. Centesimal scale, designated by C, involves dilutions of 1:100 for each attenuation step taken to make the desired C potency. (Reprinted with permission from *Introduction to Homeopathic Medicines for Pharmacists*. New Town Square, Pa: Boiron Institute; 2001:9.)

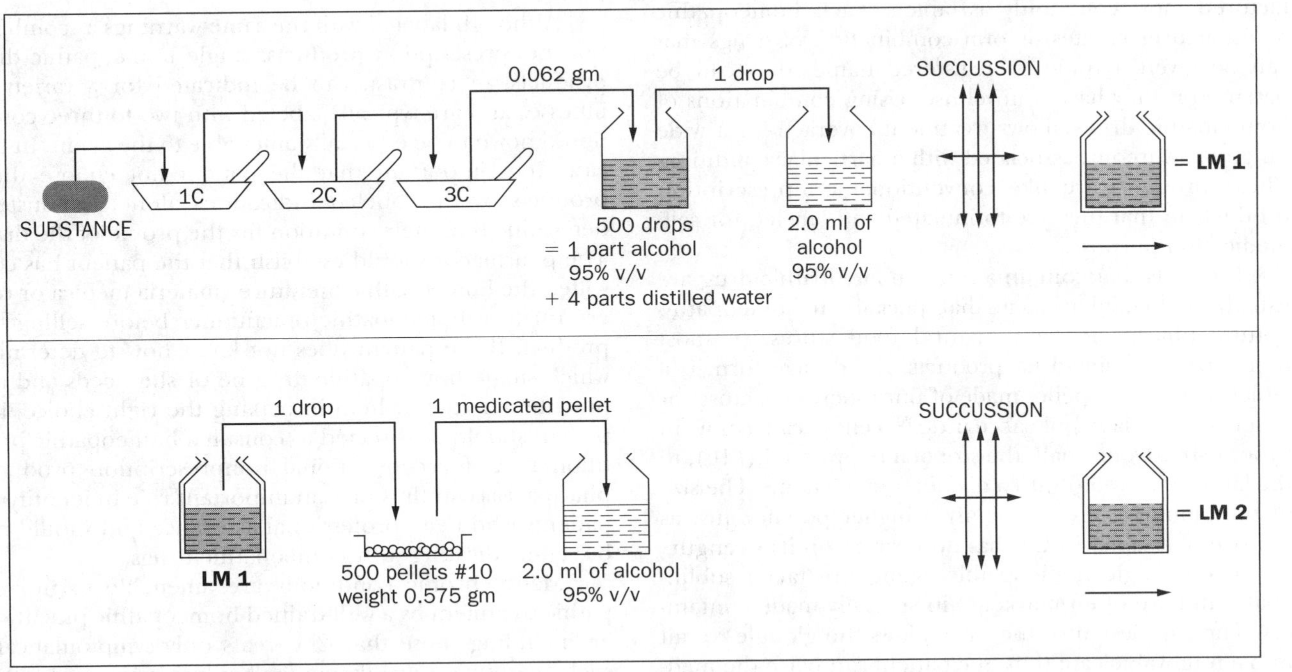


**FIGURE 55-3** Method for making LM potencies. 50-Millesimal scale, designated by LM or Q, involves a complex attenuation process using incremental dilutions of 1:50,000 with succussion. (Reprinted with permission from *The Homeopathic Pharmacopoeia of the United States*. Southeastern, Pa: The Homeopathic Pharmacopoeia Convention of the United States Revision Service; December 2004:40.)

The process for making 50 millesimal (1:50,000 dilutions) or LM (also known as Q) potencies is complex (Figure 55-3). LM potencies are less well known than centesimals because Hahnemann described them in the sixth edition of the *Organon*, which was not published until nearly a century after his death.[15] Professional homeopaths today are using them with increasing frequency. Generally, they are dispensed as a liquid, or less commonly as globules, and can be found at pharmacies that specialize in homeopathic medicines or obtained directly from a homeopathic manufacturer.

### Manufacture of Homeopathic Medications in the United States

Each homeopathic drug's *HPUS* monograph lists the class(es) designated for the approved method of its preparation.[20] As shown in Table 55-8, the technique for making a homeopathic medicine differs in relation to the substance's solubility and content characteristics.

### Homeopathic Dosage Forms

The final attenuation of the substance, prepared according to the specifications of its class, is added to a vehicle or "impregnated" into a matrix according to specifications in HPUS to make a variety of dosage forms.[20] Some of these dosage forms—such as compressed tablets, nasal and ophthalmic solutions, and injectables—are familiar to clinicians, whereas others such as globules (pellets) and tablet triturates are not so well known. Drugs such as Calendula and Hypericum for first-aid treatment of skin conditions are incorporated into dosage forms for external application similar to lotions, sprays, ointments, and gels.

Clinicians are most likely to encounter patients using homeopathy as a combination drug product. These products are marketed for general consumer use and usually contain drug ingredients in attenuations below 30C (i.e., of low potency, safe for self-medication). They are manufactured most commonly as tablets. Each homeopathic manufacturer creates its own combination of drugs that can be given a trade or registered name; they can be patented if they have a novel use. Using combinations of homeopathic drugs allows treatment coverage for a wide range of symptoms associated with a particular condition. These products are like conventional nonprescription products in that they are formulated and labeled for self-medication purposes.

Products that contain a single homeopathic drug are usually found in pharmacies that specialize in homeopathy, natural pharmacies, and natural food stores. In most homeopathic single-drug products, the dosage form is a tablet, globule, or pellet made of pure sucrose, lactose, or other appropriate polysaccharide.[20] Pellets can come in various sizes from small, the size of a poppy seed (#10), to the largest size (#55) with a diameter of 5.5 mm.[20] The size of the globule does not signify a higher potency, just as the size of a tablet in CM has no bearing on its strength.

These single homeopathic agents are taken sublingually and are often marketed in specially made containers. The cap design of the tube allows the globule to fall into a removable cap; thus, the patient can place the medication directly under the tongue without touching it. Globules are very porous, so touching them may potentially interfere with drug delivery, especially if the hands are not clean. However, no studies have measured whether touching globules has an effect on the medication's efficacy. Because of their porous nature, patients should also be advised to keep these medications in their original container. Single-drug products sold on the common retail market in the United States generally contain drugs in the lower potency ranges, rarely above 30C. The higher potencies of 200C and greater are commonly sold directly to homeopathic practitioners or can occasionally be purchased from natural pharmacies and some natural health food stores. Many stores do not stock these potencies on their shelves but keep them "behind the counter" because they consider them unsuitable for nonprescription sale except to highly self-educated consumers experienced in homeopathy or when recommended by a certified homeopath.

## Homeopathic Therapeutics

Combination homeopathic products are formulated for self-prescribing to treat self-limiting conditions such as cuts and bruises; colds, coughs, and flu symptoms; sunburn and insect bites; nausea, vomiting, and diarrhea; vaginitis; and occasional (not chronic) headaches or seasonal allergies. These combination products are labeled for the treatment of a distinct, self-limiting condition, similar to conventional nonprescription products on the market that treat physical symptoms of these everyday illnesses. Many have no published research on their effectiveness, but they pose very little risk to patients if taken as recommended on the package label. For many homeopathic combination products, unpublished clinical trials can be obtained from the manufacturer. As with conventional nonprescription products, they are labeled to warn patients to consult a primary care provider if symptoms persist for more than 3 days or worsen.

Although labeled with the same warnings as combination nonprescription products, single homeopathic drug products, in contrast, can be indicated for a variety of illnesses and are typically labeled with two to three conditions known to be especially amenable to the agent. In this case, it is important that the patient not choose these products by the labeled indications alone, but instead determine that their condition fits the profile of the drug. The pharmacist should establish that the patient has consulted the homeopathic literature (materia medica or repertory) or a homeopathic practitioner before selling the product. If the patient does not know how to determine which single homeopathic drug he or she needs and the practitioner cannot help in making the right choice, the patient should be directed to consult a homeopathic practitioner. As for conventional nonprescription products, pharmacists can thus play an important role in identifying patients who need professional assistance and should not be self-medicating with homeopathic drugs.

Many chronic conditions are amenable to homeopathic treatment by a well-trained homeopathic practitioner, including those that CM treats only symptomatically, such as asthma, acne, dysmenorrhea, migraine, and arthritis.[26] Homeopathy has also been reported to be useful as adjunctive therapy to CM care, providing relief of the specific symptoms of a serious illness and reducing or eliminating CM treatment–induced side effects. For example, homeopathic medicines are reported to mitigate the nausea, vomiting, fatigue, and stomatitis associated with radiation and chemotherapy, as well as (in an RCT trial) the pruritus associated with hemodialysis.[27] Homeopathic medicines are also reported to be useful in palliative therapy for terminal diseases, relieving physical symptoms, such as pain, and emotional states, such as the fear of dying.[26]

**TABLE 55-8 Methods of Preparation of Homeopathic Drugs According to Class**

| HPUS Class | Class Title | Substance Characteristics/Preparation Methods |
|---|---|---|
| A & B | Liquid Attenuations of Soluble Substances | 1. Substance is a soluble material.<br>2. It is made into a solution 10% (class A) or variable dilution (class B) for the first dilution of 1X or 1C. Subsequent 1:10 or 1:100 dilutions are succussed to produce higher attenuations of X or C potencies, respectively. |
| C & D (Tr., or MT [1X]) | Homeopathic Tinctures of Botanical Substances | 1. Substance is a crude, fresh, or dried botanical specimen.<br>2. It is macerated or percolated in the process of being made into a tincture 10% (class C) or 5% (class D) for the first dilution of 1X. Subsequent 1:10 or 1:100 dilutions are succussed to produce higher attenuations of X or C potencies, respectively. |
| E | Homeopathic Tinctures of Zoologic Substances | 1. Substance is a fresh or dried zoologic specimen.<br>2. It is macerated or percolated in the process of being made into a tincture 5% for the first dilution of 1X or 1C. Subsequent preparation is the same as for class C and D substances. |
| F | Triturations of Solid Substances | 1. Substance is a dry, crude, insoluble material.<br>2. It is triturated with lactose USP to make a powder 10% or 1% for the first dilution of 1X or 1C. Subsequent 1:10 or 1:100 triturations produce higher attenuations of X or C potencies, respectively. The process of trituration potentizes in place of succussion. |
| G | Trituration of Insoluble Liquid Substances | 1. Substance is an insoluble liquid material.<br>2. It is triturated with lactose USP to make a powder 10% or 1% for the first dilution of 1X or 1C. Subsequent preparation is the same as for class F substances. |
| H | Conversion of Triturations of Insoluble Basic Substances into Liquid Attenuations | 1. Substance is one used in classes F and G.<br>2. It is prepared by succussing one part of the lowest soluble trituration of the substance (usually 6X or 3C) with sufficient distilled water or other appropriate menstruum to produce a 1:10 or 1:100 dilution of the next higher attenuation of X or C potency, respectively. |
| I | Nosodes | 1. Substance is a diseased organ or tissue, infectious organisms, or product of a disease (excretions or secretions).<br>2. It is prepared in X and C potencies according to specifications of classes A, B, F, and H, in respect to the solubility characteristics of the substance.<br>3. It may not be dispensed in attenuations below 5X, and all potencies require a prescription.<br>4. The first attenuation must be rendered sterile. |
| J | Allersodes | 1. Substance is an antigen (induces formation of antibodies).<br>2. It is prepared the same as described for class I.<br>3. It may not be dispensed in attenuations below 6X or 3C. |
| K | Isodes, Detoxodes | 1. Substance is botanical, zoologic, or chemical and is capable of producing a disease (toxicity) that interferes with homeostasis.<br>2. It is prepared the same as described for class I.<br>3. It may not be dispensed in attenuations below 6X or 3C. |
| L | Sarcode | 1. The substance is a wholesome organ, gland, tissue, or metabolic factor obtained from a healthy subject.<br>2. It is prepared the same as described for class I. |
| M | Homeopathic Tinctures of Fresh and Fermented Botanical Substances | 1. The substance is a preparation of fresh and fermented botanical substances not covered in other classes. |

The term *acute* is used by homeopaths to refer to a self-limiting condition of recent onset and not to its severity, which is addressed as a separate factor. Professional homeopaths without CM training can be expected to refer patients who have serious or life-threatening conditions to appropriate CM practitioners for treatment. Therefore, in the homeopathic literature, acute prescribing can involve the treatment of mild acute conditions, such as colds, coughs, sprains, and strains, or severe acute conditions that require concurrent conventional medical attention, such as a broken bone.

Professional homeopaths use homeopathic medicines not only to treat acute and chronic conditions but also in what is sometimes called constitutional prescribing.[21] In these cases, the medicine is given to strengthen the patient's underlying constitution to help prevent recurrence of ear infections in children, vaginitis in women, or other commonly recurring conditions. This process is analogous to strengthening the immune system although the homeopathic medicine is believed to work by strengthening the body's underlying vital force or healing energy, rather than by pharmacologically strengthening the immune system. With the homeopathic treatment of simple, acute, common everyday illnesses in the otherwise healthy patient, monitoring is straightforward, as is discussed later, and follow-up is usually not required. However, for patients with chronic illnesses or multiple illnesses in their current or past medical histories, the situation is much different; these patients will need to be monitored by a skilled homeopathic practitioner, who is also well versed in CM.

Hering's law, one of the fundamental principles of homeopathy, is used by homeopaths along with CM measures of therapeutic response to monitor the patient's progress in the healing process. The principle includes the following observations: cure proceeds from above downward, from within outward, from the most important to the least important organs, and in the reverse order of appearance of symptoms.[18] It is beyond the scope of this chapter to describe each of these items in detail; however, the clinician should be aware of the connotations of Hering's law relating to responses a patient may have to homeopathic drug therapy.

For instance, according to the idea that cure proceeds from inward to outward, the appearance of a discharge (nasal, vaginal, bronchial) or skin eruption (rash) in response to a homeopathic drug therapy for an internal problem, together with improvement in the deeper complaint (e.g., asthma, colitis), is a sign that healing is proceeding. Clinicians familiar only with the reactions caused by conventional drug therapy may misinterpret these as an adverse reaction, side effect, or allergy. The homeopathic drug–induced reactions are different, however, and can be distinguished by the relative absence of any signs of inflammation, fever, angioedema, or malaise. Characteristically, patients have a heightened sense of well-being as the discharge or skin eruption takes place and their original problem has resolved substantially. Because homeopathic drugs contain very dilute amounts of a substance, an actual adverse effect by pharmacologic mechanisms is highly unlikely, and virtually impossible with potencies greater than 24X or 12C.

Many homeopaths discuss the possibility of this kind of reaction with their patients before initiating therapy and counsel them to limit their intake of pharmacologic agents, such as antihistamines, or not to use topical corticosteroid drugs, which some believe may interfere with the vital force's efforts to remove the illness and restore health. They also believe that, by the nature of Hering's law, if healing is not allowed to progress, the disease process will reverse and the original problem will return. Clinicians encountering a patient who is complaining about a severe homeopathic drug–induced discharge reaction ideally should refer the patient to a certified homeopathic practitioner, preferably one who also has CM training. For mild to moderate reactions that patients are willing to tolerate, it is best to support the homeopathic tradition and encourage the patient to allow the discharge to resolve by itself.

The clinician who is interested in reading more about homeopathic therapeutics (case studies and discussions of philosophical issues involving homeopathic practices) can refer to the professional homeopathic journals listed in Table 55-1. Many articles in these journals, are authored by licensed MDs, RNs, and NDs, and describe case studies of patients who have responded to a homeopathic therapy and were subsequently able to reduce or discontinue their pharmaceutical medication(s). The following information will help the reader interpret the literature found in homeopathic journals; however, to fully comprehend them, the reader will need to study homeopathy in more depth.

### *Diagnostic Procedures: Taking the Case*

Similar to conventional nonprescription products, combination homeopathic products are formulated for patients' use without medical supervision, and case taking is usually not required. In some circumstances, however, a little case taking can optimize use of these agents. Knowing how a professional homeopath determines which single homeopathic medication is best for a patient can provide clinicians with the insight they need to help patients use the combination products effectively and improve their ability to communicate with homeopathic practitioners.[8,21]

Since the success of a single homeopathic agent rests on its having the same characteristics as the individual patient's mental, emotional, and physical manifestations of illness, the practitioner needs to obtain detailed information about the patient's illness to correctly choose a homeopathic drug.[18] This process includes information that the person provides and information about the person that can be observed. The homeopathic history includes a conventional medical history (including appropriate laboratory studies), with special emphasis on obtaining the etiology, localization, sensations, and modalities or modifying factors of each symptom described by the patient. In most acute conditions or minor first-aid situations, this kind of information is enough for an experienced homeopathic practitioner to find the most suitable homeopathic agent for any of these kinds of cases.[18,21]

**TABLE 55-9 Comparison of Three Combination Products for Allergy Relief With Potency Indicated for Each Medication**

| Drug | Zicam Allergy Relief Nasal Solution | Boiron Sabadil Tablets | Similasan Hay Fever Relief Tablets |
|---|---|---|---|
| Allium cepa | | 5C | |
| Ambrosia artemisiifolia | | 5C | |
| Cardiospermum | | | 6X |
| Euphrasia officinalis | | 5C | |
| Galphimia glauca | 12X, 30X | | 6X |
| Histaminum | 12X, 30X, 200X | 9C | |
| Luffa operculata | 4X, 12X, 30X | | 6X |
| Sabadilla | | 5C | 6X |
| Solidago virgaurea | | 5C | |
| Sulphur | 12X, 30X, 200X | | |

For chronic and complex acute conditions or for constitutional prescribing, more extensive case taking and analysis are necessary. The general physiologic function of patients is examined by inquiring about their appetite, food cravings and aversions, thirst, sleep and dreams, temperature preference, reactions to weather conditions, and periodicity of recurring symptoms. An examination of the patient's mental state is also important. Patients are asked how they would describe themselves and how others describe them. Cognitive function (concentration, memory, thoughts, and delusions) and emotional symptoms (anxieties, fears, phobias, anger, and lack of self-confidence) are also important elements about which patients are asked, as is their desire for company and consolation; emotional reactions to confrontation, contradiction, and criticism; and their feelings related to jealousy and sexuality.

The time needed to take a homeopathic case varies in relation to the kind of condition being assessed. Taking the case of a person with a simple acute condition or first-aid situation can be conducted in a few minutes; however, for constitutional prescribing or chronic cases, the process can take 2 hours or more.

### *Selection of a Homeopathic Drug*

For the majority of single homeopathic drugs, selecting the right drug and dosing regimen for chronic or severe conditions is extremely challenging for anyone who does not have formal training. Using a homeopathic combination product for a particular condition may be worthwhile considering in cases involving patients who are contemplating taking a conventional nonprescription drug, but are taking conventional pharmaceuticals that will interact with it or have suffered intolerable side effects from it.

The allergy formulas listed in Table 55-9 illustrate how combination products may contain different medicines or the same medicine in different potencies. Each product has drugs that do not appear in the others and represents a homeopathic agent that covers a broad range of symptoms commonly exhibited by people with hay fever: spastic sneezing, itching of the nose, watery nasal discharge, and burning and redness of the eyes, which lacrimate whenever sneezing occurs.

The majority of patients with hay fever will likely respond to any one of the three common drugs contained in these products, but a minority of the patients will have more distinct or unusual combinations of symptoms. In these cases, the dissimilar drugs in each of the products become important to consider. A patient who has watery eyes that excoriate the lower lids, a symptom indicating Euphrasia, will respond only to the one product that contains it. On the other hand, a patient with excoriating nasal discharge, indicating Allium cepa, will respond only to the one product that contains it. Keeping this in mind, the clinician should realize when a patient reports that a particular homeopathic nonprescription combination product was not effective that another homeopathic nonprescription combination could contain the drug the patient needs.

As with conventional nonprescription combination products, homeopathic combination products will not be effective if the formulation does not contain the ingredient needed to treat a patient's specific symptoms. In both cases, the clinician who gets detailed information about the patient's symptoms will be able to make a better recommendation. Pharmacists who have homeopathic nonprescription combination drugs in their floor stock can become familiar with the ingredients each one contains and recommend them with greater success, especially if their store carries more than one product for the same condition. Instead of using a text such as *Drug Facts and Comparisons*, clinicians can find the drugs' indications in a homeopathic materia medica, which is discussed in the next section. As with conventional nonprescription products, recommendations should not be based on cost alone. It is far more important to choose the product with ingredients that best suit the patient's expressed needs.

Some homeopathic drugs are ideally suited for patients and clinicians who want to start using single-drug homeopathic products. These drugs are effective for injuries and common ailments that usually provoke similar symptoms in everyone. Table 55-10 lists some of these medications and provides information about the symptoms and conditions for each drug. Patients who want to try homeopathy for a common condition but have atypical or complex symptoms should be referred to a qualified professional homeopath.

## Using the Repertory and Materia Medica

The materia medica and repertory are two fundamental types of reference books used in the selection of the right homeopathic agent to treat an illness. Early texts were written by individual homeopaths who used archaic terminology common to their time. More recent materia medicas and repertories are based on these older works, updated with modern English usage, and expanded with information from ongoing proving and verification trials, toxicology reports, and clinical experience (Table 55-1).

The materia medica provides monographs of homeopathic drugs listed alphabetically, describing each drug's healing characteristics in detail. Symptoms are arranged anatomically (head, eyes, back, and so forth) and according to human conditions (vertigo, chill, perspiration, and so forth). Symptoms that are especially well established and proven are usually found in bold or italic type; those in bold type are considered keynote symptoms. Table 55-11 shows the keynote descriptions of Staphysagria by two authors, Boericke and Morrison, for two symptom categories—mental/emotional and female urogenital—to illustrate the contrast between an old-fashioned and modern materia medica.[28,29]

The repertory organizes information contained in the materia medica in a way similar to the white and yellow pages of the telephone book. Symptoms are listed in alphabetical order within chapters on the basis of anatomic regions and human conditions (Figure 55-4). After each symptom, drugs that apply to it are listed in a systematic fashion called a rubric. Subrubrics are listed below the main rubric as a means of indexing more specific characteristics of the symptom. Some rubrics contain over 100 drugs, so abbreviations are used instead of the common name. Repertories contain a table that provides the full name of each abbreviated homeopathic drug.

This kind of text allows the user to look up all the patient's symptoms and find all possible appropriate drugs without having to memorize the materia medica. Once all the drugs have been identified in all the rubrics that encompass the patient's condition, those drugs that appear most frequently in the case are then compared for the closest match to the individual patient's needs. The process of analyzing the drugs found in rubrics is termed "repertorization."

For example, the case of a child who has otitis media and thick discharges from his ear, with pain at night, and who is not thirsty despite a high fever could be repertorized using the following rubrics:

1. Ear, inflammation, media, *Arn.*, *Bell.*, **Calc.**, **Cham.**, Gels., **Lyc.**, **Merc.**, **Puls.**, Rhus-t., **Sil.**, **Sulph.**, Zinc-m.
2. Ear, pain, at night: Alum., *Bry.*, **Dulc**, *Hep.*, *Kali-bi*, *Lach.*, **Merc.**, Nux-v., **Puls**, *Rhus-t.*, *Sil.*, *Tub.*
3. Ear, discharges, thick, **Calc.**, *Carbo-v.*, **Hydr.**, **Kali-bi.**, *Lyc.*, Nat.-m., **Puls.**, Sep., **Sil.**
4. Fever, intense heat, **Acon.**, *Apis*, **Arn.**, **Ars.**, **Bell.**, Cact., **Gels.**, *Lyc.*, **Puls.**, **Rhus-t.**, *Sil.*
5. Stomach, thirstless, **Apis**, *Ars.*, **Gels.**, *Lyc.*, **Ph-ac.**, **Puls.**, Sulph.

*Note:* Most repertories use regular, bold, and italic type to indicate the usefulness or strength of the drug in a particular condition. For the sake of brevity, all drugs listed in these rubrics are not given, and drug names are abbreviated as they would be in the repertory.

The resulting information is compiled in the form of a chart; Table 55-12 shows the highest-scoring drugs in this case. From the top-scoring drugs indicated by the chart, a drug is chosen on the basis of how it covers the patient's individual experience of the illness including physical symptoms, the patient's personality, and other relevant factors. Although Pulsatilla scores higher than Lycopodium, the second highest scoring drug in this chart, both should be considered because the repertory is used as a guide to suggest possible drugs rather than a mechanical means to determine the prescription. In the earlier example of otitis media, Lycopodium would be given to a child who is described as a little tyrant, "always in a power struggle" with his parents and possibly suffering from intestinal gas, while children who need Pulsatilla tend to cling to their mother, whine and cry easily, and then cheer up quickly.

Repertorization requires training and practice, and is usually the province of the professional homeopath in severe or chronic illnesses although a drug can be chosen for a common self-limiting condition simply by consulting a self-help book, such as those listed in Table 55-1. Repertorization can be a long and tedious process, especially with complicated cases involving a large number of rubrics, some of which could contain over 500 drugs. The benefits of computerization are obvious. Computer programs not only add the repertorizations quickly, but they also provide instant access to the vast literature of homeopathy.[30,31] Once the most significant drugs are determined, the case is reanalyzed to find the drug that best fits the patient's needs by investigating symptoms that were not considered in the repertorization.

### *Selection of a Dosing Regimen*

In the case of homeopathic combination nonprescription products, the potency of each drug is fixed, and patients should be instructed to take the medication as directed on the package. These products typically contain drugs in the 3, 6, or 12 or, less often, 30C or X potency, and they are generally taken three to four times daily.[22] Because combination homeopathic nonprescription products have fixed potencies, an intensified effect can be achieved only by taking the product more frequently, up to the limit stated on the label. These drugs are usually taken as a tablet and should be discontinued when symptoms subside and repeated only if symptoms return.

**TABLE 55-10 Homeopathic Drugs Used in OTC Products for First Aid and Common Self-limiting Illnesses**

| Drug Names* | Common OTC Uses | Qualifying Principles |
|---|---|---|
| Aconite<br>Aconitum napellus<br>Monkshood | Fever; colds; sore throat; cough | Sudden onset; any acute condition caused by dry, cold wind or sudden fright; anxiety, fear, restlessness, sudden fright (e.g., almost hit by car) |
| Apis<br>Apis mellifica<br>Honey bee | Insect bites, hives; herpes, shingles; sore throat with swollen uvula; sunburn with itching, burning, or stinging feeling; edema, especially lower eyelid; swelling of arthritic knee; PMS with water retention | Any condition with swelling, redness, itching or stinging, as if stung by a bee |
| Arnica<br>Arnica montana<br>Leopard's bane | Soft tissue trauma: bruises, pulled muscles, sports injuries; hemorrhoids; flu; jet lag; immediately after head trauma, especially if hematoma; for infant after childbirth, especially if forceps or vacuum extraction were used<br>Before and after tooth extraction<br>Hoarseness from overuse of voice | Any extravasation (black eyes); any condition with a bruised, sore feeling (e.g., with a feeling of being beaten up or bruised); person says, "I am fine" and "I do not need to go to the hospital" after head trauma; sensation that bed is too hard (in insomnia, flu) |
| Arsenicum<br>Arsenicum album<br>Arsenic | First stage of cold with "nose running like a faucet"; Traveler's diarrhea; insomnia; fever; flu; sore throat; shingles | Anxiety, especially about health; restlessness; burning sensation; extreme exhaustion |
| Belladonna<br>Deadly nightshade | Fever, sore throat, ear infections; colds; boils when they first appear, but have not yet come to a head; burns and sunburn; mumps, measles, chickenpox; diaper rash; hot flashes; heavy menstrual flow with bright red, hot blood | Acute conditions with sudden onset, high fever, red face, glassy eyes; blood seems to go to one part of body (Person may feel pulse throbbing in that part; it may appear red and swollen, or feel warm.) |
| Calendula<br>Calendula officinalis<br>Pot marigold | Any skin laceration: cuts, abrasions, surgical incisions, acne, ulcers; first-degree burns; pulled muscles, if Arnica does not work | Antiseptic and promotes wound healing, promotes granulation |
| Chamomilla<br>German chamomile | Teething and ear infections; menstrual cramps or labor pains; diarrhea (green like chopped spinach); headaches from caffeine withdrawal | Intense pain; extreme irritability (Person becomes extremely peevish and impossible to please.) |
| Gelsemium<br>Gelsemium sempervirens<br>Yellow jasmine | Flu; performance anxiety; stage fright; occipital headache | Feeling totally drained of energy: "as if a truck ran over me"; fear with trembling |
| Hypericum<br>Hypericum perforatum<br>St. John's wort | Fingertip crushed in a door; neuralgic pains (shooting along the path of a nerve), including dental pains, sciatica; puncture wounds or animal bites | Any injury to an area rich with nerves |
| Kali-bic<br>Kali bichromium<br>Bichromate of potash | Later stages of colds; sinusitis, sinus headaches; cough; blocked eustachian tubes; vaginitis; postnasal drip | Any condition with thick, sticky, green or yellow-green mucus or discharge |
| Nux vomica<br>Poison-nut | Indigestion, heartburn; constipation, hemorrhoids; flu; headaches; insomnia; hay fever; hangovers; snoring | People who are rushed, active, irritable, overworked, ambitious, sedentary; use stimulants; indulge in excesses; eat rich foods; have violent temper; are chilly and overly sensitive to noise, odors, light |
| Rhus tox<br>Rhus toxicodendron<br>Poison oak | Poison ivy, herpes, chickenpox, scabies; rheumatic pains, arthritis, bursitis; sprains; flu; sciatica; hoarseness | Restless, both physically and mentally; joint symptoms are worse when first starting to move, then limber up ("rusty gate syndrome"); joints are stiff in damp weather; itchy fluid-filled vesicles, such as poison ivy |
| Ruta<br>Ruta graveolens<br>Garden rue | Sprains, joint pains; rheumatic pains; shin splints; carpal tunnel syndrome; eye strain, floaters | Injuries to connective tissue, periosteum; stringy pain" (pain along the line of a tendon or ligament) |

Key: OTC, over-the-counter; PMS, premenstrual syndrome.

* Names include common and official homeopathic drug names (which are the same for Belladonna, Chamomilla, and Nux vomica) and the common name of the drug's origin.

**TABLE 55-11 Comparison of Two Materia Medicas for Information Regarding Staphysagria[28,29]**

| Staphysagria* | Boericke† | Morrison† |
|---|---|---|
| Mental/emotional symptoms | Very sensitive to what others say about her; child cries for many things and refuses them when offered; impetuous, violent outbursts of passion, sad, hypochondriacal; dwells on sexual matters and prefers solitude; peevish; nervous affections with marked irritability; sexual sins and excesses | Sweet suppressed patients who draw our sympathy; weeps during interview; tendency to throw things when very angry; ailments from grief or suppressed anger; rage in very late stages; ailments after insults or humiliation; low self-esteem; depression; constant and often distressingly frequent sexual fantasies; in patients with a history of incest or abuse or with alcoholic parents |
| Female urogenital symptoms | Ineffectual urging to urinate in newly married women; irritable bladder in young married women; urging and pain after urination; parts very sensitive, worse sitting down; sensation as if a drop of urine were rolling continuously along the channel | Urethritis, frequent urging for urine; cystitis, which begins from the first intercourse or may happen after every intercourse; enuresis; painful genital condylomata; masturbation, many sexual fantasies; high sexual desire, weak resistance, sometimes promiscuous |

* Selected keynotes of important mental/emotional and female urogenital symptoms found for patients needing Staphysagria.

† Each materia medica has additional symptoms for each major organ system. Boericke's is one of the standard turn-of-the century reference works. Morrison's is an excellent materia medica, which presents material in modern language.

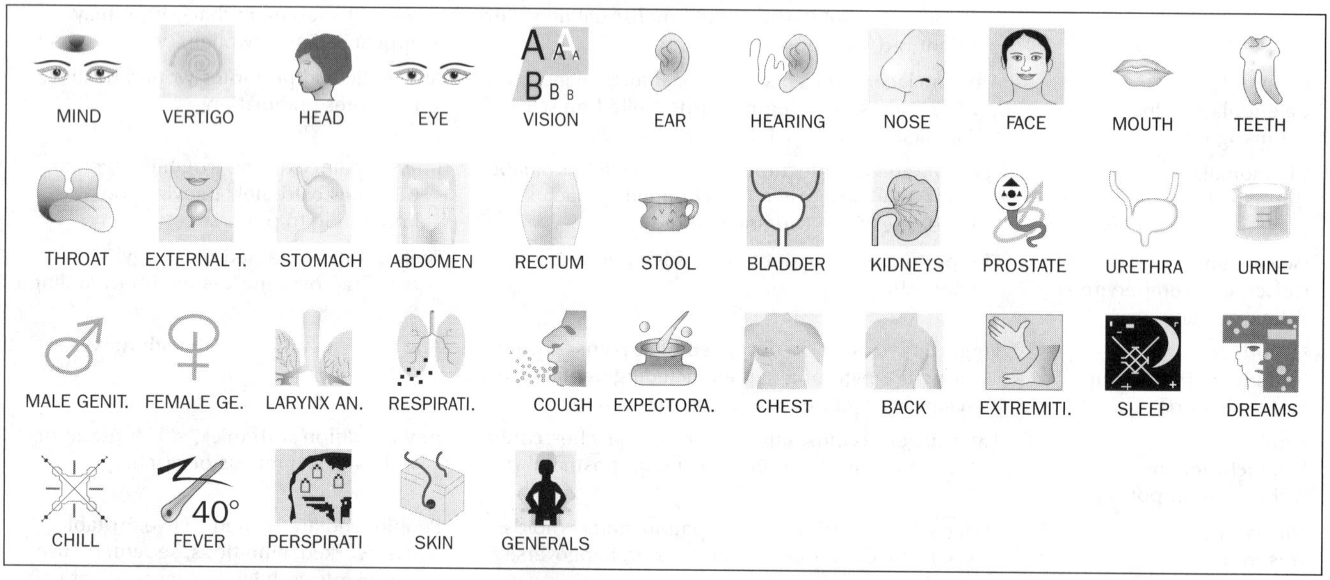


**FIGURE 55-4** Pictorial illustration of chapter headings in a repertory. (Reprinted with permission from *Radar* for Windows [computer program], Version 9, Worcester, Mass: Archibel SA; 2004.)

As for single-drug dosing, the great majority of patients can safely benefit by following the directions on the package. These agents are generally taken in the tablet or globule form. Two tablets or three to five globules are taken sublingually for one dose. Taking more globules for each dose will not increase the strength of the dose because the potency or energetic strength of each globule is not additive as with CM drugs. In other words, taking two globules of a 6C potency medicine does not provide a 12C dose. This contrasts with conventional pharmacy where two tablets of a 6 mg strength would yield a 12 mg dose. To increase a dose of a homeopathic agent, a higher attenuation of the substance must be used. Therefore, if a patient has 6C globules and needs to increase the potency to 12C, they cannot use up the 6C globules by taking twice the amount of globules as they could with a conventional pharmaceutical. Single homeopathic drugs are commonly available in 6, 12, 30C or X, and 200C potencies.

Dosing regimens given on the single homeopathic drug packages are general and usually suggest taking the first dose at the onset of symptoms, repeating the dose three to four times per day. A specific dosing interval is not given because it will vary in relation to the severity and

**TABLE 55-12 Repertorization for Case of Otitis Media**

| Homeopathic Drug | Rubric 1 | Rubric 2 | Rubric 3 | Rubric 4 | Rubric 5 | Total |
|---|---|---|---|---|---|---|
| Calcarea carbonica | 3 | | 3 | | | 2/6 |
| Gelsemium | 1 | | | 3 | 3 | 3/7 |
| Lycopodium | 3 | | 2 | 2 | 2 | 4/11 |
| Pulsatilla | 3 | 3 | 3 | 3 | 3 | 5/15 |
| Silica | 3 | 2 | 3 | 2 | | 4/8 |
| Sulphur | 3 | | | | 1 | 3/6 |

*Note:* Numbers correlate with the typeface of each homeopathic drug in each of the five rubrics listed in using the repertory and materia medica. Drugs listed in bold type are given 3 points; italic type, 2 points; and plain type, 1 point. The total score has two parts: the first is the number of rubrics in which each drug appeared, and the second is the sum of the numbers of each drug in all the rubrics in which it is listed.

nature of the condition being treated. Professional homeopathic experts use a wide variety of potencies and dosages even for the same condition. This variability exists in part because a certain condition will require a different potency, depending on its severity and impact on physical, emotional, and mental aspects of the body. A high fever will require a higher potency than a low one; the pounding pain of one person's headache will need a higher potency than someone else's mild headache. Furthermore, different people can have widely different sensitivities to homeopathic drugs. People and children with strong healing energy or vital force can tolerate a higher potency than a frail, overly sensitive, or debilitated person.

The frequency of administration of a specific potency is increased in relation to the severity of the condition being treated. Typically, lower potencies can be given more frequently than higher ones and are generally used to treat physical symptomatology. As the symptoms become less intense, the homeopathic medication is taken less frequently. As long as there is improvement, the patient can keep increasing the interval between doses, taking just enough to keep the momentum going until there is complete cessation of the symptoms. If improvement plateaus or a relapse of the symptoms occurs, the medicine can be taken again or more frequently. Homeopathic drugs should be discontinued as soon as symptoms resolve.

A reaction, called an aggravation, can occur. It is characterized by a temporary intensification of the symptoms being treated. This reaction can happen if homeopathic medicines are taken too frequently or when high potencies (200C or greater) are used; however, in the rare individual who is extremely sensitive, this reaction may occur with lower potencies. Management of an aggravation is discussed in greater detail in the next section. Pharmacies that want to sell high-potency homeopathic medicine should have contact information for at least one certified homeopathic practitioner.

### *Monitoring Patient's Response to Therapy: Common Scenarios*[32]

#### Symptoms Improved After Taking Medicine

This outcome is the desired scenario, of course; however, it is important to teach the patient to stop taking the medicine when improvement sets in and not repeat it until the symptoms start to relapse. The clinician must emphasize to the patient that homeopathic medicines are not administered like antibiotics or blood pressure medications, which must be repeated even after symptoms have resolved. Medicines *must not be repeated* when improvement is underway, because it may overstimulate the patient's system and lead to an aggravation.

#### Patient Became Drowsy After Taking Medicine

Drowsiness is not a side effect of homeopathic medicines. However, any medicine can cause drowsiness *initially* as the body starts to focus its energy on healing. Later doses of the same medicine will not have the same effect. For example, if a child screaming with pain from teething falls asleep immediately after being given a medicine, the child should not be woken up for another dose. The medicine has already begun to act, and the child is likely to be much improved on awakening. This immediate sleepiness should be taken as a very positive and encouraging sign of the medicine's effective action.

#### Symptoms Became Worse Soon After Taking Medicine

This scenario probably either represents homeopathic aggravation or may mean that the medicine failed to halt the natural worsening of the disease condition. A practitioner will consider an aggravation a good sign that the correct remedy has been selected, and that determining the potency and frequency of administration is now the major consideration. The patient should stop taking the medicine and wait for the aggravation to subside, at which point the patient will probably continue to improve until the condition is better than it was before taking the medicine. In a simple acute condition, the patient may even be cured without any further medication. If symptoms recur after the aggravation has subsided, the same drug can be readministered because this is not an allergic reaction; however, the drug should be taken much less frequently. If the patient experienced an aggravation after only a single dose, the same medicine should be taken in a lower potency if symptoms recur. If a reaction escalates to a life-threatening intensity, the patient should seek medical attention, preferably from a practitioner versed in both conventional and homeopathic medicine.

If the patient stops the medicine and continues to get worse after 24 hours, it means something different. In this case, the medicine was incorrect and failed to prevent the condition from progressing. The condition, such as a cold or flu, was going to get worse anyway, and the incorrect medicine did nothing to halt the progress. These two scenarios can easily be differentiated by the patient's reaction on stopping the medicine. As the medicine wears off in the patient's system, any symptoms it caused will tend to disappear, and any symptoms that existed independently of the medicine will continue or even intensify.

#### Medicine Did Not Work

This could mean that the medicine was not correct or was not strong enough. First, whether the medicine was the correct choice is assessed by comparing the patient's symptoms with those of the medicine as described in the materia medica. Was there a close match between the medicine and its symptoms, including several "keynote" (striking and typical) symptoms of the medicine? If it seemed to be the correct medicine, the practitioner should determine whether the patient tried it sufficiently. Was it repeated frequently enough? Was it a relatively low potency (6 or 12), medium (30), or high potency (200)?

If the medicine seemed to be the right choice, the patient can take a higher potency. A low 6 or 12 potency can be replaced with a 30. If the patient took a higher 30 potency frequently, without any improvement, it is likely that the medicine was not the correct choice or the case is complex and a professional homeopath is needed to find the correct medicine.

## Precautions and Interactions Regarding Homeopathic Drugs

### *Drug Interactions*

Homeopathic medicines generally do not interact with pharmaceuticals; one study of homeopathic medications for mild traumatic brain injury showed that concurrent use of conventional medications had no significant influence on outcomes of homeopathic treatment.[33] Direct interaction of homeopathic drugs can be ruled out confidently when potencies of greater than 12C or 24X are used because these potencies contain virtually no molecules of material substance to interact with a pharmaceutical drug. Even if a patient took a whole tube (3.8 g, which equals about 90 size-38 globules) of a 3X potency drug, they would be taking less than 2% of a $10^3$ solution of the material substance in the homeopathic drug. Therefore, a patient who took 20 globules per day would not ingest enough material substance to likely elicit a direct interaction with a pharmaceutical drug.

Even though homeopathic medications taken in therapeutic amounts have not been shown to interact with pharmaceutical drugs, anecdotal evidence indicates that dosage levels of pharmaceuticals may need to be adjusted as the homeopathic medicines become effective. For example, patients being treated for depression or hypothyroidism may require less Prozac or Synthroid, respectively, not because the homeopathic medicine has potentiated the pharmaceutical drug effects but because the underlying condition has improved.

### *Antidoting*

Some older materia medicas list homeopathic drugs that can antidote each other. However, this belief is not considered valid by many practicing homeopaths today and conflicts with widespread use of homeopathic combinations, whose elements are often listed as antidotes to each other. No formal research has been conducted on this matter or on other kinds of antidotes to homeopathic drugs. Certain substances, notably coffee, camphor, and mint, are also believed to inhibit the action of homeopathic drugs although no data support this. Professional homeopaths sometimes advise their patients to avoid coffee, mint-flavored candy or toothpaste, mouthwashes, and camphor-containing products such as Vicks VapoRub Cream, Ben Gay, and Tiger Balm. Many professional homeopaths also recommend that patients avoid other substances and conditions, including aromatherapy oils, electric blankets, microwaves, airport X-ray detectors, dental work, acupuncture, extreme stresses, and smoking lest they antidote the drug. Historically, homeopaths have warned against potential antidotes in chronic prescribing, in which a single dose is intended to last for weeks or months; however, modern patients who ignore the precautions often find their remedies still work. Antidoting is less of a concern in acute prescribing, in which the drug is repeated several times per day.

In any case, most homeopaths agree that research studies are needed to determine the true incidence of antidoting for any given substance or condition. This research will be difficult to conduct because the phenomenon does not appear to be something all patients experience, and only very sensitive individuals may be susceptible to the antidoting effects of certain drugs and/or conditions. Until more is learned about this phenomenon, the patient will ultimately have to determine if any drugs or situations disrupt their homeopathic drug therapy. Common sense would dictate that, if the patient finds something antidotes his or her homeopathic medication, it should be avoided throughout the course of therapy.

### *Precautions and Side Effects*

The claim is often made that homeopathic drugs do not cause side effects. Yet, as discussed previously in Homeopathic Therapeutics, people do have reactions to homeopathic medications for various reasons. In contrast to conventional medications, however, side effects from homeopathic drugs are not generally life threatening and are associated with various aspects of the healing process.

As discussed previously in greater detail, an aggravation is a temporary, sometimes intense worsening of the symptoms being treated, which can occur when the homeopathic drug has been taken too frequently or in too high a potency. The reaction usually resolves in a short period of time and is typically followed by a complete resolution of the original problem. The homeopathic medication should not be repeated as long as the original condition continues to improve after an aggravation. Patients who suffer from a severe, long-lasting aggravation are best referred to a certified homeopathic practitioner or CM practitioner, depending on the nature of the reaction.

Another reaction discussed previously involves a discharge or skin eruption that occurs when a homeopathic drug acts according to Hering's law, moving an interior condition to the surface or exterior of the body. This reaction occurs as the condition being treated improves. Patients who experience this reaction generally have an overall sense of well-being and can tolerate it well once they know that the reaction is part of the normal healing process. When a reaction of this kind is severe or long lasting, the patient should be directed to consult a certified homeopathic or CM practitioner, as with aggravations.

A true allergic reaction to a homeopathic agent is unlikely, especially when potencies of greater than 24X or 12C have been used. However, very sensitive individuals could conceivably react to low-potency drugs (less than 6C), even when these homeopathic agents do not contain enough substance to provoke a true pharmacologic drug reaction.

A nonprescription homeopathic medicine is labeled with a warning that pregnant or nursing mothers should seek the advice of a health professional before using the product. This is a standard warning label, and no research has indicated potential harm in these circumstances. Holistic midwives and naturopathic physicians specializing in obstetrics commonly use homeopathic drugs in their practices and would be the best source of advice.

## Research in Homeopathy

Much of the research on homeopathy has been conducted overseas and published in journals that are difficult for American clinicians to access or translate. The clinician should keep in mind that homeopathic drugs have undergone proving trials that are conducted as randomized, placebo-controlled studies (Table 55-3) and that a homeopathic drug is not included in *HPUS* unless verification trials and other published documentation (Table 55-5) have been reviewed. Designing scientific studies that maintain the integrity of homeopathy's fundamental laws and principles can be challenging, especially in regard to individualizing drug therapy and the variety of dosing regimens used. However, good studies can overcome these challenges, as has been reported in two meta-analyses.

Since the first meta-analysis, published by Kleijnen and coworkers in 1991, at least six more have been published. Two meta-analyses span results of homeopathic placebo-controlled trials conducted before 1997 up to December of 2002.[34] The analysis conducted by Linde and coworkers (*Lancet* 1997) found that homeopathic clinical effects were not attributable solely to placebo but efficacy could not be clearly established for any single medical condition. Mathie's meta-analysis of clinical trials, published from 1975 to 2002, concluded that the weight of evidence favors homeopathic treatment effectiveness in eight conditions: childhood diarrhea, fibromyalgia, hay fever/allergic rhinitis, influenza, pain (of various origins), side effects of radio-/chemotherapy, sprains, and upper respiratory tract infection. No effect above that of placebo was apparent in three medical conditions: headache, stroke, and warts.

One of the challenges involved with individualizing drug therapy is that 10 patients with the same chief complaint will likely receive 10 different drugs from a homeopath, on the basis of the etiology and specific symptoms, as well as aspects of the patient's temperament. Therefore, an RCT, which tests a single homeopathic drug for a particular diagnostic category, is likely to fail because that drug will match the symptoms of only a small percentage of patients. Homeopaths have devised two approaches to surmount this obstacle. One approach is to test the homeopathic process itself by giving patients a drug agreed on by two professional homeopaths, rather than a predetermined trial drug. The second approach involves performing the study on a diagnostic category for which a single homeopathic drug is likely to be effective, as was the case for a study of Rhus toxicodendron for fibromyalgia. Patients were accepted for the trial only if their symptoms matched the remedy; the result showed homeopathy to be twice as effective as placebo.[35]

In addition, the homeopathic drug must be administered in a potency and dosage schedule likely to be effective for that condition. The correct drug may have no apparent action if the potency is too low or given too late to be effective. A study of Arnica for postoperative pain and swelling, for example, may have failed to show effectiveness because the first dose was not given until the day after the operation, whereas the recommended schedule is to give the first dose *before* the operation and the second dose immediately afterward.[36] Crossover trials are also problematic because the action of a drug may last for weeks, months, or even years, depending on the potency used and the patient's sensitivity. Thus, a drug given in the first phase may still be acting in the second phase, even with a month-long washout period.

Some early trials of homeopathy attempted to allow for individualization by randomizing patients either to placebo or to a professional homeopath, who prescribed an individualized drug after a lengthy interview. These trials failed to account for the placebo effect of the individual attention given in the interview.[37] Homeopaths have learned from these critiques, and subsequent studies have randomized patients after the homeopathic interview process. An example is the first National Institutes of Health–funded study of homeopathy on mild traumatic brain injury, in which a homeopathic physician prescribed a drug for each patient after a full homeopathic interview. A study nurse who had no other access to the patients gave them the chosen homeopathic drug or placebo, on the basis of randomization provided by a statistician with no other access to the patients. The code designating who received the active drug and who received the placebo was kept in a locked safe on the manufacturer's premises until after the results were compiled.[33]

Critiques of homeopathic research have led to refining it in other ways. The first study demonstrating the effectiveness of homeopathy for diarrhea to be published in an American peer-reviewed journal was criticized on the basis that the drugs could have been contaminated with antibiotics. This possibility would never occur to a homeopath or anyone who had handled a homeopathic drug because the drug pellets are so small that it would be impossible to mix in an effective dose of a pharmaceutical. Nevertheless, subsequent studies are providing for independent laboratory testing of the drug pellets to guarantee against contamination.

Perhaps the most frequent criticism leveled against studies of homeopathy, including many which would otherwise demonstrate its effectiveness, is the small size of the sample. Another is the lack of replication of positive studies. Large studies and replication depend on research funds, to which homeopaths historically have had limited access. Pharmaceutical companies are able to invest hundreds of millions of dollars in research, whereas homeopathic manufacturers cannot afford to fund research because almost all the drugs are nonpatentable. One manufacturer has been successful in researching its combination homeopathic products by conducting research abroad. Heel, Inc, has conducted an RCT including 119 patients at 15 study centers in Germany, where homeopathy is more widely practiced than in the United States.[38] The study showed that the homeopathic medication Vertigoheel is therapeutically equivalent to betahistine hydrochloride.

### RCTs and Outcome Studies of Homeopathic Medicine

Allergic rhinitis and childhood diarrhea have been investigated by repeated RCTs. A randomized placebo-controlled study conducted in 2000 reproduced the results of four previous studies testing the effects of homeopathically prepared allergens (30C) in patients with allergic rhinitis or asthma.[39] Similar to the previous three studies, improvement was significant. The homeopathic group of patients with perennial allergic rhinitis tested in this study had improved nasal airflow compared with the placebo group ($p = .0001$), and patients reported more improvement in symptoms in four of five practice settings. Lewith and others[40] have challenged this work by conducting an RCT similar to the third study reported in the preceding series involving 28 patients with allergic asthma. Their study involved 242 asthmatic patients, who received homeopathically prepared house dust or placebo. The authors found homeopathic treatment no better than placebo, but also found some differences between the homeopathic treatment and placebo they could not explain. This study elicited numerous letters to the editor of the *British Medical Journal* from supporters of homeopathy; the interested reader can find them in the July 6, 2002, issue of the journal.

Childhood diarrhea has been studied in a series of three high-quality double-blind, placebo-controlled studies by Jacobs and coworkers.[41] The meta-analysis showed that homeopathic treatment reduced the duration of diarrhea from 4.1 days to 3.3 ($p = .008$), and the authors recommended it as an adjunct to oral rehydration for this leading cause of child mortality worldwide.

Outcome research provides perhaps the most realistic evidence of homeopathy's effectiveness, reflecting the results of homeopathy used in everyday practice by experienced homeopaths. A pilot study was conducted in two homeopathic practices reporting the response of 24 children with acute otitis media to individualized homeopathic therapy.[5] Only two children required antibiotic therapy, giving homeopathy a 92% success rate. A Belgian observational study of 782 homeopathic patients with diseases of all major organ systems reported high patient satisfaction and improved physical conditions with significantly lowered health care costs; prescription costs (including both homeopathic and conventional medicines) averaged only one third that of the general practice.[42] Homeopathic treatment was also effective in reducing both physical and emotional symptoms of estrogen withdrawal in a Scottish observational study of 40 women with breast cancer.[43]

Preliminary results from a multicenter, multinational study in Europe compared 281 patients treated homeopathically with 175 treated conventionally within three common diagnostic categories (upper and lower respiratory tract and ear complaints).[44] The response to treatment, measured by primary outcome criteria, for patients receiving homeopathy was 82.6%. Patients using CM had a 56.6% response rate. The incidence of adverse events for those treated with CM was 22.3% versus 7.8% for homeopathic medicine. Seventy-nine percent of patients treated with homeopathy were very satisfied versus 65.1% of patients who received CM.

The clinician who is interested in exploring RCT and outcome studies of homeopathy can refer to publications by Gray[45] as well as to the National Center for Homeopathy Web site at www.homeopathic.org and the National Center for Complementary and Alternative Medicine Web site at nccam.nih.gov/health/homeopathy/index.htm.

### Research on a Possible Mechanism of Action

Perhaps the most controversial research demonstrating the effects of homeopathy has been the multicenter study under the guidance of Jacques Benveniste, conducted in collaboration with four other laboratories, showing that doses of immunoglobulin E diluted far beyond Avogadro's number (i.e., more dilute than a 12C homeopathic remedy) could promote basophil degranulation. This work caused an international storm of controversy when it was published in *Nature* in 1988. While his work was initially refuted, subsequent studies by independent researchers have replicated the work of Benveniste's group. The most recent work in this area was conducted by Belon and others.[46] These researchers reported findings similar to those of a series of studies showing that the activation of human basophils by immunoglobulin E is strongly and significantly inhibited by dilutions of histamine beyond Avogadro's number.

The notion that homeopathy cannot possibly work because the drugs do not contain even one molecule of the active ingredient is based on a mechanistic, Newtonian view of the universe in which matter is ultimately reducible to submicroscopic bits of matter in the form of atoms. Ever since Einstein, scientists have viewed matter as also being represented by different patterns of energy. The leading research on homeopathy's mechanism of action has focused on water's capacity to record patterns of energy shifts, demonstrated by the formation of different possible configurations of water molecules expressed as icelike crystalline structures within liquid water. Various investigators have called these icelike crystalline structures clathrates[47] or $I_E$ crystals[48] (ice in an electrical field).

These researchers believe that each original drug substance, when diluted and successed in water, stimulates the formation of a unique crystalline structure, much as snowflakes represent "biochemically identical, but biophysically different forms" of water, as David Reilly expressed it in Kayne's *Homeopathic Pharmacy*.[37] As more kinetic energy is added to the system by further succussions, more water molecules are attracted into the pattern, and more information is thus stored in the water. Anagnostatos and coworkers[47] used depolarization thermocurrent and differential scanning calorimetry measurements, whereas Lo and Bonavida[48] used transmission electron micrography, fluorescence spectrophotometry, and ultraviolet spectroscopy to detect evidence of the crystalline structures identified. Changes in potentized drug water have also been measured by nuclear magnetic resonance imaging.[49]

The interested reader can find more detailed information on research discussed in this section and other models being investigated to explain a mechanism of action for homeopathic drugs in publications by Bellavite and Signorini[50] and Gray.[44]

## Assessment of Use of Homeopathic Medicines: A Case-based Approach

Cases 55-1 and 55-2 illustrate the approach to determining whether use of preformulated homeopathic products without medical supervision is appropriate or referral to a homeopathic practitioner for case taking is required.

### CASE 55-1

| Relevant Evaluation Criteria | Scenario/Model Outcome |
|---|---|
| **Information Gathering** | |
| 1. Gather essential information about the patient's symptoms, including: | |
| a. description of symptom(s) (i.e., nature, onset, duration, severity, associated symptoms) | Patient is suffering a fulminate case of poison ivy on both arms, with trails of vesicles, great pain, and intolerable itching. Associated symptoms include extreme restlessness, agitation, and insomnia. |
| b. description of any factors that seem to precipitate, exacerbate, and/or relieve the patient's symptoms. | Symptoms appeared soon after the patient was weeding her yard with her bare hands and were presumably caused by exposure to poison ivy. Itching is temporarily relieved by hot water. |
| c. description of the patient's efforts to relieve the symptoms | Frequent applications of calamine have failed to relieve the itching substantially. |
| 2. Gather essential patient history information: | |
| a. patient's identity | Frances |
| b. age, sex, height, and weight | 72 y/o F |
| c. patient's occupation | Retired |
| d. patient's dietary habits | N/A |
| e. patient's sleep habits | N/A |
| f. concurrent medical conditions, prescription and nonprescription medications, and dietary supplements | Trazodone 50 mg as needed at bedtime for sleep; ketoconazole 200 mg once daily for tinea pedis; multivitamin for seniors, and calcium carbonate 1000 mg once daily |
| g. allergies | |
| h. history of other adverse reactions to medications | Dry mouth the mornings after taking trazodone for sleep |
| i. other (describe)_______ | |

## CASE 55-1 (continued)

| Relevant Evaluation Criteria | Scenario/Model Outcome |
|---|---|
| **Assessment and Triage** | |
| 3. Differentiate the patient's signs/symptoms and correctly identify the patient's primary problem(s). | Frances is suffering from a severe outbreak of poison ivy after known exposure while gardening, confirmed by a linear pattern of extremely itchy vesicular eruptions consistent with poison ivy. |
| 4. Identify exclusions for self-treatment. | If patient is immunocompromised because of concerns about secondary infection, if rash is extensive covering a large area of the body or disseminated (later onset of symptoms), or if patient does not respond to self-care treatment within 2 to 3 days, patient may need referral to a dermatologist. |
| 5. Formulate a comprehensive list of therapeutic alternatives for the primary problem to determine if triage to a medical practitioner is required, and share this information with the patient. | Options include:<br>(1) Refer Frances to a professional homeopath for an individualized drug therapy (see box Patient Education for Homeopathic Medicines to differentiate between options 2 and 3; see box Patient Education for Allergic Contact Dermatitis in Chapter 35 for option 4<br>(2) Recommend a homeopathic combination drug for poison ivy.<br>(3) Recommend a single homeopathic drug.<br>(4) Suggest that Frances relieve her itching with topical products such as oatmeal baths, aloe vera, Calendula cream, or hydrocortisone cream 1%; or oral diphenhydramine.<br>(5) Refer Frances to a dermatologist if self-treatment is unsuccessful.<br>(6) Take no action. |
| **Plan** | |
| 6. Select an optimal therapeutic alternative to address the patient's problem, taking into account patient preferences. | The single homeopathic drug Rhus tox 30C (pellet or tablet) will be appropriate for Frances' condition. Frances can use oatmeal baths and topical aloe vera or Calendula cream as adjunctive therapy. Frances has expressed a strong preference for natural methods whenever possible. |
| 7. Describe the recommended therapeutic approach to the patient. | Take Rhus tox 30C hourly until symptoms begin to abate, then up to 3 times/day until lesions are almost gone, at which point it can be taken once a day until they are cleared completely. |
| 8. Explain to the patient the rationale for selecting the recommended therapeutic approach from the considered therapeutic alternatives. | Seeking a dermatologist or professional homeopath is unnecessary because a simple homeopathic drug will address your symptoms. A single homeopathic drug rather than a combination product is appropriate in this case because the former is likely to provide better results, and your symptoms clearly indicate a well-known single drug, easily available in most health food stores and many pharmacies. An hourly dosage is more appropriate than the 3 times/day dosage schedule on the product label because of the severity and sudden onset of your symptoms. Antihistamine OTC products to treat itching can interact with your other medications so they cannot be recommended. It is not advisable to use hydrocortisone cream as it could possibly block or suppress positive effects of the homeopathic medication. Herbal products for topical relief are more compatible with homeopathic medications, and Calendula cream is usually made homeopathically. |
| **Patient Education** | |
| 9. When recommending self-care with nonprescription medications and/or nondrug therapy, convey accurate information to the patient, including: | |
| a. appropriate dose and frequency of administration | Take Rhus tox 30C hourly (waking hours only) until symptoms begin to abate, then stop until the following day. Take it 3 times/day thereafter until symptoms are almost completely cleared, then once a day to complete the healing. It is not necessary to wake up during the night to take the drug. |

## CASE 55-1 (continued)

| Relevant Evaluation Criteria | Scenario/Model Outcome |
|---|---|
| b. maximum number of days the therapy should be employed | It is safe to take the drug as long as necessary to complete the healing process. If there is no relief after 1 day of hourly doses, the drug should be discontinued the following day. If there is still no relief, another homeopathic drug or therapeutic option should be sought. |
| c. product administration procedures | Dissolve 3-5 pellets in the mouth. |
| d. expected time to onset of relief | Partial relief may occur immediately after the first dose and should occur within 24 hours. |
| e. degree of relief that can be reasonably expected | Complete relief is to be expected. |
| f. most common side effects | A transient intensification of symptoms is highly unlikely but possible in individuals who are extremely sensitive to medications in general. |
| g. side effects that warrant medical intervention should they occur | The drug will not have side effects that would require medical intervention. See Precautions and Interactions Regarding Homeopathic Drugs. |
| h. patient options in the event that condition worsens or persists | If the condition worsens and discontinuing the drug fails to provide relief, or if it persists and the drug fails to provide any relief in 2 days, you should see a homeopathic practitioner if you want to continue being treated with homeopathic drugs. |
| i. product storage requirements | Keep in a tightly closed container away from direct sunlight, children, pets, and heat over 100°F (37.8°C). |
| j. specific nondrug measures | Identify poison ivy in garden and destroy plants. |
| 10. Solicit follow-up questions from patient. | (1) May I double the dose to get better more quickly?<br>(2) Would it be better to take the drug 3 times/day from the beginning since that is what the label recommends?<br>(3) If the symptoms start to go away, can I keep taking the drug every hour to help it get better faster? |
| 11. Answer patient's questions. | (1) Doubling the number of pellets/tablets does not double the rate of healing. Doubling the frequency will speed healing and is safe to do if you experience partial relief that subsequently relapses.<br>(2) No. The dosage schedule on the label is just a suggestion and does not take into account the individual situation. When the symptoms are very severe, intense, and sudden, the drug needs to be taken more often than the label's stated dosage.<br>(3) No. This will risk inducing a temporary worsening of your symptoms and could slow down the healing process because you will then have to discontinue the drug temporarily. |

Key: OTC, over-the-counter; N/A, not applicable.

## CASE 55-2

| Relevant Evaluation Criteria | Scenario/Model Outcome |
|---|---|
| **Information Gathering** | |
| 1. Gather essential information about the patient's symptoms, including: | |
| a. description of symptom(s) (i.e., nature, onset, duration, severity, associated symptoms) | Patient has symptoms characteristic of a beginning sinus infection that has been recurring over the past 2 years: an itchy nose and scratchy throat, postnasal drip, building pressure and pain at the root of the nose and above and below the eyes, and moderate pressure in her head. Nasal discharge has a green to yellow tint. She also has some nasal congestion developing that is starting to make it difficult for her to breathe through the nose. Patient looks stressed and run down and started to run a low-grade temperature of 99.8°F (37.9°C) today. |

## CASE 55-2 (continued)

| Relevant Evaluation Criteria | Scenario/Model Outcome |
|---|---|
| b. description of any factors that seem to precipitate, exacerbate, and/or relieve the patient's symptoms. | Symptoms typically recurred within 60 days of completing a course of antibiotics for the previous sinus infections. Patient tends to get an infection after studying long hours for midterm and finals or after working a lot of overtime hours. Condition improves faster when she can take off 2-3 days from work to rest and recover, and regains tight control of her diabetes. |
| c. description of the patient's efforts to relieve the symptoms | Patient has consulted an ENT specialist, who has ruled out structural abnormalities and allergies and recommended antibiotic treatment. Patient has had 9 rounds of antibiotics in 2 years without permanent relief. Patient has tried NSAID OTC analgesics but they upset her stomach. Pseudoephedrine and acetaminophen provide some relief. |
| 2. Gather essential patient history information: | |
| a. patient's identity | Debra |
| b. age, sex, height, and weight | 27 y/o F, 5'4", 100 lb |
| c. patient's occupation | Full-time administrative assistant and part-time law school student |
| d. patient's dietary habits | Lately, eats mostly "fast food" or frozen prepared meals because of her work and school commitments |
| e. patient's sleep habits | Sleeps okay when not experiencing bad sinus infections; gets an average of 4 hours sleep a day |
| f. concurrent medical conditions, prescription and nonprescription medications, and dietary supplements | Debra has been an insulin-dependent diabetic (Type 1) since 7 y/o and admits being lax in measuring her blood glucose over the last couple of weeks. Medications include insulin 14 U Regular/30 U NPH sq before breakfast and 10 U Regular/ 12 U NPH sq before dinner, multivitamin; pseudoephedrine 30 mg 3 times/day or 4 times/day to help relieve pressure in the sinus cavities; acetaminophen 600 mg occasionally for sinus pain. |
| g. allergies | No known allergies to drugs, foods, or animals |
| h. history of other adverse reactions to medications | Pseudoephedrine causes jitters and insomnia. |
| i. other (describe)_______ | Patient does not want to keep taking antibiotics and was told by her classmate that homeopathy may provide longer-lasting effects. |
| **Assessment and Triage** | |
| 3. Differentiate the patient's signs/symptoms and correctly identify the patient's primary problem(s). | Patient's primary problem is the development of another sinus infection. The patient's diabetes is most likely not well controlled. |
| 4. Identify exclusions for self-treatment. | Uncontrolled diabetes with acute sinus infection |
| 5. Formulate a comprehensive list of therapeutic alternatives for the primary problem to determine if triage to a medical practitioner is required, and share this information with the patient. | Options include:<br>(1) Refer Debra to her endocrinologist and ENT specialist.<br>(2) Refer Debra to a homeopathic practitioner (see Table 55-4) trained as a medical doctor for individualized homeopathic therapy and control of her diabetes.<br>(3) Recommend a combination homeopathic product that is specifically indicated for sinus disorders for initial relief, along with rigorous management of her blood glucose and diet.<br>(4) Recommend a single individualized homeopathic medicine along with rigorous management of her blood glucose and diet. |
| **Plan** | |
| 6. Select an optimal therapeutic alternative to address the patient's problem, taking into account patient preferences. | Even though Debra desires treatment with homeopathy for relief of her sinus symptoms, she is at risk for developing a serious infection because of her apparent poorly managed diabetes. |
| 7. Describe the recommended therapeutic approach to the patient. | N/A |

**CASE 55-2 (continued)**

| Relevant Evaluation Criteria | Scenario/Model Outcome |
|---|---|
| 8. Explain to the patient the rationale for selecting the recommended therapeutic approach from the considered therapeutic alternatives. | Seeing her endocrinologist and/or ENT specialist is necessary because sinus infections can lead to serious problems, especially in poorly controlled diabetics. Homeopathy can be helpful in treating sinus problems, but it is not effective in treating Type 1 diabetes. |
| **Patient Education** | |
| 9. When recommending self-care with nonprescription medications and/or nondrug therapy, convey accurate information to the patient. | Criterion does not apply in this case. |
| 10. Solicit follow-up questions from patient. | Is homeopathy an option for my sinus infections if my diabetes is controlled? |
| 11. Answer patient's questions. | It may be possible to treat a sinus infection using homeopathy, but that should be attempted only by a homeopathic practitioner or naturopath (see Table 55-4) trained as a medical doctor, who can determine the correct individualized homeopathic therapy and maintain careful control of your diabetes. |

Key: ENT, ear, nose, and throat; NSAID, nonsteroidal anti-inflammatory drug; OTC, over-the-counter; NPH, neutral protamine Hagedorn; N/A, not applicable.

## Patient Counseling for Homeopathic Medicines

The role of the pharmacist will vary depending on whether the patient is filling a prescription from a professional practitioner, in which case the pharmacist should encourage the patient to follow the practitioner's individual instructions for use, or looking for an acute nonprescription drug for self-treatment. In the latter case, some patients will be well-educated and experienced, whereas many others will be new to homeopathy, requiring the type of information listed in Table 55-1. For the best results, patients new to homeopathy should be steered toward a combination product, a first-aid medicine (i.e., one that is universally useful and does not require individualization), or a book on acute prescribing that will help narrow the choice of single drugs (Table 55-1).

Homeopathic drugs come in many forms and are used in many ways, making it difficult to construct general counseling guidelines that cover all the aspects in this chapter. Because the alleged antidoting effects of many aromatic substances, microwaves, X-rays, and so forth have not been scientifically proven, only the antidoting substances commonly reported in homeopathic journals (e.g., strong perfume, coffee, camphor, mothballs) are used in the patient education information found in the box Patient Education for Homeopathic Medicines. In any case, nonprescription products for acute conditions are taken several times per day, so most homeopaths are not concerned with possible antidotes in these conditions.

## Key Points for Homeopathic Medicines

- Homeopathy is a system of medicine used and accepted widely around the world.
- Homeopathic medicines, commonly known as remedies, are extremely safe to use, rarely causing reactions such as side effects or adverse reactions.
- Homeopathic medicines can be used to treat a wide variety of acute and chronic illnesses.
- Homeopathic remedies for nonprescription use can be self-prescribed safely by the patient using self-care guidelines recommended in this chapter.
- Chronic illnesses can be treated with homeopathy only under the care of a professional homeopath, who may also be a conventional health care practitioner (MD, DO, NP, etc.).
- Research on homeopathy has been conducted primarily in Europe and has shown homeopathy to be more effective than placebo in meta-analyses.
- Homeopathy's mechanism of action is still not understood although recent research in nanopharmacology and ultra-high dilutions is beginning to shed light on it.
- Patient education includes instructing the patient to repeat the remedy until the healing process is underway, then to refrain from further dosing to avoid an aggravation (temporary worsening of symptoms).

## References

1. National Center for Complementary and Alternative Medicine. Major domains of complementary and alternative medicine. Available at: http://nccam.nih.gov/health/backgrounds/wholemed.htm. Accessed February 22, 2005.
2. Boiron T. Economic perspective on homeopathic pharmacy. Paper presented at: American Institute of Homeopathy, Homeopathy 2000 Rededication and Celebration; June 21, 2000; Washington, DC.

## PATIENT EDUCATION FOR HOMEOPATHIC MEDICINES

### Choosing a Homeopathic Drug

- Combination homeopathic products can be taken for indicated self-limiting conditions when it is not possible to self-assess the condition for individualized therapy with a single-remedy product.
- For single-remedy products, depending on experience and knowledge, a reference book, a clinician trained in homeopathy, or a professional homeopath should be consulted before taking a remedy. A person with little knowledge should consult a homeopath.
- Single-remedy homeopathic product labels have room to list only one or two indications or conditions. For any one condition, more than one possible homeopathic drug may be indicated depending on the individual's specific symptoms. Having a condition listed on its label does not mean a product is the correct one for every person. By the same token, a drug may be correct for a condition that is not listed on the label.
- Taking the wrong homeopathic drug will not cause any harmful effects (unless the patient is extremely hypersensitive; see Assessing Sensitivity), but it will not help the patient and will keep the patient from benefiting from the correct drug.

### Choosing a Potency

- Potencies up to 30C are safe and effective for almost everyone for most acute (i.e., sudden-onset, self-limiting) conditions.
- Combination products have set potencies for the condition they are formulated to treat and should be taken as directed on the product package.
- If the condition has been occurring for more than a few months, it is better to seek professional homeopathic care rather than to self-treat. If it began recently, talk to a pharmacist or health care practitioner about whether it is safe to self-treat when in doubt.
- If the acute condition has strong symptoms (severe pain, high fever, etc.), the higher 30C potency should be used for better results (unless patient is extremely sensitive; see below). For mild conditions and hypersensitive people, 12C is more appropriate.

### Assessing Sensitivity

- Hypersensitive people should use homeopathic drugs with caution until they are familiar with homeopathic remedies and know how they are likely to react. Sensitive persons typically have environmental allergies, multiple chemical sensitivities, or many food allergies, react to fumes and chemicals, and tend to get side effects from usual doses of conventional medication.
- Sensitive individuals should use the lowest potency available at first (6C, if possible; otherwise, 12C) and put a single pellet in their mouth, waiting to observe the effects before taking any more. If an undesirable reaction occurs, some people have reported being able to halt it with caffeinated coffee or strong mint- or camphor-containing substances.

### Taking the Homeopathic Drug

- Follow the dosing recommendation found on the drug's package. These guidelines should not be exceeded without consulting a health care practitioner who specializes in homeopathy.
- Take globular dosage forms under the tongue or allow them to completely dissolve in the mouth. Place them directly into the mouth without touching them. Keep the medicine in the original container and avoid exposing the globules to strong smells, such as coffee, mothballs, camphor, and perfumes.
- Take homeopathic drugs before or after eating, not with food. For best results, make sure the mouth is clean and free of residual smoke, food, toothpaste, or mouthwash. Some homeopaths advise avoiding mint, camphor, and coffee throughout the duration of treatment; anecdotal evidence but no research substantiates these precautions.
- Avoid touching the pellets with your fingers. The pellets should be poured into the remedy cap and placed directly under the tongue without being touched. No research substantiates this precaution, but it is best to avoid introducing possible contamination.
- Do not stop taking conventional prescription drugs unless the prescriber has authorized it.
- Discuss discontinuing or decreasing dosages of prescription medications with the prescriber. The need to continue an OTC product can be discussed with a pharmacist or health care practitioner.
- Reactions to homeopathic drugs may be intense but are typically of short duration. Because they are managed differently from conventional pharmaceutical drugs, it is best to consult a health care provider who is trained in homeopathy or the manufacturer of the product for the best treatment approach. In the rare event of a severe, life-threatening reaction, seek medical attention.
- Store the homeopathic drug out of direct sunlight, away from extreme temperatures and strong odors, and out of the reach of children.


3. Barnes PM, Powell-Griner E, McFann K, et al. Complementary and Alternative Medicine Use Among Adults: United States, 2002. *Advance Data.* 2004;343:1-19.
4. Barnett ED, Levatin JL, Chapman EH, et al. Challenges of evaluating homeopathic treatment of acute otitis media. *Pediatr Infect Dis J.* 2000;19:273-5.
5. Viksveen P. Antibiotics and the development of resistant microorganisms. Can homeopathy be an alternative? *Homeopathy.* 2003; 92:99-107.
6. Sayer-Flusche A, Gupchup GV, Dole EF. Homeopathy: attitudes and opinions of members of the American Pharmaceutical Association. *J Am Pharm Assoc (Wash).* 2000;40:259-61.
7. Leckridge B. *Homeopathy in Primary Care.* New York: Churchill Livingstone; 1997.
8. Jonas, WB, Linde K, Ramirez G. Homeopathy and rheumatic disease. *Rheum Dis Clin North Am.* 2000;26: 117-23.
9. Jonas WB, Jacobs J. *Healing with Homeopathy: The Doctors' Guide.* New York: Warner Books; 1996:43.
10. Brinkhaus B, Schindler G, Lindner M, et al. Socioeconomic aspects of homeopathy as seen by decision-takers and service providers in the public health system. In: Ernst E, Hahn EG, eds. *Homeopathy: A Critical Appraisal.* Oxford, England: Butterworth Heinemann; 1998:221.
11. Homeopathy Council for Classical Homeopathy. The Recognition and Regulation of the Practice of Homeopathy in Europe: An ECCH Report. August 2003. Available at: http://www.homeopathy-ecch.org/images/stores/pdf/recognition%20&520regulation. Accessed February 22, 2005.

12. Grossinger R. *Homeopathy: The Great Riddle.* Berkeley, Calif: North Atlantic Books; 1998:11-46.
13. Lewith G. The homeopathic conundrum revisited. *Alternative Therapies.* 1999;5:32.
14. Yasgur J. *Yasgur's Homeopathic Dictionary and Holistic Health Reference.* 4th ed. Greenville, Pa: Van Hoy Publishers; 1998.
15. O'Reilly WB, ed. *Organon of the Medical Art.* Hahnemann S, trans, ed. Redmond, Wash: Birdcage Books; 1996.
16. Vithoulkas G. *The Science of Homeopathy.* New York: Grove Weidenfeld; 1980.
17. Cook T. *Samuel Hahnemann: His Life and Times.* Staines, Middlesex, England: Homeopathic Studies Ltd; 1993.
18. Kent JT. *Lectures on Homeopathic Materia Medica.* New Delhi: B. Jain Publishers, Ltd; 1996 [reprint].
19. Sankaran R. *The Soul of Remedies.* Bombay: Homeopathic Medical Publishers; 1997.
20. *Homeopathic Pharmacopoeia of the United States.* Southeastern, Pa: Homeopathic Pharmacopoeia Convention of the United States; 2004.
21. Swayne J. Homeopathic Method: Implications for Clinical Practice and Medical Sciences. New York: Churchill Livingstone; 1998:20-2.
22. Cummings S, Ullman D. *Everybody's Guide to Homeopathic Medicines.* 3rd ed. New York: G.P. Putnam's Sons; 1997.
23. Council on Homeopathic Education Summit Meeting. Standards and competencies for the professional practice of homeopathy in North America. Available at: http://www.chedu.org/standards.htm. Accessed February 22, 2005.
24. Borneman JA III, Borneman JP. *Practical Homeopathic Pharmacy.* National Center for Homeopathy Summer Homeopathy Courses, John Hopkins University; June 25, 2001; Baltimore, Md.
25. FDA/ORA CPG 7132.15. Sec. 400.400. Conditions under which homeopathic drugs may be marketed (CPG 7132.15). Available at: http://www.fda.gov/ora/compliance_ref/cpg/cpgdrg/cpg400-400.html. Accessed February 22, 2005.
26. Skinner SE. *An Introduction to Homeopathic Medicine in Primary Care.* Gaithersburg, Md: Aspen Publishers, Inc; 2001.
27. Cavalcanti AMS, Rocha LM, Carillo R, et al. Effects of homeopathic treatment on pruritus of haemodialysis patients: a randomized placebo-controlled double-blind trial. *Homeopathy.* 2003;92:177-81.
28. Morrison R. *Desktop Guide to Keynotes and Confirmatory Symptoms.* Albany, Calif: Hahnemann Clinic Publishing; 1993.
29. Boericke W. *Pocket Manual of Homeopathic Materia Medica and Repertory and a Chapter on Rare and Uncommon Remedies.* New Delhi: B. Jain Publishers, Ltd; 1995 [reprint].
30. Radar Software & Encyclopedia Homeopathica. Available at: http://www.wholehealthnow.com. Accessed February 22, 2005.
31. MacRepertory and Reference Works. Available at: http://www.kenthomeopathic.com. Accessed February 22, 2005.
32. De Schepper L. *Hahnemann Revisited.* Santa Fe, NM: Full of Life Publishing, 1999.
33. Chapman EH, Weintraub RJ, Milburn MA, et al. Homeopathic treatment of mild traumatic brain injury: a randomized, double-blind, placebo-controlled clinical trial. *J Head Trauma Rehabil.* 1999;14:521-42.
34. Mathie R. The research evidence base for homeopathy: a fresh assessment of the literature. *Homeopathy.* 2003;92:84-91.
35. Fisher P, Greenwood A, Huskisson EC, et al. Effect of homeopathic treatment on fibrositis. *BMJ.* 1989;299:365-6.
36. Sebastian I. *Efficacy of Homeopathic Arnica on Ecchymosis and Pain after Liposuction.* Paper presented at: American Institute of Homeopathy Conference; June 21-24, 2000; Washington, DC.
37. Kayne S. *Homeopathic Pharmacy: An Introduction and Handbook.* Edinburgh: Churchill Livingstone; 1997.
38. Weiser M, Strõsser W, Klein P. Homeopathic vs conventional treatment of vertigo: a randomized double-blind controlled clinical study. *Arch Otolaryngol Head Neck Surg.* 1998;124:879-85.
39. Taylor MA, Reilly DT, Llewellyn-Jones RH, et al. Randomized controlled trial of homoeopathy versus placebo in perennial allergic rhinitis with overview of four trial series. *BMJ.* 2000;321:471-6.
40. Lewith GT, Watkins AD, Hyland ME, et al. Use of ultramolecular potencies of allergen to treat asthmatic people allergic to house dust mite: double blind randomized controlled clinical trial. *BMJ.* 2002;324: 520-4.
41. Jacobs J, Jonas WB, Jiménez-Perez M, et al. Homeopathy for childhood diarrhea: combined results and metaanalysis from three randomized, controlled clinical trials. *Pediatr Infect Dis J.* 2003;22(3):229-34.
42. Van Wassenhoven M, Ives G. An observational study of patients receiving homeopathic treatment. *Homeopathy.* 2004;93:3-11.
43. Thompson EA, Reilly D. The homeopathic approach to the treatment of symptoms of oestrogen withdrawal in breast cancer patients. A prospective observational study. *Homeopathy.* 2003;92:131-4.
44. Riley D, Fischer M, Singh B, et al. Homeopathy and conventional medicine: an outcomes study comparing effectiveness in a primary care setting. *J Altern Complement Med.* 2001;7:149-59.
45. Gray B. *Homeopathy: Science or Myth?* Berkeley, Calif: North Atlantic Books; 2000.
46. Belon P, Cumps J, Ennis M, et al. Histamine dilutions modulate basophil activity. *Inflamm Res.* 2004;53:181-8.
47. Anagnostatos GS, Pissis P, Viras K, et al. Theory and experiments on high dilutions. In: Ernst E, Hahn EG, eds. *Homeopathy: A Critical Appraisal.* Oxford, England: Butterworth Heinemann; 1998:221.
48. Lo S-Y, Bonavida B. Proceedings of the First International Symposium on Physical, Chemical and Biological Properties of Stable Water [$I_E$] Clusters. Singapore: World Scientific Publishing; 1998.
49. Weingartner O. What is the therapeutically active ingredient of homeopathic potencies? *Homeopathy.* 2003;92:145-51.
50. Bellavite P, Signorini A. The Emerging Science of Homeopathy: Complexity, Biodynamics and Nanopharmacology. Berkeley, Calif: North Atlantic Books; 2002.

APPENDIX

# Pregnancy and Lactation Risk Categories for Selected Nonprescription Medications and Nutritional Supplements

Drug therapy during pregnancy may sometimes be necessary. However, because most drugs cross the placenta to some extent, a mother who takes a drug might expose her fetus to it. Medications should be used during pregnancy only under the supervision of a physician and only when the potential benefits outweigh the potential risks.

Data concerning the use of nonprescription medications while breast-feeding are limited. Many nonprescription medications do not enter breast milk to a significant degree and are often undetectable. However, this should not be interpreted as an indication that nonprescription medications are safe to use during breast-feeding.

The table on the following pages contains FDA categories for evaluating the safety of drugs during pregnancy and breastfeeding for many of the nonprescription medications discussed in this book. The listed categories pertain to the particular strengths or formulations in which the nonprescription medications are available. Prescription strengths or formulations of a medication may have different pregnancy risk categories, and pregnancy risk categories may vary slightly based on the source reference used. Subscripts on particular product listings (e.g., $C_X$) may provide additional information. The majority of the remaining pregnancy risk categories are based on available clinical information from drug information resources, with *Drugs in Pregnancy and Lactation: A Reference Guide to Fetal and Neonatal Risks* being the primary information source. The lactation risk categories are based primarily on information from *Medications and Mother's Milk.* The pregnancy risk categories and lactation risk categories are defined as follows:

**A** Adequate studies in pregnant women have not demonstrated a risk to the fetus in the first trimester of pregnancy, and there is no evidence of risk in later trimesters.

**B** Animal studies have not demonstrated a risk to the fetus, but there are no adequate studies in pregnant women...or...Animal studies have shown an adverse effect, but adequate studies in pregnant women have not demonstrated a risk to the fetus during the first trimester of pregnancy, and there is no evidence of risk in later trimesters.

**C** Animal studies have shown an adverse effect on the fetus, but there are no adequate studies in humans; the benefits from the use of the drug in pregnant women may be acceptable despite its potential risks... or...There are no animal reproduction studies and no adequate studies in humans.

**D** There is evidence of human fetal risk, but the potential benefits from the use of the drug in pregnant women may be acceptable despite its potential risks.

**X** Studies in animals or humans demonstrate fetal abnormalities, or adverse reaction reports indicate evidence of fetal risk. The risk of use in a pregnant woman clearly outweighs any possible benefit. Use of drugs with this rating is contraindicated in women who are or may become pregnant.

**L1** **Safest:** Drug has been taken by a large number of breast-feeding mothers without any observed increase in adverse effects in the infant. Controlled studies in breast-feeding women fail to demonstrate a risk to the infant, and the possibility of harm to the breast-feeding infant is remote. Or, the product is not orally bioavailable in an infant.

**L2** **Safer:** Drug has been studied in a limited number of breast-feeding women and no increase in adverse effects in the infant has been seen. And/or, the evidence of a demonstrated risk that is likely to follow use of this medication in a breast-feeding woman is remote.

**L3** **Moderately Safe:** There are no controlled studies in breast-feeding women; however, the risk of untoward effects to a breastfed infant are possible; Or, controlled studies show only minimal nonthreatening adverse effects. Drugs should be given only if the potential benefit justifies the potential risk to the infant.

**L4** **Hazardous:** There is positive evidence of risk to a breast-fed infant or to breast milk production, but the benefits from use in breast-feeding mothers may be acceptable despite the risk to the infant (e.g., if the drug is needed in a life-threatening situation or for a serious disease for which safer drugs cannot be used or are ineffective).

**L5 Contraindicated:** Studies in breast-feeding mothers have demonstrated there is significant and documented risk to the infant based on human experience. Or, it is a medication that has a high risk of causing significant damage to an infant. The risk of using the drug in breast-feeding women clearly outweighs any possible benefit from breast-feeding. The drug is contraindicated in women who are breast-feeding an infant.

### FDA Pregnancy Risk Categories for Selected Nonprescription Medications

| Agent | FDA Pregnancy Risk Category | Lactation Risk Category |
|---|---|---|
| Acetaminophen | B | L1 |
| Aluminum hydroxide | C[a,b] | |
| Aminobenzoic acid (PABA) | C[b] | |
| Ammonium chloride | B | |
| Ascorbic acid | A (C if doses > RDA)[c] | L1 |
| Aspartame | B (C in women with phenylketonuria)[c] | L1 (L5 in infants with phenylketonuria) |
| Aspirin | C (D if full-doses taken in 3rd trimester) | L3 |
| Bacitracin | C | |
| Benzocaine | C[b] | |
| Benzoyl peroxide | C[b] | |
| β-Carotene | C | |
| Bisacodyl | B[b] | L2 |
| Bismuth | C (D in 3rd trimester) | L3 |
| Brompheniramine | $C_M$[a] | L3 |
| Butoconazole | $C_M$ (for use only in 2nd or 3rd trimester) | |
| Caffeine | B | L2 |
| Calcium carbonate | C[a,c] | |
| Calcium gluconate | C[b] | |
| Camphor | C | |
| Capsaicin | No rating[d] | L3 |
| Carbamide peroxide | C[b] | L1 |
| Casanthranol | C | |
| Cascara sagrada | C | L3 |
| Castor oil | X | |
| Charcoal, activated | C[a] | |
| Chlorhexidine gluconate | B | L2 |
| Chlorpheniramine | B | L3 |
| Chlortetracycline | D | |
| Choline salicylate | C[b] (D in 3rd trimester) | |
| Chondroitin sulfate–glucosamine | No rating[d] | L3 |
| Cimetidine | $B_M$ | L2 |
| Clemastine | $B_M$ | L4 |
| Clotrimazole | B (topical/vaginal preparation); C (troches) | L1 |
| Coal tar | C[b] | |
| Codeine | C (D if used for prolonged periods or in high doses at term) | L3 |
| Cromolyn | $B_M$ | L1 |
| Cyanocobalamin | A (C if doses > RDA) | |
| Cyclizine | B | L3 |
| Dexbrompheniramine | C | |
| Dexpanthenol | C | |
| Dextromethorphan | C | L1 |
| Dimenhydrinate | $B_M$ | L2 |
| Diphenhydramine | $B_M$ | L2 |
| Docusate calcium | C | L2 |
| Docusate potassium | C | L2 |
| Docusate sodium | C | L2 |
| Doxylamine | A | L4 |
| Dyclonine | C[b] | |
| Ephedrine | C | L4 |
| Epinephrine | C | L1 |
| Ethanol | D (X if used in large amounts or for prolonged periods)[c] | L3 |
| Famotidine | $B_M$ | L1 |
| Ferrous fumarate | C[a,b] | |
| Ferrous gluconate | C[a,b] | |
| Ferrous sulfate | C[a,b] | |
| Folic acid | A (C if doses > RDA)[c] | L1 |
| Glycerin | C | |
| Guaifenesin | C | L2 |
| Hydrocortisone | C (D if used in 3rd trimester) | L2 |
| Hydroquinone | C[b] | L3 |
| Ibuprofen | $B_M$ (D if used in 3rd trimester or near delivery) | L1 |
| Insulin | B | L1 |
| Iodine | D | L4 |
| Ipecac syrup | C[b] | |

## FDA Pregnancy Risk Categories for Selected Nonprescription Medications (continued)

| Agent | FDA Pregnancy Risk Category | Lactation Risk Category |
|---|---|---|
| Iron | See ferrous fumarate, ferrous gluconate, ferrous sulfate | L1 |
| Kaolin | C | L1 |
| Ketoconazole | $C_M$ | L2 |
| Ketoprofen | $B_M$ (D if used in 3rd trimester or near delivery) | L3 |
| Lidocaine | $B_M$ | L2 |
| Loperamide | $B_M$ | L2 |
| Loratadine | $B_M$ | L1 |
| Lysine | C | |
| Magnesium citrate | B | |
| Magnesium hydroxide | C[a,b] | L1 |
| Magnesium oxide | C[a,b] | |
| Manganese | C[b] | |
| Meclizine | $B_M$ | L3 |
| Methylcellulose | $B_M$ (Metamucil) | |
| Miconazole | $C_M$ | L2 |
| Mineral oil | C | |
| Minoxidil | $C_M$ | L3 (oral) L2 (topical) |
| Naphazoline | C[b] | |
| Naproxen sodium | $B_M$ (D if used in 3rd trimester or near delivery)[c] | L3 (L4 in chronic use) |
| Neomycin | C | |
| Niacin | A (C if doses > RDA) | L3 |
| Niacinamide (Nicotinamide) | A (C if doses > RDA)[c] | L3 |
| Nicotine transdermal system | $D_M$[b] | L2 |
| Nicotine polacrilex gum | $C_M$[b] | L2 |
| Nizatidine | $B_M$ | L2 |
| Nonoxynol-9 | C | |
| Octoxynol-9 | C | |
| Omeprazole | $C_M$ | L2 |
| Oxymetazoline | C | L2 |
| Pantothenic acid | A (C if doses > RDA)[c] | |
| Permethrin | $B_M$ | L2 |
| Phenazopyridine | $B_M$ | L3 |
| Pheniramine | C | |
| Phenylephrine hydrochloride | C | L3 |
| Phenyltoloxamine | C | |
| Polyethylene glycol | $C_M$[b] | L3 |
| Polymyxin B | B | |
| Povidone–iodine | D | L4 |
| Pseudoephedrine | C | L3 (acute use) L4 (chronic) |
| Psyllium hydrocolloid | B | |
| Pyrantel pamoate | C | |
| Pyrethrins | C | |
| Pyridoxine | A (C if doses > RDA) | L2 (L4 in high doses) |
| Pyrilamine | C | |
| Ranitidine | $B_M$ | L2 |
| Riboflavin | A (C if doses > RDA) | L1 |
| Saccharin | C | L3 |
| Salicylic acid | C[b] | |
| Selenium sulfide | C[b] | L3 |
| Senna | C | L3 |
| Simethicone | C[a] | |
| Sodium bicarbonate | C[b] | |
| Sodium chloride | C[b] | |
| Sodium citrate | No rating[d] | |
| Sodium fluoride | C | |
| Sodium phosphate | C[b] | |
| Sodium salicylate | C[b] | |
| Terbinafine | $B_M$ | L2 |
| Terpin hydrate | D | |
| Tetracaine | $C_M$[b] | |
| Thiamin | A (C if doses > RDA) | L1 |
| Tioconazole | $C_M$[b] | |
| Tolnaftate | No rating[d] | |
| Triethanolamine | C[b] | |
| Triprolidine | $C_M$ | L1 |
| Urea | C | |
| Vitamin A | A (X if doses > RDA)[c] | |
| Vitamin $B_1$ (thiamin) | See Thiamin | L1 |
| Vitamin $B_2$ (riboflavin) | See Riboflavin | L1 |
| Vitamin $B_3$ (niacin) | See Niacin | L3 |
| Vitamin $B_6$ (pyridoxine) | A (C if doses > RDA)[c] | |
| Vitamin $B_{12}$ (cyanocobalamin) | A (C if doses > RDA)[c] | |
| Vitamin C (ascorbic acid) | A (C if doses > RDA)[c] | |
| Vitamin D (calcitriol) | A (D if doses > RDA)[c] | |
| Vitamin $D_2$ (ergocalciferol) | A (C if doses > RDA)[c] | |

## FDA Pregnancy Risk Categories for Selected Nonprescription Medications (continued)

| Agent | FDA Pregnancy Risk Category | Lactation Risk Category |
|---|---|---|
| Vitamin $D_3$ (cholecalciferol) | A (D if doses > RDA)[c] | |
| Vitamin E (tocopherols) | A (C if doses > RDA)[c] | |
| Vitamins, multiple | A (risk factor varies for amounts > RDAs)[c] | |
| Xylometazoline | C[b] | |

*Note:* A subscript "m" denotes a pregnancy risk category assigned by the manufacturer.

[a] Pregnancy risk categories may vary based on source reference. Recommendation based on most conservative rating.
[b] Agent is referenced in only *Drugs in Pregnancy and Lactation: A Reference Guide to Fetal and Neonatal Risk*. 7th ed.
[c] Source references did not provide pregnancy risk category. Category is instead based on available clinical information.
[d] Source references did not provide pregnancy risk category. Insufficient clinical information is available to support a rating.

*Source:*

Briggs GG, Freeman RK, Yaffe SJ. *Drugs in Pregnancy and Lactation: A Reference Guide to Fetal and Neonatal Risk*. 7th ed. Philadelphia: Lippincott Williams & Wilkins; 2005.

Briggs GG, Freeman RK, Yaffe SJ. Drugs in Pregnancy and Lactation: *A Reference Guide to Fetal and Neonatal Risk*. 6th ed. Philadelphia: Lippincott Willliams and Wilkins; 2002.

Reilly CH, publisher. *Drug Facts & Comparisons* [database online].Version 4.0. St. Louis: Wolters Kluwer Co; 2005.

*Clinical Reference Library Online* [database online]. Hudson, Ohio: Lexi-Comp Online; 2005-6.

*Micromedex Healthcare Series* [database online]. Vol 110. Greenwood Village, Colo: Micromedex, Inc; 2005.

Pagliaro LA, Pagliaro AM. Drugs as human teratogens and fetotoxins. In: *Problems in Pediatric Drug Therapy*. 4th ed. Washington, DC: American Pharmaceutical Association; 2002.

*Mosby's Drug Consult*. St. Louis: Elsevier Mosby; 2005.

*USP-DI Volume I: Drug Information for the Health Professional* [book on CD ROM]. 25th ed. Englewood, Colo: Thomson Healthcare; 2005.

Nice FJ, Snyder JL, Kotansky BC. Breastfeeding and Over-the-Counter Medications. *J Hum Lact*. 16(4);2000:319–31.

Hale T. *Medications and Mother's Milk*. 11th ed. Amarillo, Tex: Pharmasoft Publishing; 2004.

APPENDIX II

# Botanical Medicines to Avoid in Pregnancy and Lactation

| Herb | | Commission E Monographs[a] | Botanical Safety Handbook[a] | |
|---|---|---|---|---|
| | | Herbs to Avoid in Pregnancy and Lactation | Herbs to Avoid in Pregnancy (Category 2b) | Herbs to Avoid in Lactation (Category 2c) |
| **Common Name** | **Scientific Name** | | | |
| Alkanet | *Alkanna tinctoria* | | √ | √ |
| Aloe vera | *Aloe vera, Aloe ferox, Aloe perryi* | | √ | √ |
| American pennyroyal | *Hedeoma pulegioides* | | √ | |
| Andrographis | *Andrographis paniculata* | | √ | |
| Angelica | *Angelica archangelica* | √ | √ | |
| Arnica | *Arnica montana* | | √ | |
| Ashwaganda | *Withania somnifera* | | √ | |
| Basil | *Ocimum basilicum* | | √ | √ |
| Black cohosh | *Cimicifuga racemosa* | √ | √ | |
| Bladderwrack | *Fucus vesiculosus* | | √ | √ |
| Blessed thistle | *Cnicus benedictus* | √ | √ | |
| Blood root | *Sanguinaria canadensis* | | √ | |
| Blue cohosh | *Caulophyllum thalictroides* | | √ | |
| Borage | *Borago officinalis* | | √ | √ |
| Buckthorn | *Rhamnus frangula* | √ | √ | |
| Bugleweed | *Lycopus americanus, Lycopus europaeus, Lycopus virginicus* | | √ | √ |
| California poppy | *Eschscholzia caifornica* | | √ | |
| Cascara sagrada | *Rhamnus purshiana* | √ | √ | √ |
| Castor bean | *Ricinus communis* | | √ | |
| Catnip | *Nepeta cataria* | | √ | |
| Chastetree berry | *Vitex agnus castus* | √ | √ | |
| Chinese motherwort | *Leonurus cardiaca* | | √ | |
| Chinese rubarb | *Rheum officinale, Rheum palmatum, Rheum tanguticum* | | √ | √ |
| Cinnamon bark | *Cinnamonum verum, Cinnamonum aromaticum* | √ | √ | |
| Coffee | *Coffea arabica* | | √ | |
| Coltsfoot | *Tussilago farfara* | | √ | √ |
| Comfrey | *Symphytum asperum, Symphytum x uplandicum, Symphytum officinale* | | √ | √ |
| Dong quai | *Angelica sinensis* | | √ | |

| Herb | | Commission E Monographs[a] | Botanical Safety Handbook[a] | |
|---|---|---|---|---|
| | | Herbs to Avoid in Pregnancy and Lactation | Herbs to Avoid in Pregnancy (Category 2b) | Herbs to Avoid in Lactation (Category 2c) |
| **Common Name** | **Scientific Name** | | | |
| Echinacea purpurea | *Echinacea purpurea* | ✓ | ✓ | |
| Elecampane | *Inula britannica* | | ✓ | ✓ |
| Ephedra[b] | *Ephedra sinica* | ✓ | ✓ | ✓ |
| European pennyroyal | *Mentha pulegium* | | ✓ | |
| Fennel | *Foeniculum vulgare* | ✓ | ✓ | |
| Fenugreek | *Trigonella foenum-graecum* | ✓ | ✓ | |
| Feverfew | *Tanacetum parthenium* | | ✓ | |
| Forsythia | *Forsythia suspensa* | | ✓ | |
| Garlic | *Allium sativum* | ✓ | ✓ | ✓ |
| Ginger | *Zingiber officinale* | ✓ | ✓ | |
| Ginseng | *Panax ginseng* | ✓ | ✓ | |
| Goldenseal | *Hydrastis canadensis* | | ✓ | |
| Guggul | *Commiphora mukul* | | ✓ | |
| Horehound | *Marrubium vulgare* | ✓ | ✓ | |
| Horseradish | *Armoracia rusticana* | ✓ | ✓ | |
| Ipecac | *Cephaelis ipecacuanha* | | ✓ | |
| Joe Pye weed | *Eupatorium purpureum* | | ✓ | ✓ |
| Juniper | *Juniperus communis* | ✓ | ✓ | |
| Kava | *Piper methysticum* | ✓ | ✓ | |
| Lemongrass | *Cymbopogon citratus* | | ✓ | |
| Licorice | *Glycyrrhiza glabra* | ✓ | ✓ | |
| Lobelia | *Lobelia inflata, Lobelia siphilitica* | | ✓ | ✓ |
| Lycium | *Lycium barbarum, Lycium chinense* | | ✓ | |
| Male fern | *Dryopteris filix mas* | | ✓ | ✓ |
| Motherwort | *Leonurus cardiaca* | ✓ | ✓ | |
| Myrrh | *Commiphora molmol* | ✓ | ✓ | |
| Orange peel, bitter | *Citrus aurantium* | ✓ | ✓ | |
| Oregon grape | *Mahonia aquifolium, Mahonia nervosa, Mahonia repens* | | ✓ | |
| Parsley | *Petroselinum crispum* | ✓ | ✓ | |
| Prickly ash | *Zanthoxylum americanum, Zanthoxylum clava-herculis* | | ✓ | |
| Purging buckthorn | *Rhamnus catharticus, Rhamnus frangula* | | ✓ | ✓ |
| Purslane | *Portulaca oleracaea* | | ✓ | |
| Quinine | *Cinchona officinalis, Cinchona pubescens, Cinchona calisaya, Cinchona ledgeriana* | | ✓ | |
| Rosemary | *Rosmarinus officinalis* | ✓ | ✓ | |
| Red clover | *Trifolium pratense* | | ✓ | |
| Roman chamomile | *Chamaemelum nobile* | | ✓ | |
| Sage | *Salvia officinalis* | ✓ | ✓ | |
| Senna | *Senna alexandrina* | ✓ | ✓ | ✓ |
| Shepard's purse | *Capsella bursa pastoris* | ✓ | ✓ | |

| Herb | | Commission E Monographs[a] | Botanical Safety Handbook[a] | |
|---|---|---|---|---|
| Common Name | Scientific Name | Herbs to Avoid in Pregnancy and Lactation | Herbs to Avoid in Pregnancy (Category 2b) | Herbs to Avoid in Lactation (Category 2c) |
| Stillingia | *Stillingia sylvatica* | | | √ |
| Thyme | *Thymus vulgaris* | √ | √ | |
| Thuja | *Thuja occidentalis* | | √ | |
| Tree peony bark | *Paeonia suffruticosa* | | √ | |
| Tumeric | *Curcuma longa* | √ | √ | |
| Uva-ursi | *Arctostaphylos uva ursi* | √ | √ | |
| Watercress | *Nasturtium officinale* | √ | √ | |
| Wormwood | *Artemisia absinthium* | | √ | √ |
| Yarrow | *Achillea millefolium* | √ | √ | |

[a] This table is adapted from information presented in the *Botanical Safety Handbook* (1997) and *Herbal Medicine: Expanded Commission E Monographs* (2000). It is not all inclusive. According to the editors of *Herbal Medicine: Expanded Commission E Monographs*, safety studies have not been done on some of the herbs listed in the monographs, so there are no known restrictions. All herbs should be used with caution during pregnancy and lactation and, then, only under the supervision of a knowledgeable health care provider.

[b] FDA ban on ephedra sales pending. For further information, see F-D-C Reports, Inc. FDA regulatory framework for ephedra ban expected to get court review. *The Tan Sheet*. January 5, 2004;12:3–4.

*Source:* McGuffin M, Hobbs C, Upton R, Goldberg A. *Botanical Safety Handbook*, Boca Raton, Fla: CRC Press; 1997; Blumenthal M, Goldberg A, Brinckmann J. *Herbal Medicine: Expanded Commission E Monographs*. Newton, Mass: Integrative Medicine Communications; 2000.

# Index

*Note:* Page numbers followed by "f" or "t" denote figures or tables, respectively. The numbers following the designation "CP" denote the color plates, which follow page 680.

## B

## E

## F

## G

## H

## M

## N

## Q



## R



## S

## V



## W

## X



## Y



## Z